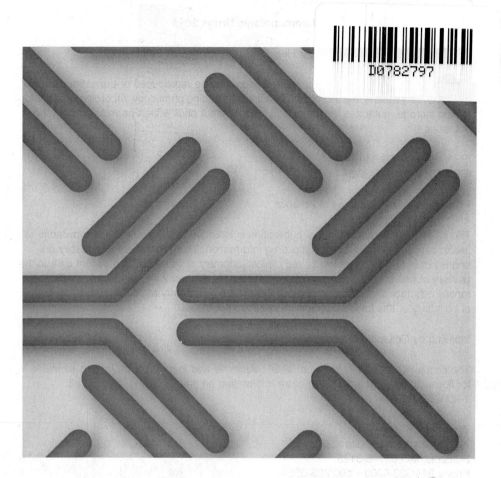

John D. Grabenstein, RPh, PhD, FAPhA

ImmunoFacts®

VACCINES AND IMMUNOLOGIC DRUGS

2013

Facts & Comparisons®

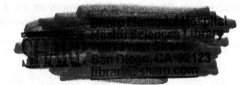

ImmunoFacts®: Vaccines and Immunologic Drugs 2013

ISBN-10: 1-57439-344-8
ISBN-13: 978-1-57439-344-6

Printed in the United States of America

The information contained in this publication is intended to supplement the knowledge of health care professionals regarding drug information. This information is advisory only and is not intended to replace sound clinical judgment or individualized patient care in the delivery of health care services. Wolters Kluwer Health and the author disclaim all warranties, whether expressed or implied, including any warranty as to the quality, accuracy, or suitability of this information for any particular purpose.

Indexing by Columbia Indexing Group, Reno, Nevada.

The content contained in *ImmunoFacts®: Vaccines and Immunologic Drugs* is available for licensing as source data. For more information on data licensing, please call 1-800-223-0554.

Wolters Kluwer Health
77 Westport Plaza, Suite 450
St. Louis, MO 63146-3125
Phone 314/392-0000 • 800/223-0554
Fax 314/392-0160
factsandcomparisons.com

About the Design: The front cover and chapter head pages of *ImmunoFacts* display an artist's rendition of an immunoglobulin molecule. The image of a double-stranded "Y" represents both the antibody products described in this book and the antibodies induced by vaccines described herein, as well as the entire pharmacopeia of immunologic drugs featured in *ImmunoFacts*.

Suggested Citation:
  Grabenstein JD. *ImmunoFacts: Vaccines and Immunologic Drugs* - 2013
  (38th revision). St. Louis, MO: Wolters Kluwer Health, 2012.

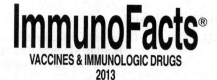

ImmunoFacts®

VACCINES & IMMUNOLOGIC DRUGS
2013

John D. Grabenstein, RPh, PhD, FAPhA

Facts and Comparisons® Publishing Group

Senior Director Content Development	Scot E. Walker, PharmD, MS, BCPS, BCACP
Senior Clinical Managers	Paul B. Johnson, RPh Cathy A. Meives, PharmD
Clinical Manager	Kim S. Dufner, PharmD
Senior Clinical Editor	Andrea L. Williams, RPh
Clinical Editors	Christine M. Cohn, PharmD, BCPS Esta Razavi, PharmD Patricia L. Spenard, PharmD
Product Manager	Melissa Kennedy, PharmD, BCPS
President and CEO, Clinical Solutions	Arvind Subramanian, MBA
Senior Managing Editors	Angela J. Bush Sarah W. Gremillion
Senior Editor	Jennifer E. Rolfes
Managing Technical Editor	Wendy M. Bell
Managing Editor, Quality Control	Susan H. Sunderman
Senior Composition Specialist	Jennifer M. Love
Inventory Analyst	Barbara J. Hunter

Facts and Comparisons® Editorial Advisory Panel

Thomas L. Whitsett, MD   Professor of Medicine and Pharmacology
Vascular Medicine Program
OU Regents Professor
University of Oklahoma Health Sciences
   Center
Oklahoma City, Oklahoma

Acknowledgements

It is not physically or intellectually possible to complete a work of this magnitude alone. I am indebted to a large number of people, only a few of whom I can list here. Michael S. Edwards, PharmD, introduced me to the world of immunology at Walter Reed Army Medical Center. Renata M. Engler, MD, and Master Sergeant Gerald J. Wallace first showed me how an up-to-date compilation of information about vaccines might be helpful to clinicians. Neil M. Davis, MS, PharmD, FASHP, gave me my start as a semi-professional journalist. Each of my bosses in various Army hospitals over the years allowed me to explore immunopharmacy and exercise my curiosity. Of course, my many teachers in Cumberland, Pittsburgh, Bremerhaven, Chapel Hill, and the Army worldwide enlightened me to the wonders of science.

Our editorial advisory panel provided a wealth of beneficial suggestions to improve the book and the publishing crew at Facts and Comparisons performed eminently. The pharmaceutical manufacturers whose products are described herein contributed innumerable pieces of data. Captain L. Clay Sisk (USPHS, Ret.) provided copies of various FDA advisory committee reports. Countless librarians humored my search for articles from the *Journal of Obscure & Irreproducible Research*.

The publishing professionals at Facts & Comparisons are both colleagues and friends. Readers have challenged me to make this book successively better. To these people and many others, I am very grateful.

J.D.G.

To my wonderful wife, Laurie Ann, with love and thanks; to Emily Christine, to Andrea Lynn, to Erica Katherine, and to Peter Christopher (each fully vaccinated), with hope, and to Mom & Dad, in gratitude.
Emily's contribution to this book at age 13 months: gH jjqq j hui jj1r5c WU23TYT2T12R1 'R11R516T712UU

NOTE: The author is a pharmacist and epidemiologist employed by Merck & Co., Inc. He writes and edits this book in his private capacity, beginning more than 15 years before he joined Merck. No endorsement by any party is intended nor should it be inferred. Merck & Co., Inc. is not involved with and takes no responsibility for this work. The publisher coordinates independent review to ensure all content is presented in an objective manner.

Table of Contents

Table of Contents

Facts & Comparisons is very proud to bring you *ImmunoFacts®: Vaccines and Immunologic Drugs*, authored by John D. Grabenstein. This book continues Facts & Comparisons' unequaled reputation in publishing timely, current, and comprehensive references for the health professional.

ImmunoFacts® is a unique publication, providing detailed information on vaccines, antibodies, and other immunologic drugs. It is the most comprehensive source available in this field. Not only does it provide extensive information on vaccine products, there is also a great deal of information about related topics, such as investigational and international drugs, immunization documents, manufacturer addresses/phone numbers, drug interactions, and vaccine indications by risk group.

This publication also covers interferons, interleukins, immunomodulators/mediators, and monoclonal antibodies, to name a few. As new developments in the field of immunology continue to emerge, you can expect to find them discussed in detail in *ImmunoFacts®*. *ImmunoFacts®* will be of importance to any health professional who is concerned with prescribing, administering, dispensing, or monitoring patients receiving any immunologic drug.

This impressive compilation of immunologic information is largely the work of John D. Grabenstein, a pharmacist and renowned expert in this area. He, along with an equally dedicated and talented editorial panel of pharmacists and physicians, as well as the publishing staff, continue to provide the most up-to-date information in this field.

We are confident that this publication will be valuable to your practice. Please feel free to contact us with any comments, questions, or suggestions for *ImmunoFacts®*. We can only make it better with your input.

"The literature of immunity, moreover, grows so amazingly that the analysis even of current works is a task of no mean proportions."
- H.T. Ricketts, 1906

Ricketts could never have imagined the advances in immunology we appreciate today. But he was correct about the complexity of the science. The goal of *ImmunoFacts®: Vaccines and Immunologic Drugs* is to provide comprehensive drug information about this specific category of drugs. The format is intended to allow quick, reliable access to discrete pieces of information, while also helping readers compare and contrast information for similar products or uses.

ImmunoFacts® was first to bring together detailed information about the pharmaceutic and pharmacologic characteristics of immunologic drugs, along with authoritative recommendations for their use.

What is an immunologic drug? This deceptively simple question is the core issue in a series of decisions on which drugs to describe in this publication and which to exclude. The rationale for these decisions considers the following factors.

Inclusion Criteria

All licensed drugs whose action is wholly or largely immunological in nature are included. Also selected are unlicensed investigational drugs in human clinical trials, based on clinical significance and availability of information.

Immunologic drugs appear whether they are derived from biological sources or not. The construct of "biological" drugs is a fuzzy one that suffers from confusion over source and action. Biologicals are included only if their action is immunologic (eg, vaccines), but excluded if their action is not immunologic (eg, insulin, *Lactobacillus acidophilus*).

Several nonimmunologic drugs also have been included based on their close relationship to immunologic drugs. For example, epinephrine is included because it is the drug of choice for treating acute anaphylactoid hypersensitivity reactions associated with immunologic drugs. Histamine is a frequent positive-control reagent for allergen skin-test batteries. Botulinum toxin, while a microbial (and hence biological) product, is a neurotoxic drug, not an immunologic one; nonetheless, it is included to allow comparison with botulinum toxoid and antitoxin.

Exclusion Criteria

Drugs produced using biotechnology are excluded from this book unless their primary action is immunologic in nature. For example, epoetin (erythropoietin) is an erythrocyte colony-stimulating factor and is produced using recombinant DNA technology. Nonetheless, epoetin is indicated for stimulating hematopoiesis of red blood cells, whose primary actions are not immunologic.

This rationale leads to the inclusion of myeloid colony-stimulating factors (eg, filgrastim, sargramostim), but the exclusion of coagulation factors and alteplase (ie, tPA). Using this same approach, the human insulins, produced by recombinant DNA technology, also are excluded.

Organization

Immunologic drugs are grouped by major pharmacologic categories (eg, vaccines, antibodies, diagnostic reagents). Whenever a drug may logically fit into two or more categories, the ultimate location was chosen on the basis of the primary use of the drug. For example, IGIV is primarily an anti-infective drug, although it also can be used for hematologic purposes for the treatment of immune thrombocytopenic purpura (ITP).

Unfortunately, this scheme led to the separation of the two BCG products. Tice-strain BCG vaccine is included with the vaccines because of its long-standing indication for prevention of tuberculosis, but *TheraCys* and *Tice BCG* for intravesical use appear with the immunostimulants because it is licensed only for the treatment of bladder cancer, not tuberculosis prophylaxis.

Content

Most of the products listed in this publication are protected by letters of patent and their names may be trademarked or registered by the enterprise listed. The product distributor may or may not be the actual manufacturer or fabricator of the final dose-form. Listing of specific products is an indication only of availability on the market and does not constitute an endorsement or recommendation. Drug product interchange is regulated by state laws; the listing of products together does not imply that they are therapeutically equivalent or legally interchangeable.

Use information derived from this book in conjunction with other clinical and printed data sources. The author and publisher have taken care to ensure that indications, contraindications, doses, and treatment schedules are correct and compatible with standards generally accepted at the time of publication. Readers are cautioned to apply their clinical judgment to individual patients for whom they care.

Editorial Review

The editorial panel of *ImmunoFacts*® includes recognized experts in clinical immunology, therapeutics, vaccinology, and drug information. Panelists review monographs and provide direction for the revision of *ImmunoFacts*®. In addition to the editorial panel, other authorities in government, academia, and the pharmaceutical industry are consulted as needed to provide information of the highest quality and reliability.

Background

Immunology is the study of the body's defenses against infectious agents and other pathogens. The human immune system protects the body by eliminating or neutralizing materials recognized as different than the self. The wide range of immunologic responses and reactions affect essentially every organ, tissue, and cell of the body. The diversity of immune responses includes, but is certainly not limited to, antibody production, allergy, inflammation, phagocytosis, cytotoxicity, transplant and tumor rejection, and the myriad of signals that turn these responses off and on. Immunity is the state of being immune or protected from a disease. Immunologic drugs include any drug that stimulates, mimics, contributes, triggers, blocks, or modifies any kind of immune response.

The following sections provide a concise review of immunology, immunopharmacology, and immunopharmaceutics. First, the key participants and theories of immunology are briefly reviewed. The following two parts discuss immunopharmacology (the study of the effects of immunologic drugs on living organisms) and immunopharmaceutics (the study of the characteristics of immunologic doseforms and immunologic drug delivery).

This section is intended to satisfy readers' basic questions about the immune system. Consult detailed references for complete descriptions of human immunity and immune responses.

The Immune Response

The immune system is an intricate regulatory and defense system within the human body. Immune cells, tissues, mediators, and antibodies are involved in rejecting tumors; inactivating viruses, bacteria, and other microbes; neutralizing toxins; and performing other defense functions. In addition to these capabilities, the immune system is capable of remembering previous encounters with immunogens and mounting even stronger responses upon rechallenge. For example, once you have had measles, you will most likely never get it again. This section reviews the structure and function of the major arms of the immune response.

Immunogens, Antigens, and Allergens: Any substance that can evoke an immune response (eg, production of antibody) is called an immunogen. Vaccines must be immunogenic to be effective. Certain immunogens that can combine with antibodies are called antigens. The exposed 3-dimensional parts or chemical groupings on antigens to which antibodies attach are called determinant groups, haptens, or epitopes. Haptens also include certain low molecular weight compounds, nonimmunogenic by themselves, that can evoke an immune response when they combine with a larger carrier molecule.

For any organic molecule to be immunogenic, it must be recognized as foreign by the host. Most immunogens have molecular weights greater than 10,000 daltons, and most are proteins. Smaller molecules (eg, insulin, penicillin) may function as haptens if they combine with a carrier protein. For example, penicillin alone is antigenic, but poorly immunogenic. However, penicillin coupled to a protein can be highly immunogenic. Both antigenicity and immunogenicity are dependent on the 3-dimensional shape of the epitope. Changes to the conformation or accessibility of an epitope can increase, decrease, or negate that epitope's ability to combine with an antibody.

B-lymphocytes, macrophages, and other antigen-presenting cells (APCs) phagocytize immunogens. Immunogens are modified within those cells by denaturation, unfolding, and proteolysis. Eventually, epitopes of the immunogen are expressed on the surface of the APC. This allows activation of T-helper lymphocytes that, through the action of cytokines, activate

3

other B cells. These B-lymphocytes differentiate either into antibody-producing plasma cells specific for that epitope or into long-lived memory B-lymphocytes.

An allergen is an antigen (something recognized by the immune system) that causes allergy, the collection of diseases in which immune responses cause tissue inflammation and organ dysfunction. Antibody-mediated allergens induce the syndrome known as immediate hypersensitivity, which includes anaphylaxis. T-lymphocyte–mediated allergens induce delayed hypersensitivity, such as dermal reactions to tuberculin skin tests. Allergenic illness on exposure to an allergen requires an initial sensitization episode, where antigen-specific immunoglobulin E (IgE) antibodies are produced that attach to Fc (fragment, crystallizable [of immunoglobulin]) receptors on mast cells and basophils. Upon a second exposure, allergens combine with IgE bound to mast cells (followed by release of mediators such as histamine), form immune complexes with immunoglobulin G (IgG) or immunoglobulin M (IgM) (followed by complement activation), or combine with T-effector cells (followed by lymphokine release). Any of these 3 pathways can lead to inflammation. Allergists may use the term allergen to refer specifically to a substance that induces IgE production.

Antibodies: An antibody, synonymous with an immunoglobulin or immune globulin, is a glycoprotein molecule that produces the effects of humoral or circulating immunity. Although antibodies can act in a nonspecific fashion (eg, complement fixation, histamine release by mast cells), their most potent effects result from their specific interactions with antigens and with the host's own immune cells.

Humans possess 5 distinct classes or isotypes of immunoglobulins: IgG, immunoglobulin A (IgA), IgM, immunoglobulin D (IgD), and IgE. Characteristics of each isotype are described in the following table. "Gamma globulin" is an obsolete term for immunoglobulins, especially IgG. The term refers to the presence of immunoglobulins in the gamma region of serum separated by electrophoresis. It is a misnomer because some antibodies are found in the beta region and, hence, are beta globulins. IgG and IgA primarily exist as gamma globulins, although some are beta globulins. To further confound the issue, although most IgM and IgD molecules are beta globulins, some are gamma globulins. Nonetheless, common usage usually equates gamma globulin with IgG and often with intramuscular immune globulin (IgIM).

IgG is the most abundant of the immunoglobulins. It consists of 2 heavy polypeptide chains and 2 light chains, which, in 2 dimensions, looks like the capital letter Y on the cover of this book. In 3-dimensional actuality, an IgG molecule appears globular until it recognizes an antigen, at which time it looks more like a coiled spring resembling a Y. Specificity for a given antibody resides in the variable region at the 2 upper tips of the Y. This area comprises the first 100 amino acids from the amino-terminal end of each chain and is called the antigen-binding site. The whole molecule contains about 1,200 amino acids.

If the Y-shaped IgG molecule is enzymatically cleaved at the point of interchain disulfide bonds (at the junction of the Y), 2 antigen-binding fragments (Fab) and 1 cell-binding fragment (Fc, called the constant region of an IgG molecule) are produced. For example, the commercial product *Digibind* is composed of Fab fragments specific for digoxin molecules. If the Fc fraction is removed from IgG but both Fab fragments remain attached to each other, the combination is called a $F(ab)_2$ molecule.

IgG production represents one of the largest single forms of response to vaccination. Two different types of IgG response to an antigen can be noted. Upon first exposure to an antigen, circulating IgG antibodies are first detected in human serum after about 6 days, peaking after about 12 to 14 days. Antibody levels then plateau at a considerably lower level. But upon rechallenge or subsequent exposure to that same antigen, a strikingly quicker and larger IgG response results, with IgG concentrations tapering off only gradually. This secondary response is also called a booster, memory, or anamnestic response to an antigen. Consider the dosing strategy for the products containing tetanus toxoid: 5 doses are given to children as a basic series to induce adequate antitoxin titers. Booster doses are then needed only every 10 years to maintain adequate immunity.

Most physical features of IgG are also generally possessed by the other 4 isotypes. IgA, like IgG, usually occurs in a monomeric form. But in human secretions, 2 IgA monomers may be linked by a J-chain to a compound called secretory component to form a complex called secretory IgA (sIgA). IgA is most notable for its role in immune defenses at mucosal barriers (eg, nose, mouth, GI tract).

IgM typically exists in a pentameric form. After initial exposure to a novel antigen or vaccination, an elevation in specific IgM will be noted, in addition to the better known IgG response. The first IgM medication, fanolesomab, was licensed in 2004.

Properties of Human Immunoglobulins					
Isotype	IgG	IgA	IgM	IgD	IgE
Adult serum concentration (mg/mL)	8 to 16	1.4 to 4	0.4 to 2	0.03	Nanogram amounts
Molecular weight (kilodaltons)	143 to 160	159 to 447	900	117 to 185	188 to 200
Mean half-life (days)	23	6	5	3	< 3
% of total body immunoglobulin	80	13	6	1	0.002
Unit	Monomer	Monomer, dimer, trimer	Pentamer	Monomer	Monomer
Subclasses	4	2	2		
Distribution	Serum, transplacental	Mucus membranes, secretions, serum	Serum	Serum	Serum
Function	Complement fixation, opsonization	Portal defense	Complement fixation, agglutination	Undetermined (differentiation of B lymphocytes)	Defense against parasites, mediator of allergic reactions

Biologists estimate that a typical human being has 1 trillion B cells capable of producing IgG antibodies with more than 10 million different antigenic specificities. That is, humans have antibodies capable of specifically combining with 10 million distinct antigens.

This diversity represents one of the wonders of the human body, but the diversity of antibodies is an evolved response to the diversity of antigens in the environment. For example, more than 200 distinct viruses are responsible for causing the common cold. It is beyond our present capacity to develop one vaccine that will induce the production of 200 distinct, safe, and effective antibodies to protect humans from each of these viruses at even a finite point in time, let alone consider the natural antigenic changes of these viruses over time. Specificity, it seems, is a double-edged sword.

IgE is implicated in many allergic diseases. Its beneficial role may have protected humans from parasites in living conditions less sanitary than commonly enjoyed today. The role of IgD is currently undetermined, but may involve some aspect of differentiation of B-lymphocytes.

Immunologic Cells: Like all blood cells, cells destined to become lymphocytes and phagocytes are produced in the bone marrow, the soft tissue primarily found in the hollow shafts of long bones. Early in life, B lymphocytes complete their maturation in the bone marrow, while T lymphocytes migrate to the thymus for maturation. Mature lymphocytes may either circulate through the vascular system, lymph vessels, and tissues or congregate in the spleen, lymph nodes, tonsils, adenoids, appendix, and the Peyer patches of the intestinal tract.

Lymphatic vessels carry lymph (the clear fluid containing lymphocytes), macrophages, and foreign antigens retrieved from the tissues. Lymph drains out of the tissues, seeps into the lymphatic vessels and is then transported to lymph nodes, where the antigens can be presented to immune cells. Lymphocytes reenter the blood stream at the thoracic duct to continue their cyclic patrol for foreign antigens.

B lymphocytes, after exposure to an antigen, are transformed into plasma cells, which are factories for secretion of antibodies, as discussed above. Antibodies generally bind with circulating antigens, but do not penetrate cells. Each B cell secretes an antibody with just one unique specificity, but it secretes millions of copies of that antibody. It is this phenomenon that is harnessed to mass-produce monoclonal antibodies.

T lymphocytes, on the other hand, interact directly with antigens. T cells interacting with antigens may secrete lymphokines, chemical mediators of the immune response. Each of the various types of cells will be reviewed.

Helper/inducer T cells activate B cells, natural killer cells (NKC), and macrophages. Helper T cells bear the T4 (CD4) antigen (or surface-identifying marker) on their cell surfaces.

Suppressor/cytotoxic T cells turn off or suppress cells activated by helper T cells. They may also attack infected or malignant cells directly and are responsible for rejection of transplanted tissue and organs. These T cells bear the T8 (CD8) surface-identifying antigen on their cell surfaces.

The third type of lymphocyte includes the NKCs. Like cytotoxic T cells, NKCs bear granules of cytotoxic chemicals to kill tumor cells and microorganisms on contact. But unlike cytotoxic T lymphocytes, NKCs do not need to recognize a specific antigen to produce this effect.

Phagocytes are a diverse class of white blood cells that engulf and digest microorganisms and other antigenic particles. Some phagocytes can present antigens to lymphocytes. Major groups of phagocytes include monocytes, macrophages, and granulocytes. Monocytes circulate in the blood, scavenging foreign cells. When monocytes migrate into tissue, they develop into macrophages and rid the body of worn-out cells and other debris. After digesting and processing antigens, monocytes and macrophages present antigens to lymphocytes. Both monocytes and macrophages also secrete monokines (messengers or mediators analogous to lymphokines), complement proteins, enzymes, and other chemicals.

Granulocytes are also known as polymorphonuclear leukocytes. These cells contain granules filled with potent chemicals (eg, histamine, myeloperoxidase). Within the broad category of granulocytes, mast cells are found in tissues, while neutrophils, eosinophils, and basophils reside in the circulation.

Macrophages and other APCs initiate a cell-mediated immune response by ingesting an antigen and then displaying antigen fragments on their own surfaces. Cell-mediated immunity (CMI) and delayed hypersensitivity (DH) represent the same phenomenon, but the choice of the term is usually based on whether the effect of the response is beneficial or harmful. In either case, an antigen fragment is bound on the macrophage surface to a class II molecule of the major histocompatibility complex (MHC). This combination attracts the attention of a specific T lymphocyte.

Once stimulated, T lymphocytes respond with a cascade of lymphokines (eg, various interleukins) to amplify the response and recruit nonspecific lymphocytes and other inflammatory cells. CMI is manifested by vasodilation, chemotaxis, fibrin deposition, and granuloma formulation. When the immune insult is under control, suppressor T cells turn off the response.

Complement: Complement is the collective term used for a set of at least 25 plasma and cellmembrane proteins. Once activated through a cascade of steps, complement coats foreign particles and microorganisms. This coating renders the object susceptible to opsonization and phagocytosis or to destruction (or lysis) of the offending agent. The complement cascade can also produce an acute inflammatory response and attract circulating leukocytes to the site of intrusion.

The complement-activation cascade may follow either of 2 major pathways, commonly named the classic pathway and the alternate pathway. The classic pathway is activated by antigen-antibody complex. Various complement proteins bind specifically to the antigen-antibody complexes. The alternate pathway does not require such complexes for activation. The complexes form during complement activation; the complexes formed cause smooth-muscle contraction and degranulation of mast cells and basophils, variously stimulate or inhibit CMI, and induce other effects. Membrane attack mediated by complement may cause cell death through lysis.

Immune Classification: In 1963, Combs & Gell proposed a categorization system to describe and differentiate immunopathologic hypersensitivity reactions. The system is somewhat simplistic in that many immunologic diseases involve a combination of these reaction types. Nonetheless, this system is a helpful means of understanding immunopathologic events.

Type I: Immediate (often within 15 minutes) or allergic hypersensitivity, primarily mediated by IgE and IgG, basophils, or mast cells. Mast cells bind IgE at their Fc receptors, inducing degranulation and release of histamine and other mediators. Examples include atopy (eg, hay fever, urticaria, food and pollen allergy, insect venom hypersensitivity, drug hypersensitivity, atopic dermatitis, eczema), bronchospasm and allergic asthma, and anaphylaxis.

Type II: Cytotoxic reaction, primarily mediated by IgG, IgM, and complement. Cytotoxicity results from antibodies directed against intrinsic cell surface antigens or antigens adsorbed onto a cell surface. Such reactions are characterized by complement-mediated lysis, phagocytosis of circulating antigens, or killer cell activity, with acute inflammation of tissues. Examples include autoimmune hemolytic anemia, erythroblastosis fetalis (hemolytic disease of the newborn), Goodpasture syndrome, Graves disease, immune thrombocytopenia purpura, myasthenia gravis, and transfusion reactions.

Type III: Immune-complex reactions, primarily mediated by IgG, IgM, IgA, and complement. Such reactions are characterized by accumulation of polymorphonuclear leukoctyes and macrophages. When antigen-antibody complexes form in large quantities that cannot be cleared adequately by the mononuclear phagocyte system (primarily in liver, spleen, and lungs), type III reactions develop. Complexes are deposited on endothelial or other tissue surfaces, causing inflammation (eg, vasculitis, lymphadenopathy). Examples include serum sickness, rheumatoid arthritis, Arthus reactions, hypersensitivity pneumonitis, post-streptococcal glomerulonephritis, and systemic lupus erythematosus.

Type IV: DH, CMI, primarily mediated by T lymphocytes and lymphokines. Such reactions are characterized by a delayed (after 24 to 72 hours) mononuclear cell infiltrate. When an antigen is trapped in a macrophage and cannot be cleared, T lymphocytes may be stimulated to produce lymphokines that mediate inflammatory responses. Examples include Jones-Mote reactions, contact dermatitis, tuberculosis and tuberculin reactions, granulomatous diseases, sarcoidosis, schistosomiasis, graft and organ rejection, and polymyositis.

Immunologic Contrasts

Immunologic drugs offer a study of contrasts. The classic dichotomy between active and passive immunity and between prevention and treatment of infections is well known, but it can benefit the student of immunology to consider a number of other contrasts in the body of knowledge that make up immunopharmacology and immunopharmaceutics. These contrasts involve the physical products themselves, their mechanisms of action, their modes of use, and other characteristics.

Their diversity of uses makes immunologic drugs a fascinating class. Further comparison and contrasting of these agents are later considered in 2 categories: differential pharmacology and differential pharmaceutics. Each of these contrasts is highlighted below in a wide-ranging (albeit superficial) essay that reflects the diversity of immunologic drugs.

Utilization: Clinicians employ immunologic drugs to serve a wide range of purposes, including the full range of prevention, diagnosis, and treatment.

Prevention: Vaccines, *Hymenoptera* venoms, immunoantidotes, and similar agents are all administered to prevent infection, disease, or illness, but the types of prevention vary considerably. Vaccines prevent disease months, years, or decades in the future, while antibodies are generally used with more acute benefit in mind. Hepatitis B immune globulin (HBIg) is used for prophylaxis in acute cases of needle-stick injury; $Rh_o(D)$ immune globulin prevents disease not in the recipient but in subsequent offspring of the recipient.

Diagnosis: Immunologic drugs are used in the detection of infections (eg, tuberculin), the diagnosis of allergy (eg, allergen extracts, benzylpenicilloyl polylysine) or other diseases (eg, a radiolabeled antibody), the staging of a disease (eg, lepromin for leprosy, anergy tests for HIV), or the assessment of general immune function (eg, anergy tests).

Treatment: Immunotherapy may include intravenous immune globulin, an antitoxin, an antivenin, an allergen extract, digoxin Fab, an interferon, or a colony-stimulating factor.

Some immunologic drugs are used in several modes simultaneously. Postexposure rabies vaccination in any given patient can be construed as prevention of rabies disease or as presumptive treatment of rabies infection. Several products can be used for distinctly different purposes depending on the case. The various antilymphocyte immune globulins can be used either for prevention or treatment of acute organ-rejection episodes. BCG vaccine can be used either for prevention of tuberculosis or treatment of certain bladder cancers. Tetanus toxoid is useful either in inducing antitoxin antibodies or diluted as an intradermal test to assess CMI. Preexposure hepatitis B immunization is an example of primary prevention, while postexposure vaccination is a form of secondary prevention.

All or some?: A nation's individual vaccination policies vary according to many factors, including the epidemiology of the diseases involved, the immunologic characteristics of the vaccines, the sociologic characteristics of patients and clinicians, the likelihood and consequences of adverse effects, and the costs associated with each factor. For some vaccines, universal vaccination of a whole population (eg, tetanus toxoid) or age cohort (eg, *Haemophilus influenzae* type b) is recommended. In some cases, immunization is so important to society that it is required before employment or admission into schools or nursing homes (eg, measles, rubella, tetanus, influenza).

In other cases, select high-risk groups are targeted for selective immunization (eg, yellow fever vaccine for travelers, meningococcal vaccine for military recruits). Recommendations for hepatitis B vaccine changed in 1991 from select use in people potentially exposed to contaminated blood or body fluids to a dual strategy of targeted immunization for high-risk groups plus universal vaccination of all American infants. Among adults, special efforts are made to assess pregnant and postpartum women for immunity to rubella.

Before, during, or after?: Rabies vaccine may be used for preexposure protection of veterinarians and others with predictable risk. Postexposure rabies prophylaxis is given to other persons only after they have been bitten or otherwise exposed. Among health care workers, it is common practice to emphasize preexposure vaccination with hepatitis B vaccine, rather than postexposure "needle-stick" protection with HBIg.

Differential Pharmacology:

Cellular vs humoral immunity: Mechanisms of immune responses are often categorized into humoral and cell-mediated types. Humoral immunity involves antibodies; cell-mediated immunity involves macrophages, other antigen-presenting cells, and T lymphocytes. The pathology of these 2 types of immune response can also be distinguished by their speed of onset: immediate (ie, within minutes) or delayed (ie, within 24 to 72 hours). See also the Coombs & Gell classification described previously in this section.

Consider the dichotomy between mumps vaccine and mumps skin test antigen (MSTA) (no longer distributed). Both are immunogens and both contain viral proteins, yet their effects are very different. Immunogens in MSTA interact with T lymphocytes to produce the characteristic Koch-type (delayed-type) hypersensitivity response similar to tuberculin. Live viruses in mumps vaccine, on the other hand, evoke specific circulating antimumps antibodies that help defend the body against infection. Tetanus toxoid is used in both of those modes: induction of antitoxin antibodies when used as a vaccine or evocation of a DH response when used intradermally as an anergy-test reagent.

The differences between benzylpenicilloyl polylysine (*Pre-Pen*) and tuberculin are noteworthy. Both are immunodiagnostic products, but one predicts drug allergy and the other detects infection. The first assesses the presence of antipenicillin antibodies, while the other signals the presence of sensitized T lymphocytes. A similar comparison can be made between allergen-extract skin tests (assessing immediate hypersensitivity) and histoplasmin (assessing DH).

Active vs passive immunity: Active immunity develops in a person in response to infection or after administration of a vaccine or toxoid. Sufficient active immunity to protect the host may take several weeks or months to induce, but active immunity is generally long-lasting. Alternatively, passive immunity is temporary immunity provided in the form of performed, donated antitoxins or antibodies (ie, immune globulins) from another living host (either human or animal). Passive immunity protects almost immediately, but only persists with the biological half-life of IgG, measured in days or weeks.

Hepatitis B vaccine and HBIg illustrate this dichotomy well. The vaccine actively induces a host's own circulating antibodies against the hepatitis B virus, as well as stimulates the production of memory B cells that permit an accelerated response upon rechallenge. Giving HBIg, on the other hand, is essentially the temporary donation of someone else's antibodies. If an HBIg recipient does not develop any of his or her own specific anti–HBV antibody-producing plasma cells, the loaned antibodies are eventually catabolized and not replaced. In this respect, the immunity provided is only temporary. In some cases of post-exposure prophylaxis, both vaccine and HBIg are given to provide immediate, transient protection while the delayed, long-lasting immunity develops.

In some cases, simultaneous administration of active and passive immunity may induce a drug-drug interaction that interferes with development of active immunity. For example, measles vaccine should be given at least 4 weeks before and several weeks or months after administration of any immune globulin or other blood product that might contain antimeasles antibodies. Hepatitis B vaccine and HBIg do not appear to interfere with each other.

Clostridium botulinum is a bacterium that has contributed 3 completely distinct drugs to the American pharmacopoeia: a toxin, a toxoid, and an antitoxin. The toxin, a bacterial poison, is used ophthalmically to treat strabismus and blepharospasm. The toxoid induces active immunity to protect recipients against the toxin. The antitoxin, like other antibody preparations, contributes passive protection against intoxication.

Comparing Vaccines and Antibodies	
Vaccines	Antibodies
Active immunity	Passive immunity
Evoke personal protection	Provide borrowed protection
For prevention (typically before exposure)	For treatment (typically after exposure)
Onset $\approx$ 2 wk	Rapid onset (h)
Prolonged effect (y)	Temporary effect (wk)
Vaccine - A medication containing antigens that causes someone to make antibodies.	
Antigen - A microbe or a molecule (eg, protein, polysaccharide) capable of evoking antibody production.	
Antibody - A specific kind of protein produced by B lymphocytes (plasma cells) that attack and help destroy an antigen.	

Killed vs live vaccines: Killed or inactivated vaccines consist of killed, whole microbes or isolated microbial components. These nonreplicating immunogens induce active immunity. Live, attenuated vaccines contain altered, weakened, or avirulent microorganisms (either bacteria or viruses) and also induce active immunity. Live vaccines can be dangerous in an immunocompromised patient who cannot mount an effective defense against even avirulent microorganisms. Attenuated vaccines are often more immunogenic than inactivated vaccines and may induce serum antibody protection of longer duration. For example, a single dose of live yellow fever vaccine induces immunity for 10 years, while the inactivated Japanese encephalitis vaccine requires a 3-dose series that protects for several years.

Consider the dichotomy between the enhanced injectable inactivated poliovirus vaccine (eIPV) and oral poliovirus vaccine (OPV), the most famous pair of killed ("Salk") and attenuated ("Sabin") vaccines. OPV was administered orally so that it would mimic natural poliovirus infection. But very rarely, OPV would actually cause poliomyelitis instead of protecting against it. Typhoid and influenza are other examples where both attenuated and inactivated vaccines are available.

Local vs circulating antibodies: Think again about the differences between eIPV and OPV. The greatest advantage of OPV was its ability to induce localized secretory IgA antibodies in the gastric mucosa. These antibodies provide the strongest immune defense at the microorganism's portal of entry into the human body. Both eIPV and OPV induce effective levels of circulating antipoliovirus IgG.

Intranasal administration of influenza vaccine and oral administration of typhoid vaccine can provide immune defenses at a microbe's portal of entry, taking advantage of secretory immunity. Such a strategy is effective for a variety of veterinary vaccines. For example, commercial fish can be vaccinated through their gills by immersion of the fish in water containing dissolved vaccine.

Toxoids vs vaccines: A vaccine is a formulation of whole or fractional microorganisms (eg, bacteria, viruses) or portions of them. Toxoids are a subset of vaccines. Toxoids are modified bacterial toxins, rendered nontoxic themselves while retaining the ability to stimulate antitoxin formation (ie, specific antibodies against the natural toxin).

Diphtheria, tetanus toxoid, and acellular pertussis vaccine provides examples of both, because it is a combination of diphtheria and tetanus toxoids plus pertussis vaccine. The toxoids cause recipients to manufacture their own antidiphtheria and antitetanus antitoxin antibodies. Antitoxins have no direct effect on the *Corynebacterium diphtheriae* and *Clostridium tetani* bacteria themselves; antibiotics are needed to eradicate them. Whole-cell pertussis vaccine, on the other hand, induces antibodies directed against the actual pertussis bacteria. Acellular pertussis vaccines contain known quantities of both bacterial components (eg, filamentous hemagglutinin [FHA], fimbrae) and pertussis toxoid.

Diseases vs infection: Vaccines provide differing kinds of protection, depending on the pathogenic characteristics of the microorganism. Toxoids prevent intoxication through antigen-antibody neutralization. Measles vaccination prevents infection by that virus. Pertussis and *Haemophilus influenzae* type b (Hib) vaccines prevent the manifestations of infection, or reduce disease severity, to a greater extent than they prevent infection or colonization itself.

Antiviral immune globulins (eg, cytomegalovirus immune globulin intravenous) attack invading microbes directly. But antitoxin antibodies neutralize circulating toxins primarily, not toxins that have already fixed to nerve tissue (eg, tetanus immune globulin, antivenins).

Polysaccharide vs protein vaccines: Polysaccharide vaccines contain sugar fragments purified from the capsules of certain bacteria. Protein vaccines, on other hand, consist of whole or fragmented bacteria or viruses. Protein vaccines generally induce immunity of longer duration than polysaccharide vaccines. T-cell memory response to booster doses of polysaccharide vaccines may be reduced or absent in young children or in immunodeficient hosts compared with proteinaceous antigens.

Polysaccharide vaccines (eg, Hib, meningococcal, pneumococcal) are T cell–independent immunogens, in contrast to protein vaccines, which induce a T-cell effect.

T-helper–lymphocytes regulate maturation, differentiation, and proliferation of antibody-producing B-cell subpopulations. Children younger than 2 years do not mount as effective a response to polysaccharide vaccines as they do to proteinaceous ones.

The differences among the various vaccines against Hib are instructive. Polysaccharide Hib vaccines were licensed as early as April 1985. Second-generation Hib vaccines, first licensed in December 1987, contain the same polysaccharide, but are conjugated (or chemically coupled) to various carrier proteins. This combination of polysaccharide and protein provides enhanced immunogenicity in infants by inducing a T-cell response, compared with the initial Hib vaccine containing the polysaccharide alone. Because subsequent conjugated doses boost the effects of early doses, routine immunization now starts at 2 months of age, compared with 1 dose at 24 months of age for the original vaccine.

Human vs animal antibodies: Rabies immune globulin (RIg), harvested from human serum, and equine antirabies serum (ARS), harvested from horses, are both effective in the prevention of rabies. RIg has entirely replaced ARS in the United States and Canada because giving human immune globulins to human patients causes far fewer side effects (eg, hypersensitivity, serum sickness) than giving whole immune globulins harvested from animals. In addition, animal, or heterologous, IgG has a shorter biological half-life in humans (8 to 15 days), compared with 20 to 35 days for human IgG.

Most licensed snake and spider antivenins are equine products and present comparable differences in safety and pharmacokinetics compared with human antibodies. Similarly, equine tetanus antitoxin has been superseded by human tetanus immune globulin (TIg). The only licensed diphtheria antitoxins are derived from equine serum. In 2003, a human botulism immune globulin was licensed in the United Sates for the first time, joining the licensed equine-derived product. Several antilymphocyte globulins are harvested in various ways from horses, rabbits, mice, or genetically engineered chimeric organisms.

Usually, administration of animal immune globulins poses no problem because patients are rarely rechallenged with a subsequent dose of the same animal immune globulin. Not many people receive a snake antivenin once, let alone twice. But in the interval following a dose of animal immune globulin, the human host develops antibodies against these foreign proteins, even though they were administered benevolently. Because antibodies are themselves proteins, they act in this case as foreign antigens that offend the human host. When next exposed to that same foreign protein, the human host can respond with an adverse reaction or less obviously by quietly neutralizing and inactivating the animal immune globulin. This inactivation might retard the drug's intended effect as an antidote, an intentional immunosuppressant (eg, lymphocyte immune globulin), or a radioimaging agent (eg, satumomab). Researchers are working to minimize this problem by amalgamating animal and human antibodies into chimeric ones.

Whole vs fragmented antibodies: Unlike other immunoglobulins harvested from animals, *Digibind* is relatively innocuous because it consists of fragments of sheep anti-digoxin IgG, rather than whole antibodies. This drug consists solely of antigen-binding fragments (Fab), which provide an antibody's specificity against one unique immunogen.

The smaller molecular size of the Fab fragments allows more rapid distribution into tissues and more rapid elimination of digoxin-Fab complexes through renal excretion. Lack of the cell-binding constant portion (Fc), an inherent part of intact immunoglobulin molecules, decreases the risk of allergic reactions common to most animal immunoglobulin products. This fragmentation also reduces the biological half-life from the 8 to 15 days characteristic of animal IgG to about 15 to 20 hours.

Drugs composed of Fab fragments may be preferred as antidotes or for use in radioimaging because of their rapid penetration of extravascular spaces, reversal of toxicity, and renal elimination. However, drugs composed of Fc fragments may be preferred in other settings if bacterial opsonization or clearance of antibody-antigen complexes is important for disease therapy. Whole IgG molecules have already proven their safety and efficacy in infections, hematologic disorders, envenomations, and other uses.

Primary vs booster responses: Following any initial or primary immunization, IgM antibodies appear after about 4 days and peak about 4 days later. IgG antibodies appear after about 7 days and peak after 10 to 14 days. IgG titers decline slowly as the antibodies are naturally catabolized or bind to antigen.

But after a period of time passes and specific memory B lymphocytes develop, a subsequent immunization yields an immune response that is qualitatively and quantitatively quite different. The secondary, or booster, challenge induces specific IgG production against the immunogen that appears earlier, persists longer, and reaches a higher titer (ie, concentration). IgM titers increase slightly, but IgG antibodies clearly predominate after booster immunizations.

In practice, several vaccine doses may be needed for a basic immunizing series to induce sufficient memory B cells. Subsequently, less frequent booster doses are needed to maintain protective antibody levels. For diphtheria and tetanus toxoids, 5 doses are given as a basic series to induce adequate antitoxin titers in young children. Booster doses are then needed only every 10 years to maintain adequate immunity.

Biologics vs drugs: Many of the immunologic drugs used today are also referred to as biologics, biologicals, or biological drugs. Even though the Food and Drug Administration (FDA) divides the responsibility for regulation of human drug products between the Center for Drug Evaluation and Research (CDER) and the Center for Biologics Evaluation and Research (CBER), biologics are themselves drugs. The classic definition of a drug is an agent intended for use in the diagnosis, cure, mitigation, treatment, or prevention of disease. At least 1 of the vaccines, immune globulins, immunodiagnostic reagents, or other immunologic agents described in this book certainly fits each of these uses.

Biologics, though, are very special drugs. Biologic drugs arise from some living process. This poses special challenges in manufacturing and quality control. Often, we expect biologic drugs (eg, vaccines) to act with an extremely high degree of certainty (often greater than 90% or 95%) over a very long period of time (eg, 10 years or more) after just 1 or a handful of doses. Very few chemical drugs can meet these expectations. In many cases, we know that the biologic drug as a whole is effective, but we cannot say which of the myriad components (eg, epitopes) does the work.

Federal legislation to control vaccines, antitoxins, and similar drugs was enacted in 1902, even before chemical drugs were federally regulated. Entitled "An act to regulate the sale of viruses, serums, toxins, and analogous products," the Act is more commonly called the Biologics Control Act, although the word "biologics" does not appear anywhere in the text or title. The term "biologics" arose as bureaucratic shorthand to differentiate drugs derived in some manner from microbes, animals, blood, or allergens from drugs more traditionally derived from plants or chemicals.

However, biologics can accurately describe insulin as well as tetanus toxoid. For accuracy, the term "immunologic drugs" should be specified whenever this mode of action applies.

Process vs outcome: Sticking a needle into someone's arm and marking an immunization record does not guarantee that the recipient is immune from disease. Even if we go to the trouble to draw an antibody titer and find it adequate, we cannot be assured of protection. Are the antibodies measured neutralizing or protective antibodies? Are there enough antibodies? Are all the other necessary components of this person's immune system competent to orchestrate an overall effective defense against disease?

It is proper for clinicians to focus on a patient's health outcomes (eg, death, disability, disease), rather than merely working to improve process indicators (eg, laboratory values, culture results) for their own sake. In a strict sense, vaccinations are process indicators of the delivery of health care. But our contemporary focus on outcomes has not yet come to grips with how to clearly measure disease avoidance for the individual. Indeed, the word choice between "vaccination" and "immunization" helps illustrate this point. One useful semantic rule is to use vaccination to refer to the physical delivery of a vaccine product, reserving immunization for the presumptive or confirmed induction of immunity.

It may be appropriate for clinicians to consider vaccinations as surrogate outcomes. If you have received the proper number of doses of measles vaccine, you have taken prudent steps to avoid measles. It has some similarities to taking the prudent steps of buying insurance, brushing your teeth, or fastening your seat belt. Your affairs are in order. You have assembled the appropriate defenses.

Of course, it remains for our society's public-health scientists to continually measure the efficacy and epidemiology of various immunization products and strategies and constantly improve them. To these professionals, the act of vaccination will always remain a process that contributes to the health outcome of a community, that is, its rates of preventable infections.

Differential Pharmaceutics:

Solutions vs suspensions: Tetanus toxoid offers the best comparison between fluid and adsorbed doseforms. Complexing the tetanus immunogens onto various forms of aluminum in the adsorbed state using aluminum phosphate or aluminum hydroxide induces a stronger response than a similar product produced without aluminum as a true solution. The antigen-alum complexes more readily mobilize macrophages.

The only product for which a choice is currently available between fluid (ie, solution) and adsorbed (ie, suspension) forms is tetanus toxoid. Both products induce an adequate immune response, but a dose of aluminum-adsorbed suspension elicits higher antitoxin concentrations and, hence, more persistent antitoxin levels than the fluid form. In the vast majority of circumstances, combined tetanus-diphtheria toxoids are preferred for wound tetanus prophylaxis. Combined tetanus and diphtheria toxoids in pediatric or adult concentrations are the proper agents for standard wound prophylaxis; both of these combination products are adsorbed formulations. The only rational remaining use of fluid tetanus toxoid is when it is diluted as a DH reagent (see Tetanus Toxoid Fluid monograph).

Subunit vs whole vaccines: Microbial vaccines can be produced either from whole microorganisms or subunits of the organisms. The most commonly known examples are the split-virion and whole-virion influenza vaccines. The split vaccine consists of chemically disrupted viruses. The smaller viral particle size of split vaccines reduces the incidence of adverse reactions in children. Whole-virus influenza vaccines, on the other hand, were composed of intact, albeit inactivated, viruses. Modern split- and whole-virus influenza vaccines are immunogenic to an equal extent.

So why were both whole- and split-virus vaccines produced for many years? Tradition may have a great deal to do with it. Until the late 1970s, influenza vaccine potency was calibrated in chick-cell agglutinating units, and whole vaccines were thought to be more immunogenic, although more reactogenic, in children than their split-virion counterparts. Current influenza vaccine potency is standardized by the more reliable immunodiffusion method, which measures the actual mass of antigen and is thought to obviate any significant difference in efficacy between the 2 formulations. By 2001, few customers asked for whole-virus vaccine; manufacturers achieved greater production efficiency by dropping whole-virus influenza vaccine from their product lines.

Other vaccines are, or have previously been, available in subunit form. Hepatitis B vaccine is a purified preparation of the hepatitis B surface antigen, to which protective antibodies develop. A split rabies vaccine from Wyeth Laboratories (*Wyvac*) was removed from the market in February 1985 because of insufficient antibody induction. Whole-virus products (eg, *Imovax Rabies*, *RabAvert*) are the only rabies vaccines currently available in the United States.

Polyclonal vs monoclonal antibodies: The dichotomy between the antilymphocytic drugs *Atgam* and muromonab CD3 is remarkable. The polyclonal nature of *Atgam* and the monoclonal nature of muromonab CD3 suggest the difference between a shotgun and a rifle. *Atgam* is a polyclonal, equine preparation of anti-thymocyte globulins. In contrast, muromonab-CD3 (*Orthoclone OKT3*) is a monoclonal, murine preparation of anti–T3-antigen antibodies. Both *Atgam* and *OKT3* act as antilymphocyte immunosuppressants but vary in their specificity, uniformity, route of administration, dose, and adverse effects.

Both polyclonal and monoclonal antibodies can be effective unless extreme specificity is needed. Such specificity is needed in radioimaging, as with the monoclonal antibody capromab (*ProstaScint*) used to deliver the indium-111 radioisotope to certain tumor sites as a diagnostic aid. Specificity is similarly important with antibody-delivered radiotherapy (eg, *Bexxar*, *Zevalin*). Too much specificity might exclude protective antibodies from an anti-infective immune globulin preparation.

Polymeric vs monomeric antibodies: The dichotomy between intramuscular and intravenous immune globulins is noteworthy. IgIM contains aggregates (ie, dimers and other polymers) and other serum components. If introduced directly into human circulation, IgIM can spontaneously activate the complement system, causing anaphylaxis. Thus, it is only administered intramuscularly, so that its use is safe. IgIV contains a comparable fraction of pure IgG per unit of protein, but far less in aggregated form, allowing it to be infused directly into the bloodstream.

Standard vs hyperimmune antibodies: Immune globulins are concentrated solutions of antibodies frequently used for treatment of certain immunodeficiencies or for passive immunization. They attack infections in both a specific (eg, neutralization) and nonspecific (ie, induction of the complement system) manner. Efficacy for many indications depends on the specificity or specificities of the antibody in the product.

Consider the dichotomy between broad-spectrum IgIM and HBIg. IgIM is useful against measles and hepatitis A because the pool of volunteer blood donors from which it is harvested has significant concentrations of circulating antibodies against these two, as well as other, microbes. Most lots of IgIM have little activity against hepatitis B virus because, on average, the pool has little of this specific antibody. Conversely, HBIg is a hyperimmune product with a known level of biological activity against the hepatitis B virus, harvested from a select population of people known to have high HBIg titers.

To help ensure broad-spectrum efficacy, each lot of IgIM requires a serum pool of at least 1,000 donors. IgIM harvested in the United States has little demonstrable activity against yellow fever virus because the volunteer pool has generally had no exposure to this agent. Batches of immune globulins available in the United States vary in their activity against unevenly distributed infectious agents (eg, cytomegalovirus, Epstein-Barr virus). Some manufacturers have responded to clinicians' requests for product labeling with specific activity against a litany of microorganisms to guide anti-infective therapy. Similarly, some manufacturers are willing to provide lot-specific information about specific antibody titers of a given production batch.

Hyperimmune globulins can be produced by assembling volunteer donors who happen to have large circulating quantities of the desired antibody, by screening units of blood about to expire (eg, cytomegalovirus immune globulin), or by intentionally hyperimmunizing volunteers to a specific antigen (eg, $Rh_o(D)$ immune globulin). Equine antitoxins and antivenins are hyperimmune globulins in the sense that they are high-titer antibody products specially evoked to neutralize certain toxins or venoms.

Standardized vs unstandardized products: The FDA divides responsibility for regulation of human drug products between CDER and CBER, in large part because of the unique requirements involved in standardizing biological products. Almost all biologic drugs are complex mixtures whose identity, uniformity, and potency are difficult to measure.

This problem is especially evident among products whose labels must bear the proviso, "No US Standard of Potency." Allergen extracts are good examples of such products. The manufacturers take all efforts possible to ensure that each lot is produced just like previous lots, but there is no reference standard of potency to compare against a batch produced today. The contents of the vials went through the same process as all preceding batches, but without a reference standard, we have no assurance that the contents will act safely, effectively, and consistently. Will today's batch be more or less potent? Without a standard, there is no way of knowing.

Only recently have biologically assayed standardization systems been developed for some allergen extracts. Allergen extracts standardized in allergy units are more reliably potent and more consistent than the traditional weight-to-volume (w/v) or protein nitrogen unit labeling systems. In contrast, *Hymenoptera* venoms are standardized by venom protein content and doses are measured in micrograms of dried venom.

Even IgIV, a well-respected product, is defined only in terms of total antibody content, not individual antigenic specificities. Batches vary in activity against specific infectious agents, as previously discussed. Some manufacturers will provide lot-specific information about antibody titers of a given production batch.

Source and production media: Source materials and production methods can have real and imagined effects on the immunologic drugs produced. Consider the dichotomy between the original hepatitis B vaccine (*Heptavax-B*) and the 2 current vaccines (*Recombivax HB*, *Engerix-B*). *Heptavax-B* was produced using purified plasma donated by human volunteers who were infected with hepatitis B virus. Despite scientific evidence to the contrary, many people, including scientists and health care workers, feared disease transmission from the source plasma used for *Heptavax-B*. The other 2 vaccines are manufactured by collecting hepatitis B surface antigen produced by yeast cells modified by recombinant DNA biotechnology. Thus far, clinical trials have shown the 2 source types (plasma and yeast) to be comparably effective in immunoprophylaxis. Duration of protection appears to be very long.

Other source differences exist or existed for rubella and rabies vaccines. HPV-77 and Cendehill strains of attenuated rubella vaccine were originally produced in dog-kidney, duck-embryo, or rabbit-kidney media. The current RA 27/3 strain is grown in human diploid-cell culture. Early rabies vaccines were variously produced in mouse brain or duck-embryo media. Rabies nerve tissue vaccines (NTVs) have a relatively high adverse reaction rate and provided incomplete protection. The current rabies vaccines are grown either in human diploid-cell or diploid fetal-rhesus lung culture media. Rabies NTVs required 23 doses compared with 14 doses for duck-embryo vaccines and 5 doses for modern cell-culture vaccines.

Production processes vary among the drugs produced from elements of human blood. For example, IgIV preparations are prepared by the Cohn-Oncley cold-ethanol fractionation process, a process that inactivates most viruses, including HIV and hepatitis B virus. Recently, solvent-detergent treatment of immune globulin products became available, promoted as an added measure of safety through inactivation of lipid-enveloped viruses (eg, hepatitis C). Heat treatment of an alpha$_1$-proteinase inhibitor (*Prolastin*), used in the management of congenital panacinar emphysema, does not completely eliminate the possibility of hepatitis B virus transmission. Hepatitis B immunization is recommended for persons expected to receive *Prolastin*.

The clinical significance of the differences in these production processes has not yet been completely defined. It is differences such as those discussed in this section that make regulation and standardization of biological drugs so much more intricate than other chemical drugs.

The Bottom Line: Clinical Equivalence

Any consideration of the differential pharmacology or pharmaceutics of an immunologic drug must address the health outcome of the drug's recipient. Did the vaccine prevent the disease? Did the immune globulin treat the disease? Did the test detect the disease? Was the patient's care affected by changing brands, sources, or types of an immunologic drug during prophylaxis, diagnosis, or therapy? The term "therapeutic equivalence" has been used to imply comparable clinical effect among chemical drugs. However, assessment of some immunologic drugs may require the corollary concepts of prophylactic equivalence or diagnostic equivalence.

Each monograph in this text includes a summary assessment of comparability for similar products. In the case of hepatitis B vaccines, the products are prophylactically equivalent (adjusting for the proper delivered dose). For Bacille Calmette-Guérin vaccine, the two products have not been shown to be equivalent for prevention of tuberculosis; unfortunately, their relative efficacy for treatment of bladder cancer in situ has not yet been assessed. The antilymphocyte products and the interferons are not therapeutically equivalent, given their varying doses, adverse-effect profiles, and routes of administration. Refer to each monograph for details on that product category.

Immunologic drugs have many similarities, but also many peculiarities. The data presented in the monographs are intended to provide the reader with an understanding of the properties, actions, and effects of each agent in order to best prevent, diagnose, or treat disease. The public health requires nothing less.

References: Adkinson NF Jr, Busse WW, Holgate ST, Bochner BS, Simons FER, eds. *Middleton's Allergy: Principles and Practice*, 7th ed. Elsevier, 2008.

Advisory Committee on Immunization Practices. General recommendations on immunization: Recommendations of the Advisory Committee on Immunization Practices (ACIP). *MMWR*. 2011;60(RR-2):1-61.

Atkinson W, Wolfe S, Hamborsky J, eds. *Epidemiology and Prevention of Vaccine-Preventable Diseases*, 12th ed. Washington DC: Public Health Foundation, 2011.

Coombs RRA, Gell PGH. The classification of allergic reactions underlying disease. In: Gell PGH, Coombs RRA, ed. *Clinical Aspects of Immunology*. Philadelphia: FA Davis, 1963:317-337.

Grabenstein JD. Don't say "biologics" if you mean "immunologics." *Am J Hosp Pharm*. 1988;45:1941-1942.

Male D, Brostoff J, Roth D, Roitt I. *Immunology*, 7th ed. Edinburgh; New York: Elsevier, 2006.

National Institute of Allergy & Infectious Diseases. Understanding the immune system: how it works. NIH Publication 07-5423. September 2007. http://www.niaid.nih.gov/topics/immuneSystem/PDF/theImmunesystem.pdf.

National Institute of Allergy & Infectious Diseases. *The Jordan Report: Accelerated Development of Vaccines 2012*. Bethesda, MD: NIH, January 2012. http://www.niaid.nih.gov/topics/vaccines/documents/JordanReport2012.pdf.

National Institute of Allergy & Infectious Diseases. Understanding vaccines: What they are, how they work. NIH Publication 08–4219, January 2008. http://www.niaid.nih.gov/topics/vaccines/Documents/undvacc.pdf.

Plotkin SA, Orenstein WA, Offit PA. *Vaccines*, 6th ed. Philadelphia: Elsevier, 2012.

This section reviews common features of many immunologic drugs. Specific information about individual products is described in each monograph.

In the United States, federal law (the Food, Drug, & Cosmetic Act, 21 USC 353, 21 CFR 610.60 [a] [6]) prohibits dispensing any human vaccine, immune globulin, or other immunologic drug without a prescription from a licensed prescriber. In common practice, immunization programs have been sponsored by organizations or institutions with the concurrence of a physician (explicit or implicit cases of standing orders), but where traditional individual physician/patient relationships do not exist. Increasingly, the Centers for Disease Control and Prevention (CDC), the Center for Medicare & Medicaid Services (CMS), and other health authorities recommend use of standing orders from a prescriber to enhance immunization delivery.

Use Characteristics

Indications: This section describes product uses for which the Food and Drug Administration (FDA) has confirmed safety and efficacy. These uses are included in the FDA-approved product labeling or accepted in common practice.

Unlabeled Uses: This section describes product uses for which a consensus is emerging or investigation is underway, but for which FDA approval has not yet been issued.

Under provisions of the Food, Drug, & Cosmetic Act, manufacturers may only print in the package insert (ie, product labeling) uses of a drug for which adequate information scientifically establishing safety and efficacy has been gathered and for which FDA approval has been obtained. The FDA does not literally approve the use of drugs, nor does it regulate the practice of medicine or how prescribers use licensed drugs. When it grants a license, the FDA's role is to confirm safety and efficacy; it has the authority to limit promotion of a given drug to information listed in the FDA-approved product labeling.

Valid uses for a drug may become evident and accepted before these uses are included in the product labeling. Because the FDA has not yet officially affirmed such uses, it is the responsibility of individual clinicians to ensure that use of the drug is likely to benefit the patient and that the benefits outweigh the risks.

Inclusion of an unlabeled use in this book does not imply that safety and efficacy for that use have been scientifically established. In some cases, randomized controlled trials to scientifically establish efficacy may be unethical (eg, botulinum toxoid). In other cases, pivotal studies of efficacy are under way, but have not yet been concluded and reported. Clinicians must use their best judgment along with published and other sources of information.

Limitations: No prophylactic immunologic drug will protect 100% of recipients against corresponding infections. Similarly, no therapeutic drug is 100% effective, and all diagnostic drugs can render false-negative or false-positive results. In addition, a number of factors beyond the manufacturer's control can reduce the efficacy of an immunologic product or result in an adverse effect from its use. Such factors include improper storage and handling of the product after it leaves the manufacturer, dosage, method of administration, patient diagnosis, and biological and other differences in individual patients.

Contraindications: History of a serious allergic reaction to a vaccine component or after a prior dose of this vaccine. Exercise caution and appropriate care in administering any vaccine to an individual with severely compromised cardiopulmonary status or to others in whom a febrile or systemic reaction could pose a significant risk. Any serious active infection is reason for delaying use of a vaccine except when, in the opinion of the physician, withholding the vaccine entails a greater risk. Generally, do not administer immunologic drugs to patients with fever, unless the cause of the fever is determined and evaluated. If the fever is due to an infection, withhold the immunologic drug until the patient is afebrile, unless the risk of withholding the drug outweighs the risks inherent in drug administration.

Patients with selective immunoglobulin A (IgA) deficiency may develop anti-IgA antibodies and could have anaphylactoid reactions to subsequent administration of blood products (including immune globulin preparations) that contain IgA.

Immunodeficiency:

Inactivated products: Inactivated vaccines used in patients with impaired immune responsiveness may not yield the expected antibody response. This may occur whether the immunocompromise is due to the use of immunosuppressive therapy (eg, irradiation, antimetabolites, alkylating agents, cytotoxic agents, large doses of corticosteroids), a genetic defect, HIV infection, leukemia, lymphoma, generalized malignancy, or other causes. Short-term corticosteroid therapy (less than 2 weeks) or intra-articular, bursal, or tendon injections of corticosteroids are usually not immunosuppressive. Inactivated vaccines pose no additional risk to immunocompromised individuals, although their efficacy may be substantially reduced.

Because patients with immunodeficiencies may not respond sufficiently to immunizing agents, they may remain susceptible despite appropriate vaccination. If feasible, measure specific serum antibody titers or other immunologic response at an appropriate time interval after immunization to assess immunity.

Some immunocompromised patients may be identified following negative response to anergy-test batteries. Vaccine recipients among this group may remain susceptible despite immunization, but immunization is nonetheless frequently recommended for them with the intent that they develop at least partial immunity. If the immunocompromise is temporary in nature, it may be appropriate to defer immunization until several months after immunosuppressive treatment is discontinued if infection risk is not acute. Consider disease threats and risk-benefit ratios for individual patients, and consult current authoritative guidelines.

Live, attenuated products: Immunization with live bacterial or viral organisms in immunocompromised patients is generally contraindicated because of the risk of vaccine-induced infection. This may occur whether the immunocompromise is due to the use of immunosuppressive therapy (eg, irradiation, antimetabolites, alkylating agents, cytotoxic agents, large doses of corticosteroids), a genetic defect, HIV infection, leukemia, lymphoma, generalized malignancy, or other causes. Short-term corticosteroid therapy (less than 2 weeks) or intra-articular, bursal, or tendon injections of corticosteroids are usually not immunosuppressive.

For example, do not give live vaccinia (smallpox) vaccine to immunocompromised patients or their household contacts. However, trivalent measles, mumps, rubella (MMR) vaccination is recommended for asymptomatic children infected with HIV, and should be considered for use in symptomatic HIV-positive children. MMR vaccination in such children has not been associated with serious or unusual adverse effects, but antibody responses have been variable.

Immunodiagnostic skin tests: Immunocompromised patients may have a diminished skin-test response to immediate- and delayed-hypersensitivity antigens. Skin test responsiveness may also be suppressed by active tuberculosis, other bacterial or viral infection, malnutrition, malignancy, and immunosuppression.

Elderly: Response to immunologic drugs may be slightly or significantly impaired in patients with advancing age. For this reason, give some vaccines (eg, pneumococcal) as risk increases but before immune response is impaired too greatly (eg, promptly at age 65).

Pregnancy: Approximately 1 in 6 of clinically recognized pregnancies result in spontaneous miscarriage; another 23% of conceptions result in other forms of preclinical embryo loss. Recognizable congenital malformations occur in approximately 2% to 5% of live births. Chance appearance of either of these types of events after vaccination or use of any drug does not necessarily imply that the drug caused the event.

The FDA's Pregnancy Categories (21 CFR 201.57) are based on the degree to which available information has ruled out a drug's risk to the fetus balanced against the drug's potential benefits to the mother:

Category A: Controlled studies showed no risk. Adequate, well-controlled studies in pregnant women failed to demonstrate risk to the fetus.

Category B: No evidence of risk in humans. Either animal findings showed risk, but human findings did not, or, if no adequate human studies have been conducted, animal findings are negative.

Category C: Risk cannot be ruled out. Human studies are lacking, and animal studies are either positive for fetal risk or lacking as well. However, potential benefits of the drug may justify the risk.

Category D: Positive evidence of risk. Investigational or postmarketing data show risk to the fetus. Nevertheless, potential benefits may outweigh the risk. The "D" rating is generally reserved for drugs without safe alternatives.

Category X: Contraindicated in pregnancy. Studies in animals or humans and investigational or postmarketing reports have shown fetal risk that clearly outweighs any possible benefit to the patient.

Immunoglobulin G (IgG) antibody passage across the placenta generally begins during the first trimester of pregnancy, but the vast majority occurs during the third trimester. Neonatal serum IgG levels correlate with gestational age. Other immunoglobulin isotypes (eg, immunoglobulin A [IgA], immunoglobulin M [IgM]) do not traverse the placenta.

Recommendations for Immunization During Pregnancy	
Vaccine	Recommendation
Live virus vaccines	
Adenovirus types 4 & 7 vaccine	Contraindicated (hazard is theoretical, not proven)
Influenza A & B (*FluMist*)	Contraindicated (hazard is theoretical, not proven)
Measles	Contraindicated (hazard is theoretical, not proven)
Mumps	Contraindicated (hazard is theoretical, not proven)
Poliovirus	OPV was formerly preferred when immediate protection was needed. Use IPV when OPV is not available[a]
Rotavirus	Inappropriate population; contraindicated (hazard is theoretical, not proven)
Rubella	Contraindicated (hazard is theoretical, not proven)
Smallpox (vaccinia)	Contraindicated unless high likelihood of exposure (hazard is fetal vaccinia, very rare)
Varicella and zoster	Contraindicated (hazard is theoretical, not proven)
Yellow fever	Contraindicated, unless exposure to yellow fever is unavoidable (hazard is theoretical, not proven)
Live bacterial vaccines	
BCG[b]	Avoid use. Use only if clearly needed.
Typhoid (capsules)	Consider actual risks of disease and probable benefits of vaccine. Vi polysaccharide vaccine may be preferred on theoretical basis

Guidelines on Use of Immunologic Drugs

Recommendations for Immunization During Pregnancy	
Vaccine	Recommendation
Inactivated virus vaccines	
Hepatitis A	Use in women at risk
Hepatitis B	Use in women at risk
Human papillomavirus	Contraindicated (hazard is theoretical, not proven)
Influenza A & B	Recommended for pregnant women during influenza season. Consult current recommendations
Japanese encephalitis	Use only if clearly needed
Poliovirus	OPV was formerly preferred when immediate protection was needed. Use IPV when OPV is not available
Rabies	Use if there is substantial risk of viral exposure
Inactivated bacterial vaccines	
Anthrax	Use only if clearly needed
*Haemophilus influenza*e type b	Use in women at risk
Meningococcal	Use in outbreak situations
Pneumococcal	Use in women at risk
Typhoid (injections)	Consider actual risks of disease and probable benefits of vaccine. Vi polysaccharide vaccine may be preferred on theoretical basis
Toxoids	
Td bivalent or with Tdap[c]	Vaccinate if woman lacks primary series or if no booster administered within past 10 y
Immune globulins	
Pooled or hyperimmune globulins	Use for exposure or anticipated, unavoidable exposure to $Rh_o(D)$ antigen, measles, hepatitis A, hepatitis B, rabies, or tetanus

a IPV = inactivated poliovirus vaccine; OPV = oral poliovirus vaccine.
b BCG = Bacille Calmette-Guérin.
c Td = tetanus-diphtheria; Tdap = combined tetanus, diphtheria, and pertussis vaccine.

For recommendations on other infrequently used vaccines, refer to individual monographs.

Lactation: It is not known whether many drugs, including immunologic agents, are excreted in breast milk. Because many drugs are excreted in breast milk, exercise caution when administering any drug to a breast-feeding woman. Secretory IgA antibodies are found in the feces of breast-fed infants by the second day of life, whereas only 30% of formula-fed infants demonstrate IgA in the feces by 1 month of age. IgM and IgG may also be present in breast milk, although in lower concentrations than IgA. Breast-feeding is not a specific contraindication to immunization.

Rather, various nutritional, immunologic, and other advantages of breast-feeding have been described. Goldman (1993) reviewed the contributions of breast milk to human health. Secretory IgA is the prevalent immunoglobulin in human milk; IgG predominates in bovine milk. Secretory IgA protects infants against *Escherichia coli, Shigella, Salmonella, Campylobacter, Haemophilus influenzae, Streptococcus pneumoniae, Klebsiella pneumoniae*, polioviruses, rotaviruses, respiratory syncytial virus, influenza virus, cytomegalovirus, and numerous other microbes. Maternal contribution of IgA is especially important until endogenous production matures in infants at 4 to 12 months of age. The enteromammary and bronchomammary pathways of IgA production are discussed, as are the numerous other chemical and cellular agents of microbial, inflammatory, and immunomodulatory protection.

Children: Published information about safety and efficacy is provided. In some cases, there have been no specific studies evaluating safety and efficacy in children. Weigh the benefit of drug use against the risk to the child from drug administration or omission.

Comfort measures can help children cope with discomfort associated with vaccination. These measures include distraction (eg, playing music, pretending to blow away the pain), ingestion of sweet liquids, cooling of the injection site, and topical or oral analgesia. Pretreatment 30 to 60 minutes before injection with lidocaine-prilocaine 5% topical emulsion can decrease the pain of vaccination among infants by causing superficial anesthesia. This product should not be used with infants treated with methemoglobin-inducing agents (eg, sulfonamides, lidocaine) because of the possible development of methemoglobinemia. Acetaminophen has been used among children to reduce discomfort and fever associated with vaccination. However, acetaminophen can cause formation of methemoglobin and thus, might interact with lidocaine-prilocaine cream if used concurrently. Ibuprofen or another nonaspirin analgesic can be used, if needed. Use of a topical refrigerant (vapocoolant) spray can reduce the short-term pain associated with injections. Administering sweet-tasting fluid orally immediately before injection can result in a calming or analgesic effect among infants.

Adverse Reactions: Not all adverse events after vaccination or drug administration have a cause-and-effect relationship with the vaccine. See detailed references for a more complete discussion of causality. Before injection of any immunologic drug, take all reasonable precautions to prevent adverse events. This includes a review of the patient's history with respect to possible hypersensitivity to the vaccine or its components. For pediatric vaccines, inform parents or guardians about any significant adverse reaction(s) that may occur with vaccine administration. CDC-sponsored Vaccine Information Statements are available for all licensed vaccines (see Immunization Documents in the Resources section, http://www.cdc.gov/vaccines/pubs/vis/default.htm, or http://www.immunize.org). Ask parents or guardians to inform the clinician of any events that do occur. As part of any child's immunization record, record the date, lot number, and manufacturer of the vaccine administered in compliance with the National Childhood Vaccine Injury Act. Refer to Immunization Documents in the Resources section for complete information.

Exercise caution in patients at risk of hemorrhage following intramuscular (IM) injection. For people with clotting-factor disorders at risk of hematoma after IM injection, the Advisory Committee on Immunization Practices (ACIP) recommends that appropriate vaccines be administered IM if in the opinion of the physician familiar with the patient's bleeding risk, the vaccine can be given with reasonable safety by this route. If the patient receives antihemophilia or similar therapy, IM vaccinations can be scheduled shortly thereafter. A fine needle (ie, 23 gauge or less) can be used for vaccination, with firm pressure applied to the site, without rubbing, for 2 minutes or more. The patient or family should be instructed about the risk of hematoma after injection.

Aluminum-containing vaccines may occasionally produce a palpable nodule at the injection site for several weeks. Sterile abscess formation or subcutaneous atrophy at the injection site may also occur. These reactions typically resolve on their own.

Systemic reactions may result from allergic hypersensitivity. With any biological product, have adequate treatment provisions, including epinephrine solution 1:1,000, readily available for immediate use in the event an anaphylactoid reaction occurs. Other products that may be helpful include antihistamines (eg, diphenhydramine [*Benadryl*]), parenteral corticosteroids (eg, hydrocortisone sodium succinate [*Solu-Cortef*]), an injectable pressor amine (eg, dopamine), syringes and needles, oxygen, IV fluids, and airways. Naturally, health care workers fully trained in the use of these products should be readily available as well. Volume expanders and vasopressor agents may be required to reverse hypotension. Inhaled bronchodilators and parenteral aminophylline may be required to reverse bronchospasm. Severe airway obstruction unresponsive to bronchodilators may require tracheal intubation.

Treatment of serum sickness usually involves symptomatic treatment with antihistamines, corticosteroids, and aspirin. Postvaccinal neurologic disorders, although uncommon, have followed injection of almost all biological products.

It is possible, although highly improbable, that any immunologic product derived from or manufactured with blood components may transmit or support the growth of infectious agents or prions.

A cause-and-effect relationship between some adverse effects and associated immunologic drugs has not been established. In some cases, the adverse effects may merely be temporally associated, and not causally associated, with the drug in question.

Response to a systemic reaction: Rarely will all of the following measures be necessary. Promptness in beginning emergency treatment is of utmost importance. Apply a tourniquet above the injection site and inject 0.3 to 0.5 mL epinephrine 1:1,000, preferably IM or, alternatively, subcutaneously into the other arm. It may be necessary to repeat the dose every 5 to 15 minutes because a succession of small doses may be more effective and less dangerous than a single, large dose. Loosen the tourniquet at least every 10 minutes. Also inject a maximum of 0.1 mL epinephrine 1:1,000 at the site of the allergen injection to delay allergen absorption. If more than 1 allergen injection was given, distribute the 0.1 mL evenly among the sites.

In children, base the dose of subcutaneous epinephrine 1:1,000 on age and weight. See table in the Epinephrine monograph.

In general, the pediatric dose is 10 mcg (0.01 mL of a 1:1,000 w/v solution) per kg body weight or 300 mcg (0.3 mL) per m^2 of body surface area, up to 500 mcg (0.5 mL).

After adequate epinephrine has been given and in cases where symptoms of angioedema, urticaria, rhinitis, or conjunctivitis do not respond rapidly, inject an antihistamine (eg, diphenhydramine [*Benadryl*]) intravenously (IV) or IM, according to the manufacturer's directions.

Patients receiving beta-adrenergic antagonists (ie, beta-blockers) may be refractory to the effects of epinephrine.

Other measures that may be necessary include inhaled or parenteral bronchodilators or oxygen for cyanosis; endotracheal intubation, tracheotomy, cricothyrotomy, or trans-tracheal catheterization for laryngeal edema; resuscitation, defibrillation, IV sodium bicarbonate, and other proper medication(s) for cardiac arrest; mechanical airway use if the patient becomes unconscious; and oral or IV corticosteroids if it is likely that the reactions may be prolonged. Monitor hypotension and, if necessary, give vasopressors along with adequate plasma volume replacement.

Syncope after immunization: FDA analysts reviewed 697 cases of syncope after immunization reported to the Vaccine Adverse Events Reporting System (VAERS). The 2 most common age groups were 10 to 19 years of age and 4 to 6 years of age. The vast majority of cases occurred within 15 minutes of administration. Six patients suffered skull fracture, cerebral bleeding, or cerebral contusion from falls; 3 required neurosurgery. Make sure your injection area will allow for fainting without injury.

Immunogenicity: The observed incidence of antibody positivity in immunogenicity assays may be influenced by several factors, including sample handling, timing of sample collection, concomitant medications, and underlying disease. For these reasons, comparison of the incidence of antibodies to one immunologic drug with the incidence of antibodies to other products may be misleading.

Pharmacologic & Dosing Characteristics

Route & Site: Subcutaneous injections are absorbed more slowly than an equivalent volume injected IM. This may slightly reduce the antibody concentrations ultimately obtained. Subcutaneous injections are usually administered into the thigh of infants or the deltoid area of older children and adults. Inject a ⅝- to ¾-inch, 23- to 25-gauge needle into the tissues below the dermal layer of the skin.

Subcutaneous fat in the gluteal area may interfere with the immunogenicity of an adsorbed vaccine. Adults and children should receive these vaccines in the deltoid area. Also avoid injection into the gluteus maximus because of the potential for damage to the sciatic nerve, especially in infants. Take care to avoid major peripheral nerve trunks. If the gluteal region is used, avoid the central region; use only the upper, outer quadrant.

Generally, killed vaccines and vaccines with an adjuvant are injected IM. Subcutaneous or intradermal (ID) injection of these vaccines may cause local irritation, induration, skin discoloration, inflammation, or granuloma formation. Preferred sites of IM injection are the anterolateral aspect of the upper thigh muscle and the deltoid muscle of the upper arm. Select a needle long enough to reach the muscle mass and prevent vaccine from seeping into subcutaneous tissue, but not long enough to endanger underlying neurovascular structures or bone. Base needle size and site of injection on the patient's age, volume of the drug, size of the muscle, and depth below the muscle surface into which the drug is to be injected.

For infants younger than 12 months, the anterolateral aspect of the thigh muscle provides the largest muscle mass. The deltoid muscle can also be used, such as when multiple vaccines are administered during the same visit. In most cases, a ⅞- to 1-inch, 22- to 25-gauge needle is sufficient to penetrate the thigh muscle of an infant 4 months of age.

For toddlers and older children, needle size for the deltoid can range from 22 to 25 gauge and from ⅝ and 1¼ inches. For the anterolateral thigh, use a longer needle (⅞ to 1¼ inches).

For adults, the deltoid muscle is preferred, with a needle size 20 to 25 gauge and 1 to 1½ inches. Analysis of deltoid fat pad thickness in adults suggests the following needle selections: for men, 1- to 1½-inch needles; for women less than 70 kg, 1-inch needles; for women more than 70 kg, 1½-inch needles; for women more than 100 kg and obese men, consider a 2-inch needle. Another study showed that a ⅝-inch, 25-gauge needle for IM injections did not significantly differ from a 1-inch, 25-gauge needle in immunogenicity to hepatitis B vaccine.

Recommendations for IM Injections			
Age group	Site	Needle length	Needle gauge
Infants	thigh	⅝" to 1"	22 to 23
Older children	deltoid	⅞" to 1¼"	22 to 25
	thigh	⅞" to 1"	22 to 25
Adult men	deltoid	1" to 1½"	20 to 25
Women < 60 kg	deltoid	1"	20 to 25
Women 60 to 90 kg	deltoid	1" to 1½"	20 to 25
Women > 90 kg	deltoid	1½"	20 to 25
Obese men and women	deltoid	consider 2"	20 to 25

ID injections are commonly administered on the volar surface of the forearm. With the bevel facing upward, insert a ⅜- to ¾-inch, 25- to 27-gauge needle into the epidermis at an angle parallel to the long axis of the forearm. Insert the needle so the entire bevel penetrates the skin and the injected solution raises a small bleb. Considering the small volume of antigen given in ID injections, take care not to inject the vaccine subcutaneously because this may result in suboptimal immunologic response.

The traditional practice of aspiration is not necessary before subcutaneous or IM immunization because there are no large blood vessels at preferred injection sites.

Preliminary Tests: Perform hypersensitivity tests each time administration of animal serum-based products is anticipated, unless it is being given daily. Carefully review the patient's history, including any report of asthma, hay fever, urticaria or other allergic manifestations, allergic reactions upon exposure to horses or other relevant animals, or prior injections of equine or other heterogeneous serum.

Compounding: For a standard set of 10-fold serial dilutions, compound the most concentrated vial first. Then compound each dilution by drawing a 1 mL aliquot (portion) and adding it to a 9 mL vial of suitable diluent. Refer to Compounding Dilutions Accurately in this section for detailed instructions.

Overdosage: Although little data are available, clinical experience with IV immune globulin preparations suggests that the major manifestations of overdosage would be related to fluid volume overload.

Missed Doses: In general, resume recommended dosage schedules as soon as possible. Additional doses are generally not needed. Refer to individual monographs for specific recommendations (for example, substitute adult-strength Td bivalent or with Tdap for diphtheria and tetanus toxoids with pertussis vaccine (DTaP) if immunization is delayed past the seventh birthday).

Waste Disposal: After administering live, attenuated bacterial or viral products, treat all equipment and materials used (eg, syringes, needles, containers, catheters) as infectious waste, and incinerate, sterilize, or otherwise dispose of as biohazardous waste. Discard disposable needles and syringes in labeled, puncture-proof containers to prevent inadvertent needlestick injury or reuse.

Efficacy: No drug is completely effective. No therapeutic drug is 100% effective. All diagnostic drugs can render false-negative or false-positive results. Vaccination may not result in a protective antibody response in 100% of patients given the vaccine. Efficacy measures may be based on antibody titers induced or, preferably, on the degree of clinical protection (ie, disease avoidance) in community settings.

Onset: An estimate of the onset of the action of the drug.

Duration: An estimate of the duration of the effect of the drug.

Mechanism: A discussion of the mechanism(s) of the action of the drug.

Drug Interactions: Refer to the individual monographs. Short-term corticosteroid therapy (less than 2 weeks) or intra-articular, bursal, or tendon injections of corticosteroids are usually not immunosuppressive. Give immunologic drugs administered IM with caution to patients on anticoagulant therapy or those with bleeding tendencies. IM hepatitis B immunization of 153 hemophiliacs with a 23-gauge needle, followed by steady pressure (without rubbing) to the injection site for 1 to 2 minutes, resulted in a 4% bruising rate; no patients required clotting factor supplementation.

Vaccines: Administration of inactivated vaccines to immunosuppressed patients may result in insufficient response to immunization. Inactivated vaccines are not a risk to immunosuppressed patients, although their efficacy may be substantially reduced. Such patients may remain susceptible to infection despite receiving an appropriate vaccine. If feasible, measure specific serum antibody titers or other immunologic response at an appropriate time interval after immunization to assess immunity. Immunization with live bacterial or viral vaccines in immunosuppressed patients is generally contraindicated because of the risk of vaccine-induced infection. To avoid inactivation of the live microorganism, administer such vaccines 14 to 30 days before or several months after administration of any immune globulin or other blood product. Reconstitute live vaccines with diluents that do not contain antimicrobial preservatives (eg, phenol, thimerosal).

Immune globulins: To avoid inactivation of microorganisms in live bacterial or viral vaccines, administer such vaccines 2 weeks before or 3 to 11 months after administration of any immune globulin or other blood product. Blood products that contain appreciable quantities of IgG include whole blood, packed red cells, plasma, and platelet products.

Immunodiagnostic reagents: Reactivity to immediate-hypersensitivity reagents may be suppressed by drugs with antihistaminic effects and topical corticosteroids. Use a positive-control reagent (eg, histamine) to confirm absence of inhibiting action. Reactivity to delayed-hypersensitivity reagents may be suppressed by systemic corticosteroids and other immunosuppressive drugs or in patients recently immunized with live virus vaccines.

Patient Information: Give a puncture-resistant container for safe disposal of used syringes and needles to patients prescribed immunologic drugs for home parenteral administration. Caution them against reusing syringes and needles.

Pharmaceutical Characteristics

Quality Assay: Potency and safety of immunological products are controlled by various physical and biological means. See individual monographs. Since 1977, each unit of plasma used in production of any immune globulin product must be nonreactive for hepatitis B surface antigen. Similarly, all lots produced since April 1985 must be free of detectable HIV-1 antibodies. All plasma must be obtained from an FDA-approved source, the majority of which harvest blood from American donors. Transmission of non–A, non–B hepatitis (eg, hepatitis C) has been linked with investigational products, but not with commercial products available in the United States. The possibility of transmission of hepatitis B from immune products prepared by Cohn-Oncley cold-ethanol fractionation is extraordinarily remote. Nonetheless, additional virucidal processing steps are also conducted.

Doseform: Immunologic drugs take a variety of forms, including tablets, capsules, solutions, suspensions, powders for reconstitution, pastes, and others. Some are joined with devices (eg, multiple-puncture devices). Always gently agitate suspensions before withdrawing each dose to ensure a uniform suspension.

Appearance: Visually inspect parenteral drug products for particulate matter and discoloration prior to administration whenever solution and container permit. If particulate matter or abnormal discoloration are noted, discard that container. Submit appropriate drug product quality reports to manufacturers or the United States Pharmacopeia.

Diluent: Use the specific recommended diluent for any dilution or infusion to avoid physical or chemical incompatibility and inactivation of the drug. Use the specific quantity called for to obtain the proper concentration.

Adjuvant: Adjuvants are chemicals used to increase the immunogenicity of some vaccines. Salts of aluminum (eg, hydroxide, hydroxyphosphate sulfate, phosphate) are the adjuvants most commonly used in humans.

Preservative: If the drug product includes no preservative, discard unused portions of the container after a single use. The most commonly used preservatives are benzyl alcohol, parabens (eg, methylparaben, propylparaben), phenol, sulfites (eg, metabisulfite), and thimerosal.

The safety issues related to ethyl-mercury content in thimerosal have been scientifically addressed. For details, see the following resources:

Canadian National Advisory Committee on Immunization. Updated recommendations on the use of thimerosal-containing vaccines in Canada. *Can Comm Dis Rep.* 2005;31:(ACS-12):1-4. Available at: http://www.phac-aspc.gc.ca/publicat/ccdr-rmtc/05vol31/asc-dcc-12/index.html.

CDC. Thimerosal. Available at www.cdc.gov/vaccinesafety/Concerns/thimerosal. Accessed May 15, 2011.

Institute of Medicine. *Immunization and Safety Review: Vaccines and Autism*. Washington, DC: National Academy of Sciences; May 2004.

Allergens: If the patient has a known or suspected hypersensitivity to any allergen included in the formulation, administer the drug cautiously, if at all.

When an immunologic drug contains residual neomycin, the amount is usually less than that used for the skin test to determine hypersensitivity. Most often, neomycin allergy is a contact dermatitis, a manifestation of cell-mediated immunity, rather than anaphylaxis, and does not contraindicate administration.

Excipients: Excipients are the inactive ingredients in a drug product needed to physically hold the dose form together, to keep the active ingredient stable and potent, or to perform functions other than the pharmacologic effect of the active ingredient. See Vaccine Excipient and Media Summary for details.

Since 1981, any product containing tartrazine (FD&C yellow dye #5) must be so labeled. The only immunologic drugs containing tartrazine were the adenovirus type 4 and type 7 vaccines through the 1990s (but not present in the 2011 formulation). The Type 7 tablet also contains FD&C Yellow #6 aluminum lake dye.

Shelf Life: Potency expirations are determined by a certain interval after release of the finished product from the manufacturer's cold storage or after successful potency test. Do not use any immunologic drug after the expiration date printed on the container label. In emergency cases, where no in-date product is available, consider the risk-benefit ratio or contact the manufacturer for guidance.

Storage/Stability: Failure to store and handle immunologic products as recommended can degrade potency and may harm patients through lack of clinical effect. Subpotent vaccines may not prevent infection, may not protect against disease, and may yield inaccurate test results, leading to erroneous clinical decisions.

Many immunologic drugs are proteins that can be denatured by heat and, thus, should be refrigerated. When traveling away from home, patients may transport these drugs in household coolers or insulated containers. To avoid freezing, do not place drug vials in direct contact with ice or another frozen coolant, which may inactivate some immunologic drugs. In such cases, vials can be separated from the coolant with a small towel, cardboard, or plastic bubble wrap.

Accelerated degradation of vaccines and other temperature-sensitive drugs may occur if they are stored on shelves in refrigerator doors, rather than in the core of the refrigerator. If space allows, it may be prudent to place coolant packs or containers of water in the refrigerator to reduce temperature fluctuations and serve as a coolant reserve if the refrigerator fails mechanically. These requirements are not idle issues; measles vaccinees whose vaccine was stored in the refrigerator door were more likely to develop the disease than if the vaccine was stored in the heart of the refrigerator. See Handling, Shipping, and Storing Guidelines for details.

Test and document refrigerator (2° to 8°C [35° to 46°F]) and freezer (−20° to −0°C [−4° to 14°F]) temperatures periodically (eg, daily). Do not store refrigerated drugs outside of the refrigerator uninsulated for prolonged intervals. Refrigerators that include an integral recording temperature graph may be purchased; alarm systems are also available. Make coordination of proper vaccine storage the specific responsibility of a staff member. Then train all staff members in proper handling procedures periodically.

Handling: Gloves are not required when administering vaccinations unless the people who administer the vaccine will come into contact with potentially infectious body fluids or have open lesions on their own hands. Gloving may be considered prudent in other settings as well.

Dose preparation: Treat the stoppers of parenteral drug containers with an appropriate disinfectant (eg, isopropyl alcohol 70%). Optimally, allow the disinfectant to work 5 minutes before opening or piercing the container with a needle (most caregivers wait for alcohol to evaporate before proceeding). Gently agitate suspensions. Draw a volume of air into a sterile syringe equal to the volume of liquid drug to be withdrawn. Next, pierce the center of the rubber stopper in the vial, invert the vial, and slowly inject the air in the syringe into the vial. Keeping the tip of the needle immersed, withdraw the desired volume of liquid drug. Alternatively, use a negative-pressure method by retracting the plunger to withdraw the product, and then allowing air in the syringe to flow into the vial to offset the vacuum created. Then, holding the syringe plunger steady, withdraw the needle from the vial. Double-check all vial labels and volume measurements for accuracy.

Thoroughly agitate suspensions before withdrawing each dose to disperse the contents and obtain a uniform suspension. Promptly inject the drug to avoid settling of the suspension in the syringe. To avoid foaming and protein denaturation, do not shake protein solutions (eg, immune globulins, antitoxins, antivenins, interferons). Gentle rotation or swirling will achieve thorough mixing. Recognize the potential contamination hazards, and exercise special precautions to maintain the sterility and potency of each product. Using aseptic techniques and proper storage are essential prior to and after any reconstitution of the vaccine and subsequent withdrawal of individual doses.

Injection site: Cleanse skin overlying the intended injection site with an appropriate antiseptic agent (eg, soap and water, povidone-iodine [*Betadine*], isopropyl alcohol 70%). Optimally, 5 minutes should elapse before injection to allow the germicide to work (most caregivers wait for alcohol to evaporate before proceeding).

Follow usual precautions to avoid injection into or near blood vessels and nerves. After insertion of the needle through the skin, aspiration can ensure that the needle has not entered a blood vessel. If blood or any suspicious discoloration appears in the syringe, do not inject. Rather, discard the contents of the syringe, and repeat these procedures with a new dose at a different site.

Syringe handling: Use a separate needle and syringe for each patient to avoid transmission of hepatitis B and other infectious agents from patient to patient. Use disposable needles and syringes only once. Sterilize reusable glass syringes and needles by autoclaving at 121°C (250°F) for 30 minutes or by use of appropriate dry heat. Sterilization by means of alcohol is not effective. Hepatitis B has been transmitted via common-source contamination of multidose vials.

Jet injection: Jet injectors are needle-free devices that drive liquid medication through a nozzle opening, creating a narrow stream under high pressure that penetrates skin to deliver a medication into intradermal, subcutaneous, or IM tissues. Jet injectors have the potential to reduce the frequency of needle-stick injuries to health care workers and to overcome the improper reuse and other drawbacks of needles and syringes in developing countries. Jet injectors have been reported safe and effective in administering live and inactivated vaccines for viral and bacterial diseases. The immune responses generated are usually equivalent to, and occasionally greater than, those induced by needle injection. However, local reactions or injury (eg, redness, induration, pain, bleeding, ecchymosis at the injection site) can be more frequent for jet injectors compared with needle injection. Jet injectors with multiple-use nozzles have caused transmission of blood-borne pathogens (eg, hepatitis B).

A new generation of jet injectors that use disposable cartridges for both dose chambers and nozzle are now available. Using a new sterile cartridge for each patient and following manufacturers' instructions, these devices avoid the safety concerns described with multi-use nozzle jet injectors.

Guidelines on Use of Immunologic Drugs

Other Information

Perspective:
1657: Christopher Wren performs first IV injection.
1856: In London, Wood and Hunter popularize the hypodermic syringe.
1886: Limousin invents the ampule.
1896: Luer introduces all-glass syringes.
1947: Frank Figge and Robert Hingson develop early forms of jet injectors.

National Policy: Specific policy recommendations issued by the CDC are provided in individual monographs as applicable. The CDC determines national policies through the recommendations of ACIP.

Similarly, any policy statement of the American Academy of Pediatrics issued since the most recent printing of the *Report of the Committee on Infectious Diseases* is also listed. Key Canadian and World Health Organization documents are cited when appropriate. If no national policy exists, pertinent review articles are cited.

ACIP. General recommendations on immunization: Recommendations of the Advisory Committee on Immunization Practices (ACIP). MMWR 2011;60(RR-2):1-61. www.cdc.gov/vaccines/recs/acip/default.htm.

References: Key references. In addition, a bibliography and other detailed references are provided in the References section.

Compounding Dilutions Accurately

Parenteral immunologic drugs are sterile products that should be reconstituted or diluted, if necessary, using aseptic technique, optimally in a vertical laminar air-flow hood. The advantages and disadvantages of specific diluents are discussed in the Diluents monograph in the Non-immunologics section.

For a standard set of 10-fold serial dilutions, compound the most concentrated vial first. Then compound each dilution by withdrawing a 1 mL aliquot (portion) and adding it to a 9 mL vial of suitable diluent. Repeat this procedure serially to yield the proper number of dilutions.

Alternatively, add 0.2 mL of concentrate to 1.8 mL of diluent, or add 0.5 mL to 4.5 mL. Pre-filled 1.8, 4.5, and 9 mL vials are commercially available from allergen-extract manufacturers to facilitate compounding dilutions.

Alternatively, to prepare a 5-fold dilution, add 2 mL concentrate to 8 mL diluent. Comparable concentrations can be achieved by adding 1 mL to 4 mL, adding 0.5 mL to 2 mL, or adding 0.4 mL to 1.6 mL.

Quality control procedures during compounding should emphasize the following:

(1) Maintenance of sterility during manipulation of sterile components, needles, syringes, and containers;

(2) confirmation of identity and volume of each drug and diluent involved;

(3) accurate product labeling; and

(4) complete compounding documentation, including manufacturer and lot number.

Many immunologic drugs are complex products for which end-product testing of identity is not feasible. Because the consequences of a compounding error may include anaphylaxis or death, personnel should emphasize error prevention. Use double-check systems at each compounding step to minimize transcription errors, inaccurate calculations or measurements, and transposition (or reversing) of vials or labels. Check for label reversal in many situations by ensuring that the most concentrated label appears on the vial with the contents of the darkest color.

Inadvertently challenging a hypersensitive patient directly with a full-strength antigen may result in anaphylaxis and death.

Hypersensitivity Testing

The following instructions provide general guidance for performing hypersensitivity tests. Refer to the monographs and product literature for individual immunologic drugs for details.

General Considerations: The back or the inner volar aspect of the forearm is generally the preferred site of hypersensitivity skin testing. The most satisfactory areas of the back range from the posterior axillary fold to the point 2.5 cm from the spinal column and then from the top of the scapula to the lower rib margins. Use skin of the posterior thigh or abdomen if necessary. Avoid hairy areas where possible, because reactions there tend to be smaller and more difficult to interpret.

To Apply a Scratch Skin Test: Apply a scratch test before progressing to an ID test. After suitably preparing the skin surface, use a sterile 20-gauge needle to make a 3 to 5 mm scratch across the epidermis; very little pressure is needed. If bleeding occurs, prepare a second site and scratch more lightly. Apply a small drop of the skin test reagent to the scratch, without touching the dropper to the skin. Rub gently with an applicator, toothpick, or the side of the needle. Alternatively, scratch through a drop of reagent already placed on the skin. Observe the patient for induration, erythema, and itching at the test site during the succeeding 15 minutes. A positive reaction consists of a pale induration, usually with pseudopods, surrounding the scratch site and varying in diameter from 5 to 15 mm or more, most often occurring within 10 minutes. This induration may be surrounded by a variable diameter of erythema and accompanied by a variable degree of itching. Wipe off the solution over the scratch after 15 minutes or as soon as a positive response is clearly evident.

If the scratch test is either negative or equivocally positive (less than 5 mm induration, little or no erythema, and no itching), an ID test may be performed.

To Apply a Prick or Puncture Test: Prick tests (also known as puncture tests) are similar in many ways to scratch tests. Apply a prick test before progressing to an ID test. Insert a suitable prick test needle (eg, a sterile disposable ½-inch, 26-gauge needle) with the bevel up through a drop of allergen superficially into the skin, lift the skin slightly, and then withdraw the needle. No bleeding should be produced. After approximately 1 minute, wipe away the allergen. Wipe needles used for prick tests in a suitable manner after each skin puncture to avoid cross-contamination of skin test sites.

Observe the patient for induration, erythema, and itching at the test site during the succeeding 15 minutes. A positive reaction consists of a pale induration, usually with pseudopods, surrounding the scratch site and varying in diameter from 5 to 15 mm or more, most often within 10 minutes. This induration may be surrounded by a variable diameter of erythema and accompanied by a variable degree of itching.

If the prick or puncture test is either negative or equivocally positive (less than 5 mm induration, little or no erythema, and no itching), an ID test may be performed.

To Apply an ID Test: In most cases, apply a scratch or prick test before progressing to an ID test.

Using a syringe graduated in units of 0.01 mL and a ⅜- to ⅝-inch, 26- to 30-gauge, short-bevel needle, withdraw the contents of the container. Prepare a sterile skin test area on the upper outer arm sufficiently below the deltoid muscle to permit proximal application of a tourniquet later, if needed. Alternatively, use the volar surface of the forearm several inches from any previous test site. Eject all air from the syringe through the needle. Insert the needle, bevel up, immediately below the skin surface. Inject an amount of the skin test reagent sufficient to raise the smallest perceptible bleb. This amount will be from 0.02 to 0.1 mL. Using a separate syringe and needle, inject a like amount of sodium chloride 0.9% as a negative control at least 1.5 inches from the reagent test site. A positive-control reagent (eg, histamine) may be appropriate when applying a battery of allergen-extract skin tests. Most reactions will develop within 5 to 15 minutes. A positive response consists of itching and marked increase in the size of the original bleb. Induration may exceed 20 mm in diameter and exhibit pseudo-pods. An ambiguous response occurs when the induration is only slightly larger than the initial injection bleb, with or without accompanying erythematous flare, yet larger than the negative-control site. A negative response demonstrates no increase in size of the original bleb or no greater reaction than the negative-control site.

The negative-control site should demonstrate no induration or erythema. If it exhibits induration more than 2 to 3 mm, repeat the test. If the same reaction is observed, consult with a specialist experienced in allergy skin testing.

Hypersensitivity Management

Several immunologic drugs contain residual egg proteins remaining from the drug's production process (eg, influenza, yellow fever vaccines). In rare cases, patients who are hypersensitive to these antigens may develop immediate hypersensitivity reactions after drug administration. Use analogous procedures for other allergenic immunologic products. Appropriate patient management may include referral to an allergist or other specialist.

A quick but valid screening procedure to identify egg-hypersensitive patients is to ask about the patient's response to eating egg products. If the patient can tolerate egg ingestion, no hypersensitivity reaction is likely. If a reaction to egg ingestion is reported, the clinical situation may occasionally call for a skin test for hypersensitivity. A variety of procedures have been proposed. Most published reports, including the consensus statement of the American Academy of Pediatrics, involve a procedure similar to the following:

Prick skin testing with:

(1) 1:10 v/v dilutions of influenza vaccine or other drug of interest, and

(2) Sodium chloride 0.9% as a negative control.

A positive prick skin test is generally considered to involve induration 3 mm greater in diameter than the reaction to the negative-control solution.

If these tests are negative, ID tests are applied with:

(1) 0.05 mL of 1:100 v/v dilutions of influenza vaccine or other drug of interest, and

(2) 0.05 mL of sodium chloride 0.9% as a negative control.

A positive ID skin test is generally considered to involve induration 5 mm greater in diameter than the reaction to the negative-control solution.

Generally, the preferred diluent is sodium chloride 0.9%.

Several clinicians have skin tested with egg-white allergen, egg-yolk allergen, or whole-egg allergen mix, but routine application of these reagents in assessing egg hypersensitivity does not seem to add any information for the diagnosis or intervention plan.

If either skin test is positive and the patient's need for the immunologic drug outweighs the risk of not administering the drug, the patient may be desensitized using the following schedule, with subcutaneous injections at 15- to 20-minute intervals if no reactions occur:

(1) 0.05 mL of a 1:100 v/v dilution of the drug of interest;

(2) 0.05 mL of a 1:10 v/v dilution of the drug;

(3) 0.05 mL of the drug undiluted;

(4) 0.1 mL of the drug undiluted;

   (5) 0.15 mL of the drug undiluted;

   (6) 0.2 mL of the drug undiluted.

Repeat this procedure if subsequent doses are needed more than a few days after the last full dose of the drug.

Vaccines & Toxoids

Summary of Vaccines Available in the United States				
Type of Vaccine	Proprietary Names	Viability	Route	Typical Dose
Adenovirus types 4 and 7	Generic	Live	Oral	1 white tablet + 1 peach tablet
Anthrax	*BioThrax*	Inactivated	IM	0.5 mL
BCG	Vaccine (*Tice*)	Live	Scarification	Punctures
Diphtheria-tetanus and acellular pertussis (DTaP)	*Daptacel, Infanrix*	Inactivated	IM	0.5 mL
Diphtheria & tetanus toxoids with acellular pertussis adsorbed, hepatitis B (recombinant), & inactivated poliovirus (DTaP-Hep B-IPV)	*Pediarix*	Inactivated	IM	0.5 mL
Diphtheria & tetanus toxoids with acellular pertussis adsorbed & inactivated poliovirus (DTaP-IPV)	*Kinrix*	Inactivated	IM	0.5 mL
Diphtheria & tetanus toxoids with acellular pertussis adsorbed, inactivated poliovirus, and *Haemophilus influenzae* type b conjugate (DTaP-IPV-Hib)	*Pentacel*	Inactivated	IM	0.5 mL
Diphtheria-tetanus toxoids (DT)	Generic	Inactivated	IM	0.5 mL
Haemophilus influenzae type b conjugate	*ActHIB, Hiberix, PedvaxHIB*	Inactivated	IM	0.5 mL
Haemophilus influenzae type b conjugate & hepatitis B	*Comvax*	Inactivated	IM	0.5 mL
Haemophilus influenzae type b & meningococcal C and Y conjugate (Hib-Men CY)	*Menhibrix*	Inactivated	IM	0.5 mL
Hepatitis A	*Havrix, Vaqta*	Inactivated	IM	1 mL; 0.5 mL if 2 to 18 years of age
Hepatitis A & Hepatitis B	*Twinrix*	Inactivated	IM	1 mL
Hepatitis B	*Engerix-B, Recombivax HB*	Inactivated	IM	Varies

Summary of Vaccines Available in the United States

Summary of Vaccines Available in the United States				
Type of Vaccine	Proprietary Names	Viability	Route	Typical Dose
Influenza A & B				
• Intramuscular	*Afluria, Fluarix, FluLaval, Fluvirin, Fluzone*	Inactivated	IM	0.5 mL
• Intradermal	*Fluzone*	Inactivated	Intradermal	0.1 mL
• Intranasal	*FluMist*	Live	Nasal	0.25 mL in each nostril
Japanese encephalitis	*Ixiaro*	Inactivated	IM	0.5 mL
Measles-mumps-rubella	*M-M-R II*	Live	Subcutaneous	0.5 mL
Measles, mumps, rubella, and varicella	*ProQuad*	Live	Subcutaneous	0.5 mL
Meningococcal A, C, Y, W-135				
• Polysaccharide	*Menomune-A/C/Y/W-135*	Inactivated	Subcutaneous	0.5 mL
• Conjugated	*Menactra, Menveo*	Inactivated	IM	0.5 mL
Papillomavirus, types 6, 11, 16, 18	*Gardasil*	Inactivated	IM	0.5 mL
Papillomavirus, types 16, 18	*Cervarix*	Inactivated	IM	0.5 mL
Pneumococcal, 13-valent	*Prevnar 13*	Inactivated	IM	0.5 mL
Pneumococcal, 23-valent	*Pneumovax 23*	Inactivated	Subcutaneous, IM	0.5 mL
Poliovirus inactivated	*Ipol*	Inactivated	Subcutaneous	0.5 mL
Rabies (various culture media)	*Imovax Rabies, RabAvert*	Inactivated	IM	1 mL
Rotavirus	*Rotarix, RotaTeq*	Live	Oral	1 mL (*Rotarix*), 2 mL (*Rotateq*)
Tetanus-diphtheria with acellular pertussis (Tdap)	*Adacel, Boostrix*	Inactivated	IM	0.5 mL
Tetanus toxoid (adsorbed) (TT)	Generic	Inactivated	IM	0.5 mL
Tetanus-diphtheria toxoids (Td)	Generic, *Decavac*	Inactivated	IM	0.5 mL
Typhoid (oral)	*Vivotif Berna*	Live	Oral	4 capsules
Typhoid Vi (parenteral, polysaccharide)	*Typhim Vi*	Inactivated	IM	0.5 mL

Summary of Vaccines Available in the United States				
Type of Vaccine	Proprietary Names	Viability	Route	Typical Dose
Vaccinia (smallpox)	*ACAM2000*	Live	Scarification	15 punctures
Varicella	*Varivax*	Live	Subcutaneous	0.5 mL
Yellow fever	*YF-Vax*	Live	Subcutaneous	0.5 mL
Zoster	*Zostavax*	Live	Subcutaneous	0.65 mL

Anthrax Vaccine

Bacterial Vaccines & Toxoids

Name: *Manufacturer:*
  BioThrax   Emergent Biosolutions

Synonyms: VISI abbreviation: ANT. The vaccine is also known as anthrax vaccine adsorbed (AVA). The disease is also known as woolsorters' disease, ragpickers' disease, malignant pustule, and charbon.

Immunologic Characteristics

Microorganism: Bacterium, *Bacillus anthracis*, endospore-forming gram-positive rod. The organism possesses 2 virulence factors: A bacterial capsule and a 3-part toxin complex, consisting of protective antigen (PA), lethal factor (LF), and edema factor (EF). PA is cleaved at certain cell receptors, binding with either LF or EF to produce active lethal toxin or edema toxin. Lethal and edema toxins inhibit the function of macrophages and neutrophils. The poly-D-glutamic acid capsule inhibits phagocytosis.

Viability: Inactivated

Antigenic Form: Cell-free microaerobic culture filtrate containing PA, the common feature of disease-causing anthrax strains

Antigenic Type: Protein

Strains: Avirulent, nonencapsulated, nonproteolytic V770-NP1-R strain of *B. anthracis*

Use Characteristics

Indications: Induction of active immunity against anthrax. Need for vaccination is based on exposure to *B. anthracis* or its spores, especially in imported hides, hairs, or bones that come from endemic areas (eg, Africa, Asia). Anthrax spores have been found on Haitian goatskin crafts, which can no longer be imported, and skins used to make drumheads. Protection against occupational risk for people engaged in diagnostic or investigational activities, including veterinarians and other people handling potentially infected animals. In the pivotal human field trial, vaccine recipients were less likely to contract either cutaneous anthrax or inhalational anthrax compared with those not vaccinated.

Although not explicitly reflected in product labeling, anthrax vaccine is used for immunization against malicious exposure to *B. anthracis* or its spores in warfare or terrorist events.

Limitations: Anthrax immunization alone after exposure may not protect against infection. Select appropriate antibiotics to treat or prevent active infections (eg, ciprofloxacin, doxycycline, penicillin G with either streptomycin or gentamicin). After exposure, immunization may still be needed to protect against later germination of spores into vegetative cells within the body.

No vaccine is completely effective. Hypothetically, the protection afforded by anthrax vaccine may be overwhelmed by exposure to massive doses of this bacterium.

Contraindications:

Absolute: History of anthrax infection or severe adverse reaction, including a serious allergic reaction to a vaccine component or after a prior dose of this vaccine.

Relative: Defer immunization in the event of acute respiratory disease or other active infection, unless delay would pose a greater threat to health.

Immunodeficiency: Patients receiving immunosuppressive therapy or those with other immunodeficiencies may have diminished antibody response to active immunization and remain susceptible to the disease.

Elderly: Although there is no evidence of lack of efficacy, it is not currently recommended by the manufacturer for use in patients older than 65 years because no studies have been conducted in that population. Nonetheless, immunization may be prudent in emergency situations.

Fertility Impairment: Anthrax-vaccinated women were as likely to conceive and to deliver offspring as unvaccinated women (Wiesen & Littell, 2002). At an assisted reproduction clinic, anthrax-vaccinated and -unvaccinated men had comparable values for semen parameters (concentration, motility, morphology), fertilization rate, embryo quality, and clinical pregnancy rates (Catherino, et al. 2005).

Pregnancy: Category D. Use only if clearly needed. It is not known if anthrax vaccine or corresponding antibodies cross the placenta. Generally, most IgG passage across the placenta occurs during the third trimester.

Lactation: It is not known if anthrax vaccine or corresponding antibodies are excreted in breast milk. Problems in humans have not been documented and are unlikely, as with other vaccines.

Children: Not currently recommended for use in patients younger than 18 years because no studies of safety or efficacy have been conducted in that population. Nonetheless, immunization may be prudent in emergency situations.

Adverse Reactions: Anthrax vaccine can cause soreness, redness, itching, swelling, and lumps (nodules) when injected subcutaneously at the injection site. Mild injection-site reactions, including local erythema and tenderness, are reported by approximately 30% of men and 60% of women. Such reactions usually occur within 24 hours and begin to subside by 48 hours. Moderate local reactions, defined as erythema more than 5 mm, may occur after a second injection (4%), occasionally with pruritus. For both genders, between 1% and 5% report moderate reactions of 1 to 5 inches in diameter. Larger reactions occur in approximately 1 in 100 vaccinees. Subcutaneous nodules may occur at the injection site and persist for several weeks. These reactions may also occur if patients with a history of natural anthrax infection are vaccinated.

Systemic reactions, usually characterized by malaise or lassitude, may occur. Chills and fever are rare. In severe cases, discontinue the immunization regimen unless needed for post-exposure prophylaxis. Based on survey data, 5% to 35% of anthrax vaccine recipients report muscle aches, joint aches, chills, fever, headaches, nausea, loss of appetite, malaise, or related symptoms. These symptoms typically go away within a few days. There are no known long-term patterns of adverse effects from anthrax vaccine.

In a record-linkage study spanning 4.2 years of experience, anthrax-vaccinated soldiers were evaluated for occupational disability claims at the same rate as unvaccinated soldiers. Subset analyses similarly found no differences for men alone, women alone, permanent disability, temporary disability, musculoskeletal disability, or neurologic disability.

Although anthrax vaccine has been alleged to contribute to "Gulf War illnesses," independent review panels convened by the Institute of Medicine (1995), the Presidential Advisory Committee on Gulf War Veterans' Illnesses (1996), the National Institute of Health (1994), and the Defense Science Board Task Force on Persian Gulf War Health Effects (1994) concluded that there is no credible evidence of any such link. For example, studies conducted by the Centers for Disease Control and Prevention (CDC) found no association between vaccination and "Gulf War" symptoms.

Anthrax Vaccine

Pharmacologic & Dosing Characteristics

Dosage: The primary immunizing series consists of 3 doses at 0, 1, and 6 months, with booster doses at 12 and 18 months after starting the primary series, with annual booster doses thereafter. Shake well before withdrawing each dose.

For postexposure prophylaxis, a regimen of 3 subcutaneous doses of 0.5 mL at 2-week intervals has been suggested, based on nonhuman primate studies, with antibiotic therapy until a few weeks after the third dose is received. This regimen is not licensed at this printing.

Route: IM. Historically, the subcutaneous route was the licensed route for many years, although it was more reactogenic.

Overdosage: Although few data are available, clinical experience with similar products suggests that the major manifestations of overdosage would be pain and tenderness at the injection site.

Booster Doses: 0.5 mL at 1-year intervals if continued immunity is needed.

Missed Doses: Prolonging the interval between vaccine doses does not interfere with immunity achieved after the concluding dose of the basic series, but may delay the induction of immunity. Resume the dosing regimen as soon as possible. Calculate the dates for subsequent doses based on the proper interval between doses, not by time elapsed from the first dose.

Efficacy: A 92.5% reduction in disease incidence (95% CI, 65% to 100%) was observed after a basic series of 6 doses of a related vaccine in a study of 1,249 New England mill workers. The 92.5% value was based jointly on protection from cutaneous anthrax and inhalational anthrax. In this study, 18 cases of cutaneous anthrax developed among patients who had received no vaccine, 2 cases developed among patients who had received 3 doses of vaccine, and 1 developed in a patient who had received 2 doses of vaccine. Five cases of inhalational anthrax occurred in unimmunized subjects but none in immunized subjects. Inhalational anthrax occurred too rarely in the study population for protective efficacy to be statistically assessed separately.

To assess the value of anthrax immunization from aerosol exposure, such as might be seen in warfare or a terrorist attack, nonhuman-primate inhalation-challenge studies have been performed by the US Army Medical Research Institute of Infectious Diseases. After 1 or 2 doses of anthrax vaccine, 62 of 65 rhesus monkeys survived challenge with the virulent Ames strain of anthrax or other strains, whereas none of 18 unvaccinated monkeys survived. Similarly, 114 of 117 vaccinated rabbits survived, whereas none of 28 unvaccinated rabbits survived.

Onset: Escalating protection after each dose

Duration: At least 1 year, after a basic series of doses

Mechanism: Induces protective antibodies that neutralize components of *B. anthracis*, particularly targeting the toxin component known as factor II or the PA.

Drug Interactions: Like all inactivated vaccines, administration of anthrax vaccine to patients receiving immunosuppressant drugs (eg, high-dose corticosteroids) or radiation therapy may result in an insufficient response to immunization. They may remain susceptible despite immunization.

Inactivated vaccines are not generally affected by circulating antibodies or administration of exogenous antibodies. Vaccination may occur at any time before or after antibody administration.

Pharmaceutical Characteristics

Concentration: Contains 5 to 20 mcg/mL of total protein, at least 35% of which is 83-kilodalton PA protein. Comparable with US Reference Anthrax Vaccine. Potency in humans is inferred from protection against an intracutaneous challenge of 1,000 spores of the virulent Vollum strain in guinea pigs.

Quality Assay: Guinea pig potency test for comparability with US Reference Anthrax Vaccine. Current product content standards require 5 to 20 mcg/mL of total protein, of which at least 35% is the 83-kilodalton PA protein, measured by densitometric analysis on sodium dodecyl sulfate-polyacrylamide gel electrophoresis (SDS-PAGE), after pooling 12 sublots. Polyacrylamide gel electrophoresis reveals a faintly detectable band for lethal factor and no detectable band for edema factor. USP monograph.

Packaging: Ten 0.5 mL doses per 5 mL multidose vial.

NDC Number: 64678-0211-05

Doseform: Suspension

Appearance: After shaking, product forms an opaque, white suspension.

Solvent: 0.85% sodium chloride

Adjuvant: Aluminum hydroxide, containing aluminum 0.8 to 1.5 mg/mL

Preservative: Formaldehyde 0.02% or less, benzethonium chloride 0.0015% to 0.003%

Allergens: The vial stopper may contain dry natural latex rubber.

Excipients: Sodium chloride 0.75% to 0.95%

pH: 7.5 to 8.5

Shelf Life: Expires within 48 months

Storage/Stability: Store at 2° to 8°C (35° to 46°F). Do not freeze. Contact manufacturer regarding prolonged exposure to room temperature or elevated or freezing temperatures. Shipped in insulated containers with coolant packs and temperature monitors.

Production Process: Prepared from filtrates of microaerophilic cultures of an avirulent, non-encapsulated strain of *B. anthracis*. These filtrates from the culture fluid are cell free and contain the factor known as PA, elaborated by the bacteria during the growth period. Aluminum hydroxide gel adsorption is used to isolate PA from the culture filtrate. This component is concentrated 10-fold and resuspended in physiologic saline. Formaldehyde and benzethonium chloride are added later in processing as preservatives.

Media: Synthetic protein-free liquid medium containing amino acids, vitamins, inorganic salts, and sugars, comparable with Puziss-Wright 1095 medium

Disease Epidemiology

Anthrax is an infection of the skin, lungs, and intestines, caused by *B. anthracis*. These bacteria can cause severe complications and death. If untreated, 5% to 20% of people infected through the skin may die; nearly all of those infected through the lungs may die. Anthrax involves fever, malaise, cough, abdominal and muscle pain, diarrhea, labored breathing, and headache. Skin infections begin as a red-brown bump that gradually enlarges. The site will also have redness, blistering, ulceration, and swollen lymph nodes. The case-fatality rate of GI anthrax is estimated at 50%. The case-fatality rate of recognized inhalation anthrax ranges from 45% to 80%; if undetected, inhalational anthrax is nearly always fatal.

Incidence: Only 6 reported cases from 1980 through 1992 in the United States. Eighteen people (confirmed, plus 4 more probable cases) were infected with anthrax during terror attacks in fall 2001.

Susceptible Pools: Estimates of the world incidence of anthrax in 1962 ranged from 20,000 to 100,000 cases per year, primarily because of agricultural exposure. In the 1980s, the estimate had fallen to approximately 2,000 cases annually, plus isolated epidemics.

Anthrax Vaccine

Transmission: Contact with diseased tissue, contaminated soil, hair, wool, or hides, or products containing contaminated materials. Anthrax is not generally transmissible from person to person. The infective dose ranges from 8,000 to 50,000 natural spores by the aerosol route. Spread of anthrax spores is considered a biological warfare or terrorism threat. The World Health Organization estimates that 50 kg of aerosolized anthrax spores, dispensed from an airplane in suitable weather conditions, could kill or incapacitate 220,000 people; other casualty estimates are higher.

Incubation: 2 to 5 days

Communicability: No evidence of transmission from person to person, except for rare instances with cutaneous anthrax.

Other Information

Perspective: Anthrax may have been the "Fifth Plague" described in Exodus.

1849: Pollender discovers *B. anthracis.*

1881: Pasteur administers live, attenuated anthrax vaccine to 24 sheep, 1 goat, and 6 cows. All the animals survived challenge 26 days later with virulent bacteria, while control animals died.

1895: Sclavo and Marchoux independently develop anthrax antisera.

1942: Biological warfare experiments contaminate island of Gruinard, off the western coast of Scotland. Island decontaminated in 1990 with a mixture of sea water and formaldehyde.

1948: Gladstone develops an acellular vaccine for human use.

1950: Wright, Puziss, and colleagues develop culture filtrate as effective vaccine. Merck, Sharp, and Dohme prepares inactivated vaccine for US Army researchers at Fort Detrick, Maryland.

1962: Brachman and colleagues publish results of 1950s field trial of anthrax vaccine in textile mill workers.

1970: MDPH vaccine licensed on November 4.

1979: Accident in Soviet biological warfare laboratory infects 96 and kills at least 66 people near Sverdlovsk (now called Yekaterinburg).

1991: One or 2 doses of anthrax vaccine administered to approximately 150,000 of the 500,000 American troops deployed for the Persian Gulf War; some immunization records listed the product as "Vaccine A."

1995: Iraq admits to United Nations officials that it had developed and deployed Scud missile warheads containing anthrax spores in 1991.

1998: Immunization of American soldiers, sailors, airmen, marines, and coast guardsmen against anthrax begins. By mid-2010, 2.5 million people vaccinated with more than 9.8 million doses of vaccine.

2001: Eighteen people (confirmed, plus 4 more probable cases) were infected with anthrax during terror attacks in the eastern United States.

National Policy: ACIP. Use of anthrax vaccine in the United States. *MMWR.* 2010;59(RR-6):1-30. www.cdc.gov/mmwr/PDF/rr/rr5906.pdf.

References: Brachman PS, Gold H, Plotkin SA, Fekety FR, Werrin M, Ingraham NR. Field evaluation of a human anthrax vaccine. *Am J Public Health Nations Health.* 1962;52(4):632-645.

Catherino WH, Levi A, Kao TC, Leondires MP, McKeeby J, Segars JH. Anthrax vaccine does not affect semen parameters, embryo quality, or pregnancy outcome in couples with a vaccinated male military service member. *Fertil Steril.* 2005;83(2):480-483.

Dixon TC, Meselson M, Guillemin J, Hanna PC. Anthrax. *N Engl J Med.* 1999;341(11):815-826.

Food & Drug Administration. Biological products; bacterial vaccines and toxoids; implementation of efficacy review. *Fed Reg.* 1985;50(240):51002-51117.

Food & Drug Administration. Biological products; bacterial vaccines and toxoids; implementation of efficacy review; anthrax vaccine adsorbed; final order. *Fed Reg.* 2005;70(242):75180-75198.

Holty JE, Bravata DM, Liu H, Olshen RA, McDonald KM, Owens DK. Systematic review: a century of inhalational anthrax cases from 1900 to 2005. *Ann Intern Med.* 2006;144(4):270-280.

Inglesby TV, O'Toole T, Henderson DA, et al; Working Group on Civilian Biodefense. Anthrax as a biological weapon, 2002: updated recommendations for management. *JAMA.* 2002;287(17):2236-2252. http://jama.ama-assn.org/issues/v287n17/fpdf/jst20007.pdf.

Jollenbeck LM, Zwanziger L, Durch JS, Strom BL, eds. *The Anthrax Vaccine: Is It Safe? Does It Work?* Washington, DC: National Academy Press; 2002. http://www.nap.edu/catalog/10310.html.

Wiesen AR, Littell CT. Relationship between prepregnancy anthrax vaccination and pregnancy and birth outcomes among US Army women. *JAMA*. 2002;287(12):1556-1560.

Anthrax Vaccine Summary Table	
Generic name	Anthrax vaccine adsorbed
Brand name	*BioThrax*
Synonyms	ANT, AVA
Manufacturer	Emergent BioSolutions
Viability	Bacterial subunit vaccine
Indication	To prevent infection with *Bacillus anthracis*.
Strain	V770-NP1-R
Concentration	5 to 20 mcg/mL protein, $\geq$ 35% protective antigen
Adjuvant	Aluminum hydroxide, 0.8 to 1.5 mg Al per mL
Preservative	Benzethonium chloride 0.0025%, formaldehyde $\leq 0.02\%$
Production medium	Synthetic medium
Doseform	Suspension
Solvent	Isotonic sodium chloride
Packaging	5 mL multidose vial
Routine storage	2° to 8°C
Dosage, route	0.5 mL IM
Standard schedule	3 doses: 0, 1, and 6 months, then booster doses at 12 and 18 months after starting primary series, plus annual boosters
CPT Code	90581

Bacillus Calmette-Guérin (BCG) Vaccine

Bacterial Vaccines & Toxoids

Name:
BCG Vaccine

Manufacturer:
Merck

Synonyms: Bacille or Bacillus Calmette-Guérin, BCG. In French, Vaccin BCG. BCG is not synonymous with tuberculosis. The disease tuberculosis has been called by various names, including consumption, phthisis, the "white plague" (Oliver Wendell Holmes, Sr.), and the "captain of all these men of death" (John Bunyan).

Comparison: BCG products are not generically equivalent because of differences in potency, route of administration, and indications. The various strains of BCG are microbiologically distinct. Intradermal vaccination may cause fewer local reactions than subcutaneous injection. A compilation of global BCG vaccination policies appears at www.bcgatlas.org. For information about BCG for treatment of bladder cancer, see the BCG monograph in the Mediators/ Modulators section.

Immunologic Characteristics

Microorganism: Bacterium, *Mycobacterium bovis*, aerobic gram-positive rod, acid-fast bacillus (AFB), family Mycobacteriaceae. Also called *M. tuberculosis* variant *bovis*.

Viability: Live, attenuated

Antigenic Form: Whole bacterium

Antigenic Type: Protein

Strains: *Tice* substrain of BCG strain of *M. tuberculosis*. *Tice* strain was developed at the University of Illinois beginning in 1934 from a BCG strain of *M. bovis* originating at the Pasteur Institut in Paris.

Use Characteristics

Indications: For the induction of active immunity against *M. tuberculosis* variant *hominus* in people not previously infected with tuberculosis who are at high risk for exposure; to lower the risk of serious complications of tuberculosis. BCG vaccination is recommended for tuberculin purified protein derivative (PPD) skin test–negative infants and children at high risk of intimate and prolonged exposure to persistently treated or ineffectively treated patients with infectious pulmonary tuberculosis who cannot be removed from the source of exposure, nor be placed on long-term preventive therapy.

BCG vaccination is recommended for people who are continuously exposed to tuberculosis patients who have mycobacteria resistant to isoniazid and rifampin and who cannot be removed from the source of exposure.

BCG vaccination is recommended on an individual basis for health care workers in whom 3 conditions are met:

• A high proportion of *M. tuberculosis* isolates are resistant to both isoniazid and rifampin
• There is a strong likelihood of transmission and infection
• Comprehensive infection control precautions have failed

Counsel health care workers and other vaccine candidates about the risks and benefits of both BCG vaccination and preventive chemotherapy. Advise them of the uncertainties associated with measuring BCG efficacy (especially among adults) and interference between BCG vaccination and tuberculin skin tests (but not with interferon gamma–release assays [IGRAs]).

BCG probably confers protection against serious forms of disease (eg, miliary and meningeal tuberculosis), but data on pulmonary disease are unclear. BCG does not appear to prevent infection but may reduce transmission.

BCG vaccination can protect well-defined communities against tuberculosis where the rate of new infection is more than 1% per year. It can also protect those for whom the usual surveillance and treatment programs have been attempted but are not operationally feasible. These groups include people without regular access to health care, those for whom usual health care is culturally or socially unacceptable, and groups who have demonstrated an inability to effectively use existing accessible care.

Induction of active immunity against tuberculosis in certain international travelers is recommended. However, the Centers for Disease Control and Prevention (CDC) suggests that BCG vaccination be considered only for travelers with an insignificant reaction to tuberculin skin tests who will be in a high-risk environment for prolonged periods of time without access to tuberculin skin test surveillance.

Unlabeled Uses: BCG vaccine induces antibodies that bind to *M. leprae* and may be effective in the prevention of leprosy. The Advisory Committee on Immunization Practices (ACIP) no longer recommends BCG vaccination of health care workers at risk of repeated exposure to tuberculosis, but it recommends that these individuals receive periodic tuberculin skin tests and isoniazid prophylaxis in case of tuberculin skin test conversion. The CDC does not recommend routine BCG vaccination of health care workers, but it does urge increased compliance with existing screening programs and antituberculosal prophylaxis.

Limitations: The primary strategy for preventing and controlling tuberculosis in the United States is to minimize the risk for transmission by early identification and treatment of patients who have active infectious tuberculosis. The second most important strategy is the identification of people who have latent *M. tuberculosis* infection and, if indicated, the use of chemotherapy to prevent the latent infection from progressing to active tuberculosis disease. BCG has only limited efficacy against infection and can confound the interpretation of tuberculin skin tests, but not IGRAs. BCG is less effective among people vaccinated as adults, compared with people vaccinated as children.

Contraindications:

Absolute: Immunodeficient patients. Patients with a history of a serious allergic reaction to a vaccine component or after a prior dose of this vaccine. Avoid BCG use in asymptomatic carriers with a positive HIV serology and in patients receiving corticosteroids at immunosuppressive doses or other immunosuppressive therapies because of the possibility of systemic BCG infection.

Relative: A positive IGRA or intradermal tuberculin skin test to 5-TU of PPD is a contraindication to vaccination against tuberculosis, but a contraindication to use for treatment of bladder cancer only if an active tuberculosis infection is in progress or suspected. If the patient exhibits a significant reaction to a 5-TU PPD test, use a physical examination, including chest radiograph, to assess tuberculosis infection.

Immunodeficiency: Do not use in immunodeficient patients, including patients with congenital or acquired immune deficiencies, whether due to genetics, disease, or drug or radiation therapy. Contains live bacteria. Several cases of disseminated BCG infection occurred in HIV-positive infants immunized during the first year of life and in adults with AIDS. In African epidemiologic studies, there is no apparent increased risk of adverse effects from BCG immunization in infants of HIV-positive mothers.

Elderly: Clinical studies of BCG vaccine did not include sufficient subjects 65 years and older to determine whether they respond differently from younger subjects. Other reported clinical experience has not identified differences in response between elderly and younger patients. An intact immune system is a prerequisite for BCG vaccination. If the immune status of an eld-

Bacillus Calmette-Guérin (BCG) Vaccine

erly patient, or any patient, is in question, hold BCG vaccination until the immune status of the patient has been evaluated.

Pregnancy: Category C. Contraindicated on hypothetical grounds. Avoid use. Use only if clearly needed. It is not known if BCG vaccine or corresponding antibodies cross the placenta.

Lactation: It is not known if BCG vaccine or corresponding antibodies are excreted in breast milk. Problems in humans have not been documented. A Canadian study suggests that breast-feeding enhanced cell-mediated immune response to BCG when it was administered at birth, but it had no significant effect if the vaccine was given at least 1 month after birth.

Children: BCG vaccination is widely used in infants and children in many countries. To vaccinate infants, give half the adult immunizing dose by diluting the vaccine powder with 2 mL of diluent rather than 1 mL.

Adverse Reactions: Although BCG vaccination often causes local reactions, serious or long-term complications are rare. Reactions expected after vaccination include moderate axillary or cervical lymphadenopathy and induration and subsequent pustule formation at the injection site; these reactions can persist for up to 3 months after vaccination. More serious local reactions include ulceration at the vaccination site, regional suppurative lymphadenitis with draining sinuses, and caseous lesions or purulent draining at the puncture site. These manifestations may occur up to 5 months after vaccination and persist for several weeks. Intensity and duration of the local reaction depend on depth of penetration of the multiple-puncture device and individual variation. Tenderness at the puncture site may occur, as well as itching. The initial skin lesions usually appear within 10 to 14 days and consist of small red papules. The papules reach maximum diameter (about 3 mm) after 4 to 6 weeks, after which they may scale and then slowly subside. Systemic adverse events lasting 1 to 2 days (eg, fever, anorexia, myalgia, neuralgia) often reflect hypersensitivity reactions. Symptoms such as fever greater than or equal to 103°F or acute localized inflammation persisting longer than 2 to 3 days suggest active infections. If a BCG infection is suspected, consult promptly with an infectious disease expert before starting therapy. In patients who develop persistent fever or experience an acute febrile illness consistent with BCG infection, administer 2 or more antimycobacterial agents while diagnostic evaluation, including cultures, is conducted. Negative cultures do not necessarily rule out infection.

The most serious complication of BCG vaccination is disseminated BCG infection. The most frequent disseminated infection is BCG osteomyelitis (0.01 to 43 cases per million doses of vaccine administered), which usually occurs 4 months to 2 years after vaccination. Fatal disseminated BCG infection has occurred at a rate of 0.06 to 1.56 cases per million doses; these deaths occurred primarily among immunocompromised people.

Consultation: Prescribers considering the use of BCG vaccine for their patients are encouraged to consult the tuberculosis control program in their area.

Lab interference: BCG does not interfere with IGRAs.

Treatment of disseminated infection: Isoniazid (INH), rifampin, streptomycin, or other antituberculous medication may be used to treat disseminated BCG infection. All BCG strains are resistant to pyrazinamide, which is of no value in this setting. Management of BCG adenitis varies from no treatment to surgical drainage or antitubercular medications, or both.

Occupational exposure: PPD- or IGRA-negative health care personnel who routinely handle BCG vaccine should record annual PPD or IGRA skin test results. In case BCG vaccine splashes into an eye, flush the affected eye(s) with large volumes of water for 15 minutes while holding the eyelid(s) open. In case of accidental self-inoculation, give a PPD skin test at the time of the accident and 6 weeks later to detect any skin test conversion. Asymptomatic skin test conversion attributable to BCG exposure is equivalent to BCG vaccination and does not require antituberculous medication.

Bacillus Calmette-Guérin (BCG) Vaccine

Pharmacologic & Dosing Characteristics

Dosage: Cleanse the skin site with an alcohol or acetone sponge and allow to dry thoroughly. Position the arm to maintain a horizontal surface. Drop 0.2 to 0.3 mL onto the cleansed surface of the skin and spread over a 1 inch by 2 inch area using the edge of the multiple puncture device. Grasp the arm firmly from underneath, tensing the skin. Center the multiple-puncture device over the vaccine and apply firm downward pressure, so that the device points are well buried in the skin. Maintain pressure for 5 seconds. Do not "rock" the device. Release pressure underneath the arm and remove the device. In a successful procedure, the points puncture the skin. If the points merely indent the skin, repeat the procedure. After successful puncture, spread vaccine as evenly as possible over the puncture area with the edge of the device. An additional 1 to 2 drops of BCG vaccine may be added to ensure a very wet vaccination site. Use a multiple-puncture device once only, then discard it in standard biohazard containers. No dressing is required; however, the site should be loosely covered and kept dry for 24 h. Advise the patient that the vaccine contains live organisms. Although the vaccine will not survive in a dry state for long, infection of others is possible.

Children: Give children 1 month of age or younger half the adult immunizing dose by diluting the vaccine powder with 2 mL of diluent rather than 1 mL.

Normal reactions to tuberculosis vaccination consist of skin lesions of small red papules appearing within 10 to 14 days. The papules may reach a maximum diameter of approximately 3 mm after 4 to 6 weeks, after which they may scale and then slowly subside.

Keep the vaccination site clean until the local reaction disappears. Usually, no visible sign of vaccination persists 6 months later, although a discernible pattern of puncture points may remain in people prone to keloid formation. Such marks are typically a permanent, slightly excavated, round scar 4 to 8 mm in diameter.

Route & Site: Order multiple-puncture devices for tuberculosis vaccination from Organon Teknika (800-662-6842). The device consists of a wafer-like, stainless-steel plate, 7/8-inch wide and 1 1/8-inch long, from which 36 points protrude. The anatomic site of vaccination is not standardized and may appear at various locations on the body, although the product labeling suggests the upper arm.

Dose preparation: Draw 1 mL of sterile, preservative-free sodium chloride 0.9% injection into a small syringe and add to 1 vial of *Tice BCG* vaccine to resuspend. Gently swirl the vial until a homogenous suspension is obtained. Avoid forceful agitation that may cause clumping of the mycobacteria.

Additional Doses: Repeat vaccination against tuberculosis after 2 to 3 months for those patients who remain negative to a 5-TU tuberculin skin test. If a vaccinated infant remains tuberculin negative to 5-TU PPD, and if indications for vaccination persist, give a full dose after the first birthday. Immunity to tuberculosis is generally considered long-lasting; routine booster immunizations are not recommended. The probability of tuberculin reactivity diminishes as the time since BCG exposure increases.

Waste Disposal: Autoclave, incinerate, or otherwise properly discard all materials contaminated during use of BCG vaccine.

Efficacy: The efficacy of currently available BCG vaccine is inferred. A meta-analysis suggests that BCG vaccines reduce disease incidence 51%. If only randomized trials are considered, the efficacy rate is 63%. Among children, the efficacy of BCG against serious forms of tuberculosis is more than 80%. Clinical trials have yielded inconsistent results, with vaccine-efficacy estimates ranging from near zero in trials in India to 14% in the southern United States, to 80% in Europe and Canada.

Likely explanations for these discrepancies in efficacy seen in field trials include differences in BCG strains, regional mycobacterial ecology, trial methods, stages of mycobacterial

Bacillus Calmette-Guérin (BCG) Vaccine

infection and disease, and other factors. Ironically, BCG may be the most widely used vaccine in the world, yet has the least scientific evidence of efficacy, mechanism of action, and utility. BCG probably confers protection against serious forms of disease (eg, miliary and meningeal tuberculosis), but data on pulmonary disease is unclear. BCG does not appear to prevent infection, but may reduce transmission.

In a prospective trial using *Tice* strain of BCG, Rosenthal studied 1,716 vaccinated and 1,665 nonvaccinated infants, all born at Chicago's Cook County Hospital and followed for 12 to 23 years. The diagnosis of tuberculosis was based on chest x-ray results and clinical findings. There were 17 cases of tuberculosis among those vaccinated (0.43/1,000 per year) and 65 cases in those nonvaccinated (1.7/1,000 per year), a 75% reduction ($P < 0.001$). One death was attributed to tuberculosis among vaccinees, compared to 6 deaths among controls, a reduction of 83%. There were 639 families with a sibling in both the vaccine and control groups. Eight of 790 vaccinees (1%) developed tuberculosis, compared with 30 of 945 controls (3.2%, $P < 0.001$). Thirteen cases of nonfatal tuberculosis developed in the control group who were 2 years or younger, with none in the vaccinated group. Three deaths from tuberculosis occurred in the control group younger than 2.5 years (all with miliary tuberculosis with meningitis), with one death in the vaccinated group (meningitis). The vaccinated infant who died had not converted to a positive PPD skin test at 6 months of age and was not subsequently revaccinated. Following a single vaccination, 99.3% of all infants studied became PPD positive, with 84.2% still being positive after 8 years.

In a 1995 study of vaccine potency, tuberculin-negative subjects were vaccinated with *Tice BCG* vaccine and subsequent tuberculin conversion was monitored. Conversion from a negative to a positive skin test may be considered a surrogate indicator of potency and efficacy of BCG vaccines; however, the correlation between PPD conversion and vaccine effectiveness has not been established. Twenty-two of 24 subjects (92%) who returned for follow-up testing with 10-TU PPD 8 weeks after vaccination converted to positive (skin test reading greater than 5 mm induration at 48 hours) and 2 remained negative. The mean positive skin test reading was 15.5 mm induration. In a second study, 22 volunteers 18 to 40 years of age who were not health care workers, were not foreign born, were HIV negative, and were negative responders to a 10-TU PPD skin test were vaccinated with the standard dose of *Tice BCG* vaccine. Eight weeks after vaccination, the subjects returned for a 10 TU PPD skin test. Twenty-one of 22 (95%) converted to PPD positive at greater than 5 mm induration.

Leprosy: Estimates range from a 20% to 80% reduction in disease incidence among contacts of leprosy patients.

Onset: Vaccinated patients typically become skin test positive to PPD within 8 to 14 weeks. In a study of PPD-negative and HIV-negative health care workers, indurated papules developed at the vaccination site with a mean maximal diameter of 9 mm (typically 5 to 15 mm), which resolved over a mean of 48 days (range, 2 to 10 weeks). A crust forms at the center of the papule, which falls off between the second and fourth week after vaccination, leaving a central ulceration. The mean maximal ulceration diameter is 5 mm (range, 1 to 10 mm), resolving over a mean of 35 days. A permanent scar of 5 to 15 mm usually develops.

Duration: Induced immunity to tuberculosis is generally considered long-lasting; routine booster immunizations are not recommended. The probability of tuberculin reactivity diminishes as the time since BCG exposure increases.

Mechanism: Induces cell-mediated immunity against tuberculosis. It is unclear if BCG induces antitubercular antibodies.

Drug Interactions: As with all live bacterial vaccines, administration of BCG to patients receiving immunosuppressant drugs (eg, high-dose corticosteroids) or radiation therapy may predispose them to disseminated infection or insufficient response to vaccination. They may remain susceptible despite vaccination. BCG vaccine does not interfere with oral poliovirus vaccine.

BCG vaccination or therapy usually induces hypersensitivity to tuberculin skin tests, typically within 8 to 14 weeks after exposure to BCG. This false-positive effect diminishes in probability as the time since BCG exposure increases.

Antitubercular therapy (eg, isoniazid) will antagonize disseminated BCG infections. Antitubercular or other antimicrobial therapy can interfere with the efficacy of BCG therapy for bladder cancer. Some BCG strains available in other countries may be resistant to isoniazid.

When a patient requires more than 1 live vaccine, the general rule is to give them simultaneously or wait at least 4 weeks between immunizations.

BCG vaccination can decrease the elimination of theophylline, increasing its biological half-life. Observe theophylline patients who receive BCG vaccine for theophylline toxicity, and advise them to seek assistance if symptoms of toxicity appear (eg, nausea, vomiting, palpitations).

Pharmaceutical Characteristics

Concentration: 1 to 8 x 10^8 CFU per 50 mg wet weight per vial, after reconstitution.

Quality Assay: Potency is assessed through colony counts derived from a serial dilution assay.
USP requirements: Meets guinea pig avirulence and potency standards.

Packaging: 2 mL single-dose vial (without diluent) (NDC#: 00052-0603-02)

Doseform: Powder for suspension

Appearance: Beige, creamy white, buff, or light gray powder, yielding a cloudy suspension

Diluent:
For reconstitution: Store diluents at a temperature ranging from 2° to 25°C (35° to 77°F). 1 mL sterile water for injection, when injected percutaneously. For neonatal doses, dilute the vaccine powder with 2 mL of diluent rather than 1 mL.

Adjuvant: None

Preservative: None

Allergens: None

Excipients: Lactose 125 mg/vial

pH: Data not specified

Shelf Life: Expires within 18 months if stored at 2° to 8°C (35° to 46°F).

Storage/Stability: Store at 2° to 8°C (35° to 46°F). Protect from direct sunlight. Lyophilized product can be stored frozen and then reconstituted and used effectively. After reconstitution, refrigerate product until used. There is no data to support freezing and thawing of reconstituted product. Shipped in insulated containers with dry ice. Discard within 2 hours after reconstitution.

Production Process: Bacteria are cultured and then lyophilized.

Media: Medium consists of glycerin, asparagine, citric acid, potassium phosphate, magnesium sulfate, and iron ammonium citrate.

Disease Epidemiology

Incidence: In the mid-19th century, tuberculosis was a leading cause of death. Disease incidence has been declining in industrialized nations since the late 19th century. Only a limited amount of the decline in tuberculosis can be attributed to chemotherapy and BCG vaccination; much of the decline resulted from improved sanitation, less-crowded urban living and working areas, improved nutrition, and related social conditions. Traditionally, people of low socioeconomic status are at greatest risk for tuberculosis (eg, migrant workers, certain immigrants, the homeless).

Bacillus Calmette-Guérin (BCG) Vaccine

Approximately 18,360 cases were reported in the United States in 1998 (6.8 cases per 100,000 population), continuing a decline from the peak in a trend of increasing disease incidence in 1992. The incidence reported in 1998 was 8% less than in 1997. The proportion of tuberculosis cases among foreign-born people steadily increased, from 27% in 1992 to 42% in 1998.

Approximately 10 million to 15 million Americans have a latent tuberculosis infection (1995 CDC estimate). Among the adult population of the United States, approximately 5% to 10% will react positively to a 5 TU tuberculin PPD test. Higher proportions are likely to test positive among high-risk populations.

Half of the world's population is infected with *M. tuberculosis*. As many as 10 million new cases of active tuberculosis occur throughout the world each year, with 2 million to 3 million deaths. More than 3 billion doses of BCG vaccine have been administered worldwide, and more than 70% of the world's children receive BCG vaccination. A compilation of global BCG vaccination policies appears at www.bcgatlas.org.

Susceptible Pools: Patients infected with HIV comprise the pool of people in the United States most susceptible to tuberculosis. They experience a 10% per year rate of active disease when infected, compared with 10% per lifetime in non-HIV-infected people. Medically underserved populations, including racial and ethnic minorities and foreign-born people, are also at increased risk.

Transmission: Exposure to bacilli in airborne droplet nuclei produced by people with pulmonary or laryngeal tuberculosis during expiratory efforts (eg, coughing, singing, sneezing). Bovine tuberculosis most often results in humans from ingestion of unpasteurized dairy products.

Incubation: From infection to primary lesion or significant tuberculin reaction, incubation time is approximately 4 to 12 weeks. While the risk of tuberculosis peaks within the first 1 to 2 years after infection, the risk of activation persists throughout life. Among immunocompetent adults, active tuberculosis disease will develop in 5% to 15% during their lifetimes. The risk is greatest in the first 2 years, then declines markedly. The likelihood that latent infection will progress to active disease in infants or children is substantially greater than for most other age groups. The risk for active tuberculosis disease among HIV-infected patients may remain high for an indefinite period of time or may even increase as immuno-suppression progresses.

Active tuberculosis disease is fatal in 50% of people or less who have not been treated. Chemotherapy has helped reduce the fatality rate by 94%, to a mortality rate of 0.6 deaths per 100,000 population in 1993. The rate in 1954 was 12.4 deaths per 100,000 population.

Communicability: Prolonged close contact with an infectious person can lead to infection. Communicability persists as long as viable tubercle bacilli are discharged in the sputum. The status of the acid-fast bacillus smear of the source case may be the strongest predictor of which patients are most contagious.

Other Information

Perspective:

1882: Koch identifies the tubercle bacillus as the cause of tuberculosis, subsequently called Koch's bacillus.

1921: First BCG vaccine, administered orally, developed at Pasteur Institut, Lille, France, by Leon Calmette and Camille Guérin. The drug was developed beginning in 1906, used experimentally in newborns from 1921 to 1924, and then used in mass vaccinations beginning around 1950.

1934: Tice strain developed from BCG strain brought to the Institution for Tuberculosis Research at the University of Illinois from the Pasteur Institut in Paris. Frederick Tice was president of the board of directors of the Chicago Municipal Tuberculosis Sanitorium.

1946: Streptomycin chemotherapy of tuberculosis begins in the United States. Other drugs soon followed (para-aminosalicylic acid in 1949, isoniazid in 1952, ethambutol in 1961, rifampin in 1963). Chemotherapy, especially isoniazid, allowed entire tuberculosis hospitals to close or change missions during the 1960s.

1985: Incidence of tuberculosis begins to rise in the United States, after declining for decades. The number of cases of multiple drug-resistant tuberculosis also begins to increase.

1990: Organon Teknika licensed to produce BCG on August 24, 1990. Versions of same Tice strain were licensed to the University of Illinois (July 7, 1950) and Bionetics Research (May 29, 1987).

Discontinued Products: Generic Danish substrain 1077 (from Glaxo and later Quad), methanol-extracted residue fraction of killed tubercle bacilli (MER-BCG, from National Cancer Institute or Merck, Sharp and Dohme). Sanofi Pasteur's BCG was licensed in the United States from 1967 until May 1990, when it was voluntarily withdrawn by the manufacturer. It was reinstated in late 1998.

National Policy: Taylor Z, Nolan CM, Blumberg HM; American Thoracic Society; Center for Disease Control and Prevention; Infectious Diseases Society of America. Controlling tuberculosis in the United States. Recommendations from the American Thoracic Society, CDC, and the Infectious Diseases Society of America. *MMWR*. 2005;54(RR-12):1-81. Erratum in: *MMWR*. 2005;54(45):1161. www.cdc.gov/mmwr/PDF/rr/rr5412.pdf.

CDC. Progress toward the elimination of tuberculosis—United States, 1998. *MMWR*. 1999;48:732-736.

ACIP. The role of BCG vaccine in the prevention and control of tuberculosis in the United States: A joint statement by the Advisory Council for the Elimination of Tuberculosis and the Advisory Committee on Immunization Practices. *MMWR*. 1996;45(RR-4):1-18.

References: CDC. Decrease in reported tuberculosis cases—United States, 2009. *MMWR*. 2010;59(10):289-294. www.cdc.gov/mmwr/pdf/wk/mm5910.pdf.

Colditz GA, Brewer TF, Berkey CS, et al. Efficacy of BCG vaccine in the prevention of tuberculosis. Meta-analysis of the published literature. *JAMA*. 1994;271(9):698-702. Letters, *JAMA*. 1994;272:765-766.

Colditz GA, Berkey CS, Mostellar F, et al. The efficacy of bacillus Calmette-Guérin vaccination of newborns and infants in the prevention of tuberculosis: meta-analyses of the published literature. *Pediatrics*. 1995;96(1, pt 1):29-35.

Fine PE. Bacille Calmette-Guérin vaccines: a rough guide. *Clin Infect Dis*. 1995;20(1):11-14.

Fine PE. Variation in protection by BCG: implications of and for heterologous immunity. *Lancet*. 1995;346(8986):1339-1345.

Groves MJ. BCG: The past, present, and future of a tuberculosis vaccine. *J Pharm Pharmacol*. 1997;49(suppl 1):7-15.

Oettinger T, Jørgensen M, Ladefoged A, Hasløv K, Andersen P. Development of the *Mycobacterium bovis* BCG vaccine: review of the historical and biochemical evidence for a genealogical tree. *Tuber Lung Dis*. 1999;79(4):243-250.

Snider GL. Tuberculosis then and now: a personal perspective on the last 50 years. *Ann Intern Med*. 1997;126(3):237-243.

Walker KB, Brennan MJ, Ho MM, et al. The second Geneva Consensus: Recommendations for novel live TB vaccines. *Vaccine*. 2010;28(11):2259-2270.

WHO. BCG vaccine. *Weekly Epidemiol Rec*. 2004;79(4):27-38.

Zwerling A, Behr MA, Verma A, Brewer TF, Menzies D, Pai M. The BCG World Atlas: a database of global BCG vaccination policies and practices. *PLoS Med*. 2011;8(3):e1001012.

A general discussion of tuberculosis appears above this section.

For a general discussion of bladder cancer, refer to the *TheraCys* monograph.

Bacillus Calmette-Guérin (BCG) Vaccine

Comparison Table of BCG Products			
Generic name:	Bacillus Calmette-Guérin		
Brand name	*BCG Vaccine (Tice)*	*Tice BCG*	*TheraCys*[a] (United States), *ImmuCyst* (Canada)
Manufacturer	Merck	Merck	Sanofi Pasteur
Availability	United States	United States, Canada	United States, Canada
Viability	Live bacterial vaccine	Live bacterial	Live bacterial
Indications	Tuberculosis prevention, treatment of bladder carcinoma in situ	Treatment of bladder cancer in situ only	Treatment of bladder carcinoma in situ only
Substrain	Tice substrain	Tice substrain	Connaught substrain
Concentration	1 to 8 $\times$ 10^8 CFU or 50 mg/vial	1 to 8 x 10^8 CFU or 50 mg/vial	1.7 to 19.2 $\times$ 10^8 CFU or 81 mg/vial
Adjuvant	None	None	None
Preservative	None	None	None
Doseform	Powder for suspension	Powder for suspension	Powder for suspension
Diluent	1 mL sterile water/vial	1 mL preservative-free sodium chloride 0.9% per vial	3 mL phosphate-buffered saline/vial for reconstitution; 50 mL saline for instillation
Packaging	2 mL vial with powder (no diluent provided)	2 mL vial with powder (no diluent provided)	Vial of powder plus 3 mL vial of diluent; 50 mL vials of diluent for instillation available
Routine storage	2° to 8°C, discard within 2 hours of reconstitution	2° to 8°C, discard within 2 hours of reconstitution	2° to 8°C, discard within 2 hours of reconstitution
Dose & Route	0.2 to 0.3 mL percutaneously	1 vial diluted in 50 mL preservative- free sodium chloride 0.9% given through urinary catheter (intravesical) for bladder carcinoma	1 vial diluted in 50 mL of sodium chloride 0.9% given through urinary catheter (intravesical) for bladder carcinoma
CPT Code	90585	90586	90586

a For complete prescribing information for *TheraCys* refer to the individual monograph.

Bacterial Vaccines & Toxoids

The following tables summarize the various formulations of diphtheria, tetanus, and pertussis and related information. Detailed discussions of these formulations can be found in the individual monographs that follow the Overview section.

Comparison Table of DTP and DT Products		
Generic name	Diphtheria and tetanus toxoids & acellular pertussis vaccine	Diphtheria and tetanus toxoids (pediatric)
Brand name (manufacturer)	*Daptacel* (Sanofi Pasteur), *Infanrix* (GlaxoSmithKline)	Generic (Sanofi Pasteur)
Synonyms	DTaP, DTPa	DT
Viability	Bacterial subunit vaccines	
Indication	To prevent infection with *Corynebacterium diphtheriae* and *Clostridium tetani*. Preferred formulations prevent infection by *Bordetella pertussis*.	
Concentration (per 0.5 mL)		
Diphtheria	6.7 to 25 Lf units	6.7 Lf units
Tetanus	5 to 10 Lf units	5 Lf units
Pertussis	Various, see next table or monographs	None
Adjuvant	*Daptacel*: Aluminum phosphate *Infanrix*: Aluminum hydroxide	Aluminum potassium sulfate
Preservative	None	None
Doseform	Suspension	Suspension
Packaging	0.5 mL vial, 0.5 mL syringe	5 mL vial
Routine storage	2° to 8°C	2° to 8°C
Dosage, route	0.5 mL IM	0.5 mL IM
Standard schedule	2, 4, and 6 months, at intervals of 6 to 8 weeks, fourth dose given at 15 to 20 months, fifth dose at 4 to 6 years of age	2, 4, and 10 to 16 months of age, with reinforcing dose 6 to 12 months after third dose.
Appropriate age range	2 months to < 7 years of age	2 months to < 7 years of age
CPT codes	90700	90701

Comparison Table of Acellular DTP Vaccines		
Generic	Diphtheria and tetanus toxoids with acellular pertussis vaccine (DTaP, DTPa)	
Brand name	*Infanrix*	*Daptacel*
Manufacturer	GlaxoSmithKline	Sanofi Pasteur
Viability	Bacterial subunit vaccines	
Indication	To prevent infection with *Corynebacterium diphtheriae*, *Clostridium tetani*, and *Bordetella pertussis*.	
Concentration (per 0.5 mL)		
Diphtheria	25 Lf units	15 Lf units
Tetanus	10 Lf units	5 Lf units
Pertussis	Pertussis toxin 25 mcg, filamentous hemagglutinin 25 mcg, pertactin 8 mcg	Pertussis toxoid 10 mcg, filamentous hemagglutinin 5 mcg, pertactin 3 mcg, types 2 and 3 fimbriae 5 mcg
Adjuvant	Aluminum hydroxide (0.625 mg aluminum per dose)	Aluminum phosphate (0.33 mg aluminum per dose)
Preservative	None	None
Doseform	Suspension	Suspension
Packaging	0.5 mL vial	0.5 mL vial
Routine storage	2° to 8°C	2° to 8°C
Dosage, route	0.5 mL IM	0.5 mL IM
Standard schedule	2, 4, and 6 months, at intervals of 6 to 8 weeks, fourth dose given at 15 to 20 months, fifth dose at 4 to 6 years of age	
CPT codes	90700	90700
Viability	Inactivated bacterial vaccine	

Comparison Table of Quadrivalent Vaccines Based on DTP		
Generic name	Diphtheria and tetanus toxoids with acellular pertussis and Hib vaccines	Diphtheria and tetanus toxoids with acellular pertussis and inactivated poliovirus vaccines
Brand name (manufacturer)	*TriHIBit*[a] (Sanofi Pasteur)	*Kinrix* (GlaxoSmithKline)
Synonyms	DTaP-Hib, DTPa-Hib	DTaP-IPV
Viability	Bacterial subunit vaccines	Bacterial subunit and inactivated virus vaccine
Indication: To prevent these diseases	Diphtheria Tetanus Pertussis *Haemophilus influenzae* type b	Diphtheria Tetanus Pertussis Poliomyelitis
Comments	Equivalent to *Tripedia* plus *ActHIB* brand of Hib vaccine	Comparable to combination of constituent vaccines
Concentration (per 0.5 mL)		
Diphtheria	6.7 Lf units	25 Lf units
Tetanus	5 Lf units	10 Lf units
Pertussis	Pertussis toxin 23.4 mcg and filamentous hemagglutinin 23.4 mcg	Pertussis toxin 25 mcg, filamentous hemagglutinin 25 mcg, pertactin 8 mcg
H. influenzae type b	10 mcg	None
Hepatitis B	None	None
Poliovirus	None	Type 1: 40 D-antigen units (DU) Type 2: 8 DU Type 3: 32 DU
Adjuvant	Aluminum potassium sulfate	Aluminum hydroxide
Preservative	None	None
Doseform	Suspension plus powder	Suspension
Packaging	0.5 mL vial	0.5 mL vial, 0.5 mL syringe
Routine storage	2° to 8°C	2° to 8°C
Dosage, route	0.5 mL IM	0.5 mL IM
Standard schedule	2, 4, 6, and 12 to 18 months of age (followed by other formulations later in life)	4 to 6 years of age (preceded and followed by other formulations)
Appropriate age range	2 to 18 months of age	4 to 6 years of age
CPT codes	90721	90696

a Product no longer distributed; content provided for historical record.

Comparison Table of Pentavalent Vaccines Based on DTP		
Generic name	Diphtheria and tetanus toxoids with acellular pertussis, hepatitis B, and inactivated poliovirus vaccines	Diphtheria and tetanus toxoids with acellular pertussis, inactivated poliovirus, and Hib vaccines
Brand name (manufacturer)	*Pediarix* (GlaxoSmithKline)	*Pentacel* (Sanofi Pasteur)
Synonyms	DTaP-HepB-IPV, DTPa-HBV-IPV	DTaP-IPV-Hib
Viability	Bacterial and viral subunit vaccines	Bacterial subunit and inactivated virus vaccine
Indication: To prevent these diseases	Diphtheria Tetanus Pertussis Hepatitis B Poliomyelitis	Diphtheria Tetanus Pertussis *Haemophilus influenzae* type b Poliomyelitis
Comments	Comparable to combination of constituent vaccines	Comparable to combination of constituent vaccines
Concentration (per 0.5 mL)		
Diphtheria	25 Lf units	15 Lf
Tetanus	10 Lf units	5 Lf
Pertussis	Pertussis toxin 25 mcg, filamentous hemagglutinin 25 mcg, pertactin 8 mcg	Pertussis toxin 20 mcg, filamentous hemagglutinin 20 mcg, pertactin 3 mcg, fimbriae types 2 and 35 mcg
H. influenzae type b	None	10 mcg
Hepatitis B	10 mcg	None
Poliovirus	Type 1: 40 D-antigen units (DU), Type 2: 8 DU, Type 3: 32 DU	Type 1: 40 D-antigen units (DU), Type 2: 8 DU, Type 3: 32 DU
Adjuvant	Aluminum hydroxide and aluminum phosphate	Aluminum phosphate
Preservative	None	None
Doseform	Suspension	Suspension plus powder
Packaging	0. 5 mL vial, 0.5 mL syringe	5-dose package of vials
Routine storage	2° to 8°C	2° to 8°C
Dosage, route	0.5 mL IM	0.5 mL IM
Standard schedule	2, 4, and 6 months of age (followed by other formulations later in life)	2, 4, 6, and 15 to 18 months of age (followed by other formulations later in life)
Appropriate age range	2 to 6 months of age (or older, for young children not vaccinated according to schedule)	2 to 18 months of age
CPT codes	90723	90698

Table of Adult Td, Tdap, and TT Products			
Generic name	Tetanus and diphtheria toxoids	Tetanus and diphtheria toxoids with acellular pertussis vaccine	Tetanus toxoid adsorbed
Brand name	Generic, *Decavac*	*Adacel*, *Boostrix*	Generic
Synonyms	Td	Tdap	TT
Manufacturer	Generic—Massachusetts Biological Laboratories; *Decavac*—Sanofi Pasteur	*Adacel*—Sanofi Pasteur; *Boostrix*—GlaxoSmith-Kline	Sanofi Pasteur
Viability	Bacterial subunit vaccines		
Indication	To prevent infection with *Clostridium tetani*. Preferred formulations also prevent infection with *Corynebacterium diphtheriae* and *Bordetella pertussis*.		
Comments	Td or Tdap is preferred over TT	Tdap is preferred over Td	Td or Tdap is preferred over TT
Concentration (per 0.5 mL) Diphtheria	2 Lf units	2 Lf units (SP), 2.5 Lf units (GSK)	None
Tetanus	2 to 5 Lf units	5 Lf units	5 Lf units
Pertussis	None	*Boostrix*: 2.5 mcg pertactin, 8 mcg FHA, 8 mcg pertussis toxin; *Adacel*: 3 mcg pertactin, 5 mcg FHA, 2.5 mcg pertussis toxin, 2.5 mcg each of fimbriae types 2 and 3	None
Adjuvant	Aluminum phosphate	*Boostrix*: Aluminum hydroxide *Adacel*: Aluminum phosphate	Aluminum potassium sulfate
Preservative	None	None	Thimerosal 0.01% in multidose vial, otherwise preservative free
Doseform	Suspension	Suspension	Suspension
Packaging	0.5 mL vial, 5 mL vial, 0.5 mL syringe	0.5 mL vial, 0.5 mL syringe	0.5 mL vial, 5 mL vial
Routine storage	2° to 8°C	2° to 8°C	2° to 8°C
Dosage, route	0.5 mL IM	0.5 mL IM	0.5 mL IM
Standard schedule	Three 0.5 mL doses: the second 4 to 8 weeks after the first, the third 6 to 12 months after the second. Then every 10 years throughout life.	Single dose (at present)	Three 0.5 mL doses: the second 4 to 8 weeks after the first, the third 6 to 12 months after the second. Then every 10 years throughout life.
Appropriate age range	7 years to adult	*Adacel*—11 to 64 years; *Boostrix*—≥ 10 years	7 years to adult
CPT	90718	90715	90703

CDC Wound-Management Guidelines				
History of adsorbed tetanus toxoid	Clean, minor wounds		All other wounds[a]	
Toxoid (doses)	Td or Tdap[b]	TIG	Td or Tdap[b]	TIG
Unknown or < 3 doses	Yes	No	Yes	Yes
≥ 3 doses[c]	No[d]	No	No[e]	No

a Including, but not limited to, wounds contaminated with dirt, feces, soil, or saliva; puncture wounds; avulsions; or wounds resulting from missiles, crushing, burns, or frostbite.

b For children younger than 7 years of age, diphtheria-tetanus-pertussis (DTP) vaccine is preferred to tetanus toxoid alone. Use DT (pediatric-strength diphtheria and tetanus toxoids) if pertussis vaccine is validly contraindicated. For people 7 years of age and older, Td bivalent or with acellular pertussis vaccine (Tdap) is preferred.

c If the patient has received only 3 doses of fluid toxoid, then give a fourth dose of toxoid, preferably an adsorbed toxoid.

d Yes, if more than 10 years have elapsed since the last dose of tetanus toxoid.

e Yes, if more than 5 years have elapsed since the last dose of tetanus toxoid.

Note: More frequent booster doses are not needed and may increase the incidence and severity of adverse effects.

TIG = Tetanus immune globulin.

Bacterial Vaccines & Toxoids

Names:
Daptacel
Infanrix

Manufacturers:
Sanofi Pasteur
GlaxoSmithKline. The pertussis component is produced by GlaxoSmithKline and combined with diphtheria and tetanus toxoids manufactured by Novartis.

Synonyms: DTP, DPT, DTPa, DTaP, APDT. *Daptacel* is marketed in Canada as *Tripacel*.

Comparison: The various acellular DTaP products are generally considered prophylactically equivalent, despite some differences in contents and methods of standardization. Whole-cell and acellular DTP (DTwP and DTaP) products are not generically equivalent because of differences in composition and side effect incidence. DTaP results in fewer common side effects than DTwP vaccines. The ACIP considers available data regarding safety and clinical efficacy to be insufficient to express a preference between the various formulations of DTaP available in the United States. Using the same brand of DTaP for a child's vaccination series is generally preferred, but any of the licensed DTaP vaccines may be used to complete the vaccination series.

> **Note:** Trivalent vaccines against diphtheria, tetanus, and pertussis are the preferred immunizing agents for most people. Tetanus and diphtheria toxoids for adult use (Td) bivalent or with acellular pertussis vaccine (Tdap) is the preferred immunizing agent for adults and older children.
>
> Specific information about the individual components of this drug appear in the individual monographs on diphtheria toxoid, tetanus toxoid, and pertussis vaccine.

Immunologic Characteristics

Microorganism: Bacteria, *Corynebacterium diphtheriae*, *Clostridium tetani*, and *Bordetella pertussis*

Viability: Inactivated

Antigenic Form: Toxoid mixture with acellular pertussis bacterial vaccine

GSK: The acellular pertussis component contains 25 mcg inactivated pertussis toxin, 8 mcg pertactin (69-kilodalton outer membrane protein), and 25 mcg FHA per 0.5 mL dose.

Sanofi Pasteur (Daptacel): The acellular pertussis component contains pertussis toxoid 10 mcg, filamentous hemagglutinin 5 mcg, pertactin 3 mcg, types 2 and 3 fimbriae 5 mcg each per 0.5 mL.

Antigenic Type: Protein

Strains:

GSK: Toxigenic strains of *Corynebacterium diphtheriae* and *Clostridium tetani*. Unspecified strain of *Bordetella pertussis*.

Sanofi Pasteur: *Corynebacterium diphtheriae* strain L34T1, derived from Park-Williams #8 strain; *Bordetella pertussis* strain 10536 obtained from Michigan Department of Health.

Diphtheria & Tetanus Toxoids & Acellular Pertussis Vaccine (DTaP)

Use Characteristics

Indications: Induction of active immunity against diphtheria, tetanus, and pertussis in infants and children from 6 weeks of age up to the seventh birthday.

Refer to the CDC's wound-management guidelines in the DTP Overview.

Limitations: Diphtheria toxoid immunization decreases but does not eliminate colonization of toxigenic strains of *Corynebacterium diphtheriae* in the pharynx, nose, or on the skin. Do not use diphtheria toxoid for the treatment of actual diphtheria infections. Select appropriate antibiotics (eg, erythromycin, penicillin) to treat active infections. Give diphtheria antitoxin if the patient is unlikely to have adequate active immunity to diphtheria toxin.

Tetanus toxoid is indicated for tetanus prevention and is not intended for the treatment or diagnosis of that disease. For treatment of tetanus infection and for passive prophylaxis, consider use of tetanus immune globulin and appropriate antibiotics (eg, penicillin G, a tetracycline).

Pertussis vaccine does not stimulate local secretory antibody production to prevent attachment of the microorganism to the respiratory epithelium. Pertussis vaccine is indicated for the prevention of pertussis and is not intended for the treatment or diagnosis of that disease. Select appropriate antibiotics (eg, erythromycin) to treat active infections.

Contraindications:

Absolute: Do not give further doses of a vaccine containing pertussis antigens to children who have recovered from culture-confirmed pertussis. Do not vaccinate patients with a history of serious adverse reactions to a previous dose of a pertussis-containing vaccine. Do not vaccinate patients with a history of a serious allergic reaction to a vaccine component or after a prior dose of this vaccine.

The following events are contraindications to administration of any pertussis-containing vaccine:

- Encephalopathy (eg, coma, decreased level of consciousness, prolonged seizures) within 7 days of administration of a previous dose of a pertussis-containing vaccine not attributable to another identifiable cause.

- Progressive neurologic disorder, including infantile spasms, uncontrolled epilepsy, or progressive encephalopathy. Do not administer pertussis vaccine to people with such conditions until a treatment regimen has been established and the condition has stabilized.

If a contraindication to the pertussis-vaccine component is present, substitute diphtheria and tetanus toxoids for pediatric use (DT) for each of the remaining doses.

Relative: Defer immunization during the course of any febrile illness or acute infection. A minor respiratory illness such as a mild upper respiratory tract infection is not usually reason to defer immunization. Give DTaP with caution to children with thrombocytopenia or any coagulation disorder that would contraindicate IM injection.

Several events were previously listed as contraindications but are now listed simply as precautions, warranting careful consideration: Temperature higher than 40.5°C (105°F) within 48 hours after DTP administration not caused by another identifiable cause; collapse or shock-like state (ie, hypotonic-hyporesponsive episode) within 48 hours; persistent inconsolable crying lasting 3 hours or more within 48 hours; convulsions with or without fever within 3 days. There may be circumstances, such as a high local incidence of pertussis, in which the potential benefits outweigh possible risks, particularly because these events are not associated with permanent sequelae.

The occurrence of any type of neurological symptoms or signs, including 1 or more convulsions following DTaP administration, is generally a contraindication to further use. The presence of any evolving or changing disorder affecting the CNS contraindicates administration of pertussis vaccine regardless of whether the suspected neurological disorder is associated with occurrence of any type of seizure activity.

The ACIP and AAP recognize certain circumstances in which children with stable CNS disorders, including well-controlled seizures or satisfactorily-explained single seizures, may receive pertussis vaccine. The ACIP and AAP do not consider a family history of seizures to be a contraindication to pertussis vaccine. Studies suggesting that infants and children with a history of convulsions in first-degree family members (eg, siblings, parents) have an increased risk for neurologic events, compared with those without such histories, may be flawed by selection bias or genetic confounding.

Immunodeficiency: Patients receiving immunosuppressive therapy or who have other immunodeficiencies may have a diminished antibody response to active immunization. Consider deferral of vaccine administration. Nonetheless, routine immunization of symptomatic and asymptomatic HIV-infected patients is recommended.

Elderly: DTaP is generally contraindicated after the seventh birthday.

Adults: DTaP is generally contraindicated after the seventh birthday. Tetanus and diphtheria toxoids for adult use (Td) bivalent or with acellular pertussis vaccine (Tdap) is the preferred immunizing agent for adults and older children. The benefit of routine pertussis immunization of adults to reduce their role as community disease reservoirs is being investigated.

Pregnancy: Category C. DTaP is generally contraindicated after the seventh birthday. It is not known if DTP antigens or corresponding antibodies cross the placenta. Generally, most IgG passage across the placenta occurs during the third trimester. Problems in humans have not been documented and are unlikely.

Lactation: DTaP generally is contraindicated after the seventh birthday. It is unknown if DTP antigens or corresponding antibodies cross into human breast milk. Problems in humans have not been documented and are unlikely.

Children: Do not reduce or divide the DTaP dose for preterm infants or any other children. DTaP is contraindicated in children younger than 6 weeks of age because the product may not be immunogenic. DTaP also is contraindicated in children after the seventh birthday because of their decreased risk of pertussis and increased likelihood of adverse effects. Trivalent DTaP is the preferred immunizing agent for most children younger than 7 years of age. Tetanus and diphtheria toxoids for adult use (Td) bivalent or with acellular pertussis vaccine (Tdap) is the preferred immunizing agent for adults and older children.

Children who have recovered from culture-confirmed pertussis do not need further doses of a pertussis-containing vaccine. Tetanus and diphtheria toxoids for adult use (Td) bivalent or with acellular pertussis vaccine (Tdap) is the preferred immunizing agent for adults and older children.

Adverse Reactions: Some adverse reactions following DTaP administration occur less frequently than those seen in recipients of DTwP, especially pain and tenderness, erythema, induration, swelling, and warmth at the injection site. Less drowsiness, fretfulness or irritability, and fever followed DTaP use compared with DTwP. *Infanrix* cites less erythema, swelling, tenderness, fever higher than 38°C (100.4°F), irritability, drowsiness, prolonged crying, and seizures within 48 hours of vaccination. The relative frequency of rare events can only be determined in large postmarketing surveillance studies currently underway.

Among children 1 year of age and older, fever 38°C or higher (100.4°F) occurred in 7% to 19% of recipients within 72 hours of DTaP administration. Fever higher than 39°C (102.2°F) occurred in 1.5% to 3% of recipients. Other occasional reactions included upper respiratory tract infection or rhinitis (6%), diarrhea or loose stools (3.5%), vomiting (2%), or rash (1.2%). As with other aluminum-containing vaccines, a nodule may occasionally be palpable at the injection site for several weeks. Sterile abscess formation or subcutaneous atrophy at the injection site also may occur.

Diphtheria & Tetanus Toxoids & Acellular Pertussis Vaccine (DTaP)

Among infants 2 to 6 months of age, *Infanrix* is associated with erythema (5% to 16%), swelling (5% to 15%), tenderness (4% to 5%), fever (7% to 9%), irritability (29% to 36%), drowsiness (11% to 35%), loss of appetite (11.5% to 16.5%), vomiting (3% to 6%), and crying 1 hour or more (2% to 4%); rates of erythema, swelling, and fever increased after 4 successive doses of *Infanrix*.

Reactions not noted with DTaP in clinical trials but noted coincidentally with broader use of other drugs containing diphtheria, tetanus, or pertussis antigens included urticaria, erythema multiforme, other rashes, arthralgias, or, more rarely, a severe anaphylactic reaction (eg, urticaria with swelling of the mouth, difficult breathing, hypotension, shock). Other coincidental reactions included neurological complications, such as convulsions, encephalopathy, various mono- or polyneuropathies, including Guillain-Barré syndrome. Permanent neurological disability and death occurred rarely in temporal association to immunization with a pertussis antigen.

An expert panel assembled by the Institute of Medicine has concluded that no causal association exists between pertussis vaccination and autism, infantile spasms, hypsarrhythmia, Reye syndrome, SIDS, aseptic meningitis, chronic neurologic damage, erythema multiforme or other rash, Guillain-Barré syndrome, hemolytic anemia, juvenile diabetes, learning disabilities, attention deficit disorder, peripheral mononeuropathy, or thrombocytopenia.

The panel found evidence consistent with a causal association between DTwP and acute encephalopathy, shock and "unusual shock-like state," anaphylaxis, and protracted, inconsolable crying.

When a child returns for the next dose in a series of either pertussis or DTaP vaccine injections, question the adult accompanying the child about possible side effects following the prior dose. If any of the effects that contraindicate additional pertussis-vaccine doses occur, continue childhood immunization with bivalent diphtheria and tetanus toxoids for pediatric use (DT).

Pharmacologic & Dosing Characteristics

Dosage: Shake vial well to obtain a uniform suspension before withdrawing each dose. Any brand may be used for the doses of a primary immunizing series. In the absence of specific information about interchanging various DTaP vaccines, using the same brand in a given patient is preferred. Although safety and efficacy data have not been specifically evaluated, any DTaP vaccine can be used to complete the immunizing series in a child previously given DTwP or another DTaP.

Primary immunizing series: Typically, 4 doses are given at 2, 4, 6, and 15 to 18 months of age. Give 0.5 mL at 6 to 8 weeks of age, a second 0.5 mL dose 4 to 8 weeks later, a third 0.5 mL dose 4 to 8 weeks later, and a fourth reinforcing 0.5 mL dose 1 year after the third dose. Observe a minimum interval between the third and fourth doses of at least 6 months. Give a fifth reinforcing dose at 4 to 6 years of age, at least 6 months after the fourth dose. If the fourth primary dose (ie, the reinforcing dose) is given after a child's fourth birthday, a booster dose (fifth dose) prior to school entry is not necessary.

DTaP may be used for doses in series begun with DTwP. In such cases, give a total of 5 DTP doses.

Do not use partial or fractional doses of DTaP because the immunogenicity and clinical efficacy of such practices have not been adequately studied. Give preterm infants a full 0.5 mL dose at the normal chronologic age after birth. Do not dilute. Do not count doses within the minimum interval because too short an interval may interfere with antibody response and protection from disease.

Refer to the CDC's wound-management guidelines in the DTP Overview.

Route & Site: IM; use no other route. The anterolateral aspect of the thigh or the deltoid muscle of the upper arm is preferred. Do not inject DTaP in the gluteal area or other areas where there may be a major nerve trunk.

Documentation Requirements: Federal law requires that the following information be documented in the recipient's permanent medical record or in a permanent office log: (1) The manufacturer and lot number of this vaccine, (2) the date of its administration, and (3) the name, address, and title of the person administering the vaccine.

Certain adverse events must be reported to the VAERS system ([800] 822-7967). Refer to Immunization Documents in the Resources section for complete information.

Overdosage: Although few data are available, clinical experience with similar products suggests that the major manifestations of overdosage would be pain and tenderness at the injection site.

Booster Doses: No doses of DTaP are recommended after the seventh birthday. Tetanus and diphtheria toxoids for adult use (Td) bivalent or with acellular pertussis vaccine (Tdap) is the preferred immunizing agent for adults and older children.

Missed Doses: Interrupting the recommended schedule or delaying subsequent doses does not require restarting the series. Use Td or Tdap, rather than DTaP, for doses needed after the seventh birthday. Increasing the interval beyond the recommended time does not affect the ultimate efficacy of immunization, but waiting does delay achieving adequate protection from infection.

Related Interventions: There are no data on whether prophylactic use of antipyretic drugs (eg, acetaminophen) can decrease the risk of febrile convulsions. Data suggest that acetaminophen will reduce the incidence of postvaccination fever. The ACIP and AAP suggest administering an appropriate dose of acetaminophen based on age at the time of vaccination and every 4 to 6 hours to children at higher risk for seizures than the general population (eg, children with personal or family history of seizures).

Efficacy: Acellular pertussis vaccines have been used in Japan since 1981, mostly in children 2 years of age. The decline in pertussis with routine use of acellular vaccines in this setting provides evidence of the efficacy of these vaccines as a group. The vaccines were rated 88% effective among household contacts in protecting against clinical pertussis.

In Swedish and German studies of the Sanofi Pasteur formulation among children 5 to 11 months of age, the estimated vaccine efficacy was 69% for all cases of culture-confirmed pertussis and 80% for culture-confirmed cases with cough persisting more than 30 days. The role of specific serum antibodies in clinical protection is not known at present. Antibody responses to PT and FHA were significantly higher after *Tripedia* than after Connaught's brand of DTwP.

GlaxoSmithKline's brand of DTaP vaccine was compared with a whole-cell DTwP vaccine and DT in a randomized, double-blind Italian study. The mean length of follow-up was 17 months after the third vaccine dose. After 3 doses, the protective efficacy of *Infanrix* against typical pertussis (at least 21 days of paroxysmal cough with confirmed infection) was 84% compared with 36% for DTwP from Connaught. If the case definition was loosened, the calculated efficacy was 71% for more than 7 days of any cough and 73% for more than 14 days of any cough. In a German study of household pertussis infections, this brand of DTaP was 89% effective compared with 98% for DTwP from Behringwerke. Using the less conservative definition of pertussis gave similar efficacies.

Onset: Escalating protection with each sequential dose

Duration: Adequate immunization against diphtheria and tetanus generally persists for 10 years. Protection against pertussis in children persists approximately 4 to 6 years.

Protective Level: Serum diphtheria and tetanus antitoxin levels of 0.01 unit/mL are the lowest levels giving some degree of protection. Antitoxin levels 0.1 unit/mL and higher are regarded as protective. Efficacy of the pertussis component does not have a well-established correlate of protection.

Mechanism: *Corynebacterium diphtheriae* may cause a localized or generalized disease. Diphtheria exotoxin, an extracellular protein metabolite of toxigenic strains of *C. diphtheriae*, causes systemic intoxication. Complete immunization induces protective antitoxin antibodies against diphtheria toxin and significantly reduces the risk of developing diphtheria. Immunized patients who develop disease have milder illnesses.

Tetanus toxoid induces specific protective antibodies against the exotoxin excreted by *Clostridium tetani*.

The aluminum salt, a mineral adjuvant, prolongs and enhances the antigenic properties of tetanus toxoid by retarding the rate of absorption. Pertussis vaccine exerts an adjuvant effect on the diphtheria and tetanus toxoids. The role of circulating pertussis antibodies is not clear at present.

Drug Interactions: Like all inactivated vaccines, administration of DTP to patients receiving immunosuppressant drugs (eg, high-dose corticosteroids) or radiation therapy may result in an insufficient response to immunization. They may remain susceptible despite immunization.

Delay diphtheria toxoid administration until 3 to 4 weeks after diphtheria antitoxin use to avoid the hypothetical possibility of antitoxin-toxoid interference.

Several routine pediatric vaccines may be safely and effectively administered simultaneously at separate injection sites (eg, DTP, MMR, e-IPV, Hib, hepatitis B, varicella). National authorities recommend simultaneous immunization at separate sites as indicated by age or health risk.

Inactivated vaccines are not generally affected by circulating antibodies or administration of exogenous antibodies. Vaccination may occur at any time before or after antibody administration.

Coadministration of tetanus toxoid and tetanus immune globulin may delay development of active immunity by several days through partial antigen-antibody antagonism, but this interaction is not clinically significant and does not preclude coadministration of both drugs if both are needed.

Systemic chloramphenicol therapy may impair anamnestic response to tetanus toxoid. Avoid concurrent use of these 2 drugs.

As with other drugs administered by IM injection, give DTaP with caution to patients on anticoagulant therapy.

Pharmaceutical Characteristics

Concentration:
> *GSK:* 25 Lf units of diphtheria toxoid, 10 Lf units of tetanus toxoids, 25 mcg inactivated pertussis toxin, 8 mcg pertactin, and 25 mcg FHA per 0.5 mL dose.
>
> *Sanofi Pasteur (Daptacel):* 15 Lf units of diphtheria toxoid, 5 Lf units of tetanus toxoid, pertussis toxoid 10 mcg, FHA 5 mcg, pertactin (PRN) 3 mcg, types 2 and 3 fimbriae 5 mcg per 0.5 mL.

Quality Assay:
> *GSK:* Each toxoid induces 2 units or more of antitoxin per mL in guinea-pig potency tests. The potency of the pertussis component is evaluated by measurement of antibody levels

against FHA, pertussis toxin, and pertactin by the ELISA method in immunized mice. The inactivated acellular pertussis components contribute less than 5 endotoxin units (EU) per 0.5 mL dose.

Sanofi Pasteur (Daptacel): Diphtheria and tetanus toxoids each induce 2 or more units of antitoxin per mL in guinea-pig potency tests. The potency of the pertussis component is evaluated by measuring antibody levels against pertussis toxin, FHA, pertactin, and fimbriae types 2 and 3 by ELISA.

Packaging:
GSK: Single-dose 0.5 mL vials (each: 58160-0810-01, 10 vials: 58160-0810-11). Prefilled 0.5 mL syringes (tip cap and plunger contain latex) without needles (each: 58160-0810-41; 5s: 58160-0810-46; 10s: 58160-0810-51; 25s: 58160-0810-50). Prefilled 0.5 mL syringes (tip cap may contain latex; plunger contains no latex) without needles (each: 58160-0810-43; 10s: 58160-0810-52).

Sanofi Pasteur (Daptacel): Box of 10 single-dose 0.5 mL vials (49281-0286-10).

Doseform: Suspension

Appearance: After shaking, a homogeneous white suspension

Solvent: Phosphate-buffered saline

Adjuvant:
GSK: Aluminum hydroxide containing no more than 0.625 mg aluminum per 0.5 mL
Sanofi Pasteur (Daptacel): Aluminum phosphate containing 0.33 mg aluminum per 0.5 mL

Preservative:
GSK: None
Sanofi Pasteur (Daptacel): 3.3 mg (0.6% v/v) 2-phenoxyethanol per 0.5 mL

Allergens: The vial stopper or syringe components may contain dry natural latex rubber. Check package labeling.

Excipients:
GSK: 5 mg/mL sodium chloride, no more than 0.02% w/v residual formaldehyde, polysorbate 80.
Sanofi Pasteur (Daptacel): Residual free formaldehyde 0.1 mg/0.5 mL or less and residual glutaraldehyde less than 5 ng/0.5 mL.

pH: Data not provided

Shelf Life: Expires within 36 months

Storage/Stability: Store at 2° to 8°C (35° to 46°F). Discard frozen vaccine. Contact manufacturers regarding exposures to elevated temperatures. Temperature extremes may adversely affect resuspendability of this vaccine. Shipped in insulated containers with coolant packs.

Production Process: *Corynebacterium diphtheriae* and *Clostridium tetani* grow in media according to the method of Mueller and Miller (1947). Their exotoxins are detoxified with formaldehyde. The toxoids are refined by the Pillemer alcohol-fractionation method (1946). The acellular pertussis vaccines are prepared by growing Phase 1 *Bordetella pertussis* in Stainer-Scholte-defined medium and harvesting the culture fluid.

GSK: The 3 acellular pertussis antigens are isolated from phase 1 *Bordetella pertussis* culture grown in modified Stainer-Scholte liquid medium. Pertussis toxin and filamentous hemagglutinin (FHA) are extracted from the fermentation broth by adsorption on hydroxyapatite gel and purified by hydrophobic, affinity, and size-exclusion chromatography. Pertactin is extracted from the cells by heat treatment and flocculation using barium chloride and detoxified with formaldehyde and glutaraldehyde. FHA and pertactin are treated with formaldehyde. Diphtheria toxin is produced by growing *Corynebacterium diphtheriae* in Linggoud and Fenton medium containing a bovine extract. Tetanus toxin is produced by growing *Clostridium tetani* in a modified Lathmam medium.

Diphtheria & Tetanus Toxoids & Acellular Pertussis Vaccine (DTaP)

Sanofi Pasteur (Daptacel): Bordetella pertussis cultures are grown in Stainer-Scholte medium modified by the addition of casamino acids and dimethyl-beta-cyclodextrin. The fimbriae types 2 and 3 are extracted from the bacterial cells, and the pertussis toxin, FHA, and pertactin are prepared from the supernatant. These proteins are purified by sequential filtration, salt-precipitation, ultrafiltration, and chromatography. Pertussis toxin is inactivated with glutaraldehyde, and FHA is treated with formaldehyde. The individual antigens are adsorbed separately onto aluminum phosphate.

Disease Epidemiology

See DT and Td monographs for details about diphtheria and tetanus.

Incidence: An estimated 265,269 cases of pertussis occurred in 1934 with 5,000 deaths; about 120,000 cases in 1950 with 1,100 deaths. From 1985 through 1991, the number of pertussis cases reported in the United States ranged from 2575 in 1991 to 4570 in 1990. From 1985 through 1988, an average 3,300 hospitalizations and 25 deaths occurred each year. Worldwide, pertussis used to kill 850,000 infants each year. The WHO's Expanded Programme on Immunization has reduced this toll to 350,000 deaths per year.

Approximately 12% of reported pertussis cases affect individuals 15 years of age and older, probably an underestimate. Some 50 million American adults are susceptible to pertussis. An estimated 60 million pertussis cases and 700,000 related deaths occur annually around the world. Precise data do not exist, because bacteriological confirmation of pertussis can be obtained in less than half of suspected cases. Most reported illness occurs in infants and young children. Two-thirds of reported deaths occur in children younger than 1 year of age. Older children and adults, in whom classic signs are often absent, may escape diagnosis and serve as disease reservoirs. Of 10,749 patients younger than 1 year of age reported nationally from 1980 to 1989, 69% were hospitalized, 22% had pneumonia, 3% had at least 1 seizure, 0.9% had encephalopathy, and 0.6% died.

Susceptible Pools:
Pertussis: As many as 40% of preschool children may be inadequately vaccinated, although by the time of entry into elementary school, more than 95% of American school children are adequately protected.

Transmission:
Pertussis: Direct contact with discharges from respiratory mucous membranes of infected people by the airborne route, probably by droplets. Frequently brought home by an older sibling and sometimes by a parent. Attack rate in unimmunized populations exceeds 90%.

Incubation:
Pertussis: Generally, 7 to 10 days, rarely exceeding 14 days.

Communicability:
Pertussis: Highly communicable in the early catarrhal stage before the paroxysmal cough stage. The attack rate in unimmunized household contacts can exceed 90%. Thereafter, communicability gradually decreases and becomes negligible for ordinary nonfamilial contacts in approximately 3 weeks, despite persisting spasmodic cough with whoop. The communicable stage extends from the early catarrhal stage to 3 weeks after onset of typical paroxysms in patients not treated with antibiotics. When treated with erythromycin, the period of infectiousness usually extends only 5 days or less after onset of therapy.

Other Information

Perspective: See DT and Td monographs for details about diphtheria and tetanus.
1906: Bordet and Gengou isolate the causative bacterium, initially called *Hemophilus pertussis.*
1914: Pertussis vaccine licensed in the United States to the Massachusetts Public Health Biological Laboratories.
1933: Sauer develops pertussis vaccine.
1940: Strean develops pertussis antiserum.

1948: Eldering and Kendrick conduct large field trials at Michigan Department of Public Health's Grand Rapids laboratory. Their formula, using an intracerebral mouse-protection test, was used for decades for whole-cell pertussis vaccines.

1949: Diphtheria and tetanus toxoids with whole-cell pertussis vaccine licensed in the United States.

1967: MDPH vaccine licensed in October 1967.

1977-1980: A reduction of pertussis vaccine acceptance in Great Britain from 79% in 1973 to 31% in 1978 resulted in an epidemic of 102,500 pertussis cases and 36 pertussis deaths between late 1977 and 1980 (with 1440 cases per week reported during the winter of 1981 to 1982). A similar situation occurred in Japan.

1996: *Tripedia* licensed for vaccination of infants in July.

First Licensed:

GlaxoSmithKline (Previously SmithKline Beecham): January 30, 1997 (for infants and children)

Sanofi Pasteur (Daptacel): May 14, 2002

Sanofi Pasteur (Tripedia, previously Pasteur-Mérieux-Connaught and Aventis Pasteur): August 21, 1992 (July 31, 1996, for infants). Discontinued 2011.

Discontinued Products: *Pertussis Serobacterin* parenteral vaccine (Sharp and Dohme); *Pertussis Topagen* intranasal vaccine (Sharp and Dohme); *Solgen* extracted pertussis vaccine (Eli Lilly and Co). *Solgen* was reported to contain less protein nitrogen than other contemporary whole-cell vaccines, inducing fewer adverse reactions; it was available from 1962 through 1977.

DTaP: Acel-Imune (Wyeth-Lederle, 1991 to 2001). *Certiva* (Baxter Hyland, July 28, 1998, to 2000), *Tripedia* (Sanofi Pasteur, 1996 to 2011).

DTaP-Hib: Trihibit (Sanofi Pasteur, previously Pasteur-Merieux-Connaught), a package containing *Tripedia* (DTaP) solution plus *ActHib* powder (available September 1996 until 2012).

DTwP: Dip-Pert-Tet (Cutter); *Infagen Adsorbed* (Pitman-Moore; Dow); *Tridipigen* (Eli Lilly); *Tri-Immunol* (Wyeth-Lederle); *Trinavac Adsorbed* (Merck, Sharp and Dohme); *Triogen Adsorbed* (Parke-Davis); *Triple Antigen Adsorbed* (Wyeth); *Solgen Adsorbed* (Eli Lilly; its pertussis component was described as extracted pertussis antigen, available from 1962 to 1977). Acellular extract vaccine (Lederle, 1940s).

DTwP-Hib: Tetramune (Wyeth-Lederle); *ActHib/DTP* (Pasteur-Mérieux-Connaught).

National Policy: ACIP. Pertussis vaccination: Use of acellular pertussis vaccines among infants and young children. *MMWR.* 1997;46(RR-7):1-25. ftp.cdc.gov/pub/Publications/mmwr/rr/rr4607.pdf.

ACIP. Use of diphtheria toxoid-tetanus toxoid-acellular pertussis vaccine as a five-dose series. *MMWR.* 2000;49(RR-13):1-8. erratum 1074.

Canadian National Advisory Committee on Immunization. Prevention of pertussis in adolescents and adults. *Can Comm Dis Rep.* 2003;29(ACS-5):1-9.

CDC. Diphtheria, tetanus, and pertussis: Recommendations for vaccine use and other preventive measures: Recommendations of the Immunization Practices Advisory Committee. *MMWR.* 1991;40(RR-10):1-28.

References: CDC. Tetanus surveillance, United States, 1998-2000. *MMWR.* 2003;52(SS-03):1-8.

WHO. Diphtheria vaccine. *Weekly Epidemiol Rec.* 2006;81:24-32. http://www.who.int/wer/2006/wer8103.pdf.

WHO. Pertussis vaccines: WHO position paper — Recommendations. *Vaccine.* 2011;29(13):2355-2356.

WHO. Tetanus vaccine. *Weekly Epidemiol Rec.* 2006;81:198-208. http://www.who.int/wer/2006/wer8004.pdf.

Wintermeyer SM, et al. Whole-cell and acellular pertussis vaccines. *Ann Pharmacother.* 1994;28:925-939.

Diphtheria & Tetanus Toxoids with Acellular Pertussis Adsorbed & Inactivated Poliovirus Vaccine (DTaP-IPV)

Bacterial Vaccines & Toxoids

Name:
Kinrix

Manufacturer:
GlaxoSmithKline

Synonyms: DTaP-IPV

Comparison: Therapeutically equivalent to various combinations of constituent vaccines. The diphtheria, tetanus, and pertussis components of *Kinrix* are the same as those in *Infanrix* and *Pediarix*; the poliovirus component is the same as that in *Pediarix*. The various acellular DTaP products are generically equivalent, recognizing their differences in contents and methods of standardization. The ACIP considers available data regarding safety and clinical efficacy to be insufficient to express a preference between the various formulations of DTaP available in the United States. Using the same brand of DTaP for a child's vaccination series is generally preferred, but any licensed DTaP vaccine may be used to complete the vaccination series.

> **Note:** Vaccines containing diphtheria, tetanus, and pertussis antigens are the preferred immunizing agents for most people. Tetanus and diphtheria toxoids for adult use (Td) bivalent or with acellular pertussis vaccine (Tdap) is the preferred immunizing agent for adults and older children.
>
> Specific information about the individual components of this drug appear in the individual monographs for diphtheria and tetanus toxoids with acellular pertussis vaccine (DTaP) and inactivated poliovirus vaccine (IPV).

Immunologic Characteristics

Microorganism: Bacteria, *Corynebacterium diphtheriae, Clostridium tetani, Bordetella pertussis.* Viruses, polioviruses types 1, 2, and 3.

Viability: Inactivated

Antigenic Form: Mixture of 2 toxoids with 3 acellular pertussis antigens (detoxified pertussis toxin, filamentous hemagglutinin [FHA], and pertactin [69-kilodalton outer membrane protein]) and 3 types of poliovirus vaccine

Antigenic Type: Proteins

Strains: Toxigenic strains of *C. diphtheriae* and *C. tetani*; unspecified strain of *B. pertussis*; poliovirus type 1 (Mahoney strain), type 2 (MEF-1 strain), and type 3 (Saukett strain)

Use Characteristics

Indications: For active immunization against diphtheria, tetanus, pertussis, and poliomyelitis as the fifth dose in the DTaP series and the fourth dose in the IPV series in children 4 through 6 years of age whose previous DTaP vaccine doses have been with *Infanrix* and/or *Pediarix* for the first 3 doses and *Infanrix* for the fourth dose.

Refer to CDC's wound management guidelines in the DTP Overview.

Limitations: Diphtheria toxoid immunization decreases, but does not eliminate, colonization of toxigenic strains of *C. diphtheriae* in the pharynx, nose, or on the skin. Do not use diphtheria toxoid for the treatment of actual diphtheria infections. Select appropriate antibiotics (eg, erythromycin, penicillin) to treat active infections. Give diphtheria antitoxin if the patient is not likely to have adequate active immunity to diphtheria toxin.

Tetanus toxoid is not intended for the treatment or diagnosis of tetanus. For treatment of tetanus infection and for passive prophylaxis, consider use of tetanus immune globulin and appropriate antibiotics (eg, penicillin G, a tetracycline).

Pertussis vaccine does not stimulate local secretory antibody production to prevent attachment of the microorganism to the respiratory epithelium. Pertussis vaccine is not intended for the treatment of the disease. Select appropriate antibiotics (eg, erythromycin) to treat active infections.

Outmoded Practices: Do not use reduced volumes (fractional doses) of vaccines. The effect of such practices on the frequency of serious adverse events and protection against disease has not been determined.

Contraindications:

Absolute: Do not give further doses of a vaccine containing pertussis antigens to children who have recovered from culture-confirmed pertussis. A severe allergic reaction (eg, anaphylaxis) after a previous dose of any ingredient of this vaccine (including the latex in relevant containers) is a contraindication to administration of *Kinrix*. Because of uncertainty as to which ingredient of the vaccine may be responsible, none of the ingredients should be administered. Alternatively, such individuals may be referred to an allergist for evaluation if further immunizations are considered.

The following events are contraindications to administration of any pertussis-containing vaccine, including *Kinrix*.

- Encephalopathy (eg, coma, decreased level of consciousness, prolonged seizures) within 7 days of a previous dose of a pertussis-containing vaccine not attributable to another cause.

- Progressive neurologic disorder, including infantile spasms, uncontrolled epilepsy, or progressive encephalopathy. Do not administer pertussis vaccine to people with such conditions until a treatment regimen has been established and the condition has stabilized.

Relative: Defer vaccination during the course of a moderate or severe illness with or without fever. Vaccinate such children as soon as they have recovered from the acute phase of the illness. If any of the following events occur within the specified period after administration of a whole-cell pertussis or acellular pertussis-containing vaccine, base the decision to administer *Kinrix* or any pertussis-containing vaccine on potential benefits and possible risks.

- Temperature of 40.5°C or higher (105°F or higher) within 48 hours, not attributable to another cause

- Collapse or shock-like state (hypotonic-hyporesponsive episode) within 48 hours

- Persistent, inconsolable crying lasting 3 hours or more within 48 hours

- Seizure with or without fever within 3 days

A review by the Institute of Medicine found evidence for a causal relation between tetanus toxoid and brachial neuritis, Guillain-Barré syndrome, or anaphylaxis. If Guillain-Barré syndrome occurred within 6 weeks of a prior vaccination containing tetanus toxoid, base the decision to give *Kinrix* or any vaccine containing tetanus toxoid on potential benefits and possible risks.

There may be circumstances, such as a high local incidence of pertussis, in which the potential benefits outweigh possible risks, particularly because these events are not associated with permanent sequelae.

The occurrence of any type of neurological symptoms or signs, including 1 or more convulsions following DTaP administration, is generally a contraindication to further use. The presence of any evolving or changing disorder affecting the CNS contraindicates administration of pertussis vaccine, regardless of whether the suspected neurological disorder is associated with occurrence of any type of seizure activity.

Diphtheria & Tetanus Toxoids with Acellular Pertussis Adsorbed & Inactivated Poliovirus Vaccine (DTaP-IPV)

If a decision is made to withhold pertussis vaccine, provide vaccination against diphtheria, tetanus, and poliomyelitis.

The decision to administer a pertussis-containing vaccine to children with stable CNS disorders must be made by the clinician on an individual basis, considering all relevant factors and assessing potential risks and benefits for that individual. The ACIP and AAP have issued guidelines for such children.

Immunodeficiency: Patients receiving immunosuppressive therapy or who have other immunodeficiencies may have a diminished antibody response to active immunization. Consider deferral of vaccine administration. Nonetheless, routine immunization of symptomatic and asymptomatic HIV-infected patients is recommended.

Elderly: DTaP is generally contraindicated after the seventh birthday.

Adults: DTaP is generally contraindicated after the seventh birthday. Td or Tdap is the preferred immunizing agent for adults and older children.

Carcinogenicity: *Kinrix* has not been evaluated for carcinogenic potential.

Mutagenicity: *Kinrix* has not been evaluated for mutagenic potential.

Fertility Impairment: *Kinrix* has not been evaluated for impairment of fertility.

Pregnancy: Category C. Animal reproduction studies have not been conducted with *Kinrix*. DTaP is generally contraindicated after the seventh birthday. It is not known if *Kinrix* antigens or corresponding antibodies cross the placenta. Generally, most IgG passage across the placenta occurs during the third trimester. Problems in humans have not been documented and are unlikely.

Lactation: DTaP is generally contraindicated after the seventh birthday. It is not known if *Kinrix* antigens or corresponding antibodies cross into breast milk. Problems in humans have not been documented and are unlikely.

Children: Safety and effectiveness of *Kinrix* in children younger than 4 years of age not been evaluated. *Kinrix* is not approved for use in children in this age groups. Do not reduce or divide the DTaP dose for preterm infants or other children. Use Td, Tdap, and IPV for people after the seventh birthday. Children who have recovered from culture-confirmed pertussis do not need further doses of a pertussis-containing vaccine.

Adverse Reactions: The most frequently reported solicited local reaction (greater than 50%) was injection-site pain. Other common solicited local reactions (25% or more) were redness, increase in arm circumference, and swelling. Common solicited general adverse events (15% or more) were drowsiness, fever (99.5°F or higher), and loss of appetite.

A total of 3,537 children were vaccinated with a single dose of *Kinrix* in 3 clinical trials. Of these, 381 children received a non-US formulation of *Kinrix* (containing 2-phenoxyethanol 2.5 mg or less per dose as preservative). The primary study (study 048), conducted in the United States, was a randomized, controlled clinical trial in which children 4 to 6 years of age received *Kinrix* (N = 3,156) or control vaccines (*Infanrix* + *Ipol*) (N = 1,053) as a fifth DTaP vaccine dose following 4 doses of *Infanrix* and as a fourth IPV dose following 3 doses of *Ipol*. Subjects also received the second dose of the US-licensed measles-mumps-rubella (MMR) vaccine administered concomitantly at separate sites. Data on adverse events were collected by parents/guardians using standardized forms for 4 consecutive days after children received *Kinrix* or control vaccines (ie, day of vaccination and the next 3 days). The reported frequencies of solicited local reactions and general adverse events in study 048 appear in the following table. In 3 studies (studies 046, 047, and 048), children were monitored for unsolicited adverse events, including serious adverse events, that occurred in the 31-day period following vaccination. In 2 studies (studies 047 and 048), parents/guardians were actively queried about changes in their child's health status, including the occurrence of serious adverse events, through 6 months after vaccination.

Diphtheria & Tetanus Toxoids with Acellular Pertussis Adsorbed & Inactivated Poliovirus Vaccine (DTaP-IPV)

<table>
<thead>
<tr><th colspan="3">Percentage of Children 4 to 6 Years of Age Reporting Solicited Local Reactions or General Adverse Events Within 4 Days of Vaccination[a] With Kinrix or Separate Concomitant Administration of Infanrix and IPV When Coadministered With MMR Vaccine (Study 048) (Total Vaccinated Cohort)</th></tr>
<tr><th></th><th>Kinrix</th><th>Infanrix + IPV</th></tr>
</thead>
<tbody>
<tr><td>Local[b]</td><td>N = 3,121 to 3,128</td><td>N = 1,039 to 1,043</td></tr>
<tr><td>Pain, any</td><td>57[c]</td><td>53.3</td></tr>
<tr><td>Pain, grade 2 or 3[d]</td><td>13.7</td><td>12</td></tr>
<tr><td>Pain, grade 3[e]</td><td>1.6[c]</td><td>0.6</td></tr>
<tr><td>Redness, any</td><td>36.6</td><td>36.6</td></tr>
<tr><td>Redness, ≥ 50 mm</td><td>17.6</td><td>20</td></tr>
<tr><td>Redness, ≥ 110 mm</td><td>2.9</td><td>4.1</td></tr>
<tr><td>Arm circumference increase, any</td><td>36</td><td>37.8</td></tr>
<tr><td>Arm circumference increase, > 20 mm</td><td>6.9</td><td>7.4</td></tr>
<tr><td>Arm circumference increase, > 30 mm</td><td>2.4</td><td>3.2</td></tr>
<tr><td>Swelling, any</td><td>26</td><td>27</td></tr>
<tr><td>Swelling, ≥ 50 mm</td><td>10.2</td><td>11.5</td></tr>
<tr><td>Swelling, ≥ 110 mm</td><td>1.4</td><td>1.8</td></tr>
<tr><td>General</td><td>N = 3,037 to 3,120</td><td>N = 993 to 1,036</td></tr>
<tr><td>Drowsiness, any</td><td>19.1</td><td>17.5</td></tr>
<tr><td>Drowsiness, grade 3[e]</td><td>0.8</td><td>0.8</td></tr>
<tr><td>Fever, ≥ 99.5°F</td><td>16</td><td>14.8</td></tr>
<tr><td>Fever, ≥ 100.4°F</td><td>6.5[c]</td><td>4.4</td></tr>
<tr><td>Fever, ≥ 102.2°F</td><td>1.1</td><td>1.1</td></tr>
<tr><td>Fever, ≥ 104°F</td><td>0.1</td><td>0</td></tr>
<tr><td>Loss of appetite, any</td><td>15.5</td><td>16</td></tr>
<tr><td>Loss of appetite, grade 3[f]</td><td>0.8</td><td>0.6</td></tr>
</tbody>
</table>

N = number of children with evaluable data.
a Day of vaccination and the next 3 days.
b Local reactions at the injection site for *Kinrix* or *Infanrix*.
c Statistically higher than comparator group ($P < 0.05$).
d Grade 2 defined as painful when the limb was moved; grade 3 defined as preventing normal daily activities.
e Grade 3 defined as preventing normal daily activities.
f Grade 3 defined as not eating at all.

In study 048, *Kinrix* was noninferior to *Infanrix* with regard to swelling that involved more than 50% of the injected upper arm length and was associated with a greater than 30 mm increase in mid-upper arm circumference within 4 days following vaccination.

Serious adverse events: Within the 31-day period after study vaccination in studies 046, 047, and 048, in which all subjects received concomitant MMR vaccine (US-licensed MMR vaccine in studies 047 and 048; non–US-licensed MMR vaccine in study 046), 3 subjects (0.1% [3/3,537]) who received *Kinrix* reported serious adverse events (dehydration and hypernatremia, cerebrovascular accident, dehydration and gastroenteritis) and 4 subjects (0.3% [4/1,434]) who received *Infanrix* and IPV reported serious adverse events (cellulitis, constipation, foreign body trauma, fever without identified etiology).

Diphtheria & Tetanus Toxoids with Acellular Pertussis Adsorbed & Inactivated Poliovirus Vaccine (DTaP-IPV)

Postlicensing experience: In addition to reports in clinical trials, the following adverse events, for which a causal relationship to components of *Kinrix* is plausible, have been reported since market introduction of *Kinrix* outside the United States.

Cutaneous: Pruritus.

General: Injection-site vesicles.

Other: Additional adverse events reported following postlicensing use of *Infanrix*, for which a causal relationship to vaccination is plausible, are: allergic reactions, including anaphylactoid reactions, anaphylaxis, angioedema, and urticaria; apnea; collapse or shock-like state (hypotonic-hyporesponsive episode); convulsions (with or without fever); lymphadenopathy; and thrombocytopenia.

Pharmacologic & Dosing Characteristics

Dosage: 0.5 mL, as the fifth dose in the DTaP series and the fourth dose in the IPV series in children 4 to 6 years of age (before the seventh birthday) whose previous DTaP doses have been with *Infanrix* and/or *Pediarix* for the first 3 doses and *Infanrix* for the fourth dose.

Route & Site: Intramuscular (IM). Do not administer subcutaneously or intravenously. Preferred sites include the deltoid muscle of the upper arm. Do not inject in the gluteal area or areas where there may be a major nerve trunk.

Documentation Requirements: Federal law requires that the following information be documented in the recipient's permanent medical record or in a permanent office log: (1) the manufacturer and lot number of this vaccine, (2) the date of administration, and (3) the name, address, and title of the person administering the vaccine.

Certain adverse events must be reported to VAERS (1-800-822-7967). Refer to Immunization Documents in the Resources section.

Overdosage: No specific data are available. A larger-than-recommended volume of vaccine may increase the risk of injection-site reactions but is unlikely to have other consequences.

Booster Doses: Complete the diphtheria, tetanus, pertussis, and poliovirus vaccination series with other vaccines, as necessary.

Missed Doses: Interrupting the recommended schedule or delaying subsequent doses does not require restarting the series. Use Td or Tdap, rather than DTaP, for doses after the seventh birthday. Interrupting the recommended schedule with a delay between doses should not interfere with the final immunity achieved with *Kinrix*, but waiting does delay achieving adequate protection from infection. There is no need to start the series over, regardless of time elapsed between doses.

Related Interventions: For infants or children at higher risk for seizures than the general population, an appropriate dosage of antipyretic (eg, acetaminophen) may be administered at the time of vaccination and for the following 24 hours to reduce the possibility of postvaccination fever.

Efficacy: In a US multicenter study (study 048), 4,209 children were randomized 3:1 to receive either *Kinrix* or *Infanrix* + IPV administered concomitantly at separate sites. Subjects also received MMR vaccine administered concomitantly at a separate site. Subjects were children 4 to 6 years of age who had received 4 doses of *Infanrix*, 3 doses of IPV, and 1 dose of MMR vaccine. Among subjects in both vaccine groups combined, 49.6% were girls; 45.6% of subjects were white, 18.8% Hispanic, 13.6% Asian, 7% black, and 15% were of other ethnic groups.

Levels of antibodies to the diphtheria, tetanus, pertussis (pertussis toxin, FHA, and pertactin), and poliovirus antigens were measured in sera obtained immediately before vaccination and 1 month (range, 31 to 48 days) after vaccination. The co-primary immunogenicity end points were antidiphtheria toxoid, antitetanus toxoid, antipertussis toxin, anti-FHA, and anti-pertactin booster responses, and antipoliovirus types 1, 2, and 3 geometric mean antibody titers (GMTs) 1 month after vaccination. *Kinrix* was shown to be noninferior to *Infanrix* and IPV administered separately, in terms of booster responses to DTaP antigens and postvaccination GMTs for antipoliovirus antibodies.

The efficacy of the pertussis component of *Kinrix* was determined in clinical trials of *Infanrix* administered as a 3-dose series in infants.

Onset: Escalating protection with each sequential dose.

Duration: After adequate immunization against diphtheria and tetanus, protection persists for 10 years or longer. After immunization against pertussis, protection persists for approximately 4 to 6 years. After immunization against poliovirus, protection persists for many years.

Protective Level:

Diphtheria: Serum antitoxin level of 0.01 international unit/mL is the lowest level giving some degree of protection. Antitoxin levels of at least 0.1 international unit/mL are regarded as protective. Levels of 1 international unit/mL have been associated with long-term protection.

Tetanus: A serum tetanus antitoxin level of 0.01 international unit/mL is considered the minimum protective level. More recently, a level of at least 0.1 to 0.2 international unit/mL has been considered protective.

Pertussis: Efficacy of the pertussis component does not have a well-established correlate of protection.

Poliovirus: Any detectable neutralizing antibody (in practice a titer greater than 1:4).

Mechanism: *C. diphtheriae* may cause a localized or generalized disease. Diphtheria exotoxin, an extracellular protein metabolite of toxigenic strains of *C. diphtheriae*, causes systemic intoxication. Complete immunization induces protective antitoxin antibodies against diphtheria toxin and significantly reduces the risk of developing diphtheria. Immunized patients who develop disease have milder illnesses.

Tetanus toxoid induces specific protective antibodies against the exotoxin excreted by *C. tetani*.

Pertussis vaccine exerts an adjuvant effect on the diphtheria and tetanus toxoids. The role of circulating pertussis antibodies is not clear.

Poliovirus vaccine induces neutralizing antibodies, reducing pharyngeal excretion of poliovirus through a mucosal secretory-IgA response at that site. This helps block respiratory transmission. Some immunity in the mucosa of the GI tract develops, but it is inferior to that induced by oral poliovirus vaccine. If patients vaccinated with IPV swallow viable polioviruses, the viruses can be shed in their stools.

Drug Interactions:

Concomitant vaccination: In a US study (study 047) among recipients of DTaP-IPV (same formulation as *Kinrix* but also containing 2-phenoxyethanol) and the second dose of MMR vaccine who had prevaccination sera tested for antibodies to measles, mumps, and rubella (N = 175-181), 99% of subjects were seropositive for antibodies to measles, mumps, and rubella before vaccination. Data are not available on concomitant use of *Kinrix* and varicella vaccine.

Immunosuppressive therapies, including irradiation, antimetabolites, alkylating agents, cytotoxic drugs, and corticosteroids (used in higher than physiologic doses), may reduce the immune response to vaccines. Recipients may remain susceptible despite immunization. Although no specific *Kinrix* data are available, if immunosuppressive therapy will be discontinued shortly, defer immunization until the patient is off therapy for 3 months; otherwise, vaccinate while still on therapy.

Diphtheria & Tetanus Toxoids with Acellular Pertussis Adsorbed & Inactivated Poliovirus Vaccine (DTaP-IPV)

Inactivated vaccines are not generally affected by circulating antibodies or administration of exogenous antibodies. Vaccination may occur at any time before or after antibody administration.

As with other IM injections, do not give *Pentacel* to children on anticoagulant therapy, unless the potential benefit clearly outweighs the risk of administration.

Pharmaceutical Characteristics

Concentration: Each 0.5 mL dose contains diphtheria toxoid 25 Lf, tetanus toxoid 10 Lf, detoxified pertussis toxin 25 mcg, FHA 25 mcg, pertactin (69-kilodalton outer membrane protein) 8 mcg, type 1 poliovirus (Mahoney) 40 D-antigen units (DU), type 2 poliovirus (MEF-1) 8 DU, and type 3 poliovirus (Saukett) 32 DU.

Quality Assay: Diphtheria and tetanus toxoid potency is determined by measuring the amount of neutralizing antitoxin in previously immunized guinea pigs. The potency of the acellular pertussis components (detoxified pertussis toxin, FHA, and pertactin) is determined by enzyme-linked immunoabsorbent assay (ELISA) on sera from immunized mice. The potency of the inactivated poliovirus component is determined by using the D-antigen ELISA and by a poliovirus-neutralizing cell culture assay on sera from immunized rats.

Packaging: Single 0.5 mL single-dose vial without latex (NDC #: 58160-0812-01), package of ten 0.5 mL single-dose vials without latex (58160-0812-11), single 0.5 mL prefilled syringe without needle (tip cap and plunger contain latex) (58160-0812-41), package of five 0.5 mL single-dose prefilled syringes without needles (tip cap and plunger contain latex) (58160-0812-46), package of ten 0.5 mL single-dose prefilled syringes without needles (tip cap and plunger contain latex) (58160-0812-51), single 0.5 mL prefilled syringe without needle without latex (58160-0812-43), package of ten 0.5 mL prefilled syringes without needles without latex (58160-0812-52)

Doseform: Suspension

Appearance: Homogeneous, turbid, white suspension

Solvent: Sodium chloride 4.5 mg per 0.5 mL dose

Adjuvant: Aluminum hydroxide (not more than 0.6 mg aluminum per 0.5 mL by assay).

Preservative: None

Allergens: Neomycin 0.05 ng or less and polymyxin B 0.01 ng or less per 0.5 mL dose. Consult package labeling regarding latex content.

Excipients: Formaldehyde 100 mcg or less and polysorbate 80 (*Tween 80*) 100 mcg or less per 0.5 mL dose

pH: Not described

Shelf Life: Expires within an unspecified period of time.

Storage/Stability: Store at 2° to 8°C (36° to 46°F). Discard if frozen. Contact the manufacturer regarding exposure to elevated temperatures. Shipping data not provided.

Handling: Do not mix *Kinrix* with any other vaccine in the same syringe or vial. Shake thoroughly but gently to obtain a homogeneous, turbid, white suspension. Do not use if resuspension does not occur.

Production Process: Both diphtheria and tetanus toxins are detoxified with formaldehyde, concentrated by ultrafiltration, and purified by precipitation, dialysis, and sterile filtration. The acellular pertussis antigens (pertussis toxin, FHA, and pertactin) are isolated from fermentation broth; pertactin is extracted from the cells by heat treatment and flocculation. The antigens are purified in successive chromatographic and precipitation steps. Pertussin toxin is detoxified using glutaraldehyde and formaldehyde. FHA and pertactin are treated with formaldehyde. Diphtheria and tetanus toxoids and pertussis antigens (detoxified pertussis toxin, FHA, and pertactin) are individually adsorbed onto aluminum hydroxide.

The inactivated poliovirus component is an enhanced potency component. After clarification, each poliovirus suspension is purified by ultrafiltration, diafiltration, and successive chromatographic steps, and inactivated with formaldehyde. The purified viral strains are then pooled to form a trivalent concentrate.

Media: *C. diphtheriae* bacteria are grown in Fenton medium containing a bovine extract. *C. tetani* bacteria are grown in a modified Latham medium derived from bovine casein. *B. pertussis* bacteria are grown in modified Stainer-Scholte liquid medium. Each of the 3 strains of poliovirus is individually grown in Vero cells, cultivated on microcarriers. Calf serum and lactalbumin hydrolysate are used during Vero cell culture and/or virus culture. Bovine materials used are sourced from countries that the USDA has determined neither have nor are at risk of bovine spongiform encephalopathy.

Disease Epidemiology

See monographs for individual vaccine components.

Other Information

Perspective: See monographs for individual vaccine components.

First Licensed: June 24, 2008

National Policy: See recommended childhood vaccination schedule, revised each January.

Diphtheria & Tetanus Toxoids with Acellular Pertussis Adsorbed, Inactivated Poliovirus, and *Haemophilus influenzae* Type b Conjugate Vaccine (DTaP-IPV-Hib)

Bacterial Vaccines & Toxoids

Name:
Pentacel

Manufacturer:
Sanofi Pasteur

Synonyms: DTaP-IPV-Hib

Comparison: Therapeutically equivalent to various combinations of constituent vaccines. The various DTaP products are generically equivalent, recognizing their differences in contents and methods of standardization. The ACIP considers available data regarding safety and clinical efficacy to be insufficient to express a preference between the various formulations of DTaP available in the United States. Using the same brand of DTaP for a child's vaccination series is generally preferred, but any licensed DTaP vaccine may be used to complete the vaccination series. The Hib antigen is the same as that in *ActHib*-brand Hib vaccine.

> **Note:** Vaccines containing diphtheria, tetanus, and pertussis antigens are the preferred immunizing agents for most people. Tetanus and diphtheria toxoids for adult use (Td) bivalent or with acellular pertussis vaccine (Tdap) is the preferred immunizing agent for adults and older children.
>
> Specific information about the individual components of this drug appear in the individual monographs on diphtheria and tetanus toxoids with acellular pertussis vaccine, inactivated poliovirus vaccine (IPV), and *Haemophilus influenzae* type b vaccine.

Immunologic Characteristics

Microorganism: Bacteria, *Corynebacterium diphtheriae*, *Clostridium tetani*, *Bordetella pertussis*, Hib. Viruses, polioviruses types 1, 2, and 3.

Viability: Inactivated

Antigenic Form: Mixture of 2 toxoids with 5 acellular pertussis antigens (detoxified pertussis toxin, filamentous hemagglutinin [FHA], pertactin [69-kilodalton outer membrane protein], and fimbriae types 2 and 3), 3 types of poliovirus vaccine, and Hib conjugated to tetanus toxoid.

Antigenic Type: Proteins; the Hib vaccine component consists of Hib capsular polysaccharide (polyribosyl ribitol phosphate [PRP]) covalently bound to tetanus toxoid.

Strains: Toxigenic strains of *C. diphtheriae* and *C. tetani*; unspecified strain of *B. pertussis*; poliovirus type 1 (Mahoney strain), type 2 (MEF-1 strain), and type 3 (Saukett strain); Hib strain 1482.

Use Characteristics

Indications: For active immunization against diphtheria, tetanus, pertussis, poliomyelitis, and invasive Hib disease in children 6 weeks through 4 years of age (before fifth birthday).

Refer to CDC's wound management guidelines in the DTP Overview.

Limitations: Diphtheria toxoid immunization decreases, but does not eliminate, colonization of toxigenic strains of *C. diphtheriae* in the pharynx, nose, or on the skin. Do not use diphtheria toxoid for the treatment of actual diphtheria infections. Select appropriate antibiotics (eg, erythromycin, penicillin) to treat active infections. Give diphtheria antitoxin if the patient is not likely to have adequate active immunity to diphtheria toxin.

Tetanus toxoid is not intended for the treatment or diagnosis of tetanus. For treatment of tetanus infection and for passive prophylaxis, consider use of tetanus immune globulin and appropriate antibiotics (eg, penicillin G, a tetracycline).

Diphtheria & Tetanus Toxoids with Acellular Pertussis Adsorbed, Inactivated Poliovirus, and *Haemophilus influenzae* Type b Conjugate Vaccine (DTaP-IPV-Hib)

Pertussis vaccine does not stimulate local secretory antibody production to prevent attachment of the microorganism to the respiratory epithelium. Pertussis vaccine is not intended for the treatment of the disease. Select appropriate antibiotics (eg, erythromycin) to treat active infections.

Outmoded Practices: Do not use reduced volumes (fractional doses) of vaccines. The effect of such practices on the frequency of serious adverse events and protection against disease has not been determined.

Contraindications:

Absolute: Do not give further doses of a vaccine containing pertussis antigens to children who have recovered from culture-confirmed pertussis. A severe allergic reaction (eg, anaphylaxis) after a previous dose of any ingredient of this vaccine is a contraindication to administration of *Pentacel*. Because of uncertainty as to which ingredient of the vaccine may be responsible, none of the ingredients should be administered. Alternatively, such individuals may be referred to an allergist for evaluation if further immunizations are considered.

The following events are contraindications to administration of any pertussis-containing vaccine, including *Pentacel*:

- Encephalopathy (eg, coma, decreased level of consciousness, prolonged seizures) within 7 days of a previous dose of a pertussis-containing vaccine not attributable to another cause.

- Progressive neurologic disorder, including infantile spasms, uncontrolled epilepsy, or progressive encephalopathy. Do not administer pertussis vaccine to persons with such conditions until a treatment regimen has been established and the condition has stabilized.

Relative: Defer vaccination during the course of a moderate or severe illness with or without fever. Vaccinate such children as soon as they have recovered from the acute phase of the illness. If any of the following events occur within the specified period after administration of a whole-cell pertussis or acellular pertussis-containing vaccine, base the decision to administer *Pentacel* or any pertussis-containing vaccine on potential benefits and possible risks.

- Temperature of 40.5°C or higher (105°F or higher) within 48 hours, not attributable to another cause

- Collapse or shock-like state (hypotonic-hyporesponsive episode) within 48 hours

- Persistent, inconsolable crying lasting 3 hours or more within 48 hours

- Seizure with or without fever within 3 days

A review by the Institute of Medicine found evidence for a causal relation between tetanus toxoid and brachial neuritis, Guillain-Barré syndrome, or anaphylaxis. If Guillain-Barré syndrome occurred within 6 weeks of a prior vaccination containing tetanus toxoid, base the decision to give *Pentacel* or any vaccine containing tetanus toxoid on potential benefits and possible risks.

There may be circumstances, such as a high local incidence of pertussis, in which the potential benefits outweigh possible risks, particularly because these events are not associated with permanent sequelae.

The occurrence of any type of neurological symptoms or signs, including 1 or more convulsions following DTaP administration, is generally a contraindication to further use. The presence of any evolving or changing disorder affecting the CNS contraindicates administration of pertussis vaccine, regardless of whether the suspected neurological disorder is associated with occurrence of any type of seizure activity.

If a decision is made to withhold pertussis vaccine, provide vaccination against diphtheria, tetanus, poliomyelitis, and invasive Hib disease.

Diphtheria & Tetanus Toxoids with Acellular Pertussis Adsorbed, Inactivated Poliovirus, and *Haemophilus influenzae* Type b Conjugate Vaccine (DTaP-IPV-Hib)

The decision to administer a pertussis-containing vaccine to children with stable CNS disorders must be made by the clinician on an individual basis. Consider all relevant factors, and assess the potential risks and benefits for that individual. The ACIP and AAP have issued guidelines for such children.

Immunodeficiency: Patients receiving immunosuppressive therapy or who have other immunodeficiencies may have a diminished antibody response to active immunization. Consider deferral of vaccine administration. Nonetheless, routine immunization of symptomatic and asymptomatic HIV-infected patients is recommended.

Elderly: DTaP is generally contraindicated after the seventh birthday.

Adults: DTaP is generally contraindicated after the seventh birthday. Td or Tdap is the preferred immunizing agent for adults and older children.

Carcinogenicity: *Pentacel* has not been evaluated for carcinogenic potential.

Mutagenicity: *Pentacel* has not been evaluated for mutagenic potential.

Fertility Impairment: *Pentacel* has not been evaluated for impairment of fertility.

Pregnancy: Category C. Animal reproduction studies have not been conducted with *Pentacel*. DTaP is generally contraindicated after the seventh birthday. It is not known if *Pentacel* antigens or corresponding antibodies cross the placenta. Generally, most IgG passage across the placenta occurs during the third trimester. Problems in humans have not been documented and are unlikely.

Lactation: DTaP is generally contraindicated after the seventh birthday. It is not known if *Pentacel* antigens or corresponding antibodies cross into breast milk. Problems in humans have not been documented and are unlikely.

Children: Do not reduce or divide the DTaP dose for preterm infants or other children. Safety and efficacy of *Pentacel* in infants younger than 6 weeks of age have not been evaluated. *Pentacel* is not recommended for patients after the seventh birthday. Use Td, Tdap, Hib, and IPV for patients after the seventh birthday. Children who have recovered from culture-confirmed pertussis do not need further doses of a pertussis-containing vaccine.

Adverse Reactions: In studies 494-01, 494-03, 5A9908, and P3T06, 5,980 participants received at least 1 dose of *Pentacel*, including 4,198 participants enrolled in 1 of 3 US studies that evaluated the safety of 4 consecutive doses of *Pentacel* administered at 2, 4, 6, and 15 to 16 months of age. Two of the US studies, studies 494-01 and P3T06, included a control group that received separately administered vaccines. In study 5A9908, conducted in Canada, 1,782 participants previously vaccinated with 3 doses of *Pentacel* received a fourth dose at 15 to 18 months of age. Across the 4 studies, 51% of participants were girls. Among participants in the 3 US studies, 65% were white, 9% were black, 13% were Hispanic, 4% were Asian, and 10% were of other ethnic groups. Following doses 1 to 3 combined, the proportion of temperature measurements taken by axillary, rectal, or other routes, or not recorded were 46%, 53%, 1%, and 0%, respectively, for *Pentacel* and 45%, 54%, 1%, and 0.1%, respectively, for *Daptacel + Ipol + ActHIB*. After dose 4, the proportion of temperature measurements taken by axillary, rectal, or other routes, or not recorded were 63%, 34%, 2%, and 0.5%, respectively, for *Pentacel*, and 61%, 37%, 2% and 0.5%, respectively, for *Daptacel + ActHIB*.

Serious adverse events: In study P3T06, within 30 days after doses 1 to 3 of *Pentacel* or control vaccines, 19 of 484 (3.9%) participants who received *Pentacel* and 50 of 1,455 (3.4%) participants who received *Daptacel + Ipol + ActHIB* experienced a serious adverse event. Within 30 days after dose 4 of *Pentacel* or control vaccines, 5 of 431 (1.2%) participants who received *Pentacel* and 4 of 418 (1%) participants who received *Daptacel + ActHIB* experienced a serious adverse event. In study 494-01, within 30 days after doses 1 to 3 of *Pentacel* or control vaccines, 23 of 2,506 (0.9%) participants who received *Pentacel*

Diphtheria & Tetanus Toxoids with Acellular Pertussis Adsorbed, Inactivated Poliovirus, and *Haemophilus influenzae* Type b Conjugate Vaccine (DTaP-IPV-Hib)

and 11 of 1,032 (1.1%) participants who received HCPDT (a non–US-licensed DTaP vaccine identical to the DTaP component of *Pentacel*, marketed in some countries as *Quadracel*) + *Poliovax* + *ActHIB* experienced a serious adverse event. Within 30 days after dose 4 of *Pentacel* or control vaccines, 6 of 1,862 (0.3%) participants who received *Pentacel* and 2 of 739 (0.3%) participants who received HCPDT + *Poliovax* + *ActHIB* experienced a serious adverse event. Across studies 494-01, 494-03, and P3T06, within 30 days after doses 1 to 3 of *Pentacel* or control vaccines, overall, the most frequently reported serious adverse events were bronchiolitis, dehydration, pneumonia, and gastroenteritis. Across studies 494-01, 494-03, 5A9908, and P3T06, within 30 days after dose 4 of *Pentacel* or control vaccines, overall, the most frequently reported serious adverse events were dehydration, gastroenteritis, asthma, and pneumonia. Across studies 494-01, 494-03, 5A9908, and P3T06, 2 cases of encephalopathy were reported, both in participants who had received *Pentacel* (n = 5,979). One case occurred 30 days postvaccination and was secondary to cardiac arrest after cardiac surgery. One infant who had onset of neurologic symptoms 8 days postvaccination was later found to have structural cerebral abnormalities and was diagnosed with congenital encephalopathy. Five deaths occurred during studies 494-01, 494-03, 5A9908, and P3T06: 4 in children who had received *Pentacel* (n = 5,979) and 1 in a participant who had received *Daptacel* + *Ipol* + *ActHIB* (n = 1,455). There were no deaths reported in children who received HCPDT + *Poliovax* + *ActHIB* (n = 1,032). Causes of death among children who received *Pentacel* were asphyxia caused by suffocation, head trauma, sudden infant death syndrome, and neuroblastoma (8, 23, 52, and 256 days postvaccination, respectively). One participant with ependymoma died secondary to aspiration 222 days after *Daptacel* + *Ipol* + *ActHIB*.

Hypotonic-hyporesponsive episodes: In study P3T06, diary cards included questions pertaining to hypotonic-hyporesponsive episodes. In studies 494-01, 494-03, and 5A9908, a question about the occurrence of fainting or change in mental status was asked during postvaccination phone calls. Across these 4 studies, no hypotonic-hyporesponsive episodes, as defined in a report of a US Public Health Service workshop were reported among participants who received *Pentacel* (n = 5,979), separately administered HCPDT + *Poliovax* + *ActHIB* (n = 1,032), or separately administered *Daptacel* + *Ipol* + *ActHIB* (n = 1,455). Hypotonia not fulfilling hypotonic-hyporesponsive episodes criteria within 7 days after vaccination was reported in 4 participants after administration of *Pentacel* (1 on the same day as the first dose; 3 on the same day as the third dose) and in 1 participant after administration of *Daptacel* + *Ipol* + *ActHIB* (4 days after the first dose).

Seizures: Across studies 494-01, 494-03, 5A9908, and P3T06, 8 participants experienced a seizure within 7 days after either *Pentacel* (4 participants; n = 4,197 for at least one of doses 1 to 3; n = 5,033 for dose 4), separately administered HCPDT + *Poliovax* + *ActHIB* (3 participants; n = 1,032 for at least one of doses 1 to 3; n = 739 for dose 4), separately administered *Daptacel* + *Ipol* + *ActHIB* (1 participant; n = 1,455 for at least one of doses 1 to 3), or separately administered *Daptacel* + *ActHIB* (0 participants; n = 418 for dose 4). Among the 4 participants who experienced a seizure within 7 days following *Pentacel*, 1 participant in study 494-01 had an afebrile seizure 6 days after the first dose, 1 participant in study 494-01 had a possible seizure the same day as the third dose, and 2 participants in study 5A9908 had a febrile seizure 2 and 4 days, respectively, after the fourth dose. Among the 4 participants who experienced a seizure within 7 days after control vaccines, 1 participant had an afebrile seizure the same day as the first dose of *Daptacel* + *Ipol* + *ActHIB*, 1 participant had an afebrile seizure the same day as the second dose of HCPDT + *Poliovax* + *ActHIB*, and 2 participants had a febrile seizure 6 and 7 days, respectively, after the fourth dose of HCPDT + *Poliovax* + *ActHIB*.

Diphtheria & Tetanus Toxoids with Acellular Pertussis Adsorbed, Inactivated Poliovirus, and *Haemophilus influenzae* Type b Conjugate Vaccine (DTaP-IPV-Hib)

Postlicensing experience: The following additional adverse events have been spontaneously reported between 1997 and 2007 during the postmarketing use of *Pentacel* outside of the United States, primarily in Canada.

Cardiac: Cyanosis.

CNS: Depressed level of consciousness, hypotonic-hyporesponsive episodes, somnolence.

Cutaneous: Erythema, skin discoloration.

GI: Diarrhea, vomiting.

General: Extensive swelling of injected limb, injection-site reactions (eg, inflammation, mass, abscess, sterile abscess), vaccination failure (invasive Hib disease).

Immune system: Hypersensitivity (eg, rash, urticaria).

Infections: Meningitis, rhinitis, viral infection.

Metabolism: Decreased appetite.

Psychiatric disorders: Screaming.

Respiratory: Apnea, cough.

Vascular: Pallor.

Pharmacologic & Dosing Characteristics

Dosage: Four 0.5 mL doses, typically at 2, 4, 6, and 15 to 18 months of age. Administer the first 3 doses at 6- or preferably 8-week intervals. The customary age for the first dose is 2 months of age, but it may be given starting at 6 weeks of age. Four doses of *Pentacel* comprise a primary immunization course against pertussis. Three doses of *Pentacel* constitute a primary immunization course against diphtheria, tetanus, poliomyelitis, and invasive Hib disease; the fourth dose provides booster vaccination against diphtheria, tetanus, poliomyelitis, and invasive Hib disease.

Children who have completed a 4-dose series with *Pentacel* should receive a fifth dose of DTaP vaccine at 4 to 6 years of age. Because the pertussis antigens in *Daptacel* are the same as those in *Pentacel* (although with different amounts of detoxified pertussis toxin and FHA), these children should receive *Daptacel* as their fifth dose of DTaP. Data are not available to evaluate the safety of *Daptacel* after 4 previous doses of *Pentacel*.

Children previously vaccinated with 1 or more doses of Daptacel: *Pentacel* may be used to complete the first 4 doses of the DTaP series in infants and children who have received 1 or more doses of *Daptacel* and are also scheduled to receive the other antigens of *Pentacel*. However, the safety and efficacy of *Pentacel* in such infants have not been evaluated.

Children previously vaccinated with 1 or more doses of IPV: *Pentacel* may be used to complete the 4-dose IPV series in infants and children who have received 1 or more doses of another licensed IPV vaccine and are also scheduled to receive the other antigens of *Pentacel*. However, the safety and efficacy of *Pentacel* in such infants have not been evaluated.

Children previously vaccinated with 1 or more doses of Hib vaccine: *Pentacel* may be used to complete the vaccination series in infants and children previously vaccinated with 1 or more doses of a Hib conjugate vaccine, who are also scheduled to receive the other antigens of *Pentacel*. However, the safety and efficacy of *Pentacel* in such infants have not been evaluated. If different brands of Hib conjugate vaccines are administered to complete the series, 3 primary immunizing doses are needed, followed by a booster dose.

Route: Intramuscular (IM). Do not administer subcutaneously or intravenously. Preferred sites are anterolateral aspects of the thigh or the deltoid muscle of the upper arm. Do not inject in the gluteal area or areas where there may be a major nerve trunk.

Diphtheria & Tetanus Toxoids with Acellular Pertussis Adsorbed, Inactivated Poliovirus, and *Haemophilus influenzae* Type b Conjugate Vaccine (DTaP-IPV-Hib)

Documentation Requirements: Federal law requires that the following information be documented in the recipient's permanent medical record or in a permanent office log: (1) the manufacturer and lot number of this vaccine, (2) the date of administration, and (3) the name, address, and title of the person administering the vaccine.

Certain adverse events must be reported to VAERS (1-800-822-7967). Refer to Immunization Documents in the Resources section.

Overdosage: No specific data are available. A larger-than-recommended volume of vaccine may increase the risk of injection-site reactions but is unlikely to have other consequences.

Booster Doses: Complete the diphtheria, tetanus, pertussis, poliovirus, and Hib vaccination series with other vaccines, as necessary.

Missed Doses: Interrupting the recommended schedule or delaying subsequent doses does not require restarting the series. Use Td or Tdap, rather than DTaP, for doses after the seventh birthday. Interrupting the recommended schedule with a delay between doses should not interfere with the final immunity achieved with *Pentacel*, but waiting does delay achieving adequate protection from infection. There is no need to start the series over, regardless of time elapsed between doses.

Related Interventions: For infants or children at higher risk for seizures than the general population, an appropriate dosage of antipyretic (eg, acetaminophen) may be administered at the time of vaccination and for the following 24 hours to reduce the possibility of postvaccination fever.

Efficacy: The safety and effectiveness of *Pentacel* was established in children 6 weeks through 18 months of age on the basis of clinical studies. The safety and effectiveness of *Pentacel* in children 19 months through 4 years of age is supported by evidence in children 6 weeks through 18 of age. The safety and effectiveness of *Pentacel* in infants younger than 6 weeks of age and in children 5 to 16 years of age have not been established.

The efficacy of *Pentacel* is based on the immunogenicity of the individual antigens compared with separately administered vaccines. Serological correlates of protection exist for diphtheria, tetanus, poliomyelitis, and invasive Hib disease. *Pentacel* met noninferiority criteria for diphtheria, tetanus, and poliovirus responses. Efficacy against pertussis, for which there is no well-established serological correlate of protection, was based on comparing pertussis immune responses after *Pentacel* in US children to responses after *Daptacel* in an efficacy study conducted in Sweden (Sweden I efficacy trial). While *Pentacel* and *Daptacel* contain the same pertussis antigens, manufactured by the same process, *Pentacel* contains twice as much detoxified pertussis toxin and 4 times as much FHA as *Daptacel*.

Based on comparisons of the immune responses to *Daptacel* in US infants (postdose 3) and Canadian children (postdose 4) relative to infants who participated in the Sweden I efficacy trial, 4 doses of *Daptacel* vaccine were needed for primary immunization against pertussis in US children.

In a serology bridging analysis, immune responses to FHA, pertactin (PRN), and fimbriae types 2 and 3 (FIM) in a subset of infants who received 3 doses of *Daptacel* in the Sweden I efficacy trial were compared with the postdose 3 and 4 responses in a subset of US children from study 494-01 who received *Pentacel*. Available stored sera from infants who received *Daptacel* in the Sweden I efficacy trial and sera from children who received PCV7 concomitantly with the first 3 doses of *Pentacel* in study 494-01 were assayed in parallel. Data on levels of antibody to pertussis toxin using an adequately specific assay were not available.

For anti-FHA and anti-FIM, the noninferiority criteria were met for seroconversion rates and for anti-FHA, anti-PRN, and anti-FIM, the noninferiority criteria were met for geometric mean concentrations (GMCs), after dose 4 of *Pentacel*, relative to dose 3 of *Daptacel*. The noninferiority criterion for anti-PRN seroconversion after dose 4 of *Pentacel*, relative to dose 3 of *Daptacel*, was not met (upper limit of 95% confidence interval for difference in rate [*Daptacel* − *Pentacel*] = 13.24%]. Whether the lower anti-PRN seroconversion rate after dose 4 of *Pentacel* in US children relative to dose 3 of *Daptacel* in Swedish infants correlates with diminished efficacy of *Pentacel* against pertussis is unknown.

In study P3T06, US infants were randomized to receive either *Pentacel* or *Daptacel* + *Ipol* + *ActHIB* at 2, 4, 6, and 15 to 16 months of age. The pertussis immune responses (GMCs and seroconversion rates) 1 month after the third and fourth doses were compared. Seroconversion was defined as a 4-fold rise in antibody level. Data on anti-pertussis toxin responses obtained from an adequately specific assay were available on only a nonrandom subset of study participants. For each of the pertussis antigens, noninferiority criteria were met for seroconversion rates and GMCs after *Pentacel* dose 3, relative to *Daptacel* dose 3. After *Pentacel* dose 4, relative to *Daptacel* dose 4, noninferiority criteria were met for all comparisons, except for anti-PRN GMCs. Whether the lower anti-PRN GMC after *Pentacel* dose 4, relative to *Daptacel* dose 4, in US children correlates with diminished efficacy of *Pentacel* against pertussis is unknown.

In study 494-01, noninferiority criteria were not met for the proportion of participants who achieved an anti-PRP level of 1 mcg/mL or more and for anti-PRP GMCs after *Pentacel*, compared with separately administered *ActHIB*. In each of studies P3T06 and M5A10, the noninferiority criterion was met for the proportion of participants who achieved an anti-PRP level of 1 mcg/mL or more after *Pentacel*, compared with separately administered *ActHIB*. In study M5A10, the noninferiority criterion was met for anti-PRP GMCs after *Pentacel*, compared with separately administered *ActHIB*.

In study 494-01, at 15 months of age before receipt of dose 4 of study vaccines, 69% of *Pentacel* recipients (n = 829) and 81% of separately administered *ActHIB* vaccine recipients (n = 276) had an anti-PRP level of 0.15 mcg/mL or more. After dose 4 of study vaccines, 98% of *Pentacel* recipients (n = 874) and 99% of separately administered *ActHIB* vaccine recipients (n = 291) had an anti-PRP level of 1 mcg/mL or more.

In study P3T06, at 15 months of age before receipt of dose 4 of study vaccines, 65% of *Pentacel* recipients (n = 335) and 61% of separately administered *ActHIB* vaccine recipients (n = 323) had an anti-PRP level of 0.15 mcg/mL or more. After dose 4 of study vaccines, 98% of *Pentacel* recipients (n = 361) and 96% of separately administered *ActHIB* vaccine recipients (n = 340) had an anti-PRP level of 1 mcg/mL or more.

Onset: Escalating protection with each sequential dose.

Duration: After adequate immunization against diphtheria and tetanus, protection persists for 10 years or longer. After immunization against pertussis, protection persists for approximately 4 to 6 years. After immunization against poliovirus and Hib, protection persists for many years.

Protective Level:

Diphtheria: Serum antitoxin level of 0.01 international unit/mL is the lowest level giving some degree of protection. Antitoxin levels of 0.1 international unit/mL or more are regarded as protective. Levels of 1 international unit/mL have been associated with long-term protection.

Tetanus: A serum tetanus antitoxin level of 0.01 international unit/mL is considered the minimum protective level. More recently, a level of 0.1 to 0.2 or more international unit/mL has been considered as protective.

Pertussis: Efficacy of the pertussis component does not have a well-established correlate of protection.

Poliovirus: Any detectable neutralizing antibody (in practice a titer greater than 1:4).

Diphtheria & Tetanus Toxoids with Acellular Pertussis Adsorbed, Inactivated Poliovirus, and *Haemophilus influenzae* Type b Conjugate Vaccine (DTaP-IPV-Hib)

Hib: Antibody concentrations of 0.15 mcg/mL or more correlate with clinical protection from disease. Antibody concentrations higher than 1 mcg/mL 3 weeks after vaccination correlate with prolonged protection from disease, generally implying several years of protection.

Mechanism: *C. diphtheriae* may cause a localized or generalized disease. Diphtheria exotoxin, an extracellular protein metabolite of toxigenic strains of *C. diphtheriae*, causes systemic intoxication. Complete immunization induces protective antitoxin antibodies against diphtheria toxin and significantly reduces the risk of developing diphtheria. Immunized patients who develop disease have milder illnesses.

Tetanus toxoid induces specific protective antibodies against the exotoxin excreted by *C. tetani*.

Pertussis vaccine exerts an adjuvant effect on the diphtheria and tetanus toxoids. The role of circulating pertussis antibodies is not clear at present.

Poliovirus vaccine induces neutralizing antibodies, reducing pharyngeal excretion of poliovirus through a mucosal secretory-immunoglobulin A response at that site. This helps block respiratory transmission. Some immunity in the mucosa of the GI tract develops, but it is inferior to that induced by oral polio vaccine. If patients vaccinated with IPV swallow viable polioviruses, the viruses can be shed in their stools.

Hib vaccine induces specific protective antibodies against type b strains of *Haemophilus influenzae*.

Drug Interactions: Do not mix *Pentacel* with any other vaccine or immune globulin in the same syringe or vial. When coadministration with other vaccines is required, give with separate syringes and at different injection sites.

Concomitant vaccination: In study P3T06, there was no evidence for reduced antibody responses to hepatitis B vaccine (percent with anti-HBsAg of 10 milli-international unit/mL or more and GMCs) or PCV7 (percent with antibody levels of 0.15 mcg/mL or more and 0.5 mcg/mL or more and GMCs to each serotype) administered concomitantly with *Pentacel* (n = 321 to 325) relative to these vaccines administered concomitantly with *Daptacel* + *Ipol* + *ActHIB* (n = 998 to 1,029). The immune responses to hepatitis B vaccine and PCV7 were evaluated 1 month after the third dose. In study 494-03, there was no evidence for interference in the immune response to the fourth dose of PCV7 (percent with antibody levels of 0.15 mcg/mL or more and 0.5 mcg/mL or more and GMCs to each serotype) administered at 15 months of age concomitantly with *Pentacel* (n = 155) relative to this vaccine administered concomitantly with measles-mumps-rubella (MMR) and varicella vaccines (n = 158). There was no evidence for interference in the immune response to MMR and varicella vaccines (percent with prespecified seroresponse level) administered at 15 months of age concomitantly with *Pentacel* (n = 154) relative to these vaccines administered concomitantly with PCV7 (n = 144). The immune responses to MMR, varicella vaccine, and the fourth dose of PCV7 were evaluated 1 month postvaccination.

Immunosuppressive therapies, including irradiation, antimetabolites, alkylating agents, cytotoxic drugs, and corticosteroids (used in greater-than-physiologic doses), may reduce the immune response to vaccines. Recipients may remain susceptible despite immunization. Although no specific *Pentacel* data are available, if immunosuppressive therapy will be discontinued shortly, defer immunization until the patient is off therapy for 3 months; otherwise, vaccinate while still on therapy.

Inactivated vaccines are not generally affected by circulating antibodies or administration of exogenous antibodies. Vaccination may occur at any time before or after antibody administration.

Diphtheria & Tetanus Toxoids with Acellular Pertussis Adsorbed, Inactivated Poliovirus, and *Haemophilus influenzae* Type b Conjugate Vaccine (DTaP-IPV-Hib)

As with other IM injections, do not give *Pentacel* to children on anticoagulant therapy, unless the potential benefit clearly outweighs the risk of administration.

Lab Interference: Antigenuria has been detected in some instances after receipt of *ActHIB* vaccine. Urine antigen detection may not have definite diagnostic value in suspected Hib disease within 1 week after receipt of *Pentacel*.

Pharmaceutical Characteristics

Concentration: Each 0.5 mL dose contains diphtheria toxoid 15 Lf, tetanus toxoid 5 Lf, detoxified pertussis toxin 20 mcg, FHA 20 mcg, PRN 3 mcg, FIM 5 mcg, type 1 poliovirus (Mahoney) 40 D-antigen units (DU), type 2 poliovirus (MEF-1) 8 DU, type 3 poliovirus (Saukett) 32 DU, and 10 mcg PRP of Hib covalently bound to tetanus toxoid 24 mcg.

Quality Assay: Both diphtheria and tetanus toxoids induce at least 2 neutralizing units per mL in the guinea pig potency test. The potency of the acellular pertussis antigens is evaluated by the antibody response of immunized mice to pertussis toxin, FHA, PRN, and FIM, as measured by enzyme-linked immunosorbent assay (ELISA). The immunogenicity of the inactivated polioviruses is evaluated by the antibody response in monkeys measured by virus neutralization. Potency of the Hib component is specified on each lot by limits on the content of PRP polysaccharide and protein per dose and the proportion of polysaccharide and protein characterized as high molecular weight conjugate.

Packaging: Five-dose package containing 5 vials of DTaP-IPV component to be used to reconstitute 5 single-dose vials of lyophilized *ActHIB* vaccine.

NDC Number: 49281-0510-05

Doseform: Suspension used to reconstitute lyophilized powder

Appearance: Uniform, cloudy, white to off-white (yellow tinge) suspension

Solvent: Isotonic sodium chloride

Diluent:
For reconstitution: The DTaP-IPV component is used to reconstitute the lyophilized Hib vaccine powder

Adjuvant: Each 0.5 mL dose contains aluminum phosphate 1.5 mg (aluminum 0.33 mg)

Preservative: None

Allergens: Each 0.5 mL dose contains less than 4 pg of neomycin and less than 4 pg polymyxin B sulfate.

Excipients: Each 0.5 mL dose contains polysorbate 80 (approximately 10 ppm by calculation), formaldehyde 5 mcg or less, glutaraldehyde less than 50 ng, bovine serum albumin 50 ng or less, 2-phenoxyethanol 3.3 mg (0.6% v/v) (not as a preservative).

pH: Not described

Shelf Life: Expires within an unspecified period of time.

Storage/Stability: Store at 2° to 8°C (36° to 46°F). Discard if frozen. Contact the manufacturer regarding exposure to elevated temperatures. Shipping data not provided.

Use immediately after reconstitution.

Handling: Thoroughly but gently shake the vial of DTaP-IPV component, withdraw the entire liquid content, and inject into the vial of *ActHIB* powder. Shake the vial now containing *Pentacel* thoroughly until a cloudy, uniform suspension results. Do not use if a uniform suspension does not result.

Production Process: After purification by ammonium sulfate fractionation, the diphtheria toxin is detoxified with formaldehyde and diafiltered.

Diphtheria & Tetanus Toxoids with Acellular Pertussis Adsorbed, Inactivated Poliovirus, and *Haemophilus influenzae* Type b Conjugate Vaccine (DTaP-IPV-Hib)

Tetanus toxin is detoxified with formaldehyde and purified by ammonium sulfate fractionation and diafiltration. Tds are individually adsorbed onto aluminum phosphate.

The acellular pertussis vaccine antigens pertussis toxin, FHA, and PRN are isolated separately from the supernatant culture medium. FIM are extracted and copurified from the bacterial cells. The pertussis antigens are purified by sequential filtration, salt precipitation, ultrafiltration, and chromatography. Pertussis toxin is detoxified with glutaraldehyde. FHA is treated with formaldehyde, and the residual aldehydes are removed by ultrafiltration. The individual antigens are adsorbed separately onto aluminum phosphate.

After clarification and filtration, the poliovirus suspensions are concentrated by ultrafiltration and purified by liquid chromatography steps. The monovalent viral suspensions are inactivated with formaldehyde. Monovalent concentrates of each inactivated poliovirus are combined to produce a trivalent poliovirus concentrate.

The adsorbed diphtheria, tetanus, and acellular pertussis antigens are combined into an intermediate concentrate. The trivalent poliovirus concentrate is added and the DTaP-IPV component is diluted to its final concentration.

Hib PRP is isolated as a high molecular weight polymer. The tetanus toxoid for conjugation to PRP is prepared by ammonium sulfate purification and formalin inactivation of the toxin. The toxoid is filter sterilized before conjugation.

Media: *C. diphtheriae* is grown in modified Mueller's growth medium. *C. tetani* is grown in modified Mueller-Miller casamino acid medium. *B. pertussis* cultures are grown in Stainer-Scholte medium modified by the addition of casamino acids and dimethyl-beta-cyclodextrin. Poliovirus types 1, 2, and 3 are each grown in separate cultures of MRC-5 cells by the microcarrier method. The cells are grown in Connaught Medical Research Laboratories 1969 medium, supplemented with calf serum. For viral growth, the culture medium is replaced by Medium 199 without calf serum. Hib bacteria are grown in a semisynthetic medium.

Disease Epidemiology

See monographs for individual vaccine components.

Other Information

Perspective: See monographs for individual vaccine components.

First Licensed: June 20, 2008

National Policy: See recommended childhood vaccination schedule, revised each January.

Diphtheria & Tetanus Toxoids with Acellular Pertussis Adsorbed, Hepatitis B (Recombinant) & Inactivated Poliovirus Vaccine (DTaP-Hep B-IPV)

Bacterial Vaccines & Toxoids

Name:
Pediarix

Manufacturers:
Diphtheria and tetanus toxoids manufactured by Novartis (Marburg, Germany).
Pertussis antigens, HBsAg, and poliovirus antigens manufactured by GlaxoSmithKline (Rixensart, Belgium).
Distributed by GlaxoSmithKline

Synonyms: DTaP-HBV-IPV

Comparison: Prophylactically equivalent to various combinations of constituent vaccines. The diphtheria toxoid, tetanus toxoid, and pertussis antigens are the same as those in *Infanrix*-brand DTaP vaccine. The various acellular DTaP products are generally considered prophylactically equivalent, despite some differences in contents and methods of standardization. The ACIP considers available data regarding safety and clinical efficacy to be insufficient to express a preference between the various formulations of DTaP available in the United States. Using the same brand of DTaP for a child's vaccination series is generally preferred, but any licensed DTaP vaccine may be used to complete the vaccination series. The hepatitis B surface antigen is the same as that in *Engerix-B*-brand hepatitis B vaccine.

> **Note:** Vaccines containing diphtheria, tetanus, and pertussis antigens are the preferred immunizing agents for most people. Tetanus and diphtheria toxoids for adult use (Td) bivalent or with acellular pertussis vaccine (Tdap) is the preferred immunizing agent for adults and older children.
>
> Specific information about the individual components of this drug appear in the individual monographs on diphtheria and tetanus toxoids with acellular pertussis vaccine, hepatitis B vaccine, and inactivated poliovirus vaccine.

Immunologic Characteristics

Microorganism: Bacteria, *Corynebacterium diphtheriae*, *Clostridium tetani*, *Bordetella pertussis*. Viruses, hepatitis B virus, polioviruses type 1, 2, and 3.

Viability: Inactivated

Antigenic Form: Mixture of 2 toxoids with 3 acellular pertussis antigens (inactivated pertussis toxin [PT], filamentous hemagglutinin [FHA], and pertactin [69-kilodalton outer membrane protein]), hepatitis B surface antigen (HBsAg), and 3 types of poliovirus vaccine

Antigenic Type: Proteins

Strains: Toxigenic strains of *Corynebacterium diphtheriae* and *Clostridium tetani*. Unspecified strain of *Bordetella pertussis*. Hepatitis B adw_2 subtype. Poliovirus type 1 (Mahoney strain), type 2 (MEF-1 strain), and type 3 (Saukett strain).

Use Characteristics

Indications: For active immunization against diphtheria, tetanus, pertussis, all known subtypes of hepatitis B virus, and 3 types of poliomyelitis, as a 3-dose primary series in infants born of HBsAg-negative mothers, beginning as early as 6 weeks of age.

Reduced risk of hepatocellular carcinoma: Hepatitis B vaccine is recognized as the first anticancer vaccine, because it can prevent primary liver cancer. A clear link has been demonstrated between chronic hepatitis B infection and the occurrence of hepatocellular carcinoma.

Diphtheria & Tetanus Toxoids with Acellular Pertussis Adsorbed, Hepatitis B (Recombinant) & Inactivated Poliovirus Vaccine (DTaP-Hep B-IPV)

As hepatitis D (caused by the delta virus) does not occur in the absence of hepatitis B infection, vaccination with *Pediarix* will also prevent hepatitis D.

Refer to the CDC's wound-management guidelines in the DTP Overview.

Limitations: *Pediarix* is not indicated for use as a booster dose after a 3-dose primary series of *Pediarix*. Licensed combination vaccines may be used when any components of the combination are indicated and the vaccine's other components are not contraindicated. Give children who receive a 3-dose primary series of *Pediarix* a fourth dose of DTaP vaccine at 15 to 18 months of age and a fourth dose of IPV at 4 to 6 years of age. Because the pertussis antigen components of *Infanrix* are the same as in *Pediarix*, give these children *Infanrix* as their fourth dose of DTaP.

Give infants born of HBsAg-positive mothers HBIG and monovalent hepatitis B vaccine within 12 hours of birth and complete the hepatitis B vaccination series.

Give infants born of mothers of unknown HBsAg status monovalent hepatitis B vaccine within 12 hours of birth and complete the hepatitis B vaccination series.

Pediarix will not prevent hepatitis caused by other agents, such as hepatitis A, C, and E viruses, or other pathogens known to infect the liver. Hepatitis B has a long incubation period. Vaccination with *Pediarix* may not prevent hepatitis B infection in people who had an unrecognized hepatitis B infection during vaccine administration.

Diphtheria toxoid immunization decreases, but does not eliminate, carriage of *C. diphtheriae* in the pharynx, nose, or on the skin. Do not use diphtheria toxoid for the treatment of actual diphtheria infections. Select appropriate antibiotics (eg, erythromycin, penicillin) to treat active infections. Give diphtheria antitoxin if the patient is unlikely to have adequate active immunity to diphtheria toxin.

Tetanus toxoid is not intended for the treatment of that disease. For treatment of tetanus infection and for passive prophylaxis, consider use of tetanus immune globulin and appropriate antibiotics (eg, a penicillin, a tetracycline).

Pertussis vaccine does not stimulate local secretory antibody production to prevent attachment of the microorganism to the respiratory epithelium. Pertussis vaccine is not intended for the treatment of the disease. Select appropriate antibiotics (eg, erythromycin) to treat active infections.

Outmoded Practices: Do not use reduced volumes (fractional doses) of vaccines. The effect of such practices on the frequency of serious adverse events and protection against disease has not been determined.

Contraindications:

Absolute: Do not give further doses of a vaccine containing pertussis antigens to children who have recovered from culture-confirmed pertussis. This vaccine is also contraindicated in people with a hypersensitivity to any component of the vaccine, including yeast, neomycin, and polymyxin B.

The following events are contraindications to administration of any pertussis-containing vaccine, including *Pediarix*:

- Encephalopathy (eg, coma, decreased level of consciousness, prolonged seizures) within 7 days of administration of a previous dose of a pertussis-containing vaccine not attributable to another identifiable cause.
- Progressive neurologic disorder, including infantile spasms, uncontrolled epilepsy, or progressive encephalopathy. Do not administer pertussis vaccine to people with such conditions until a treatment regimen has been established and the condition has stabilized.

Diphtheria & Tetanus Toxoids with Acellular Pertussis Adsorbed, Hepatitis B (Recombinant) & Inactivated Poliovirus Vaccine (DTaP-Hep B-IPV)

Relative: Defer vaccination during the course of a moderate or severe illness with or without fever. Vaccinate such children as soon as they have recovered from the acute phase of the illness.

If any of these events occur in temporal relation to receipt of a vaccine containing a pertussis component, base the decision to give subsequent doses of a vaccine containing a pertussis component on careful consideration of potential benefits and possible risks:

- Temperature 40.5°C (105°F) and higher within 48 hours not caused by another identifiable cause;
- Collapse or shock-like state (hypotonic-hyporesponsive episode) within 48 hours;
- Persistent, inconsolable crying lasting 3 hours or more, occurring within 48 hours;
- Seizures with or without fever, occurring within 3 days.

There may be circumstances, such as a high local incidence of pertussis, in which the potential benefits outweigh possible risks, particularly because these events are not associated with permanent sequelae.

The occurrence of any type of neurological symptoms or signs, including 1 or more convulsion following DTaP administration, is generally a contraindication to further use. The presence of any evolving or changing disorder affecting the CNS contraindicates administration of pertussis vaccine regardless of whether the suspected neurological disorder is associated with occurrence of any type of seizure activity.

When a decision is made to withhold pertussis vaccine, continue immunization with DT vaccine, hepatitis B vaccine, and IPV. If Guillain-Barré syndrome occurs within 6 weeks of receipt of tetanus toxoid, base the decision to give subsequent doses of any vaccine containing tetanus toxoid on careful consideration of potential benefits and possible risks.

The decision to administer a pertussis-containing vaccine to children with stable CNS disorders must be made by the physician on an individual basis, considering all relevant factors, and assessing potential risks and benefits for that individual. The ACIP and AAP have issued guidelines for such children.

Immunodeficiency: Patients receiving immunosuppressive therapy or who have other immunodeficiencies may have a diminished antibody response to active immunization. Consider deferral of vaccine administration. Nonetheless, routine immunization of symptomatic and asymptomatic HIV-infected patients is recommended.

Elderly: DTaP is generally contraindicated after the seventh birthday.

Adults: DTaP is generally contraindicated after the seventh birthday. Tetanus and diphtheria toxoids for adult use (Td) bivalent or with acellular pertussis vaccine (Tdap) is the preferred immunizing agent for adults and older children.

Carcinogenicity: *Pediarix* has not been evaluated for carcinogenic potential.

Mutagenicity: *Pediarix* has not been evaluated for mutagenic potential.

Fertility Impairment: *Pediarix* has not been evaluated for the potential for impairment of fertility.

Pregnancy: Category C. DTaP is generally contraindicated after the seventh birthday. It is not known if *Pediarix* antigens or corresponding antibodies cross the placenta. Generally, most IgG passage across the placenta occurs during the third trimester. Problems in humans have not been documented and are unlikely.

Lactation: DTaP is generally contraindicated after the seventh birthday. It is not known if *Pediarix* antigens or corresponding antibodies cross into human breast milk. Problems in humans have not been documented and are unlikely.

Diphtheria & Tetanus Toxoids with Acellular Pertussis Adsorbed, Hepatitis B (Recombinant) & Inactivated Poliovirus Vaccine (DTaP-Hep B-IPV)

Children: Do not reduce or divide the DTaP dose for preterm infants or other children. Safety and efficacy of *Pediarix* in infants younger than 6 weeks of age have not been evaluated. *Pediarix* is not recommended for people after the seventh birthday. Use Td, Tdap, IPV, and hepatitis B vaccine for people after the seventh birthday. Children who have recovered from culture-confirmed pertussis do not need further doses of a pertussis-containing vaccine.

Adverse Reactions: *Pediarix* is associated with higher rates of fever, compared with separately administered vaccines. In 1 study that evaluated medically attended fever after the first dose of *Pediarix* or separately administered vaccines, infants who received *Pediarix* had a higher rate of medical encounters for fever within the first 4 days after vaccination.

A total of 20,739 doses of *Pediarix* have been administered to 7,028 infants as a 3-dose primary series. The most common adverse reactions observed in clinical trials were local injection-site reactions (eg, pain, redness, swelling), fever, and fussiness. In comparative studies, administration of *Pediarix* was associated with higher rates of fever relative to separately administered vaccines. The prevalence of fever was highest on day of vaccination and the following day. More than 98% of fever episodes resolved within the 4-day period after vaccination (ie, vaccination day and the next 3 days). Rates of most other solicited adverse events after *Pediarix* were comparable with rates observed after separately administered vaccines.

In a German study, data were collected for 4,666 infants who received *Pediarix* concomitantly at separate sites with 1 of 4 Hib vaccines and for 768 infants in the control group that received separate *Infanrix*, Hib, and OPV vaccines. Unlike the *Pediarix* group, infants in the separate-administration group did not receive hepatitis B vaccine. Data on adverse events were collected by parents using standardized diary cards for 4 consecutive days after each vaccine dose (ie, vaccination day and next 3 days). The primary end point was any Grade 3 solicited symptom (ie, redness or swelling more than 20 mm, fever higher than 103.1°F, or crying, pain, vomiting, diarrhea, loss of appetite, or restlessness that prevented normal daily activities) over the 3-dose primary series. Of 3,773 infants for whom safety data were available, 16.2% (95% CI, 14.9% to 17.5%) of 3,029 infants who received *Pediarix* and Hib vaccine compared with 20.3% (95% CI, 17.5% to 23.4%) of 744 infants who received separate vaccines were reported to have had at least one Grade 3 solicited symptom within 4 days of vaccination. The difference between groups in the rate of Grade 3 symptoms was 4.1% (90% CI, 1.4% to 7.1%).

In this study, infants also were monitored for unsolicited adverse events that occurred within 30 days after vaccination using diaries, supplemented by spontaneous reports and a medical history as reported by parents. Over the entire study period, 6 subjects in the group that received *Pediarix* reported seizures. Two of these subjects had a febrile seizure, 1 of whom also developed afebrile seizures. The remaining 4 subjects had afebrile seizures, including 2 with infantile spasms. Two subjects reported seizures within 7 days after vaccination (1 subject had febrile and afebrile seizures, and 1 subject had afebrile seizures), corresponding to a rate of 0.22 seizures per 1,000 doses (febrile seizures, 0.07 per 1,000 doses; afebrile seizures, 0.14 per 1,000 doses). No subject who received concomitant *Infanrix*, Hib, and OPV reported seizures. No cases of hypotonic-hyporesponsiveness, encephalopathy, or anaphylaxis were reported.

In a separate German study that evaluated the safety of *Infanrix* in 22,505 infants who received 66,867 doses of *Infanrix* administered as a 3-dose primary series, the rate of seizures within 7 days of vaccination with *Infanrix* was 0.13 per 1,000 doses (febrile seizures, 0 per 1,000 doses; afebrile seizures, 0.13 per 1,000 doses).

Postdose 1 safety data are available from a US study initiated in December 2001, designed to assess *Pediarix* administered concomitantly with Hib and pneumococcal conjugate vaccines, relative to separately administered *Infanrix*, *Engerix-B*, IPV, Hib, and 7-valent pneumococcal conjugate vaccines at 2, 4, and 6 months of age. The study was powered to evaluate fever higher than 101.3°F. Enrollment for this study is complete, with 673 infants in the group that received *Pediarix* and 335 infants in the separate vaccines group. Safety data after the second and third doses are expected in 2003. Data for fever within 4 days after dose 1 (ie, vaccination day and next 3 days) are presented in the following table.

Infants in a US Study with Fever within 4 Days of Dose 1[a] at 2 Months of Age with *Pediarix* Administered Concomitantly with Hib Vaccine and Pneumococcal Conjugate Vaccine or with Separate Coadministration of *Infanrix*, *Engerix-B*, IPV, Hib Vaccine, and Pneumococcal Conjugate Vaccine			
	Pediarix, Hib, and Pneumococcal Conjugate (N = 667)	*Infanrix*, *Engerix-B*, IPV, Hib, and Pneumococcal Conjugate (N = 333)	Separate Vaccine Group Minus Combination Vaccine Group
Fever[b]	%	%	Difference (95% CI)
≥ 100.4°F[c]	27.9	19.8	-8.07 (-13.54, -2.60)
> 101.3°F	7.0	4.5	-2.54 (-5.50, 0.41)
> 102.2°F[c]	2.2	0.3	-1.95 (-3.22, -0.68)
> 103.1°F	0.4	0.0	-0.45 (-0.96, 0.06)
M.A.[d]	1.2	0.0	-1.20 (-2.03, -0.37)

N Number of infants for whom at least 1 symptom sheet was completed, excluding 3 infants for whom temperature was not measured and 3 infants whose temperature was measured by the tympanic method.
a Within 4 days of dose 1 defined as day of vaccination and the next 3 days.
b Rectal temperatures.
c The group that received *Pediarix* compared with separate vaccine group, $P < 0.05$ (2-sided Fisher Exact test) or the 95% confidence interval on the difference between groups does not include 0.
d M.A. = medically attended (a visit to or from medical personnel).

In this study, medical attention for fever within 4 days after vaccination was sought for 8 infants who received *Pediarix* (1.2%) and no infants who received separately administered vaccines. Four infants were seen by medical personnel in an office setting; no diagnostic tests were performed in 2 infants and a complete blood count (CBC) was done in the other 2 infants. Of 3 infants who were seen in an emergency room, all had a CBC and a blood and urine culture performed; chest x-rays were done in 2 infants and a nasopharyngeal specimen was tested for RSV in 1 infant. One infant was hospitalized for a workup that included a CBC, blood and urine cultures, a lumbar puncture, and a chest x-ray. All episodes of medically attended fever resolved within 4 days postvaccination.

In 12 clinical trials, 5 deaths were reported in 7,028 (0.07%) recipients of *Pediarix* and 1 death was reported in 1764 (0.06%) recipients of comparator vaccines. Causes of death in the group that received *Pediarix* included 2 cases of sudden infant death syndrome (SIDS) and one case of each of the following: Convulsive disorder, congenital immunodeficiency with sepsis, and neuroblastoma. One case of SIDS was reported in the comparator group. The rate of SIDS among all recipients of *Pediarix* across the 12 trials was 0.3/1,000. The rate of SIDS observed for recipients of *Pediarix* in the German safety study was 0.2/1,000 infants (reported rate of SIDS in Germany in the latter part of the 1990s was 0.7/1,000 newborns). The reported rate of SIDS in the United States from 1990 to 1994 was 1.2/1,000 live births. By chance alone, some cases of SIDS can be expected to follow receipt of pertussis-containing vaccines.

Limited data are available on the safety of administering *Pediarix* after a birth dose of hepatitis B vaccine. In a study conducted in Moldova, 160 infants received a dose of hepatitis B vaccine within 48 hours of birth followed by 3 doses of *Pediarix* at 6, 10, and 14 weeks of age.

No information was collected on the HBsAg status of mothers of enrolled infants. Although there was no comparator group who received *Pediarix* without a birth dose of hepatitis B vaccine, available data suggest that some local adverse events may occur at a higher rate when *Pediarix* is administered after a birth dose of hepatitis B vaccine.

Rarely, an anaphylactic reaction (ie, hives, swelling of the mouth, difficulty breathing, hypotension, or shock) has been reported after receiving preparations containing diphtheria, tetanus, and/or pertussis antigens. Arthus-type hypersensitivity reactions, characterized by severe local reactions, may follow receipt of tetanus toxoid. A review by the Institute of Medicine (IOM) found evidence for a causal relationship between receipt of tetanus toxoid and both brachial neuritis and Guillain-Barré syndrome. A few cases of demyelinating diseases of the CNS have been reported after some tetanus toxoid-containing vaccines or tetanus and diphtheria toxoid-containing vaccines, although the IOM concluded that the evidence was inadequate to accept or reject a causal relationship. A few cases of peripheral mononeuropathy and of cranial mononeuropathy have been reported after tetanus toxoid administration, although the IOM concluded that the evidence was inadequate to accept or reject a causal relationship.

Worldwide voluntary reports of adverse events received for *Infanrix* and *Engerix-B* in children younger than 7 years of age since market introduction of these US-licensed vaccines are listed below. This list includes adverse events for which 20 or more reports were received, except for intussusception, idiopathic thrombocytopenic purpura, thrombocytopenia, anaphylactic reaction, angioedema, encephalopathy, hypotonic-hyporesponsive episode, and alopecia for which less than 20 reports were received. These latter events are included either because of the seriousness of the event or the strength of causal connection to components of this or other vaccines or drugs.

An expert panel assembled by the IOM concluded that no causal association exists between pertussis vaccination and autism, infantile spasms, hypsarrhythmia, Reye syndrome, SIDS, aseptic meningitis, chronic neurologic damage, erythema multiforme or other rash, Guillain-Barré syndrome, hemolytic anemia, juvenile diabetes, learning disabilities, attention deficit disorder, peripheral mononeuropathy, or thrombocytopenia.

The panel found evidence consistent with a causal association between DTwP and acute encephalopathy, shock and "unusual shock-like state," anaphylaxis, and protracted, inconsolable crying.

When a child returns for the next dose in a series of either pertussis or DTaP vaccinations, question the adult accompanying the child about possible side effects following the prior dose. If any of the effects that contraindicate additional pertussis vaccine doses occur, continue childhood immunization with bivalent DT toxoids, rather than DTaP.

In the following list, abbreviations were used to note the vaccines associated with adverse reactions: after *Infanrix* (a); after *Engerix-B* (b); after either *Infanrix* or *Engerix-B* (a+b).

Body as a whole: Asthenia (b), fever (a+b), lethargy (b), malaise (b), SIDS (a+b).

Cardiovascular: Cyanosis (a+b), edema (b), pallor (b).

CNS: Convulsions (a+b), encephalopathy (a), headache (b), hypotonia (a+b), hypotonic-hyporesponsive episode (a), somnolence (a+b).

Dermatologic: Alopecia (b), erythema (a+b), erythema multiforme (b), petechiae (b), pruritis (a+b), rash (a+b), urticaria (a+b).

GI: Abdominal pain (b), anorexia (b), diarrhea (a+b), intussusception (a+b), nausea (b), vomiting (a+b).

Hematologic/Lymphatic: Idiopathic thrombocytopenic purpura (a+b), lymphadenopathy (a), thrombocytopenia (a+b).

Diphtheria & Tetanus Toxoids with Acellular Pertussis Adsorbed, Hepatitis B (Recombinant) & Inactivated Poliovirus Vaccine (DTaP-Hep B-IPV)

Hepatic: Jaundice (b), liver function tests abnormal (b).

Hypersensitivity: Anaphylactic reaction (a+b), angioedema (b), hypersensitivity (a).

Immunologic: Cellulitis (a).

Local: Injection-site reactions (a+b).

Musculoskeletal: Arthralgia (b), limb swelling (a+b).

Psychiatric: Crying (a+b), irritability (a+b).

Respiratory: Respiratory tract infection (a).

Special Senses: Ear pain (a).

Pharmacologic & Dosing Characteristics

Dosage: Three 0.5 mL doses, at 6- to 8-week intervals (preferably 8 weeks).

The customary age for the first dose is 2 months of age, but it may be given starting at 6 weeks of age. Only monovalent hepatitis B vaccine can be used for the birth dose.

Infants born of HBsAg-positive mothers should receive HBIG and hepatitis B vaccine within 12 hours of birth at separate sites and complete the hepatitis B vaccination series. Infants born of mothers of unknown HBsAg status should receive hepatitis B vaccine within 12 hours of birth and complete the hepatitis B vaccination series.

Vaccinate preterm infants according to their chronological age from birth.

Children previously vaccinated with 1 or more doses of hepatitis B vaccine: Infants born of HBsAg-negative mothers and who received a dose of hepatitis B vaccine at or shortly after birth may be administered 3 doses of *Pediarix* according to the recommended schedule. There are no data to support the use of a 3-dose series of *Pediarix* in infants who have previously received more than one dose of hepatitis B vaccine. *Pediarix* may be used to complete a hepatitis B vaccination series in infants who received 1 or more doses of hepatitis B vaccine and who are also scheduled to receive the other vaccine components of *Pediarix*.

Children previously vaccinated with 1 or more doses of Infanrix: *Pediarix* may be used to complete the first 3 doses of the DTaP series in infants who have received 1 or 2 doses of *Infanrix* and are also scheduled to receive the other vaccine components of *Pediarix*.

Children previously vaccinated with 1 or more doses of IPV: *Pediarix* may be used to complete the first 3 doses of the IPV series in infants who have received 1 or 2 doses of IPV and are also scheduled to receive the other vaccine components of *Pediarix*.

Interchangeability of Pediarix and licensed DTaP, IPV, or hepatitis B vaccines: *Pediarix* can be given for all 3 doses because data are limited regarding the safety and efficacy of using acellular pertussis vaccines from different manufacturers for successive doses of the pertussis vaccination series. *Pediarix* is not recommended for completion of the first 3 doses of the DTaP vaccination series initiated with a DTaP vaccine from a different manufacturer because no data are available regarding the safety or efficacy of using such a regimen.

Pediarix may be used to complete a hepatitis B vaccination series initiated with a hepatitis B vaccine from a different manufacturer.

Pediarix may be used to complete the first 3 doses of the IPV vaccination series initiated with IPV from a different manufacturer.

If any recommended dose of pertussis vaccine cannot be given, give DT, hepatitis B, and inactivated poliovirus vaccines as needed to complete the series.

Route & Site: IM injection. Do not administer subcutaneously or IV. Preferred sites are anterolateral aspects of thigh or deltoid muscle of upper arm. Do not inject in gluteal area or areas where there may be a major nerve trunk. Gluteal injections may result in suboptimal hepatitis B immune response.

Diphtheria & Tetanus Toxoids with Acellular Pertussis Adsorbed, Hepatitis B (Recombinant) & Inactivated Poliovirus Vaccine (DTaP-Hep B-IPV)

Documentation Requirements: Federal law requires that the following information be documented in the recipient's permanent medical record or in a permanent office log: (1) The manufacturer and lot number of this vaccine, (2) the dates of its administration, and (3) the name, address, and title of the person administering the vaccine. Certain adverse events must be reported to VAERS ([800] 822-7967). Refer to Immunization Documents in the Resources section for complete information.

Overdosage: No specific data are available. Larger-than-recommended volume of vaccine may increase the risk of injection-site reactions, but are unlikely to have other consequences.

Booster Doses: Complete the diphtheria, tetanus, pertussis, hepatitis B, and poliovirus vaccination series with other vaccines, as necessary.

Missed Doses: Interrupting the recommended schedule or delaying subsequent doses does not require restarting the series. Use Td or Tdap, rather than DTaP, for doses after the seventh birthday. Interrupting the recommended schedule with a delay between doses should not interfere with the final immunity achieved with *Pediarix*, but waiting does delay achieving adequate protection from infection. There is no need to start the series over, regardless of time elapsed between doses.

Related Interventions: For children at higher risk for seizures than the general population, an appropriate antipyretic may be administered at time of vaccination with an acellular pertussis component and for the ensuing 24 hours to reduce the possibility of postvaccination fever.

Efficacy: *Pediarix* efficacy is based on immunogenicity of individual antigens compared with licensed vaccines. Efficacy of the pertussis component, which does not have a well-established correlate of protection, was determined in clinical trials of *Infanrix*. Efficacy of HBsAg was determined in clinical studies of *Engerix-B*. Serological correlates of protection exist for the diphtheria, tetanus, hepatitis B, and poliovirus components.

Efficacy of a 3-dose primary series of *Infanrix* has been assessed in 2 clinical studies, 1 in Italy and 1 in Germany. A double-blind, randomized, DT-controlled trial conducted in Italy, assessed *Infanrix* when administered at 2, 4, and 6 months of age. After 3 doses, the absolute protective efficacy of *Infanrix* against WHO-defined typical pertussis (21 days or more of paroxysmal cough with infection confirmed by culture and/or serologic testing) was 84% (95% CI, 76% to 89%). When the definition of pertussis was expanded to include clinically milder disease with respect to type and duration of cough, with infection confirmed by culture and/or serologic testing, the efficacy of *Infanrix* was 71% (95% CI, 60% to 78%) against longer than 7 days of any cough and 73% (95% CI, 63% to 80%) against 14 or more days of any cough. A second follow-up period to a mean age of 33 months was conducted in a partially unblinded cohort, showing that after 3 doses and with no booster dose in the second year of life, the efficacy of *Infanrix* against WHO-defined pertussis was 86% (95% CI, 79% to 91%) among children followed to 6 years of age.

A prospective efficacy trial was conducted in Germany, employing a household-contact study design. In preparation for this study, 3 doses of *Infanrix* were administered at 3, 4, and 5 months of age to more than 22,000 children living in 6 areas of Germany. Infants who did not participate in the safety and immunogenicity study could have received a whole-cell DTP vaccine or DT vaccine. Index cases were identified by spontaneous presentation to a physician. Households with at least 1 other member aged 6 through 47 months were enrolled. Household contacts of index cases were monitored for incidence of pertussis by a physician who was blinded to the vaccination status of the household. Calculation of vaccine efficacy was based on attack rates of pertussis in household contacts classified by vaccination status. Of the 173 household contacts who had not received a pertussis vaccine, 96 developed WHO-defined pertussis, as compared to 7 of 112 contacts vaccinated with *Infanrix*. The protective efficacy of *Infanrix* was 89% (95% CI, 77% to 95%), with no indication of waning of protection up until the time of the booster vaccination. When the definition of pertussis was expanded to include clinically milder disease with infection confirmed by culture and/or serologic testing, the efficacy of *Infanrix* against 7 or more days of any cough was 67% (95% CI, 52% to 78%) and against 7 or more days of paroxysmal cough was 81% (95% CI, 68% to 89%). The corresponding efficacy rates of *Infanrix* against 14 or more days of any cough or paroxysmal cough were 73% (95% CI, 59% to 82%) and 84% (95% CI, 71% to 91%), respectively.

Protective efficacy with *Engerix-B* was demonstrated in a clinical trial in neonates at high risk of hepatitis B infection. Fifty-eight neonates born of mothers who were both HBsAg-negative and HBsAg-positive were given *Engerix-B* (10 mcg at 0, 1, and 2 months) without concomitant HBIG. Two infants became chronic carriers in the 12-month follow-up period after initial inoculation. Assuming an expected carrier rate of 70%, the protective efficacy rate against the chronic carrier state during the first 12 months of life was 95%.

Pediarix formulation: In a US study, immune responses to each antigen in *Pediarix* 1 month after the third vaccination were compared to those after administration of US-licensed vaccines (*Infanrix*, *Engerix-B*, and OPV [*Orimune*, Lederle]). Both groups received *Haemophilus influenzae* type b (Hib) vaccine (Sanofi Pasteur) concomitantly. One month after the third dose of *Pediarix*, vaccine response rates for each of the pertussis antigens (except FHA), geometric mean antibody concentrations for each pertussis antigen, and seroprotection rates for diphtheria, tetanus, hepatitis B, and the polioviruses were noninferior to those achieved after separately administered vaccines. The vaccine response to FHA marginally exceeded the 10% limit for noninferiority.

Antibody Responses to Antigens in *Pediarix* Compared with *Infanrix*, *Engerix-B*, and OPV in US Infants Vaccinated at 2, 4, and 6 Months of Age			
		Pediarix (N = 86 to 91)	*Infanrix*, *Engerix-B*, OPV (N = 73 to 78)
Anti-Diphtheria	% ≥ 0.1 unit/mL[a]	98.9	100
Anti-Tetanus	% ≥ 0.1 unit/mL[a]	100	100
Anti-PT	% VR[a]	98.9	98.7
	GMC[b]	97.1	47.5
Anti-FHA	% VR	95.6	100
	GMC[b]	119.1	153.2
Anti-Pertactin	% VR[a]	95.6	91.0
	GMC[b]	150.4	108.6
Anti-HBsAg	% ≥ 10 milliunits/mL[a]	100	100
	GMC[b]	1,661.2	804.9
Anti-Polio 1	% ≥ 1:8[a,c]	100	98.6
Anti-Polio 2	% ≥ 1:8[a,c]	98.8	100
Anti-Polio 3	% ≥ 1:8[a,c]	100	100

VR Vaccine response: In initially seronegative infants, appearance of antibodies (concentration greater than or equal to 5 ELU/mL); in initially seropositive infants, at least maintenance of prevaccination concentration.

GMC: Geometric mean antibody concentration.

a Seroprotection rate or vaccine response rate to *Pediarix* not inferior to separately administered vaccines (upper limit of 90% CI on the difference for separate administration minus *Pediarix* less than 10%).

b GMC in the group that received *Pediarix* not inferior to separately administered vaccines (upper limit of 90% CI on the ratio of GMC for separate administration/*Pediarix* less than 1.5 for anti-PT, anti-FHA, and anti-pertactin, and less than 2 for anti-HBsAg).

c Poliovirus neutralizing antibody titer.

Onset: Escalating protection with each sequential dose.

Diphtheria & Tetanus Toxoids with Acellular Pertussis Adsorbed, Hepatitis B (Recombinant) & Inactivated Poliovirus Vaccine (DTaP-Hep B-IPV)

Duration: After adequate immunization against diphtheria and tetanus, protection persists for 10 or more years. After immunization against pertussis, protection persists for approximately 4 to 6 years. After immunization against hepatitis B and poliovirus, protection persists for many years.

Protective Level:

Diphtheria: Serum antitoxin level of 0.01 unit/mL is the lowest level giving some degree of protection. Antitoxin levels at least 0.1 unit/mL are regarded as protective.

Tetanus: A serum tetanus antitoxin level of 0.01 unit/mL is considered the minimum protective level. More recently, a level at least 0.1 to 0.2 unit/mL has been considered as protective.

Pertussis: Efficacy of the pertussis component does not have a well-established correlate of protection.

Hepatitis B: People who develop anti-HBs antibodies after active infection are usually protected against subsequent infection. Antibody concentrations at least 10 milliunits/mL against HBsAg are recognized as conferring protection against hepatitis B.

Poliovirus: Any detectable neutralizing antibody, in practice a titer greater than 1:4.

Mechanism: *Corynebacterium diphtheriae* may cause a localized or generalized disease. Diphtheria exotoxin, an extracellular protein metabolite of toxigenic strains of *C. diphtheriae*, causes systemic intoxication. Complete immunization induces protective antitoxin antibodies against diphtheria toxin and significantly reduces the risk of developing diphtheria. Immunized patients who develop disease have milder illnesses.

Tetanus toxoid induces specific protective antibodies against the exotoxin excreted by *Clostridium tetani*.

Pertussis vaccine exerts an adjuvant effect on the diphtheria and tetanus toxoids. The role of circulating pertussis antibodies is not clear at present.

Hepatitis B vaccine induces specific antibodies against the surface antigen of hepatitis B virus.

Poliovirus vaccine induces neutralizing antibodies, reducing pharyngeal excretion of poliovirus through a mucosal secretory-IgA response at that site. This helps block respiratory transmission. Some immunity in the mucosa of the GI tract develops, but it is inferior to that induced by OPV. If patients vaccinated with IPV swallow viable polioviruses, the viruses can be shed in their stools.

Drug Interactions: Do not mix *Pediarix* with any other vaccine or immune globulin in the same syringe or vial. When coadministration of other vaccines is required, give with separate syringes and at different injection sites.

Concomitant vaccine administration: In clinical trials, *Pediarix* was routinely administered concomitantly, at separate sites, with Hib vaccine. Safety data are available after the first dose of *Pediarix* administered concomitantly, at separate sites, with Hib and pneumococcal conjugate vaccines.

Immunosuppressive therapies, including irradiation, antimetabolites, alkylating agents, cytotoxic drugs, and corticosteroids (in greater than physiologic doses), may reduce the immune response to vaccines. Recipients may remain susceptible despite immunization. Although no specific *Pediarix* data are available, if immunosuppressive therapy will be discontinued shortly, defer immunization until off-therapy for 3 months; otherwise, vaccinate while still on therapy.

Inactivated vaccines are not generally affected by circulating antibodies or administration of exogenous antibodies. Vaccination may occur at any time before or after antibody administration.

Diphtheria & Tetanus Toxoids with Acellular Pertussis Adsorbed, Hepatitis B (Recombinant) & Inactivated Poliovirus Vaccine (DTaP-Hep B-IPV)

As with other IM injections, do not give *Pediarix* to children on anticoagulant therapy, unless the potential benefit clearly outweighs the risk of administration.

Pharmaceutical Characteristics

Concentration: Each 0.5 mL dose contains 25 Lf units of diphtheria toxoid, 10 Lf units of tetanus toxoid, 25 mcg of inactivated PT, 25 mcg of FHA, 8 mcg of pertactin, 10 mcg of HBsAg, 40 D-antigen Units (DU) of type 1 poliovirus, 8 DU of type 2 poliovirus, and 32 DU of type 3 poliovirus.

Quality Assay: Diphtheria and tetanus toxoid potency is determined by measuring neutralizing antitoxin in previously immunized guinea pigs. The potency of PT, FHA, and pertactin is determined by enzyme-linked immunosorbent assay (ELISA) on sera from previously immunized mice. Hepatitis B potency is established by HBsAg ELISA. Poliovirus potency is determined by D-antigen ELISA and by a poliovirus-neutralizing cell-culture assay on sera from previously immunized rats.

Packaging: Package of 10 single-dose vials (NDC #: 58160-0811-11), package of 5 single-dose prefilled *Tip-Lok* syringes without needles (58160-0811-46), package of 25 single-dose prefilled *Tip-Lok* syringes without needles (58160-0811-50).

Doseform: Suspension

Appearance: Turbid white suspension after shaking

Solvent: Saline

Adjuvant: Aluminum, not more than 0.85 mg aluminum per 0.5 mL by assay. The diphtheria, tetanus, and pertussis antigens are individually absorbed onto aluminum hydroxide; hepatitis B component is absorbed onto aluminum phosphate.

Preservative: None

Allergens: The vial stopper is latex-free. The tip cap and the rubber plunger of needleless, prefilled syringes contain dry natural latex rubber that may cause allergic reactions in latex-sensitive people.

Excipients: 4.5 mg of NaCl per 0.5 mL. Each dose also contains up to 100 mcg of residual formaldehyde and up to 100 mcg of polysorbate 80 (Tween 80). Neomycin sulfate and polymyxin B are used in poliovirus manufacturing and may be present at up to 0.05 ng neomycin and up to 0.01 ng polymyxin B per 0.5 mL dose. Procedures in HBsAg manufacture result in a product that contains up to 5% yeast protein.

pH: 5.8 to 6.8

Shelf Life: 24 months when stored between 2° to 8°C (36° to 46°F).

Storage/Stability: Store at 2° to 8°C (36° to 46°F). Discard frozen vaccine. *Pediarix* has been shown to be stable when held at temperatures between 68° and 77°F (20° to 25°C) for up to 24 hours. If accidently left at temperatures between 47° and 77°F, return the vaccine as soon as possible. Shipping data not provided.

Handling: Vaccine must be well shaken before administration. Do not use if resuspension does not occur with vigorous shaking.

Production Process: Diphtheria toxin is produced by growing *Corynebacterium diphtheriae* in Fenton medium containing a bovine extract. Tetanus toxin is produced by growing *Clostridium tetani* in modified Latham medium derived from bovine casein. Bovine materials used in these extracts are sourced from countries USDA determined neither have nor are at risk of bovine spongiform encephalopathy (BSE). Both toxins are detoxified with formaldehyde, concentrated by ultrafiltration, and purified by precipitation, dialysis, and sterile filtration.

Diphtheria & Tetanus Toxoids with Acellular Pertussis Adsorbed, Hepatitis B (Recombinant) & Inactivated Poliovirus Vaccine (DTaP-Hep B-IPV)

The 3 acellular pertussis antigens (PT, FHA, and pertactin) are isolated from *Bordetella pertussis* culture grown in modified Stainer-Scholte liquid medium. PT and FHA are isolated from fermentation broth; pertactin is extracted from cells by heat treatment and flocculation. The antigens are purified in successive chromatographic and precipitation steps. PT is detoxified using glutaraldehyde and formaldehyde. FHA and pertactin are treated with formaldehyde.

Hepatitis B surface antigen (HBsAg) is obtained by culturing genetically engineered *Saccharomyces cerevisiae* cells, which carry the surface antigen gene of hepatitis B virus, in synthetic medium. The surface antigen expressed in *S. cerevisiae* cells is purified by several physiochemical steps, including precipitation, ion-exchange chromatography, and ultrafiltration.

To yield enhanced-potency inactivated poliovirus components, each of the 3 strains of poliovirus is individually grown in Vero cells, a continuous line of monkey kidney cells cultivated on microcarriers. Calf serum and lactalbumin hydrolysate are used during Vero cell culture and/or virus culture. Calf serum is sourced from countries USDA determined neither have nor are at risk of BSE. After clarification, each viral suspension is purified by ultrafiltration, diafiltration, and successive chromatographic steps, and inactivated with formaldehyde. Each purified viral strain is then pooled to form a trivalent concentrate.

Diphtheria, tetanus, and pertussis antigens are individually adsorbed onto aluminum hydroxide. Hepatitis B component is adsorbed onto aluminum phosphate. All 5 antigens are then diluted and combined to produce the final formulated vaccine.

Disease Epidemiology

See monographs for individual vaccine components.

Other Information

Perspective: See monographs for individual vaccine components.

First Licensed: December 13, 2002

National Policy: See recommended childhood vaccination schedule, revised each January.

Diphtheria & Tetanus Toxoids Adsorbed, for Pediatric Use (DT)

Bacterial Vaccines & Toxoids

Name:
Generic

Manufacturer:
Sanofi Pasteur

Synonyms: DT
Comparison: Generically equivalent

> **Note:** Trivalent vaccines against diphtheria, tetanus, and pertussis are the preferred immunizing agent for most people. Tetanus and diphtheria toxoids for adult use (Td) bivalent or with acellular pertussis vaccine (Tdap) is the preferred immunizing agent for most adults and older children.
>
> Specific information about the individual components of this drug appear in the individual monographs on diphtheria toxoid and tetanus toxoid.

Immunologic Characteristics

Microorganism: Bacteria, *Corynebacterium diphtheriae* and *Clostridium tetani*
Viability: Inactivated
Antigenic Form: Toxoid mixture
Antigenic Type: Protein
Strains: Tetanus: S120-6; diphtheria: C58, C59

Use Characteristics

Indications: Selective induction of active immunity against both tetanus and diphtheria in infants and children from age 2 months up to the seventh birthday. All people should maintain tetanus immunity by means of booster doses throughout life because tetanus spores are ubiquitous. Trivalent DTP is the preferred immunizing agent for most children up to their seventh birthday. Use diphtheria and tetanus toxoids for pediatric use (DT) only for children for whom pertussis vaccination alone is contraindicated.

Refer to CDC's wound-management guidelines in the DTP Overview.

Limitations: Diphtheria toxoid immunization decreases, but does not eliminate, colonization of toxigenic strains of *Corynebacterium diphtheriae* in the pharynx, nose, or on the skin. Do not use diphtheria toxoid for the treatment of actual diphtheria infections. Select appropriate antibiotics (eg, erythromycin, penicillin) for treatment of active infections. Give diphtheria antitoxin if the patient is not likely to have adequate active immunity to diphtheria toxin.

Tetanus toxoid is not intended for the treatment or diagnosis of tetanus. For treatment of tetanus infection and for passive prophylaxis, consider use of tetanus immune globulin and appropriate antibiotics (eg, penicillin G, a tetracycline).

Outmoded Practices: Do not conduct a Schick or diphtheria-toxoid-sensitivity test of susceptibility prior to administration.

Contraindications:
Absolute: People after the seventh birthday; people with a history of serious allergic reaction to a vaccine component or after a prior dose of this vaccine.
Relative: An acute infection is reason for deferring administration of routine primary immunizing or recall booster doses but not emergency recall booster doses.

Immunodeficiency: Patients receiving immunosuppressive therapy or those with other immunodeficiencies may have diminished antibody response to active immunization. This is a reason for deferring primary diphtheria immunization until discontinuing treatment, or for injecting an additional dose at least 1 month after discontinuing treatment. Nonetheless, routine immunization of symptomatic and asymptomatic HIV-infected patients is recommended.

Elderly: Use of DT is contraindicated after the seventh birthday. Tetanus and diphtheria toxoids for adult use (Td) bivalent or with acellular pertussis vaccine (Tdap) is the preferred immunizing agent for most adults and older children.

Adults: Use of DT is contraindicated after the seventh birthday. Tetanus and diphtheria toxoids for adult use (Td) bivalent or with acellular pertussis vaccine (Tdap) is the preferred immunizing agent for most adults and older children.

Pregnancy: Use of DT is contraindicated after the seventh birthday.

Lactation: It is not known if DT antigens or corresponding antibodies are excreted in breast milk. Problems in humans have not been documented.

Children: DT is indicated for children older than 6 weeks and before the seventh birthday in whom pertussis vaccination is contraindicated. Trivalent DTaP is the preferred immunizing agent for most children up to their seventh birthday. Td bivalent or with acellular pertussis vaccine (Tdap) is the preferred immunizing agent for most adults and children after the seventh birthday.

Adverse Reactions: The most likely side effect of DT is redness, pain, or mild fever at the injection site (35% to 55%). A small amount of erythema, induration, pain, tenderness, heat, and edema surrounding the injection site and persisting for a few days is not unusual. Temperatures higher than 38°C (100°F) following DT administration are unusual. A nodule may be palpable at the injection site for a few weeks. Allow such nodules to recede spontaneously and do not incise. Sterile abscesses (incidence, 6 to 10 cases per million doses) and subcutaneous atrophy may also occur. Adverse reactions often associated with multiple prior booster doses may be manifested by erythema, boggy edema, pruritus, lymphadenopathy, and induration surrounding the point of injection, 2 to more than 12 hours after administration. Pain and tenderness, if present, are usually not the primary complaints.

Systemic manifestations: Transient low-grade fever, chills, malaise, generalized aches and pains, headache, flushing, generalized urticaria or pruritus, tachycardia, anaphylaxis, hypotension, neurologic complications. Although the cause is unknown, hypersensitivity to the toxin or bacillary protein of the tetanus organism itself is assumed to be possible. In other people, interaction between the injected antigen and high levels of preexisting tetanus antibody from prior booster doses seems to be the most likely cause of the Arthus-like response. Do not give these people even emergency doses of tetanus toxoid more frequently than every 10 years.

Pharmacologic & Dosing Characteristics

Dosage: Shake well before withdrawing each dose.

Primary immunizing series: For children beginning at 6 to 8 weeks of age, two 0.5 mL doses at an interval of 4 to 8 weeks followed by a third reinforcing 0.5 mL dose 6 to 12 months later. The third dose is an integral part of the primary series. Do not consider basic immunization complete until the third dose has been given.

When immunization with DT begins in the first year of life (rather than immunization with DTaP), the primary series consists of three 0.5 mL doses 4 to 8 weeks apart followed by a fourth reinforcing 0.5 mL dose 6 to 12 months after the third dose.

Immunization of infants normally starts at 6 weeks to 2 months of age; always start immunization at once if diphtheria is present in the community. Give unimmunized children 1 year of age or older in whom pertussis immunization is contraindicated two 0.5 mL DT doses 4 to 8 weeks apart, followed by a third 0.5 mL dose 6 to 12 months after the second dose, to complete the primary series.

Separate doses of DT by at least 4 weeks. Do not count doses within the minimum interval because too short an interval may interfere with antibody response and protection from disease. Typically, 6 months should elapse between the next-to-last and the last dose of a DT series. Increasing the interval beyond the recommended timing does not affect the ultimate efficacy of immunization, but waiting does delay achieving adequate protection from infection.

Refer to the CDC's wound-management guidelines in the DTP Overview.

Route & Site: IM. Give injections in the deltoid area of the upper arm or the midlateral muscle of the thigh (the vastus lateralis). Take care to avoid major peripheral nerve trunks. Do not inject the same muscle site more than once during the course of primary immunization. To avoid deposition of this product along the needle track, expel the antigen slowly and terminate the dose with a small bubble of air (0.1 to 0.2 mL) before withdrawing the needle. Do not inject ID or into superficial subcutaneous tissues.

Documentation Requirements: Federal law requires that the following information be documented in the recipient's permanent medical record or in a permanent office log: (1) The manufacturer and lot number of the vaccine, (2) the date of administration, and (3) the name, address, and title of the person administering the vaccine.

Certain adverse events must be reported to the VAERS system ([800] 822-7967). Refer to Immunization Documents in the Resources Section for complete information.

Overdosage: Although few data are available, clinical experience with similar products suggests that the major manifestations of overdosage would be pain and tenderness at the injection site.

Booster Doses: Give routine recall (booster) 0.5 mL doses of tetanus and diphtheria toxoids for adult use (Td) bivalent or with acellular pertussis vaccine (Tdap) at 10-year intervals throughout life to maintain immunity. Upon intimate exposure to diphtheria, an emergency recall booster dose of 0.5 mL (based on age) may be indicated. If emergency tetanus prophylaxis is indicated during the period between the third primary dose and the reinforcing dose, give a 0.5 mL dose of monovalent tetanus toxoid adsorbed. If given before 6 months have elapsed, count this dose as a primary dose. If given after 6 months, regard it as a reinforcing dose.

Missed Doses: Prolonging the interval between primary immunizing doses for 6 months or longer does not interfere with the final immunity. Count any dose of diphtheria and tetanus toxoids, even if received a decade earlier, as one of the immunizing injections.

Efficacy: Extremely high, more than 99% after a complete immunizing series and proper booster doses

Onset: After third dose

Duration: Approximately 10 years, if a complete primary immunizing series was given

Protective Level: Specific antitoxin levels more than 0.01 antitoxin units/mL for each antigen are generally regarded as protective. More recently, a level of 0.1 to 0.2 or more units/mL has been considered protective.

Mechanism: *Corynebacterium diphtheriae* may cause either a localized or a generalized disease. Diphtheria exotoxin, an extracellular protein metabolite of toxigenic strains of *diphtheriae*, causes systemic intoxication. Complete immunization induces protective antitoxin antibodies against diphtheria toxin and significantly reduces the risk of developing diphtheria. Immunized persons who develop disease have milder illnesses.

Tetanus toxoid induces specific protective antibodies against the exotoxin excreted by *Clostridium tetani*.

The aluminum salt, a mineral adjuvant, prolongs and enhances the antigenic properties of tetanus toxoid by retarding the rate of absorption.

Drug Interactions: Like all inactivated vaccines, administration of DT to people receiving immunosuppressant drugs (eg, high-dose corticosteroids) or radiation therapy may result in an insufficient response to immunization. They may remain susceptible despite immunization.

Several routine pediatric vaccines may safely and effectively be administered simultaneously at separate injection sites (eg, DTP or DT, MMR, e-IPV, Hib, hepatitis B, varicella). National authorities recommend simultaneous immunization at separate sites as indicated by age or health risk, if return of a vaccine recipient for a subsequent visit is doubtful. Delay diphtheria toxoid administration until 3 to 4 weeks after diphtheria antitoxin use to avoid the hypothetical possibility of antitoxin-toxoid interference.

Inactivated vaccines are not generally affected by circulating antibodies or administration of exogenous antibodies. Vaccination may occur at any time before or after antibody administration.

Concurrent administration of tetanus toxoid and tetanus immune globulin may delay development of active immunity by several days through partial antigen-antibody antagonism. This interaction is not clinically significant and does not preclude concurrent administration of both drugs if both are needed.

Systemic chloramphenicol therapy may impair anamnestic response to tetanus toxoid. Avoid concurrent use of these 2 drugs.

As with other drugs administered by IM injection, give DT with caution to people receiving anticoagulant therapy.

Pharmaceutical Characteristics

Concentration: 6.7 Lf units diphtheria toxoid and 5 Lf units tetanus toxoid/0.5 mL

Quality Assay: Each toxoid induces 2 units or more of each specific antitoxin/mL in guinea-pig potency tests.

USP requirement: No more than 0.02% residual formaldehyde

Packaging: Box of ten 0.5 mL single-dose vials (49281-0278-10)

Doseform: Suspension

Appearance: Turbid liquid, white, slightly gray- or cream-colored suspension

Solvent: Variously formulated with sodium chloride, with or without phosphate buffers

Adjuvant: Aluminum potassium sulfate, containing no more than 0.25 mg aluminum/0.5 mL

Preservative: Single-dose containers are formulated without preservative, but do contain a trace amount of thimerosal (no more than 0.3 mcg mercury per 0.5 mL dose).

Allergens: None

Excipients: No more than 0.02% residual free formaldehyde. Variously formulated with glycine, sodium phosphate, sodium acetate, hydrochloric acid, or sodium hydroxide.

pH: Data not provided

Shelf Life: Expires within 24 months

Storage/Stability: Store at 2° to 8°C (35° to 46°F). Discard frozen toxoids. Contact manufacturer regarding prolonged exposure to room temperature or elevated temperatures. Shipped in insulated containers with coolant packs.

Product can tolerate 4 days at 37°C (100°F) or lower.

Production Process: *Corynebacterium diphtheriae* and *Clostridium tetani* bacteria grow in separate media according to the method of Mueller and Miller (1947). Each toxoid is produced by detoxification of exotoxin with formaldehyde and refined by the Pillemer alcohol-fractionation method (1946).

Media: Modified Mueller and Miller medium and peptone-based medium containing bovine extract from a US source

Disease Epidemiology

Incidence:

Diphtheria: 206,000 cases of diphtheria with 10,000 deaths were reported in 1921, primarily among children (200 cases per 100,000 people, 5% to 10% case-fatality rate). Between 1980 and 1992, only 37 cases of diphtheria were reported in the United States, but the case-fatality rate remained constant at about 5% to 10%. Diphtheria is rare in modern times because of high levels in immunization and an apparent reduction in the circulation of toxigenic strains of the bacterium. Case-fatality rates are highest in very young persons and in the elderly.

Tetanus: Peak reported: 601 cases of tetanus in 1948 (0.39 cases/100,000 people). About 50 cases are reported each year in the United States (0.03 cases/100,000 people), primarily among older Americans; 68% of reported cases were at least 50 years old. Overall, the case-fatality rate was 21%. An estimated 770,000 neonatal tetanus deaths occur around the world each year.

Susceptible Pools:

Diphtheria: 49% to 66% of those 50 years of age and older.

Tetanus: 41% to 84% of Americans 60 years of age and older; especially men and women who have not served in the armed forces.

Transmission:

Diphtheria: Contact with a patient or carrier or articles soiled with their discharges. Raw milk may transmit infection.

Tetanus: Tetanus is an intoxication manifested primarily by neuromuscular dysfunction caused by a potent exotoxin elaborated by *Clostridium tetani*. Tetanus spores introduced into the body, usually through a puncture wound contaminated with soil, street dust, or animal or human feces; through lacerations, burns, and trivial or unnoticed wounds; by injection of contaminated illicit drugs. Tetanus occasionally follows surgery. Presence of necrotic tissue or foreign bodies favors growth of the anaerobic pathogen.

Incubation:

Diphtheria: 2 to 5 days, occasionally longer

Tetanus: 3 to 21 days (range: 1 day to several months), depending on character, extent, and location of the wound. In general, short incubation periods correspond with more heavily contaminated wounds, more severe disease, and a worse prognosis.

Communicability:

Diphtheria: Isolate until nose and throat clear, usually 2 weeks or less, seldom longer than 4 weeks. Effective antibiotic therapy promptly terminates shedding. Chronic carriers may rarely shed organisms for 6 months or longer.

Tetanus: Not directly transmitted from person to person

Other Information

Perspective:

1883: Loeffler & Klebs isolate and describe *Corynebacterium diphtheriae*.

1884: Nicolaier discovers *Clostridium tetani*.

1923: Ramon modifies diphtheria toxin with formaldehyde to produce "anatoxin," French for toxoid.

1923: Ramon & Zoeller at Pasteur Institute report use of tetanus toxoid to induce active immunity.

1926: Glenny, et al report that alum-precipitated toxoid enhances activity. Diphtheria toxoid licensed in the United States. Widespread childhood vaccination programs begin in the United States.

1937: Adsorbed form of tetanus toxoid licensed in the United States.

1947: Combination diphtheria and tetanus toxoids for pediatric use licensed in the United States.

1948: Adsorbed form of diphtheria toxoid licensed in the United States.

1950: Witte peptone eliminated from production medium, resulting in a lower adverse-reaction rate.

1953: Combination tetanus & diphtheria toxoids for adult use licensed in the United States, with reduced concentration of diphtheria toxoid to reduce injection-site reactions.

1963: Sclavo's diphtheria toxoid licensed on January 4, 1963.

NB: The Moloney test was formerly conducted with ID injection of fluid diphtheria toxoid on the forearm. The appearance in 12 to 24 hours of induration more than 12 mm in diameter was a positive reaction implying immunity.

First Licensed:

Massachusetts: May 1950
Michigan: May 1951
Lederle: January 3, 1954
Wyeth: May 1961
Connaught: January 1978 (now Sanofi Pasteur)
Sclavo: March 1978

National Policy: CDC. Diphtheria, tetanus, and pertussis: Recommendations for vaccine use and other preventive measures: Recommendations of the Immunization Practices Advisory Committee. *MMWR.* 1991;40(RR-10):1-28.

References: CDC. Tetanus surveillance, United States, 1998-2000. *MMWR.* 2003;52(SS-03):1-8.

Tetanus & Diphtheria Toxoids with Acellular Pertussis Vaccine Adsorbed (Tdap)

Bacterial Vaccines & Toxoids

Names:
Boostrix

Adacel
Synonyms: Tdap

Manufacturers:
GlaxoSmithKline (diphtheria and tetanus components manufactured by Novartis)
Sanofi Pasteur

Comparison: Prophylactically equivalent, but the two brands have different licensed age ranges and different pertussis antigens.

> **Note:** Trivalent vaccines against diphtheria, tetanus, and pertussis are the preferred immunizing agent for most people. Tetanus and diphtheria toxoids for adult use bivalent (Td) or with acellular pertussis vaccine (Tdap) is the preferred immunizing agent for most adults and older children.

Immunologic Characteristics

Antigen Source: Bacteria, *Clostridium tetani*, *Corynebacterium diphtheriae*, and *Bordetella pertussis*

Viability: Inactivated (subunit)

Antigenic Form: Toxoid mixture plus various acellular pertussis antigens

Antigenic Type: Protein

Strains:

GSK: Data not provided

Sanofi Pasteur: Tetanus: S120-6; diphtheria: C58, C59; pertussis: strain 10536

Use Characteristics

Indications: As a booster dose, to induce active immunity against tetanus, diphtheria, and pertussis. The ACIP recommends routine use of Tdap for adults 19 years and older, to replace the next booster dose of Td, including adults who have close contact with infants younger than 12 months of age. ACIP also recommended Tdap for health care workers (especially those with direct patient contact) as soon as feasible.

GSK: For booster immunization against tetanus, diphtheria, and pertussis in people 10 years of age or older.

Sanofi Pasteur: For booster immunization against tetanus, diphtheria, and pertussis in people 11 to 64 years of age.

Tetanus and diphtheria toxoids for adult use bivalent (Td) or with acellular pertussis vaccine (Tdap) is the preferred immunizing agent for most adults and older children. All people should maintain tetanus immunity by means of booster doses throughout life because tetanus spores are ubiquitous. Tetanus immunity is especially important for military personnel, farm and utility workers, those working with horses, firemen, and all people whose occupation or avocation renders them susceptible to even minor lacerations and abrasions. Advise travelers to developing nations to maintain active tetanus immunity to obviate any need for therapy with equine tetanus antitoxin and, thus, avoid associated complications.

Refer to CDC's wound-management guidelines in the DTP Overview.

Limitations: The use of Tdap as a primary immunizing series or to complete a primary series has not been studied.

Tetanus toxoid is not intended for the treatment or diagnosis of tetanus. To treat tetanus infection and for passive prophylaxis, consider use of tetanus immune globulin and appropriate antibiotics (eg, penicillin G, a tetracycline).

Diphtheria toxoid immunization decreases, but does not eliminate, colonization of toxigenic strains of *C. diphtheriae* in the pharynx or nose or on the skin. Do not use diphtheria toxoid to treat actual diphtheria infections. Select appropriate antibiotics (eg, an erythromycin, a penicillin) to treat active infections. Give diphtheria antitoxin if the patient is not likely to have adequate active immunity to diphtheria toxin.

Pertussis vaccine does not stimulate local secretory antibody production to prevent attachment of the microorganism to the respiratory epithelium. Pertussis vaccine is not intended for the treatment of that disease. Select appropriate antibiotics (eg, erythromycin) to treat active infections.

Outmoded Practices: Do not conduct a Schick or diphtheria-toxoid-sensitivity test for susceptibility before administration.

Contraindications:

Absolute: People with a history of serious allergic reaction to a vaccine component or after a prior dose of this vaccine. The following events are contraindications to administration of any pertussis-containing vaccine, including Tdap:

- Encephalopathy (eg, coma, decreased level of consciousness, prolonged seizures) within 7 days of administration of a previous dose of a pertussis-containing vaccine not attributable to another identifiable cause;
- Progressive neurologic disorder, uncontrolled epilepsy, or progressive encephalopathy. Do not administer pertussis vaccine to people with these conditions until a treatment regimen has been established and the condition has stabilized.

Relative: Consider the decision to give Tdap based on potential benefits and possible risks if any of the following events occurred in temporal relation to previous receipt of DTwP or a vaccine containing an acellular pertussis component: temperature 40.5°C (105°F) or higher within 48 hours not due to another identifiable cause; collapse or shock-like state (hypotonic-hyporesponsive episode) within 48 hours; persistent, inconsolable crying lasting 3 or more hours, occurring within 48 hours; seizures with or without fever occurring within 3 days.

People who experienced serious Arthus-type hypersensitivity reactions after a prior dose of tetanus toxoid usually have high serum tetanus antitoxin levels and should not be given Td or Tdap vaccines or even emergency doses of Td more frequently than every 10 years, even if the wound is neither clean nor minor.

If Guillain-Barré syndrome occurred within 6 weeks of receipt of vaccine containing tetanus toxoid, base the decision to give any vaccine containing tetanus toxoid on potential benefits and risks.

Make decisions to administer a pertussis-containing vaccine to people with stable central nervous system (CNS) disorders on an individual basis, assessing potential risks and benefits.

As with other IM injections, do not give Tdap to people with bleeding disorders such as hemophilia or thrombocytopenia, or to people on anticoagulant therapy unless the potential benefit outweighs the risk of administration. If the decision is made to administer Tdap in such cases, take steps to avoid the risk of hematoma after injection.

A family history of seizures or other CNS disorders is not a contraindication to pertussis vaccine.

An acute infection is reason for deferring administration of routine primary immunizing or routine recall doses, but not emergency recall doses.

If a decision is made to withhold pertussis vaccine, immunize with Td.

Immunodeficiency: People receiving immunosuppressive therapy or with other immunodeficiencies may have diminished antibody response to active immunization. This is a reason for deferring primary diphtheria immunization until treatment is discontinued or for injecting an additional dose 1 month or longer after treatment is discontinued. Nonetheless, routine immunization of symptomatic and asymptomatic HIV-infected people is recommended.

Elderly: No specific information is available about geriatric use of Tdap. The elderly develop lower to normal antitoxin levels after tetanus immunization compared with younger people. No specific information is available about geriatric use of diphtheria toxoid.

Adults: Tetanus and diphtheria toxoids for adult use bivalent (Td) or with acellular pertussis vaccine (Tdap) is the preferred immunizing agent for most adults and older children.

Carcinogenicity: Tdap has not been evaluated for carcinogenic potential.

Mutagenicity: Tdap has not been evaluated for mutagenic potential.

Fertility Impairment: Tdap has not been evaluated for impairment of fertility.

Pregnancy: Category C. Use if needed. It is not known if Tdap crosses the placenta. Generally, most IgG passage across the placenta occurs during the third trimester. Problems in humans have not been documented and are unlikely. Based on extensive human experience, there is no evidence that tetanus toxoid is teratogenic. For a previously unimmunized pregnant woman who may deliver her child under nonhygienic conditions, give 2 properly spaced doses of a product containing tetanus toxoid (eg, Td), preferably during the last 2 trimesters. Incompletely immunized pregnant women should complete the 3-dose series. Give those immunized more than 10 years previously a booster dose. Generally, most IgG passage across the placenta occurs during the third trimester.

GSK: In a developmental toxicity study, the effect of *Boostrix* on embryo-fetal and preweaning development was evaluated in pregnant rats. Animals were administered *Infanrix* before gestation and *Boostrix* during the period of organogenesis (gestation days 6, 8, 11) and later in pregnancy (gestation day 15), 0.1 mL/rat/occasion (a 45-fold increase compared with the human dose of *Boostrix* on a body weight basis). No adverse effect on pregnancy and lactation parameters, embryo-fetal or preweaning development was observed. There were no fetal malformations or other evidence of teratogenesis noted in this study. Health care providers are encouraged to register pregnant women who receive *Boostrix* in a pregnancy registry by calling (888)-825-5249.

Sanofi Pasteur: Animal reproduction studies have not been conducted with *Adacel*. In a developmental toxicity study, the effect of *Adacel* on embryo-fetal and preweaning development was evaluated in pregnant rabbits. Animals were administered *Adacel* twice before gestation, during the period of organogenesis (gestation day 6), and later in pregnancy (gestation day 29), 0.5 mL/rabbit/occasion IM (a 17-fold increased compared to the human dose of *Adacel* on a body weight basis). No adverse effect on pregnancy, parturition, or lactation parameters, or embryo-fetal or preweaning development was observed. There were no vaccine-related fetal malformations or other evidence of teratogenesis noted in this study. Health care providers are encouraged to register pregnant women who receive *Adacel* in a pregnancy registry by calling 800-822-2463.

Lactation: It is not known if Tdap crosses into human breast milk. Problems in humans have not been documented and are unlikely.

Children: Trivalent DTaP is the preferred immunizing agent for most children up to their seventh birthday. If pertussis vaccination is contraindicated, use diphtheria and tetanus toxoids for pediatric use (DT) until the child's seventh birthday. From 7 years of age through adulthood, tetanus and diphtheria toxoids for adult use bivalent (Td) or with acellular pertussis vaccine (Tdap, for those 10 years of age or older) is the preferred immunizing agent.

Adverse Reactions: Rarely, an anaphylactic reaction (ie, hives, swelling of the mouth, difficulty breathing, hypotension, or shock) has been reported after receiving preparations containing diphtheria, tetanus, and/or pertussis antigens. Death after vaccine-caused anaphylaxis has been reported. Arthus-type hypersensitivity reactions, characterized by severe local reactions, may follow receipt of tetanus toxoid. A review by the IOM found evidence for a causal relationship between receipt of tetanus toxoid and both brachial neuritis and Guillain Barré syndrome. A few cases of demyelinating diseases have been reported after some tetanus toxoid-containing vaccines or tetanus and diphtheria toxoid-containing vaccines, although the IOM concluded that the evidence was inadequate to accept or reject a causal relationship. A few cases of peripheral mononeuropathy and of cranial mononeuropathy have been reported after tetanus toxoid administration, although the IOM concluded that the evidence was inadequate to accept or reject a causal relationship.

GSK: The primary safety study, conducted in the United States, was a randomized, observer-blinded, controlled study in which 3,080 adolescents 10 to 18 years of age received a single dose of *Boostrix* and 1,034 received Td. Approximately 98% of participants had received 4 or 5 doses of either DTwP or a combination of DTwP and DTaP in childhood. No serious adverse events were reported within 31 days of vaccination. During the 6-month extended safety evaluation period, no serious adverse events that were of potential autoimmune origin or new onset and chronic in nature were reported. The most common local adverse events within 15 days after administration of *Boostrix* were pain (74%), redness (23%), and swelling at the injection site (21%). The most common general adverse events were headache (43%), fatigue (37%), fever (higher than 38°C: 5%), and GI symptoms (any: 26%). Most of these events were reported at a similar frequency in recipients of either *Boostrix* or Td. Any pain (74%), grade 2 or 3 pain (51%) [but not grade 3 alone], and grade 2 or 3 headache (16%) [but not grade 3 alone] were reported at a higher rate in *Boostrix* recipients. The primary safety end point of the US study was the incidence of grade 3 pain (spontaneously painful and/or prevented normal activity) at the injection site within 15 days of vaccination. Grade 3 pain was reported in 4.6% of those who received *Boostrix*, compared with 4% of those who received Td. The difference in rate of grade 3 pain was within the predefined clinical limit for noninferiority. Mid-upper arm circumference was measured before and daily for 15 days after vaccination. There was no significant difference between *Boostrix* recipients and Td recipients in the proportion of subjects reporting an increase in mid-upper arm circumference in the vaccinated arm.

Sanofi Pasteur: The primary safety studies were randomized, blinded, controlled studies which contrasted adolescents 11 to 17 years of age or adults 18 to 64 years of age receiving a single dose of *Adacel* with people of similar age receiving Td. The most common local adverse events within 15 days after administration of *Adacel* were pain (66% to 78%), redness (21% to 25%), and swelling at the injection site (21%). The most common general adverse events were headache (34% to 44%), fatigue (24% to 30%), body ache (22% to 30%), and fever (higher than 38°C: 1% to 5%). Most of these events were reported at a similar frequency in recipients of either *Adacel* or Td. Any pain (78%) among adolescents was reported at a higher rate in *Adacel* recipients. The primary safety end points were within the predefined clinical limit for noninferiority. Generally, the rates of adverse events occurred more frequently among women than men, an effect more pronounced in adults than adolescents. No associations between diphtheria, tetanus, or pertussis antitoxin levels and severe injection-site reactions were evident. There was no apparent relationship between limb-circumference swelling (3 cm or more) and size of injection-site swelling.

Pharmacologic & Dosing Characteristics

Dosage: Shake vial well before withdrawing each dose. Limited data are available on the use of Tdap after administration of Td, but the safety of an interval as short as 2 years is supported by a Canadian study of children and adolescents. The principal risk of short-interval dosing is injection-site swelling.

Refer to CDC's wound-management guidelines in the DTP Overview.

GSK: A single 0.5 mL injection in people 10 years and older.

Sanofi Pasteur: A single 0.5 mL injection in people 11 to 64 years of age.

Route & Site: IM, typically into the deltoid muscle.

Documentation Requirements: Federal law requires that the following information be documented in the recipient's permanent medical record or in a permanent office log: (1) the manufacturer and lot number of the vaccine, (2) the date of administration, and (3) the name, address, and title of the person administering the vaccine.

Certain adverse events must be reported to the VAERS system (800)-822-7967. Refer to Immunization Documents in the Resources section.

Overdosage: Although few data are available, clinical experience with similar products suggests that the major manifestations of overdosage would be pain and tenderness at the injection site.

Booster Doses: At present, there are no data to support repeat administration of Tdap.

Missed Doses: Interrupting the recommended schedule or delaying subsequent doses does not require restarting the series.

Efficacy: Efficacy of the tetanus and diphtheria toxoid components of Tdap is based on the immunogenicity of these antigens, compared to Td, using established serologic correlates of protection. Efficacy of the pertussis components of Tdap is based on comparison of the immune response of adolescents after a single dose of Tdap to the immune response of infants after a primary series of DTaP. In addition, the ability of Tdap to induce a booster response to each of the antigens was evaluated. One month after a single dose, the seroprotection rate (0.1 units/mL or more) or booster response rate to Tdap (either *Boostrix* or *Adacel*) was non-inferior to Td (upper limit of two-sided 95% CI on the difference for Td minus Tdap 10% or less). Starting from a baseline rate of approximately 30% to 40%, the proportion of people with tetanus antitoxin concentrations 1 units/mL or more rose to 63% to 99% after a single dose of Tdap. With a booster response to pertussis antigens defined as 4-fold or more increase in the prevaccination antibody concentration, 78% to 99% of vaccinees responded to Tdap.

GSK: The geometric mean concentrations (GMCs) to each of the three pertussis antigens 1 month after a single dose of *Boostrix* in the US adolescent study were compared to the GMCs of infants after a 3-dose primary series of *Infanrix* administered at 3, 4, and 5 months of age. GMCs to the various pertussis antigens were 1.9 to 7.4 times higher in *Boostrix*-vaccinated adolescents, compared with *Infanrix*-vaccinated infants.

Sanofi Pasteur: The geometric mean concentrations (GMCs) to each of the 5 pertussis antigens 1 month after a single dose of *Adacel* in both adolescents and adults were consistently higher than among infants given a 3-dose primary series of *Daptacel* administered at 3, 4, and 5 months of age. GMCs to the various pertussis antigens were 1.9 to 5.4 times higher in *Adacel*-vaccinated adolescents and adults, compared with *Daptacel*-vaccinated infants.

Onset: Within a few weeks, when given as a booster dose in people who previously received a primary immunizing series.

Duration: Protection against tetanus and diphtheria persists for at least 10 years, when given as a booster dose in people who previously received a primary immunizing series. The duration of protection against pertussis is uncertain.

Protective Level: A serum tetanus antitoxin level of 0.01 unit/mL or more, measured by neutralization assays, is considered the minimum protective level. A level 0.1 to 0.2 unit/mL or more has been considered protective. A serum diphtheria antitoxin level of 0.01 unit/mL is the lowest level giving some degree of protection; a level of 0.1 unit/mL is regarded as protective. Levels 1 unit/mL or more are associated with long-term protection. A serologic correlate of protection for pertussis has not been established.

Mechanism: *C. diphtheriae* may cause either a localized or a generalized disease. Diphtheria exotoxin, an extracellular protein metabolite of toxigenic strains of *C. diphtheriae*, causes systemic intoxication. Complete immunization induces antitoxin antibodies against diphtheria toxin and significantly reduces the risk of developing diphtheria. Immunized people who develop disease have milder illnesses. Immunization with diphtheria toxoid does not, however, eliminate carriage of *C. diphtheriae* in the pharynx or nares or on the skin. Tetanus toxoid induces specific protective antibodies against the exotoxin excreted by *C. tetani*. The role of the different components produced by *B. pertussis* in either the pathogenesis of, or the immunity to, pertussis is not well understood, but the pertussis components in Tdap have been shown to prevent pertussis in clinical trials of DTaP vaccines.

The aluminum salt, a mineral adjuvant, prolongs and enhances antigenic properties of tetanus toxoid by retarding the rate of absorption.

Drug Interactions: Like all inactivated (subunit) vaccines, administration of Tdap to people receiving immune-suppressing drugs, including high-dose corticosteroids (in greater than physiologic doses), or radiation therapy may result in an insufficient response to immunization. They may remain susceptible despite immunization.

Several routine vaccines may safely and effectively be administered simultaneously at separate injection sites (eg, meningococcal, influenza, hepatitis B). Minor interferences with tetanus antitoxin levels and responses to pertactin were noted when *Adacel* and influenza vaccine were coadministered, but these effects are not expected to affect protective efficacy. National authorities recommend simultaneous immunization at separate sites as indicated by age or health-risk, if return of a vaccine recipient for a subsequent visit is doubtful.

As with other IM injections, do not give Tdap to people on anticoagulant therapy, unless the potential benefit outweighs the risk of administration. If the decision is made to administer Tdap in such cases, take steps to avoid the risk of hematoma after injection.

Delay diphtheria toxoid administration until 3 to 4 weeks after diphtheria antitoxin use, to avoid the hypothetical possibility of antitoxin-toxoid interference.

Concurrent administration of tetanus toxoid and tetanus immune globulin may delay development of active immunity by several days through partial antigen-antibody antagonism; however, this interaction is not clinically significant and does not preclude concurrent administration of both drugs if both are needed.

Otherwise, subunit vaccines are not generally affected by circulating antibodies or administration of other exogenous antibodies. Vaccination may occur at any time before or after antibody administration.

Systemic chloramphenicol therapy may impair anamnestic response to tetanus toxoid. Avoid concurrent use of these drugs.

Pharmaceutical Characteristics

Concentration:

GSK: Each 0.5 mL dose contains 5 Lf units tetanus toxoid, 2.5 Lf units diphtheria toxoid, 2.5 mcg pertactin (69 kilodalton outer membrane protein), 8 mcg filamentous hemagglutinin (FHA), and 8 mcg inactivated pertussis toxin (PT).

Sanofi Pasteur: Each 0.5 mL dose contains 5 Lf units tetanus toxoid, 2 Lf units diphtheria toxoid, 3 mcg pertactin (69 kilodalton outer membrane protein), 5 mcg FHA, 2.5 mcg inactivated PT, and 2.5 mcg each of fimbriae types 2 and 3.

Tetanus & Diphtheria Toxoids with Acellular Pertussis Vaccine Adsorbed (Tdap)

Quality Assay: Tetanus and diphtheria toxoid potency is determined by measuring the amount of neutralizing antitoxin in immunized guinea pigs. The potency of the acellular pertussis components is determined by enzyme-linked immunosorbent assay (ELISA) on sera from previously immunized mice.

Packaging:

GSK: Ten single-dose 0.5 mL vials (NDC #: 58160-0842-11). One single-dose 0.5 mL prefilled *Tip-Lok* syringes without needles (58160-0842-32), five syringes (58160-0842-46).

Sanofi Pasteur: Ten single-dose 0.5 mL vials (49281-0400-10). Five single-dose 0.5 mL prefilled syringes without needles (49281-0400-15).

Doseform: Suspension

Appearance: After shaking, a homogeneous, turbid, white suspension.

Solvent:

GSK: Isotonic sodium chloride

Sanofi Pasteur: Sterile water for injection

Adjuvant:

GSK: Aluminum hydroxide (0.39 mg/0.5 mL or less aluminum by assay)

Sanofi Pasteur: 1.5 mg aluminum phosphate (0.33 mg/0.5 mL aluminum by assay)

Preservative: None

Allergens:

GSK: The tip cap and rubber plunger of the needleless prefilled syringes contain dry natural latex rubber. The vial stopper is latex-free.

Sanofi Pasteur: The vial stopper is latex-free.

Excipients:

GSK: 4.5 mg NaCl, up to 100 mcg formaldehyde, and up to 100 mcg of polysorbate 80 (Tween 80) per 0.5 mL.

Sanofi Pasteur: Residual formaldehyde up to 5 mcg/0.5 mL and up to 5 ng/0.5 mL glutaraldehyde, and 3.3 mg (0.6% v/v) 2-phenoxyethanol (not as a preservative).

pH: Data not provided.

Shelf Life: Expires within 36 months.

Storage/Stability: Store at 2° to 8°C (36° to 46°F). Discard if frozen. Contact the manufacturer regarding exposure to freezing or elevated temperatures. Shipping data not provided.

Handling: Do not mix Tdap with any other product in the same syringe or vial.

GSK: The recommended needle size for administration of *Boostrix* is a 22- to 25-gauge needle, 1 to 1¼ inches in length.

Production Process:

GSK: Diphtheria and tetanus toxins are detoxified with formaldehyde, concentrated by ultrafiltration, and purified by precipitation, dialysis, and sterile filtration. The three acellular pertussis antigens are the same as those contained in *Infanrix* brand of DTaP. PT and FHA are isolated from the fermentation broth; pertactin is extracted from the cells by heat treatment and flocculation. The antigens are purified in successive chromatographic and precipitation steps. PT is detoxified using glutaraldehyde and formaldehyde. FHA and pertactin are treated with formaldehyde. Each antigen is individually adsorbed onto aluminum hydroxide. All antigens are then diluted and combined to produce the final formulated vaccine.

Sanofi Pasteur: Diphtheria and tetanus toxins are detoxified with formaldehyde, concentrated, and purified by ammonium sulfate fractionation. Tetanus toxoid is also diafiltered. The five acellular pertussis antigens are the same as those contained in *Daptacel* brand of DTaP. The fimbriae types 2 and 3 are extracted from the bacterial cells and the pertussis toxin, FHA, and pertactin are prepared from the supernatant. These proteins are

Tetanus & Diphtheria Toxoids with Acellular Pertussis Vaccine Adsorbed (Tdap)

purified by sequential filtration, salt-precipitation, ultrafiltration, and chromatography. Pertussis toxin is inactivated with glutaraldehyde, FHA is treated with formaldehyde, and residual aldehydes are removed by ultrafiltration. The individual antigens are adsorbed separately onto aluminum phosphate.

Media:

GSK: Tetanus toxin is produced by growing *C. tetani* in a modified Latham medium derived from bovine casein. The diphtheria toxin is produced by growing *C. diphtheriae* in Fenton medium containing a bovine extract. The bovine materials used in these extracts are sourced from countries that the USDA determined neither have nor are at risk of bovine spongiform encephalopathy (BSE). The pertussis antigens (PT, FHA, and pertactin) are isolated from *B. pertussis* culture grown in modified Stainer-Scholte liquid medium.

Sanofi Pasteur: Tetanus toxin is produced by growing *C. tetani* in modified Mueller-Miller casamino-acid medium without beef heart infusion. Diphtheria toxin is produced by growing *C. diphtheriae* in modified Mueller's growth medium. After purification, *B. pertussis* cultures are grown in Stainer-Scholte medium modified by the addition of casamino acids and dimethyl-beta-cyclodextrin.

Disease Epidemiology

Incidence: The reported incidence of pertussis in the United States has been rising since 1990, with a marked increase since 2002. The increase in cases has principally been reported among teenagers and adults. Pertussis in adolescents and adults can involve prolonged coughing, vomiting, missed school or work, and various complications. Infected adolescents and adults can transmit pertussis bacteria to unimmunized or partially immunized infants and young children, who are more vulnerable to serious pertussis-related complications or death.

See also Td and DTaP monographs.

Other Information

Perspective: See Td and DTaP monographs.

First Licensed:
GSK: May 3, 2005
Sanofi Pasteur: June 10, 2005

National Policy: Committee on Obstetric Practice. ACOG Committee Opinion No. 521: Update on immunization and pregnancy: tetanus, diphtheria, and pertussis vaccination. *Obstet Gynecol.* 2012;119(3):690-691.

ACIP. Updated recommendations for use of tetanus toxoid, reduced diphtheria toxoid and acellular pertussis (Tdap) vaccine from the Advisory Committee on Immunization Practices, 2010. *MMWR.* 2011;60(1):13-15. http://www.cdc.gov/mmwr/PDF/wk/mm6001.pdf.

ACIP. Updated recommendations for use of tetanus toxoid, reduced diphtheria toxoid and acellular pertussis vaccine (Tdap) in pregnant women and persons who have or anticipate having close contact with an infant aged < 12 months—Advisory Committee on Immunization Practices (ACIP), 2011. *MMWR.* 2011;60(41):1424-1426. http://www.cdc.gov/mmwr/pdf/wk/mm6041.pdf.

ACIP. Prevention of pertussis, tetanus, and diphtheria among pregnant and postpartum women and their infants. *MMWR.* 2008;57(RR-4):1-51, erratum 723. http://www.cdc.gov/mmwr/PDF/rr/rr5704.pdf.

ACIP. Preventing tetanus, diphtheria, and pertussis among adolescents: use of tetanus toxoid, reduced diphtheria toxoid, and acellular pertussis vaccines. *MMWR.* 2006;55(RR-3):1-17. http://www.cdc.gov/mmwr/PDF/rr/rr5503.pdf.

ACIP. Preventing tetanus, diphtheria, and pertussis among adults: use of tetanus toxoid, reduced diphtheria toxoid, and acellular pertussis vaccines. *MMWR.* 2006;55(RR-17):1-37. http://www.cdc.gov/mmwr/PDF/rr/rr5517.pdf.

Tetanus & Diphtheria Toxoids with Acellular Pertussis Vaccine Adsorbed (Tdap)

References: WHO. Diphtheria vaccine. *Weekly Epidemiol Rec*. 2006;81:24-32. http://www.who.int/wer/2006/wer8103.pdf.

WHO. Tetanus vaccine. *Weekly Epidemiol Rec*. 2006;81:198-208. http://www.who.int/wer/2006/wer8120.pdf.

WHO. Pertussis vaccines: WHO position paper — Recommendations. *Vaccine*. 2011;29(13):2355-2356.

Tetanus & Diphtheria Toxoids Adsorbed, for Adult Use (Td)

Bacterial Vaccines & Toxoids

Names:
Decavac
Generic

Manufacturers:
Sanofi Pasteur
Massachusetts Biological Laboratories, distributed by Merck

Synonyms: Td, *Tenivac* (Sanofi Pasteur)
Comparison: Generically equivalent

> **Note:** Trivalent vaccines against diphtheria, tetanus, and pertussis are the preferred immunizing agent for most people. Tetanus and diphtheria toxoids for adult use (Td) bivalent or with acellular pertussis vaccine (Tdap) is the preferred immunizing agent for most adults and older children.
>
> Specific information about the individual components of this drug appear in the individual monographs on diphtheria toxoid and tetanus toxoid.

Immunologic Characteristics

Microorganism: Bacteria, *Clostridium tetani* and *Corynebacterium diphtheriae*
Viability: Inactivated
Antigenic Form: Toxoid mixture
Antigenic Type: Protein
Strains:

Massachusetts: Data not provided
Sanofi Pasteur: Tetanus: S120-6; diphtheria: C58, C59

Use Characteristics

Indications: Induction of active immunity against tetanus and diphtheria. Tetanus and diphtheria toxoids for adult use (Td) bivalent or with acellular pertussis vaccine (Tdap) is the preferred immunizing agent for most adults and children after their seventh birthday. All people should maintain tetanus immunity by means of booster doses throughout life because tetanus spores are ubiquitous. Tetanus immunity is especially important for military personnel, farm and utility workers, those working with horses, firemen, and all individuals whose occupation or vocation renders them susceptible to even minor lacerations and abrasions. Advise travelers to developing nations to maintain active tetanus immunity to obviate any need for therapy with equine tetanus antitoxin and thus avoid associated complications.

Refer to CDC's wound-management guidelines in the DTP Overview.

Limitations: Tetanus toxoid is not intended for the treatment or diagnosis of tetanus. For treatment of tetanus infection and for passive prophylaxis, consider use of tetanus immune globulin and appropriate antibiotics (eg, penicillin G, a tetracycline).

Diphtheria toxoid immunization decreases, but does not eliminate, colonization of toxigenic strains of *Corynebacterium diphtheriae* in the pharynx, nose, or on the skin. Do not use diphtheria toxoid for the treatment of actual diphtheria infections. Select appropriate antibiotics (eg, erythromycin, penicillin) to treat active infections. Give diphtheria antitoxin if the patient is not likely to have adequate active immunity to diphtheria toxin.

Outmoded Practices: Do not conduct a Schick or diphtheria-toxoid-sensitivity test for susceptibility prior to administration.

Contraindications:

Absolute: Patients with a history of serious allergic reaction to a vaccine component or after a prior dose of this vaccine.

Relative: An acute infection is reason for deferring administration of routine primary immunizing or routine recall doses but not emergency recall doses.

Immunodeficiency: Patients receiving immunosuppressive therapy or those with other immunodeficiencies may have diminished antibody response to active immunization. This is reason for deferring primary diphtheria immunization until treatment is discontinued or for injecting an additional dose at least 1 month after treatment is discontinued. Nonetheless, routine immunization of symptomatic and asymptomatic HIV-infected patients is recommended.

Elderly: Following tetanus immunization, the elderly may develop lower antitoxin levels than younger patients. No specific information is available about geriatric use of diphtheria toxoid.

Adults: Tetanus and diphtheria toxoids for adult use (Td) bivalent or with acellular pertussis vaccine (Tdap) is the preferred immunizing agent for most adults and older children.

Pregnancy: Category C. Use only if clearly needed. Based on extensive human experience, there is no evidence that tetanus or diphtheria toxoid is teratogenic. Give a previously unimmunized pregnant woman who may deliver her child under nonhygienic conditions 2 properly spaced doses of a product containing tetanus toxoid (eg, Td, Tdap), preferably during the last 2 trimesters. Incompletely immunized pregnant women should complete the 3-dose series. Give a booster dose to those immunized more than 10 years previously. Generally, most IgG passage across the placenta occurs during the third trimester.

Lactation: It is not known if Td antigens or corresponding antibodies are excreted in breast milk. Problems in humans have not been documented and are unlikely.

Children: Trivalent DTaP is the preferred immunizing agent for most children up to their seventh birthday. If pertussis vaccination is contraindicated, use diphtheria and tetanus toxoids for pediatric use (DT) until the child's seventh birthday. From 7 years of age through adulthood, tetanus and diphtheria toxoids for adult use (Td) bivalent or with acellular pertussis vaccine (Tdap) is the preferred immunizing agent.

Adverse Reactions: The most likely side effect of Td is redness or pain at the injection site (approximately 40% to 50%). A small amount of erythema, induration, pain, tenderness, heat, and edema surrounding the injection site and persisting for a few days is not unusual. Temperatures higher than 38°C (100°F) following Td administration are unusual. A nodule may be palpable at the injection site for a few weeks. Allow such nodules to recede spontaneously and do not incise. Sterile abscesses (incidence, 6 to 10 cases per million doses) and subcutaneous atrophy may also occur. Adverse reactions often associated with multiple prior booster doses may be manifested 2 to more than 12 hours after administration by erythema, boggy edema, pruritus, lymphadenopathy, and induration surrounding the point of injection. Pain and tenderness, if present, are usually not the primary complaints.

Systemic manifestations: Transient low-grade fever, chills, malaise, generalized aches and pains, headaches, flushing, generalized urticaria or pruritus, tachycardia, anaphylaxis, hypotension, neurological complications. Although the cause is unknown, hypersensitivity to the toxin or bacillary protein of the tetanus organism itself is assumed to be possible. In other people, interaction between the injected antigen and high levels of preexisting tetanus antibody from prior booster doses seems to be the most likely cause of the Arthus-like response. Do not give these people even emergency doses of tetanus toxoid more frequently than every 10 years.

Tetanus & Diphtheria Toxoids Adsorbed, for Adult Use (Td)

Pharmacologic & Dosing Characteristics

Dosage: Shake vial gently before withdrawing each dose. Assuming 5 initial DTP doses earlier in life, the standard schedule is to give the first dose of Td or Tdap at 11 to 12 years of age if 5 years have elapsed since last vaccination. Additional doses are then given at 10-year intervals.

Primary immunizing series: For adults and children after their seventh birthday, two 0.5 mL doses, at an interval of 4 to 8 weeks, followed by a third reinforcing 0.5 mL dose 6 to 12 months later. The third dose is an integral part of the primary series. Do not consider immunization complete until the third dose has been given. Start immunization at once if diphtheria is present in the community.

Separate doses of Td by at least 4 weeks. Do not count doses within the minimum interval because too short an interval may interfere with antibody response and protection from disease. Typically, 6 months should elapse between the next-to-last and the last dose of a Td series. Increasing the interval beyond the recommended timing does not affect the ultimate efficacy of immunization, but waiting does delay achieving adequate protection from infection.

Refer to the CDC's wound-management guidelines in the DTP Overview.

Route & Site: IM. Give IM injections in the deltoid area of the upper arm or the midlateral muscle of the thigh (the vastus lateralis). Take care to avoid major peripheral nerve trunks. Do not inject the same muscle site more than once during the course of primary immunization. To avoid deposition of this product along the needle track, expel the antigen slowly and terminate the dose with a small bubble of air (0.1 to 0.2 mL) before withdrawing the needle. Do not inject ID or into superficial subcutaneous tissues.

Documentation Requirements: Federal law requires that the following information be documented in the recipient's permanent medical record or in a permanent office log: (1) The manufacturer and lot number of the vaccine, (2) the date of administration, and (3) the name, address, and title of the person administering the vaccine.

Certain adverse events must be reported to the VAERS system ([800] 822-7967). Refer to Immunization Documents in the Resources section.

Overdosage: Although few data are available, clinical experience with similar products suggests that the major manifestations of overdosage would be pain and tenderness at the injection site.

Booster Doses: Give routine 0.5 mL recall (booster) doses at 10-year intervals throughout life to maintain immunity.

In the event of injury for which tetanus prophylaxis is indicated, refer to the CDC's wound-management guidelines in the DTP Overview. If emergency tetanus prophylaxis is indicated during the period between the third primary dose and the reinforcing dose, give a 0.5 mL dose. If given before 6 months have elapsed, count it as a primary dose. If given after 6 months, regard it as a reinforcing dose.

Upon intimate exposure to diphtheria, an emergency recall booster dose of 0.5 mL may be indicated.

Missed Doses: Prolonging the interval between primary immunizing doses for 6 months or more does not interfere with the final immunity. Count any dose, even if received a decade earlier, as one of the immunizing injections.

Efficacy: Extremely high (more than 99%) after a complete immunizing series and proper booster doses.

Onset: Within a few weeks, when given as a booster dose in people who previously received a primary immunizing series.

Duration: Protection against tetanus and diphtheria persists for at least 10 years, when given as a booster dose in people who previously received a primary immunizing series.

Protective Level: Specific antitoxin levels more than 0.01 antitoxin units/mL for each antigen are generally regarded as protective. More recently, a level of 0.1 to 0.2 or more units/mL for each antitoxin has been considered protective.

Mechanism: *Corynebacterium diphtheriae* may cause either a localized or a generalized disease. Diphtheria exotoxin, an extracellular protein metabolite of toxigenic strains of *Corynebacterium diphtheriae*, causes systemic intoxication. Complete immunization induces antitoxin antibodies against diphtheria toxin and significantly reduces the risk of developing diphtheria. Immunized people who develop disease have milder illnesses.

Tetanus toxoid induces specific protective antibodies against the exotoxin excreted by *Clostridium tetani*.

The aluminum salt, a mineral adjuvant, prolongs and enhances antigenic properties of tetanus toxoid by retarding the rate of absorption.

Drug Interactions: Like all inactivated vaccines, administration of Td to people receiving immunosuppressant drugs (eg, high-dose corticosteroids) or radiation therapy may result in an insufficient response to immunization. They may remain susceptible despite immunization.

Several routine vaccines may safely and effectively be administered simultaneously at separate injection sites (eg, Td, MMR, e-IPV, Hib, hepatitis B). National authorities recommend simultaneous immunization at separate sites as indicated by age or health risk if return of a vaccine recipient for a subsequent visit is doubtful.

Delay diphtheria toxoid administration until 3 to 4 weeks after diphtheria antitoxin use, to avoid the hypothetical possibility of antitoxin-toxoid interference.

Concurrent administration of tetanus toxoid and tetanus immune globulin may delay development of active immunity by several days through partial antigen-antibody antagonism. But this interaction is not clinically significant and does not preclude concurrent administration of both drugs if both are needed.

Otherwise, subunit vaccines are not generally affected by circulating antibodies or administration of other exogenous antibodies. Vaccination may occur at any time before or after antibody administration.

Systemic chloramphenicol therapy may impair anamnestic response to tetanus toxoid. Avoid concurrent use of these 2 drugs.

As with other drugs administered by IM injection, give Td with caution to people receiving anticoagulant therapy.

Pharmaceutical Characteristics

Concentration:
Massachusetts: 2 Lf units tetanus toxoid and 2 Lf units diphtheria toxoid/0.5 mL
Sanofi Pasteur: 5 Lf units tetanus toxoid and 2 Lf units diphtheria toxoid/0.5 mL

Quality Assay: The tetanus and diphtheria toxoids induce at least 2 units and 0.5 units of antitoxin per mL of serum, respectively, in guinea pig potency tests.
USP requirements: Contains one-tenth of the pediatric dose of diphtheria toxoid. Contains 0.02% or less residual-free formaldehyde.
Massachusetts: Purified to a specific activity of 1,500 Lf diphtheria units/mL total nitrogen or more.

Packaging:
>*Massachusetts:* Package of 10 single-dose 0.5 mL vials (distributed by MBL: 17478-0131-01; distributed by Merck: 00006-4133-41)
>
>*Sanofi Pasteur (Decavac):* Package of 10 single-dose 0.5 mL vials (49281-0291-83), package of 10 single-dose 0.5 mL prefilled syringes (49281-0291-10)

Doseform: Suspension

Appearance: Turbid liquid, whitish-gray in color

Solvent: Variously formulated with sodium chloride, with or without phosphate buffers.

Adjuvant:
>*Massachusetts:* 2 mg aluminum phosphate (0.45 mg aluminum)/0.5 mL
>
>*Sanofi Pasteur:* Aluminum phosphate 1.5 mg/0.5 mL, containing not more than 0.33 mg aluminum/0.5 mL

Preservative:
>*Massachusetts:* 0.0033% thimerosal
>
>*Sanofi Pasteur (Decavac):* None; the preservative-free formulations contain a trace amount of thimerosal from manufacturing, with 0.3 mcg/0.5 mL mercury or less per dose.

Allergens: None

Excipients:
>*Sanofi Pasteur:* No more than 0.02% residual formaldehyde. Variously formulated with glycine, sodium acetate, sodium phosphate, aluminum chloride, hydrochloric acid, or sodium hydroxide.

pH:
>*Massachusetts:* 5.9 to 6.1
>
>*Sanofi Pasteur:* Data not provided

Shelf Life: Expires within 24 months

Storage/Stability: Store at 2° to 8°C (35° to 46°F). Discard frozen toxoids. Contact manufacturer regarding prolonged exposure to room temperature or elevated temperatures. Shipped in insulated containers with coolant packs.
>*Sanofi Pasteur:* Product can tolerate 4 days at 37°C (100°F) or lower.

Production Process: *Corynebacterium diphtheriae* and *Clostridium tetani* bacteria grow in separate media according to the method of Mueller and Miller (1947). *Clostridium tetani* are grown in a peptone-based medium containing a bovine extract, from a US source. Each toxoid is produced by detoxification of exotoxin with formaldehyde and refined by the Pillemer alcohol-fractionation method (1946) or serial ammonium-sulfate fractionation and diafiltration.

Disease Epidemiology

Incidence:
>*Diphtheria:* 206,000 cases of diphtheria with 10,000 deaths were reported in 1921, primarily among children (200 cases per 100,000 people), 5% to 10% case-fatality rate). Between 1980 and 1992, only 37 cases of diphtheria were reported in the United States, but the case-fatality rate remained constant at about 5% to 10%. Diphtheria is rare in modern times because of high levels in immunization and an apparent reduction in the circulation of toxigenic strains of the bacterium. Case-fatality rates are highest in very young persons and in the elderly.
>
>*Tetanus:* Peak reported: 601 cases of tetanus in 1948 (0.39 cases/100,000 people). About 50 cases are reported each year in the United States (0.03 cases/100,000 people), primarily among older Americans; 68% of reported cases were at least 50 years of age. Overall, the case-fatality rate was 21%. An estimated 770,000 neonatal tetanus deaths occur around the world each year.

Susceptible Pools:
>*Diphtheria:* 49% to 66% of those 50 years and older.

Tetanus & Diphtheria Toxoids Adsorbed, for Adult Use (Td)

Tetanus: 41% to 84% of Americans 60 years and older; especially men and women who have not served in the armed forces.

Transmission:

Diphtheria: Contact with a patient or carrier or articles soiled with their discharges. Raw milk may transmit infection.

Tetanus: Tetanus is an intoxication manifested primarily by neuromuscular dysfunction caused by a potent exotoxin elaborated by *Clostridium tetani.* Tetanus spores introduced into the body, usually through a puncture wound contaminated with soil, street dust, or animal or human feces; through lacerations, burns, and trivial or unnoticed wounds; by injection of contaminated illicit drugs. Tetanus occasionally follows surgery. Presence of necrotic tissue or foreign bodies favors growth of the anaerobic pathogen.

Incubation:

Diphtheria: 2 to 5 days, occasionally longer.

Tetanus: 3 to 21 days (range: 1 day to several months), depending on character, extent, and location of the wound. In general, short incubation periods correspond with more heavily contaminated wounds, more severe disease, and a worse prognosis.

Communicability:

Diphtheria: Isolate until nose and throat clear, usually 2 weeks or less, seldom longer than 4 weeks. Effective antibiotic therapy promptly terminates shedding. Chronic carriers may rarely shed organisms for 6 months or longer.

Tetanus: Not directly transmitted from person to person.

Other Information

Perspective:

1883: Loeffler & Klebs isolate and describe *Corynebacterium diphtheriae.*

1884: Nicolaier discovers *Clostridium tetani.*

1923: Ramon modifies diphtheria toxin with formaldehyde to produce "anatoxin," French for toxoid.

1923: Ramon & Zoeller at Pasteur Institute report use of tetanus toxoid to induce active immunity.

1926: Glenny et al. report that alum-precipitated toxoid enhances activity. Diphtheria toxoid licensed in the United States. Widespread childhood vaccination programs begin in the United States.

1937: Adsorbed form of tetanus toxoid licensed in the United States.

1941: US Army Surgeon General receives authority from the War Department to administer tetanus toxoid to American troops. A record of each dose of tetanus toxoid administered was stamped on soldiers' identification tags. Only 12 tetanus cases and 6 tetanus deaths were reported throughout the war, in all theaters of operations, despite more than 12 million Americans in uniform who incurred more than 2.7 million hospital admissions for wounds or injuries. All 12 cases were in unimmunized or incompletely immunized troops. The German Army (the Wehrmacht) did not give tetanus toxoid to its troops, relying instead on tetanus antitoxin. It suffered high rates of morbidity and mortality from tetanus. In contrast, the German Air Force (the Luftwaffe) immunized its men with toxoid and suffered much less morbidity and mortality.

1947: Combination diphtheria and tetanus toxoids for pediatric use licensed in the United States.

1948: Adsorbed form of diphtheria toxoid licensed in the United States.

c. 1950: Witte peptone eliminated from production medium, resulting in a lower adverse-reaction rate.

1953: Combination tetanus & diphtheria toxoids for adult use licensed in the United States, with reduced concentration of diphtheria toxoid to reduce injection-site reactions.

1963: Sclavo's diphtheria toxoid licensed on January 4, 1963.

2004: *Decavac* adopted as proprietary name, March 24, 2004.

NB: The Moloney test was formerly conducted with ID injection of fluid diphtheria toxoid on the forearm. The appearance in 12 to 24 hours of induration more than 12 mm in diameter was a positive reaction implying immunity.

First Licensed:

Wyeth: December 1954
Lederle: April 1962
Massachusetts: October 1967
Connaught: January 1978 (now Sanofi Pasteur)
Sclavo: February 1979

National Policy: ACIP. Preventing tetanus, diphtheria, and pertussis among adolescents: Use of tetanus toxoid, reduced diphtheria toxoid, and acellular pertussis vaccines. *MMWR*. 2006;55(RR-3):1-43. http://www.cdc.gov/mmwr/PDF/rr/rr5503.pdf.

ACIP. Preventing tetanus, diphtheria, and pertussis among adults: Use of tetanus toxoid, reduced diphtheria toxoid, and acellular pertussis vaccines. *MMWR*. 2006;55(RR-17):1-37. http://www.cdc.gov/mmwr/PDF/rr/rr5517.pdf.

ACIP. Prevention of pertussis, tetanus, and diphtheria among pregnant and postpartum women and their infants. *MMWR*. 2008;57(RR-4):1-51, erratum 723. http://www.cdc.gov/mmwr/PDF/rr/rr5704.pdf.

References: CDC. Tetanus surveillance, United States, 1998-2000. *MMWR*. 2003;52(SS-03):1-8.

WHO. Diphtheria vaccine. *Wkly Epidemiol Rec*. 2006;81:24-32.

WHO. Tetanus vaccine. *Wkly Epidemiol Rec*. 2006;81:198-208.

Tetanus Toxoid Adsorbed

Bacterial Vaccines & Toxoids

Name:
Generic

Manufacturer:
Sanofi Pasteur

Synonyms: T, TT, tetanus vaccine. The disease is also known as lockjaw.

Comparison: Generically equivalent. While the rate of seroconversion and promptness of antibody response are essentially equivalent for both the fluid and adsorbed forms of tetanus toxoid, adsorbed toxoids induce higher antitoxin titers and, hence, more persistent antitoxin levels. Therefore, adsorbed tetanus toxoid is strongly recommended for both primary and booster immunizations. Use fluid tetanus toxoid to immunize the rare patient who is hypersensitive to the aluminum adjuvant. The only other rational use remaining for fluid tetanus toxoid is in compounding dilutions of a reagent for delayed-hypersensitivity skin-testing (refer to product information).

> **Note:** Trivalent vaccines against diphtheria, tetanus, and pertussis are the preferred immunizing agent for most people. Tetanus and diphtheria toxoids for adult use (Td) bivalent or with acellular pertussis vaccine (Tdap) is the preferred immunizing agent for most adults and older children.

Immunologic Characteristics

Microorganism: Bacterium, *C. tetani*, anaerobic endospore-forming gram-positive rod
Viability: Inactivated
Antigenic Form: Toxoid
Antigenic Type: Protein
Strains: S120-6

Use Characteristics

Indications: Selective induction of active immunity against tetanus in selected patients. Tetanus and diphtheria toxoids for adult use (Td) bivalent or with acellular pertussis vaccine (Tdap) is the preferred immunizing agent for most adults and children after their seventh birthday. All people should maintain tetanus immunity by means of booster doses throughout life because tetanus spores are ubiquitous. Tetanus immunity is especially important for military personnel, farm and utility workers, those working with horses, firemen, and all individuals whose occupation or vocation renders them liable to even minor lacerations and abrasions. Advise travelers to developing nations to maintain active tetanus immunity to obviate any need for therapy with equine tetanus antitoxin and thus avoid associated complications.

While the rate of seroconversion and promptness of antibody response are essentially equivalent for both the fluid and adsorbed forms of tetanus toxoid, adsorbed toxoids induce higher antitoxin titers and, hence, more persistent antitoxin levels. Therefore, selection of tetanus toxoid adsorbed is strongly recommended for both primary and booster immunizations. Use fluid tetanus toxoid to immunize the rare patient who is hypersensitive to the aluminum adjuvant.

Limitations: Tetanus toxoid is not intended for the treatment or diagnosis of tetanus. For treatment of tetanus infection and for passive prophylaxis, consider use of tetanus immune globulin and appropriate antibiotics (eg, penicillin G, a tetracycline).

Contraindications:

Absolute: Patients with a history of serious allergic reaction to a vaccine component or after a prior dose of this vaccine.

Relative: An acute infection is reason for deferring administration of routine primary immunizing or routine recall doses but not emergency recall doses.

The FDA recommends that elective tetanus immunization be deferred during any outbreak of poliomyelitis because injections are an important cause of provocative poliomyelitis. This recommendation presupposes that the patient has not sustained an injury that increases the risk of tetanus. The caution has largely been superseded, as poliomyelitis has been controlled in the United States by universal vaccination, but the warning persists in some drug labeling.

Immunodeficiency: People receiving immunosuppressive therapy or with other immunodeficiencies may have a diminished antibody response to active immunization. This is a reason for deferring primary diphtheria immunization until treatment is discontinued or for injecting an additional dose at least 1 month after treatment is ceased. Nonetheless, routine immunization of symptomatic and asymptomatic HIV-infected people is recommended.

Elderly: Tetanus and diphtheria toxoids for adult use (Td) bivalent or with acellular pertussis vaccine (Tdap) is the preferred immunizing agent for most adults and older children. The elderly develop lower to normal antitoxin levels following tetanus immunization than younger people.

Adults: Tetanus and diphtheria toxoids for adult use (Td) bivalent or with acellular pertussis vaccine (Tdap) is the preferred immunizing agent for most adults and older children.

Pregnancy: Category C. Use only if clearly needed; Td or Tdap is preferred. Based on extensive human experience, there is no evidence that tetanus toxoid is teratogenic. Give a previously unimmunized pregnant woman who may deliver her child under nonhygienic conditions 2 properly spaced doses of a product containing tetanus toxoid adsorbed (eg, Td, Tdap), preferably during the last 2 trimesters. Incompletely immunized pregnant women should complete a 3-dose primary series. Give those immunized more than 10 years ago a booster dose. It is not known if tetanus toxoid or corresponding antibodies cross the placenta. Generally, most IgG passage across the placenta occurs during the third trimester.

Lactation: It is not known if tetanus toxoid or corresponding antibodies are excreted in human breast milk. Problems in humans have not been documented.

Children: Safety and efficacy of tetanus toxoid are known for children as young as 2 months. Nonetheless, trivalent DTaP is the preferred immunizing agent for most children until their seventh birthday.

Tetanus and diphtheria toxoids for adult use (Td) bivalent or with acellular pertussis vaccine (Tdap) is the preferred immunizing agent for most adults and older children.

Adverse Reactions: A small amount of erythema and induration surrounding the injection site and persisting for a few days is not unusual. A nodule may be palpable at the injection site for a few weeks. Allow such nodules to recede spontaneously and do not incise. Sterile abscesses (incidence, less than 6 to 10 cases per million doses) and subcutaneous atrophy may also occur. Adverse reactions often associated with multiple prior booster doses may be manifested 2 to more than 12 hours after administration by erythema, boggy edema, pruritus, lymphadenopathy, and induration surrounding the site of injection. Pain and tenderness, if present, are usually not the primary complaints.

Systemic manifestations: Low-grade fever, chills, malaise, generalized aches and pains, headaches, flushing, generalized urticaria or pruritus, tachycardia, anaphylaxis, hypotension, neurological complications.

Although the cause is unknown, hypersensitivity to the exotoxin or bacillary protein of the tetanus organism itself is assumed to be possible. In other people, interaction between the injected antigen and high levels of preexisting tetanus antibody from prior booster doses seems to be the most likely cause of these Arthus-like responses. Do not give these people even emergency doses of tetanus toxoid more frequently than every 10 years.

Pharmacologic & Dosing Characteristics

Dosage: Shake vial gently before withdrawing each dose.

Primary immunizing series: For adults and children beginning at 6 to 8 weeks of age, two 0.5 mL doses, at an interval of 4 to 8 weeks, followed by a third reinforcing 0.5 mL dose 6 to 12 months after the second dose. The third dose is an integral part of the primary series. Do not consider basic immunization complete until the third dose has been given. The dosage is the same for children and adults. Shake the vial vigorously before withdrawing each dose.

Separate doses of diphtheria toxoid by at least 4 weeks. Do not count doses within the minimum interval because too short an interval may interfere with antibody response and protection from disease. Typically, 6 months should elapse between the next-to-last and the last dose of a series. Increasing the interval beyond the recommended timing does not affect the ultimate efficacy of immunization, but waiting does delay achieving adequate protection from infection.

However, when immunization with tetanus toxoid adsorbed begins in the first year of life (rather than immunization with DTaP), the primary series consists of three 0.5 mL doses, 4 to 8 weeks apart, followed by a fourth reinforcing 0.5 mL dose 6 to 12 months after the third dose.

If doubt exists about the patient's tolerance of tetanus toxoid and if an emergency booster dose is indicated, give a small dose (eg, 0.05 to 0.1 mL) subcutaneously as a test dose. If no reaction occurs, give the balance of the full 0.5 mL dose 12 hours later. If a marked reaction does occur, further toxoid injections at that time may safely be omitted because reducing the dose of tetanus toxoid does not proportionately reduce the magnitude of the response obtained.

Route & Site: IM. Give IM injections in the deltoid area of the upper arm or the midlateral muscle of the thigh (the vastus lateralis). Take care to avoid major peripheral nerve trunks. Do not inject the same muscle site more than once during the course of primary immunization. Expel the antigen slowly and terminate the dose with a small bubble of air (0.1 to 0.2 mL) to reduce the risk of nodules. Do not inject ID or into superficial subcutaneous tissues.

Documentation Requirements: Federal law requires that the following information be documented in the recipient's permanent medical record or in a permanent office log: (1) The manufacturer and lot number of this vaccine, (2) the date of its administration, and (3) the name, address, and title of the person administering the vaccine.

Certain adverse events must be reported to the VAERS system ([800] 822-7967). Refer to Immunization Documents in the Resources section.

Overdosage: Although few data are available, clinical experience with similar products suggests that the major manifestations of overdosage would be pain and tenderness at the injection site.

Booster Doses: Give routine recall (booster) doses of 0.5 mL at 10-year intervals throughout life to maintain immunity. In event of injury for which tetanus prophylaxis is indicated, refer to CDC wound-management guidelines in the DTP Overview. If emergency tetanus prophylaxis is indicated between the third primary dose and the reinforcing dose, give a 0.5 mL dose. If given before 6 months have elapsed, count it as a primary dose. If given after 6 months, regard it as a reinforcing dose.

Missed Doses: Prolonging the interval between primary immunizing doses for at least 6 months does not interfere with the final immunity. Count any dose of tetanus toxoid, even if received a decade earlier, as one of the immunizing injections.

Efficacy: Nearly perfect after a complete immunizing series and proper booster doses.

Onset: After multiple doses

Duration: Approximately 10 years

Protective Level: Specific antitoxin levels more than 0.01 antitoxin units/mL are generally regarded as protective. More recently, a level of 0.1 to 0.2 or more units/mL has been considered protective.

Mechanism: Induces specific protective antibodies against the exotoxin excreted by *C. tetani*. The aluminum salt, a mineral adjuvant, prolongs and enhances the antigenic properties of tetanus toxoid by retarding the rate of absorption.

Drug Interactions: Like all inactivated vaccines, tetanus toxoid adsorbed given to people receiving immunosuppressant drugs (eg, high-dose corticosteroids) or radiation therapy may result in an insufficient response to immunization. They may remain susceptible despite immunization.

Several routine vaccines may safely and effectively be administered simultaneously at separate injection sites (eg, DTP or Td, MMR, e-IPV, Hib, hepatitis B). National authorities recommend simultaneous immunization at separate sites as indicated by age or health risk, if return of a vaccine recipient for a subsequent visit is doubtful.

Delay diphtheria toxoid administration until 3 to 4 weeks after diphtheria antitoxin use to avoid the hypothetical possibility of antitoxin-toxoid interference.

Concurrent administration of tetanus toxoid adsorbed and tetanus immune globulin may delay active immunity by several days through partial antigen-antibody antagonism. But this interaction is not clinically significant and does not preclude concurrent administration of both drugs if both are needed.

Otherwise, subunit vaccines are not generally affected by circulating antibodies or administration of other exogenous antibodies. Vaccination may occur at any time before or after antibody administration.

Systemic chloramphenicol therapy may impair anamnestic response to tetanus toxoid. Avoid concurrent use of these 2 drugs.

As with other drugs administered IM, give with caution to people on anticoagulant therapy.

Pharmaceutical Characteristics

Concentration: 5 Lf units/0.5 mL

Quality Assay: Toxoid induces at least 2 units of antitoxin per mL in mouse or guinea-pig potency tests. A guinea-pig detoxification test is conducted.

USP requirement: No more than 0.02% residual-free formaldehyde.

Packaging: Box of ten 0.5 mL vials (49281-0820-10).

Doseform: Suspension

Appearance: Turbid, white, slightly gray or slightly pink suspension

Solvent: Variously formulated with sodium chloride, with or without phosphate buffers.

Adjuvant: Aluminum potassium sulfate, with no more than 0.25 mg aluminum/0.5 mL

Preservative: 0.01% thimerosal in the multidose vial. The single-dose preservative-free vials contain a trace amount of thimerosal from manufacturing, with 0.3 mcg/0.5 mL mercury or less per dose.

Allergens: The multidose vial stopper may contain dry natural latex rubber. The single-dose vial package is latex free.

Excipients: No more than 0.02% residual formaldehyde. Manufacturers variously use glycine, sodium acetate, hydrochloric acid, or sodium hydroxide.

pH: Data not provided

Shelf Life: Expires within 24 months

Storage/Stability: Store at 2° to 8°C (35° to 46°F). Discard frozen toxoid. Contact manufacturer regarding prolonged exposure to room temperature or elevated temperatures. Shipped in insulated containers with coolant packs.
Sanofi Pasteur: Product can tolerate 4 days at 37°C (100°F) or lower.

Production Process: *C. tetani* grows in media according to the method of Mueller and Miller (1947). Toxoid is produced by detoxification of tetanus exotoxin with formaldehyde and refined by the Pillemer alcohol-fractionation method (1946).

Disease Epidemiology

Incidence: 601 cases in 1948 (0.39 cases/100,000 people). The record low was 36 reported cases in 1994.

From 50 to 90 cases are reported each year in the United States (0.03 cases/100,000 people), primarily among older Americans; 68% of reported cases were 50 years of age and older. Overall, the case-fatality rate was 21%. The global incidence of tetanus is estimated at 1 million cases annually, with a case-fatality ratio of 20% to 50%. At least half the deaths occur in neonates, often resulting from unsanitary treatment of umbilical stumps.

Susceptible Pools: Unvaccinated children, primarily those younger than 1 year of age; 30% to 40% of preschool children may be susceptible. Also, 41% to 84% of Americans older than 60 years of age, especially men and women who have not served in the armed forces.

Transmission: Tetanus is an intoxication manifested primarily by neuromuscular dysfunction caused by a potent exotoxin elaborated by *C. tetani*. Tetanus spores introduced into the body, usually through a puncture wound contaminated with soil, street dust, or animal or human feces; through lacerations, burns, and trivial or unnoticed wounds; by injection of contaminated illicit drugs. Tetanus occasionally follows surgery. Presence of necrotic tissue or foreign bodies favors growth of the anaerobic pathogen.

Incubation: 3 to 21 days (range, 1 day to several months), depending on the character, extent, and location of the wound. In general, short incubation periods correspond with more heavily contaminated wounds, more severe disease, and a worse prognosis.

Communicability: Not directly transmitted from person to person.

Other Information

Perspective:
1884: Nicolaier discovers *C. tetani*.
1923: Ramon and Zoeller at Pasteur Institute report use of tetanus toxoid to induce active immunity.
1937: Adsorbed form of tetanus toxoid licensed in the United States.
1941: US Army Surgeon General receives authority from the War Department to administer tetanus toxoid to American troops. A record of each dose of tetanus toxoid administered was stamped on soldiers' identification tags. Only 12 tetanus cases and 6 tetanus deaths were reported throughout the war, in all theaters of operations, despite more than 12 million Americans in uniform who incurred more than 2.7 million hospital admissions for wounds or injuries. All 12 cases were in unimmunized or incompletely immunized troops. The German Army (the Wehrmacht) did not give tetanus toxoid to its troops, relying instead on tetanus antitoxin. It suffered high rates of morbidity and mortality from tetanus. In contrast, the German Air Force (the Luftwaffe) immunized its men with toxoid and suffered much less morbidity and mortality.
1950: Witte peptone eliminated from production medium, resulting in a lower adverse reaction rate.

First Licensed:
Berna: February 11, 1970
Lederle: October 1954
Massachusetts: May 1967
Michigan: September 1955
Connaught: October 1970 (now Sanofi Pasteur)
Wyeth: June 1955

National Policy: ACIP. Preventing tetanus, diphtheria, and pertussis among adolescents: Use of tetanus toxoid, reduced diphtheria toxoid, and acellular pertussis vaccines. *MMWR.* 2006;55(RR-3):1-43. http://www.cdc.gov/mmwr/PDF/rr/rr5503.pdf.

ACIP. Preventing tetanus, diphtheria, and pertussis among adults: Use of tetanus toxoid, reduced diphtheria toxoid, and acellular pertussis vaccines. *MMWR.* 2006;55(RR-17):1-37. http://www.cdc.gov/mmwr/PDF/rr/rr5517.pdf.

ACIP. Prevention of pertussis, tetanus, and diphtheria among pregnant and postpartum women and their infants. *MMWR.* 2008;57(RR-4):1-51, erratum 723. http://www.cdc.gov/mmwr/PDF/rr/rr5704.pdf.

References: CDC. Tetanus surveillance, United States, 1998-2000. *MMWR.* 2003;52(SS-03):1-8.

WHO. Tetanus vaccine. *Wkly Epidemiol Rec.* 2006;81:198-208.

Haemophilus influenzae Type B Conjugate Vaccine

Bacterial Vaccines & Toxoids

Names:
Meningococcal Protein Conjugate,
Liquid *PedvaxHIB*,
PRP-OMP (outer membrane
protein), PRP-OMPC (outer
membrane protein conjugate)
Tetanus Toxoid Conjugate, *ActHIB*,
PRP-T
Tetanus Toxoid Conjugate, *Hiberix*,
PRP-T

Manufacturers:
Merck

Sanofi Pasteur

GlaxoSmithKline

Synonyms: Hib vaccine, HBcV. The bacterium was previously known as the influenza bacillus.

Comparison: Not generically equivalent, based on immunogenicity and dosage schedule. Each Hib vaccine is immunogenically unique. PRP-OMP induces higher antibody titers after the first dose than other Hib vaccines, but the extent of clinical protection is comparable for all licensed products.

OmniHIB (formerly distributed by GSK) and *ActHIB* are the same vaccine. *ActHIB* is marketed with *Tripedia* brand of DTaP vaccine under the trade name *TriHIBit*, a name that may be confused with *ProHIBiT*.

Immunologic Characteristics

Microorganism: Bacterium, *Haemophilus influenzae* type b, facultative anaerobic gram-negative rod, family Pasteurellaceae

Viability: Inactivated

Antigenic Form: Capsular polysaccharide fragments, conjugated to various protein carriers

Antigenic Type: Polysaccharide conjugated to protein. The polysaccharide is a polymer of ribose, ribitol, and phosphate (polyribosyl-ribitol-phosphate, PRP).

Strains:
GSK: Strain 20,752
Merck: Hib strain: Ross; *Neisseria meningitidis* serogroup B strain: B11
Sanofi Pasteur: Strain 1482

Use Characteristics

Indications: Induction of active immunity against invasive diseases caused by encapsulated *H. influenzae* type b. Routine immunization of all infants beginning at 2 months of age is recommended in the United States, using either *HibTITER*, *PedvaxHIB*, or *ActHIB*. Risk groups with increased susceptibility to disease include children attending day care facilities, people of low socioeconomic status, blacks (especially those lacking the Km [1] Ig allotype), whites lacking the G2m (n or 23) Ig allotype, Native Americans, household contacts of Hib disease cases, and individuals with asplenia, sickle-cell disease, and antibody-deficiency syndromes.

Children who have invasive Hib disease when younger than 24 months may not develop adequate anticapsular antibody concentrations and remain at risk for a second episode of disease. Vaccinate these children according to current age, ignoring previous Hib doses. Do not immunize children whose disease occurred at older than 24 months because they are likely to develop a protective immune response.

Adolescents and adults who may benefit from a single dose of any brand of Hib vaccine include patients without functioning spleens, patients with cancer, recipients of organ transplants, and other patients with severe immunosuppression. Consider vaccinating patients infected with HIV. Whenever possible, give Hib vaccine before immunosuppression occurs.

Limitations: Hib vaccines do not protect against *H. influenzae* other than type b strains, nor does vaccination prevent infection with other microorganisms that cause meningitis or septic disease. Do not use Hib vaccine to prevent recurrent sinusitis or bronchitis in adults because *Haemophilus* organisms associated with these conditions are almost always nontypeable, nonencapsulated strains unaffected by anti-Hib antibody.

There is insufficient evidence to suggest that Hib vaccine given immediately after exposure to natural Hib will prevent illness. Cases of Hib disease may occur in vaccine recipients prior to the onset of the protective effects of the vaccine. Select appropriate antibiotics (eg, cefotaxime, ceftriaxone) to treat active Hib infections.

Vaccination is not effective in preventing secondary cases of invasive disease. Instead, rifampin prophylaxis is often recommended. Rifampin prophylaxis is no longer indicated for management of households where all contacts younger than 48 months are fully immunized. Give rifampin prophylaxis to all members of a household with a case of invasive Hib disease if a child contact younger than 12 months is present who has not yet received the booster or reinforcing dose, regardless of the vaccination status of the child. In households with a child 1 to 3 years of age who is inadequately vaccinated, all household contacts should receive rifampin following a case of invasive Hib disease that occurs in any family member. Nonetheless, the risk of secondary disease is very low among children who completed the primary 2- or 3-dose series.

Some antibody response to the carrier protein occurs with each of these vaccines, but immunization with Hib vaccine does not substitute for routine diphtheria or tetanus (eg, DTP, Td, DT) immunization, nor does *PedvaxHIB* protect against *Neisseria* infections.

Contraindications:

Absolute: People with a history of serious allergic reaction to a vaccine component or after a prior dose of this vaccine.

Relative: Any febrile illness or acute infection is reason for delaying immunization with this vaccine. A mild afebrile illness, such as a mild upper respiratory infection, is not usually reason to defer immunization.

Immunodeficiency: If this vaccine is used in patients deficient in producing antibody, whether because of genetic defect, illness, or immunosuppressive therapy, the expected immune response may not result.

The ACIP recommends Hib immunization of children who are immunosuppressed in association with AIDS or any other immunodeficiency disease. Administration of Hib vaccine to adults early in the course of HIV infection will produce presumably protective antibody titers, although their excess risk of Hib infection may be slight.

Children with sickle-cell disease, IgG_2 immunoglobulin deficiency, HIV infection, bone-marrow transplants, splenectomy, those receiving chemotherapy for malignancies, and others with immunologic impairment may benefit from an additional dose of Hib vaccine, beyond the usual number of doses. This may be delivered as 2 doses of any conjugate vaccine after 12 months of age, separated by 2 months, or 1 additional dose for children who received 2 doses before 12 months of age. Unvaccinated children older than 59 months with these underlying diseases should receive 1 or 2 doses of any Hib vaccine, separated by 1 to 2 months.

Hib disease longer than 2 weeks after immunization may reflect an evolving immunodeficient state. Children who manifest disease despite immunization at 15 months of age or older may warrant immunologic evaluation. Infants with Hib disease despite immunization and other factors suggesting increased susceptibility to infection should similarly be evaluated.

Elderly: No specific information is available about geriatric use of Hib vaccine.

Adults: The American College of Physicians (1994) suggests vaccination of older children and adults who have underlying conditions associated with increased susceptibility to infection with encapsulated bacteria. These conditions include splenectomy, sickle-cell disease, Hodgkin disease and other hematologic neoplasms, and immunosuppression. Do not use Hib vaccine to prevent recurrent sinusitis or bronchitis in adults because *Haemophilus* organisms associated with these conditions are almost always nontypeable, nonencapsulated strains unaffected by anti-Hib antibody. Hib vaccination is not necessary for health care personnel or day care workers who frequently come in contact with children with invasive disease.

Carcinogenicity: Hib vaccine has not been evaluated for carcinogenic potential.

Mutagenicity: Hib vaccine has not been evaluated for mutagenic potential.

Fertility Impairment: Hib vaccine has not been evaluated for impairment of fertility.

Pregnancy: Category C. Use is not generally recommended, but is not contraindicated. It is not known if Hib vaccine or corresponding antibodies cross the placenta. Generally, most IgG passage across the placenta occurs during the third trimester.

Lactation: It is not known if Hib vaccine or corresponding antibodies are excreted in breast milk. Problems in humans have not been documented and are unlikely.

Children: Routine immunization of all infants beginning at 2 months of age is recommended in the United States. Routinely vaccinate children as old as 5 years of age. Use in children younger than 6 weeks may lead to immune tolerance (impaired ability to respond to subsequent exposure to the PRP antigen).

Adverse Reactions: A fever higher than 38.3°C (101°F) occurred at least once in up to 18% of recipients during clinical trials. Other possible reactions include erythema, swelling, induration, pain, soreness, or tenderness, which are generally infrequent, mild, transient, with no serious sequelae. Other adverse events reported include irritability, sleepiness, restless sleep, crying, unusual high-pitched crying, prolonged crying, otitis media, rash, urticaria, angioedema, upper respiratory infection, lymphadenopathy, sterile injection-site abscess, diarrhea, vomiting, loss of appetite, rash, hives, thrombocytopenia, convulsions (including febrile seizures), renal failure, or Guillain-Barré syndrome. A cause-and-effect relationship between Hib vaccination and these experiences has not been established.

Pharmacologic & Dosing Characteristics

Dosage: Each Hib conjugate vaccine is immunogenically unique. Dosage schedules vary for each product. The standard schedule is to give 3 or 4 doses at 2, 4, 6, and 12 to 15 months of age. For *PedvaxHIB*, the dose at 6 months of age may be omitted. If possible, give the entire immunizing series with the same brand of Hib vaccine. If this is not possible, permutations of the vaccine brands are immunogenic.

Adolescent and adult dose: For adults and adolescents who need Hib vaccine, give a single 0.5 mL dose of any brand.

GSK: Give as a 0.5 mL booster dose for the prevention of invasive disease caused by *H. influenzae* type b in children 15 months though 4 years of age (prior to fifth birthday).

Merck: Give infants 2 to 14 months of age a 0.5 mL dose, optimally at 2 months of age, followed by 0.5 mL 2 months later, or as soon as possible thereafter. When the primary 2-dose regimen is completed before 12 months of age, a 0.5 mL booster dose is needed at 12 months of age, but not earlier than 2 months after the second dose. Give a single 0.5 mL dose to children at least 15 months of age who were previously unvaccinated against Hib disease.

Sanofi Pasteur: In infants 2 to 6 months of age, give 3 separate 0.5 mL doses at 2-month intervals. Give all vaccinated children a single booster at 15 to 18 months of age.

Only limited data regarding interchange of brands of Hib vaccines to complete a dosage schedule are available. For booster doses, using the product used for the first dose is generally preferred. Nonetheless, the sequences PRP-OMP/PRP-T/PRP-T, PRP-OMP/HbOC/HbOC, HbOC/PRP-OMP/PRP-OMP, or HbOC/PRP-T/PRP-T, at 2-month intervals, are known to be immunogenic after the primary series is completed; other sequences may be effective as well. It is not necessary to give more than 3 doses to any child to complete the primary series.

Increasing the interval beyond the recommended timing does not affect the ultimate efficacy of immunization, but waiting does delay achieving adequate protection from infection.

Route & Site: IM, preferably in the outer aspect of the vastus lateralis, mid-thigh, or the outer aspect of the upper arm. Do not administer IV or ID, nor into the gluteal area or areas where there may be a nerve trunk.

Sanofi Pasteur: In patients with coagulation disorders, PRP-T may be given subcutaneously in the mid-lateral aspect of the thigh.

Documentation Requirements: Federal law requires that (1) the manufacturer and lot number of this vaccine, (2) the dates of its administration, and (3) the name, address, and title of the person administering the vaccine be documented in the recipient's permanent medical record or in a permanent office log.

Certain adverse events must be reported to VAERS (800-822-7967). Refer to Immunization Documents in the Resources section for complete information.

Overdosage: Although few data are available, clinical experience with similar products suggests that the major manifestations of overdosage would be pain and tenderness at the injection site.

Booster Doses: Several doses of Hib vaccine are needed to complete a primary immunization series. The intervals between the initial doses are preferably 2 months or longer, although an interval of 1 month is acceptable, if necessary.

Booster doses after 15 months of age are not currently recommended. However, children with sickle-cell disease, IgG_2 immunoglobulin deficiency, HIV infection, bone-marrow transplants, splenectomy, those receiving chemotherapy for malignancies, and others with immunologic impairment may benefit from an additional dose of Hib vaccine. This may be delivered as 2 doses of any conjugate vaccine after 12 months of age, separated by 2 months, or 1 additional dose for children who received 2 doses before 12 months of age. Unvaccinated children older than 59 months with these underlying diseases should receive 1 or 2 doses of any Hib vaccine, separated by 1 to 2 months.

Missed Doses: Prolonging the interval between doses does not interfere with immunity achieved after the concluding dose of the basic series, but waiting does delay achieving adequate protection from infection.

Efficacy: The initial unconjugated polysaccharide Hib vaccines produced roughly 45% to 88% reduction in disease incidence among children at least 18 to 24 months of age, although some published reports failed to demonstrate efficacy.

GSK: In clinical studies, the immune response to *Hiberix* administered as a booster dose was evaluated in 415 children 12 to 23 months of age. At the time of vaccination, 30 children were 12 to 24 months of age, 316 children were 15 to 18 months of age, and 69 children were 19 to 23 months of age. Antibodies to PRP were measured in sera obtained immediately before and 1 month after booster vaccination. Geometric mean concentrations ranged from 47 to 96 mcg/mL. All children received anti-PRP concentrations of at least 0.15 mcg/mL and 97% to 100% achieved concentration of at least 1 mcg/mL (seroprotection rates) after this booster dose.

Merck: In a study of 3,486 Navajo infants, vaccination provided a 93% reduction in disease incidence. After the first dose, 88% and 52% of infants, respectively, developed antibody responses more than 0.15 mcg/mL or more than 1 mcg/mL. After the second dose, those proportions rose to 91% and 60%, respectively.

Sanofi Pasteur: Of infants receiving PRP-T doses at 2, 4, and 6 months of age, 90% develop a GMT of anti-Hib antibody more than 1 mcg/mL. More than 98% of infants exceeded this level after a booster dose.

Onset:

GSK: Within 1 month after booster dose

Merck: Greater than 1 week after the dose at 2 months of age

Sanofi Pasteur: As much as 2 weeks after the last recommended dose

Duration: Antibody titers exceeding 1 mcg/mL correlate with prolonged protection from disease, generally implying several years of protection.

Protective Level: Antibody titers of 0.15 mcg/mL or more correlate with clinical protection from disease.

Mechanism: Induction of specific protective antibodies against type b strains of *H. influenzae*. Vaccination may decrease nasopharyngeal colonization and produce lower rates of acquisition of colonization by unvaccinated infants.

The immune response depends on the type of cells producing the response and the antigens stimulating the process. Protein antigens induce B lymphocytes to produce antibody, aided by thymus-derived lymphocytes (T-helper cells); thus, they are called thymus-dependent antigens. This immune response is potentially boostable and IgG antibody predominates. In contrast, polysaccharide antigens stimulate B cells directly without T-cell help, producing a nonboostable response of both IgG and IgM antibodies; these antigens are known as thymus-independent antigens. Linkage of Hib saccharides to a protein can convert the thymus-independent saccharide to a thymus-dependent antigen and can result in an enhanced antibody response to the saccharide and immunologic memory.

IgG_1 subclass predominates in the response to *PedvaxHIB*. IgG_1 also predominates after administration of *ActHIB* and *OmniHIB* to children younger than 2 years, but IgG_2 is induced after vaccination of older children and adults. IgG_2 is associated with natural infection. There is some evidence suggesting natural increases in antibody levels over time after vaccination.

Drug Interactions: Like all inactivated vaccines, administration of Hib vaccine to patients receiving immunosuppressant drugs (eg, high-dose corticosteroids) or radiation therapy may result in an insufficient response to immunization. They may remain susceptible despite immunization. Hib vaccine does not impair immunogenicity of DTP, e-IPV, hepatitis B, influenza, or MMR vaccines. Rates of adverse reactions when Hib vaccine was administered concurrently with DTP and either OPV or e-IPV were comparable with rates when DTP was given alone. Hib, meningococcal, and pneumococcal vaccines may safely and effectively be administered simultaneously at separate injection sites.

Inactivated vaccines are not generally affected by circulating antibodies or administration of exogenous antibodies. Vaccination may occur at any time before or after antibody administration.

Concurrent administration of PRP-T and a DTP vaccine formulation that is not licensed in the United States resulted in decreased antibody response to the pertussis component in a trial in Chile. The implications for PRP-T use in the United States have yet to be determined.

As with other drugs administered IM, give Hib vaccine with caution to patients receiving anticoagulant therapy.

Lab Interference: Antigenuria has been detected following receipt of Hib vaccines; therefore, antigen detection (eg, with latex agglutination kits) may have no diagnostic value in suspected Hib disease within a short period after immunization (GSK: 1 to 2 weeks; Merck:

30 days; Sanofi Pasteur: 3 days). False-positive latex agglutination tests of cerebrospinal fluid have also been reported 1 to 21 days following Hib vaccination.

Pharmaceutical Characteristics

Concentration:
GSK: 10 mcg Hib polysaccharide/0.5 mL
Merck: 7.5 mcg Hib polysaccharide/0.5 mL
Sanofi Pasteur: 10 mcg Hib polysaccharide/0.5 mL

Quality Assay:
Merck: Assay of PRP by HPLC. Coupling to the OMP protein is confirmed by analysis of components of the conjugate following chemical treatment that yields a unique amino acid [S-(carboxymethyl)-homocysteine].
Sanofi Pasteur: Potency is specified by limits on the content of PRP polysaccharide and protein and the proportion of polysaccharide and protein characterized as high molecular weight conjugate.

Packaging:
GSK: Package of ten 1-dose vials of lyophilized vaccine, package with 0.7 mL vials of preservative free sodium chloride 0.9% diluent in prefilled Tip-Lok syringes without needles (NDC#: 58160-0806-05)
Merck: Box of ten 0.5 mL single-dose vials (00006-4897-00)
Sanofi Pasteur: Five single-dose vials of lyophilized vaccine, packaged with 0.6 mL vials of preservative-free sodium chloride 0.4% diluent (49281-0545-05)

Doseform:
GSK: Powder for suspension
Merck: Suspension
Sanofi Pasteur: Powder for suspension

Appearance:
GSK: Powder, yielding a clear and colorless solution
Merck: Slightly opaque, white suspension
Sanofi Pasteur: White powder, yielding a clear and colorless solution

Solvent:
GSK: 0.9% sodium chloride
Merck: 0.9% sodium chloride

Diluent:
For reconstitution: Sanofi Pasteur: 0.6 mL of 0.4% sodium chloride. Alternatively, Sanofi Pasteur's *Tripedia* (DTaP) vaccine may be used as the diluent for the fourth DTaP dose.

Adjuvant:
GSK: 25 mcg tetanus toxoid per 0.5 mL
Merck: 125 mcg *N. meningitidis* OMP and 225 mcg aluminum as aluminum hydroxyphosphate sulfate/0.5 mL
Sanofi Pasteur: 24 mcg tetanus toxoid per 0.5 mL

Preservative: None

Allergens: Package stoppers may contain dry natural rubber (a latex derivative).

Excipients:
GSK: Lactose 12.6 mg and residual formaldehyde at least 0.5 mcg per 0.5 mL
Merck: None
Sanofi Pasteur: 8.5% sucrose, ammonium sulfate, formalin

pH: Data not provided

Haemophilus influenzae Type B Conjugate Vaccine

Shelf Life: Expires within 24 months

Storage/Stability: Store at 2° to 8°C (35° to 46°F). Discard frozen vaccine. Contact manufacturer regarding exposures to prolonged room temperature or elevated temperatures.

GSK: After reconstitution, refrigerate and discard within 24 hours. If the vaccine is not administered promptly, shake the solution vigorously again before injection. Discard vaccine if frozen.

Merck: Discard vaccine if frozen. Shipped in an insulated container at a temperature between 2° to 8°C (35° to 46°F).

Sanofi Pasteur: Shipped from the manufacturer in insulated containers with temperature monitors. Use or discard within 24 hours of reconstitution.

Production Process:

GSK: H. influenzae type b bacteria are grown in a synthetic medium that undergoes heat inactivation and purification. The tetanus toxin, prepared from *Clostridium tetani* grown in a semisynthetic medium, is detoxified with formaldehyde and purified. The capsular polysaccharide is covalently bound to the tetanus toxoid. After purification, the conjugate is lyophilized in the presence of lactose as a stabilizer.

Merck: Polysaccharide purified by a series of phenol extractions and selective ethanol precipitations. OMPC is purified by a series of detergent-extraction, centrifugation, diafiltration, and sterile filtration steps. Hib polysaccharides are covalently bound to an OMP complex of *N. meningitidis* serogroup B. Each molecule consists of polysaccharide, a bigeneric thioether spacer, and the meningococcal B OMP protein. After conjugation, the aqueous bulk antigen is then absorbed onto aluminum hydroxyphosphate sulfate.

Sanofi Pasteur: Conjugated by a 6-carbon spacer to tetanus toxoid.

Media:

GSK: Synthetic medium

Merck: Complex fermentation media, phenol inactivated, primarily consisting of yeast extract, nicotinamide adenine dinucleotide, hemin chloride, soy peptone, dextrose, and mineral salts. The *N. meningitidis* bacteria are grown in a medium primarily consisting of yeast extract, amino acids, and mineral salts.

Sanofi Pasteur: Semisynthetic medium

Disease Epidemiology

Incidence: In the mid-1980s in the United States, disease incidence of 0.1% per year of all children younger than 5 years was common, accounting for 20,000 cases, including 12,000 cases of meningitis and 1,000 deaths annually. Risk of disease was 1:200 overall by 5 years of age prior to vaccine availability; 47% of disease occurred in children younger than 1 year, 53% occurred in children 1 to 5 years of age.

In 1991, after infant vaccination was widely implemented, the number of Hib meningitis cases fell to 1,900. Adams and colleagues (1993) reported that the incidence of meningitis fell from 99 per 100,000 children younger than 15 months in 1989 to 29 per 100,000 in 1991; almost no cases occurred in vaccinated children.

The case fatality rate is 5%; 35% of survivors have neurologic sequelae. Around the world, some 800,000 cases with 145,000 deaths may occur annually.

Susceptible Pools: Unvaccinated children, primarily those younger than 1 year; 30% to 40% of preschool children may be susceptible.

Transmission: By droplet infection and discharges from nose and throat during the infectious period. The portal of entry is usually nasopharyngeal.

Incubation: Probably short, 2 to 4 days

Communicability: As long as organisms are present, which may be for a prolonged period of time, even without nasal discharge. Patients are rendered noncommunicable within 24 to 48 hours after starting effective antibiotic therapy.

Other Information

Perspective:

1892: Pfeiffer discovers *H. influenzae* in Berlin; mistakenly attributes the bacterium as the cause of an influenza virus epidemic.

c.1920: Polyvalent respiratory bacterial vaccines licensed but demonstrate limited efficacy.

1920s: Landsteiner, Goebel, and Avery develop the technique of protein conjugation of saccharides to enhance immunogenicity.

1941-1970s: Hib antiserum available in the United States.

c.1960: Squibb markets an anti-Hib immune serum, derived from rabbit plasma. Withdrawn by the early 1970s.

1970s: Smith and Anderson develop first *Haemophilus* polysaccharide vaccine.

1985: Unconjugated polysaccharide Hib vaccines licensed in the United States, for all children at 24 months of age, plus children 18 to 23 months of age if in day care or other high-risk groups; immunizing children 25 to 60 months of age suggested.

1987: Protein-conjugated Hib vaccine licensed in the United States for children older than 14 months. Technology based on work of Robbins and Schneerson. Connaught licensed on December 22, 1987.

1988: In January, Connaught's *ProHIBiT* recommended for use in all children at 18 months of age. Wyeth's *HibTITER* licensed on December 21.

1989: In January, Lederle's *HibTITER* recommended for use in children at 18 months of age. Merck's *PedvaxHIB* licensed on December 20.

1990: In April, the ACIP recommends routine use of *ProHIBiT*, *HibTITER*, and *PedvaxHIB* for children as young as 15 months of age. "Some" differences noted in immunogenicity among these 3 formulations. In October, the ACIP recommends *HibTITER* for use at 2, 4, 6, and 15 months of age. In December, the ACIP recommends *PedvaxHIB* for use in infants at 2, 4, and 12 months of age.

1993: Connaught/SKB's *OmniHIB* licensed on March 30 for use at 2, 4, 6, and 15 months of age.

1996: Liquid formulation of *PedvaxHIB* licensed on August 12.

2009: *Hiberix* licensed on August 19.

Discontinued Products: *b-CAPSA-I* (Praxis/Mead Johnson, licensed April 12, 1985), *HIB-Vax* (Connaught, licensed December 20, 1985), *HIB-Immune* (Wyeth, licensed December 20, 1985); all unconjugated polysaccharide vaccines; *ProHIBiT* (Diphtheria-toxoid conjugate, PRP-D, Pasteur-Mérieux Connaught, licensed 1987); *HibTITER* (CRM197–conjugate, Wyeth).

National Policy: ACIP. Recommendations for use of *Haemophilus* b conjugate vaccines and a combined diphtheria, tetanus, pertussis, and *Haemophilus* b vaccine. Recommendations of the Advisory Committee on Immunization Practices. *MMWR.* 1993;42(RR-13):1-15.

References: Robbins JB, Schneerson R, Anderson P, Smith DH. Prevention of systemic infections, especially meningitis, caused by *H. influenzae* type b: Impact on public health and implications for other polysaccharide-based vaccines. *JAMA.* 1996;276:1181-1185.

WHO Position Paper on *H. influenzae* type b conjugate vaccines. *Weekly Epidemiol Rec.* 2006;81:445-452. http://www.who.int/wer/2006/wer8147.pdf.

Comparison Table of *Haemophilus* b Conjugate Vaccines[a]			
Generic name	*H. influenzae* type b conjugate vaccine		
Brand name	*PedvaxHIB*	*ActHIB* (also called *OmniHIB*)	*Hiberix*
Synonyms	PRP-OMP	PRP-T	PRP-T
Manufacturer	Merck	Sanofi Pasteur	GlaxoSmithKline
Viability	Bacterial subunit vaccine, conjugated	Bacterial subunit vaccine, conjugated	Bacterial subunit vaccine, conjugated
Indication	To prevent Hib infection		
Strains	Ross	1482	20,752
Polysaccharide concentration	7.5 mcg/0.5 mL	10 mcg/0.5 mL	10 mcg/0.5 mL
Conjugating protein	Meningococcal outer membrane protein 125 mcg/0.5 mL	Tetanus toxoid 24 mcg/0.5 mL	Tetanus toxoid 25 mcg/0.5 mL
Adjuvant	Aluminum 225 mcg per 0.5 mL as aluminum hydroxyphosphate sulfate	None	None
Preservative	None	None	None
Doseform	Suspension	Powder for solution	Powder for suspension
Diluent	n/a	0.4% NaCl (*Tripedia* DTaP vaccine may also be used as diluent)	Sodium chloride 0.9%
Packaging	0.5 mL vial	One vial of lyophilized vaccine packaged with 0.6 mL vial containing diluent	Vial with 0.7 mL syringe of diluent
Routine storage	2° to 8°C	2° to 8°C	2° to 8°C
Stability	n/a	Discard within 24 hours of reconstitution	Discard within 24 hours of reconstitution
Dosage, route	0.5 mL IM	0.5 mL IM	0.5 mL IM
Standard schedule	2, 4, and 12 to 15 months	2, 4, 6, and 15 to 18 months	Booster dose: 15 months to 4 years
CPT Code	90647	90648	90648

a A fourth Hib vaccine, *ProHIBiT*, is no longer distributed by Sanofi Pasteur. *ProHIBiT* has the disadvantage of being licensed for people 12 months and older, but not licensed for infants.

Recommended Administration Schedules for Conjugated *Haemophilus* Vaccines				
Vaccine formulation	Age at first dose (months)	Primary series	Age sequence	Age for booster dose[a]
PRP-OMP (*PedvaxHIB*, Merck)	2 to 10	2 doses, 2 months apart	—	12 to 15 months[c]
	11 to 14	2 doses, 2 months apart	—	None
	15 to 71	1 dose	—	None
PRP-T[b] (*ActHIB*, Sanofi Pasteur)	2 to 6	3 doses, 2 months apart	2, 4, 6 months	15 to 18 months[c]
	7 to 11	2 doses, 2 months apart		15 to 18 months[c]
	12 to 14	1 dose		15 months[c]
	15 to 59	1 dose		None
PRP-T (*Hiberix*, Glaxo-SmithKline)				Use in multidose series as booster dose at 15 months to 4 years

a Use any of the licensed vaccines for the booster dose, although continuing with the product used for the first dose is generally preferred. Nonetheless, it is not necessary to give more than 3 doses to any child to complete the primary series.
b PRP-T is also available in combination with DTaP vaccine (*TriHIBit*, Sanofi Pasteur). For Hib immunity, the same schedule described here applies; additional DTP, DT, Td, or Tdap doses may be needed for immunity to diphtheria, tetanus, and pertussis.
c At least 2 months after previous dose.

Haemophilus influenzae Type B Conjugate & Hepatitis B Vaccine

Bacterial Vaccines & Toxoids

Name:
Comvax

Manufacturer:
Merck

Synonyms: *Procomvax*

Comparison: This vaccine is a combination of Merck's liquid *PedvaxHIB* and *Recombivax HB* vaccines. Additional information is included in each of the separate monographs.

Immunologic Characteristics

Microorganism: Bacterium, *Haemophilus influenzae* type b, facultative anaerobic gram-negative rod, family Pasteurellaceae. Virus (double-stranded DNA), family Hepadnaviridae.

Viability: Inactivated

Antigenic Form: Hib vaccine consists of capsular polysaccharide fragments, conjugated to a *Neisseria meningitidis* protein carrier. Hepatitis B vaccine consists of the purified hepatitis B surface antigen (HBsAg), a 226-amino acid polypeptide, 22 nm particles possessing antigenic epitopes of the hepatitis B virus surface-coat (S) protein. The S protein contains the principal envelope antigen, HBsAg.

Antigenic Type: Hib vaccine consists of polysaccharide conjugated to protein; the polysaccharide is a polymer of ribose, ribitol, and phosphate (polyribosyl-ribitol-phosphate, PRP). Hepatitis B vaccine consists of a lipoprotein complex containing the S protein.

Strains: Hib strain: Ross; *N. meningitidis* serogroup B strain: B11. Hepatitis B *adw* subtype, *Saccharomyces cerevisiae* strain 2150-2-3.

Use Characteristics

Indications: For active immunization of infants 6 weeks to 15 months of age born of HBsAg-negative mothers who need protection against both *H. influenzae* type b and hepatitis B virus.

Children who have invasive Hib disease when younger than 24 months may not develop adequate anticapsular antibody concentrations and remain at risk of a second episode of disease. Vaccinate these children according to current age, ignoring previous Hib doses. Do not immunize children whose disease occurred at older than 24 months because they are likely to have developed a protective immune response via infection.

Because hepatitis D virus (delta hepatitis, the delta agent) can only infect and cause illness in patients infected with hepatitis B, and because hepatitis D virus requires a coat of hepatitis B surface antigen to become infectious, immunity to hepatitis B also protects against hepatitis D. Hepatitis D virus is a circular RNA-containing virus.

Limitations: Hib vaccines do not protect against *H. influenzae* other than type b strains, nor does vaccination prevent infection with other microorganisms that cause meningitis or septic disease. Do not use Hib vaccine to prevent recurrent sinusitis or bronchitis in adults because *Haemophilus* organisms associated with these conditions are almost always nontypeable, nonencapsulated strains unaffected by anti-Hib antibody.

There is insufficient evidence to suggest that Hib vaccine given immediately after exposure to natural Hib will prevent illness. Cases of Hib disease may occur in vaccine recipients before the onset of the protective effects of the vaccine. Select appropriate antibiotics (eg, cefotaxime, ceftriaxone) to treat active Hib infections.

Vaccination is not effective in preventing secondary cases of invasive Hib disease among unvaccinated patients. Instead, rifampin prophylaxis may be recommended. Rifampin prophylaxis is no longer indicated for management of households where all contacts younger than 48 months are fully immunized. Give rifampin prophylaxis to all members of a household with a case of invasive Hib disease if a child contact younger than 12 months is present who has not yet received the booster or reinforcing dose, regardless of the vaccination status of the child. In households with a child 1 to 3 years of age who is inadequately vaccinated, give all household contacts rifampin after a case of invasive Hib disease in any family member. Nonetheless, the risk of secondary disease is very low among children who complete the primary 2- or 3-dose series.

Some antibody response to the carrier protein occurs, but this vaccine does not protect against *Neisseria* infections.

This vaccine does not contain sufficient HBsAg to protect adults, adolescents, or infants born of HBsAg-positive mothers. Use an appropriate dose of hepatitis B vaccine with HBIG for postexposure prophylaxis and for infants born of HBsAg-positive mothers. For detailed information about postexposure prophylaxis, refer to the HBIG monograph. No hepatitis B vaccine will protect against hepatitis A virus, non-A/non-B hepatitis viruses, hepatitis C virus, hepatitis E virus, or other viruses known to infect the liver.

Hepatitis B has a long incubation period. Hepatitis B vaccination may not prevent hepatitis B infection in individuals who had an unrecognized hepatitis B infection at the time of immunization. Additionally, it may not prevent infection in individuals who do not achieve protective antibody titers.

Contraindications:
Absolute: People with a history of serious allergic reaction to a vaccine component or after a prior dose of this vaccine.
Relative: Any unexplained febrile illness or acute infection is reason for delaying immunization with this vaccine. A mild afebrile illness, such as a mild upper respiratory infection, is not usually reason to defer immunization.

Immunodeficiency: If this vaccine is used in patients deficient in producing antibody, whether caused by genetic defect, illness, or immunosuppressive therapy, the expected immune response may not result.

Hib disease longer than 2 weeks after immunization may reflect an evolving immunodeficient state. Children who manifest disease despite immunization at 15 months of age or older may warrant immunologic evaluation. Similarly, evaluate infants with Hib disease despite immunization or other factors suggesting increased susceptibility to infection.

Elderly: This vaccine is intended for children 6 weeks to 15 months of age.

Carcinogenicity: Hib-hepatitis B vaccine has not been evaluated.

Mutagenicity: Hib-hepatitis B vaccine has not been evaluated for mutagenic potential.

Fertility Impairment: Hib-hepatitis B vaccine has not been evaluated for impairment of fertility.

Pregnancy: Category C. This vaccine is intended for children 6 weeks to 15 months of age.

Lactation: This vaccine is intended for children 6 weeks to 15 months of age.

Children: These vaccines are well tolerated and highly immunogenic in newborns, infants, and children. Maternal antibodies do not interfere with pediatric immunogenicity. This vaccine is intended for children 6 weeks to 15 months of age. Use in children younger than 6 weeks may lead to immune tolerance (impaired ability to respond to subsequent exposure to the PRP antigen).

Adverse Reactions: This bivalent vaccine, like its constituent parts, is generally well tolerated. No serious vaccine-related adverse experiences were observed during clinical trials involving 2,612 infants. Observed reactions did not differ substantially from rates seen with *Pedvax HIB* and *Recombivax-HB* administered at separate sites. Reactions to *Comvax* included these:

Injection-site reactions: Pain or soreness (24% to 35%), erythema more than 1 inch (22% to 27%), swelling or induration more than 1 inch (27% to 30%).

Systemic complaints: Irritability (32% to 57%); somnolence (21% to 50%); fever of 38.3° to 39.4°C (101° to 102.9°F) rectally (11% to 14%); unusual crying (1% to 11%); anorexia (1% to 4%); vomiting, otitis media, fever higher than 39.4°C (103°F) (1% to 3%); diarrhea (1% to 2%); upper respiratory tract infection, rash, rhinorrhea, respiratory congestion, cough, oral candidiasis (1%). Other adverse events after vaccination reported since vaccine licensing include urticaria, erythema multiforme, and seizures. Other adverse events seen with the component vaccines but not with *Comvax* in clinical trials include the following: Anaphylaxis and other forms of hypersensitivity, angioedema, lymphadenopathy, febrile seizures, sterile injection-site abscess, tachycardia, syncope, elevation of liver enzymes, increased erythrocyte sedimentation rate, thrombocytopenia, arthritis, Bell palsy, Guillain-Barré syndrome, agitation, Stevens-Johnson syndrome, alopecia, conjunctivitis, and visual disturbances. Serious events judged not to be related to vaccination included the following: Viral infection, bacterial infection, febrile seizure, asthma, hypoglycemia, bronchiolitis, apnea, reflux esophagitis, and vitreous hemorrhage.

Pharmacologic & Dosing Characteristics

Dosage: Shake product well before withdrawing each dose. Give a 0.5 mL dose to infants 2 to 14 months of age, optimally at 2 months of age. Follow this initial dose with another 0.5 mL 2 months later or as soon as possible thereafter. When the primary 2-dose regimen is completed before 12 months of age, a 0.5 mL booster dose is needed at 12 to 15 months of age but not earlier than 2 months after the second dose. Make the interval between the second and third doses as close to 8 to 11 months as possible for the best response to the hepatitis B vaccine component. *Comvax* may be used to continue or complete immunization schedules begun with separate Hib or hepatitis B vaccines.

Give children 15 months of age or older previously unvaccinated against Hib disease a single 0.5 mL dose of Hib vaccine. Three doses of a vaccine containing HBsAg are required for complete vaccination against hepatitis B, regardless of age.

Route & Site: IM, preferably in the outer aspect of the vastus lateralis (anterolateral thigh). Use a needle sufficiently long to deposit the vaccine into the muscle (eg, ⅞- to 1 inch). Do not administer IV or ID into the gluteal area, or into areas where there may be a nerve trunk.

Documentation Requirements: Federal law requires that (1) the manufacturer and lot number of this vaccine, (2) the dates of its administration, and (3) the name, address, and title of the person administering the vaccine be documented in the recipient's permanent medical record or in a permanent office log.

Certain adverse events must be reported to VAERS (800-822-7967). Refer to Immunization Documents in the Resources section for complete information.

Overdosage: Although few data are available, clinical experience with similar products suggests that the major manifestations of overdosage would be pain and tenderness at the injection site.

Booster Doses: Several doses of Hib and hepatitis B vaccines are needed to complete a primary immunization series. The intervals between the initial doses are preferably 2 months or more, although a 1-month interval is acceptable, if necessary. Booster doses of either vaccine after a primary immunizing series are not recommended.

Missed Doses: Interrupting the recommended schedule or delaying subsequent doses does not require restarting the series. Increasing the interval beyond the recommended timing does not affect the ultimate efficacy of immunization, but waiting does delay adequate protection from infection.

Efficacy: In a study of this Hib vaccine among 3,486 Navajo infants, a 2-dose vaccination series reduced disease incidence by 93% (95% CI, 57% to 98%). After the first dose, 88% and 52% of infants, respectively, developed antibody responses more than 0.15 mcg/mL or more than 1 mcg/mL. After the second dose, those proportions rose to 91% and 60%, respectively.

For hepatitis B vaccine, 98% to 99% of infants, children, and adolescents develop protective levels of anti-HBs after immunization with three 2.5 mcg doses of *Recombivax HB*.

In a multicenter, randomized, open-label study, 882 infants approximately 2 months old, who had not previously received any Hib or hepatitis B vaccine, were assigned to receive a 3-dose regimen of either *Comvax* or *PedvaxHIB* plus *Recombivax HB* at approximately 2, 4, and 12 to 15 months of age. The proportions of evaluable vaccinees developing clinically important levels of anti-PRP (greater than 1 mcg/mL after the second dose, n = 762) and anti-HBs (greater than 10 milliunits/mL after the third dose, n = 750) were similar in children given *Comvax* or concurrent *PedvaxHIB* and *Recombivax HB*. The anti-PRP response after the second dose among infants given *Comvax* was 72% (95% CI, 69% to 76%) greater than 1 mcg/mL with a GMT of 2.5 mcg/mL (95% CI, 2.5 to 2.8), comparable to infants given concurrent vaccinations, which was 76% (95% CI, 70% to 82%) with a GMT of 2.8 mcg/mL (95% CI, 2.2 to 3.5). These responses exceed the response of Native American (Navajo) infants in a previous study of lyophilized *PedvaxHIB* (60% greater than 1 mcg/mL; GMT = 1.43 mcg/mL) associated with a 93% reduction in incidence of invasive Hib disease. The anti-HBs response after the third dose among infants given *Comvax* was 98% at least 10 milliunits/mL (95% CI, 97%, 99%) with a GMT of 4,468 (95% CI, 3,786 to 5,271) compared with 100% (95% CI, 98%, 100%) with a GMT of 6,944 (95% CI, 5,556, 8,679) among infants given *Comvax* or concurrent vaccinations. Although the difference in anti-HBs GMT is statistically significant ($P = 0.011$), both values are much greater than the level of 10 milliunits/mL previously established as marking a protective response to hepatitis B. These GMTs are higher than those observed in young infants who received the currently licensed 5 mcg regimen of *Recombivax HB* administered on the standard 0, 1, and 6-month schedule (GMT = 1,360 milliunits/mL). Two clinical studies assessed antibody responses to a 3-dose series of *Comvax* in 128 evaluable infants previously given a birth dose of hepatitis B vaccine. The antibody responses were clinically comparable to those observed in the pivotal trial of *Comvax*.

Onset: For Hib vaccine, most recipients are protected within 1 week after the dose at 2 months of age. For hepatitis B vaccine, 70% to 80% of recipients are protected after the second dose and more than 95% after the third dose.

Duration: Hib antibody concentrations more than 1 mcg/mL correlate with prolonged protection from disease, generally implying several years of protection. Duration of protection against hepatitis B is undetermined but apparently lasts more than 5 to 7 years in most healthy recipients. Several studies suggest that clinical protection may persist even after circulating anti-HBs antibodies can no longer be detected.

Protective Level: Hib antibody concentrations 0.15 mcg/mL or more correlate with clinical protection from disease. An anti-HBs titer at least 10 milliunits/mL or 10 sample ratio units (SRU) by RIA is considered protective. In some studies, antibody titers among successful vaccinees have fallen below the protective level, yet clinical protection has continued. In some cases, vaccinees developed anti-HBc antibodies, indicative of viral infection, without becoming clinically ill.

Mechanism: Induction of specific protective antibodies against type b strains of *H. influenzae* and hepatitis B virus. Hib vaccination may decrease nasopharyngeal colonization and produce lower rates of acquisition of colonization by unvaccinated infants. Linking Hib polysaccharides to a protein can convert the thymus-independent polysaccharide to a thymus-dependent antigen and result in an enhanced antibody response and immunologic memory.

Drug Interactions: As with all inactivated vaccines, administration of Hib-hepatitis B vaccine to patients receiving immunosuppressant drugs (eg, high-dose corticosteroids) or radiation therapy may result in an insufficient response to immunization. Patients may remain susceptible despite immunization.

Hib-hepatitis B vaccine does not impair immunogenicity of DTwP, DTaP, e-IPV, MMR, or varicella vaccine. Rates of adverse reactions when Hib-hepatitis B vaccine was administered concurrently with DTP and e-IPV were comparable with rates when DTP was given alone. Meningococcal and pneumococcal vaccines may be safely and effectively administered simultaneously at separate injection sites.

Inactivated vaccines are not generally affected by circulating antibodies or administration of exogenous antibodies. Vaccination may occur at any time before or after antibody administration. There is no significant interaction between hepatitis B vaccines and HBIG, if administered at separate sites. Maternal antibodies do not interfere with immunogenicity in newborn infants.

Concurrent vaccination against hepatitis B and yellow fever viruses in 1 study reduced the antibody titer otherwise expected from yellow fever vaccine. Separate these vaccines by 1 month if possible.

As with other drugs administered by IM injection, give Hib-hepatitis B vaccine with caution to patients receiving anticoagulant therapy.

Lab Interference: Antigenuria has been detected following administration of Hib vaccines; therefore, antigen detection (eg, with latex agglutination kits) may have no diagnostic value in suspected Hib disease within 30 days after immunization with *PedvaxHIB* or, presumably, *Comvax*. False-positive latex agglutination tests of cerebrospinal fluid have also been reported 1 to 21 days following Hib vaccination.

Pharmaceutical Characteristics

Concentration: 7.5 mcg Hib polysaccharide and 5 mcg hepatitis B surface antigen per 0.5 mL.

Quality Assay:

Hib: Assay of PRP by HPLC. Coupling to the OMP protein is confirmed by analysis of components of the conjugate following chemical treatment that yields a unique amino acid [S-(carboxymethyl)-homocysteine].

Hepatitis B: Potency measured relative to a standard by an in vitro immunoassay

Packaging: Box of 10 single-dose vials (00006-4898-00)

Doseform: Suspension

Appearance: A fine, white deposit with clear, colorless supernatant may develop during storage. When shaken, product forms a slightly opaque, white suspension.

Solvent: 0.9% sodium chloride

Adjuvant: 125 mcg *N. meningitidis* OMP and 225 mcg aluminum as aluminum hydroxyphosphate sulfate per 0.5 mL

Preservative: None

Allergens: The package stopper contains dry natural rubber (a latex derivative).

Excipients: 35 mcg/0.5 mL sodium borate decahydrate, no more than 1% yeast protein but no detectable yeast DNA. No more than 0.0004% w/v residual formaldehyde.

pH: Data not provided

Shelf Life: Expires within 36 months

Storage/Stability: Store at 2° to 8°C (35° to 46°F). Discard frozen vaccine. Contact the manufacturer regarding exposure to prolonged room temperate or elevated temperatures. Shipped in an insulated container at a temperature between 2° to 8°C (35° to 46°F).

Production Process:

Hib: Polysaccharide purified by a series of phenol extractions, selective ethanol precipitations, enzyme digestion, and diafiltration. OMPC is purified by a series of detergent extraction, centrifugation, diafiltration, and sterile filtration steps. Hib polysaccharides are covalently bound to an OMP complex of *N. meningitidis* serogroup B. Each molecule consists of polysaccharides, a bigeneric thioether spacer, and the meningococcal B OMP protein. After conjugation, the aqueous bulk antigen is then adsorbed onto aluminum hydroxyphosphate sulfate.

Hepatitis B: DNA sequence of Dane particles obtained using endogenous DNA-polymerase activity. Gene derived from a hybrid *Escherichia coli* clone; 19 amino acids cloned at aminoterminus of hepatitis B surface antigen. Gene cloned into *Saccharomyces cerevisiae*. The 22 nm HBsAg particles are released from the yeast cells by mechanical cell disruption and detergent extraction, then purified by a series of physical and chemical methods, including ion and hydrophobic-interaction chromatography and diafiltration. Purified protein is treated in phosphate buffer with formaldehyde, then coprecipitated with potassium aluminum sulfate, to form bulk vaccine adjuvanted with amorphous aluminum hydroxyphosphate sulfate. The antigen is uniformly nonglycosylated.

Bivalent vaccine: After all the component vaccines are adsorbed onto aluminum hydroxyphosphate sulfate, they are combined.

Media:

Hib: Complex fermentation media, phenol inactivated, primarily consisting of yeast extract, nicotinamide adenine dinucleotide, hemin chloride, soy peptone, dextrose, and mineral salts. The *N. meningitidis* bacteria are grown in a medium primarily consisting of yeast extract, amino acids, and mineral salts.

Hepatitis B: S. cerevisiae, grown in a complex fermentation medium consisting of yeast extract, soy peptone, dextrose, amino acids, and mineral salts.

Disease Epidemiology

See individual monographs.

Other Information

Perspective: See individual monographs.

First Licensed: October 2, 1996

National Policy: ACIP. Updated recommendations for use of H. influenzae type b (Hib) vaccine: Reinstatement of the booster dose at ages 12-15 months. *MMWR*. 2009;58:673-674.

CDC. FDA approval for infants of a *H. influenzae* type b conjugate and hepatitis B (recombinant) combined vaccine. *MMWR*. 1997;46:107-109.

H. *influenzae* type b and Hepatitis B Vaccine Summary Table	
Generic name	*H. influenzae* type b conjugate vaccine and hepatitis B vaccine
Brand name	*Comvax*
Manufacturer	Merck
Viability	Bacterial and viral subunit vaccines
Indication	To prevent infection with *H. influenzae* type b and hepatitis B virus
Components	Hib conjugate vaccine and HBsAg vaccine
Concentration	Hib 7.5 mcg and 5 mcg HBsAg per 0.5 mL
Conjugating protein	Meningococcal outer membrane protein (OMP) 125 mcg/0.5 mL
Adjuvant	225 mcg aluminum as aluminum hydroxyphosphate sulfate per 0.5 mL
Preservative	None
Doseform	Suspension
Packaging	Single-dose vials
Routine storage	2° to 8°C
Dosage, route	0.5 mL IM
Standard schedule	When both *H. influenzae* type b vaccine and hepatitis B vaccines are indicated

Haemophilus influenzae Type B & Meningococcal Groups C and Y Conjugate Vaccine (Hib-Men CY)

Bacterial Vaccines & Toxoids

Name:
Menhibrix
Synonyms: Hib-Men CY

Manufacturer:
GlaxoSmithKline

Immunologic Characteristics

Microorganism: Bacteria, *Haemophilus influenzae* type b (Hib) and *Neisseria meningitidis* serogroups C and Y

Viability: Inactivated

Antigenic Form: Capsular polysaccharide fragments individually conjugated to tetanus toxoid

Antigenic Type: Polysaccharides linked to protein. *Haemophilus* b capsular polysaccharide (polyribosyl-ribitol-phosphate [PRP]) and *N. meningitidis* serogroups C and Y capsular polysaccharide antigens.

Strains: Hib strain 20,752. Meningococcal strains not specified.

Use Characteristics

Indications: To prevent invasive disease caused by Hib and *N. meningitidis* serogroups C and Y in children 6 weeks through 18 months of age.

Limitations: Meningococcal serogroup C and Y vaccines do not protect against other serogroups of *N. meningitidis*. Hib vaccines do not protect against *H. influenzae* strains other than type b, nor does vaccination prevent infection with other microorganisms that cause meningitis or septic disease. Do not use Hib vaccine to prevent recurrent sinusitis or bronchitis in adults because *Haemophilus* organisms associated with these conditions are almost always nontypeable, nonencapsulated strains unaffected by anti-Hib antibody. Use of Hib-Men CY vaccine does not substitute for routine tetanus immunization. Select appropriate antibiotics (eg, cefotaxime, ceftriaxone) to treat active Hib infections.

Contraindications: Severe allergic reaction (eg, anaphylaxis) after a previous dose of any meningococcal-, Hib-, or tetanus toxoid–containing vaccine or allergy to any component of this vaccine.

Immunodeficiency: Immunosuppressive therapies, including irradiation, antimetabolites, alkylating agents, cytotoxic drugs, and corticosteroids (used in higher than physiologic doses), may reduce the immune response to Hib-Men CY vaccine. Safety and effectiveness in immunosuppressed children have not been evaluated.

Elderly: No specific information is available about use of Hib-Men CY vaccine in the elderly population.

Carcinogenicity: Hib-Men CY vaccine has not been evaluated for carcinogenic potential.

Mutagenicity: Hib-Men CY vaccine has not been evaluated for mutagenic potential.

Fertility Impairment: Hib-Men CY vaccine has not been evaluated for impairment of fertility.

Pregnancy: Category C. Generally, most IgG passage across the placenta occurs during the third trimester. Problems in humans have not been documented and are unlikely.

Lactation: It is not known if Hib-Men CY vaccine crosses into human breast milk. Problems in humans have not been documented and are unlikely.

Children: Safety and effectiveness of Hib-Men CY vaccine in children younger than 6 weeks of age and in children 19 months to 16 years of age have not been established.

145

Haemophilus influenzae Type B & Meningococcal Groups C and Y Conjugate Vaccine (Hib-Men CY)

Adverse Reactions: Data on solicited adverse events were collected by parents or guardians using standardized forms for 4 consecutive days after vaccination with Hib-Men CY or Hib (control) vaccines (ie, day of vaccination and next 3 days). Children were monitored for unsolicited adverse events that occurred in the 31-day period after vaccination and for serious adverse events, new-onset chronic disease, rash, and conditions prompting emergency department visits or physician office visits during the entire study period (6 months after the last vaccine administered).

Solicited adverse events: The reported frequencies of solicited local and systemic adverse events from US participants in Study 009/010 are presented in the following table.

Percentage of US Children From Study 009/010 With Solicited Local and General Adverse Events Within 4 Days of Vaccination[a] With Hib-Men CY Vaccine or Hib Conjugate Vaccine (Total Vaccinated Cohort)[b]								
	Hib-Men CY vaccine[c]				Hib conjugate vaccine[c,d]			
	Dose 1	Dose 2	Dose 3	Dose 4	Dose 1	Dose 2	Dose 3	Dose 4
Local[e]								
n[f]	2,009	1,874	1,725	1,533	659	612	569	492
Pain, any	46.2%	44.6%	41.4%	42.1%	61.6%	52.8%	49.9%	50.4%
Pain, grade 3[g]	3.7%	3.3%	2.3%	1.6%	11.4%	5.1%	3%	5.3%
Redness, any	20.6%	31%	35.5%	34.6%	27.9%	33.7%	42.2%	46.7%
Redness, > 30 mm	0.1%	0.3%	0.1%	0.7%	1.8%	0.3%	0.4%	1.2%
Swelling, any	14.7%	20.4%	23.8%	25.4%	20.5%	20.8%	28.6%	31.7%
Swelling, > 30 mm	0.5%	0.3%	0.3%	0.6%	1.5%	0.2%	0.4%	0.8%
Systemic								
n	2,008 to 2,009	1,871	1,723	1,535 to 1,536	659	609 to 610	569	493 to 494
Irritability	67.5%	70.8%	65.8%	62.1%	76.9%	75.1%	65.4%	66.1%
Irritability, grade 3[h]	3.7%	4.8%	3.3%	2.5%	7.4%	5.6%	4.2%	4.3%
Drowsiness, any	62.8%	57.7%	49.5%	48.7%	66.9%	61.8%	52.4%	48.5%
Drowsiness, grade 3	2.7%	3.2%	1.7%	2.1%	2.7%	2.6%	1.4%	2%
Loss of appetite, any	33.8%	32.1%	30.1%	32.1%	37.6%	33.6%	30.2%	32.5%
Loss of appetite, grade 3	0.5%	0.7%	0.5%	1.1%	0.3%	0.7%	1.1%	2.2%
Fever ≥ 100.4°F	18.9%	25.9%	23%	11%	21.4%	28.2%	23.7%	12.6%
Fever ≥ 102.2°F	1.1%	1.9%	3.2%	1.5%	0.9%	2.6%	2.8%	2%
Fever > 104°F	0%	0.1%	0.3%	0.3%	0%	0%	0.4%	0.2%

a Within 4 days of vaccination, defined as day of vaccination and the next 3 days.
b Total vaccinated cohort = all participants who received at least 1 dose of either vaccine.
c Coadministered with DTaP-Hep B-IPV and PCV7 at doses 1, 2, and 3 and PCV7, MMR, and varicella vaccines at dose 4.
d US-licensed monovalent Hib conjugate vaccine manufactured by Sanofi Pasteur for doses 1, 2, and 3 (PRP-T) and by Merck for dose 4 (PRP-OMP).
e Local reactions at the injection site for Hib-Men CY vaccine or Hib conjugate vaccine.
f n = number of children who completed the symptom sheet for a given symptom at the specified dose.
g Cried when limb was moved, or spontaneously painful.
h Crying that could not be comforted or that prevented normal daily activities.

Unsolicited adverse events: Among children who received Hib-Men CY vaccine or Hib control vaccine coadministered with US-licensed vaccines at 2, 4, 6, and 12 to 15 months of age, the incidence of unsolicited adverse events reported within the 31-day period following study vaccination (doses 1, 2, and 3) was comparable between Hib-Men CY vaccine (62%) and PRP-T (63%). The incidence of unsolicited adverse events reported within the 31-day period following dose 4 was also comparable between Hib-Men CY vaccine (43%) and PRP-OMP (41%).

Serious adverse events: Following doses 1, 2, and 3, 1.8% of children who received Hib-Men CY vaccine and 2.1% of children who received PRP-T reported at least one serious adverse event within the 31-day period. Up to 6 months following the last vaccine administered (doses 1, 2, and 3) or until administration of dose 4, 4.8% of children who received Hib-Men CY vaccine and 5% of children in the PRP-T group reported at least one serious adverse event. Following dose 4, 0.5% of children who received Hib-Men CY vaccine and 0.5% of children who received PRP-OMP reported at least one serious adverse event within the 31-day period. Up to 6 months following the last vaccine administered (dose 4), 2.5% of children who received Hib-Men CY vaccine and 2% of children who received PRP-OMP reported at least one serious adverse event.

Guillain-Barré syndrome: If Guillain-Barré syndrome has occurred within 6 weeks of receipt of a prior vaccine containing tetanus toxoid, consider the potential benefits and possible risks of giving Hib-Men CY vaccine.

Syncope: Syncope (fainting) can occur in association with administration of injectable vaccines, including Hib-Men CY vaccine. Syncope can be accompanied by transient neurological signs, such as visual disturbance, paresthesia, and tonic-clonic limb movements. Use procedures to avoid falling injury and to restore cerebral perfusion after syncope.

Apnea in premature infants: Apnea following intramuscular (IM) vaccination has been observed in some infants born prematurely. Base decisions regarding when to administer an IM vaccine, including Hib-Men CY vaccine, to infants born prematurely on the infant's medical status, as well as the potential benefits and possible risks of vaccination.

Consultation: Clinicians involved with meningococcal outbreak situations should consult with their state or local public health department or call the Centers for Disease Control and Prevention (CDC).

Pharmacologic & Dosing Characteristics

Dosage: 0.5 mL in a 4-dose series, with each dose given at 2, 4, 6, and 12 through 15 months of age. The first dose may be given as early as 6 weeks of age. The fourth dose may be given as late as 18 months of age.

Route & Site: IM. Do not administer intravenously, intradermally, or subcutaneously. For most infants younger than 1 year, the anterolateral aspect of the thigh is preferred. In older children, the deltoid muscle is usually large enough for IM injection.

Documentation Requirements: Federal law requires that the following information be documented in the recipient's permanent medical record or in a permanent office log: (1) the manufacturer and lot number of this vaccine, (2) the date of administration, and (3) the name, address, and title of the person administering the vaccine.

Certain adverse events must be reported to the Vaccine Adverse Event Reporting System (VAERS) (1-800-822-7967). Refer to immunization documents in the Resources section.

Overdosage: Although few data are available, clinical experience with similar products suggests that the major manifestations of overdosage would be pain and tenderness at the injection site.

Missed Doses: Interrupting the recommended schedule or delaying subsequent doses does not require restarting the series.

Haemophilus influenzae Type B & Meningococcal Groups C and Y Conjugate Vaccine (Hib-Men CY)

Efficacy: In Study 009/0105, the immune response to Hib-Men CY vaccine and control vaccines was evaluated in a subset of US participants. In this clinical study, Hib-Men CY vaccine and Hib control vaccines were coadministered with routinely recommended US-licensed vaccines. Among participants in the according-to-protocol immunogenicity cohort for both vaccine groups combined, 47% were female and 81% were white, 8% were black, 4% were Hispanic, 1% was Asian, and 6% were of other racial/ethnic groups. Study objectives included evaluation of *N. meningitidis* serogroups C (MenC) and Y (MenY), as measured by serum bactericidal assay using human complement (hSBA) and antibodies to PRP as measured by enzyme-linked immunosorbent assay (ELISA) in sera obtained approximately 1 month (range, 21 to 48 days) after dose 3 of Hib-Men CY vaccine or PRP-T, and approximately 6 weeks (range, 35 to 56 days) after dose 4 of Hib-Men CY vaccine or PRP-OMP. The hSBA-MenC and hSBA-MenY geometric mean antibody titers (GMTs) and the percentage of children with hSBA-MenC and hSBA-MenY levels of 1:8 or greater are presented in the following table. Anti-PRP geometric mean antibody concentrations (GMCs) and the percentage of children with anti-PRP levels of 0.15 mcg/mL or greater and 1 mcg/mL or greater are presented subsequently.

Bactericidal Antibody Responses Following Hib-Men CY Vaccine (1 Month After Dose 3 and 6 Weeks After Dose 4) in US Children Vaccinated at 2, 4, 6, and 12 to 15 Months of Age (According-to-Protocol Cohort for Immunogenicity)		
	Hib-Men CY vaccine (postdose 3)	Hib-Men CY vaccine (postdose 4)
hSBA-MenC	n^a = 491	n = 331
Percentage ≥ 1:8 (95% CI)[b]	98.8 (97.4, 99.6)	98.5[c] (96.5, 99.5)
GMT (95% CI)	968 (864, 1,084)	2,040 (1,746, 2,383)
hSBA-MenY	n = 481	n = 342
Percentage ≥ 1:8 (95% CI)	95.8 (93.7, 97.4)	98.8[c] (97, 99.7)
GMT (95% CI)	237 (206, 272)	1,390 (1,205, 1,602)

a n = number of US children eligible for inclusion in the according-to-protocol immunogenicity cohort for whom serological results were available for the postdose 3 and postdose 4 immunological evaluations.
b CI = confidence interval.
c Acceptance criteria were met (lower limit of 95% CI for the percentage of children with hSBA-MenC and hSBA-MenY titers ≥ 1:8 ≥ 90% following 4 doses).

Comparison of anti-PRP Responses Following Hib-Men CY Vaccine or Hib Conjugate Vaccine[a] (1 Month After Dose 3 and 6 Weeks After Dose 4) in US Children Vaccinated at 2, 4, 6, and 12 to 15 Months of Age (According-to-Protocol Cohort for Immunogenicity)				
	Postdose 3		Postdose 4	
	Hib-Men CY vaccine	PRP-T	Hib-Men CY vaccine	PRP-OMP
Anti-PRP[b]	n^c = 518	n = 171	n = 361	n = 126
Percentage ≥ 0.15 mcg/mL (95% CI)	100 (99.3, 100)	98.2 (95, 99.6)	100 (99, 100)	100 (97.1, 100)
Percentage ≥ 1 mcg/mL (95% CI)	96.3[d] (94.3, 97.8)	91.2 (85.9, 95)	99.2[d] (97.6, 99.8)	99.2 (95.7, 100)

Haemophilus influenzae Type B & Meningococcal Groups C and Y Conjugate Vaccine (Hib-Men CY)

Comparison of anti-PRP Responses Following Hib-Men CY Vaccine or Hib Conjugate Vaccine[a] (1 Month After Dose 3 and 6 Weeks After Dose 4) in US Children Vaccinated at 2, 4, 6, and 12 to 15 Months of Age (According-to-Protocol Cohort for Immunogenicity)				
	Postdose 3		Postdose 4	
	Hib-Men CY vaccine	PRP-T	Hib-Men CY vaccine	PRP-OMP
GMC (mcg/mL)	11	6.5	34.9	20.2
(95% CI)	(10, 12.1)	(5.3, 7.9)	(30.7, 39.6)	(16.4, 24.9)

a US-licensed monovalent *Haemophilus* b conjugate vaccine for doses 1, 2, and 3 (PRP-T), and for dose 4 (PRP-OMP).

b Anti-PRP = antibody concentrations to *H. influenzae* capsular polysaccharide.

c n = number of US children eligible for inclusion in the according-to-protocol immunogenicity cohort for whom serological results were available for the postdose 3 and postdose 4 immunological evaluations.

d Noninferiority was demonstrated (lower limit of 95% CI on the group difference of Hib-Men CY vaccine minus *Haemophilus* b conjugate vaccine ≥ −10%).

Mechanism:

Hib: Specific levels of anti-PRP antibodies correlate with protection against invasive Hib disease. Based on passive antibody studies and a clinical efficacy study with unconjugated Hib polysaccharide vaccine, an anti-PRP concentration of 0.15 mcg/mL has been accepted as a minimal protective level. Data from an efficacy study with unconjugated Hib polysaccharide vaccine indicate that an anti-PRP concentration of 1 mcg/mL or greater predicts protection through at least 1 year. These antibody levels have been used to evaluate the effectiveness of Hib-containing vaccines, including Hib-Men CY vaccine.

Meningococcal: The presence of bactericidal anticapsular meningococcal antibodies has been associated with protection from invasive meningococcal disease. Hib-Men CY vaccine induces production of bactericidal antibodies specific to the capsular polysaccharides of serogroups C and Y.

Drug Interactions: In clinical studies, Hib-Men CY vaccine was coadministered with routinely recommended pediatric US-licensed vaccines (DTaP-Hep B-IPV, PCV7, MMR, varicella) without evidence of reduced antibody responses. Data are insufficient to evaluate potential interference when a fourth PCV7 dose is coadministered with Hib-Men CY vaccine at 12 to 15 months of age.

Lab Interference: *Haemophilus* b capsular polysaccharide derived from *Haemophilus* b conjugate vaccines has been detected in the urine of some vaccinees. Urine antigen detection may not have a diagnostic value in suspected disease due to Hib within 1 to 2 weeks after receipt of a Hib-containing vaccine, including Hib-Men CY vaccine.

Pharmaceutical Characteristics

Concentration: After reconstitution, each 0.5 mL dose contains 5 mcg of *N. meningitidis* serogroup C capsular polysaccharide conjugated to approximately 5 mcg of tetanus toxoid, 5 mcg of *N. meningitidis* serogroup Y capsular polysaccharide conjugated to approximately 6.5 mcg of tetanus toxoid, and 2.5 mcg of *Haemophilus* b capsular polysaccharide conjugated to approximately 6.25 mcg of tetanus toxoid.

Packaging: Single-dose vials of lyophilized vaccine, with 0.85 mL vials of saline diluent (packaged without syringes or needles). Package of 10 doses (NDC#: 58160-0801-11). Vial of lyophilized vaccine (58160-0809-01), package of 10 vials (58160-0809-05). Vial of saline diluent (58160-0813-01), package of 10 vials (58160-0813-05).

Doseform: Powder to yield solution

Appearance: Powder yielding clear and colorless solution

Haemophilus influenzae Type B & Meningococcal Groups C and Y Conjugate Vaccine (Hib-Men CY)

Diluent:
For reconstitution: Sodium chloride 0.9%

Adjuvant: None

Preservative: None

Allergens: The vial stoppers do not contain latex.

Excipients: Each dose contains *Tris* (trometamol)-hydrochloride 96.8 mcg, sucrose 12.6 mg, and residual formaldehyde 0.72 mcg or less.

pH: Not described

Shelf Life: Data not provided.

Storage/Stability: Store lyophilized vaccine at 2° to 8°C (36° to 46°F). Protect vials from light. Diluent may be stored refrigerated or at room temperature. Discard diluent if frozen. Contact the manufacturer regarding exposure to freezing or elevated temperatures. Shipping data not provided.

Handling: After reconstitution, administer Hib-Men CY vaccine immediately. Discard vaccine if frozen.

Production Process: The PRP is a high molecular weight polymer prepared from Hib strain 20,752 grown in a synthetic medium that undergoes heat inactivation and purification. *N. meningitidis* C strain and Y strain are grown in semisynthetic media and undergo heat inactivation and purification. The tetanus toxin, prepared from *Clostridium tetani* grown in a semisynthetic medium, is detoxified with formaldehyde and purified. Each capsular polysaccharide is individually covalently bound to the inactivated tetanus toxoid. After purification, the conjugate is lyophilized in the presence of sucrose as a stabilizer.

Media:
Hib: Synthetic medium
Meningococcal: Semisynthetic media
Clostridium tetani: Semisynthetic medium

Disease Epidemiology

See Hib and Meningococcal monographs.

Other Information

Perspective: See Hib and Meningococcal monographs.
First Licensed: June 14, 2012

Haemophilus influenzae Type B & Meningococcal Groups C and Y Conjugate Vaccine (Hib-Men CY)

Hib-Men CY Vaccine Summary Table	
Generic name	*Haemophilus influenzae* type b & meningococcal CY conjugate vaccine
Brand name	*Menhibrix*
Synonyms	Hib-Men CY
Manufacturer	GlaxoSmithKline
Viability	Bacterial subunit vaccine
Indication	To prevent invasive disease caused by Hib and *N. meningitidis* serogroups C and Y in children 6 weeks through 18 months of age.
Components	Hib and *N. meningitidis* serogroups C and Y
Concentration	Each 0.5 mL dose contains 5 mcg of *N meningitidis* serogroup C capsular polysaccharide, 5 mcg of *N. meningitidis* serogroup Y capsular polysaccharide, and 2.5 mcg of *Haemophilus* b capsular polysaccharide
Conjugating protein	Tetanus toxoid 17.25 mcg per 0.5 mL dose
Adjuvant	None
Preservative	None
Production medium	Synthetic and semisynthetic media
Doseform	Powder yielding solution
Diluent	Sodium chloride 0.9%
Packaging	Single-dose vials
Routine storage	2° to 8°C (36° to 46°F)
Stability	Administer immediately after reconstitution
Dosage, route	0.5 mL IM
Standard schedule	Four doses given at 2, 4, 6, and 12 through 15 months of age

Meningococcal Vaccines

Bacterial Vaccines & Toxoids

Comparison Table of Meningococcal Vaccines			
Generic name	Meningococcal Polysaccharide Vaccine A/C/Y/W-135	Meningococcal Conjugate Vaccine A/C/Y/W-135	Meningococcal Conjugate Vaccine A/C/Y/W-135
Brand name	*Menomume-A/C/Y/W-135*	*Menactra*	*Menveo*
Synonyms	MENps, MPSV4, MPV	MENcn, MCV4	MENcn, MCV4
Manufacturer	Sanofi Pasteur	Sanofi Pasteur	Novartis
Viability	Bacterial subunit vaccine, polysaccharide	Bacterial subunit vaccine, protein-conjugated	Bacterial subunit vaccine, protein-conjugated
Indications	People 2 years and older needing protection, principally military basic trainees, outbreak settings, college students	People 9 months to 55 years needing protection, principally military basic trainees, outbreak settings, adolescents 11 to 18 years or college students	People 2 to 55 years of age needing protection, principally military basic trainees, outbreak settings, adolescents 11 to 18 years of age, or college students.
Components	Combination of 4 polysaccharide antigens	Combination of 4 polysaccharide antigens conjugated to diphtheria toxoid proteins	Combination of 4 polysaccharide antigens conjugated to diphtheria CRM197 protein
Serogroup valence	Four: A, C, Y, W-135	Four: A, C, Y, W-135	Four: A, C, Y, W-135
Concentration	50 mcg of each serogroup polysaccharide per 0.5 mL	4 mcg of each serogroup polysaccharide per 0.5 mL	10 mcg of serogroup A and 5 mcg each of serogroups C, Y, and W-135 polysaccharides per 0.5 mL
Conjugating protein	None	≈ 48 mg of diphtheria toxoid protein per 0.5 mL	Diphtheria CRM197 protein 32.7 to 64.1 mcg per 0.5 mL
Adjuvant	None	None	None
Preservative	None in single-dose vials; thimerosal in 10-dose vials	None	None
Doseform	Powder yielding solution	Solution	Powder and liquid to yield composite solution
Diluent	Sterile water for injection	n/a	Men CYW-135 liquid
Solvent	n/a	Sodium phosphate-buffered saline solution	n/a
Packaging	Single-dose, 10-dose vials	Single-dose vials	Package of 5 vials of lyophilized MenA powder and 5 vials of MenCYW-135 liquid
Routine storage	2° to 8°C	2° to 8°C	2° to 8°C
Stability	Discard multidose vial within 35 days of reconstitution	n/a	Discard within 8 hours after reconstitution
Dosage, route	0.5 mL subcutaneous	0.5 mL intramuscular	0.5 mL intramuscular
Standard schedule	Single dose	9 to 23 months of age: Two doses, 3 months apart 2 to 55 years of age: Single dose	Single dose
CPT Code	90733	90734	90734

Meningococcal Polysaccharide Vaccine, Groups A, C, Y, and W-135

Bacterial Vaccines & Toxoids

Name:
Menomune-A/C/Y/W-135

Manufacturer:
Sanofi Pasteur

Synonyms: VISI abbreviation: MENps, MGC, MPSV4, MPV

Immunologic Characteristics

Microorganism: Bacterium, *Neisseria meningitidis*, aerobic gram-negative diplococci, family Neisseriaceae

Viability: Inactivated

Antigenic Form: Capsular polysaccharide fragments

Antigenic Type: Polysaccharide mixture. The group A polysaccharide consists of a polymer of N-acetyl-O-acetyl mannosamine phosphate. The group C polysaccharide is primarily N-acetyl-O-acetylneuraminic acid (partly O-acetylated repeating units of sialic acid). The group Y polysaccharide consists of partly O-acetylated alternating units of sialic acid and D-glucose. The group W-135 polysaccharide consists of partly O-acetylated alternating units of sialic acid and D-galactose. Immunogenicity is correlated with molecular weight; the group C antigen weighs more than 100 kilodaltons.

Strains: A-1, C-11, 6306Y, W-135-6308

Use Characteristics

Indications: Induction of active immunity against select serogroups of *N. meningitidis*. Patients warranting immunization include military recruits during basic training, those with anatomic or functional asplenia (because of their increased risk of developing meningococcal disease of high severity), and travelers to countries with epidemic meningococcal disease, particularly travelers who will have prolonged contact with the local populace (eg, travelers to sub-Saharan Africa, pilgrims to the Hajj or Umrah in Saudi Arabia). In addition, consider this vaccine for household or institutional contacts of patients with meningococcal disease as an adjunct to antibiotic chemotherapy; medical, research, industrial, and laboratory personnel at risk of aerosol exposure to meningococcal disease; and immunosuppressed patients, including those with defects in the terminal common complement pathway (C3, C5 to C9) or deficiency of properdin.

Other children, adolescents, and adults who may benefit from meningococcal vaccine include patients with other diseases associated with immune suppression (eg, HIV, *Streptococcus pneumoniae*). Whenever possible, vaccinate before immunosuppression occurs.

To reduce the risk of meningococcal disease among college students, especially freshman students and those living in dormitories or other close conditions.

Meningococcal vaccine is used to quell certain meningococcal serogroup C outbreaks. The group to be offered vaccine may follow organizational lines (eg, students and faculty of a school) or demographic patterns (eg, people 2 to 19 or 2 to 29 years of age in a defined locale). It may be appropriate to limit the group offered vaccine to those with the highest attack rate.

Limitations: Meningococcal vaccine is not as likely to be effective in children younger than 2 years because of its polysaccharide nature. This vaccine is not effective against serogroup B, another form of meningococcal infection. Select appropriate antibiotics to treat active infections (eg, rifampin, ciprofloxacin, ceftriaxone). Because of the delay in developing protec-

153

tive antibody titers, vaccine does not substitute for chemoprophylaxis in individuals exposed to meningococcal disease.

Contraindications:

Absolute: People with a history of serious allergic reaction to a vaccine component or after a prior dose of this vaccine.

Relative: Defer immunization during the course of any acute illness.

Immunodeficiency: Patients receiving immunosuppressive therapy or with other immunodeficiencies may have diminished antibody response to active immunization. Nonetheless, this vaccine is indicated for asplenic patients.

Elderly: No specific information is available about geriatric use of meningococcal vaccine.

Pregnancy: Category C. Use only if clearly needed. The manufacturer recommends that this vaccine should not be used in pregnant women, especially in the first trimester, on theoretical grounds. The use of this vaccine in many pregnant women during an epidemic in Brazil resulted in no attributable adverse reproductive effects. Vaccinate pregnant women if a substantial risk of infection exists. High antibody levels develop in maternal and umbilical cord blood after vaccination during pregnancy. Most IgG crosses the placenta during the third trimester. Problems have not been documented and are unlikely. Antibody levels in the infants decreased during the first few months after birth.

Lactation: Problems have not been documented and are unlikely.

Children: Not routinely recommended for children younger than 2 years because they are unlikely to develop an adequate antibody response. Children 3 to 24 months of age may be vaccinated to induce short-term protection against serogroup A meningococcal disease (use 2 doses 3 months apart for children 3 to 18 months of age). Serogroup A polysaccharide induces antibody in some children as young as 3 months of age, although a response comparable to that seen in adults is not achieved until 4 or 5 years of age. Serogroup A and C vaccines demonstrate clinical efficacies of 85% to 100% in older children and are useful in controlling epidemics. Serogroup Y and W-135 vaccines are safe in children older than 2 years and induce bactericidal antibodies.

Adverse Reactions: Reactions to vaccination are generally mild and infrequent, consisting of localized erythema lasting 1 to 2 days. Up to 2% of young children develop fever transiently after vaccination. Reported side effects included: Headache (1% to 5%), malaise (less than 3%), chills (no more than 2.5%), temperature higher than 37.2°C (99°F; 1% to 3%), and injection-site reactions, including pain (17% to 43%), redness (1% to 33%), and induration (5% to 13%).

Consultation: Clinicians involved with outbreak situations should consult with their state or local public health departments or call the National Immunization Program ([800] 232-2522).

Pharmacologic & Dosing Characteristics

Dosage: 0.5 mL as a single dose

Route & Site: Subcutaneously. Do not inject ID, IM, or IV.

Subsequent Doses: For children 3 to 18 months of age, give 2 doses 3 months apart. Revaccination may be indicated, particularly in children at high risk who were first immunized at younger than 4 years. Revaccinate such children after 2 or 3 years if they remain at high risk. Subsequent doses will reinstate the primary immune response, but will not evoke an accelerated booster response. Although the need for revaccination of older children and adults has not been determined, antibody levels decline rapidly over 2 to 3 years. If indications persist of immunization, consider revaccination within 3 to 5 years.

Documentation Requirements: Federal law requires that (1) the manufacturer and lot number of this vaccine, (2) the dates of its administration, and (3) the name, address, and title of the person administering the vaccine be documented in the recipient's permanent medical record or in a permanent office log.

Certain adverse events must be reported to VAERS (800-822-7967). Refer to Immunization Documents in the Resources section for complete information.

Overdosage: Although few data are available, clinical experience with similar products suggests that the major manifestations of overdosage would be pain and tenderness at the injection site.

Efficacy: Groups A and C vaccines reduce disease incidence by 85% to 95%. Clinical protection from the Y and W-135 strains have not been determined directly, but immunogenicity has been demonstrated in adults and children older than 2 years.

Onset: 7 to 10 days

Duration: Antibodies against group A and C polysaccharides decline markedly over the first 3 years after vaccination. This decline is more rapid in infants and young children than in adults; in a group of children older than 4 years, elevated antibody concentrations declined from more than 90% to 67% three years after vaccination. In the same interval, antibody levels fell from more than 90% to less than 10% among children younger than 4 years at time of vaccination. In a New Zealand study, children 2 to 13 years of age received a single dose of monovalent group A polysaccharide vaccine. After 2.5 years of active surveillance, there were no cases of invasive group A disease in children vaccinated at 2 years of age or older.

Protective Level: Meningococcal bactericidal antibody 2 mcg/mL after polysaccharide vaccination, perhaps less after protein-conjugated vaccination.

Mechanism: Induction of protective bactericidal antibodies. Subsequent doses will reinstate the primary immune response, but not evoke an accelerated booster response.

Drug Interactions: Like all inactivated vaccines, administration of meningococcal vaccine to patients receiving immunosuppressant drugs (eg, high-dose corticosteroids) or radiation therapy may result in an insufficient response to immunization. Patients may remain susceptible despite immunization.

Inactivated vaccines are not generally affected by circulating antibodies or administration of exogenous antibodies. Vaccination may occur at any time before or after antibody administration.

Combining attenuated measles virus (Schwarz strain) and meningococcal groups A and C polysaccharides into a single vaccine resulted in depressed measles vaccine effectiveness in 110 Parisian children. Measles seroconversion was only 80% in combination with meningococcal group A vaccine and 69% in combination with a combined groups A and C vaccine. Meningococcal seroconversion was unaffected. Conversely, researchers found no interaction between attenuated measles and meningococcal A vaccines in 87 Sudanese children receiving an extemporaneous combination of measles, tetanus, and meningococcal A immunogens. Neither of these 2 studies should be considered conclusive; they provide preliminary data only. Public health authorities do not recommend any separation of measles and meningococcal vaccines if both are needed by a patient.

Hib, meningococcal, and pneumococcal vaccines may safely and effectively be administered simultaneously at separate injection sites.

Pharmaceutical Characteristics

Concentration: 50 mcg of each serogroup polysaccharide per 0.5 mL

Quality Assay: Exhibits 90% or more immunogenicity in at least 25 subjects, defined as a 4-fold increase in antibody titers. USP standards are published for the A and C polysaccharide components. Product is assayed for O-acetyl, sialic acid, protein, and other chemical content and molecular size. Guinea-pig safety tests and rabbit pyrogenicity and serologic tests are conducted. The product should be free of detectable human blood-group substances.

Packaging: Package of 1 single-dose vial with 0.78 mL preservative-free diluent vial (NDC#: 49281-0489-01).

Doseform: Powder for solution

Appearance: White powder, yielding a clear, colorless liquid

Diluent: Sterile water for injection (with thimerosal for 10-dose vials only). Single-dose vials contain no preservative.

Adjuvant: None

Preservative: 0.01% thimerosal (10-dose vials only)

Allergens: The stopper to the vial contains dry natural latex rubber.

Excipients: 2.5 to 5 mg lactose per 0.5 mL

pH: Data not provided

Shelf Life: Expires within 18 months

Storage/Stability: Store at 2° to 8°C (35° to 46°F) Discard if frozen. Powder can tolerate 12 weeks at 37°C (98.6°F) and 6 to 8 weeks at 45°C (113°F). Shipped in insulated containers with coolant packs via overnight or next-day courier. Reconstitute gently. Discard single-dose vial within 30 minutes after reconstitution. Refrigerate the multidose vial after reconstitution and discard within 35 days.

Production Process: Polysaccharide precipitated with cationic detergent, purified by centrifugation and ethanol fractionation, then lyophilized.

Media: Casamino acid medium and medium 199. *N. meningitidis* are cultivated with Mueller Hinton agar and Watson Scherp media.

Disease Epidemiology

Incidence: The last major epidemic of meningococcal disease occurred in the United States in 1946; the outbreak was due to serogroup A. *N. meningitidis* is now the leading cause of bacterial meningitis in children and young adults in the United States. Meningococcal disease peaks in February and March, reaching its lowest point each September. The rate of endemic serogroup C meningococcal disease is approximately 0.5 cases/100,000 population per year. Most of these cases are sporadic and not associated with outbreaks.

On average, 2,600 cases of meningococcal meningitis occur per year in the United States. Disease also can take the form of meningococcemia, which can progress rapidly to *Purpura fulminans*, shock, and death. During 1989 to 1991, serogroup B accounted for 46% of cases, serogroup C for 45%, with serogroups W-135, Y, and untypable serogroups accounting for the balance. The proportion of meningococcal cases caused by serogroup Y increased from 2% during 1989 to 1991 to 37% during 1997 to 2002. Serogroups B, C, and Y are the major causes of meningococcal disease in the United States, each being responsible for approximately one third of cases. The proportion of cases caused by each serogroup varies by age group. Among infants younger than 1 year, more than 50% of cases are caused by serogroup B, for which no vaccine is licensed or available in the United States. Of all cases of meningococcal disease among people 11 years of age or older, 75% are caused by serogroups (C, Y, or W-135). Since the early 1990s, outbreaks of meningococcal disease have occurred with increasing frequency in the United States. From July 1994 to June 2002, 76 outbreaks were identified: 63% caused by serogroup C, 25% by serogroup B, and 12% by serogroup Y.

Mortality ranges from 10% to 30%, despite appropriate antimicrobial therapy. Serogroups represented in this vaccine protect against approximately 50% of these cases. The incidence of endemic meningococcal disease peaks in late winter or early spring. Attack rates are highest among children 6 to 12 months of age and then steadily decline. An estimated 310,000 cases occur annually around the world, with 35,000 deaths. Serogroup A is the most common cause of epidemics in Africa and Asia, but rarely causes diseases in the United States. The so-called sub-Saharan meningitis belt stretches from Senegal to Ethiopia. Epidemics are most common during the dry season, from December to June. Epidemics have also occurred in Saudi Arabia, Kenya, Tanzania, Burundi, and Mongolia.

Susceptible Pools: Military basic trainees, asplenic and certain other immunosuppressed patients, travelers to meningococcal-endemic areas, laboratory workers, college freshmen, and people living in dormitories.

Transmission: Direct contact, including respiratory droplets

Incubation: 2 to 10 days

Communicability: Carriage is usually asymptomatic until meningococci are no longer present in oral and nasal discharges. If sensitive to sulfonamides, meningococci usually disappear from the nasopharynx within 24 hours after institution of treatment. Outbreaks are defined as at least 3 confirmed or probable cases of meningococcal disease during a period of at least 3 months in patients who are not close contacts of one another, with a primary attack rate of at least 10 cases/100,000 people.

Outbreak Evaluation: Establish a diagnosis of meningococcal disease. Administer chemoprophylaxis to appropriate contacts. Enhance surveillance, save isolates, and review historical data. Investigate links between cases. Consider subtyping. Exclude secondary and coprimary cases. Determine if the suspected outbreak is organization- or community-based. Define population at risk and determine its size. Calculate the attack rate. Select the target group for vaccination.

Other Information

Perspective:
1884: Marchiafava and Celli isolate *N. meningitidis*.
1905: Jochmann treats patients with equine *N. meningitidis* antiserum.
1968: Scientists at Walter Reed Army Institute of Research develop serogroup C vaccine. Widespread use of group C polysaccharide among military recruits begins in 1971.
1972: Institut Mérieux develops serogroup A vaccine.
1974: 100 million doses of serogroup A vaccine distributed in Brazilian epidemic. Merck's group C vaccine licensed in the United States on April 2.
1978: Connaught monovalent group A vaccine, monovalent group C vaccine, and bivalent A/C vaccine licensed on January 3, 1978.
1981: Connaught's quadrivalent Menomune A-C-Y-W135 licensed in November 1981.

Discontinued Products: *Meningovax* (Merck, Sharp and Dohme; licensed in 1974-75, 1982). In 1925, meningococcus vaccines containing the bacterium *Diplococcus intracellularis meningitidis* were manufactured by Lederle, Mulford, Sherman, and Squibb.

National Policy: CDC. Prevention and control of meningococcal disease: recommendations of the Advisory Committee on Immunization Practices (ACIP). *MMWR.* 2005;54(RR-7):1-21. http://www.cdc.gov/mmwr/preview/mmwrhtml/rr5407a1.htm.

ACIP. Revised recommendations of the Advisory Committee on Immunization Practices to vaccinate all persons aged 11-18 years with meningococcal conjugate vaccine. *MMWR.* 2007;56:794-795. http://www.cdc.gov/mmwr/PDF/wk/mm5631.pdf.

References: Peltola H. Meningococcal vaccines: Current status and future possibilities. *Drugs.* 1998;55:347-366.

Rosenstein NE, Perkins BA, Stephens DS, Popovic T, Hughes JM. Meningococcal disease. *N Engl J Med.* 2001;344(18):1378-1388.

WHO. Meningococcal vaccines: Polysaccharide and polysaccharide conjugate vaccines. *Weekly Epidemiol Rec.* 2002;77:331-339.

Meningococcal (Groups A, C, Y, and W-135) Conjugate Vaccine

Bacterial Vaccines & Toxoids

Names:
Menactra
Menveo

Manufacturers:
Sanofi Pasteur
Novartis

Synonyms: VISI abbreviation: MENcn. Meningococcal (Groups A, C, Y and W-135) Polysaccharide Diphtheria Toxoid Conjugate Vaccine, MCV4

Immunologic Characteristics

Microorganism: Bacterium, *Neisseria meningitidis*, aerobic gram-negative diplococci, family *Neisseriaceae*

Viability: Inactivated

Antigenic Form: Capsular polysaccharide fragments individually conjugated to diphtheria toxoid protein.

Antigenic Type: Polysaccharides linked to protein. The group A polysaccharide consists of a polymer of N-acetyl-O-acetyl mannosamine phosphate; the group C polysaccharide is primarily N-acetyl-O-acetylneuraminic acid. Immunogenicity is correlated with molecular weight; the group C antigen weighs more than 100 kilodaltons.

Strains:

Novartis: Not described.

Sanofi Pasteur: A-strain 1, C-strain 11, Y-strain 6306Y, W-135-strain 6308

Use Characteristics

Indications: For active immunization of children and adults to prevent invasive meningococcal disease caused by *N. meningitidis* serogroups A, C, Y and W-135.

Novartis: 2 to 55 years of age

Sanofi Pasteur: 9 months to 55 years of age

Populations warranting immunization include the following: military recruits during basic training; college students (especially freshmen and those living in dormitories); adolescents 11 to 18 years of age; people with anatomic or functional asplenia (because of an increased risk of developing meningococcal disease of high severity); and travelers to countries with epidemic meningococcal disease, particularly travelers who will have prolonged contact with the local populace (eg, travelers to sub-Saharan Africa, pilgrims to the Hajj or Umrah in Saudi Arabia). In addition, consider this vaccine for household or institutional contacts of people with meningococcal disease as an adjunct to antibiotic chemotherapy; medical and laboratory personnel at risk of exposure to meningococcal disease; and immunosuppressed people, including those with terminal complement defects or deficiency of properdin.

Limitations: MCV4 will not prevent meningitis caused by other microorganisms or prevent invasive meningococcal disease caused by *N. meningitidis* serogroup B. Do not use MCV4 to treat meningococcal infections. Do not use MCV4 to immunize against diphtheria. Select appropriate antibiotics to treat active infections (eg, penicillin G, chloramphenicol, sulfonamides, rifampin). Because of the delay in developing protective antibody titers, this vaccine does not substitute for chemoprophylaxis in individuals exposed to meningococcal disease.

Contraindications:

Absolute: People with a history of serious allergic reaction to a vaccine component or after a prior dose of this vaccine. People with known hypersensitivity to dry natural rubber latex, a component of the vial stopper in some packages.

Relative: The manufacturer recommends that people with a history of Guillain-Barré syndrome not receive *Menactra*.

Immunodeficiency: The immune response to MCV4 among immunosuppressed people has not been studied. People receiving immunosuppressive therapy or who have other immunodeficiencies may have diminished antibody response to active immunization. Nonetheless, this vaccine is indicated for asplenic patients.

Elderly: Safety and efficacy of MCV4 in adults older than 55 years have not been established.

Carcinogenicity: MCV4 has not been evaluated in animals for its carcinogenic potential.

Mutagenicity: MCV4 has not been evaluated in animals for its mutagenic potential.

Fertility Impairment: MCV4 has not been evaluated in animals for its potential to impair fertility.

Pregnancy: Register pregnant women who receive MCV4 in the manufacturer's pregnancy registry. Inform women of childbearing potential that the manufacturer maintains a pregnancy registry to monitor fetal outcomes of pregnant women exposed to MCV4. If they are pregnant or become aware they were pregnant at the time of immunization, they should contact their healthcare professional or the manufacturer.

Novartis: Category B. Reproduction studies were performed in female rabbits at approximately 20 times the human dose that revealed no evidence of impaired fertility or harm to the fetus due to *Menveo*. There are, however, no adequate and well-controlled studies in pregnant women. Give *Menveo* to a pregnant woman only if clearly needed. The effect of *Menveo* on embryo-fetal and post-natal development was evaluated in pregnant rabbits. Animals were administered *Menveo* IM 3 times before gestation, during organogenesis (gestation day 7), and later in pregnancy (gestation day 20), 0.5 mL/rabbit per occasion (approximately 20-fold higher than the human dose on a mg/kg basis). There were no adverse effects attributable to vaccine on mating, female fertility, pregnancy, or embryo-fetal development. There were no vaccine related fetal malformations or other evidence of teratogenesis noted. To enroll in the pregnancy registry, call 1-877-311-8972.

Sanofi Pasteur: Category C. Animal reproduction studies were performed in mice using 0.2 mL of *Menactra* (900 times the human dose, adjusted by body weight). There were no effects on fertility, maternal health, embryo/fetal survival, or postnatal development. Skeletal examinations revealed one fetus (1 of 234 examined) in the vaccine group with a cleft palate. None were observed in the concurrent control group (0 of 174 examined). No data suggest this isolated finding is vaccine related, and no other skeletal and organ malformations were observed. There are no adequate and well-controlled studies in pregnant women. Generally, most IgG passage across the placenta occurs during the third trimester. Because animal studies are not always predictive of human response, use *Menactra* during pregnancy only if clearly needed.

Lactation: It is not known if MCV4 or corresponding antibodies cross into human breast milk. Problems in humans have not been documented and are unlikely.

Children: Safety and efficacy in children younger than the labeled age range have not been established.

Adverse Reactions: The safety of *Menactra* was evaluated in 6 clinical studies that enrolled 7,642 participants 11 to 55 years of age who received *Menactra* and 3,041 participants who received *Menomune-A/C/Y/W-135*. The most frequently reported solicited local and systemic adverse reactions in US children 2 to 10 years of age were injection-site pain and irritability. Diarrhea, drowsiness, and anorexia were also common. Serious adverse events reported within a 6-month period after vaccination occurred at the same rate (1.3%) in the *Menactra* and *Menomune-A/C/Y/W-135* groups. The events reported were consistent with events expected in healthy adolescent and adult populations. The most commonly reported solicited adverse reactions in adolescents 11 to 18 years of age, and adults 18 to 55 years of age were local pain, headache, and fatigue. Except for redness in adults, local reactions were more frequently reported after *Menactra* than after *Menomune-A/C/Y/W-135*. Most local and systemic reactions after *Menactra* or *Menomune-A/C/Y/W-135* vaccination were reported as mild in intensity. No important differences in rates of anorexia, diarrhea, rash, or vomiting were observed between the vaccine groups.

The most common adverse events reported in children who received *Menactra* at 9 and 12 months of age were injection-site tenderness and irritability. Rates of fever were comparable with other vaccines routinely recommended for young children.

The safety of *Menveo* was evaluated in 5 randomized clinical trials in which 6,185 participants, 11 to 55 years of age received *Menveo* (5,286 received *Menveo* alone, and 899 received *Menveo* concomitant with other vaccine(s) [eg, *Boostrix* or *Boostrix* plus *Gardasil*]) and 1,966 participants who received either *Menomune* or *Menactra*. In clinical trials, the most frequently occurring adverse events in all subjects who received *Menveo* were pain at the injection site (41%), headache (30%), myalgia (18%), malaise (16%), and nausea (10%). In a randomized multicenter study in the United States, the most commonly reported solicited adverse events after administration of *Menveo* to adolescents and adults were injection-site pain and headache. The rates of these solicited adverse events were comparable to those reported following *Menactra*. The reported frequency and severity of local reactions and systemic adverse events that occurred within 7 days after administration of *Menveo* or *Menactra* to adolescents and adults appear in the following tables. Neither study vaccine was administered with concomitant vaccines.

Participants 11 to 18 Years of Age Reporting Solicited Symptoms Within 7 Days After Vaccination						
	Menveo N = 1,631 %			*Menactra* N = 539 %		
Reaction	Any	Moderate	Severe	Any	Moderate	Severe
Local						
Injection-site pain[a]	44	9	1	53	11	1
Erythema[b]	15	2	<1	16	1	0
Induration[b]	12	2	<1	11	1	0
Systemic						
Headache[a]	29	8	2	28	7	1
Myalgia[a]	19	4	1	18	5	<1
Nausea[a]	12	3	1	9	2	1
Malaise[a]	11	3	1	12	5	1
Chills[a]	8	2	1	7	1	<1
Arthralgia[a]	8	2	<1	6	1	0
Rash[c]	3	-	-	3	-	-
Fever[d]	1	<1	0	1	0	0

a Moderate: Some limitation in normal daily activity; severe: Unable to perform normal daily activity.
b Moderate: > 50 to 100 mm; severe: > 100 mm.
c Assessed only as present or not present, without grading for severity.
d Moderate: 39° to 39.9°C; severe: ≥ 40°C.

Participants 19 to 55 Years of Age Reporting Solicited Symptoms Within 7 Days After Vaccination						
	Menveo (n = 1,018) %			*Menactra* (n = 336) %		
Reaction	Any	Moderate	Severe	Any	Moderate	Severe
Local						
Injection-site pain[a]	38	7	<1	41	6	0
Erythema[b]	16	2	1	12	1	0
Induration[b]	13	1	<1	9	<1	0
Systemic						
Headache[a]	25	7	2	25	7	1
Myalgia[a]	14	4	<1	15	3	1
Malaise[a]	10	3	1	10	2	1
Nausea[a]	7	2	<1	5	1	<1
Arthralgia[a]	6	2	<1	6	1	1
Chills[a]	4	1	<1	4	1	0
Rash[c]	2	-	-	1	-	-
Fever[d]	1	<1	0	1	<1	0

a Moderate: Some limitation in normal daily activity; Severe: Unable to perform normal daily activity
b Moderate: > 50 to 100 mm; severe: > 100 mm
c Assessed only as present or not present, without grading for severity.
d Moderate: 39° to 39.9°C; severe: ≥ 40°C

During the 6 months after immunization, SAEs reported by more than one subject were as follows:

Menveo: appendicitis (3 subjects), road traffic accident (3 subjects), and suicide attempt (5 subjects)

Menactra: intervertebral disc protrusion (2 subjects)

Menomune: none

Serious adverse events that occurred within 30 days of vaccination were reported by 7 of 6,185 (0.1%) of subjects in the *Menveo* group, 4 of 1,757 (0.2%) of subjects in the *Menactra* group, and no *Menomune* subjects.

The events that occurred during the first 30 days after immunization with *Menveo* were: vitello-intestinal duct remnant, Cushing syndrome, viral hepatitis, pelvic inflammatory disease, intentional multiple drug overdose, simple partial seizure, and suicidal depression.

The events that occurred during the first 30 days after immunization with *Menactra* were: herpes zoster, fall, intervertebral disc protrusion, and angioedema.

Hematologic: Because of a risk of hemorrhage, only give this vaccine to people with a bleeding disorder (eg, hemophilia, thrombocytopenia), or to people on anticoagulant therapy if the potential benefit outweighs the risk of bleeding after IM administration. Take steps to avoid the risk of bleeding or hematoma formation after IM injection.

Neurologic: Cases of Guillain-Barré syndrome (GBS) and transverse myelitis have been reported after *Menactra* administration. A cause-and-effect relationship between these events has not been established. The manufacturer recommends that people with a history of GBS not receive *Menactra*.

With Td: Local and systemic reactions when given with Td vaccine were similar to the separate-administration group in frequency of local pain, induration, redness, and swelling at the *Menactra* injection site, as well as the Td injection site. Pain was the most frequent local reaction reported at both the *Menactra* and Td injection sites. More participants experienced pain after Td than after *Menactra* (71% vs 53%). Most local solicited reactions for both groups (66% to 77%) at either injection site were reported as mild and resolved within 3 days postvaccination. The overall rate of systemic adverse events was higher when *Menactra* and Td vaccines were given concomitantly than when *Menactra* was administered 28 days after Td. In both groups, the most common reactions were headache (*Menactra* + Td, 36%; Td + placebo, 34%; *Menactra* alone, 22%) and fatigue (*Menactra* + Td, 32%; Td + placebo, 29%; *Menactra* alone, 17%). No important differences in rates of malaise, diarrhea, anorexia, vomiting, or rash were observed between the groups. Fever 40°C or higher occurred at 0.5% or less in all groups. No seizures occurred in either group.

With Typhim Vi: Local and systemic reactions when given with *Typhim Vi* were similar to the separate-administration group in frequency of local pain, induration, redness and swelling at the *Menactra* injection site, as well as the *Typhim Vi* injection site. Pain was the most frequent local reaction reported at both the *Menactra* and *Typhim Vi* injection sites. More participants experienced pain after *Typhim Vi* than after *Menactra* (76% vs 47%). Most local solicited reactions for both groups (70% to 77%) at either injection site were reported as mild and resolved within 3 days postvaccination. In both groups, the most common systemic reactions were headache (*Menactra* + *Typhim Vi*, 41%; *Typhim Vi* + placebo, 42%; *Menactra* alone, 33%) and fatigue (*Menactra* + *Typhim Vi*, 38%; *Typhim Vi* + placebo, 35%; *Menactra* alone, 27%). No important differences in rates of malaise, diarrhea, anorexia, vomiting, or rash were observed between the groups. Fever 40°C or higher and seizures were not reported in either group.

With Tdap + Gardasil: The safety of *Menveo* administered concomitantly with *Boostrix* and *Gardasil* was evaluated in a single-center study conducted in Costa Rica. Solicited local and systemic adverse events were recorded and reported as noted above. Subjects 11 to 18 years of age received *Menveo* concomitantly with *Boostrix* and *Gardasil* (N = 540), or *Menveo* followed 1 month later by *Boostrix* and then 1 month later by *Gardasil* (N = 541), or *Boostrix* followed 1 month later by *Menveo* and then 1 month later by *Gardasil* (N = 539). Some solicited systemic adverse events were more frequently reported in the group that received *Menveo, Boostrix*, and *Gardasil* concomitantly (headache 40%, malaise 25%, myalgia 27%, and arthralgia 17%) compared to the group that first received *Menveo* alone (headache 36%, malaise 20%, myalgia 19%, and arthralgia 11%). Among subjects administered *Menveo* alone (1 month before *Boostrix*), 36% reported headache, 20% malaise, and 16% myalgia. Among subjects administered *Menveo* 1 month after *Boostrix*, 27% reported headache, 18% malaise, and 16% myalgia.

Consultation: Clinicians involved with meningococcal outbreak situations should consult with their state or local public health departments or call the CDC National Immunization Program.

Pharmacologic & Dosing Characteristics

Dosage:
Novartis: 2 to 55 years of age: A single 0.5 mL injection
Sanofi Pasteur: 9 to 23 months of age: Two 0.5 mL injections 3 months apart
    2 to 55 years of age: A single 0.5 mL injection

Route & Site: IM, preferably in the deltoid region.

Documentation Requirements: Federal law requires that the following information be documented in the recipient's permanent medical record or in a permanent office log: (1) The manufacturer and lot number of this vaccine, (2) the date of administration, and (3) the name, address, and title of the person administering the vaccine.

Certain adverse events must be reported to the VAERS system ([800] 822-7967). Refer to the Immunization Documents in the Resources section.

Overdosage: No specific data are available. Larger than recommended volumes of vaccine may increase the risk of injection-site reactions, but they are unlikely to have other consequences.

Additional Doses: The ACIP recommends that people previously vaccinated with either *Menactra* or meningococcal polysaccharide vaccine who are at prolonged increased risk for meningococcal disease should be revaccinated with *Menactra*. Revaccinate people previously vaccinated at 7 years of age or older and at prolonged increased risk 5 years after the previous meningococcal vaccination. Revaccinate people previously vaccinated at 2 to 6 years of age and at prolonged increased risk 3 years after their previous meningococcal vaccination. Because of the limited period of increased risk, ACIP currently does not recommend that college freshman living in dormitories who were previously vaccinated with *Menactra* be revaccinated. However, college freshman living in dormitories who were vaccinated with meningococcal polysaccharide vaccine 5 or more years previously are recommended to be vaccinated with MCV4.

Efficacy:

Sanofi Pasteur: Vaccine efficacy for *Menactra* was inferred by demonstrating immunologic equivalence to a meningococcal polysaccharide vaccine, *Menomune-A/C/Y/W-135*. The primary measure of immune response was induction of serogroup-specific anticapsular antibody with bactericidal activity. The antibody response to vaccination was evaluated by determining the proportion of participants with a 4-fold or greater increase in serum bactericidal antibody to each serogroup. Sera from clinical trial participants were tested for these antibodies with a serum bactericidal assay (SBA) using baby rabbit complement (SBA-BR). Immunogenicity was evaluated in 3 randomized clinical trials that enrolled male and female children, adolescents, and adults, respectively. Participants received *Menactra* or *Menomune-A/C/Y/W-135*. Sera were obtained before and approximately 28 days after vaccination.

Children: The response to vaccination in children 2 to 10 years old was evaluated by the proportion of subjects having an SBA-H antibody titer of 1:8 or greater for each serogroup. The median age of participants was 3 years old; 95% completed the study. Of 1,408 enrolled children 2 to 10 years old, immune responses evaluated in a subset of *Menactra* and *Menomune-A/C/Y/W-135* recipients were comparable for all 4 serogroups. Among participants 2 to 3 years old with undetectable prevaccination titers (ie, less than 4 at day 0), seroconversion rates (defined as at least 8 at day 28) were similar between *Menactra* and *Menomune-A/C/Y/W-135* recipients. *Menactra* recipients achieved seroconversion rates of 57% for serogroup A (n = 12/21), 62% for serogroup C (n = 29/47), 84% for serogroup Y (n = 26/31), and 53% for serogroup W-135 (n = 20/38). The seroconversion rates for *Menomune-A/C/Y/W-135* vaccine recipients were 55%, 30%, 57%, and 26%, respectively. among participants 4 to 10 years old, percentages of patients who seroconverted were similar between the groups. *Menactra* recipients achieved seroconversion rates of 69% for serogroup A (n = 11/16), 81% for serogroup C (n = 50/62), 98% for serogroup Y (n = 45/46), and 69% for serogroup W-135 (n = 27/39). The seroconversion rates for *Menomune-A/C/Y/W-135* vaccine recipients were 45%, 38%, 84%, and 68%, respectively.

Adolescents: Results in 881 adolescents 11 to 18 years of age (median = 14 years) showed that the immune responses to *Menactra* and *Menomune-A/C/Y/W-135* were similar for all 4 serogroups. In participants with undetectable titers (ie, less than 8 at day 0), seroconversion rates (defined as at least a 4-fold rise in day 28 titers) were similar between the 2 groups. *Menactra* recipients achieved seroconversion rates of: 100% for serogroup A (n = 81/81), 99% for serogroup C (n = 153/155), 93% for serogroup Y (n = 60/61), and 99% for serogroup W-135 (n = 161/164). The seroconversion rates for *Menomune-A/C/Y/W-135* were

100% for serogroup A (n = 93/93), 99% for serogroup C (n = 151/152), 100% for serogroup Y (n = 47/47), and 99% for serogroup W-135 (n = 138/139).

Adults: Results in 2,554 adults 18 to 55 years of age (median = 24 years) showed that the immune responses to *Menactra* and *Menomune-A/C/Y/W-135* were similar for all 4 serogroups. In participants with undetectable titers (ie, less than 8 at day 0), seroconversion rates (defined as at least a 4-fold rise in day 28 titers) were similar between *Menactra* and *Menomune-A/C/Y/W-135* groups. *Menactra* recipients achieved seroconversion rates of: 100% for serogroup A (n = 156/156), 99% for serogroup C (n = 343/345), 91% for serogroup Y (n = 253/279), and 97% for serogroup W-135 (n = 360/373). The seroconversion rates for *Menomune-A/C/Y/W-135* recipients were 99% for serogroup A (n = 143/144), 98% for serogroup C (n = 297/304), 97% for serogroup Y (n = 221/228), and 99% for serogroup W-135 (n = 325/328).

Novartis: Vaccine efficacy for *Menveo* was inferred by demonstrating noninferiority of the serum bactericidal antibody (SBA) responses to those of *Menactra.*

Immunogenicity was evaluated in a randomized, multicenter clinical trial that enrolled adolescents (11 to 18 years of age) and adults (19 to 55 years of age). The trial enrolled 3,539 participants, randomized to receive *Menveo* (N = 2,663) or *Menactra* (n = 876). Sera were obtained both before vaccination and 28 days after vaccination.

Adolescents: In participants 11–18 years of age, noninferiority of *Menveo* to *Menactra* was demonstrated for all four serogroups based on SBA seroresponse. The percentages of subjects with SBA seroresponse were statistically higher for serogroups A, W, and Y in the *Menveo* group compared to *Menactra*, however, the clinical relevance of higher postvaccination immune responses is not known.

Bactericidal Antibody Responses[a] to *Menveo* and *Menactra* 28 Days After Vaccination of Subjects 11 to 18 Years of Age				
	Bacterial Antibody Response[a]		Comparison of *Menveo* and *Menactra*	
End point	*Menveo* (95% CI)	*Menactra* (95% CI)	*Menveo/Menactra* (95% CI)	*Menveo - Menactra* (95% CI)
Serogroup A	n = 1,075	n = 359		
% seroresponse[b]	75 (72, 77)	66 (61, 71)		8 (3, 14)[c,d]
% ≥ 1:8	75 (73, 78)	67 (62, 72)		8 (3, 14)
GMT	29 (24, 35)	18 (14, 23)	1.63 (1.31, 2.02)	
Serogroup C	n = 1,483	n = 501		
% seroresponse[b]	75 (73, 77)	73 (69, 77)		2 (-2, 7)[d]
% ≥ 1:8	84 (82, 86)	84 (80, 87)		1 (-3, 5)
GMT	59 (48, 73)	47 (36, 61)	1.27 (1.01, 1.6)	
Serogroup W-135	n = 1,024	n = 288		
% seroresponse[b]	75 (72, 77)	63 (57, 68)		12 (6, 18)[c,d]
% ≥ 1:8	96 (95, 97)	88 (84, 92)		8 (4, 12)
GMT	87 (74, 102)	44 (35, 54)	2 (1.66, 2.42)	

Meningococcal (Groups A, C, Y, and W-135) Conjugate Vaccine

	Bactericidal Antibody Responses[a] to *Menveo* and *Menactra* 28 Days After Vaccination of Subjects 11 to 18 Years of Age			
	Bacterial Antibody Response[a]		Comparison of *Menveo* and *Menactra*	
End point	*Menveo* (95% CI)	*Menactra* (95% CI)	*Menveo/Menactra* (95% CI)	*Menveo - Menactra* (95% CI)
Serogroup Y	n = 1,036	n = 294		
% seroresponse[b]	68 (65, 71)	41 (35, 47)		27 (20, 33)[c,d]
% ≥ 1:8	88 (85, 90)	69 (63, 74)		19 (14, 25)
GMT	51 (42, 61)	18 (14, 23)	2.82 (2.26, 3.52)	

a Serum Bactericidal Assay with exogenous human complement source (hSBA).
b Defined as a postvaccination titer greater than or equal to 1:8 for subjects with a prevaccination titer less than 1:4, or a post vaccination titer at least 4-fold higher than baseline for subjects with a prevaccination titer of greater than or equal to 1:4.
c Seroresponse was statistically higher (the lower limit of the two-sided 95% CI greater than 0% for vaccine group differences).
d Noninferiority criterion for primary end point met (the lower limit of the two-sided 95% CI greater than -10% for vaccine group differences).

> *Adults:* In participants 19-55 years of age, noninferiority of *Menveo* to *Menactra* was demonstrated for all four serogroups based on SBA seroresponse. The percentage of subjects with SBA seroresponse was statistically higher for serogroups C, W, and Y in the *Menveo* group, compared to *Menactra*; however, the clinical relevance of higher postvaccination immune responses is not known.

	Bactericidal Antibody Responses[a] to *Menveo* and Menactra 28 Days After Vaccination of Subjects 19 to 55 Years of Age			
	Bacterial Antibody Response[a]		Comparison of *Menveo* and *Menactra*	
End point	*Menveo* (95% CI)	*Menactra* (95% CI)	*Menveo/Menactra* (95% CI)	*Menveo-Menactra* (95% CI)
Serogroup A	n = 963	n =321		
% seroresponse[b]	67 (64, 70)	68 (63, 73)		1 (-7, 5)[d]
% ≥ 1:8	69 (66, 72)	71 (65,76)		2 (-7, 4)
GMT	31 (27, 36)	30 (24, 37)	1.06 (0.82, 1.37)	
Serogroup C	n = 961	n = 318		
% seroresponse[b]	67 (64, 70)	58 (53, 64)		9 (3, 15)[c,d]
% ≥ 1:8	80 (77, 83)	72 (67, 77)		8 (3, 14)
GMT	52 (44, 60)	32 (25, 40)	1.63 (1.24, 2.13)	
Serogroup W-135	n = 484	n = 292		
% seroresponse[b]	50 (46,55)	41 (35, 47)		9 (2, 17)[c,d]
% ≥ 1:8	94 (91, 96)	90 (86, 93)		4 (0, 9)
GMT	111 (93, 132)	69 (55, 85)	1.61(1.24, 2.1)	
Serogroup Y	n = 503	n = 306		
% seroresponse[b]	56 (51, 60)	40 (34, 46)		16 (9, 23)[c,d]
% ≥ 1:8	79 (76, 83)	70 (65, 75)		9 (3, 15)
GMT	44 (37, 52)	21 (17, 26)	2.1 (1.6, 2.75)	

a Serum Bactericidal Assay with exogenous human complement source (hSBA).
b Defined as a postvaccination titer greater than or equal to 1:8 for subjects with a prevaccination titer less than 1:4, or a post vaccination titer at least 4-fold higher than baseline for subjects with a prevaccination titer of greater than or equal to 1:4.
c Seroresponse was statistically higher (the lower limit of the two-sided 95% CI greater than 0% for vaccine group differences).
d Noninferiority criterion for primary end point met (the lower limit of the two-sided 95% CI greater than − 10% for vaccine group differences).

Meningococcal (Groups A, C, Y, and W-135) Conjugate Vaccine

Onset: Typically within 7 to 10 days.

Duration: The need for, or timing of, a booster dose of MCV4 has not yet been determined. Because of the protein-conjugated characteristics of this vaccine, duration is expected to be 5 years or longer.

Protective Level: Meningococcal bactericidal antibody 2 mcg/mL after polysaccharide vaccination, perhaps less after protein-conjugated vaccination.

Mechanism: Bactericidal anticapsular meningococcal antibodies are associated with protection from invasive meningococcal disease. This vaccine induces the production of bactericidal antibodies specific to the capsular polysaccharides of serogroups A, C, Y, and W-135.

Drug Interactions: Like all inactivated vaccines, administration of meningococcal vaccine to people receiving immunosuppressant drugs, including high-dose corticosteroids, or radiation therapy may result in an insufficient response to immunization. They may remain susceptible despite immunization.

Inactivated vaccines are not generally affected by circulating antibodies or administration of exogenous antibodies. Vaccination may occur at any time before or after antibody administration.

Td: The concomitant use of *Menactra* and tetanus-diphtheria toxoids (Td) was evaluated in a double-blind, randomized trial in 1,021 participants 11 to 17 years of age. One group received Td and *Menactra* (at separate injection sites) at day 0 and a saline placebo 28 days later (N = 509). The other group received Td and a saline placebo at day 0 and *Menactra* 28 days later (N = 512). Sera were obtained approximately 28 days after each vaccination. The proportion of participants with a 4-fold or greater rise in SBA-BR titer was higher when *Menactra* was given concomitantly with Td than when *Menactra* was given 1 month after Td. The clinical relevance of this finding has not been evaluated fully. No interference was observed in the immune response to the tetanus and diphtheria components after either concomitant or sequential vaccination.

Typhim Vi: The concomitant use of *Menactra* and *Typhim Vi* capsular polysaccharide vaccine was evaluated in a double-blind, randomized trial conducted in 945 participants 18 to 55 years of age. One group received *Typhim Vi* and *Menactra* (at separate injection sites) at day 0 and a saline placebo 28 days later (N = 469). The other group received *Typhim Vi* and a saline placebo at day 0 and *Menactra* 28 days later (N = 476). Sera were obtained approximately 28 days after each vaccination. The immune responses to *Menactra* and to *Typhim Vi* when given concurrently were comparable to the immune response(s) when given alone.

Pharmaceutical Characteristics

Concentration:

Novartis: 10 mcg of serogroup A and 5 mcg each of serogroups C, Y, and W-135 polysaccharides per 0.5 mL, conjugated to diphtheria CRM197 protein 32.7 to 64.1 mcg per 0.5 mL.

Sanofi Pasteur: Each 0.5 mL dose contains 4 mg each of meningococcal A, C, Y, and W-135 polysaccharides conjugated to approximately 48 mg of diphtheria toxoid protein carrier.

Quality Assay: Potency is determined by quantifying the amount of each polysaccharide antigen conjugated to diphtheria toxoid protein and the amount of unconjugated polysaccharide present. Product is assayed for O-acetyl, sialic acid, protein, and other chemical constituents and molecular size.

Packaging:

Novartis: Package of 5 glass vials of lyophilized MenA powder and 5 glass vials of MenCYW-135 liquid (NDC #: 46028-0208-01)

Sanofi Pasteur: Package of 5 single-dose vials (NDC #: 49281-0589-05)

Meningococcal (Groups A, C, Y, and W-135) Conjugate Vaccine

Doseform:
> *Novartis:* Powder and liquid to yielded composite solution
> *Sanofi Pasteur:* Solution

Appearance:
> *Novartis:* After reconstitution, the vaccine is clear and colorless
> *Sanofi Pasteur:* Clear to slightly turbid liquid

Solvent:
> *Sanofi Pasteur:* Sodium phosphate-buffered isotonic sodium chloride solution

Diluent: For Reconstitution
> *Novartis:* Men CYW-135 liquid, to reconstitute the MenA powder

Adjuvant: None

Preservative: None

Allergens: None

Excipients:
> *Novartis:* Residual formaldehyde less than or equal to 0.3 mcg per dose
> *Sanofi Pasteur:* Sodium phosphate-buffered sodium chloride solution

pH: 6.3 to 7.3

Shelf Life: Expires within 18 months.

Storage/Stability:
> *Novartis:* Store at 2° to 8°C (36° to 46°F). Protect vials from light. Discard if frozen. Contact the manufacturer regarding exposure to freezing or elevated temperatures. Shipped at 2° to 8°C (36° to 46°F).
> Use the MenCYW-135 liquid component to reconstitute the MenA powder. Gently invert or swirl the reconstituted vial until the vaccine is dissolved. use promptly, but may be held at up to 25°C (77°F) for up to 8 hours after reconstitution.
> *Sanofi Pasteur:* Store at 2° to 8°C (36° to 46°F). Protect vials from light. Discard if frozen. Contact the manufacturer regarding exposure to freezing or elevated temperatures. Shipped in insulated containers with coolant packs.

Production Process:
> *Novartis:* The polysaccharides are extracted from *N. meningitidis* cells and purified. *Corynebacterium diphtheriae* cultures are detoxified with formaldehyde. Serogroup A, Y, and W-135 polysaccharides are purified by several extraction and precipitation steps. Serogroup C polysaccharide is purified by a combination of chromatography and precipitation steps. The diphtheria protein is purified by a series of chromatography and ultrafiltration steps. Oligosaccharides are prepared for conjugation from purified polysaccharides by hydrolysis, sizing, and reductive amination. After activation, each oligosaccharide is covalently linked to CRM197 protein. The resulting glycoconjugates are purified to yield the four drug substances, which compose the final vaccine.
> *Sanofi Pasteur:* The polysaccharides are extracted from *N. meningitidis* cells and purified by centrifugation, detergent precipitation, alcohol precipitation, solvent extraction, and diafiltration. To prepare the polysaccharides for conjugation, they are depolymerized, derivatized, and purified by diafiltration. *C. diphtheriae* cultures are detoxified with formaldehyde. The diphtheria toxoid protein is purified by ammonium sulfate fractionation and diafiltration. The derivatized polysaccharides are covalently linked to diphtheria toxoid and purified by serial diafiltration. The four meningococcal components, present as individual serogroup-specific glycoconjugates, compose the final formulated vaccine.

Meningococcal (Groups A, C, Y, and W-135) Conjugate Vaccine

Media:

Novartis: N. meningitidis A, C, Y and W-135 strains are cultured on Franz complete medium. *C. diphtheriae* cultures are grown on CY medium containing yeast extracts and amino acids.

Sanofi Pasteur: N. meningitidis A, C, Y, and W-135 strains are cultured on Mueller-Hinton agar and grown in Watson-Scherp media. *C. diphtheriae* cultures are grown in a modified Mueller and Miller medium.

Disease Epidemiology

Incidence: Meningococcal bacteria, *N. meningitidis*, cause both endemic and epidemic disease, principally meningitis and meningococcemia. At least 13 meningococcal serogroups have been identified, based on antigenic differences in their capsular polysaccharides. Five serogroups (A, B, C, Y, and W-135) are responsible for nearly all cases of meningococcal disease worldwide. Early clinical manifestations of meningococcal disease are often difficult to distinguish from other, more common but less serious, illnesses. Onset and progression of disease can be rapid; in 60% of cases, infected individuals are symptomatic for less than 24 hours before seeking medical care. Even with antibiotic treatment and adjunctive therapy, the case fatality rate has remained at approximately 10%. In cases of fulminant septicemia, the case fatality rate may reach 40%. About 11% to 19% of meningococcal disease survivors have sequelae such as hearing loss and neurologic disability, or loss of skin, digits, or limbs because of ischemia.

In the United States, overall rates of meningococcal disease from 1967 to 2002 have remained stable, with yearly case counts varying from 1,323 to 3,525, reflecting a cyclical pattern with peaks occurring every 10 to 15 years. The age-specific incidence of meningococcal disease continues to be highest among infants younger than 1 year, among whom serogroup B predominates. The rate of meningococcal disease also peaks during adolescence and early adulthood. The incidence of endemic meningococcal disease peaks in late winter or early spring (eg, February, March). Attack rates are highest among children 6 to 12 months of age and then decline steadily.

From 1989 to 2002, the proportion of all meningococcal cases caused by serogroup Y increased from 2% to 29%, while serogroups B and C decreased from 46% and 45% of cases to 24% and 34%, respectively. The remaining cases were caused by serogroup W-135 and other strains. In 2002, serogroups C and Y accounted for 42% and 24% of meningococcal cases, respectively, in adolescents and adults 18 to 49 years of age. From July 1994 to June 2002, 76 outbreaks were identified: 63% caused by serogroup C, 25% by serogroup B, and 12% by serogroup Y.

Serogroup A is the most common cause of epidemics in Africa and Asia, but is a rare cause of disease in the United States. The so-called sub-Saharan meningitis belt stretches from Senegal to Ethiopia. Epidemics are most common during the dry season, from December to June. Epidemics have also occurred in Saudi Arabia, Kenya, Tanzania, Burundi, and Mongolia. Outbreaks of serogroup W-135 have been reported among pilgrims returning from the Hajj or Umrah to Saudi Arabia in 2000 and 2001. An estimated 310,000 cases of meningococcal disease occur annually around the world, with 35,000 deaths.

Susceptible Pools: Military basic trainees, college students, adolescents, asplenic and certain other immunosuppressed people, travelers to meningococcal-endemic areas, laboratory workers.

Transmission: Direct contact, including respiratory droplets

Incubation: 2 to 10 days

Communicability: Until meningococci are no longer present in oral and nasal discharges. If sensitive to sulfonamides, meningococci usually disappear from the nasopharynx within 24 hours after institution of treatment.

Outbreaks are defined as at least 3 confirmed or probable cases of meningococcal disease during a periods of 3 months or more in patients who are not close contacts of one another, with a primary attack rate of ate least 10 cases per 100,00 people.

Outbreak Evaluation: Establish a diagnosis of meningococcal disease. Administer chemoprophylaxis to appropriate contacts. Enhance surveillance, save clinical specimens, and review historical data.

Investigate links between cases. Consider bacteriologic subtyping. Exclude secondary and coprimary cases. Determine if the suspected outbreak is organization- or community-based. Define population at risk and determine its size. Calculate an attack rate. Select a target group for vaccination.

Other Information

Perspective:

1884: Marchiafava & Celli isolate *N. meningitidis.*

1905: Jochmann treats patients with equine *N. meningitidis* antiserum.

1946: Last major epidemic of meningococcal disease (serogroup A) in the United States.

1968: Scientists at Walter Reed Army Institute of Research (WRAIR) develop serogroup C vaccine. Widespread use of group C polysaccharide among military recruits begins in 1971.

1972: Institut Mérieux adapts WRAIR technology to produce serogroup A vaccine.

1974: 100 million doses of serogroup A vaccine distributed in Brazilian epidemic. Group C vaccine licensed in the United States.

1978: Connaught vaccine licensed on January 3, 1978.

1981: Connaught's quadrivalent *Menomune A/C/Y/W-135* licensed in November 1981.

2005: Sanofi Pasteur's *Menactra* licensed on January 17, 2005.

2010: Menveo licensed to Novartis on February 19.

Discontinued Products: *Meningovax* (Merck Sharp & Dohme; licensed in 1974-75, 1982). In 1925, meningococcus vaccines containing the bacterium *Diplococcus intracellularis meningitidis* were manufactured by Lederle, Mulford, Sherman, and Squibb.

National Policy: ACIP. Recommendation of the Advisory Committee on Immunization Practices (ACIP) for use of quadrivalent meningococcal conjugate vaccine (MenACWY-D) among children aged 9 through 23 months at increased risk for invasive meningococcal disease. *MMWR.* 2011;60(40):1391-1392. http://www.cdc.gov/mmwr/pdf/wk/mm6040.pdf.

ACIP. Licensure of a meningococcal conjugate vaccine for children aged 2 through 10 years and updated booster dose guidance for adolescents and other persons at increased risk for meningococcal disease—Advisory Committee on Immunization Practices (ACIP), 2011. *MMWR.* 2011;60(30):1018-1019. http://www.cdc.gov/mmwr/pdf/wk/mm6030.pdf.

ACIP. Updated recommendations for use of meningococcal conjugate vaccines, Advisory Committee on Immunization Practices (ACIP), 2010. *MMWR.* 2011;60(3):72-76. http://www.cdc.gov/mmwr/pdf/wk/mm6003.pdf.

ACIP. Updated recommendation from the ACIP for revaccination of persons at prolonged increased risk for meningococcal disease. *MMWR.* 2009;58:1042-1043.

Canadian National Advisory Committee on Immunization. Update on the invasive meningococcal disease and meningococcal vaccine conjugate recommendations. *Can Comm Dis Rep.* 2009;35(ACS-3):1-39.

Committee to Advise on Tropical Medicine and Travel (CATMAT). Statement on meningococcal vaccination for travellers. *Can Comm Dis Rep.* 2009;35(ACS-4):1-22.

ACIP. Decision not to recommend routine vaccination of all children aged 2-10 years with quadrivalent meningococcal conjugate vaccine (MCV4). *MMWR.* 2008;57(17):462-465. http://www.cdc.gov/mmwr/PDF/wk/mm5717.pdf.

ACIP. Revised recommendations of the Advisory Committee on Immunization Practices to vaccinate all persons aged 11-18 years with meningococcal conjugate vaccine. *MMWR.* 2007;56:794-795. http://www.cdc.gov/mmwr/PDF/wk/mm5631.pdf.

Canadian National Advisory Committee on Immunization. Meningococcal C conjugate vaccination recommendations for infants. *Can Comm Dis Rep.* 2007;33(ACS-11):1-12.

References: WHO. Meningococcal vaccines: WHO position paper, November 2011. *Weekly Epidem Rec.* 2011;86(47):521-539.

Bacterial Vaccines & Toxoids

Comparison Table of Pneumococcal Vaccines		
Generic name	Pneumococcal Conjugate Vaccine, 13-valent	Pneumococcal Polysaccharide Vaccine, 23-valent
Brand name	*Prevnar 13*	*Pneumovax 23*
Synonyms	PCV, PCV13, PNUc13	PNUps23, PPV, PPV23
Manufacturer	Pfizer	Merck
Viability	Bacterial subunit vaccine, protein-conjugated	Bacterial subunit vaccine, polysaccharides
Indication	All children < 72 months of age; adults ≥ 50 years of age (package insert)	Everyone ≥ 50 years of age (package insert) or 65 years of age (ACIP), plus those with certain chronic diseases
Serotype valence	13-valent	23-valent
Components	Types 1, 3, 4, 5, 6A, 6B, 7F, 9V, 14, 18C, 19F, 19A, and 23F	Types 1, 2, 3, 4, 5, 6B, 7F, 8, 9N, 9V, 10A, 11A, 12F, 14, 15B, 17F, 18C, 19F, 19A, 20, 22F, 23F, and 33F
Coverage of serotypes	80% of invasive pneumococcal disease among children < 6 years	90% of blood isolates in adults
Concentration	2.2 or 4.4 mcg of each type	25 mcg of each type
Conjugating protein	Diphtheria CRM_{197} protein 34 mcg per 0.5 mL	None
Adjuvant	Aluminum 0.125 mg per 0.5 mL as aluminum phosphate	None
Preservative	None	Phenol 0.25%
Doseform	Suspension	Solution
Packaging	0.5 mL single-dose vials	0.5 mL and 2.5 mL vials
Routine storage	2° to 8°C	2° to 8°C
Dose	0.5 mL for infants at 2, 4, 6, and 12 to 15 months of age. Older children should receive 1 to 3 doses depending on age. For adults ≥ 50 years, 0.5 mL once.	0.5 mL once or twice in a lifetime
Route	IM	IM or subcutaneously
CPT codes	90670	90732

Pneumococcal Conjugate Vaccine, 13-Valent

Bacterial Vaccines & Toxoids

Name:
Prevnar 13

Manufacturer:
Pfizer

Synonyms: PCV13, PNUc13. In some countries, this vaccine was known as *Prevenar 13*.

Comparison: Pneumococcal polysaccharide and conjugate vaccines each induce antibody responses in people 2 years and older. Some, but not all, head-to-head clinical studies find superior antibody responses for PCV13 compared with PPV23 for some serotypes 1 month after vaccination, but this differential tends to dissipate in following months. No protective threshold for antibody response has been established in adults. Consider the separate components in the 2 products when selecting a pneumococcal vaccine.

Immunologic Characteristics

Microorganism: Bacterium, *Streptococcus pneumoniae* (also known as pneumococcus or diplococcus), homofermentative gram-positive cocci

Viability: Inactivated

Antigenic Form: Saccharides of the capsular antigens of 13 distinct *S. pneumoniae* serotypes, individually conjugated to diphtheria CRM_{197} protein

Antigenic Type: Protein-polysaccharide mixture

Strains: Types 1, 3, 4, 5, 6A, 6B, 7F, 9V, 14, 18C, 19F, 19A, and 23F

Use Characteristics

Indications: To induce active immunity in infants and toddlers against invasive disease caused by *S. pneumoniae* serotypes represented in the vaccine. Base the decision to administer *Prevnar 13* primarily on its efficacy in preventing invasive pneumococcal disease. *Prevnar 13* is also indicated for active immunization of infants and toddlers against otitis media caused by serotypes 4, 6B, 9V, 14, 18C, 19F, and 23F. However, for vaccine serotypes, protection against otitis media is expected to be substantially lower than protection against invasive disease. The ACIP recommends this vaccine for all infants up to 71 months of age.

To induce active immunity against *S. pneumoniae* in adults 50 years of age and older, based largely on noninferior immune responses relative to *Pneumovax 23*. No controlled trials in adults demonstrating a decrease in pneumococcal pneumonia or invasive disease after vaccination with *Prevnar 13* have been reported.

Cochlear implant recipients: To reduce the risk of pneumococcal meningitis, people with cochlear implants should use the age-appropriate vaccine according to ACIP schedules for people at high risk.

Limitations: Pneumococcal vaccines are not expected to protect against pneumococcal types not represented in the vaccine. Because many organisms other than *S. pneumoniae* cause otitis media, vaccination will not protect against all causes of otitis media. Vaccination does not warrant discontinuation of penicillin or other antibiotic prophylaxis against pneumococcal infection. This vaccine is not intended for treatment of active infection. Select appropriate antibiotics to treat active infections (eg, penicillin G or V or an erythromycin). Immunization with *Prevnar 13* is not a substitute for routine diphtheria immunization.

Patients with impaired immune responsiveness (ie, from genetic defect, splenectomy or functional asplenia, immunosuppressive chemotherapy or radiotherapy, HIV infection) may have a reduced antibody response to active immunization.

Pneumococcal Conjugate Vaccine, 13-Valent

Contraindications:
Absolute: Patients with severe hypersensitivity to any component of the vaccine, including diphtheria toxoid.

Relative: Temporarily defer vaccination in patients with an active infection.

Immunodeficiency: Patients receiving immunosuppressive therapy or who have otherwise impaired immune responses (eg, from genetic defect, splenectomy or functional asplenia, immunosuppressive chemotherapy or radiotherapy, HIV infection) may have a diminished antibody response to active immunization. They may remain susceptible despite immunization.

Elderly: Antibody responses to PCV13 were lower in persons older than 65 years compared with persons 50 through 59 years of age.

Carcinogenicity: *Prevnar 13* has not been evaluated for carcinogenic potential.

Mutagenicity: *Prevnar 13* has not been evaluated for mutagenic potential.

Fertility Impairment: *Prevnar 13* has not been evaluated for impairment of fertility.

Pregnancy: Category B. Use only if clearly needed. It is not known if pneumococcal conjugate vaccine or corresponding antibodies cross the placenta. Generally, most IgG passage across the placenta occurs during the third trimester. A developmental and reproductive toxicity study has been performed in female rabbits at a dose approximately 20 times the human dose (on a mg/kg basis) and revealed no evidence of impaired female fertility or harm to the fetus due to PCV13. There are, however, no adequate and well-controlled studies in pregnant women. Problems in humans have not been documented and are unlikely.

Lactation: It is not known if pneumococcal conjugate vaccine or corresponding antibodies cross into human breast milk. Problems in humans have not been documented and are unlikely.

Children: The safety and efficacy of *Prevnar 13* in children younger than 6 weeks have not been established. Immune responses elicited by *Prevnar 13* among infants born prematurely have not been studied.

Children older than 24 months who have sickle cell disease, asplenia, HIV infection, chronic illness, or who are immunocompromised should complete an age-appropriate PCV13 regimen and then receive PPV23 to provide broad serotype protection. Data on sequential vaccination with PCV13 followed by PPV23 are limited.

Adverse Reactions: The safety of *Prevnar 13* was evaluated in 13 clinical trials in which 4,729 infants and toddlers received at least one dose of *Prevnar 13* and 2,760 infants and toddlers received at least one dose of *Prevnar* active control. There were no substantive differences in demographic characteristics between the vaccine groups. Three studies evaluated the safety of *Prevnar 13* when administered concomitantly with routine US pediatric vaccinations at 2, 4, 6, and 12 to 15 months of age. Overall, the safety data show a similar proportion of *Prevnar 13* and *Prevnar* subjects reporting serious adverse events. Among US study subjects, a similar proportion of *Prevnar 13* and *Prevnar* recipients reported solicited local and systemic adverse reactions as well as unsolicited adverse events.

Serious adverse events: Serious adverse events were collected throughout the study period for all 13 clinical trials. Serious adverse events reported following vaccination in infants and toddlers occurred in 8.2% of *Prevnar 13* recipients and 7.2% of *Prevnar* recipients. The most commonly reported serious adverse events were in the infections and infestations class, including bronchiolitis (0.9%, 1.1%), gastroenteritis, (0.9%, 0.9%), and pneumonia (0.9%, 0.5%) for *Prevnar 13* and *Prevnar*, respectively.

Adults 50 years and older: Commonly reported solicited adverse events were pain at injection site (greater than 50%), fatigue (greater than 30%), headache (greater than 20%), muscle pain (greater than 20%), joint pain (greater than 10%), decreased appetite (greater than 10%), injection-site redness (greater than 10%), injection-site swelling (greater than 10%), limited arm movement (greater than 10%), chills (greater than 5%), or rash (greater than 5%).

Infant and toddler studies: 1,907 subjects received at least 1 dose of *Prevnar 13* and 701 subjects received at least 1 dose of *Prevnar* in 3 US studies. The most common solicited adverse events after *Prevnar 13* were redness (24% to 42% per dose), swelling (20% to 32%), tenderness (58% to 63%), fever (24% to 37%), decreased appetite (48% to 51%), irritability (80% to 86%), increased sleep (49% to 72%), and decreased sleep (43% to 47%). The following symptoms were determined to be adverse drug reactions based on experience with *Prevnar 13* in clinical trials:

Reactions in greater than 1% of infants and toddlers: diarrhea, vomiting, and rash.

Reactions in less than 1% of infants and toddlers: crying, hypersensitivity reaction (including face edema, dyspnea, and bronchospasm), seizures (including febrile seizures), and urticaria or urticaria-like rash.

Older children: In a catch-up study conducted in Poland, 354 children (7 months through 5 years of age) receiving at least one dose of *Prevnar 13* were also monitored for safety. The most common solicited adverse events that occurred within 4 days following each dose of *Prevnar 13* administered to pneumococcal vaccine–naive children 7 months through 5 years of age were redness (38% to 70%, varying by dose and age), swelling (25% to 45%), tenderness (15% to 44%), fever (1% to 8%), decreased appetite (16% to 26%), irritability (14% to 35%), increased sleep (3% to 13%), decreased sleep (7% to 24%).

Experience with Prevnar: The safety experience with 7-valent *Prevnar* is relevant to *Prevnar 13* because the 2 vaccines share common components. Generally, the adverse reactions reported in clinical trials with *Prevnar 13* were also reported with *Prevnar*. Overall, the safety of *Prevnar* was evaluated in a total of 5 clinical studies in the United States, in which 18,168 infants and children received a total of 58,699 doses of vaccine at 2, 4, 6, and 12 to 15 months of age. Adverse events reported in clinical trials with *Prevnar* include bronchiolitis, urinary tract infection, acute gastroenteritis, asthma, aspiration, breath holding, influenza, inguinal hernia repair, viral syndrome, upper respiratory tract infection, croup, thrush, wheezing, choking, conjunctivitis, pharyngitis, colic, colitis, congestive heart failure, roseola, and sepsis. The following adverse events have been reported through passive surveillance since market introduction of *Prevnar* and, therefore, are considered adverse reactions for *Prevnar 13* as well. Because these events are reported voluntarily from a population of uncertain size, it is not possible to reliably estimate frequency or establish a causal relationship to the vaccine: injection-site dermatitis, injection-site pruritus, injection-site urticaria, lymphadenopathy localized to the region of the injection site, anaphylactic/anaphylactoid reaction including shock, angioneurotic edema, erythema multiforme, and apnea.

Concomitant vaccination: The safety of *Prevnar* given concomitantly with other vaccines as part of routine care was assessed in a 3-year observational study in which 65,927 children received 3 doses of *Prevnar* in the first year of life. Primary safety outcomes analyses included an evaluation of predefined adverse events occurring in temporal relationship to immunization. Rates of adverse events occurring within various time periods postvaccination were compared to a control time window. The primary safety outcomes analyses did not demonstrate a consistently elevated risk of healthcare utilization for croup, gastroenteritis, allergic reactions, seizures, wheezing diagnoses, or breath-holding across doses, healthcare settings, or multiple time windows. As in prelicensure trials, fever was associated with *Prevnar* administration. In analyses of secondary safety outcomes, the adjusted relative risk of hospitalization for reactive airways disease was 1.23 (95% CI, 1.11-1.35). Potential confounders, such as differences in concomitantly administered vaccines, yearly variation in respiratory infections, or secular trends in reactive airway disease incidence, could not be controlled. Extended follow-up of subjects originally enrolled in the efficacy trial revealed no increased risk of reactive airway disease among *Prevnar* recipients. In general, the study results support the previously described safety profile of *Prevnar*.

Pharmacologic & Dosing Characteristics

Dosage: 0.5 mL

Adults 50 years and older: One 0.5 mL dose

Infants: Give 3 doses of 0.5 mL each at approximately 2-month intervals, typically at 2, 4, and 6 months of age, followed by a fourth dose of 0.5 mL at 12 to 15 months of age. The customary age for the first dose is 2 months, but it can be given as young as 6 weeks of age. The recommended dosing interval is 4 to 8 weeks. Give the fourth dose at least 2 months after the third dose and after the first birthday.

Older infants and children: For previously unvaccinated older infants and children beyond the age of the routine infant schedule, the following schedule applies:

Prevnar 13 Dosing Schedule for Older Infants and Children	
Age at first dose	Total number of 0.5 mL doses
7 to 11 months of age	3 (2 doses ≥ 4 weeks apart; third dose after the 1-year birthday, separated from the second dose by ≥ 2 months)
12 to 23 months of age	2 (each dose ≥ 2 months apart)
> 24 months to 71 months of age	1[a]

a Children older than 24 months who have sickle cell disease, asplenia, HIV infection, chronic illness, or who are immunocompromised also receive PPV23 for broad serotype protection.

Route & Site: IM, preferably in the anterolateral aspect of the thigh in infants or the deltoid muscle of the upper arm in toddlers, young children, and adults. Do not inject in the gluteal area or areas where there may be a major nerve trunk or blood vessel.

Documentation Requirements: Federal law requires that the following information be documented in the recipient's permanent medical record or in a permanent office log: (1) the manufacturer and lot number of the vaccine, (2) the date of administration, and (3) the name, address, and title of the person administering the vaccine.

Certain adverse events must be reported to the Vaccine Adverse Event Reporting System (VAERS) ([800] 822-7967). Refer to Immunization Documents in the Resources section for more information.

Overdosage: There have been reports of overdose with *Prevnar 13*, including administration of a higher than recommended dose, as well as subsequent doses administered closer than recommended to the previous dose. Most patients were asymptomatic. In general, adverse events reported with overdose have also been reported with recommended single doses of *Prevnar 13*.

Booster Doses: Booster doses are not currently recommended, beyond the recommended multidose schedule based on age.

Missed Doses: Interrupting the recommended schedule or delaying subsequent doses does not require restarting the series. Resume the series as soon as practical.

Related Interventions: Children older than 24 months who have sickle cell disease, asplenia, HIV infection, chronic illness, or who are immunocompromised should complete an age-appropriate PCV13 regimen and then receive PPV23 to provide broad serotype protection. Data on sequential vaccination with PCV13 followed by PPV23 are limited.

Efficacy:

Invasive pneumococcal disease: Prevnar was licensed in the United States in 2000, based on a randomized, double-blind clinical trial in a multiethnic population at Northern California Kaiser Permanente (NCKP) from 1995 through 1998, in which 37,816 infants received either *Prevnar* or a control vaccine (an investigational meningococcal group C conjugate vaccine [MnCC]) at 2, 4, 6, and 12 to 15 months of age. In this study, the efficacy of *Prevnar* against invasive disease due to *S. pneumoniae* in cases accrued during this period was 100% in both the per-protocol and intent-to-treat analyses (95% CI, 75%-100% and 82%-100%, respectively). Data accumulated through an extended follow-up period to April 1999 resulted in similar efficacy estimates of 97.4% in the per-protocol analysis and 93.9% in the intent-to-treat analysis (95% CI, 83%-99.9% and 80%-98.5%, respectively).

Acute otitis media: The efficacy of *Prevnar* against otitis media was assessed in 2 clinical trials: a trial in Finnish infants and the pivotal-efficacy trial in United States infants at NCKP. The Finnish Otitis Media (FinOM) trial was a randomized, double-blind trial in which 1,662 infants received either *Prevnar* or a *Recombivax HB* at 2, 4, 6, and 12 to 15 months of age. In this study, conducted between 1995 and 1999, parents were asked to bring children to study clinics if the child had respiratory infections or symptoms suggesting acute otitis media (AOM). If AOM was diagnosed, tympanocentesis was performed, and the middle-ear fluid was cultured and serotyped. In the NCKP trial, the efficacy of *Prevnar* against otitis media was assessed from 1995 through 1998. The otitis media analysis included 34,146 infants randomized to receive either *Prevnar* (n = 17,070), or MnCC (n = 17,076) at 2, 4, 6, and 12 to 15 months of age. In this trial, no routine tympanocentesis was performed, and no standard definition of otitis media was used. Vaccine efficacy against AOM episodes due to vaccine serotypes assessed in the Finnish trial was 57% (95% CI, 44%-67%) in the per-protocol population and 54% (95% CI, 41%-64%) in the intent-to-treat population. The vaccine efficacy against AOM episodes due to vaccine-related serotypes (6A, 9N, 18B, 19A, 23A), also assessed in the Finnish trial, was 51% (95% CI, 27-67) in the per-protocol population and 44% (95% CI, 20-62) in the intent-to-treat population. There was a nonsignificant increase in AOM episodes caused by serotypes unrelated to the vaccine in the per-protocol population, compared to children who received the control vaccine, suggesting that children who received *Prevnar* appeared to be at increased risk of otitis media due to pneumococcal serotypes not represented in the vaccine. However, vaccination with *Prevnar* reduced pneumococcal otitis media episodes overall. In the NCKP trial, in which the end point was all otitis media episodes regardless of etiology, vaccine efficacy was 7% (95% CI, 4%-10%) and 6% (95% CI, 4%-9%), respectively, in the per-protocol and intent-to-treat analyses. Several other otitis media end points were also assessed in the 2 trials. Recurrent AOM, defined as 3 episodes in 6 months or 4 episodes in 12 months, was reduced by 9% in both the per-protocol and intent-to-treat populations (95% CI, 3%-15% and 4%-14%) in the NCKP trial; a similar trend was observed in the Finnish trial. The NCKP trial also demonstrated a 20% reduction (95% CI, 2-35) in the placement of tympanostomy tubes in the per-protocol population and a 21% reduction (95% CI, 4-34) in the intent-to-treat population. Data from the NCKP trial accumulated through an extended follow-up period to April 1999, in which a total of 37,866 children were included (18,925 *Prevnar* and 18,941 MnCC), resulted in similar otitis media efficacy estimates for all end points.

Prevnar 13 effectiveness: *Prevnar 13* effectiveness against invasive pneumococcal disease (IPD) was inferred from comparative studies to *Prevnar*, assessing immune responses as measured by antipolysaccharide binding and functional opsonophagocytic activity (OPA) antibodies. The pivotal US noninferiority study was a randomized, double-blind, active-controlled trial in which 2-month-old infants were randomly assigned to receive either *Prevnar 13* or *Prevnar*. The vaccine groups were well balanced with respect to race, ethnicity, and age and weight at enrollment. Responses to the 7 common serotypes in *Prevnar 13* and *Prevnar* recipients were compared directly. Responses to the 6 additional serotypes in *Prevnar 13* recipients were each compared to the lowest response observed among the *Prevnar* serotypes in *Prevnar* recipients.

Responses after 3 doses: In the pivotal US noninferiority study, the noninferiority criterion for the proportion of subjects with pneumococcal anticapsular polysaccharide IgG antibody concentrations greater than or equal to 0.35 mcg/mL 1 month after the third dose was met for 10 of the 13 serotypes. The exceptions were serotypes 6B, 9V, and 3. Although the response to serotypes 6B and 9V did not meet the prespecified noninferiority criterion, the differences were marginal. The clinical relevance of these differences, if any, is unknown. The percentage of infants achieving pneumococcal anticapsular polysaccharide IgG antibody concentrations 0.35 mcg/mL or more 1 month after the third dose appears in this table.

Subjects With Anticapsular Antibody Concentration ≥ 0.35 mcg/mL 1 Month After Dose 3[a,b]			
Serotype	*Prevnar 13* (n = 249 to 252) % (95% CI)	*Prevnar* (n = 250 to 252) % (95% CI)	Difference in % responders (95% CI)
Prevnar serotypes			
4	94.4 (90.9, 96.9)	98 (95.4, 99.4)	−3.6 (−7.3, −0.1)
6B	87.3 (82.5, 91.1)	92.8 (88.9, 95.7)	−5.5 (−10.9, −0.1)
9V	90.5 (86.2, 93.8)	98.4 (96, 99.6)	−7.9 (−12.4, −4)
14	97.6 (94.9, 99.1)	97.2 (94.4, 98.9)	0.4 (−2.7, 3.5)
18C	96.8 (93.8, 98.6)	98.4 (96, 99.6)	−1.6 (−4.7, 1.2)
19F	98 (95.4, 99.4)	97.6 (99.4, 99.1)	0.4 (−2.4, 3.4)
23F	90.5 (86.2, 93.8)	94 (90.4, 96.6)	−3.6 (−8.5, 1.2)
Additional serotypes[c]			
1	95.6 (92.3, 97.8)	c	2.8 (−1.3, 7.2)
3	63.5 (57.1, 69.4)	c	−29.3 (−36.2, −22.4)
5	89.7 (85.2, 93.1)	c	−3.1 (−8.3, 1.9)
6A	96 (92.8, 98.1)	c	3.2 (−0.8, 7.6)
7F	98.4 (96, 99.6)	c	5.6 (1.9, 9.7)
19A	98.4 (96, 99.6)	c	5.6 (1.9, 9.7)

a Noninferiority was met when the lower bound of the 95% CI for the difference between groups (*Prevnar 13* minus *Prevnar*) was greater than −10%.

b Antibody measured by a standardized ELISA involving preabsorption of the test sera with pneumococcal C-polysaccharide and serotype 22F polysaccharide to reduce nonspecific background reactivity.

c Comparison for the 6 additional serotypes was to the lowest responder of the 7 common serotypes in *Prevnar* recipients, which for this analysis was serotype 6B (92.8%; 95% CI, 88.9-95.7).

OPA antibody responses were elicited for all 13 serotypes, as shown in the following table.

Pneumococcal OPA Geometric Mean Titers 1 Month After the Third Dose-Evaluable Immunogenicity Population, US Pivotal Noninferiority Study[a]		
Serotype	*Prevnar 13* n = 91-94 (95% CI)	*Prevnar* n = 89-94 (95% CI)
Prevnar serotypes		
4	359 (276, 468)	536 (421, 681)
6B	1,055 (817, 1,361)	1,514 (1,207, 1,899)
9V	4,035 (2,933, 5,553)	3,259 (2,288, 4,641)
14	1,240 (935, 1,646)	1,481 (1,133, 1,934)

Pneumococcal OPA Geometric Mean Titers 1 Month After the Third Dose-Evaluable Immunogenicity Population, US Pivotal Noninferiority Study[a]		
Serotype	Prevnar 13 n = 91-94 (95% CI)	Prevnar n = 89-94 (95% CI)
18C	276 (210, 361)	376 (292, 484)
19F	54 (40, 74)	45 (34, 60)
23F	791 (605, 1,034)	924 (709, 1,204)
Additional serotypes		
1	52 (39, 69)	4 (4, 5)
3	121 (92, 158)	7 (5, 9)
5	91 (67, 123)	4 (4, 4)
6A	980 (783, 1226)	100 (66, 152)
7F	9,494 (7,339, 12,281)	128 (80, 206)
19A	152 (105, 220)	7 (5, 9)

a The OPA assay measures the ability of immune sera, in conjunction with complement, to mediate the uptake and killing of *S. pneumoniae* by phagocytic cells.

Responses after 4 doses: In the pivotal US noninferiority study, postdose 4 antibody concentrations were higher for all 13 serotypes than those achieved after the third dose. The noninferiority criterion for pneumococcal anticapsular polysaccharide GMCs after 4 doses was met for 12 of the 13 pneumococcal serotypes. The noninferiority criterion was not met for the response to serotype 3. After the fourth dose, the functional OPA response for each serotype was quantitatively greater than the response following the third dose.

Onset: Not specifically determined; immunity increases with successive doses.

Duration: Not determined

Pharmacokinetics: See antibody data provided in Efficacy section.

Protective Level: In all studies in which the immune responses to *Prevnar 13* were compared with control, a significant antibody response was seen to all vaccine serotypes following 3 or 4 doses, although geometric mean concentrations of antibody varied among serotypes. The World Health Organization (WHO) accepts the minimum serum antibody concentration necessary for protection against invasive pneumococcal disease to be 0.35 mcg/mL in children for each of the 7 serotypes in the original *Prevnar*. *Prevnar 13* induces functional antibodies to all vaccine serotypes, as measured by opsonophagocytosis following 3 doses.

For adults, a protective level or correlate of immunity has not been established.

Mechanism: Induction of specific protective antibodies. Type-specific antibody facilitates bacterial destruction by complement-mediated lysis.

Drug Interactions: Like all inactivated vaccines, administration of pneumococcal vaccine to patients receiving immunosuppressant drugs (eg, high-dose corticosteroids), antimetabolites, alkylating agents, cytotoxic agents, or radiation therapy may result in an insufficient response to immunization. These patients may remain susceptible despite immunization. In patients anticipating immunosuppression, response to pneumococcal vaccine is best if administered 10 to 14 days prior to immunosuppressive chemotherapy or radiation.

As with other IM injections, administer *Prevnar 13* with caution to children on anticoagulant therapy.

During clinical studies, *Prevnar 13* was administered simultaneously with DTaP plus Hib, IPV; hepatitis B; MMR; and varicella vaccines. The safety experience with *Prevnar 13* reflects the use of this product as part of the routine immunization schedule. The immune response to routine vaccines when administered with *Prevnar 13* (at separate sites) was assessed in clinical studies in which there was a control group for comparison. Immune responses to concomitant vaccine antigens were compared in infants receiving *Prevnar* and *Prevnar 13*. Responses to diphtheria toxoid, tetanus toxoid, pertussis, polio types 1, 2, and 3, hepatitis B, PRP-T, PRP-OMP, measles, and varicella antigens in *Prevnar 13* recipients were similar to those in *Prevnar* recipients. Based on limited data, responses to mumps and rubella antigens in *Prevnar 13* recipients were similar to those in *Prevnar* recipients. Enhancement of antibody response to *Hib* in the infant series was observed with 7-valent *Prevnar*. Some suppression of *Haemophilus influenzae* type b (Hib) response was seen at the fourth dose, but more than 97% of children achieved titers more than 1 mcg/mL. Although some inconsistent differences in response to pertussis antigens were observed, the clinical relevance is unknown. The response to 2 doses of IPV given concomitantly with *Prevnar* (assessed 3 months after the second dose) was equivalent to controls for poliovirus types 2 and 3, but lower for type 1. *Havrix* brand of hepatitis A vaccine has been administered simultaneously with *Prevnar* and did not interfere with immune responses to either vaccine.

Pharmaceutical Characteristics

Concentration: Each 0.5 mL dose contains 2.2 mcg of each saccharide for serotypes 1, 3, 4, 5, 6A, 7F, 9V,14, 18C, 19F, 19A, and 23F, and 4.4 mcg of serotype 6B per dose (16 mg total saccharide).

Quality Assay: Individual polysaccharides are purified through centrifugation, precipitation, ultrafiltration, and column chromatography. The individual glycoconjugates are purified by ultrafiltration and column chromatography and are analyzed for saccharide-to-protein ratios, molecular size, free saccharide, and free protein. Potency of the formulated vaccine is determined by quantification of each of the saccharide antigens, and by the saccharide-to-protein ratios in the individual glycoconjugates.

Packaging: Package of 10 single-dose 0.5 mL prefilled syringes.

NDC Number: 00005-1971-02

Doseform: Suspension

Appearance: After shaking, the vaccine is a homogeneous, white suspension.

Solvent: Succinate buffer solution

Adjuvant: Approximately 34 mcg diphtheria CRM_{197} protein per 0.5 mL, plus 0.125 mg of aluminum per 0.5 mL as aluminum phosphate

Preservative: None

Allergens: None.

Excipients: Succinate buffer 295 mcg and polysorbate 80 100 mcg per 0.5 mL

pH: Not described.

Shelf Life: Expires within 18 months

Storage/Stability: Store at 2° to 8°C (36° to 46°F). Discard frozen vaccine. Contact the manufacturer regarding exposure to extreme temperatures. Shipped in insulated containers with coolant packs and temperature monitor via overnight courier.

Handling: Shake vigorously to obtain a uniform suspension immediately before withdrawing the dose. Do not use the vaccine if it cannot be resuspended.

Production Process: The individual polysaccharides are purified through centrifugation, precipitation, ultrafiltration, and column chromatography. The polysaccharides are chemically activated to make saccharides, which are directly conjugated by reductive amination to the protein carrier CRM_{197} to form the glycoconjugate. CRM_{197} is a nontoxic variant of diphtheria toxin isolated from cultures of *Corynebacterium diphtheriae* strain C7 (β197) grown in a casamino acids- and yeast extract-based medium. CRM_{197} is purified through ultrafiltration, ammonium sulfate precipitation, and ion-exchange chromatography. The individual glycoconjugates are purified by ultrafiltration and column chromatography and are analyzed for saccharide-to-protein ratios, molecular size, free saccharide, and free protein.

The individual glycoconjugates are compounded to formulate the vaccine. Potency of the formulated vaccine is determined by quantification of each of the saccharide antigens, and by the saccharide-to-protein ratios in the individual glycoconjugates.

Media: Soy peptone broth

Disease Epidemiology

Incidence: *Streptococcus pneumoniae* is an important cause of morbidity and mortality in people of all ages worldwide. The organism causes invasive infections, including bacteremia and meningitis, pneumonia, and upper respiratory tract infections, including otitis media and sinusitis. More than 90 serotypes of *S. pneumoniae* have been identified based on antigenic differences in their capsular polysaccharides. The distribution of serotypes responsible for disease differs with age and geographic location.

Susceptible Pools: Children in group child care have an increased risk for invasive pneumococcal disease. Immunocompromised individuals with neutropenia, asplenia, sickle cell disease, disorders of complement and humoral immunity, HIV infections, or chronic underlying disease are also at increased risk for invasive pneumococcal disease. Daycare attendance, a history of ear infection, and a recent history of antibiotic exposure have also been associated with invasive infections with PNSP in children 2 to 59 months of age.

Transmission: By droplet spread or oral contact

Incubation: 1 to 3 days

Communicability: Until oral and nasal discharges are free of virulent pneumococci. Penicillin will render the patient noninfectious within 24 to 48 hours.

Other Information

Perspective: See Pneumococcal Vaccine, 23-valent monograph.

First Licensed:
Prevnar 13: February 24, 2010
Prevnar (7-valent): February 17, 2000

National Policy: ACIP. Licensure of a 13-valent pneumococcal conjugate vaccine (PCV13) and recommendations for use among children (ACIP), 2010. *MMWR*. 2010;59:258-261.

ACIP. Prevention of pneumococcal disease among infants and children — use of 13-valent pneumococcal conjugate vaccine and 23-valent pneumococcal polysaccharide vaccine. *MMWR*. 2010;59(RR-11):1-19. www.cdc.gov/mmwr/pdf/rr/rr5911.pdf.

Canadian National Advisory Committee on Immunization. Update on the use of conjugate pneumococcal vaccines in childhood. *Can Comm Dis Rep.* 2010;36(ACS-12):1-21. www.phac-aspc.gc.ca/publicat/ccdr-rmtc/10vol36/acs-12/acs-12-eng.pdf.

Canadian National Advisory Committee on Immunization. Statement on the recommended use of pneumococcal conjugate vaccine: Addendum. *Can Comm Dis Rep.* 2003;29(ACS-8):14-15.

References: CDC. Direct and indirect effects of routine vaccination of children with 7-valent pneumococcal conjugate vaccine on incidence of invasive pneumococcal disease—United States, 1998-2003. *MMWR*. 2005;54:893-897. www.cdc.gov/mmwr/PDF/wk/mm5436.pdf.

WHO. Pneumococcal vaccines: WHO position paper—2012. *Wkly Epidemiol Rec.* 2012;87(14):129-144.

Pneumococcal Polysaccharide Vaccine, 23-Valent

Bacterial Vaccines & Toxoids

Name:
Pneumovax 23

Manufacturer:
Merck

Synonyms: PPV23, PPSV23. In other countries, *Pneumovax 23* is known as *Pneumovax II*, *Pneumovax NP*, *Prodiax 23*, and *Pulmovax*.

Comparison: Polysaccharide vaccine varies considerably from protein-conjugated formulations of pneumococcal vaccine.

Pneumococcal polysaccharide and conjugate vaccines each induce antibody responses in people 2 years and older. Some, but not all, head-to-head clinical studies find superior antibody responses for PCV13 compared with PPV23 for some serotypes 1 month after vaccination, but this differential tends to dissipate in following months. No protective threshold for antibody response has been established in adults. Consider the separate components in the 2 products when selecting a pneumococcal vaccine.

Immunologic Characteristics

Microorganism: Bacterium, *Streptococcus pneumoniae* (also known as pneumococcus or diplococcus), homofermentative gram-positive cocci

Viability: Inactivated

Antigenic Form: Capsular polysaccharide fragments

Antigenic Type: Polysaccharide mixture

Strains:
US system: Types 1, 2, 3, 4, 5, 8, 9, 12, 14, 17, 19, 20, 22, 23, 26, 34, 43, 51, 54, 56, 57, 68, 70
Danish nomenclature: Types 1, 2, 3, 4, 5, 6B, 7F, 8, 9N, 9V, 10A, 11A, 12F, 14, 15B, 17F, 18C, 19F, 19A, 20, 22F, 23F, 33F

Use Characteristics

Indications: For induction of active immunity against pneumococcal disease caused by those pneumococcal types included in the vaccine. Vaccination offers protection against invasive pneumococcal disease, pneumococcal bacteremia, and other pneumococcal infections. Evidence for efficacy against pneumococcal pneumonia is less consistent, but confirmed by meta-analysis (Moberley et al, 2008).

Adults: Vaccinate all adults 65 years of age and older, emphasizing immunization of the older adult while still in good health. The vaccine is licensed for people 50 years of age or older. Vaccinate all immunocompetent adults who are at increased risk of pneumococcal disease or its complications because of chronic illnesses (eg, cardiovascular or pulmonary disease, impaired hepatic or renal systems, diabetes mellitus, alcoholism, cirrhosis, chronic cerebrospinal fluid leaks, adults who smoke cigarettes). Examples of cardiopulmonary disease warranting pneumococcal immunization include congestive heart failure, cardiomyopathy, chronic obstructive pulmonary disease, or emphysema. Asthma complicated by chronic bronchitis, emphysema, or long-term use of systemic corticosteroids is another indication. Refer to the tables of pertinent diagnoses and related indicator medications in Annex B. Vaccinate immunocompromised adults at increased risk of pneumococcal disease or its complications (eg, splenic dysfunction or anatomic asplenia, sickle cell anemia and other severe hemoglobinopathies, Hodgkin disease, lymphoma, multiple myeloma, chronic renal failure, nephrotic syndrome, conditions such as organ transplantation associated with immunosuppression).

Children: Vaccinate children 2 years and older with chronic illness specifically associated with increased risk of pneumococcal disease or its complications (eg, splenic dysfunction or anatomic asplenia, sickle cell disease, nephrotic syndrome, cerebrospinal fluid leaks). Pneumococcal immunization is specifically recommended for children 2 years and older with renal failure, diabetes, or severe immunosuppression.

Members of closed groups: Pneumococcal vaccination is also indicated for adults or children living in closed groups (eg, residential schools, nursing homes, other institutions) to decrease the likelihood of acute outbreaks of pneumococcal disease where there is increased risk that the disease may be severe.

Cochlear implant recipients: To reduce the risk of pneumococcal meningitis, people with cochlear implants should use the age-appropriate vaccine according to Advisory Committee on Immunization Practices (ACIP) schedules for people at high risk.

Native populations: Routine use of PPV23 after PCV13 is not recommended for Alaska Native or American Indian children 24 to 59 months of age. However, in special situations, public health authorities may recommend the use of PPV23 after PCV13 for Alaska Native or American Indian children living in areas where risk of invasive pneumococcal disease is increased. Routine use of PPV23 is not recommended for Alaska Native or American Indians younger than 65 years unless they have underlying medical conditions that are PPV23 indications. However, in special situations, public health authorities may recommend PPV23 for Alaska Native or American Indians 50 to 64 years of age living in areas where the risk of invasive pneumococcal disease is increased.

Limitations: Pneumococcal vaccine is not effective for prophylaxis against pneumococcal disease caused by pneumococcal types not represented in the vaccine. Vaccination does not warrant discontinuation of penicillin or other antibiotic prophylaxis against pneumococcal infection. Select appropriate antibiotics to treat active infections (eg, penicillin G or V, an erythromycin).

Patients with impaired immune responsiveness (ie, from genetic defect, splenectomy or functional asplenia, immunosuppressive chemotherapy or radiotherapy, HIV infection) may have a reduced antibody response to active immunization.

The vaccine may not be effective in preventing infection resulting from basilar skull fracture or from external communication with cerebrospinal fluid.

Contraindications:

Absolute: People with a history of serious allergic reaction to a vaccine component or after a prior dose of this vaccine.

Relative: A febrile respiratory illness or active infection. Do not vaccinate patients younger than 2 years because they are less likely to respond to the vaccine.

Immunodeficiency: Patients receiving immunosuppressive therapy or those with other immunodeficiencies may have a diminished antibody response to active immunization. They may remain susceptible despite immunization. Patients with AIDS may have an impaired antibody response to pneumococcal vaccine. However, asymptomatic patients infected with HIV or those with generalized lymphadenopathy generally respond to pneumococcal vaccine. Routine immunization of symptomatic and asymptomatic HIV-infected patients is recommended.

The ACIP specifically recommends influenza immunization for children 6 months of age and older and pneumococcal-conjugate immunization for children 2 months and older with renal failure, diabetes, or severe immunosuppression. Severe immunosuppression may result from congenital immunodeficiency, HIV infection, leukemia, lymphoma, aplastic anemia, generalized malignancy, or therapy with alkylating agents, antimetabolites, radiation, or large, sustained doses of corticosteroids.

Patients without functioning spleens have a reduced ability to clear encapsulated bacteria from the bloodstream. They are at highest risk for pneumococcal infection. Those 2 years of age and older respond to immunization with antibody concentrations comparable with those of healthy people of the same age.

Pneumococcal vaccine may be given as early as several months after completing chemotherapy or radiation therapy for neoplastic disease. In Hodgkin disease, immune response to vaccination may be impaired for 2 years or longer after intensive chemotherapy. During those 2 years, antibody responses improve in some patients as the interval between end of treatment and vaccination increases.

Elderly: Immune response in the elderly is generally good, although immunosuppressed elderly patients may exhibit an impaired response. The elderly may exhibit a lower IgM antibody response. Published data support giving pneumococcal vaccine to the "young elderly," before advancing age impairs immune response to vaccines such as this one.

Pregnancy: Category C. Not recommended unless substantial risk exists. It is not known if pneumococcal vaccine or corresponding antibodies cross the placenta. Generally, most IgG passage across the placenta occurs during the third trimester.

Lactation: It is not known if pneumococcal vaccine or corresponding antibodies are excreted in breast milk. Problems in humans have not been documented.

Children: All children 2 months of age or older should receive routine immunization with PCV13. Children younger than 2 years respond poorly to most capsular types in polysaccharide vaccines. Children younger than 5 years may not respond to some antigens. Nonetheless, children 2 years of age and older with anatomical or functional asplenia and otherwise intact lymphoid function generally respond to pneumococcal vaccines with a serological conversion comparable with that observed in healthy individuals of the same age.

Children older than 24 months who have sickle cell disease, asplenia, HIV infection, chronic illness, or who are immunocompromised should complete an age-appropriate PCV13 regimen and then receive PPV23 to provide broad serotype protection. Data on sequential vaccination with PCV13 followed by PPV23 are limited.

Adverse Reactions: Local erythema, warmth, swelling, and soreness at the injection site, usually lasting less than 48 hours in duration, occur commonly (approximately 33%). Local induration occurs less commonly. Rash, arthralgia, adenitis, fever higher than 39°C (102°F), malaise, myalgia, urticaria, cellulitis-like reactions, and asthenia occur rarely. Low-grade fever (lower than 38.3°C [100.9°F]) occurs occasionally and usually subsides within 24 hours.

Compared with primary vaccination, an elevated rate of self-limited injection-site reactions may occur with revaccination at 3 to 5 years after primary vaccination.

Patients with otherwise stabilized idiopathic thrombocytopenic purpura have, on rare occasions, experienced a relapse in their thrombocytopenia, occurring 2 to 14 days after vaccination and lasting up to 2 weeks.

Systemic reactions of greater severity, duration, or extent are unusual, although anaphylactoid reactions have been reported. Neurological disorders, such as paresthesias and acute radiculoneuropathy, including Guillain-Barré syndrome, have been rarely reported in temporal association with administration of pneumococcal vaccine, but no cause-and-effect relationship has been established. Other adverse events reported in clinical trials or postlicensing experience include fever greater than 39°C (102°F), chills, nausea, vomiting, lymphadenitis, hemolytic anemia (in patients who had other hematologic disorders), serum sickness, angioneurotic edema, arthritis, headache, and paresthesia.

Patients who have had episodes of pneumococcal pneumonia or other pneumococcal infection may have high levels of preexisting pneumococcal antibodies to certain types of the bacteria that may result in increased reactions to pneumococcal vaccine. These reactions are usually localized to the injection site, but occasionally may be systemic.

Pharmacologic & Dosing Characteristics

Dosage: 0.5 mL. When elective splenectomy, cancer chemotherapy, or other immunosuppression is planned, give pneumococcal vaccine at least 2 weeks before surgery or immunosuppression, if possible. With unplanned splenectomy, vaccinate after the immediate postoperative period.

Route & Site: Subcutaneous or IM injection, preferably in the deltoid muscle or lateral midthigh. IM may be less painful. Severe reactions may follow intradermal or intravenous administration; do not use these routes.

Overdosage: Although few data are available, clinical experience with similar products suggests that the major manifestations of overdosage would be pain and tenderness at the injection site.

Monitor: Following immunization of healthy adults, antibody levels remain elevated for at least 5 years, but in some individuals, antibody levels may fall to preimmunization levels within 10 years. A more rapid decline may occur in children, particularly those who have undergone splenectomy and those with sickle cell disease or nephrotic syndrome, in whom antibodies for some pneumococcal types can fall to preimmunization levels 3 to 5 years after immunization.

Booster Doses: Revaccinate patients at highest risk of fatal disease (eg, asplenia) or rapid decline in antibody levels (eg, nephrotic syndrome) 5 years or more after the initial dose. This category includes anyone with an immunosuppressive disorder or on immunosuppressive therapy.

Revaccinate patients 65 years and older if they were younger than 65 years when they received their first dose and if that dose was at least 5 years ago.

For children, give a single revaccination if 5 years or more have elapsed.

If immunization records are not readily available, vaccinate the patient. Among patients given a second dose of pneumococcal vaccine within 2 years after the first dose, adverse injection-site reactions are more severe after the second dose than after the first dose. However, giving a second dose 4 years or more after an initial dose is not associated with an increased incidence of adverse events. Localized adverse effects from too-frequent dosing are overshadowed by the risk of fatal pneumococcal infections.

Efficacy of pneumococcal vaccine did not decline with increasing interval after vaccination in an indirect cohort analysis of patients with confirmed pneumococcal isolates: 5 to 8 years after vaccination, it was 71% (95% CI, 24%-89%); 9 years or more after vaccination, it was 80% (95% CI, 16%-95%).

Efficacy: Vaccination will reduce disease incidence 60% to 80%. Strains represented in the 23-valent vaccine account for 90% of blood isolates and 85% of isolates from other normally sterile sites.

Seroconversion: More than 90% of healthy adults, including the elderly, demonstrate a 2-fold or more rise in type-specific geometric mean antibody titers within 2 to 3 weeks after immunization. Similar antibody responses occurred in patients with alcoholic cirrhosis and diabetes mellitus. In elderly individuals with chronic pulmonary disease and immunocompromised patients, the response to immunization may be lower.

Clinical protection:

Pneumonia: In Austrian's 1976 report of a 13-valent pneumococcal vaccine among young, healthy gold miners, pneumonias caused by the capsular types present in the vaccine were reduced 79%. Randomized clinical trials have been inconsistent in detecting a protective effect for pneumococcal vaccine in high-risk groups, perhaps because of a lack of specific and sensitive diagnostic tests for nonbacteremic pneumococcal pneumonia.

Bacteremia: Case-control studies show the vaccine to prevent invasive diseases, with point estimates of efficacy (reduction in disease incidence) of 56% to 81%. Vaccine effectiveness of 65% to 84% was demonstrated among specific patient groups, including patients with diabetes mellitus, coronary vascular disease, congestive heart failure, chronic pulmonary disease, and anatomic asplenia. Effectiveness among immunocompetent patients 65 years of age and older was 75%.

Onset: 14 days to 3 weeks. Vaccinate more than 2 weeks before elective splenectomy or planned immunosuppressive therapy, if possible.

Duration: Protective antibody levels decline over 5 to 10 years. A more rapid decline may occur in some groups (eg, children, elderly).

Protective Level: Not established because differences in measuring antibody yield differing results. Antibody function or avidity may be a more important measure of immunity than antibody concentrations.

Mechanism: Induction of serotype-specific antibodies. Type-specific antibody facilitates bacterial destruction by opsonization and phagocytosis and killing by leukocytes and other phagocytic cells.

Drug Interactions: In patients anticipating immunosuppression, response to pneumococcal vaccine is best if administered 10 to 14 days prior to immunosuppressive chemotherapy or radiation. Like all inactivated vaccines, administration of pneumococcal vaccine to patients receiving immunosuppressant drugs (eg, high-dose corticosteroids) or radiation therapy may result in an insufficient response to immunization. Patients may remain susceptible despite immunization.

Pneumococcal and influenza vaccines may safely and effectively be administered simultaneously at separate injection sites. While influenza vaccine is given annually, PPV23 is given once to all but those at highest risk of fatal disease. Hib, meningococcal, and pneumococcal vaccines may safely and effectively be administered simultaneously at separate injection sites.

In a study of 6 patients, PPV23 had no effect on the pharmacokinetics of theophylline.

As with other drugs administered IM, give pneumococcal vaccine with caution to patients receiving anticoagulant therapy.

Inactivated vaccines are not generally affected by circulating antibodies or administration of exogenous antibodies. Vaccination may occur at any time before or after antibody administration.

In a double-blind study, 473 adults 60 years or older were randomized to receive zoster vaccine and PPV23 concomitantly (N = 237), or PPV23 alone followed 4 weeks later by zoster vaccine alone (N = 236). Four weeks after vaccination, the VZV antibody levels following concomitant use were significantly lower than the VZV antibody levels following nonconcomitant administration (geometric mean titers [GMTs] of 338 vs 484 gpELISA units/mL, respectively; GMT ratio = 0.7 (95% CI, 0.61-0.8). The manufacturer recommends against coadministration. However, IgG levels against varicella-zoster virus may not directly correlate with clinical protection against zoster. A study in a large managed-care database did not find a clinically significant difference in the incidence of herpes zoster among people who received PPV23 and zoster vaccine either on the same day or separated by 30 to 365 days.

Lab Interference: Three of 9 children immunized with pneumococcal polysaccharide vaccine had urine positive for pneumococcal antigen 2 days after vaccination, based on the *Wellcogen* kit (Murex Biologicals).

Three of 10 urine samples from men and women 75 to 97 years of age vaccinated with pneumococcal polysaccharide vaccine were positive on the first day after vaccination, using the NOW *S. pneumoniae* urinary antigen test (*Binax*, Portland, Maine).

Pharmaceutical Characteristics

Concentration: 25 mcg each of 23 polysaccharides per 0.5 mL

Quality Assay: Product is assayed for O-acetyl, uronic acid, methyl pentose, hexosamine, protein, and other chemical content and molecular size. Guinea pig safety tests and rabbit pyrogenicity and serologic tests are conducted. At least 80% of more than 25 volunteers demonstrate a 2-fold or more increase in antipneumococcal polysaccharide type-specific antibodies for each capsular type.

Packaging: 2.5 mL 5-dose vial (NDC#: 00006-4739-00); box of ten 5-dose vials (00006-4739-50); box of ten 0.5 mL single-dose vials (00006-4943-00); package of 1,000 0.5 mL vials (00006-4741-01)

Doseform: Solution

Appearance: Clear, colorless solution

Solvent: Sodium chloride 0.9%

Adjuvant: None

Preservative: Phenol 0.25%

Allergens: None

Excipients: None

pH: 4.5 to 7.4

Shelf Life: Expires within 30 months

Storage/Stability: Store at 2° to 8°C (35° to 46°F). Do not freeze. Shipped in insulated containers with coolant packs.

Production Process: Each polysaccharide type is produced separately to ensure a high degree of purity. After an individual pneumococcal type is cultured, the polysaccharide is separated from the cell and purified by a series of steps, including ethanol fractionation. Each lot requires 1 year to produce.

Media: Suitable media, containing bovine proteins and other macromolecular components

Disease Epidemiology

Incidence: At least 5,500 deaths due to invasive pneumococcal disease occur per year in the United States, resulting from an estimated 175,000 cases of pneumococcal pneumonia, 50,000 cases of pneumococcal bacteremia, 3,000 to 6,000 cases of pneumococcal meningitis, and 250,000 or more hospitalizations per year. Pneumococcal pneumonia accounts for 25% to 35% of cases of community-acquired pneumonia among patients who are hospitalized (and approximately 35,000 deaths) per year in the United States, although the degree to which vaccination can prevent pneumococcal pneumonia is unclear. Annual rates of pneumococcal bacteremia range from 15 to 30 cases per 100,000 for the total population and 50 to 83 cases per 100,000 for people 65 years of age and older. Among adults with pneumococcal bacteremia, 60% to 87% develop pneumonia. Among adults with pneumococcal pneumonia, 25% to 30% manifest bacteremia. The overall mortality rate for bacteremia is about 20%, but among some high-risk patients, mortality may exceed 40% for bacteremic disease (60% in elderly patients) and 30% for meningitis (80% in elderly patients), despite appropriate antimicrobial therapy; 60% of all deaths among patients with pneumococcal bacteremia treated with penicillin or tetracycline occur within 5 days of illness onset. People without a functioning spleen who develop bacteremia may experience a fulminant clinical course. The incidence of *S. pneumoniae* infections resistant to penicillin and other antibiotics is increasing. American Indians, blacks, and certain other population groups may have considerably higher rates of disease incidence.

Mortality is highest in patients with bacteremia or meningitis, patients with underlying medical conditions, and the elderly. The case-fatality rate is generally 15% to 20%. However, among elderly patients, that rate is 30% to 40%. An estimated 100 million cases occur annually around the world, with 10 million deaths.

In children 2 years of age or younger, bacteremia without a known site of infection is the most common invasive clinical presentation, accounting for approximately 70% of invasive pneumococcal disease (IPD) in this age group. Bacteremic pneumonia accounts for 12% to 16% of IPD in this age group. With the decline of invasive Hib disease, *S. pneumoniae* became the leading cause of bacterial meningitis among children younger than 5 years in the United States. Before routine use of pneumococcal conjugate vaccine, an estimated 17,000 cases of IPD occurred annually, of which 13,000 were bacteremia without a known site of infection and about 700 were meningitis. In 1998, the rate of IPD in children younger than 2 years was 188 per 100,000 population, accounting for 20% of all cases of IPD. An estimated 200 children died each year from IPD.

Pneumococci are a common cause of acute otitis media, detected in 25% to 55% of middle-ear aspirates. An estimated 5 million cases of acute otitis media occurred each year among children younger than 5 years.

Susceptible Pools: Approximately 35% of people 65 years of age and older are unvaccinated. Younger people with chronic diseases that warrant pneumococcal immunization are even more likely to be unvaccinated.

Transmission: By droplet spread, by oral contact

Incubation: 1 to 3 days

Communicability: Until oral and nasal discharges are free of virulent pneumococci. Penicillin will render the patient noninfectious within 24 to 48 hours.

Other Information

Perspective:

1880: Army Major George M. Sternberg discovers *S. pneumoniae*, the pneumococcus.

1881: Pasteur discovers the pneumococcus.

1891: Klemperer and Klemperer use rabbit immune serum in treatment of pneumonia.

1911: Wright tests a pneumococcal vaccine with little success. Whole bacterial pneumococcal vaccines continue to be used through the 1930s.

1920: Heidelberger establishes that rabbit antibodies bind to capsular polysaccharides of *S. pneumoniae*.

1933: Francis, Finland, Tillett, and colleagues conduct test of soluble pneumococcal polysaccharide.

1945: Multivalent pneumococcal polysaccharide vaccine tested at Army Air Corps Technical School, Sioux Falls, South Dakota.

1947: Hexavalent polysaccharide vaccine available from E.R. Squibb until 1954. Squibb's vaccine was not widely accepted because of widespread confidence in the newly introduced drug, penicillin. The vaccine was withdrawn because of lack of acceptance and low sales.

1960s: Austrian conducts trials of 14-valent pneumococcal vaccine.

1977: 14-valent vaccine licensed in the United States on November 21. Booster doses at 3-year intervals recommended in product labeling approved by the US Food and Drug Administration.

1980: Public Law 96-611 mandates reimbursement of pneumococcal vaccination by Medicare (effective in 1981).

1981: The Centers for Disease Control and Prevention (CDC) specifically recommends against booster doses.

1983: 23-valent vaccine licensed in the United States (Lederle: July 21; Merck: July 7). Product labeling recommends not giving booster doses.

1988: The ACIP recommends booster doses every 6 years for patients at highest risk of disease.

1997: The ACIP recommends 1 repeat dose 5 years after the initial dose for patients at highest risk of disease.

Discontinued Products: *Pneumonia Bacterin* (Abbott), *Pneumonia Phylacogen* (Parke-Davis), *Pneumo-Serobacterin* (Mulford, National Drug Company). *Pnu-Imune* (14-valent product, Lederle, 1977-1983), *Pnu-Imune 23* (Wyeth-Lederle, 1983-2002).

National Policy: ACIP. Prevention of pneumococcal disease among infants and children — use of 13-valent pneumococcal conjugate vaccine and 23-valent pneumococcal polysaccharide vaccine. *MMWR*. 2010;59(RR-11):1-19. www.cdc.gov/mmwr/pdf/rr/rr5911.pdf.

ACIP. Updated recommendations for prevention of invasive pneumococcal disease among adults using the 23-valent pneumococcal polysaccharide vaccine (PPSV23). *MMWR*. 2010;59(34):1102-1106. www.cdc.gov/mmwr/pdf/wk/mm5934.pdf.

Canadian National Advisory Committee on Immunization. Statement on the recommended use of pneumococcal 23-valent polysaccharide vaccine in homeless persons and injection drug users. *Can Comm Dis Rep*. 2008;34(ACS-5):1-12.

Canadian National Advisory Committee on Immunization. Immunization recommendation for cochlear implant recipients. *Can Comm Disp Rep*. 2003;29(ACS-2):1-4.

ACIP. Prevention of pneumococcal disease: Recommendations of the Advisory Committee on Immunization Practices (ACIP). *MMWR* . 1997;46(RR-8):1-24.

References: Butler JC, Breiman RF, Capmpbell JF, Lipman HB, Broome CV, Facklam RR. Pneumococcal polysaccharide vaccine efficacy. An evaluation of current recommendations. *JAMA*. 1993;270(15):1826-1831.

Filice GA. Pneumococcal vaccines and public health policy. Consequences of missed opportunities. *Arch Intern Med*. 1990;150(7):1373-1375.

Moberley SA, Holden J, Tatham DP, Andrews RM. Vaccines for preventing pneumococcal infection in adults. *Cochrane Database Syst Rev*. 2008:(1):CD000422.

WHO. 23-valent pneumococcal polysaccharide vaccine. WHO position paper. *Wkly Epidemiol Rec*. 2008;83(42):373-384.

Pharmacoeconomics: Pneumococcal vaccine is reimbursed by Medicare (CPT code 90732, diagnosis code V03.82). Use HCPCS procedure code G0009 to report the administration fee to Medicare. If a physician visit is rendered in conjunction with vaccination, it may be reimbursed as well.

Typhoid Fever Vaccines

Bacterial Vaccines & Toxoids

Comparison Table of Typhoid Vaccines		
Generic name	Vi Capsular Polysaccharide (ViCPs) Vaccine	Oral Ty21a Vaccine
Brand name	*Typhim Vi*	*Vivotif*
Synonyms	ViCPs	
Manufacturer	Sanofi Pasteur	Berna Products/Crucell
Viability	Bacterial subunit vaccine	Live, attenuated bacterial vaccine
Indication	To prevent typhoid fever, primarily in endemic areas	To prevent typhoid fever, primarily in endemic areas
Strain	Ty2	Ty21a
Concentration	25 mcg/0.5 mL	2 to 6 billion CFU/capsule
Adjuvant	None	None
Preservative	Phenol 0.25%	None
Manufacturing process	Precipitation with hexadecyl-trimethylammonium	Live, attenuated bacteria
Doseform	Solution	Oral capsule
Packaging	0.5 mL syringe, 20-dose vials	Blister package of 4 light pink and white capsules
Routine storage	2° to 8°C	2° to 8°C
Dosage	0.5 mL	4 capsules, 1 every other day
Route	IM	Oral
Standard schedule	Single dose	1 capsule every other day for 4 doses
Booster doses	1 dose every 2 years	4-capsule regimen every 5 years
CPT codes	90691	90690

Bacterial Vaccines & Toxoids

Name:
Typhim Vi

Manufacturer:
Sanofi Pasteur

Synonyms: Typhoid Vi capsular polysaccharide vaccine may be abbreviated ViCPs. Typhoid fever is also known as enteric fever and typhus abdominalis.

Comparison: Acetone-killed and dried (AKD) and heat-phenol (HP) inactivated whole-cell typhoid vaccines are no longer produced in the United States. The Vi polysaccharide inactivated injectable vaccine and the live, attenuated typhoid vaccine for oral administration are not equivalent. The Vi polysaccharide vaccine reduces disease incidence 49% to 87%, while the capsules reduce disease 60% to 77%. Each typhoid vaccine induces comparable immunity.

Direct comparisons of various typhoid vaccines have not yet been performed. A meta-analysis indicates that the 3-year cumulative efficacy of 73% for 2 doses of whole-cell vaccine (no longer available), 55% for 1 dose of Vi vaccine, 51% for 3 doses of oral vaccine might be expected; note that the conditions for this analysis differ from recommended use for travelers from the United States.

Immunologic Characteristics

Microorganism: Bacterium, *Salmonella enterica serovar typhi* (also known as *Salmonella typhi* or *Salmonella typhosa*), facultative anaerobic gram-negative rod, family Enterobacteriaceae

Viability: Inactivated

Antigenic Form: Bacterial polysaccharide

Antigenic Type: Vi polysaccharide, partly 3-O-acetylated repeated units of 2-acetylamino-2-deoxy-D-galactopyranuronic acid with α-(1→4) linkages.

Strains: Ty-2

Use Characteristics

Indications: For induction of active immunity against typhoid fever in people 2 years of age or older. The vaccine regimen should be completed 2 weeks before potential exposure to typhoid bacteria. People at greatest risk include:

- Travelers to endemic areas (especially Africa, Asia, and South and Central America), especially if prolonged exposure to potentially contaminated food and water is likely;
- People with intimate exposure (eg, prolonged household contact) to a known typhoid carrier;
- Laboratory personnel who work frequently with *S. typhi*.

For specific locations, consult specialty references, the Disease Epidemiology section in this monograph, or call one of CDC's travel hotlines.

Unlabeled Uses: Parenteral typhoid vaccine may offer some cross-protection against *S. paratyphi A*. These bacteria share a common O antigen factor 12 with *S. typhi*.

Limitations: Effectiveness of protective immunity appears to be dependent on the size of the bacterial inoculum that the patient consumes. Counsel travelers to take standard food and water precautions to avoid typhoid fever. Select appropriate antibiotics to treat active infections (eg, chloramphenicol, ampicillin). Consider cholecystectomy or ciprofloxacin therapy for chronic carriers. No evidence indicates that typhoid vaccine is useful in controlling common-source outbreaks. Typhoid vaccine will not prevent infection or disease caused by other species of *Salmonella* or other bacteria that cause enteric disease.

Outmoded Practices: In the middle of the twentieth century, typhoid immunization was suggested for people attending rural summer camps or for residents of areas where flooding had occurred, but there are no data to support continuation of such practices. Routine vaccination for sewage sanitation workers is not warranted in the United States.

Contraindications:

Absolute: A previous severe systemic or allergic reaction is a contraindication to future use. Do not vaccinate a patient with typhoid fever or a chronic typhoid carrier.

Relative: Defer administration in the presence of acute respiratory or other active infection, or intensive physical activity (particularly when environmental temperatures are high).

Immunodeficiency: Patients receiving immunosuppressive therapy or with other immunodeficiencies may have a diminished antibody response to active immunization.

Elderly: No specific information is available about geriatric use of typhoid vaccine.

Pregnancy: Category C. Specific information about use of typhoid vaccine during pregnancy is not available. Parenteral vaccination is not specifically contraindicated. Nonetheless, use typhoid vaccine only if clearly needed (ie, if disease risk exceeds vaccination risks). It is not known if typhoid vaccine or corresponding antibodies cross the placenta. Generally, most IgG passage across the placenta occurs during the third trimester. Problems in humans have not been documented and are unlikely.

Lactation: It is not known if typhoid vaccine or corresponding antibodies cross into human breast milk. Problems in humans have not been documented and are unlikely.

Children: Vi vaccine is not currently recommended for children younger than 2 years because no safety or efficacy data are available for that age group.

Adverse Reactions: Most adverse reactions to Vi polysaccharide are minor and transient local reactions. Local reactions may include erythema (4% to 11%) or induration (5% to 18%) at the injection site. Many recipients experience pain (26% to 56%) or tenderness (more than 93%) at the site. These almost always resolve within 48 hours. Systemic effects may include: Fever 37.8°C or higher (100°F or higher; 0% to 2%), malaise (4% to 37%), myalgia (2% to 7%), nausea (2% to 8%), or headache (11% to 27%). Rarely, lymphadenopathy, cervical pain, vomiting, diarrhea, abdominal pain, tremor, hypotension, loss of consciousness, allergic reactions including urticaria, and other events have been reported. Because Vi vaccine contains negligible amounts of bacterial lipopolysaccharide, it produces reactions less than 50% as frequently as H-P or AKD vaccines. No statistically significant difference in reaction rates were seen between first and subsequent doses of Vi polysaccharide.

Pharmacologic & Dosing Characteristics

Dosage: A single 25 mcg dose in 0.5 mL for people 2 years of age and older.

Route & Site: IM. Inject adults in the deltoid muscle. Inject children in either the deltoid or vastus lateralis. Do not inject in the gluteal area or where there may be a nerve trunk.

Overdosage: Although few data are available, clinical experience with similar products suggests that the major manifestations of overdosage would be pain and tenderness at the injection site.

Booster Doses: A single 25 mcg dose every 2 years under conditions of repeated or continued exposure. Booster doses do not elicit higher antibody levels than primary immunization with the polysaccharide antigen.

No data are available about boosting patients with a vaccine different from the one they were originally vaccinated against. CDC accepts use of Vi vaccine or vaccine capsules as a reasonable choice for boosting any patient.

Missed Doses: Administer the next dose as soon as feasible. Prolonging the interval between doses does not interfere with immunity achieved, but it does delay that immunity.

Efficacy: A 25 mcg dose produced a 4-fold rise in antibody titers in 88% to 96% of healthy American adults. The Vi polysaccharide vaccine reduced disease incidence 49% to 87% in a trial among adults and children in Nepal. In a pediatric study in South Africa, blood culture-confirmed cases of typhoid fever were reduced 61%, 52%, and 50% in the first, second, and third years, respectively, after a single dose of Vi polysaccharide vaccine.

Onset: Protective antibody titers develop within 2 weeks after a single dose.

Duration: Approximately 2 years

Protective Level: For Vi antigen: 1 mcg/mL is presumed to be protective.

Mechanism: Induction of specific protective antibodies

Drug Interactions: Like all inactivated vaccines, administration of typhoid vaccine to patients receiving immunosuppressant drugs (eg, high-dose corticosteroids) or radiation therapy may result in an insufficient response to immunization. They may remain susceptible despite immunization.

Avoid concurrent administration with other reactogenic parenteral vaccines (eg, cholera, plague) if possible, to avoid the theoretical risk of additive adverse effects.

Concomitant therapy with phenytoin decreased antibody response to subcutaneous whole-cell typhoid vaccination in a small study. This effect has not been reported with the Vi polysaccharide typhoid vaccine.

As with other drugs administered by IM injection, give Vi polysaccharide vaccine with caution to patients receiving anticoagulant therapy.

Patient Information: Advise vaccine recipients to take standard food and water precautions to avoid typhoid fever and other enteric infections. Vaccine protection can be overwhelmed by swallowing a large dose of typhoid bacteria.

Pharmaceutical Characteristics

Concentration: 25 mcg of purified Vi polysaccharide per 0.5 mL

Quality Assay: Potency of purified polysaccharide is assessed by molecular size and O-acetyl content.

Packaging: 0.5 mL single-use syringe without needle (NDC #: 49281-0790-51). Vials are available on a special contract basis: 20 doses per 10 mL vial (49281-0790-20), 50 doses per 25 mL vial (49281-0790-50).

Doseform: Solution

Appearance: Clear, colorless solution

Solvent: Isotonic phosphate-buffered saline

Adjuvant: None

Preservative: 0.25% phenol

Allergens: None

Excipients: Sodium chloride 8.3 mg/mL, disodium phosphate 0.13 mg/mL, monosodium phosphate 0.046 mg/mL, residual polydimethylsilozane-based antifoam agents

pH: 6.7 to 7.3

Shelf Life: Expires within 30 months

Storage/Stability: Store at 2° to 8°C (35° to 46°F). Discard frozen vaccine. Contact the manufacturer regarding exposure to extreme temperatures. Shipped in insulated containers with coolant packs.

Typhoid Vi Polysaccharide Vaccine

Production Process: *S. typhi* Ty-2 strain bacteria are grown in a semisynthetic medium without animal proteins. The capsular polysaccharide is precipitated from the concentrated culture supernatant by addition of hexadecyltrimethylammonium bromide (cetrimonium bromide). The product is purified by differential centrifugation and precipitation. The potency of the purified polysaccharide is assessed by molecular size and O-acetyl content.

Media: Semisynthetic medium without animal proteins

Disease Epidemiology

Incidence: Typhoid-fever incidence peaked in the United States at the end of the 19th century, before effective sanitation systems became commonplace.

Four hundred to 600 cases are reported each year in the United States, approximately 0.2 cases per 100,000 people. Most cases are associated with foreign travel, especially to Latin America, Asia, and Africa. Of American cases from 1977 to 1979, 62% originated outside the continental United States and 38% within the United States. Of cases originating during international travel, 50% were imported from Mexico, 20% from Asian countries, and 15% from India. Of US-acquired cases, 23% were associated with typhoid carriers, 24% with food outbreaks, 23% with ingestion of contaminated food or water, 6% with household contact, and 4% with laboratories.

Endemic areas include many parts of Mexico, Central and South America, the Caribbean basin, Africa, Portugal, Spain, Italy, Eastern Europe, India, the Far East, and the Philippines. Multidrug-resistant strains are now common on the Indian subcontinent, the Arabian peninsula, and other places. An estimated 30 million cases occur annually around the world, with 581,000 deaths. Outbreaks of typhoid fever are often traced to food handlers who are asymptomatic carriers.

Classic cases involve fever, myalgia, anorexia, abdominal discomfort, and headaches. Constipation is common in older children and adults, while diarrhea may occur in younger children. Disease complications can include intestinal perforation and hemorrhage. Approximately 2% to 4% of typhoid-fever cases develop a chronic carrier state. Infection of the gallbladder can lead to a chronic carrier state. Typhoid can be fatal if improperly treated. Without antibiotics, the case-fatality rate is approximately 10% to 20%.

Susceptible Pools: Most Americans are susceptible, although exposure is usually negligible.

Transmission: By food and water contaminated by feces or urine of patients or carriers

Incubation: 7 to 14 days (range, 3 to 38 days)

Communicability: Isolate until bacilli no longer appear in stool or urine.

Other Information

Perspective:

1837: Gerhard distinguishes typhoid and typhus fevers.

1880: Eberth discovers causative organism, initially called *Bacillus typhosus*, later *Eberthella typhosa* and *S. typhosa*.

c.1896: Pfeiffer and Kolle develop a typhoid vaccine for human use. At the same time, Wright is independently developing his own vaccine.

1898: Wright conducts trial of inactivated vaccine among the British Army stationed in India. Spanish-American War, US Army Typhoid Board lead by Major Walter Reed improves camp sanitation, shows cause of outbreak and carrier state.

1907: First verified case of a healthy microbial carrier who infects others: "Typhoid Mary" Mallon.

1907: Chantemesse develops an antityphoid serum.

1908: Russell develops typhoid vaccine in the United States. By 1911, all American soldiers are routinely vaccinated against typhoid fever.

1909: Dreyer develops paratyphoid vaccine.

1914: Typhoid vaccine licensed in the United States.

1916: Paratyphoid A and B antigens combined with typhoid vaccine, called the TAB vaccine.

1934: Felix and Pitt describe the capsular polysaccharide of *S. typhi*, calling it the virulence (Vi) antigen.

1938: Grasset uses anti-O antiserum to treat cases of typhoid fever.

1944: Acetone-killed and dried (AKD) typhoid vaccine licensed (May).

1950s: Landy and Webster develop typhoid Vi polysaccharide vaccine.

1952: Heat-phenol (HP) inactivated typhoid vaccine licensed (July 16).

1972: Wong develops typhoid Vi polysaccharide vaccine.

1975: Germanier develops oral typhoid vaccine Ty21a.

1989: Vivotif Berna licensed in December 1989.

1994: Typhim Vi licensed in November 1994.

2000: Production of whole-cell typhoid vaccines suspended by Wyeth-Lederle Vaccines. Two formulations were suspended: An AKD whole-cell typhoid vaccine and a heat- and phenol-inactivated (HP) vaccine. The AKD and HP vaccines were commonly considered generically equivalent, although the HP vaccine may have contained little of the important Vi antigen. Efficacy of the AKD vaccine varied from 75% to 94%; efficacy of the HP vaccine varied from 61% to 77% over 2.5 to 3 years.

2001: Wyeth discontinues distribution of AKD and HP typhoid vaccines.

First Licensed:

AKD and H-P: May 1944 and July 16, 1952. Production suspended in 2000.

Vi: November 28, 1994

Discontinued Products: Typho-Bacterin. Whole-cell AKD typhoid vaccine (Wyeth and others). Whole-cell heat-phenol inactivated typhoid vaccine (Wyeth and others).

National Policy: ACIP. Typhoid immunization. *MMWR.* 1994;43(RR-14):1-7.

References: Engels EA, et al. Typhoid fever vaccines: A meta-analysis of studies on efficacy and toxicity. *BMJ.* 1998;316(7125):110-116.

WHO. Typhoid vaccines. *Wkly Epidemiol Rec.* 2008;83(6):49-60.

Typhoid Vaccine (Oral)

Bacterial Vaccines & Toxoids

Name:
Typhoid Vaccine, Live, Oral, Ty21a
Capsules: *Vivotif*

Manufacturer:
Crucell Vaccines, distributed by Berna Products

Synonyms: Ty21a. Typhoid fever is also known as enteric fever and typhus abdominalis.

Comparison: AKD & H-P parenteral vaccines are not equivalent to the Vi polysaccharide vaccine or live, attenuated typhoid vaccine for oral administration. The Vi polysaccharide vaccine reduces disease incidence 49% to 87%, while the capsules reduce disease 60% to 77%.

Although each typhoid vaccine induces comparable immunity, the vaccines vary considerably in the side effects they induce. The AKD vaccine causes the most cases of pain at the injection site, while the oral vaccine causes the fewest adverse effects. Direct comparisons of various typhoid vaccines have not yet been performed. A meta-analysis indicates that the 3-year cumulative efficacy of 73% for 2 doses of whole-cell vaccine, 55% for 1 dose of Vi vaccine, 51% for 3 doses of oral vaccine might be expected. Note that these conditions differ from recommended use in the United States.

Immunologic Characteristics

Microorganism: Bacterium, *Salmonella typhi* (also known as *Salmonella typhosa*), facultative anaerobic gram-negative rod, family Enterobacteriaceae

Viability: Live, attenuated bacteria, plus nonviable cells

Antigenic Form: Whole bacterium

Antigenic Type: Protein and polysaccharide

Strains: Ty21a strain, also called the Ty21a gal E mutant strain. The main characteristic of the strain is a defect of the enzyme uridine diphosphate-galactose-4-epimerase.

Use Characteristics

Indications: Induction of active immunity against typhoid fever in people 2 years of age or older. People at greatest risk include:

- Travelers to endemic areas (especially Latin America, Asia and Africa);
- People with intimate exposure (eg, household contact) to a known typhoid carrier;
- Laboratory personnel who work frequently with *S. typhi*.

For specific locations, consult specialty references, the Disease Epidemiology section in this monograph, or call one of CDC's travel hotlines.

Limitations: Advise travelers to take standard food and water precautions to avoid typhoid fever. Select appropriate antibiotics to treat active infections (eg, ampicillin, chloramphenicol, ciprofloxacin). Consider cholecystectomy or ciprofloxacin therapy for chronic carriers. No evidence indicates that typhoid vaccine is useful in controlling common-source outbreaks. Typhoid vaccine will not prevent infection or disease caused by other species of *Salmonella* or other bacteria that cause enteric disease.

Outmoded Practices: At one time, typhoid immunization was suggested for people attending rural summer camps or for residents of areas where flooding had occurred, but there are no data to support such practices. Routine vaccination for sewage sanitation workers is not warranted in the United States.

Contraindications:

Absolute: Patients with a history of hypersensitivity to any component of the vaccine or the capsule. Do not vaccinate a person with typhoid fever or a chronic typhoid carrier.

Relative: Do not give typhoid vaccine capsules during an acute febrile illness or during an acute GI illness (eg, persistent diarrhea, vomiting). Vaccine efficacy may be diminished or absent in people who had some or all of their intestinal tract surgically removed. Vaccine efficacy would be expected to diminish in proportion to the proportion of the intestines removed.

Immunodeficiency: Do not give typhoid vaccine capsules to immunocompromised people, including people with congenital or acquired immune deficiencies, whether because of genetics, disease, or drug or radiation therapy, regardless of possible benefits from vaccination. This product contains live bacteria. Avoid use in HIV-positive people. Use a parenteral inactivated typhoid vaccine instead.

Elderly: No specific information is available about geriatric use of typhoid vaccine capsules.

Pregnancy: Category C. Use only if clearly needed. It is not known if attenuated typhoid vaccine or corresponding antibodies cross the placenta. Generally, most IgG passage across the placenta occurs during the third trimester. Consider using parenteral inactivated typhoid vaccine in pregnant women at risk of typhoid fever.

Lactation: It is not known if attenuated typhoid vaccine or corresponding antibodies cross into breast milk. Problems in humans have not been documented.

Children: Typhoid vaccine capsules are not recommended for children younger than 6 years, because no safety or efficacy data are available for that age group.

Adverse Reactions: Nausea (5.8%), abdominal pain (6.4%), headache (4.8%), fever (3.3%), diarrhea (2.9%), vomiting (1.5%), skin rash (1%), or urticaria on trunk or extremities may occur, although they are generally self-resolving. At 5 times the recommended dose, no significant reactions were noted. Bacteria are not shed in feces at the normal dose, but overdosages increase the possibility of shedding.

Pharmacologic & Dosing Characteristics

Dosage: Four capsules, given as one capsule orally every other day on days 0, 2, 4, and 6.

Swallow each capsule whole, 1 hour before meals, with cold or lukewarm water (not to exceed body temperature). Do not consume alcohol within 1 hour before or after swallowing capsules, because alcohol will prematurely break the enteric-coated capsule and not allow the capsule to reach the intestinal tract intact. Do not chew capsules. Swallow as soon as possible after placing in mouth. Encourage compliance with complete regimen.

Route: Oral

Overdosage: At 5 times the recommended dose, no significant reactions were noted.

Booster Doses: Four capsules taken on alternate days every 5 years, under conditions of repeated or continued exposure.

Missed Doses: Prolonging the interval between doses by 2 to 4 days does not interfere with immunity achieved after the concluding dose of the basic series. Ingest all 4 capsules within a period of 10 days or less.

Efficacy: Vaccination reduces disease incidence by 60% to 70%. Counsel vaccinated travelers to take all necessary precautions to avoid contact or ingestion of potentially contaminated food or water. Ty21a trials were conducted in Alexandria, Egypt; Santiago, Chile; and Plaju, Indonesia.

Onset: Finish the fourth capsule at least 1 week before travel or potential exposure to *S. typhi.*

Duration: At least 5 years

Typhoid Vaccine (Oral)

Protective Level: Unknown

Mechanism: Induction of specific protective antibodies directed against *S. typhi* lipopolysaccharide. This bacterial strain is restricted in its ability to produce complete lipopolysaccharide, which impairs its ability to cause disease but not to induce an immune response.

Drug Interactions: Like all live bacterial vaccines, administration to patients receiving immunosuppressant drugs (eg, steroids) or radiation therapy may predispose patients to disseminated infections or insufficient response to immunization. They may remain susceptible despite immunization.

Sulfonamides and other antibiotics (eg, amoxicillin, chloramphenicol, ciprofloxacin) may be active against the Ty21a vaccine strain and may reduce vaccine efficacy. Therefore, give the vaccine capsules at least 24 hours before or after the antibiotic.

Several antimalarial drugs (eg, mefloquine, chloroquine, proguanil) possess antibacterial activity that may interfere with the immunogenicity of typhoid Ty21a vaccine. When healthy adults receiving these drugs were given typhoid Ty21a vaccine, mefloquine or chloroquine did not result in a significant reduction in immune response to vaccination, compared with people who received vaccine only. But simultaneous administration of proguanil did affect a significant decrease in immune responsiveness. Administer proguanil (including combination products containing proguanil, such as Malarone) only if 10 or more days have elapsed since the fourth dose of typhoid Ty21a vaccine. Proguanil (not available in the United States) reduces the fraction of recipients responding with antityphoid antibodies; wait at least 10 days between the last dose of oral typhoid vaccine and the first dose of proguanil. Chloroquine, mefloquine (*Lariam*), and pyrimethamine-sulfadoxine (*Fansidar*) can be taken simultaneously with the vaccine.

Immune globulin (eg, IGIM) and other live vaccines (eg, poliovirus, yellow fever) can be taken simultaneously with this vaccine without loss of antibody response.

Concomitant therapy with phenytoin may decrease antibody response to parenteral typhoid vaccination, although no effect on oral vaccination has been reported. Anticipate suboptimal antibody response and consider risk/benefit ratios for each drug. Counsel these people to especially observe good food and water discipline.

No evidence of interaction between simultaneous administration of live virus vaccines (eg, MMR, OPV, yellow fever vaccines) and oral live typhoid (Ty21a) vaccine has been documented. Oral cholera vaccine (CVD103-HgR) and oral typhoid vaccine do not interfere with the antibody response to each other. If both drugs are needed (eg, prior to international travel), both vaccines may be administered simultaneously or at any interval between each other.

Although no formal interaction studies have been performed, proton-pump inhibitors (eg, omeprazole) would not be expected to interfere with typhoid Ty21a vaccine, because the vaccine itself contains a buffer to reduce gastric acidity.

Alcohol can break the enteric-coated capsule of typhoid Ty21a vaccine, so that the capsule dissolves in the stomach rather than the intestinal tract. In addition, tests show that alcohol can kill the live, attenuated bacteria in the vaccine. Therefore, advise patients not to consume alcohol within 2 hours of taking vaccine capsules.

Patient Information: Store unused capsules in the refrigerator between doses. Advise patients not to consume alcohol within 2 hours of taking vaccine capsules. Advise vaccine recipients to take standard food and water precautions to avoid typhoid fever and other enteric infections.

Pharmaceutical Characteristics

Concentration: 2 to 6 $\times$ 10^9 CFU of viable *S. typhi* organisms per capsule, plus 5 to 50 $\times$ 10^9 nonviable bacterial cells

Quality Assay: Vaccine potency, in viable cells per capsules, is determined by inoculation of agar plates with dilutions of vaccine suspended in physiologic saline. The bacteria are assessed for galactose metabolism, biosynthesis of lipopolysaccharide, and biochemical markers. Whatever the growth conditions, the strain does not contain Vi antigen. The strain agglutinates to anti-O:9 antiserum only if grown in medium containing galactose. It contains the flagellar H:d antigen. Cells of strain Ty21a lyse if grown in the presence of 1% galactose.

Packaging: Unit-dose blister package of 4 capsules

NDC Number: 58337-0003-01

Doseform: Enteric-coated oral capsules

Appearance: Salmon pink and white capsules; without imprinted characters.

Adjuvant: None

Preservative: None

Allergens: 100 to 180 mg lactose per capsule

Excipients: Each capsule contains 26 to 130 mg sucrose, 1.4 to 7 mg amino-acid mixture, 3.6 to 4.4 mg magnesium stearate, and 1 to 5 mg ascorbic acid.

pH: Not applicable

Shelf Life: Expires within 15 months

Storage/Stability: Store at 2° to 8°C (35° to 46°F) prior to use and between doses. If frozen, thaw the capsules before administration. Shipped at 2° to 8°C (36° to 46°F).

Production Process: Bacteria are grown in fermenters, then collected by centrifugation, mixed with stabilizer (a mixture of sucrose, ascorbic acid, and amino acids), lyophilized, mixed with lactose and magnesium stearate, filled into gelatin capsules, and coated with an organic solution to make the capsules resistant to dissolution in stomach acid. The freeze-drying process ensures survival of 10% or more of the bacteria involved.

Media: Digest of bovine tissue, an acid digest of casein, dextrose, and galactose.

Disease Epidemiology

Incidence: Typhoid-fever incidence peaked in the United States at the end of the 19th century, before effective sanitation systems became commonplace.

Four hundred to 600 cases are reported each year in the United States, approximately 0.2 cases per 100,000 people. Most cases are associated with foreign travel, especially to Latin America, Asia, and Africa. Of American cases from 1977 to 1979, 62% originated outside the continental United States and 38% within the United States. Of cases originating during international travel, 50% were imported from Mexico, 20% from Asian countries, and 15% from India. Of US-acquired cases, 23% were associated with typhoid carriers, 24% with food outbreaks, 23% with ingestion of contaminated food or water, 6% with household contact, and 4% with laboratories.

Endemic areas include many parts of Mexico, Central and South America, the Caribbean basin, Africa, Portugal, Spain, Italy, Eastern Europe, India, the Far East, and the Philippines. Multidrug-resistant strains are now common on the Indian subcontinent, the Arabian peninsula, and other places. An estimated 30 million cases occur annually around the world, with 581,000 deaths. Outbreaks of typhoid fever are often traced to food handlers who are asymptomatic carriers.

Classic cases involve fever, myalgia, anorexia, abdominal discomfort, and headaches. Constipation is common in older children and adults, while diarrhea may occur in younger children. Disease complications can include intestinal perforation and hemorrhage. Approximately 2% to 4% of typhoid-fever cases develop a chronic carrier state. Infection of the gallbladder can lead to a chronic carrier state. Typhoid can be fatal if improperly treated. Without antibiotics, the case-fatality rate is approximately 10% to 20%.

Susceptible Pools: Most Americans are susceptible, although exposure is usually negligible.

Transmission: By food and water contaminated by feces or urine of patients or carriers

Incubation: 7 to 14 days (range, 3 to 38 days)

Communicability: Isolate until bacilli no longer appear in stool or urine.

Other Information

Perspective:

1837: Gerhard distinguishes typhoid and typhus fevers.

1880: Eberth discovers causative organism, initially called *Bacillus typhosus*, later *Eberthella typhosa*, and *S. typhosa*.

c.1896: Pfeiffer and Kolle develop a typhoid vaccine for human use. At the same time, Wright is independently developing his own vaccine.

1898: Wright conducts trial of inactivated vaccine among the British Army stationed in India.

1907: First verified case of a healthy microbial carrier who infects others: "Typhoid Mary" Mallon.

1907: Chantemesse develops an antityphoid serum.

1908: Russell develops typhoid vaccine in the United States. By 1911, all American soldiers are routinely vaccinated against typhoid fever.

1909: Dreyer develops paratyphoid vaccine.

1914: Typhoid vaccine licensed in the United States.

1916: Paratyphoid A and B antigens combined with typhoid vaccine, called the TAB vaccine.

1934: Felix and Pitt describe the capsular polysaccharide of *S. typhi*, calling it the virulence (Vi) antigen.

1938: Grasset uses anti-O antiserum to treat cases of typhoid fever.

1944: Acetone-killed and dried (AKD) typhoid vaccine licensed (May).

1950s: Landy and Webster develop typhoid Vi polysaccharide vaccine.

1952: Heat-phenol (HP) inactivated typhoid vaccine licensed (July 16).

1972: Wong develops typhoid Vi polysaccharide vaccine.

1975: Germanier develops oral typhoid vaccine Ty21a.

1989: *Vivotif Berna* licensed in December 1989.

1994: *Typhim Vi* licensed in November 1994.

2000: Production of whole-cell typhoid vaccines suspended by Wyeth-Lederle Vaccines. Two formulations were suspended: An acetone-killed and dried (AKD) whole-cell typhoid vaccine and a heat- and phenol-inactivated (HP) vaccine. The AKD and HP vaccines were commonly considered generically equivalent, although the HP vaccine may have contained little of the important Vi antigen. Efficacy of the AKD vaccine varied from 75% to 94%; efficacy of the HP vaccine varied from 61% to 77% over 2.5 to 3 years.

2001: Wyeth discontinues distribution of AKD and HP typhoid vaccines.

Discontinued Products: *Typho-Bacterin* injection (Mulford)

National Policy: ACIP. Typhoid immunization. *MMWR*. 1994;43(RR-14):1-7.

References: Engels EA, et al. Typhoid fever vaccines: A meta-analysis of studies on efficacy and toxicity. *BMJ*. 1998;316(7125):110-116.

WHO. Typhoid vaccines. *Weekly Epidemiol Rec*. 2008;83(6):49-60.

Adenovirus Type 4 and Type 7 Vaccine Live Oral Tablets

Viral Vaccines

Names:
Generic

Manufacturers:
Manufactured by Barr Laboratories, distributed by Teva Pharmaceuticals

Immunologic Characteristics

Microorganism: Virus (double-stranded DNA), adenovirus, subgroup E, genus *Mastadenovirus*, family Adenoviridae

Viability: Live, but not attenuated

Antigenic Form: Whole virus

Antigenic Type: Protein

Strains: Serotype 4 and serotype 7; strain data not provided. The strains are not attenuated. The viral seeds used by Teva/Barr have the same genetic sequence as vaccine viruses obtained from earlier Wyeth vaccine tablets.

Use Characteristics

Indications: For induction of active immunity against adenovirus serotypes 4 and 7. Vaccination helps prevent adenovirus-associated acute respiratory disease (ARD). Serotype 4 and 7 vaccines are licensed for use in military populations 17 through 50 years of age.

Contraindications: Do not administer to pregnant women, people with a history of severe allergic reaction to any component of the vaccine, or people with an inability to swallow.

Postpone vaccination in people with vomiting or diarrhea because effectiveness depends on multiplication of orally administered live adenovirus within the intestinal tract.

Immunodeficiency: Live adenovirus vaccination is theoretically contraindicated in immunodeficient patients because the vaccine consists of live viruses.

Avoid use in HIV-infected people.

Elderly: No specific information is available about use of adenovirus vaccines in elderly patients.

Carcinogenicity: Adenovirus serotypes 4 and 7 are not oncogenic.

Pregnancy: Contraindicated. It is not known whether adenovirus vaccines can cause fetal harm or affect reproductive capacity. It is not known if live adenoviruses or corresponding antibodies cross the placenta. Naturally occurring infection with adenoviruses has been associated with fetal harm. Avoid pregnancy for 6 weeks after vaccination.

Lactation: It is not known if adenoviruses or corresponding antibodies cross into human breast milk. Problems in humans have not been documented.

Children: No data on safety or immunogenicity are available.

Adverse Reactions: Safety was evaluated in a multicenter, double-blind study of 3,031 subjects who received the vaccine and 1,009 who received placebo (lactose tablets). The study was conducted among healthy male (63%) and female (37%) US Army and Navy recruits during basic training. The mean age was 21 years (range, 17 to 42 years of age). Subjects in both groups also received other vaccines concomitantly. The specific vaccines each subject received varied based on personal immunization history and included hepatitis A vaccine; hepatitis B vaccine; human papillomavirus vaccine type 4; influenza intranasal vaccine; influenza intramuscular vaccine; measles, mumps, and rubella vaccine; meningococcal conjugate vaccine (MCV4); meningococcal polysaccharide vaccine (MPSV4); poliovirus inactivated vaccine; tetanus toxoid and diphtheria toxoid with acellular pertussis vaccine; typhoid Vi polysaccharide vaccine; varicella vaccine; and/or yellow fever vaccines. Overall, 91.2% of vaccine recipients and 93.9% of placebo recipients reported at least 1 adverse event during the 56-day study period.

Serious events: Serious events in vaccine recipients included hematuria, gastroenteritis, febrile gastroenteritis, gastritis, pneumonia, and hematochezia. No deaths occurred during the trial. The same proportion (1.2%) of the vaccine and placebo groups reported serious events. A vaccine strain of adenovirus type 4 was detected from posterior pharyngeal and tonsillar swabbing in a placebo recipient who developed febrile ARD.

Solicited Adverse Events Reported by ≥ 5% of Subjects								
	Adenovirus type 4 and 7 vaccine				Placebo			
	0 to 7 days (N = 3,031)		8 to 14 days (n = 660)		0 to 7 days (N =1,009)		8 to 14 days (n = 218)	
Adverse event	n	%	n	%	n	%	n	%
Headache	894	30%	38	7%	31	31%	11	6%
Nasal congestion (stuffy nose)	463	15%	49	8%	141	14%	12	6%
Pharyngolaryngeal pain (sore throat)	391	13%	72	12%	124	12%	24	12%
Cough	375	12%	59	10%	130	13%	14	7%
Nausea	412	14%	29	5%	137	13%	11	6%
Diarrhea	310	10%	18	3%	84	8%	10	5%

Oral temperature of at least 100.5°F within 7 days was reported by 1.4% of vaccine recipients and 0.5% of placebo recipients not diagnosed with ARD. During the 8 to 14 days after vaccination, the rates were 0.6% and 1.1%, respectively.

Shedding and transmission: Oral adenovirus type 4 and type 7 vaccines contain live viruses that are shed in the stool and can cause disease if transmitted. Vaccine virus strains were shed as early as 7 days after vaccination. No shedding was detected in any subjects by 28 days after vaccination. Of 30 vaccine recipients, 8 (27%) tested positive for shedding type 4 at least once; for type 7, 60% tested positive at least once. Vaccine strain virus was not detected in the throat of any subject.

This vaccine is intended for individuals undergoing cohorted military training who have limited contact with pregnant women, children younger than 7 years, and people with a compromised immune system. During the 28-day period of viral shedding, vaccinated individuals should use caution when in close contact with pregnant women, children younger than 7 years, and people with compromised immune systems, as well as other vaccinees. Use caution when in close contact with pregnant women during the 28-day period of viral shedding. To minimize the risk of transmission, observe proper personal hygiene (eg, frequent hand washing, especially after bowel movements).

Pharmacologic & Dosing Characteristics

Dosage: One tablet of type-4 vaccine plus 1 tablet of type 7 vaccine

Route: Oral. To avoid releasing the virus into the upper respiratory tract, do not chew tablets. Keep tablets in the mouth as briefly as possible.

Booster Doses: None.

Efficacy: The pivotal study assessed efficacy against type 4 adenovirus–associated febrile ARD and the ability to induce neutralizing antibody to type 7 adenovirus. A seroconversion end point, rather than prevention of clinical disease, was used to assess efficacy of type 7 vaccine because the incidence of febrile ARD due to type 7 adenovirus was not anticipated to be high enough to permit a meaningful statistical assessment of clinical effect. At baseline, 64% were seronegative to type 4 (titer < 1:4) and 38% were seronegative to type 7 (titer less than 1:4).

One case of wild-type adenovirus type 4 febrile ARD occurred among 3,031 vaccine recipients compared with 48 cases among 1,009 placebo recipients, yielding 99% vaccine efficacy (95% confidence interval, 96%-99.9%). Cases were defined as 1 or more clinical signs and symptoms of ARD (sore throat, cough, rhinorrhea, nasal congestion, rales, or rhonchi), oral temperature greater than 100.5°F, and throat culture positive for wild-type adenovirus type 4 by polymerase chain reaction testing. Seroconversion to type 4 (titer at least 1:8) occurred in 95% of vaccine recipients and 11% of placebo recipients by day 26.

No type 7 febrile or afebrile ARD cases occurred in either the vaccine or placebo groups. Seroconversion to adenovirus type 7 (titer at least 1:8) occurred in 94% of vaccine recipients and 5% of placebo recipients by day 26.

Onset: 1 or more weeks.

Duration: At least 60 days.

Mechanism: Adenovirus type 4 and type 7 replicate in the intestinal tract and induce immunity in people with low or no preexisting neutralizing antibodies. Vaccination induces specific protective serum and secretory intestinal antibodies.

Drug Interactions: Type 4 and type 7 vaccines do not appear to interact. As with all live viral vaccines, administration to patients receiving immunosuppressant drugs, including steroids, or radiation may predispose them to disseminated infections or insufficient response to immunization and they may remain susceptible despite immunization. Vaccine recipients received multiple other vaccines during the pivotal study, but no immunogenicity assessments of the other vaccines were conducted.

Pharmaceutical Characteristics

Concentration: Not less than 32,000 tissue culture infective doses ($TCID_{50}$) ($10^{4.5}$ $TCID_{50}$) of type 4 or type 7 virus per tablet

Packaging: Carton containing 2 bottles of 100 tablets of each component vaccine (NDC #: 051285-0138-50). The type 4 component bottle carries NDC # 051285-0174-02. The type 7 component bottle carries NDC # 051285-0175-02.

Doseform: Enteric-coated tablets. The inner core contains virus and excipients, covered with a layer of starch and inert binders; a dry protective coating is added on top of the core.

Appearance:
Type 4: White to off-white, round, coated tablet with stylized b imprinted on one side
Type 7: Light peach, round, coated tablet with stylized b imprinted on one side

Adjuvant: None

Preservative: None

Allergens: Calf serum, human albumin, lactose

Excipients: Sucrose, D-mannose, D-fructose, dextrose, human serum albumin (less than 0.3 mg/tablet), potassium phosphate, and plasdone C. Each tablet is designed to pass intact through the stomach and release the live virus in the intestine. Each enteric-coated tablet contains an inner-core tablet containing anhydrous lactose, microcrystalline cellulose, polacrilin potassium, magnesium stearate, and live adenovirus. The outer tablet layer contains microcrystalline cellulose, magnesium stearate, and anhydrous lactose, with an enteric coating consisting of cellulose acetate phthalate, alcohol, acetone, and castor oil. The type 7 tablet also contains FD&C yellow #6 aluminum lake dye.

Adenovirus Type 4 and Type 7 Vaccine Live Oral Tablets

Shelf Life: Expires within 24 months

Storage/Stability: Store between 2° and 8°C (36° and 46°F). Do not freeze. Keep bottle tightly closed and protect from moisture. Do not remove desiccant canister from bottle. Shipping data not provided. Contact the manufacturer regarding exposure to freezing temperatures.

Production Process: The virus is harvested, freed of particulate cellular material by filtration, formulated, and lyophilized before tableting.

Media: WI-38 human diploid-cell culture grown on Dulbecco's modified Eagle's medium, fetal bovine serum, and sodium bicarbonate.

Disease Epidemiology

Incidence: 600 to 800 ARD hospitalizations occurred per week at northern military basic-training sites in the early 1960s, disabling 40% to 50% of the closed community. At that time, adenovirus infection represented the leading cause of military hospitalizations in the United States. Between 2000 and 2010, when no adenovirus vaccines were available to the US Department of Defense (DoD), adenoviruses affected about 15,000 military basic trainees annually, with 3 to 4 days of illness per event and 1 to 2 deaths. Recruits may arrive as hosts or with mild cases of respiratory infections endemic to their own region of the country; they are housed in close contact with individuals from other parts of the country who may be susceptible. New recruits may also be exposed to respiratory infections that are endemic to the recruit training center. Close contact, coupled with the unique stressors of military operations, often put military recruits at a greater risk for respiratory disease than other cohorts.

Transmission: Oral contact or droplet spread

Incubation: 1 to 10 days

Communicability: 6% to 8% per week during basic training

Other Information

Perspective:

1957: Inactivated adenovirus vaccine types 3, 4, and 7 (Parke-Davis) licensed in the United States.

1959: Combined adenovirus-influenza adsorbed vaccine licensed by Parke-Davis (Resprogen). No lots were released for sale by the US Food and Drug Administration after October 1964 because of concern over oncogenic simian virus SV-40 contamination. License formally revoked in 1980.

1964: Clinical trials of live, attenuated type 4 vaccine begin at the Walter Reed Army Institute of Research. Trials of type 7 begin in 1969 and type 21 in 1971.

1980: Wyeth licensed to produce type 4 and type 7 vaccines on July 1, 1980.

1984: Adenovirus vaccines routinely given to Army recruits year-round until 1999.

1999: Last production run of Wyeth's vaccines. Because DoD declined Wyeth's request for additional funding to upgrade manufacturing facilities , production was discontinued.

2011: Adenovirus vaccine production licensed to Barr Laboratories on March 16.

References: Lyons A, Longfield J, Kuschner R, et al. A double-blind, placebo-controlled study of the safety and immunogenicity of live, oral type 4 and type 7 adenovirus vaccines in adults. *Vaccine.* 2008;26(23):2890-2898.

Tucker SN, Tingley DW, Scallan CD. Oral adenoviral-based vaccines: historical perspective and future opportunity. *Expert Rev Vaccines.* 2008;7(1):25-31.

Adenovirus Type 4 and Type 7 Vaccine Summary	
Generic name	Adenovirus type 4 and 7 vaccine
Brand name	Generic
Manufacturer	Manufactured by Barr Laboratories, distributed by Teva Pharmaceuticals
Viability	Live
Indication	To prevent acute respiratory disease
Strain	Data not provided
Concentration	Not < 32,000 $TCID_{50}$ per tablet
Adjuvant	None
Preservative	None
Production medium	WI-38 human diploid-cell culture
Doseform	Tablets: Type 4 – white; type 7 – peach
Diluent	Not applicable
Packaging	Bottles of 100 tablets
Routine storage	2° to 8°C
Stability	24 months under refrigeration
Dosage, route	1 of each tablet, oral
Standard schedule	1 of each tablet

Hepatitis A Vaccine (HAV)

Viral Vaccines

Names:
Havrix
Vaqta

Manufacturers:
GlaxoSmithKline
Merck

Synonyms: HAV. The disease is also known as infectious hepatitis, epidemic jaundice, and catarrhal jaundice.

Comparison: Hepatitis A vaccine is considered more effective than IGIM in reducing the frequency and severity of hepatitis A infection. Hepatitis A vaccine provides more persistent protection, although induction of protective antibody levels may be delayed several days after levels are obtained with IGIM.

Havrix and *Vaqta* are comparably safe and effective. They can be considered prophylactically equivalent, although their potencies are measured in differing systems, using units with different bases.

Immunologic Characteristics

Microorganism: Virus (single-stranded RNA), human enterovirus 72, genus *Enterovirus*, family Picornaviridae

Viability: Inactivated

Antigenic Form: Lysed whole viruses

Antigenic Type: Protein

Strains: Only 1 serotype of hepatitis A virus has been described.
GSK: HM-175 strain
Merck: Attenuated CR326F′ strain

Use Characteristics

Indications: For induction of active immunity against infection caused by hepatitis A virus in adults and children at least 1 year of age. The quality of antibodies induced by hepatitis A vaccine is indistinguishable from the quality found in human immune globulin products by in vitro assays. The quantity of antibodies induced by immunization is considerably higher than that induced after a standard dose of IGIM or clinical infection. People who are or will be at increased risk of infection or transmission of hepatitis A virus include:

- People traveling to areas of higher endemicity for hepatitis A (eg, Africa, Asia [except Japan], the Mediterranean basin, eastern Europe, the Middle East, Central and South America, Mexico, parts of the Caribbean). Consult specialty references for exact locations, call one of the CDC's travel hotlines, or visit the CDC's Web site at http://www.cdc.gov/travel. Hepatitis A prophylaxis is not needed by travelers to Australia, Canada, Japan, New Zealand, and countries in western Europe and Scandinavia.
- Military personnel.
- People living in or relocating to areas of high endemicity (eg, missionaries, diplomats, engineers).
- Certain ethnic or geographical populations that experience cyclic hepatitis A epidemics (eg, native peoples of Alaska, the Americas, and the Pacific Islands).
- People with chronic liver disease persisting 6 months or more, including alcoholic cirrhosis, chronic hepatitis B or hepatitis C infection, autoimmune hepatitis, or primary biliary cir-

rhosis. People with chronic liver disease are not more likely to be infected with hepatitis A virus, but they are more likely to develop fulminant hepatitis and die if infected.

- People engaging in high-risk sexual activity (eg, homosexual males); users of illicit injectable drugs; residents of a community experiencing an outbreak of hepatitis A; patients with hemophilia A or B receiving plasma-derived clotting factors (the solvent-detergent production method does not reliably inactivate hepatitis A virus, a nonenveloped virus).

- People who work as food handlers can contract hepatitis A and transmit the virus to others. To decrease the evaluation frequency of food handlers for hepatitis A and the need for post-exposure prophylaxis of patrons, vaccination may be considered if cost-effective.

- People exposed to hepatitis A through household and sexual contacts with hepatitis A-infected people. For those desiring both immediate and long-term protection, hepatitis A vaccine may be administered concomitantly with IGIM.

- The ACIP recommends routine vaccination of all children at 1 year of age (ie, 12 to 23 months old).

- For prophylaxis within 2 weeks of exposure for healthy people aged 12 months to 40 years, the ACIP recommendations acknowledge use of either IGIM or hepatitis A vaccine (based on a study of *Vaqta*).

Although the epidemiology of hepatitis A does not permit the identification of other specific populations at high risk for the disease, outbreaks of hepatitis A or exposure to hepatitis A virus have been described in a variety of populations in which hepatitis A vaccination may be useful: Certain institutional workers (eg, caretakers for the developmentally challenged), employees of child day care centers, laboratory workers who handle live hepatitis A virus, or handlers of primate animals that may be harboring hepatitis A virus.

Unlabeled Uses: The value of vaccination for people described below is less clear:

- Other people for whom hepatitis A is an occupational hazard, including the following: Individuals in frequent contact with human fecal matter as a result of their occupationally-related activities (eg, sewage workers, certain hospital workers such as neonatal ICU workers).

- Other people who, if infected, could transmit the disease to others (eg, children in day care settings).

Preliminary data for each brand of hepatitis A vaccine suggest that vaccination may help reduce the risk of disease after exposure to hepatitis A virus. Experiences in Alaska, California, and elsewhere suggest that hepatitis A vaccination may quell community epidemics. This may result because the relatively long incubation period for hepatitis A allows induction of active immunity before the disease manifests.

People with severe congenital protein C deficiency repeatedly given human plasma-derived protein C concentrate, to prevent or treat venous thrombosis and purpura fulminans, should be considered for vaccination against hepatitis A and hepatitis B, to guard against bloodborne pathogens.

Limitations: Hepatitis A vaccine may not prevent hepatitis A infection in people who have an unrecognized hepatitis A infection at the time of immunization. Treatment of hepatitis A infection is primarily supportive; antiviral therapy is not typically needed.

Hepatitis A vaccine will not prevent infection caused by other agents such as hepatitis B virus, hepatitis C virus, hepatitis E virus, or other pathogens that may infect the liver.

People who smoke are slightly less likely to respond to hepatitis A vaccine than nonsmokers.

Contraindications:

Absolute: Patients with known hypersensitivity to any component of the vaccine. Patients who experience hypersensitivity reactions to hepatitis A vaccine should not receive further injections.

Relative: Defer administration of hepatitis A vaccine, if possible, in patients with any febrile illness or active infection. Administer with caution to patients with thrombocytopenia or a bleeding disorder; bleeding may occur following an IM injection.

Immunodeficiency: Patients receiving immunosuppressive therapy or those with other immunodeficiencies may have a diminished antibody response to active immunization. Consider deferring vaccination in patients receiving immunosuppressive therapy. Alternatively, these patients may require administration of additional doses of vaccine. Immunodeficient patients are not apparently predisposed to hepatitis A infection.

Elderly: No specific information is available about geriatric use of hepatitis A vaccine. People born prior to 1945 are more likely to be immune to this disease already, but those who are infected later in life will have greater morbidity and mortality.

Adults:

GSK: In 3 clinical studies of more than 400 adults given a single 1,440 ELU dose of hepatitis A vaccine, specific anti-HAV antibodies developed in more than 96% of subjects when measured 1 month after vaccination. By day 15, 80% to 98% of vaccinees had already seroconverted (defined as anti-HAV at least 20 milliunits/mL). GMTs among seroconverters varied from 264 to 339 milliunits/mL at day 15 and increased to 335 to 637 milliunits/mL by 1 month after immunization.

Merck: In clinical trials, 98% of adults seroconverted at 24 weeks after an approximately 50 unit dose, with a GMT of 134 milliunits/mL. They were then given an approximately 50 unit booster dose. Four weeks later, 100% of adults had seroconverted, with a GMT of 6,010 milliunits/mL.

Carcinogenicity: Hepatitis A vaccine has not been evaluated for carcinogenic potential.

Mutagenicity: Hepatitis A vaccine has not been evaluated for mutagenic potential.

Fertility Impairment: Hepatitis A vaccine has not been evaluated for impairment of fertility.

Pregnancy: Category C. Use only if clearly needed. It is not known if hepatitis A vaccine or corresponding antibodies cross the placenta. Generally, most IgG passage across the placenta occurs during the third trimester. Problems in pregnant women have not been documented and are unlikely.

Lactation: It is not known if hepatitis A vaccine or corresponding antibodies cross into human breast milk. Problems in humans have not been documented and are unlikely.

Children: Safety and efficacy in children younger than 1 year of age have not been established. Hepatitis A antibodies in infants that were contributed from the mother's circulation may interfere with the immune response to hepatitis A immunization. These children appear to be immunologically primed for future viral exposures, but the antibody titers they achieve are lower than those of children without circulating maternal antibodies.

GSK: In 6 clinical trials around the world, involving 762 children ranging from 1 to 18 years of age, the GMT following two 360 ELU doses of hepatitis A vaccine given 1 month apart ranged from 197 to 660 milliunits/mL. Seroconversion occurred in 99% of subjects after the second dose. When the second dose was administered 6 months after the first, all subjects were seropositive at month 7, with GMTs ranging from 3,388 to 4,643 milliunits/mL. In 1 study of children followed for 6 more months, all subjects remained seropositive.

Merck: In clinical trials, 97% of children and adolescents seroconverted at 24 weeks after an approximately 25 unit dose, with a GMT of 109 milliunits/mL. They were then given an approximately 25 unit booster dose. Four weeks later, 100% of them had seroconverted, with a GMT of 10,609 milliunits/mL. Another group showed 91% seroconversion, with a GMT of 48 milliunits/mL, when they received a booster dose 52 weeks after initial vaccination. Four weeks later, 100% had seroconverted, with a GMT of 12,308 milliunits/mL. A third group showed 90% seroconversion, with a GMT of 50 milliunits/mL, when they received a booster dose 78 weeks after initial vaccination. Four weeks later, 100% had sero-converted, with a GMT of 9591 milliunits/mL.

Adverse Reactions:

GSK: Generally well tolerated during clinical trials involving more than 26,000 subjects receiving doses from 360 to 1,440 ELU. The frequency of solicited adverse events tends to decrease with successive doses of vaccine. Most events reported were rated by subjects as mild and did not last more than 24 hours. The most frequent reactions reported were injection-site soreness (56% of adults and 15% of children; less than 0.5% of soreness was reported as severe) and headache (14% of adults and less than 5% of children).

Incidence 1% to 10% of injections: Induration, redness, or swelling at injection site; fatigue; fever (higher than 37.5°C [100°F]); malaise; anorexia; or nausea.

Incidence less than 1 % of injections: Hematoma at injection site; pruritus, rash, or urti-caria; pharyngitis or other upper respiratory tract symptoms; abdominal pain; diar-rhea, dysgeusia, or vomiting; arthralgia, elevated creatinine phosphokinase, or myalgia; lymphadenopathy; hypertonic episode, insomnia, photophobia, or vertigo.

While no causal relationship has been established, spontaneous voluntary reports of adverse events include: Localized edema, anaphylaxis or anaphylactoid reactions, somno-lence, syncope, jaundice, hepatitis, erythema multiforme, Guillain-Barré syndrome, hyperhydrosis, angioedema, dyspnea, convulsions, transient encephalopathy, dizziness, neuropathy, myelitis, paresthesia, multiple sclerosis, and a report of a child born with a deformed ear to a mother vaccinated during pregnancy.

Merck: In combined clinical trials, 16,252 doses were given to 9,181 healthy children, ado-lescents, and adults. No serious vaccine-related adverse experiences were observed dur-ing clinical trials. In the Monroe Efficacy Study, subjects were observed for 5 days for fever and local complaints and for 14 days for systemic complaints. Injection-site complaints, generally mild and transient, were the most frequently reported complaints. There were no significant differences in the rates of any complaints between vaccine and placebo recipi-ents.

Among children 12 to 23 months of age, who received hepatitis A and other routine pedi-atric vaccinations, reported adverse events included pain, tenderness, or soreness (3.1% to 3.5%), erythema (1.3% to 1.6%), swelling (1.3% to 1.6%), warmth (0.8% to 0.9%), measles- or rubella-like rash (1%), varicella-like rash (0.9%), oral temperature at least 38°C (100.4°F) (9.1% to 11.3%), oral temperature at least 38.8°C (102°F) (3.1% to 3.8%). Unsolicited adverse reactions occurring in at least 1% of children included ecchymosis (1%), diarrhea (6%), vomiting (4%), decreased appetite (1%), irritability (11%), upper res-piratory infection (10%), rhinorrhea (6%), cough (5%), respiratory congestion (2%), nasal congestion (1%), laryngotracheobronchitis (1%), rash (5%), viral exanthema (1%), oti-tis media (8%), otitis (2%), and conjunctivitis (1%). Rare serious events reported tempo-rally after vaccination included seizures, bronchiolitis, dehydration, pneumonia, asthma, and asthma exacerbation.

Local or systemic allergic reactions that occurred in less than 1% of children, adoles-cents, or adults in clinical trials, regardless of causality, included injection-site pruritus and/or rash, bronchial constriction, asthma, wheezing, edema/swelling, rash, generalized erythema, urticaria, pruritus, eye irritation/itching, thrombocytopenia, Guillain-Barré syndrome, cerebellar ataxia, encephalitis, and dermatitis.

In a cohort study of *Vaqta* recipients, outpatient visits for diarrhea/gastroenteritis were the only novel vaccine-related adverse event recognized.

Among children and adolescents in all studies, these are the events reported (1% or more) without regard to causality: Pain (18.7%); tenderness (16.8%); warmth (8.6%); erythema (7.5%); swelling (7.3%); fever (102°F or higher, oral) (3.1%); headache (2.3%); abdomi-nal pain (1.6%); pharyngitis (1.5%); ecchymosis (1.3%); upper respiratory infection

(1.1%); cough, diarrhea, vomiting (1%). Laboratory abnormalities included isolated reports of elevated liver function tests, eosinophilia, and increased urine protein (very few).

Among adults in all studies, these are the events reported (1% or more) without regard to causality: Tenderness (52.6%, generally mild and transient); pain (51.1%); warmth (17.3%); headache (16.1%); swelling (13.6%); erythema (12.9%); asthenia/fatigue (3.9%); upper respiratory infection (2.8%); pharyngitis (2.7%); fever (101°F or higher, oral) (2.6%); diarrhea (2.4%); nausea (2.3%); myalgia (2%); ecchymosis (1.5%); abdominal pain, arm pain (1.3%); pain/soreness (1.2%); back pain, nasal congestion, menstruation disorder (1.1%); stiffness (1%).

Local or systemic allergic reactions that occurred in less than 1% of children, adolescents, or adults in clinical trials, regardless of causality, included injection-site pruritus or rash, bronchial constriction, asthma, wheezing, edema/swelling, rash, generalized erythema, urticaria, pruritus, eye irritation/itching, and dermatitis.

Pharmacologic & Dosing Characteristics

Dosage: Shake product gently before withdrawing a dose. Separate doses of hepatitis A vaccine by at least 4 weeks. Do not count doses within the minimum interval listed below, because too short an interval may interfere with antibody response and protection from disease. Increasing the interval beyond the recommended timing does not affect the ultimate efficacy of immunization, but waiting does delay achieving adequate protection from infection.

GSK: Adult: 1,440 ELU on day 0. In Europe, other schedules have been used, including 720 ELU on days 0 and 30. Most countries have now adopted the single 1,440 ELU-dose. A single 1,440 ELU/mL booster dose is recommended 6 to 12 months later, if persistent antibody titers are desired. A 1- to 1½-inch needle is recommended.

Pediatric: For children 2 to 18 years of age, give 1 dose of 720 ELU. The initial recommendation was to give 360 ELU on days 0 and 30. A single booster dose of 720 ELU is recommended 6 to 12 months later, if persistent antibody titers are desired. Children started on the 360 ELU dose should complete a 3-dose series at that dose.

Merck: Adult: 50 units on day 0. A single 50 units/1 mL booster dose is recommended 6 months later, if persistent antibody titers are desired.

Pediatric: 25 units on day 0. A single 25 unit/0.5 mL booster dose is recommended 6 to 18 months later, if persistent antibody titers are desired. A ⅞- to 1-inch needle is recommended.

Route & Site: IM. In adults, inject into the deltoid region. Do not inject into the gluteal region to avoid a suboptimal immune response. Do not inject IV, ID, or subcutaneously. Jet injection induces higher antibody responses for the first 8 months after immunization; immune responses are similar to IM administration thereafter. Patients may experience arm soreness following jet injection.

Documentation Requirements: Federal law requires that (1) the manufacturer and lot number of this vaccine, (2) the dates of its administration, and (3) the name, address, and title of the person administering the vaccine be documented in the recipient's permanent medical record or in a permanent office log.

Certain adverse events must be reported to VAERS (800-822-7967). Refer to Immunization Documents in the Resources section for complete information.

Overdosage: Although few data are available, clinical experience with similar products suggests that the major manifestations of overdosage would be pain and tenderness at the injection site.

Booster Doses:

GSK: A booster dose is recommended 6 to 18 months after the initial dose, if persistent antibody titers are desired.

Merck: A booster dose is recommended 6 months (for adults) or 6 to 18 months (for children and adolescents) after the initial dose, if persistent antibody titers are desired.

Accelerated Schedules: Although not recommended in product labeling, several accelerated dosing schedules produce antibody responses that persist approximately 6 months: Two doses on day 0, one dose on days 0 and 14, or one dose on days 0 and 30.

Missed Doses: Interrupting the recommended schedule or delaying subsequent doses does not require restarting the series. Resume the schedule as soon as possible.

Efficacy:

GSK: In an efficacy trial of 40,119 children at high risk of hepatitis A infection, 41 cases of clinical hepatitis A occurred in the control group, compared with 2 markedly attenuated cases in the vaccinated group. The rate of disease prevention was 94%. A 96% efficacy rate for protection against unapparent or subclinical infection was observed. In outbreak investigations during the study, protection against symptomatic and asymptomatic hepatitis A infection was 97%.

Merck: In combined clinical studies, 97% of 1,214 healthy children and adolescents 2 to 17 years of age seroconverted with a GMT of 43 milliunits/mL within 4 weeks after a single dose of approximately 25 units/0.5 mL IM. Similarly, 95% of 1428 adults 18 years of age and older seroconverted with a GMT of 37 milliunits/mL within 4 weeks after a single dose of approximately 50 units/mL IM. Two weeks after a single dose, 69% (n = 744) of adults seroconverted with a GMT of 16 milliunits/mL. Immune memory was demonstrated by an anamnestic antibody response in patients who received a booster dose.

A high degree of protection was shown after a single dose in children and adolescents. In a randomized, double-blind, placebo-controlled study of 1,037 susceptible healthy children and adolescents 2 to 16 years of age in a US community with recurrent outbreaks of hepatitis A (Monroe Efficacy Study), each received an IM dose (approximately 25 units) or placebo. Protective efficacy of a single dose of vaccine was 100%, with 21 cases of hepatitis A in the placebo group and none in the vaccine group ($P < 0.001$). No cases of confirmed hepatitis A occurred in the vaccine group after day 16.

Onset: Protective antibody titers develop within 15 to 30 days after immunization. By day 15, 80% to 98% of vaccinees seroconvert (anti-HAV at least 20 milliunits/mL, the lower limit of the antibody assay).

Duration:

GSK: In 89 vaccinees, a single 1,440 ELU dose of hepatitis A vaccine elicited anti-HAV neutralizing antibodies in more than 94% of vaccinees when measured 1 month after vaccination. These antibodies persisted for 6 months or more. After a second dose given at month 6, 100% of vaccinees had neutralizing antibodies when measured at month 7.

In 2 clinical trials in which a booster dose of 1,440 ELU was given 6 months after the initial dose, 100% of vaccinees (n = 269) were seropositive 1 month after the booster dose, with GMTs ranging from 3,318 to 5,925 milliunits/mL. The titers obtained from the second dose approximate those observed several years after natural infection.

Merck: Seropositivity persisted 18 months or more after a single approximately 25 unit dose in a cohort of 35 out of 39 children and adolescents who participated in the Monroe Efficacy Study; 95% of this cohort responded anamnestically following a booster at 18 months. To date, no cases of hepatitis A disease have occurred within 250 days after vaccination in those vaccinees from the Monroe Efficacy Study who were monitored for up to 4 years.

Pharmacokinetic models of anti-hepatitis A antibodies suggest that clinical protection may persist for 10 to 20 years. More data are needed to make definitive recommendations about booster doses for lifelong immunity.

Protective Level: The lowest titer needed to confer protection against infection is unknown but may be 10 to 20 milliunits/mL or more. GMTs after a single HAV dose are at least several times greater than those expected after an appropriate dose of IGIM. The presence of antibodies to HAV, as detected in a standardized assay (HAVAB), is an indication of the presence of protective antibodies against hepatitis A disease. Natural infection provides lifelong immunity even when antibodies to hepatitis A are undetectable.

Mechanism: Neutralizing anti-HAV antibodies protect against infection.

Drug Interactions: Giving hepatitis A vaccine to patients receiving immunosuppressant drugs (eg, high-dose corticosteroids) or radiation therapy may result in inadequate response to immunization. Patients may remain susceptible despite immunization.

Inactivated vaccines are not generally affected by circulating antibodies or administration of exogenous antibodies. Vaccination may occur at any time before or after antibody administration.

For patients desiring both immediate and long-term protection, hepatitis A vaccine may be administered concomitantly with IGIM, with separate syringes and at different injection sites. Simultaneous administration of hepatitis A vaccine and parenteral immune globulin products may reduce the ultimate antibody titer obtained from vaccination compared with vaccine alone. In a study using 2.5 to 5 times the standard IGIM dose, the anti-hepatitis A GMT was 146 milliunits/mL 5 days after IGIM administration, 77 milliunits/mL after 1 month, and 63 milliunits/mL 2 months after IGIM. Lower antibody titers might result in protection of less duration than without IGIM administration.

Havrix brand of hepatitis A vaccine has been administered simultaneously with *Engerix-B* (hepatitis B vaccine) without impairing immune response to either. Concomitant administration with other inactivated vaccines (eg, tetanus-diphtheria, Hib, rabies, pneumococcal conjugate vaccine, poliovirus, typhoid) has not interfered with immune responses to either vaccine.

In a series of small studies, recipients of yellow fever vaccine were generally as likely to seroconvert if they also received hepatitis A vaccine, compared with separated vaccinations. Yellow fever vaccine does not interfere with the antibody response to hepatitis A vaccine. Hepatitis A vaccine did not affect the immunogenicity of, nor was it affected by, oral poliovirus vaccine or oral typhoid vaccine.

Vaqta may be given concomitantly with typhoid and yellow-fever vaccines. The GMTs for hepatitis A when *Vaqta*, typhoid, and yellow-fever vaccines were administered concomitantly were reduced when compared with *Vaqta* alone. After the booster dose of *Vaqta*, the GMTs for hepatitis A in the 2 groups were comparable.

As with other drugs administered IM, administer hepatitis A vaccine with caution to patients receiving anticoagulant therapy.

Patient Information: Advise vaccine recipients that food and water precautions are essential to avoid infection. Refer to the section on Recommendations for International Travel.

Pharmaceutical Characteristics

Concentration:
GSK: Adult: 1,440 ELU/mL
   Pediatric: 360 or 720 ELU/0.5 mL
Merck: Adult: 50 units/mL
   Pediatric: 25 units/0.5 mL

Quality Assay:

GSK: Antigen activity is assayed in reference to a standard using an enzyme-linked immunosorbent assay (ELISA). Potency is expressed in ELISA units (ELU). Contains less than 1 ng/mL bovine albumin; WHO standard is no more than 50 ng/mL.

Merck: 25 units were previously described as 400 ng of virus antigen. In the current *Vaqta* formulation, 1 unit of *Vaqta* is approximately 1 ng of purified hepatitis A virus protein. Antigen is measured by enzyme immunoassay. Each adult 50 unit dose contains no more than 100 ng nonviral protein, approximately 10 ng RNA, approximately 10 ng glucose, and less than 4 pg DNA at the level of sensitivity of the assay.

Packaging:

GSK: Adult: 1,440 ELU/1 mL single-dose vial (10 vials: NDC # 58160-0826-11), disposable, prefilled single-dose 1 mL *Tip-Lok* syringe of 1,440 ELU with no needle (5s: 58160-0826-46; 10s: 58160-0835-51).

   Pediatric: 720 ELU/0.5 mL single-dose vial (10 vials: 58160-0825-11), disposable, prefilled, single-dose 0.5 mL *Tip-Lok* syringe of 720 ELU with no needle (1 syringe: 58160-0837-32; 5s: 58160-0825-46).

Merck: Adult: 50 units/1 mL single-dose vial (00006-4841-00); box of 10 single-dose vials (00006-4841-41); 6 prefilled, single-dose 50 units/mL syringes without needles (00006-4096-09)

   Pediatric/adolescent: Box of 10 single-dose 25 units per 0.5 mL vials (00006-4831-41); 6 single-dose 25 units per 0.5 mL syringes without needles (00006-4095-09).

Doseform: Suspension

Appearance:

GSK: A fine, white precipitate; a clear, colorless supernatant may form during storage. The suspension is slightly milky.

Merck: Slightly opaque, white suspension

Solvent:

GSK: Phosphate-buffered saline solution

Merck: Solution of sodium borate 70 mcg/mL and sodium chloride 0.9%

Adjuvant:

GSK: 0.5 mg aluminum (as aluminum hydroxide) per 1 mL adult dose; 0.25 mg aluminum (as aluminum hydroxide) per 0.5 mL pediatric dose

Merck: 0.45 mg aluminum (as aluminum hydroxyphosphate sulfate) per 1 mL adult dose; 0.225 mg aluminum (as aluminum hydroxyphosphate sulfate) per 0.5 mL pediatric dose

Preservative:

GSK: None

Merck: None

Allergens:

GSK: The tip cap and the syringe plunger of prefilled syringes contain dry natural rubber (a latex derivative). The vial stopper is latex free.

Merck: The vial stopper and syringe plunger stopper contain dry natural rubber (a latex derivative).

Excipients:

GSK: Amino acid supplement 0.3% w/v with polysorbate-20 0.05 mg/mL, formalin 0.1 mg/mL or less, bovine albumin less than 1 ng/mL, MRC-5 cellular protein 5 mcg or less, neomycin sulfate 40 ng/mL or less, per each adult dose.

Merck: The 50 unit dose contains less than 0.1 mcg of nonviral protein, less than 4×10^{-6} mcg DNA, less than 10^{-4} bovine albumin, and less than 0.8 mcg formaldehyde. Other process chemical residuals are present at less than 10 parts per billion.

Hepatitis A Vaccine (HAV)

pH:
>   *GSK:* 6.8 to 7.5
>   *Merck:* 5.5 to 7.5

Shelf Life:
>   *GSK:* Expires within 2 years
>   *Merck:* Expires within 36 months

Storage/Stability: Store at 2° to 8°C (35° to 46°F). Discard frozen vaccine.

>   *GSK:* In 1 study, immunogenicity was not affected by storage for 7 days at 37°C (98.6°F). Shipped in insulated containers with coolant packs and temperature monitoring strips.

>   *Merck:* Contact manufacturer regarding prolonged exposure to room temperature or elevated temperatures. Shipped in an insulated container to maintain temperature 2° to 8° C (36° to 46°F). Product can tolerate 72 hours at temperatures up to 37°C (99°F) during shipment.

Production Process:

>   *GSK:* After removal of the cell-culture medium, the cells are lysed to form a suspension, then purified and concentrated by ultrafiltration and gel chromatography. Treatment of this lysate with formalin ensures viral inactivation. The lysate is then adsorbed to aluminum hydroxide.

>   *Merck:* Grown in MRC-5 diploid cell fibroblasts; purified by physical techniques and high performance liquid chromatography; inactivated with formalin, octoxynol-9 (*Triton X-100*), and chloroform; and adsorbed to 300 mcg aluminum as aluminum hydroxyphosphate sulfate.

Media:
>   *GSK:* MRC-5 human diploid cell culture
>   *Merck:* MRC-5 human diploid cell culture

Disease Epidemiology

Incidence: Disease incidence peaked in the United States prior to widespread improvements in sanitation systems. From 1981 through 1992, 21,000 to 36,000 cases were reported annually in the United States. But the true rate is probably substantially higher, perhaps 75,000 to 143,000 cases per year, at a cost of $200 million. Approximately 100 people die of fulminant hepatitis A in the United States each year. The disease rate in the United States is approximately 15 cases per 100,000 population, but 100 cases per 100,000 for American Indians. Throughout the world, more than 10 million clinical cases occur each year, with an estimated 14,000 deaths.

Hepatitis A in adulthood is more severe and more likely to be fatal. The case-fatality rate is approximately 0.3% overall but may reach 2.7% in people 49 years of age and older. Although 67% of cases occur in children, more than 70% of deaths occur in people 49 years of age and older. Up to 22% of adults who contract hepatitis A are hospitalized and approximately 100 patients die annually in the United States from complications of hepatitis A. Hepatitis A accounts for as many as 50% of all US hepatitis cases each year.

In Canada, from 1,000 to 3,000 cases of hepatitis A are reported annually. Since 1987, the reported incidence rate has varied from 4.4 to 11.2 per 100,000 population. Risk groups in Canada are comparable with those in the United States.

Prolonged infection does not occur; there is no chronic carrier state. The virus replicates in the liver and is excreted in bile. Recovery is generally complete, followed by protection from further infection.

In developing countries with poor hygiene and sanitation practices, 90% of children are infected by 5 years of age.

Susceptible Pools: The primary risk of hepatitis A disease among Americans is from international travel to countries with inadequate sanitation. The risk of acquiring hepatitis A during international travel is 10 to

100 times greater than contracting typhoid fever or cholera. The incidence of hepatitis A infection among a typical group of American travelers, assuming 40% of them are already immune, is 3 cases per 1,000 travelers per month of stay. People eating and drinking under poor hygienic conditions have a disease rate of 20 cases per 1,000 per month. Unprotected travelers who stay in endemic areas for long periods (eg, missionaries, other volunteers) may have disease rates of 1.6% to 5.4% per year. Hepatitis A is the most common infection of travelers that can be prevented by immunization.

The seroprevalence of protective anti-hepatitis A antibodies is approximately 38% of the population, but that rate is higher among people born before 1945 and lower among younger people (5% to 20%). As sanitation improves, the number of susceptible adults increases.

Approximately 5 million people in the United States have chronic liver disease, including alcoholic cirrhosis, chronic hepatitis B, chronic hepatitis C, autoimmune hepatitis, or primary biliary cirrhosis. These people are not more likely to be infected with hepatitis A virus, but they are more likely to develop fulminant hepatitis and die if infected.

Transmission: Person-to-person by the fecal-oral route. The infectious agent is found in the feces, reaching peak levels 1 to 2 weeks before onset of symptoms. It diminishes rapidly within the week after liver dysfunction or symptoms appear, concurrent with appearance of circulating antibodies to hepatitis A virus. Common-source outbreaks may be related to contaminated food or water, often via infected food handlers. Uncooked or undercooked mollusks (eg, oysters, clams, mussels, scallops) harvested from contaminated waters have been the source of many outbreaks. Other cases may occur after breakdown in sanitary sewage disposal and in the supply of clean water, or after floods or natural disasters. Infection may occur among institutionalized children or adults, or in day care centers where children have not been toilet trained. Parenteral transmission via blood transfusions or sharing needles with infected people has been observed. Direct transmission can occur among male homosexuals or those whose sexual practices involve the fecal-oral route of viral transmission.

As countries improve sanitation, the endemicity of hepatitis A decreases and the mean age of exposure to hepatitis A virus increases. Because icteric disease is more common among older infected people, the number of symptomatic cases of hepatitis A may increase as sanitation improves, despite a net reduction in the incidence of this infection.

Chronic shedding of hepatitis A virus in feces has not been demonstrated, but relapses of hepatitis A can occur in as many as 20% of patients and fecal shedding of virus may recur at this time. About 70% of pediatric patients younger than 6 years of age infected with hepatitis A are asymptomatic and serve as a reservoir for infection among adults.

Incubation: Depending on the dose ingested, incubation time is 15 to 50 days (mean, 28 to 30 days). Infection may be asymptomatic, but 76% to 97% of adults exhibit symptoms. Disease onset is often abrupt, with fever, malaise, anorexia, nausea, vomiting, diarrhea, and abdominal discomfort during the prodromal phase. Jaundice typically follows within a few days in up to 88% of adults, often with hepatomegaly and biochemical evidence of hepatocellular damage. Severity may range from a mild illness lasting 1 to 2 weeks to a disabling disease (icteric hepatitis) lasting several months. Generally, severity increases with the age of the patient, but complete recovery without sequelae or relapses is common. Many cases are mild and without jaundice, especially in children, and are recognized only through liver function tests. Relapses of hepatitis A can occur in up to 20% of patients and fecal shedding of the virus can recur at this time.

Hepatitis A infection in children younger than 2 years of age is often asymptomatic. Nonetheless, these children may excrete the virus in their stool and be a source of infection for others.

Communicability: Maximum infectivity occurs during the latter half of the incubation period, continuing for a few days after onset of jaundice. The highest concentrations of hepatitis A virus are found in stools of infected people during the 2-week period immediately before the onset of jaundice and decline after jaundice appears. Children and infants may shed the virus for longer periods than adults, up to several weeks after the onset of clinical illness. Most cases are probably noninfectious after the first week of jaundice. In 1 study of point-source outbreaks, an average of 11 contacts received IGIM for each index case reported by health authorities.

Other Information

Perspective:

1942: Hepatitis A and B viruses differentiated, based on a manufacturing defect involving yellow fever vaccine.

1945: Stokes and Neefe publish study demonstrating the efficacy of IGIM in preventing hepatitis A.

1972: Feinstone and colleagues identify hepatitis A virus by electron microscopy.

1978: Provost and Hilleman replicate hepatitis A virus in cell culture, develop vaccine candidate by 1982.

1984: Hepatitis A virus isolated and grown in primate cell culture.

1985: Formalin-inactivated hepatitis A vaccine first prepared by Binn and colleagues at the Walter Reed Army Institute of Research.

1991: Innis conducts efficacy trial in Thai school children.

1992: Werzberger reports efficacy trial in a Hasidic Jewish community in upstate New York.

1999: ACIP recommends routine pediatric hepatitis A vaccination in high-risk (largely Western) states.

2006: ACIP recommends routine pediatric hepatitis A vaccination in all states.

First Licensed:

GSK: February 22, 1995. A lower adult dose was initially used in Canada and Europe, but 1,440 ELU is now considered the standard adult dose.

Merck: March 29, 1996

National Policy: ACIP. Prevention of hepatitis A after exposure to hepatitis A virus and in international travelers. *MMWR.* 2007;56(41):1080-1084. http://www.cdc.gov/mmwr/PDF/wk/mm5641.pdf.

ACIP. Prevention of hepatitis A through active or passive immunization. *MMWR.* 2006;55(RR-7):1-23. http://www.cdc.gov/mmwr/PDF/rr/rr5507.pdf.

ACIP. Updated recommendations from the Advisory Committee on Immunization Practices (ACIP) for use of hepatitis A vaccine in close contacts of newly arriving international adoptees. *MMWR.* 2009;58(Sep 18):1006-1007.

References: Innis BL, et al. Protection against hepatitis A by an inactivated vaccine. *JAMA.* 1994;271(17):1328-1334.

Victor JC, Monto AS, Surdina TY, et al. Hepatitis A vaccine versus immune globulin for post exposure prophylaxis. *N Engl J Med.* 2007;357(17):1685-1694.

Werzberger A, et al. A controlled trial of a formalin-inactivated hepatitis A vaccine in healthy children. *N Engl J Med.* 1992;327(7):453-457.

WHO. Hepatitis A vaccines. *Weekly Epidemiol Rec.* 2000;75(5):38-44.

Pharmacoeconomics: Preliminary screening for the presence of anti-hepatitis A antibodies is only needed if economic considerations make such screening cost-effective. Vaccinating an immune person is not harmful. Screening for preexisting immunity will seldom be practical, unless a large fraction of the population to be screened is likely to be anti-HAV positive. Such populations might include people with a history of jaundice, people who emigrated to North America after spending their early childhoods in a developing country, and people raised in communities with endemic HAV infections.

Comparison Table of Hepatitis A Vaccines		
Generic name	Hepatitis A vaccine inactivated	
Brand name	*Havrix*	*Vaqta*
Manufacturer	GlaxoSmithKline	Merck
Viability	Whole inactivated virus vaccine	Whole inactivated virus vaccine
Indication	To prevent hepatitis A infection	To prevent hepatitis A infection
Strain	HM-175 strain	Attenuated CR326F' strain
Concentration	360 ELU/0.5 mL, 720 ELU/0.5 mL, 1,440 ELU/1 mL	50 units/mL
Adjuvant	Aluminum 500 mcg/mL as aluminum hydroxide	Aluminum 450 mcg/mL as aluminum hydroxyphosphate sulfate
Preservative	None	None
Production medium	MRC-5 cell culture	MRC-5 cell culture
Doseform	Suspension	Suspension
Packaging	Single-dose vial or syringe	Single-dose vial or syringe
Routine storage	2° to 8°C	2° to 8°C
Booster dose	6 to 12 months after initial dose	6 to 18 months after initial dose
Route	IM	IM
Standard schedule Children (2 to 18 years) Adults	Single dose 720 ELU (or 2 doses of 360 ELU) 1,440 ELU	Single dose 25 units 50 units
CPT code	Adult: 90632 Pediatric/adolescent (3-dose): 90634	Adult: 90632 Pediatric/adolescent (3-dose): 90634 Pediatric/adolescent (2-dose): 90633

Hepatitis A and Hepatitis B Vaccine

Viral Vaccines

Name: *Manufacturer:*

   Twinrix   GlaxoSmithKline

Comparison: *Twinrix* is a simple combination of 720 ELISA units of *Havrix* hepatitis A vaccine and 20 mcg of *Engerix-B* hepatitis B vaccine. It is administered on a 3-dose schedule, unlike the 2-dose adult schedule with the 1,440 ELISA units formulation of *Havrix*. Also see hepatitis A vaccine and hepatitis B vaccine monographs for more detail.

Immunologic Characteristics

Microorganism: Hepatitis A virus (single-stranded RNA), genus *Enterovirus*, family Picornaviridae. Hepatitis B virus (double-stranded RNA), family Hepadnaviridae.

Viability: Inactivated

Antigenic Form: Hepatitis A: Lysed whole viruses. Hepatitis B: Purified 226-amino acid polypeptide possessing antigenic epitopes of the hepatitis B virus surface-coat (S) protein (hepatitis B surface antigen [HBsAg]).

Antigenic Type: Protein

Strains:

   Hepatitis A: HM-175 strain

   Hepatitis B: Adw$_2$ subtype

Use Characteristics

Indications: To induce active immunity against infections caused by either hepatitis A virus (HAV) or hepatitis B virus (HBV) in patients 18 years of age and older. As hepatitis D (caused by the delta virus) does not occur in the absence of HBV infection, hepatitis D will also be prevented by this vaccine. Immunization is recommended for all susceptible people 18 years of age and older who are or will be at risk of exposure to hepatitis A and B viruses, including but not limited to the following:

- Travelers to areas of high or intermediate endemicity for both HAV and HBV who are at increased risk of HBV infection because of behavioral or occupational factors.
- Patients with chronic liver disease, including alcoholic cirrhosis, chronic hepatitis C infection, autoimmune hepatitis, or primary biliary cirrhosis.
- People at risk through their work, such as laboratory workers who handle live hepatitis A and hepatitis B virus; police and other personnel who render first-aid or medical assistance; workers who come in contact with feces or sewage; health care personnel who render first-aid or emergency medical assistance; or personnel employed in day care centers and correctional facilities.
- Residents of drug and alcohol treatment centers.
- Patients and staff of hemodialysis units.
- People living in or relocating to areas of high/intermediate endemicity of HAV and who have risk factors for HBV.
- Men who have sex with men, as well as other people at increased risk of disease because of their sexual practices.
- Patients frequently receiving blood products, including patients who have clotting-factor disorders (eg, hemophiliacs and other recipients of therapeutic blood products).
- Military basic trainees and other military personnel at increased risk for HBV.

- Users of injectable illicit drugs.
- People at increased risk for HBV infection and who are close household contacts of patients with acute or relapsing hepatitis A, and individuals who are at increased risk for HAV infection and who are close household contacts of individuals with acute or chronic hepatitis B infection.

Unlabeled Uses: People with severe congenital protein C deficiency repeatedly given human plasma-derived protein C concentrate, to prevent or treat venous thrombosis and purpura fulminans, should be considered for vaccination against hepatitis A and hepatitis B, to guard against bloodborne pathogens.

Limitations: *Twinrix* will not prevent hepatitis caused by other agents such as hepatitis C virus, hepatitis E virus, or other pathogens known to infect the liver. Hepatitis A and hepatitis B infections have relatively long incubation periods. The vaccine may not prevent HAV or HBV infection in people who have unrecognized hepatitis A or hepatitis B infection at the time of vaccination. Additionally, it may not prevent infection in individuals who do not achieve protective antibody titers.

Contraindications:

Absolute: Patients with known hypersensitivity to any component of the vaccine. Patients who experience serious hypersensitivity reactions to this vaccine (or one of the component monovalent vaccines) should not receive further injections.

Relative: Defer administration of this vaccine, if possible, in patients with a febrile illness or active infection. But minor illnesses, such as mild upper respiratory infections with or without low-grade fever, are not contraindications. Administer with caution to patients with thrombocytopenia or a bleeding disorder, as bleeding may occur following an intramuscular (IM) injection.

Immunodeficiency: Patients receiving immunosuppressive therapy or with other immunodeficiencies may have a diminished antibody response to active immunization. Consider deferring vaccination in patients receiving immunosuppressive therapy. Alternatively, these patients may require administration of additional doses of vaccine. Immunodeficient patients are not apparently predisposed to hepatitis A or B infections.

Elderly: Clinical studies of this vaccine did not include sufficient subjects 65 years of age and older to determine whether they respond differently from younger subjects. People born before 1945 are more likely to be already immune to hepatitis A, but those who are infected later in life will have greater morbidity and mortality.

Adults: The effect of age on immune response to *Twinrix* was studied in trials comparing subjects older than 40 years of age (mean age, 48 to 50) with those 40 years of age and younger (mean age, 32.5). The response to the hepatitis A component of *Twinrix* declined slightly with age, but more than 99% of subjects achieved protective antibody levels in both age groups, and antibody titers were comparable with 2 doses of hepatitis A vaccine alone in age-matched controls.

The response to hepatitis B immunization is known to decline in vaccinees older than 40 years of age. *Twinrix* elicited a seroprotective response to hepatitis B in 97% of younger subjects and 93% to 94% of the older subjects, as compared with 92% of older subjects given hepatitis B vaccine alone. Geometric mean titers (GMT) elicited by *Twinrix* were 2,285 in the younger subjects and 1,890 or 1,038 for the older subjects in the 2 trials. Hepatitis B vaccine alone gave titers of 2,896 in younger subjects and 1,157 in those older than 40 years of age.

Carcinogenicity: This vaccine has not been evaluated for carcinogenic potential.

Mutagenicity: This vaccine has not been evaluated for mutagenic potential.

Fertility Impairment: This vaccine has not been evaluated for fertility impairment.

Pregnancy: Category C. Use only if clearly needed. Animal reproduction studies have not been conducted with *Twinrix*. It is not known if this vaccine crosses the placenta. Generally, most

IgG passage across the placenta occurs during the third trimester. Problems in humans have not been documented and are unlikely.

Lactation: It is not known if this vaccine crosses into human breast milk. Problems in humans have not been documented and are unlikely.

Children: Safety and efficacy of this vaccine in children younger than 18 years of age have not been established.

Adverse Reactions: In clinical trials involving 6,594 doses administered to 2,165 people and during routine clinical use outside the United States, *Twinrix* has been generally well tolerated. In a trial comparing *Twinrix* with separate but simultaneous injections of *Havrix* and *Engerix-B*, adverse events after *Twinrix* were similar to those observed after vaccination with the monovalent components. The frequency of solicited adverse events did not increase with successive doses. Subjects reported most events to be mild and self-limiting, lasting 48 hours or more.

	Rate of Solicited Adverse Events Reported After Administration of *Twinrix* or *Engerix-B* and *Havrix* (%)							
	Twinrix			*Engerix-B*			*Havrix*	
Adverse event	Dose 1 (n = 385)	Dose 2 (n = 382)	Dose 3 (n = 374)	Dose 1 (n = 382)	Dose 2 (n = 376)	Dose 3 (n = 369)	Dose 1 (n = 382)	Dose 2 (n = 369)
Local								
Soreness	37	35	41	41	25	30	53	47
Redness	8	9	11	6	7	9	7	9
Swelling	4	4	6	3	5	5	5	5

	Twinrix			*Engerix-B* and *Havrix*		
Adverse event	Dose 1 (n = 385)	Dose 2 (n = 382)	Dose 3 (n = 374)	Dose 1 (n = 382)	Dose 2 (n = 376)	Dose 3 (n = 369)
General						
Headache	22	15	13	19	12	14
Fatigue	14	13	11	14	9	10
Diarrhea	5	4	6	5	3	3
Nausea	4	3	2	7	3	5
Fever	4	3	2	4	2	4
Vomiting	1	1	0	1	1	1

Among 2,165 subjects in 14 clinical trials, the following adverse experiences were reported to occur within 30 days after vaccination:

Incidence 1% to 10%:
  Local reactions at injection site: Induration.
  Respiratory system: Upper respiratory tract infections.
Incidence less than 1%:
  Local reactions at injection site: Pruritus, ecchymoses.
  Body as a whole: Sweating, weakness, flushing, influenza-like symptoms.
  Cardiovascular system: Syncope.
  GI system: Abdominal pain, anorexia, vomiting.
  Musculoskeletal system: Arthralgia, myalgia, back pain.
  Nervous system: Migraine, paresthesia, vertigo, somnolence, insomnia, irritability, agitation, dizziness.
  Respiratory system: Respiratory tract illnesses.
  Skin and appendages: Rash, urticaria, petechiae, erythema.
Postmarketing reports: More than 61 million doses of *Havrix* and more than 600 million doses of *Engerix-B* have been distributed worldwide. Voluntary reports of adverse events

in patients receiving *Engerix-B* or *Havrix* reported since market introduction of the vaccines include the following:

Body as a whole: Anaphylaxis/anaphylactoid reactions and allergic reactions.

Hypersensitivity: Erythema multiforme including Stevens-Johnson syndrome, angioedema, arthritis, serum-sickness-like syndrome days to weeks after vaccination including arthralgia/arthritis (usually transient), fever, urticaria, erythema multiforme, ecchymoses, and erythema nodosum.

Cardiovascular system: Tachycardia/palpitations.

Skin and appendages: Erythema multiforme, hyperhydrosis, angioedema, eczema, herpes zoster, erythema nodosum, alopecia.

GI system: Jaundice, hepatitis, abnormal liver function tests, dyspepsia.

Hematologic/lymphatic: Thrombocytopenia.

Nervous system: Convulsions, paresis, encephalopathy, neuropathy, myelitis, Guillain-Barré syndrome, multiple sclerosis, Bell palsy, transverse myelitis, optic neuritis.

Respiratory system: Dyspnea, bronchospasm including asthma-like symptoms.

Special senses: Conjunctivitis, keratitis, visual disturbances, tinnitus, earache.

Other: Congenital abnormality.

Multiple sclerosis: Results from 2 clinical studies indicate that there is no association between hepatitis B vaccination and the development of multiple sclerosis and that vaccination with hepatitis B vaccine does not appear to increase the short-term risk of relapse in multiple sclerosis.

Pharmacologic & Dosing Characteristics

Dosage: Primary immunization for adults consists of 3 doses, given on a 0-, 1-, and 6-month schedule. Each 1 mL dose contains 720 ELISA units of inactivated hepatitis A virus and 20 mcg of HBsAg. Alternately, a 4-dose schedule may be used, with doses on days 0, 7, and 21 to 30, followed by a booster dose around day 365.

Route & Site: IM. In adults, inject in the deltoid region. Do not administer in the gluteal region; such injections may result in a suboptimal response.

If the patient receives antihemophilia or similar therapy, IM vaccination can be scheduled shortly after such therapy is administered. A fine needle (23 gauge or smaller) can be used, followed by firm pressure applied to the site (without rubbing) for at least 2 minutes. Instruct the patient about the risk of hematoma from the injection.

Documentation Requirements: Federal law requires that (1) the manufacturer and lot number of this vaccine, (2) the dates of its administration, and (3) the name, address, and title of the person administering the vaccine be documented in the recipient's permanent medical record or in a permanent office log.

Certain adverse events must be reported to VAERS (800-822-7967). Refer to Immunization Documents in the Resources section for complete information.

Overdosage: Although few data are available, clinical experience with similar products suggests that the major manifestations of overdosage would be pain and tenderness at the injection site.

Booster Doses: Routine revaccination is not recommended for hepatitis A or hepatitis B vaccine at this time, except for predialysis and dialysis patients. See hepatitis B vaccine monograph for details.

Missed Doses: Interrupting the recommended schedule or delaying subsequent doses does not require restarting the series.

Efficacy: Sera from 1,551 healthy adult volunteers ages 17 to 70, including 555 male subjects and 996 female subjects, in 11 clinical trials were analyzed after administration of 3 doses of *Twinrix* on a 0-, 1-, and 6-month schedule. Seroconversion for antibodies against HAV occurred in 99.9% of vaccinees, and protective antibodies against HBV developed in 98.5%, 1 month after completing the 3-dose series.

Onset: After the first dose, 94% of vaccinees seroconverted to hepatitis A. Protective antibody concentrations against HBV developed in 31% of vaccinees after the first dose, 78% after the second dose, and 98.5% after the third dose.

Duration: Antibodies to both HAV and HBV persisted for at least 4 years after the first vaccine dose in a 3-dose series of *Twinrix*, given on a 0-, 1-, and 6-month schedule. For comparison, after the recommended immunization regimens for *Havrix* and *Engerix-B*, similar studies show that seropositivity to HAV and HBV also persists for 4 years or more.

Pharmacokinetics: One trial compared either *Twinrix* (given on a 0-, 1-, 6-month schedule) or *Havrix* (0-, 6-month schedule) and *Engerix-B* (0-, 1-, 6-month schedule). The monovalent vaccines were given concurrently in opposite arms. Among 553 adults (ages 18 to 70 years) who completed the study according to protocol, the *Twinrix*-induced immune responses to hepatitis A and hepatitis B were noninferior to the monovalent vaccines. Thus, efficacy is expected to be similar to the efficacy for each of the monovalent vaccines.

Geometric Mean Titers (GMT) in the *Twinrix* US Clinical Trial				
Vaccine	N	Time-point	GMT to Hep A (95% CI)	GMT to Hep B (95% CI)
Twinrix	263	Month 1	335	8
	259	Month 2	636	23
	264	Month 7	4,756 (4,152-5,448)	2,099 (1,663-2,649)
Havrix and *Engerix-B*	268	Month 1	444	6
	269	Month 2	257	18
	269	Month 7	2,948 (2,638-3,294)	1,871 (1,428-2,450)

Antibody levels achieved 1 month after the final dose of *Twinrix* were higher than titers achieved 1 month after the final dose of *Havrix* in these clinical trials. This may have been due to a difference in the recommended dosage regimens for these 2 vaccines; *Twinrix* vaccinees received 3 doses of 720 ELISA units of hepatitis A antigen at 0, 1, and 6 months, and *Havrix* vaccinees received 2 doses of 1,440 ELISA units (at 0 and 6 months). However, these differences in peak titer have not been shown to be clinically significant.

Protective Level:

Hepatitis A: The lowest antibody concentration needed to confer protection against HAV infection is unknown, but may be approximately 20 milliunits/mL. GMT after a single HAV dose are at least several times greater than that expected after an appropriate dose of immunoglobulin IM.

Hepatitis B: Antibody concentrations at least 10 milliunits/mL against HBsAg are recognized as conferring prolonged protection against HBV. Seroconversion is defined as an antibody concentration at least 1 milliunit/mL.

Mechanism: Neutralizing anti-HAV and anti-HBV antibodies protect against infection. Cellular immunity may play some role in protection from clinically apparent disease.

Drug Interactions: Like all inactivated vaccines, administration of this vaccine to patients receiving immunosuppressant drugs (eg, high-dose corticosteroids) or radiation therapy may result in an inadequate response to immunization. They may remain susceptible despite immunization.

There have been no studies of concomitant administration of *Twinrix* with other vaccines. Nonetheless, neither hepatitis A nor hepatitis B vaccines have been shown to interfere with other vaccinations in any clinically significant way.

As with other drugs administered by IM injection, give this vaccine with caution to patients receiving anticoagulant therapy, because bleeding may occur following IM injection.

Patient Information: No vaccine is perfect. Advise vaccine recipients that precautions against food-, water-, or blood-borne diseases are essential to avoid infection.

Pharmaceutical Characteristics

Concentration: Hepatitis A: At least 720 ELISA units of inactivated hepatitis A virus per 1 mL

Hepatitis B: 20 mcg of recombinant HBsAg protein per 1 mL

Packaging: Single-dose 1 mL vials: package of 10 vials (NDC # 58160-0815-11). Single-dose prefilled 1 mL *Tip-Lok* syringes with no needles; package of 5 syringes (58160-0850-46).

Doseform: Suspension

Appearance: After shaking, a homogenous, white turbid suspension

Solvent: Phosphate-buffer sodium chloride

Adjuvant: Aluminum 0.45 mg/mL in the form of aluminum phosphate and aluminum hydroxide

Preservative: None

Allergens: The tip cap and syringe plunger of prefilled syringes contain dry natural rubber (a latex derivative). The vial stopper is latex-free.

Excipients: Amino acids and polysorbate 20. Trace amounts of several materials used in manufacturing may remain in the finished product after purification: Formalin (no more than 0.1 mg/mL), residual MRC-5 cellular proteins (no more than 2.5 mcg/mL), no more than 5% yeast protein, neomycin sulfate (no more than 20 ng/mL).

pH: 6.4 to 7.5

Shelf Life: Expires within 36 months

Storage/Stability: Store at 2° to 8°C (36° to 46°F). Discard frozen vaccine. Stable at controlled room temperature (20° to 25°C, 68° to 77°F) for at least 4 days. Contact the manufacturer regarding exposure to elevated temperatures. Shipped in insulated containers with coolant packs.

Handling: Shake vial or syringe well before withdrawal and use. After removing the appropriate volume from a single-dose vial, discard any vaccine remaining in the vial.

Production Process: Hepatitis A virus (strain HM-175) is propagated in MRC-5 cells and then inactivated. Purified hepatitis B surface antigen (HBsAg) is obtained by culturing genetically engineered *Saccharomyces cerevisiae* cells (strain RIT 4376), which carry the surface antigen gene of the hepatitis B virus, in synthetic media containing inorganic salts, amino acids, dextrose, and vitamins. Bulk preparations of each antigen are adsorbed separately onto aluminum salts and then pooled during formulation.

Media: MRC-5 cells (hepatitis A component) and *S. cerevisiae* cells (strain RIT 4376; hepatitis B component) in synthetic media.

Disease Epidemiology

See hepatitis A vaccine and hepatitis B vaccine monographs for details.

Other Information

Perspective: See hepatitis A vaccine and hepatitis B vaccine monographs for details.

First Licensed: May 11, 2001

National Policy: See hepatitis A vaccine and hepatitis B vaccine monographs for details.

Hepatitis A and Hepatitis B Vaccine

Hepatitis A and Hepatitis B Vaccine Summary Table	
Generic name	Hepatitis A and hepatitis B vaccine
Brand name	*Twinrix*
Manufacturer	GlaxoSmithKline
Viability	Whole inactivated virus and viral subunit vaccine
Indication	To prevent infection with hepatitis A and hepatitis B viruses
Concentration	Each mL contains 720 ELISA units of *Havrix* brand hepatitis A vaccine and 20 mcg of *Engerix B* brand hepatitis B vaccine
Adjuvant	Aluminum 450 mcg/mL as aluminum phosphate and aluminum hydroxide
Preservative	None
Production medium	MRC-5 cells and *Saccharomyces cerevisiae*
Doseform	Suspension
Packaging	1 mL vial, 1 mL syringe
Routine storage	2° to 8°C
Dosage, route	1 mL IM
Standard schedule	Days 0, 30, 180, when both hepatitis A and hepatitis B vaccines indicated for people 18 years of age and older. Alternately, days 0, 7, 21 to 30, and 365

Names:
Engerix-B
Recombivax HB

Manufacturers:
GlaxoSmithKline
Merck

Synonyms: Hepatitis B surface antigen (HBsAg) is also called the "Dane particle" and the "Australia antigen." Hepatitis B was initially called "serum hepatitis," to differentiate it from "infectious hepatitis" (IH, hepatitis A). The acronym HBV may refer either to hepatitis B virus or hepatitis B vaccine, depending on context. In other countries, *Recombivax HB* is known as *Gen H-B-Vax*, *HB-Vax DNA*, *HB-Vax II*, *HB-Vax II DNA*, *HB-Vax Pro*, *Heptavax-II*, or *r-HB* vaccine.

Comparison: Either hepatitis B vaccine is prophylactically interchangeable with the other (including the original plasma-derived vaccine, *Heptavax-B*, Merck) for completion of a basic immunization series or for booster doses, but the quantity of antigen or the dosage volume will vary between the comparably potent *Recombivax HB* and *Engerix-B*. Immunogenic potency of the 2 current products varies because of antigenic differences in their 3-dimensional epitopes, effects of the purification process on the hepatitis B surface antigen particles, and other factors. Although the 2 vaccines contain the same aluminum concentration, *Recombivax HB* has a higher ratio of hepatitis B surface antigen to aluminum.

Immunologic Characteristics

Microorganism: Virus (double-stranded DNA), family Hepadnaviridae

Viability: Inactivated

Antigenic Form: Purified antigen, a 226-amino acid polypeptide, 22 nm virus-like particles (VLPs, in contrast to 42 nm infectious virions of HBV) possessing antigenic epitopes of the hepatitis B virus surface-coat (S) protein

Antigenic Type: Lipoprotein complex containing the small envelope (S) protein. The S protein contains the principal envelope antigen, hepatitis B surface antigen (HBsAg). Other envelope proteins, pre-S1 and pre-S2, are not included in vaccines licensed in the United States, but are under study for enhanced immunogenicity.

Strains:

GSK: Hepatitis B adw_2 subtype, *Saccharomyces cerevisiae* strain RIT4376

Merck: Hepatitis B *adw* subtype, *Saccharomyces cerevisiae* strain 2150-2-3

Use Characteristics

Indications: Induction of active immunity against hepatitis B virus among patients of all ages who are currently or will be at increased risk of infection with hepatitis B. By preventing hepatitis B infection, hepatitis B vaccine prevents primary liver cancer.

Because hepatitis D virus (delta hepatitis, the delta agent) can only infect and cause illness in people infected with hepatitis B, and because hepatitis D virus requires a coat of hepatitis B surface antigen to become infectious, immunity to hepatitis B also protects against hepatitis D. Hepatitis D virus is a circular RNA-containing virus.

The CDC, ACIP, AAP, Canada's National Advisory Committee on Immunization (NACI), and Canadian Paediatric Society recommend routine vaccination of all infants against hepatitis B with 3 doses either:

(1) At birth (prior to discharge from a hospital), at 1 to 2 months of age, and at 6 to 18 months of age; or

(2) at 1 to 2 months of age, at 4 months of age, and at 6 to 18 months of age.

Vaccines that do not contain thimerosal as a preservative are preferred for newborns and very young infants.

Make special efforts to vaccinate all children younger than 11 years of age who are Alaskan natives, Pacific islanders, or who reside in households of first-generation immigrants from countries where hepatitis B virus is of high or intermediate endemicity.

Vaccinate all children not vaccinated earlier in childhood. Vaccination of adolescents is most important in high-risk settings, including communities where use of illicit injectable drugs, teenage pregnancy, or sexually transmitted diseases are common. These steps are important to quickly control the rate of hepatitis B infection among young adults.

Vaccination is indicated for several major groups of people:

(1) Health care workers exposed to blood or blood products, such as the following: Dentists and oral surgeons; physicians and surgeons; nurses; podiatrists; paramedical personnel; dental hygienists and nurses; laboratory personnel; students in these occupations; and cleaning staff who handle potentially infectious waste. Routine postvaccination assessment of antibody titers among immunized health care workers can help differentiate people who do not respond to hepatitis B vaccine from people whose level of anti-hepatitis B antibodies later falls below detectable limits.

(2) Selected patients and patient contacts, such as the following: Patients and staff of hemodialysis and hematology/oncology units; people with hemophilia, thalassemia, or similar conditions requiring large-volume transfusions of blood or blood products; residents and staff in institutions for the mentally handicapped; classroom contacts of deinstitutionalized mentally handicapped people with persistent hepatitis B antigenemia who demonstrate aggressive behavior; and household and other intimate contacts of people with persistent hepatitis B antigenemia.

(3) Social groups with a known high incidence of disease, such as Alaskan Eskimos, Indochinese refugees, and Haitian refugees.

(4) People at increased risk because of their sexual practices, such as the following: People who have heterosexual activity with multiple partners (eg, more than 1 partner in a 6-month period); people who repeatedly contract sexually transmitted diseases; homosexual males; and female prostitutes.

(5) Other people at increased risk, including the following: Certain military personnel; morticians and embalmers; blood bank and plasma fractionation workers; prisoners; children adopted from countries of high hepatitis-B endemicity; and users of contaminated injectable drugs (eg, through needle sharing).

(6) People who have been sexually assaulted should receive a 3-dose regimen of hepatitis B vaccine (without need for hepatitis B immune globulin) if they have not previously been vaccinated.

OSHA requires that hepatitis B vaccine be offered for occupational protection to anyone at risk from blood-borne pathogens. For all employees who have the potential for occupational exposure to blood, the vaccine must be made available within 10 working days of initial assignment at no cost to the employee, at a reasonable time and place, under the supervision of a health care professional, and according to the latest recommendations of the US PHS; antibody screening may not be required as a condition of receiving the vaccine.

Unlabeled Uses: Hepatitis B vaccination is appropriate for patients expected to receive human alpha$_1$-proteinase inhibitor (*Prolastin*). If insufficient time is available for the development of adequate antibody responses to active vaccination, give a single dose of HBIG with the initial dose of vaccine. *Prolastin* is produced from heat-treated, pooled human plasma that may contain the causative agents of hepatitis and other viral diseases. Manufacturing procedures at plasma collection centers, plasma testing laboratories, and fractionation facilities are designed to reduce the risk of transmitting viral infection, but the risk cannot be totally eliminated. Hepatitis B vaccination will further reduce the risk of this disease but not of other hepatic viral diseases that might be transmitted by *Prolastin.*

People with severe congenital protein C deficiency repeatedly given human plasma-derived protein C concentrate, to prevent or treat venous thrombosis and purpura fulminans, should be considered for vaccination against hepatitis A and hepatitis B, to guard against bloodborne pathogens.

Limitations: No hepatitis B vaccine will protect against hepatitis A virus, non-A/non-B hepatitis viruses, hepatitis C virus, hepatitis E virus, or other viruses known to infect the liver.

Hepatitis B has a long incubation period. Hepatitis B vaccination may not prevent hepatitis B infection in individuals who had an unrecognized hepatitis B infection at the time of immunization. Additionally, it may not prevent infection in individuals who do not achieve protective antibody titers.

Adult predialysis and dialysis patients do not respond as well to hepatitis B vaccines and require higher doses. Increasing age, increasing skin-fold thickness (a marker of obesity), and cigarette smoking were independently associated with lower antibody responses in patients receiving buttock injections, but not in patients receiving arm injections. Preliminary reports of other unpublished retrospective studies suggest that increasing age and body mass, smoking, and male gender may be risk factors for failure to seroconvert to deltoid immunization.

Use hepatitis B vaccine with HBIG for postexposure prophylaxis. For detailed information about postexposure prophylaxis, refer to the HBIG monograph.

Interferon alfa and perhaps other drugs are effective in treating some forms of hepatitis B, hepatitis C, and possibly other viral hepatitis infections.

Contraindications:

Absolute: People with a history of serious allergic reaction to a vaccine component or after a prior dose of this vaccine.

Relative: Defer vaccination until after resolution of any serious active infection. Vaccines that do not contain thimerosal as a preservative are preferred for newborns and very young infants.

Immunodeficiency: Patients receiving immunosuppressive therapy or with other immunodeficiencies may have a diminished antibody response to active immunization. Response may be impaired, especially in HIV-positive homosexual men. Give dialysis patients and other immunocompromised patients a 40 mcg dose.

Elderly: Immunogenicity of hepatitis B vaccines is somewhat reduced in people older than 40 years of age.

Carcinogenicity: Hepatitis B vaccine has not been evaluated for carcinogenic potential.

Mutagenicity: Hepatitis B vaccine has not been evaluated for mutagenic potential.

Fertility Impairment: Hepatitis B vaccine has not been evaluated for impairment of fertility.

Pregnancy: Category C. Use if clearly needed. It is not known if hepatitis B vaccine or corresponding antibodies cross the placenta. Generally, most IgG passage across the placenta occurs during the third trimester. Problems have not been documented and are unlikely. Give this vaccine to pregnant women if indicated.

Lactation: It is not known if hepatitis B vaccine or corresponding antibodies are excreted in breast milk. Problems in humans have not been documented and are unlikely.

Children: Hepatitis B vaccine is well tolerated and highly immunogenic in newborns, infants, and children. Maternal antibodies do not interfere with pediatric immunogenicity. For low-

Hepatitis B Vaccines (HBV)

birth-weight infants, give the first vaccine dose after the infant weighs more than 2 kg. Otherwise, give low-birth-weight infants 1 additional dose of vaccine.

Adverse Reactions: Adverse effects are comparable for the two hepatitis B vaccines. Injection site (17% to 22%) and systemic complaints (14% to 15%) may involve pain, tenderness, soreness, pruritus, induration, erythema, ecchymosis, swelling, warmth, or nodule formation.

Systemic reactions: Fatigue, weakness, irritability, headache, fever higher than 37.5°C (100°F), malaise, nausea, diarrhea, dizziness, rhinitis, pharyngitis, upper respiratory infection, abnormal liver functions, thrombocytopenia, eczema, purpura, tachycardia or palpitations, erythema multiforme (eg, Stevens-Johnson syndrome) by temporal association.

Reactions following less than 1% of injections: Sweating, achiness, chills, lightheadedness, insomnia, disturbed sleep, agitation, somnolence, migraine, syncope, tachycardia, tingling, hypertension, anorexia, abdominal pain or cramps, dyspepsia, dysuria, elevated liver enzymes, elevated erythrocyte sedimentation rate, thrombocytopenia, constipation, flushing, vomiting, paresthesia, rash, angioedema, urticaria, herpes zoster, alopecia, petechiae, eczema, keratitis, arthralgia, arthritis, myalgia, back pain, neck pain, shoulder pain, pain in extremity, neck stiffness, lymphadenopathy, hypotension, anaphylaxis, bronchospasm, cough, vertigo, dizziness, hypotension, earache, systemic lupus erythematosus, lupus-like syndrome, vasculitis, polyarteritis nodosa, optic neuritis, tinnitus, conjunctivitis, visual disturbances, multiple sclerosis (or exacerbation of), myelitis (including transverse myelitis), seizure, febrile seizure, peripheral neuropathy, Bell palsy, muscle weakness, hypesthesia, encephalitis, radiculopathy, Guillain-Barré syndrome. Some of these events may have been only temporally associated with immunization.

Anaphylaxis and symptoms of immediate hypersensitivity have been reported within the first few hours of vaccination.

An apparent serum sickness-like syndrome of delayed onset has been reported days to weeks after vaccination. The syndrome has included arthralgia/arthritis (usually transient), fever, and dermatologic reactions such as urticaria, erythema multiforme, ecchymoses, and erythema nodosum.

When the National Academy of Sciences evaluated the evidence for demyelinating neurologic disorders after hepatitis B vaccination in 2002, it concluded that the evidence favors rejection of a cause-and-effect relationship between hepatitis B vaccine administered to adults and multiple sclerosis (both incident and relapse).

Pharmacologic & Dosing Characteristics

Dosage: Shake product gently before withdrawing each dose. Separate doses of hepatitis B vaccine by at least 4 weeks. Do not count doses given less than 4 weeks apart because too short an interval may interfere with antibody response and protection from disease. Increasing the interval beyond the recommended timing does not affect the ultimate efficacy of immunization, but waiting does delay achieving adequate protection from infection. Dosage (both quantity of antigen and fluid volume) varies between the licensed products. The harmonized pediatric schedule is as follows: Give the first dose from birth to 2 months of age, the second dose from 1 to 4 months of age, and the third dose from 6 to 18 months of age. Either brand may be used on this schedule. At least 4 weeks between doses is needed for proper immune response.

Preexposure prophylaxis:

GSK: Give patients 3 doses, with the second dose 1 month after the first and the third dose 6 months after the first (ie, at 0, 1, and 6 months). At each dose, give recipients an amount of vaccine corresponding to their age (see table).

An alternative schedule of doses at 0, 1, and 2 months will provide rapid induction of immunity (eg, in neonates born of hepatitis B infected mothers, others who may have been exposed to the virus, travelers to high-risk areas wanting prompt attention). On this alternative schedule, give an additional dose 12 months after the first dose to infants born of infected mothers and to others for whom prolonged protection is desired. Also give these infants 0.5 mL of HBIG at birth and 10 mcg/0.5 mL of vaccine within 7 days of birth, with additional 10 mcg/0.5 mL vaccine doses either 1 and 6 months later or 1, 2, and 12 months later.

Give dialysis patients and other immunocompromised patients 40 mcg/2 mL, with additional doses 1, 2, and 6 months after the first dose. Although not described in labeling from either manufacturer, the most persistently elevated antibody titers may result from a 3-dose series in months 0, 1, and 12. Such a schedule may be appropriate for health care students whose current risk is small but who will need prolonged immunity.

Merck: Give patients 3 doses, with the second dose 1 month after the first and the third dose 6 months after the first (ie, at 0, 1, and 6 months). At each dose, give recipients an amount of vaccine corresponding to their age (see table).

Give dialysis patients and other immunocompromised patients 40 mcg at each dose.

Although not described in the product labeling, *Recombivax HB* may be administered on an alternative schedule with doses at 0, 1, and 2 months to provide rapid induction of immunity. On this alternative schedule, give an additional dose 12 months after the first dose if prolonged protection is needed.

For adolescents 11 to 15 years of age, a 2-dose schedule of 10 mcg at 0 and 4 to 6 months results in antibody responses comparable with the standard 3-dose regimen of 5 mcg at 0, 1, and 6 months. With this 2-dose regimen, 98% developed a protective antibody level 1 month after the second dose.

Hepatitis B Vaccine Dose Based on Age		
	Recombivax HB	*Engerix-B*
Dialysis and immunocompromised patients	40 mcg/1 mL (0, 1, 6 mo)	40 mcg/2 mL (0, 1, 2, 6 mo)
Adults (20 years of age and older)	10 mcg/1 mL	20 mcg/1 mL
Adolescents (11 to 19 years of age)	5 mcg/0.5 mL	10 mcg/0.5 mL
Infants and children (birth to 10 years of age)	5 mcg/0.5 mL[a]	10 mcg/0.5 mL[b]

a Unless the infant is born of an HBsAg-positive mother. Give these infants 0.5 mL HBIG at birth and 5 mcg *Recombivax HB* within 7 days of birth, with an additional 5 mcg vaccine dose 1 month and 6 months later.

b Unless the infant is born of an HBsAg-positive mother. Give these infants 0.5 mL HBIG at birth and 10 mcg *Engerix-B* within 7 days of birth, with an additional 10 mcg vaccine dose 1 and 6 months later. The vaccine can also be given on a schedule of 0, 1, 2, and 12 months.

Postexposure prophylaxis: Also see the HBIG monograph.

In response to known or presumed exposure to hepatitis B surface antigen (eg, needle-stick, ocular, or mucous-membrane exposure; human bites that penetrate the skin; sexual contact; infants born of HBsAg-positive mothers), give previously unvaccinated patients postexposure prophylaxis. This consists of 0.06 mL/kg HBIG as soon as possible or within 24 hours after exposure, if possible (within 14 days in the case of sexual contact). Give the appropriate volume of either hepatitis B vaccine based on age within 7 days of exposure with additional vaccine doses either 1 and 6 months after the first dose or 1, 2, and 12 months after the first dose.

Patients who have been sexually assaulted should receive a 3-dose regimen of hepatitis B vaccine (without need for hepatitis B immune globulin), if they have not previously been vaccinated.

Route & Site: IM in deltoid muscle or, for infants and young children, in the anterolateral thigh. Avoid gluteal injection into the buttock, which may result in less than optimal immune response because of vaccine deposition in fatty tissue rather than muscle. Never inject IV. Subcutaneous injection may be used in patients at risk for hemorrhage following IM injection (eg, patients with hemophilia or thalassemia), but the subcutaneous route may produce a less than optimal response and may lead to an increased incidence of local reactions, including nodules.

Merck and GSK recommend against administering a reduced (usually $\frac{1}{10}$) dose of hepatitis B vaccine via the ID route. The CDC has reported several programs in which suboptimal immune response followed ID injection, probably because of improper technique. Some practitioners have successfully used the ID route to immunize large groups of patients when appropriate attention was paid to proper technique. Inadvertent subcutaneous injection into fat will impair the immune response. Proper ID technique may not achieve antibody titers as high (or perhaps as persistent) as IM injection of either plasma-derived or recombinant vaccines. Additionally, the likelihood of seroconversion may be reduced when using recombinant vaccines ID. Delayed hypersensitivity reactions at the injection site may follow ID administration.

Nonresponders: Give additional doses of vaccine to patients who do not develop protective levels of anti-HBs antibodies after an initial 3-dose series. Various approaches have been published involving 1 to 3 extra doses, typically at 1- to 5-month intervals. Approximately 30% to 75% of patients will respond to the second vaccination series. To differentiate nonresponders from patients who have lost detectable antibody concentrations, measure anti-HBs antibodies a few months after the third vaccine dose.

Documentation Requirements: Federal law requires that (1) the manufacturer and lot number of this vaccine, (2) the dates of its administration, and (3) the name, address, and title of the person administering the vaccine be documented in the recipient's permanent medical record or in a permanent office log.

Certain adverse events must be reported to VAERS (800-822-7967). Refer to Immunization Documents in the Resources section for complete information.

Overdosage: Although few data are available, clinical experience with similar products suggests that the major manifestations of overdosage would be pain and tenderness at the injection site.

Booster Doses: Consider revaccination of predialysis and dialysis patients with an additional 40 mcg dose if their anti-HBs level is less than 10 milliunits/mL 1 to 2 months after the third dose. No booster doses are recommended for healthy patients at risk of infection.

Missed Doses: Resume the recommended dosage schedule as soon as possible. Waiting delays achieving adequate protection from infection. However, prolonging the interval between doses does not interfere with immunity achieved after the concluding dose of the basic series.

Efficacy:

GSK: In healthy adults and adolescents who received 3 doses at months 0, 1, and 6, seroprotection (defined as titers 10 milliunits/mL or more) of 79% was seen at month 6 and 96% at month 7; the geometric mean antibody titer for seroconverters at month 7 was 2,204 milliunits/mL.

On the alternative month 0, 1, and 2 schedule, 99% of recipients were seroprotected at month 3 and remained protected through month 12. An additional dose after 12 months produced a geometric mean titer (GMT) of 9,163 milliunits/mL for seroconverters at month 13.

Immunization at 0, 1, and 6 months of age resulted in 100% seroconversion of infants by month 7, with a GMT of 713 milliunits/mL and a seroprotection rate of 97%. In a study of clinical protection, only 3.4% of 58 infants became chronic carriers in the 12-month follow-up period (a protective efficacy rate of 95% compared with an expected rate of 70%).

Among older subjects given 20 mcg at months 0, 1, and 6, 88% seroprotection resulted 1 month after the third dose. In adults older than 40 years of age, the GMT among seroconverters 1 month after the third dose was 610 milliunits/mL.

Hemodialysis patients respond to hepatitis B vaccine with lower titers that remain at protective levels for shorter durations than healthy subjects. Among chronic hemodialysis patients who received 40 mcg of *Heptavax-B* at months 0, 1, and 6, only approximately 50% of patients were seroprotected.

Merck: 94% to 98% immunogenicity in adults 20 to 39 years of age 1 to 2 months after the third dose; 89% immunogenicity in adults 40 years of age and older.

In children, three 5 mcg doses of vaccine induced a protective level of antibody in 100% of 92 infants, 99% of 129 children, and in 99% of 112 adolescents. Protective efficacy of three 5 mcg doses was demonstrated in neonates born of mothers positive for both HBsAg and HBeAg. In a clinical study of infants who received one dose of HBIG at birth followed by the recommended 3-dose regimen, chronic infection had not occurred in 96% of 130 infants after nine months of follow-up. The estimated efficacy in prevention of chronic hepatitis B infection was 95% compared with the infection rate in untreated historical controls. HBIG, administered simultaneously at separate body sites, did not interfere with the induction of protective antibodies against hepatitis B virus elicited by the vaccine.

For adolescents 11 to 15 years of age, the immunogenicity of a 2-dose regimen (10 mcg at 0 and 4 to 6 months) was compared with a 3-dose regimen (5 mcg at 0, 1, and 6 months) in a randomized, multicenter study. Adolescents receiving the 2-dose regimen who developed a protective level of antibody one month after the last dose (99% of 255 subjects) as often as adolescents who received the 3-dose regimen (98% of 121 subjects). After these adolescents received the first 10 mcg dose of the 2-dose regimen, the proportion who developed a protective level of antibody was approximately 72%.

Seroprotection rates in individuals with chronic HCV infection given the standard regimen was approximately 70%. In another study of IV drug users given an accelerated schedule, infection with HCV did not affect the immune response.

Predialysis and dialysis adult patients respond less well to hepatitis B vaccines than do healthy individuals. But vaccination of adult patients early in the course of their renal disease produces higher seroconversion rates than vaccination after dialysis has begun. Response to vaccination may be lower if vaccine is administered as a buttock injection. When 40 mcg was administered in the deltoid muscle, 89% of 28 participants developed anti-HBs with 86% achieving levels at least 10 milliunits/mL. But when the same dosage was administered inappropriately either in the buttock or a combination of buttock and deltoid, 62% of 47 participants developed anti-HBs with 55% achieving levels of at least 10 milliunits/mL. A booster dose or revaccination with the dialysis formulation may be considered in predialysis/dialysis patients if the anti-HBs level is less than 10 milliunits/mL.

Onset: 70% to 80% of recipients are protected after the second dose and more than 95% after the third dose.

Duration: Duration of protection is undetermined but apparently lasts more than 5 to 7 years in most healthy recipients. Studies of Alaskan Eskimos suggest that clinical protection may persist even after circulating anti-HBs antibodies can no longer be detected.

Protective Level: Seroconversion is usually defined as a change from less than 1 milliunit/mL to an antibody titer greater than that threshold. An anti-HBs titer of at least 10 milliunits/mL or 10 SRU by RIA is considered protective. In some studies, antibody titers among successful vaccinees fell below the protective level, yet clinical protection continued. In some cases, vaccinees developed anti-HBs antibodies, indicative of viral infection, without becoming clinically ill.

Mechanism: Induction of specific antibodies against the hepatitis B virus.

Drug Interactions: As with all inactivated vaccines, giving hepatitis B vaccine to patients receiving immunosuppressant drugs (eg, high-dose corticosteroids) or radiation therapy may result in an inadequate response to immunization. Patients may remain susceptible despite immunization.

Several routine vaccines may safely and effectively be administered simultaneously at separate injection sites (eg, DTP, MMR, e-IPV, Hib, hepatitis B, influenza). National authorities recommend simultaneous immunization at separate sites as indicated by age or health risk, if return of a vaccine recipient for a subsequent visit is doubtful.

Inactivated vaccines are not generally affected by circulating antibodies or administration of exogenous antibodies. Vaccination may occur at any time before or after antibody administration.

If administered at separate sites, no significant interaction between hepatitis B vaccines and HBIG occurs. Maternal antibodies do not interfere with immunogenicity in newborn infants. The *Havrix* brand of hepatitis A vaccine has been administered simultaneously with the *Engerix-B* brand of hepatitis B vaccine without impairing immune response.

Concurrent vaccination against hepatitis B and yellow fever in 1 study reduced the antibody titer otherwise expected from yellow fever vaccine. Separate vaccines by 1 month if possible.

As with other drugs administered IM, give hepatitis B vaccine with caution to patients receiving anticoagulant therapy.

Natural interleukin-2 may boost systemic immune response to HBsAg in immunodeficient nonresponders to hepatitis B vaccination, but the recombinant interleukin-2, known as teceleukin, did not augment response to hepatitis B vaccine in healthy adults in another study.

IM hepatitis B immunization of 153 hemophiliacs with a 23-gauge needle followed by steady pressure (without rubbing) to the injection site for 1 to 2 minutes resulted in a 4% bruising rate with no patients requiring factor supplementation.

Pharmaceutical Characteristics

Concentration:
GSK: 20 mcg/mL
Merck: 10 or 40 mcg/mL, depending on package
Quality Assay:
GSK: 97% pure by electrophoresis. Contains less than 2 mcg polysaccharide per dose.
Merck: Potency measured relative to a standard by an in vitro immunoassay.
Packaging:
GSK: Adult formulation (20 mcg/mL, with orange caps): 1 mL single-dose vial (box of 10 vials: 58160-0821-11); one 1 mL *Tip-Lok* syringe (tip cap and plunger contain latex) without needle (NDC #: 58160-0821-32); one 1 mL syringe (tip cap may contain latex) (each: 58160-0821-43; 5s: 58160-0821-48; 10s: 58160-0821-52).

Pediatric/adolescent formulation (10 mcg/0.5 mL, with blue caps): 0.5 mL single-dose vial (each: 58160-0820-01); 0.5 mL prefilled *Tip-Lok* syringes (tip cap and plunger contain latex) without needles (each: 58160-0820-32; 5s: 58160-0820-46; 10s: 58160-0820-51); 0.5 mL prefilled syringe (tip cap may contain latex) (each: 58160-0820-43; 10s: 58160-0820-52).

Merck: Adult formulation (preservative free) (10 mcg/mL with green caps and orange banners stating "preservative free"): 1 mL single-dose vial (each: 00006-4995-00; box of 10 vials: 00006-4995-41); six 10 mcg per 1 mL single-dose *Luer-Lok* syringes without needles (00006-4094-09).

Pediatric/adolescent formulation (preservative free) (5 mcg/0.5 mL with yellow caps and orange banners stating "preservative free" on labels and cartons): 0.5 mL single-dose vial (each: 00006-4980-00; box of 10 vials: 00006-4981-00); six 5 mcg per 0.5 mL single-dose *Luer-Lok* syringes without needles (00006-4093-09).

Dialysis formulation (40 mcg/mL with blue caps): 1 mL single-dose vial (00006-4992-00).

Doseform: Suspension

Appearance: A fine, white deposit with clear, colorless supernatant may develop during storage. When shaken, each product forms a slightly opaque, white suspension.

Solvent: Do not dilute prior to administration.

GSK: 0.9% sodium chloride and phosphate buffers

Merck: Sterile water

Adjuvant:

GSK: Aluminum hydroxide, containing no more than 0.5 mg/mL aluminum

Merck: Aluminum hydroxyphosphate sulfate, containing no more than 0.5 mg/mL aluminum

Preservative: None

Allergens:

GSK: Less than 5% yeast protein or plasmid DNA; contains no substances of human origin. The tip cap and syringe plunger of prefilled syringes may contain dry natural rubber (a latex derivative); check package labeling. The vial stopper is latex-free.

Merck: No more than 1% yeast protein; contains no detectable yeast DNA

Excipients:

GSK: Buffered with disodium phosphate dihydrate 0.98 mg/mL and sodium dihydrogen phosphate 0.71 mg/mL

Merck: Phosphate buffer with trace formaldehyde, no more than 1% yeast protein but no detectable yeast DNA

pH:

GSK: 6.4 to 7.4

Merck: 5.5 to 7.2

Shelf Life: Expires within 36 months

Storage/Stability: Store at 2° to 8°C (36° to 46°F). Discard vaccine if frozen; freezing destroys potency. Discard preservative-free packages promptly after piercing the seal 1 time.

GSK: Product can tolerate 37°C (98.6°F) for 7 days according to the Belgian package insert. Shipped by overnight courier in insulated containers with coolant packs and temperature monitor.

Merck: Product can tolerate 7 days at room temperature without significant loss of potency when prefilled into syringes. Shipped by routine courier in insulated containers with coolant packs.

Production Process:

GSK: The expression plasmid was derived from a hybrid *E. coli* clone (pACYC 184). The plasmid (pRIT12363) was cloned into *S. cerevisiae* and contains the coding sequence of the major HBsAg protein (P24), flanked by the promoter sequences from a glycolytic gene and by the transcription-termination region of the ARG3 gene. The P24 protein is recovered from yeast by precipitation, ion-exchange, gel-permeation chromatography, and caesium chloride ultracentrifugation. Adsorbed onto aluminum hydroxide. The antigen is uniformly nonglycosylated.

Merck: DNA sequence of Dane particles obtained using endogenous DNA-polymerase activity. Gene derived from a hybrid *Escherichia coli* clone; 19 amino acids cloned at aminoterminus of hepatitis B surface antigen. Gene cloned into *Saccharomyces cerevisiae*. The 22 nm HBsAg particles are released from the yeast cells by mechanical cell disruption and detergent extraction, then purified by a series of physical and chemical methods, including ion and hydrophobic chromatography and diafiltration. The antigen is uniformly non-glycosylated. Purified protein is treated in phosphate buffer with formaldehyde, then coprecipitated with potassium aluminum sulfate, to form bulk vaccine adjuvanted with amorphous aluminum hydroxyphosphate sulfate.

Media:

GSK: *S. cerevisiae*

Merck: *S. cerevisiae* grown in a fermentation medium consisting of an extract of yeast, soy peptone, dextrose, amino acids, and mineral salts

Disease Epidemiology

Incidence: The estimated incidence rate of acute hepatitis B in the United States is approximately 65 cases/100,000 people. Approximately 1 to 1.25 million chronic carriers currently reside in the United States, a pool that is growing 2% to 3% per year. At least 30% of reported adult hepatitis B cases are not associated with an identifiable risk factor (eg, sexual activity, parenteral drug use).

In the United States, 150,000 cases and 5,000 deaths occur per year, 85% among adults and 45% through heterosexual contact. These include 100,000 asymptomatic cases, 16,000 hospitalizations, 4,000 cirrhosis deaths, 800 liver cancer deaths, and 400 fulminant hepatitis B deaths per year. Most hepatitis B cases occur among young adults. The lifetime risk of hepatitis B infection in the United States varies from approximately 100% for the highest-risk groups to 5% for the population as a whole. Of infected people, 60% to 80% of neonates and 6% to 10% of adults become chronic carriers. An estimated 200 to 300 million people around the world are chronically infected ("chronic carriers") with the hepatitis B virus, which is responsible for 250,000 deaths. There are 5 million new cases annually.

Susceptible Pools: Eighty percent of American adults at risk (an estimated 20 million Americans) are unvaccinated. Infant vaccination programs have not yet become commonplace.

Transmission: Hepatitis B surface antigen is found in virtually all body secretions and excretions, but only blood, serum-derived fluids, saliva, semen, and vaginal fluids are infectious. The most common modes of transmission are needle-stick accidents, contaminated IV drug use, perinatal exposure, and sexual exposure.

Incubation: Usually 60 to 90 days (range, 45 to 180 days). The variation is related in part to the amount of virus in the inoculum, the mode of transmission, and host factors.

Communicability: Blood may be infective many weeks before the onset of first symptoms and remain infective through the acute clinical course of the disease and during the chronic carrier state.

Other Information

Perspective:

1939: Findlay and MacCallum implicate a virus as the likely cause of homologous serum hepatitis.

1942: Yellow fever vaccine lots contaminated with hepatitis B virus present in human albumin added during production.

1970: Dane images hepatitis B virus by electron microscopy.

1977: Hyperimmune hepatitis B immune globulin (HBIG) licensed in the United States.

1978: Hepatitis B virus shown to cause liver cancer.

1981: Plasma-derived hepatitis B vaccine, *Heptavax-B* from Merck, Sharp and Dohme, licensed in the United States on November 16.

1983: Hepatitis B surpasses hepatitis A as the most common viral cause of hepatitis.

1991: Universal immunization of all infants against hepatitis B recommended as US policy.

1999: Preservative-free formulations licensed by Merck (September 1999) and SmithKline (March 2000).

First Licensed:
Recombivax HB: July 23, 1986.
Engerix-B: August 28, 1989.

Discontinued Products: *Heptavax-B* (Merck, Sharp and Dohme)

National Policy: ACIP. Use of hepatitis B vaccination for adults with diabetes mellitus: recommendations of the Advisory Committee on Immunization Practices (ACIP). *MMWR*. 2011;60(50):1709-1711. http://www.cdc.gov/mmwr/pdf/wk/mm6050.pdf.

CDC. A comprehensive immunization strategy to eliminate transmission of hepatitis B virus infection in the United States, Part 2: Immunization of adults. *MMWR*. 2006;55(RR-16):1-33.

CDC. A comprehensive immunization strategy to eliminate transmission of hepatitis B virus infection in the United States, Part 1: Immunization of infants, children, and adolescents. *MMWR*. 2005;54(RR-16):1-32.

References: WHO. Hepatitis B vaccines. *Wkly Epidemiol Rec*. 2004;79:255-264.

WHO. Hepatitis B vaccines. *Wkly Epidemiol Rec*. 2009;84(Oct 2):405-419.

Pharmacoeconomics: Hepatitis B vaccine is reimbursed by several procedure codes: Birth to 10 years of age, 90744; 11 to 19 years of age, 90745; adult, 90731 or 90746; dialysis or immunosuppressed patients, 90747. Use ICD-9-CM diagnosis code V05.3. Use procedure code G0010 to report the administration fee. If a physician visit is rendered in conjunction with vaccination, it may be reimbursed as well.

Dosage Recommendations of FDA, CDC, ACIP, & AAP (for both preexposure and postexposure prophylaxis)			
	Heptavax-B[a]	*Recombivax HB*	*Engerix-B*
Infants of HBsAg-positive mothers	10 mcg/0.5 mL	5 mcg/0.5 mL	10 mcg/0.5 mL
Other infants/children			
< 11 years of age	10 mcg/0.5 mL	5 mcg/0.5 mL	10 mcg/0.5 mL
11 to 19 years of age	20 mcg/1 mL	5 mcg/0.5 mL[b]	10 mcg/0.5 mL
Adults (20 years of age and older)	20 mcg/1 mL	10 mcg/1 mL	20 mcg/1 mL
Dialysis patients and other immunocompromised patients	40 mcg/2 mL (3 doses)	40 mcg/1 mL (3 doses)	40 mcg/2 mL (4 doses)
Administration schedules			
Labeled	0, 1, 6 months	0, 1,6 months	0, 1, 6 months 0, 1, 2 (12) months
Unlabeled	0, 1, 2 (12) months 0, 1, 12 months	0, 1, 2 (12) months 0, 1, 12 months	0, 1, 12 months
Measures of immunogenicity			
Seroconversion[c] (titer ≥ 1 milliunit/mL)	97% to 100%	99% to 100%	98% to 100%
Seroprotection[b] (titer ≥ 10 milliunits/mL)	95% to 100%	94% to 98%	96% to 100%
Antibody titers[b] (GMT, milliunit/mL)	1,288 to 1,318	3,154 to 3,846	944 to 7,488

a Distribution of *Heptavax-B* was discontinued in 1990. Information is provided for historical comparison only.

b For adolescents 11 to 15 years of age, a 2-dose schedule of 10 mcg at 0 and 4 to 6 months results in antibody responses comparable to the standard 3-dose regimen of 5 mcg at 0, 1, and 6 months.

c Among healthy adults, younger than 40 years of age, using a 0-, 1-, and 6-month schedule.

Recommended Schedule for Prophylaxis of Perinatal Hepatitis B		
Infant born to mother known to be HBsAg-positive		
Age of infant	Vaccine dose	HBIG dose
Birth (within 12 hours)	First	First
1 month	Second	
6 months[a]	Third	
Infant born of mother not screened or known to be HBsAg-negative		
Age of infant	Vaccine dose	HBIG dose[b]
Birth to 2 months of age	First	
1 to 4 months[c]	Second	
6 to 18 months[a]	Third	

a If the 4-dose schedule for *Engerix-B* is used, give the third dose at 2 months of age and the fourth dose at 12 to 18 months.
b If mother is later found to be HBsAg-positive, administer HBIG to infants as soon as possible, not later than 1 week after birth.
c Vaccinate infants of women who are HBsAg-negative, beginning at birth or at 2 months of age.

Hepatitis B Blood Test Result Implications		
Tests	Test result	Implications
HBsAg	negative	susceptible, never infected
anti-HBc	negative	
anti-HBs	negative	
HBsAg	negative	immune
anti-HBc	neg. or pos.	
anti-HBs	positive	
HBsAg	positive	currently infected; either acutely infected or a chronic hepatitis B carrier; if HBsAg-positive, patient is highly infectious
anti-HBc	neg. or pos.	
anti-HBs	negative	
HBsAg	negative	various: recovering from HB infection, waning immunity; false-positive/uninfected or chronic carrier
anti-HBc	positive	
anti-HBs	negative	

Summary Table for Hepatitis B Vaccines		
Generic name	Hepatitis B vaccine	
Brand name	*Recombivax-HB*	*Engerix-B*
Manufacturer	Merck	GlaxoSmithKline
Viability	Viral subunit vaccine	
Indication	To prevent infection with hepatitis B virus	
Concentration	10 mcg/mL, 40 mcg/mL	20 mcg/mL
Adjuvant	≤ 0.5 mg/mL aluminum, as aluminum hydroxyphosphate sulfate	≤ 0.5 mg/mL aluminum, as aluminum hydroxide
Preservative	None	None
Production medium	Antigen expressed by *Saccharomyces cerevisiae*	Antigen expressed by *Saccharomyces cerevisiae*
Doseform	Suspension	Suspension
Packaging	5 mcg/0.5 mL, 10 mcg/1 mL, 40 mcg/1 mL	10 mcg/0.5 mL, 20 mcg/1 mL
Routine storage	2° to 8°C	2° to 8°C
Dosage		
Dialysis and immunocompromised people	40 mcg/1 mL (3 doses)	40 mcg/2 mL (4 doses)
Adults (20 years of age and older)	10 mcg/1 mL	20 mcg/1 mL
Adolescents (11 to 19 years of age)	5 mcg/0.5 mL	10 mcg/0.5 mL
Children (birth to 10 years of age)	5 mcg/0.5 mL	10 mcg/0.5 mL
Route	IM	IM
Standard schedule		
Infants	Birth to 2 months, 1 to 4 months, 6 to 18 months	
Others	Days 0, 30, 180	
Administration Schedules		
Labeled	0, 1, 6 months	0, 1, 6 months; 0, 1, 2[a] months, 0, 12, 24 months
Unlabeled	0, 1, 2[a] months	
Comment	For adolescents 11 to 15 years of age, two 10 mcg doses may be given 4 to 6 months apart	

a Optionally, give a 12-month dose for prolonged immunity.

Guide to Postexposure Prophylaxis for Hepatitis B	
Type of exposure	Immunoprophylaxis
Perinatal	HBIG and vaccine
Infants (< 12 months) (acute case in primary caregiver)	HBIG and vaccine
Household contact—exposed to acute case	None, unless known exposure
Household contact—exposed to acute case, known exposure	HBIG with or without vaccine
Household contact—exposed to chronic carrier	Vaccine
HBIG—Hepatitis B immune globulin	HBIG dose: 0.06 mL/kg IM

Recommendations for Hepatitis B Prophylaxis Following Percutaneous or Permucosal Exposure in the Occupational Setting			
	Treatment of exposed person when source is found to be:		
	HBsAg-positive	HBsAg-negative	Source not tested or unknown
Unvaccinated	HBIG[a] × 1 then initiate vaccine series[b]	Initiate vaccine series[b]	Initiate vaccine series[b]
Previously vaccinated			
Known responder	Test exposed person for anti-HBs antibody. 1. If adequate,[c] no treatment. 2. If inadequate, give vaccine booster dose.	No treatment	No treatment
Known nonresponders	HBIG[a,d] × 2 or HBIG × 1 plus one dose of vaccine	No treatment	If known high-risk source, may treat as if source were HBsAg-positive.
Response unknown	Test exposed person for anti-HBs antibody. 1. If adequate,[c] no treatment. 2. If inadequate, HBIG × 1[a] plus vaccine booster dose.	No treatment	Text exposed person for anti-HBs antibody. 1. If adequate,[c] no treatment. 2. If inadequate, HBIG × 1[a] plus vaccine booster dose.

a HBIG dose: 0.06 mL/kg IM
b Hepatitis B vaccine: give age-specific dose appropriate for each vaccine brand.
c Adequate anti-HBs antibody concentration is ≥ 10 SRU by RIA or positive by EIA.
d Give second dose 30 days after first dose.

Guidelines for Postexposure Prophylaxis[a] of People Exposed[b] to Blood or Body Fluids that Contain Blood Outside of Occupational Settings		
	Treatment	
Exposure	Unvaccinated person[c]	Previously vaccinated person[d]
HBsAg[e]-positive source		
Percutaneous (eg, bite or needlestick) or mucosal exposure to HBsAg-positive blood or body fluids	Hepatitis B vaccine series and HBIG	Hepatitis B vaccine booster dose
Sex or needle-sharing contact of an HBsAg-positive person	Hepatitis B vaccine series and HBIG	Hepatitis B vaccine booster dose
Victim of sexual assault/abuse by a perpetrator who is HBsAg positive	Hepatitis B vaccine series and HBIG	Hepatitis B vaccine booster dose
Source with unknown HBsAg status		
Victim of sexual assault/abuse by a perpetrator with unknown HBsAg status	Hepatitis B vaccine series	No treatment
Percutaneous (eg, bite or needlestick) or mucosal exposure to potentially infectious blood or body fluids from a source with unknown HBsAg status	Hepatitis B vaccine series	No treatment
Sex or needle-sharing contact of person with unknown HBsAg status	Hepatitis B vaccine series	No treatment

a When indicated, start immunoprophylaxis as soon as possible, preferably within 24 hours. Studies are limited on the maximum interval after exposure during which postexposure prophylaxis is effective, but the interval is unlikely to exceed 7 days for percutaneous exposures or 14 days for sexual exposures. The hepatitis B vaccine series should be completed.

b These guidelines apply to nonoccupational exposures. Guidelines for management of occupational exposures appear in a separate table and also can be used to manage nonoccupational exposures, if feasible.

c A person who is in the process of being vaccinated but who has not completed the vaccine series should complete the series and receive treatment as indicated.

d A person who has written documentation of a complete hepatitis B vaccine series and who did not receive postvaccination testing.

e Hepatitis B surface antigen.

Human Papillomavirus Vaccine, Types 6, 11, 16, 18

Viral Vaccines

Name:
  Gardasil

Manufacturer:
  Merck

Synonyms: HPV4, HPV 6/11/16/18 vaccine, *Silgard*

Immunologic Characteristics

Microorganism: Virus (double-stranded DNA, non-enveloped), human papillomavirus, genus *Papillomavirus*, family Papillomaviridae

Viability: Inactivated

Antigenic Form: Noninfectious, recombinant virus-like particles (VLPs) of the major capsid (L1) protein of HPV types 6, 11, 16, and 18

Antigenic Type: Protein

Strains: HPV types 6, 11, 16, and 18

Use Characteristics

Indications: For girls and women 9 to 26 years of age to prevent the following diseases caused by HPV types included in the vaccine:

- Cervical, vulvar, vaginal, and anal cancer caused by HPV types 16 and 18
- Genital warts (condyloma acuminata) caused by HPV types 6 and 11
- The following precancerous or dysplastic lesions: cervical adenocarcinoma in situ (AIS); cervical intraepithelial neoplasia (CIN) grades 1, 2, and 3; vulvar intraepithelial neoplasia (VIN) grade 2 and grade 3; vaginal intraepithelial neoplasia (VaIN) grade 2 and grade 3; anal intraepithelial neoplasia (AIN) grades 1, 2, and 3.

HPV4 vaccine is indicated in boys and men 9 to 26 years of age to prevent the following diseases caused by HPV types included in the vaccine:

- Anal cancer caused by HPV types 16 and 18
- Genital warts (condyloma acuminata) caused by HPV types 6 and 11

And the following precancerous or dysplastic lesions caused by HPV types 6, 11, 16, and 18:
- AIN grades 1, 2, and 3.

Limitations: There was no clear evidence of protection from disease caused by HPV types for which subjects were polymerase chain reaction (PCR) positive and/or seropositive at baseline.

This vaccine is not intended as treatment of active genital warts; cervical, vulvar, vaginal, or anal cancers; CIN; VIN; VaIN; or AIN.

This vaccine will not protect against diseases that are caused by the HPV types not present in the vaccine.

Not all vulvar and vaginal cancers are caused by HPV, and HPV vaccine protects only against those vulvar and vaginal cancers caused by HPV 16 and 18.

Contraindications:

Absolute: People with a history of serious allergic reaction to a vaccine component or after a prior dose of this vaccine.

Relative: Gardasil is not recommended for use in pregnant women.

Immunodeficiency: People with impaired immune responsiveness, whether due to immuno-suppressive therapy, a genetic defect, HIV infection, or other causes, may have reduced antibody response to active immunization.

Elderly: No specific information is available about the safety and efficacy of HPV vaccine in adults older than 26 years of age.

Carcinogenicity: HPV vaccine has not been evaluated for carcinogenic potential.

Mutagenicity: HPV vaccine has not been evaluated for mutagenic or genotoxic potential.

Fertility Impairment: HPV vaccine administered to female rats at a dose of 120 mcg total protein, which corresponds to approximately 300-fold excess relative to the projected human dose, had no effects on mating performance, fertility, or embryonic/fetal survival.

The effect of HPV vaccine on male fertility was studied in male rats at an IM dose of 0.5 mL/rat/occasion (120 mcg total protein, equivalent to the human dose). One group of male rats was administered HPV vaccine once, 3 days before cohabitation, and a second group was administered HPV vaccine 3 times, at 6 weeks, 3 weeks, and 3 days before cohabitation. There were no treatment-related effects on reproductive performance, including fertility, sperm count, and sperm motility. There were no treatment-related gross or histomorphologic and weight changes on the testes.

Pregnancy: Category B. Reproduction studies performed in female rats at doses up to 300 times the human dose (on a mg/kg basis) revealed no evidence of impaired female fertility or harm to the fetus due to HPV vaccine. Use only if clearly needed. It is not known if HPV vaccine or corresponding antibodies cross the placenta. Generally, most IgG passage across the placenta occurs during the third trimester. Problems in humans have not been documented and are unlikely. Patients and health care providers are encouraged to report exposure to HPV vaccine during pregnancy to a registry monitoring fetal outcomes by calling (800) 986-8999.

An evaluation of the effect of HPV vaccine on embryo-fetal, pre- and postweaning development was conducted using rats. One group of rats was administered HPV vaccine twice before gestation, during the period of organogenesis (gestation day 6), and on lactation day 7. A second group of pregnant rats was administered HPV vaccine during the period of organogenesis (gestation day 6) and on lactation day 7 only. HPV vaccine was administered at 0.5 mL/rat/occasion (approximately 300-fold excess relative to the projected human dose on a mg/kg basis) by intramuscular (IM) injection. No adverse effects on mating, fertility, pregnancy, parturition, lactation, embryo-fetal, or pre- and postweaning development were observed. There were no vaccine-related fetal malformations or other evidence of teratogenesis noted in this study. In addition, there were no treatment-related effects on developmental signs, behavior, reproductive performance, or fertility of the offspring. The effect of HPV vaccine on male fertility has not been studied.

In clinical studies, women underwent urine pregnancy testing before administration of each dose of HPV vaccine. Women found to be pregnant before completing a 3-dose regimen of HPV vaccine were instructed to defer completion of their vaccination regimen until resolution of the pregnancy.

During clinical trials, 2,266 women (1,115 received vaccine; 1,151 received placebo) reported at least 1 pregnancy each. Overall, the proportion of pregnancies with an adverse outcome were comparable in subjects who received HPV vaccine or placebo. Overall, 40 and 41 subjects in the group that received HPV vaccine or placebo, respectively (corresponding to 3.6% and 3.6% of subjects who reported a pregnancy in each group), experienced a serious adverse experience during pregnancy. The most common events reported were conditions that can result in Caesarean section (eg, cephalopelvic disproportion, failure of labor, malpresentation), premature onset of labor (eg, premature rupture of membranes, threatened abortions), and pregnancy-related medical problems (eg, hyperemesis, preeclampsia). The proportions of pregnant subjects who experienced such events were comparable between the groups.

There were 15 cases of congenital anomaly in pregnancies that occurred in HPV vaccine recipients and 16 such cases in the placebo group.

Further subanalyses were conducted to evaluate pregnancies with estimated onset within 30 days or more than 30 days from administration of a dose of HPV vaccine or placebo. For pregnancies with estimated onset within 30 days of vaccination, 5 cases of congenital anomaly were observed in the HPV vaccine group, compared with 0 cases in the placebo group. The congenital anomalies seen in pregnancies with estimated onset within 30 days of vaccination included pyloric stenosis, congenital megacolon, congenital hydronephrosis, hip dysplasia, and club foot. Conversely, in pregnancies with onset more than 30 days after vaccination, 10 cases of congenital anomaly were observed in the group that received HPV vaccine compared with 16 cases in the placebo group. The types of anomalies observed were consistent (regardless of when pregnancy occurred in relation to vaccination) with those generally observed in pregnancies in women 16 to 26 years of age.

Lactation: It is not known if HPV vaccine antigens or corresponding antibodies cross into human breast milk.

A total of 995 breast-feeding women (500 vaccine; 495 placebo) were given HPV vaccine or placebo during clinical trials. The geometric mean titers (GMTs) in breast-feeding women were 595.9 (95% CI, 522.5, 679.5) for anti-HPV 6; 864.3 (95% CI, 754, 990.8) for anti-HPV 11; 3,056.9 (95% CI, 2,594.4, 3,601.8) for anti-HPV 16; and 527.2 (95% CI, 450.9, 616.5) for anti-HPV 18. The GMTs for women who did not breast-feed during vaccine administration were 540.1 (95% CI, 523.5, 557.2) for anti-HPV 6; 746.3 (95% CI, 720.4, 773.3) for anti-HPV 11; 2,290.8 (95% CI, 2,180.7, 2,406.3) for anti-HPV 16; and 456 (95% CI, 438.4, 474.3) for anti-HPV 18.

Overall, 17 and 9 infants of women who received HPV vaccine or placebo (representing 3.4% and 1.8% of the subjects breast-feeding during the period in which they received injections), respectively experienced a serious adverse event. None were judged to be vaccine related. In clinical studies, a higher number of breast-feeding infants (n = 6) whose mothers received HPV vaccine had acute respiratory illnesses within 30 days after vaccination of the mother, compared with infants (n = 2) whose mothers received placebo. In these studies, the rates of other adverse experiences in the mother and the breast-feeding infant were comparable between the groups.

Children: Safety and efficacy of HPV vaccine have not been evaluated in children younger than 9 years of age.

Adverse Reactions: In 5 clinical trials (4 placebo-controlled), subjects were administered HPV vaccine or placebo on the day of enrollment, and approximately 2 and 6 months thereafter. Few subjects (0.1%) discontinued because of adverse experiences. In 4 of the clinical trials, safety was evaluated using vaccination report card (VRC)-aided surveillance for 14 days after each injection of HPV vaccine or placebo (5,088 vaccine; 3,790 placebo).

Common experiences: The vaccine-related adverse experiences observed among female recipients of HPV vaccine at a frequency of 1% or more and also more often than observed among placebo recipients are shown in the following table:

Vaccine-related Injection-site and Systemic Adverse Experiences (%)			
Adverse experience (1 to 5 days after vaccination)	HPV vaccine (N = 5,088)	Aluminum-containing placebo (N = 3,470)	Saline placebo (N = 320)
Injection site			
Pain	83.9	75.4	48.6
Swelling	25.4	15.8	7.3
Erythema	24.6	18.4	12.1
Pruritus	3.1	2.8	0.6
Adverse experience (1 to 15 days after vaccination)	HPV vaccine (N = 5,088)	Placebo (N = 3,790)	
Systemic			
Fever	10.3	8.6	

The injection-site reactions observed among males 9 to 26 years of age at a frequency of at least 1% and also at a greater frequency than that observed among recipients of the aluminum-adjuvant control or saline placebo appear in the following table.

Injection-Site Reactions in Males 9 To 26 Years of Age			
Adverse reaction (1 to 5 days postvaccination)	HPV vaccine (n = 3,092)	Aluminum control[a] (n = 2,029)	Saline placebo (n = 274)
Pain	61.5%	50.8%	41.6%
Erythema	16.7%	14.1%	14.5%
Swelling	13.9%	9.6%	8.2%

a Amorphous aluminum hydroxyphosphate sulfate.

All-cause systemic adverse experiences: All-cause systemic adverse experiences in female subjects observed at a frequency of 1% or greater where the incidence in the vaccine group was greater than or equal to the incidence in the placebo group are shown in the following table:

All-cause Common Systemic Adverse Experiences (%)		
Adverse experiences (1 to 15 days after vaccination)	HPV vaccine (N = 5,088)	Placebo (N = 3,790)
Pyrexia	13	11.2
Nausea	6.7	6.6
Nasopharyngitis	6.4	6.4
Dizziness	4	3.7
Diarrhea	3.6	3.5
Vomiting	2.4	1.9
Myalgia	2	2
Cough	2	1.5
Toothache	1.5	1.4
Upper respiratory tract infection	1.5	1.5
Malaise	1.4	1.2
Arthralgia	1.2	0.9
Insomnia	1.2	0.9
Nasal congestion	1.1	0.9

Adverse events observed among HPV vaccine recipients, at a frequency of at least 1% where incidence in the HPV vaccine group was greater than or equal to the control group, are shown in the following table.

Common Systemic Adverse Reactions in Boys and Men 9 To 26 Years of Age		
Adverse events (1 to 15 days postvaccination)	HPV vaccine (n = 3,092)	Aluminum-adjuvant or saline control group (n = 2,303)
Headache	12.3	11.2
Pyrexia	8.2	6.5
Pharyngolaryngeal pain	2.8	2.1
Diarrhea	2.7	2.2
Nasopharyngitis	2.6	2.6
Nausea	2	1
Upper respiratory tract infection	1.5	1
Abdominal pain upper	1.4	1.4
Myalgia	1.3	0.7
Dizziness	1.2	0.9
Vomiting	1	0.8

Injection-site experiences by dose: An analysis of adverse injection-site experiences in female subjects by dose is shown in the following table. Overall, 94.3% of subjects who received HPV vaccine judged their injection-site adverse experience to be mild or moderate in intensity.

Fever experiences by dose: An analysis of fever in girls and women by dose is shown in the following table:

Evaluation of Fever by Dose						
	Vaccine (% occurrence)			Placebo (% occurrence)		
Temperature (°F)	After dose 1	After dose 2	After dose 3	After dose 1	After dose 2	After dose 3
≥ 100 to < 102	3.7	4.1	4.4	3.1	3.8	3.6
≥ 102	0.3	0.5	0.5	0.3	0.4	0.6

An analysis of fever in boys and men by dose provided similar findings.

Serious adverse experiences: Across the clinical studies, 255 out of 29,323 people reported a serious systemic adverse reaction (HPV vaccine, n = 126 of 15,706, or 0.8%; placebo, n = 129 of 13,617, or 1%). Of the entire study population (29,323 individuals), 0.04% of the reported serious systemic adverse reactions were judged to be vaccine-related by the study investigator. The most frequently reported serious systemic adverse reactions (with at least 4 cases reported among all the groups), regardless of causality, were headache (0.02% HPV vaccine vs 0.02% aluminum control), gastroenteritis (0.02% HPV vaccine vs 0.02% aluminum control), appendicitis (0.03% HPV vaccine vs 0.01% aluminum control), pelvic inflammatory disease (0.02% HPV vaccine vs 0.03% aluminum control), urinary tract infection (0.01% HPV vaccine vs 0.02% aluminum control), pneumonia (0.01% *Gardasil* vs 0.02% aluminum control), pyelonephritis (0.01% HPV vaccine vs 0.02% aluminum control), and pulmonary embolism (0.01% HPV vaccine vs 0.02% aluminum control). One case (0.006% HPV vaccine, 0% aluminum control or saline placebo) of bronchospasm and 2 cases (0.01% HPV vaccine, 0.0% aluminum control or saline placebo) of asthma were reported as serious systemic adverse reactions that occurred following any vaccination visit. In addition, 1 individual in the HPV vaccine group reported 2 injection-site serious adverse reactions (injection-site pain and injection-site joint movement impairment).

Deaths: Across the clinical studies, 37 deaths (HPV vaccine, n= 18, or 0.1%; placebo, n = 19, or 0.1%) were reported in 29,323 (HPV vaccine, n = 15,706; aluminum control, n = 13,023; saline placebo, n = 594) individuals. The events reported were consistent with events expected in healthy adolescent and adult populations. The most common cause of death was motor vehicle accident (5 who received HPV vaccine and 4 who received aluminum control), followed by drug overdose/suicide (2 who received HPV vaccine and 6 who received aluminum control), gunshot wound (1 who received HPV vaccine and 3 who received aluminum control), and pulmonary embolus/deep vein thrombosis (1 who received HPV vaccine and 1 who received aluminum control). In addition, there were 2 cases of sepsis, and 1 case each of pancreatic cancer, arrhythmia, pulmonary tuberculosis, hyperthyroidism, postoperative pulmonary embolism and acute renal failure, traumatic brain injury/cardiac arrest, and systemic lupus erythematosus in the group that received HPV vaccine; 1 case each of asphyxia, acute lymphocytic leukemia, chemical poisoning, and myocardial ischemia in the aluminum control group; and 1 case of medulloblastoma in the saline placebo group.

Systemic autoimmune disorders: In clinical studies, girls and women 9 to 26 years of age were evaluated for new medical conditions that occurred over the course of follow-up. New medical conditions potentially indicative of a systemic autoimmune disorder seen in the group that received HPV vaccine or aluminum control or saline placebo are shown below. This population includes all girls and women who received at least 1 dose of HPV vaccine or aluminum control or saline placebo, and had safety data available.

Females 9 to 26 Years of Age Who Reported an Incident Condition Potentially Indicative of a Systemic Autoimmune Disorder After Enrollment in Clinical Trials, Regardless of Causality		
Conditions	HPV vaccine (n = 10,706) n (%)	Aluminum control or saline placebo (n = 9,412) n (%)
Arthralgia, arthritis, arthropathy[a]	120 (1.1)	98 (1)
Autoimmune thyroiditis	4 (0)	1 (0)
Celiac disease	10 (0.1)	6 (0.1)
Diabetes mellitus, insulin-dependent	2 (0)	2 (0)
Erythema nodosum	2 (0)	4 (0)
Hyperthyroidism[b]	27 (0.3)	21 (0.2)
Hypothyroidism[c]	35 (0.3)	38 (0.4)
Inflammatory bowel disease[d]	7 (0.1)	10 (0.1)
Multiple sclerosis	2 (0)	4 (0)
Nephritis[e]	2 (0)	5 (0.1)
Optic neuritis	2 (0)	0 (0)
Pigmentation disorder[f]	4 (0)	3 (0)
Psoriasis[g]	13 (0.1)	15 (0.2)
Raynaud phenomenon	3 (0)	4 (0)
Rheumatoid arthritis[h]	6 (0.1)	2 (0)
Scleroderma, morphea	2 (0)	1 (0)
Stevens-Johnson syndrome	1 (0)	0 (0)
Systemic lupus erythematosus	1 (0)	3 (0)
Uveitis	3 (0)	1 (0)

Females 9 to 26 Years of Age Who Reported an Incident Condition Potentially Indicative of a Systemic Autoimmune Disorder After Enrollment in Clinical Trials, Regardless of Causality		
Conditions	HPV vaccine (n = 10,706) n (%)	Aluminum control or saline placebo (n = 9,412) n (%)
All conditions	245 (2.3)	218 (2.3)

a Includes arthralgia, arthritis, arthritis reactive, and arthropathy.
b Includes Basedow disease, goiter, toxic nodular goiter, and hyperthyroidism.
c Includes hypothyroidism and thyroiditis.
d Includes colitis ulcerative, Crohn disease, and inflammatory bowel disease.
e Includes nephritis, glomerulonephritis minimal lesion, and glomerulonephritis proliferative.
f Includes pigmentation disorder, skin depigmentation, and vitiligo.
g Includes psoriasis, pustular psoriasis, and psoriatic arthropathy.
h Includes juvenile rheumatoid arthritis. One woman counted in the rheumatoid arthritis group reported rheumatoid arthritis as an adverse experience at day 130.

Similarly, boys and men 9 to 26 years of age were evaluated for new medical conditions that occurred over the course of follow-up. New medical conditions potentially indicative of a systemic autoimmune disorder are presented in the following table.

Males 9 to 26 Years of Age Who Reported an Incident Condition Potentially Indicative of a Systemic Autoimmune Disorder After Enrollment in Clinical Trials, Regardless of Causality		
Conditions	HPV vaccine (n = 3,092) n (%)	Aluminum control or saline placebo (n = 2,303) n (%)
Alopecia areata	1 (0)	0 (0)
Ankylosing spondylitis	1 (0)	2 (0.1)
Arthralgia, arthritis, reactive arthritis	30 (1)	17 (0.7)
Autoimmune thrombocytopenia	1 (0)	0 (0)
Diabetes mellitus type 1	3 (0.1)	2 (0.1)
Hyperthyroidism	0 (0)	1 (0)
Hypothyroidism	3 (0.1)	0 (0)
Inflammatory bowel disease	0 (0)	2 (0.1)
Myocarditis	1 (0)	1 (0)
Proteinuria	1 (0)	0 (0)
Psoriasis	0 (0)	2 (0.1)
Vitiligo	2 (0.1)	5 (0.2)
All conditions	43 (1.4)	32 (1.4)

Post-licensing experience: The following adverse events have been spontaneously reported during post-approval use of *Gardisil*.

Blood and lymphatic: Autoimmune hemolytic anemia, idiopathic thrombocytopenic purpura, lymphadenopathy.

CNS: Acute disseminated encephalomyelitis, dizziness, Guillain-Barré syndrome, headache, motor neuron disease, paralysis, seizures, syncope (sometimes associated with tonic-clonic movements or other seizure-like activity) sometimes resulting in falling with injury, transverse myelitis.

GI: Nausea, pancreatitis, vomiting.

Musculoskeletal: Arthralgia, myalgia.

General disorders: Asthenia, fatigue, malaise, chills, death.

Immune system: Autoimmune diseases, hypersensitivity reactions, including anaphylactic/anaphylactoid reactions, bronchospasm, and urticaria.

Respiratory: Pulmonary embolus.

Vascular disorders: Deep venous thrombosis.

Pharmacologic & Dosing Characteristics

Dosage: Shake well immediately before use to maintain suspension of the vaccine. Three doses of 0.5 mL each, preferably on days 0, 60, and 180. That is, with the second dose given 2 months after the first dose, and the third dose given 4 months after the second dose.

Route & Site: IM, preferably in the deltoid region of the upper arm or the higher anterolateral area of the thigh. Subcutaneous and intradermal administration have not been studied and therefore are not recommended.

Documentation Requirements: Federal law requires that the following information be documented in the recipients's permanent medical record or in a permanent office log: (1) The manufacturer and lot number of this vaccine, (2) the date of administration, and (3) the name, address, and title of the person administering the vaccine.

Certain adverse events must be reported to the VAERS system ([800] 822-7696). Refer to the Immunization Documents in the Resources Section.

Overdosage: Although few data are available, clinical experience with similar products suggests that the major manifestations of overdosage would be pain and tenderness at the injection site.

Missed Doses: Interrupting the recommended schedule or delaying subsequent doses does not require restarting the series.

Related Interventions: Because no vaccine is 100% effective and HPV vaccine does not protect against HPV types not present in the vaccine nor against existing HPV infections, routine Pap screening remains critically important to detect precancerous changes in the cervix and allow treatment before cervical cancer develops. Do not discontinue anal cancer screening if it has been recommended by a health care provider.

Efficacy: Moderate to high-grade cervical intraepithelial neoplasia (CIN 2/3) and adenocarcinoma in situ (AIS) are the immediate and necessary precursors of squamous cell carcinoma and adenocarcinoma of the cervix, respectively. Their detection and removal has been shown to prevent cancer; thus, they serve as surrogate markers for prevention of cervical cancer.

Efficacy was assessed in 4 placebo-controlled, double-blind, randomized phase 2 and 3 clinical studies. The first phase 2 study evaluated the HPV-16 component of HPV vaccine (Protocol 005, N = 2,391), and the second evaluated all 4 components of HPV vaccine (Protocol 007, N = 551). The phase 3 studies, termed FUTURE (Females United to Unilaterally Reduce Endo/Ectocervical Disease), evaluated HPV vaccine in 5,442 (FUTURE I, Protocol 013) and 12,157 (FUTURE II, Protocol 015) volunteers. Together, these 4 studies evaluated 20,541 women 16 to 26 years of age at enrollment. The median duration of follow-up was 4, 3, 2.4, and 2 years for Protocol 005, Protocol 007, FUTURE I, and FUTURE II, respectively. Subjects received vaccine or placebo on the day of enrollment and 2 and 6 months thereafter.

HPV vaccine is designed to prevent HPV 6-, 11-, 16-, or 18-related cervical cancer, cervical dysplasias, vulvar or vaginal dysplasias, or genital warts. HPV vaccine was administered without prescreening for presence of HPV infection, and the efficacy trials allowed enrollment of subjects regardless of baseline HPV status (ie, by PCR or serology). Subjects infected with a particular vaccine HPV type (and who may already have had disease caused by that infection) were not eligible for prophylactic efficacy evaluations for that type.

Primary analyses of efficacy were conducted in the per-protocol efficacy (PPE) population, consisting of women who received all 3 doses within 1 year of enrollment, did not have major deviations from the study protocol, and were naive (PCR negative in cervicovaginal specimens and seronegative) to relevant HPV types before dose 1 and through 1 month after dose 3 (month 7). Efficacy was measured starting after the month 7 visit.

Overall, 73% of subjects were naive to all 4 vaccine HPV types at enrollment; 27% of subjects had evidence of prior exposure to or ongoing infection with at least 1 of the 4 vaccine HPV types. Among these latter subjects, 74% had evidence of prior exposure to or ongoing infection with only 1 of the 4 vaccine HPV types and were naive to the remaining 3 types.

HPV vaccine reduced the incidence of CIN (any grade, including CIN 2/3); AIS; genital warts; VIN (any grade); and VaIN (any grade) related to vaccine HPV types in those who were PCR negative and seronegative at baseline.

Primary Analysis of Efficacy of HPV Vaccine					
	HPV vaccine		Placebo		
Population	n	# of cases	n	# of cases	% Efficacy (95% CI)[a]
HPV 16- or 18-related CIN 2/3 or AIS[b]					
Protocol 005[c]	755	0	750	12	100 (65.1, 100)
Protocol 007	231	0	230	1	100 (−3,734.9, 100)
FUTURE I	2,200	0	2,222	19	100 (78.5, 100)
FUTURE II	5,301	0	5,258	21	100[d] (80.9, 100)
Combined protocols	8,487	0	8,460	53	100[d] (92.9, 100)
HPV 6-, 11-, 16-, 18-related CIN (CIN 1, CIN 2/3) or AIS					
Protocol 007	235	0	233	3	100 (−137.8, 100)
FUTURE I	2,240	0	2,258	37	100[d] (89.5, 100)
FUTURE II	5,383	4	5,370	43	90.7 (74.4, 97.6)
Combined protocols	7,858	4	7,861	83	95.2 (87.2, 98.7)
HPV 6-, 11-, 16-, or 18-related genital warts					
Protocol 007	235	0	233	3	100 (−139.5, 100)
FUTURE I	2,261	0	2,279	29	100 (86.4, 100)
FUTURE II	5,401	1	5,387	59	98.3 (90.2, 100)
Combined protocols	7,897	1	7,899	91	98.9 (93.7, 100)

n = Number of subjects with at least 1 follow-up visit after month 7.

a Note: Point estimates and confidence intervals are adjusted for person-time of follow-up.

b The first listed analysis (ie, HPV 16- or 18-related CIN 2/3, AIS or worse) was the primary end point.

c Evaluated only the HPV-16 L1 VLP vaccine component.

d $P < 0.001$, indicating efficacy against HPV 16/18-related CIN 2/3 is > 0% (FUTURE II); efficacy against HPV 16/18-related CIN 2/3 is > 25% (combined protocols); and efficacy against HPV 6/11/16/18-related CIN is > 20% (FUTURE I).

HPV vaccine was efficacious against HPV disease caused by each of the 4 vaccine HPV types. Efficacy against HPV 16/18-related disease was 100% (95% CI, 87.9% to 100%) for CIN 3 or AIS and 100% (95% CI, 55.5% to 100%) for VIN 2/3 or VaIN 2/3. Efficacy against HPV 6-, 11-, 16-, and 18-related VIN 1 or VaIN 1 was 100% (95% CI, 75.8% to 100%). Women already infected with one or more vaccine-related HPV type before vaccination were protected from clinical disease caused by the remaining vaccine HPV types.

The general population of young American women includes women who are HPV naive and women who are not HPV naive, some of whom have HPV-related disease. The clinical-trials population resembled the general population of American women with respect to prevalence of HPV infection and disease at enrollment. Analyses were conducted to evaluate the overall effect of HPV vaccine with respect to HPV 6-, 11-, 16-, and 18-related cervical and genital disease in the general population. Analyses included events arising from HPV infections present at the start of vaccination as well as events that arose from infections acquired after the start of vaccination.

The effect of HPV vaccine in the general population was measured starting 1 month after dose 1. Prophylactic efficacy denotes the vaccine's efficacy in women who are naive to the relevant HPV types at vaccination onset. General population impact denotes vaccine effect among women regardless of baseline PCR status and serostatus. Most cases of CIN, genital warts, VIN, and VaIN detected in the group that received HPV vaccine occurred as a consequence of HPV infection with the relevant HPV type already present at day 1.

General Population Impact for Vaccine HPV Types[a]						
		Gardasil or HPV 16 L1 VLP vaccine		Placebo		% Reduction
End points	Analysis	N	Cases	N	Cases	(95% CI)
HPV 16- or 18-related CIN 2/3 or AIS	Prophylactic efficacy[b]	9,342	1	9,400	81	98.8 (92.9, 100)
	HPV 16 and/or 18 positive at day 1	—	121	—	120	—
	General population impact[c]	9,831	122	9,896	201	39 (23.3, 51.7)
HPV 16- or 18-related VIN 2/3 and VaIN 2/3	Prophylactic efficacy[b]	8,641	0	8,667	24	100 (83.3, 100)
	HPV 16 and/or 18 positive at day 1	—	8	—	2	—
	General population impact[c]	8,954	8	8,962	26	69.1 (29.8, 87.9)
HPV 6-, 11-, 16-, 18-related CIN (CIN 1, CIN 2/3) or AIS	Prophylactic efficacy[b]	8,625	9	8,673	143	93.7 (87.7, 97.2)
	HPV 6, 11, 16, and/or 18 positive at day 1	—	161[d]	—	174[d]	—
	General population impact[c]	8,814	170	8,846	317	46.4 (35.2, 55.7)
HPV 6-, 11-, 16-, or 18-related genital warts	Prophylactic efficacy[b]	8,760	9	8,786	136	93.4 (87, 97)
	HPV 6, 11, 16, and/or 18 positive at day 1	—	49	—	48[e]	—
	General population impact[c]	8,954	58	8,962	184	68.5 (57.5, 77)

a Note: The HPV 16- and 18-related CIN 2/3 or AIS composite end point included data from studies 005, 007, 013, and 015. All other end points only included data from studies 007, 013, and 015. Positive status at day 1 denotes PCR-positive or sero-positive for the respective type at day 1. Percent reduction includes the prophylactic efficacy of HPV vaccine as well as the effect of HPV vaccine on the course of infections present at the start of the vaccination. This table does not include disease due to nonvaccine HPV types.
b Includes all subjects who received at least 1 vaccination and who were naive to HPV 6, 11, 16, and/or 18 at day 1. Case counting started at 1 month after dose 1.
c Includes all subjects who received at least 1 vaccination (regardless of baseline HPV status at day 1). Case counting started at 1 month after dose 1.
d Includes 2 subjects (1 in each group) who underwent colposcopy for reasons other than an abnormal Pap and 1 placebo subject with missing serology/PCR data at day 1.
e Includes 1 subject with missing serology/PCR data at day 1.

HPV vaccine does not prevent infection with the HPV types not contained in the vaccine. Cases of disease caused by nonvaccine types were observed among recipients of HPV vaccine and placebo in phase 2 and phase 3 efficacy studies.

Among cases of CIN 2/3 or AIS caused by vaccine or nonvaccine HPV types in subjects in the general population who received HPV vaccine, 79% occurred in subjects who had an abnormal Pap test at day 1 or who were positive (PCR positive or seropositive) for HPV 6, 11, 16, and/or 18 at day 1.

An interim analysis of the general population impact for HPV vaccine was performed from studies 007, 013, and 015 that had a median duration of follow-up of 1.9 years. HPV vaccine reduced the overall rate of CIN 2/3 or AIS caused by vaccine or nonvaccine HPV types by 12.2% (95% CI, −3.2% to 25.3%) compared with placebo.

An analysis of overall population impact for the HPV 16 L1 VLP vaccine was conducted from study 005 that had a median duration of follow-up of 3.9 years. The HPV 16 L1 VLP vaccine reduced the overall incidence of CIN 2/3 caused by vaccine or nonvaccine HPV types by 32.7% (95% CI, −34.7% to 67.3%) through a median duration of follow-up of 1.9 years (fixed case analysis) and by 45.3% (95% CI, 10.9% to 67.1%) through a median duration of follow-up of 3.9 years (end of study).

HPV vaccine reduced the incidence of definitive therapy (eg, cold knife conization, laser conization, loop electrosurgical excision procedure) by 16.5% (95% CI, 2.9% to 28.2%) and surgery to excise external genital lesions by 26.5% (95% CI, 3.6% to 44.2%) compared with placebo for all HPV-related diseases. These analyses were performed in the general population of women, including women regardless of baseline HPV PCR status or serostatus. HPV vaccine has not been shown to protect against the diseases caused by all HPV types and will not treat existing disease caused by the HPV types contained in the vaccine. The overall efficacy of HPV vaccine, described above, will depend on the baseline prevalence of HPV infection related to vaccine HPV types in the population vaccinated and the incidence of HPV infection due to types not included in the vaccine.

Efficacy in males: The primary analyses of efficacy were conducted in the per-protocol efficacy (PPE) population, boys and men who received all 3 vaccinations within 1 year of enrollment, did not have major deviations from the study protocol, and were naive (PCR negative and seronegative) to HPV types 6, 11, 16, and 18 before dose 1 and through 1 month after dose 3 (month 7). Efficacy was measured starting after the month 7 visit. HPV vaccine was efficacious in reducing the incidence of genital warts related to HPV types 6 and 11 in those boys and men who were PCR negative and seronegative at baseline. Efficacy against penile, perineal, and perianal intraepithelial neoplasia (PIN) grades 1/2/3, or penile, perineal, and perianal cancer was not demonstrated, because the number of cases was too limited to reach statistical significance.

Efficacy in the PPE Population of Boys and Men 16 to 26 Years of Age for Vaccine HPV Types					
	HPV vaccine		Aluminum control		% efficacy
End point	N	Number of cases	N	Number of cases	(95% CI)
External genital lesions HPV 6-, 11-, 16-, or 18-related					
External genital lesions	1,397	3	1,408	31	90.4 (69.2, 98.1)
Condyloma	1,397	3	1,408	28	89.4 (65.5, 97.9)
PIN 1/2/3	1,397	0	1,408	3	100 (−141.2, 100)

The impact of HPV vaccine in a population of boys and men who have not been screened for current or prior exposure to a vaccine HPV type is shown in the following table. Prophylactic efficacy denotes the vaccine's efficacy in boys and men who are naive to the relevant HPV types at day 1. Vaccine impact in boys and men who were positive for vaccine-type HPV infection, as well as vaccine impact among boys and men regardless of baseline vaccine HPV status, are also presented. Most genital disease related to a vaccine HPV type in the vaccinated group involved an HPV infection already present at day 1. There was no clear evidence that vaccination protected from disease caused by infections already underway before vaccination.

Effectiveness in Preventing HPV Types 6-, 11-, 16-, or 18-Related Genital Disease in Boys and Men 16 To 26 Years of Age, Regardless of Current or Prior Exposure to Vaccine HPV Types		HPV vaccine		Aluminum control		% reduction
End point	Analysis	N	Cases	N	Cases	(95% CI)
External genital lesions	Prophylactic efficacy	1,775	13	1,770	52	75.5 (54.3, 87.7)
	HPV 6-, 11-, 16-, and/or 18-positive at day 1	168	14	167	25	—[a]
	Boys and men regardless of current or prior exposure to vaccine or nonvaccine HPV types	1,943	27	1,937	77	65.5 (45.8, 78.6)[b]
Condyloma	Prophylactic efficacy	1,775	10	1,770	48	79.6 (59.1, 90.8)
	HPV 6-, 11-, 16-, and/or 18-positive at day 1	168	14	167	24	—[a]
	Boys and men regardless of current or prior exposure to vaccine or nonvaccine HPV types	1,943	24	1,937	72	67.2 (47.3, 80.3)[b]
PIN 1/2/3	Prophylactic efficacy	1,775	4	1,770	4	1.2 (−431, 81.6)
	HPV 6-, 11-, 16-, and/or 18-positive at day 1	168	2	167	1	—[a]
	Boys and men regardless of current or prior exposure to vaccine or nonvaccine HPV types	1,943	6	1,937	5	−19.2 (−394, 69.7)[b]

a There is no expected efficacy since HPV vaccine has not been demonstrated to provide protection against disease from vaccine HPV types to which a person has previously been exposed through sexual activity.
b Percent reduction for these analyses includes the prophylactic efficacy of HPV vaccine as well as the impact of HPV vaccine on the course of infections present at the start of vaccination.

The impact of HPV vaccine against the overall burden of HPV-related genital disease (ie, disease caused by any HPV type) results from a combination of prophylactic efficacy against vaccine HPV types, disease contribution from vaccine HPV types present at time of vaccination, and the disease contribution from HPV types not contained in the vaccine. Additional efficacy analyses were conducted in 2 populations: (1) a generally HPV-naive population that consisted of boys and men who are seronegative and PCR negative to HPV 6, 11, 16, and 18 and PCR negative to HPV 31, 33, 35, 39, 45, 51, 52, 56, 58, and 59 at day 1, approximating a population of sexually naive boys and men, and (2) the general study population of boys and men regardless of baseline HPV status, some of whom had HPV-related disease at day 1. Among generally HPV naive boys and men and among all boys and men (including boys and men with HPV infection at day 1), HPV vaccine reduced the overall incidence of genital disease. These reductions were primarily due to reductions in lesions caused by HPV types 6, 11, 16, and 18 in boys and men naive (seronegative and PCR negative) for the specific relevant vaccine HPV type. Infected boys and men may already have genital disease at day 1 and some will develop genital disease during follow-up, either related to a vaccine or nonvaccine HPV type present at the time of vaccination or related to a nonvaccine HPV type not present at the time of vaccination.

		HPV vaccine		Aluminum control		% reduction
End point	Analysis	N	Cases	N	Cases	(95% CI)
External genital lesions	Generally HPV naive	1,275	6	1,270	36	83.8 (61.2, 94.4)
	Boys and men regardless of current or prior exposure to vaccine or nonvaccine HPV types	1,943	36	1,937	89	60.2 (40.8, 73.8)[a]
Condyloma	Generally HPV naive	1,275	5	1,270	33	85.3 (62.1, 95.5)
	Boys and men regardless of current or prior exposure to vaccine or nonvaccine HPV types	1,943	32	1,937	83	62.1 (42.4, 75.6)[a]
PIN 1/2/3	Generally HPV naive	1,275	1	1,270	3	67.4 (−307, 99.4)
	Boys and men regardless of current or prior exposure to vaccine or nonvaccine HPV types	1,943	7	1,937	6	−15.9 (−318, 66.6)[a]

Table title (spanning header): **Effectiveness in Preventing Any HPV Type-Related Genital Disease in Boys and Men 16 To 26 Years of Age, Regardless of Current or Prior Infection With Vaccine or Nonvaccine HPV Types**

a Percent reduction includes prophylactic efficacy of HPV vaccine as well as the impact of HPV vaccine on course of infections present at start of vaccination.

Onset: Protection against infection begins within 1 month after the third dose.

Duration: The duration of protection via immunization against HPV is not yet known.

Protective Level: Not established.

Mechanism: HPV only infects humans, but animal studies with animal papillomaviruses suggest that the efficacy of L1 VLP vaccines is mediated by antibody-based immune responses.

Because there were few disease cases in subjects naive (ie, PCR negative and seronegative) to vaccine HPV types at baseline in the group that received HPV vaccine, it has not been possible to establish minimum anti-HPV 6, 11, 16, and 18 antibody levels that protect against clinical disease caused by HPV 6, 11, 16, and/or 18.

Immunogenicity was assessed in 8,915 women (HPV vaccine N = 4,666; placebo N = 4,249) 18 to 26 years of age and female adolescents 9 to 17 years of age (HPV vaccine N = 1,471; placebo N = 583). Type-specific competitive immunoassays with type-specific standards were used to assess immunogenicity to each vaccine HPV type. These assays measured antibodies against neutralizing epitopes for each HPV type. The scales for these assays are unique to each HPV type; thus, comparisons across types and to other assays are not appropriate.

The primary immunogenicity analyses were conducted in a per-protocol immunogenicity (PPI) population. This population consisted of individuals who were seronegative and PCR negative to the relevant HPV type(s) at enrollment, remained HPV PCR negative to the relevant HPV type(s) through 1 month after dose 3 (month 7), received all 3 vaccinations, and did not deviate from the study protocol in ways that could interfere with the effects of the vaccine.

Overall, 99.8%, 99.8%, 99.8%, and 99.5% of girls and women who received HPV vaccine became anti-HPV 6, 11, 16, and 18 seropositive, respectively, by 1 month after dose 3 across all age groups tested. Anti-HPV 6, 11, 16, and 18 GMTs peaked at month 7. GMTs declined through month 24 and then stabilized through month 36 at levels above baseline. The duration of immunity following a complete schedule of immunization with HPV vaccine has not been established.

Anti-HPV cLIA Geometric Mean Titers in the PPI Population (Protocol 007)				
		HPV vaccine $N^a = 276$		Aluminum-containing placebo $N = 275$
		Geometric mean titer (95% CI)		Geometric mean titer (95% CI)
Study time	n^b	mMU/mL^c	n	mMU/mL
Anti-HPV 6				
Month 7	208	582.2 (527.2, 642.8)	198	4.6 (4.3, 4.8)
Month 24	192	93.7 (82.2, 106.9)	188	4.6 (4.3, 5)
Month 36	183	93.8 (81, 108.6)	184	5.1 (4.7, 5.6)
Anti-HPV 11				
Month 7	208	696.5 (617.8, 785.2)	198	4.1 (4, 4.2)
Month 24	190	97.1 (84.2, 112)	188	4.2 (4, 4.3)
Month 36	174	91.7 (78.3, 107.3)	180	4.4 (4.1, 4.7)
Anti-HPV 16				
Month 7	193	3,889 (3,318.7, 4,557.4)	185	6.5 (6.2, 6.9)
Month 24	174	393 (335.7, 460.1)	175	6.8 (6.3, 7.4)
Month 36	176	507.3 (434.6, 592)	170	7.7 (6.8, 8.8)
Anti-HPV 18				
Month 7	219	801.2 (693.8, 925.4)	209	4.6 (4.3, 5)
Month 24	204	59.9 (49.7, 72.2)	199	4.6 (4.3, 5)
Month 36	196	59.7 (48.5, 73.5)	193	4.8 (4.4, 5.2)

a Number of subjects randomized to the respective group who received at least 1 injection.
b Number of subjects in the per-protocol analysis with data at the specified study time point.
c mMU = milli-Merck units.

The following table shows anti-HPV GMTs 1 month after dose 3 among subjects who received dose 2 between month 1 and month 3, compared with subjects who received dose 3 between month 4 and month 8.

GMTs for Variation of Dosing Regimen								
Variation of dosing regimen		Anti-HPV 6		Anti-HPV 11		Anti-HPV 16		Anti-HPV 18
	N	GMT^a (95% CI)	N	GMT^a (95% CI)	N	GMT^a (95% CI)	N	GMT (95% CI)
Dose 2								
Early^b	883	570.9 (542.2, 601.2)	888	824.6 (776.7, 875.5)	854	2,625.3 (2,415.1, 2,853.9)	926	517.7 (482.9, 555)
On time^b	1,767	552.3 (532.3, 573.1)	1,785	739.7 (709.3, 771.5)	1,737	2,400 (2,263.9, 2,544.3)	1,894	473.9 (451.8, 497.1)
Late^b	313	447.4 (405.3, 493.8)	312	613.9 (550.8, 684.2)	285	1,889.7 (1,624.4, 2,198.5)	334	388.5 (348.3, 433.3)
Dose 3								
Early^c	495	493.1 (460.8, 527.8)	501	658.9 (609.5, 712.2)	487	2,176.6 (1,953.4, 2,425.3)	521	423.4 (388.8, 461.2)
On time^c	2,081	549.6 (531.1, 568.8)	2,093	752.8 (723.8, 782.9)	2,015	2,415 (2,286.3, 2,550.9)	2,214	486 (464.7, 508.2)

Human Papillomavirus Vaccine, Types 6, 11, 16, 18

GMTs for Variation of Dosing Regimen							
Variation of	Anti-HPV 6		Anti-HPV 11		Anti-HPV 16		Anti-HPV 18
dosing		GMT[a]		GMT[a]		GMT[a]		GMT
regimen	N	(95% CI)	N	(95% CI)	N	(95% CI)	N	(95% CI)
Dose 3 (*cont.*)								
Late[c]	335	589 (537, 645.9)	339	865.3 (782.6, 956.7)	326	2,765.9 (2,408.7, 3,176.2)	361	498.5 (446.2, 557)

a GMT in mMU (milli-Merck units).
b Early = 36 to 50 days after dose 1; On time = 51 to 70 days after dose 1; Late = 71 to 84 days after dose 1.
c Early = 80 to 105 days after dose 2; On time = 106 to 137 days after dose 2; Late = 138 to 160 days after dose 2.

To bridge the efficacy data on HPV vaccine among young adult women to adolescent girls, a clinical study compared anti-HPV 6, 11, 16, and 18 GMTs in girls 10 to 15 years of age with responses in adolescent and young adult women 16 to 23 years of age. Among subjects who received HPV vaccine, 99.1% to 100% became anti-HPV 6, 11, 16, and 18 seropositive by 1 month after dose 3.

The following table compares the 1 month anti-HPV 6, 11, 16, and 18 GMTs after dose 3 in girls 9 to 15 years of age with those in adolescent and young adult women 16 to 26 years of age.

Immunogenicity Bridging Between Female Adolescents 9 to 15 Years of Age and Adult Women 16 to 26 Years of Age						
	Female adolescents 9 to 15 years of age (Protocols 016 and 018) N = 1,121			Adult women 16 to 26 years of age (Protocols 013 and 015) N = 4,229		
Assay (cLIA)	n	GMT[a]	(95% CI)	n	GMT[a]	(95% CI)
Anti-HPV 6	927	931.3	(876.9, 989.2)	2,827	542.4	(526.6, 558.7)
Anti-HPV 11	927	1,305.7	(1,226.2, 1,390.4)	2,827	766.1	(740.5, 792.6)
Anti-HPV 16	929	4,944.9	(4,583.5, 5,334.8)	2,707	2,313.8	(2,206.2, 2,426.7)
Anti-HPV 18	932	1,046	(9,71.2, 1,126.5)	3,040	460.7	(443.8, 478.3)

a mMU = milli-Merck units.

Anti-HPV responses 1 month after dose 3 among girls 9 to 15 years of age were non-inferior to anti-HPV responses in adolescent and young adult women 16 to 26 years of age in the combined database of immunogenicity studies for HPV vaccine. On the basis of this immunogenicity bridging, the efficacy of HPV vaccine in girls 9 to 15 years of age is inferred.

Drug Interactions: Like all inactivated vaccines, administration of HPV vaccine to people receiving immunosuppressant drugs (eg, high-dose corticosteroids) or radiation therapy may result in an insufficient response to immunization. They may remain susceptible despite immunization.

The safety and immunogenicity of HPV vaccine administered concomitantly with hepatitis B vaccine (recombinant) was evaluated in a placebo-controlled study of 1,871 women 16 to 24 years of age at enrollment. There were no statistically significant higher rates in systemic or injection-site adverse experiences among subjects who received concomitant vaccination compared with those who received HPV vaccine or hepatitis B vaccine alone. Immune response to both HPV vaccine and hepatitis B vaccine was non-inferior whether they were administered at the same visit or at a different visit.

The safety and immunogenicity of HPV vaccine administered concomitantly with MCV4 and Tdap was evaluated in a randomized study of 1,040 boys and girls (mean age, 12.6 y). The rate of injection-site swelling at the HPV vaccine injection site increased when HPV vaccine was administered concomitantly with MCV4 and Tdap compared with nonconcomitant vaccination. Most of these swelling experiences were reported as mild to moderate in intensity. Coadministration did not interfere with the antibody response to any of the vaccine antigens in this study.

Coadministration of HPV vaccine with other vaccines has not been specifically studied.

Inactivated vaccines are not generally affected by circulating antibodies or administration of exogenous antibodies. Vaccination may occur at any time before or after antibody adminis-tration.

As with other drugs given by IM injection, give HPV vaccine with caution to people receiv-ing anticoagulant therapy. Do not give HPV vaccine to people with bleeding disorders such as hemophilia or thrombocytopenia, unless the potential benefits clearly outweigh the risk of administration. If HPV vaccine is given to such persons, take steps to avoid the risk of hema-toma after injection.

Hormonal contraceptives: In clinical studies, 13,293 subjects (vaccine = 6,644; placebo = 6,649) who had post-month 7 follow-up used hormonal contraceptives for a total of 17,597 person-years (65.1% of the follow-up time for these subjects). Use of hor-monal contraceptives or lack of use of hormonal contraceptives among study participants did not alter vaccine efficacy in the PPE population.

Patient Information: Vaccination does not substitute for routine cervical-cancer screening. Women who receive HPV vaccine should continue to undergo cervical cancer screening per standard of care. Completing the immunization series unless contraindicated is important to protection.

Pharmaceutical Characteristics

Concentration: Each 0.5 mL dose contains approximately 20 mcg of HPV-6 L1 protein, 40 mcg of HPV-11 L1 protein, 40 mcg of HPV-16 L1 protein, and 20 mcg of HPV-18 L1 pro-tein.

Packaging: One 0.5 mL single-dose vial (NDC #: 00006-4045-00); carton of ten 0.5 mL single-dose vials (00006-4045-41). Carton of six 0.5 mL single-dose *Luer Lock* syringes, prefitted with *UltraSafe Passive* delivery system, plus six 1-inch, 25-gauge needles (00006-4109-06). Carton of six 0.5 mL single-dose prefilled *Luer Lock* syringes without needles (00006-4109-09).

If a different needle is chosen, it should fit securely on the syringe and be no longer than 1 inch to ensure proper functioning of the needle-guard device. Two detachable labels are pro-vided that can be removed after the needle is guarded.

Doseform: Suspension

Appearance: After agitation, a white, cloudy liquid

Solvent: Buffered water for injection

Adjuvant: 225 mcg aluminum (as amorphous aluminum hydroxyphosphate sulfate) per 0.5 mL dose

Preservative: None

Allergens: None

Excipients: Each 0.5 mL dose contains sodium chloride 9.56 mg, L-histidine 0.78 mg, polysorbate-80 50 mcg, sodium borate 35 mcg, and water for injection.

pH: Data not provided

Shelf Life: Expires within 36 months.

Storage/Stability: Store at 2° to 8°C (36° to 46°F). Protect product from light. Do not freeze. Contact the manufacturer regarding exposure to freezing or elevated temperatures. Product can tolerate temperatures at or below 25°C (77°F) for a total time of not more than 72 hours. Shipping data not provided.

Human Papillomavirus Vaccine, Types 6, 11, 16, 18

Handling: Depress both anti-rotation tabs to secure syringe and attach Luer needle by twisting in clockwise direction. Remove needle sheath. Administer IM injection as usual. Depress plunger while grasping the finger flange until the entire dose has been given. The needle-guard device will not activate to cover and protect the needle unless the entire dose has been given. Remove needle from the vaccine recipient. Release plunger and allow syringe to move up until the entire needle is guarded. To document immunization, remove detachable labels by pulling slowly on them. Dispose of syringe unit in approved sharps container.

Production Process: L1 proteins are produced by 4 separate fermentations in recombinant *Saccharomyces cerevisiae*. The proteins form pentamers and then 72 pentamers self-assemble into VLPs. The fermentation process involves growth of *S. cerevisiae* on chemically defined fermentation media that include vitamins, amino acids, mineral salts, and carbohydrates. The VLPs are released from the yeast cells by cell disruption and purified by a series of chemical and physical methods. The purified VLPs are adsorbed on preformed aluminum-containing adjuvant (amorphous aluminum hydroxyphosphate sulfate). The quadrivalent HPV VLP vaccine is a sterile liquid suspension prepared by combining the adsorbed VLPs of each HPV type with additional amounts of the aluminum-containing adjuvant and the final purification buffer.

Media: *S. cerevisiae* in a defined fermentation medium that includes vitamins, amino acids, mineral salts, and carbohydrates.

Disease Epidemiology

Incidence: More than 100 different human papillomavirus (HPV) types have been identified. As with rabbit papillomaviruses, some human HPV types can cause cancer, most notably cervical cancer.

HPV is the most common sexually transmitted infection in the United States. The CDC estimates that approximately 6.2 million Americans become infected with genital HPV each year and that over half of all sexually active men and women become infected at some time in their lives.

HPV causes squamous cell cervical cancer (and its histologic precursor lesions cervical intraepithelial neoplasia [CIN] 1 or low-grade dysplasia and CIN 2/3 or moderate to high-grade dysplasia) and cervical adenocarcinoma (and its precursor lesion adenocarcinoma in situ [AIS]). HPV also causes approximately 35% to 50% of vulvar and vaginal cancers. Vulvar intraepithelial neoplasia (VIN) grade 2/3 and vaginal intraepithelial neoplasia (VaIN) grade 2/3 are immediate precursors to these cancers.

Cervical cancer prevention focuses on routine screening (eg, Pap tests) and early intervention. This strategy has reduced cervical cancer rates by approximately 75% in compliant individuals by monitoring and removing premalignant dysplastic lesions. HPV also causes genital warts (condyloma acuminata) that are growths of the cervicovaginal, vulvar, and the external genitalia that rarely progress to cancer. HPV 6, 11, 16, and 18 are common HPV types.

HPV 16 and 18 cause 70% of cervical cancer, AIS, CIN 3, VIN 2/3, and VaIN 2/3 cases; and 50% of CIN 2 cases.

HPV 6, 11, 16, and 18 cause approximately 35% to 50% of all CIN 1, VIN 1, and VaIN 1 cases; and 90% of genital wart cases.

In the United States each year, HPV infections result in 500,000 to 1 million cases of genital warts caused by HPV, 10 million HPV infections without cytologic abnormality, 1 million cases of low-grade dysplasia, 300,000 cases of high-grade dysplasia, 12,200 cases of cervical cancer, and 4,100 deaths due to cervical cancer. The death rate may be higher among black women than white women.

Other Information

Perspective:

1932: Richard E. Shope identifies papillomaviruses, by showing that skin warts (ie, papillomas) could be transmitted between rabbits via a filterable infectious agent. Peyton Rous went on to show that the Shope papillomavirus could cause skin cancer in infected rabbits, the first demonstration that a virus could cause cancer in mammals.

1943: Georgios Papanikolaou, considered the father of cytopathology, describes a large series of cases of uterine cancer diagnosed by vaginal smear. "Pap" is an abbreviation for Papanikolaou.

1970s: zur Hausen identifies relationship between cervical cancer and human papillomavirus.

1991: Zhou and Frazer discover novel way to produce L1 protein of HPV, so that the protein spontaneously folds and forms pentamers and then virus-like particles (VLPs).

First Licensed: June 8, 2006

National Policy: ACIP. Recommendations on the use of quadrivalent human papillomavirus vaccine in males—Advisory Committee on Immunization Practices (ACIP), 2011. *MMWR.* 2011;60(50):1705-1708. http://www.cdc.gov/mmwr/pdf/wk/mm6050.pdf.

ACIP. Quadrivalent human papillomavirus vaccine. *MMWR.* 2007;56(RR-2):1-24. http://www.cdc.gov/mmwr/PDF/rr/rr5602.pdf.

References: Block SL, Nolan T, Sattler C, et al. Comparison of the immunogenicity and reactogenicity of a prophylactic quadrivalent human papillomavirus (types 6, 11, 16, and 18) L1 virus-like particle vaccine in male and female adolescents and young adult women. *Pediatrics.* 2006;118(5):2135-2145.

Garnett GP. Role of herd immunity in determining the effect of vaccines against sexually transmitted disease. *J Infect Dis.* 2005;191(Suppl 1):S97-S106.

Shi L, Sings HL, Bryan JT, et al. *Gardasil:* Prophylactic human papillomavirus vaccine development-From bench top to bedside. *Clin Pharm Ther.* 2007;81(2):259-264.

Taira AV, Neukermans CP, Sanders GD. Evaluating human papillomavirus vaccination programs. *Emerg Infect Dis.* 2004;10:1915-1923.

Villa LL, Costa RL, Petta CA, et al. Prophylactic quadrivalent human papillomavirus (types 6, 11, 16, and 18) L1 virus-like particle vaccine in young women: a randomised double-blind placebo-controlled multicentre phase II efficacy trial. *Lancet Oncol.* 2005;6:271-278.

WHO. WHO consultation on human papillomavirus vaccines. *Wkly Epidemiol Rec.* 2005;80:299-302. http://www.who.int/wer/2005/wer8035.pdf

Human Papillomavirus Vaccine, Types 6, 11, 16, 18

Human Papillomavirus Vaccine Summary Table		
Generic name	Human papillomavirus vaccine quadrivalent (types 6, 11, 16, 18)	Human papillomavirus vaccine bivalent (types 16 and 18)
Brand name	*Gardasil*	*Cervarix*
Synonym	HPV4	HPV2
Manufacturer	Merck	GlaxoSmithKline
Viability	Viral subunit vaccine	Viral subunit vaccine
Indication	To prevent cervical, vulvar, vaginal, and anal cancer and genital warts in girls and women 9 to 26 years of age To prevent anal cancer and genital warts in boys and men 9 to 26 years of age	To prevent cervical cancer in girls and women 9 to 26 years of age
Components	Types 6, 11, 16, and 18	Types 16 and 18
Concentration	HPV-6 L1 protein 20 mcg, HPV-11 L1 protein 40 mcg, HPV-16 L1 protein 40 mcg, and HPV-18 L1 protein 20 mcg each per 0.5 mL	HPV-16 L1 protein 20 mcg and HPV-18 L1 protein 20 mcg each per 0.5 mL
Adjuvant	225 mcg aluminum, as aluminum hydroxyphosphate sulfate per 0.5 mL	AS04 adjuvant system, containing aluminum hydroxide 500 mcg and 3-O-desacyl-4'-monophosphoryl lipid A 50 mcg per 0.5 mL
Preservative	None	None
Production medium	*Saccharomyces cerevisiae*	L1-encoding recombinant baculoviruses that replicate in *Trichoplusia ni* insect cells
Dosage, route	0.5 mL IM	0.5 mL IM
Standard schedule	0, 2, and 6 months	0, 1, and 6 months
Doseform	Suspension	Suspension
Packaging	0.5 mL vial, 0.5 mL syringe	0.5 mL vial, 0.5 mL syringe
Routine storage	2° to 8°C	2° to 8°C
CPT code	90649	90650

Name:
  Cervarix
Synonyms: HPV2

Manufacturer:
  GlaxoSmithKline

Immunologic Characteristics

Microorganism: Virus (double-stranded DNA, nonenveloped), human papillomavirus (HPV), genus *Papillomavirus*, family Papillomaviridae

Viability: Inactivated

Antigenic Form: Noninfectious, recombinant viruslike particles (VLPs) of the major capsid (L1) protein of HPV types 16 and 18

Antigenic Type: Protein

Strains: HPV types 16 and 18

Use Characteristics

Indications: To prevent the following diseases caused by oncogenic HPV types 16 and 18 in girls and women 10 to 25 years of age:

- Cervical cancer
- Cervical intraepithelial neoplasia (CIN) grade 2 or higher and adenocarcinoma in situ (AIS)
- CIN grade 1

Limitations: There is no clear evidence of protection from disease caused by HPV types for which patients were polymerase chain reaction (PCR) positive and/or seropositive at baseline.

This vaccine is not intended as treatment of cervical cancer or CIN.

This vaccine will not protect against diseases that are caused by the HPV types not present in the vaccine.

Contraindications: Severe allergic reactions (eg, anaphylaxis) to any component of this vaccine.

Immunodeficiency: The immune response to HPV vaccine may be diminished in immunocompromised people.

Elderly: Clinical studies of HPV vaccine did not include sufficient numbers of patients 65 years of age and older to determine whether they respond differently from younger patients.

Carcinogenicity: HPV vaccine has not been evaluated for carcinogenic potential.

Mutagenicity: HPV vaccine has not been evaluated for mutagenic potential.

Fertility Impairment: HPV vaccine has not been evaluated for impairment of fertility in humans. Vaccination of female rats with HPV vaccine at doses shown to be significantly immunogenic in rats had no effect on human fertility.

Pregnancy: Category B. There are no adequate and well-controlled studies in pregnant women. Because animal reproduction studies are not always predictive of human response, use this drug during pregnancy only if clearly needed. Patients and health care providers are encouraged to register pregnant women who inadvertently receive HPV vaccine in the GlaxoSmithKline *Cervarix* pregnancy registry by calling 1-888-452-9622.

Reproduction studies in rats at a dose approximately 47 times the human dose revealed no evidence of harm to the fetus caused by HPV vaccine. One group of rats was administered HPV vaccine 30 days before gestation and during organogenesis (gestation days 6, 8, 11, and 15). A second group of rats was administered saline 30 days before gestation followed by HPV vaccine on days 6, 8, 11, and 15 of gestation. Two additional groups of rats received saline or adjuvant following the same dosing regimen. HPV vaccine was administered at 0.1 mL/rat/occasion (approximately 47-fold excess relative to the projected human dose on a mg/kg basis) by intramuscular (IM) injection. No adverse effects on mating, fertility, pregnancy, parturition, lactation, embryo-fetal, or pre- or postnatal development were observed. There were no vaccine-related fetal malformations or other evidence of teratogenesis.

In clinical studies, pregnancy testing was performed before each vaccination; vaccination was discontinued if a patient had a positive pregnancy test. In all trials, volunteers were instructed to avoid pregnancy until 2 months after the last vaccination. During prelicensure clinical development, 7,276 pregnancies were reported among 3,696 women receiving HPV vaccine and 3,580 women receiving a control (hepatitis A vaccine 360 extended length of utterance [ELU], hepatitis A vaccine 720 ELU, or aluminum hydroxide 500 mcg). The overall proportions of pregnancy outcomes were similar between treatment groups. Most women gave birth to healthy infants (62% and 63% of recipients of HPV vaccine and control, respectively). Other outcomes included spontaneous abortion (11% and 11%), elective termination (6% and 6%), abnormal infant other than congenital anomaly (2.8% and 3.2%), and premature birth (2% and 1.7%). Other outcomes (eg, congenital anomaly, stillbirth, ectopic pregnancy, therapeutic abortion) were reported in 0.1% to 0.8% of pregnancies in both groups. Subanalyses were conducted to describe pregnancy outcomes in 761 women (n = 396 for HPV vaccine and n = 365 for control groups) who had their last menstrual period within 30 days before or 45 days after a vaccine dose and for whom pregnancy outcome was known. Most women gave birth to healthy infants (65% and 69%). Spontaneous abortion was reported in 12% (13.6% for HPV vaccine and 9.6% for control) and elective termination in 9.7% (9.9% and 9.6%). Abnormal infant other than congenital anomaly was reported in 4.9% (5.1% and 4.7%) and premature birth was reported in 2.5% (2.5% of each group). Other outcomes (eg, congenital anomaly, stillbirth, ectopic pregnancy, therapeutic abortion) were reported in 0.3% to 1.8% of pregnancies among recipients of HPV vaccine and in 0.3% to 1.4% of pregnancies among control recipients.

It is not known whether the observed numerical imbalance in spontaneous abortions in pregnancies that occurred around the time of vaccination is due to a vaccine-related effect.

Lactation: It is not known if HPV vaccine antigens or corresponding antibodies cross into human breast milk. In nonclinical studies in rats, serological data suggest a transfer of anti–HPV-16 and anti–HPV-18 antibodies via milk during lactation in rats. Excretion of vaccine-induced antibodies in human milk has not been studied for HPV vaccine. Because many drugs are excreted in human milk, use caution when HPV vaccine is administered to a breast-feeding woman.

Children: Safety and effectiveness in children younger than 10 years of age have not been established. The safety and effectiveness of HPV vaccine were evaluated in 1,193 patients 10 to 14 years of age and 6,316 patients 15 to 17 years of age.

Adverse Reactions: The most common injection-site adverse reactions (at least 20% of patients) were pain, redness, and swelling. The most common general adverse events (at least 20% of patients) were fatigue, headache, myalgia, GI symptoms, and arthralgia.

Safety was evaluated by pooling data from controlled and uncontrolled clinical trials involving 23,713 girls and women 10 to 25 years of age. In these studies, 12,785 girls and women received at least 1 dose of this vaccine and 10,928 girls and women received at least 1 dose of a control (hepatitis A vaccine containing 360 ELU [10 to 14 years of age], hepatitis A vaccine containing 720 ELU [15 to 25 years of age], or aluminum hydroxide 500 mcg [15 to

25 years of age]). Overall, most patients were white (59%), with Asian (26%), Hispanic (9%), black (3%), and other racial/ethnic groups (3%). Injection-site reactions were reported more frequently with HPV vaccine than with control groups; in at least 84% of HPV vaccine recipients, these reactions were mild to moderate in intensity. Compared with dose 1, pain was reported less frequently after doses 2 and 3 of HPV vaccine; however, there was a small increased incidence of redness and swelling. There was no increase in the frequency of general adverse events with successive doses.

The pattern of solicited injection-site reactions and general adverse events after HPV vaccine was similar between the age cohorts (10 to 14 years of age and 15 to 25 years of age).

Unsolicited adverse events: The frequency of unsolicited adverse events within 30 days of vaccination (at least 1% for HPV vaccine and greater than any of the control groups) in girls and women 10 to 25 years of age appears in the following table.

Unsolicited Adverse Events in Women and Girls 10 to 25 Years of Age Within 30 Days of Vaccination (Total Vaccinated Cohort)[a]			
Adverse event	*Cervarix* (N = 6,654)	HAV 720[b] (N = 3,186)	HAV 360[c] (N = 1,032)	Aluminum hydroxide control[d] (N = 581)
Headache	5.3%	7.6%	3.3%	9.3%
Nasopharyngitis	3.6%	3.4%	5.9%	3.3%
Influenza	3.2%	5.6%	1.3%	1.9%
Pharyngolaryngeal pain	2.9%	2.7%	2.2%	2.2%
Dizziness	2.2%	2.6%	1.5%	3.1%
Upper respiratory infection	2%	1.3%	6.7%	1.5%
Chlamydia infection	2%	4.4%	0%	0%
Dysmenorrhea	2%	2.3%	1.9%	4%
Pharyngitis	1.5%	1.8%	2.2%	0.5%
Injection-site bruising	1.4%	1.8%	0.7%	1.5%
Vaginal infection	1.4%	2.2%	0.1%	0.9%
Injection-site pruritus	1.3%	0.5%	0.6%	0.2%
Back pain	1.1%	1.3%	0.7%	3.1%
Urinary tract infection	1%	1.4%	0.3%	1.2%

a Total vaccinated cohort included patients with at least 1 dose administered (N).
b Hepatitis A vaccine (720 ELU of antigen and aluminum hydroxide 500 mcg).
c Hepatitis A vaccine (360 ELU of antigen and aluminum hydroxide 250 mcg).
d Aluminum hydroxide 500 mcg.

New-onset autoimmune diseases: The pooled safety database, including girls and women 10 to 25 years of age, was searched for new medical conditions indicative of potential new-onset autoimmune diseases. Overall, the incidence of potential new-onset autoimmune diseases, as well as new-onset autoimmune diseases, in HPV vaccine recipients was 0.8% (95/12,533), comparable with the pooled control group (0.8%, 87/10,730) during the 4.3 years of follow-up (mean, 3 years). In the largest randomized, controlled trial (study 2) that enrolled girls and women 15 to 25 years of age with active surveillance for potential new-onset autoimmune diseases, the incidence of potential new-onset autoimmune diseases and new-onset autoimmune diseases was 0.8% among HPV vaccine recipients (78/9,319) and 0.8% among patients who received hepatitis A vaccine or aluminum hydroxide control (77/9,325).

New Medical Conditions Indicative of Potential New-Onset Autoimmune Disease and New-Onset Autoimmune Disease During Follow-up Period, Regardless of Causality, in Women and Girls 10 to 25 Years of Age (Total Vaccinated Cohort)[a]		
	Cervarix (n = 12,533) n (%)[c]	Pooled control group[b] (n = 10,730) n (%)[c]
Total with at least 1 medical condition	95 (0.8)	87 (0.8)
Arthritis[d]	9 (0)	4 (0)
Celiac disease	2 (0)	5 (0)
Dermatomyositis	0 (0)	1 (0)
Diabetes mellitus insulin-dependent (Type 1 or unspecified)	5 (0)	5 (0)
Erythema nodosum	3 (0)	0 (0)
Hyperthyroidism[e]	14 (0.1)	15 (0.1)
Hypothyroidism[f]	30 (0.2)	28 (0.3)
Inflammatory bowel disease[g]	8 (0.1)	4 (0)
Multiple sclerosis	4 (0)	1 (0)
Myelitis transverse	1 (0)	0 (0)
Optic neuritis/Optic neuritis retrobulbar	3 (0)	1 (0)
Psoriasis[h]	8 (0.1)	11 (0.1)
Raynaud phenomenon	0 (0)	1 (0)
Rheumatoid arthritis	4 (0)	3 (0)
Systemic lupus erythematosus[i]	2 (0)	3 (0)
Thrombocytopenia[j]	1 (0)	1 (0)
Vasculitis[k]	1 (0)	3 (0)
Vitiligo	2 (0)	2 (0)

a Includes patients with at least 1 documented dose (N).
b Hepatitis A vaccine 720 ELU of antigen and aluminum hydroxide 500 mcg, hepatitis A vaccine 360 ELU of antigen and aluminum hydroxide 250 mcg, or aluminum hydroxide 500 mcg.
c n (%) = number and percentage of patients with medical condition.
d Includes reactive arthritis and arthritis.
e Includes Basedow disease, goiter, and hyperthyroidism.
f Includes thyroiditis, autoimmune thyroiditis, and hypothyroidism.
g Includes colitis ulcerative, Crohn disease, proctitis ulcerative, and inflammatory bowel disease.
h Includes psoriatic arthropathy, nail psoriasis, guttate psoriasis, and psoriasis.
i Includes systemic lupus erythematosus and cutaneous lupus erythematosus.
j Includes idiopathic thrombocytopenic purpura and thrombocytopenia.
k Includes leukocytoclastic vasculitis and vasculitis.

Serious adverse events: In the pooled safety database, including controlled and uncontrolled studies of girls and women 10 to 72 years of age, 5.3% (862/16,142) of patients who received HPV vaccine and 5.9% (814/13,811) of patients who received control reported at least 1 serious adverse event, without regard to causality, during the entire follow-up period (up to 7.4 years). Among girls and women 10 to 25 years of age enrolled in these clinical studies, 6.4% of patients who received HPV vaccine and 7.2% of patients who received the control reported at least 1 serious adverse event during the entire follow-up period (up to 7.4 years).

Deaths: In completed and ongoing studies that enrolled 57,323 girls and women 9 to 72 years of age, 37 deaths were reported during the 7.4 of follow-up: 20 in patients who received HPV vaccine (0.06%, 20/33,623) and 17 in patients who received control (0.07%, 17/23,700). Causes of death among patients were consistent with those reported in adolescent and adult female populations. The most common causes of death were motor vehicle accident (5, HPV vaccine; 5, control) and suicide (2 and 5), followed by neoplasm (3 and 2), autoimmune disease (3 and 1), infectious disease (3 and 1), homicide (2 and 1), cardiovascular disorders (2 HPV vaccine), and death of unknown cause (2 control). Among girls and women 10 to 25 years of age, 31 deaths were reported (0.05%, 16/29,467 of HPV vaccine recipients; 0.07%, 15/20,192 of control).

Immune system: Allergic reactions (including anaphylactic and anaphylactoid reactions), angioedema, erythema multiforme.

Nervous system: Syncope or vasovagal responses to injection (sometimes accompanied by tonic-clonic movements). Because syncope, sometimes associated with tonic-clonic movements and other seizure-like activity, has been reported after vaccination, observe vaccinees for at least 15 minutes after administration. Syncope associated with tonic-clonic movements is usually transient and typically responds to restoring cerebral perfusion by maintaining a supine or Trendelenburg position.

Pharmacologic & Dosing Characteristics

Dosage: Three 0.5 mL doses at 0, 1, and 6 months.

Route & Site: IM, preferably the deltoid region of the upper arm.

Documentation Requirements: Federal law requires that the following information be documented in the recipient's permanent medical record or in a permanent office log: the manufacturer and lot number of this vaccine; the date of administration; and the name, address, and title of the person administering the vaccine.

Certain adverse events must be reported to the Vaccine Adverse Event Reporting System (800-822-7967). Refer to immunization documents in the Resources Section.

Overdosage: Although few data are available, clinical experience with similar products suggests that the major manifestations of overdosage would be pain and tenderness at the injection site.

Missed Doses: Interrupting the recommended schedule or delaying subsequent doses does not require restarting the series.

Related Interventions: Because no vaccine is 100% effective and HPV vaccines do not protect against HPV types not present in the vaccine nor against existing HPV infections, routine Pap screening remains critically important to detect precancerous changes in the cervix to allow treatment before cervical cancer develops.

Efficacy: Cervical AIS CIN grade 2 and 3 lesions are the immediate and necessary precursors of squamous cell carcinoma and adenocarcinoma of the cervix, respectively. Their detection and removal have been shown to prevent cancer. Therefore, CIN 2/3 and AIS (precancerous lesions) serve as surrogate markers for the prevention of cervical cancer. In clinical studies of HPV vaccine, the end points were cases of histopathologically-confirmed CIN 2/3 and AIS associated with HPV-16, HPV-18, and other oncogenic HPV types. Persistent infection with HPV-16 and HPV-18 that lasts for 12 months was also an end point.

Efficacy to prevent CIN 2/3 or AIS was assessed in 2 double-blind, randomized, controlled clinical studies that enrolled 19,778 girls and women 15 to 25 years of age. In both studies, PCR testing was conducted to detect HPV DNA in archived biopsy samples.

Study 1 enrolled women negative for oncogenic HPV DNA (HPV types 16, 18, 31, 33, 35, 39, 45, 51, 52, 56, 58, 59, 66, and 68) in cervical samples, seronegative for HPV-16 and HPV-18 antibodies, and with normal cytology, representing a population presumed naive (without current HPV infection at vaccination and without prior exposure to either HPV-16 or HPV-18). Patients (N = 776) were enrolled in an extended follow-up study and were followed for up to 6.4 years (mean, 5.9 years). Efficacy in preventing HPV-16 or HPV-18 incidence and persistent infections was compared with aluminum hydroxide control in 1,113 girls and women 15 to 25 years of age. Efficacy against CIN 2/3 or AIS associated with HPV-16 or HPV-18 was 100% (98.67% confidence interval [CI], 28.4-100). Efficacy against 12-month persistent infection with HPV-16 or HPV-18 was 100% (98.7% CI, 74.4-100). The CI reflected in this final analysis results from statistical adjustment for analyses previously conducted.

In study 2, women were vaccinated regardless of baseline HPV DNA status, serostatus, or cytology. This study reflects a population of women naive (without current infection and without prior exposure) or nonnaive (with current infection and/or with prior exposure) to HPV. Before vaccination, cervical samples were assessed for oncogenic HPV DNA (HPV types 16, 18, 31, 33, 35, 39, 45, 51, 52, 56, 58, 59, 66, and 68) and serostatus of HPV-16 and HPV-18 antibodies. The trial enrolled 18,665 healthy girls and women 15 to 25 years of age who received HPV vaccine or hepatitis A vaccine on a 0-, 1-, and 6-month schedule. Before vaccination, 73.6% were naive (without current infection [DNA-negative] and without prior exposure [seronegative]) to HPV-16 and/or HPV-18. The mean follow-up after the first dose was approximately 39 months. The according to protocol cohort for efficacy analyses for HPV-16 and/or HPV-18 included all patients who received 3 doses of vaccine, for whom efficacy end point measures were available, and who were HPV-16 and/or HPV-18 DNA-negative and seronegative at baseline and HPV-16 and/or HPV-18 DNA negative at month 6 for the HPV type considered in the analysis. Case counting for the according to protocol cohort started on day 1 after the third dose of vaccine. This cohort included women who had normal or low-grade cytology (cytological abnormalities including atypical squamous cells of undetermined significance [ASCUS] or low-grade squamous intraepithelial lesions [LSIL]) at baseline and excluded women with high-grade cytology.

The total vaccinated cohort for each efficacy analysis included all patients who received at least 1 dose of the vaccine, for whom efficacy end point measures were available, regardless of their HPV DNA status, cytology, and serostatus at baseline. This cohort included women with or without current HPV infection and/or prior exposure. Case counting for the total vaccinated cohort started on day 1 after the first dose. The total vaccinated cohort naive subset is a subset of the total vaccinated cohort that had normal cytology and were HPV DNA-negative for 14 oncogenic HPV types and seronegative for HPV-16 and HPV-18 at baseline.

HPV vaccine was efficacious in preventing precancerous lesions or AIS associated with HPV-16 or HPV-18.

Efficacy Against Histopathological Lesions Associated With HPV-16 or HPV-18 in Women and Girls 15 To 25 Years of Age (According to Protocol Cohort)[a] (Study 2)					
	Cervarix		Control[b]		
	N	Number of cases	N	Number of cases	% efficacy (96.1% CI)[c]
CIN 2/3 or AIS	7,344	4	7,312	56	92.9 (79.9-98.3)
CIN 1/2/3 or AIS	7,344	8	7,312	96	91.7 (82.4-96.7)

a Patients who received 3 doses of vaccine and were HPV DNA-negative and seronegative at baseline and HPV DNA-negative at month 6 for the corresponding HPV type (N). The mean follow-up was approximately 35 months.
b Hepatitis A vaccine (720 ELU of antigen and aluminum hydroxide 500 mcg).
c 96.1% CI results from statistical adjustment for previous interim analysis.

Because CIN 3 or AIS represents a more immediate precursor to cervical cancer, cases of CIN 3 or AIS associated with HPV-16 or HPV-18 were evaluated. In the according to protocol cohort, HPV vaccine was efficacious in the prevention of CIN 3 or AIS associated with HPV-16 or HPV-18 (vaccine efficacy = 80.0%; 96.1% CI, 0.3-98.1).

Patients already infected with 1 vaccine HPV type (16 or 18) before vaccination were protected from precancerous lesions or AIS and infection caused by the other vaccine HPV type.

Efficacy of HPV vaccine against 12-month persistent infection with HPV-16 or HPV-18 was also evaluated. In the according to protocol cohort, HPV vaccine reduced the incidence of 12-month persistent infection with HPV-16 and/or HPV-18 by 91.2% (96.1% CI, 85.9-94.8).

Immune response after natural infection does not reliably confer protection against future infections. Among patients who received 3 doses of HPV vaccine and who were seropositive at baseline and DNA-negative for HPV-16 or HPV-18 at baseline and month 6, HPV vaccine reduced the incidence of 12-month persistent infection by 91.5% (96.1% CI, 64-99.2%). However, the number of cases of CIN 2/3 or AIS was too few to determine efficacy against histopathological end points in this population.

Study 2 included women regardless of HPV DNA status (current infection) and serostatus (prior exposure) to vaccine types HPV-16 or HPV-18 at baseline. HPV vaccine was efficacious in preventing precancerous lesions or AIS associated with HPV-16 or HPV-18. However, among women HPV DNA–positive regardless of serostatus at baseline, there was no clear evidence of efficacy against precancerous lesions or AIS associated with HPV-16 or HPV-18.

Efficacy Against Disease Associated With HPV-16 or HPV-18 in Women and Girls 15 to 25 Years of Age, Regardless of Current or Prior Exposure to Vaccine HPV Types (Study 2)[a]					
	Cervarix		Control		
	N	Number of cases[b]	N	Number of cases	% efficacy (96.1% CI)[c]
CIN 1/2/3 or AIS					
Prophylactic efficacy[d]	5,449	3	5,436	85	96.5 (89-99.4)
HPV-16 or HPV-18 DNA-positive at baseline[e]	641	90	592	92	–
Regardless of current infection or prior exposure to HPV-16 or HPV-18[f]	8,667	107	8,682	240	55.5[g] (43.2-65.3)
CIN 2/3 or AIS					
Prophylactic efficacy[d]	5,449	1	5,436	63	98.4 (90.4-100)
HPV-16 or HPV-18 DNA-positive at baseline[e]	641	74	592	73	–
Regardless of current infection or prior exposure to HPV-16 or HPV-18[f]	8,667	82	8,682	174	52.8[g] (37.5-64.7)
CIN 3 or AIS					
Prophylactic efficacy[d]	5,449	0	5,436	13	100 (64.7-100)
HPV-16 or HPV-18 DNA-positive at baseline[e]	641	41	592	38	–
Regardless of current infection or prior exposure to HPV-16 or HPV-18[f]	8,667	43	8,682	65	33.6[g] (−1.1-56.9)

a Table does not include disease caused by nonvaccine HPV types.
b Histopathological cases associated with HPV-16 and/or HPV-18.
c 96.1% CI results from statistical adjustment for previous interim analysis.
d Total vaccinated cohort naive includes all vaccinated patients (who received at least 1 dose of vaccine) who had normal cytology, were HPV DNA-negative for 14 oncogenic HPV types, and seronegative for HPV-16 and HPV-18 at baseline (N). Case counting started on day 1 after the first dose.
e Total vaccinated cohort subset includes all vaccinated patients (who received at least 1 dose of vaccine) who were HPV DNA–positive for HPV-16 or HPV-18 regardless of serostatus at baseline (N). Case counting started on day 1 after the first dose.
f Total vaccinated cohort includes all vaccinated patients (who received at least 1 dose of vaccine) regardless of HPV DNA status and serostatus at baseline (N). Case counting started on day 1 after the first dose.
g Includes prophylactic efficacy and effect of HPV vaccine on course of infections present at first vaccination.

The effect of HPV vaccine against the overall burden of HPV-related cervical disease results from a combination of prophylactic efficacy against, and disease contribution of, HPV-16, HPV-18, and nonvaccine HPV types. In the population naive to oncogenic HPV (total vaccinated cohort naive), HPV vaccine reduced the overall incidence of CIN 1/2/3 or AIS, CIN 2/3 or AIS, and CIN 3 or AIS, regardless of the HPV DNA type in the lesion. In the population of women naive and nonnaive (total vaccinated cohort), vaccine efficacy against CIN 1/2/3 or AIS, CIN 2/3 or AIS, and CIN 3 or AIS was demonstrated in all women regardless of HPV DNA type in the lesion.

Efficacy in Preventing CIN or AIS Regardless of Any HPV Type in Women and Girls 15 To 25 Years of Age, Regardless of Current or Prior Infection with Vaccine or Nonvaccine Types (Study 2)

	Cervarix		Control		
	N	Number of cases	N	Number of cases	% efficacy (96.1% CI)[a]
CIN 1/2/3 or AIS					
Prophylactic efficacy[b]	5,449	106	5,436	211	50.1 (35.9-61.4)
Regardless of HPV DNA at baseline[c]	8,667	451	8,682	577	21.7 (10.7-31.4)
CIN 2/3 or AIS					
Prophylactic efficacy[b]	5,449	33	5,436	110	70.2 (54.7-80.9)
Regardless of HPV DNA at baseline[c]	8,667	224	8,682	322	30.4 (16.4-42.1)
CIN 3 or AIS					
Prophylactic efficacy[b]	5,449	3	5,436	23	87.0 (54.9-97.7)
Regardless of HPV DNA at baseline[c]	8,667	77	8,682	116	33.4 (9.1-51.5)

a 96.1% CI results from statistical adjustment for previous interim analysis.
b Total vaccinated cohort naive includes all vaccinated patients (who received at least 1 dose of vaccine) who had normal cytology, were HPV DNA-negative for 14 oncogenic HPV types (including HPV-16 and HPV-18) and seronegative for HPV-16 and HPV-18 at baseline (N). Case counting started on day 1 after the first dose.
c Total vaccinated cohort includes all vaccinated patients (who received at least 1 dose of vaccine) regardless of HPV DNA status and serostatus at baseline (N). Case counting started on day 1 after the first dose.

In exploratory analyses, HPV vaccine reduced definitive cervical therapy procedures (includes loop electrosurgical excision procedure, cold-knife cone, and laser procedures) by 24.7% (96.1% CI, 7.4-8.9) in the total vaccinated cohort and by 68.8% (96.1% CI, 50-81.2) in the total vaccinated cohort naive.

To assess reductions in disease caused by nonvaccine HPV types, 2 analyses were conducted combining 12 nonvaccine oncogenic HPV types, including and excluding lesions in which HPV-16 or HPV-18 were also detected. In these analyses, among females who received 3 doses of HPV vaccine and were DNA-negative for the specific HPV type at baseline and month 6, HPV vaccine reduced the incidence of CIN 2/3 or AIS by 54% (96.1% CI, 34-68.4) and 37.4% (96.1% CI, 7.4-58.2), respectively.

Post hoc analyses, adjusted for multiplicity, were conducted to assess the impact of HPV vaccine on CIN 2/3 or AIS caused by specific nonvaccine HPV types. Protocol cohort for these analyses included all patients regardless of serostatus who received 3 doses of HPV vaccine and were DNA-negative for the specific HPV type at baseline and month 6. These post hoc analyses were also conducted in the total vaccinated cohort naive population. In analyses including lesions in which HPV-16 or HPV-18 were also detected, vaccine efficacy in preventing CIN 2/3 or AIS associated with HPV-31 was 92% (99.7% CI, 49-99.8) and 100% (99.7% CI, 62.3-100), respectively. In analyses excluding lesions in which HPV-16 or HPV-18 were detected, vaccine efficacy in preventing CIN 2/3 or AIS associated with HPV-31 was 89.4% (99.7% CI, 29-99.7) and 100% (99.7% CI, 36.3-100), respectively.

Onset: Protection against infection occurs within 1 month after the third dose.

Duration: The duration of protection via immunization against HPV is not yet known.

Protective Level: Not established.

Mechanism: Animal studies suggest that the efficacy of L1 VLP vaccines may be mediated by eliciting immunoglobulin G–neutralizing antibodies directed against HPV-L1 capsid proteins generated as a result of vaccination.

Immunogenicity was evaluated in 2 clinical studies involving 1,193 girls 10 to 14 years of age who received HPV vaccine. Based on these data, the efficacy of HPV vaccine is inferred in girls 10 to 14 years of age.

Study 3 was a double-blind, randomized, controlled study in which 1,035 patients received HPV vaccine and 1,032 patients received hepatitis A vaccine 360 ELU as control, with a subset of patients evaluated for immunogenicity. All initially seronegative patients in the group that received HPV vaccine were seropositive after vaccination (ie, antibody levels greater than limit of detection of assay to both HPV-16 [at least 8 ELU/mL] and HPV-18 [at least 7 ELU/mL] antigens).

In study 4, immunogenicity of HPV vaccine administered to girls 10 to 14 years of age was compared with that in girls and women 15 to 25 years of age. The immune response in girls 10 to 14 years of age measured 1 month after dose 3 was noninferior to that seen in girls and women 15 to 25 years of age for both HPV-16 and HPV-18 antigens.

Immunogenicity at Month 7 for Initially Seronegative Women and Girls 10 to 14 Years of Age Compared With 15 to 25 Years of Age (According to Protocol Cohort for Immunogenicity)[a] (Study 4)						
	10 to 14 years of age			15 to 25 years of age		
Antibody assay	N	GMT ELU/mL (95% CI)	Seropositive rate	N	GMT ELU/mL (95% CI)	Seropositive rate
Anti–HPV-16	143	17, 273 (15,118, 19,734)	100%	118	7,439 (6,325, 8,750)	100%
Anti–HPV-18	141	6,864 (5,976, 7,883)	100%	116	3,070 (2,600, 3,625)	100%

a Patients who received 3 doses of vaccine for whom assay results were available for at least 1 postvaccination antibody measurement (N); GMT = geometric mean titer.

Drug Interactions: Like all inactivated vaccines, administration of HPV vaccine to patients receiving immunosuppressant drugs (eg, high-dose corticosteroids) or radiation therapy may result in an insufficient response to immunization. Patients may remain susceptible despite immunization.

Coadministration of HPV vaccine with other vaccines has not been specifically studied.

Inactivated vaccines are not generally affected by circulating antibodies or administration of exogenous antibodies. Vaccination may occur at any time before or after antibody administration.

As with other drugs given by IM injection, administer HPV vaccine with caution to patients receiving anticoagulant therapy. Do not give HPV vaccine to patients with bleeding disorders, such as hemophilia or thrombocytopenia, unless the potential benefits clearly outweigh the risk of administration. If HPV vaccine is given to these patients, take steps to avoid the risk of hematoma after injection.

Hormonal contraceptives: Among 7,693 patients 15 to 25 years of age in study 2 who used hormonal contraceptives for a mean of 2.8 years, observed efficacy was similar to that among patients who did not report use of hormonal contraceptives.

Patient Information: Vaccination does not substitute for routine cervical cancer screening. Women who receive HPV vaccine should continue to undergo cervical cancer screening per standard of care. Completing the immunization series unless contraindicated is important to protection.

Human Papillomavirus Vaccine, Types 16, 18

Pharmaceutical Characteristics

Concentration: Each 0.5 mL dose contains HPV-16 L1 protein 20 mcg and HPV-18 L1 protein 20 mcg.

Packaging: Ten 0.5 mL single-dose vials (NDC #: 58160-0830-11); 1 prefilled syringe without needle (58160-0830-32); 5 prefilled syringes without needles (58160-0830-46).

Doseform: Suspension

Appearance: After thorough agitation, product is a homogeneous, turbid, white suspension

Solvent: Water with sodium chloride, sodium dihydrogen phosphate dihydrate

Adjuvant: AS04 adjuvant system, containing aluminum hydroxide 500 mcg and 3-O-desacyl-4'-monophosphoryl lipid A (MPL) 50 mcg per 0.5 mL

Preservative: None

Allergens: The tip cap and the rubber plunger of the needleless prefilled syringes contain dry natural latex rubber that may cause allergic reactions in latex-sensitive individuals. The vial stopper does not contain latex.

Excipients: Sodium chloride 4.4 mg and sodium dihydrogen phosphate dihydrate 0.624 mg per dose. Each dose may also contain residual amounts of insect cell and viral protein (less than 40 ng) and bacterial cell protein (less than 150 ng) from the manufacturing process.

pH: Data not provided

Shelf Life: Data not provided

Storage/Stability: Store at 2° to 8°C (36° to 46°F). Protect vials from light. Discard if frozen. Upon storage, a fine, white deposit with a clear, colorless supernatant may be observed. This does not constitute a sign of deterioration. Contact the manufacturer regarding exposure to freezing or elevated temperatures. Shipping data not provided.

Handling: Shake vial or syringe well before withdrawal and use.

Production Process: The L1 proteins are produced in separate bioreactors using a recombinant baculovirus expression-vector system in a serum-free culture media composed of chemically defined lipids, vitamins, amino acids, and mineral salts. Baculoviruses are rod-shaped, double-stranded DNA viruses. The L1-encoding recombinant baculoviruses replicate in *Trichoplusia ni* insect cells (a member of the moth family *Noctuidae*). The L1 protein accumulates in the cytoplasm of the cells. The L1 proteins are released by cell disruption and purified by a series of chromatographic and filtration methods. Assembly of the L1 proteins into VLPs occurs at the end of the purification process. The purified, noninfectious VLPs are then adsorbed on to aluminum (as hydroxide salt). The adjuvant system, AS04, is composed of 3-O-desacyl-4'-monophosphoryl lipid A (MPL) adsorbed onto aluminum (as hydroxide salt).

Media: L1-encoding recombinant baculoviruses that replicate in *Trichoplusia ni* insect cells

Disease Epidemiology

See monograph for Human Papillomavirus Vaccine, Types 6, 11, 16, 18.

Other Information

First Licensed: October 16, 2009

National Policy: ACIP. FDA licensure of bivalent human papillomavirus (HPV2, *Cervarix*) for use in females and updated HPV vaccination recommendations from the Advisory Committee on Immunization Practices (ACIP) [published correction appears in *MMWR*. 2010;59(36):1184]. *MMWR*. 2010;59(20):626-629, erratum 1184. http://www.cdc.gov/mmwr/pdf/wk/mm5920.pdf.

Comparison Table of Influenza Vaccines		
Generic name	Inactivated injectable vaccines	Live, attenuated intranasal vaccine
Brand name (Manufacturer)	*Afluria* (CSL Biotherapies, Merck), *Fluarix* (GlaxoSmithKline), *FluLaval* (GlaxoSmithKline), *Fluvirin* (Novartis), *Fluzone* (Sanofi Pasteur) *Fluzone High Dose* (Sanofi Pasteur)[a] *Fluzone Intradermal* (Sanofi Pasteur)[b]	*FluMist* (MedImmune/AstraZeneca)
Synonyms	INFi, TIIV, TIV	INFn, CAIV-T, LAIV
Viability	Viral subunit vaccine	Live, cold-adapted, temperature-sensitive, attenuated viruses
Indication	To prevent influenza disease	To prevent influenza disease
Labeled age range	6 months or older (lower age varies by brand)	2 to 49 years, healthy
Special populations	People at high risk for complications due to influenza, close contacts of immunosuppressed people	Preferred for people at elevated risk for exposure
Components	Three viral strains (A/H1N1, A/H3N2, B)	Three viral strains (A/H1N1, A/H3N2, B)
Concentration	Traditional: 15 mcg each antigen/0.5 mL High-Dose: 60 mcg each antigen/0.5 mL Intradermal: 9 mcg each antigen/0.1 mL	$10^{6.5-7.5}$ FFU of each reassortant virus type per 0.2 mL
Adjuvant	None	None
Preservative	None in single-dose containers, thimerosal in multidose containers	None
Production medium	Allantoic fluid of fertilized chicken eggs	Reassortant viruses grown in chick kidney cells. Virus then mass produced in allantoic fluid of fertilized chicken eggs
Doseform	Solution	Solution
Packaging	0.5 mL syringe, 0.5 mL vial, 5 mL vial. Intradermal: 0.1 mL device	Package of 10 single-use sprayers
Routine storage	Refrigerate, 2° to 8°C (36° to 46°F)	Refrigerate, 2° to 8°C (36° to 46°F)
Dose	Up to 35 months: 0.25 mL 36 months or older: 0.5 mL Intradermal: 0.1 mL	0.1 mL in each nostril
Route	IM or intradermal	Intranasal
Standard schedule	1 dose per season, except 2 doses for children < 9 years of age in first season	1 dose per season, except 2 doses for children < 9 years of age in first season
Frequency	Annual	Annual

a *Fluzone High Dose* contains 60 mcg per 0.5 mL of each antigen and is indicated for people at least 65 years of age.
b *Fluzone Intradermal* contains 9 mcg per 0.1 mL of each antigen and is indicated for people 18 to 64 years of age.

Viral Vaccines

Names:
Afluria split-virion vaccine
Fluarix split-virus vaccine
FluLaval split-virion vaccine
Fluvirin purified surface antigen
Fluzone subvirion vaccine
Fluzone High Dose
Fluzone Intradermal

Manufacturers:
CSL Biotherapies, distributed by Merck
GlaxoSmithKline
GlaxoSmithKline
Novartis
Sanofi Pasteur
Sanofi Pasteur
Sanofi Pasteur

Synonyms: VISI abbreviation: INFi. Flu vaccine. Split-virion, split-virus, subvirion, and purified surface antigen are comparable terms.

Comparison: Split-virion influenza vaccines are generically equivalent to each other; whole-virion influenza vaccines are generically equivalent to each other. Split vaccines are slightly less reactogenic in children than whole vaccines, although they demonstrate comparable immunogenicity in both adults and children. Use only split vaccines in children younger than 13 years of age. Distribution of whole-viron vaccines ceased in the United States in 2001. Preliminary data suggest live, attenuated influenza vaccine (LAIV) may offer clinical advantages over traditional injectable influenza vaccine (TIIV) in some groups; additional information is needed.

Immunologic Characteristics

Microorganism: Virus (single-stranded RNA), influenza virus, genus *Influenzavirus*, family Orthomyxoviridae

Viability: Inactivated. Influenza vaccine cannot cause influenza, despite this common myth. Occasional cases of respiratory disease following vaccination represent coincidental viral infection unrelated to vaccination or lethargy associated with any vaccination.

Antigenic Form: Viral subunits, called subvirion or purified surface antigens.

Antigenic Type: Protein

Strains: Revised annually. Influenza A viruses are categorized on the basis of 2 cell-surface antigens: Hemagglutinin (H) and neuraminidase (N). Each of these antigens is further divided into subtypes (eg, H1, H2, or H3; N1 or N2). Specific strains within a subtype are named for the location, sequence number, and year of their isolation (eg, A/Taiwan/1/86 [H1N1]). For example, the 2012-13 formula includes the following antigens: A/California/7/2009-like (H1N1), A/Victoria/361/2011 (H3N2), and B/Wisconsin/1/2010. Strains are selected each year in the spring for the northern hemisphere; that year's vaccine is released by manufacturers each autumn.

Use Characteristics

Indications: Induction of active immunity against influenza viruses corresponding to the strains in the vaccine formula. Routine vaccination of all persons 6 months of age or older is recommended beginning in fall 2010. A universal vaccination recommendation for all persons 6 months of age or older eliminates the need to determine whether each person has an indication for vaccination and emphasizes the importance of preventing influenza among person of all ages. Expansion of vaccination recommendations reflects the need to remove potential barriers to receipt of influenza vaccine, including lack of awareness about vaccine indications among persons at higher risk for influenza complications and their close contacts.

The Advisory Committee on Immunization Practices (ACIP) recommends that vaccination efforts in October and earlier be focused primarily on people 50 years of age and older; people younger than 50 years of age at increased risk of influenza-related complications (including children 6 to 23 months of age); household contacts of high-risk people (including out-of-home caregivers and household contacts of children 0 to 23 months of age); and health care workers. Strongly encourage people of all ages with high-risk conditions and people 50 years of age and older who are hospitalized at any time from September to March to receive influenza vaccine before discharge. People planning organized vaccination campaigns should schedule these events after mid-October.

If influenza vaccine is used in an immunization program sponsored by an organization where a traditional physician/patient relationship does not exist, advise each participant or guardian of the possible risks associated with influenza vaccination.

Limitations: Influenza vaccine is not effective against unrelated viral strains not represented in the vaccine formula, although there may be some degree of cross-protection with strains of similar viral subtypes (eg, various strains of subtype H1N1).

Contraindications:

Absolute: Do not vaccinate patients with a history of anaphylactoid or other immediate reactions (eg, hives, swelling of the mouth or throat, difficulty breathing, hypotension, shock) following a prior dose of influenza vaccine.

Relative: Several studies have documented safe receipt of influenza vaccine in persons with egg allergy, in some cases after desensitization. Using a dilution of the vaccine as the antigen, perform a skin test on patients suspected of being hypersensitive to egg protein. Refer to detailed instructions in the Introduction section. Do not vaccinate patients with adverse reactions to such testing unless benefits outweigh risks. Patients are apparently not at risk if they have egg allergies that are not anaphylactoid in nature; vaccinate such patients in the usual manner. There is no evidence that patients with allergies to chickens or feathers are at an increased risk of reaction to the vaccine. For influenza vaccine brands containing residual neomycin, the residual amount would be less than used in a skin test to assess hypersensitivity. Neomycin allergy is usually a contact dermatitis, a manifestation of cell-mediated immunity rather than anaphylaxis, and does not contraindicate administration.

Do not routinely vaccinate patients with acute febrile illness until their symptoms abate. Delay vaccination in patients with an active neurological disorder characterized by changing neurological findings, but reconsider vaccination after the disease process has stabilized. The occurrence of any neurological signs or symptoms after vaccination with this product is a contraindication to further use. Conflicting advice is offered regarding vaccination of patients with a history of Guillain-Barré syndrome. The US Food and Drug Administration (FDA) and manufacturers include this contraindication in product labeling, but it is not included in the ACIP recommendations. According to the ACIP, for most patients with a history of Guillain-Barré syndrome who are at high risk for severe complications from influenza, the established benefits of influenza immunization justify annual vaccination.

Immunodeficiency: Patients receiving immunosuppressive therapy or those with other immunodeficiencies may have a diminished antibody response to active immunization. They may remain susceptible despite immunization. Chemoprophylaxis of influenza A with an amantadine or a neuraminidase inhibitor may be indicated in such patients.

The ACIP specifically recommends influenza and pneumococcal immunization for children older than 24 months of age with renal failure, diabetes, or severe immunosuppression. Operationally defined, severe immunosuppression may result from congenital immunodeficiency, HIV infection, leukemia, lymphoma, aplastic anemia, generalized malignancy, or therapy with alkylating agents, antimetabolites, radiation, or large, sustained doses of corticosteroids.

Little information exists about the frequency and severity of influenza illness in HIV-infected patients, but recent reports suggest that symptoms may be prolonged and the risk of complications increased for this high-risk group. Vaccination of patients infected with HIV is a prudent measure and will result in protective antibody levels in many recipients. However, the antibody response to the vaccine may be low in people with advanced HIV-related illnesses. A booster dose has not improved the immune response in these individuals.

Elderly: Elderly patients and patients with certain chronic diseases may develop lower postvaccination antibody titers than healthy young adults and, therefore, remain susceptible to influenza upper respiratory tract infections. Nevertheless, even if such people develop influenza illness, vaccination is effective in preventing lower respiratory tract involvement or other complications, thereby reducing the risk of hospitalization and death.

Pregnancy: Category C. Immunize women who are pregnant during the influenza season (at least 14 weeks gestation). Influenza-associated excess mortality among pregnant women has not been documented, except in the largest pandemics of 1918-19, 1957-58, and 2009-10. However, limited studies suggest that pregnancy may increase the risk for serious medical complications of influenza because of increased heart rate, stroke volume, and oxygen consumption; decreased lung capacity; and changes in immunologic function. The ACIP estimates that 1 to 2 hospitalizations among pregnant women related to influenza can be averted for each 1,000 pregnant women vaccinated. Vaccinate pregnant women with medical complications that increase their risk of complications, regardless of the pregnancy stage.

Studies of influenza immunization of more than 2,000 pregnant women showed no adverse fetal effects associated with this vaccine. Influenza vaccine is an inactivated vaccine and is considered safe during any stage of pregnancy. Because spontaneous abortion is common in the first trimester and unnecessary exposures have traditionally been avoided during that time, some clinicians prefer to give influenza vaccine beginning in the second trimester to avoid coincidental association of immunization with early pregnancy loss. However, additional case reports and limited studies suggest that women in the third trimester of pregnancy and shortly after pregnancy, including women without underlying risk factors, may be at increased risk for serious complications from influenza. It is not known if influenza vaccine or corresponding antibodies cross the placenta. Generally, most IgG passage across the placenta occurs during the third trimester.

Fluzone Intradermal: Category B. A developmental and reproductive toxicity study performed in female rabbits at a dose approximately 20 times the human dose on a mg/kg basis revealed no evidence of impaired female fertility or harm to the fetus.

Lactation: It is not known if influenza vaccine or corresponding antibodies are excreted in breast milk. Problems in humans have not been documented and are unlikely.

Children: Give previously unvaccinated children younger than 9 years of age 2 doses at least 1 month apart. Give the second dose before December, if possible. Use only split-virion vaccine in children younger than 13 years of age.

Vaccinate children and teenagers (6 months to 18 years of age) who are receiving long-term aspirin therapy and who are therefore at risk of developing Reye syndrome after influenza infection. For children 6 months to 4 years of age, use only split- or subvirion types. For children 4 to 13 years of age, any split-virus vaccine (split, subvirion, or purified surface antigen) may be used. Split-virus vaccines cause fewer febrile adverse reactions than whole-virus vaccines.

Fluzone Intradermal: Safety and effectiveness in persons younger than 18 years have not been established. In a clinical trial, 97 infants and toddlers 6 to 35 months of age and 160 children 3 to 8 years of age received 2 injections of *Fluzone Intradermal.* Infants and children in a control group received 2 injections of standard *Fluzone. Fluzone Intradermal* was associated with increased local reactogenicity relative to *Fluzone.* The size of the study was not adequate to reliably evaluate serious adverse events or the immune response elicited by *Fluzone Intradermal* relative to *Fluzone*.

Adverse Reactions: Influenza vaccine contains only noninfectious, inactivated viruses. It cannot cause influenza. The most likely adverse effect of influenza vaccine is fever or tenderness at the injection site (20% to 30%).

Adverse effects of influenza vaccine are generally inconsequential in adults and occur at low frequency, but adverse effects may be more common in younger recipients. As many as 66% of recipients experience soreness around the vaccination site for 2 days. Fever, malaise, myalgia, and other systemic symptoms occur infrequently and usually affect patients with no prior exposure to the antigens in the vaccine (eg, young children). The effects usually begin 6 to 12 hours after vaccination and persist 1 to 2 days. Immediate, probably allergic, reactions such as hives, angioedema, allergic asthma, or systemic anaphylaxis occur extremely rarely after influenza vaccination. Do not vaccinate patients with severe egg allergy (eg, hives, swelling of lips or tongue, acute respiratory distress, collapse).

Influenza vaccination of patients with relapsing/remitting multiple sclerosis in a randomized, placebo-controlled study did not affect exacerbation rates or disease progression over 6 months. Prevention of febrile illness in these patients is desirable.

Increased risk of Guillain-Barré syndrome was noted among recipients of the 1976-77 A/New Jersey/76 (swine flu) influenza vaccine. An active surveillance system for Guillain-Barré syndrome was initiated in 1978 and data were collected for 3 years. A statistically significant excess risk of contracting Guillain-Barré syndrome after receipt of the 1978-79, 1979-80, and 1980-81 influenza vaccine formulations could not be demonstrated. Unlike the 1976 swine influenza vaccine, most subsequent influenza vaccines prepared from other influenza virus strains have not been associated with an increased frequency of Guillain-Barré syndrome. The risk of Guillain-Barré syndrome attributable to the 1992-93 and 1993-94 influenza vaccines was 1.1 cases per million influenza vaccinations during those years. It is prudent to avoid vaccinating people who are not at high risk for severe influenza complications and who are known to have developed Guillain-Barré syndrome within 6 weeks after a previous influenza vaccination. Although data are limited, for most people who have a history of Guillain-Barré syndrome and who are at risk for severe complications from influenza, the established benefits of influenza vaccinations justify yearly vaccinations.

Before modern purification techniques were adopted, split-virion vaccine induced fewer adverse effects than whole-virion vaccine, although possibly at the cost of reduced immunogenicity. Modern split- and whole-virion vaccines are comparably immunogenic and reactogenic in adults. Use split vaccine in children to reduce the likelihood of inducing fever.

When the National Academy of Sciences evaluated the evidence for neurologic complications after influenza vaccination in 2004, it concluded that the evidence favors rejection of a cause-and-effect relationship between influenza vaccine administered to adults and relapse of multiple sclerosis.

In a comparison of standard and high-dose *Fluzone*, the comparative incidence of various events was as follows: injection-site pain (36% high dose, 24% standard), erythema (15%, 11%), swelling (9%, 6%), myalgia (21%, 18%), malaise (18%, 14%), headache (17%, 14%), and fever (3.6%, 2.3%). The rates of serious adverse events were comparable between the 2 groups: 6.1% for high dose and 7.4% for standard.

Assessing *Fluzone Intradermal* in adults 18 to 64 years of age, the most common injection-site reactions were erythema (more than 75%); induration, swelling, and pain (more than 50%); and pruritus (more than 40%). Erythema, induration, swelling, and pruritus occurred more frequently after *Fluzone Intradermal* than standard *Fluzone*. The most common solicited systemic adverse events were headache, myalgia, and malaise (more than 20%).

Influenza Virus Vaccines, Trivalent, Types A & B (Injection)

Pharmacologic & Dosing Characteristics

Dosage: Shake well before withdrawing each dose.

Skin test for egg hypersensitivity: Refer to detailed protocol in the Introduction.

Vaccination, IM: Give adults and children 9 years of age and older one 0.5 mL dose annually, so long as indications persist. Give children 12 years of age and younger only the split-virion vaccine.

Give previously unvaccinated children 8 years of age and younger 2 doses at least 1 month apart. Give the second dose before December 1, if possible. For children 6 to 35 months of age, give 0.25 mL at each injection. For children 3 to 8 years of age, give two 0.5 mL injections. If the child received only 1 dose in the first season, administer 2 doses in the next season. Give children 9 to 12 years of age one 0.5 mL injection.

Offer the annual vaccine formula to high-risk individuals, such as those presenting for routine care or hospitalization, from September through March. Organized vaccination campaigns where high-risk people are routinely accessible (eg, nursing homes) are optimally undertaken between October and November each year. Continue to offer the vaccine to both children and adults up to and even after influenza virus activity is documented in a community, as late as April in some years.

Vaccination, intradermal: Give adults 18 to 64 years of age 0.1 mL using the prefilled device.

Route & Site: IM: Use the deltoid muscle for adults and older children. For infants and young children, the anterolateral aspect of the thigh is preferred. Do not inject IV.

Intradermal: Hold the device between thumb and middle finger. Insert needle rapidly, perpendicular to the skin, in the region of the deltoid. Once the needle is inserted, push on the plunger. Do not aspirate. Remove the needle from the skin. Push very firmly with the thumb on the plunger to activate the needle shield.

Documentation Requirements: Federal law requires that (1) the manufacturer and lot number of this vaccine, (2) the dates of its administration, and (3) the name, address, and title of the person administering the vaccine be documented in the recipient's permanent medical record or in a permanent office log.

Certain adverse events must be reported to the Vaccine Adverse Event Reporting System (VAERS) (800-822-7967). Refer to Immunization Documents in the Resources section for complete information.

Overdosage: Although few data are available, clinical experience with similar products suggests that the major manifestations of overdosage would be pain and tenderness at the injection site.

Booster Doses: Give previously unvaccinated children younger than 9 years of age 2 doses, at least 30 days apart, optimally before December 1.

Because of waning immunity and changing antigenicity of prevalent viral strains, give patients at risk of influenza a booster dose annually.

Related Interventions: Several antiviral drugs are effective against influenza A for pre- and postexposure prophylaxis, but are not active against influenza B. Consider chemoprophylaxis in addition to influenza vaccination during the 2-week period immediately after vaccination when anti-influenza A antibody titers are not yet protective. Chemoprophylaxis can be given simultaneously with influenza vaccine without impairing the effect of either drug or inducing increased adverse reactions. Also consider chemoprophylaxis against influenza A in patients who cannot or will not accept influenza vaccination.

Efficacy: Vaccination will reduce disease incidence approximately 70%. Influenza vaccine is more effective at preventing mortality than at preventing morbidity.

In a comparison of standard and high-dose *Fluzone*, the high-dose group achieved higher hemagglutinin-inhibition titers for 2 of 3 influenza strains among volunteers at least 65 years of age, and higher seroconversion rates for 3 of 3 strains: 49% vs 23% seroconversion for A/H1N1, 69% vs 51% for A/H3N2, and 42% vs 30% for B. There are no data establishing clinically relevant prevention of culture-confirmed influenza or its complications.

Fluzone Intradermal: Adults 18 to 64 years of age were randomized to receive *Fluzone Intradermal* or *Fluzone* (year 2008-2009 formulation) in a multicenter trial. In each group, the mean age was 43 years (age range, 18 to 65 years). Hemagglutinin-inhibition antibody geometric mean titers (GMTs) after *Fluzone Intradermal* were noninferior to those after *Fluzone* for all 3 strains. Seroconversion rates after *Fluzone Intradermal* were noninferior to those after *Fluzone* for all A/H1N1 and A/H3N2 strains, but not for the B strain. At 28 days after vaccination with either formulation, the proportion of subjects with a serum hemagglutination inhibition (HI) antibody titer of at least 1:40 ranged from 87% to 92%, depending on the strain.

Onset: 2 to 4 weeks

Duration: Declines during the year following immunization.

Protective Level: HI antibody titers greater than or equal to 1:40 correlate with clinical protection.

Mechanism: Induction of protective serum and mucosal IgG and IgA antibodies against influenza viral surface glycoproteins (hemagglutinins and neuraminidases) represented in the vaccine formula. Antihemagglutinin antibodies inhibit viral attachment to cell membrane receptors and neutralize viral infectivity. Antineuraminidase antibodies target an enzyme necessary for the release and spread of influenza virus from infected cells to other cells in the respiratory tract.

Drug Interactions: Like all inactivated vaccines, administration of influenza vaccine to patients receiving immunosuppressant drugs (eg, high-dose corticosteroids) or radiation therapy may result in an insufficient response to immunization. They may remain susceptible despite immunization. Chemoprophylaxis may be indicated in such patients.

Pneumococcal and influenza vaccines may safely and effectively be administered simultaneously at separate injection sites. While influenza vaccine is given annually, pneumococcal vaccine is given only once to all but those at highest risk of fatal pneumococcal disease.

Although no studies are published, influenza vaccine is not expected to diminish immunogenicity or enhance adverse reactions with other routine pediatric vaccines (eg, e-IPV, Hib, MMR, hepatitis B).

Inactivated vaccines are not generally affected by circulating antibodies or administration of exogenous antibodies. Vaccination may occur at any time before or after antibody administration.

Several vaccine-drug interactions have been attributed to influenza vaccine, although independent researchers have often been unable to corroborate the interactions. The vaccine-drug interaction may be clinically significant only in a few isolated individuals. Influenza vaccine, like some other vaccines and drugs, may be able to depress drug-metabolizing pathways by induction of endogenous interferon production. Influenza vaccine can decrease elimination and increase the biological half-life of aminopyrine, a probe chemical not used therapeutically, by inhibiting the P-450 metabolic pathway in the liver.

Theophylline elimination, which includes the P-450 pathway, has been noted by several clinicians to decline following influenza vaccination, but their work has been contradicted by others. This effect may be greatest in patients with higher prevaccination theophylline metabolism. Watch patients on chronic theophylline therapy for symptoms of theophylline toxicity (eg, nausea, vomiting, palpitations).

A few patients treated with warfarin have shown prolonged prothrombin time after influenza vaccination (incidence, 10 of 208 patients reported). None of the studies preclude the possibility of isolated cases of significant bleeding events, but there is insufficient evidence to substantiate a systematic interaction between warfarin and influenza vaccine. Watch patients on chronic warfarin therapy for symptoms of toxicity. As with other drugs administered by IM injection, give influenza vaccine with caution to patients receiving anticoagulant therapy.

Phenytoin steady-state plasma concentrations rose, fell, or remained unchanged after influenza vaccination in several studies. Carbamazepine and phenobarbital levels rose after influenza vaccination in one study. Phenytoin and phenobarbital are metabolized by the P-450 pathway, but carbamazepine is not. Watch patients on chronic anticonvulsant therapy for symptoms of drug toxicity.

Methacholine inhalation challenge may be falsely positive for a few days after influenza or other immunization. This effect appears to mimic the bronchospastic effect associated with acute respiratory infections. The effect has been observed in 44% to 90% of asthmatic patients but apparently not among normal subjects.

Lab Interference: The 1991 influenza vaccine formulation was associated with a transient slight increase in the incidence of false-positive serologic tests for HIV, human T-cell lymphotrophic virus type 1 (HTLV-1), and hepatitis C virus. No infections occurred as a result of vaccination, and there is no apparent need to defer vaccinees from blood donation. This effect has not been seen with more recent influenza vaccine formulations.

Pharmaceutical Characteristics

Concentration:

Standard dose: 3 hemagglutinin antigens, each at a concentration of 15 mcg per 0.5 mL dose

High dose: 3 hemagglutinin antigens, each at 60 mcg per 0.5 mL dose

Intradermal: 3 hemagglutinin antigens, each at 9 mcg per 0.1 mL dose

Quality Assay: Antigenicity determined in specific radial-immunodiffusion tests relative to the US Reference Standard Influenza Vaccine.

Packaging:

CSL: Package of ten 0.5 mL prefilled syringes; 5 mL multidose vial

GSK: (Fluarix): Package of five 0.5 mL single-dose syringes without needles

GSK: (FluLaval): 10 doses per 5 mL multidose vial

Novartis (Fluvirin): 0.5 mL prefilled single-dose syringe with ⅝-inch, 25-gauge needle, 10 doses per 5 mL multidose vial

Sanofi Pasteur (standard): 0.25 mL prefilled single-dose syringe without needle (with pink plunger), 0.5 mL prefilled single-dose syringe without needle (with clear plunger), single-dose 0.5 mL vial, 10 dose 5 mL multidose vial

Sanofi Pasteur (high dose): 0.5 mL prefilled single-dose syringe without needle (with gray plunger)

Sanofi Pasteur (intradermal): 0.1 mL prefilled device with 0.06-inch (1.5 mm) 30-gauge needle

NDC Number: Revised annually with each new formula

Doseform: Solution

Appearance: Essentially clear and slightly opalescent; slightly turbid, slightly yellow- or red-tinged

Solvent: Isotonic sodium chloride with sodium or potassium phosphate buffer 0.1 molar

Adjuvant: None

Preservative: 0.01% thimerosal (except for some packages of single-dose containers)

Allergens: Residual egg proteins. Check package labeling regarding presence of latex rubber in packaging.

GSK (Fluarix): Gentamicin added during processing, not more than 0.15 mcg per 0.5 mL remains in the final product.

GSK (FluLaval): No antibiotics are used in the production process.

Novartis (Fluvirin): Neomycin and polymyxin B added during processing, but neither can be detected in the final product.

Sanofi Pasteur (standard): Gelatin 0.05%. No antibiotics are used in the production process.

Sanofi Pasteur (high dose): None. No antibiotics used in production.

Sanofi Pasteur (intradermal): None. No antibiotics used in production.

Excipients:

CSL: Each 0.5 mL dose contains sodium chloride 4.1 mg, monobasic sodium phosphate 80 mcg, dibasic sodium phosphate 300 mcg, monobasic potassium phosphate 20 mcg, potassium chloride 20 mcg, calcium chloride 1.5 mcg, and ovalbumin (0.1 mcg or less).

GSK (Fluarix): Each 0.5 mL dose contains up to 85 mcg of octoxynol-10 (*Triton X-100*), up to 100 mcg of α-tocopheryl hydrogen succinate, up to 415 mcg of polysorbate 80, less than 1.25 mcg of mercury, up to 0.0016 mcg of hydrocortisone, up to 0.15 mcg of gentamicin, up to 1 mcg of ovalbumin, up to 50 mcg of formaldehyde, and up to 50 mcg of sodium deoxycholate.

GSK (FluLaval): Each dose may contain residual egg proteins (1 mcg of ovalbumin or less), formaldehyde (25 mcg or less), and sodium deoxycholate (50 mcg or less).

Novartis (Fluvirin): Triton N101, phosphate-buffered saline 0.01 M, beta-propiolactone undetectable in the final product

Sanofi Pasteur (standard): Octylphenol ethoxylate (*Triton X-100*) 0.02% or less, residual formaldehdye 100 mcg per 0.5 mL or less

Sanofi Pasteur (high dose): Octylphenol ethoxylate (*Triton X-100*) 250 mcg per 0.5 mL or less, residual formaldehyde 100 mcg per 0.5 mL or less

Sanofi Pasteur (intradermal): Octylphenol ethoxylate (*Triton X-100*) 50 mcg per 0.1 mL or less, residual formaldehyde 20 mcg per 0.1 mL or less

pH: Approximately 7.2

Shelf Life: Expires nominally by June 30 at the end of influenza season in the northern hemisphere, to minimize errors in administering the wrong annual formulation. Physicochemical stability may last 3 years if stored at 4°C (39°F).

Storage/Stability: Store at 2° to 8°C (36° to 46°F). Discard frozen vaccine. Contact manufacturer regarding prolonged exposure to room temperature or elevated temperatures. Shipped in insulated containers with coolant packs.

Production Process: Influenza viruses are grown in the extraembryonic, allantoic fluid of fertilized hen eggs. Tens of millions of eggs are processed each year to produce the nation's influenza vaccine supply. Each egg yields 1 to 2 doses of vaccine.

CSL: Virus is purified in a sucrose density gradient using a continuous flow zonal centrifuge. The inactivated virus is inactivated with beta-propiolactone, and the virus particles are disrupted using sodium taurodeoxycholate to produce a split virion. The disrupted virus is further purified and suspended in a phosphate buffered isotonic solution.

GSK (Fluarix): Viruses are concentrated and purified by zonal centrifugation using a linear sucrose density gradient solution containing detergent (ie, octoxynol-10) to disrupt the viruses. After dilution, the vaccine is further purified by diafiltration. Virus solution is inactivated by consecutive effects of sodium deoxycholate and formaldehyde leading to split virus.

GSK (FluLaval): Viruses are inactivated with ultraviolet light, followed by formaldehyde treatment, purified by centrifugation, and disrupted with sodium deoxycholate.

Novartis (Fluvirin): Clarified by centrifugation and filtration prior to inactivation with beta-propiolactone. Inactivated virus is concentrated and purified by zonal centrifugation. Purified surface antigens are obtained by centrifugation with *Triton N101*, which removes most internal proteins.

Sanofi Pasteur: Viruses inactivated with formaldehyde, then concentrated and purified in linear sucrose density gradient solution using continuous-flow (isopyknic) centrifuge. For the split-virion vaccine, the virus is chemically disrupted using glycol p-isooctylphenyl ether *(Triton X-100-A)*. The split antigen is further purified by chemical means.

Sanofi Pasteur (high dose and intradermal): Same process as standard dose product, except for additional concentration after ultrafiltration, to obtain a higher hemagglutinin concentration.

Media: Extraembryonic (allantoic) fluids of specific pathogen-free (SPF) embryonated chicken eggs. Each egg yields 1 to 2 doses of vaccine.

Disease Epidemiology

Incidence:

1889: Global influenza pandemic (an H2 subtype).

1918: More than 50 million deaths worldwide, 500,000 deaths in the United States (400/100,000 people). The worldwide pandemic killed more people than all military casualties of World War I and World War II combined: 500 million cases, 50 million deaths, 1% of the world population. Strain designated A_0 (H1N1).

1933: Prevalent strain designated A (H1N1).

1933-1947, 1977-present: Prevalent strain designated A_0 (H1N1).

1947-1957: Prevalent strain designated A' or A_1 (H1N1).

1957-1958: Asian influenza (A_2 or H2N2) pandemic in the United States: 60,000 deaths (because of high attack rate, not high virulence). From 1957 to 1960: 86,000 excess deaths.

1968-1969: Hong Kong influenza (H3N2) epidemic. Morbidity 20%, 50 million cases, 33,000 deaths (14/100,000 people).

2009-2010: H1N1 pandemic that originated in Mexico and California.

In the last 2 decades an average 36,000 deaths occurred each year, after infecting 10% to 20% of the general population each year.

Approximately 90% of deaths caused by influenza occur among the elderly. The death toll is even higher in epidemic years. For example, in 1991, approximately 77,000 influenza deaths were recorded. To compound the problem, influenza may precipitate other deaths that are attributed to cardiac, pulmonary, or other causes. From 1969 through 1994, between 20,000 and just over 300,000 influenza-associated hospitalizations occurred with each annual epidemic. The average was 130,000 to 170,000 per epidemic.

Susceptible Pools: Influenza immunization campaigns are targeted at 34 million people 65 years of age and older and 30 million people under 65 years of age who are at high risk for influenza-associated complications. Influenza immunization delivery among people 65 years of age and older increased from 23% in 1985 to 58% in 1995, but immunization among younger people at high risk trails far behind at less than 30%.

Greater morbidity and mortality occurs following periodic major antigenic changes (or "shifts") in prevalent influenza strains. Continuous and progressive antigenic variation within a given virus subtype over time (antigenic "drifts") causes infection or immunization with any one strain to not induce immunity to distantly related strains. Both types of antigenic variability necessitate new vaccine formulations almost every year.

Transmission: Airborne spread among crowded populations in enclosed spaces, also by direct contact through droplet spread

Incubation: 1 to 3 days

Communicability: Probably 3 to 5 days from clinical onset in adults, 7 days or less in young children

Other Information

Perspective:

1918: Worldwide pandemic of influenza A (H1N1, formerly referred to as Hsw0N1).

1933: Laidlaw isolates influenza virus type A.

1940: Francis isolates influenza virus type B.

1943: Studies of inactivated influenza vaccine commissioned by Surgeon General of the US Army.

1945: Influenza vaccine licensed in the United States.

1948: World Influenza Centre established in London.

1967: Maassab describes cold-adapted live influenza viruses.

1968: Improved rate-zonal centrifugation techniques allow more purified, less reactogenic vaccines to be produced. Parke-Davis produces first split vaccine.

1976: Swine influenza vaccine: Based on a perceived threat of an H1N1 pandemic similar to 1918, over 43.3 million vaccine doses were administered in the United States and territories (plus doses given in VA and DoD hospitals). The remarkable delivery rate was overshadowed by the occurrence of several cases of Guillain-Barré syndrome. The Guillain-Barré syndrome risk from swine influenza vaccine was 1 case per 110,000 vaccinations (case-fatality rate, 3.5%).

Before 1976, no association between Guillain-Barré syndrome and influenza vaccine was recognized. However, that year Guillain-Barré syndrome appeared with excess frequency among people who had received the A/New Jersey/76 (swine flu) influenza vaccine. For the 10 weeks following vaccine administration, the excess risk was found to be approximately 10 cases of Guillain-Barré syndrome for every million recipients, an incidence 7 times higher than that in unimmunized people. People younger than 25 years of age had a lower relative risk than others and also had a lower case-fatality rate.

An active surveillance system for Guillain-Barré syndrome was initiated in 1978 and data were collected for 3 years. A statistically significant excess risk of contracting Guillain-Barré syndrome after receipt of the 1978-79, 1979-80, and 1980-81 influenza vaccine formulations could not be demonstrated. Unlike the 1976 swine influenza vaccine, subsequent influenza vaccines prepared from other virus strains generally have not been clearly associated with an increased frequency of Guillain-Barré syndrome. The 1992-93 and 1993-94 influenza vaccine formulations were attributable to causing 1 Guillain-Barré syndrome case per million influenza vaccinations, but this effect has not been observed in other influenza seasons.

1978: Standardized system for influenza virus vaccines changes from chick-cell agglutination (CCA) units to mass of hemagglutinin antigen.

1993: Influenza vaccine nationally reimbursed by Medicare for the first time.

First Licensed:

Connaught (now Sanofi Pasteur): January 3, 1978

CSL Biotherapies: September 30, 2007

Evans (now Novartis): 1993

GlaxoSmithKline (Fluarix): August 31, 2005

GlaxoSmithKline (FluLaval): October 5, 2006

Novartis (Agriflu): November 27, 2009

Sanofi Pasteur (Fluzone High Dose): December 23, 2009

Sanofi Pasteur (Fluzone Intradermal): May 10, 2011

Discontinued Products: *Fluax* (Merck, Sharp and Dohme); *Flu-Immune* (Lederle); *Influenza Irado-gen* (Parke-Davis); *Zonomune* (Eli Lilly); *Fluogen*(Parke-Davis licensed November 26, 1946, and later Parkedale Pharmaceuticals).

National Policy: ACIP. Prevention and control of influenza with vaccines: recommendations of the Advisory Committee on Immunization Practices (ACIP), 2012-13 influenza season. *MMWR.* 2012;61(32):613-618.

American College of Obstetricians and Gynecologists Committee on Obstetric Practice. ACOG Committee Opinion No. 468: Influenza vaccination during pregnancy. *Obstet Gynecol.* 2010;116(4):1006-1007.

References: Institute of Medicine. *Immunization Safety Review: Influenza Vaccines and Neurological Complications.* Washington, DC: National Academy Press; 2004.

WHO. Influenza vaccines. *Wkly Epidemiol Rec.* 2005;80(33):279-287.

Influenza Virus Vaccines, Trivalent, Types A & B (Injection)

Pharmacoeconomics: Influenza vaccine is reimbursed by Medicare (procedure code 90657 for split-virus vaccine for children 6 to 35 months of age; 90658 for split-virus vaccine for older people; and 90659 for whole-virus vaccine for older people). Use diagnosis code V04.8. Use procedure code G0008 to report the administration fee. If a physician visit is rendered in conjunction with vaccination, it may be reimbursed as well.

Influenza Vaccine, Trivalent, Types A & B, Live (Nasal)

Viral Vaccines

Name:
FluMist

Manufacturer:
MedImmune/AstraZeneca

Synonyms: VISI abbreviation: INFn. Live, attenuated influenza vaccine (LAIV). The refrigerator-stable product is known as CAIV-T (cold-adapted influenza vaccine-trivalent).

Comparison: Preliminary data suggest live, attenuated influenza vaccine (LAIV) may offer clinical advantages over traditional injectable influenza vaccine (TIIV); additional information is needed. The two types of influenza vaccines contain the same strains of influenza viruses, selected annually, and both are grown industrially in chicken eggs. LAIV contains attenuated influenza viruses, whereas TIIV contains inactivated viral subunits.

In February 2012, the FDA licensed a quadrivalent form of *FluMist*, but it is not expected to be distributed during the 2012-13 influenza season. The vaccine will contain 2 type-A strains (A/H1N1 and A/H3N2) and 2 type-B strains (one each from the B/Yamagata/16/88 and B/Victoria/2/87 lineages).

Immunologic Characteristics

Microorganism: Virus (single-stranded RNA), influenza virus, genus *Influenzavirus*, family Orthomyxoviridae

Viability: Live, attenuated, reassortant influenza viruses. The virus strains included in the vaccine are cold-adapted (CA) (ie, replicate efficiently at 25°C, a temperature conducive to replication in human upper airway passages but restrictive for replication of many wild-type viruses), temperature-sensitive (TS) (ie, restricted in replication at 37°C [Type B strains] or 39°C [Type A strains], temperatures similar to human lower airways, at which many wild-type influenza viruses grow efficiently), and attenuated (ATT) so as not to produce classic influenza-like illness in the ferret model of human influenza infection. The cumulative effect of the antigenic properties and the CA, TS, and ATT phenotype is that the vaccine viruses replicate in the nasopharynx to produce protective immunity. No evidence of reversion has been observed in the recovered vaccine strains that have been tested (135 of 250 possible recovered isolates).

Antigenic Form: Whole, live viruses

Antigenic Type: Protein

Strains: Revised annually. Influenza A viruses are categorized on the basis of 2 cell-surface antigens: hemagglutinin (H) and neuraminidase (N). Each of these antigens is further divided into subtypes (eg, H1, H2, or H3; N1 or N2). Specific strains with a subtype are named for the location, sequence number, and year of their isolation (eg, A/Taiwan/1/86 [H1N1]). For example, the 2012-13 formula includes the following antigens: A/California/7/2009-like (H1N1), A/Victoria/361/2011 (H3N2), and B/Wisconsin/1/2010. Strains are selected each year in the spring for the northern hemisphere; that year's vaccine is released by manufacturers each autumn.

Each of the 3 influenza virus strains contained in *FluMist* is a genetic reassortant of a master donor virus (MDV) and a wild-type influenza virus. The MDVs (A/Ann Arbor/6/60 and B/Ann Arbor/1/66) were developed by serial passage at sequentially lower temperatures in specific pathogen-free (SPF) primary chick kidney cells. During this process, the MDVs acquired the CA, TS, and ATT phenotype and multiple mutations in the gene segments that encode viral proteins other than the surface glycoproteins. The individual contribution of the genetic sequences of the 6 non-glycoprotein MDV genes ("internal gene segments") to the

Influenza Vaccine, Trivalent, Types A & B, Live (Nasal)

CA, TS, and ATT phenotype is not completely understood. But at least 5 genetic loci in 3 different internal gene segments of the Type A MDV and at least 3 genetic loci in 2 different internal gene segments of the Type B MDV contribute to the TS property. For each of the 3 strains in *FluMist*, the 6 internal gene segments responsible for CA, TS, and ATT phenotypes are derived from the MDV, and the 2 segments that encode the 2 surface glycoproteins, hemagglutinin (H) and neuraminidase (N), are derived from corresponding antigenically relevant wild-type influenza viruses included in the annual vaccine formulation. Thus, the 3 viruses contained in *FluMist* maintain the replication characteristics and phenotypic properties of the MDV and express the H and N of wild-type viruses that are related to strains expected to circulate during the corresponding influenza season.

Use Characteristics

Indications: For active immunization for the prevention of disease caused by influenza A and B viruses in healthy children and adolescents, 2 to 17 years of age, and healthy adults, 18 to 49 years of age.

Limitations: *FluMist* is not indicated for immunization of people younger than 2 years of age, or 50 years of age and older, or for therapy of influenza, nor will it protect against infections and illness caused by infectious agents other than influenza A or B viruses.

The terms "healthy children, adolescents, and adults" exclude people with underlying medical conditions that may predispose them to severe disease following wild-type influenza infection. Such people include, but are not limited to, adults and children with chronic disorders of the cardiovascular and pulmonary systems, including asthma; pregnant women in their second or third trimesters during influenza season; adults and children who required regular medical follow-up or hospitalization during the preceding year because of chronic metabolic diseases (including diabetes), renal dysfunction, or hemoglobinopathies; and adults and children with congenital or acquired immunosuppression caused by underlying disease or immunosuppressive therapy. Injectable influenza vaccine is recommended to immunize high-risk people and the close contacts of immunocompromised people.

Contraindications:

Absolute: None

Relative: People with a history of hypersensitivity, especially anaphylactic reactions, to any component of *FluMist*, including eggs or egg products.

Desensitization with injectable influenza vaccine is possible.

FluMist should not be administered to people with asthma and children younger than 5 years of age with recurrent wheezing because of the potential for increased risk of wheezing after vaccination, unless the potential benefit outweighs the potential risk. Do not administer *FluMist* to people with severe asthma or active wheezing because these individuals have not been studied in clinical trials. Injectable influenza vaccine is available for these people.

FluMist is contraindicated in children and adolescents 2 to 17 years of age receiving aspirin therapy or aspirin-containing therapy, because of the association of Reye syndrome with aspirin and wild-type influenza infection. Injectable influenza vaccine is recommended for these people.

If Guillain-Barré syndrome has occurred within 6 weeks of any prior influenza vaccination, base the decision to give *FluMist* on careful consideration of the potential benefits and risks.

Base administration of *FluMist*, a live virus vaccine, to immunocompromised persons on careful consideration of potential benefits and risks. Although *FluMist* was studied in 57 asymptomatic or mildly asymptomatic adults with HIV infection, data supporting the safety and effectiveness of *FluMist* administration in immunocompromised individuals are limited. Injectable influenza vaccine is an alternative for these people.

Postpone administration of *FluMist* until after the acute phase (at least 72 hours) of febrile and/or substantial respiratory illnesses.

Immunodeficiency: Do not administer *FluMist* to people with known or suspected immune deficiency diseases such as combined immunodeficiency, agammaglobulinemia, and thymic abnormalities and conditions such as human immunodeficiency virus infection, malignancy, leukemia, or lymphoma. *FluMist* is also contraindicated in patients who may be immunosuppressed or have altered or compromised immune status as a consequence of treatment with systemic corticosteroids, alkylating drugs, antimetabolites, radiation, or other immunosuppressive therapies. Injectable influenza vaccine is recommended for these people.

Elderly: *FluMist* is not indicated for use in people 65 years of age and older. Volunteers 65 years of age and older with underlying high-risk medical conditions (n = 200) were studied for safety. Compared with controls, *FluMist* recipients had a higher rate of sore throat. *FluMist* is not indicated for use in people 50 to 64 years of age. In study AV009, effectiveness was not demonstrated in 641 people 50 to 64 years of age. Solicited adverse events were similar in type and frequency to those reported in younger adults.

Carcinogenicity: *FluMist* has not been evaluated for carcinogenic potential.

Mutagenicity: *FluMist* has not been evaluated for mutagenic potential.

Fertility Impairment: *FluMist* has not been evaluated for impairment of fertility.

Pregnancy: Category C. Contraindicated on hypothetical grounds. Animal reproduction studies have not been conducted with *FluMist*. It is not known whether *FluMist* can cross the placenta or cause fetal harm when administered to a pregnant woman. Therefore, *FluMist* should not be administered to pregnant women. Injectable influenza vaccine is explicitly recommended for certain pregnant women.

The effect of the vaccine on embryo-fetal and pre-weaning development was evaluated in a developmental toxicity study using pregnant rats receiving the frozen formulation. Animals received the vaccine either once (during organogenesis on gestation day 6) or twice (before gestation and during organogenesis on gestation day 6), 250 mcL/rat/occasion (approximately 110 to 140 human dose equivalents based on $TCID_{50}$), by intranasal instillation. No adverse effects on pregnancy, parturition, lactation, embryo-fetal, or pre-weaning development were observed. There were no vaccine-related fetal malformations or other evidence of teratogenesis noted in this study.

Lactation: It is not known if *FluMist* crosses into human breast milk. Therefore, as some viruses are excreted in human milk and, additionally, because of the possibility of shedding of vaccine virus and the close proximity of a nursing infant and mother, caution should be exercised if *FluMist* is administered to nursing mothers.

Children: Do not administer *FluMist* to children younger than 24 months of age. In clinical trials, an increased risk of wheezing postvaccination and an increase in hospitalizations was observed in *FluMist* recipients younger than 24 months of age.

Adverse Reactions: In 5 randomized, placebo-controlled studies, 9,537 children and adolescents 1 to 17 years of age and 3,041 adults 18 to 64 years of age received *FluMist*. In addition, 4,179 children 6 to 59 months of age received *FluMist* in a randomized, active-controlled trial. Among pediatric *FluMist* recipients 6 months to 17 years of age, 50% were female; in the study of adults, 55% were female. The most common adverse reactions (10% or more with *FluMist* and 5% or greater than in control) were runny nose or nasal congestion in all ages, temperature higher than 100°F in children 2 to 6 years of age, and sore throat in adults.

Children and adolescents: In a placebo-controlled safety study (AV019) conducted in a large health maintenance organization (HMO) in children 1 to 17 years of age (n = 9,689), an increase in asthma events, identified by review of diagnostic codes, was observed in children younger than 5 years of age (relative risk 3.53, 90% CI: 1.1 to 15.7). This observation was prospectively evaluated in study MI-CP111. In MI-CP111, an active-controlled study, increases in wheezing and hospitalization (for any cause) were observed in children younger than 24 months of age, as shown in the following table.

Percentages of Children with Hospitalizations and Wheezing from Study MI-CP111			
Adverse Reaction	Age Group	*FluMist*	Active Control[a]
Hospitalizations[b]	6 to 23 months (n = 3,967)	4.2%	3.2%
	24 to 59 months (n = 4,385)	2.1%	2.5%
Wheezing[c]	6 to 23 months (n = 3,967)	5.9%	3.8%
	24 to 59 months (n = 4,385)	2.1%	2.5%

a Trivalent injectable influenza vaccine.
b From randomization through 180 days after last vaccination.
c Wheezing requiring bronchodilator therapy or with significant respiratory symptoms evaluated from randomization through 42 days after last vaccination.

Most hospitalizations observed involved GI or respiratory infections and occurred more than 6 weeks after vaccination. In post hoc analysis, hospitalization rates in children 6 to 11 months of age (n = 1,367) were 6.1% and 2.6% in *FluMist* and active-control recipients.

The following table shows an analysis of pooled solicited events, occurring in at least 1% of *FluMist* recipients and at a higher rate compared with placebo after dose 1 in studies D153-P501 and AV006 and solicited events after dose 1 in study MI-CP111. Solicited events were those about which parents/guardians were specifically queried after *FluMist* vaccination. Solicited events were documented for 10 days postvaccination. Solicited events after dose 2 for *FluMist* were similar to those after dose 1 and generally observed at a lower frequency.

Summary of Solicited Events Observed Within 10 Days After Dose 1 for Vaccine[a] and Either Placebo or Active Control Recipients; Children 2 to 6 Years of Age				
	D153-P501 and AV006		MI-CP111	
Event	*FluMist* (N = 876 to 1,764)[c]	Placebo (N = 424 to 1,036)[c]	*FluMist* (N = 2,170)[c]	Active Control[b] (N = 2,165)[c]
Runny nose/nasal congestion	58%	50%	51%	42%
Decreased appetite	21%	17%	13%	12%
Irritability	21%	19%	12%	11%
Decreased activity (lethargy)	14%	11%	7%	6%
Sore throat	11%	9%	5%	6%
Headache	9%	7%	3%	3%
Muscle aches	6%	3%	2%	2%
Chills	4%	3%	2%	2%
Fever 100° to 101°F Oral	9%	6%	6%	4%
101° to 102°F Oral	4%	3%	4%	3%

a Frozen formulation used in AV006. Refrigerated formulations used in D153-P501 and MI-CP111.
b Trivalent injectable influenza vaccine.
c Number of evaluable subjects (those who returned diary cards) for each event. Range reflects differences in data collection between the 2 pooled studies.

In studies D153-P501 and AV006, other adverse reactions in children occurring in 1% or more of *FluMist* recipients and at a higher rate compared with placebo were abdominal pain (2%; 0%) and otitis media (3%; 1%).

An additional adverse reaction identified in trial MI-CP111 occurring in 1% or more of *FluMist* recipients and at a higher rate compared with active control was sneezing (2%; 1%).

In a separate trial (MI-CP112) that compared the refrigerated and frozen formulations of *FluMist* in children and adults ages 5 to 49 years of age, the solicited events and other adverse events were consistent with observations from previous trials. Temperature higher than 103°F was observed in 1% to 2% of children 5 to 8 years of age.

In a separate placebo-controlled trial (D153-P526) using the refrigerated formulation in a subset of older children and adolescents 9 to 17 years of age who received 1 dose of *FluMist*, the solicited events and other adverse events were generally consistent with observations from previous trials. Abdominal pain was reported in 12% of *FluMist* recipients compared with 4% of placebo recipients and decreased activity was reported in 6% of *FluMist* recipients compared with 0% of placebo recipients.

Adults: In adults 18 to 49 years of age in study AV009, solicited adverse events occurring in 1% or more of *FluMist* recipients and at a higher rate compared with placebo included runny nose, (44%; 27%), headache (40%; 38%), sore throat (28%; 17%), tiredness/weakness (26%; 22%), muscle aches (17%; 15%), cough (14%; 11%), and chills (9%; 6%). Other adverse reactions from study AV009 occurring in 1% or more of *FluMist* recipients and at a higher rate compared with placebo were nasal congestion (9%; 2%) and sinusitis (4%; 2%).

Post-licensing surveillance: The following adverse reactions were identified during post-licensing use of *FluMist*. These events were reported voluntarily from a population of uncertain size, so it is not possible to reliably estimate their frequency or establish a causal relationship to vaccine exposure: Guillain-Barré syndrome, Bell palsy, rash, nausea, vomiting, diarrhea, hypersensitivity reactions (including anaphylactic reaction, facial edema, and urticaria), epistaxis.

Pharmacologic & Dosing Characteristics

Dosage: Approximately 0.1 mL (ie, half the contents of a single sprayer) is administered into each nostril while the recipient is in an upright position. Insert the tip of the sprayer just inside the nose and depress the plunger to spray. Remove the dose-divider clip from the sprayer to administer the second half of the dose (approximately 0.1 mL) into the other nostril.

For healthy children 2 to 8 years of age, not previously vaccinated with any influenza-virus vaccine, give one 0.5 mL dose followed by a second 0.5 mL dose given at least 6 weeks later (preferably 60 ± 14 days apart), for the initial influenza season. Only limited data are available on the degree of protection in children who receive 1 dose. If the child received only 1 dose in the first season, administer 2 doses in the next season.

For healthy children 2 to 8 years of age, previously vaccinated with any influenza-virus vaccine, give one 0.5 mL dose per season.

For healthy children and adults 9 to 49 years of age, give one 0.5 mL dose per season.

If the vaccine recipient sneezes after vaccine administration, the dose should not be repeated.

Route: Intranasal only, do not inject parenterally

Documentation Requirements: Federal law requires that (1) the manufacturer and lot number of this vaccine, (2) the dates of its administration, and (3) the name, address, and title of the person administering the vaccine be documented in the recipient's permanent medical record or in a permanent office log.

Certain adverse events must be reported to VAERS (800-822-7967). Refer to Immunization Documents in the Resources section for complete information.

Overdosage: No data available

Booster Doses: Give previously unvaccinated children 2 to 9 years of age 2 doses, at least 30 days apart, optimally before December 1. Because the duration of protection induced by *FluMist* is not known and yearly antigenic variation in circulating influenza strains is possible, annual revaccination increases the likelihood of protection.

Waste Disposal: Dispose of the used sprayer according to standard procedures for biohazardous waste products.

Efficacy: *FluMist* was administered to approximately 35,000 subjects in clinical studies. The population evaluated included 10,297 healthy children 5 to 17 years of age and 3,297 healthy adults 18 to 49 years of age who received 1 or more dose of *FluMist*. Second and third annual doses have been given to 1,766 and 128 children 5 to 17 years of age, respectively. In randomized, placebo-controlled trials, 4,719 healthy children 5 to 17 years of age and 2,864 healthy adults 18 to 49 years of age received *FluMist*.

The efficacy of *FluMist* against culture-confirmed influenza disease for Types A/H3N2 and B was assessed in a field trial in children. The effectiveness of *FluMist* against Types A/H3N2 and B, defined as a reduction in influenza-like illness and illness-associated health care utilization, was assessed in a field trial in adults. Type A/HlN1 did not circulate during either trial, and no field efficacy data against this strain are available.

Pediatrics: The Pediatric Efficacy Study was a placebo-controlled trial performed in healthy US children to evaluate *FluMist* over 2 seasons. The primary end point was prevention of culture-confirmed influenza illness due to antigenically matched wild-type influenza in healthy children who received 2 doses of vaccine. During the first year of the study a subset of 312 children 60 to 71 months of age were randomized 2:1 to vaccine or placebo. All children with culture-confirmed influenza experienced respiratory symptoms (cough, runny nose, or sore throat) and most experienced fever (68%), health care provider visits (68%), and missed school days (74%).

Compared with placebo recipients, *FluMist* recipients 60 to 71 months of age who received 2 doses of vaccine (n = 238) experienced fewer cases of culture-confirmed influenza (efficacy 87%, 95% CI, 59% to 98%). In the 60 to 71 months-of-age group, children who received 1 dose of *FluMist* experienced a significant reduction in the incidence of culture-confirmed influenza (0 of 54 *FluMist* recipients vs 3 of 20 placebo recipients; efficacy 100%, 95% CI, 47% to 100%).

Approximately 85% of participants returned for the second year of the Pediatric Efficacy Study, including 544 children 60 to 84 months of age. During the second year, the H3N2 strain included in the vaccine was A/Wuhan/359/95. However, the H3N2 strain that primarily circulated was A/Sydney/05/97, which differed antigenically from A/Wuhan/359/95. Type A/Wuhan/359/95 (H3N2) also circulated, as did type B strains. Children remained in the same treatment group as in year 1 and received a single dose of *FluMist* or placebo. The primary end point was the prevention of culture-confirmed influenza illness due to antigenically matched wild-type influenza after a single annual revaccination dose of *FluMist*.

In the subset of 544 children 60 to 84 months of age, illness in the second year was similar in scope and severity to the first year. The overall efficacy of *FluMist* against culture-confirmed wild-type influenza, regardless of antigenic match, was 87% (95% CI, 71% to 94%).

Pediatric comparative study (MI-CP111): A multinational, randomized, double-blind, active-controlled trial was performed to assess the efficacy and safety of *FluMist* compared with an injectable influenza vaccine (active control) in children, using the refrigerated formulation. During the 2004 to 2005 influenza season, 3,916 children younger than 5 years of age and without severe asthma, without use of bronchodilator or steroids, and without wheezing within the prior 6 weeks were randomized to *FluMist* and 3,936 were randomized to active control. Participants were followed through the influenza season to identify illness caused by influenza virus. As the primary end point, culture-confirmed modified CDC-defined influenza-like illness (CDC-ILI) was defined as a positive culture for a wild-type influenza virus associated within ± 7 days of modified CDC-ILI. Modified CDC-ILI was defined as fever (oral temperature 100°F or higher or equivalent) plus cough, sore throat, or runny nose/nasal congestion on the same or consecutive days. In the primary efficacy analysis, *FluMist* demonstrated a 44.5% (95% CI: 22.4 to 60.6) reduction in influenza rate compared with active control as measured by culture-confirmed modified CDC-ILI caused by wild-type strains antigenically similar to those contained in the vaccine.

Pediatric study (D153-P501): A randomized, double-blind, placebo-controlled trial evaluated the efficacy of *FluMist* in children 12 to 35 months of age without high-risk medical conditions against culture-confirmed influenza illness, using the refrigerated formulation. A total of 3,174 children were randomized 3:2 (vaccine:placebo) to receive 2 doses of study vaccine or placebo at least 28 days apart in year 1. Vaccine efficacy was 81% for A/H1N1, 90% for A/H3N1, 44% for B, and 73% overall.

Adults: The Adult Effectiveness Study was a placebo-controlled trial of healthy adults, including 3,920 adults 18 to 49 years of age (2,150 women, 1,770 men). Participants were randomized 2:1 to vaccine or placebo. The trial evaluated effectiveness in reduction of influenza-like illness during the peak influenza outbreak period at each site, based on community surveillance. Efficacy against culture-confirmed influenza was not assessed. The predominant circulating strain of influenza virus during the trial period was A/Sydney/05/97 (H3N2), a strain that differed antigenically from the A/Wuhan/359/95 (H3N2) strain contained in *FluMist*. Type A/Wuhan (H3N2) and type B strains also circulated in the United States during the study period. The primary end point was reduction in proportion of participants with 1 or more episodes of any febrile illness (AFI). Two other, more specific febrile influenza-like illness definitions were also prospectively assessed: severe febrile illness (SFI), and febrile upper respiratory illness (FURI). AFI was defined as symptoms for at least 2 consecutive days with fever on at least 1 day and 2 or more symptoms (fever, chills, headache, runny nose, sore throat, cough, muscle aches, tiredness/weakness) on at least 1 day. SFI was defined as at least 3 consecutive days of symptoms, at least 1 day of fever, and 2 or more symptoms on at least 3 days. FURI was defined as at least 2 consecutive days of upper respiratory infection (URI) symptoms (runny nose, sore throat, or cough), fever on at least 1 day, and at least 2 URI symptoms on at least 1 day. Adults meeting the illness definitions often had associated health care provider visits (25% to 31%), used antibiotics (28% to 32%), and missed at least 1 day of work (51% to 58%).

During the 7-week, site-specific outbreak period among subjects age 18 to 49 years, *FluMist* recipients did not experience a significant reduction in AFI; significant reductions were observed for SFI and FURI. *FluMist* recipients experienced significant reductions in days of health care provider visits associated with SFI (18%, 95% CI, 2% to 31%) and FURI (37%, 95% CI, 24% to 47%) when compared with placebo recipients. However, no significant reduction in days of health care provider visits associated with AFI was observed among *FluMist* recipients when compared with placebo recipients.

Challenge study: The ability of *FluMist* to protect adults from influenza illness after challenge with wild-type influenza was assessed in a placebo-controlled trial in healthy adults 18 to 41 years of age sero-susceptible to at least 1 strain included in the vaccine. Adults were randomized to receive *FluMist* (n = 29) or placebo (n = 31). Each subject was challenged intranasally with 1 strain of wild-type virus (A/H3N2, A/H1N1, or B) to which he/she was sero-susceptible, and the results were pooled for all 3 strains combined within each treatment group. Laboratory-documented influenza illness due to all 3 strains combined was reduced compared with placebo by 85% (95% CI, 28% to 100%) in *FluMist* recipients. A third arm of the study involving the traditional injectable influenza vaccine demonstrated 71% efficacy, which was not statistically different from *FluMist*'s efficacy.

HIV-infected adults: Safety and shedding of vaccine virus following *FluMist* administration were evaluated in 57 HIV-infected (median CD4 cell count 541 cells/mm^3) and 54 HIV-negative adults 18 to 58 years of age in a randomized, double-blind, placebo-controlled trial using the frozen formulation. No serious adverse events were reported during the 1-month follow-up period. Vaccine strain (type B) virus was detected in 1 of 28 HIV-infected subjects on day 5 and none of the HIV-negative *FluMist* recipients. No adverse effects on HIV viral load or CD4 counts were identified following *FluMist*. The effectiveness of *FluMist* in preventing influenza illness in HIV-infected individuals has not been evaluated.

Onset: Not established, probably within 2 weeks

Duration: Not established

Pharmacokinetics:

Distribution: A biodistribution study of intranasally administered radio-labeled placebo was conducted in 7 healthy adult volunteers. The mean percentage of the delivered doses detected were as follows: nasal cavity 89.7%, stomach 2.6%, brain 2.4%, and lung 0.4%. The clinical significance of these findings is unknown.

Transmission: FluMist contains live attenuated influenza viruses that replicate in the nasopharynx of the recipient and are shed in respiratory secretions. Assessing the probability that these shed vaccine viruses will be transmitted from a vaccinated individual to a non-vaccinated individual was the primary objective of a placebo-controlled trial in a daycare setting in Finland. Children enrolled in the study attended daycare at least 3 days per week for 4 hours/day, and were in a playroom with at least 4 children, at least 1 of whom was vaccinated with *FluMist*. A total of 197 children 8 to 36 months of age were randomized to receive 1 dose of *FluMist* (n = 98) or placebo (n = 99). Virus shedding was evaluated for 21 days by culture of nasal swabs obtained from each subject approximately 3 times per week. Wild-type A (H3N2) influenza virus was documented to have circulated in the community and in the study population during the trial, whereas type A (H1N1) and type B strains did not.

Eighty percent of *FluMist* recipients shed at least 1 vaccine strain, with a mean duration of shedding of 7.6 days (range, 1 to 21 days). The cold-adapted (CA) and temperature-sensitive (TS) phenotypes were preserved in all shed viruses tested (n = 135). Seven placebo subjects shed 10 influenza isolates, including 1 placebo subject who shed a type B virus confirmed to be a vaccine strain. This type B isolate retained the CA, TS, and ATT phenotypes of the vaccine strain, and had the same genetic sequence when compared with a type B virus shed by a vaccine recipient within the same play group. Six placebo subjects shed 9 isolates identified as type A. Two of these subjects had 2 cultures that grew type A strains (4 isolates) confirmed as wild-type A/Panama (H3N2). The remaining 4 placebo subjects shed type A isolates that could not be further characterized, and thus vaccine strains could not be excluded.

Assuming that a single transmission event occurred (isolation of the type B vaccine strain), the probability of a young child acquiring vaccine virus following close contact with a single *FluMist* vaccinee in this daycare setting was 0.58% (95% CI, 0% to 1.7%) based on the Reed-Frost model. With documented transmission of one type B in one placebo subject and possible transmission of type A viruses in 4 placebo subjects, the probability of acquiring a transmitted vaccine virus was estimated to be 2.4% (95% CI, 0.13% to 4.6%), using the Reed-Frost model.

The frequency and duration of shedding *FluMist* viral strains by people 5 to 49 years of age has not been established. Preliminary data suggest adults may shed *FluMist* viruses for as long as 1 week.

Shed viruses recovered during efficacy trials exhibited genotypic stability, retaining the LAIV genotype and the CA and TS phenotype.

Protective Level: Hemagglutination inhibition (HI) antibody titers of at least 1:40 correlate with clinical protection. There is no single laboratory measurement that correlates with immunity induced by LAIV.

Mechanism: The vaccine viruses replicate efficiently in the mucosa of the nasopharynx. Immune mechanisms conferring protection against influenza after vaccination with *FluMist* are not fully understood, but include production of IgG and IgA antibodies. Likewise, naturally acquired immunity to wild-type influenza has not been completely elucidated. Serum antibodies, mucosal (ie, secretory) antibodies, and influenza-specific T cells may play a role in prevention and recovery from infection. Vaccination with *FluMist* induces influenza strain-specific serum antibodies.

Drug Interactions: Concurrent use of *FluMist* with antiviral compounds active against influenza A and/or B viruses has not been evaluated. Based upon the potential for interference, do not administer *FluMist* until 48 hours after ceasing antiviral therapy. Do not administer antiviral agents until 2 weeks after administration of *FluMist*, unless medically indicated.

There are no data regarding coadministration of *FluMist* with other intranasal preparations, including steroids.

As with other live virus vaccines, do not administer *FluMist* to people who may be immunosuppressed or have altered or compromised immune status as a consequence of treatment with systemic corticosteroids, alkylating drugs, antimetabolites, radiation, or other immunosuppressive therapies. Injectable influenza vaccine is recommended for these people.

Do not administer *FluMist* to children or adolescents receiving aspirin therapy or aspirin-containing therapy. Injectable influenza vaccine is recommended for these people.

The safety and immunogenicity of *FluMist* when administered concurrently with inactivated vaccines have not been determined. Concurrent administration of *FluMist* with MMR vaccine and varicella vaccine was studied in 1,245 children 12 to 15 months of age. Adverse events were similar to those seen in other clinical trials with *FluMist*. No evidence of interference with immune responses to measles, mumps, rubella, varicella, and *FluMist* vaccines was observed; however, *FluMist* is not indicated for use in children younger than 24 months of age. The ACIP recommends that standard recommendations for spacing of live-virus vaccines be observed: no restrictions on timing of inactivated vaccinations and administration of multiple live-virus vaccines either simultaneously or 4 or more weeks apart.

Lab Interference: Data related to shedding of *FluMist* in children and adults are limited. Nasopharyngeal secretions or swabs collected from vaccinees may test positive for influenza virus for up to 3 weeks.

Patient Information: Before administering *FluMist*, ask recipients or their parent or guardian about current health status, personal medical history and the medical history of household and close contacts, including immune status, to determine the existence of any contraindications to immunization with *FluMist*. *FluMist* recipients should avoid close contact (eg, within the same household) with immunocompromised people for at least 21 days.

Pharmaceutical Characteristics

Concentration: Each 0.2 mL dose contains $10^{6.5-7.5}$ fluorescent focus units (FFU) of live attenuated influenza virus reassortants of each of 3 strains recommended by the US Public Health Service for the annual season.

Quality Assay: Each lot of viral harvest is tested for cold-adapted, temperature-sensitive, and attenuated characteristics and also tested extensively by in vitro and in vivo methods to detect adventitious agents.

Influenza Vaccine, Trivalent, Types A & B, Live (Nasal)

Packaging: Package of 10 prefilled, single-use glass sprayers (NDC #: revised annually). The *Teflon* tip attached to the sprayer is equipped with a one-way valve that produces a fine mist primarily deposited in the nose and nasopharynx.

Doseform: Solution. Some proteinaceous particulates may be present but do not affect the use of the product.

Appearance: A colorless to pale yellow liquid, clear to slightly cloudy

Solvent: Allantoic egg fluid, sucrose, potassium phosphate, monosodium glutamate (0.47 mg/dose)

Adjuvant: None

Preservative: None

Allergens: Gentamicin sulfate is added early in the manufacturing process during preparation of reassortant viruses at a calculated concentration of approximately 1 pg/mL. Later steps of the manufacturing process do not use gentamicin, resulting in a diluted residual concentration in the final product of less than 0.015 mcg/mL (limit of detection of the assay).

Excipients: Each 0.2 mL dose contains monosodium glutamate 0.188 mg, hydrolyzed porcine gelatin 2 mg, arginine 2.42 mg, sucrose 13.68 mg, dibasic potassium phosphate 2.26 mg, and monosodium phosphate 0.96 mg.

pH: Data not provided

Shelf Life: Expires 18 weeks from the date of manufacture of the final filled container, but not beyond June 30 at the end of influenza season in the northern hemisphere, to minimize errors in administering the wrong annual formula formulation.

Storage/Stability: Refrigerate, 2° to 8°C (36° to 46°F).

Handling:

(1) Remove rubber tip protector.

(2) While the patient is in an upright position with head tilted back, place the tip just inside the nostril to ensure *FluMist* is delivered into the nose.

(3) Depress plunger as rapidly as possible.

(4) Pinch and remove dose-divider clip.

(5) Place the tip just inside the other nostril and depress plunger as rapidly as possible to deliver remaining vaccine.

Production Process: Each of the 3 influenza virus strains contained in *FluMist* is a genetic reassortant of a master donor virus (MDV) and a wild-type influenza virus. The MDVs were developed by serial passage at sequentially lower temperatures in specific pathogen-free (SPF) primary chick kidney cells. During this process, the MDVs acquired the phenotype and multiple mutations in the gene segments that encode viral proteins other than the surface glycoproteins.

Viral harvests used in the production of *FluMist* are produced by inoculating each of the 3 reassortant viruses into specific pathogen-free (SPF) eggs incubated to allow for vaccine virus replication. The allantoic fluid of these eggs is harvested, pooled, and then clarified by filtration. The virus is concentrated by ultracentrifugation and diluted with stabilizing buffer to obtain the final sucrose and potassium phosphate concentrations. In addition, EDTA is added to the dilution buffer for H3N2 strains. The viral harvests are then sterile filtered to produce the monovalent bulks. Each lot is tested for *ca*, *ts*, and *att* phenotypes and is also tested extensively by in vitro and in vivo methods to detect adventitious agents. Monovalent bulks from the 3 strains are subsequently blended and diluted as required to obtain the desired potency with stabilizing buffers to produce the trivalent bulk vaccine. The bulk vaccine is then filled directly into individual sprayers for nasal administration.

Influenza Vaccine, Trivalent, Types A & B, Live (Nasal)

Media: Extraembryonic (allantoic) fluids of specific pathogen-free (SPF) embryonated chicken eggs.

Disease Epidemiology

See description under monograph for traditional injectable influenza vaccine.

Other Information

Perspective: See description under monograph for traditional injectable influenza vaccine.

First Licensed: June 17, 2003 (frozen formulation), January 5, 2007 (refrigerator-stable formulation)

National Policy: ACIP. Prevention and control of influenza with vaccines: recommendations of the Advisory Committee on Immunization Practices (ACIP), 2012-2013 influenza season. *MMWR.* 2012;61(32):613-618.

HICPAC, ACIP. Influenza vaccination of health care personnel. *MMWR.* 2007;56(RR-5):1-54.

References: Belshe RB, et al. The efficacy of live attenuated, cold-adapted, trivalent, intranasal influenza virus vaccine in children. *N Engl J Med.* 1998;338(20):1405-1412.

Belshe RB, et al. Efficacy of vaccination with live attenuated, cold-adapted, trivalent, intranasal influenza virus vaccine against a variant (A/Sydney) not contained in the vaccine. *J Pediatr.* 2000;136(2):168-175.

Murphy BR, Coelingh KC. Principles underlying the development and use of live attenuated cold-adapted influenza A and influenza B virus vaccines. *Viral Immunol.* 2002;15(2):295-323.

Nichol KL, et al. Effectiveness of live, attenuated intranasal influenza virus vaccine in healthy, working adults: a randomized controlled trial. *JAMA.* 1999;282(2):137-144.

Treanor JJ, et al. Evaluation of trivalent, live, cold-adapted (CAIV-T) and inactivated (TIV) influenza vaccines in prevention of virus infection and illness following challenge of adults with wild-type influenza A (H1N1), A (H3N2), and B viruses. *Vaccine.* 1999;18(9-10):899-906.

Pharmacoeconomics: Sullivan KM. Health impact of influenza in the United States. *Pharmacoeconomics.* 1996;9(suppl 3):26-33.

Japanese Encephalitis Vaccine

Viral Vaccines

Name:
  Ixiaro

Manufacturer:
  Intercell, distributed by Novartis Vaccine and
  Diagnostics

Synonyms: JE vaccine, *Jespect*. The disease was previously called Japanese encephalitis type B.

Immunologic Characteristics

Microorganism: Japanese encephalitis virus (JEV), single-stranded RNA virus, family Flaviviridae

Viability: Inactivated

Antigenic Form: Inactivated, whole virus

Antigenic Type: Protein

Strains: SA14-14-2

Use Characteristics

Indications: To induce active immunity to prevent disease caused by JEV in persons 17 years of age and older. In general, vaccination is recommended for people who plan to reside in or travel to areas where JEV is endemic or epidemic during a transmission season, principally those who will spend at least 1 month doing extensive outdoor activities in rural areas, which places them at high risk for exposure.

Consider the incidence of JEV in the location of the intended stay, the conditions of housing, nature of activities, duration of stay, and the possibility of unexpected travel to high-risk areas before vaccinating. Consult current references with regard to JEV endemicity for specific locations.

Laboratory-acquired JEV has been reported in 22 cases. JEV may be transmitted in research laboratories through needle sticks and other accidental exposures. Vaccine-derived immunity presumably protects against exposure through these percutaneous routes. Exposure to aerosolized JEV and particularly to high concentrations of virus, which may occur during viral purification, could lead to infection through mucous membranes and possibly directly into the CNS through the olfactory mucosa. It is unknown whether vaccine-derived immunity protects against such exposures, but all laboratory workers with a potential for exposure to infectious JEV should be immunized.

Limitations: Vaccinees who receive only 1 dose may have a suboptimal response and may therefore incur a higher risk if exposed to JEV, compared with vaccinees who receive both doses. *Ixiaro* will not protect against encephalitis caused by pathogens other than JEV.

JEV vaccine is not recommended for all people traveling to or residing in Asia. In the decision to vaccinate, balance the risk of exposure to the virus and for developing illness, the availability and acceptability of mosquito repellents and other alternative protective measures, and the adverse effects of vaccination. Risk of JEV in highly endemic areas during the transmission season can reach 1 of 5,000 per month of exposure; risk for most short-term travelers may be 1 of 1,000,000.

Contraindications: People with a history of serious allergic reaction to a vaccine component or after a prior dose of this vaccine. This vaccine contains protamine sulfate, a compound known to cause hypersensitivity reactions in some individuals.

Immunodeficiency: Patients receiving immunosuppressive therapy or with other immunodeficiencies may have a diminished antibody response to active immunization. They may remain susceptible despite immunization.

Elderly: Clinical studies of *Ixiaro* did not include sufficient subjects at least 65 years of age to determine whether they respond differently than younger subjects. Among 24 *Ixiaro*-vaccinated subjects at least 65 years of age, the seroconversion rate was 95.8% and geometric mean titer was 255.2. In subjects at least 65 years of age vaccinated in any of 5 trials included in a pooled dataset (N = 161), adverse events were reported in 62% (73/118) of *Ixiaro* recipients, 58% (15/26) of *JE-Vax* recipients, and 71% (12/17) among controls. Five serious adverse events were reported.

Carcinogenicity: *Ixiaro* has not been evaluated for carcinogenic potential.

Mutagenicity: *Ixiaro* has not been evaluated for mutagenic potential.

Fertility Impairment: The effect of *Ixiaro* vaccine on embryo-fetal and preweaning development was evaluated in a developmental toxicity study using pregnant rats. One group of rats was administered *Ixiaro* twice before gestation and once during the period of organogenesis (gestation day 6). A second group of pregnant rats was administered *Ixiaro* once before gestation and once during the period of organogenesis (gestation day 6). *Ixiaro* was administered intramuscularly (IM) at 0.5 mL per rat per occasion (approximately 300-fold higher than the human dose on a mg/kg basis). No adverse effects on mating, fertility, pregnancy, parturition, lactation, embryo-fetal or preweaning development were observed. There was a statistically significant finding of incomplete ossification in a few fetuses derived from the second group of pregnant rats. However, there are no data to suggest that this finding is vaccine related. There were no vaccine-related fetal malformations or other evidence of teratogenesis noted in this study.

The effect of *Ixiaro* on male fertility has not been evaluated.

Pregnancy: Category B. Reproduction studies were performed in female rats at doses approximately 300-fold higher than the human dose (on a mg/kg basis) and revealed no evidence of impaired fertility or harm to the fetus caused by *Ixiaro*. However, there are no adequate and well-controlled studies in pregnant women. Because animal reproduction studies are not always predictive of human response, use *Ixiaro* during pregnancy only if clearly needed. It is not known if JEV-neutralizing antibodies cross the placenta. Generally, most immunoglobulin G (IgG) passage across the placenta occurs during the third trimester. Problems in humans have not been documented and are unlikely. Consider that JE acquired during pregnancy carries the potential for intrauterine infection and fetal death. To enter a woman inadvertently vaccinated during pregnancy in a prospective registry, contact Novartis Vaccines at 800-244-7668.

Lactation: It is not known if JEV-neutralizing antibodies cross into human breast milk. Problems in humans have not been documented and are unlikely. It is not known whether this vaccine is excreted in human milk.

Children: Safety and efficacy of *Ixiaro* in children younger than 17 years of age have not been established.

Adverse Reactions: The most common (at least 10%) systemic adverse events were headache and myalgia. The most common (at least 10%) injection-site reactions were pain and tenderness. In 5 clinical studies conducted in North America, Europe, Australia, and New Zealand, 3,558 adults 18 to 86 years received at least 1 dose of *Ixiaro* (92% completed the 2-dose series) and were followed for safety for at least 6 months after the first dose. In this pooled dataset, 1 death occurred in a subject with metastatic lung adenocarcinoma 4 months after completing the 2-dose regimen. Approximately 1% of subjects experienced a serious adverse event, including 1 case of multiple sclerosis. Approximately 1% of subjects discontinued because of adverse events.

Safety was evaluated in a randomized, controlled, double-blind clinical trial in healthy men and women. *Ixiaro* was compared with a control product containing phosphate-buffered saline with aluminum hydroxide 0.1%. A total of 2,675 subjects were randomized in a 3:1 ratio to receive *Ixiaro* 0.5 mL IM on days 0 and 28 or the control product on the same schedule. Analysis was carried among 1,993 subjects receiving at least 1 dose of *Ixiaro* and 657 subjects receiving at least 1 dose of control product (mean age, 33.8 years [range, 18 to 86 years]; 55% women; 92% white, 2% Asian, 3% black, 3% other). Subjects recorded adverse events on a diary card for the first 7 days after each vaccination. In addition, the study investigator took a medical history and performed a physical exam to evaluate for adverse events on the day of each vaccination and at a visit 4 weeks after the second vaccination.

Serious adverse events: No deaths occurred during this trial. Sixteen serious adverse events were reported during the study period (10 in *Ixiaro* recipients and 6 in control recipients). The serious adverse events in the *Ixiaro* group included dermatomyositis, appendicitis, rectal hemorrhage, limb abscess (contralateral to injected arm), chest pain, ovarian torsion, ruptured corpus luteal cyst, and 3 orthopedic injuries.

Systemic adverse events: Overall, the percentage of subjects who experienced at least 1 adverse event during the study period was 59% in the *Ixiaro* group, compared with 57% in the control group. The severity of adverse events was as follows: mild in 34% (*Ixiaro*) and 34% (control), moderate in 20% (*Ixiaro*) and 17% (control), and severe in 5% (*Ixiaro*) and 5% (control). Adverse events of any severity occurring in at least 1% of subjects are shown in the following table.

Common Systemic Adverse Events After *Ixiaro* or Control						
	Incidence (% of subjects)					
	Days 0 to 28		Days 28 to 56		Days 0 to 56	
Adverse event	*Ixiaro* (n = 1,993)	Control (n = 657)	*Ixiaro* (n = 1,968)	Control (n = 645)	*Ixiaro* (n = 1,993)	Control (n = 657)
Headache[a]	21.6	20.2	13.4	13	27.9	26.2
Myalgia[a]	13.3	12.9	5.6	5.3	15.6	15.5
Fatigue[a]	8.6	8.7	5.2	5.9	11.3	11.7
Influenza-like illness[a]	8.2	8.5	5.8	4.3	12.3	11.7
Nausea[a]	4.7	5.3	2.6	3.7	6.6	7.5
Nasopharyngitis	2.3	1.8	2.6	2.3	4.7	4
Pyrexia[a]	1.9	2.1	1.5	1.7	3.2	3
Rhinitis	1	0.8	0.5	0.6	1.4	1.4
Upper respiratory infection	0.9	0.9	0.8	0.9	1.7	2
Back Pain	0.8	0.9	0.6	0.2	1.3	1.1
Pharyngolaryngeal pain	0.8	0.9	1	0.5	1.6	1.4
Rash[a]	0.8	0.9	0.7	0.8	1.3	1.5
Diarrhea	0.8	0.8	0.7	0.3	1.5	1.1
Cough	0.8	0.8	0.6	0.6	1.2	1.2
Vomiting[a]	0.6	0.8	0.8	0.9	1.4	1.7

a These symptoms were solicited in a subject diary card. Percentages include unsolicited events that occurred after the 7-day period covered by the diary card.

Injection-site reactions: The severity of injection-site reactions observed after either dose was as follows: mild in 42% (*Ixiaro*) and 44% (control), moderate in 10% (*Ixiaro*) and 8% (control), and severe in 3% (*Ixiaro*) and 3% (control). The frequency of injection-site reactions of any severity appears in the following table.

Solicited Injection-Site Reactions[a] After *Ixiaro* or Control					
	Incidence after dose 1 (% of subjects[b])		Incidence after dose 2 (% of subjects[b])		Incidence overall (% of subjects[b])
Adverse reaction	*Ixiaro* (n = 1,963[c])	Control (n = 645[c])	*Ixiaro* (n = 1,951[c])	Control (n = 638[c])	*Ixiaro* (n = 1,963[c])	Control (n = 645[c])
Any reaction	48.5	47.7	32.6	32.2	55.4	56.2
Pain	27.7	28.2	17.7	18.2	33	35.8
Tenderness	28.8	26.9	22.5	18.1	35.9	32.6
Erythema	6.8	5.4	4.6	4.1	9.6	7.4
Induration	4.8	5.3	4	3	7.5	7.4
Edema	2.4	3.3	2.3	1.6	4.2	4.6
Pruritus	2.6	3.3	1.6	1.9	3.8	4.5

a Injection-site reactions were assessed for 7 days after each dose.
b Denominators used to calculate percentages are based on the number of evaluable diary card entries (defined as documented presence on any day [ie, entry of "yes"] or absence on all days [ie, entry of "no"]) for each individual symptom and observation period.
c n = number of subjects who returned diary cards after each dose

Adverse events compared with JE-Vax: The safety of *Ixiaro* compared with another inactivated JEV vaccine (*JE-Vax*, Sanofi Pasteur) was evaluated in a randomized, double-blind clinical trial. No deaths occurred during this trial. One serious adverse event occurred in a subject with a history of myocardial infarction (MI) who experienced an MI 3 weeks after receiving the second dose of *Ixiaro*. The most common adverse events after immunization occurring in at least 1% of subjects were headache, myalgia, fatigue, influenza-like illness, nausea, nasopharyngitis, pyrexia, pharyngolaryngeal pain, cough, rash, diarrhea, sinusitis, upper respiratory tract infection, back pain, migraine, vomiting, and influenza, which occurred with similar frequency in both treatment groups. Injection-site reactions solicited in diary cards were observed at a rate of 54% in the *Ixiaro* group (n = 428) compared with 69% in the *JE-Vax* group (n = 435).

Safety in concomitant use with hepatitis A vaccine: The safety of *Ixiaro* administered concomitantly with hepatitis A vaccine (*Havrix*, GSK) was evaluated in a controlled trial in which subjects were assigned randomly to 1 of 3 treatment groups: group A (n = 62) received *Ixiaro* plus *Havrix*; group B (n = 65) received *Ixiaro* plus control; group C (n = 65) received *Havrix* plus control. One serious adverse event occurred in this trial in a subject with a history of alcoholism and seizure disorder who experienced a seizure 3 weeks after receiving the second dose of *Ixiaro* plus control. The percentages of subjects who experienced at least 1 adverse event were as follows: 39% in group A, 42% in group B, and 48% in group C. The most frequently reported injection-site reaction on the day of the first vaccination in all 3 groups was injection-site pain: 59% in group A, 48% in group B, and 48% in group C.

Pharmacologic & Dosing Characteristics

Dosage: Two 0.5 mL doses administered 28 days apart

Route: IM. Do not inject intravenously, intradermally, or subcutaneously.

Booster Doses: If the primary series was administered more than 1 year previously, a booster dose may be given before potential re-exposure. The immunogenicity of booster doses was assessed in seronegative subjects following 3 primary immunization regimens (2 × 6 mcg [the licensed dose], 1 × 12 mcg, or 1 × 6 mcg). Booster doses were administered at 11 or 23 months after the first dose to subjects with JE-neutralizing antibody titers less than 1:10. Results showed that the second injection can be given up to 11 months after the first one. When a second dose was given 11 months after the first dose, the seroconversion rate was 99% (99/100; GMT of 504; 95% CI, 367-692) 4 weeks later, and by month 24 was 89% (85/96; GMT of 121; 95% CI, 87-168) without any further doses. In the group with 2-dose primary immunization, the rates of subjects with persistent JE-neutralizing antibody titers of at least 1:10 without a booster dose at months 12 and 24 were 58% (95% CI, 49-67) and 48% (95% CI, 39-57), respectively, and GMTs were 18 (95% CI, 14-23) and 16 (95% CI, 13-21). After a booster dose to subjects with JE-neutralizing antibodies titers less than 1:10 in the group with complete primary immunization, SCRs 4 weeks after the booster at months 11 and 23 were 100% (17/17; 95% CI, 82-100) and 100% (27/27; 95% CI, 88-100), respectively, and GMTs were 674 (95% CI, 379-1,198) and 2,537 (95% CI, 1,468-4,384), respectively.

Missed Doses: Interrupting the recommended schedule or delaying subsequent doses does not require restarting the series.

Efficacy: Clinical trials of JEV vaccines found that neutralizing antibody, as measured by a plaque-reduction neutralization test, is protective against JEV infection. Therefore, *Ixiaro* was evaluated for immunogenicity using plaque-reduction neutralization test as a serological correlate of protection. Immunogenicity was evaluated in a randomized, active-controlled, observer-blinded clinical trial conducted in the United States, Germany, and Austria in 867 healthy men and women 18 to 80 years of age (mean age, 41 years; 61% women; 81% white, 1% Asian, 13% black, 5% other). *Ixiaro* recipients received 3 IM doses: *Ixiaro* on day 0, control product on day 7, and *Ixiaro* on day 28. The comparator group received *JE-Vax* 1 mL on days 0, 7, and 28. The coprimary end points were seroconversion rate, defined as anti-JEV antibody titer at least 1:10, and geometric mean titer at day 56 in the per protocol population. The immune responses elicited by *Ixiaro* met predefined statistical criteria for noninferiority compared with those induced by *JE-Vax*.

Immune Responses After *Ixiaro* or *JE-Vax*, Per Protocol Population			
	Seroconversion Rates		
Time point	*Ixiaro* seroconversion rate (n/N) (95% CI)	*JE-Vax* seroconversion rate (n/N) (95% CI)	Rate difference (95% CI)
Prevaccination screen	0	0	
Day 56 (28 days after vaccine dose 2)	96.4% (352/365) (94%-97.9%)	93.8% (347/370) (90.9%-95.8%)	2.6% (−0.5%-6%)[a]
	GMTs		
Time point	*Ixiaro* n = 365 n (GMT) (95% CI)	*JE-VAX* n = 370 n (GMT) (95% CI)	GMT ratio estimator (95% CI)
Prevaccination screen	365 (5[b])	370 (5[b])	
Day 56 (28 days after vaccine dose 2)	361 (243.6) (216.4-274.1)	364 (102) (90.3-115.2)	2.33 (1.97-2.75)[c]

a Seroconversion rates: noninferiority of *Ixiaro* compared with *JE-Vax* for seroconversion rates was demonstrated if lower bound of 2-sided 95% confidence interval [CI] for seroconversion rate difference (*Ixiaro* minus *JE-Vax*) was greater than 10% at day 56.

b Prevaccination titers were negative by definition in per-protocol population and have been imputed to 5.

c Geometric mean titers (GMTs): noninferiority of *Ixiaro* compared with *JE-Vax* for GMTs was demonstrated if lower bound of 2-sided 95% CI for GMT ratio (*Ixiaro/JE-VAX*) was grater than 1 of 1.5 at day 56.

Onset: Receive the second dose at least 1 week before potential exposure to JEV.

Duration: The full duration of protection following immunization is not known.

Pharmacokinetics:

Long-term immunogenicity: The persistence of JE-neutralizing antibody was evaluated in subjects recruited after participation in 1 of 2 clinical trials. In the intent-to-treat (ITT) population of subjects randomized to *Ixiaro* (N = 181), seroconversion rates at 6 and 12 months after starting the 2-dose series were 95% [95% CI, 90.8-97.4%] and 83.4% [95% CI, 77.3-88.1%], respectively. GMTs at 6 and 12 months after starting the 2-dose series were 83.5 [95% CI, 70.9-98.4] and 41.2 [95% CI, 34.4-49.3], respectively.

Temporal immunogenicity: In a randomized, dosing regimen, observer-blinded clinical trial in 374 healthy subjects 18 to 76 years, the immunogenicity of *Ixiaro* was evaluated on days 10, 28, 35, and 56. Seroconversion rates at each time point for the subjects randomized to the standard dosing regimen (*Ixiaro* on days 0 and 28) are displayed in the following table.

Seroconversion Rates During the Vaccination Series (*Ixiaro* on Days 0 and 28), Per-Protocol Population			
Day 10 (10 days after dose 1)	Day 28 (28 days after dose 1)	Day 35 (7 days after dose 2)	Day 56 (28 days after dose 2)
Seroconversion rate (n/N) (95% CI)	Seroconversion rate (n/N) (95% CI)	Seroconversion rate (n/N) (95% CI)	Seroconversion rate (n/N) (95% CI)
21.1% (24/114) (13.6%-28.5%)	39.8% (45/113) (30.8%-48.8%)	97.3% (110/113) (94.4%-100%)	97.3% (110/113) (94.4%-100%)

Protective Level: Based on challenge experiments in passively protected mice, neutralizing antibody levels at least 1:10 protected against a 105 median lethal dose (LD_{50}), the viral dose thought to be transmitted by an infected mosquito.

Mechanism: Induction of antibodies that neutralize live JEV

Drug Interactions: Inactivated vaccines are not generally affected by circulating antibodies or administration of exogenous antibodies. Vaccination may occur at any time before or after antibody administration. Like all inactivated vaccines, administration of JEV vaccines to patients receiving immunosuppressant drugs (eg, high-dose corticosteroids) or radiation therapy may result in an insufficient response to immunization. They may remain susceptible despite immunization.

Ixiaro was administered concomitantly with hepatitis A vaccine (*Havrix*, GSK) in a randomized clinical trial in 192 healthy subjects 18 to 61 years. There was no evidence for interference with the immune response to *Ixiaro* or to *Havrix* when *Havrix* was administered concomitantly with dose 1 of *Ixiaro*. Data are not available on concomitant administration of *Ixiaro* with other US-licensed vaccines or other drugs (eg, chloroquine, mefloquine). Anti-JEV GMT at day 56 and anti-HAV GMT at day 28 in the concomitant group met noninferiority criteria compared with groups receiving the vaccines separately.

Patient Information: This vaccine may not fully protect recipients. Take personal precautions to reduce exposure to mosquito bites (eg, adequate clothing, repellents, mosquito nets).

Pharmaceutical Characteristics

Concentration: 6 mcg of purified, inactivated JEV proteins per 0.5 mL

Packaging: 0.5 mL single-dose syringe (NDC #: 42515-0001-01); package of two 0.5 mL single-dose syringes (42515-0001-02)

Doseform: Suspension

Appearance: During storage, a clear liquid with a white precipitate. After shaking, a white, opaque, homogeneous suspension. Do not administer if coarse particulate matter remains after shaking or if discoloration is observed

Solvent: Aqueous

Adjuvant: Aluminum hydroxide 250 mcg per 0.5 mL

Preservative: None

Allergens: Protamine sulfate 1 mcg/mL or less. The plunger stopper contains chlorobutyl elastomer. None of the syringe or packaging materials contain latex.

Excipients: Formaldehyde 200 ppm or less, bovine serum albumin 100 ng/mL or less, host-cell DNA 200 pg/mL or less, sodium metabisulphite 200 ppm or less, host-cell proteins 300 ng/mL or less

pH: Not described

Shelf Life: Expires within an unspecified period of time.

Storage/Stability: Store at 2° to 8°C (36° to 46°F). Do not freeze. Store in the original package to protect from light. Contact manufacturer regarding exposure to freezing or elevated temperatures. Shipping data not provided.

Production Process: JE viruses are propagated in Vero cells. Multiple viral harvests are performed, which are pooled, clarified, and concentrated. The virus suspension is treated with protamine sulfate to remove contaminating DNA and proteins. The resulting partially purified virus is processed through a sucrose density-gradient centrifugation step and fractionated. Each fraction is analyzed for the presence of virus, and fractions with the highest virus activity are pooled to give a purified virus suspension. The purified virus is then inactivated by treatment with formaldehyde. The preparation is adjusted to a specified protein concentration and formulated by addition of aluminum hydroxide.

Media: Vero cells

Disease Epidemiology

Incidence: Encephalitis caused by JEV is the most common form of epidemic viral encephalitis in the world, causing an estimated 30,000 to 50,000 cases and 7,000 deaths annually. In China alone, 10,000 cases of Japanese encephalitis occur annually, despite childhood immunization. In areas where JEV is endemic, annual incidence ranges from 1 to 10 infections per 10,000 people. Cases occur primarily in children younger than 15 years of age.

Most cases are asymptomatic. Viral infection induces overt encephalitis, a potentially fatal inflammation of the brain, in 1 per 20 to 1,000 cases. Illness is usually severe, with a case-fatality ratio of 25% to 30% and residual brain disorders in an additional 50% of cases. A higher case-fatality ratio affects the elderly, but serious sequelae are more frequent in the very young, possibly because they are more likely to survive a severe infection.

Countries that have had major epidemics in the past, but that have controlled the disease primarily by vaccination, include China, Korea, Japan, Taiwan, and Thailand. Other countries that still have periodic epidemics include Vietnam, Cambodia, Myanmar, India, Nepal, and Malaysia.

Prevalence: Seroprevalence studies in these endemic areas indicate nearly universal exposure by adulthood. Calculating from a ratio of asymptomatic to symptomatic infections of 200 to 1, approximately 10% of the susceptible population is infected per year. In addition to children 10 years of age and younger, an increase in JEV incidence has been observed in the elderly.

Susceptible Pools: Virus is endemic in parts of Japan, other Pacific islands, and Far East Asia. Each element of the transmission cycle is prevalent in rural areas of Asia, and human infections occur principally in this setting. Because vertebrate-amplifying hosts and agricultural activities may be situated within and at the periphery of cities, human cases occasionally are reported from urban locations.

Transmission: Various species of Culex mosquito, including *Culex tritaeniorhynchus* and the *Culex vishnui* complex. The virus is transmitted in an enzootic cycle among mosquitoes and vertebrate-amplifying hosts, chiefly domestic pigs and, in some areas, wild Ardeid (warfing) birds. Viral infection rates in mosquitoes range from 1% to 3%. These species are prolific in rural areas where their larvae breed in ground pools and flooded rice fields.

JEV is transmitted seasonally in most areas of Asia. Seasonal patterns of viral transmission correlate with abundance of vector mosquitoes and vertebrate-amplifying hosts. Although abundance of mosquitoes fluctuates with the amount of rainfall in some tropical locations, irrigation associated with agricultural practices is a more important factor affecting vector abundance, so transmission may occur year-round. The periods of greatest risk for JE viral transmission vary regionally and from year to year.

Incubation: Usually 5 to 15 days

Communicability: Not directly transmitted from person to person.
Other products: Live, attenuated vaccines are produced in China.

Other Information

Perspective:
1935: Virus isolated from brain of patient dying from encephalitis in Japan.
1943: US scientists produce vaccine based on Russian vaccine in the Far Eastern theater; used in Okinawa in 1945.
1965: Purified Nakayama-NIH strain developed.
1983: Centers for Disease Control and Prevention distributes vaccine in the United States as an investigational new drug until 1987.
1992: *JE-Vax* (Connaught Laboratories) licensed on December 18, 1992. Last doses expired May 2011.

First Licensed: March 30, 2009

National Policy: ACIP. Japanese encephalitis vaccines: Recommendations of the ACIP. *MMWR.* 2010;59(RR-1):1-27.

ACIP. Recommendations for use of a booster dose of inactivated Vero cell culture–derived Japanese encephalitis vaccine: Advisory Committee on Immunization Practices, 2011. *MMWR.* 2011;60(May 27):661-663.

Canadian Committee to Advise on Tropical Medicine and Travel (CATMAT). Statement on protection against Japanese encephalitis vaccine.*Can Comm Dis Rep.* 2008;34(ACS-4):1-14.

WHO. Japanese encephalitis vaccines. *Wkly Epidemiol Rec.* 2006;81:331-340.

References: CDC. Update on Japanese encephalitis vaccine for children — United States, May 2011. *MMWR.* 2011;60(May 27):664-665.

Duggan ST, Plosker GL. Japanese encephalitis vaccine (inactivated, adsorbed) [*Ixiaro*]. *Drugs.* 2009;69:115-122.

Erlanger TE, Weiss S, Keiser J, Utzinger J, Wiedenmayer K. Past, present, and future of Japanese encephalitis. *Emerg Infect Dis.* 2009;15(Jan):1-7.

Hoke CH, Nisalak A, Sangawhipa N, et al. Protection against Japanese encephalitis by inactivated vaccines. *N Engl J Med.* 1988;319:608-614.

Hombach J, Solomon T, Kurane I, et al. Report on a WHO consultation on immunological endpoints for evaluation of new Japanese encephalitis vaccines. *Vaccine.* 2005;23:5205-5211.

Vaughn DW, Hoke CH Jr. The epidemiology of Japanese encephalitis: Prospects for prevention. *Epidemiol Rev.* 1992;14:197-221.

Japanese Encephalitis Vaccine Summary Table		
Indication	To induce immunity against Japanese encephalitis virus.	
Brand name	*JE-Vax*[a]	*Ixiaro*
Manufacturer	Sanofi Pasteur	Intercell, Novartis
Viability	Inactivated vaccine	Inactivated vaccine
Strain	Nakayama-NIH	SA14-14-2
Dosage	1 mL (0.5 mL if < 3 years)	0.5 mL
Route	Subcutaneous	IM
Standard schedule	Days 0, 7, and 30	Days 0 and 28
Licensed ages	1 year and older	17 years and older
Booster schedule	Boost after 24 to 36 months	Interval not yet determined
Concentration	2 to 3 mcg nitrogen per mL	6 mcg JEV proteins per 0.5 mL
Doseform	Powder for suspension	Suspension
Diluent	Sterile water	n/a
Adjuvant	None	Aluminum hydroxide 250 mcg per 0.5 mL
Preservative	Thimerosal 0.007%	None
Excipients	Mouse protein, gelatin, formaldehyde, polysorbate 80	Protamine sulfate, formaldehyde, bovine albumin, host-cell proteins, sodium metabisulphite
Medium	Mouse brains	Vero cells
Packaging	Three 1 mL vials plus diluent, 10-dose vial plus diluent	Prefilled 0.5 mL syringes
Routine storage	2° to 8°C	2° to 8°C
Stability	Discard within 8 hours after reconstitution.	n/a

a Distributed in the US from 1992 to 2011. Information provided for historical perspective.

Comparison Table of Measles, Mumps, Rubella, and Varicella Vaccines		
Generic name	Measles-mumps-rubella vaccine	Measles-mumps-rubella-varicella vaccine
Brand name	*M-M-R II*	*ProQuad*
Synonyms	MMR	MMRV
Manufacturer	Merck	Merck
Viability	Live viral vaccine	Live viral vaccine
Indication	To prevent infection with measles, mumps, rubella, and/or varicella viruses	
Components	Measles, mumps, rubella vaccine	Measles, mumps, rubella, varicella vaccine
Concentration	Measles: > 1,000 $TCID_{50}$ Mumps: > 20,000 $TCID_{50}$ Rubella: > 1,000 $TCID_{50}$ each per 0.5 mL	Measles: > 1,000 $TCID_{50}$ Mumps: > 20,000 $TCID_{50}$ Rubella: > 1,000 $TCID_{50}$ Varicella: > 10,000 PFU each per 0.5 mL
Adjuvant	None	None
Preservative	None	None
Doseform	Powder for solution	Powder for solution
Diluent	Sterile water without preservative	Sterile water without preservative
Packaging	Single-dose vials	Single-dose vials
Routine storage	2° to 8°C	≤ −15°C (5°F)
Stability	Discard within 8 hours of reconstitution	Discard within 30 minutes of reconstitution
Dosage, route	0.5 mL subcutaneously	0.5 mL subcutaneously
Standard schedule	12 to 18 months old and 4 to 6 years of age	12 to 18 months of age and 4 to 6 years of age

Measles, Mumps, & Rubella Virus Vaccine Live

Viral Vaccines

Name:
M-M-R II

Manufacturer:
Merck

Synonyms: In other countries, *M-M-R II* is known as *M-M-Rvax* or *Virivac*.

Immunologic Characteristics

Microorganism: Viruses (single-stranded RNA), measles, mumps, and rubella viruses
Viability: Live, attenuated
Antigenic Form: Whole viruses
Antigenic Type: Protein
Strains:

Measles: Moraten strain (More-attenuated line of Enders' attenuated Edmonston A strain)
Mumps: Jeryl Lynn (B Level) strain
Rubella: Wistar Institute RA 27/3 strain

Use Characteristics

Indications: For simultaneous active immunization against measles, mumps, and rubella and to prevent congenital rubella syndrome (CRS) among offspring of women who contract rubella during pregnancy. Trivalent measles-mumps-rubella (MMR) vaccine or the quadrivalent product containing varicella vaccine is the preferred immunizing agent for most children and many adults. Almost all children and some adults need more than 1 dose of MMR vaccine.

Prior to international travel, vaccinate individuals susceptible to measles, mumps, or rubella.

Limitations: If attenuated measles vaccine is given immediately after exposure to natural measles, some protection may be provided. However, if the vaccine is given a few days before exposure, substantial protection may still result.

Attenuated mumps vaccine does not protect when given after exposure to natural mumps.

There is no evidence that attenuated rubella vaccine given after exposure to natural rubella virus will prevent illness. However, there is no contraindication to vaccinating children already exposed to natural rubella.

Contraindications:

Absolute: Pregnant patients; patients with a personal history of a hypersensitivity reaction to this vaccine or its components (eg, gelatin); patients receiving immunosuppressive therapy.

Relative: Patients with a blood dyscrasia, leukemia, lymphoma of any type, or other malignant neoplasms affecting the bone marrow or lymphatic systems; patients with primary or acquired immunodeficiency, any febrile illness or infection, or active untreated tuberculosis; and patients with a family history of congenital or hereditary immunodeficiency, until the immune competence of the potential vaccine recipient is demonstrated. Refer to individual monographs for details.

Do not vaccinate people who are immunosuppressed in association with AIDS or other clinical manifestations of HIV infection, cellular immune deficiencies, and hypogammaglobulinemic and dysgammaglobulinemic states. Nonetheless, vaccinate asymptomatic children with HIV infection.

Traditionally, experts recommended to not vaccinate people with a history of anaphylactoid or other immediate reactions (eg, hives, swelling of the mouth or throat, difficulty breathing, hypotension, shock) following egg ingestion. The recommendation had been to give people suspected of being hypersensitive to egg protein a skin test using a dilution of the vaccine as the antigen and to not vaccinate people with adverse reactions to such testing.

More recent information indicates that allegedly egg-allergic people almost always fail to react to vaccines containing eggs. This includes people with positive oral-egg challenges or egg skin tests. More anaphylaxis has been reported in patients without allergy to eggs than with the allergy. Patients do react severely to MMR in extraordinarily rare cases, but egg hypersensitivity does little to predict it.

People also are not at risk if they have egg allergies that are not anaphylactoid in nature; vaccinate these people in the usual manner. There is no evidence to indicate that people with allergies to chickens or feathers are at increased risk of reaction to the vaccine.

Immunodeficiency: Do not use in immunodeficient people, including people with congenital or acquired immune deficiencies, whether because of genetics, disease, or drug or radiation therapy. The vaccine contains live viruses. Nonetheless, routine immunization with MMR is recommended for symptomatic and asymptomatic HIV-infected people.

Elderly: Most people born in 1956 or earlier are likely to have been infected naturally and generally are considered not susceptible.

Adults: Vaccinate people born more recently than 1956, unless they have a personal contraindication to vaccination, because they are considered susceptible. Vaccinate people who may be immune but who lack adequate documentation of immunity as evidenced by physician diagnosis, laboratory evidence of immunity, or adequate immunization with live vaccine on or after the first birthday.

Pregnancy: Category C. Contraindicated on hypothetical grounds.

Measles: Contracting natural measles during pregnancy enhances fetal risk. There are no adequate studies of attenuated measles vaccine in pregnant women. Do not intentionally give measles vaccine to pregnant women because the possible effects of the vaccine on fetal development are unknown at this time. If postpubertal women are vaccinated, counsel these women to avoid pregnancy for 1 month following vaccination. It is not known if attenuated measles virus or corresponding antibodies cross the placenta.

Mumps: Although mumps virus can infect the placenta and fetus, there is a lack of good evidence that it can cause congenital malformations in humans. Attenuated mumps-vaccine virus can infect the placenta, but the virus has not been isolated from fetal tissues of susceptible women who were vaccinated and underwent elective abortions. Nonetheless, do not intentionally give attenuated mumps vaccine to pregnant women. If postpubertal women are vaccinated, counsel these women to avoid pregnancy for 1 month following vaccination.

Rubella: Natural rubella infection of the fetus may result in congenital rubella syndrome (CRS). There is evidence suggesting transmission of attenuated rubella virus to the fetus, although the vaccine is not known to cause fetal harm when administered to pregnant women. Nonetheless, do not intentionally give attenuated rubella vaccine to pregnant females. If postpubertal females are vaccinated, counsel these women to avoid pregnancy for 1 month following vaccination. It may be convenient to vaccinate rubella-susceptible women in the immediate postpartum period.

In counseling women who are inadvertently vaccinated when pregnant or who become pregnant within 28 days of vaccination, the following information may be useful. In a 10-year survey of more than 700 pregnant women who received rubella vaccine within 3 months before or after conception (of whom 189 received the Wistar RA 27/3 strain), no newborns had abnormalities compatible with congenital rubella syndrome. Generally, most IgG passage across the placenta occurs during the third trimester.

The Vaccine in Pregnancy Study conducted by the CDC from 1971 to 1989 examined the risk of congenital rubella syndrome in children born to women vaccinated early in pregnancy. Of 324 live births to these mothers, no cases of CRS were observed. No risk of fetal damage is evident after more than 25 years of using this vaccine. To screen a woman of childbearing age, ask if she is pregnant or likely to become pregnant in the next 28 days. Do not vaccinate her if she answers "yes." In this case, encourage vaccination as soon as possible after pregnancy. Otherwise, explain the theoretical risk, recommend avoiding pregnancy, and vaccinate.

Lactation: It is not known if attenuated measles virus or corresponding antibodies are excreted in breast milk. Problems in human mothers or children have not been documented.

It is not known if the mumps virus or corresponding antibodies are excreted in breast milk. Problems in humans have not been documented.

Vaccine-strain rubella virus has been found in breast milk and may be transmitted to infants in this manner. In the infants with serologic evidence of rubella infection, none exhibited severe disease. However, one exhibited mild clinical illness typical of acquired rubella.

Children: Trivalent MMR vaccine is safe and effective for children 12 months of age and older. Vaccination is not recommended for children younger than 12 months of age because remaining maternal virus-neutralizing antibody may interfere with the immune response.

Adverse Reactions: Burning or stinging of short duration at the injection site has occurred. Local pain, induration, and erythema may occur at the site of injection. Reactions are usually mild and transient. Moderate fever (38.3° to 39.4°C; 101° to 102.9°F) occurs occasionally; high fever (higher than 39.4°C; 103°F, 5 to 12 days after vaccination) occurs less commonly (5% to 15%).

Symptoms of the same kind as seen following natural measles or rubella infection may occur after vaccination: Mild regional lymphadenopathy, urticaria, rash, malaise, sore throat, fever, headache, dizziness, nausea, vomiting, diarrhea, polyneuritis, arthralgia or arthritis (usually transient and rarely chronic).

Rarely, erythema multiforme or Stevens-Johnson syndrome has followed vaccination, as have allergic reactions at the injection site, urticaria, diarrhea, febrile and afebrile convulsions or seizures, thrombocytopenia, purpura, and optic neuritis. Very rarely, encephalitis and encephalopathy have occurred within 30 days after measles vaccination, but no cause-and-effect relationship has been established. The risks of encephalitis and encephalopathy are far less after vaccination than after natural measles infection. A similar relationship has been seen between attenuated measles vaccine and risk of subacute sclerosing panencephalitis (SSPE).

Rarely, parotitis or orchitis occur. In most cases, prior exposure to natural mumps was established.

Local reactions characterized by swelling, redness, and vesiculation at the injection site and systemic reactions (including atypical measles) have occurred in people who previously received killed measles vaccine. Rarely, more severe reactions requiring hospitalization, including prolonged high fever, panniculitis, and extensive local reactions, have occurred. There have been no published reports of transmission of attenuated measles virus from vaccinees to susceptible contacts.

Children under treatment for tuberculosis have not experienced exacerbation of that disease when immunized with attenuated measles vaccine. No studies have reported the effect of attenuated measles vaccine on untreated tuberculosis in children.

Isolated cases of polyneuropathy, including Guillain-Barré syndrome, have been reported after immunization with rubella-containing vaccines.

Encephalitis, encephalopathy, measles inclusion-body encephalitis (MIBE), and other nervous system reactions have occurred very rarely in subjects given this vaccine, but a cause-and-effect relationship has not been established.

In view of reported decreases in platelet counts, thrombocytopenic purpura is a theoretical hazard of rubella vaccination. Individuals with current thrombocytopenia may develop more severe thrombocytopenia after vaccination. People who experienced thrombocytopenia with the first dose of MMR vaccine (or its component vaccines) may develop thrombocytopenia with repeat doses. Evaluate the risk-benefit ratio before vaccination in such cases.

Chronic arthritis is associated with natural rubella infection. Only rarely have vaccine recipients developed chronic joint symptoms, but an Institute of Medicine (IOM) report classified the association as consistent with a causal relation. Following vaccination in children, reactions in joints are uncommon (0% to 3%) and generally of brief duration. In adult women, incidence rates for arthritis and arthralgia are higher (12% to 20%) and reactions tend to be more marked and of longer duration. Symptoms may persist for months or, rarely, for years. In adolescent girls, reactions appear to be intermediate in incidence between those in children and in adult women. Even in older women (35 to 45 years of age), reactions are generally well tolerated and rarely interfere with normal activities. Myalgia and paresthesia have been reported rarely. Advise postpubertal females of the frequent occurrence of generally self-limited arthralgia or arthritis 2 to 4 weeks after vaccination.

There have been no published reports of transmission of attenuated mumps virus from vaccinees to susceptible contacts.

Excretion of small amounts of attenuated rubella virus from the nose or throat has occurred in the majority of susceptible individuals 7 to 28 days after vaccination. There is no firm evidence that vaccine virus is transmitted to susceptible people in contact with vaccinees. Transmission through close personal contact, while accepted as a theoretical possibility, is not considered a significant risk. Transmission of attenuated rubella virus to infants through breast milk has been documented.

Other adverse events (without regard to causality) reported during clinical trials, with use of the marketed vaccine, or with use of the vaccine's three components include: Panniculitis, syncope, irritability, vasculitis, pancreatitis, diabetes mellitus, leukocytosis, angioneurotic edema, bronchospasm, myalgia, ataxia, ocular palsies, aseptic meningitis, sore throat, cough, rhinitis, nerve deafness, otitis media, retinitis, papillitis, retrobulbar neuritis, conjunctivitis, and death.

The National Academy of Sciences and the American Academy of Pediatrics both reported in 2001 and in 2004 reports that no scientific evidence exists for a cause-and-effect relationship between MMR vaccination and autism spectrum disorder. The groups found that (1) the epidemiological evidence shows no association between MMR and autism; (2) case studies based on small numbers of children with autism and bowel disease do not provide enough evidence to draw a conclusion about a cause-and-effect relationship between these symptoms and vaccination; (3) biological models linking MMR and autism are fragmentary; and (4) there is no relevant animal model linking MMR and autism. The groups recommended maintaining current policies on MMR licensure and utilization.

Pharmacologic & Dosing Characteristics

Dosage: 0.5 mL for children and adults, preferably at 12 to 15 months of age. A booster dose is recommended under certain conditions (see Booster Doses).

In some other countries, measles vaccine is routinely administered at 9 months of age, even though seroconversion rates are lower than at ages 12 to 15 months. Revaccinate children who were vaccinated against measles before their first birthday.

The minimum interval between 2 MMR doses is 4 weeks. Do not count doses within the minimum interval, because too short an interval may interfere with antibody response and protection from disease. Increasing the interval beyond that recommended does not affect the ultimate efficacy of immunization, but waiting does delay achieving adequate protection from infection.

Route & Site: Subcutaneously, preferably in the outer aspect of the upper arm, with a 25-gauge, ⅝-inch needle. Do not inject IV.

Documentation Requirements: Federal law requires that the following information be documented in the recipient's permanent medical record or in a permanent office log: (1) The manufacturer and lot number of the vaccine, (2) the date of administration, and (3) the name, address, and title of the person administering the vaccine.

Certain adverse events must be reported to the VAERS system ([800]) 822-7967). Refer to the Resources section for complete information.

Booster Doses: Almost all children and adults born since 1957 should receive an additional dose of MMR vaccine, in addition to a primary dose given after the age of 12 months. Routine revaccination with trivalent MMR vaccine is recommended by the ACIP and AAP as children enter kindergarten or first grade, because the second dose is less painful at that age than if given later. Those who have not previously received the second dose should receive it no later than the routine visit to a health care provider at 11 to 12 years of age.

Unnecessary doses are best avoided by preserving written documentation of vaccination and giving a copy to each vaccinee or the vaccinee's agent.

Missed Doses: Give missed doses as soon as practical. Waiting delays protection from infection.

Efficacy: Induces measles hemagglutination-inhibiting (HI) antibodies in 97%, mumps-neutralizing antibodies in 97%, and rubella HI antibodies in 97% of children. Seroconversion is somewhat less in adults. Disease incidence is typically reduced 95% in family and classmates.

Onset: 2 to 6 weeks

Duration: Antibody levels persist 11 years or longer in most recipients without substantial decline.

Protective Level:

Measles: 0.2 unit/mL

Mumps: Unknown

Rubella: Specific rubella hemagglutination-inhibiting antibody titer of at least 1:8 is considered immune.

Mechanism: Attenuated measles vaccine induces a modified measles infection in susceptible people. Fever and rash may appear. Antibodies induced by this infection protect against subsequent infection.

Attenuated mumps vaccine produces a modified, noncommunicable mumps infection in susceptible people. These induced antibodies protect against subsequent infection.

Attenuated rubella vaccine induces a modified, noncommunicable rubella infection in susceptible patients. RA 27/3 strain elicits higher immediate postvaccination HI, complement-fixing, and neutralizing antibody levels than other strains of rubella vaccine and will induce a broader profile of circulating antibodies, including anti-theta and anti-iota precipitating antibodies. RA 27/3 strain immunologically simulates natural infection more closely than other rubella virus strains. The increased levels and broader profile of antibodies produced by RA 27/3 strain appear to correlate with greater resistance to subclinical reinfection by the wild virus.

Drug Interactions: Reconstitute trivalent MMR vaccine with the diluent provided. Addition of a diluent with an antimicrobial preservative may inactivate the attenuated viruses.

Like all live viral vaccines, administration to patients receiving immunosuppressant drugs (eg, steroids) or radiation therapy may predispose patients to disseminated infections or insufficient response to immunization. They may remain susceptible despite immunization.

To avoid inactivation of the attenuated virus, administer live virus vaccines at least 14 to 30 days before or several months after administration of any immune globulin or other blood product. Alternatively, check antibody titers or repeat the vaccine dose 3 months after immune globulin administration. Base the interval on the dose of IgG administered: 3 months for 3 to 10 mg IgG/kg, 4 months for 20 mg/kg, 5 months for 40 mg/kg, 6 months for 60 to 100 mg/kg, 7 months for 160 mg/kg, 8 months for 300 to 400 mg/kg, 10 months for 1 g/kg, 11 months for 2 g/kg.

To avoid the hypothetical concern over antigenic competition, administer measles vaccine after or at least 1 month before administration of other virus vaccines, except those given simultaneously. This caution does not apply to coadministration of MMR and OPV vaccines. Several routine vaccines may safely and effectively be administered simultaneously at separate injection sites (eg, DTP, MMR, OPV or e-IPV, Hib, hepatitis B, varicella, influenza). National authorities recommend simultaneous immunization at separate sites as indicated by age or health risk.

Live virus vaccines may cause delayed-hypersensitivity skin tests (eg, tuberculin, histoplasmin) to appear falsely negative. Evaluate such tests knowingly. The effect may persist for several weeks after vaccination. The ACIP and AAP recommend that tuberculin tests be given prior to live-virus vaccination, simultaneously, or at least 6 weeks after vaccination.

Administration of a live-virus vaccine and an interferon product may inhibit antibody response to the vaccine, although this is poorly studied. Avoid concurrent use.

Combining attenuated measles virus (Schwarz strain) and meningococcal groups A and C polysaccharides into a single vaccination resulted in depressed measles vaccine effectiveness in 110 Parisian children. Measles seroconversion was only 80% in combination with meningococcal group A vaccine and 69% in combination with a combined groups A and C vaccine. Meningococcal seroconversion was unaffected. Conversely, another study found no interaction between attenuated measles and meningococcal A vaccines in 87 Sudanese children receiving an extemporaneous combination of measles, tetanus, and meningococcal A immunogens. Neither of these 2 studies should be considered conclusive, as they provide preliminary data only. Public health authorities do not recommend any separation of measles and meningococcal vaccines if both are needed by a patient.

Anti-Rh_o(D) immune globulin does not appear to impair rubella vaccine efficacy. Susceptible postpartum women who received blood products or anti-Rh_o(D) immune globulin may receive attenuated rubella vaccine prior to discharge, provided that a repeat HI titer is drawn 6 to 8 weeks after vaccination to ensure seroconversion.

Methacholine inhalation challenge may be falsely positive for a few days after influenza, measles, or other immunization, but not after rubella vaccine. This effect appears to mimic the bronchospastic effect associated with acute respiratory infections. The effect has been observed in 44% to 90% of asthmatic patients, but apparently not among healthy subjects.

Simultaneous administration of large doses of vitamin A impaired the response to Schwarz-strain measles vaccine in a group of Indonesian infants at 6 months of age.

Interval Between Antibodies & Measles or Varicella-Containing Vaccine	
Antibody source	Delay before vaccination
Hepatitis B, tetanus, or $Rh_o(D)$ immune globulins (HBIG, TIG, RhIG)	3 mo for measles, 5 mo for varicella
IGIM, 0.02 to 0.06 mL/kg	3 mo for measles, 5 mo for varicella
IGIM, 0.25 mL/kg	5 mo
IGIM, 0.5 mL/kg	6 mo
IGIV, 400 mg/kg	8 mo
IGIV, high-dose for ITP or Kawasaki disease	8 to 11 mo
Packed RBCs	5 mo
Plasma or platelet	7 mo
Rabies immune globulin	4 mo for measles, 5 mo for varicella
RBCs with adenine-saline added	3 mo for measles, 5 mo for varicella
Vaccinia immune globulin IV	3 mo (Cangene)
Washed red blood cells (RBCs)	No wait
Whole blood	6 mo

Pharmaceutical Characteristics

Concentration: At least 1,000 (3 $\log_{10}$) $TCID_{50}$ of measles virus; at least 12,500 (4.3 $\log_{10}$) $TCID_{50}$ of mumps virus; and at least 1,000 (3 $\log_{10}$) $TCID_{50}$ of rubella virus, each per 0.5 mL dose.

Quality Assay: Produced in conformance with USP monograph.

Packaging: Single-dose package of separate vials of powder and diluent (NDC #: 00006-4749-00), box of 10 single-dose vial sets (00006-4681-00).

Doseform: Powder for solution

Appearance: Light-yellow compact crystalline plug, yielding a clear, yellow solution

Diluent: Sterile water for injection without preservative

Adjuvant: None

Preservative: None

Allergens: Gelatin, residual egg proteins, 25 mcg neomycin per dose. Measles and mumps viruses are grown in vitro, in chick embryo fibroblast cultures. As a result, only picogram or nanogram quantities of egg protein remain in each dose of vaccine.

Excipients: Sorbitol 14.5 mg/dose and hydrolyzed gelatin 14.5 mg/dose added as stabilizers, plus sodium phosphate, sodium chloride, sucrose 1.9 mg/dose, human albumin 0.3 mg/dose, fetal bovine serum (less than 1 ppm), other buffer and media ingredients.

pH: 6.2 to 6.6

Shelf Life: Expires within 24 months

Storage/Stability: Store at 2° to 8°C (35° to 46°F). Freezing does not harm this vaccine, but diluent vials may crack. Store diluent at room temperature or refrigerate. Shipped in an insulated container with dry ice, to maintain a temperature of 10°C (50°F) or colder. Freezing during shipment will not affect potency.

Protect vaccine from light. Contact manufacturer regarding prolonged exposure to room temperature or elevated temperatures. Reconstituted vaccine can tolerate 8 hours in the refrigerator.

Production Process:

Measles: Further attenuation of the virus strain in this vaccine was achieved by multiple passage of Edmonston strain virus in cell cultures of chick embryo at low temperature.

Mumps: Virus is cultured in egg cultures, purified, and packaged.

Rubella: Virus is cultured in cell cultures, purified, and packaged.

Media:

Measles and mumps: Chicken-embryo cell culture, grown in Medium 199, a buffered salt solution containing vitamins and amino acids, supplemented with fetal bovine serum and neomycin. Medium 199 is stabilized with sucrose, phosphate, glutamate, and human albumin.

Rubella: Human-diploid WI-38 cell culture, grown in Minimum Essential Medium, a buffered salt solution containing vitamins and amino acids, fetal bovine serum, human albumin, and neomycin. Sorbitol and hydrolyzed gelatin stabilizer are added to the individual viral harvests.

Disease Epidemiology

Measles:

Incidence: In the United States, 894,134 cases were reported in 1941. Before the vaccine era, each year's entire birth cohort was assumed to contract measles eventually. The rationale for a 2-dose national policy is based on several factors, in descending order of significance: failure of approximately 5% of vaccinees to seroconvert to the first dose, delays in delivering properly timed doses to young children, vaccine impairment by maternal antibodies if administered too early, suboptimal early vaccine formulations, and waning immunity. Failure to vaccinate contributes more to disease incidence than vaccine failures. Almost 2 million children die of measles annually around the world.

Transmission: Airborne by droplet spread or direct contact with nasal or throat secretions of infected patients. There have been no published reports of transmission of live attenuated measles virus from vaccinees to susceptible contacts.

Incubation: 7 to 18 days from exposure to onset of fever, usually 14 days until rash appears. Immune globulin, if given for passive protection later than the third day of incubation, may extend the incubation period to 21 days instead of preventing disease.

Communicability: Measles is 1 of the most communicable of all diseases, and a herd immunity of at least 94% may be needed to interrupt community transmission. Communicability extends from slightly before the beginning of the prodromal period to 4 days after appearance of the rash.

Mumps:

Incidence: A peak 185,691 cases were reported in 1967, with an estimated total incidence of 2 million cases that year. Mumps occurs around the world.

Transmission: By droplet spread or by direct contact with saliva of an infected person. There have been no published reports of transmission of live attenuated mumps virus from vaccinees to susceptible contacts.

Incubation: Commonly 18 days (range, 12 to 26 days)

Communicability: Consider exposed, nonimmune patients infectious from the twelfth through the twenty-fifth day after exposure. Maximum infectiousness occurs approximately 48 hours before onset of illness.

Rubella:

Incidence: In the United States, the 1963 to 1964 rubella pandemic produced 12.5 million rubella cases and 2,000 cases of encephalitis; it affected 30,000 infants (1% of all pregnancies), with 6,250 spontaneous abortions and 2,100 excess neonatal deaths.

Transmission: Contact with nasopharyngeal secretions of infected patients, droplet spread, or direct contact with patients. Infants with congenital rubella shed large quantities of virus in their pharyngeal secretions and urine and may infect contacts. Excretion of small amounts of attenuated rubella virus from the nose or throat occurred in most susceptible individuals 7 to 28 days after vaccination. There is no firm evidence that such virus is transmitted to susceptible people in contact with vaccinees. Transmission of attenuated rubella virus to infants through breast milk has been documented.

Incubation: For natural infection, 16 to 18 days (range: 10 to 23 days).

Communicability: Natural infection is communicable approximately 1 week before and at least 4 days after onset of rash. Infants with congenital rubella may shed the virus for months after birth.

Other Information

Perspective:

1971: *M-M-R* licensed on April 22, 1971.

1973: Measles-mumps bivalent vaccine (Merck's *M-M-Vax*) licensed in the United States on July 18.

1977: MMR first recommended for routine use.

1978: Reformulated with new stabilizer and RA 27/3 rubella strain on September 18; name changes to *M-M-R II.*

1980: *M-M-R II* recommended explicitly as preferred agent for children.

Measles:

1960: Katz, Enders, and colleagues attenuate the Edmonston strain of virus. Further attenuation of the Edmonston A strain eventually yielded the Schwarz strain. The Moraten and Edmonston-Zagreb strains are eventually derived from the Edmonston B strain.

1963: The first measles vaccines licensed in the United States on March 21, 1963, with doses recommended as young as 9 months of age. Early versions of attenuated Edmonston B measles vaccines are given with broad-spectrum IGIM or specific measles immune globulin to reduce the incidence of adverse reactions. The other type is a killed measles vaccine (KMV), which ceased production in 1967. After January 1, 1969, only the various attenuated vaccines are available.

1965: "Further attenuated" Schwarz strain licensed in the United States, produced until 1976. The recommended age for routine administration changes from 9 to 12 months of age.

1968: "More attenuated" (Moraten) strain licensed in the United States; used without IGIM.

1971: *Rubeovax* reformulated in April 1971.

1976: Routine administration recommendations for MMR vaccine change from 12 to 15 months of age.

1979: Moraten vaccine reformulated with new stabilizer; name changes to Attenuvax. The pH and tonicity are also changed, increasing the pain associated with an injection.

1982: Unmet target date for elimination of indigenous measles from the United States.

1989: Sharp increase in measles incidence begins. ACIP and AAP recommend 2-dose vaccination schedule.

Mumps:

1934: Johnson and Goodpasture isolate mumps virus.

1948: Weller and Enders grow mumps virus in tissue culture.

1949: Gordon and Kilham prepare mumps vaccine inactivated with either ether or ultraviolet radiation.

1951: Inactivated mumps vaccine licensed in US.

1963: Jeryl Lynn strain of mumps virus isolated in March from the daughter of researcher Maurice Hilleman.

1967: *Mumpsvax* licensed on December 28, 1967.

1977: First ACIP recommendation for routine use of mumps vaccine, delayed to allow limited resources to be directed toward poliovirus and measles vaccination.

1978: New stabilizer licensed on September 8.

2006: ACIP and AAP recommend 2-dose vaccination strategy.

Rubella:

1941: Gregg identifies congenital rubella syndrome through association with an unusually high incidence of cataracts in infants of mothers who contracted rubella during pregnancy.

1947: Pregnant women exposed to rubella begin receiving convalescent serum or IGIM to prevent infection.

1962: Rubella pandemic strikes Europe, reaching the United States in 1963 to 1964. Rubella virus isolated by Parkman and colleagues at Walter Reed Army Institute of Research, followed shortly afterward by Weller and Neva at Harvard University, and by Sever and colleagues at NIH.

1969: Three rubella vaccine strains licensed in the United States: HPV-77 strain grown in dog-kidney culture (DK-12: Rubelogen, Parke-Davis), HPV-77 grown in duck-embryo culture (DE-5: Meruvax, MSD), and Cendehill strain grown in rabbit-kidney culture (Cendevax, RIT-SKF; a component of Lirubel, and Lirutrin, Dow). HPV-77 was initially called M-33 strain. DK-12 is eventually withdrawn because of a higher incidence of arthritic side effects; Cendehill is later voluntarily withdrawn.

1979: Merck vaccine reformulated with new stabilizer and RA 27/3 rubella strain on September 18; name changes to *Meruvax II.*

1989: ACIP and AAP recommend 2-dose vaccination schedule.

Discontinued Products: *Lirutrin* (Schwarz, Jeryl Lynn, and Cendehill strains; Dow)

National Policy: ACIP. Control and prevention of rubella: Evaluation and management of suspected outbreaks, rubella in pregnant women, and surveillance for congenital rubella syndrome. *MMWR.* 2001;50(RR-12):1–23. http://www.cdc.gov/mmwr/PDF/rr/rr5012.pdf.

ACIP. Measles, mumps, and rubella—Vaccine use and strategies for elimination of measles, rubella, and congenital rubella syndrome and control of mumps. *MMWR.* 1998;47(RR-8):1-57. ftp.cdc.gov/pub/Publications/mmwr/rr/rr4708.pdf.

ACIP. Revised ACIP Recommendations for avoiding pregnancy after receiving a rubella-containing vaccine. *MMWR.* 2001;50:1117. http://www.cdc.gov/mmwr/preview/mmwrhtml/mm5049a5.htm.

ACIP. Updated recommendations of the ACIP for the control and elimination of mumps. *MMWR.* 2006;55:629-630. http://www.cdc.gov/mmwr/PDF/wk/mm5522.pdf.

Canadian National Advisory Committee on Immunization. Statement on mumps vaccine. *Can Comm Dis Rep.* 2007;33(ACS-8):1-9.

WHO. Measles vaccines. *Wkly Epidemiol Rec.* 2009;84(Aug 28):349-360.

References: CDC. Progress toward control of rubella and prevention of congenital rubella syndrome, worldwide, 2009. *MMWR.* 2010;59(40) ;1307-1310. http://www.cdc.gov/mmwr/pdf/wk/mm5940.pdf.

Institute of Medicine. *Immunization Safety Review: Vaccines and Autism.* Washington, DC: National Academy Press, 2004.

WHO. Mumps virus vaccines. *Weekly Epidemiol Rec.* 2007;82:50-60. http://www.who.int/wer/2007/wer8207.pdf.

WHO. Rubella vaccines. *Wkly Epidemiol Rec.* 2000;75:161-69.

Measles, Mumps, Rubella, & Varicella Virus Vaccine Live

Viral Vaccines

Name:
  ProQuad

Manufacturer:
  Merck

Synonyms: MMRV vaccine

Immunologic Characteristics

Antigen Source: Viruses; measles, mumps, and rubella viruses are single-stranded RNA viruses; varicella is a double-stranded RNA virus

Viability: Live, attenuated

Antigenic Form: Whole viruses

Antigenic Type: Protein

Strains:

Measles: Moraten strain (a more attenuated line of Enders' attenuated Edmonston A strain)
Mumps: Jeryl Lynn (B Level) strain
Rubella: Wistar Institute RA 27/3 strain
Varicella: Oka/Merck strain

Use Characteristics

Indications: To simultaneously induce active immunity against measles, mumps, rubella, and varicella viruses in children 12 months to 12 years of age. May be used in children 12 months to 12 years of age if a second dose of measles, mumps, and rubella vaccine is to be administered.

Limitations: If attenuated measles vaccine is given immediately after exposure to natural measles, some protection may be provided. However, if measles vaccine is given a few days before exposure, substantial protection may still result.

Attenuated mumps vaccine does not protect when given after exposure to natural mumps.

Attenuated rubella vaccine does not prevent illness when given after exposure to natural rubella. There is, however, no contraindication to vaccinating children already exposed to natural rubella.

The efficacy of varicella vaccine after exposure to varicella virus has not been established.

Contraindications:

Absolute: Pregnant women; people with a history of hypersensitivity reaction to this vaccine or any of its components (eg, gelatin, neomycin); people receiving immunosuppressive therapy; people with a blood dyscrasia, leukemia, lymphoma of any type, or other malignant neoplasms affecting the bone marrow or lymphatic systems; people with primary or acquired immunodeficiency, any febrile illness or infection, or active untreated tuberculosis; and people with a family history of congenital or hereditary immunodeficiency, until the immune competence of the potential vaccine recipient is demonstrated. Refer to individual monographs for details.

Do not vaccinate people who are immunosuppressed because of AIDS or other clinical manifestations of infection with HIV, cellular immune deficiencies, and hypogammaglobulinemic and dysgammaglobulinemic states. Nonetheless, national authorities recommend MMR immunization of asymptomatic children with HIV infection.

Traditionally, experts recommended not immunizing people with a history of anaphylactoid or other immediate reactions (eg, hives, swelling of the mouth or throat, difficulty breathing, hypotension, shock) after egg ingestion. The recommendation had been to give people suspected of being hypersensitive to egg protein a skin test using a dilution of the vaccine as the antigen. More recent information indicates that allegedly egg-allergic people almost always fail to react to vaccines containing egg proteins. This includes people with positive oral-egg challenges or egg skin tests. More anaphylaxis cases have been reported in people without allergy to eggs than in those with such an allergy. People do react severely to MMR in extraordinarily rare cases, but egg hypersensitivity does little to predict it. People also are not at risk if they have egg allergies that are not anaphylactoid in nature; vaccinate such people in the usual manner. There is no evidence to indicate that people with allergies to chickens or feathers are at increased risk of reaction to the vaccine. Children with egg allergy are at low risk for anaphylactic reactions to measles-containing vaccines (including MMR), and skin testing of children allergic to eggs is not predictive of reactions to MMR vaccine. People with allergies to chickens or feathers are not at increased risk of reaction to the vaccine. Conduct any immunization in a setting where emergency services can be promptly provided.

Relative: Defer immunization during the course of any acute illness. Do not give to people with a family history of congenital or hereditary immunodeficiency unless the immune competence of the potential vaccine recipient is demonstrated.

Do not give to people with active untreated tuberculosis, to people with an active febrile illness with fever higher than 101.3°F (higher than 38.5°C), or to women who are pregnant.

Immunodeficiency: Do not use in immunodeficient people, including people with congenital or acquired immune deficiencies, whether due to genetics, disease, or drug or radiation therapy. The vaccine contains live viruses. Nonetheless, routine immunization with MMR is recommended for symptomatic and asymptomatic HIV-infected people. Measles inclusion-body encephalitis, pneumonitis, and death as a direct consequence of disseminated measles vaccine virus infection have been reported in severely immunocompromised people inadvertently immunized with measles-containing vaccine. Immunization with a live, attenuated vaccine, such as varicella, can result in a more extensive vaccine-associated rash or disseminated disease in people on immunosuppressive drugs.

Elderly: Most people born in 1956 or earlier are likely to have been infected naturally and generally are considered not susceptible. MMRV is not indicated for use in the geriatric population.

Adults: Vaccinate people born more recently than 1956, unless they have a personal contraindication to immunization, because they are considered susceptible. Vaccinate people who may be immune but who lack adequate documentation of immunity as evidenced by physician diagnosis, laboratory evidence of immunity, or adequate immunization with live vaccine on or after the first birthday.

Carcinogenicity: MMRV has not been evaluated for carcinogenic potential.

Mutagenicity: MMRV has not been evaluated for mutagenic potential.

Fertility Impairment: MMRV has not been evaluated for impairment of fertility.

Pregnancy: Category C. Contraindicated on hypothetical grounds.

Measles: Contracting natural measles during pregnancy enhances fetal risk. Increased rates of spontaneous abortion, stillbirth, congenital defects, and prematurity have been observed subsequent to natural measles during pregnancy. There are no adequate studies of attenuated measles vaccine in pregnant women. Do not intentionally give measles vaccine to pregnant women because the possible effects of the vaccine on fetal development are unknown. If postpubertal women are immunized, counsel these women to avoid pregnancy for 1 month after immunization. It is not known if attenuated measles virus or corresponding antibodies cross the placenta.

Mumps: Although mumps virus can infect the placenta and fetus, there is a lack of good evidence that it causes congenital malformations in humans. Mumps infection during the first trimester of pregnancy may increase the rate of spontaneous abortion. Attenuated mumps-vaccine virus can infect the placenta and fetus, but there is no evidence that it causes congenital malformations in humans. Nonetheless, do not intentionally give attenuated mumps vaccine to pregnant women. If postpubertal women are immunized, counsel these women to avoid pregnancy for 1 month after immunization.

Rubella: Natural rubella infection of the fetus may result in congenital rubella syndrome (CRS). There is evidence suggesting transmission of attenuated rubella virus to the fetus, although the vaccine is not known to cause fetal harm when administered to pregnant women. Nonetheless, do not intentionally give attenuated rubella vaccine to pregnant women. If postpubertal women are immunized, counsel these women to avoid pregnancy for 1 month after immunization. It may be convenient to vaccinate rubella-susceptible women in the immediate postpartum period. In counseling women who are inadvertently immunized when pregnant or who become pregnant shortly after immunization, the following information may be useful: in a 10-year survey of more than 700 pregnant women who received rubella vaccine within 3 months before or after conception (of whom 189 received the Wistar RA 27/3 strain), no newborns had abnormalities compatible with CRS.

Varicella: Wild-type varicella can sometimes cause congenital varicella infection. Of 129 seronegative women and 423 women of unknown serostatus who received varicella vaccine during pregnancy or within 3 months before pregnancy, none had newborns with abnormalities compatible with congenital varicella syndrome.

General: Most IgG passage across the placenta occurs during the third trimester. Patients and health care providers are encouraged to report any exposure to varicella-containing vaccine (Oka/Merck) during pregnancy by calling (800) 986-8999.

Lactation: It is not known if attenuated measles virus, mumps virus, or corresponding antibodies cross into human breast milk. Problems in human mothers or children have not been documented.

Vaccine-strain rubella virus can be secreted in milk and may be transmitted to infants in this manner. In the infants with serologic evidence of rubella infection, none exhibited severe disease. However, one exhibited mild clinical illness typical of acquired rubella.

Limited evidence in the literature suggests that virus, viral DNA, or viral antigen could not be detected in the breast milk of women immunized postpartum with the vaccine strain of varicella virus.

Children: MMRV is safe and effective for children 12 months to 12 years of age. Immunization is not recommended for children younger than 12 months of age because remaining maternal virus neutralizing antibody may interfere with the immune response.

Adverse Reactions: Fever (102°F and higher, 38.9°C and higher oral; 21.5% vs 14.9%) and measles-like rash (3% vs 2.1%) were the adverse experiences that occurred more frequently in recipients of a single dose of MMRV compared with recipients of single doses of MMR and *Varivax*. Fever and measles-like rash usually occurred within 5 to 12 days after immunization, were of short duration, and resolved with no long-term sequelae. Pain/tenderness/soreness at the injection site was reported less often in people who received MMRV than people who received MMR and *Varivax* concomitantly (22% vs 26.7%). The only vaccine-related injection-site adverse experience more frequent among recipients of MMRV than recipients of MMR and *Varivax* was rash at the injection site (2.3% vs 1.5%).

In children who received 2 doses of MMRV, the rates of adverse experiences after the second dose were generally similar to, or lower than, those seen with the first dose. The fever rate was lower after the second dose than the first dose.

In healthy 4- to 6-year-old children receiving MMRV after previous MMR and varicella immunization, the rates of adverse experiences, including the most commonly reported adverse experiences of injection-site reactions, nasopharyngitis and cough, were similar among treatment groups.

Febrile seizures: Febrile seizures have been reported in children receiving MMRV. Consistent with clinical study data on the timing of fever and measles-like rash, an interim analysis of a postmarketing observational study in children (N = 14,263) receiving their first dose of vaccine has shown that febrile seizures occurred more frequently 5 to 12 days following vaccination with MMRV (0.5/1,000) when compared with data from children in a historical, age- and gender-matched, control group vaccinated with *M-M-R II* and *Varivax* (N = 14,263) concomitantly (0.2/1,000). In the 0 to 30 day time period after vaccination, the incidence of febrile seizures with *ProQuad* (1/1,000) was not greater than that observed in children receiving *M-M-R II* and *Varivax* concomitantly (1.3/1,000).

Herpes zoster: In clinical trials, 2 cases of herpes zoster were reported among 2,108 healthy subjects 12 to 23 months of age immunized with MMRV and followed for 1 year. Both cases were unremarkable and no sequelae were reported. The reported rate of zoster in recipients of *Varivax* appeared not to exceed that previously determined in a population-based study of healthy children who had experienced wild-type varicella. In clinical trials, 8 cases of herpes zoster were reported in 9,454 immunized people 12 months to 12 years of age during 42,556 person-years of follow-up. This resulted in a calculated incidence of at least 18.8 cases per 100,000 person-years. All 8 cases reported after *Varivax* were mild and no sequelae were reported. The long-term effect of varicella immunization on incidence of herpes zoster is not yet known.

Transmission: Excretion of small amounts of the live, attenuated rubella virus from the nose or throat occurred in most susceptible people 7 to 28 days after immunization. There is no confirmed evidence to indicate that such virus is transmitted to susceptible people who are in contact with recently immunized people. Consequently, transmission through close personal contact, while accepted as a theoretical possibility, is not regarded as a significant risk. Experience with *Varivax* suggests that transmission of varicella vaccine virus may occur rarely between healthy vaccine recipients who develop a varicella-like rash and contacts susceptible to varicella, as well as high-risk people susceptible to varicella. Vaccine recipients should attempt to avoid close association with high-risk people (eg, immunocompromised people, susceptible pregnant women, newborn infants of susceptible mothers) susceptible to varicella for up to 6 weeks after immunization. In circumstances where contact with high-risk people susceptible to varicella is unavoidable, weigh the potential risk of transmission of the varicella vaccine virus against the risk of acquiring and transmitting wild-type varicella virus.

Autism: The National Academy of Sciences and the American Academy of Pediatrics both reported that no scientific evidence exists for a cause-and-effect relationship between MMR immunization and autism spectrum disorder in an April 2001 report. The groups found that (1) the epidemiological evidence shows no association between MMR and autism, (2) case studies based on small numbers of children with autism and bowel disease do not provide enough evidence to draw a conclusion about a cause-and-effect relationship between these symptoms and immunization, (3) biological models linking MMR and autism are fragmentary, and (4) there is no relevant animal model linking MMR and autism. The groups recommended maintaining current policies on MMR licensure and utilization (*JAMA* 2001;285:2567-2569).

CNS: Exercise caution administering MMRV to people with a history of cerebral injury, individual or family history of convulsions, or any other condition in which stress due to fever should be avoided. Be alert to temperature elevations that may occur after immunization. Encephalitis and encephalopathy have been reported once for every approximately 3 million doses of MMR. Postmarketing surveillance of more than 400 million doses distributed worldwide from 1978 to 2003 indicates that serious adverse reactions such as encephalitis and encephalopathy continue to be rarely reported. In no case has it been shown conclusively that reactions were caused by the vaccine; however, the data suggest the possibility that some of these cases may have been caused by measles vaccines. The risk of such serious neurological disorders after live measles virus vaccine administration remains far less than that for encephalitis and encephalopathy with wild-type measles (1 per 2,000 reported cases). There have been reports of subacute sclerosing panencephalitis (SSPE) in children who did not have a history of infection with wild-type measles but did receive measles vaccine. Some of these cases may have resulted from unrecognized measles in the first year of life or possibly from measles immunization. Based on estimated measles vaccine distribution in the United States, the association of SSPE cases to measles immunization is about 1 case per million vaccine doses distributed. This is far less than the association with infection with wild-type measles— 6 to 22 cases of SSPE per 1 million cases of measles. The results of a retrospective case-control study suggest that the overall effect of measles vaccine has been to protect against SSPE by preventing measles with its inherently higher risk of SSPE. Cases of aseptic meningitis have been reported after measles, mumps, and rubella immunization. Although a causal relationship between other strains of mumps vaccine and aseptic meningitis has been shown, there is no evidence to link Jeryl Lynn-strain mumps vaccine to aseptic meningitis.

Febrile seizures have been reported in children receiving MMRV. Consistent with clinical study data on the timing of fever and measles-like rash, an interim analysis of a postmarketing observational study in children (N = 14,263) receiving their first dose of vaccine has shown that febrile seizures occurred more frequently 5 to 12 days after MMRV vaccination (0.5 per 1,000) when compared with data from children in a historical, age-, and gender-matched control group vaccinated with *M-M-R II* and *Varivax* (N = 14,263) concomitantly (0.2 per 1,000). In the 0- to 30-day time period after vaccination, the incidence of febrile seizures with MMRV (1 per 1,000) was not greater than that observed in children receiving *M-M-R II* and *Varivax* concomitantly (1.3 per 1,000).

Hematologic: No clinical data are available regarding the development or worsening of thrombocytopenia in people immunized with MMRV. Cases of thrombocytopenia have been reported after use of measles vaccine, MMR vaccine, and varicella vaccine. Postmarketing experience with MMR vaccine indicates that people with current thrombocytopenia may develop more severe thrombocytopenia after immunization. In addition, people who experienced thrombocytopenia after the first dose of MMR vaccine may develop thrombocytopenia with repeat doses. Consider serologic testing for antibody to measles, mumps, or rubella to determine if additional doses of vaccine are needed. Evaluate the risk-to-benefit ratio before considering immunization with MMRV in such cases.

Musculoskeletal: Arthralgia and/or arthritis (usually transient and rarely chronic) and polyneuritis are features of infection with wild-type rubella and vary in frequency and severity with age and gender; occurrence is greatest in adult women and least in prepubertal children. After immunization in children, reactions in joints are uncommon (0% to 3%) and of brief duration. In women, incidence rates for arthritis and arthralgia are generally higher than those seen in children (12% to 26%), and the reactions tend to be more marked and of longer duration. Symptoms may persist for a matter of months or, on rare occasions, for years. In adolescent girls, the reactions appear to be intermediate in incidence between those in children and adult women. In women 35 to 45 years of age these reactions are generally well tolerated and rarely interfere with normal activities. Chronic arthritis has been associated with wild-type rubella infection and has been related to persistent virus and/or viral antigen isolated from body tissues. Only rarely have vaccine recipients developed chronic joint symptoms.

Measles, Mumps, Rubella, & Varicella Virus Vaccine Live

Pharmacologic & Dosing Characteristics

Dosage: 0.5 mL, for both children and adults, preferably at 12 to 15 months of age. A booster dose is recommended under certain conditions (see Booster Doses).

Route & Site: Subcutaneous, preferably in the outer aspect of the deltoid region of the upper arm or in the higher anterolateral area of the thigh, with a 25-gauge, ⅝-needle. Do not inject IV.

Documentation Requirements: Federal law requires that the following information be documented in the recipient's permanent medical record or in a permanent office log: (1) the manufacturer and lot number of the vaccine, (2) the date of its administration, and (3) the name, address, and title of the person administering the vaccine. Certain adverse events must be reported to the VAERS system, 800-822-7967. Refer to the Resources section for complete information.

Booster Doses: At least 1 month should elapse between a dose of a measles-containing vaccine (eg, MMR) and a dose of MMRV. If a second dose of varicella-containing vaccine is required, at least 3 months should elapse between administration of the 2 doses.

Missed Doses: Give missed doses as soon as is practical, observing the minimum intervals discussed above. Waiting delays protection from infection.

Efficacy: The presence of detectable antibody was assessed by an appropriately sensitive enzyme-linked immunosorbent assay (ELISA) for measles, mumps (wild type and vaccine type strains), and rubella, and by gpELISA for varicella. For evaluation of vaccine response rates, a positive result in the measles ELISA corresponded to measles antibody concentrations of at least 255 milliunits/mL. Children were positive for mumps antibody if the antibody level was at least 10 ELISA units/mL. A positive result in the rubella ELISA corresponded to concentrations of at least 10 units rubella antibody/mL. Children with varicella antibody levels at least 5 gpELISA units/mL were considered seropositive.

In 4 randomized clinical trials, 5,446 healthy children 12 to 23 months of age were administered MMRV, and 2,038 children were immunized with MMR and *Varivax* given concomitantly at separate injection sites. After a single dose of MMRV, the vaccine response rates were 97.4% for measles, 95.8% to 98.8% for mumps, 98.5% for rubella, and 91.2% for varicella. These results were similar to the immune response rates induced by coadministration of single doses of MMR and *Varivax* at separate injection sites.

In a subanalysis, 1,035 children received a second dose of MMRV approximately 3 months after the first dose. The proportion of initially seronegative vaccinees with positive serological responses after 2 doses were 99.4% for measles, 99.9% for mumps, 98.3% for rubella, and 99.4% for varicella. The geometric mean titers (GMTs) after the second dose of MMRV increased approximately 2-fold each for measles, mumps, and rubella, and approximately 41-fold for varicella.

In a trial involving 799 healthy 4- to 6-year-old children who had received MMR and *Varivax* at least 1 month before study entry, 399 received MMRV and placebo, while 205 received MMR and placebo concomitantly at separate injection sites. Another 195 healthy children were administered MMR and *Varivax* concomitantly at separate injection sites. After the dose of MMRV, seropositivity rates were 99.2% for measles, 99.5% for mumps, 100% for rubella, and 98.9% for varicella. Geometric mean fold-rises in antibody titers for measles, mumps, rubella, and varicella were 1.2, 2.4, 3, and 12, respectively. Post-immunization GMTs for recipients of MMRV were similar to those after a second dose of MMR and *Varivax* administered concomitantly. Additionally, GMTs for measles, mumps, and rubella were similar to those after a second dose of MMR given concomitantly with placebo.

Onset: 2 to 6 weeks

Measles, Mumps, Rubella, & Varicella Virus Vaccine Live

Duration: The duration of protection from measles, mumps, rubella, and varicella infections after immunization with MMRV is unknown. Experience with MMR demonstrates that antibodies to measles, mumps, and rubella viruses are detectable in most people 11 to 13 years after primary immunization. Varicella antibodies were present for up to 10 years post-immunization in most people who received 1 dose of *Varivax*.

Protective Level: See separate MMR and varicella monographs.

Mechanism: Attenuated measles vaccine induces a modified measles infection in susceptible people. Fever and rash may appear. Antibodies induced by this infection protect against subsequent infection.

Attenuated mumps vaccine produces a modified, noncommunicable mumps infection in susceptible people. Antibodies induced by this infection protect against subsequent infection.

Attenuated rubella vaccine induces a modified, noncommunicable rubella infection in susceptible people. RA 27/3 strain elicits higher immediate post-immunization hemagglutination inhibition (HI), complement-fixing, and neutralizing antibody levels than other strains of rubella vaccine and will induce a broader profile of circulating antibodies, including anti-theta and anti-iota precipitating antibodies. RA 27/3 strain immunologically simulates natural infection more closely than other rubella virus strains. The increased levels and broader profile of antibodies produced by RA 27/3 strain appear to correlate with greater resistance to subclinical reinfection by the wild virus.

Attenuated varicella vaccine induces antibody responses against varicella virus at least 5 units/mL in gpELISA assay (not commercially available) correlated with long-term protection.

A single dose of MMRV elicited rates of antibody responses against measles, mumps, and rubella similar to those observed after immunization with a single dose of MMR, and seroresponse rates for varicella virus were similar to those observed after immunization with a single dose of *Varivax*.

Drug Interactions: Reconstitute MMRV vaccine with the diluent provided. Addition of a diluent with an antimicrobial preservative may inactivate the attenuated viruses.

Like all live viral vaccines, administration to people receiving immunosuppressant drugs (eg, steroids) or radiation therapy may predispose them to disseminated infections or insufficient response to immunization. They may remain susceptible despite immunization.

To avoid inactivation of the attenuated virus, administer live-virus vaccines at least 14 to 30 days before or several months after administration of any immune globulin or other blood product. Alternately, check antibody titers or repeat the vaccine dose 3 months after IG administration. Base the interval on the dose of IgG administered: 3 months for 3 to 10 mg/kg, 4 months for 20 mg/kg, 5 months for 40 mg/kg, 6 months for 60 to 100 mg/kg, 7 months for 160 mg/kg, 8 months for 300 to 400 mg/kg, 10 months for 1g/kg, and 11 months for 2 g/kg.

To avoid the hypothetical concern over antigenic competition, administer measles vaccine after or at least 1 month before administration of other virus vaccines, except those given simultaneously. Several routine vaccines may safely and effectively be administered simultaneously at separate injection sites (eg, DTP, MMR, IPV, Hib, hepatitis B). National authorities recommend simultaneous immunization at separate sites as indicated by age or health risk.

Based on a clinical trial involving 1,913 healthy children 12 to 15 months of age who received various sequences of DTaP, Hib, and hepatitis B vaccines with either MMRV or separate MMR or *Varivax* immunizations, seroconversion rates and antibody titers for measles, mumps, rubella, varicella, anti-polyribosyl-ribitol-phosphate and hepatitis B were comparable among the groups at approximately 6 weeks after immunization. This indicates that MMRV, Hib, and hepatitis B vaccines may be administered concomitantly without interference. There are

316

insufficient data to support concomitant immunization with DTaP, but no clinically significant differences in adverse experiences were reported between treatment groups.

Live virus vaccines may cause delayed-hypersensitivity skin tests (eg, tuberculin, histoplasmin) to appear falsely negative. Evaluate such tests knowingly. The effect may persist for several weeks after immunization. The ACIP and the American Academy of Pediatrics recommend that tuberculin tests be given before live-virus immunization, simultaneously, or 6 or more weeks after immunization.

Coadministration of a live-virus vaccine and an interferon product may inhibit antibody response to the vaccine, although this is poorly studied. Avoid concurrent use.

Combining attenuated measles virus (Schwarz strain) and meningococcal groups A and C polysaccharides into a single immunization resulted in depressed measles vaccine effectiveness in 110 Parisian children as reported by Ajjan et al (*Dev Biol Stand*. 1978;41:209-216). Measles seroconversion was only 80% in combination with meningococcal group A vaccine and 69% in combination with a combined groups A and C vaccine. Meningococcal seroconversion was unaffected. Conversely, Lapeyssonnie et al (*Med Trop [Mars]*. 1979;39:71-79), found no interaction between attenuated measles and meningococcal A vaccines in 87 Sudanese children receiving an extemporaneous combination of measles, tetanus, and meningococcal A immunogens. Neither of these 2 studies should be considered conclusive because they provide preliminary data only. Public health authorities do not recommend any separation of measles and meningococcal vaccines if both are needed by a patient.

Anti-Rh$_o$(D) immune globulin does not appear to impair rubella vaccine efficacy. Susceptible postpartum women who received blood products or anti-Rh$_o$(D) immune globulin may receive attenuated rubella vaccine before discharge, provided that a repeat HI titer is drawn 6 to 8 weeks after immunization to assure seroconversion.

Methacholine inhalation challenge may be falsely positive for a few days after influenza, measles, or other immunization (but not rubella vaccine). This effect appears to mimic the bronchospastic effect associated with acute respiratory infections. The effect has been observed in 44% to 90% of asthmatic patients, but apparently not among normal subjects.

Simultaneous administration of large doses of vitamin A impaired the response to Schwarz-strain measles vaccine in a group of Indonesian infants at 6 months of age.

Interval Between Antibodies & Measles- or Varicella-Containing Vaccine	
Antibody source	Delay before immunization
Hepatitis B, tetanus, or Rh$_o$(D) immune globulins (HBIG, TIG, RhIG)	3 months for measles, 5 months for varicella
IGIM 0.02 to 0.06 mL/kg	3 months for measles, 5 months for varicella
IGIM, 0.25 mL/kg	5 months
IGIM, 0.5 mL/kg	6 months
IGIV, 400 mg/kg	8 months
IGIV, high-dose for ITP or Kawasaki disease	8 to 11 months
Packed RBCs	5 months
Plasma or platelet	7 months
Rabies immune globulin	4 months for measles, 5 months for varicella
RBCs with adenine-saline added	3 months for measles, 5 months for varicella
Vaccinia immune globulin IV	3 months
Washed red blood cells (RBCs)	No wait
Whole blood	6 months

Measles, Mumps, Rubella, & Varicella Virus Vaccine Live

Patient Information: Advise the parent or guardian that the vaccine recipient should avoid use of salicylates for 6 weeks after immunization with MMRV to avoid the risk of Reye syndrome.

Pharmaceutical Characteristics

Concentration: At least 1,000 (3 $\log_{10}$) $TCID_{50}$ of measles virus; at least 20,000 (4.3 $\log_{10}$) $TCID_{50}$ of mumps virus; at least 1,000 (3 $\log_{10}$) $TCID_{50}$ of rubella virus; and at least 10,000 (3.99 $\log_{10}$) plaque-forming units (PFUs) of Oka/Merck varicella virus, each per 0.5 mL dose.

Quality Assay: The cells, virus pools, bovine serum, and human albumin used in manufacturing are all tested to provide assurance that the final product is free of potential adventitious agents. This product contains albumin, a derivative of human blood. Based on effective donor screening and product manufacturing processes, it carries an extremely remote risk for transmission of viral diseases. Although there is a theoretical risk for transmission of Creutzfeld-Jakob disease (CJD), no cases of transmission of CJD or viral disease have ever been identified that were associated with the use of albumin.

Packaging: Package of 10 single-dose vials of vaccine powder (NDC #: 00006-4999-00) with separate package of 10 vials of sterile water diluent.

Doseform: Powder for solution

Appearance: White to pale yellow colored powder, yielding a clear, pale yellow to light pink liquid

Diluent:

For reconstitution: Sterile water for injection without preservative

Adjuvant: None

Preservative: None

Allergens: Hydrolyzed gelatin 11 mg per 0.5 mL

Excipients: Sucrose up to 21 mg, sodium chloride 2.4 mg, sorbitol 1.8 mg, monosodium L-glutamate 0.4 mg, sodium phosphate dibasic 0.34 mg, human albumin 0.31 mg, sodium bicarbonate 0.17 mg, potassium phosphate monobasic 72 mcg, potassium chloride 60 mcg; potassium phosphate dibasic 36 mcg; residual components of MRC-5 cells including DNA and protein; neomycin less than 16 mcg, bovine calf serum 0.5 mcg, and other buffer and media ingredients per 0.5 mL

pH: Data not provided.

Shelf Life: Expires within 18 months, if stored properly.

Storage/Stability: Before reconstitution, store the vaccine powder continuously in a freezer (eg, chest, frost-free) for up to 18 months, at an average temperature of –15°C (5°F) or colder. Any freezer that reliably maintains an average temperature of 5°F or colder and has a separate sealed freezer door is acceptable for storing MMRV. If vaccine powder is inadvertently stored in the refrigerator, discard it. Protect vials from light. During shipment, to ensure no loss of potency, the vaccine must be maintained at a temperature of 20°C (–4°F) or colder.

Store diluent separately at room temperature (20° to 25°C [68° to 77°F]), or in a refrigerator (2° to 8°C [36° to 46°F]).

After reconstitution, discard vaccine if not used within 30 minutes. Do not freeze reconstituted vaccine.

Production Process: See separate MMR and varicella monographs.

Media:

Measles: Propagated in chick embryo cell culture
Mumps: Propagated in chick embryo cell culture
Rubella: Propagated in WI-38 human diploid lung fibroblasts
Varicella: Propagated in MRC-5 cells

Disease Epidemiology

See separate MMR and varicella monographs.

Other Information

Perspective: See separate MMR and varicella monographs.

Licensed Measles, Mumps, Rubella & Varicella Vaccines		
Generic name	Proprietary name	Licensed
Measles, mumps, & rubella vaccine	*M-M-R II*	September 18, 1978
Measles, mumps, rubella & varicella vaccine	*ProQuad*	September 6, 2005
Measles & rubella vaccine	*M-R-Vax II*[a]	April 22, 1971, revised September 18, 1978
Mumps & rubella vaccine	*Biavax II*[a]	August 3, 1970, revised September 18, 1978
Measles & mumps vaccine	*M-M Vax*[a]	July 18, 1973
Measles vaccine	*Attenuvax*	November 26, 1968, revised September 7, 1977
Mumps vaccine	*Mumpsvax*	December 28, 1967, revised September 8, 1978
Rubella vaccine	*Meruvax II*	June 9, 1969, revised September 18, 1978
Varicella vaccine	*Varivax*	March 17, 1995

a No longer distributed in the United States.

First Licensed: September 6, 2005

National Policy: ACIP. Updated recommendations of the ACIP for the control and elimination of mumps. *MMWR.* 2006;55:629-630. http://www.cdc.gov/mmwr/PDF/wk/mm5522.pdf.

ACIP. Measles, mumps, and rubella–vaccine use and strategies for elimination of measles, rubella, and congenital rubella syndrome and control of mumps. *MMWR.* 1998;47(RR-8):1-57.

ACIP. Prevention of varicella: Updated recommendations of the ACIP. *MMWR.* 1999;48(RR-6):1-5.

ACIP. Use of combination measles, mumps, rubella, and varicella vaccine: Recommendations of the ACIP. *MMWR.* 2010;59(RR-3):1-12.

Canadian National Advisory Committee on Immunization. Statement on mumps vaccine. *Can Comm Dis Rep.* 2007;33(ACS-8):1-9.

References: WHO. Measles vaccines. *Wkly Epidemiol Rec.* 2004;79:130-141.

WHO. Mumps virus vaccines. *Wkly Epidemiol Rec.* 2007;82:50-60.

WHO. Rubella vaccines. *Wkly Epidemiol Rec.* 2000;75:161-169.

WHO. Varicella vaccines. *Wkly Epidemiol Rec.* 1998;73:241-248.

Poliovirus Vaccine Inactivated

Viral Vaccines

Name: *Manufacturer:*

Ipol   Sanofi Pasteur

Synonyms: IPV, enhanced-potency IPV, e-IPV, ep-IPV, Salk vaccine

Comparison: Enhanced-potency inactivated poliovirus vaccine (e-IPV) is more potent and consistently immunogenic than previous IPV formulations that may still be available in other countries. Oral poliovirus vaccine (OPV) and e-IPV are generically different. OPV is no longer recommended for routine immunization of infants and children in the United States because of rare cases of OPV-associated paralytic poliomyelitis (VAPP). Currently, e-IPV is recommended for all 4 infant doses. e-IPV is used for vaccination of adults and immunocompromised patients and their contacts. e-IPV is preferred for adults because they are slightly more likely to develop OPV-induced poliomyelitis than children.

Immunologic Characteristics

Microorganism: Virus (single-stranded RNA), poliovirus, genus *Enterovirus*, family Picornaviridae

Viability: Inactivated

Antigenic Form: Whole viruses

Antigenic Type: Protein

Strains: Serotype 1—Mahoney strain; serotype 2—MEF-1 strain; serotype 3—Saukett strain

Use Characteristics

Indications: For induction of active immunity in infants, children, and adults against poliovirus types 1, 2, and 3 to prevent poliomyelitis. e-IPV is recommended for routine use with all 4 immunizing doses in infants and children.

Immunization of adults residing in the continental United States is not usually necessary because of the extremely low probability of exposure. Vaccinate adults traveling to regions where poliomyelitis is endemic or epidemic (eg, developing countries); health care workers in close contact with patients who may be excreting polioviruses; laboratory workers handling specimens that may contain polioviruses; and members of communities or specific population groups with disease caused by wild polioviruses.

In a household with an immunocompromised member, or among other close contacts, or in a household with an unimmunized adult, use only e-IPV for all those requiring poliovirus immunization.

Previous clinical poliomyelitis (usually caused by only a single poliovirus type) or incomplete immunization are not contraindications to completing the primary series of immunization.

Unlabeled Uses: Alternative immunization schedules for children using both OPV and e-IPV have been shown to be safe and immunogenic.

Limitations: e-IPV is not effective in modifying or preventing cases of existing or incubating poliomyelitis.

Contraindications:

Absolute: Patients with a history of hypersensitivity to any component of the vaccine. If anaphylaxis or anaphylactic shock occurs within 24 hours of administration, give no further doses.

Relative: Defer immunization during the course of any acute illness.

Immunodeficiency: e-IPV is the preferred product for polio immunization of people who reside with an immunodeficient person. The benefit of e-IPV use in HIV-infected children outweighs the undocumented risk of adverse immunologic effects. Patients receiving immunosuppressive therapy or those with other immunodeficiencies may have diminished antibody response to active immunization with e-IPV.

Elderly: No specific information is available regarding geriatric use of e-IPV.

Pregnancy: Category C. Use only if clearly needed. It is not specifically known if e-IPV or corresponding antibodies cross the placenta. Generally, most IgG passage across the placenta occurs during the third trimester. Problems in humans have not been documented and are unlikely.

Lactation: It is not known if e-IPV or corresponding antibodies cross into breast milk. Problems in humans have not been documented and are unlikely.

Children: e-IPV is safe and effective in children 6 weeks of age and older.

Adverse Reactions: No paralytic reactions to e-IPV are known to have occurred since a 1955 manufacturing incident in which live polioviruses escaped inactivation. e-IPV administration may result in erythema, induration, and pain at the injection site. With traditional (not enhanced) IPV, these symptoms occurred in 3.2%, 1%, and 13%, respectively, of vaccine recipients within 48 hours after vaccination. Temperatures 39°C and higher (102°F and higher) were reported in 38% of e-IPV vaccinees. Other symptoms included irritability, sleepiness, fussiness, and crying.

Additional data show that injection-site and systemic reactions after e-IPV administered in combination with DTaP vaccine to children 2 to 18 months of age are similar to reactions when DTaP was administered alone. These data reported erythema more than 1 inch (0% to 1.4%), swelling (0% to 11%), tenderness (0% to 29%), fever higher than 102.2°F (0% to 4.2%), irritability (7% to 65%), tiredness (4% to 61%), anorexia (1% to 17%), vomiting (0% to 3%), and persistent crying (0% to 1.4%).

Pharmacologic & Dosing Characteristics

Dosage: A primary series consists of three 0.5 mL doses of poliovirus vaccine. The multiple doses in the primary series are not administered as boosters, but rather to ensure that immunity to all 3 types of virus has been achieved. A booster dose is given several years after the primary series.

Children: The national policy consensus is to give 4 doses of e-IPV. Typically, this would include e-IPV doses at 2 months, 4 months, 6 to 18 months, and 4 to 6 years of age. Separate the first 2 doses by at least 4 weeks (preferably 8 weeks). Give the third dose at least 4 weeks (preferably 8 to 12 months) after the second dose.

If the third dose of poliovirus vaccine is given after the fourth birthday, a fourth dose is not needed.

Adults: For unvaccinated adults at increased risk of exposure to poliovirus, give a primary series of e-IPV: 2 doses 4 to 8 weeks apart, with a third dose given 6 to 12 months later. If 2 to 3 months remain before protection is needed, give 3 doses of e-IPV at least 4 weeks apart. Likewise, if only 1 or 2 months remain, give 2 doses of e-IPV 4 weeks apart. If less than 4 weeks remain, give a single dose of either OPV or e-IPV.

Give a single dose of e-IPV to adults who have completed a primary series with any poliovirus vaccine and who are at increased risk of exposure to poliovirus.

Do not count doses within the minimum interval, because too short an interval may interfere with antibody response and protection from disease. Increasing the interval beyond the recommended timing does not affect the ultimate efficacy of immunization, but waiting does delay achieving adequate protection from infection.

Poliovirus Vaccine Inactivated

Route & Site: Subcutaneously or IM in the deltoid region. In infants and children, the preferred site is the anterolateral thigh.

Documentation Requirements: Federal law requires that the following information be documented in the recipient's permanent medical record or in a permanent office log: (1) The manufacturer and lot number of the vaccine, (2) the date of its administration, and (3) the name, address, and title of the person administering the vaccine.

Certain adverse events must be reported to the VAERS system ([800] 822-7967). Refer to Immunization Documents in the Resources section for complete information.

Booster Doses: A total of 4 doses is needed to complete a series of primary and booster doses. Give incompletely immunized children and adolescents sufficient additional doses to reach this number. The need to routinely administer additional doses is not apparent at this time.

Adult travelers to polio-endemic areas who received 4 childhood doses as children or adolescents may receive an additional IPV dose prior to travel. Travelers who have not received 4 childhood doses should complete as much of the age-appropriate basic series as possible before arrival in the endemic area.

Missed Doses: Longer than recommended intervals between doses do not necessitate additional doses beyond the standard total of 4 doses, but waiting does delay achieving adequate protection from infection.

Efficacy: 97.5% to 100% seroconversion to each type after 2 doses. This formulation is more potent and more consistently immunogenic than previous IPV formulations.

Onset: Antibodies develop within 1 to 2 weeks following several doses.

Duration: Many years

Protective Level: Any detectable neutralizing antibody, in practice a titer more than 1:4.

Mechanism: Induces antipoliovirus neutralizing antibodies, reducing pharyngeal excretion of poliovirus through a mucosal secretory-IgA response at that site. This helps block respiratory transmission. Some immunity in the mucosa of the GI tract develops, but it is inferior to that induced by OPV. If patients vaccinated with IPV swallow viable polioviruses, the viruses can be shed in their stools.

Drug Interactions: As with all inactivated vaccines, administration of e-IPV to patients receiving immunosuppressant drugs (eg, high-dose corticosteroids) or radiation therapy may result in an insufficient response to immunization. They may remain susceptible despite immunization.

Several routine pediatric vaccines may safely and effectively be administered simultaneously at separate injection sites (eg, DTP, MMR, OPV, e-IPV, Hib, hepatitis A, hepatitis B, influenza). National authorities recommend simultaneous immunization at separate sites as indicated by age or health risk, if return of a vaccine recipient for a subsequent visit is doubtful.

Inactivated vaccines are not generally affected by circulating antibodies or the administration of exogenous antibodies. Vaccination may occur at any time before or after antibody administration.

Pharmaceutical Characteristics

Concentration: 40, 8, and 32 D-antigen units per 0.5 mL dose of poliovirus types 1, 2, and 3, respectively. The D-antigen is 1 of 2 major antigenic components of polioviruses.

Quality Assay: Assessed by tissue, mouse, guinea pig, rabbit, and monkey tests for safety and by monkey potency test for neutralizing antibody production. Poliovirus cultures are tested to ensure the absence of B virus, SV-40 virus, lymphocyte choriomeningitis virus, *Mycobacterium tuberculosis*, and other microbes.

Packaging: Ten 0.5 mL single-dose syringes without needle (NDC #: 49281-0860-55); 10-dose vial (49281-0860-10)

Doseform: Suspension (the product appears clear)

Appearance: Clear and colorless

Solvent: Phosphate-buffered saline

Adjuvant: None

Preservative: 0.5% 2-phenoxyethanol and no more than 0.02% formaldehyde

Allergens: No detectable antibiotics remain but may be present below detectable limits: less than 5 ng neomycin, 200 ng streptomycin, or 25 ng polymyxin B, each per 0.5 mL. The stopper to the vial contains no rubber of any kind. The needle cover of the syringe contains dry natural latex rubber, but the plunger for the syringe contains no rubber of any kind.

Excipients: Newborn calf serum, originating from countries free of bovine spongiform encephalopathy, less than 1 ppm in the final vaccine

pH: Data not provided

Shelf Life: Expires within 18 months

Storage/Stability: Store at 2° to 8°C (35° to 46°F). Discard if frozen. Contact manufacturer regarding prolonged exposure to elevated or room temperature. Shipped by second-day courier in insulated containers with coolant packs.

Production Process: Produced by a microcarrier-culture technique, clarified and filtered, concentrated by ultrafiltration, purified by 3 liquid chromatography steps (anion exchange, gel filtration, anion exchange), then inactivated at 37°C for at least 12 days with formalin 1:4,000.

Media: Vero cells, a continuous line of monkey kidney cells of Vervet or African green monkeys. The cells are grown in Eagle MEM modified medium, supplemented with newborn calf serum tested for adventitious agents before use. For viral growth, the culture medium is replaced by M-199, without calf serum.

Disease Epidemiology

Incidence: Some 57,000 cases (21,269 paralytic) and 3100 deaths occurred in 1952 in the United States.

No indigenous cases of paralytic poliomyelitis associated with wild virus have been reported in the United States since 1980. All indigenous US cases reported since 1980 have been vaccine associated. No wild virus case has been reported in the Western Hemisphere since mid-1990. More than 100,000 children around the world are paralyzed annually by poliomyelitis, down from more than 500,000 a decade ago.

The ratio of cases of inapparent infection to paralytic disease ranges from 100-to-1 to 1,000-to-1. Paralytic poliomyelitis is fatal in 2% to 10% of cases.

Polio-free zones exist or are developing in the Americas; northern, southern, and eastern Africa; the Arabian peninsula; western and central Europe; and the western Pacific. Poliomyelitis remains endemic in the Indian subcontinent. It also occurs in sub-Saharan Africa, Asia, and the republics of the former Soviet Union. Outbreaks have occurred in Oman, Jordan, Malaysia, and the Netherlands and after importation of cases from the Indian subcontinent.

Susceptible Pools: 20% to 40% of preschool children. In a study of 233 American citizens preparing for international travel, 12% were seronegative to serotype 1 or 3; all were immune to serotype 2. A national serosurvey of 1,547 US Army recruits born from 1954 to 1972 suggests that 2.3% are susceptible to serotype 1, 0.6% to serotype 2, and 14.6% to serotype 3.

Transmission: Direct contact through close association; fecal-oral is the main route of transmission in areas with poor sanitation. During epidemics and where sanitation is good, pharyngeal spread becomes relatively more important. In the United States, almost all cases are caused by vaccine-associated virus.

Incubation: Commonly 7 to 14 days for paralytic cases (range, 3 to 35 days).

Poliovirus Vaccine Inactivated

Communicability: Poliovirus is demonstrable in throat secretions as early as 36 hours and in the feces 72 hours after exposure to infection. The virus persists in the throat for 1 week and in the feces for 3 to 6 weeks or longer. Cases are most infectious during the first few days before and after the onset of symptoms.

Other Information

Perspective:

1909: Landsteiner shows viral etiology of poliomyelitis.

1916: Poliomyelitis outbreak in the northeastern United States, centered around New York City: 27,000 cases and 6,000 deaths.

1935: Kolmer tests an insufficiently-attenuated live poliovirus vaccine in 12,000 children: 6 die, 3 are paralyzed. Brodie and Park test formaldehyde-treated IPV in 9,000 children: 1 dies, 3 are paralyzed, probably due to inadequate inactivation.

1949: Robbins grows polioviruses in cell culture.

1953: Hammon develops polio immune globulin.

1954: National field trial of Salk's IPV. To this day, it ranks as the largest human experiment ever conducted: 440,000 children received vaccine and 210,000 received placebo. Another 1,180,000 children served in an unvaccinated comparison group. Licensure of Salk's IPV followed in 1955 (April 12), after a commission chaired by Thomas Francis determined efficacy in the national field trial.

1955: "Cutter incident": Inadequate viral inactivation, contrary to Salk's instructions, allows some live virus to persist in the IPV formulation. No paralytic reactions to IPV are known to have occurred since this manufacturing accident. To preclude insufficient inactivation, all IPV lots since 1955 have been filtered before inactivation.

1956: Sabin tests OPV.

1961: OPV types 1 and 2 licensed in the United States.

1962: OPV type 3 licensed in the United States (March 27). Three separate doses of monovalent OPV (MOPV) are routinely administered on separate occasions through 1964, when the trivalent formulation comes into widespread use. Originally, type 1 was given at 2 months, type 3 at 3 months, and type 2 at 4 months of age.

1963: OPV used for routine pediatric immunization almost exclusively. Trivalent OPV licensed in the United States on June 25.

1974: Landmark Reyes vs Davis Laboratories case: Manufacturer liable for poliomyelitis attributed to an OPV dose.

1988: Enhanced-potency human diploid-cell vaccine replaces original monkey-kidney IPV in the United States.

1990: Enhanced-potency Vero-cell culture IPV licensed in the United States on December 21.

1996: National policy changes to a combined regimen of e-IPV and OPV, in an effort to reduce the already rare likelihood of OPV-associated paralytic poliomyelitis. Such a strategy is desirable as natural poliovirus infection becomes rare and the risk of VAPP becomes less acceptable.

1999: National policy changes to a regimen of 4 doses of e-IPV, with OPV restricted to unusual circumstances.

Other Licensed Products: Sanofi Pasteur still has an FDA license for another form of e-IPV, *Poliovax*. *Poliovax* would be distributed in the event of any shortage of *Ipol*. The 2 e-IPV formulations are similar in most respects, including safety and efficacy. *Poliovax* is produced in MRC-5 human-diploid cell culture by a microcarrier technique. Trace amounts of neomycin, streptomycin, or bovine serum may persist from the manufacturing processes. It is packaged in 0.5 mL ampules, standardized in the same D-antigen system used for *Ipol*. *Poliovax* contains 27 ppm formaldehyde, 0.5% 2-phenoxyethanol, 0.5% human albumin, and 20 ppm polysorbate 80. It was first licensed on December 22, 1987; distribution began in March 1988; *Poliovax* was superseded in the United States by *Ipol* in 1991.

Discontinued Products: *Purivax* (monkey kidney-cell culture, Merck, Sharp and Dohme)

National Policy: ACIP. Poliomyelitis prevention in the United States: Updated recommendations. *MMWR.* 2000;49(RR-5):1-22. http://ftp.cdc.gov/pub/Publications/mmwr/rr/rr4905.pdf.

ACIP. Updated recommendations of the Advisory Committee on Immunization Practices (ACIP) regarding routine poliovirus vaccination. *MMWR*. 2009;58:829-830.

Canadian Committee to Advise on Tropical Medicine and Travel. Poliomyelitis vaccination for international travelers. *Can Comm Dis Rep*. 2003;29(ACD-10):1-8.

References: CDC. 50th anniversary of the first effective polio vaccine-April 12, 2005. *MMWR*. 2005;54:335-336. http://www.cdc.gov/mmwr/PDF/wk/mm5413.pdf.

WHO. Polio vaccines and polio immunization in the pre-eradication era: WHO position paper — recommendations. *Vaccine*. 2010;28(Oct 8):6943-6944.

Comparison Table of Poliovirus Vaccines		
Generic name	Poliovirus vaccine inactivated	Poliovirus vaccine live, attenuated
Brand name	*Ipol*	*Orimune*[a]
Synonyms	IPV, e-IPV, ep-IPV, Salk vaccine	OPV, Sabin vaccine
Manufacturer	Sanofi Pasteur	Wyeth-Lederle
Viability	Whole inactivated viral vaccine	Live, attenuated viral vaccine
Indications	Adults; immunocompromised patients and their household contacts, including HIV-infected patients; all 4 doses in routine immunizations of children	No longer recommended for routine immunization of infants, children, or adults
Strains	Type 1 (Mahoney), type 2 (MEF-1), type 3 (Saukett)	Sabin strains 1, 2, 3
Concentration	40, 8, and 32 D-antigen units of poliovirus types 1, 2, and 3 per 0.5 mL	800,000, 100,000, and 500,000 particles of poliovirus types 1, 2, and 3 per 0.5 mL
Adjuvant	None	None
Preservative	2-phenoxyethanol 0.5%	None
Production medium	Vero cells	Monkey-kidney cell culture
Doseform	Liquid suspension	Frozen suspension
Packaging	0.5 mL prefilled syringe, 10-dose vial	Single-dose disposable pipettes (1s, 10s, 50s)
Routine storage	Refrigerate	Freeze
Dosage, route	0.5 mL IM or subcutaneously	0.5 mL oral
Efficacy	95% to 100%	95% to 100%
Systemic immunity	High	High
GI mucosal immunity	Low	High
Comments	Preferred vaccine for all ages	No longer preferred
Standard schedule	2, 4, 6 to 18 months, and 4 to 6 years of age	2, 4, 6 to 18 months, and 4 to 6 years of age
Ability to induce poliomyelitis	No risk	Overall, 1 case per 2.4 million OPV doses distributed, ≈ 8 to 9 cases per year. Among patients given OPV as the initial vaccination, the risk is higher with first doses (1 per 750,000 doses) than with subsequent doses (1 per 5.1 million doses). The risk in immunodeficient infants is 3,200 to 6,800 times the risk in immunocompetent infants. The risk for recipients (1 per 6.2 million doses) is comparable with the risk for household contacts (1 per 7.6 million doses).

a No longer distributed in the United States; information provided for historical perspective.

Rabies Vaccines

Viral Vaccines

Names: *Manufacturers:*

Rabies Vaccine (Human Diploid Cell):   Pasteur-Mérieux Sérums and Vaccins in France,
  Imovax Rabies   distributed by Sanofi Pasteur

Rabies Vaccine (Purified Chicken   Novartis
  Embryo Cell): *RabAvert*

Rabies Vaccine (Vero Cell): Generic   Sanofi Pasteur (not marketed in the United
                                                                 States)

Synonyms: VISI abbreviation: RAB. *Sanofi Pasteur:* Human diploid-cell vaccine, HDCV. *Novartis:* Purified chicken embryo cell, PCEC. *RabAvert* is marketed in Europe under the name *Rabipur*. Rabies is also called hydrophobia, related to a fear of swallowing among its victims (not to a fear of water, a common misconception). Archaic: rabic vaccine.

Comparison: IM dosage forms are generically equivalent and are considered interchangeable. Until there are data on the use of different brands within a series, use the same brand whenever possible. Data are accumulating on the use of one brand to successfully boost immunity developed with another brand.

Immunologic Characteristics

Microorganism: Virus (single-stranded RNA), genus *Lyssavirus*, family Rhabdoviridae

Viability: Inactivated

Antigenic Form: Whole virus

Antigenic Type: Protein

Strains:

Novartis: Fixed-virus strain Flury LEP-C 25 (low-egg-passage)

Sanofi Pasteur-Diploid: PM-1503-3M (Pitman Moore) strain obtained from the Wistar Institute, derived from a Pasteur strain

---

Use Characteristics

Indications: Induction of active immunity against rabies virus, either before or after viral exposure.

Preexposure immunization: Vaccinate people with greater than usual risk of exposure to rabies virus by reason of occupation or avocation, including veterinarians, certain laboratory workers, animal handlers, forest rangers, spelunkers, and people staying longer than 1 month in other countries (eg, India) where rabies is a constant threat (see tables at the end of the monograph).

Postexposure prophylaxis: If a bite from a carrier animal is unprovoked, the animal is not apprehended, and rabies is present in that species in the area, administer RIG and vaccine as indicated in tables at the end of the monograph. Consider vaccine recipients adequately immunized if they have completed pre- or postexposure prophylaxis with any current rabies vaccine or have a documented adequate antibody response to duck-embryo rabies vaccine (DEV).

Limitations: Preexposure immunization does not eliminate the need for prompt postexposure prophylaxis; it only eliminates the need for RIG and reduces the number of injections of rabies vaccine needed for postexposure prophylaxis.

Contraindications:

Absolute: There are essentially no absolute contraindications to rabies vaccination when used for postexposure prophylaxis. Consult an allergist regarding desensitization for people with a history of serious allergic reaction to a vaccine component or after a prior dose of this vaccine.

Relative: No antirabies treatment is indicated unless the skin is broken or a mucosal surface has been contaminated with the animal's saliva. Rabies vaccine may theoretically be contraindicated in people who have had a life-threatening allergic reaction to rabies vaccine or any of its components. Carefully consider a patient's risk of developing rabies before deciding to discontinue vaccination. Local or mild postvaccination reactions are not a contraindication to continuing immunization.

Give no further doses of rabies vaccine to people who experience immune-complex-like (or serum-sickness-like) hypersensitivity reactions during preexposure prophylaxis unless they are exposed to rabies or they are likely to be unapparently or unavoidably exposed to rabies virus and have unsatisfactory antibody titers.

Immunodeficiency: Immunosuppression and immunodeficiency can interfere with development of active immunity and may predispose the patient to developing rabies following exposure to rabies virus. Do not give immunosuppressive agents during postexposure therapy unless essential for treatment of other conditions.

Elderly: No specific information is available about geriatric use of rabies vaccine.

Pregnancy: Category C. Use is not contraindicated, but use only if clearly needed. It is not known if rabies vaccine or corresponding antibodies cross the placenta. Generally, most IgG passage across the placenta occurs during the third trimester. Problems in humans have not been documented and are unlikely.

Lactation: It is not known if rabies vaccine or corresponding antibodies cross into breast milk. Problems in humans have not been documented and are unlikely.

Children: Pediatric and adult doses are the same. Safety and efficacy are established in children. Safe and effective use of the BioPort vaccine is established for people older than 6 years of age.

Adverse Reactions:

Novartis: Transient pain at the injection site (34% to 84%), localized lymphadenopathy (15%). The most common systemic reactions were myalgia (53%), headache (15% to 52%), malaise (15% to 20%), dizziness (15%). Uncommon reactions included fever higher than 38°C (100°F) and GI complaints. In rare cases, severe headache, fatigue, circulatory reactions, sweating, chills, monoarthritis, allergic reactions, transient paresthesias, and suspected urticaria pigmentosa were noted. None of the adverse events were serious and almost all were of mild or moderate intensity. No cases of type III hypersensitivity (serum-sickness-like or immune-complex-like) reactions have been reported with use of *RabAvert*, nor have antibodies to chick-cell proteins been reported. For 11.8 million doses of *RabAvert* distributed worldwide, 10 cases of encephalitis or meningitis, 7 cases of transient paralysis (including 2 cases of Guillain-Barré syndrome), 1 case of myelitis, 1 case of retrobulbar neuritis, 2 cases of anaphylaxis, and 2 cases of suspected multiple sclerosis have been temporarily associated with use of *RabAvert*.

Sanofi Pasteur-Diploid: Transient pain, erythema, swelling, or itching at the injection site (25%). Treat such reactions with simple analgesics.

Mild systemic reactions (20%): Headache, nausea, abdominal pain, muscle aches, and dizziness. In general, ID administration results in fewer adverse reactions, except for a slight increase in transient local reactions.

Serum-sickness-like reaction: Occurred 2 to 21 days after injection in 6% of those receiving ID booster doses. These reactions may be caused by albumin in the vaccine formula rendered allergenic by beta-propiolactone during the manufacturing process.

Consultation: Clinicians with limited experience with rabies vaccine should consult with their state or local public health department.

Pharmacologic & Dosing Characteristics

Dosage:

Preexposure prophylaxis: Vaccine doses on days 0, 7, and 21 to 28, and then every 2 to 5 years based on antibody titers. Give 1 mL IM (any manufacturer).

Postexposure prophylaxis: Do not inject postexposure vaccine ID. Give rabies immune globulin (RIG, 20 units/kg, refer to specific monograph in the Immune Globulins section) as soon after exposure as possible, followed by IM vaccine doses (any manufacturer) on days 0, 3, 7, 14, and 28.

For patients who have received preexposure prophylaxis, give 1 mL IM only of any vaccine brand on days 0 and 3. Do not give RIG.

Notwithstanding the labeled dosage for rabies vaccine, the ACIP recommended four 1 mL doses of rabies vaccine for postexposure prophylaxis in June 2009.

Route & Site: The deltoid area is the only acceptable site for postexposure vaccination of adults and older children. For younger children, use the outer aspect of the thigh. Never administer rabies vaccine in the gluteal area because of erratic absorption and variable immunogenicity.

Novartis: IM only. Do not inject subcutaneously, ID, or IV.

Sanofi Pasteur-Diploid: IM. Use only the IM route for postexposure prophylaxis.

Previously, intradermal rabies vaccination had been accepted for preexposure prophylaxis, using a 0.1 mL dose. Manufacturers no longer distribute ID formulations. Care must be taken to avoid inadvertent subcutaneous injection into adipose tissue, which could impair the immune response.

Booster Doses: For occupational or other continuing risk, every 2 to 5 years based on antibody titers in a single 1 mL IM injection.

Preexposure booster immunization: Test people who work with live rabies virus in research laboratories, in vaccine production, or with diagnostic tests for serum rabies antibody titer every 6 months. Give booster vaccine doses as needed to maintain an adequate titer. Give workers (ie, veterinarians, animal control, and wildlife officers in areas where animal rabies is epizootic) booster doses every 2 years or have their serum rabies antibody titer determined every 2 years. If the titer is insufficient, give a booster dose. Veterinarians and similar workers in areas of low rabies endemicity do not require routine booster doses of rabies vaccine after completion of primary preexposure immunization or postexposure prophylaxis.

Missed Doses:

Preexposure prophylaxis: Prolonging the interval between doses does not interfere with immunity achieved after the concluding dose of the basic series.

Postexposure prophylaxis: Prolonging the interval between doses may seriously delay achieving protective antibody titers, with potentially fatal consequences.

Efficacy: Essentially 100%, when administered according to ACIP recommendations.

Onset: After IM injection, antibodies appear in 7 days and peak within 30 to 60 days. Adequate titers usually develop within 2 weeks after the third preexposure dose. Antibody kinetics after ID injection (no longer recommended) were presumably comparable, if administered correctly, although slightly delayed.

Duration: Antibodies persist 1 year or longer.

Protective Level: Two alternative definitions are used for minimally acceptable antibody titers in vaccinees. These definitions vary among laboratories, based on the type of test performed. The CDC considers a 1:5 titer by rapid fluorescent-focus inhibition test (RFFIT) to indicate an adequate response to preexposure vaccination. The WHO specifies an antibody titer of 0.5 unit/mL (comparable with a dilution titer of 1:25) as adequate for postexposure vaccination.

Mechanism: Rabies vaccine induces neutralizing antibody, cellular immunity, and perhaps interferon.

Drug Interactions: Like all inactivated vaccines, rabies vaccine administered to patients receiving immunosuppressant drugs (eg, high-dose corticosteroids) or radiation therapy may result in an insufficient response to immunization. They may remain susceptible despite immunization.

Do not give immunosuppressive agents during postexposure therapy unless essential for treatment of other conditions. Exercise caution, especially with corticosteroids used to treat life-threatening neuroparalytic reactions, as they may inhibit the development of active immunity to rabies. It may be helpful to test steroid-treated patients for development of antirabies antibodies.

Simultaneous administration of RIG may slightly delay the antibody response to rabies vaccine through partial antigen-antibody antagonism. Because of this possibility, follow the CDC recommendations exactly and give no more than the recommended dose of RIG.

Long-term therapy with chloroquine may suppress the immune response to low-dose HDCV administered ID. This effect may also occur with other structurally-related antimalarial drugs, such as mefloquine. Complete preexposure rabies vaccination 1 to 2 months before antimalarial administration begins. If this is not feasible, perform serologic tests several weeks after vaccination to determine the magnitude of the recipient's antibody response.

Rabies immunogenicity was not impaired by simultaneous vaccination with yellow fever, OPV, MMR, DT, cholera, meningococcal, and hepatitis B vaccines in 1 study.

As with other drugs administered IM, administer rabies vaccine with caution to patients receiving anticoagulant therapy.

Pharmaceutical Characteristics

Concentration: At least 2.5 units/mL

Quality Assay: Tissue and animal safety tests. Potency assayed in comparison with US Reference Standard Rabies Vaccine by mouse protection test. USP monograph for diploid vaccine.
Novartis: Residual chicken protein assayed by ELISA

Packaging:
Novartis: Single-dose package containing vial of powder; a disposable syringe; 1 mL vial of sterile water for injection; 21-gauge, 1.5-inch needle for reconstitution; and 25-gauge, 1-inch needle for injection (NDC #: 53901-0501-01)
Sanofi Pasteur-Diploid: Single-dose package containing vial of powder; syringe containing diluent; a separate plunger for insertion and use; and disposable needle for reconstitution (54281-0250-51)

Doseform:
Novartis: Powder for suspension
Sanofi Pasteur-Diploid: Powder for suspension

Appearance:
Novartis: White lyophilized powder, yielding a clear or slightly opaque, colorless suspension
Sanofi Pasteur-Diploid: Creamy white-to-orange powder, yielding a pink-to-red solution

Diluent:
Novartis: Sterile water for injection. Mix gently to avoid foaming.
Sanofi Pasteur-Diploid: Sterile water for injection. Gently swirl until completely dissolved.

Adjuvant:
Novartis: None
Sanofi Pasteur-Diploid: None

Preservative:
Novartis: None
Sanofi Pasteur-Diploid: None

Allergens:
Novartis: Per 1 mL dose, neomycin less than 1 mcg, chlortetracycline less than 20 ng, amphotericin B less than 2 ng, ovalbumin less than 3 ng
Sanofi Pasteur-Diploid: IM: Neomycin no more than 150 mcg; human serum albumin (HSA) no more than 100 mg/mL dose. Residual HSA may be antigenically altered by beta-propiolactone treatment during processing.

Excipients:
Novartis: Per 1 mL dose, 1 mg potassium glutamate, less than 12 mg processed bovine gelatin (polygeline), and 0.3 mg sodium ethylenediamine tetra-acetic acid (EDTA). Small quantities of bovine serum are used in the cell-culture process. Bovine components originate only from source countries known to be free of bovine spongiform encephalopathy.
Sanofi Pasteur-Diploid: 20 mcg phenolsulfonphthalein (phenol red), fetal calf serum, vitamins

pH:
Novartis: 7.4 to 7.8 after reconstitution
Sanofi Pasteur-Diploid: 7.4 to 8.5

Shelf Life:
Novartis: Expires within 36 months
Sanofi Pasteur-Diploid: IM package expires within 48 months

Storage/Stability: Store at 2° to 8°C (35° to 46°F). Discard if frozen.
Novartis: Protect from light during storage. Use immediately after reconstitution. Contact manufacturer regarding exposure to extreme temperatures. Shipped via overnight courier in insulated containers with coolant packs.
Sanofi Pasteur-Diploid: Powder can presumably tolerate 30 days at room temperature. Lots produced by the same process for distribution in Europe can tolerate 1 month at 37°C (98.6°F). Contact the manufacturer regarding exposure to freezing temperatures. Use vaccine immediately after reconstitution. Shipped in insulated containers with coolant packs by overnight or next-day courier.

Production Process:
Novartis: Rabies viruses are grown in chicken embryonic fibroblasts. The virus is inactivated with beta-propiolactone. It is purified by zonal centrifugation in a sucrose density-gradient to remove cell-culture allergens, including beta-propiolactone-modified albumin. The vaccine is then lyophilized after addition of a stabilizer solution containing buffered potassium glutamate and processed bovine gelatin (polygeline).
Sanofi Pasteur-Diploid: Concentrated by ultrafiltration, inactivated with 0.0025% beta-propiolactone, then lyophilized.

Media:
Novartis: Synthetic cell-culture medium including human albumin, processed bovine gelatin, and antibiotics
Sanofi Pasteur-Diploid: MRC-5 human diploid-cell line

Disease Epidemiology

Incidence: At its peak, 22 human cases occurred per year from 1946 to 1950. From 1981 to 1992, 0 to 3 human cases occurred per year, while 4,600 to 7,850 animal cases were reported.

According to the WHO, some 40,000 to 70,000 deaths result from rabies around the world each year. Approximately 10 million people receive postexposure treatments each year after exposure to suspect animals. Neural tissue vaccines, long ago abandoned in the United States because of adverse effects, are still the most widely used vaccines in developing nations.

Susceptible Pools: There were 40,000 to 50,000 deaths per year in India during the late 1980s. In the United States, an estimated 100,000 doses of rabies vaccine are administered annually to approximately 25,000 people, 85% for postexposure prophylaxis and 15% for preexposure prophylaxis. Rabies vaccine has been described as the only overused vaccine in the United States.

Transmission: Virus-laden saliva of a rabid animal introduced by or through a bite, scratch, abrasion, open wound, or mucous membrane. Corneal transplants have transmitted undiagnosed infections from donor to recipient. Rarely, airborne exposure in laboratories or bat-infested caves has resulted in rabies infection. Progress of rabies virus after exposure is believed to follow a neural pathway, and the time between exposure and clinical rabies is a function of the proximity of the bite or abrasion to the CNS and the dose of virus injected. In North America, the prime reservoirs of virus are dogs, foxes, coyotes, wolves, skunks, raccoons, feral cats, and certain bats. Rabbits, squirrels, chipmunks, rats, and mice are rarely infected, and their bites rarely, if ever, indicate rabies prophylaxis.

Incubation: 14 to 56 days (range, 5 to at least 180 days), depending on severity of the wound, site of the wound with respect to the richness of the nerve supply, and its distance from the brain; amount of virus introduced; and other factors.

Communicability: In dogs and cats, infection is communicable beginning 3 to 10 days before onset of clinical signs and throughout the course of the disease. Some wild animals may shed virus for 8 to 12 days before onset of symptoms and for at least 18 days afterward.

Other Information

Perspective:

1885: Pasteur tests antirabies vaccine (an attenuated strain weakened by desiccation) in 9-year-old Joseph Meister, brought from Alsace for treatment. Patient survived despite 14 bites on hands, legs, and thighs.

1908: Rabies *Iradogen* vaccine available in the United States.

1911: Semple develops phenol-inactivated rabies vaccine cultured in rabbit brain tissue. Semple- or Hempt-type vaccines are still prepared in developing countries from infected adult rabbit, sheep, or goat brains, inactivated with phenol.

1914: Rabies vaccine licensed in the United States.

1926: Fermi combines phenolized vaccine with equine antiserum.

1940: Leach and Johnson isolate a strain of rabies vaccine from a girl named Flury. After attenuation, this strain is used widely as a canine vaccine. It is also developed into low-egg-passage (LEP) and high-egg-passage (HEP) strains for human use.

1954: Wolf attacks Iranian village of Sahan and bites 29 people. Some of the victims were treated with RIG and vaccine, some with vaccine alone. Survival was 92% among those given RIG and vaccine and 40% among those given vaccine only.

1956: Powell, Culbertson and colleagues, and Peck and colleagues develop the safer but poorly immunogenic inactivated duck-embryo vaccine (DEV). Standard dose: 1 subcutaneous injection daily for 14 or 23 days. This was 1 of the Fuenzalida-type vaccines produced in newborn animals that have not developed myelin; others are cultured in suckling mouse brains.

1964: Wiktor and colleagues develop HDCV at Wistar Institute.

1975-76: Efficacy of HDCV demonstrated among 45 Iranian villagers bitten by rabid wolves and dogs.

1980: HDCVs from both Mérieux and Wyeth licensed in the United States.

1984: Purified chick-embryo culture vaccines first licensed in Europe.

1985: Wyeth withdraws *Wyvac* (a split-virion HDCV) from the US market because of low neutralizing antibody titers following postexposure prophylaxis. Until this time, the United States government had considered *Wyvac* and Mérieux's *Imovax Rabies* to be interchangeable.

1988: RVA licensed to Michigan Department of Public Health.

First Licensed:

Connaught (now Sanofi Pasteur)-Diploid: June 9, 1980
Michigan (now Emergent): March 19, 1988
Connaught (now Sanofi Pasteur)-Vero cell culture: December 27, 1991, but not yet marketed
Chiron (now Novartis): October 20, 1997

National Policy: ACIP. Human rabies prevention-United States, 2008. MMWR. 2008;57(RR-3):1-28. http://www.cdc.gov/mmwr/PDF/rr/rr5703.pdf.

Canadian National Advisory Committee on Immunization. Update on rabies vaccines. *Can Commun Dis Rep.* 2005;31(ACS-5):1-7.

References: National Association of State Public Health Veterinarians. Compendium of animal rabies prevention and control, 2008. *MMWR.* 2008;57(RR-2):1-9. http://www.cdc.gov/mmwr/PDF/rr/rr5702.pdf.

Rupprecht CE, Gibbons RV. Prophylaxis against rabies. *N Engl J Med.* 2004;351:2626-2635.

WHO. Rabies vaccines: WHO position paper—recommendations. *Vaccine.* 2010;28(Oct 18):7140-7142.

Comparison Table of Rabies Vaccines			
Generic name	Rabies vaccine adsorbed	Rabies vaccine (purified chicken embryo cell)	Rabies vaccine (human diploid cell)
Brand name	*BioRab*[a]	*RabAvert*	*Imovax Rabies*
Manufacturer	Emergent BioSolutions	Novartis	Sanofi Pasteur
Viability	Whole inactivated viral vaccine	Whole inactivated viral vaccine	Whole inactivated viral vaccine
Indication	Pre- and postexposure prophylaxis	Pre- and postexposure prophylaxis	Pre- and postexposure prophylaxis
Strain	Kissling/M PH strain	Flury LEP-C 25	PM-1503-3M
Concentration	≥ 2.5 units/mL	≥ 2.5 units/mL	≥ 2.5 units/mL
Adjuvant	Aluminum phosphate ≤ 2 mg/mL	None	None
Preservative	Thimerosal 0.01%	None	None
Production medium	Diploid fetal rhesus lung-2 cell culture	Chicken embryonic fibroblasts	MRC-5 human diploid cell culture
Doseform	Suspension	Powder for suspension	Powder for suspension
Diluent	n/a	Sterile Water	Sterile Water
Packaging	1 mL IM package	1 mL IM package	1 mL IM package
Routine storage	2° to 8°C	2° to 8°C	2° to 8°C
Stability	n/a	Use promptly after reconstitution	Use promptly after reconstitution
Allergens	None	Trace neomycin chlortetracycline, amphotericin B, ovalbumin	Human albumin and neomycin
Dosage	1 mL	1 mL	1 mL
Route	IM	IM	IM

Comparison Table of Rabies Vaccines			
Generic name	Rabies vaccine adsorbed	Rabies vaccine (purified chicken embryo cell)	Rabies vaccine (human diploid cell)
Incidence of serum sickness-like reaction	< 1%	Rare	6%
Shelf life	24 months	36 months	30 months

a Distributed in the US from 1988 to approximately 1998. Information provided for historical perspective.

Criteria for Preexposure Rabies Prophylaxis			
Risk category	Nature of risk	Typical populations	Preexposure risk recommendations
Continuous	Virus present continuously, often in high concentrations. Aerosol, mucous membrane, bite, or nonbite exposure. Specific exposures may go unrecognized.	Rabies research laboratory workers; rabies vaccine or immune globulin production workers.	Primary series. Serologic tests every 6 months; booster vaccination when antibody titer falls below an acceptable level.[a]
Frequent	Exposure usually episodic, with source recognized, but exposure may also be unrecognized. Aerosol, mucous membrane, bite, or nonbite exposure.	Rabies diagnostic laboratory workers, spelunkers, veterinarians and staff, and animal-control and wildlife workers in rabies enzootic areas. Travelers visiting foreign areas of enzootic-rabies for ≥ 30 days.	Primary series. Serologic tests or booster vaccination every 2 years.[a]
Infrequent, but greater than general population	Exposure nearly always episodic, with source recognized. Mucous membrane, bite, or nonbite exposure.	Veterinarians and animal-control and wildlife workers in areas of low rabies enzooticity. Veterinary students.	Primary series. No serologic testing or booster vaccination.
Rare, same as general population	Exposure always episodic. Mucous membrane or bite with source unrecognized.	US population at large, including people in rabies epizootic areas.	No vaccination necessary.

a Minimum acceptable antibody level is complete virus neutralization at a 1:5 serum dilution by RFFIT. Administer a booster vaccine dose if the titer falls below this level.

Rabies Vaccines

Treatment Schedule for Preexposure Rabies Prophylaxis		
Type of vaccination	Route	Regimen
Primary	IM	1 mL in the deltoid area on days 0, 7, and 21 or 28 (any licensed vaccine).
Booster	IM	One 1 mL dose in the deltoid area (any licensed vaccine).

Criteria for Postexposure Rabies Prophylaxis		
Animal species	Condition of animal at time of attack	Treatment[a]
Domestic dogs, cats, and ferrets	Healthy and available for 10 days of observation	None, unless animal develops rabies[b]
	Rabid or suspected rabid	Vaccinate immediately. Give RIG if not previously vaccinated.[c]
	Unknown, escaped	Consult public health officials.
Bats, wild carnivores (eg, raccoon, skunk, fox, coyote, bobcat)	Regard as rabid unless proven negative by laboratory tests[d]	Consider immediate vaccination. Consider RIG if not previously vaccinated.[c]
Livestock, small rodents, lagomorphs (eg, rabbits, hares), large rodents (eg, woodchucks, beavers), other mammals	Consider individually. Consult public health official. Bites of squirrels, hamsters, guinea pigs, gerbils, chipmunks, rats, mice, other rodents, rabbits, and hares almost never call for rabies prophylactic treatment.	Consult public health officials.

a Immediately cleanse all animal bites and wounds thoroughly with soap and water. If indicated, give vaccine or vaccine plus RIG[c] as soon as possible, regardless of the interval since possible rabies exposure.

b During the usual 10-day holding period, give vaccine or vaccine plus RIG[c] at the first sign of rabies in a dog or cat that has bitten a human. Kill the symptomatic animal immediately and test to confirm the diagnosis.

c Local reactions to vaccination do not contraindicate continuing treatment. Discontinue vaccine if direct fluorescent or immunofluorescent antibody (FA) tests of the animal are negative.

d Kill the animal and perform tests to confirm the diagnosis as soon as possible. Observation is not recommended. Postexposure prophylaxis is recommended for all people with a bite, scratch, or mucous membrane exposure to a bat, unless the bat tests negative for rabies. When a bat is found in close proximity to humans, it should be submitted to a public health laboratory for diagnostic testing, if it can be captured safely. If the animal is not available for testing, administer postexposure prophylaxis if a strong probability exists that exposure occurred.

Treatment Schedule for Postexposure Rabies Prophylaxis	
Vaccination status	Treatment[a]
Not previously vaccinated	*Local wound cleansing:* Begin all postexposure treatment with immediate, thorough cleansing of each wound with soap (preferably a virucidal agent such as povidone- iodine) and water.
	Rabies immune globulin: Give 20 units/kg body weight. Infiltrate the wound site with the full dose of RIG, if the nature and location of the wound site permit. Administer the balance of the dose IM at a different site and in a different extremity from rabies vaccine. Suitable sites may include deltoid muscle or gluteal muscle (upper, outer quadrant only). Do not give RIG through the same syringe or into the same anatomical site as rabies vaccine. Because RIG may partially suppress active induction of anti-rabies antibody, give no more than the recommended dose.
	Rabies vaccine: Give 1 mL IM in the deltoid area on days 0, 3, 7, 14, and 28.[b]
Previously vaccinated[c]	*Local wound cleansing:* Begin all postexposure treatment with immediate, thorough cleansing of each wound with soap (preferably a virucidal agent such as povidone-iodine) and water.
	Do not administer RIG.
	Rabies vaccine: Give 1 mL IM in the deltoid area on days 0 and 3.[b]

a These regimens apply to all age groups, including children. Young children may be vaccinated in the anterolateral aspect of the thigh, rather than the deltoid muscle. Vaccine should not be administered in the gluteal area.

b Day 0 is the day the first dose of vaccine is administered.

c Any patient with a history of pre- or postexposure vaccination with a licensed vaccine or with both a history of prior vaccination with any other type of rabies vaccine and a documented history of antibody response to that vaccination.

Rotavirus Vaccine Live Oral

Viral Vaccines

Name:
Rotarix
RotaTeq

Manufacturer:
GlaxoSmithKline
Merck

Immunologic Characteristics

Microorganism: Virus (double-stranded RNA), rotavirus, genus Rotavirus, family Reoviridae. Human rotaviruses are classified based on 10 G (G protein, VP7) types and 11 P (P protein, VP4) types from the outer capsid; this classification is analogous to the H and N system used to subtype influenza A viruses.

Viability: Live, attenuated

Antigenic Form: Whole viruses

Antigenic Type: Protein, G refers to glycoprotein type, P refers to protease type

Strains:

GSK: Human 89-12 strain of the G1P[8] type (also called RIX4414)

Merck: RotaTeq contains 5 live reassortant rotaviruses, each consisting of human outer surface proteins placed on a bovine viral backbone. The rotavirus parent strains of the reassortants were isolated from human and bovine hosts. Four reassortant rotaviruses express one of the outer capsid proteins (G1, G2, G3, or G4) from the human rotavirus parent strain and the attachment protein (P7) from the bovine rotavirus parent strain. The fifth reassortant virus expresses the attachment protein named P1A (genotype P[8]), hereafter referred to as P1[8], from the human rotavirus parent strain and the outer capsid protein G6 from the bovine rotavirus parent strain. WC3 refers to Wistar calf-3.

Name of reassortant virus in *RotaTeq*	Human rotavirus parent strains and outer surface protein compositions	Bovine rotavirus parent strain and outer surface protein composition	Reassortant outer surface protein composition (human component italicized)
G1	WI79 - G1, P1[8]	WC3 - G6, P7[5]	*G1*, P7[5]
G2	SC2 - G2, P2[6]	WC3 - G6, P7[5]	*G2*, P7[5]
G3	WI78 - G3, P1[8]	WC3 - G6, P7[5]	*G3*, P7[5]
G4	BrB - G4, P2[6]	WC3 - G6, P7[5]	*G4*, P7[5]
P1[8]	WI79 - G1, P1[8]	WC3 - G6, P7[5]	G6, *P1[8]*

Use Characteristics

Indications:

GSK: To prevent rotavirus gastroenteritis in infants and children caused by serotypes G1, G3, G4, and G9.

Merck: To prevent rotavirus gastroenteritis in infants and children caused by serotypes G1, G2, G3, and G4.

Limitations: The level of protection provided by less than the full dosing series was not studied in clinical trials. Regarding postexposure prophylaxis, no clinical data are available for rotavirus vaccination administered after exposure to rotavirus. Rotavirus vaccination does not protect against nonrotaviral diarrhea.

GSK: Safety and effectiveness of *Rotarix* in infants with chronic GI disorders have not been evaluated.

Contraindications:

Absolute: People with a history of serious allergic reaction to a vaccine component or after a prior dose of this vaccine. Do not vaccinate infants with severe combined immunodeficiency disease (SCID). Do not vaccine infants with a history of intussusception or uncorrected congenital malformation of the GI tract that would predispose the infant to intussusception. Gastroenteritis, including severe diarrhea and prolonged shedding of vaccine-type rotaviruses, has been reported in infants given live oral rotavirus vaccines and later identified as having SCID.

Relative: Febrile illness may be a reason for delaying use of rotavirus vaccine, except when withholding the vaccine entails a greater risk. Low-grade fever (less than 38.1°C [100.5°F]) and mild upper respiratory infection do not preclude vaccination.

No safety or efficacy data are available on rotavirus vaccination of infants with a history of GI disorders, including infants with active acute GI illness, infants with chronic diarrhea and failure to thrive, and infants with a history of congenital abdominal disorders and abdominal surgery. Use caution when considering rotavirus vaccination of such infants. Data from clinical studies support rotavirus vaccination in infants with controlled gastroesophageal reflux disease.

Use caution when considering rotavirus vaccination of infants with immunodeficient close contacts (ie, people with malignancies, those receiving immunosuppressive therapy, those with other forms of immunocompromise). There is a theoretical risk that live rotaviruses can be transmitted to nonvaccinated contacts. Weigh the potential risk of transmission of vaccine virus against the risk of acquiring and transmitting natural rotavirus.

GSK: History of uncorrected congenital malformation of the GI tract (eg, Meckel diverticulum) that would predispose the infant for intussusception. Delay administration of *Rotarix* in infants suffering from acute diarrhea or vomiting.

Immunodeficiency: Few safety or efficacy data are available regarding rotavirus vaccination of infants who are potentially immunocompromised (eg, blood dyscrasias, leukemia, lymphomas of any type, malignant neoplasms affecting bone marrow or lymphatic system, HIV/AIDS or other clinical manifestations of infection with HIV, cellular immune deficiencies, hypo- or dysgammaglobulinemic states, immunosuppressive therapy). Gastroenteritis, including severe diarrhea and prolonged shedding of vaccine-type rotaviruses, occurred in infants given live oral rotavirus vaccines and later identified as having SCID. There are insufficient data from the clinical trials to support rotavirus vaccination of infants with indeterminate HIV status who are born to mothers with HIV/AIDS. Rotavirus vaccine has been administered to infants who are being treated with topical corticosteroids or inhaled steroids.

Elderly: No information is available about geriatric use of rotavirus vaccine.

Carcinogenicity: Rotavirus vaccine has not been evaluated for carcinogenic potential.

Mutagenicity: Rotavirus vaccine has not been evaluated for mutagenic potential.

Fertility Impairment: Rotavirus vaccine has not been evaluated for impairment of fertility.

Pregnancy: Category C. Rotavirus vaccine is not recommended for adults. It is not known if rotavirus vaccine viruses cross the placenta. Generally, most IgG passage across the placenta occurs during the third trimester. Problems in humans have not been documented.

Lactation: There are no restrictions on an infant's consumption of food or liquid, including breast milk, either before or after vaccination with rotavirus vaccine. Breast milk is known to contain anti-rotavirus IgA antibodies and other nonspecific viral inhibitors, but multiple studies indicate that there is no significant interaction between breast-feeding and the efficacy of various rotavirus vaccines.

Children: Safety and efficacy in infants younger than 6 weeks or older than 24 weeks (*Rotarix*) or 32 weeks (*RotaTeq*) of age have not been established.

GSK: The effectiveness of *Rotarix* in preterm infants has not been established. Safety data are available in preterm infants (*Rotarix*, n = 134; placebo, n = 120) with a reported gestational age of 36 weeks or younger who were followed for serious adverse events up to 30 to 90 days after dose 2. Serious adverse events were observed in 5.2% of *Rotarix* recipients, compared with 5% of placebo recipients. No deaths or cases of intussusception were reported in this population.

Merck: Data from clinical studies support *RotaTeq* vaccination of preterm infants according to their age in weeks since birth.

Adverse Reactions:

GSK: Safety data were collected in 8 clinical studies evaluating 71,209 infants who received *Rotarix* (n = 36,755) or placebo (n = 34,454). The racial distribution for these studies was Hispanic (73.4%), white (16.2%), black (1%), and other (9.4%); 51% were male. Solicited adverse events among *Rotarix* and placebo recipients occurred at similar rates.

	Dose 1		Dose 2	
Solicited Adverse Events Within 8 Days After Doses 1 and 2 of *Rotarix* or Placebo (Total Vaccinated Cohort)[a]				
	Rotarix n = 3,284	Placebo n = 2,013	*Rotarix* n = 3,201	Placebo n = 1,973
Fussiness/irritability[b]	52%	52%	42%	42%
Cough/runny nose[c]	28%	30%	31%	33%
Fever[d]	25%	33%	28%	34%
Loss of appetite[e]	25%	25%	21%	21%
Vomiting	13%	11%	8%	8%
Diarrhea	4%	3%	3%	3%

a Total vaccinated cohort = all vaccinated infants for whom safety data were available.
b Defined as crying more than usual.
c Data not collected in 1 of 7 studies; dose 1: *Rotarix*, n = 2,583; placebo, n = 1,897; dose 2: *Rotarix*, n = 2,522; placebo, n = 1,863.
d Defined as temperature of 38°C (100.4°F) or higher rectally or 37.5°C (99.5°F) or higher orally.
e Defined as eating less than usual.

Infants were monitored for serious adverse events in the 31-day period after vaccination in 8 clinical studies. Serious adverse events occurred in 1.7% of *Rotarix* recipients (n = 36,755) and 1.9% of placebo recipients (n = 34,454). Among placebo recipients, diarrhea (placebo, 0.07%; *Rotarix*, 0.02%), dehydration (placebo, 0.06%; *Rotarix*, 0.02%), and gastroenteritis (placebo, 0.3%; *Rotarix*, 0.2%) occurred at a statistically higher incidence (95% confidence interval [CI] of relative risk [RR], excluding 1) than in *Rotarix* recipients. Infants were monitored for unsolicited adverse events in the 31-day period after vaccination in 7 clinical studies. Adverse events occurring at a statistically higher incidence among *Rotarix* recipients (n = 5,082) than in placebo recipients (n = 2,902) included irritability (*Rotarix*, 11.4%; placebo, 8.7%) and flatulence (*Rotarix*, 2.2%; placebo, 1.3%).

Merck: In 3 placebo-controlled clinical trials, 71,725 infants were evaluated with 36,165 infants in the *RotaTeq* cohort and 35,560 infants in the placebo cohort. On days 7, 14, and 42 after each dose, parents/guardians were contacted regarding intussusception and any other serious adverse events. Serious adverse events occurred in 2.4% of *RotaTeq* recipients, compared with 2.6% of placebo recipients within the 42-day period of a dose in the phase 3 clinical studies. The most frequently reported serious adverse events for *RotaTeq* compared with placebo were bronchiolitis (*RotaTeq*, 0.6% vs placebo, 0.7%), gastroenteritis (0.2% vs 0.3%), pneumonia (0.2% vs 0.2%), fever (0.1% vs 0.1%), and urinary tract infection (0.1% vs 0.1%). Detailed safety information was collected from 11,711 infants (including 6,138 *RotaTeq* recipients), including a subset of subjects in the Rotavirus Efficacy and Safety Trial (REST) and all subjects from Studies 007 and 009 (referred to as the Detailed Safety Cohort). Events reported appear in the following table.

Solicited Adverse Experiences Within the First Week After Doses 1, 2, and 3 (Detailed Safety Cohort)						
	Dose 1		Dose 2		Dose 3	
Adverse experience	*RotaTeq*	Placebo	*RotaTeq*	Placebo	*RotaTeq*	Placebo
Elevated temperature[a]	n = 5,616 17.1%	n = 5,077 16.2%	n = 5,215 20%	n = 4,725 19.4%	n = 4,865 18.2%	n = 4,382 17.6%
	n = 6,130	n = 5,560	n = 5,703	n = 5,173	n = 5,496	n = 4,989
Vomiting	6.7%	5.4%	5%	4.4%	3.6%	3.2%
Diarrhea	10.4%	9.1%	8.6%	6.4%	6.1%	5.4%
Irritability	7.1%	7.1%	6%	6.5%	4.3%	4.5%

a Temperature $\geq 38.1°C$ (100.5°F), rectal equivalent obtained by adding 1°F to otic and oral temperatures and 2°F to axillary temperatures.

Parents/guardians of the 11,711 infants also reported other events for 42 days after each dose. Fever was observed at similar rates in vaccine (n = 6,138) and placebo (n = 5,573) recipients (42.6% vs 42.8%). Adverse events that occurred at a statistically higher incidence (ie, 2-sided P value < 0.05) within the 42 days of any dose among recipients of *RotaTeq* compared with placebo recipients appear in the following table.

Adverse Events That Occurred at a Statistically Higher Incidence Within 42 Days of Any Dose Among Recipients of *RotaTeq* as Compared With Placebo Recipients		
Adverse event	*RotaTeq* n = 6,138 n (%)	Placebo n = 5,573 n (%)
Diarrhea	1,479 (24.1%)	1,186 (21.3%)
Vomiting	929 (15.2%)	758 (13.6%)
Otitis media	887 (14.5%)	724 (13%)
Nasopharyngitis	422 (6.9%)	325 (5.8%)
Bronchospasm	66 (1.1%)	40 (0.7%)

Intussusception: After administration of a previously licensed live rhesus rotavirus-based vaccine (*RotaShield*, Wyeth-Lederle), an increased risk of intussusception (a type of bowel obstruction in which the bowel folds in on itself) was observed.

GSK: The risk of intussusception with *Rotarix* was evaluated in a safety study (including 63,225 infants: *Rotarix*, n = 31,673; placebo, n = 31,552) conducted in Latin America and Finland. No increased risk of intussusception after *Rotarix* was observed within a 31-day period after any dose, and rates were comparable with the placebo group after a median of 100 days. In a subset of 20,169 infants followed up to 1 year after dose 1, there were 4 cases of intussusception with *Rotarix* compared with 14 cases of intussusception with placebo (RR, 0.28; 95% CI, 0.1-0.81). Each of the infants who developed intussusception recovered without sequelae. Among vaccine recipients, there were no confirmed cases of intussusception within the 0- to 14-day period after the first dose, which was the period of highest risk for the previously licensed oral live rhesus rotavirus-based vaccine.

Merck: In REST (N = 69,625), the data did not show an increased risk of intussusception for *RotaTeq* compared with placebo. In REST, 34,837 vaccine recipients and 34,788 placebo recipients were monitored by active surveillance to identify potential cases of intussusception at 7, 14, and 42 days after each dose and every 6 weeks thereafter for 1 year after the first dose. For the primary safety outcome (cases of intussusception occurring within 42 days of any dose), there were 6 cases among *RotaTeq* recipients and 5 cases among placebo recipients (RR, 1.6; 95% CI, 0.4-6.4). Within 365 days of dose 1, there were 13 cases among *RotaTeq* recipients and 15 cases among placebo recipients (RR, 0.9; 95% CI, 0.4-1.9). Among vaccine recipients, there were no confirmed cases of intussusception within the 42-day period after the first dose, the period of highest risk for the rhesus rotavirus-based product distributed from 1998 to 1999. Additional cases of intussusception after rotavirus vaccination have been reported since vaccine licensing, but not at a rate higher than expected based on background incidence among unvaccinated children.

Shedding and transmission:

    GSK: Rotavirus shedding in stool occurs after *Rotarix* vaccination, with peak excretion occurring around day 7 after dose 1. Live rotavirus shedding was evaluated in 2 studies among a subset of infants at day 7 after dose 1. In these studies, the proportion of *Rotarix* recipients who shed live rotavirus were 26% (95% CI, 10%-41%) and 27% (95% CI, 16%-38%), respectively. Transmission of virus was not evaluated. There is a possibility that the live vaccine virus can be transmitted to nonvaccinated contacts. Weigh the potential for transmission of vaccine virus after vaccination against the possibility of acquiring and transmitting natural rotavirus.

    Merck: Shedding was evaluated among a subset of subjects in REST 4 to 6 days after each dose and among all subjects who submitted an antigen rotavirus-positive stool sample at any time. *RotaTeq* was shed in the stools of 32 of 360 (9%; 95% CI, 6%-12%) vaccine recipients tested after dose 1; 0 of 249 (0%; 95% CI, 0%-1.5%) vaccine recipients tested after dose 2; and in 1 of 385 (0.3%; 95% CI, less than 0.1%-1.4%) vaccine recipients after dose 3. In phase 3 studies, shedding was observed as early as 1 day and as late as 15 days after a dose. Transmission was not evaluated.

Hematochezia:

    GSK: One or more cases of hematochezia (bloody stools) after *Rotarix* administration has been reported since product introduction.

    Merck: Hematochezia (bloody stools) reported as an adverse event occurred in 0.6% (39/6,130) of vaccine recipients and 0.6% (34/5,560) of placebo recipients within 42 days of any dose. As a serious adverse event, hematochezia occurred in less than 0.1% (4/36,150) of vaccine recipients and less than 0.1% (7/35,536) of placebo recipients within 42 days of any dose. Additional cases of hematochezia after rotavirus vaccination have been reported since vaccine licensing, but not at a rate higher than expected based on background incidence among unvaccinated children.

Kawasaki disease:

    GSK: Kawasaki disease was reported in 18 (0.035%) *Rotarix* recipients and 9 (0.021%) placebo recipients from 16 completed or ongoing clinical trials. Of the 27 cases, 5 occurred after *Rotarix* in clinical trials that were either not placebo controlled or 1:1 randomized. In placebo-controlled trials, Kawasaki disease was reported in 17 *Rotarix* recipients and 9 placebo recipients (RR, 1.71; 95% CI, 0.71-4.38). Three of the 27 cases were reported within 30 days after vaccination: 2 cases (*Rotarix* = 1, placebo = 1) were from placebo-controlled trials, and 1 case after *Rotarix* was from a non–placebo-controlled trial. Among *Rotarix* recipients, the time of onset after study dose ranged from 3 days to 19 months.

    Merck: In phase 3 clinical trials, infants were followed for up to 42 days after vaccine dose. Kawasaki disease was reported in 5 of 36,150 vaccine recipients and 1 of 35,536 placebo recipients with unadjusted RR of 4.9 (95% CI, 0.6-239.1).

Seizures:
   Merck: Seizures reported as serious adverse experiences occurred in 27 of 36,150 *RotaTeq*
   recipients and 18 of 35,536 placebo recipients (not a statistically significant difference). Ten febrile seizures were reported as serious adverse experiences; 5 were
   observed in vaccine recipients and 5 in placebo recipients. All seizures reported in the
   phase 3 trials of *RotaTeq* (by vaccination group and interval after dose) were as follows: days 1 to 7: *RotaTeq*-10, placebo-5; days 1 to 14: *RotaTeq*-15, placebo-8; days 1 to 42:
   RotaTeq-33, placebo-24.

Deaths:
   GSK: During the 8 clinical studies, there were 68 (0.19%) deaths after administration of
   Rotarix (n = 36,755) and 50 (0.15%) deaths after placebo (n = 34,454). The most com-
   monly reported cause of death after vaccination was pneumonia, observed in 19 (0.05%)
   Rotarix recipients and 10 (0.03%) placebo recipients (RR, 1.74; 95% CI, 0.76-4.23).
   Merck: Across the clinical studies, 52 deaths were reported. There were 25 deaths among
   RotaTeq recipients, compared with 27 deaths in placebo recipients. The most com-
   monly reported cause of death was sudden infant death syndrome (SIDS), observed in
   8 *RotaTeq* recipients and 9 placebo recipients.

Postlicensed experience:
   GSK: Idiopathic thrombocytopenic purpura, misadministration.

Preterm infants:
   GSK: The effectiveness of *Rotarix* in preterm infants has not been established. Safety data
   are available in preterm infants (*Rotarix*, n = 134; placebo, n = 120) with a reported gestational age of 36 weeks. These preterm infants were followed for serious adverse
   events up to 30 to 90 days after dose 2. Serious adverse events were observed in 5.2%
   of recipients of *Rotarix* compared with 5% of placebo recipients. No deaths or cases
   of intussusception were reported in this population.
   Merck: *RotaTeq* or placebo was administered to 2,070 preterm infants (25 to 36 weeks gestational age; median, 34 weeks) according to their age in weeks since birth in REST.
   All preterm infants were followed for serious adverse experiences; a subset of
   308 infants was monitored for all adverse experiences. There were 4 deaths throughout the study, 2 among vaccine recipients (1 SIDS and 1 motor vehicle accident) and
   2 among placebo recipients (1 SIDS and 1 unknown cause). No cases of intussusception were reported. Serious adverse experiences occurred in 5.5% of vaccine recipients and 5.8% of placebo recipients. The most common serious adverse experience was
   bronchiolitis, occurring in 1.4% of vaccine and 2% of placebo recipients. Parents/
   guardians were asked to record their children's temperatures and any episodes of vomiting and diarrhea daily for the first week following vaccination. The frequencies of
   these adverse experiences and irritability within the week after dose 1 appear in the following table.

Solicited Adverse Experiences Within the First Week of Doses 1, 2, and 3 among Preterm Infants						
	Dose 1		Dose 2		Dose 3	
Adverse event	*RotaTeq*	Placebo	*RotaTeq*	Placebo	*RotaTeq*	Placebo
Elevated temperature[a]	n = 127	n = 133	n = 124	n = 121	n = 115	n = 108
	18.1%	17.3%	25%	28.1%	14.8%	20.4%
	n = 154	n = 154	n = 137	n = 137	n = 135	n = 129
Vomiting	5.8%	7.8%	2.9%	2.2%	4.4%	4.7%
Diarrhea	6.5%	5.8%	7.3%	7.3%	3.7%	3.9%
Irritability	3.9%	5.2%	2.9%	4.4%	8.1%	5.4%

a Temperature was approximately 38.1°C (100.5°F); rectal equivalent obtained by adding 1°F to otic and oral temperatures
and 2°F to axillary temperatures.

Pharmacologic & Dosing Characteristics

Dosage:

GSK: Two 1 mL doses, starting at 6 weeks of age, with at least 4 weeks between the first and second dose. Complete the 2-dose series by 24 weeks of age. A standard schedule of 2 and 4 months of age may be followed.

Merck: Three 2 mL doses, starting at 6 to 12 weeks of age, with later doses at 4- to 10-week intervals. A standard schedule of 2, 4, and 6 months of age may be followed.

Route: Oral administration only. Do not inject.

GSK: Reconstitute the product according to directions provided. Seat infant in a reclining position. Administer orally the entire contents of the oral applicator on the inside of the cheek.

Merck: Administer the dose by gently squeezing liquid into the infant's mouth toward the inner cheek until the dosing tube is empty. A residual drop may remain in the tip of the tube. Do not mix *RotaTeq* with any other vaccine or solution. Do not dilute.

Documentation Requirements: Federal law requires that the following information be documented in the recipient's permanent medical record or in a permanent office log: (1) The manufacturer and lot number of this vaccine, (2) the date of administration, and (3) the name, address, and title of the person administering the vaccine.

Certain adverse events must be reported to the Vaccine Adverse Event Reporting System (VAERS) ([800] 822-7967). Refer to the Immunization Documents in the Resources section.

Booster Doses:

GSK: The *Rotarix* vaccination series consists of an oral dose beginning at 6 weeks of age, with a second dose after an interval of at least 4 weeks. Do not give the second dose after 24 weeks of age.

Merck: The *RotaTeq* vaccination series consists of an oral dose at 6 to 12 weeks of age, with subsequent doses at 4- to 10-week intervals. Do not give the third dose after 32 weeks of age.

Missed Doses: Interrupting the recommended schedule or delaying subsequent doses does not require restarting the series.

GSK: If an incomplete dose is administered (eg, infant spits or regurgitates the vaccine), a single replacement dose may be considered at the same vaccination visit.

Merck: If an incomplete dose is administered (eg, infant spits or regurgitates the vaccine), a replacement dose is not recommended because such dosing was not studied in the clinical trials. The infant should continue to receive any remaining doses in the recommended series.

Related Interventions: There are no restrictions on the infant's consumption of food or liquid, including breast milk, either before or after vaccination with rotavirus vaccine.

Waste Disposal: Discard vaccine tubes in appropriate biological waste containers according to local regulations.

Efficacy:

GSK: Data demonstrating *Rotarix* efficacy come from 24,163 infants randomized in 2 placebo-controlled studies conducted in 17 countries in Europe and Latin America. In these studies, oral polio vaccine (OPV) was not coadministered. A randomized, double-blind, placebo-controlled study was conducted in 6 European countries. A total of 3,994 infants were enrolled to receive *Rotarix* (n = 2,646) or placebo (n = 1,348). Vaccine or placebo was given to healthy infants as a 2-dose series, with the first dose given orally from 6 to 14 weeks of age, followed by a second dose administered at least 4 weeks after the first dose. The 2-dose series was completed by 24 weeks of age. For both vaccination groups, 98.3% of infants were white and 53% were male. The clinical case definition of rotavirus gastroenteritis was an episode of diarrhea (passage of 3 or more loose or watery stools within a day), with or without vomiting, where rotavirus was identified in a stool sample. Analyses were also done to evaluate efficacy among infants who received at least one vaccination (total vaccinated cohort [TVC]). Scores range from 0 to 20, where higher scores indicate greater severity. An episode of gastroenteritis with a score of 11 or higher was considered severe. Efficacy of *Rotarix* against any grade of severity of rotavirus gastroenteritis through 1 rotavirus season was 87% (95% CI, 80-92); TVC efficacy was 87% (95% CI, 80-92). Efficacy against severe rotavirus gastroenteritis through one rotavirus season was 96% (95% CI, 90-99); TVC efficacy was 96% (95% CI, 90-99). The protective effect of *Rotarix* against any grade of severity of rotavirus gastroenteritis observed immediately after dose 1 and before dose 2 was 90% (95% CI, 9-99.8). Efficacy of *Rotarix* in reducing hospitalizations for rotavirus gastroenteritis through one rotavirus season was 100% (95% CI, 82-100); TVC efficacy was 100% (95% CI, 82-100). *Rotarix* reduced hospitalizations for all-cause gastroenteritis regardless of presumed etiology by 75% (95% CI, 46-89).

A randomized, double-blind, placebo-controlled study was conducted in 11 countries in Latin America and Finland. A total of 63,225 infants received *Rotarix* (n = 31,673) or placebo (n = 31,552). An efficacy subset of these infants consisting of 20,169 infants from Latin America received *Rotarix* (n = 10,159) or placebo (n = 10,010). Vaccine or placebo was given to healthy infants as a 2-dose series, with the first dose administered orally from 6 through 13 weeks of age followed by 1 additional dose administered at least 4 weeks after the first dose. The 2-dose series was completed by 24 weeks of age. For both vaccination groups, the racial distribution of the efficacy subset was as follows: Hispanic 86%, white 8%, black 1%, and other 5%; 51% were male. The clinical case definition of severe rotavirus gastroenteritis was an episode of diarrhea (passage of 3 or more loose or watery stools within a day), with or without vomiting, where rotavirus was identified in a stool sample, requiring hospitalization and/or rehydration therapy equivalent to World Health Organization plan B (oral rehydration therapy) or plan C (IV rehydration therapy) in a medical facility. Efficacy of *Rotarix* against severe rotavirus gastroenteritis through 1 year was 85% (95% CI, 72-92); TVC efficacy was 81% (95% CI, 69-89). Efficacy of *Rotarix* in reducing hospitalizations for rotavirus gastroenteritis through 1 year was 85% (95% CI, 70-94); TVC efficacy was 81% (95% CI, 66-90).

The type-specific efficacy against any grade of severity and severe rotavirus gastroenteritis caused by G1P[8], G3P[8], G4P[8], G9P[8], and combined non-G1 (G2, G3, G4, G9) types was statistically significant through 1 year. Additionally, type-specific efficacy against any grade of severity and severe rotavirus gastroenteritis caused by G1P[8], G2P[4], G3P[8], G4P[8], G9P[8], and combined non-G1 (G2, G3, G4, G9) types was statistically significant through 2 years.

Type-Specific Efficacy of *Rotarix* Against Any Grade of Severity and Severe Rotavirus Gastroenteritis (According to Protocol)						
	Through 1 rotavirus season Number of cases			Through 2 rotavirus seasons Number of cases		
Type identified[a]	*Rotarix* n = 2,572	Placebo n = 1,302	% efficacy (95% CI)	*Rotarix* n = 2,572	Placebo n = 1,302	% efficacy (95% CI)
Any grade of severity						
G1P[8]	4	46	95.6%[b] (87.9-98.8)	18	89[c,d]	89.8%[b] (82.9-94.2)
G2P[4]	3	4[c]	NS	14	17[c]	58.3%[b] (10.1-81)
G3P[8]	1	5	89.9%[b] (9.5-99.8)	3	10	84.8%[b] (41-97.3)

Type-Specific Efficacy of *Rotarix* Against Any Grade of Severity and Severe Rotavirus Gastroenteritis (According to Protocol)						
	Through 1 rotavirus season Number of cases			Through 2 rotavirus seasons Number of cases		
Type identified[a]	*Rotarix* n = 2,572	Placebo n = 1,302	% efficacy (95% CI)	*Rotarix* n = 2,572	Placebo n = 1,302	% efficacy (95% CI)
Any grade of severity (*cont.*)						
G4P[8]	3	13	88.3%[b] (57.5-97.9)	6	18	83.1%[b] (55.6-94.5)
G9P[8]	13	27	75.6%[b] (51.1-88.5)	38	71[d]	72.9%[b] (59.3-82.2)
Combined non-G1 (G2, G3, G4, G9, G12) types[e]	20	49	79.3%[b] (64.6-88.4)	62	116	72.9%[b] (62.9-80.5)
Severe						
G1P[8]	2	28	96.4%[b] (85.7-99.6)	4	57	96.4%[b] (90.4-99.1)
G2P[4]	1	2[c]	NS	2	7[c]	85.5%[b] (24-98.5)
G3P[8]	0	5	100%[b] (44.8-100)	1	8	93.7%[b] (52.8-99.9)
G4P[8]	0	7	100%[b] (64.9-100)	1	11	95.4%[b] (68.3-99.9)
G9P[8]	2	19	94.7%[b] (77.9-99.4)	13	44[d]	85%[b] (71.7-92.6)
Combined non-G1 (G2, G3, G4, G9, G12) types[f]	3	33	95.4%[b] (85.3-99.1)	17	70	87.7%[b] (78.9-93.2)

a Statistical analyses done by G type; if more than one rotavirus type was detected from a rotavirus gastroenteritis episode, the episode was counted in each of the detected rotavirus type categories.
b Statistically significant vs placebo ($P < 0.05$).
c The P genotype was not typeable for one episode.
d P[8] genotype was not detected in one episode.
e Two cases of G12P[8] were isolated in the second season (one in each group).

Merck: Overall, 72,324 infants were randomized in 3 placebo-controlled, phase 3 studies conducted in 11 countries on 3 continents. Data demonstrating efficacy in preventing rotavirus gastroenteritis come from 6,983 of these infants in the United States and Finland enrolled in REST and Study 007. The third trial, Study 009, provided clinical evidence supporting consistency of manufacture and contributed data to the safety evaluation.

The vaccine was given as a 3-dose series to healthy infants, with the first dose administered between 6 and 12 weeks of age and followed by 2 additional doses administered at 4- to 10-week intervals. The age of infants receiving the third dose was 32 weeks of age or less. Oral polio vaccine administration was not permitted; however, other childhood vaccines could be administered concomitantly. Breast-feeding was permitted in all studies.

The case definition for rotavirus gastroenteritis used to determine vaccine efficacy required at least 3 watery or looser-than-normal stools within a 24-hour period and/or forceful vomiting and rotavirus antigen detection by enzyme immunoassay in stool within 14 days of onset of symptoms. The severity of acute gastroenteritis was determined by a clinical scoring system that took into account the intensity and duration of fever, vomiting, diarrhea, and behavioral changes.

REST: Efficacy against any grade of severity of rotavirus gastroenteritis caused by naturally occurring serotypes G1, G2, G3, or G4 that occurred at least 14 days after the third dose through the first rotavirus season after vaccination was 74% (95% CI, 67-80). Efficacy assessed by an intent-to-treat (ITT) analysis from the first dose through the first rotavirus season after vaccination among infants who received at least 1 vaccination was 60% (95% CI, 51-67). Efficacy against severe gastroenteritis through the first rotavirus season after vaccination was 98% (95% CI, 88-100); the ITT efficacy was 96% (95% CI, 86-100). Vaccination reduced hospitalizations for rotavirus gastroenteritis caused by serotypes G1, G2, G3, and G4 through the first 2 years after the third dose by 96% (95% CI, 90-98); the ITT efficacy in reducing hospitalizations was 95% (95% CI, 89-97).

Study 007: Efficacy against any grade of severity of rotavirus gastroenteritis caused by naturally occurring serotypes G1, G2, G3, or G4 through the first rotavirus season after vaccination was 73% (95% CI, 51-86); the ITT efficacy was 58% (95% CI, 34-75). Efficacy against severe gastroenteritis through the first rotavirus season after vaccination was 100% (95% CI, 13-100); the ITT efficacy against severe disease was 100% (95% CI, 31-100).

Disease regardless of serotype: The rotavirus serotypes identified in the efficacy subset of REST and Study 007 were G1, P1[8]; G2, P1[4]; G3, P1[8]; G4, P1[8]; and G9, P1[8]. In REST, efficacy against any grade of severity regardless of serotype was 72% (95% CI, 65-78), and efficacy against severe disease was 98% (95% CI, 88-100). The ITT efficacy starting at dose 1 was 51% (95% CI, 42-59) for any grade of severity and was 96% (95% CI, 86-100) for severe disease. In Study 007, efficacy against any grade of severity regardless of serotype was 73% (95% CI, 52-85), and efficacy against severe disease was 100% (95% CI, 13-100). The ITT efficacy starting at dose 1 was 48% (95% CI, 22-66) for any grade of severity of rotavirus disease and was 100% (95% CI, 31-100) for severe disease.

G9P1A[8] gastroenteritis: In a post hoc analysis of health care utilization data from 68,038 infants (*RotaTeq,* 34,035; placebo, 34,003) in REST, using a case definition that included culture confirmation, hospitalization, and emergency department visits because of G9P1A[8] rotavirus gastroenteritis were reduced (*RotaTeq,* 0 cases; placebo, 14 cases) by 100% (95% CI, 69.6%-100%).

Onset:

GSK: Not described.

Merck: Full protection is presumed to begin within 2 weeks after the third dose; this was the basis for efficacy in clinical trials.

Duration: The duration of immunity has not been fully determined.

GSK: The efficacy of *Rotarix* persisting through 2 rotavirus seasons was evaluated in 2 studies. In the European study, the efficacy of *Rotarix* against any grade of severity of rotavirus gastroenteritis through 2 rotavirus seasons was 79% (95% CI, 73-84). Efficacy in preventing any grade of severity of rotavirus gastroenteritis cases occurring only during the second season after vaccination was 72% (95% CI, 61-80). The efficacy of *Rotarix* against severe rotavirus gastroenteritis through 2 rotavirus seasons was 90% (95% CI, 85-94). Efficacy in preventing severe rotavirus gastroenteritis cases occurring only during the second season after vaccination was 86% (95% CI, 76-92). The efficacy of *Rotarix* in reducing hospitalizations for rotavirus gastroenteritis through 2 rotavirus seasons was 96% (95% CI, 84-99.5). In the Latin American study, the efficacy of *Rotarix* against severe rotavirus gastroenteritis through 2 years was 81% (95% CI, 71-87). Efficacy in preventing severe rotavirus gastroenteritis cases occurring only during the second year after vaccination was 79% (95% CI, 66-87). The efficacy of *Rotarix* in reducing hospitalizations for rotavirus gastroenteritis through 2 years was 83% (95% CI, 73-90). The efficacy of *Rotarix* beyond the second season after vaccination was not evaluated.

Merck: Efficacy through a second rotavirus season was evaluated in REST. Efficacy against any grade of severity of rotavirus gastroenteritis caused by rotavirus serotypes G1, G2, G3, and G4 through the 2 rotavirus seasons after vaccination was 71% (95% CI, 65-77). Efficacy in preventing cases occurring only during the second rotavirus season after vaccination was 63% (95% CI, 44-75). Efficacy beyond the second season after vaccination was not evaluated.

Pharmacokinetics: Not described.

Protective Level:

GSK: A relationship between antibody responses to rotavirus vaccination and protection against rotavirus gastroenteritis has not been established. Seroconversion was defined as the appearance of antirotavirus IgA antibodies (concentration, 20 units/mL or more) after vaccination in the serum of infants previously negative for rotavirus. In 2 safety and efficacy studies, 1 to 2 months after a 2-dose series, 86.5% of 787 *Rotarix* recipients seroconverted, compared with 6.7% of 420 placebo recipients; 76.8% of 393 *Rotarix* recipients seroconverted, compared with 9.7% of 341 placebo recipients.

Merck: In phase 3 studies, 93% to 100% of 439 recipients of *RotaTeq* achieved a 3-fold or more rise in serum antirotavirus IgA after a 3-dose regimen, compared with 12% to 20% of 397 placebo recipients.

Mechanism: The exact immunologic mechanism by which rotavirus vaccine protects against rotavirus gastroenteritis is unknown. Rotavirus vaccine is a live viral vaccine that replicates in the small intestine and induces immunity.

Drug Interactions: Like all live viral vaccines, administration to people or contacts of people receiving immune-suppressing therapies (eg, irradiation, antimetabolites, alkylating agents, cytotoxic drugs, greater than physiologic doses of corticosteroids) may reduce the immune response to vaccines. These patients may remain susceptible despite immunization.

No safety or efficacy data are available regarding rotavirus vaccination of infants who received a blood transfusion or blood products (eg, immune globulins) within 42 days.

GSK: In clinical trials, *Rotarix* was administered concomitantly with US-licensed and non–US-licensed vaccines. In a US study in 484 infants, there was no evidence of interference in immune responses to any of the antigens when DTaP-Hep B-IPV, PCV7, and Hib conjugate vaccines were coadministered with *Rotarix*, compared with separate administration.

Merck: In clinical trials, *RotaTeq* was routinely administered concomitantly with DTaP, IPV, Hib, hepatitis B, and PCV7 vaccines. There was no evidence of reduced antibody responses to the vaccines coadministered.

Pharmaceutical Characteristics

Concentration:

GSK: Each 1 mL dose contains at least 10^6 median cell culture infective doses ($CCID_{50}$) of G1P[8].

Merck: Each 2 mL dose contains at least the following concentrations in infectious units: 2.2×10^6 of G1, 2.8×10^6 of G2, 2.2×10^6 of G3, 2×10^6 of G4, 2.3×10^6 of P1[8].

Packaging:

GSK: Package of 10 units, each containing a vial of lyophilized vaccine, a prefilled 1 mL oral applicator of liquid diluent with a plunger stopper, and a transfer adapter for reconstitution (NDC#: 58160-0 805-11)

Merck: Ten individually pouched 2 mL tubes (00006-4047-41).

Doseform:

GSK: Powder yielding suspension

Merck: Suspension

Appearance:

GSK: The shaken diluent suspension appears as a turbid liquid with a slowly settling, white deposit. The reconstituted vaccine appears more turbid than diluent alone.

Merck: Pale yellow, clear liquid that may have a pink tint.

Solvent:

    Merck: Buffered stabilizer solution containing sucrose, sodium citrate, sodium phosphate monobasic monohydrate, sodium hydroxide, and polysorbate 80.

Diluent:

    GSK: Calcium carbonate (an antacid), xanthan, and water.

Adjuvant: None

Preservative: None

Allergens:

    GSK: The tip cap and rubber plunger of the oral applicator contain dry natural latex rubber. The vial stopper and transfer adapter are latex free.

    Merck: None. The package is latex free.

Excipients:

    GSK: The lyophilized vaccine contains amino acids, dextran, Dulbecco's Modified Eagle Medium (DMEM), sorbitol, and sucrose. DMEM contains sodium chloride, potassium chloride, magnesium sulfate, ferric (III) nitrate, sodium phosphate, sodium pyruvate, D-glucose, concentrated vitamin solution, L-cystine, L-tyrosine, amino acids solution, L-glutamine, calcium chloride, sodium hydrogenocarbonate, and phenol red.

    Merck: The viruses are suspended in a buffered stabilizer solution. Each vaccine dose contains sucrose, sodium citrate, sodium phosphate monobasic monohydrate, sodium hydroxide, polysorbate 80, cell-culture media, and trace amounts of fetal bovine serum.

pH: Not described

Shelf Life: Expires within 24 months.

Storage/Stability:

    GSK: Store and transport vaccine powder at 2° to 8°C (36° to 46°F). Diluent may be stored at 20° to 25°C (68° to 77°F). Protect vials from light. Reconstituted vaccine may be stored refrigerated at 2° to 8°C (36° to 46°F) or at room temperature up to 25°C (77°F) for up to 24 hours. Discard unused vaccine in biohazard waste container. Discard if vaccine is frozen at any stage. Do not mix *Rotarix* with other vaccines or solutions.

    Merck: Store and transport at 2° to 8°C (36° to 46°F). Protect tubes from light. Do not freeze. Contact the manufacturer (800-MERCK-90) regarding exposure to freezing or elevated temperatures. Shipping data is not provided.

    Administer as soon as possible after removing tube from refrigeration.

Handling:

    GSK: Reconstitute only with accompanying diluent. Connect transfer adapter onto vial by pushing downward until transfer adapter is securely in place. Shake oral applicator containing the liquid diluent vigorously. Remove protective tip cap from oral applicator. Connect oral applicator to the transfer adapter by pushing it firmly on the device. Transfer the entire contents into the vial of lyophilized vaccine. With oral applicator attached, shake the vial and examine for complete suspension. The reconstituted vaccine will appear more turbid than the diluent alone. Withdraw entire mixture back into oral applicator. Remove oral applicator from transfer adapter. Seat infant in a reclining position. Administer orally the entire contents of the oral applicator on the inside of the cheek.

    Merck: Remove the dosing tube from the pouch. Clear any fluid from the dispensing tip by holding tube vertically and tapping the cap. Open the dosing tube in 2 easy motions: (a) Puncture the dispensing tip by screwing cap clockwise until it becomes tight, and (b) remove the cap by turning it counterclockwise. Discard vaccine tubes in appropriate biological waste containers according to local regulations.

Rotavirus Vaccine Live Oral

Production Process:
GSK: Vaccine-strain viruses are grown in Vero cells using standard cell-culture techniques.

Merck: Each reassortant virus consists of a bovine rotavirus genome backbone engineered to express a gene encoding an outer surface protein representing 1 of 5 human rotavirus serotypes.

Media:
GSK: Vaccine-strain viruses are grown in Vero cells using standard cell-culture techniques, including use of trypsin.

Merck: Reassortant viruses are grown in Vero cells using standard cell-culture techniques, including use of trypsin, in the absence of antifungal agents.

Disease Epidemiology

Incidence: Rotaviruses are, by far, the leading cause of severe gastroenteritis and dehydrating diarrheal disease among infants and young children in both developed and developing nations. In both settings, rotaviral gastroenteritis causes 5% of diarrheal disease in the community but nearly 40% of severe dehydrating illness. Untreated severe rotaviral diarrhea in infants can be rapidly fatal, unless dehydration is corrected with oral or IV fluid replacement. The most severe cases occur among infants and young children between 6 and 24 months of age.

Rotavirus is the most important cause of pediatric gastroenteritis in the United States. Four serotypes designated G1, G2, G3, and G4 are epidemiologically important and account for more than 90% of rotavirus cases in the United States. Before vaccine licensure, approximately 2.7 million children developed acute rotaviral diarrhea annually in this country. Approximately half of these young children developed severe diarrhea. Before vaccine licensure, rotavirus infections resulted in 55,000 to 70,000 hospitalizations in the United States each year, 4% to 6% of all pediatric hospitalizations. The number of emergency department visits was estimated at 205,000 to 272,000 per year. Rotavirus infections accounted for approximately one-third of all hospitalizations for diarrhea among children younger than 5 years of age, evenly distributed geographically and by socioeconomic status. Approximately 1 in 8 children required medical treatment for rotavirus gastroenteritis, and 1 in 50 US infants was hospitalized with rotaviral gastroenteritis. A large children's hospital determined that rotaviral disease accounted for 3% of all hospital days. On average, rotaviral infections led to the deaths of 20 to 60 children annually in this country.

Around the world, hundreds of millions of cases of rotaviral diarrhea occur annually among children younger than 5 years of age, with over 2 million hospitalizations. Rotaviruses are believed to be responsible for 440,000 to 2 million deaths each year from diarrhea in young children, with at least 1,200 children dying per day. Rotaviruses represent the most frequently detected pathogen among the 5 to 10 million childhood deaths from diarrhea annually. This disease burden is equivalent to 25% of all diarrheal deaths and 5% of all childhood deaths before the fifth birthday.

Rotaviral infections of adults are usually asymptomatic. Outbreaks have occurred in geriatric units and among the elderly in day care settings. Rotaviruses can cause diarrhea in adult travelers or in immunocompromised patients and can infect parents of children with rotaviral diarrhea.

Prevalence: Before vaccine licensure, over 95% of US children were infected by the time they reached 5 years of age.

Susceptible Pools: Children are both the primary sufferers of rotaviral disease and the principal means of rotavirus transmission. Most disease occurs among children 6 to 36 months of age and persists for 3 to 9 days. Children younger than 6 months of age have the second highest incidence rate.

Transmission: Rotaviruses are spread through close contact, especially fecal-oral transmission. Respiratory spread may play a role as well. The disease peaks in fall and winter in temperate climates; no seasonality is seen in most tropical settings. Morbidity because of rotaviral diarrhea results primarily from severe dehydration.

Incubation: Ingested viruses infect cells in the villi of the small intestine. Acute watery diarrhea occurs after an incubation period of 1 to 2 days.

Other Information

Perspective:
1974: Kapikian identifies rotavirus by electron microscopy.
1980: Offit, Clark, and Plotkin develop rotavirus vaccine candidate. This invention eventually becomes *RotaTeq.*
1989: Ward and Bernstein develop rotavirus vaccine candidate from strain circulating in Cincinnati. This invention, later licensed to Avant, eventually becomes *Rotarix.*
1993: Merck begins first trial leading toward the product *RotaTeq.*
1997: Avant licenses technology for *Rotarix* to GlaxoSmithKline.
1998: Wyeth-Lederle's rhesus rotavirus tetravalent vaccine (*RotaShield*) licensed on August 31.
1999: Wyeth-Lederle's *RotaShield* withdrawn on October 15, 1999 because of elevated risk of intussusception, primarily in the 2 weeks after the first and second doses. Estimates of the risk ranged from 1 per 2,500 to 32,000 vaccinees.
2000: *RotaTeq* study design endorsed by Food and Drug Administration (FDA) advisory committee.

First Licensed:
GSK: April 3, 2008
Merck: February 3, 2006

Discontinued Products: *RotaShield* (Wyeth-Lederle, available August 1998 to October 1999)

National Policy: ACIP. Prevention of rotavirus gastroenteritis among infants and children. *MMWR.* 2009;58(RR-2):1-25. www.cdc.gov/mmwr/PDF/rr/rr5802.pdf.

CDC. Reduction in rotavirus after vaccine introduction—United States, 2000-2009. *MMWR.* 2009;58(41):1146-1149.

Canadian National Advisory Committee on Immunization. Statement on the recommended use of pentavalent human-bovine reassortant rotavirus vaccine. *Can Comm Dis Rep.* 2008;34(ACS-1):1-32.

References: Vesikari T, Matson DO, Dennehy P, et al; Rotavirus Efficacy and Safety Trial (REST) Study Team. Safety and efficacy of a pentavalent human-bovine (WC3) reassortant rotavirus vaccine. *N Engl J Med.* 2006;354(1):23-33.

Parashar UD, Hummelman EG, Bresee JS, Miller MA, Glass RI. Global illness and deaths caused by rotavirus disease in children. *Emerg Infect Dis.* 2003;9(5):565-572.

WHO. Rotavirus vaccines: an update. *Wkly Epidemiol Rec.* 2009;84(50):533-540.

Rotavirus Vaccine Summary Table		
Generic name	Rotavirus vaccine live oral [monovalent]	Rotavirus vaccine live oral [pentavalent]
Brand name	*Rotarix*	*RotaTeq*
Manufacturer	GlaxoSmithKline	Merck Vaccines & Infectious Diseases
Viability	Live viral vaccine	Live viral vaccine
Indication	To prevent rotavirus gastroenteritis caused by serotypes G1, G3, G4, and G9	To prevent rotavirus gastroenteritis caused by serotypes G1, G2, G3, G4
Components	Rotavirus type G1P[8]	Rotavirus types G1, G2, G3, G4, P1[8]
Concentration	At least 10^6 median cell culture infective doses ($CCID_{50}$) of G1P[8]	Infectious units: 2.2×10^6 of G1, 2.8×10^6 of G2, 2.2×10^6 of G3, 2×10^6 of G4, 2.3×10^6 of P1[8]
Adjuvant	None	None
Preservative	None	None
Production medium	Vero cells	Vero cells
Doseform	Powder yielding suspension	Suspension
Diluent or solvent	Diluent: Calcium carbonate, xanthan, and water	Solvent: Buffered sucrose stabilizer solution
Packaging	Powdered vaccine with 1 mL diluent in prefilled oral applicator	2 mL, single-dose plastic tubes
Routine storage	2° to 8°C	2° to 8°C
Dosage, route	1 mL, oral	2 mL, oral
Standard schedule	2 and 4 months of age. Do not administer after 24 weeks of age.	2, 4, and 6 months of age. Do not administer after 32 weeks of age.
CPT code	90681	90680

Viral Vaccines

Comparison Table of Smallpox Vaccines (Vaccinia Vaccines)		
Generic name	Vaccinia vaccine dried calf-lymph type	Vaccinia vaccine live (Vero cell)
Brand name	*Dryvax*[a]	*ACAM2000*
Manufacturer	Wyeth Laboratories	Acambis
Viability	Live viral vaccine	Live viral vaccine
Indication	To prevent infection with variola virus, the cause of smallpox	To prevent infection with variola virus, the cause of smallpox
Strain	NYCBOH	NYCBOH
Concentration	1×10^8 pock-forming units/mL	1 to 5×10^8 plaque-forming units/mL
Adjuvant	None	None
Preservative	None	None
Production medium	Calf lymph	Vero (African green monkey kidney) cells
Doseform	Powder for suspension	Powder for suspension
Diluent	50% glycerin in water, 0.25 mL per 100-dose vial	50% glycerin in water, 0.25 mL per 100-dose vial
Packaging	100-dose vial	100-dose vial
Routine storage	Store powder at 2° to 8°C or colder	Freeze or refrigerate powder
Stability after reconstitution	If refrigerated, use within 90 days	If stored at room temperature, use within 6 to 8 hours. If refrigerated, use within 30 days.
Route	Percutaneous jabs, known as scarification	Percutaneous jabs, known as scarification
Dosage	3 jabs for primary (first) vaccination, 15 jabs for revaccination	15 jabs for both primary (first) and revaccination
Standard schedule	Single dose, confirmed by lesion 6 to 8 days after vaccination. Repeat approximately 3 to 10 years later.	Single dose, confirmed by lesion 6 to 8 days after vaccination. Repeat approximately 3 to 10 years later.

a No longer distributed in the United States; information provided for reference value.

Smallpox Vaccinia Vaccine, Live

Viral Vaccines

Name:
ACAM2000

Manufacturer:
Acambis

Synonyms: VISI abbreviation: SMA. Vaccinia vaccine, vaccinia virus, vaccine virus, Jennerian vaccine. Although this product is classically called smallpox vaccine, this term is a misnomer because it contains no smallpox (variola) virus. Vaccinia is sometimes referred to as cowpox, although this is also a misnomer.

Immunologic Characteristics

Microorganism: Virus (double-stranded DNA), vaccinia virus, genus *Orthopoxvirus*, family Poxviridae

Viability: Live, attenuated

Antigenic Form: Whole virus

Antigenic Type: Protein

Strains: New York City Board of Health (NYCBOH) strain

Use Characteristics

Indications: For induction of active immunity against smallpox disease (caused by variola virus) for people at high risk for smallpox infection.

For induction of active immunity against vaccinia and smallpox among military personnel. Vaccination of select military personnel resumed in 2002.

Unlabeled Uses: For induction of active immunity against vaccinia among health care workers involved with clinical trials of recombinant vaccinia viruses. Such workers might be exposed to vaccinia while changing dressings or during other cutaneous exposure.

Limitations:

Inappropriate uses: There is no evidence that vaccinia vaccination has therapeutic value in treating or preventing recurrent herpes simplex infection, warts, or any other disease. Misuse of vaccinia vaccine to treat herpes infections can cause severe complications.

Contraindications: There are very few absolute contraindications to this vaccine for those who are at high risk for smallpox. The risk of experiencing serious vaccination complications must be weighed against the risks of experiencing a potentially fatal smallpox infection. People at greatest risk of experiencing serious vaccination complications are often those at greatest risk for death from smallpox.

Absolute: People with severe immunodeficiency who are not expected to benefit from the vaccine. These may include people undergoing bone-marrow transplantation or with primary or acquired immunodeficiency states who require isolation.

Relative: Some risks of adverse reactions after vaccinia vaccination are increased in vaccinees with certain disease states, theoretically or based on experience. This increase may be based on increased frequency or increased consequence. People with cardiac disease may be more likely to progress to dilated cardiomyopathy or other cardiac problems. People with eye disease treated with topical steroids may be less able to tolerate ocular vaccinia, and this may increase the risk of progressive vaccinia. Congenital or acquired immune deficiency disorders may increase the risk of eczema vaccinatum. Infants younger than 12 months of age may have an increased risk of encephalitis. Pregnant women have a very rare risk of complications involving fetal vaccinia. People hypersensitive to neomycin or polymyxin B may develop allergic reactions after vaccination. Persons with eczema of any description (eg, atopic dermatitis, neurodermatitis, other eczematous conditions), regardless of severity, or persons who have a history of these conditions at any time in the past, are at higher risk of developing eczema vaccinatum. Vaccinees with close contacts who have eczematous conditions may be at increased risk because live vaccinia virus can be transmitted to these close contacts. Vaccinees with other active acute, chronic, or exfoliative skin disorders (eg, burns, impetigo, varicella-zoster, acne vulgaris with open lesions, Darier disease, psoriasis, seborrheic dermatitis, erythroderma, pustular dermatitis) or vaccinees with household contacts having such skin disorders might also be at higher risk for eczema vaccinatum.

Defer vaccination during the course of an acute illness, except in an outbreak. Do not vaccinate patients of any age who have exfoliative skin conditions (eg, impetigo, varicellazoster, wounds, burns, uncontrolled acne) until the condition resolves or is under control; also do not vaccinate household contacts of such patients because of an increased risk of eczema vaccinatum.

Several cases of ischemia after smallpox vaccination led the Advisory Committee on Immunization Practices (ACIP) to recommend deferral of people with cardiac risk factors, but further analysis showed that the risk of ischemia is essentially the same in unvaccinated and recently smallpox-vaccinated people.

Immunodeficiency: Except in the case of a smallpox outbreak, do not administer vaccinia (smallpox) vaccine to immunodeficient patients, including patients with congenital or acquired immune deficiencies, whether due to genetics, disease, or drug or radiation therapy, because of the risk of severe localized or systemic infection with vaccinia (eg, progressive vaccinia). Similarly, do not vaccinate household contacts of such patients. Exposure of immunocompromised HIV-infected patients to smallpox vaccine has led to disseminated vaccinia infection. Do not give to HIV-infected patients or to those residing in a household with an HIV-infected patient.

Elderly: No specific information is available about geriatric use of *ACAM2000*. Historically, smallpox vaccine was given to the elderly when indicated.

Carcinogenicity: *ACAM2000* has not been evaluated for carcinogenic potential.

Mutagenicity: *ACAM2000* has not been evaluated for mutagenic potential.

Fertility Impairment: *ACAM2000* has not been evaluated for impairment of fertility.

Pregnancy: Category D. Contraindicated, except in an outbreak in which the woman has been exposed to variola virus. On rare occasions, usually after primary vaccination, vaccinia virus has caused fetal infection (fetal vaccinia), principally during the first trimester. Fetal vaccinia usually results in stillbirth or death of the infant shortly after delivery. The NYCBOH strain of vaccinia is not known to cause congenital malformations. It is not known if corresponding antibodies cross the placenta. Generally, most IgG passage across the placenta occurs during the third trimester.

Lactation: Live vaccinia virus may be transmitted from a lactating mother to her infant, mainly through proximity to the vaccination site, causing complications in the infant from inadvertent inoculation. It is not known whether vaccine virus or antibodies are secreted in human milk.

Children: Current indications are based on occupational exposure only, except in an outbreak. Vaccinia vaccine may be associated with an increased risk of serious complications in children, especially infants younger than 12 months of age. The use of *ACAM2000* in pediatric age groups is supported by evidence from studies of *ACAM2000* in adults and by historical data on vaccinia vaccines in children. Before the eradication of smallpox disease, live vaccinia vaccine was administered routinely in all pediatric age groups, including neonates and infants, and was effective in preventing smallpox disease. During that time, live vaccinia virus was occasionally associated with serious complications in children, the highest risk being in infants.

Adverse Reactions: In *ACAM2000* clinical studies, 97% and 92% of vaccinia-naïve and previously vaccinated subjects, experienced one or more adverse event. Common events included vaccination-site reactions (eg, erythema, pruritus, pain, swelling) and constitutional symptoms (eg, fatigue, malaise, hot feeling, rigors, decreased exercise tolerance). Across all *ACAM2000* studies, 10% of vaccinia-naïve and 3% of previously vaccinated subjects experienced at least one severe adverse event that interfered with normal daily activities.

Two randomized, controlled, multicenter phase 3 trials enrolled 2,244 subjects who received *ACAM2000* and 737 who received *Dryvax*. Adverse events reported by at least 5% of subjects in either the *ACAM2000* or the *Dryvax* group are presented in the following table. Severe vaccine-related adverse events, defined as interfering with normal daily activities, in vaccinia-naïve subjects were reported by 10% of subjects in the *ACAM2000* group and 13% in the comparison group. In the previously vaccinated subjects, the incidence of severe vaccine-related adverse events was 4% for the *ACAM2000* groups and 6% for the comparison group.

Adverse Events Reported by ≥ 5% of Subjects				
	Study 1: Vaccinia-naive subjects		Study 2: Previously vaccinated subjects	
	ACAM2000 N = 873 n (%)	*Dryvax* N = 289 n (%)	*ACAM2000* N = 1,371 n (%)	*Dryvax* N = 447 n (%)
At least 1 adverse event	864 (99)	288 (100)	1,325 (97)	443 (99)
Blood and lymphatic system disorders	515 (59)	204 (71)	302 (22)	133 (30)
Lymph node pain[a]	494 (57)	199 (69)	261 (19)	119 (27)
Lymphadenopathy	72 (8)	35 (12)	78 (6)	29 (6)
Gastrointestinal disorders	273 (31)	91 (31)	314 (23)	137 (31)
Nausea[a]	170 (19)	65 (22)	142 (10)	63 (14)
Diarrhea[a]	144 (16)	34 (12)	158 (12)	77 (17)
Constipation[a]	49 (6)	9 (3)	88 (6)	31 (7)
Vomiting[a]	42 (5)	10 (3)	40 (3)	18 (4)
General disorders and administration site conditions	850 (97)	288 (100)	1,280 (93)	434 (97)
Injection site pruritus[a]	804 (92)	277 (96)	1,130 (82)	416 (93)
Injection site erythema[a]	649 (74)	229 (79)	841 (61)	324 (72)
Injection site pain[a]	582 (67)	208 (72)	505 (37)	209 (47)
Fatigue[a]	423 (48)	161 (56)	468 (34)	184 (41)
Injection site swelling	422 (48)	165 (57)	384 (28)	188 (42)
Malaise[a]	327 (37)	122 (42)	381 (28)	147 (33)
Hot feeling [a]	276 (32)	97 (34)	271 (20)	114 (25)
Rigors[a]	185 (21)	66 (23)	171 (12)	76 (17)
Exercise tolerance decreased[a]	98 (11)	35 (12)	105 (8)	50 (11)
Musculoskeletal and connective tissue disorders	418 (48)	153 (53)	418 (30)	160 (36)

Adverse Events Reported by ≥ 5% of Subjects				
	Study 1: Vaccinia-naive subjects		Study 2: Previously vaccinated subjects	
	ACAM2000 N = 873 n (%)	*Dryvax* N = 289 n (%)	*ACAM2000* N = 1,371 n (%)	*Dryvax* N = 447 n (%)
Myalgia[a]	404 (46)	147 (51)	374 (27)	148 (33)
Nervous system disorders	444 (51)	151 (52)	453 (33)	174 (39)
Headache[a]	433 (50)	150 (52)	437 (32)	166 (37)
Respiratory, thoracic, and mediastinal disorders	134 (15)	40 (14)	127 (9)	42 (9)
Dyspnea[a]	39 (4)	16 (6)	41 (3)	18 (4)
Skin and subcutaneous tissue disorders	288 (33)	103 (36)	425 (31)	139 (31)
Erythema[a]	190 (22)	69 (24)	329 (24)	107 (24)
Rash[a]	94 (11)	30 (10)	80 (6)	29 (6)

a Event was listed on a checklist included in subject diaries.

Transfer: Vaccinia vaccine contains live vaccinia virus that can be transmitted to other body sites or to people who have close contact with the vaccinee. Inadvertent inoculation of other sites most commonly involves the face, nose, mouth, lips, genitalia, and anus. Accidental infection of the eye (ocular vaccinia) may result in ocular complications (eg, keratitis, corneal scarring, blindness). Among vaccinees from 2002 to 2005 in the contemporary vaccination programs, the principal risk of contact transfer of vaccinia virus has been to spouses and adult intimate contacts (ie, bed partners) and, to a lesser extent, to sports partners and children. The risks in contacts largely are the same as those stated for vaccinees.

Virus is shed from the vaccination site during the period starting with the development of a papule (days 2 to 5); shedding ceases when the scab separates and the lesion is re-epithelialized, about 14 to 28 or more days after vaccination. Use infection-control measures to reduce the risk of accidental transfer.

Serious events: Myocarditis and pericarditis, encephalitis, encephalomyelitis, encephalopathy, progressive vaccinia, generalized vaccinia, severe vaccinial skin infections, erythema multiforme major (including Stevens-Johnson syndrome), eczema vaccinatum resulting in permanent sequelae or death, ocular complications and blindness, and fetal death have occurred after either primary vaccination or revaccination with live vaccinia vaccines. These may result in severe disability, permanent neurological sequelae and/or death. Death is most often the result of sudden cardiac death, postvaccinial encephalitis, progressive vaccinia, or eczema vaccinatum. Estimates of the risks of occurrence of serious complications after primary vaccination and revaccination, based on safety surveillance studies conducted when *Dryvax* was routinely recommended, appear in the following table.

Rates of Reported Complications[a] Associated With Vaccination With *Dryvax* (Cases/Million Vaccinations)[b]					
Primary vaccination					
Age (y)	< 1	1 to 4	5 to 19	≥ 20	Overall rates[c]
Inadvertent inoculation[d]	507	577.3	371.2	606.1	529.2
Generalized vaccinia	394.4	233.4	139.7	212.1	241.5
Eczema vaccinatum	14.1	44.2	34.9	30.3	38.5
Progressive vaccinia[e]	—[f]	3.2	—[f]	—[f]	1.5

Rates of Reported Complications[a] Associated With Vaccination With *Dryvax* (Cases/Million Vaccinations)[b]					
Primary vaccination					
Age (y)	< 1	1 to 4	5 to 19	≥ 20	Overall rates[c]
Postvaccinial encephalitis	42.3	9.5	8.7	—[f]	12.3
Death[g]	5	0.5	0.5	unknown	—
Total[h]	1,549.3	1,261.8	855.9	1,515.2	1,253.8
Revaccinations					
Age (y)	< 1	1 to 4	5 to 19	≥ 20	Overall rates[c]
Inadvertent inoculation[d]	—[f]	109.1	47.7	25	42.1
Generalized vaccinia	—[f]	—[f]	9.9	9.1	9
Eczema vaccinatum	—[f]	—[f]	2	4.5	3
Progressive vaccinia[e]	—[f]	—[f]	—[f]	6.8	3
Postvaccinial encephalitis	—[f]	—[f]	—[f]	4.5	2
Death[g]	—	—	—	—	—
Total[h]	—[f]	200	85.5	113.6	108.2

a See article for descriptions of complications.
b Adapted from Lane JM, et al. *J Infect Dis.* 1970;122(4):303-309.
c Overall rates include persons of unknown age.
d Referenced as accidental implantation.
e Referenced as vaccinia necrosum.
f No instances were identified during the 1968 10-state survey.
g Death from all complications.
h Rates of overall complications include complications not itemized in this table, including severe local reactions, bacterial superinfection of the vaccination site, and erythema multiforme.

Data on adverse events among U.S. military personnel and civilian workers vaccinated with *Dryvax* during vaccination programs initiated in December 2002 appear in the following table. The incidence of preventable adverse events (eg, eczema vaccinatum, contact transmission, autoinoculation) were notably lower in these programs compared with data collected in the 1960s, presumably because of better vaccination screening procedures and routine use of protective bandages over the inoculation site. Myocarditis and pericarditis were not commonly reported after vaccinia vaccination in the 1960s but emerged as a more frequent event based on more active surveillance of adult vaccinees in military and civilian programs.

Serious Adverse Events after Vaccination with *Dryvax* in 2002-2005				
	Department of Defense Program as of January 2005[a] (n = 730,580)		Department of Health and Human Services Program as of January 2004[b] (n = 40,422)	
Adverse event	N	Incidence/million	N	Incidence /million
Myocarditis/pericarditis	86	117.7	21	519.5
Postvaccinial encephalitis	1	1.4	1	24.7
Eczema vaccinatum	0	0	0	0
Generalized vaccinia	43	58.9	3	74.2
Progressive vaccinia	0	0	0	0
Fetal vaccinia	0	0	0	0
Contact transmission	52	71.2	0	0
Autoinoculation (nonocular)	62	84.9	20	494.8
Ocular vaccinia	16	21.9	3	74.2

a 36% primary vaccinees; 36% male; median age 47.1 y.
b 71% primary vaccinees; 89% male; median age 28.5 y.

Cardiovascular: In clinical trials, 10 cases of suspected myocarditis were identified, 7 among 2,983 subjects (0.2%) who received *ACAM2000* and 3 among 868 subjects (0.3%) who received *Dryvax*. The mean time to onset of suspected myocarditis and/or pericarditis from vaccination was 11 days, with a range of 9 to 20 days. All subjects who experienced these cardiac events were naive to vaccinia. Of the 10 subjects, 2 were hospitalized. None of the remaining 8 cases required hospitalization or treatment with medication. Of the 10 cases, 8 were subclinical and were detected only by electrocardiogram (ECG) abnormalities, with or without associated elevations of cardiac troponin I. All cases resolved within 9 months, except one female *Dryvax* vaccinee, who had persistent borderline abnormal left ventricular ejection fraction on echocardiogram. Among vaccinees naive to vaccinia, 8 cases were identified across both treatment groups, or 6.9 per 1,000 vaccinees. The rate for the *ACAM2000* treatment group was similar (5.7 [95% CI, 1.9 to 13.3] per 1,000 vaccinees) to the *Dryvax* group (10.4 [95% CI, 2.1 to 30] per 1,000 vaccinees). No cases of myocarditis and/or pericarditis were identified in 1,819 previously vaccinated subjects. The long-term outcome of myocarditis and pericarditis after *ACAM2000* vaccination is currently unknown. Ischemic cardiac events, including fatalities, have been reported after vaccinia vaccination; the relationship of these events, if any, to vaccination has not been established. In addition, cases of nonischemic, dilated cardiomyopathy have been reported after vaccinia vaccination; the relationship of these cases to vaccinia vaccination is unknown.

Dermatologic: Major cutaneous reactions at the site of inoculation, characterized by large area of erythema and induration and streaking inflammation of draining lymphatics may resemble cellulitis. Benign and malignant lesions have been reported to occur at the vaccinia vaccination site. Erythema and rash were noted in 18% and 8% of subjects, respectively. In *ACAM2000* subjects, 1% of vaccinia-naïve and less than 1% of previously vaccinated subjects experienced at least one severe adverse event. Except for one case of contact dermatitis and one case of urticaria, erythema and rash accounted for all severe events. Generalized rashes (eg, erythematous, papulovesicular, urticarial, folliculitis, nonspecific) are not uncommon after vaccinia vaccination and are presumed to be hypersensitivity reactions occurring among persons without underlying illnesses. These rashes are generally self-limited and require little or no therapy, except among patients whose conditions appear to be systemic or who have serious underlying illnesses. Self-limited skin rashes not associated with vaccinia replication in skin, including urticaria and folliculitis, may occur after vaccination. Progressive vaccinia (vaccinia necrosum), severe vaccinial skin infections, erythema multiforme major (including Stevens-Johnson syndrome), and eczema vaccinatum have been reported rarely.

GI: Commonly reported GI disorders among *ACAM2000*-treated subjects included nausea and diarrhea (14%), constipation (6%), and vomiting (4%). Severe abdominal pain, nausea, vomiting, constipation, diarrhea, and toothache accounted for all severe adverse events reported, occurring in less than 1% of subjects.

Immunologic: Severe localized or systemic infection with vaccinia (progressive vaccinia) may occur in persons with weakened immune systems, including patients with leukemia, lymphoma, organ transplantation, generalized malignancy, HIV/AIDS, cellular or humoral immune deficiency, radiation therapy, or treatment with antimetabolites, alkylating agents, or high-dose corticosteroids (more than 10 mg prednisone/day or equivalent for at least 2 weeks). Vaccinees with close contacts who have these conditions may be at increased risk because live vaccinia virus can be shed and transmitted to close contacts.

Lymphatic: The only adverse events occurring in at least 5% of subjects were lymph-node pain and lymphadenopathy. The incidence of severe lymph-node pain and lymphadenopathy was less than 1%.

Musculoskeletal: Across all *ACAM2000* studies, severe, vaccine-related myalgia was seen in 1% of vaccinia-naive subjects and less than 1% of previously vaccinated subjects. Other

357

adverse events included back pain, arthralgia, and pain in extremity; none occurred with a frequency of more than 2%.

CNS: Fifty-one percent and 35% of vaccinia-naive subjects and previously vaccinated subjects reported headaches in *ACAM2000* studies. Although less than 1% of the subjects in the *ACAM2000* program experienced severe headaches, none required hospitalization. Neurological events temporally associated with vaccinia vaccination and assessed among the 2002 to 2005 military and Department of Health and Human Services programs included headache (95 cases), nonserious limb paresthesias (17 cases) or pain (13 cases), and dizziness or vertigo (13 cases). Serious neurologic adverse events included 13 cases of suspected meningitis, 3 cases of suspected encephalitis or myelitis, 11 cases of Bell palsy, 9 seizures (including 1 death), and 3 cases of Guillain-Barré syndrome. Among these 39 events, 27 (69%) occurred in primary vaccinees, and all but 2 occurred within 12 days of vaccination. There have also been cases of photophobia after vaccinia vaccination, some of which required hospitalization.

GU: Vaccinia virus rarely may cause fetal infection (fetal vaccinia), usually resulting in stillbirth or death.

Ophthalmic: Accidental infection of the eye (ocular vaccinia) may result in ocular complications, including keratitis, corneal scarring, and blindness. Patients who are using corticosteroid eye drops may be at increased risk of ocular complications with *ACAM2000* if they develop ocular vaccinia.

Consultation: The Centers for Disease Control and Prevention (CDC) and the Department of Defense can assist clinicians in diagnosis and management of patients with suspected complications of vaccinia vaccination. Vaccinia immune globulin (VIG) is indicated for certain complications of vaccination live vaccinia vaccine. If VIG is needed or additional information is required, contact the CDC at (404) 639-3670 during business hours or (404) 639-2888 at other times.

Pharmacologic & Dosing Characteristics

Dosage: Shake or stir product well before withdrawing a dose. A droplet of *ACAM2000* is administered using 15 jabs of a bifurcated needle. The droplet (0.0025 mL) of reconstituted vaccine is picked up with a bifurcated needle by dipping the needle into the *ACAM2000* vial.

Route & Site: Administration of vaccinia vaccine requires specific training for the percutaneous route (scarification). The preferred site of vaccination is the upper arm over the insertion of the deltoid muscle. *ACAM2000* should not be injected by the intradermal, subcutaneous, intramuscular, or intravenous routes. A residual scar indicates prior vaccination. Historically, women and girls were sometimes vaccinated at sites other than the upper arm (eg, inner thigh, outer thigh, buttocks, ankle) for cosmetic reasons.

Cutaneous response to vaccination: A papule typically develops at the site of vaccination 2 to 5 days after administration to a nonimmune patient. The papule becomes vesicular. Successful vaccination results in a "major reaction," defined by the CDC and World Health Organization (WHO) as a vesicular (blistery) or pustular (pus-filled) lesion or area of definite palpable induration or congestion surrounding a central lesion that might be a crust or an ulcer. Any other reaction at days 6 to 8 is defined as "equivocal"; check vaccination procedures and repeat vaccination. The vesicle (often surrounded by a red areola) becomes a pustule, becomes umbilicated (with a collapsed center), and reaches its maximum size in 8 to 10 days. The pustule dries and forms a scab, which separates within 14 to 28 or more days after vaccination, leaving a typical scar that at first is pink in color but eventually becomes flesh colored. The scab may persist longer if it is kept covered and not allowed to air dry. Primary vaccination can produce swelling and tenderness of regional lymph nodes beginning 3 to 10 days after vaccination and persisting for 2 to 4 weeks after the skin lesion has healed. Maximum viral shedding occurs 4 to 14 days after vaccination, but vaccinia can be recovered from the site of vaccination until the scab separates from the skin.

Special Handling: Do not prepare the skin unless the intended site of vaccination is obviously dirty, in which case an alcohol swab(s) may be used to clean the area. If alcohol is used, allow the skin to dry thoroughly to prevent inactivation of the live virus by the alcohol.

Remove the vaccine vial cap. Remove the bifurcated needle from the individual wrapping. Submerge the bifurcated end of needle in the reconstituted vaccine solution. The needle will pick up a droplet of vaccine (0.0025 mL) within the fork of the bifurcation. Use aseptic technique. Do not insert the upper part of the needle that has been in contact with fingers into the vaccine vial. Never re-dip the needle into the vaccine vial if the needle has touched skin.

Deposit the droplet of vaccine onto clean, dry skin of the arm prepared for vaccination. Hold the needle between thumb and first finger perpendicular to the skin. Rest the wrist of the hand holding the vaccination needle against the patient's arm. Rapidly make 15 jabs of the needle perpendicular to the skin through the vaccine droplet to puncture the skin, within a diameter of approximately 5 mm. Make the jabs vigorous enough so that a spot of blood appears at the vaccination site.

Wipe any excess droplets of vaccine or blood from the skin using a dry gauze pad. Discard the needle and gauze in a biohazard sharps container. Close the vaccine vial by reinserting the rubber cap. Return vial to a refrigerator or cooling tray, unless it will be used immediately to vaccinate another patient.

Cover the vaccination site loosely with a gauze bandage, using medical tape to keep it in place. This bandage provides a barrier to protect against spread of the vaccinia virus. Do not use a bandage that blocks air from the vaccination site. This may cause the skin at the vaccination site to soften and wear away. If the vaccinee is involved in direct patient care, cover the gauze with a semipermeable (semiocclusive) dressing as an additional barrier. A semipermeable dressing is one that allows for the passage of air but does not allow for the passage of fluids. Do not put salves or ointments on the vaccination site.

Keep the vaccination site dry. While bathing, cover the site with an impermeable bandage. The most important measure to prevent inadvertent inoculation and contact transfer is thorough hand washing after changing bandages or any contact with the vaccination site.

To remove virus from hands and prevent contact spread, wash hands with soap and warm water or with alcohol-based hand rubs such as gels or foams after direct contact with the vaccination site, the bandage, or clothes, towels, or sheets that might be contaminated with virus from the vaccination site.

Additional Doses: Individuals who are not successfully vaccinated (ie, vaccination failures) after primary vaccination may be vaccinated again in an attempt to achieve a satisfactory take. Check vaccination procedures and repeat vaccination with vaccine from another vial or vaccine lot, employing the same technique. Vaccine failure may be due to impotent vaccine, inadequate vaccination technique, or host factors in the vaccinee. If such a repeat vaccination fails to produce a major reaction, consult the CDC, DoD, or a state health department before giving another vaccination.

Revaccinate people at continued high risk of exposure to smallpox (eg, research laboratory workers handling variola virus) every 3 years. Successful revaccination reaction manifests as a vesicular or pustular lesion or area of definite palpable induration surrounding a central lesion that may be a crust or ulcer. After revaccination, skin reactions may be less pronounced and may progress and heal more rapidly compared with primary vaccination but the vaccinee still may exhibit an immune response to the vaccine. Any other reaction is considered equivocal. Response to vaccinia may be blunted by immunity, insufficiently potent vaccine, or vaccination technique failure. Previously vaccinated individuals who do not have a cutaneous response on revaccination do not require revaccination to try to elicit a cutaneous response.

If repeat vaccination using vaccine from another vial fails to elicit a major reaction, consult public health authorities before attempting another vaccination of that person.

Day after vaccination	Major reaction, for primary (first) vaccination	Major reaction, for revaccinated people[a]	Equivocal: delayed hypersensitivity reaction	Equivocal: all other reactions
Response to Smallpox Vaccination				
Day 1			Erythema	
2			Erythema[b]	
3	Papule	Papule		
4	(bump, pimple)	Vesicle		
5	Vesicle (blister)			
6		Pustule, induration or congestion around		
7	Pustule			
8	pus-filled blister			
9	(center collapses)	Scab or ulcer		
10	(if previously			
11	vaccinated, may		No further reaction	Requires revaccination
12	show "induration"			
13	[hard swelling] only)		Requires revaccination	
14	Scab			
15	(dark, then			
16	flesh-colored).			
17	Scab falls off			
18	(day 14 to 21 or later			
19	if frequently			
20	covered).			
21				

a Greatest erythema occurs after 3 days following revaccination; implies viral propagation.
b Vesicles occur infrequently.

Obsolete terms, no longer used, but included in older health records:
- Accelerated reactions (Vaccinoid): Accelerated vesicular reactions appear between the fifth and eighth days, inclusive, or if a typical pustular vaccinial reaction occurs.
- Immediate or early reactions, which peak approximately 48 hours after vaccination, likely represented delayed-hypersensitivity reactions not associated with protective immunity from infection.
- Immune, Reaction of immunity, Typical primary vaccinia. Modified: Terms not recommended because they are ambiguous or ill-defined.

Waste Disposal: Discard vaccine vial, stopper, diluent syringe, vented needle, bifurcated needle, and any gauze or cotton that came in contact with the vaccine in leak-proof, puncture-proof biohazard containers. Bandages and vaccination scabs in health care settings should be treated as biohazardous materials. At home, bandages and scabs can be placed in a sealed bag and discarded with other trash.

Wash separately clothing, towels, bedding, or other items that may have come in direct contact with the vaccination site or drainage from the site, using hot water with detergent and/or bleach. Wash hands afterwards.

Efficacy: Efficacy of *ACAM2000* was assessed by comparing immunologic response to *ACAM2000* with *Dryvax* in 2 randomized, multicenter, active-controlled clinical trials. One study involved people not previously given vaccinia vaccine (ie, vaccinia-naive). The other involved people given vaccinia vaccine more than 10 years previously (ie, previously vaccinated). Successful primary vaccination was defined as a major cutaneous reaction on days 6 to 11. Successful revaccination was defined as development of any cutaneous lesion of a measurable size on days 6 to 8. The statistical method was a test of noninferiority of *ACAM2000* to *Dryvax*, for both successful vaccination and neutralizing antibody geometric mean antibody titer (GMT).

In study 1, 1,037 male and female vaccinia-naive subjects, aged 18 to 30 years, primarily white (76%), were randomized in a 3:1 ratio to receive *ACAM2000* (n = 780) or *Dryvax* (n = 257). The *ACAM2000* subjects were stratified to receive 1 of 3 lots.

In study 2, 1,647 male and female previously vaccinated subjects, aged 31 to 84 years, primarily white (81%), were randomized in a 3:1 ratio to receive *ACAM2000* (n = 1242) or *Dryvax* (n = 405). The *ACAM2000* subjects were stratified to receive 1 of 3 lots.

The results of the primary efficacy analyses for both studies appear in this table.

Cutaneous Response (Vaccination Success) and Neutralizing Antibody Response in Subjects Given *ACAM2000* or *Dryvax*				
	Study population / Treatment group			
	Study 1: Vaccinia-naive subjects		Study 2: Previously vaccinated subjects	
	ACAM2000	*Dryvax*	*ACAM2000*	*Dryvax*
Cutaneous response (vaccination success)				
Evaluable population[a]	776	257	1,189	388
Vaccination successes (%)	747 (96)[b]	255 (99)	998 (84)[c]	381 (98)
97.5% 1-sided CI by normal approximation on percent difference between *ACAM2000* and *Dryvax*	-4.67%[d]		-17%[e]	
Noninferior to *Dryvax*?	Yes		No	
Neutralizing antibody response (based on $PRNT_{50}$[f] titer on day 30)				
Evaluable population[g]	565	190	734	376
GMT[h]	166	255	286	445
Log_{10} mean	2.2	2.4	2.5	2.6
97.5% 1-sided CI by analysis of variance (ANOVA) on difference between *ACAM2000* and *Dryvax*	-0.307[i]		-0.275[j]	
Noninferior to *Dryvax*?	No		Yes	

a Subjects who received study vaccine and were evaluated for a local cutaneous reaction within the protocol-designated timeframe.
b Results for 3 *ACAM2000* lots were 95%, 98%, and 96%.
c Results for 3 *ACAM2000* lots were 79%, 87%, and 86%.
d Because critical value for evaluation was -5%, *ACAM2000* is considered noninferior to *Dryvax* for this parameter.
e Because critical value for evaluation was -10%, *ACAM2000* is not considered noninferior to *Dryvax* for this parameter.
f $PRNT_{50}$ vaccinia 50% plaque-reduction neutralization test.
g A random sample of subjects who received study vaccine and had samples collected for neutralizing antibody response at baseline and designated time point posttreatment.
h GMT = Geometric mean neutralizing antibody titer.
i Because critical value for evaluation was -0.301, *ACAM2000* is not considered noninferior to *Dryvax* for this parameter.
j Because critical value for evaluation was -0.301, *ACAM2000* is considered noninferior to *Dryvax* for this parameter.

The primary determinant for an effective immune response in those naive to vaccinia is a major cutaneous reaction. *ACAM2000* was noninferior to *Dryvax* in this population with regards to eliciting a major cutaneous reaction. The measure of the strength of the generated antibody response was similar but did not meet the predefined criterion for noninferiority. Among subjects previously vaccinated, development of a major cutaneous response after revaccination with vaccinia-based smallpox vaccines may not provide an accurate measure of the strength of the immune response because the preexisting immunity modifies the scope of the cutaneous response. In previously vaccinated subjects, *ACAM2000* was noninferior to *Dryvax* with regards to the strength of the neutralizing antibody immune response.

Onset: With previous vaccinia vaccines, antibody appears in 4 to 5 days and peaks within 4 weeks.

Duration: Three to 30 years. Neutralizing antibody titer 1:10 or more persist in 75% of people 10 years after receiving a second dose of vaccinia vaccine and approximately 30 years after receiving a third dose.

In a European study, smallpox case-fatality rates were studied as a function of time since the most recent vaccination. In contrast to a traditional case-fatality rate of 30% among unvaccinated people, the risk of dying from smallpox infection was 11% among people vaccinated at least 21 years earlier, 7% among people vaccinated 11 to 20 years earlier, and 1.4% in people vaccinated 1 to 10 years earlier. Most people in the United States 30 years of age and older were vaccinated against smallpox at least 20 years ago.

Protective Level: Neutralizing antibodies are known to mediate protection against smallpox. Neutralizing or hemagglutination-inhibiting antibodies against vaccinia develop in more than 95% of individuals after primary vaccination, rise rapidly (by day 15 to 20 after vaccination), and may be boosted on revaccination. Antibody titers are highly variable. Titers may remain high for longer periods after 2 or more vaccinations than after a primary vaccination. The level of the neutralizing antibody response after primary vaccination is generally in proportion to the intensity of the cutaneous reaction. The level of neutralizing antibody required to protect against smallpox has not been clearly established, although some studies indicate that persons with antibody titers more than 1:32 are protected.

Mechanism: Induction of antivaccinia neutralizing antibodies that also protect against variola. Cell-mediated immune responses are also elicited by vaccination and are believed to contribute to protection and immunological memory. Vaccinia (smallpox) vaccine does not contain smallpox virus (variola) and cannot spread or cause smallpox.

Vaccinia virus is a member of the same taxonomic group (the Orthopox genus) as smallpox (variola) virus, and immunity induced by vaccinia virus cross-protects against variola virus. Vaccinia virus causes a localized virus infection of the epidermis at the site of inoculation, surrounding dermal and subcutaneous tissues and draining the lymph nodes. Virus may be transiently present in the blood and may infect reticuloendothelial and other tissues. Langerhans cells in the epidermis are specific targets for the early stage of virus replication. The formation of a pustule ("pock" or "take") at the site of inoculation provides evidence of protective immunity. The virus replicates within cells and viral antigens are presented to the immune system. Neutralizing antibodies and B and T cells provide long-term memory.

Drug Interactions: There are no data evaluating the simultaneous administration of *ACAM2000* with other vaccines. In general, live-virus vaccines may be administered simultaneously with inactivated vaccines or at any interval. Varicella and vaccinia vaccines should be separated by 28 or more days to prevent causal confusion related to cutaneous lesions after vaccination. Other live virus vaccines may be administered simultaneously with inactivated vaccines or at any interval.

VIG is the antidote to disseminated vaccinia infection resulting from vaccinia (smallpox) vaccine. Refer to the VIG monograph in the Immune Globulins section. If sufficient VIG is available to allow prophylactic use, consider administering VIG along with the vaccinia vaccine to people with contraindications who require vaccination. This use of VIG aims to attenuate the expected replication of vaccinia viruses within the vaccine recipient.

As with all live viral vaccines, administration to patients receiving immunosuppressant drugs (eg, steroids) or radiation therapy may predispose patients to disseminated infections or insufficient response to immunization. They may remain susceptible despite immunization.

Simultaneous administration of an earlier vaccinia vaccine and indomethacin caused an exaggerated cutaneous response in an isolated case. Avoid concurrent use. It is not known if this effect occurs with other nonsteroidal anti-inflammatory drugs.

Concurrent administration of exogenous interferon products may inhibit viral replication and, thus, inhibit antibody response to the vaccine. Avoid concurrent use.

As a general rule, smallpox vaccination is not affected by administration of blood, exogenous antibodies, or other blood products, probably because of the superficial route of vaccine administration. Defer blood and organ donation for 30 days or more after vaccination with *ACAM2000*.

Lab Interference: *ACAM2000* may induce temporary false-negative results for tuberculin skin tests using purified protein derivative (PPD) and, possibly, blood tests for tuberculosis. Delay tuberculin testing if possible for 1 month after vaccinia vaccination.

ACAM2000 may induce false-positive tests for syphilis. Confirm positive rapid plasma reagin (RPR) tests results using a more specific test, such as the fluorescent treponemal antibody (FTA) assay.

Patient Information: Give each vaccinee a Medication Guide before administering the vaccine. In the event of a smallpox outbreak, follow educational instructions from the manufacturer, such as how to educate vaccinees without a Medication Guide.

Inform patients of the major serious adverse events associated with vaccination, including myocarditis and/or pericarditis, progressive vaccinia in immunocompromised persons, eczema vaccinatum in persons with skin disorders, autoinoculation and accidental inoculation, generalized vaccinia, urticaria, and erythema multiforme major (including Stevens-Johnson syndrome), and fetal vaccinia in pregnant women. Advise them to avoid contact with people at high risk of serious adverse effects of vaccinia virus (eg, those with past or present eczema; immunodeficiency states, including HIV infection, pregnancy, and infancy). Advise them that virus is shed from the site of inoculation from approximately day 3 until scabbing occurs. Vaccinia virus may be transmitted by direct physical contact. Accidental infection of skin at sites other than the site of intentional vaccination (self-inoculation) may occur by trauma or scratching. Contact spread may also result in accidental inoculation of household members or other close contacts. The result of accidental infection is a pock lesion(s) at an unwanted site(s) in the vaccinee or contact and resembles the vaccination site. Self-inoculation occurs most often on the face, eyelid, nose, and mouth, but lesions at any site of traumatic inoculation can occur. Self-inoculation of the eye may result in ocular vaccinia, a potentially serious complication.

Advise vaccinees to keep the vaccination site covered until the scab falls off on its own and to keep the vaccination site dry. Normal bathing may continue, but patients should cover the vaccination site with waterproof bandages when bathing. Patients should not scrub the site and should cover the vaccination site with loose gauze bandage after bathing. Instruct patients not to scratch the vaccination site and not to scratch or pick at the scab. Tell patients not to touch the lesion or soiled bandages and subsequently touch other parts of their bodies. Instruct patients to wash hands thoroughly with soap and water or more than 60% alcohol-based handrub solutions after changing the bandage or touching the site.

To prevent transmission to contacts, instruct patients to avoid the physical contact of objects that have come into contact with the lesion (eg, soiled bandages, clothing, fingers). Advise patients to wash separately clothing, towels, bedding, or other items that may have come in direct contact with the vaccination site or drainage from the site, using hot water with detergent and/or bleach, and to wash their hands afterwards. Instruct patients to place soiled and contaminated bandages in plastic bags for disposal.

Advise patients to wear shirts with sleeves that cover the vaccination site as an extra precaution to prevent spread of the vaccinia virus. This is particularly important in situations of close physical contact. Advise patients to change the bandage every 1 to 3 days. This will keep skin at the vaccination site intact and minimize softening. Instruct patients not to put salves or ointments on the vaccination site. Instruct each patient that when the scab falls off, he or she should throw it away in a sealed plastic bag and wash his or her hands afterwards.

Pharmaceutical Characteristics

Concentration: After reconstitution, each vial contains approximately 100 doses of 0.0025 mL of live vaccinia virus containing 1 to 5 $\times$ 10^8 plaque-forming units (PFU)/mL or 2.5 to 12.5 $\times$ 10^5 PFU/dose.

Quality Assay: Standardized by plaque assay in Vero cells

Packaging: Package containing 3 mL clear-glass vial of vaccine powder, 3 mL vial of diluent, a box of 100 bifurcated stainless steel needles, and a 1 mL syringe with 25-gauge, ⅝-inch needle for reconstitution.

NDC Number: Each vial: 24992-0330-01. Box of 50 vials: 24992-0330-02. Carton of 400 vials: 24992-0330-03.

Doseform: Powder yielding a suspension

Appearance: Yellowish to grayish pellet. Reconstituted vaccine should be a clear to slightly hazy, colorless to straw-colored liquid free from extraneous matter.

Diluent:
For reconstitution: 0.6 mL of 50% v/v glycerin in sterile water in a 3 mL vial. Use 0.25 mL to reconstitute the 100 dose vial.

Adjuvant: None

Preservative: Phenol 0.25%

Allergens: Trace amounts of neomycin and polymyxin B

Excipients: 4-(2-hydroxyethyl)-1-piperazineethanesulfonic acid (HEPES) 6 to 8 millimolar (mM), human serum albumin 2%, sodium chloride 0.5% to 0.7%, mannitol 5%.

pH: 6.5 to 7.5

Shelf Life: Expires within 72 months when powder is stored at $-15°$ to $-25°$C (5° to $-13°$F). Powder expires within 18 months after removal from the freezer, unless extended based on repeat potency tests.

Storage/Stability: Long-term storage of freeze-dried vaccine in a freezer with an average temperature of $-15°$ to $-25°$C (5° to $-13°$F). Before reconstitution, *ACAM2000* retains a potency of 1×10^8 PFU or higher per dose for at least 18 months when refrigerated (2° to 8°C, 36° to 46°F).

Protect vaccine vials from light. Contact the manufacturer regarding exposure to elevated temperatures. During shipment, maintain at a temperature of $-15°$C (5°F) or colder. Store diluent vials at room temperature (15° to 30°C, 59° to 86°F).

If stored at room temperature (20° to 25°C, 68° to 77°F) after reconstitution, administer *ACAM2000* vaccine within 6 to 8 hours, then discard it as a biohazardous material. If refrigerated (2° to 8°C, 36° to 46°F) after reconstitution, *ACAM2000* vaccine may be stored in a refrigerator for up to 30 days, after which it should be discarded as a biohazardous material. Minimize exposure of reconstituted vaccine to room temperature during vaccination sessions by placing it in a refrigerator or in a cooling tray between patient administrations.

Handling: Remove the vaccine vial from cold storage and bring it to room temperature before reconstitution. To reconstitute *ACAM2000*, add 0.3 mL of diluent to the vaccine vial. Use only 0.3 mL of the diluent provided. Remove the flip-cap seals of the vaccine and diluent vials. Wipe each rubber stopper with an isopropyl alcohol swab and allow it to dry thoroughly. Using aseptic technique and a sterile 1 mL syringe fitted with a 25-gauge, ⅝-inch needle, draw up 0.3 mL of diluent and transfer it to the vial. Gently swirl to mix, but do not get product on the rubber stopper.

Personnel preparing or administering *ACAM2000* should wear protective gloves and avoid contact of the vaccine with skin, eyes, or mucous membranes.

Production Process: Live vaccinia virus in *ACAM2000* is derived from plaque-purification cloning from *Dryvax* vaccine (the NYCBOH strain of vaccinia), grown in African green monkey kidney (Vero) cells, and tested to be free of adventitious agents.

Media: Vero (African green monkey kidney) cells

Disease Epidemiology

Incidence: During its peak in the 18th century, smallpox infected a large portion of the population. In 1980, WHO declared smallpox (variola) to have been eradicated from the planet. No cases of endemic smallpox have occurred in the United States since 1949.

Susceptible Pools: Most people born since 1970, unless vaccinated since 2002

Transmission: By close contact with respiratory discharges and, less frequently, with skin lesions of patients or material they had recently contaminated

Incubation: 12 to 14 days (range, 7 to 17 days)

Communicability: Smallpox disease is transmitted through the air or by touch.

Other Information

Perspective:
c.1000: Chinese develop prophylactic inoculation with smallpox virus (variolation) as a means to minimize the effects of smallpox.

1500s: More than 3.5 million people die after Europeans introduce smallpox into Mexico.

1777: Washington directs the variolation of the entire Continental Army.

1796: Jenner intentionally transfers cowpox scabs from milkmaid Sarah Nelmes to 8-year-old James Phipps in Berkeley, Gloustershire, England on May 14. Experiences published in 1798.

1813: Madison signs an "Act to encourage vaccination," the first federal legislation for the control of a drug, establishing a National Vaccine Agency.

1949: Last outbreak of smallpox in the United States, in Hidalgo County, Texas.

1960: WHO begins worldwide smallpox eradication program.

1965: Bifurcated needle introduced.

1976: Last case of variola major in Bangladesh. The patient's name was Rahima Banu.

1977: Last case of variola minor in southern Somalia. The patient's name was Ali Maow Maalin.

1978: Two cases of smallpox result from Birmingham, England, laboratory accidents, one fatal.

1980: WHO declares the Earth free of smallpox.

1983: Production and distribution of vaccinia vaccine for the US civilian population discontinued.

1984: Routine military smallpox vaccinations limited to trainees entering basic training. Between 1984 and 1989, some trainees were immunized and others were not, due to a shortage of vaccinia immune globulin. In 1990, the DoD discontinued routine smallpox vaccination of military basic trainees, until December 2002.

2000-2002: Studies of dilution of remaining *Dryvax* stocks conducted to find a way to protect additional people in an outbreak, given the limited inventory.

2002: FDA relicenses *Dryvax* with diluent devoid of brilliant green dye on October 25. President Bush restarts national smallpox vaccination program on December 13.

Smallpox Vaccinia Vaccine, Live

First Licensed: *ACAM2000*: August 31, 2007. Earlier forms of vaccine: August 21, 1903 and May 1944 (*Dryvax*, Wyeth).

National Policy: ACIP, Healthcare Infection Control Practices Advisory Committee. Recommendations for using smallpox vaccine in a pre-event vaccination program: Supplemental recommendations. *MMWR*. 2003;53(RR-7):1-16.

ACIP. Vaccinia (smallpox) vaccine. *MMWR*. 2001;50(RR-10):125. http://www.cdc.gov/mmwr/PDF/rr/rr5010.pdf.

Canadian National Advisory Committee on Immunisation. Statement on smallpox vaccination. *Can Comm Dis Rep*. 2002;28(ACS-1):1-12.

CDC. Newly licensed smallpox vaccine to replace old smallpox vaccine. *MMWR*. 2008;56:207-208. http://www.cdc.gov/mmwr/PDF/wk/mm5708.pdf.

References: Arness MK, Eckart RE, Love SS, et al. Myopericarditis following smallpox vaccination. *Am J Epidemiol*. 2004;160(7):642-651.

Casey C, Vellozzi C, Mootrey GT, et al. Vaccinia Case Definition Development Working Group; Advisory Committee on Immunization Practices-Armed Forces Epidemiological Board Smallpox Vaccine Safety Working Group. Surveillance guidelines for smallpox vaccine (vaccinia) adverse reactions. *MMWR*. 2006;55(RR-1):1-16. http://www.cdc.gov/MMWR/PDF/rr/rr5501.pdf.

CDC. Smallpox vaccination and adverse events: Guidance for clinicians. *MMWR*. 2003;52(RR-4):1-30.

CDC. Women with smallpox vaccine exposure during pregnancy reported to the National Smallpox Vaccine in Pregnancy Registry—United States, 2003. *MMWR*. 2003;52:386-388.

Eckart RE, et al. Incidence and follow-up of inflammatory cardiac complications following smallpox vaccination. *J Am Coll Cardiol*. 2004;44(1):201-205.

Fenner F, Henderson DA, Arita I, Jezek Z, Ladnyi ID. Smallpox and Its Eradication. Geneva: World Health Organization; 1988. http://www.who.int/emc/diseases/smallpox/Smallpoxeradication.html.

Grabenstein JD, Winkenwerder W Jr. US military smallpox vaccination program experience. *JAMA*. 2003;289(24):3278-3282.

Henderson DA, Inglesby TV, Bartlett JG, et al. Smallpox as a biological weapon: Medical and public health management. Working Group on Civilian Biodefense. *JAMA*. 1999;281(22):2127-2137. http://jama.ama-assn.org/issues/v281n22/ffull/jst90000.html.

WHO. Smallpox. *Weekly Epidemiol Rec*. 2001;76(44):337-344.

Comparison Table of Varicella-Zoster Virus Vaccines		
Generic name	Varicella vaccine live	Zoster vaccine live
Brand name	*Varivax*	*Zostavax*
Manufacturer	Merck	Merck
Viability	Live viral vaccine	Live viral vaccine
Indications	To prevent chickenpox in people 12 months or older	To prevent herpes zoster (shingles) in people 50 years or older
Strain	Oka/Merck	Oka/Merck
Concentration	$\geq 1,350$ PFU per 0.5 mL	$\geq 19,400$ PFU per 0.65 mL
Adjuvant	None	None
Preservative	None	None
Production medium	MRC-5 cell culture	MRC-5 cell culture
Doseform	Powder yielding suspension	Powder yielding suspension
Diluent	Sterile water without preservative	Sterile water without preservative
Packaging	Vial, box of 10 vials	Vial, box of 10 vials
Routine storage	Freeze at $-15°C$ (5°F) or colder. May refrigerate for up to 72 continuous hours before reconstitution. Stable 30 minutes after reconstitution.	Freeze at $-15°C$ (5°F) or colder. May refrigerate for up to 72 continuous hours before reconstitution. Stable 30 minutes after reconstitution.
Dosage, route	0.5 mL subcutaneously	0.65 mL subcutaneously
Standard schedule	2 doses at least 4 to 8 weeks apart	Single dose
CPT code	90716	90736

Varicella Virus Vaccine Live

Viral Vaccines

Name:
Varivax

Manufacturer:
Merck, licensed from the Research Foundation
for Microbial Disease of Osaka University
(Biken).

Synonyms: VISI abbreviation: VAR. Varicella virus infection is also known as chickenpox. The delayed manifestations are known as herpes zoster or shingles.

Immunologic Characteristics

Microorganism: Virus (double-stranded DNA), varicella-zoster virus, human herpes virus 3, genus *Varicellavirus*, subfamily Alphaherpesvirinae, family Herpesviridae

Viability: Live, attenuated

Antigenic Form: Whole virus

Antigenic Type: Protein

Strains: Oka/Merck strain, named for the Japanese boy from whom the virus was isolated.

Use Characteristics

Indications: Induction of active immunity against infections caused by varicella-zoster virus in patients 12 months of age and older.

Data from household, hospital, and community settings indicate that varicella vaccine is effective in preventing illness or modifying varicella severity if used within 3 days, and possibly up to 5 days, after exposure. The ACIP recommends varicella vaccination in susceptible people in these circumstances. If exposure to varicella does not cause infection, postexposure vaccination should induce protection against subsequent exposure. If the exposure results in infection, no evidence indicates that administration of varicella vaccine during the presymptomatic or prodromal stage of illness increases the risk for vaccine-associated adverse events.

Limitations: There are insufficient data to assess the rate of protection against the complications of chickenpox (eg, encephalitis, hepatitis, pneumonia, pneumonitis) in children or adults or during pregnancy (congenital varicella syndrome).

It is not known whether *Varivax* given immediately after exposure to natural varicella virus will prevent illness. Preliminary data using other vaccine formulations suggest at least 90% protection when children were vaccinated within 3 days of exposure. Acyclovir, given at the earliest signs or symptoms of disease, can reduce the duration of chickenpox symptoms slightly.

Contraindications:

Absolute: A history of hypersensitivity to any component of the vaccine, including gelatin. A history of anaphylactoid reaction to neomycin. Patients with a blood dyscrasia, leukemia, lymphomas of any type, or other malignant neoplasms affecting the bone marrow or lymphatic systems. Patients receiving immunosuppressive therapy, because they are more susceptible to infections than healthy people; vaccination with live attenuated varicella vaccine can result in a more extensive vaccine-associated rash or disseminated disease in patients on immunosuppressant doses of corticosteroids (at least 2 mg/kg prednisone or equivalent). Patients with certain primary and acquired immunodeficiency states (eg, blood dyscrasias, leukemia, lymphomas of any type, other malignant neoplasms) or cellular immune deficiencies. Active untreated tuberculosis. Pregnancy.

Relative: A family history of congenital or hereditary immunodeficiency, until the immune competence of the potential vaccine recipient is evaluated. Any febrile respiratory illness or other active febrile infection.

Immunodeficiency: Do not use in immunodeficient patients, including patients with congenital or acquired cellular immune deficiencies, whether caused by genetics, disease, or drug or radiation therapy. Contains live viruses. Because children infected with HIV are at an increased risk for morbidity from varicella and herpes zoster compared with healthy children, the ACIP recommends that, after weighing potential risks and benefits, varicella vaccine should be considered for asymptomatic or mildly symptomatic HIV-infected children in CDC class N1 (no signs or symptoms) or A1 (mild signs and symptoms with no evidence of immune suppression) with age-specific CD4+ T-lymphocyte percentages 25% or more. Eligible children should receive 2 doses of varicella vaccine with a 3-month interval between doses. Because patients with impaired cellular immunity are potentially at a greater risk for complications after vaccination with a live vaccine, these vaccinees should be encouraged to return for evaluation if they experience a postvaccination varicella-like rash. The use of varicella vaccine in other HIV-infected children is being investigated further. Recommendations regarding use of varicella vaccine in patients with other conditions associated with altered immunity (eg, immunosuppressive therapy) or in patients receiving steroid therapy have not changed.

Elderly: Early studies suggest that varicella vaccine may boost immunity to varicella-zoster virus in the elderly and may prevent or attenuate herpes zoster ("zoster" or "shingles") in that group. Randomized, clinical trials are underway to assess this possibility.

Adults: Varicella vaccine is safe and effective in adults. Vaccination is recommended for susceptible people in close contact with others at high risk for serious complications (eg, health care workers and family contacts of immunocompromised patients). Consider vaccinating susceptible people in the following settings:

- People who live or work in environments where varicella transmission is likely (eg, teachers of young children, day care employees, residents and staff in institutional settings).
- People who live or work in environments in which transmission can occur (eg, college students, inmates and staff of correctional institutions, military personnel).
- Nonpregnant women of childbearing age, to reduce the risk of viral transmission to the fetus.
- International travelers, especially if the traveler expects to have close personal contact with local populations.

Carcinogenicity: Varicella vaccine has not been evaluated for carcinogenic potential.

Mutagenicity: Varicella vaccine has not been evaluated for mutagenic potential.

Fertility Impairment: Varicella vaccine has not been evaluated for impairment of fertility.

Pregnancy: Category C. Contraindicated on hypothetical grounds. It is not known if attenuated varicella virus or corresponding antibodies cross the placenta. Generally, most IgG passage across the placenta occurs during the third trimester. The possible effects of the vaccine on fetal development are unknown at this time. However, natural varicella is known to sometimes cause fetal harm. If vaccination of postpubertal females is undertaken, pregnancy should be avoided for 1 month following each vaccination. To assess any effects of *Varivax* on fetal development, clinicians are encouraged to register any patient vaccinated within 3 months before pregnancy or any time during pregnancy by calling (800) 986-8999.

Lactation: It is not known if attenuated varicella virus or corresponding antibodies cross into human breast milk. Problems in humans have not been documented. Varicella vaccination may be considered for a nursing mother.

Children: Safe and effective in immunocompetent children 12 months of age and older. Safety and efficacy of varicella vaccine in children younger than 12 months of age have not been established. There is a 17% transmission rate of disease from vaccinated leukemic children to healthy, seronegative individuals if the vaccinated leukemic child develops a rash. Children and adolescents with acute lymphoblastic leukemia (ALL) in remission can receive the vaccine under an investigational protocol.

Adverse Reactions: In clinical trials, varicella vaccine was given to 11,102 healthy children, adolescents, and adults. The vaccine was generally well tolerated.

In a double-blind, placebo-controlled study of 914 healthy children and adolescents who were serologically confirmed to be susceptible to varicella, the only adverse reactions that occurred at a significantly greater rate in vaccine recipients than in placebo recipients were pain and redness at the injection site.

In clinical trials involving healthy children monitored for 42 days or less after a single dose of varicella vaccine, the frequency of fever, injection-site complaints, or rashes were reported as follows: Injection-site complaints including pain/soreness, swelling or erythema, rash, pruritis, hematoma, induration, stiffness (19.3%; peaking 0 to 2 days after vaccination); fever 39°C or higher (102°F) oral (14.7%; this rate was measured over a 6-week interval without any control group to compare it with); generalized varicella-like rash (3.8%; peaking after 5 to 26 days; median number of lesions, 5); varicella-like rash at the injection site (3.4%; peaking after 8 to 19 days; median number of lesions, 2).

The most frequently (1% or more) reported adverse experiences, without regard to causality, are listed in decreasing order of frequency: Upper respiratory illness, cough, irritability/nervousness, fatigue, disturbed sleep, diarrhea, loss of appetite, vomiting, otitis, diaper rash/contact rash, headache, teething, malaise, abdominal pain, other rash, nausea, eye complaints, chills, lymphadenopathy, myalgia, lower respiratory illness, allergic reactions (including allergic rash, hives), stiff neck, heat rash/prickly heat, arthralgia, eczema/dry skin/dermatitis, constipation, itching. Pneumonitis and febrile seizures have occurred rarely (less than 1%) in children; a causal relationship has not been established.

A chickenpox rash develops in 40% of vaccinated leukemic children, but usually consists of less than 10 lesions.

In clinical trials involving healthy adolescents, the majority of whom received 2 doses of varicella vaccine and were monitored for 42 days or less after any dose, the frequency of fever, injection-site complaints, or rashes were reported as follows: Injection-site complaints including soreness, erythema, swelling, rash, pruritis, pyrexia, hematoma, induration, numbness (24.4% to 32.5%; peaking 0 to 2 days after vaccination); generalized varicella-like rash (5.5% after the first dose, peaking after 7 to 21 days; 0.9% after the second dose; median number of lesions, 5); fever 37.7°C or higher (100°F) oral (9.5% to 10.2%); varicella-like rash at the injection site (3% after the first dose; peaking after 6 to 20 days; 1% after the second dose, peaking after 0 to 6 days; median number of lesions, 2).

The most frequently (1% or more) reported adverse experiences, without regard to causality, are listed in decreasing order of frequency: Upper respiratory illness, headache, fatigue, cough, myalgia, disturbed sleep, nausea, malaise, diarrhea, stiff neck, irritability/nervousness, lymphadenopathy, chills, eye complaints, abdominal pain, loss of appetite, arthralgia, otitis, itching, vomiting, other rashes, constipation, lower respiratory illness, allergic reactions (including allergic rash, hives), contact rash, cold/canker sore.

After vaccine licensing, between March 1995 and July 1998, 9.7 million doses of varicella vaccine were distributed in the United States. During this time, VAERS received 6,580 reports of adverse events, 4% categorized as serious. Approximately 66% of the reports involved children younger than 10 years of age. The most frequently reported event was rash (rate: 37 reports per 100,000 vaccine doses distributed). PCR analysis confirmed that wild-type viruses cause most rash events occurring within 2 weeks after vaccination. Serious adverse events reported, without regard to causality, included: Encephalitis, ataxia, erythema multiforme, Stevens-Johnson syndrome, Henoch-Schonlein purpura, pneumonia/pneumonitis, pharyngitis, secondary bacterial infections of skin and soft tissue (including impetigo and cellulitis), thrombocytopenia, seizures (febrile and nonfebrile), cerebrovascular accident, aseptic meningitis, dizziness, paresthesia, transverse myelitis, Bell palsy, Guillain-Barre syndrome, neuropathy, and herpes zoster. Three cases of anaphylaxis within 10 minutes of vaccination were reported in the first 12 months of widespread vaccine availability.

In a clinical trial assessing 2 doses of varicella vaccine given 3 months apart, 981 subjects were actively followed for 42 days after each dose. The 2-dose regimen was generally well tolerated, with a safety profile comparable to a 1-dose regimen. The incidence of injection-site clinical complaints (primarily erythema and swelling) observed in the first 4 days after vaccination was slightly higher after dose 2 (25.4%) than after dose 1 (21.7%), whereas the incidence of systemic clinical complaints in the 42-day follow-up period was lower after dose 2 (66.3%) than after dose 1 (85.8%).

Herpes zoster ("shingles"): Overall, 9,454 healthy children (1 to 12 years of age) and 1,648 adolescents and adults (3 years of age or older) have been vaccinated with Oka/Merck live attenuated varicella vaccine in clinical trials. Eight cases of herpes zoster have been reported in children during 44,994 person-years of follow-up in clinical trials, resulting in a calculated incidence of 18 cases or more per 100,000 person-years. The completeness of this reporting has not been determined. This rate is considerably less than a rate of 77 per 100,000 person-years in a separate study of healthy, unvaccinated children after natural infection. One case of herpes zoster has been reported in the adolescent and adult age group during 7,826 person-years of follow-up in clinical trials, resulting in a calculated incidence of 12.8 cases per 100,000 person-years. All 9 cases were mild and without sequelae. Two cultures (from 1 child and 1 adult) obtained from vesicles were positive, wild-type varicella-zoster virus as confirmed by restriction endonuclease analysis. The long-term effect of varicella vaccine on the incidence of herpes zoster, particularly in those vaccinees exposed to natural varicella, is unknown at present.

Transmission: In a placebo-controlled trial, transmission of vaccine virus was assessed for 8 weeks in 416 susceptible placebo recipients who were household contacts of 445 vaccine recipients. Three placebo recipients developed chickenpox and seroconverted, 9 reported a varicella-like rash and did not seroconvert, and 6 had no rash but seroconverted. If vaccine virus transmission occurred, it did so at a very low rate and possibly without recognizable clinical disease in contacts. These cases may represent either natural varicella from community contacts or a low incidence of transmission vaccine virus from vaccinated contacts. Nonetheless, advise vaccine recipients to avoid close contact with susceptible high-risk individuals (eg, newborns, pregnant women, immunocompromised people), especially if a varicella-like rash occurs in the vaccinee. The ACIP believes the value of vaccination outweighs the risk of viral transmission after vaccinating susceptible health care workers. Even so, precautions are appropriate if a worker develops a rash after vaccination or for occupational contact with highly vulnerable patients.

The risk of transmission of vaccine virus from vaccinees who are immunocompromised is higher and may be associated with rash following vaccination.

The potential risk of transmission of vaccine virus should be weighed against the risk of transmission of natural varicella virus.

Pharmacologic & Dosing Characteristics

Dosage:
> *Children (1 to 12 years of age):* 0.5 mL, typically at 15 months of age, followed by a second dose at 4 to 6 years of age or at another time. The minimum planned interval between the first and second dose is 3 months. If the second dose was administered 28 days or more after the first dose, it does not need to be repeated.

Adults and adolescents (13 years of age and older): A single 0.5 mL dose, followed by a second 0.5 mL dose 4 to 8 weeks later.

Route & Site: Subcutaneously. When some children inadvertently received varicella vaccine IM, seroconversion rates were similar to the subcutaneous route. Persistence of antibody and efficacy after IM injection are unknown.

The outer aspect of the upper arm (deltoid) is the preferred site of injection, although the anterolateral thigh may be used.

Documentation Requirements: Federal law requires that the following information be documented in the recipient's permanent medical record or in a permanent office log: (1) The manufacturer and lot number of the vaccine, (2) the date of administration, and (3) the name, address, and title of the person administering the vaccine.

Certain adverse events must be reported to the VAERS system ([800] 822-7967).

Booster Doses: Booster doses are not routinely recommended, although the duration of clinical protection is not fully known. A second dose may be administered, principally to reduce the risk of waning immunity. Such doses should be administered to children 3 months or more after the first dose. In clinical trials of teenagers and adults, higher (and presumably more persistent) antibody titers were observed with an interval of 8 weeks between vaccine doses, compared with an interval of 4 weeks.

Missed Doses: Interrupting the recommended schedule or delaying subsequent doses does not require restarting the series. Resume as soon as practical.

Efficacy: Among children 1 to 12 years of age, 83% reduction in age-adjusted incidence rates. A seroconversion rate 95% or more after a single dose was seen in healthy children. The rate in adolescents and adults is approximately 75% to 94% after the first dose. A second dose of varicella vaccine produces virtually 100% seroconversion. Seroconversion was defined as acquisition of any detectable varicella antibodies (gpELISA > 0.3). This is a highly sensitive assay that is not commercially available.

In trials of several formulations of varicella vaccine, at doses ranging from 1,000 to 17,000 plaque-forming units (PFU), the majority of subjects who received varicella vaccine and were exposed to wild-type virus were either completely protected from chickenpox or developed a milder form of the disease. The protective efficacy of varicella vaccine was evaluated in 3 different ways: 1) By comparing chickenpox rates in vaccinees vs historical controls, 2) by assessment of protection from disease following household exposure, and 3) by a placebo-controlled, double-blind clinical trial.

In 1 trial of 4,142 children, 2.1% to 3.6% of vaccinees per year reported chickenpox (breakthrough cases). This represents a 57% to 77% decrease from the total number of cases expected based on attack rates in children 1 to 9 years of age over this same period (8.3% to 9.1%). In those who developed breakthrough chickenpox after vaccination, the majority experienced mild disease (median number of lesions less than 50). In 1 study, 47% (27/58) of breakthrough cases had less than 50 lesions, compared with 8% (7/92) in unvaccinated individuals; 7% (4/58) of breakthrough cases had more than 300 lesions, compared with 50% (46/92) in unvaccinated individuals. In studies of vaccinated children who contracted chickenpox after a household exposure, 57% (31/54) of the cases reported less than 50 lesions and 1.9% (1/54) reported more than 300 lesions with an oral temperature higher than 37.8°C (100°F).

In later studies of the current vaccine, 1,164 children received 2,900 to 9,000 PFU of attenuated virus per dose and have been followed for 3 years or less after a single dose. From 0.2% to 1% of vaccinees per year reported breakthrough chickenpox for up to 3 years after vaccination. This represents a 93% decrease from the number of cases expected. In those who developed breakthrough chickenpox after vaccination, the majority experienced mild disease.

Among a subset of vaccinees who were actively followed, 259 were exposed to an individual with chickenpox in a household setting. There were no reports of breakthrough chickenpox in 80% of exposed children; 20% reported a mild form of chickenpox. This represents a 77% reduction in the expected number of cases when compared with the historical 87% attack rate of varicella following household exposure in unvaccinated individuals.

Although no placebo-controlled trial was carried out with varicella vaccine using the current vaccine formula, a placebo-controlled trial was conducted using a formulation containing 17,000 PFU per dose. In this trial, a single dose of varicella vaccine protected 96% to 100% of children 1 to 14 years of age against chickenpox over a 2-year period.

In a clinical trial, 2,216 children 12 months to 12 years of age with a negative history of varicella were randomized to receive either 1 dose (n = 1,114) of varicella vaccine or 2 doses (n = 1,102) given 3 months apart. Subjects were actively followed for varicella, any varicella-like illness, or herpes zoster and any exposures to varicella or herpes zoster on an annual basis for 10 years after vaccination. In the 1-dose group, the seroconversion rate was 98.95, with 84.9% developing varicella antibody titers 5 gpELISA units/mL or more (GMT = 12 u/mL). In the 2-dose group, 99.5% and 99.9% seroconverted after the first and second doses, respectively, with 87.3% and 99.5% reaching the 5 gpELISA u/mL threshold after the first and second doses, respectively (GMT = 12.8 and 141.5 u/mL, respectively). Persistence of VZV antibody was measured annually for 9 years. Most cases of varicella reported in recipients of 1 dose or 2 doses of vaccine were mild. The estimated vaccine efficacy for the 10-year observation period was 94% for 1 dose and 98% for 2 doses ($P < 0.001$). This translates to a 3.4-fold lower risk of developing varicella more than 42 days after vaccination during the 10-year observation period in children who received 2 doses than in those who received 1 dose (2.2% vs 7.5%, respectively). Results from this and other studies in which a second dose of vaccine was administered 3 to 6 years after the initial dose demonstrate significant boosting of the VZV antibody response with a second dose. VZV antibody levels after 2 doses given 3 to 6 years apart are comparable to those obtained when the 2 doses are given 3 months apart.

Although no placebo-controlled trial was carried out in adolescents and adults, efficacy was determined by evaluation of protection when vaccinees received 2 doses of varicella vaccine 4 or 8 weeks apart and were subsequently exposed to chickenpox in a household setting. In up to 2 years of active follow-up, 17 of 64 (27%) vaccinees reported breakthrough chickenpox following household exposure; of the 17 cases, 12 (71%) reported less than 50 lesions, 5 reported 50 to 300 lesions, and none reported more than 300 lesions with an oral temperature higher than 37.7°C (100°F). In combined clinical studies of adolescents and adults (n = 1,019) who received 2 doses of varicella vaccine and later developed breakthrough chickenpox (42 of 1019), 25 of 42 (60%) reported less than 50 lesions, 16 (38%) reported 50 to 300 lesions, and 1 of 42 (2%) reported more than 300 lesions and an oral temperature higher than 37.7°C (100°F).

The attack rate among unvaccinated adults exposed to a single contact in a household has not been previously studied. When compared with the previously reported attack rate of natural varicella of 87% following household exposure among unvaccinated children, this represents an approximately 70% reduction in the expected number of cases in the household setting.

Onset: 97% of healthy children had seroconverted when assessed 4 to 6 weeks after vaccination.

Duration: The duration of protection of *Varivax* is not precisely known at present and the need for booster doses is not fully defined. This vaccine provides 70% to 90% protection against infection and 95% protection against severe disease for 7 to 10 years after vaccination.

A boost in antibody levels has been observed in vaccinees following exposure to natural varicella and after a booster dose of *Varivax* given 4 to 6 years after vaccination. In a highly vaccinated population, immunity for some people may wane because of lack of exposure to natural varicella as a result of shifting epidemiology. Postmarketing surveillance studies are ongoing to evaluate the need and timing for booster vaccination.

Studies examining chickenpox breakthrough rates in vaccinees over 5 years showed the lowest rates (0.2% to 2.9%) in the first 2 years after vaccination, and somewhat higher but stable rates in the third through fifth year. The severity of reported breakthrough chickenpox, as measured by number of lesions and maximum temperature, appeared not to increase with time since vaccination.

In clinical studies involving healthy children who received 1 dose of vaccine, detectable varicella antibodies (gpELISA > 0.3) were present in 98.8% at 1 year, 98.9% at 2 years, 97.5% at 3 years, and 99.5% at 4 years after vaccination. Antibody levels were present at least 1 year in 97.2% of healthy adolescents and adults who received 2 doses of live varicella vaccine separated by 4 to 8 weeks. A boost in antibody levels has been observed in vaccinees following exposure to natural varicella. This could account for the apparent long-term persistence of antibody levels after vaccination in these studies. The duration of protection from varicella obtained using *Varivax* in the absence of wild-type boosting is unknown. *Varivax* also induces cell-mediated immune responses in vaccinees. The relative contributions of humoral immunity and cell-mediated immunity to protection from chickenpox are unknown.

Protective Level: Rates of breakthrough disease were significantly lower among children with VZV antibody titers at least 5 gpELISA units/mL compared with children with titers less than 5 gpELISA units/mL. Titers at least 5 gpELISA units/mL were induced in approximately 76% of children vaccinated with a single dose of vaccine at 1,000 to 17,000 PFU per dose.

Varicella vaccine also induces cell-mediated immune responses in vaccinees. The relative contributions of humoral immunity and cell-mediated immunity to protection from chickenpox are unknown.

Mechanism: Induction of neutralizing antibodies and cell-mediated immunity. The relative contributions of humoral immunity and cell-mediated immunity to protection from chickenpox are unknown.

Drug Interactions: Because varicella vaccine consists of live viruses, reconstitute it with a diluent that does not contain preservatives. Preservatives may inactivate constituent viruses and render the vaccine ineffective.

Like all live viral vaccines, administration to patients receiving immunosuppressant drugs (eg, steroids) or radiation therapy may predispose patients to disseminated infections or insufficient response to immunization. They may remain susceptible despite immunization. Immunosuppressive doses of corticosteroids are generally considered to be 20 mg/day or 2 mg/kg/day of prednisone, or an equivalent dose of other systemic steroids. Inhaled or topical corticosteroids are not immunosuppressive, nor are some alternate-day or short courses of systemic steroids. Otherwise, wait 1 to 3 months or more after discontinuing steroids before giving varicella vaccine. Withhold steroids for 2 to 3 weeks after vaccination, if possible.

Varivax can be given at the same time as MMR vaccine. Otherwise, give the vaccines at least 30 days apart. To assess any interaction between *Varivax* and *M-M-R II* (Merck's measles-mumps-rubella vaccine), children were given the vaccines either concomitantly at separate sites or 6 weeks apart. Seroconversion rates and antibody levels were comparable between the 2 groups approximately 6 weeks after vaccination to each of the virus vaccine components. No differences were noted in adverse reactions reported.

Limited data from an experimental product containing varicella vaccine suggest that varicella vaccine can be given simultaneously with diphtheria, tetanus, acellular pertussis (DTaP) vaccine, and *PedvaxHIB* (Merck's Hib vaccine) using separate sites and syringes. However, there are no data relating to simultaneous administration of varicella vaccine with DTP or oral poliovirus vaccine (OPV). In 1 study, children received an investigational vaccine (a formulation combining measles, mumps, rubella, and varicella in 1 syringe) at the same time as booster doses of DTaP and OPV or received *M-M-R II* with booster doses of DTP and OPV, followed by varicella vaccine 6 weeks later. Six weeks after vaccination, seroconversion rates for measles, mumps, rubella, and varicella, and the percentage of vaccinees whose titers were boosted for diphtheria, tetanus, pertussis, and polio, were comparable between the 2 groups. But anti-varicella levels were slightly, perhaps insignificantly, decreased when the investigational vaccine containing varicella was administered concomitantly with DTaP. No clinically significant differences were noted in adverse reactions between the 2 groups.

In another study, 1 group of children received an investigational vaccine (a formulation combining measles, mumps, rubella, and varicella in 1 syringe) at the same time as a booster dose of *PedvaxHIB*. Another group received *M-M-R II* and a booster dose of *PedvaxHIB* followed by varicella vaccine 6 weeks later. Six weeks after vaccination, seroconversion rates for measles, mumps, rubella, and varicella and geometric mean titers for *PedvaxHIB* were comparable between the 2 groups, but anti-varicella levels were decreased when the investigational vaccine containing varicella was given with *PedvaxHIB*. No clinically significant differences in adverse reactions were seen.

To avoid inactivation of the attenuated virus, give varicella vaccine at least 14 to 30 days before or 5 months after giving any immune globulin or other blood product. After giving varicella vaccine, any immune globulin, including VZIG, should not be given for 2 months thereafter, unless its use outweighs the benefits of vaccination. Alternatively, check antibody titers or repeat the vaccine dose 5 months after IG administration.

Acyclovir and perhaps other antiviral drugs antagonize disseminated varicella infection, which may rarely be induced in vaccine recipients.

No data are yet available about possible suppression of tuberculin skin tests by varicella vaccine virus. Live virus vaccines may cause delayed-hypersensitivity skin tests (eg, tuberculin, histoplasmin) to appear falsely negative. Evaluate such tests knowingly. The effect may persist several weeks after vaccination. The ACIP and AAP recommend that tuberculin tests be given prior to live-virus vaccination, simultaneously with it, or at least 6 weeks after vaccination.

Salicylates: Reye syndrome has occurred in children and adolescents following natural varicella infection. The majority of these patients had received salicylates. Caution varicella vaccine recipients, parents, or guardians not to use salicylates in vaccine recipients for 6 weeks after vaccination. There were no reports of Reye syndrome in varicella vaccine recipients during clinical trials.

Interval Between Antibodies & Measles or Varicella-Containing Vaccine	
Antibody source	Delay before vaccination
Varicella-zoster immune globulin	5 months
Hepatitis B, tetanus, or Rh$_o$(D) immune globulins (HBIG, TIG, RhIG)	3 months for measles, 5 months for varicella
IGIM, 0.02 to 0.06 mL/kg	3 months for measles, 5 months for varicella
IGIM, 0.25 mL/kg	5 months
IGIM, 0.5 mL/kg	6 months
IGIV, 400 mg/kg	8 months
IGIV, high-dose for ITP or Kawasaki disease	8 to 11 months
Packed RBCs	5 months
Plasma or platelet	7 months
Rabies immune globulin	4 months for measles, 5 months for varicella
RBCs with adenine-saline added	3 months for measles, 5 months for varicella
Vaccinia immune globulin IV	3 mg (Cangene), 6 months (DVC)
Washed red blood cells (RBCs)	No wait
Whole blood	6 months

Patient Information: Ask patients, parents, or guardians about reactions to previous doses of varicella vaccine or a similar product.

Pharmaceutical Characteristics

Concentration: At least 1,350 PFU per 0.5 mL dose 30 minutes after reconstitution at room temperature (20° to 25°C; 68° to 77°F)

Quality Assay: Varicella vaccine retains a potency level of at least 1,500 PFU per dose for at least 24 months in a frost-free freezer with an average temperature of −15°C (+5°F) or colder.

Packaging:

Freezer-stable package: A single-dose vial of freeze-dried vaccine (NDC #: 00006-4826-00, package A) with a box of 10 vials of diluent (package B).

A box of 10 single-dose vials of freeze-dried vaccine (00006-4827-00, package A) with a box of 10 vials of diluent (package B).

Doseform: Lyophilized powder for suspension

Appearance: White powder, yielding a clear, colorless to pale yellow liquid

Diluent:

For reconstitution: Sterile water for injection without preservative

Adjuvant: None

Preservative: None

Allergens: Trace amounts of neomycin.

Freezer-stable package: 12.5 mg hydrolyzed gelatin per dose.

Refrigerator-stable package: 8.9 mg hydrolyzed gelatin per dose.

Excipients: Residual components of MRC-5 cells including DNA and protein, and fetal bovine serum per dose.

Freezer-stable package: 25 mg sucrose, 3.2 mg sodium chloride, 0.5 mg monosodium L-glutamate, 0.45 mg of sodium phosphate dibasic, 0.08 mg of potassium phosphate monobasic, 0.08 mg potassium chloride, and trace quantities of sodium phosphate monobasic, ethylenediaminetetraacetic acid (EDTA) per dose.

Refrigerator-stable package: 18 mg sucrose, 3.6 mg urea, 2.3 mg sodium chloride, 0.36 mg monosodium L-glutamate, 0.33 mg sodium diphosphate dibasic, 57 mcg potassium phosphate monobasic, and 57 mcg potassium chloride per dose.

pH: 6.8 to 7.2 after reconstitution

Shelf Life: Expires within 18 to 24 months. Retains potency at least 1500 PFU per doses when stored according to labeled instructions.

Storage/Stability:

Freezer-stable package: Keep powdered vaccine frozen at an average temperature of −15°C (5°F) or colder. Any freezer (eg, chest, frost-free) that reliably maintains an average temperature of −15°C (5°F) or colder and has a separate sealed freezer door is acceptable. Before reconstitution, protect from light. Store the diluent separately at room temperature or in a refrigerator. During shipment, to ensure that there is no loss of potency, the vaccine must be maintained at a temperature of −20°C (−4°F) or colder. Ship in insulated containers with coolants. Minimal potency can be maintained if the vaccine powder is stored continuously for no more than 72 hours at 2° to 8°C (36° to 46°F). Discard vaccine stored at 2° to 8°C (36° to 46°F) if not used within 72 hours of beginning storage at 2° to 8°C (36° to 46°F).

For information regarding stability at temperatures other than those recommended for storage, call (800) 9-VARIVAX.

Administer the vaccine immediately after reconstitution to minimize loss of potency. Discard if reconstituted vaccine is not used within 30 minutes. Do not freeze reconstituted vaccine.

Handling: To reconstitute the vaccine, first withdraw 0.7 mL of diluent into a syringe. Inject all the diluent in the syringe into the vial of freeze-dried vaccine and gently agitate to mix thoroughly. Withdraw the entire contents into a syringe, change the needle, and inject the total volume (approximately 0.5 mL).

Production Process: The virus was initially obtained from a child with natural varicella, then introduced into human embryonic-lung cell cultures, adapted to and propagated in embryonic guinea-pig cell cultures, and finally propagated in human diploid cell cultures (WI-38). Further passage of the virus for varicella vaccine was performed in human diploid cell cultures (MRC-5) that were free of adventitious agents. The production cycle for each lot takes 10 months to complete.

Media: MRC-5 human diploid-cell culture

Disease Epidemiology

Incidence: Varicella is a highly communicable disease in children, adolescents, and adults caused by the varicella-zoster virus. The disease usually consists of 300 to 500 maculopapular or vesicular lesions, usually seen first on the face, scalp, or trunk. Fever (oral temperature higher than 37.8°C; higher than 100°F) accompanies the infection in up to 70% of cases. Other symptoms include malaise, loss of appetite, or headache. The disease can cause scarring of the skin where lesions have appeared.

Incidence peaks among children 5 to 9 years of age. From 1980 to 1994, the incidence rate of chickenpox was 8.3% to 9.1% per year in children 1 to 9 years of age. Seasonally, incidence peaks sharply each year during the months of March, April, and May in temperate climates. The attack rate of natural varicella following household exposure among healthy, susceptible children was 87%. Although it is generally a benign, self-limiting disease, varicella may be associated with serious complications (eg, bacterial superinfection with organisms such as group A *Streptococci*, pneumonia, encephalitis, Reye syndrome) or death.

Approximately 2% of chickenpox cases occurred in adults 20 years of age and older; adult cases are often more severe. Adults are almost 10 times more likely than children to be hospitalized with chickenpox and are at least 20 times more likely to die as a result of the infection.

An episode of chickenpox generally confers lifelong protection against subsequent attack. But after the acute illness resolves, varicella-zoster viruses remain dormant in sensory nerve roots (nerve ganglia) for life. Herpes zoster ("zoster" or "shingles") results from reactivation of that virus, usually after the age of 50, in approximately 10% to 20% of people who have had chickenpox. Shingles can affect people of all ages, but the incidence of shingles increases with advancing age. It typically begins with neurologic pain, ranging from numbness and itching to severe pain in the skin area supplied by the affected nerve roots. Clusters of blister-like lesions follow within 3 to 4 days. These lesions, generally forming on only 1 side of the body, usually disappear within 2 to 3 weeks, leaving some people with permanent scars. Up to 14% of people who develop shingles experience persistent, stabbing neurologic pain for at least 1 month after onset of the disease. In some cases, pain related to shingles may persist for years.

Essentially the entire birth cohort is eventually infected. Before varicella vaccine was available, 3.5 to 3.7 million cases of varicella and 300,000 cases of herpes zoster occurred each year in the United States, resulting in an estimated 600 cases of encephalitis and approximately 50 to 90 deaths. Varicella results in the hospitalization of approximately 9,000 previously healthy people each year, 80% of them children. Only approximately 10% of cases were reported. Among untreated leukemic children, approximately 30% develop disseminated chickenpox, with a mortality rate approaching 10%.

Susceptible Pools: Most young children are susceptible to disease, as are 5% of adults, totaling approximately 31 million Americans.

Transmission: From person to person by direct contact, droplet, or airborne spread of secretions of the respiratory tract of chickenpox cases, or of the vesicle fluid of herpes-zoster patients. Varicella scabs are not infectious.

Incubation: 14 days (range: 10 to 21 days). May be prolonged after passive immunization and in immunodeficient patients.

Communicability: The period of contagiousness begins approximately 1 to 2 days before onset of rash and ends when all lesions have crusted over. This is usually no more than 5 days after the first group of vesicles appear. People with progressive varicella may be contagious longer, perhaps because viral replication persists longer.

Consider susceptible individuals infectious 10 to 21 days after exposure. The AAP recommends that children with chickenpox be excluded from school or day care for 7 days after rash onset or until all lesions are crusted. These guidelines have been disputed as inadequate to prevent transmission.

Other Information

Perspective:
1909: Von Bokay recognizes relationship between varicella and zoster.

1970: Takahashi isolates virus from a 3-year-old boy named K. Oka.

1981: Merck begins developing *Varivax*. Earlier research into varicella at Merck dates back to the late 1960s.

1992: FDA permits distribution of *Varivax* to children with acute lymphoblastic leukemia (ALL) in remission.

1995: FDA licenses *Varivax* on March 17, the first vaccine in America against a herpes virus.

2006: ACIP and AAP recommend a 2-dose vaccination strategy.

National Policy: ACIP. Prevention of varicella. *MMWR.* 2007;56(RR-4):1-40. http://www.cdc.gov/mmwr/PDF/rr/rr5604.pdf.

Canadian National Advisory Committee on Immunization. Update on varicella. *Can Comm Dis Rep.* 2004;30(ACS-1):1-28.

References: Hardy IR, et al. Prospects for use of a varicella vaccine in adults. *Infect Dis Clin North Am.* 1990;4:159-173.

Kuter BJ, et al. Oka/Merck varicella vaccine in healthy children: Final report of a 2-year efficacy study and 7-year follow-up studies. *Vaccine.* 1991;9:643-647.

WHO. Varicella vaccines. *Weekly Epidemiol Rec.* 1998;73:241-248.

Pharmacoeconomics: According to 1 model, routine chickenpox vaccination could save $384 million each year in the United States, $5.40 for each dollar invested in the program. This model adopted a societal perspective, including costs of medical care and the cost of work loss saved by preventing chickenpox.

Because of the high proportion of adults who are immune to varicella, antibody testing for varicella immunity is likely to be cost-effective among people with a negative or uncertain history of varicella infection.

Name:
Zostavax

Manufacturer:
Merck

Immunologic Characteristics

Antigen Source: Virus (double-stranded DNA), varicella-zoster virus (VZV), human herpes virus 3, genus *Varicellavirus*, subfamily Alphaherpesvirinae, family Herpesviridae

Viability: Live, attenuated

Antigenic Form: Whole virus

Antigenic Type: Protein

Strains: Oka/Merck strain, named for the Japanese boy from whom the virus was isolated.

Use Characteristics

Indications: To prevent herpes zoster (HZ, shingles) in people 50 years or older.

Limitations: Zoster vaccine is not indicated for the treatment of zoster or postherpetic neuralgia (PHN). The use of zoster vaccine in people with a previous history of zoster has not been studied.

Contraindications:

Absolute: People with a history of anaphylactic or anaphylactoid reactions to gelatin, neomycin, or any other component of the vaccine. People with a history of primary or acquired immunodeficiency states including leukemia; lymphomas of any type, or other malignant neoplasms affecting the bone marrow or lymphatic system; or AIDS or other clinical manifestations of infection with HIV. People on immunosuppressive therapy, including high-dose corticosteroids. People with active untreated tuberculosis. Women who are or may be pregnant.

Relative: Defer vaccination during acute illness, for example, in the presence of fever higher than 38.5°C (higher than 101.3°F). Neomycin allergy commonly manifests as a contact dermatitis, which is not a contraindication to receiving this vaccine. People with a history of anaphylactic reaction to topically or systemically administered neomycin should not receive zoster vaccine.

Immunodeficiency: Do not use in immunodeficient people, including people with congenital or acquired cellular immune deficiencies, whether due to genetics, disease, or drug or radiation therapy. Contains live viruses. Avoid use in people who are HIV-positive.

Vaccination with a live attenuated vaccine, such as zoster vaccine, may result in a more extensive vaccine-associated rash or disseminated disease in individuals who are immunosuppressed. Safety and efficacy of zoster vaccine have not been evaluated in individuals on immunosuppressive therapy, nor in individuals receiving daily topical or inhaled corticosteroids or low-dose oral corticosteroids.

Elderly: The median age of subjects enrolled in the largest (N = 38,546) clinical study of zoster vaccine was 69 years (range, 59 to 99 years). Of the 19,270 subjects who received zoster vaccine, 10,378 were 60 to 69 years of age, 7,629 were 70 to 79 years of age, and 1,263 were 80 years of age or older.

Carcinogenicity: Zoster vaccine has not been evaluated for carcinogenic potential.

Mutagenicity: Zoster vaccine has not been evaluated for mutagenic potential.

Fertility Impairment: Zoster vaccine has not been evaluated for impairment of fertility.

Pregnancy: Category C. Animal reproduction studies have not been conducted with zoster vaccine. It is also not known whether zoster vaccine can cause fetal harm when administered to a pregnant woman or can affect reproduction capacity. However, naturally occurring VZV infection is known to sometimes cause fetal harm. Therefore, do not administer zoster vaccine to pregnant women. Counsel women to avoid pregnancy for 3 months after vaccination. Vaccinees and health care providers are encouraged to report any exposure to zoster vaccine during pregnancy by calling (800) 986-8999.

Lactation: Some viruses are excreted in human milk, but it is not known whether VZV is secreted in human milk. Therefore, exercise caution if zoster vaccine is administered to a woman who is breast-feeding.

Children: Zoster vaccine is not a substitute for *Varivax* (varicella virus vaccine live [Oka/Merck]) and should not be used in children.

Adverse Reactions: In clinical trials, zoster vaccine was evaluated for safety in approximately 21,000 adults. In the Shingles Prevention Study (SPS), subjects received a single dose of either zoster vaccine (n = 19,270) or placebo (n = 19,276). The racial distribution across both groups was similar: white (95%); black (2%); Hispanic (1%); and other (1%) in both vaccination groups. The gender distribution was 59% male and 41% female in both groups. The age distribution of subjects enrolled, 59 to 99 years of age, was similar in both groups.

The Adverse Event Monitoring Substudy (AEMS; 3,345 received zoster vaccine and 3,271 received placebo) used vaccination report cards (VRCs) to record adverse events occurring from days 0 to 42 after vaccination (97% of subjects completed VRCs in both groups). In addition, monthly surveillance for hospitalization was conducted through the end of the study, 2 to 5 years after vaccination.

The remainder of subjects in the SPS (15,925 received zoster vaccine and 16,005 received placebo) were actively followed for safety outcomes through day 42 after vaccination and passively followed for safety after day 42.

Serious adverse reactions: In the overall study population, serious adverse experiences (SAEs) occurred at a similar rate (1.4%) in subjects vaccinated with zoster vaccine or placebo.

Rates of hospitalizations were similar among the vaccine group and the placebo group in the AEMS throughout the entire study.

Investigator-determined, vaccine-related SAEs were reported for 2 subjects vaccinated with zoster vaccine (asthma exacerbation and polymyalgia rheumatica) and 3 subjects who received placebo (Goodpasture syndrome, anaphylactic reaction, and polymyalgia rheumatica).

Deaths: The overall incidence of death occurring 0 to 42 days after vaccination was similar between groups; 14 deaths occurred in the zoster vaccine group and 16 deaths occurred in the placebo group. The most commonly reported cause of death was cardiovascular disease (10 in the vaccine group, 8 in the placebo group). The overall incidence of death occurring at any time during the study was similar between vaccination groups: 793 deaths (4.1%) occurred in the vaccine group and 795 deaths (4.1%) in the placebo group.

Common adverse reactions: Injection-site and systemic adverse experiences reported at an incidence greater than or equal to 1% in the AEMS are shown in the following table. Most were reported as mild in intensity. The overall incidence of vaccine-related injection-site adverse experiences was significantly greater for subjects vaccinated with zoster vaccine (48% for zoster vaccine and 17% for placebo).

Adverse Experiences Reported by VRC in ≥ 1% of Adults Who Received Zoster Vaccine or Placebo (0 to 42 Days After Vaccination) in the AEMS of the SPS		Zoster vaccine (N = 3,345) %	Placebo (N = 3,271) %
Adverse experience			
Injection site	Erythema[a]	33.7	6.4
	Pain/tenderness[a]	33.4	8.3
	Swelling[a]	24.9	4.3
	Hematoma	1.4	1.4
	Pruritus	6.6	1
	Warmth	1.5	0.3
Systemic	Headache	1.4	1.4

a Designates a solicited adverse experience. Injection-site adverse experiences were solicited only from days 0 to 4 after vaccination.

The numbers of subjects with elevated temperature (higher than 38.3°C, higher than 101°F) within 42 days after vaccination were similar in both groups (27 [0.8%] for zoster vaccine vs 27 [0.9%] for placebo).

The following adverse experiences in the AEMS of the SPS (days 0 to 42 after vaccination) were reported at an incidence greater than or equal to 1% and more frequently in subjects who received zoster vaccine than in subjects who received placebo, respectively: respiratory infection (65 [1.9%] vs 55 [1.7%]), fever (59 [1.8%] vs 53 [1.6%]), viral-like syndrome (57 [1.7%] vs 52 [1.6%]), diarrhea (51 [1.5%] vs 41 [1.3%]), rhinitis (46 [1.4%] vs 36 [1.1%]), skin disorder (35 [1.1%] vs 31 [1%]), respiratory disorder (35 [1.1%] vs 27 [0.8%]), asthenia (32 [1%] vs 14 [0.4%]).

Adverse events after day 42: AEMS subjects in the SPS were monitored for hospitalizations through monthly automated telephone queries and the remainder of subjects was passively monitored for safety in this study from day 43 after vaccination through study end. Over the course of the study (4.9 years), 51 (1.5%) individuals receiving zoster vaccine were reported to have congestive heart failure (CHF) or pulmonary edema compared with 39 (1.2%) individuals receiving placebo in the AEMS; 58 (0.3%) individuals receiving zoster vaccine were reported to have CHF or pulmonary edema compared with 45 (0.2%) individuals receiving placebo in the overall study.

Clinical safety with high-potency zoster vaccine: In an additional clinical study, high-potency zoster vaccine (203,000 PFU) administered to 461 subjects was compared with a lower-potency zoster vaccine (57,000 PFU; similar to potencies studied in the SPS) administered to 234 subjects. Moderate or severe injection-site reactions were more common in recipients of the higher-potency zoster vaccine (17%) as compared with recipients of the lower-potency vaccine (9%). Among recipients of the higher-potency zoster vaccine, 4 subjects (0.9%) reported SAEs (1 case each of angina pectoris, CAD, depression, and enteritis); 1 subject (0.4%) receiving the lower-potency zoster vaccine reported an SAE (lung cancer).

VZV rashes after vaccination: Within the 42-day after-vaccination period in the SPS, non–injection-site zoster-like rashes were reported by 53 subjects (17 for zoster vaccine and 36 for placebo). Of 41 specimens that were adequate for PCR testing, wild-type VZV was detected in 25 (5 for zoster vaccine, 20 for placebo) of these specimens. The Oka/Merck strain of VZV was not detected from any of these specimens. Of reported varicella-like rashes (n = 59), 10 had specimens that were available and adequate for PCR testing. VZV was not detected in any of these specimens. In all other clinical trials in support of zoster vaccine, the reported rates of non–injection-site zoster-like and varicella-like rashes within 42 days after vaccination were also low in both zoster vaccine recipients and placebo recipients. Of the 17 reported varicella-like rashes and non–injection-site, zoster-like rashes, 10 specimens were available and adequate for PCR testing. The Oka/Merck strain was identified by PCR analysis from the lesion specimens of 2 subjects who reported varicella-like rashes (onset on day 8 and 17).

Transmission: In clinical trials with zoster vaccine, transmission of the vaccine virus has not been reported. However, postmarketing experience with varicella vaccines suggests that transmission of vaccine virus may occur rarely from vaccinees who develop a varicella-like rash to susceptible contacts. Transmission of vaccine virus from varicella-vaccine recipients without a VZV-like rash has been reported but has not been confirmed. Weigh the risk of transmitting the attenuated vaccine virus to a susceptible individual against the risk of developing natural zoster that could be transmitted to a susceptible individual.

Pharmacologic & Dosing Characteristics

Dosage: 19,400 PFU per 0.65 mL dose

Route & Site: Subcutaneous, preferably in the upper arm

Overdosage: Although few data are available, clinical experience with similar products suggests that the major manifestations of overdosage would be pain and tenderness at the injection site.

Additional Doses: None currently recommended.

Efficacy:

People 50 to 59 years of age: In the efficacy study, volunteers received a single dose of either zoster vaccine live (n = 11,211) or placebo (n = 11,228). Subjects were followed for a median of 1.3 years (range, 0 to 2 years). Compared with placebo, zoster vaccine live significantly reduced the risk of developing zoster by 69.8% (95% CI, 54-81) in subjects 50 to 59 years of age.

Efficacy of zoster vaccine was evaluated in the SPS, a placebo-controlled, double-blind clinical trial in which 38,546 subjects 60 years of age or older were randomized to receive a single dose of either zoster vaccine (n = 19,270) or placebo (n = 19,276). Subjects were followed for the development of zoster for a median of 3.1 years (range, 31 days to 4.9 years). The study excluded people who were immunocompromised or using corticosteroids on a regular basis, and anyone with a previous history of HZ. People in both groups who developed zoster were given famciclovir, and, as necessary, pain medications. The primary efficacy analysis included all subjects randomized in the study who were followed for at least 30 days after vaccination and did not develop an evaluable case of HZ within the first 30 days after vaccination (modified intent-to-treat [MITT] analysis).

Zoster vaccine significantly reduced the risk of developing zoster when compared with placebo. Vaccine efficacy for the prevention of HZ was highest for those 60 to 69 years of age and declined with increasing age.

Herpes Zoster Incidence in the Shingles Prevention Study							
	Zoster vaccine			Placebo			
Age group[a] (y)	# Subjects	# HZ cases	Incidence rate of HZ per 1,000 person-years	# Subjects	# HZ cases	Incidence rate of HZ per 1,000 person-years	Vaccine efficacy (95% CI)
Overall	19,254	315	5.4	19,247	642	11.1	51% (44%, 58%)
60 to 69	10,370	122	3.9	10,356	334	10.8	64% (56%, 71%)

Herpes Zoster Incidence in the Shingles Prevention Study							
	Zoster vaccine			Placebo			
Age group[a] (y)	# Subjects	# HZ cases	Incidence rate of HZ per 1,000 person-years	# Subjects	# HZ cases	Incidence rate of HZ per 1,000 person-years	Vaccine efficacy (95% CI)
70 to 79	7,621	156	6.7	7,559	261	11.4	41% (28%, 52%)
≥ 80	1,263	37	9.9	1,332	47	12.2	18% (−29%, 48%)

a Age strata at randomization were 60 to 69 and 70 years of age or older.

Forty-five subjects were excluded from the MITT analysis (16 in the vaccine group and 29 in the placebo group), including 24 subjects with evaluable HZ cases that occurred in the first 30 days after vaccination (6 in the vaccine group and 18 in the placebo group).

Suspected HZ cases were followed prospectively for the development of HZ-related complications. Rates of PHN, defined as HZ-associated pain (rated as 3 or greater on a 10-point scale by the study subject and occurring or persisting at least 90 days) after onset of rash in evaluable cases of HZ, appear in the following table.

Post-Herpetic Neuralgia in the Shingles Prevention Study											
	Zoster vaccine					Placebo					Vaccine efficacy against PHN in subjects who develop HZ after vaccination (95% CI)
Age group (y)	# Subjects	# HZ cases	# PHN cases	Incidence rate of PHN per 1,000 person-years	% HZ cases with PHN	# Subjects	# HZ cases	# PHN cases	Incidence rate of PHN per 1,000 person-years	% HZ cases with PHN	
Overall	19,254	315	27	0.5	8.6%	19,247	642	80	1.4	12.5%	39%[a] (7%, 59%)
60 to 69	10,370	122	8	0.3	6.6%	10,356	334	23	0.7	6.9%	5% (−107%, 56%)
70 to 79	7,621	156	12	0.5	7.7%	7,559	261	45	2	17.2%	55% (18%, 76%)
≥ 80	1,263	37	7	1.9	18.9%	1,332	47	12	3.1	25.5%	26% (−69%, 68%)

a Age-adjusted estimate based on the age strata (60 to 69 and 70 years of age or older) at randomization.

The median duration of clinically significant pain (greater than or equal to 3 on a 0 to 10 point scale) among HZ cases in the vaccine group compared with the placebo group was 20 days vs 22 days based on the confirmed HZ cases. Overall, the benefit of zoster vaccine in preventing PHN can be primarily attributed to the effect of the vaccine on the prevention of herpes zoster. Vaccination reduced the incidence of PHN in individuals 70 years of age and older who developed zoster after vaccination.

Other prespecified zoster-related complications were reported less frequently in subjects who received zoster vaccine compared with subjects who received placebo. Among HZ cases, zoster-related complications were reported at similar rates in both vaccination groups.

Specific Complications[a] of Zoster among HZ Cases in the SPS				
	Zoster vaccine (N = 19,270)		Placebo (N = 19,276)	
Complication	(n = 321)	% among zoster cases	(n = 659)	% among zoster cases
Allodynia	135	42.1	310	47
Bacterial superinfection	3	0.9	7	1.1
Dissemination	5	1.6	11	1.7
Impaired vision	2	0.6	9	1.4
Ophthalmic zoster	35	10.9	69	10.5
Peripheral nerve palsies (motor)	5	1.6	12	1.8
Ptosis	2	0.6	9	1.4
Scarring	24	7.5	57	8.6
Sensory loss	7	2.2	12	1.8

N = number of subjects randomized
n = number of zoster cases, including those cases occurring within 30 days after vaccination, with these data available
a Complications reported at a frequency of greater than or equal to 1% in at least 1 group among subjects with zoster.

Visceral complications reported by less than 1% of subjects with zoster included 3 cases of pneumonitis and 1 case of hepatitis in the placebo group, and 1 case of meningoencephalitis in the vaccine group.

Immunogenicity: Immune responses to vaccination were evaluated in a subset of subjects enrolled in the SPS (N = 1,395). VZV GMT antibody levels, as measured by gpELISA 6 weeks after vaccination, were increased 1.7-fold (95% CI, 1.6 to 1.8) in the vaccine group compared with the placebo group. The specific antibody level that correlates with protection from zoster has not been established.

Onset: Within 30 days.

Duration: The duration of protection from zoster vaccination is unknown. In the SPS, protection from zoster was demonstrated through 4 years of follow-up. The need for revaccination has not been defined.

Protective Level: VZV GMT antibody levels, as measured by gpELISA 6 weeks after vaccination, were increased 1.7-fold (95% CI, 1.6 to 1.8) in the vaccine group compared with the placebo group. The specific antibody level that correlates with protection from zoster has not been established.

Mechanism: The risk of developing zoster appears to be related to a decline in VZV-specific immunity. Zoster vaccine boosts VZV-specific immunity, believed to be the mechanism by which it protects against zoster and its complications.

Drug Interactions: Because zoster vaccine consists of live viruses, reconstitute it with the supplied diluent that does not contain preservatives. Preservatives may inactivate constituent viruses and render the vaccine ineffective.

Concurrent administration of zoster vaccine and antiviral medications known to be effective against VZV has not been evaluated.

In a double-blind study, 374 adults 60 years and older received either trivalent inactivated influenza vaccine and zoster vaccine concurrently or 4 weeks apart. The antibody responses to each vaccine 4 weeks after vaccination were similar in both groups.

In a double-blind study, 473 adults 60 years of age or older were randomized to receive zoster vaccine and PPV23 concomitantly (n = 237), or PPV23 alone followed 4 weeks later by zoster vaccine alone (n = 236). Four weeks after vaccination, the VZV antibody levels following concomitant use were significantly lower than the VZV antibody levels following nonconcomitant administration (GMTs of 338 vs 484 gpELISA units/mL, respectively; GMT ratio = 0.70 [95% CI, 0.61, 0.80]). The manufacturer recommends against concomitant administration. However, IgG levels against varicella-zoster virus may not directly correlate with clinical protection against zoster. A study in a large managed-care database did not find a clinically significant difference in the incidence of herpes zoster among people who received PPV23 and zoster vaccine either on the same day or separated by 30 to 365 days. Coadministration of zoster vaccine with other vaccines has not been evaluated.

Like all live viral vaccines, administration to patients receiving immunosuppressive drugs, including steroids, or radiation, may predispose patients to disseminated infections or insufficient response to immunization. They may remain susceptible despite immunization. Immunosuppressive doses of corticosteroids are generally considered to be 20 mg/day or 2 mg/kg/day of prednisone or an equivalent dose of other systemic steroids. Inhaled or topical corticosteroids are not considered immunosuppressive, nor are some alternate-day or short courses of systemic steroids. Nonetheless, the safety and efficacy of zoster vaccine have not been evaluated in people receiving daily topical or inhaled corticosteroids or low-dose oral corticosteroids. Otherwise, wait 1 to 3 months or more after discontinuing steroids before giving zoster vaccine. Withhold steroids for 2 to 3 weeks after vaccination, if possible.

As a general rule, to avoid inactivation of the attenuated virus, administer live virus vaccines at least 14 to 30 days before or 6 to 8 weeks after administration of any immune globulin or other blood product. Alternately, check antibody titers or repeat the vaccine dose 3 months after immune globulin administration.

No data are available about possible suppression of tuberculin skin tests by VZV vaccines. Live virus vaccines may cause delayed-hypersensitivity skin tests (eg, histoplasmin, tuberculin) to appear falsely negative. Evaluate such tests knowingly. The effect may persist for several weeks after vaccination. ACIP recommends that tuberculin tests be given before live-virus vaccination, simultaneously with it, or at least 6 weeks after vaccination.

Interval Between Antibodies & Measles- or Varicella-Containing Vaccine	
Antibody source	Delay before immunization
Hepatitis B, tetanus, or Rh_o (D) immune globulins (HBIG, TIG, RhIG)	3 months for measles, 5 months for varicella
Vaccinia immune globulin IV	3 months
Rabies immune globulin	4 months for measles, 5 months for varicella
Varicella-zoster immune globulin	5 months
IGIM 0.02 to 0.06 mL/kg	3 months for measles, 5 months for varicella
IGIM, 0.25 mL/kg	5 months
IGIM, 0.5 mL/kg	6 months
IGIV, 400 mg/kg	8 months
IGIV, high-dose for ITP or Kawasaki disease	8 to 11 months
RBCs with adenine-saline added	3 months for measles, 5 months for varicella
Plasma or platelet products	7 months
Whole blood	6 months
Packed RBCs	5 months
Washed red blood cells (RBCs)	No wait

Patient Information: Inform vaccinees of the theoretical risk of transmitting the vaccine virus to varicella-susceptible individuals, including pregnant women who have not had chickenpox. Advise women to avoid pregnancy for 3 months following vaccination.

Zoster Vaccine Live

Pharmaceutical Characteristics

Concentration: At least 19,400 PFU per 0.65 mL dose 30 minutes after reconstitution at room temperature (20° to 25°C [68° to 77°F]).

Quality Assay: The cells, virus seeds, virus bulks, and bovine serum used in the manufacturing are all tested to provide assurance that the final product is free of adventitious agents.

Packaging: A single-dose vial of freeze-dried vaccine (NDC #: 00006-4963-00, package A) with a box of 10 vials of diluent (package B).

A box of 10 single-dose vials of freeze-dried vaccine (00006-4963-41, package A) with a box of 10 vials of diluent (package B).

Doseform: Lyophilized powder for suspension

Appearance: White powder, yielding a semihazy to translucent, off-white to pale yellow liquid.

Diluent:
For reconstitution: Sterile water without preservative.

Adjuvant: None

Preservative: None

Allergens: 15.58 mg hydrolyzed porcine gelatin per dose. Trace quantities of neomycin.

Excipients: 31.16 mg sucrose, 15.58 mg hydrolyzed porcine gelatin, 3.99 mg sodium chloride, 0.62 mg monosodium L-glutamate, 0.57 mg sodium phosphate dibasic, 0.1 mg potassium phosphate monobasic, 0.1 mg potassium chloride; residual components of MRC-5 cells including DNA and protein; and trace quantities of neomycin and bovine calf serum per 0.65 mL dose.

pH: Data not available

Shelf Life: Expires within 12 months.

Storage/Stability: Store vaccine powder frozen at −15°C (5°F) or colder. Store diluent separately at room temperature or in the refrigerator. Protect vials from light before reconstitution. Contact the manufacturer regarding exposure to elevated temperatures.

This vaccine may be stored at refrigerator temperature (2° to 8°C [36° to 46°F]) for up to 72 continuous hours before reconstitution. Discard vaccine stored at 2° to 8°C (36° to 46°F) that is not used within 72 hours of removal from −15°C (5°F) storage.

Reconstitute immediately upon removal from the freezer. Discard reconstituted vaccine if not used within 30 minutes. Do not freeze reconstituted vaccine.

Production Process: The virus was initially obtained from a child with naturally occurring varicella, then introduced into human embryonic lung cell cultures, adapted to and propagated in embryonic guinea pig cell cultures, and finally propagated in human diploid cell cultures (WI-38). Further passage of the virus was performed at Merck Research Laboratories (MRL) in human diploid cell cultures (MRC-5).

Media: MRC-5 human diploid cell culture

Disease Epidemiology

Incidence: Herpes zoster (HZ), commonly known as shingles or zoster, is a manifestation of the reactivation of varicella-zoster virus (VZV). Primary VZV infection produces chickenpox (varicella). After initial infection, VZV virus remains latent in the dorsal root or cranial sensory ganglia until it reactivates, producing zoster. Zoster is characterized by a unilateral, painful, vesicular cutaneous eruption with a dermatomal distribution.

Anyone previously infected with chickenpox (more than 90% of adults in the United States) is at risk for developing shingles. As people age, it is possible for VZV virus to reappear in the form of shingles. This condition affects 2 in every 10 people in their lifetime. The incidence and severity of shingles, as well as the frequency and severity of its complications, increase with age. About 40% to 50% of the estimated 1 million cases of shingles that occur in the United States each year occur in people 60 years of age and older. Shingles can be unpredictable and can occur without warning at any time.

Shingles usually starts as an unusual or painful sensation on one side of the body or face, followed by a blistering rash. Pain from shingles can be mild to severe and may occur just before the rash appears, during the eruption of the rash, and as long-term nerve pain (postherpetic neuralgia, PHN). PHN has been described as tender, burning, throbbing, stabbing, shooting, and/or sharp pain. This pain can last months or even years.

Other complications, such as scarring, allodynia (pain from an innocuous stimulus such as the touch of soft clothing or a light breeze), pneumonia, visual impairment, and hearing loss also can occur as the result of shingles. Treating shingles and PHN can be difficult, often requiring a multifaceted approach.

Other Information

Perspective: See Varicella Virus Vaccine Live monograph.

First Licensed: May 25, 2006

National Policy: ACIP. Prevention of herpes zoster. *MMWR.* 2008;57(RR-5):1-30, erratum 779. http://www.cdc.gov/mmwr/PDF/rr/rr5705.pdf.

Canadian National Advisory Committee on Immunization. Statement on the recommended use of herpes zoster vaccine. *Can Comm Dis Rep.* 2010;36(ACS-1):1-19.

References: Oxman MN, Levin MJ, Johnson GR, et al; Shingles Prevention Study Group. A vaccine to prevent herpes zoster and postherpetic neuralgia in older adults. *N Engl J Med.* 2005;352:2271-2284.

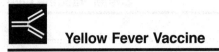

Yellow Fever Vaccine

Viral Vaccines

Name:
YF-Vax

Manufacturer:
Sanofi Pasteur. Distribution is limited to designated Yellow Fever Vaccination Centers authorized by state health departments to issue certificates of yellow fever vaccination. Contact local health departments for locations of local centers.

Synonyms: VISI abbreviation: YEL. Yellow fever is also known as fiebre amarilla and yellow jack, for the flag of quarantine that flew over infected sailing vessels.

Immunologic Characteristics

Microorganism: Virus (single-stranded RNA), yellow fever virus, family Flaviviridae

Viability: Live, attenuated

Antigenic Form: Whole virus

Antigenic Type: Protein

Strains: 17D-204, cultured in a manner to be free of avian-leukosis virus. A primary viral seed for the vaccine strain is maintained at passage 237 (subculture subcutaneous-237); the viruses in the vaccine are derived from passage 239. The lineage of this strain began with what is known as the Rockefeller or Asibi strain.

Use Characteristics

Indications: Induction of active immunity against yellow fever virus, primarily among people 9 months of age and older traveling to or living in areas of South America and Africa where yellow fever infection is officially reported, or to countries that require a certificate of vaccination against yellow fever. Vaccination is also recommended for travel outside urban areas of countries that do not officially report the disease but that lie in the yellow fever-endemic zone. In recent years, fatal cases of yellow fever have occurred among unvaccinated tourists visiting rural areas within the yellow fever-endemic zone. Vaccinate laboratory personnel who might be exposed to virulent yellow fever virus by direct or indirect contact or by aerosols.

Consider infants 4 to 9 months of age and pregnant women for vaccination if traveling to areas experiencing ongoing epidemic yellow fever when travel cannot be postponed and a high level of prevention against mosquito exposure is not feasible. In no instance should infants younger than 4 months of age receive yellow fever vaccine, because of the risk of encephalitis.

Contraindications:

Absolute: People with a history of serious allergic reaction to a vaccine component or after a prior dose of this vaccine.

Relative: Defer immunization during the course of any acute illness. Women breast-feeding infants younger than 9 months of age, who are at elevated risk of encephalitis from yellow fever vaccine.

Immunodeficiency: Do not use in immunodeficient people, including those with congenital or acquired immune deficiencies, whether because of genetics, disease, or drug or radiation therapy. Contains live viruses. Infection with yellow-fever vaccine virus poses a theoretical risk of encephalitis to patients with immune suppression in association with AIDS, leukemia, lymphoma, generalized malignancy, or those whose immunologic responses are suppressed for any reason. Such patients should not be vaccinated. If they must travel to a yellow-fever-infected zone, advise them of their risk, instruct them to avoid mosquitos, and supply them with vaccination waiver letters.

Elderly: No specific information is available about geriatric use of yellow fever vaccine. Analysis of VAERS reports suggests that people 65 years of age and older may be at increased risk for systemic adverse events after yellow fever vaccination.

Pregnancy: Category C. Contraindicated on hypothetical grounds. Avoid use unless travel to high-risk area is unavoidable. Generally, most IgG passage across the placenta occurs during the third trimester. In a study of 101 Nigerian women in various stages of pregnancy, yellow fever vaccine was not associated with adverse effects on the fetus or with risk of fetal infection. However, the percentage of pregnant women who seroconverted after vaccination was significantly less than a nonpregnant control group (39% vs 82%). Yellow-fever vaccine virus crossed the placenta to 1 newborn among 81 mothers unknowingly vaccinated during pregnancy. The child appeared unaffected by infection, but yellow fever virus is known to be neurotropic. Avoid vaccination during pregnancy if at all possible.

Lactation: At least 2 cases of vaccine-associated neurologic disease (ie, encephalitis) developed in breast-fed infants whose mothers had recently received yellow fever vaccine. Both infants were younger than 1 month of age and exclusively breast-fed. Avoid giving yellow fever vaccine to breast-feeding women. However, when travel of breast-feeding mothers to high-risk endemic zones cannot be avoided or postponed, these women should be offered vaccine, after discussion of risks and benefits.

Children: The same dose is used for children and adults. To avoid risk of encephalitis, do not administer to infants 4 to 9 months of age unless travel to high-risk area is unavoidable. Vaccinate pregnant women and infants 4 to 9 months of age only if they must travel and they cannot avoid mosquito bites. Vaccinate infants 4 to 9 months of age only if the risk of infection is high. Do not vaccinate infants younger than 4 months of age; they are especially vulnerable to swelling of the brain after vaccination. One case of fatal vaccine-associated encephalitis occurred after vaccination of an apparently healthy girl of 3 years and 3 months of age.

Adverse Reactions: Two to 5 percent of vaccine recipients have mild headaches, myalgia, low-grade fevers, or other minor symptoms for 5 to 10 days. Fewer than 0.2% of vaccinees curtail regular activities. In rare instances, encephalitis has developed, but historically only 23 cases of encephalitis temporally associated with or confirmed to be caused by 17D vaccine have been reported in the scientific literature since 1945. Of these, 16 occurred among children younger than 9 months of age. In very young infants, this usually has not been severe and recovery has ordinarily occurred without sequelae. One pediatric death was reported. Anaphylaxis may occur. Immediate hypersensitivity reactions (eg, rash, urticaria, asthma) occur after 1 per 130,000 to 250,000 doses, principally among people with a history of egg allergy.

Sepsis-like syndromes after receipt of the yellow fever vaccine were not reported, despite millions of doses administered, until identification of 7 such cases between 1996 and 2001 (6 fatal) within 2 to 5 days after vaccination. Five received the US-licensed 17D-204 strain of vaccine (range: 53 to 79 years of age), whereas 2 received the Brazilian 17DD strain (5 and 22 years of age). The syndromes included fever, hypotension, renal failure, hyperbilirubinemia, lymphocytopenia, thrombocytopenia, and elevated liver enzymes. Studies are underway to better understand the risk factors for this association.

Pharmacologic & Dosing Characteristics

Dosage: 0.5 mL

Hypersensitivity test: Apply a drop of 1:10 v/v dilution of the vaccine in sodium chloride 0.9% as a scratch, prick, or puncture test. Also apply appropriate positive (ie, histamine) and negative (ie, isotonic sodium chloride) tests. A positive test is induration 3 mm larger than that of the saline control, usually with surrounding erythema. The histamine control must be positive for valid interpretation. If the result of this test is negative, perform an ID test, as follows: Inject 0.02 mL of a 1:100 v/v dilution of the vaccine in sodium chloride 0.9% as an ID test. Again, apply appropriate positive and negative tests. A positive test is induration 5 mm larger than that of the saline control, usually with surrounding erythema. The histamine control must be positive for valid interpretation.

Desensitization: For patients with a history of severe egg sensitivity and a positive skin test to the vaccine, the vaccine may be given using a desensitization procedure if immunization is imperative. Administer the following successive doses at 15- to 20-minute intervals:

(1) 0.05 mL of 1:10 v/v dilution

(2) 0.05 mL of full-strength vaccine

(3) 0.10 mL of full-strength vaccine

(4) 0.15 mL of full-strength vaccine

(5) 0.20 mL of full-strength vaccine.

Route: Subcutaneously

Booster Doses: Every 10 years

Waste Disposal: Discard yellow-fever vaccine containers and needles in a manner that will inactivate the live virus (eg, autoclaving, incineration).

Efficacy: Essentially 100%

Onset: 7 to 10 days

Duration: 10 years or longer. International Health Regulations require revaccination at intervals of 10 years. Evidence from several studies suggests that immunity after yellow fever vaccination persists for 30 to 35 years or more and probably for life.

Protective Level: A $\log_{10}$ neutralization (plaque reduction) index of 0.7 indicates protection in Rhesus monkeys.

Mechanism: Induction of protective antibodies

Drug Interactions: Because yellow fever vaccine consists of live viruses, reconstitute it with a diluent that does not contain preservatives. Preservatives may inactivate constituent viruses and render the vaccine ineffective.

Like all live viral vaccines, administration to patients receiving immunosuppressant drugs (eg, steroids) or radiation therapy may predispose patients to disseminated infections or insufficient response to immunization. They may remain susceptible despite immunization.

As a general rule, when a patient needs live vaccines, administer them simultaneously or wait at least 4 weeks between immunizations. Measles and yellow fever vaccines have been administered in combination, with full efficacy of each component. Similarly, BCG or smallpox vaccine have been administered in combination with yellow fever vaccine without interference. Adverse events to vaccination are not amplified by concurrent administration.

Concurrent yellow fever and injectable inactivated cholera vaccination impairs the immune response to each vaccine. Separate these vaccinations by at least 3 weeks, if possible, or administer them on the same day if separation is not feasible.

In 1 study, concurrent vaccination against hepatitis B and yellow fever viruses reduced the antibody titer expected from yellow fever vaccine. The manufacturer recommends concurrent administration at separate sites.

Yellow fever vaccine does not interact with 5 mL doses of American-produced immune globulins, yet it may be prudent to maintain an interval of several weeks between these drugs if time permits.

Concurrent administration of chloroquine to yellow-fever vaccine recipients does not affect antibody response.

Patient Information: Advise vaccinated people to take personal precautions to reduce exposure to mosquito bites. Travelers should stay in screened or air-conditioned rooms, use insecticidal space sprays as necessary, and use mosquito repellents and protective clothing to avoid mosquito bites. Mosquitoes are most active at twilight hours and in the evening.

Pharmaceutical Characteristics

Concentration: At least 4.74 $\log_{10}$ plaque-forming units per 0.5 mL, at least 2,000 mouse LD_{50} units; 75% suspension of embryo particles by weight

Quality Assay: Chicks must come from avian-leukosis virus (ALV) free flocks. No human protein is added to the virus suspension at any stage.

USP requirements: Tested in monkeys for viscerotropism, immunogenicity, and neurotropism.

Packaging: Five single-dose vials with 1 mL diluents (NDC #: 49281-0915-01), 5-dose vial with 3 mL vial of diluent (49281-0915-05)

Doseform: Powder for suspension

Appearance: White powder, yielding a slightly opalescent and light orange suspension.

Diluent:

For reconstitution: 0.9% sodium chloride without preservative. Add diluent slowly. Allow to stand 1 to 2 minutes, then swirl gently until uniformly suspended. To avoid foaming and protein degradation, do not shake. Do not dilute further.

Adjuvant: None

Preservative: None

Allergens: Gelatin, residual egg proteins. Yellow fever vaccine contains a larger mass of egg protein per dose than other egg-cultured vaccines. The stopper of the vial contains dry natural latex rubber.

USP requirement: Must not contain human serum.

Excipients: Sorbitol and gelatin added as stabilizers

pH: Data not provided

Shelf Life: Expires within 12 months

Storage/Stability: Store the vaccine powder between 2° and 8°C (36° and 46°F). It should no longer be stored in the freezer.

Shipped within the US at refrigerated temperature (2° to 8°C, 36° to 46°F), rather than frozen.

Elevated-temperature studies suggest a potency half-life of 14 days at 35° to 37°C (95° to 99°F) and 3.3 to 4.5 days at 45° to 47°C (113° to 117°F).

After reconstitution, potency persists for 1 hour. Discard unused vaccine 1 hour after reconstitution.

Yellow fever vaccine is shipped to sites designated by state health departments. To obtain information about sites near you or to request designation, contact your state or territorial health department.

Yellow Fever Vaccine

Production Process: Cultured in chicken embryos. Viruses are harvested from the chick embryos themselves. The vaccine consists of the freeze-dried supernatant of centrifuged embryo homogenate. As a result, a far larger mass of egg protein per dose persists, compared with other egg-derived vaccines. The vaccine is partially purified, lyophilized, and packaged. The air in each vaccine vial is displaced with nitrogen.

Media: Embryonated chicken eggs

Disease Epidemiology

Incidence: The last sizable outbreak in the United States occurred in New Orleans in 1905. The last indigenous case of yellow fever was reported in 1911; the last imported case in 1924.

No indigenous cases occur in the United States. An estimated 200,000 cases occur annually around the world, most in sub-Saharan Africa, with more than 10,000 deaths.

Susceptible Pools: Most of the American population is susceptible, although exposure is usually negligible.

Transmission: Two types of transmission are recognized: jungle and urban. Jungle (or sylvan) transmission occurs among nonhuman primates via several mosquito species. Human infection is incidental. For urban transmission, *Aedes aegypti* mosquitoes transmit the virus from infected humans to susceptible humans. Transmission involves a 7- to 17-day period of viral replication within a female mosquito, known as "extrinsic incubation."

Incubation: 3 to 6 days. In most cases, infection involves only mild illness with fever and malaise for several days. In approximately 15% of infections, the disease may result in hemorrhagic fever, hepatitis, or nephritis, and may be fatal. Among patients with symptoms, the case-fatality rate can reach 50% to 75%, with higher proportions of death among children younger than 10 years of age.

Communicability: Blood of patients is infective for mosquitoes shortly before onset of fever and for the first 3 to 5 days of illness.

Other Information

Perspective:
1702: Outbreak in New York City kills one-tenth of the city's population.
1793: Yellow fever epidemic kills approximately 5,000 people in Philadelphia, approximately 15% of the capital city of the fledgling United States. Additional outbreaks occurred through 1799. Virus was probably imported by people fleeing the Haiti revolution.
1853: Outbreak in New Orleans kills estimated 8,000 to 11,000 people, mainly immigrants.
1878: Outbreak throughout Mississippi Valley kills 20,000.
1901: Walter Reed and colleagues in Cuba prove Finlay's hypothesis that mosquitoes are vectors of yellow fever and that the causative agent is a filterable organism, a virus.
1905: Outbreak in New Orleans causes 5,000 cases and 1,000 deaths.
1927: Theiler isolates 17D strain from an African patient named Asibi. Theiler earns the 1951 Nobel Prize for this and related work.
1934: Peltier and colleagues develop the so-called French or Dakar vaccine, a mouse passage-adapted neurotropic strain for administration by scarification, often combined with smallpox vaccine. Unfortunately, this strain is encephalitogenic, especially in children. Licensed in the United States in 1935. Discontinued globally in 1982.
1942: 49,000 American soldiers vaccinated against yellow fever become infected with hepatitis B, because of contamination of the vaccine with infected human serum.
1953: Merrell National Laboratories' yellow fever vaccine licensed in the United States on May 22.

First Licensed: YF-Vax: January 3, 1978

National Policy: ACIP. Yellow fever vaccine: Recommendations of the Advisory Committee on Immunization Practices. *MMWR.* 2010;59(RR-7):1-27. http://www.cdc.gov/mmwr/PDF/rr/rr5117.pdf.

CDC. Requirements for use of a new International Certificate of Vaccination or Prophylaxis for yellow fever vaccine. *MMWR.* 2008;56:1345-1346. http://www.cdc.gov/mmwr/PDF/wk/mm5651.pdf.

References: CDC. Adverse events associated with 17D-derived yellow fever vaccination—United States, 2001-2002. *MMWR*. 2002;51:989-993. http://www.cdc.gov/mmwr/PDF/wk/mm5144.pdf.

CDC. Fever, jaundice, and multiple organ system failure associated with 17D-derived yellow fever vaccination, 1996-2001. *MMWR*. 2001;50:643-645. http://www.cdc.gov/mmwr/preview/mmwrhtml/mm5030a3.htm.

Jentes ES, Poumerol G, Gershman MD, et al; Informal WHO Working Group on Geographic Risk for Yellow Fever. The revised global yellow fever risk map and recommendations for vaccination, 2010: consensus of the Informal WHO Working Group on Geographic Risk for Yellow Fever [published correction appears in *Lancet Infect Dis*. 2012;12(2):98]. *Lancet Infect Dis*. 2011;11(8):622-632.

WHO. Yellow fever vaccines. *Weekly Epidemiol Rec*. 2003;78:349-359. http://www.who.int/wer/2003/en/wer7840.pdf.

Pierce JR, Writer J. *Yellow Jack: How Yellow Fever Ravaged America and Walter Reed Discovered Its Deadly Secrets*. Hoboken, NJ: John Wiley and Sons; 2005.

Yellow Fever Vaccine Summary Table	
Generic name	Yellow fever vaccine live
Brand name	*YF-Vax*
Manufacturer	Sanofi Pasteur
Viability	Live viral vaccine
Indication	To prevent infection with yellow fever virus
Strain	17D-204 strain
Concentration	$\geq 4.74 \log_{10}$, PFU per 0.5 mL
Adjuvant	None
Preservative	None
Production medium	Embryonated chicken eggs
Doseform	Powder for solution
Diluent	Sodium chloride 0.9% without preservative
Packaging	Single-dose, 5-dose vials plus diluent
Routine storage	2° to 8°C (no longer frozen)
Stability	Discard within 1 hour of reconstitution
Dosage, route	0.5 mL subcutaneously
Standard schedule	1 dose (if $\geq$ 9 months old), boost every 10 years

Summary of Antibody Products

Naming Conventions

Guidelines for naming monoclonal antibodies and antibody fragments are established by the US Adopted Names (USAN) Council and the International Nonproprietary Name (INN) Working Group. The syllables in each name reveal a great deal of information about each product. The order for combining the syllables is: (1) a prefix, (2) an infix reflecting the target or disease, (3) an infix indicating the antibody source, and (4) the stem used as a suffix.

The suffix "-mab" is used for monoclonal antibodies, antibody fragments and radiolabeled antibodies. For polyclonal mixtures of antibodies, "-pab" is used. The -pab suffix applies to polyclonal pools of recombinant monoclonal antibodies, as opposed to polyclonal antibody preparations isolated from blood.

This is preceded by 1 to 3 letters describing the antibody's source: "-a-" for rat, "-axo-" for rat-murine hybrids, "-e-" for hamster, "-i-" for primate, "-o-" for mouse, "-u-" for human, "-xi-" for chimeric, "-zu-" for humanized, or "-xizu-" combinations of humanized and chimeric chains.

The target or disease state of the antibody's indication is designated with an additional internal syllable or letter (an "infix" in USAN jargon). Tumor-specific infixes have been discontinued because most monoclonal antibodies with oncology indications are investigated for more than 1 type of tumor. Target infixes include:

- "-b-", "-ba-", or "-bac-" for bacterial
- "-c-", "-ci-", or "-cir-" for cardiovascular
- "-f-" or "-fu-" for fungal
- "-k-" or "-ki-" for interleukins
- "-l-", "-li-", or "-lim -"for immunomodulator
- "-n-" or "-neu-" for neurons
- "-s-" or "-so-" for bone
- "-toxa-" for toxin as target
- "-t-", "-tu-", or "-tum-" for other tumors
- "-v-", "-vi-", or "-vir-" for viral

This infix is preceded by a "distinct, compatible syllable" to complete the name. Assemble all the parts, and words like biciromab, sevirumab, edobacumab, and nebacumab result.

If another molecule is added to the antibody, a separate word is added to the name. If a toxin is added, the letters "tox" must be part of the second word. For example, "aritox" refers to the toxic A chain of ricin, and "sudotox" to exotoxin A of *Pseudomonas aeruginosa*. Another word also is used for any linker or chelator that holds the antibody to a toxin or isotope. Examples include pendetide and pentetate. For radiolabeled products, the word order is: name of the isotope, element symbol, isotope number, and name of the monoclonal antibody. For example, technetium Tc-99m biciromab, indium In-111 altumomab pentetate.

For the USAN Council to initiate the selection of a nonproprietary name for a monoclonal antibody or fragment, the nomenclature application must provide the following information:

- The immunoglobulin class and subclass and the type of associated light chain.
- Identity of the fragment of the immunoglobulin used (if applicable).
- Species source from which the coding region for the immunoglobulin originated and specific, complete origin of all parts of chimeric, humanized, or semisynthetic immunoglobulins.
- The antigen specificity of the immunoglobulin, including its source.
- The clone designation (specify if vector or vector-cell combination).
- For conjugated monoclonal antibodies, the identity of any linkers, chelators, toxins, and/or isotopes present in the product.
- Identity of other modifications to the antibody (eg, reduction of disulfide bonds, glycosylation or deglycosylation, amino acid modification, or substitution).

Summary of Antibody Products

References

USAN Council. List #351: Monoclonal antibodies. *Clin Pharmacol Ther*. 1993;54:114-116.

WHO. General policies for monoclonal antibodies. INN Working Document 09.251, June 24, 2009.

Immune Globulins: IGIM and IGIV				
Active ingredients	Trade name	Manufacturer	Source, type	Indication(s)
Immune globulin intramuscular (IGIM)	*Gamastan S/D*	Talecris	Human, polyclonal IgG	Immune deficiency
Immune globulin intravenous (IGIV)	*Carimune NF*	CSL Behring	Human, polyclonal IgG	Various[a]
	Flebogamma	Instituto Grifols	Human, polyclonal IgG	
	Flebogamma DIF	Instituto Grifols	Human, polyclonal IgG	
	Gammagard Liquid	Baxter Healthcare	Human, polyclonal IgG	
	Gammagard S/D	Baxter Healthcare	Human, polyclonal IgG	
	Gammaplex	Bio Products Laboratory	Human, polyclonal IgG	
	Gamunex-C	Talecris	Human, polyclonal IgG	
	Octagam	Octapharma	Human, polyclonal IgG	
	Privigen	CSL Behring	Human, polyclonal IgG	
Immune globulin subcutaneous (IGSC)	*Hizentra*	CSL Behring	Human, polyclonal IgG	Immune deficiency
	Gammagard	Baxter Healthcare	Human, polyclonal IgG	

a IGIV products hold various labeled indications for B-cell chronic lymphocytic leukemia, bone-marrow transplantation, immune thrombocytopenic purpura, immunodeficiency, Kawasaki disease, multifocal motor neuropathy, and infections in children with AIDS.

Summary of Antibody Products

Interval Between Antibodies and Measles- or Varicella-Containing Vaccine	
Antibody source	Delay before vaccination
Hepatitis B, tetanus, or Rh$_o$(D) immune globulins (HBIG, TIG, RhIG)	3 mo for measles, 5 mo for varicella
IGIM 0.02 to 0.06 mL/kg	3 mo for measles, 5 mo for varicella
IGIM 0.25 mL/kg	5 mo
IGIM 0.5 mL/kg	6 mo
IGIV 400 mg/kg	8 mo
IGIV high-dose for immune thrombocytopenic purpura or Kawasaki disease	8 to 11 mo
Packed red blood cells (RBCs)	5 mo
Plasma or platelet products	7 mo
Rabies immune globulin	4 mo for measles, 5 mo for varicella
RBCs with adenine-saline added	3 mo for measles, 5 mo for varicella
Vaccinia immune globulin IV	3 mo
Varicella-zoster immune globulin	5 mo
Washed RBCs	No wait
Whole blood	6 mo

Immune Globulins for Infectious Diseases				
Active ingredients	Trade name	Manufacturer	Source, type	Indication(s)
Botulinum antitoxin types A, B, C, D, E, F, G (equine)	generic	Cangene	Equine, polyclonal IgG	*Clostridium botulinum* intoxication (IND)
Botulism immune globulin	*BabyBIG*	California Dept. of Health Services, Massachusetts Biological Laboratories, Cangene	Human, polyclonal IgG	Infant botulism types A or B
Cytomegalovirus immune globulin	*CytoGam*	CSL Behring	Human, polyclonal IgG	*Cytomegalovirus* infection
Diphtheria antitoxin (equine)	generic	Instituto Butantan [IND]	Equine, polyclonal IgG	*Corynebacterium diphtheriae* intoxication
Hepatitis B immune globulin	*HepaGam B*	Cangene	Human, polyclonal IgG	Hepatitis B infection, liver transplant
Hepatitis B immune globulin	*HyperHep B S/D*	Talecris	Human, polyclonal IgG	Hepatitis B infection
Hepatitis B immune globulin	*Nabi-HB*	NABI	Human, polyclonal IgG	Hepatitis B infection
Palivizumab	*Synagis*	MedImmune/ AstraZeneca	Humanized, monoclonal IgG1κ	RSV infection
Rabies immune globulin	*Imogam Rabies-HT*	CSL Behring, Sanofi Pasteur	Human, polyclonal IgG	Rabies infection
Rabies immune globulin	*HyperRab S/D*	Talecris	Human, polyclonal IgG	Rabies infection
Tetanus immune globulin	*HyperTet S/D*	Talecris	Human, polyclonal IgG	*Clostridium tetani* intoxication
Vaccinia immune globulin IV	generic	Cangene	Human, polyclonal IgG	Certain adverse effects of smallpox vaccination

Summary of Antibody Products

Immune Globulins: Isoantibodies				
Active ingredients	Trade name	Manufacturer	Source, type	Indication(s)
Abatacept	*Orencia*	Bristol-Myers Squibb	CTLA-4 antigen with human IgG1 Fc fragment	Rheumatoid arthritis
Abciximab	*ReoPro*	Centocor, Lilly	Chimeric, monoclonal IgG Fab	Inhibit platelet aggregation
Adalimumab	*Humira*	Abbott	Human, monoclonal IgG1κ	Rheumatoid arthritis
Aflibercept	*Eylea*	Regeneron	Vascular endothelial growth factor (VEGF) receptor linked to IgG1 Fc fragment	Neovascular (wet) age-related macular degeneration (AMD)
Alefacept	*Amevive*	Astellas	CD2 receptor with IgG1-Fc fragment	Plaque psoriasis
Alemtuzumab	*CamPath*	Millennium, Genzyme, Berlex	Humanized, monoclonal IgG	B-cell chronic lymphocytic leukemia
Bevacizumab	*Avastin*	Genentech	Humanized, monoclonal IgG1	Colorectal cancer, metastatic NSCLC, breast cancer, glioblastoma with progressive disease
Belimumab	*Benlysta*	Human Genome Sciences	Human, monoclonal IgG1λ	Systemic lupus erythematosus
Brentuximab vedotin	*Adcetris*	Seattle Genetics	Humanized IgG1 with monomethyl auristatin E (MMAE)	Hodgkin lymphoma or anaplastic large cell lymphoma
Canakinumab	*Ilaris*	Novartis	Humanized, monoclonal IgG1κ	Cryopyrin-associated periodic syndromes
Certolizumab pegol	*Cimzia*	Nektar, UCB	Humanized IgG Fab′ fragment conjugated to PEG	Crohn disease, rheumatoid arthritis
Cetuximab	*Erbitux*	ImClone, Bristol-Myers Squibb	Chimeric monoclonal IgG1	Colorectal carcinoma
Denosumab	*Prolia*	Amgen	Humanized monoclonal IgG2	Postmenopausal osteoporosis
Eculizumab	*Soliris*	Alexion	Humanized IgG2/4κ	Paroxysmal nocturnal hemoglobinuria
Etanercept	*Enbrel*	Immunex, Amgen	TNF receptor with human IgG Fc fragment	Rheumatoid arthritis, juvenile rheumatoid arthritis, ankylosing spondylitis, psoriatic arthritis, plaque psoriasis
Golimumab	*Simponi*	Centocor	Humanized, monoclonal IgG1κ	Rheumatoid arthritis, psoriatic arthritis, ankylosing spondylitis
Ibritumomab tiuxetan	*Zevalin*	Biogen Idec	Murine, monoclonal IgG	B-cell non-Hodgkin lymphoma

Immune Globulins: Isoantibodies				
Active ingredients	Trade name	Manufacturer	Source, type	Indication(s)
Infliximab	*Remicade*	Centocor	Chimeric, monoclonal IgG1κ	Crohn disease, rheumatoid arthritis, ankylosing spondylitis, psoriatic arthritis
Ipilimumab	*Yervoy*	Bristol-Myers Squibb	Human, monoclonal IgG1κ	Unresectable or metastatic melanoma
Natalizumab	*Tysabri*	Biogen Idec	Humanized, monoclonal IgG4κ	Multiple sclerosis
Ofatumumab	*Arzerra*	GlaxoSmithKline	Humanized, monoclonal IgG1κ	Chronic lymphocytic leukemia
Omalizumab	*Xolair*	Genentech, Novartis	Humanized, monoclonal IgG1κ	Persistent asthma
Panitumumab	*Vectibix*	Amgen	Humanized IgG2κ	Colorectal cancer
Pertuzumab	*Perjeta*	Genentech	Humanized IgG1	HER2-positive metastatic breast cancer
Ranibizumab	*Lucentis*	Genentech	Humanized IgG1κ Fab fragment	Wet macular degeneration
Rituximab	*Rituxan*	Genentech	Chimeric, monoclonal IgG1	Non-Hodgkin lymphoma, rheumatoid arthritis
Tocilizumab	*Actemra*	Genentech	Humanized, monoclonal IgG1κ	Rheumatoid arthritis
Trastuzumab	*Herceptin*	Genentech	Humanized, monoclonal IgG1κ	Breast cancer
Ustekinumab	*Stelara*	Centocor Ortho Biotech	Humanized, monoclonal IgG1κ	Plaque psoriasis
Ziv-aflibercept	*Zaltrap*	Sanofi-Aventis	IgG1 fused to VEGF-binding domains	Metastatic colorectal cancer

Immune Globulins to Bind Rh$_o$(D) Antigen			
Trade name	Manufacturer	Source, type	Indication(s)
HyperRho S/D (full dose)	Talecris	Human, polyclonal IgG	Prevent isoimmunization with Rh antigen
HyperRho S/D (mini dose)	Talecris	Human, polyclonal IgG	Prevent isoimmunization with Rh antigen
MICRhoGAM	Ortho Diagnostics	Human, polyclonal IgG	Prevent isoimmunization with Rh antigen
RhoGAM	Ortho Diagnostics	Human, polyclonal IgG	Prevent isoimmunization with Rh antigen
Rhophylac	CSL Behring	Human, polyclonal IgG	Prevent isoimmunization with Rh antigen or treat immune thrombocytopenic purpura
WinRho SDF	NABI	Human, polyclonal IgG	Prevent isoimmunization with Rh antigen or treat immune thrombocytopenic purpura

Summary of Antibody Products

TNF Blocking Agents					
	Adalimumab	Etanercept	Infliximab	Certolizumab pegol	Golimumab
Indication	Rheumatoid arthritis (RA)	RA, juvenile RA, ankylosing spondylitis, psoriatic arthritis, plaque psoriasis	Crohn disease, RA	Crohn disease, RA	RA, psoriatic arthritis, ankylosing spondylitis
Brand name	*Humira*	*Enbrel*	*Remicade*	*Cimzia*	*Simponi*
Synonym	—	TNFR: Fc	cA2	CDP-870	—
Manufacturer	Abbott	Immunex, Amgen	Centocor	Nektar, UCB	Centocor
Antigenic type	IgG1κ antibody	p75 receptor linked to IgG1 Fc antibody fragment	IgG1κ antibody	Humanized IgG Fab′ fragment conjugated to PEG	IgG1κ antibody
Dose	40 mg weekly or every other week	25 mg twice weekly	Crohn: 5 mg/kg, 1 to 3 times over 6 weeks RA: 3 mg/kg periodically	400 mg at wk 0, 2, 4, then every 4 wk	50 mg monthly
Route	Subcutaneous	Subcutaneous	IV infusion	Subcutaneous	Subcutaneous
Doseform	Solution	Powder for solution	Powder for solution	Powder for solution	Solution
Concentration	40 mg/0.8 mL	25 mg/vial	100 mg/vial	200 mg/mL	50 mg/0.5 mL
Packaging	Syringe, vial	Vial with syringe	Vial	Vials with syringes	Syringe, autoinjector
Diluent	—	Bacteriostatic water	Sterile water	Sterile water	—
Solvent	Buffered saline	—	—	—	Aqueous
Routine storage	2° to 8°C	2° to 8°C	2° to 8°C	2° to 8°C	2° to 8°C

Interleukin-1 beta Inhibitors		
	Anakinra	Rilonacept	Canakinumab
---	---	---	---
Brand name	*Kineret*	*Arcalyst*	*Ilaris*
Manufacturer	Amgen	Regeneron	Novartis
Indication	Rheumatoid arthritis	Cryopyrin-associated periodic syndromes	Cryopyrin-associated periodic syndromes
Antigenic type	IL-1 receptor antagonist	Fusion protein of ligand-binding domains of IL-1RI and IL-1RAcP fused to Fc portion of IgG_1	IgG1κ antibody
Concentration	100 mg per 0.67 mL	80 mg/mL	150 mg/mL
Doseform	Solution	Powder for solution	Powder for solution
Diluent/Solvent	Sterile water	Sterile water	Sterile water
Preservative	None	None	None
Packaging	1 mL syringes	220 mg vials	180 mg vial
Routine storage	2° to 8°C	2° to 8°C	2° to 8°C
Stability	n/a	After reconstitution: Discard within 3 h	After reconstitution: 60 min at 25°C or 4 h at 2° to 8°C
Dosage, route	100 mg subcutaneously daily	Adults: 320 mg once, then 160 mg subcutaneously weekly	> 40 kg: 150 mg subcutaneously every 8 weeks 15 to 40 kg: 2 mg/kg subcutaneously
Production medium	*E. coli*	CHO cells	Murine Sp2/0-Ag14 cell line

Summary of Antibody Products

Psoriasis-Treating Agents			
	Alefacept	Etanercept	Ustekinumab
Brand names	*Amevive*	*Enbrel*	*Stelara*
Manufacturer	Astellas	Immunex, Amgen	Centocor Ortho Biotech
Antigen	CD2	p75	p40 subunit of IL-12 and IL-23
Antigenic type	CD2 receptor of LFA-3 fused with Fc portion of IgG1	p75 receptor linked to IgG1 Fc antibody fragment	Humanized, monoclonal IgG1κ
Indication	Moderate to severe chronic plaque psoriasis	RA, juvenile RA, ankylosing spondylitis, psoriatic arthritis, plaque psoriasis	Moderate to severe plaque psoriasis who are candidates for phototherapy or systemic therapy
Dose, Route	7.5 mg/week IV bolus or 15 mg/week IM	25 mg twice weekly subcutaneously	45 or 90 mg, based on body mass, at various intervals, subcutaneously
Age range	≥ 18 years	≥ 18 years	≥ 18 years
Doseform	Powder for solution	Powder for solution	Solution
Concentration	IV: 7.5 mg/0.5 mL IM: 15 mg/0.5 mL	25 mg/vial	90 mg/mL
Packaging	Carton of 4 dose packs	Vial with syringe	45 mg per 0.5 mL, 90 mg/mL syringes or vials
Diluent	Sterile water (USP) 0.6 mL per vial	Bacteriostatic water	Histidine-sucrose solvent
Routine storage	15° to 30°C (59° to 86°F)	2° to 8°C (36° to 46°F)	2° to 8°C (36° to 46°F)

Immune Globulins in Transplantation			
Active ingredients	Manufacturer	Source, type	Indication(s)
Antithymocyte globulin (*Atgam*)	Pfizer	Equine, polyclonal IgG	Treat aplastic anemia, prevent or treat rejection
Antithymocyte globulin (*Thymoglobulin*)	Genzyme	Rabbit, polyclonal IgG	Treat acute rejection
Basiliximab (*Simulect*)	Novartis	Chimeric, monoclonal IgG1κ	Prevent acute rejection
Belatacept (*Nulojix*)	Bristol-Myers Squibb	CTLA-4 antigen with human IgG1 Fc fragment	Prevent acute rejection (kidney)
Daclizumab (*Zenapax*)	Roche	Humanized, monoclonal IgG1	Prevent acute rejection
Muromonab-CD3 (*Orthoclone OKT3*)	Ortho Biotech	Murine, monoclonal IgG2a	Treat acute rejection

Immune Globulins for Animal Intoxications			
Active ingredients	Manufacturer	Source, type	Indication(s)
Antivenin *Latrodectus mactans* (equine)	Merck	Equine, polyclonal IgG	Neutralize venom of widow spiders
Antivenin *Micrurus fulvius* (equine)	Pfizer	Equine, polyclonal IgG	Neutralize venom of coral snakes
Centruroides (Scorpion) Immune F(ab')$_2$ (*Anascorp*)	Accredo Health Group, Instituto Bioclon	Equine, F(ab')$_2$ fragments	Neutralize venom of *Centruroides* genus scorpions
Crotalidae polyvalent immune Fab (*CroFab*)	Protherics	Ovine, Fab fragments	Neutralize venom of crotalid snakes (vipers)
Digoxin immune Fab (*Digibind, DigiFab*)	GlaxoSmithKline, Protherics	Ovine, Fab fragments	Reverse symptoms of digoxin intoxication

Immune Globulins, Radiodiagnostic			
Active ingredients	Manufacturer	Source, type	Indication(s)
Capromab pendetide with In-111 (*ProstaScint*)	Laureate Pharma for EUSA Pharma	Murine, monoclonal IgG1κ	Prostate cancer

Immune Globulins, Radiotherapeutic			
Active ingredients	Manufacturer	Sources, type	Indication(s)
Ibritumomab tiuxetan with In-111 or Y-90 (*Zevalin* regimen)	Cell Therapeutics	Murine, monoclonal IgG1κ	B-cell non-Hodgkin lymphoma
Tositumomab (with I-131) (*Bexxar*)	Corixa, GlaxoSmithKline	Murine, monoclonal IgG2a	B-cell non-Hodgkin lymphoma

Summary of Antibody Products

Antigen-Binding Table		
Antibody name	Mechanism	Category
Abatacept (*Orencia*)	Binds CD80 and CD86, thereby blocking interaction with CD28	Isoantibodies
Abciximab (*ReoPro*)	Binds GPIIb/IIIa receptor	Isoantibodies
Adalimumab (*Humira*)	Binds TNFα	Isoantibodies
Aflibercept (*Eylea*)	Binds VEGF	Isoantibodies
Alefacept (*Amevive*)	Binds CD2 antigen	Isoantibodies
Alemtuzumab (*CamPath*)	Binds CD52 antigen	Isoantibodies
Basiliximab (*Simulect*)	Binds IL-2Ra chain (CD25 antigen)	Transplantation
Belatacept (*Nulojix*)	Binds CD80 and CD86, thereby blocking interaction with CD28	Transplantation
Belimumab (*Benlysta*)	Binds BLyS (BAFF)	Isoantibodies
Bevacizumab (*Avastin*)	Binds VEGF	Isoantibodies
Brentuximab vedotin (*Adcetris*)	Binds CD30 antigen	Isoantibodies
Canakinumab (*Ilaris*)	Binds IL-1β	Isoantibodies
Capromab (*ProstaScint*)	Binds PSMA	Diagnostic
Certolizumab pegol (*Cimzia*)	Binds TNFα	Isoantibodies
Cetuximab pegol (*Erbitux*)	Binds epidermal growth factor receptor (EGFR)	Isoantibodies
Daclizumab (*Zenapax*)	Binds IL-2Ra (CD25 antigen)	Transplantation
Denosumab (*Prolia*)	Binds human receptor activator of nuclear factor-kappa B ligand (RANK ligand)	Isoantibodies
Eculizumab (*Soliris*)	Binds complement C-5	Isoantibodies
Etanercept (*Enbrel*)	Binds to TNF	Isoantibodies
Golimumab (*Simponi*)	Binds TNFα	Isoantibodies
Ibritumomab (*Zevalin*)	Binds CD20 antigen	Radiotherapeutic
Ibritumomab tiuxetan (*Zevalin*)	Binds CD20 antigen	Isoantibodies
Infliximab (*Remicade*)	Binds TNFα	Isoantibodies
Ipilimumab (*Yervoy*)	Binds CTLA-4	Isoantibodies
Muromonab-CD3 (*Orthoclone OKT3*)	Binds CD3 antigen	Transplantation
Natalizumab (*Tysabri*)	Binds α_4-integrin	Isoantibodies
Ofatumumab (*Arzerra*)	Binds CD-20	Isoantibodies
Omalizumab (*Xolair*)	Binds FcεRI IgG receptor	Isoantibodies
Panitumumab (*Vectibix*)	Binds EGFR	Isoantibodies
Pertuzumab (*Perjeta*)	Binds subdomain II of HER2 protein	Isoantibodies
Ranibizumab (*Lucentis*)	Binds VEGF-A	Isoantibodies
Rh$_o$(D) IGs (*HypRho (D) MicRhoGam, RhoGam, Rhophylac, WinRho SDF*)	Binds Rh$_o$(D) antigen	Rh$_o$(D) antigen
Rituximab (*Rituxan*)	Binds CD20 antigen	Isoantibodies
Tocilizumab (*Actemra*)	Binds IL-6	Isoantibodies
Tositumomab (*Bexxar*)	Binds CD20 antigen	Radiotherapeutic
Trastuzumab (*Herceptin*)	Binds HER2 protein	Isoantibodies
Ustekinumab (*Stelara*)	Binds p40 subunit of IL-12 and IL-23	Isoantibodies
Ziv-aflibercept (*Zaltrap*)	Binds to VEGF domains of VEGF receptors 1 and 2	Isoantibodies

Broad-Spectrum Immune Globulins

Comparison Table of Parenteral Immune Globulins		
Generic name	Immune globulin intramuscular (IGIM)	Immune globulin intravenous (IGIV)	Immune globulin subcutaneous (IGSC)
Brand name	*Gamastan S/D*	Various, see table	*Vivaglobin, Hizentra*
Manufacturer	Talecris	Various, see table	CSL Behring
Indication(s)	Immune deficiency	Immune deficiency, CLL, ITP, Kawasaki disease, multifocal motor neuropathy, children with AIDS, bone marrow transplant	Immune deficiency
Concentration	15% to 18%; 1.5 to 1.8 g per 10 mL	3% to 12%; 0.3 to 1.2 g per 10 mL	16%: 1.6 g per 10 mL; 20%: 2 g per 10 mL
Packaging	300 mg to 1.8 g	500 mg to 20 g	480 mg per 3 mL, to 4 g per 20 mL vials
Doseform	Solution	Solution, powder for solution	Liquid
Routine storage	Refrigerator	Refrigerator or room temperature	Refrigerator (*Vivaglobin*), room temperature (*Hizentra*)
Onset	IgG peaks 2 to 5 days after injection	Immediate	IgG peaks 2.5 days after subcutaneous infusion begins
Half-life	≈ 18 to 25 days	≈ 18 to 25 days	≈ 18 to 25 days
Interval between IG and measles vaccine	3 to 6 months	8 to 11 months	≈ 3 to 6 months
Preservative	None	None	None
IgA content	150 to 680 mcg per mL	< 2 to 970 mcg per mL	Trace quantity
First licensed	September 1943	December 1981	January 2006 (*Vivaglobin*), March 2010 (*Hizentra*)
Production process	Cohn-Oncley methods 6 & 9 cold-ethanol fractionation	Cohn-Oncley methods 6 & 9 cold-ethanol fractionation or Kistler-Nitschmann technique with purification	Cohn-Oncley methods 6 & 9 cold-ethanol fractionation
Specific virucidal processing steps	Yes	Yes	Yes

Immune Globulin Intramuscular (Human)

Broad-Spectrum Immune Globulins

Name: *Manufacturer:*
Gamastan S/D   Talecris Biotherapeutics

Synonyms: IG, IGIM, IMIG, gamma globulin, GG, Cohn globulin; formerly called immune serum globulin, ISG. Human normal immunoglobulin (HNIG) is the comparable term used in the United Kingdom. Gamma globulin is a misnomer, originally based on electrophoretic mobility. IgG and IgA primarily exist as gamma globulins, although some are beta globulins. To further confound the issue, most IgM and IgD molecules are beta globulins, although some are gamma globulins. Nonetheless, the usual therapeutic meaning of the term gamma globulin refers to IgG.

Comparison: The various IGIMs are therapeutically equivalent. Hepatitis A vaccine induces more persistent immunity against hepatitis A than IGIM, although IGIM provides immunity against hepatitis A a few days sooner than does active immunization.

Immunologic Characteristics

Microorganism: Active against multiple bacteria, viruses, and fungi
Viability: Inactive, passive, transient
Antigenic Form: Human immunoglobulin, unmodified
Antigenic Type: Protein, IgG antibody, polyclonal, 20% to 30% polymeric
Strains: Polyvalent, reflecting the antibody diversity in the donor population

---

Use Characteristics

Indications: For passive prevention or modification of hepatitis A, especially if given before or soon after exposure.

For passive prevention or modification of measles infection in susceptible people exposed less than 6 days previously, especially household contacts younger than 1 year of age, in whom the risk of measles complications is highest.

For IgG-replacement therapy in certain people with hypo- or agammaglobulinemia. Prophylaxis, especially against infections caused by encapsulated bacteria, is effective in Bruton-type, sex-linked congenital agammaglobulinemia, agammaglobulinemia, and severe combined immunodeficiency.

For passive prevention of varicella in immunocompromised patients if varicella-zoster immune globulin (VZIG) is not available and IGIM can be given promptly.

To reduce the likelihood of fetal damage in susceptible women exposed to rubella in the first trimester of pregnancy who do not wish to have a therapeutic abortion. This therapy is of questionable value.

The ACIP explicitly recommends immune globulin (IV or IM, as appropriate) administration to symptomatic HIV-infected people and other severely immunocompromised people exposed to measles, regardless of immunization status. Operationally defined, severe immunosuppression may result from congenital immunodeficiency, HIV infection, leukemia, lymphoma, aplastic anemia, generalized malignancy, or therapy with alkylating agents, antimetabolites, radiation, or large, sustained doses of corticosteroids.

Limitations: IGIM provides only short-term passive immunity. Use appropriate vaccines to induce active immunity.

IGIM is not indicated for routine prophylaxis or treatment of measles, rubella, poliomyelitis, mumps, or varicella. Immune globulin, if given for passive protection later than the third day of incubation of measles, may extend the incubation period to 21 days instead of preventing the disease.

IGIM is not indicated in people with clinical manifestations of hepatitis A or in those exposed to hepatitis A longer than 2 weeks previously. Because IGIM may not suppress unapparent infection, long-lasting hepatitis A immunity and persistent antihepatitis A seroconversion may occur in IGIM recipients.

IGIM is not standardized for hepatitis B surface antibody content. Use hepatitis B immune globulin (HBIG) for passive immunization against that virus.

IGIM is not indicated for treatment of allergy or asthma in patients who have normal serum levels of immunoglobulin.

In people with immunoglobulin deficiency, IGIM may not prevent chronic infections of the external secretory tissues (eg, respiratory or gastrointestinal tracts).

Outmoded Practices: Do not perform skin tests prior to administration of IGIM (such tests were performed with immunoglobulin products harvested from animals). In most humans, intradermal (ID) injection of concentrated immune globulin with its buffers causes a localized area of inflammation that can be misinterpreted as a positive allergic reaction. This reaction is caused by localized tissue irritation of a chemical nature. Misinterpretation of such a test may cause urgently needed immunoglobulin to be withheld from a patient not actually allergic to it.

True allergic responses to IgG administered IM are rare.

Contraindications:
> *Absolute:* Patients with isolated IgA deficiency, because circulating IgE antibodies that specifically neutralize IgA may react with IgA in this product and induce an anaphylactoid reaction.

> *Relative:* Patients with thrombocytopenia or other coagulation disorders, in view of the IM route of administration. Give IGIM with caution to patients with a history of systemic allergic reactions following the administration of human IG preparations.

Immunodeficiency: IGIM may be indicated for immunoglobulin replacement therapy in certain immunocompromised people.

Elderly: Generally safe and effective.

Pregnancy: Category C. Use only if clearly needed. Intact IgG crosses the placenta from the maternal circulation increasingly after 30 weeks gestation. Problems in humans have not been documented and are unlikely.

Lactation: It is not known if IGIM antibodies are excreted in breast milk. Problems in humans have not been documented and are unlikely.

Children: Generally safe and effective.

Adverse Reactions: Local pain and tenderness at the injection site, urticaria, and angioedema may occur. Anaphylactic reactions, although rare, have been reported following injection of this product.

Pharmacologic & Dosing Characteristics

Dosage:
> *Hepatitis A:* 0.02 mL/kg for household and institutional contacts of people infected with hepatitis A. Give 0.02 mL/kg to travelers to hepatitis A-endemic areas (eg, developing countries with inadequate sanitation systems) staying shorter than 3 months. Give

0.06 mL/kg to travelers staying 3 months or longer, with booster doses every 4 to 6 months throughout their stay.

Measles: 0.5 mL/kg (maximum, 15 mL) to prevent or modify measles in susceptible people exposed less than 6 days previously. Give 0.5 mL/kg to susceptible immunocompromised children (maximum dose, 15 mL).

Immunoglobulin deficiency: IGIM may prevent serious infections in patients if circulating IgG levels are maintained around 200 mg per 100 mL plasma. Give 0.66 mL/kg (100 mg/kg or more) every 3 to 4 weeks. A larger initial dose (eg, 1.2 mL/kg) is often given at the onset of therapy. Fast metabolizers may require more frequent injections.

Varicella: If VZIG is unavailable, give 0.6 to 1.2 mL/kg IGIM.

Rubella: 0.55 mL/kg IGIM may benefit children of women who will not consider therapeutic abortion.

Route & Site: IM, preferably in the upper, outer quadrant of the gluteal region. Divide doses larger than 10 mL and inject into several muscle sites to reduce local pain and discomfort.

Do not inject IGIM IV, because its high proportion of aggregates may cause serious adverse reactions (eg, activation of the complement cascade).

Overdosage: Clinical experience with other immune globulin preparations suggest that the major manifestations of overdosage would be pain and tenderness at the injection site.

Additional Doses: Additional doses may be warranted if disease exposure continues and no other prophylactic alternatives are available.

Efficacy:

Hepatitis A: IGIM is 80% to 95% effective in preventing hepatitis A, depending on the temporal relation between administration and exposure and on the severity of exposure.

Measles: IGIM reduces the risk of clinical evidence of measles by an estimated 50%. A lower incidence of measles encephalitis also has been associated with use of IGIM.

Varicella: IGIM reduces severity of disease, as measured by temperature and number of pox.

Onset: IgG titers peak 2 to 5 days after IM injection.

Duration: Mean IgG half-life in circulation of people with normal IgG levels is 23 days.

Pharmacokinetics: Immunoglobulins are primarily eliminated by catabolism.

Protective Level: 200 mg per 100 mL of plasma is a target in immunoglobulin replacement therapy.

Mechanism: IGIM is a transient source of IgG that specifically and nonspecifically inactivates various bacteria, viruses, and fungi. IgG antibodies activate the complement system, promote opsonization, neutralize microorganisms and their toxins, and participate in antibody-dependent cytolytic reactions.

Drug Interactions: IGIM may diminish the antibody response to attenuated measles, mumps, and rubella vaccines through antigen-antibody antagonism. As a general rule, administer live virus vaccines 14 to 30 days before or 6 to 12 weeks after IGIM. Alternately, administer live virus vaccines during this interval if corresponding antibody titers are measured 3 months after IGIM administration. Base the interval on the dose of IgG administered. For varicella vaccine, wait 5 months after IGIM administration before giving the vaccine. For a vaccine containing measles virus, wait 3 months after a dose of 0.02 to 0.06 mL/kg, 5 months after a dose of 0.25 mL/kg, or 6 months after a dose of 0.5 mL/kg.

IGIM does not appear to interfere with development of immunity following oral poliovirus (OPV) or yellow fever vaccination. However, it may be prudent not to administer these vaccines shortly after IGIM administration. Exceptions include unexpected travel to, or contact with, epidemic or endemic areas or people. If OPV is given with or shortly after IG, repeat the OPV dose 3 months later if immunization is still indicated.

Immune Globulin Intramuscular (Human)

It is not known if IGIM interferes with the efficacy of other attenuated vaccines (eg, adenovirus, Bacillus Calmette-Guérin, typhoid, vaccinia). It may be prudent not to administer these vaccines shortly after IGIM administration unless such a procedure is unavoidable.

Inactivated vaccines generally are not affected by circulating antibodies or administration of exogenous antibodies. Immunization with such vaccines may occur at any time before or after antibody administration.

As with other drugs administered IM, give with caution to people receiving anticoagulant therapy.

Pharmaceutical Characteristics

Concentration: 15% to 18% protein, 90% IgG or more

Quality Assay: Standardized for antibody content to measles (at least half the potency of the US Reference Standard), diphtheria (2 antitoxin units/mL or less) and poliovirus (at least as potent as the US Reference Standard for poliovirus type 1 and type 2, and 2.5 times or more potent for type 3). Minimum measles antibody potency: 25.2 international units/mL. IGIM also is tested against diphtheria test toxin in guinea pigs. Since 1977, all plasma units have been tested to ensure the absence of hepatitis B surface antigen before pooling for manufacture. Since April 1985, all units have been tested to ensure the absence of HIV-1 antibodies. Not standardized for anti-HBs antibody titer.

Packaging: 2 mL single-dose vial (NDC#: 13533-0635-04), box of ten 2 mL vials (13533-0635-02), 10 mL single-dose vial (13533-0635-12), box of 10 single-dose vials (13533-0635-10); 2 mL prefilled syringe with 22-gauge, 1 ¼-inch needle (13533-0635-03)

Doseform: Solution

Appearance: Clear, colorless solution, slightly opalescent, viscous

Solvent: Cohn fraction II

Adjuvant: None

Preservative: None

Allergens: 150 to 680 mcg/mL IgA; an unspecified trace quantity of IgM

Excipients: 0.21 to 0.32 M glycine

pH: 6.4 to 7.2

Shelf Life: Expires within 24 months

Storage/Stability: Store at 2° to 8°C (36° to 46°F). Discard if frozen. Contact manufacturer regarding prolonged exposure to room temperature or elevated temperatures. Shipping data not provided.

Production Process: Prepared from pooled human plasma by Cohn-Oncley methods 6 & 9 cold-ethanol fractionation process at pH 7 (near IgG's isoelectric point) with repeated ethanol treatment. Each unit of blood processed yields only 2 to 3 mL of IGIM. Cohn fraction II is lyophilized to remove the ethanol before packaging. The lyophilized powder is stored until formulation. Unlike the various production processes for IGIV, the lyophilization process does not remove IgG aggregates.

Since the mid-1990s, production procedures must include a specific virucidal processing step. *Gammar-P I.M.* was pasteurized for this purpose. *Gamastan S/D* (previously *BayGam*) uses a virucidal solvent-detergent treatment step with 0.3% tri-n-butylphosphate and 0.2% sodium cholate at 30°C (86°F) for 6 hours or longer. It is incubated in the final container for 21 to 28 days at 20° to 27°C (68° to 80.6°F).

Media: 1,000 units or more of human plasma per lot

Immune Globulin Intramuscular (Human)

Disease Epidemiology

For epidemiology of hepatitis A, see the Hepatitis A Vaccine monograph.

For epidemiology of immunodeficiency, see the Immune Globulin IV (IGIV) monograph.

For epidemiology of other diseases, see the Measles Vaccine, Rubella Vaccine, or Varicella Vaccine monographs.

Other Information

Perspective:

1901: Porges and Spiro discover gamma globulin fraction of serum.

1907: Cenci uses human serum for the prevention of measles and later for mumps and pertussis.

1933: McKhann and Chu use immune globulin from human placentas against measles.

1938: Tiselius and Kabat demonstrate that antibodies are predominantly gamma globulins.

1944: Cohn, Oncley, and colleagues develop cold-ethanol fractionation method of isolating human immune globulin from human blood.

1945: IGIM used for hepatitis A prophylaxis.

1951: IGIM used for treatment and prophylaxis of poliomyelitis until Salk vaccine becomes available in 1955.

1952: Treatment of agammaglobulinemia (Bruton disease) with IGIM begins.

1954: IGIM decontrolled by the Federal Office of Defense Mobilization for the first time since World War II.

1959: Porter separates antibodies into Fab and Fc components.

1960: IgG subclasses detected by Dray.

1963: *Gammagee* introduced by Merck, Sharp and Dohme, intended for concurrent use with *Rubeovax*, Merck, Sharp and Dohme's original, partially attenuated measles vaccine.

1975: Köhler and Milstein develop method to make monoclonal antibodies.

1995: Virucidal manufacturing steps required of all antibody products.

First Licensed:

Armour (now Talecris): January 11, 1944

Discontinued Products:
Baygam (Bayer), *Gammar-P* (Centeon), *Gamastan* (Cutter, Miles), *Gamulin* (Pitman-Moore, Dow), *Gammagee* (Merck, Sharp and Dohme), *Immu-G* (Parke-Davis), *Immuglobulin* (Savage).

National Policy:
ACIP. Prevention of hepatitis A after exposure to hepatitis A virus and in international travelers. *MMWR* 2007;56:1080-1084. www.cdc.gov/mmwr/PDF/wk/mm5641.pdf.

ACIP. Prevention of hepatitis A through active or passive immunization. *MMWR* 2006;55(RR-7):1-23. www.cdc.gov/mmwr/PDF/rr/rr5507.pdf.

References:
Dwyer JM. Manipulating the immune system with immune globulin. *N Engl J Med.* 1992;326:107-116.

Immune Globulin Intravenous (Human)

Broad-Spectrum Immune Globulins

Names:
  Carimune NF
  Flebogamma DIF
  Gammagard Liquid
  Gammagard S/D
  Gammaplex
  Gamunex-C
  Octagam
  Privigen

Manufacturers:
  CSL Behring
  Instituto Grifols, Grifols Biological
  Baxter Healthcare Corporation
  Baxter Healthcare Corporation
  Bio Products Laboratory
  Talecris Biotherapeutics
  Octapharma
  CSL Behring

Synonyms: IGIV, IVIG, IVIgG, IVGG. The S/D suffix refers to solvent/detergent treatment. The NF suffix of *Carimune* refers to nanofiltered. The DIF suffix of *Flebogamma* refers to dual inactivation plus filtration. Gamma globulin is a misnomer, originally based on electrophoretic mobility. IgG and IgA primarily exist as gamma globulins, although some are beta globulins. To further confound the issue, most IgM and IgD molecules are beta globulins, although some are gamma globulins. Nonetheless, the usual therapeutic meaning of the term gamma globulin refers to IgG.

Comparison: For most purposes, the various IGIV products are therapeutically equivalent in function. There are obvious differences in concentration, method of infusion, storage, and other variables. In a very small subset of patients with anti-IgA antibodies, the quantity of IgA in the IGIV product must be minimized.

Immunologic Characteristics

Microorganism: Active against multiple bacteria, viruses, and fungi

Viability: Inactive, passive, transient

Antigenic Form: Human immunoglobulin, unmodified. The Fc portion of the IgG molecule remains functionally intact.

Antigenic Type: Protein, IgG antibody, polyclonal, primarily monomeric, permitting IV administration

Strains: Polyvalent, reflecting the antibody diversity in the donor population. One gram of IgG contains 4×10^{18} molecules with more than 10^7 unique-binding specificities.

Use Characteristics

Indications: FDA-licensed indications for each brand appear in the table at the end of the monograph. IGIV is especially useful when high levels or rapid elevation of circulating antibodies are desired or when IM injections are contraindicated, such as in patients with limited muscle mass or with a bleeding tendency. The various brands of IGIV have been licensed for one or more of the following uses:

Immunoglobulin replacement therapy: For treatment of primary immunodeficiency states with severe impairment of antibody-forming capacity, such as congenital hypo- or agammaglobulinemia, common variable immunodeficiency, X-linked immunodeficiency with hyper IgM, transient hypogammaglobulinemia of infancy, IgG subclass deficiency with or without IgA deficiency, antibody deficiency with near-normal immunoglobulin levels, severe combined immunodeficiency, X-linked lymphoproliferative syndrome, ataxia-

413

telangiectasia, and Wiskott-Aldrich syndrome. IGIV product labeling refers to these uses as "substitution therapy."

B-cell chronic lymphocytic leukemia (CLL): For passive prevention of bacterial infections in patients with hypogammaglobulinemia or recurrent bacterial infections associated with CLL.

Immune thrombocytopenic purpura (ITP, formerly called idiopathic thrombocytopenic purpura): For treatment of ITP, in situations that require a rapid rise in platelet count (eg, prior to surgery), a control of excessive bleeding, or as a measure to defer splenectomy. It presently is not possible to predict which ITP patients will respond to IGIV therapy, although the increase in platelet counts in children seems to be better than in adults. Childhood ITP may resolve spontaneously without treatment.

Kawasaki disease: For use in combination with aspirin in the treatment of Kawasaki disease, within 10 days of onset of disease, to prevent the development of coronary artery abnormalities (eg, dilation, aneurysm, ectasia) that could lead to myocardial infarction.

Multifocal motor neuropathy: As maintenance therapy to improve muscle strength and disability in adult patients with multifocal motor neuropathy (MMN).

Children with AIDS: Treatment of HIV-infected children can decrease the frequency of bacterial infections, increase the time free from serious bacterial infections, and decrease the frequency of hospitalization in children with AIDS. A double-blind, placebo-controlled trial among 394 HIV-infected children 1 month to 12 years of age was conducted, using 400 mg/kg *Gamimune N* monthly. The rate of bacterial infections fell from 56.7 infections per 100 patient-years among placebo recipients to 33.1 infections using IGIV, a 40% drop. Similarly, the frequency of hospitalizations fell 36%.

Bone marrow transplant patients: IGIV is safe and effective in reducing the incidence and severity of infections and graft-vs-host disease (GVHD) in bone marrow transplant recipients older than 20 years of age. A controlled clinical trial was conducted using 500 mg/kg *Gamimune N* weekly, reduced to monthly infusions 100 days after transplant. Among 384 patients, the frequency of GVHD was reduced from 51% in the control group to 34% in the treated group of patients older than 20 years of age. Mortality after 100 days was unaffected by IGIV. Little or no benefit was apparent among younger patients.

Chronic inflammatory demyelinating polyneuropathy (CIDP): To treat CIDP to improve neuromuscular disability and impairment and for maintenance therapy to prevent relapse.

Unlabeled Uses: An expert panel convened by the University Hospital Consortium (UHC) determined that there is documented evidence of efficacy for three indications not currently recognized by the FDA. These include posttransfusion purpura, Guillain-Barré syndrome, and chronic inflammatory demyelinating polyneuropathy (as an alternative to plasma exchange). Use might be warranted for select patients with certain other conditions for whom other interventions have been unsuccessful or intolerable, such as: patients with autoimmune hemolytic anemia, parvovirus B19 infection and severe anemia, multiple myeloma, immune-mediated neutropenia, neonatal alloimmune thrombocytopenia, thrombocytopenia refractory to platelet transfusions, acute decompensation in severe myasthenia gravis, severe active dermatomyositis or polymyositis, systemic lupus erythematosus, systemic vasculitic syndromes, West or Lennox-Gastaut forms of pediatric intractable epilepsy, cytomegalovirus (CMV)–seronegative recipients of CMV-seropositive organs, low-birth-weight infants (less than 1,500 g), or hypogammaglobulinemic infants. The UHC panel found no convincing evidence of efficacy for routine IGIV use in 35 other indications suggested in case reports or other preliminary publications, including some described in the following paragraph.

IGIV is being investigated in the prevention or treatment of the following diseases: HIV infection, autoimmune diseases (eg, rhesus hemolytic disease, factor VIII deficiencies, bullous pemphigoid, rheumatoid arthritis, Sjögren syndrome, type 1 diabetes mellitus), IgG4 subclass deficiencies, intractable epilepsy (possibly caused by IgG2 subclass deficiency), cystic fibrosis, trauma, thermal injury (eg, severe burns), CMV infection, neuromuscular disorders, prophylaxis of infections associated with bone marrow transplantation, and gastrointestinal (GI) protection (ie, oral administration).

A review of controlled trials indicates that IGIV is effective in treating Guillain-Barré syndrome, multifocal motor neuropathy, chronic inflammatory demyelinating polyneuropathy, and dermatomyositis. In other situations, IGIV helped several patients with Lambert-Eaton myasthenic syndrome and myasthenia gravis, but had variable, mild, or unsubstantiated benefit in other conditions.

A study of IGIV therapy to prevent neonatal sepsis demonstrated significant reduction in time to first nosocomial infection and length of hospital stays. Nonetheless, reservations have been expressed about IGIV use in this manner.

Oral administration of IGIV may provide some local protection of the GI tract from bacterial, viral, and fungal infections. IGIV given orally reduced the duration of rotaviral diarrhea, viral excretion, and hospitalization in a placebo-controlled trial. IgG is not extensively absorbed from the GI tract. Native IgA predominates in the GI tract with smaller amounts of IgM and IgG. Oral immune globulin supplements should be considered investigational. In one experiment of an oral dose of radiolabeled IgG, 50% of the recovered radioactivity was found in the stool in an immunologically active form, while the balance was excreted in the urine. A trial of an oral IgA-IgG preparation shows promise.

If hyperimmune tetanus immune globulin (TIG) is unavailable, IGIV may be used to provide prompt passive immunity against tetanus. Among 29 lots tested, antitetanus IgG levels varied from 4 to 90 units per mL (geometric mean, 18.6). A dose of 6 g (at 4 units per mL) is likely to provide an equivalent quantity of antitetanus IgG antibodies as a 500 unit dose of TIG, although the actual dose varies between lots. Only 1.6 g of lots with antibody levels higher than 15 units per mL would be needed.

Limitations: IGIV provides only short-term passive immunity. Use appropriate vaccines to induce active immunity. Consider appropriate antibiotic or antiviral drugs for the treatment of active infections. IGIV is not recommended for use as standard prophylaxis in low birthweight, high-risk infants.

Contraindications:

Absolute: None

Relative: IGIV is contraindicated in patients with a history of anaphylactic or severe systemic response to human IM or IV immune globulin products. IGIV products generally are contraindicated in people with IgA deficiency (serum IgA less than 0.05 g/L), 17% to 40% of whom have circulating anti-IgA antibodies, because of a risk of anaphylactic reactions. Nonetheless, low-IgA content formulations have been given to some of these patients with due caution.

CSL Behring (Privigen): Do not administer to patients with hyperprolinemia because product contains L-proline as a stabilizer.

Immunodeficiency: IGIV may be indicated as immunoglobulin replacement therapy for certain immunocompromised people. The Advisory Committee on Immunization Practices (ACIP) explicitly recommends immune globulin administration to symptomatic HIV-infected patients and other severely immunocompromised patients exposed to measles, regardless of immunization status. Operationally defined, severe immunosuppression may result from congenital immunodeficiency, HIV infection, leukemia, lymphoma, aplastic anemia, generalized malignancy, or therapy with alkylating agents, antimetabolites, radiation, or large, sustained doses of corticosteroids.

Pregnancy: Category C. Use only if clearly needed. Intact IgG crosses the placenta from the maternal circulation increasingly after 30 weeks gestation. In cases of maternal ITP, when

IGIV was administered to the mother prior to delivery, the platelet response and clinical effect were similar in the mother and neonate. Problems in humans have not been documented and are unlikely.

Lactation: It is not known if IGIV antibodies are excreted in breast milk. Problems in humans have not been documented and are unlikely.

Children: Generally safe and effective.

Adverse Reactions: Most adverse reactions are mild, transient, systemic reactions such as the following: anxiety, back pain, chills, headache, muscle pain, arthralgia, pruritus, malaise, joint pain, fever, nausea, vomiting, abdominal cramps, flushing, tightness of the chest, palpitations, diaphoresis, hypotension, hypertension, dizziness, pallor, cyanosis, dyspnea, and wheezing. Rash occurs rarely. Immediate anaphylactic and hypersensitivity reactions have been observed in exceptional cases.

Some of the infusion-related adverse effects (eg, temperature, chills, nausea, vomiting) may be caused by a reaction between administered antibodies and free antigens in the blood and tissues of recipients. When free antigen is fully bound, further administration of IGIV usually does not cause subsequent untoward side effects. These reactions may recur if the time interval since the last IGIV treatment is longer than 8 weeks or if a different brand of IGIV is used.

A detailed case of maltose-induced hyponatremia was reported following infusion of IGIV (*Gamimune N*) in 10% maltose. The authors attribute maltose accumulation to the patient's acute renal failure.

Non-A/Non-B hepatitis (hepatitis C) has occurred rarely following IGIV administration, most often in other countries. A hepatitis C outbreak in the United States was linked to IGIV products that did not include a specific viral inactivation step. All current IGIV products include one or more virucidal processing steps. One outbreak of IGIV-associated hepatitis B occurred in India, possibly because of inadequate quality-control procedures.

Blood-group antibodies in the donor population may be transferred to IGIV recipients; in isolated cases, this has been associated with confusion regarding the recipient's blood type and, rarely, hemolysis. In one case, blood-group antigens may have been transferred to an IGIV recipient.

An aseptic meningitis syndrome (AMS) has been reported infrequently in association with IGIV. AMS usually begins within several hours to two days after IGIV treatment. AMS includes signs and symptoms such as severe headache, nuchal rigidity, drowsiness, fever, photophobia, painful eye movement, nausea, and vomiting. Cerebrospinal fluid (CSF) studies frequently show pleocytosis up to several thousand cells/mm^3, mostly granulocytes, and protein levels elevated up to several hundred mg/dL. Give patients with such signs and symptoms a thorough neurological examination, including CSF studies, to rule out other causes of meningitis. AMS occurs more frequently in association with high-dose (higher than 2 g/kg) IGIV therapy. Stopping the IGIV has resulted in remission of AMS within several days without sequelae.

Several reports of acute renal failure (ARF) have been published among patients who received IGIV, particularly those with compromised renal function. IGIV products, especially those containing sucrose, may be associated with a higher risk of ARF than other IGIV products. To minimize the risk, ensure adequate hydration before IGIV infusion, and use caution in patients prone to develop ARF (eg, those with renal insufficiency, diabetes, volume depletion, sepsis, paraproteinemia, concomitant nephrotoxic drugs, or those 65 years of age and older). Higher IGIV doses may increase the risk of ARF. Monitor renal function tests (eg, BUN, serum creatinine) and urine output in patients at increased risk of ARF. Consider reducing infusion rate. If renal function deteriorates, consider discontinuing IGIV therapy.

Hematology: Thrombotic events have been reported in association with IGIV. Patients at risk may include those with a history of atherosclerosis, multiple cardiovascular risk factors, advanced age, impaired cardiac output, or known or suspected hyperviscosity. Weigh the potential risks and benefits of IGIV against those of alternative therapies. Consider baseline assessment of blood viscosity in patients at risk for hyperviscosity, including those with cryoglobulins, fasting chylomicroanemia, or markedly high triglycerides or monoclonal gammopathies. IGIV products can contain blood-group antibodies that may act as hemolysins and induce in vivo coating of red blood cells with immunoglobulin, causing a positive direct-antiglobulin reaction and, rarely, hemolysis. Hemolytic anemia may develop because of enhanced red blood cell sequestration. Monitor recipients for signs and symptoms of hemolysis.

Infection: IGIV products are made from human plasma and carry the possibility for transmission of blood-borne viral agents and, theoretically, the Creutzfeldt-Jakob disease agent. The risk of transmission of blood-borne viruses has been reduced by screening plasma donors for prior exposure to certain viruses and for the current presence of certain viral infections, and by the viral inactivation or removal properties of purification procedures. Despite these measures, some as-yet unrecognized blood-borne viruses may not be inactivated by the manufacturing processes.

Pulmonary: There have been reports of noncardiogenic pulmonary edema (transfusion-related acute lung injury [TRALI]) in patients given IGIV. TRALI is characterized by severe respiratory distress, pulmonary edema, hypoxemia, normal left ventricular function, and fever, and typically occurs one to six hours after transfusion. Patients with TRALI may be managed by using oxygen therapy with adequate ventilatory support. Monitor IGIV recipients for pulmonary adverse events. If TRALI is suspected, perform appropriate tests for antineutrophil antibodies in the product and patient serum.

Multifocal motor neuropathy: Serious adverse reactions included pulmonary embolism and blurred vision. The most common adverse reactions for MMN (in 5% or more of subjects) were headache, chest discomfort, muscle spasms, muscular weakness, nausea, oropharyngeal pain, and pain in extremity.

Pharmacologic & Dosing Characteristics

Dosage: No consensus exists on whether IGIV dosage should be based on actual, ideal, or adjusted body mass. In treating neurologic disorders, 2-day infusions, in patients who can tolerate them, may have superior efficacy over doses divided over five days.

Immunoglobulin replacement therapy: As the initial dose, give 100 to 400 mg/kg (4 to 8 mL/kg), repeated every 3 to 4 weeks. If the clinical response is inadequate or the level of serum IgG achieved is insufficient, increase the periodic dose to 300 to 800 mg/kg every 3 to 4 weeks or repeat the same dose at shorter intervals. Monthly doses up to 800 mg/kg or more have been used.

B-cell CLL: 400 mg/kg is the recommended dose, given every 3 to 4 weeks.

ITP, acute: For induction therapy, 400 to 2,000 mg/kg body weight daily for 1 to 7 consecutive days. Various protocols have used 400 mg/kg/day for 5 days, 1 g/kg/day for 1 or 2 days or daily for 3 doses on alternate days, or 2 g/kg/day for 2 to 7 consecutive days.

IGIV therapy in patients who respond to induction therapy with a platelet count of 30,000 to 50,000 cells/mm^3 may be discontinued after 2 to 7 daily doses. The extent and rapidity of platelet recovery for induction therapy and degree of success for maintenance therapy in clinical trials were independent of dose.

ITP, chronic: After induction therapy in adults and children, if the platelet count falls below 30,000 cells/mm^3 or if the patient manifests clinically significant bleeding, give 400 to 2,000 mg/kg as a single infusion every two weeks, or more frequently as needed to maintain the platelet count above 30,000 cells/mm^3 in children and above 20,000 cells/mm^3 in adults.

Kawasaki disease: Within 10 days of onset of disease, treatment with either a single dose of 2 g/kg body weight given over a 10-hour period or 400 mg/kg body weight on four consecutive days. Give concurrent aspirin therapy at a dose such as 100 mg/kg/day through the fourteenth day of illness, then 3 to 5 mg/kg/day thereafter for a period of five weeks.

Multifocal motor neuropathy: 0.5 to 2.4 g/kg per month. Adjust to achieve desired clinical response. During the clinical study, 9% of subjects experienced neurological decompensation that required an increase in dose.

Children with AIDS: Fewer bacterial infections were observed in children infected with HIV-1 who received 400 mg/kg every 28 days.

Bone marrow transplant patients: Give 500 mg/kg 7 and 2 days before transplantation (or at the time conditioning therapy for transplantation begins), then weekly through day 90 after transplant. Administer through a central line while it is in place and thereafter through a peripheral vein.

CIDP: Give 2 g/kg loading dose at an initial infusion rate of 2 mg/kg/min, which may be given in divided doses over 2 to 4 consecutive days. Follow with a maintenance dose of 1 g/kg given over 1 to 2 consecutive days every 3 weeks, at up to 8 mg/kg/min, if tolerated.

Measles: The ACIP recommends 400 mg/kg to prevent measles infection after exposures occurring within 3 weeks after IGIV administration.

Route & Site: IV infusion. In general, begin infusions at a rate of 0.01 mL/kg/min (0.6 mL/kg/h), increasing to 0.02 mL/kg/min (1.2 mL/kg/h) after 15 to 30 minutes. Most patients tolerate a gradual increase to 0.03 to 0.08 mL/kg/min (1.8 to 4.8 mL/kg/h). For a typical 70 kg person, this is equivalent to 2 to 4 mL/min (120 to 240 mL/h). If adverse reactions develop, slowing the infusion rate usually will eliminate the reaction. For patients judged to be at an increased risk for developing renal dysfunction, consider infusing IGIV at a rate slower than 0.8 mL/kg/min. Specific recommended rates of infusion appear in the table at the end of the monograph. The *Sandoglobulin* formulation (similar to *Carimune NF* formulations) has been infused as fast as 30 mL/kg/min in one study. *Gamunex-C* may be given subcutaneously for primary immunodeficiency, dose calculated initially as 1.37 times current IV dose in mg/kg/IV dose interval in weeks. Start 1 week after last IGIV infusion. Infusion rate: 20 mL/h/site. Adjust dose based on patient response. Do not administer subcutaneously in patients with ITP because of the risk of hematoma formations.

Subcutaneous administration: Gammagard 10% liquid (Baxter) is also licensed for subcutaneous injection.

Overdosage: Although few data are available, clinical experience with other immune globulin preparations suggests that the major manifestations of overdosage would be related to fluid volume overload.

Efficacy:

Immunoglobulin replacement therapy: IGIV therapy reduces the incidence of infection.

B-cell CLL: IGIV therapy reduces the incidence of bacterial infections to approximately 50% of the incidence without IGIV administration. The median time to the first bacterial infection was increased from 192 days in the control group to more than 365 days in the IGIV-treated group.

ITP, acute: In various studies, 64% to 100% of IGIV recipients attained platelet counts 100,000 cells/mL or higher within 7 days and were considered full treatment successes.

ITP, chronic: 67% to 86% of IGIV recipients responded satisfactorily to maintenance therapy.

Kawasaki disease: IGIV in conjunction with aspirin therapy can reduce the incidence of coronary artery abnormalities 65% to 78%, compared with treatment with aspirin alone.

Onset: Rapid

Duration: In general, the mean half-life in healthy people is 18 to 25 days, although there is substantial intersubject variability. Fever or infection may decrease antibody half-life because of increased catabolism or consumption, respectively. In ITP, the increase in platelets usually lasts from several days to weeks, although it may rarely persist for one year or longer. In a group of burn patients, the half-life ranged from 47 to 154 days. Reported half-lives appear in the table at the end of the monograph.

Pharmacokinetics: Immunoglobulins are primarily eliminated by catabolism. IV administration makes essentially 100% of the dose immediately available in the recipient's circulation. After infusion, IGIV shows a biphasic decay curve. The initial (α) phase includes an immediate postinfusion peak in serum IgG, followed by rapid decay due to equilibration between plasma and extravascular fluid compartments. After approximately 6 days, approximately 50% of the body pool partitions into the extravascular space, with the balance remaining in the serum. The second (β) phase involves a slower and constant rate of decay.

The half-life of IgG may vary considerably from person to person. The commonly cited half-life in healthy adults is 18 to 25 days. In patients with hypogammaglobulinemia or agammaglobulinemia, half-lives ranged from 12 to 40 days. High concentrations of IgG and hypermetabolism associated with fever and infection coincide with a shortened half-life of IgG. In pharmacokinetic studies of immunodeficient patients given high doses of IGIV, half-lives of 26 to 35 days are consistently reported.

Protective Level: The minimum serum concentration of IgG necessary for protection has not been established; 200 mg per 100 mL plasma is a common target in replacement therapy.

Mechanism: IGIV passively supplies a broad spectrum of IgG antibodies against bacterial, viral, parasitic, and mycoplasmic antigens. IGIV antibodies act through a variety of mechanisms, including antimicrobial or antitoxin neutralization. Other postulated mechanisms include the following:

- Fc receptor blockade of reticuloendothelial cell system and mononuclear phagocytes, including competitive interaction of IGIV with antiplatelet antibodies for Fc receptors
- Modulation of Fc receptor expression or affinity
- Immunomodulation, including enhancement of T-cell suppressor function or inhibition of B-cell function or antigen-processing cells via Fc receptors
- Restoration of idiotype-anti-idiotype network
- Modification of complement-dependent immune damage to tissue
- Inhibition of cytokine or interleukin production or action
- Neutralization of toxic superantigens
- Accessory presence of soluble CD4 and CD8, soluble human leukocyte antigen (HLA) class II molecules that modulate antigen processing or T-cell activation

IGIV appears to work by contributing anti-idiotypic antibodies that bind and neutralize pathogenic autoantibodies. There also may be negative feedback and down-regulation of antibody production. Other mechanisms may involve binding to CD5 receptors, interleukin-1a, interleukin-6, tumor necrosis factor-α, and T-cell receptors, suppressing pathogenic cytokines and phagocytes. IGIV also interferes with pathogenic effects of products of complement activation.

Antibodies processed by the Cohn-Oncley or Kistler-Nitschman processes are presumed to retain full biological function for the prevention or attenuation of a wide variety of infectious diseases, including their abilities to promote opsonization, fix complement, and neutralize microorganisms and their toxins. In general, therapeutic use of IGIV may involve general replacement therapy, specific passive immunotherapy, Fc receptor blockage, management of immunologic disorders, and management of inflammatory disorders.

In ITP, IGIV induces a rapid increase in platelet counts. The mechanism is not fully understood but may involve anti-idiotypic binding of the patient's own antiplatelet antibodies. Alterations in T-cell subsets and of in vitro B-cell function have occurred in patients treated with IGIV, but it is unknown if these observations are related to the mechanism of therapeutic effect.

In Kawasaki disease, IGIV plus aspirin has a striking anti-inflammatory response greater than that of aspirin alone. Reductions in fever, neutrophil counts, coronary artery abnormalities, and acute phase reactants may occur, usually within a day of IGIV therapy initiation. The mechanism may involve inhibition of complement-dependent tissue damage caused by binding of IGIV to active C3 fragments. Other possible mechanisms for these and other uses may involve Fc receptor blockade and alteration of reticuloendothelial cell system function.

Drug Interactions: IGIV may diminish the antibody response to attenuated measles, mumps, and rubella vaccines through antigen-antibody antagonism. As a general rule, administer live virus vaccines 14 to 30 days before, or 6 to 12 weeks after, IGIV. For varicella vaccine, wait five months. For a vaccine containing the measles virus, wait eight months after standard 400 mg/kg IGIV therapy. After high-dose IGIV therapy for ITP or Kawasaki disease, wait 8 to 11 months. Alternatively, administer live virus vaccines during this interval if antiviral antibody titers are measured three months after IGIV administration.

IGIV is unlikely to interfere with development of immunity following oral poliovirus or yellow fever vaccination; however, it may be prudent not to administer these vaccines shortly after IGIV administration. Exceptions include unexpected travel to, or contact with, epidemic or endemic areas or people. If oral poliovirus vaccine (OPV) is given with IGIV, or shortly after, repeat the OPV dose 3 months later if immunization is still indicated.

It is not known if IGIV interferes with the efficacy of other attenuated vaccines (eg, adenovirus, Bacillus Calmette-Guérin, typhoid, vaccinia). It may be prudent not to administer these vaccines shortly after IGIV administration unless unavoidable.

Inactivated vaccines generally are not affected by circulating antibodies or administration of exogenous antibodies. Immunization with such vaccines may occur at any time before or after antibody administration.

Lab Interference: IGIV products may contain low levels of antiblood group A and B antibodies, which may act as hemolysins and induce in vivo coating of red blood cells with IgG. As a result, direct antiglobin tests (DAT or direct Coombs tests), used in some centers as a safety check before red blood cell transfusions, may become positive temporarily. IGIV products do not contain irregular antibodies to rhesus antigens or other non-ABO red blood cell antigens. Hemolytic events (eg, anemia) may develop after IGIV therapy because of enhanced red blood cell sequestration. IGIV products containing maltose may cause misinterpretation of glucose concentrations by certain blood-glucose testing systems (eg, those based on the glucose dehydrogenase pyrroloquinolinequinone [GDH-PQQ] method). This can result in falsely elevated glucose readings and, consequently, in the inappropriate administration of insulin, resulting in life-threatening hypoglycemia. Cases of true hypoglycemia may go untreated if the hypoglycemic state is masked by falsely elevated results.

A transitory increase of passively transferred antibodies in the patient's blood may result in misleading positive results in serological testing (eg, Coombs test).

After administration, a transitory increase of passively transferred antibodies in the patient's blood may result in misleading positive results in serological testing (eg, anti-HBs).

Patient Information: Patients should report symptoms of decreased urine output, sudden weight gain, fluid retention, edema, or shortness of breath (which may suggest kidney problems) right away to their physicians.

Pharmaceutical Characteristics

Concentration:

Baxter (Gammagard Liquid): 10% solution (100 mg protein/mL), containing 98% or more IgG.

Baxter (Gammagard S/D): Powder yielding 5% or 10% solution, containing 90% or more IgG.

Bio Products (Gammaplex): 5% (50 mg/mL) solution containing 95% or more IgG.

CSL Behring (Carimune NF): 3%, 6%, 9%, or 12% solution, depending on quantity of diluent added, when reconstituted according to directions, containing 96% or more IgG and 92% monomeric (7S), with the remainder dimeric and a small portion polymeric. Fragments less than 10% (mean, 6%) and aggregates less than 3% (mean, less than 1%).

Native human IgG subclass distributions typically follow this pattern: IgG1, 60% to 70%; IgG2, 23% to 29%; IgG3, 4% to 8%; IgG4, 2% to 6%. Product-specific subclass distributions appear in the table at the end of the monograph.

CSL Behring (Privigen): 10% (100 mg/mL) solution containing 98% or more IgG. Consists primarily of monomer, with up to 12% dimers, small amounts of fragments and polymers, and albumin.

Grifols (Flebogamma): 5% or 10% solution (50 or 100 mg/mL), containing 97% or more IgG.

Grifols (Flebogamma DIF): 5% solution (100 mg/mL), containing 97% or more IgG.

Octapharma (Octagam): 5% (50 mg/mL) solution containing 96% or more IgG.

Talecris (Gamunex-C): 9% to 11% (90 to 110 mg/mL) solution containing 98% or more IgG.

Quality Assay:
All plasma units are tested to ensure the absence of hepatitis B surface antigen and HIV-1 antibodies before pooling for manufacture. Most manufacturers have begun testing plasma units for HIV-2 and hepatitis C antibodies. Standardized to meet World Health Organization requirements for antibodies against hepatitis B surface antigen, hepatitis A virus, streptolysin O, poliovirus type 1, measles, and diphtheria antitoxin. Minimum measles antibody potency: 12.3 international units/mL. In general, users may request lot-specific information from manufacturers, including IgA levels, CMV ELISA titers, hepatitis B titers, isohemagglutinin titers, and anti-D (Rh_o) levels.

Packaging:

Baxter (Gammagard Liquid): 1 g single-dose 10 mL vial (00944-2700-02), 2.5 g single-dose 25 mL vial (00944-2700-03), 5 g single-dose 50 mL vial (00944-2700-04), 10 g single-dose 100 mL vial (00944-2700-05), 20 g single-dose 200 mL vial (00944-2700-06).

Baxter (Gammagard S/D): 2.5 g single-dose vial (00944-2620-02), 5 g single-dose vial (00944-2620-03), or 10 g single-dose vial (00944-2620-04). Each package includes a suitable container of sterile water for injection, a transfer device, an administration set that contains an integral airway, and a 15-micron filter.

Low-IgA formulation: 5 g single-dose vial (00944-2655-03), 10 g single-dose vial (00944-2655-04). Each package includes a suitable container of sterile water for injection, a transfer device, an administration set that contains an integral airway, and a 15-micron filter.

Bio Products (Gammaplex): 2.5 g/50 mL single-dose vial (64208-8234-01), 5 g/100 mL single-dose vial (64208-8234-02), 10 g/200 mL single-dose vial (64208-8234-03).

Grifols (Flebogamma DIF): *5%:* 0.5 g single-dose 10 mL vial (61953-0004-01), 2.5 g single-dose 50 mL vial (61953-0004-02), 5 g single-dose 100 mL vial (61953-0004-03), 10 g single-dose 200 mL vial (61953-0004-04), 20 g single-dose 400 mL vial (61953-0004-05).

10%: 5 g single-dose 50 mL vial (61953-0005-01), 10 g single-dose 100 mL vial (61953-0005-02), 20 g single-dose 200 mL vial (61953-0005-03).

CSL Behring (Carimune NF): 1 g single-dose vial (44206-0415-01), 3 g single-dose vial (44206-0416-03), 6 g single-dose vial (44206-0417-06), 12 g single-dose vial (44206-0418-12). Each package includes a transfer spike.

CSL Behring (Privigen): 5 g per 50 mL single-dose vial (44206-0436-05), 10 g per 100 mL single-dose vial (44206-0437-10), 20 g per 200 mL single-dose vial (44206-0438-20).

Grifols (Flebogamma): 0.5 g/10 mL single-dose vial (61953-0003-01), 2.5 g/5 mL single-dose vial (61953-0003-02), 5 g/100 mL single-dose vial (61953-0003-03), 10 g/200 mL single-dose vial (61953-0003-04).

Octapharma (Octagam): 1 g/20 mL single-dose vial (67467-0843-01), 2.5 g/50 mL single-dose vial (67467-0843-02), 5 g/100 mL single-dose vial (67467-0843-03), 10 g/200 mL single-dose vial (67467-0843-04), 25 g/500 mL single-dose vial (67467-0843-05).

Talecris (Gamunex-C): 1 g/10 mL single-dose vial (13533-0800-12), 2.5 g/25 mL single-dose vial (13533-0800-15), 5 g/50 mL single-dose vial (13533-0800-20), 10 g/100 mL single-dose vial (13533-0800-71), 20 g/200 mL single-dose vial (13533-0800-24).

Doseform: See tables at the end of the monograph.

Appearance: Do not use if turbid or discolored or if particulates appear.

Solution: Clear or slightly opalescent, colorless to pale yellow liquid

Powders: White to light-beige powder, yielding clear and colorless to slightly straw-colored or slightly cloudy solutions.

Solvent:

Baxter (Gammagard Liquid): Sterile water with glycine 0.25 M

Bio Products (Gammaplex): Sterile water with D-sorbitol 50 mg/mL and glycine 6 mg/mL

CSL Behring (Privigen): Sterile water with L-proline 210 to 290 mmol/L and trace amounts of sodium

Grifols (Flebogamma): Sterile water with 50 mg/mL D-sorbitol

Grifols (Flebogamma DIF): Sterile water with D-sorbitol 50 mg/mL

Octapharma (Octagam): Sterile water with 100 mg/mL maltose

Talecris (Gamunex-C): Sterile water with 0.16 to 0.24 molar glycine

Diluent:

For reconstitution: CSL Behring (Carimune NF): Reconstitute with 0.9% sodium chloride. Alternatively, use 5% dextrose or sterile water for injection as the diluent. Usually dissolves in less than 10 minutes. Do not add other products to the final solution, especially protein-denaturing agents. Data on specific physical or chemical incompatibilities with other infused drugs have not been published.

All other powders: Sterile water for injection, without bacteriostatic agents or other preservatives. Do not add other products to the final solution, especially protein-denaturing agents. Little data on specific drug interactions or incompatibilities have been published.

For infusion: Baxter (Gammagard Liquid): 5% dextrose may be used. Do not use 0.9% sodium chloride as diluent.

CSL Behring (Carimune NF): 0.9% sodium chloride, 5% dextrose, sterile water, preferably acid or neutral fluids, pH 7.4 or less

Grifols (Flebogamma DIF): Dilution with IV fluids is not recommended.

Talecris: 5% dextrose

Adjuvant: None

Preservative: None

Allergens: See tables at the end of the monograph.

Excipients:

General: Sucrose administered IV is excreted unchanged in the urine and may be given to diabetic patients without compensatory changes in insulin dosage. IV maltose is cleared from the blood within 24 hours after administration, primarily metabolized in the renal proximal tubule, and excreted in the urine.

Baxter (Gammagard Liquid): Glycine 0.25 M

Baxter (Gammagard S/D): Based on 5% solution: Albumin human 3 mg/mL, glycine 22.5 mg/mL, glucose 20 mg/mL, polyethylene glycol 2 mg/mL, tri-n-butyl phosphate 1 mcg/mL, octoxynol 9 1 mcg/mL, and polysorbate 80 100 mcg/mL

Bio Products (Gammaplex): D-sorbitol 50 mg/mL, glycine 6 mg/mL, sodium acetate 2 mg/mL, sodium chloride 3 mg/mL, and polysorbate 80 approximately 50 ng/mL

CSL Behring (Carimune NF): Sodium chloride 20 mg/g of protein, sucrose 1.67 g/g of protein as a stabilizer, 1 to 2 mg/mL human albumin, 100 mcg/mL pepsin

CSL Behring (Privigen): Contains L-proline 210 to 290 mmol/L as a stabilizer and trace amounts of sodium. Contains no carbohydrate stabilizers (eg, maltose, sucrose)

Grifols (Flebogamma): 5%: 50 mg/mL D-sorbitol, 6 mg/mL or less PEG

    10%: D-sorbitol 5% and PEG 6 mg/mL or less

Grifols (Flebogamma DIF): D-sorbitol 5% and polyethylene glycol 3 mg/mL or less

Octapharma (Octagam): 5 mcg/mL or less polyethylene glycol p-isooctyl-phenyl ether (*Triton X-100*), 1 mcg/mL or less tri-n-butylphosphate

Talecris (Gamunex-C): 0.16 to 0.24 molar glycine, caprylate 0.216 g/L (1.3 mmol/L) or less

pH: See table at the end of the monograph. Powdered IGIV exhibits various values in the range of 6.4 to 7.2 after reconstitution to 5% concentration with the appropriate volume of diluent.

Talecris: Gamunex-C has a buffer capacity of 35 mEq/L or 0.35 mEq/g. The acid load delivered in the largest dose would be neutralized by the buffering capacity of whole blood alone, even if the dose were infused instantaneously rather than over several hours. There were no clinically important differences in mean venous pH or bicarbonate measurements in recipients of *Gamimune N* compared with those receiving a chemically modified IGIV with a pH of 6.8. In patients with limited or compromised acid-base compensatory mechanisms, consider the effect of the additional acid load that the product might present (eg, neonates, patients in renal failure).

Osmolality: See table at the end of the monograph.

Shelf Life: See table at the end of the monograph.

Storage/Stability: See table at the end of the monograph. Freezing may break diluent bottles but will not affect the potency of powdered IGIV products. Discard solution forms of IGIV if frozen. Infuse IGIV at room temperature.

Admixtures with other drugs have not been evaluated. Administer IGIV separately from other drugs or medications the patient receives. Delay in administration may be safer following reconstitution in a laminar air-flow hood (to reduce risk of bacterial contamination) if the solution was refrigerated before use.

No manufacturer data are available on stability in plastic containers. The Fc portion of IgG molecules will adhere to plastic in milligram quantities, but no clinical problems have been documented.

Baxter (Gammagard Liquid): Stable for 36 months if stored at 2° to 8°C (36° to 46°F) for the entire interval. In general, the product is stable for 9 months after transfer to room temperature, up to a total of 24 months. After 24 months from date of manufacture, product cannot be stored at room temperature. The total storage time depends on the point when the vial is transferred to room temperature. Record the new expiration date on the package when the product is transferred to room temperature. Do not freeze.

Baxter (Gammagard S/D): Contact manufacturer regarding prolonged exposure to elevated temperatures. Shipped at ambient temperature. Do not mix *Gammagard S/D* with sodium chloride solutions as a diluent.

Bio Products (Gammaplex): Store between 2° and 25°C and (36° and 77°F). Discard if frozen.

CSL Behring (Carimune NF): Do not warm above 30°C (86°F). Do not freeze solution. Shipped at ambient temperature.

CSL Behring (Privigen): Contact manufacturer regarding prolonged exposure to elevated temperatures. Shipped at ambient temperature. Discard if frozen. The infusion line may be flushed with 5% dextrose or 0.9% sodium chloride.

Grifols (Flebogamma): Can tolerate temperatures 2° to 25°C (36° to 77°F). Discard if frozen. Contact manufacturer regarding elevated temperatures. Shipped in insulated containers with coolant packs.

Grifols (Flebogamma DIF): Can tolerate temperatures 2° to 25°C (36° to 77°F). Do not freeze.

Octapharma (Octagam): Product can tolerate temperatures up to 25°C (77°F) for up to 18 months.

Talecris (Gamunex-C): Store for 36 months from date of manufacture at 2° to 8°C (36° to 46°F); AND product may be stored at temperatures at or below 25°C (77°F) for up to 6 months any time during the 36-month shelf life, after which the product must be used or discarded. Discard if frozen. Shipped in insulated containers with coolant packs.

Handling: Avoid foaming. To prevent denaturation of antibody proteins, swirl to facilitate dissolution; do not shake. Discard any unused portions. If large doses will be administered, several containers may be pooled into an empty, sterile IV solution container using aseptic technique. Administer pooled preparations within a few hours; do not store for later use. Bring IGIV solutions to room temperature before infusion.

Individual IgG molecules measure less than 0.002 microns in diameter. The American Red Cross and Baxter recommend use of a 15 micron in-line filter to preclude infusion of aggregates. Filtering of CSL Behring formulations, *Flebogamma*, *Flebogamma DIF*, and *Octagam* is acceptable but not required. Pore diameters 15 microns or wider are less likely to slow down infusion rates, especially at higher concentrations. Sterilizing filters (eg, 0.2 microns) may be used.

Recommendations to record lot numbers and manufacturers of all serum-based products are becoming common.

Production Process: The Cohn-Oncley methods 6 & 9 cold-ethanol fractionation process, developed in the 1940s, involves six steps of plasma separation, inactivation, fractional precipitation, reprecipitation, and washing. It isolates IgG of high quality and purity in the fraction II precipitate but produces low yield. In contrast, the Kistler-Nitschmann technique, first developed in 1954, is a modification of the Cohn-Oncley method that combines fractional precipitation and extraction. The Kistler-Nitschmann process involves less labor and ethanol and provides higher yields but with slightly more extraneous proteins. Further steps after fractionation are needed to produce an IgG product suitable for IV administration.

Viral-Inactivation Steps: IGIV processes include one or more inactivation steps. Solvent-detergent treatment helps inactivate lipid-enveloped viruses (eg, HIV, HBV, HCV) by destroying the lipid coat and associated virus-binding sites. Nanofiltration helps remove lipid-enveloped viruses and reduces certain nonlipid enveloped viruses (eg, HAV, parvovirus B19) by specific size exclusion. Treatment with low pH at elevated temperature helps inactivate lipid-enveloped viruses and certain nonlipid enveloped viruses. Pasteurization helps inactivate both enveloped and nonenveloped viruses.

Baxter (Gammagard Liquid): Purified from plasma pools using a modified Cohn-Oncley cold-ethanol fractionation process, as well as cation- and anion-exchange chromatography. Three independent virus inactivation/removal steps are integrated into manufacturing and formulation: solvent/detergent (S/D) treatment (tri-n-butyl phosphate, octoxynol 9, and polysorbate 80 at 18° to 25°C for 60 minutes or more), 35 nm nanofiltration, and low pH incubation at 30° to 32°C. Fc and Fab functions are maintained and prekallikrein activator activity is not detectable.

Baxter (Gammagard S/D): Prepared from pooled human plasma by Cohn-Oncley methods 6 & 9 cold-ethanol fractionation process, as well as cation and anion exchange chromatography. Viral inactivation and removal steps include solvent/detergent treatment with tri-n-butylphosphate, octoxynol-9 and polysorbate 80 at 18° to 25°C for at least 60 minutes; 35 nm nanofiltration; and incubation at low pH at 30° to 32°C. Glycine is added as a stabilizing and buffering agent. No sugar, sodium, or preservative is added. Fc and Fab functions are maintained. Pre-kallikrein activator activity is not detectable.

Bio Products (Gammaplex): Prepared from pooled human plasma by cold-ethanol fractionation and ion-exchange chromatography. Three processing steps are specifically designed to remove or inactivate viruses: solvent/detergent treatment targeted at enveloped viruses; virus filtration using Pall Ultipor DV20 to remove small viruses, including nonenveloped viruses, on a size-exclusion basis; and the terminal low-pH incubation step to contribute to overall viral clearance capacity for enveloped and nonenveloped viruses.

CSL Behring (Carimune NF): Prepared from pooled human plasma by the Cohn-Oncley methods 6 & 9 cold-ethanol fractionation process. Fraction II is nanofiltered to remove viruses, then treated with trace amounts of immobilized porcine pepsin at pH 4, the Kistler-Nitschmann modification, a process considered virucidal. The final product is lyophilized with maltose. *Carimune NF* is not exposed to a specific IgA depletion step, as this tends to remove IgG4 as well, disturbing the composition of the preparation. This is because of the electrophoretic similarity of IgG4 and IgA.

CSL Behring (Privigen): Prepared from pooled human plasma by a combination of cold-ethanol fractionation, octanoic-acid fractionation, and anion-exchange chromatography. The IgG proteins are not subjected to heating or to chemical or enzymatic modification. The IgG molecules retain Fab and Fc functions. Fab functions tested include antigen-binding capacities. Fc functions tested include complement activation and Fc-receptor-mediated leukocyte activation (determined with complexed IgG). This product does not activate the complement system or prekallikrein in an unspecific manner. Two manufacturing steps reduce the risk of virus transmission: pH 4 incubation and virus filtration. In addition, a depth-filtration step contributes to the virus-reduction capacity. Several of the production steps were shown to decrease infectivity of transmissible spongiform encephalopathy (TSE) in an experimental model. These steps include octanoic-acid fractionation, depth filtration, and virus filtration.

Grifols (Flebogamma): Prepared by Cohn-Oncley methods 6 & 9 cold-ethanol fractionation process, PEG precipitation, and ion-exchange chromatography.

Grifols (Flebogamma DIF): The purification process includes cold-alcohol fractionation, 4% PEG precipitation, ion exchange chromatography, pH 4 treatment for 4 hours at 37°C, pasteurization (at 60°C for 10 hours), solvent/detergent treatment for 6 h, and sequential nanofiltrations through 35 nm and 20 nm nanofilters connected in series. Using sorbitol as a stabilizer during pasteurization avoids denaturation of proteins and preserves antibody activity. Fc and Fab functions are maintained.

Octapharma (Octagam): Prepared from pooled human plasma by Cohn-Oncley methods 6 & 9 cold-ethanol fractionation process, followed by ultrafiltration and chromatography. The process includes virucidal treatment with a solvent/detergent mixture composed of tri-n-butylphosphate and polyethylene glycol p-isooctyl-phenyl ether (*Triton X-100*).

Talecris (Gamunex-C): Prepared by Cohn-Oncley methods 6 & 9 cold-ethanol fractionation of fractions II and III, precipitation with 20 millimolar sodium caprylate (a naturally occurring fatty acid) at pH 5.1 to remove lipoproteins, albumin, and some caprylate. The precipitate is removed by cloth filtration. The caprylate concentration is returned to 20 millimolar and the solution incubated at pH 5.1 for one hour at 25°C to inactivate lipid-enveloped viruses, followed by depth filtration. Two of the four ethanol fractionation steps of the Cohn-Oncley process have been replaced by tandem anion-exchange chromatography (Q Sepharose FF and ANX Sepharose FF) at pH 5.2 to remove non-IgG proteins, viruses, and caprylate, followed by ultra- and diafiltration. IgG proteins are not subjected to heating, chemical, or enzymatic modification steps. IgG remains in solution at each step from fraction II and III dissolution to final container. Fc and Fab functions of the IgG molecule are retained, but do not activate complement or pre-Kallikrein activity in an unspecified manner. Protein is stabilized during the process by adjusting the pH to 4 to 4.5. Isotonicity is achieved by the addition of glycine. *Gamunex-C* is incubated in the final container for further virus inactivation at pH 4 to 4.3 for at least 21 days at 23° to 27°C.

Media: Human plasma; each lot pools 1,000 to more than 50,000 donor units.

Disease Epidemiology

Incidence:

B-cell CLL: Characteristically a disease of the elderly, more than 95% of CLL cases involve B-lymphocytes, with the balance involving T-cells. This is the most common form of leukemia in adults, with incidence increasing with age to a level of 10 to 20 cases per 10,000 adults older than 70 years of age. An estimated 31,000 patients are affected in the United States, with approximately 9,000 new patients diagnosed annually.

ITP: Neonatal ITP affects between 1 in 2,000 to 1 in 5,000 fetuses. Acute ITP affects 100,000 to 150,000 Americans annually, including 10% of people infected with HIV.

Kawasaki disease: An acute febrile vasculitis of unknown cause that occurs predominantly among children younger than 4 years of age, Kawasaki disease also is known as mucocutaneous lymph node syndrome. Approximately 3,000 cases occur annually in the United States. More than 105,000 cases were reported in Japan between 1967 and 1991.

Prevalence: The prevalence of primary immunodeficiency states in the United States is 1 to 10 cases per 100,000 people, representing approximately 5,000 to 10,000 people. More than 70 forms of inherited primary immunodeficiency are known. The incidence of new cases is approximately 400 children born per year in the United States. Following are estimated prevalences of selected primary immunodeficiencies: DiGeorge syndrome (1:66,000), severe combined immunodeficiency (1:66,000), common variable immunodeficiency (1:83,000), Bruton or infantile X-linked immunodeficiency (1:103,000), chronic mucocutaneous candidiasis (1:103,000), and chronic granulomatous disease (1:181,000). Estimates of the prevalence of IgA deficiency range from 1:700 to 1:23,000 people; as many as 40% of these people have anti-IgA antibodies of the IgG or IgE subclasses in their circulation.

Among hospitalized adults in one study, 2.3% of admitted patients had a serum IgG level lower than 400 mg/dL. Of this sample, 0.3% represented a primary immunodeficiency, 0.3% denoted hypogammaglobulinemia of infancy, and 1.7% represented secondary hypogammaglobulinemia. Other immunodeficiencies involving cellular immunity are common among hospitalized patients.

Other Information

Perspective: See also the historical perspective provided in the Immune Globulin IM monograph.

1944: Cohn, Oncley, and colleagues develop cold-ethanol fractionation method of isolating human immune globulin from human blood.

1952: Bruton at Walter Reed Army Hospital first recognizes a patient with agammaglobulinemia.

1954: Kistler, Nitschmann, and colleagues modify the Cohn-Oncley methods 6 & 9 cold-ethanol fractionation process by combining fractional precipitation and extraction.

1959: Porter separates antibodies into Fab and Fc components.

1969: *Gammagee-V* licensed to Merck, Sharp and Dohme for IV use, but never marketed. Consisted of a 5% pepsin-treated solution.

1975: Köhler and Milstein develop method to make monoclonal antibodies.

1979: Immune globulin IV first developed by scientists at Cutter Laboratories. Reduction and alkylation of the proteins eliminated fragmentation, aggregation, and anticomplement activity that led to adverse reactions if the IM product was given IV. Improved techniques were introduced in succeeding years that spared the 3-dimensional shape and improved functionality of the immunoglobulin molecules.

1981: Cutter introduces *Gamimune*, the first commercial IGIV, formulated by reduction with dithiothreitol and alkylation with iodacetamide. The production process is changed in 1986 to yield an unmodified form of IgG.

1984: *Sandoglobulin*, the first commercial unmodified form of IGIV, licensed to Sandoz.

1991: Alpha produces first solvent-detergent treated, virally inactivated IGIV.

1994: *Gammagard* and *Polygam* recalled because of more than 100 cases of acute hepatitis C. Products reintroduced as *Gammagard S/D* and *Polygam S/D* with solvent-detergent virucidal steps in production.

2003: Bayer introduces *Gamunex*, first caprylate/chromatography purified form of IGIV.

First Licensed: See tables at the end of the monograph.

Discontinued Products: *Carimune* (CSL Behring), *Gamimune* (Cutter), *Gamimune N 5%* form (Bayer), *Gammagard* (Hyland), *Gammagee-V* (Merck), *Gammar-IV* (Armour), *Gammar-P I.V.* (Centeon, later CSL Behring), *Iveegam EN* (Baxter), *Panglobulin* (American Red Cross), *Polygam* (American Red Cross), *Polygam S/D*, *Sandoglobulin* (Swiss Red Cross, distributed by Sandoz, then Novartis), *Venoglobulin-I* and *Venoglobulin-S* (Alpha, "I" stood for "intact," "S" stood for "solution").

References: Ballow M. Clinical and investigational considerations for the use of IGIV therapy. *Am J Health Syst Pharm.* 2005;62(16 suppl 3):S12-S18.

Bonilla FA, Bernstein IL, Khan DA, et al. Practice parameter for the diagnosis and management of primary immunodeficiency. *Ann Allergy Asthma Immunol.* 2005;94(5 Suppl 1):S1-63.

Dalakas MC, et al. Intravenous immunoglobulin in autoimmune neuromuscular disorders. *JAMA.* 2004;291:2367-2375.

Hughes RA, Wijdicks EF, Barohn R, et al. Practice parameter: immunotherapy for Guillain-Barré syndrome: report of the Quality Standards Subcommittee of the American Academy of Neurology. *Neurology.* 2003;61(6):736-740.

Bonilla FA, Bernstein IL, Khan DA, et al. Practice parameter for the diagnosis and management of primary immunodeficiency. *Ann Allergy Asthma Immunol.* 2005;94(suppl 1):S1-S63.

Religious Implications: A 1994 issue of *Pediatrics* reports in detail the decision of 2 parents, each a Jehovah's Witness, to treat their child with IGIV. The case report discusses the scriptural basis for Jehovah's Witnesses avoiding blood transfusions. IgG freely passes through a mother's placenta to her fetus, while formed elements of blood (eg, cells) do not. This places IGIV in a "gray area" where individual Jehovah's Witnesses may exercise their own conscience. The parents agreed to treat the boy with IGIV. Church elders supported the decision, noting a discussion of the issue in the June 1, 1990, issue of *The Watchtower* (Roy-Bornstein C, et al. *Pediatrics.* 1994;93:112-113). See also:

Muramoto O. Bioethical aspects of the recent changes in the policy of refusal of blood by Jehovah's witnesses. *BMJ.* 2001;322:37-39.

Associated Jehovah's Witnesses for Reform on Blood Web site. Available at: http://www.ajwrb.org.

Watch Tower Bible and Tract Society Web site. Available at: http://www.watchtower.org.

Immune Globulin Intravenous (Human)

IGIV Comparisons

	Carimune NF	Flebogamma	Flebogamma DIF	Gammagard Liquid	Gammagard S/D	Gammaplex	Gamunex-C	Octagam	Privigen
Distributor	CSL Behring	Grifols Biologicals	Grifols Biologicals	Baxter	Baxter	Bio Products Laboratory	Talecris	Octapharma	CSL Behring
Licensed	Feb. 2003	Dec. 15, 2003	July 2007	Apr. 27, 2005	Apr. 27, 2005	Sep. 17, 2009	Aug. 28, 2003	May 21, 2004	July 26, 2007
Pharmaceutical Characteristics									
Concentration	3%, 6%, 9%, 12%	5%	5% or 10%	10%	5% or 10%	5% (50 mg/mL)	10%	5%	10%
IgG content	≥ 96%	≥ 99%	≥ 97%	≥ 98%	> 98%	> 95%	≥ 98%	≥ 96%	≥ 98%
Monomeric IgG	92%	≥ 95%	≥ 95%	96%	96%	Not provided	≥ 95%	≥ 90%	≥ 87%
IgG subclasses: (native)									
IgG1 (60%-70%)	61%	70%	67%	Similar to normal plasma	69%	64%	65%	65%	68%
IgG2 (23%-29%)	30%	25%	29%		22%	30%	26%	30%	29%
IgG3 (4%-8%)	7%	3.1%	2.7%		4%	5%	5.6%	3%	2%
IgG4 (2%-6%)	3%	1.9%	2.2%		5%	1%	2.6%	2%	1%
Package size	6 g	0.5 g, 2.5 g, 5 g, 10 g	0.5 g, 2.5 g, 5 g, 10 g, 20 g	1 g, 2.5 g, 5 g, 10 g, 20 g	2.5 g, 5 g, 10 g	2.5 g, 5 g, 10 g	1 g, 2.5 g, 5 g, 10 g, 20 g	1 g, 2.5 g, 5 g, 10 g	5 g, 10 g, 20 g
Doseform	Powder	Solution	Solution	Solution	Powder	Solution	Solution	Solution	Solution
Diluent for reconstitution	0.9% NaCl, D5W, SWFI	n/a	n/a	n/a	SWFI	n/a	n/a	n/a	n/a

IGIV Comparisons

	Carimune NF	Flebogamma	Flebogamma DIF	Gammagard Liquid	Gammagard S/D	Gammaplex	Gamunex-C	Octagam	Privigen
Time for reconstitution	5 to 9 min	n/a	n/a	n/a	≤ 5 min	n/a	n/a	n/a	n/a
Diluent for infusion	0.9% NaCl, D5W, sterile water	n/a	Not recommended	D5W	n/a		D5W	n/a	D5W, if needed
IgA content	< 970 mcg/mL	< 50 mcg/mL	Typically < 50 mcg/mL (in 5%) or 100 mcg/mL (in 10%)	mean 37 mcg/mL	mean 37 mcg/mL	< 10 mcg/mL	mean 46 mcg/mL	≤ 200 mcg/mL	≤ 25 mcg/mL
IgM content	< 20 mcg/mL	Trace	Trace	Trace	Trace	Trace	≤ limit of detection (2 mcg/mL)	≤ 100 mcg/mL	Trace
Primary excipients	NaCl, sucrose, 1 to 2 mg/mL albumin, 100 mcg/mL pepsin	50 mg/mL D-sorbitol, ≤ 6 mg/mL PEG	50 mg/mL D-sorbitol, ≤ 3 mg/mL (in 5%) or ≤ 6 mg/mL (in 10%) PEG	0.25 M glycine	Glycine, glucose	Sorbitol, glycine, polysorbate 80	10% glycine	100 mg/mL maltose	L-proline 210 to 290 mmol/L
Typical pH	6.4 to 6.8	5 to 6	5 to 6	4.6 to 5.1	6.4 to 7.2	4.8 to 5	4 to 4.5	5.1 to 6	4.6 to 5
Shelf life	36 mo	24 mo	24 mo	Up to 36 mo, less if room temperature	24 mo	24 months	36 mo	24 mo	24 mo

IGIV Comparisons

	Carimune NF	Flebogamma	Flebogamma DIF	Gammagard Liquid	Gammagard S/D	Gammaplex	Gamunex-C	Octagam	Privigen
Normal storage	≤ 30°C (≤ 86°F)	2° to 25°C (36° to 77°F)	2° to 25°C (36° to 77°F)	2° to 8°C (36° to 46°F) Room temp storage shortens stability.	2° to 8°C (36° to 46°F)	2° to 25°C (36° to 77°F)	For 36 months at 2° to 8°C (36° to 46°F) For 6 months up to 25°C (77°F)	2° to 8°C (36° to 46°F) for 24 mo, up to 25°C (77°F) for 18 mo	2° to 25°C (36° to 77°F) for 24 mo
Stability after reconstitution	Begin use within 6 to 24 h	n/a	n/a	n/a	Begin use within 2 h	n/a	n/a	n/a	n/a
Use Characteristics									
Production process	K-N fractionation, nanofiltration, pH 4 and pepsin treatment	C-O process, PEG precipitation, ion exchange chromatography	C-O process, PEG precipitation, ion exchange chromatography, low-pH treatment	C-O process, ion exchange chromatography	C-O process, ion exchange chromatography	C-O process, ion exchange chromatography	C-O process, caprylate precipitation and incubation, anion exchange chromatography	C-O process, ultrafiltration, chromatography	Cold-ethanol fractionation, octanoic-acid fractionation, anion-exchange chromatography
Viral inactivation or removal	Nanofiltration, pH 4 and pepsin treatment	Pasteurization, PEG precipitation	Pasteurization, S/D treatment, and dual nanofiltration	S/D treatment, nanofiltration, low-pH incubation at 30° to 32°C	S/D treatment	Solvent/detergent treatment, virus filtration, low-pH incubation	Caprylate precipitation and incubation, depth filtration, low-pH incubation	S/D treatment, pH 4 treatment	pH incubation, virus filtration, depth filtration

IGIV Comparisons

	Carimune NF	Flebogamma	Flebogamma DIF	Gammagard Liquid	Gammagard S/D	Gammaplex	Gamunex-C	Octagam	Privigen
Labeled indications	Immunodeficiency, ITP	Immunodeficiency	Immunodeficiency	Immunodeficiency, multifocal motor neuropathy	Immunodeficiency	Immunodeficiency	Immunodeficiency, ITP CIDP	Immunodeficiency	Immunodeficiency, chronic ITP
Pharmaceutical and Dosing Characteristics									
Infusion rates									
Initial	3% <1 mL/min, increased gradually up to 30 mg/kg min	0.5 mg/kg/min (0.01 mL/kg/min)	1 mg/kg/min (0.01 mL/kg/min)	0.8 mg/kg/min (0.5 mL/kg/min)	5%: 0.4 mg/kg/min (0.008 mL/kg/min)	0.5 mg/kg/min (0.01 mL/kg/min)	1 mg/kg/min (0.01 mL/kg/min)	30 mg/kg/h (0.01 mL/kg/min) × 30 min, then progressing to	0.5 mg/kg/h (0.005 mL/kg/min)
Eventual		5 mg/kg/min (0.1 mL/kg/min)	5%: 5 mg/kg/min (0.1 mL/kg/min) 10%: 8 mg/kg/min (0.08 mL/kg/min)	8.9 mg/kg/min (0.5 mL/kg/min)	3.3 mg/kg/min (0.07 mL/kg/min)	4 mg/kg/min (0.08 mL/kg/min)	8 mg/kg/min (0.08 mL/kg/min)	≤ 200 mg/kg/h (≤ 0.07 mL/kg/min)	4 to 8 mg/kg/h (0.04 to 0.08 mL/kg/min)
Mean half-life	23 d	30 to 45 d	5%: 30 to 32 d 10%: 21 to 58 d	31 to 42 d	35 d	41 to 42 d	35.7 d	25 to 30 d	36.6 d

CIDP = Chronic inflammatory demyelinating polyneuropathy.
CLL = Chronic leukocytic leukemia.
C-O = Cohn-Oncley methods 6 & 9 cold-ethanol fractionation.
ITP = Immune thrombocytopenia purpura.
K-N = Kistler-Nitschmann.
n/a = Not applicable.
PEG = Polyethylene glycol.
S/D = Solvent detergent.
SWFI = Sterile water for injection.

Key IGIV Parameters				
Manufacturer	Proprietary name	Packaging	IgA content	Normal storage
Baxter	*Gammagard Liquid*	Solution	mean, 37 mcg/mL	≤ 25°C (77°F) up to 9 mo; 2° to 8°C (36° to 46°F) for 36 mo
Baxter	*Gammagard S/D*	Powder	mean, 37 mcg/mL Low IgA formulation: < 1 mcg/mL at 5%	2° to 8°C (36° to 46°F)
Bio Products	*Gammaplex*	Solution	< 10 mcg/mL	2° to 25°C (36° to 77°F)
Grifols	*Flebogamma DIF*	Solution	typically < 50 mcg/mL (in 5%) or 100 mcg/mL (in 10%)	2° to 25°C (36° to 77°F)
Octapharma	*Octagam*	Solution	≤ 200 mcg/mL	2° to 8°C (36° to 46°F)
Talecris	*Gamunex-C*	Solution	mean, 46 mcg/mL	For 30 mo at 2° to 8°C (36° to 46°F). For 6 months up to 25°C (77°F).
CSL Behring	*Carimune NF*	Powder	< 970 mcg/mL	≤ 30°C (86°F)
CSL Behring	*Privigen*	Solution	≤ 25 mcg/mL	2° to 25°C (36° to 77°F)

Osmolality (mOsm/kg) and Sodium Content of IGIV at Various Concentrations[a]							
	IGIV concentration						
Manufacturer	3%	5%	6%	9%	10%	12%	NaCl content[b]
CSL Behring (*Carimune NF*)							
Diluent:							
0.9% NaCl	498		690	882		1,074	0.9%
5% Dextrose	444		636	828		1,020	0%
Sterile Water	192		384	576		768	0%
Baxter (*Gammagard Liquid*)					240-300		Not detectable
Baxter (*Gammagard S/D*)		636			1,250		1.7%
Bio Products (*Gammaplex*)		420-500					0.3%
Grifols (*Flebogamma DIF*)		240-370					< 3.2 mEq/L (< 0.02%)
Octapharma (*Octagam*)		310-380					30 mMol/L
Talecris (*Gamunex-C*)					258		trace
CSL Behring (*Privigen*)					240-440		trace

a Normal physiologic osmolality is 285 to 319 mOsm/kg.
b At 5% IgG concentration.

Considerations in Selecting an IGIV Product[a]						
Patient risk factor	Fluid volume	Sugar content	Sodium content	Osmolality	pH	IgA content
Cardiac impairment	•		•	•		
Renal dysfunction	•	•	•	•		
Anti-IgA antibodies						•
Thromboembolic risk	•		•	•		
Glucose tolerance (diabetes)		•				
Age, elderly	•	•	•	•		
Age, very young	•		•	•	•	

a Table adapted from Ballow M (*Am J Health Syst Pharm*. 2005;62[16 suppl 3]:S12-S18).

Immune Globulin Subcutaneous (Human)

Broad-Spectrum Immune Globulins

Name:
　Hizentra

Manufacturer:
　CSL Behring

Synonyms: IGSC

Comparison: For most purposes, the various IGIV and IGSC products are therapeutically equivalent in function. There are obvious differences in concentration, method of infusion, storage, and other variables. In a very small subset of patients with anti-IgA antibodies, the quantity of IgA in the IG product must be minimized.

Subcutaneous administration: Gammagard 10% liquid (Baxter) is also licensed for subcutaneous injection.

Immunologic Characteristics

Microorganism: Active against multiple bacteria, viruses, and fungi

Viability: Inactive, passive, transient

Antigenic Form: Human immunoglobulin, unmodified. The Fc portion of the IgG molecule remains functionally intact.

Antigenic Type: Protein, IgG antibody, polyclonal, primarily monomeric

Strains: Polyvalent, reflecting the antibody diversity of the donor population. One gram of IgG contains 4×10^{18} molecules with more than 10^7 unique binding specificities.

Use Characteristics

Indications: To treat patients with primary immune deficiency (PID).

Limitations: IGSC provides only short-term passive immunity. Use appropriate vaccines to induce active immunity. Consider appropriate antibiotic or antiviral drugs for the treatment of active infections.

Contraindications:

Absolute: People with a history of anaphylactic or severe systemic response to IG preparations and people with selective IgA deficiency (serum IgA less than 0.05 g/L) who have known antibody against IgA.

Relative: None.

Do not administer to people with hyperprolinemia.

Immunodeficiency: IGSC may be indicated as immunoglobulin replacement therapy for certain immunocompromised people. The Advisory Committee on Immunization Practices (ACIP) explicitly recommends IG administration to symptomatic HIV-infected patients and other severely immunocompromised people exposed to measles, regardless of immunization status. Operationally defined, severe immunosuppression may result from congenital immunodeficiency, HIV infection, leukemia, lymphoma, aplastic anemia, generalized malignancy, or therapy with alkylating agents, antimetabolites, radiation, or large, sustained doses of corticosteroids.

Elderly: The clinical study of IGSC did not include a sufficient number of subjects 65 years of age and older to determine whether they respond differently from younger subjects.

Fertility Impairment: IGSC has not been evaluated for impairment of fertility.

Pregnancy: Category C. Use only if clearly needed. Animal reproduction studies have not been conducted. Generally, most IgG passage across the placenta occurs during the third trimester. Problems in humans have not been documented and are unlikely.

Lactation: It is not known if IGSC antibodies cross into human breast milk. Problems in humans have not been documented and are unlikely.

Children: IGSC was evaluated in 3 children and 7 adolescents with primary immunodeficiency. No pediatric-specific dose requirements were necessary to achieve the desired serum IgG levels. IGSC was not evaluated in neonates or infants.

Adverse Reactions: In clinical studies, IGSC has been shown to be well tolerated in both adult and pediatric subjects. Reactions similar to those reported with other IG products may also occur with IGSC (eg, hypersensitivity, renal dysfunction or failure, thrombotic events, aseptic meningitis syndrome, hemolysis, transfusion-associated acute lung injury).

Patients who receive IG therapy for the first time, who switch from another brand, or who have not received IG therapy within the previous 8 weeks may be at risk for developing reactions, including fever, chills, nausea, and vomiting. On rare occasions, these reactions may lead to shock. Monitor such patients for these reactions in a clinical setting.

Rarely, immediate anaphylactoid and hypersensitivity reactions may occur. In exceptional cases, sensitization to IgA may result in an anaphylactic reaction. If anaphylactic or anaphylactoid reactions are suspected, discontinue administration immediately.

In the clinical study of IGSC, the most frequent reactions occurred at injections sites. Injection-site reactions (eg, swelling, redness, heat, pain, itching) comprised 98% of local reactions. Other reported adverse events included headache (27% of patients), cough (16%), diarrhea (14%), fatigue (12%), back pain (10%), nausea (10%), upper abdominal pain (10%), and rash (10%).

Injection-site reactions: Injection-site reactions consisted mostly of mild or moderate swelling, redness, and itching. Most resolved within 4 days. The number of subjects reporting injection-site reactions decreased substantially with repeated use.

Pharmacologic & Dosing Characteristics

Dosage: The manufacturer recommends that patients start treatment with IGSC 1 week after receiving a regularly scheduled IGIV infusion.

Calculate the initial weekly IGSC dose (in grams) by multiplying the previous IGIV dose by a product-specific factor (see below), then dividing this dose into weekly doses based on the patient's previous IGIV treatment interval. For example, if IGIV was administered every 3 weeks, divide by 3. This dose of IGSC will provide a systemic IgG exposure (ie, area under the curve [AUC]) comparable to the previous IGIV treatment. Weekly administration of this dose will lead to stable steady-state serum IgG levels with lower IgG peak levels and higher IgG trough levels compared with monthly IGIV treatment.

The recommended weekly dose of IGSC is 100 to 200 mg/kg administered subcutaneously.

Multiply the previous IGIV dose by 1.53, then divide by the number of weeks between IGIV doses, to obtain the initial dose.

Route & Site: For subcutaneous infusion, preferentially in the abdomen, thighs, upper arms, and/or lateral hip. Change the actual point of injection with each weekly administration. Do not inject into a blood vessel.

For first infusion, administer at up to 15 mL/h per site. This may be increased up to 25 mL/h per site as tolerated. Do not exceed a total 50 mL/h for all sites combined.

Overdosage: Although few data are available, clinical experience with other IG preparations suggests that the major manifestations of overdosage would be related to fluid volume overload.

Additional Doses: Adjust doses over time to achieve the desired clinical response and serum IgG levels. Because there can be differences in the half-life of IgG among patients with PID, the dose and dosing interval may vary.

Missed Doses: Interrupting the recommended schedule or delaying subsequent doses does not require restarting the series.

Laboratory Tests: Serum IgG levels can be sampled at any time during routine weekly IGSC treatment. Subjects on IGSC therapy maintained relatively constant IgG levels, rather than the peak and trough pattern observed with monthly IGIV therapy.

Efficacy: An open-label, multicenter, single-arm clinical study evaluated efficacy, tolerability, and safety in 38 adult and pediatric subjects with PID. Subjects previously receiving monthly IGIV treatment were switched to IGSC weekly for 15 months. Weekly doses of IGSC ranged from 72 to 379 mg/kg body weight, which was 149% (range, 114% to 180%) of the previous IGIV dose. Subjects received a total of 2,264 infusions of IGSC. The number of injection sites per infusion ranged from 1 to 12. In 73% of infusions; the number of injection sites was 4 or fewer. For the efficacy phase, 38 subjects contributed 12,697 days of observation. The annual rate of serious bacterial infections was 0 per patient-year, with an upper 99% CI of 0.132. The annual rate of any infection was 2.76 infections per patient-year (95% CI, 2.235-3.37). Of the 38 subjects, 27 (71%) used antibiotics for prophylaxis or treatment, at a rate of 48.5 days per patient-year. These patients missed a mean of 2.06 days of school or work due to infection per year.

Onset: After 18 subjects reached steady state with weekly administration of IGSC, peak serum IgG levels were observed after a mean of 2.9 days (range, 0 to 7 days).

Duration: Weekly dosing leads to a steady-state serum concentration.

Pharmacokinetics: Subcutaneous administration of IgG decreases bioavailability compared with IV administration. Various factors, such as site of administration and IgG catabolism, affect absorption. Peak serum IgG levels are lower with IGSC than with IGIV. Subcutaneous administration results in relatively stable steady-state serum IgG levels when administered on a weekly basis. This serum IgG profile is representative of that seen in a normal population.

Pharmacokinetics was evaluated in 19 PID subjects in the 15-month study. All subjects were treated previously with IGIV and were switched to weekly subcutaneous treatment with IGSC. After a 3-month wash-in/wash-out period, doses were adjusted individually with the goal of providing a systemic serum IgG exposure not inferior to that of the previous weekly equivalent IGIV dose. For the subjects completing the wash-in/wash-out period, the average dose adjustment for IGSC was 153% (range, 126% to 187%) of the previous weekly equivalent IGIV dose. After 12 weeks of treatment with IGSC at this individually adjusted dose, the final steady-state AUC determinations were made in 18 of 19 subjects. The geometric mean ratio of the steady-state AUCs, standardized to a weekly treatment period, for IGSC versus IGIV treatment was 1.002 (range, 0.77 to 1.2) with a 90% confidence limit of 0.951 to 1.055 for the 18 subjects. The study assessed the ratio of serum IgG trough levels with IGSC compared to the previous trough levels with IGIV associated with matching AUCs. The calculated IGSC:IGIV ratio of 1.3 ($\pm$15% of this value, or $\pm$0.2) can be used to assess dosing with IGSC by providing a steady-state target IgG trough level, which may be assumed to be within the range of 1.1 to 1.5 times the previous steady-state trough levels with IGIV. However, use the patient's clinical response as the primary consideration in dose adjustment. With a mean treatment dose of 152 mg/kg for IGIV (range, 86 to 254 mg/kg) and 228 mg/kg for IGSC (range, 141 to 381 mg/kg), the mean IgG peak levels were 2,564 mg/dL for IGIV (range, 2,046 to 3,456 mg/dL) and 1,616 mg/dL for IGSC (range, 1,090 to 2,825 mg/dL). The mean IgG trough levels were 1,127 mg/dL for IGIV (range, 702 to 1,810 mg/dL) and 1,448 mg/dL for IGSC (range, 952 to 2,623 mg/dL).

Protective Level: The minimum serum concentration of IgG necessary for protection against infections has not been established. Based on clinical experience, a target serum IgG trough level (ie, just before next infusion) of at least 500 mg/dL has been proposed for IGIV therapy.

Mechanism: Supplementation of a broad spectrum of opsonizing and neutralizing IgG antibodies against a wide variety of bacterial and viral agents.

Drug Interactions: IGSC may diminish the antibody response to attenuated measles, mumps, rubella, and varicella vaccines through antigen-antibody antagonism. As a general rule, administer live virus vaccines 14 to 30 days before or several months after administration of any immune globulin or other blood product. Alternately, check antibody titers or repeat the vaccine dose 3 months after IG administration. Base the interval on the dose of IgG administered: 3 months for 3 to 10 mg/kg, 4 months for 20 mg/kg, 5 months for 40 mg/kg, 6 months for 60 to 100 mg/kg, 7 months for 160 mg/kg, 8 months for 300 to 400 mg/kg, 10 months for 1 g/kg, and 11 months for 2 g/kg.

IGSC is unlikely to interfere with development of immunity following oral poliovirus or yellow fever vaccination. However, it may be prudent not to administer these vaccines shortly after IG administration.

Lab Interference: After injection of immunoglobulins, the transitory rise of the various passively transferred antibodies in the patient's blood may yield positive serological testing results, with the potential for misleading interpretation. Passive transmission of antibodies to erythrocyte antigens (eg, A, B, D) may cause a positive direct or indirect antiglobulin (Coombs) test.

Patient Information: If home administration is appropriate, provide the patient with instructions on subcutaneous infusion. This should include the type of equipment to be used along with its maintenance, proper infusion techniques, selection of appropriate infusion sites, maintaining a treatment diary, and measures to take in case of adverse reactions.

Pharmaceutical Characteristics

Concentration: 20% (200 mg/mL) protein solution, at least 98% IgG.

Quality Assay: Plasma used in manufacture is tested for HBsAg and antibodies to hepatitis C virus (HCV) and HIV-1 and -2, as well as nucleic acid testing (NAT) for hepatitis A virus (HAV), hepatitis B virus (HBV), HCV, HIV-1, and parvovirus B19 (B19). The acceptable limit for B19 in the fractionation pool is up to 10^4 IU B19 DNA per mL. IGSC may carry a risk of transmitting infectious agents (eg, viruses, and theoretically, the Creutzfeldt-Jakob disease agent). This risk has been reduced by screening plasma donors, by plasma testing, and by manufacturing processes. Report any infections thought to have been possibly transmitted by this product to CSL Behring at 800-504-5434.

Packaging: Single-use vials containing 200 mg IgG per mL: 1 g/5 mL (NDC#: 44206-0451-01), 2 g/10 mL (44206-0452-02), 4 g/20 mL (44206-0454-04)

Doseform: Liquid

Appearance: Clear and pale yellow to light brown

Solvent: Water for injection

Adjuvant: None

Preservative: None

Allergens: ≤ 50 mcg/mL IgA

Immune Globulin Subcutaneous (Human)

Excipients: L-proline 210 to 290 mmol/L, polysorbate 80 10 to 30 mg/L, trace amounts of sodium

pH: 4.6 to 5.2

Osmolality: Data not provided.

Shelf Life: Data not provided.

Storage/Stability: Store at room temperature (up to 25°C [77°F]). Discard if frozen. Do not shake. Keep in original carton to protect from light.

Handling: Before use, allow solution to reach room temperature. Do not shake. Do not mix with other medicinal products. Follow the manufacturer's instructions for filling the pump reservoir and preparing the pump, administration tubing, and Y-site connection tubing, if needed. Prime the administration tubing to ensure no air is left in the tubing or needle by filling the tubing/needle.

Production Process: Manufactured from large pools of human plasma by cold-alcohol fractionation, octanoic acid fractionation, and anion-exchange chromatography, without chemical alteration or enzymatic degradation. Viral inactivation steps include pH 4 incubation to inactivate enveloped viruses and virus filtration to remove, by size exclusion, both enveloped and nonenveloped viruses as small as approximately 20 nanometers. In addition, a depth-filtration step contributes to virus reduction. Steps to reduce agents of transmissible spongiform encephalopathy include octanoic acid fractionation, virus filtration and depth filtration. Total mean cumulative virus reductions ranged from 7.8 to 17.7 $\log_{10}$ or more against various model enveloped and nonenveloped viruses.

Media: Human plasma

Disease Epidemiology

See IGIV monograph.

Other Information

Perspective: See IGIV monograph.

First Licensed: March 1, 2010

Discontinued Products: *Vivaglobin* (CSL Behring), licensed January 9, 2006, distributed through 2011.

References: Waniewski J, Gardulf A, Hammarström L. Bioavailability of gamma-globulin after subcutaneous infusions in patients with common variable immunodeficiency. *J Clin Immunol.* 1994;14(2):90-97.

Cytomegalovirus Immune Globulin Intravenous (Human)

Anti-Infective Immune Globulins

Name:
  CytoGam

Manufacturer:
  Talecris Biotherapeutics and Baxter Pharmaceutical Solutions, distributed by CSL Behring

Synonyms: CMV-IG, CMV-IGIV

Immunologic Characteristics

Microorganism: Virus (double-stranded DNA), enveloped, human cytomegalovirus, human herpesvirus-5, genus *Cytomegalovirus*, subfamily Betaherpesviridae, family Herpesviridae

Viability: Inactive, passive, transient

Antigenic Form: Human immunoglobulin, unmodified

Antigenic Type: Protein, IgG antibody, polyclonal, primarily monomeric

Strains: Harvested without regard to viral strain, although screening assay is based on Davis strain.

Use Characteristics

Indications: For the prophylaxis of cytomegalovirus (CMV) disease associated with transplantation of kidney, lung, liver, pancreas, or heart. Consider prophylactic CMV-IGIV in combination with ganciclovir (*Cytovene*, Roche) in transplants from CMV-seropositive donors into CMV-negative recipients.

Unlabeled Uses: For prevention or attenuation of primary CMV disease in immunosuppressed recipients of organ transplants (eg, bone marrow, liver). Also used in immunocompromised patients with CMV pneumonia or to prevent CMV disease.

Limitations: CMV-IGIV provides only short-term passive immunity, primarily against CMV. Select appropriate antiviral agents (eg, foscarnet, ganciclovir) to treat active infections, such as CMV retinitis.

Combined therapy with ganciclovir and CMV-IGIV may be more effective than either drug alone.

Contraindications:

Absolute: None

Relative: Patients with a history of a severe reaction associated with administration of IM or IV human immune globulin products.

Patients with selective immunoglobulin A deficiency (IgA) have the potential for developing anti-IgA antibodies and could have anaphylactic reactions to subsequent administration of blood products (including immune globulin preparations) that contain IgA.

Immunodeficiency: No impairment of effect is likely. CMV-IGIV may be indicated in certain immunodeficient patients.

Elderly: No specific information is available about geriatric use of CMV-IGIV. Problems have not been documented and are unlikely.

Pregnancy: Category C. Use only if clearly needed. It is not specifically known if CMV antibodies cross the placenta. Intact IgG increasingly crosses the placenta from the maternal circulation after 30 weeks gestation. Problems in humans have not been documented and are unlikely.

Cytomegalovirus Immune Globulin Intravenous (Human)

Lactation: It is not known if anti-CMV antibodies are excreted in breast milk. Problems in humans have not been documented and are unlikely.

Children: CMV-IGIV generally is safe and effective in children.

Adverse Reactions: Flushing, chills, muscle cramps, back pain, fever, nausea, vomiting, and wheezing were the most common adverse reactions (less than 5% of infusions), and usually were related to infusion rates. Hypotension has not been reported. Theoretically, severe reactions such as angioedema and anaphylactic shock might occur rarely. Consider slowing the rate immediately or interrupting the infusion, according to the patient's response.

CMV-IGIV is made from human plasma. Like other plasma products, it carries the possibility for transmission of blood-borne pathogenic agents. The risk of transmission of recognized blood-borne viruses is considered to be low because of screening of plasma donors, an added viral inactivation step, and removal properties in the Cohn-Oncley 6 & 9 cold-ethanol precipitation procedure used for purification of immune globulin products. Because new blood-borne agents may yet emerge, some of which may not be inactivated or eliminated by the manufacturing process or by solvent-detergent treatment, give CMV-IGIV only if a benefit is expected.

Pharmacologic & Dosing Characteristics

Dosage: Preoperative prophylaxis is preferred. Otherwise, administer within 72 hours after transplant. Dosage depends on the organ transplanted. For kidneys, give 150 mg/kg initially. At 2, 4, 6, and 8 weeks after transplant give 100 mg/kg. At 12 and 16 weeks after transplant give 50 mg/kg.

For other organs, give 150 mg/kg initially. At 2, 4, 6, and 8 weeks after transplant give 150 mg/kg. At 12 and 16 weeks after transplant give 100 mg/kg.

Route & Site: IV infusion starting at 15 mg/kg/h, progressing to 30 mg/kg/h, and then to 60 mg/kg/h if no reaction occurs. Use an IV infusion pump for administration. In-line filters are recommended. The maximum recommended rate of infusion is 60 mg/kg/h (with total volume 75 mL/h or lower). If any reaction occurs, slow or stop the infusion until the reaction abates. Use epinephrine or an antihistamine to treat allergic symptoms.

Overdosage: Although few data are available, clinical experience with other immune globulin preparations suggests that the major manifestations of overdosage would be related to fluid volume overload.

Efficacy: In a clinical trial, the incidence of virologically confirmed, CMV-associated syndromes in renal transplant recipients at risk for primary CMV disease was reduced from 60% in 35 control patients to 21% in 24 CMV-IGIV recipients ($P < 0.01$). Marked leukopenia fell from 37% in controls to 4% in recipients ($P < 0.01$). Fungal or parasitic superinfections were not seen in recipients but occurred in 20% of controls ($P = 0.05$). Serious CMV disease dropped from 46% to 13%. The incidence of CMV pneumonia also fell, from 17% among controls to 4% among recipients, but this difference was not statistically significant. No effect on rates of viral isolation or seroconversion was seen, although the rate of viremia was less in CMV-IGIV recipients.

In a later, nonrandomized trial in 36 renal transplant recipients, the rate of virologically confirmed, CMV-associated syndrome fell to 36% of recipients. The rates of CMV-associated pneumonia, CMV-associated hepatitis, and concomitant fungal or parasitic superinfection were similar to those observed in the earlier trial.

Onset: Rapid

Duration: Mean half-life is 21 days, shorter in transplant recipients, where half-lives have been measured as 8 days immediately after transplant, or 13 to 15 days if given 60 days or longer after transplant.

Pharmacokinetics: Immunoglobulins are primarily eliminated by catabolism.

Protective Level: Unknown, and may not be clinically relevant because CMV is an intracellular pathogen.

Mechanism: CMV-IGIV can raise relevant antibody titers to levels sufficient to attenuate or reduce the incidence of serious CMV disease.

Drug Interactions: CMV-IGIV may diminish the antibody response to attenuated measles, mumps, and rubella vaccines through antigen-antibody antagonism. For a vaccine containing measles virus, wait 6 months after giving CMV-IGIV. For varicella vaccine, wait 5 months after CMV-IGIV. Alternately, administer live virus vaccines during this interval if corresponding antibody titers are measured 3 months after CMV-IGIV administration. Revaccinate if necessary.

IGIM does not appear to interfere with development of immunity following oral poliovirus (OPV) or yellow fever vaccination. However, it may be prudent not to administer these vaccines shortly after CMV-IGIV administration. Exceptions include unexpected travel to or contact with epidemic or endemic areas or people. If OPV is given with or shortly after CMV-IGIV, repeat the OPV dose 3 months later if protection is still needed.

It is not known if CMV-IGIV interferes with the efficacy of other attenuated vaccines (eg, adenovirus, Bacillus Calmette-Guérin, typhoid, vaccinia). It may be prudent to avoid administering these vaccines shortly after CMV-IGIV administration unless unavoidable.

Antibody responses to inactivated vaccines are not substantially affected by IGIVs. Consider giving a booster dose of routine childhood vaccines 3 or 4 months after the last dose of CMV-IG to ensure immunity to diphtheria, tetanus, pertussis, *Haemophilus influenzae* type b, and poliovirus.

Lab Interference: After administration, a transitory increase of passively transferred antibodies in the patient's blood may result in misleading positive results in serological testing (eg, anti-HBs).

Pharmaceutical Characteristics

Concentration: 40 to 60 mg Ig per mL, primarily IgG

Quality Assay: Plasma units screened by ELISA, using the Davis strain of virus, for anti-CMV IgG titers 1:1,000 and higher. A proprietary assay is conducted to guarantee minimum CMV antibody titers of 1:7,000 and higher in the finished product. Using that assay, *CytoGam* lots must achieve a potency ratio of 0.8. In contrast, 9 unselected commercial IGIV antibody preparations had a ratio of approximately 0.3.

Packaging: 2,500 mg ± 500 mg per 50 mL single-use vial (NDC#: 44206-0532-11).

Doseform: Solution

Appearance: Colorless and translucent

Diluent:

For infusion: Administer directly or piggyback into 0.9% sodium chloride or 2.5%, 5%, 10%, or 20% dextrose in water (with or without sodium chloride). Do not dilute the CMV-IGIV primary IV fluid higher than 1:2 (ie, 50 mL CMV-IGIV with 100 mL or lower infusion fluid).

Adjuvant: None

Preservative: None

Allergens: 30 to 200 mcg/mL IgA, trace amounts of IgM, 10 mg/mL human serum albumin

Excipients: 5% sucrose. The sodium content is 20 to 30 mEq/L (1 to 1.5 mEq/50 mL).

pH: 5.5

Cytomegalovirus Immune Globulin Intravenous (Human)

Shelf Life: Expires within 36 months

Storage/Stability: Store at 2° to 8°C (36° to 46°F). The product can tolerate up to 7 days at 27°C (80°F). Shipped in insulated containers with coolant packs, usually by overnight courier.

Begin infusion within 6 hours and complete within 12 hours after entering the vial. Do not mix CMV-IGIV with other drugs.

Handling: Do not shake; avoid foaming to prevent protein degradation.

Production Process: Purified from pooled adult human plasma selected for high titers of neutralizing antibody against CMV, using a proprietary screening assay. Pooled plasma is fractionated by cold-ethanol precipitation of the proteins according to Cohn-Oncley methods 6 & 9 cold-ethanol fractionation process. IgG is isolated from effluent III by ultrafiltration and stabilized with sucrose and albumin. A solvent-detergent viral-inactivation process is used to decrease the possibility of transmission of blood-borne pathogens. Solvent-detergent treatment is known to inactivate a wide spectrum of lipid-enveloped viruses, including HIV-1, HIV-2, hepatitis B virus, and hepatitis C virus.

Media: Human plasma, at least 2,000 to 5,000 donor units per lot

Disease Epidemiology

Incidence: Sixty percent to 80% of the population of developed countries and almost 100% of the population in developing nations are eventually infected.

From 1% to 2% of all fetuses are infected in utero, of which 10% to 15% will suffer lasting damage, usually to the brain or organ of Corti. At least 3,000 American newborn infants are believed to be damaged by intrauterine CMV infection each year, resulting in mental retardation, seizure disorders, neuromuscular dysfunction, or premature death. Approximately 30,000 to 40,000 infected infants are asymptomatic at birth and subsequently develop deafness or other neurologic handicaps during their lifetime.

The primary risk groups among adults are CMV-seronegative kidney transplant recipients, other patients receiving immunosuppressive therapy, and patients with AIDS.

Susceptible Pools: Fetuses, organ transplant recipients, and patients with AIDS.

Transmission: Intimate exposure by mucosal contact with infectious tissues, secretions, and excretions. CMV is excreted in urine, saliva, breast milk, cervical secretions, and semen. A fetus may be infected in utero.

Incubation: Illness caused by transfusion begins 3 to 8 weeks after the transfusion. Infections acquired during birth are first demonstrable 3 to 12 weeks after delivery.

Communicability: Virus is excreted in urine and saliva for many months and may persist or be episodic for years after primary infection. After neonatal infection, virus may be excreted for 5 to 6 years. Adults may excrete virus for shorter periods, but the virus persists as a latent infection. Excretion recurs with immunodeficiency and immunosuppression.

Other Information

Perspective:
1956: Rowe, Smith, and colleagues isolate causative organism, named CMV, in 1960.
1974: Elek and Stern develop AD-169 CMV-lysate vaccine strain.
1975: Plotkin and colleagues develop attenuated Towne strain on the 125th passage in WI-38 human diploid cells, using virus harvested from a congenitally infected infant named Towne.
1978: Early trials of CMV antibody preparations begin.
1987: Snydman and colleagues develop CMV immune globulin.

First Licensed: April 17, 1990 (designated an orphan drug August 3, 1987; treatment IND #1579 approved October 1987). Distributed by Connaught from November 1991 until 1994. Distributed by MedImmune from 1992 to 2006. Product sold to CSL Behring in December 2006.

Cytomegalovirus Immune Globulin Intravenous (Human)

References: Adler SP. Cytomegalovirus hyperimmune globulin: who needs it? *Pediatr Infect Dis J.* 1992;11:266-269.

Bass EB, et al. Efficacy of immune globulin in preventing complications of bone marrow transplantation: a meta-analysis. *Bone Marrow Transplant.* 1993;12:273-282.

Nigro G, Adler SP, La Torre R, Best AM; Congenital Cytomegalovirus Collaborating Group. Passive immunization during pregnancy for congenital cytomegalovirus infection. *N Engl J Med.* 2005;353:1350-1362.

Snydman DR. Cytomegalovirus immunoglobulins in the prevention and treatment of cytomegalovirus disease. *Rev Infect Dis.* 1990;12(suppl 7):S839-S848.

Snydman DR. Historical overview of the use of cytomegalovirus hyperimmune globulin in organ transplantation. *Transpl Infect Dis.* 2001;3(suppl 2):6-13.

Hepatitis B Immune Globulin (Human)

Anti-Infective Immune Globulins

Names:
HepaGam B
HyperHep B S/D
Nabi-HB

Manufacturers:
Cangene Corporation
Talecris Biotherapeutics
Biotest Pharmaceuticals

Synonyms: HBIG

Comparison: Therapeutically equivalent, except for *HepaGam B*'s use in liver transplant recipients.

Immunologic Characteristics

Microorganism: Virus (double-stranded DNA), enveloped, family Hepadnaviridae

Viability: Inactive, passive, transient

Antigenic Form: Human immunoglobulin, unmodified

Antigenic Type: Protein, IgG antibody (anti-HBsAb) to hepatitis B surface antigen (HBsAg), polyclonal, primarily monomeric

Strains: Harvested without regard to viral subtype

Use Characteristics

Indications: For passive, transient, postexposure prevention of hepatitis B infection. Such exposures may include parenteral exposure (eg, needlestick, human bites that penetrate the skin), mucous membrane contact (eg, accidental splashes), sexual contact, or oral ingestion (eg, pipetting accidents) of HBsAg-positive materials such as blood, plasma, or serum.

For passive, transient, postexposure prophylaxis of hepatitis B in infants born to HBsAg-positive mothers. Such infants are at risk of being infected with hepatitis B virus and becoming chronic carriers. The risk is especially great if the mother is HBeAg-positive.

HBIG is most effective when used within 7 days of exposure, or within 14 days in the case of sexual contact.

Cangene: For hepatitis B-positive liver transplant recipients, as prolonged therapy, to prevent hepatitis B recurrence. *HepaGam B* is recommended in patients who have no or low levels of viral replication at the time of liver transplantation.

Unlabeled Uses: HBIG continues to be evaluated for efficacy in other situations that involve nonparenteral exposure to hepatitis B, such as among dialysis patients, hospital workers, and close contacts of HBsAg-positive patients.

Hepatitis B vaccination is appropriate for patients expected to receive human alpha$_1$-proteinase inhibitor (*Prolastin*). If sufficient time is not available to develop adequate antibody responses, give a single dose of HBIG with the initial dose of vaccine. *Prolastin* is produced from heat-treated, pooled human plasma that may contain the causative agents of hepatitis and other viral diseases. Manufacturing procedures at plasma collection centers, testing laboratories, and fractionation facilities are designed to reduce the risk of transmitting viral infection, but that risk cannot be totally eliminated.

HBIG has been given in utero to fetuses of HBsAg-positive mothers during cordocentesis.

Limitations: HBIG provides only short-term passive immunity. Use hepatitis B vaccine to induce active immunity.

Liver transplant: The clinical trial evaluating *HepaGam B* in liver transplant patients selected patients with no or low replication status only. *HepaGam B* therapy has not been evaluated in combination with antiviral therapy post-transplantation.

Outmoded Practices: Unlike immunoglobulin harvested from animals, do not perform skin tests prior to administration of HBIG. In most humans, intradermal injection of concentrated immune globulin causes a localized area of inflammation that can be misinterpreted as a positive allergic reaction. This reaction is caused by localized tissue irritation of a chemical nature. Misinterpretation of such a test may cause urgently needed immunoglobulin to be withheld from a patient who is not actually allergic to it.

True allergic responses to HBIG given IM are rare.

Contraindications:

Absolute: None

Relative: Use caution in patients with a history of systemic allergic reactions following administration of human immune globulins. Patients with selective immunoglobulin A (IgA) deficiency have the potential for developing anti-IgA antibodies and could have anaphylactic reactions to subsequent administration of blood products (including immune globulins) containing IgA.

Immunodeficiency: No impairment of effect is likely. HBIG may be indicated in certain immunodeficient patients.

Elderly: No specific information is available about geriatric use of HBIG. Problems have not been documented and are unlikely.

Pregnancy: Category C. Use only if clearly needed. Clinical experience suggests that there are no known adverse effects on the fetus from immune globulins. Intact IgG increasingly crosses the placenta from the maternal circulation after 30 weeks gestation. Problems in humans have not been reported and are unlikely.

Lactation: It is not known if anti-HBs antibodies are excreted in human breast milk. Problems in humans have not been documented and are unlikely.

Children: Safe and effective in newborns, infants, and children.

Adverse Reactions: Anaphylaxis occurs rarely after immune globulin administration. With IM administration, pain and tenderness at injection site, urticaria, or angioedema may occur. In an uncontrolled pharmacokinetic trial of healthy volunteers, reported injection-site reactions included pain (12%), ache (3%), erythema (3%), burning (3%), and heat (1%). Systemic events reported included headache (26%), malaise (5%), nausea (5%), myalgia (5%), and diarrhea (3%).

With IV infusion, the most common expected adverse drug reactions are chills, fever, headaches, vomiting, allergic reactions, nausea, arthralgia, and moderate low back pain. In a clinical trial in liver transplant patients, tremor and hypotension were reported in 2 of 14 patients who received IV infusions of *HepaGam B*. Certain adverse reactions may be related to rate of infusion. Follow the recommended infusion rate closely. Carefully observe patients for symptoms throughout the infusion period and immediately after an infusion. Adverse events occurring in more than 10% of liver transplant recipients included the following: splenomegaly; presbyopia; aphthous stomatitis, diarrhea, dyspepsia, gingival hyperplasia; fatigue, peripheral edema, pyrexia; hepatobiliary disease; liver transplant rejection; infectious diarrhea, pnemonia, sepsis; hyperglycemia; back pain; amnesia, essential tremor, headache; agitation; nocturia; pleural effusion; pruritus, rash; hypertension, hypotension.

Hepatitis B Immune Globulin (Human)

Pharmacologic & Dosing Characteristics

Dosage:

Adults and children: 0.06 mL/kg (usually 3 to 5 mL). Equivalent to 10 mg IgG/kg.

Give as soon as possible after exposure, preferably within 7 days. In the case of sexual contact, give within 14 days. Repeat 28 to 30 days after exposure.

If the exposed patient fails to respond to a primary vaccine series, administer either a single dose of HBIG and another dose of vaccine as soon as possible after exposure, or two 0.06 mL/kg doses of HBIG, 1 dose as soon as possible and a second dose 1 month later.

Newborns born of HBsAg-positive mothers: 0.5 mL. Give first HBIG dose as soon as possible, preferably 12 hours or less after birth. Also give appropriate volume of either hepatitis B vaccine formulation within 7 days after birth. If the first dose of vaccine is delayed as long as 3 months, give a repeat HBIG dose of 0.5 mL at 3 months of age. If hepatitis B vaccine is declined, repeat HBIG at 3 and 6 months of age.

Liver transplant: To prevent hepatitis B recurrence, administer 20,000 units/dose to attain anti-HBs serum levels of 500 units/L or more. Give the first dose concurrently with grafting of the transplanted liver, followed by daily doses for days 1 through 7, then dosing every 2 weeks through week 12, followed by monthly dosing for month 4 and beyond. Adjust dose volume based on the concentration of the product used. Adjust dose for patients who fail to reach anti-HBs concentrations of 500 units within the first week after liver transplantation. Patients who have surgical bleeding or abdominal fluid draining of more than 500 mL, or who undergo plasmapheresis, are particularly susceptible to extensive loss of anti-HBs. In these cases, increase the dosing regimen to 10,000 units IV every 6 hours until the target anti-HBs is reached.

Route & Site: IM for postexposure prophylaxis indications, preferably in the gluteal or deltoid region in adults and children. The anterolateral thigh is preferred in newborns. Do not inject IV.

For liver transplant indications: Administer IV at 2 mL/min through a separate line using an IV administration set via an infusion pump. Decrease the rate of infusion to 1 mL/min or slower if the patient develops discomfort, infusion-related adverse events, or if there is concern about speed of infusion.

Overdosage: Although few data are available, clinical experience with other immune globulins suggests that the major manifestations of overdosage would be pain and tenderness at the injection site. Experience reported with another IGIV preparation suggests that doses of more than 1 g IG per kilogram body weight are tolerated.

Additional Doses: In adults, repeat HBIG 28 to 30 days after the first HBIG dose, if vaccine is declined. If hepatitis B vaccine is declined in infants of HBsAg-positive mothers, give HBIG at birth and at 3 and 6 months of age.

Laboratory Tests: Perform regular monitoring of serum HBsAg and anti-HBs antibody before infusion to track treatment response and allow for treatment adjustment. Regularly monitor liver transplant patients for serum anti-HBs antibody levels using a quantitative assay.

Efficacy: HBIG reduces disease incidence by 75% among sexual partners of HBsAg-positive people, if administered within 2 weeks of the last sexual exposure to a person with acute hepatitis B infection. In infants of HBsAg-positive mothers, use of HBIG and vaccine protects 85% to 98% from infection. Regimens involving either multiple doses of HBIG alone or the vaccine series alone have a 70% to 90% efficacy, while a single HBIG dose alone has 50% efficacy.

After accidental percutaneous exposures (eg, needlesticks) involving HBsAg, the incidence of both clinical and subclinical hepatitis B during the following 6 months was 0.7% in a group treated with HBIG and 6.1% in a group treated with IGIM. After 6 months, 32% of the IGIM group demonstrated anti-HBs antibodies, compared with 6% of the HBIG group.

Liver transplant: HBIG products are most effective in patients with no or low levels of HBV replication at time of transplantation. A trial examining *HepaGam B* to prevent hepatitis B recurrence after liver transplantation was conducted as a multicenter, open-label, superiority study involving HBsAg-positive/HBeAg-negative liver transplant patients. An active treatment group received *HepaGam B* during transplant and over the course of a year. With a targeted potency of 550 units/mL at the time of manufacture, the 35 mL doses of *HepaGam B* contained 17,000 to 23,000 units of anti-HBs. The retrospective untreated control group of historical patients was assessed by chart review. HBV recurrence occurred in 2 of 15 *HepaGam B* patients (13%) compared with 12 of 14 untreated control patients (86%, $P < 0.001$). Time to recurrence was 358 days for 2 *HepaGam B*-treated HBV recurrent patients. In contrast, the retrospective untreated control patients had a median time to recurrence of 88 days (95% CI: 47 to 125 days). Survival calculations showed that 93% (14 of 15) of the patients in the treatment group survived for 1 year or longer compared with 43% (6 of 14) of control patients. One patient in the active treatment group died 266 days post-transplant. The median time to death for the control patients was 339 days. The end points for HBV recurrence were supported by an observed drop in anti-HBs levels and elevated liver function tests at the time of recurrence.

Onset: Antibodies appear within 1 to 6 days after IM administration and peak in 3 to 11 days.

Duration: Mean half-life is 17 to 25 days (range, 6 to 35). Clinical protection typically persists for approximately 2 months.

Pharmacokinetics: Immunoglobulins are primarily eliminated by catabolism.

Solvent/detergent treatment does not affect the kinetics of immune globulins. Pharmacokinetic trials of *Nabi-HB* given IM to 48 healthy volunteers found a half-life of 24.8 ± 5.6 days. The clearance rate was 0.433 ± 0.144 L/day and the volume of distribution was 15.3 ± 62 L. Maximum concentration was reached in 6.6 ± 3.0 days. The maximum concentration of anti-HBs achieved was consistent with another HBIG preparation assessed in the same trial.

In a pharmacokinetic trial of *BayHep B* (comparable to *HyperHep B S/D*), peak anti-HBs serum levels were seen in the following distribution: day 3, 39%; day 7, 42%; day 14, 11%; day 21, 8%. Mean half-life values were between 17.5 and 25 days, ranging from 5.9 to 35 days.

In a pharmacokinetic trial of *HepaGam B*, 70 volunteers developed mean peak concentrations within 4 to 5 days of administration. Mean elimination half-lives after IM administration were 22 to 25 days. The mean clearance rate was 0.21 to 0.24 L/day and the volume of distribution was approximately 7.5 L.

Liver transplant: The 35 mL doses given to HBsAg-positive/HBeAg-negative liver transplant patients yielded anti-HBs trough levels of more than 500 units/L in 99% of assays. Values below the target trough were observed only in the 2 patients with HBV recurrence who had anti-HBs levels of less than 150 units/L at the time of seroconversion.

Protective Level: Anti-HBs titer of 10 milliunits/mL or more.

Mechanism: Specific neutralization of hepatitis B virus, by binding to the surface antigen and reducing the rate of hepatitis B infection. Hepatitis B virus reinfection after liver transplantation results from exposure of the new liver graft to hepatitis B virus. Reinfection may occur immediately at the time of liver reperfusion due to circulating virus or later from virus retained in extrahepatic sites. The mechanism whereby HBIG protects the transplanted liver against HBV reinfection is not well understood. HBIG may protect naive hepatocytes against infection through blockage of a putative HBV receptor. Or HBIG may neutralize circulating virions through immune precipitation and immune-complex formation or may trigger an antibody-dependent cell-mediated cytotoxicity response resulting in target cell lysis. In addition, HBIG has been reported to bind to hepatocytes and interact with HBsAg within cells. Regardless of the mechanism, there is evidence of a dose-dependent response to HBIG treatment.

Drug Interactions: There is no significant interaction between simultaneous administration of HBIG and hepatitis B vaccine if administered at separate sites.

Inactivated vaccines are not generally affected by circulating antibodies or administration of exogenous antibodies. Immunize with such vaccines at any time before or after antibody administration.

HBIG may diminish the antibody response to attenuated measles, mumps, rubella, or varicella vaccines through antigen-antibody antagonism. As a general rule, administer live virus vaccines 14 to 30 days before or 12 weeks after immune globulin administration. Alternatively, administer live virus vaccines during this interval if corresponding antibody titers are measured 3 months after HBIG administration. Revaccinate if necessary.

IGIM does not appear to interfere with development of immunity following oral poliovirus or yellow fever vaccination. However, it may be prudent not to administer these vaccines shortly after HBIG administration. Exceptions include unexpected travel to or contact with epidemic or endemic areas or people. If oral poliovirus vaccine (OPV) is given with, or shortly after, HBIG, repeat the OPV dose 3 months later if immunization is still indicated.

It is not known if HBIG interferes with the efficacy of other attenuated vaccines (eg, adenovirus, Bacillus Calmette-Guérin, typhoid, vaccinia). Interactions are unlikely, but it may be prudent to separate administration of HBIG from these attenuated vaccines by several weeks, unless coadministration is unavoidable.

As with other drugs administered by IM injection, give HBIG with caution to patients receiving anticoagulant therapy.

Lab Interference:

Cangene: Parenteral products containing maltose may cause misinterpretation of glucose concentrations by certain blood glucose testing systems (eg, those based on the glucose dehydrogenase pyrroloquinolinequinone [GDH-PQQ] method). This can result in falsely elevated glucose readings and, consequently, in the inappropriate administration of insulin, resulting in life-threatening hypoglycemia. Cases of true hypoglycemia may go untreated if the hypoglycemic state is masked by falsely elevated results. A transitory increase of passively transferred antibodies in the patient's blood may result in misleading positive results in serological testing (eg, Coombs test).

Pharmaceutical Characteristics

Concentration: Not less than 80% monomeric IgG form

Biotest: 4% to 6% protein. Each vial contains more than 312 units anti-HBs per mL, by comparison with the World Health Organization (WHO) standard.

Cangene: 5% (50 mg/mL protein, greater than 312 international units per mL)

Talecris: 15% to 18% protein

Quality Assay: Meets potency of US Reference Standard anti-HBs Immune Globulin. Contains anti-HBs titer 1:100,000 or more by radioimmunoassay (RIA) or passive hemagglutination (PHA), at least 312 units/mL. Each unit of plasma must be nonreactive for HBsAg. All lots produced since April 1985 have been free of detectable HIV-1 antibodies.

Like other specific immune globulin products, HBIG has a target potency of more than 312 units/mL to account for variability in the potency assay and changes in potency over time. The potency assay has a relative standard deviation of approximately 10%. Based on a target potency of 550 units/mL, the actual potency test result may vary from approximately 400 to 700 units/mL (3 times the relative standard deviation). The measured potency is provided on the container label. Due to the inherent variability of the potency assay, calculate doses to prevent hepatitis B recurrence after liver transplantation based on the measure potency stamped on the vial label.

USP requirement: No ultracentrifugally detectable fragments or aggregates with sedimentation coefficient greater than 12S.

Packaging:

Biotest: 1 mL single-dose vial (NDC#: 59730-4202-01), 5 mL single-dose vial (59730-4203-01)

Cangene: 1 mL single-dose vial (NDC#: 53270-0052-01), 5 mL single-dose vial (53270-0051-01)

Talecris: 0.5 mL single-dose syringe with 25-gauge, ⅝-inch needle (NDC#: 13533-0636-03), 1 mL single-dose syringe with 22-gauge, 1¼-inch needle (13533-0636-02), 1 mL, single-dose vial (13533-0636-01), 5 mL single-dose vial (13533-0636-05)

Doseform: Solution

Appearance: Do not use if turbid.

Biotest: Clear to opalescent liquid

Cangene: Clear to opalescent liquid

Talecris: Clear solution, slightly amber, moderately viscous liquid

Solvent:

Biotest: Sodium chloride and glycine

Cangene: Maltose 10%

Talecris: Glycine 0.21 to 0.32 M. Potency may be adjusted with Cohn fraction II immune globulin.

Adjuvant: None

Preservative: None

Allergens:

Biotest: IgA content not described

Cangene: Less than 40 mcg/mL IgA

Talecris: 0.1 to 1 mg/mL IgA at 16.5% protein

Excipients:

Biotest: 0.07 M sodium chloride, 0.15 M glycine, 0.01% polysorbate 80

Cangene: 0.03% polysorbate 80

Talecris: 0.21 to 0.32 M glycine, pH adjusted with sodium carbonate

pH:

Biotest: 6.25

Cangene: 5.6

Talecris: 6.4 to 7.2 at 1% protein

Shelf Life: Expires within 36 months.

Storage/Stability: Store at 2° to 8°C (36° to 46°F). Discard if frozen.

Biotest: Store between 2° and 8°C (36° and 46°F). Use within 6 hours after the vial has been entered. Contact the manufacturer regarding exposure to freezing temperatures. Shipping data not provided.

Cangene: Use within 6 hours after vial has been entered. Contact the manufacturer regarding exposure to extreme temperatures. Shipping data not provided.

Talecris: Product can tolerate 30 days at 30°C (86°F). Shipping data not provided.

Production Process: Cohn-Oncley methods 6 & 9 cold-ethanol fractionation process of plasma harvested from a small group of individuals hyperimmunized with hepatitis B vaccine to produce high levels of anti-HBsAg antibody.

Biotest: Purified by an anion-exchange column chromatography method, with 2 added viral reduction steps: treatment with tri-n-butylphosphate and Triton X-100, to inactivate known enveloped viruses, and virus filtration using a Planova 35 nm virus filter, to reduce some known enveloped and nonenveloped viruses.

Cangene: Solvent-detergent treatment with tri-n-butyl phosphate and Triton X-100, purified with anion-exchange chromatography, with filtration through a Planova 20N virus filter.

Talecris: A virucidal solvent-detergent treatment step using 0.3% tri-n-butylphosphate and 0.2% sodium cholate at 30°C (86°F) for at least 6 hours is performed. After the viral inactivation step, the reactants are removed by precipitation, filtration, ultrafiltration, and diafiltration. It is incubated in the final container for 21 to 28 days at 20° to 27°C (68° to 80°F).

Media: Human plasma, from 100 units per lot (Talecris)

Disease Epidemiology

See Hepatitis B Vaccine monograph in the Vaccines/Toxoids section.

Other Information

Perspective: See Hepatitis B Vaccine monograph in the Vaccines/Toxoids section.

Hepatitis B Immune Globulin Comparison Table			
Brand Name	*HyperHep B S/D*	*Nabi-HB*	*Nabi-HB*
Manufacturer	Talecris	Biotest	Cangene
Labeled Indications	Postexposure prophylaxis	Postexposure prophylaxis	Prevent recurrence after liver transplantation in HBsAg-positive patients, postexposure prophylaxis
Concentration	150 to 180 mg/mL	40 to 60 mg/mL	50 mg/mL
Potency	≥ 220 units/mL	> 312 units/mL	> 312 units/mL, vials specifically labeled
Preservative	None	None	None
Solvent	Glycine 0.21 to 0.32 M	Sodium chloride 0.07 M, glycine 0.15 M	Maltose 10%
Packaging	0.5 mL syringe, 1 mL vial, 5 mL vial	1 mL vial, 5 mL vial	1 mL vial, 5 mL vial
Routine Storage	2° to 8°C	2° to 8°C	2° to 8°C
Dosage, Route	Usual: 0.06 mL/kg IM; Infant: 0.5 mL IM plus vaccine	Usual: 0.06 mL/kg IM; Infant: 0.5 mL IM plus vaccine	Usual: 0.06 mL/kg IM; Infant: 0.5 mL IM plus vaccine; Transplant: 20,000 units daily, then biweekly, then monthly, to attain serum anti-HBs > 500 units /L
Viral inactivation steps	Treatment with TNBP and sodium cholate, virus filtration	Treatment with TNBP and Triton X-100, virus filtration	Treatment with TNBP and Triton X-100, virus filtration

First Licensed:
Abbott: June 1987
Cangene: January 27, 2006
Cutter (now Talecris): June 12, 1974 (revised August 1996)
NABI: March 24, 1999 (now Biotest)

Discontinued Products: *BayHep B* (Bayer), *Hep B Gammagee* (Merck), *HyperHep* (Cutter, Bayer), *H-BIG* (Abbott Laboratories)

National Policy: CDC. A comprehensive immunization strategy to eliminate transmission of hepatitis B virus infection in the United States, part 1: Immunization of infants, children, and adolescents. *MMWR.* 2005;54(RR-16):1-32.

CDC. A comprehensive immunization strategy to eliminate transmission of hepatitis B virus infection in the United States, part 2: Immunization of adults. *MMWR.* 2006;55(RR-16):1-33.

Guidelines for Postexposure Prophylaxis[a] of People Exposed[b] to Blood or Body Fluids that Contain Blood Outside of Occupational Settings		
	Treatment	
Exposure	Unvaccinated person[c]	Previously vaccinated person[d]
HBsAg[e]-positive source		
Percutaneous (eg, bite or needlestick) or mucosal exposure to HBsAg-positive blood or body fluids	Hepatitis B vaccine series and HBIG	Hepatitis B vaccine booster dose
Sex or needle-sharing contact of an HBsAg-positive person	Hepatitis B vaccine series and HBIG	Hepatitis B vaccine booster dose
Victim of sexual assault/abuse by a perpetrator who is HBsAg positive	Hepatitis B vaccine series and HBIG	Hepatitis B vaccine booster dose
Source with unknown HBsAg status		
Victim of sexual assault/abuse by a perpetrator with unknown HBsAg status	Hepatitis B vaccine series	No treatment
Percutaneous (eg, bite or needlestick) or mucosal exposure to potentially infectious blood or body fluids from a source with unknown HBsAg status	Hepatitis B vaccine series	No treatment
Sex or needle-sharing contact of person with unknown HBsAg status	Hepatitis B vaccine series	No treatment

a When indicated, start immunoprophylaxis as soon as possible, preferably within 24 hours. Studies are limited on the maximum interval after exposure during which postexposure prophylaxis is effective, but the interval is unlikely to exceed 7 days for percutaneous exposure or 14 days for sexual exposure. The hepatitis B vaccine series should be completed.

b These guidelines apply to nonoccupational exposures. Guidelines for management of occupational exposures appear in a separate table and also can be used to manage nonoccupational exposures, if feasible.

c A person who is in the process of being vaccinated but who has not completed the vaccine series should complete the series and receive treatment as indicated.

d A person who has written documentation of a complete hepatitis B vaccine series and who did not receive postvaccination testing.

e Hepatitis B surface antigen.

Recommended Schedule for Prophylaxis of Perinatal Hepatitis B	
At birth	Infants born to HBsAg-positive mothers: hepatitis B vaccine and HBIG within 12 hours of birth.
	Infants born to mothers whose HBsAg status is unknown: hepatitis B vaccine within 12 hours of birth. Then the mother should have blood drawn as soon as possible to determine her HBsAg status; if she is HBsAg-positive, give the infant HBIG as soon as possible (no later than age 1 week).
	Full-term infants who are medically stable and weigh > 2,000 g born to HBsAg-negative mothers should receive hepatitis B vaccine before hospital discharge.
	Preterm infants weighing < 2,000 g born to HBsAg-negative mothers should receive the first vaccination 1 month after birth or at hospital discharge.
After the birth dose	All infants should complete the hepatitis B vaccine series with either single-antigen vaccine or combination vaccine, according to a recommended vaccination schedule.
	Infants born to HBsAg-positive mothers should be tested for HBsAg and antibody to HBsAg after completion of the hepatitis B vaccine series at age 9 to 18 months.
Vaccination of children and adolescents	All unvaccinated children and adolescents aged < 19 years should receive the hepatitis B vaccine series.

Guide to Postexposure Prophylaxis for Hepatitis B	
Type of exposure	Immunoprophylaxis
Perinatal	HBIG and vaccine
Infant (< 12 months of age): acute case in primary caregiver	HBIG and vaccine
Household contact: exposed to acute case	None unless known exposure
Household contact: exposed to acute case, known exposure	HBIG with or without vaccine
Household contact: exposed to chronic carrier	Vaccine

Hepatitis B Postexposure Treatment Schedule				
	HBIG		Hepatitis B vaccine	
Exposure	Dose	Recommended timing	Dose	Recommended timing
Perinatal	0.5 mL IM	Within 12 hours of birth	3 doses[a]	Within 12 hours of birth[b]
Sexual	0.06 mL/kg IM	Single dose within 14 days of last sexual contact	3 doses[a]	First dose at time of HBIG treatment[b]

a Standard dose. Refer to hepatitis B vaccine monograph for appropriate age-specific doses for each marketed vaccine brand.
b The first vaccine dose can be given at the same time as the HBIG dose but at a different site. Give subsequent doses as recommended for the specific vaccine.

Recommendations for Hepatitis B Prophylaxis Following Percutaneous or Permucosal Exposure in Occupational Setting			
	Treatment of exposed person when source is found to be:		
Status of exposed person	HbsAg-positive	HbsAg-negative	Source not tested or unknown
Unvaccinated	HBIG × 1,[a] then initiate vaccine series[b]	Initiate vaccine series[b]	Initiate vaccine series[b]
Previously vaccinated: known responder	Test exposed person for anti-HBs antibody. 1. If adequate,[c] no treatment. 2. If inadequate, give vaccine booster dose.	No treatment	No treatment
Known nonresponder	HBIG × 2[a,d] or HBIG × 1 plus 1 vaccine dose	No treatment	If known high-risk source, may treat as if source were HbsAg-positive.
Response unknown	Test exposed person for anti-HBs antibody. 1. If adequate,[c] no treatment. 2. If inadequate, HBIG × 1[a] plus vaccine booster dose.	No treatment	Test exposed person for anti-HBs antibody. 1. If adequate,[c] no treatment. 2. If inadequate, HBIG × 1[a] plus vaccine booster dose.

a HBIG dose: 0.06 mL/kg IM.
b Hepatitis B vaccine dose. Refer to vaccine monograph for appropriate age-specific dose of each marketed vaccine.
c Adequate anti-HBs is at least 10 SRU by RIA or positive by EIA.
d Give second dose 30 days after first dose.

Rabies Immune Globulin (Human)

Anti-Infective Immune Globulins

Names:
HyperRab S/D
Imogam Rabies-HT

Manufacturers:
Talecris Biotherapeutics
Manufactured by CSL Behring, distributed by
Sanofi Pasteur

Synonyms: RIG. Rabies disease also is called hydrophobia. HT refers to heat treatment, a viral inactivation process.

Comparison: Therapeutically equivalent

Immunologic Characteristics

Microorganism: Virus (single-stranded RNA), genus *Lyssavirus*, family Rhabdoviridae

Viability: Inactive, passive, transient

Antigenic Form: Human immunoglobulin, unmodified

Antigenic Type: Protein, IgG antibody, polyclonal, 20% or less polymeric

Strains:

Sanofi Pasteur: PM-1503-3M strain

Talecris: Data not provided

Use Characteristics

Indications: For passive, transient, postexposure prevention of rabies infection. Administer as soon as possible after exposure, 8 days or less after the first vaccine dose. Give RIG to all patients suspected of exposure to rabies with one exception: patients who have been completely immunized with rabies vaccine and are known to have an adequate antibody titer should receive postexposure vaccine booster doses only, not RIG.

Limitations: Provides only short-term passive immunity. Use rabies vaccine to induce persistent active immunity.

Outmoded Practices: Unlike immunoglobulin products harvested from animals, do not perform skin tests prior to administration of RIG. In most humans, intradermal injection of concentrated immune globulin with its buffers causes a localized area of inflammation that can be misinterpreted as a positive allergic reaction. This reaction is caused by localized tissue irritation of a chemical nature. Misinterpretation of such a test may cause urgently needed immunoglobulin to be withheld from a patient not actually allergic to it. True allergic responses to RIG IM are rare.

Contraindications:

Absolute: Successful preexposure vaccine prophylaxis

Relative: Use with caution in patients with a history of systemic allergic reactions following administration of human immune globulin products.

Patients with selective immunoglobulin A (IgA) deficiency have the potential for developing anti-IgA antibodies and could have anaphylactic reactions to subsequent administration of blood products (including immune globulin preparations) that contain IgA.

Immunodeficiency: No impairment of effect is likely.

Pregnancy: Category C. Use only if clearly needed. Intact IgG crosses the placenta from the maternal circulation increasingly after 30 weeks gestation. Problems in humans have not been documented and are unlikely.

Lactation: It is not known whether antirabies antibodies are excreted in breast milk. Problems in humans have not been documented.

Children: RIG is generally safe and effective in children.

Adverse Reactions: Local tenderness, soreness, or stiffness at the injection site and mild temperature elevations may persist for several hours. Sensitization to repeated injections has occurred occasionally in immunoglobulin-deficient recipients. Angioedema, urticaria, skin rash, nephrotic syndrome, and anaphylactic shock have been reported rarely.

Pharmacologic & Dosing Characteristics

Dosage: Immediate and thorough washing of all bite wounds and scratches with soap and water is perhaps the most effective measure for preventing rabies. Give RIG 20 units/kg (0.133 mL/kg) as soon as possible after exposure, preferably with the first dose of vaccine. This delivers a dose of approximately 22 mg IgG/kg. To avoid vaccine antibody interaction, do not administer RIG longer than 7 days after vaccine administration.

Route & Site: Infiltrate the wound site with the full dose of RIG, if the nature and location of the wound site permit. Administer the balance of the dose IM at a different site and in a different extremity from the rabies vaccine. Suitable sites may include the deltoid muscle or gluteal muscle (upper, outer quadrant only).

Overdosage: Clinical experience with other immune globulin preparations suggests that the major manifestations of overdosage would be pain and tenderness at the injection site.

Additional Doses: No additional RIG doses are needed. Repeating the RIG dose may interfere with the development of active immunity from rabies vaccine. Follow rabies vaccination schedules exactly.

Efficacy: Nearly perfect; efficacy demonstrated in people attacked by a rabid wolf in Iran in 1955.

Onset: Adequate levels of antibody appear in serum within 24 hours and peak within 2 to 13 days. Because rabies vaccine takes approximately 1 week to induce active immunity, the importance of RIG cannot be overemphasized.

Duration: The mean serum half-life of rabies antibody is 24 days, consistent with the 21-day half-life expected of IgG.

Pharmacokinetics: Immunoglobulins are primarily eliminated by catabolism.

Protective Level: An adequate rabies antibody titer is considered to be 1:5 or more by rapid fluorescent focus inhibition test (RFFIT) or a concentration of 0.5 units/mL.

Mechanism: Neutralizes rabies virus

Drug Interactions: Simultaneous administration of RIG may slightly delay the antibody response to rabies vaccine through partial antigen-antibody antagonism. Because of this, follow Centers for Disease Control and Prevention recommendations exactly and give no more than the recommended dose of RIG.

Inactivated vaccines generally are not affected by circulating antibodies or administration of exogenous antibodies. Immunization with such vaccines may occur at any time before or after antibody administration.

RIG may diminish the antibody response to attenuated measles, mumps, and rubella vaccines through antigen-antibody antagonism. As a general rule, administer live virus vaccines 14 to 30 days before, or 6 to 12 weeks after, immune globulin. Alternately, administer live virus vaccines during this interval if corresponding antibody titers are measured 3 months after RIG administration. For varicella vaccine, wait 5 months. For a vaccine containing the measles virus, wait 4 months.

Rabies Immune Globulin (Human)

IMIG does not appear to interfere with development of immunity following oral poliovirus (OPV) or yellow fever vaccination. Nonetheless, it may be prudent not to administer these vaccines shortly after RIG. Exceptions include unexpected travel to epidemic or endemic areas. If OPV is given with, or shortly after, RIG, repeat the OPV dose 3 months later if immunization is still indicated.

It is not known whether RIG interferes with the efficacy of other attenuated vaccines (eg, adenovirus, Bacillus Calmette-Guérin, typhoid, vaccinia), but it may be prudent not to administer these vaccines shortly after RIG administration unless this is unavoidable.

As with other drugs administered IM, give with caution to patients receiving anticoagulant therapy.

Pharmaceutical Characteristics

Concentration: 150 units per mL, 10% to 18% IgG, 80% or more monomeric

Quality Assay: Contains a geometric mean lower limit (95% confidence) potency value 110 units/mL or higher. Contains no aggregates with a sedimentation coefficient more than 12S or less than 6S. Monomeric IgG exhibits a sedimentation coefficient between 6S and 7.5S.

    USP requirement: Standardized against US Reference Standard Rabies Immune Globulin. The US unit of potency is equivalent to the International Unit (IU).

Packaging:

    Sanofi Pasteur: 2 mL single-dose vial (49281-0190-20), 10 mL single-dose vial (49281-0190-10)

    Talecris: 2 mL single-dose vial (13533-0618-02), 10 mL single-dose vial (13533-0618-10)

Doseform: Solution

Appearance: Slightly opalescent and cloudy, practically colorless to light straw color

Solvent: Variously contains glycine, sodium chloride, and water for injection

Adjuvant: None

Preservative: None

Allergens:

    Sanofi Pasteur: May contain minute quantities of IgA

    Talecris: 0.1 to 1 mg/mL IgA at 16.5%

Excipients:

    Sanofi Pasteur: 0.3 molar glycine, with hydrochloric acid or sodium hydroxide to adjust pH

    Talecris: 0.21 to 0.32 molar glycine, with sodium carbonate to adjust pH

pH: 6.4 to 7.2 at 1% protein

Shelf Life: Expires within 12 months

Storage/Stability: Store at 2° to 8°C (36° to 46°F); discard if frozen.

    Sanofi Pasteur: Product can tolerate 4 days at room temperature. Shipped in insulated containers with coolant packs.

    Talecris: Product can tolerate 30 days at 30°C (86°F). Shipping data not provided.

Production Process: Cohn-Oncley methods 6 & 9 cold-ethanol fractionation process of pooled venous plasma of individuals immunized with rabies vaccine. Specific virucidal steps are performed during manufacture.

    Sanofi Pasteur: A virucidal heat-treatment process at 58° to 60°C (136.4° to 140°F) for 10 hours is performed.

    Talecris: A virucidal solvent-detergent treatment step using 0.3% tri-n-butylphosphate and 0.2% sodium cholate at 30°C (86°F) for 6 hours or longer is performed. It is incubated in the final container for 21 to 28 days at 20° to 27°C (68° to 80.6°F).

Media: Human plasma, from 100 units per lot (Talecris) to 2,000 units per lot (Sanofi Pasteur).

Disease Epidemiology

See Rabies Vaccine monograph in the Vaccine/Toxoids section.

Several charts of rabies prophylaxis guidelines appear in the Vaccines/Toxoids section.

Other Information

Perspective: See also the Rabies Vaccine monograph.

1889: Canine antirabies serum used for rabies prophylaxis.

1891: Babes treats people bitten by rabid wolves with whole blood from vaccinees.

1945: Habel develops antirabies serum, combined with rabies vaccine in a field study in Iran in 1954.

1950: Koprowski, Cox, and colleagues develop antirabies serum from rabbits and sheep for use in humans.

First Licensed:

Connaught (now CSL Behring): Original form licensed in April 1984. HT form was licensed in July 1997.

Cutter (now Talecris): June 12, 1974 (revised August 1996)

Discontinued Products: *BayRab* (Bayer), *HyperRab* (Cutter, Miles, Bayer)

National Policy: ACIP. Human rabies prevention-United States, 2008. *MMWR.* 2008;57(RR-3):1-28. www.cdc.gov/mmwr/PDF/rr/rr5703.pdf.

References: Rupprecht CE, Gibbons RV. Prophylaxis against rabies. *N Engl J Med.* 2004;351:2626-2635.

WHO. Rabies vaccines. *Wkly Epidemiol Rec.* 2007;82:425-35. www.who.int/wer/2007/wer8249_50.pdf.

Anti-Respiratory Syncytial Virus Antibodies

Anti-Infective Immune Globulins

Anti-Respiratory Syncytial Virus Antibody Comparison Table		
	Palivizumab	Respiratory Syncytial Virus Immune Globulin[a]
Synonyms	*Synagis*, MEDI-493	*RespiGam*
Manufacturer	MedImmune	Manufactured by Massachusetts Biological Laboratories; distributed by MedImmune
Antibody type	Monoclonal, 95% human, 5% murine	Polyclonal, 100% human
Half-life	20 days	22 to 28 days
Doseform	Solution	Solution
Concentration	100 mg/mL	40 to 60 mg/mL
Packaging	50 or 100 mg vial	100 ± 200 mg or 2,500 ± 500 mg vial
Diluent	Sterile water for injection	Dextrose IV solution, with or without NaCl
Preservative	None	None
Routine storage	Refrigerator	Refrigerator
Dose	15 mg/kg	750 mg/kg
Route	IM injection	2- to 4-hour IV infusion
Standard schedule	Monthly for 5 months	Monthly for 5 months
Interactions with vaccines	Not apparent, unlikely	Likely, especially with live virus vaccines
Production process	Produced in recombinant murine myeloma cell line	Harvested from human plasma units with high titers of anti-RSV antibodies
CPT code	90378	90379

a No longer marketed.

Palivizumab (Humanized)

Anti-Infective Immune Globulins

Name:
Synagis

Manufacturer:
MedImmune/AstraZeneca

Synonyms: MEDI-493

Comparison: Palivizumab differs from polyclonal respiratory syncytial virus immune globulin (RSV-IG, *RespiGam*) in potency, dosing, route of administration, packaging, and other characteristics. Palivizumab is 50 to 100 times more potent than polyclonal RSV-IG in a cotton rat model.

Immunologic Characteristics

Microorganism: Virus (single-stranded RNA), enveloped, genus *Pneumovirus*, family Paramyxoviridae

Viability: Inactive, passive, transient

Antigenic Form: Humanized IgG1κ, consisting of 95% human and 5% murine antibody sequences, directed toward an epitope in the A antigenic site of the F protein of RSV. Palivizumab is composed of two heavy chains and two light chains and has a molecular weight of approximately 148 kilodaltons. The human heavy chain sequence was derived from the constant domains of human IgG1 and the variable framework regions of the V_H genes Cor and Cess. The human light chain sequence was derived from the constant domain of Ck and the variable framework regions of the VL gene K104 with Jk-4. The murine sequences were derived from a murine monoclonal antibody, Mab 1129, by grafting the murine complementarity determining regions into the human antibody frameworks.

Antigenic Type: Protein, IgG1κ antibody, monoclonal

Strains: Neutralizes 57 clinical RSV isolates of both A and B strains.

Use Characteristics

Indications: To prevent serious lower respiratory tract disease caused by RSV in high-risk children. Safety and efficacy were established in infants with chronic lung disease (CLD) or bronchopulmonary dysplasia (BPD), infants with a history of premature birth (35 weeks or less gestational age), and children with hemodynamically significant congenital heart disease (CHD). In the IMpact-RSV trial, palivizumab reduced the incidence of RSV hospitalization by 55%. Therapy is particularly warranted for those who required supplemental oxygen or bronchodilator, diuretic, or corticosteroid therapy for CLD within 6 months before the anticipated start of RSV season. Patients with more severe CLD may benefit from prophylaxis during a second RSV season if they continue to require medical therapy for pulmonary or cardiac dysfunction. Infants born at 32 weeks gestation or earlier may benefit from RSV prophylaxis even if they do not have CLD.

Prophylaxis with palivizumab (but not RSV-IG) is appropriate for infants and children younger than 24 months of age with hemodynamically significant congenital heart disease. Palivizumab is preferred for most high-risk infants and children because of ease of IM administration. Immunoprophylaxis should be considered for infants born after 32 to 35 weeks gestation only if two or more risk factors are present (eg, child care attendance, school-aged siblings, exposure to environmental air pollutants, congenital abnormalities of airways, severe neuromuscular disease). High-risk infants should not attend child care during the RSV season when feasible, and their exposure to tobacco should be eliminated.

Palivizumab (Humanized)

Unlabeled Uses: Research in progress is assessing the role of palivizumab diluted for controlled IV infusion in transplant patients to treat RSV infection.

Limitations: Palivizumab did not alter the incidence and mean duration of hospitalization for non-RSV respiratory illness nor the incidence of otitis media. Palivizumab has not been demonstrated to aid in the treatment of established RSV disease.

Contraindications:

Absolute: None

Relative: Patients with a history of a severe reaction to palivizumab or other components of this product.

Immunodeficiency: No impairment of effect is likely. Palivizumab may be indicated in certain immunodeficient people.

Elderly: No specific information is available about the use of palivizumab in elderly patients.

Pregnancy: Category C. Palivizumab is not indicated for adult use. It is not known whether palivizumab can cause fetal harm when administered to a pregnant woman or could affect reproductive capacity. Generally, most IgG passage across the placenta occurs during the third trimester. Problems in humans have not been documented and are unlikely.

Lactation: It is not known if palivizumab crosses into human breast milk. Problems in humans have not been documented and are unlikely.

Children: Safety and efficacy of palivizumab in children older than 2 years of age have not been established.

Adverse Reactions: In studies of children with bronchopulmonary dysplasia (BPD) or prematurity, the proportions of subjects in the placebo and palivizumab groups who experienced any adverse event or any serious adverse event were similar.

Most of the safety information was derived from the IMpact-RSV trial. In this study, palivizumab was discontinued in 5 patients: 2 because of vomiting and diarrhea, 1 because of erythema and moderate induration at the site of the fourth injection, and 2 because of preexisting medical conditions that required management (congenital anemia or pulmonary venous stenosis requiring cardiac surgery). The overall fatality rate was lower in patients receiving palivizumab (0.4%) than in placebo recipients (1%). None of the fatalities was attributed to palivizumab.

Adverse events that occurred in more than 1% of 1,641 patients receiving palivizumab in clinical trials (age 3 days to 24.1 months) for which the incidence in the palivizumab group was at least 1% greater than in the placebo group appear below.

Adverse Events Occurring at Greater Frequency in the Palivizumab Group		
	Palivizumab[a] (n = 1,641)	Placebo (n = 1,148)
Upper respiratory tract infection	830 (50.6%)	544 (47.4%)
Otitis media	597 (36.4%)	397 (34.6%)
Fever	446 (27.1%)	289 (25.2%)
Rhinitis	439 (26.8%)	282 (24.6%)
Hernia	68 (4.1%)	30 (2.6%)
AST increased	49 (3%)	20 (1.7%)

a Cyanosis (9.1% palivizumab vs 6.9% placebo) and dysrhythmia (3.1% vs 1.7%) were reported during trial 2 in CHD patients.

Based on experience in more than 400,000 patients who received more than 2 million doses of palivizumab, rare severe acute hypersensitivity reactions were reported after initial or subsequent exposure. Very rare cases of anaphylaxis (less than 1 case per 100,000 patients) have also been reported after reexposure. None of the reported hypersensitivity reactions were fatal.

Hypersensitivity reactions may include dyspnea, cyanosis, respiratory failure, urticaria, pruritus, angioedema, hypotonia, and unresponsiveness.

Limited information from postmarketing reports suggests that, within a single RSV season, adverse events after a sixth or greater dose of palivizumab are similar in character and frequency to those after the initial five doses.

Other adverse events reported in more than 1% of the palivizumab group included: cough; wheezing; bronchiolitis; pneumonia; bronchitis; asthma; croup; dyspnea; sinusitis; apnea; failure to thrive; nervousness; diarrhea; vomiting; gastroenteritis; ALT increase; liver function abnormality; injection-site reactions; conjunctivitis; viral infection; oral monilia; fungal dermatitis; eczema; seborrhea; anemia; viral-like syndrome. The incidence of these adverse events was similar between the palivizumab and placebo groups.

In the IMpact-RSV trial, the incidence of antihumanized antibody after the fourth injection was 1.1% in the placebo group and 0.7% in the palivizumab group. Among 56 pediatric patients receiving palivizumab for a second season, 1 patient had transient, low-titer reactivity. This reactivity was not associated with adverse events or alteration in palivizumab serum concentrations.

Pharmacologic & Dosing Characteristics

Dosage: 15 mg/kg. The dose per month should be calculated as patient weight (kg) times 15 mg/kg divided by 100 mg/mL of palivizumab. Divide injection volumes larger than 1 mL into separate doses. Administer monthly doses throughout the RSV season to all patients, including those who develop an RSV infection. Give the first dose before the start of the RSV season. In the northern hemisphere, the RSV season typically begins in November and lasts through April, but it may begin earlier or persist later in certain communities. Give patients undergoing cardio-pulmonary bypass a dose of palivizumab as soon as possible after the bypass procedure (even if sooner than a month after the previous dose).

Route & Site: IM injection, preferably in the anterolateral aspect of the thigh. Do not routinely use the gluteal muscle as an injection site because of the risk of damage to the sciatic nerve.

Overdosage: No data from clinical studies are available on overdosage. No toxicity was observed in rabbits administered a single IM or subcutaneous injection of palivizumab at 50 mg/kg. No data are available from human subjects who received more than 5 monthly palivizumab doses during a single RSV season. Clinical experience with other immune globulin preparations suggest that the major manifestations of overdosage would be pain and tenderness at the injection site.

Additional Doses: Because a mean decrease in palivizumab serum concentration of 58% was observed after surgical procedures that use cardiopulmonary bypass, a postoperative dose of 15 mg/kg should be considered for children who still require prophylaxis as soon as the child is medically stable.

Missed Doses: Administer missed doses as soon as possible to avoid lapses in antibody-mediated protection. Administer the next dose 1 month after the preceding dose.

Related Interventions: All high-risk infants and children and their contacts should be immunized against influenza early each season.

Efficacy: In the pivotal IMpact-RSV trial, 1,502 high-risk infants received either placebo or palivizumab 15 mg/kg monthly for 5 doses or less. This trial studied patients 24 months of age and younger with BPD and patients with premature birth (35 weeks or less gestation) who were 6 months of age or younger at study entry. Subjects were followed for 150 days between November 1996 and April 1997. Palivizumab reduced the incidence of RSV-associated hospitalization by 55% (from 10.6% in the placebo arm to 4.8% in the treatment arm). The reduction of RSV hospitalization was observed both in patients enrolled with a diagnosis of BPD

(12.8% vs 7.9%) and in patients enrolled with a diagnosis of prematurity without BPD (8.1% vs 1.8%). The reduction of RSV hospitalization was observed throughout the course of the RSV season. For all infants younger than 32 weeks gestational age, the risk of hospitalization was reduced by 47% (11% vs 5.8%). For premature infants 32 to 35 weeks gestational age, the risk reduction was 80%. Palivizumab therapy also was associated with fewer RSV hospital days, ICU admissions (3% vs 1.3%), and hospital days with increased supplemental oxygen. Overall, data do not suggest that RSV illness was less severe among patients who received palivizumab and who required hospitalization because of RSV infection than among placebo patients who required hospitalization because of RSV infection.

In a second trial conducted over 4 consecutive seasons among 1,287 patients 24 months of age or younger involving infants with hemodynamically significant CHD, RSV hospitalization was reduced from 9.7% in placebo recipients to 5.3% in palivizumab recipients, a 45% reduction. Hospitalization was reduced in both acyanotic (11.8% vs 5%) and cyanotic (7.9% vs 5.6%) subsets of children.

Onset: Prompt

Pharmacokinetics: In studies in adult volunteers, palivizumab had a pharmacokinetic profile similar to a human IgG1 antibody in regard to volume of distribution and half-life (mean, 18 days). In pediatric patients younger than 24 months of age, the mean half-life of palivizumab was 20 days, and monthly IM doses of 15 mg/kg achieved mean ± SD 30-day trough serum drug concentrations of 37 ± 21 mcg/mL after the first injection, 57 ± 41 mcg/mL after the second injection, 68 ± 51 mcg/mL after the third injection, and 72 ± 50 mcg/mL after the fourth injection. In pediatric patients given palivizumab for a second RSV season, the mean ± SD serum concentrations following the first and fourth injections were 61 ± 17 mcg/mL and 86 ± 31 mcg/mL, respectively.

In 139 pediatric patients 24 months of age or younger with hemodynamically significant CHD who received palivizumab, and underwent cardio-pulmonary bypass for open-heart surgery, the mean ± SD serum concentration was 98 ± 52 mcg/mL before bypass and declined to 41 ± 33 mcg/mL after bypass, a 58% reduction. The clinical significance of this reduction is unknown.

Specific studies were not conducted to evaluate demographic parameters on palivizumab pharmacokinetics. No effects of gender, age, body weight, or race on palivizumab serum trough concentrations were observed in a clinical study with 639 pediatric patients 24 months of age or younger with CHD receiving 5 monthly IM palivizumab injections of 15 mg/kg.

Elimination: Immunoglobulins are primarily eliminated by catabolism.

Protective Level: Palivizumab serum concentrations 40 mcg/mL and larger reduced pulmonary RSV replication by 100-fold in the cotton rat model of RSV infection.

Mechanism: Palivizumab binds to the F protein, a protein necessary for the virus to infect cells, on the surface of RSV in a process called fusion. The F protein is also expressed on the surface of infected cells and is responsible for subsequent fusion with other cells, which leads to the formation of syncytia (masses of protoplasm lacking cell membranes between nuclei). Palivizumab exhibits neutralizing and fusion-inhibitory activity against RSV. These activities inhibit RSV replication in laboratory experiments.

Drug Interactions: In the IMpact-RSV trial, the proportions of patients in the placebo and palivizumab groups who received routine childhood vaccines, influenza vaccine, bronchodilators, or corticosteroids were similar, and no incremental increase in adverse reactions was observed among patients receiving these agents.

The monoclonal nature of palivizumab decreases the likelihood that it interferes with the immune response to live virus vaccines or live bacterial vaccines. Responses to inactivated vaccines are not substantially affected by circulating antibodies.

As with any IM injection, palivizumab should be given with caution to patients with thrombocytopenia or any coagulation disorder.

Pharmaceutical Characteristics

Concentration: 50 mg per 0.5 mL or 100 mg per 1 mL

Quality Assay: Purified using ion exchange and other chromatographic methods, low pH, and nanofiltration.

Packaging: 50 mg per 0.5 mL vial (NDC#: 60574-4114-01) or 100 mg per 1 mL vial (60574-4113-01)

Doseform: Solution

Appearance: The solution should appear clear or slightly opalescent.

Solvent: Glycine with histidine solution

Adjuvant: None

Preservative: None

Allergens: None

Excipients:
  50 mg vial: Histidine 1.9 mg/0.5 mL, glycine 0.6 mg/0.5 mL, and chloride 0.2 mg/0.5 mL
  100 mg vial: Histidine 3.9 mg/mL, glycine 0.1 mg/mL, and chloride 0.5 mg/mL

pH: 5 to 7 in liquid state

Shelf Life: Expires within 24 months

Storage/Stability: Store at 2° to 8°C (36° to 46°F). Do not freeze. Contact the manufacturer regarding exposure to extreme temperatures. Preliminary data suggest that palivizumab may tolerate room temperature for 1 week, 15° to 25°C (59° to 77°F) for 2 weeks, and 38° to 42°C (100° to 108°F) for up to 3 days without significant degradation. Shipped in insulated containers with coolant packs by overnight or second-day courier.

Production Process: The antibody is produced in a mouse myeloma cell line, then purified using ion exchange and other chromatographic methods. The drug is then sterile-filtered, lyophilized, and packaged in sterile vials.

Media: Stable cell lines expressing palivizumab from mouse myeloma cells, non-secreting zero (NS0), using glutamine synthetase selection and amplification using methionine sulfoximine. The cell line yields antibody at approximately 1 g/L of culture.

Disease Epidemiology

Incidence: RSV, associated with 90,000 hospitalizations and 4,500 deaths a year in the United States, is the leading cause of bronchiolitis and pneumonia in infants and can be life-threatening to high-risk infants. The fatality rate in infants with heart or lung disease hospitalized for RSV infection is 3% to 4%. RSV usually occurs in epidemics during winter and early spring. Most children are infected during the first 3 years of life. Reinfection throughout life is common.

Susceptible Pools: At greatest risk are infants with BPD, congenital heart disease, prematurity, or immune compromise. Approximately 300,000 babies are born at less than 35 weeks gestation in the United States each year. Approximately 15,000 infants develop BPD each year. Approximately 16,000 infants have congenital heart disease.

Transmission: Spread is usually by direct or close contact, perhaps involving droplets. RSV can persist on environmental surfaces for hours. Nosocomial infections are common among both infants and medical personnel.

Incubation: 2 to 8 days

Communicability: RSV can persist on the hands for 30 minutes or longer. Contact isolation can help control transmission. Hand-washing, prevention of contamination from respiratory secretions, and eye-nose goggles can decrease nosocomial spread. Viral shedding usually lasts 3 to 8 days, but in infants may persist for up to 3 to 4 weeks.

Palivizumab (Humanized)

Other Information

Perspective:

1956: Morris, Chanock, and colleagues isolate RSV from a chimpanzee.

1969: Investigational formalin-inactivated RSV vaccine causes worse bronchiolitis and pneumonia, with more severe morbidity and death, after natural infection in vaccine recipients than in placebo recipients.

1980s: Fischer, Hemming, and Prince demonstrate that polyvalent high-titer anti-RSV immune globulin is effective prophylaxis in infants.

1996: Polyclonal RSV-IG (Massachusetts Public Health Biological Laboratory, MedImmune) licensed on January 18. Granted orphan drug status on September 27, 1990.

1998: Palivizumab (MedImmune) licensed on June 19.

National Policy: Canadian National Advisory Committee on Immunization. Statement on the recommended use of monoclonal anti-RSV antibody (palivizumab). *Can Comm Dis Rep.* 2003;29(ACS-7):1-13.

Krilov LR, Weiner LB, Yogev R, Fergie J, Katz BZ, Henrickson KJ, Welliver RC Sr. The 2009 COID recommendations for RSV prophylaxis: Issues of efficacy, cost, and evidence-based medicine. *Pediatrics.* 2009;124(Dec):1682-1684.

American Academy of Pediatrics. Policy statements—Modified recommendations for use of palivizumab for prevention of respiratory syncytial virus infections. *Pediatrics.* 2009;124(Dec):1694-1701.

References: Connor EM. Palivizumab, a humanized respiratory syncytial virus monoclonal antibody, reduces hospitalization from RSV infection in high-risk infants. *Pediatrics.* 1998;102:531-537.

Johnson S, et al. Development of a humanized monoclonal antibody (MEDI-493) with potent in vitro and in vivo activity against respiratory syncytial virus. *J Infect Dis.* 1997;176:1215-1224.

Geskey JM, Thomas NJ, Brummel GL. Palivizumab in congenital heart disease: Should international guidelines be revised? *Expert Opin Biol Ther.* 2007;7(Nov):1615-1620.

Name:
Generic

Manufacturer:
Cangene Corporation

Synonyms: VIG, VIG-IV. Cangene's product is known as CNJ–016. Vaccinia is similar to cowpox but is distinct from variola (smallpox), other orthopox viruses, and varicella (chickenpox) virus (a herpes virus).

Comparison: An IM formulation of VIG had been licensed for several decades and has been available under IND protocol in recent years. The intravenous (IV) formulations offer advantages in pharmacokinetics, ease of administration, and lack of preservative. The two IV formulations are presumed to be therapeutically comparable, although they differ in concentration, dosage, and administration.

Immunologic Characteristics

Microorganism: Virus (double-stranded DNA), genus Orthopoxvirus, family Poxviridae

Viability: Inactive, passive, transient

Antigenic Form: Human immunoglobulin, unmodified

Antigenic Type: Protein, IgG antibody, polyclonal, polymeric

Strains: New York City Board of Health strain of vaccinia virus

Use Characteristics

Indications: To treat or modify certain severe complications resulting from smallpox vaccination:

- Aberrant infections induced by vaccinia virus that include its accidental implantation in eyes (except in cases of isolated keratitis), mouth, or other areas where vaccinia infection would constitute a special hazard;
- eczema vaccinatum;
- progressive vaccinia;
- severe generalized vaccinia; and
- vaccinia infections in individuals who have skin conditions, such as burns, impetigo, varicella-zoster, or poison ivy, or in individuals who have eczematous skin lesions because of the activity or extensiveness of such lesions.

Treat complications, including vaccinia keratitis with VIG-IV, with caution because a single study in rabbits demonstrated increased corneal scarring with intramuscular vaccinia immune globulin (VIG-IM) administration. The scarring presumably results from deposition of antigen-antibody complexes. The feasibility of corneal transplant may mitigate the contraindication against treatment of keratitis with VIG.

Unlabeled Uses: Although there is little evidence to support the practice, and a larger supply would be needed than is available currently, VIG could be used prophylactically while administering smallpox vaccine to people with contraindications to vaccination in the setting of a smallpox outbreak. This use of VIG would be intended to attenuate the expected replication of vaccinia viruses within the vaccinee.

Limitations: VIG is not considered effective in the treatment of postvaccinal encephalitis. VIG provides only short-term passive immunity. Use vaccinia (smallpox) vaccine to induce persistent active immunity, if appropriate. VIG has no role in the treatment of smallpox (variola) infection. For this use, a 0.3 mg/kg dose of VIG-IM has been proposed, but a dosage for VIG-IV has not been proposed.

Contraindications:

Absolute: None

Relative: While VIG-IV should be considered in the treatment of severe ocular complications caused by vaccinia virus, VIG-IV is contraindicated for use in the presence of isolated vaccinia keratitis. Do not use VIG-IV, or use caution, in people with histories of severe reactions associated with the parenteral administration of this or other human immunoglobulin preparations. VIG-IV contains trace amounts of IgA. People with selective IgA deficiency can develop antibodies to IgA and, therefore, could have anaphylactic reactions to subsequent administration of blood products that contain IgA, including VIG-IV.

Immunodeficiency: Treatment of progressive vaccinia in an immunodeficient patient may require repeated doses of VIG.

Elderly: No specific information is available about use of VIG-IV in the elderly. No impairment of effect is likely.

Carcinogenicity: VIG-IV has not been evaluated for carcinogenic potential.

Mutagenicity: VIG-IV has not been evaluated for mutagenic potential.

Fertility Impairment: VIG-IV has not been evaluated for impairment of fertility.

Pregnancy: Category C. Use only if clearly needed. It is not known if VIG-IV crosses the placenta. Generally, most IgG passage across the placenta occurs during the third trimester. Problems in humans have not been documented and are unlikely. Animal reproduction studies have not been conducted with VIG-IV.

Lactation: It is not known if VIG-IV crosses into human breast milk. Problems in humans have not been documented and are unlikely.

Children: VIG-IV has not been tested for safety or efficacy in children. No impairment of effect is likely.

Adverse Reactions: Most adverse events reported in a clinical evaluation of the pharmacokinetics of this product in healthy volunteers (who fasted overnight before administration) were mild and similar to those causally related to infusion of other protein products, such as headache, nausea, dizziness, feeling hot, feeling cold, and rigors. VIG-IV had no effect on blood pressure or heat rate during a 90-day trial. Other subjects in the 9,000 units/kg cohort experienced syncope. There was a lower incidence of adverse events when the 9,000 units/kg dose was infused at 2 mL/min (60%) than at 4 mL/min (86%).

Related Adverse Events That Occurred Within 3 Days of VIG-IV Administration (≥ 5%)				
Body system	6,000 units/kg[a] (n = 31)	9,000 units/kg[a] (n = 29)	9,000 units/kg[b] (n = 10)	Placebo[c] (n = 22)
All body systems	19 (61%)	24 (83%)	6 (60%)	4 (18%)
Eye disorders	2 (7%)	1 (3%)	0 (0%)	0 (0%)
GI disorders (eg, nausea, vomiting, dry lips)	5 (16%)	8 (28%)	3 (30%)	1 (5%)
General disorders/administration-site conditions (eg, rigors, feeling cold, pain, asthenia, feeling hot, pyrexia, fatigue, increased energy)	10 (32%)	15 (52%)	4 (40%)	1 (5%)
Metabolism/nutrition disorders (eg, decreased appetite)	2 (7%)	2 (7%)	0 (0%)	0 (0%)
Musculoskeletal/connective tissue disorders (eg, back pain, muscle cramps)	5 (16%)	7 (24%)	0 (0%)	0 (0%)

Related Adverse Events That Occurred Within 3 Days of VIG-IV Administration (≥ 5%)				
Body system	6,000 units/kg[a] (n = 31)	9,000 units/kg[a] (n = 29)	9,000 units/kg[b] (n = 10)	Placebo[c] (n = 22)
Nervous system disorders (eg, headache, dizziness, paresthesia, tremor)	18 (58%)	20 (69%)	6 (60%)	4 (18%)
Respiratory/thoracic/mediastinal disorders	0 (0%)	0 (0%)	0 (0%)	0 (0%)
Skin/subcutaneous tissue disorders (eg, increased sweating)	3 (10%)	2 (7%)	0 (0%)	0 (0%)
Vascular disorders (eg, pallor)	1 (3%)	2 (7%)	1 (10%)	1 (5%)

a 4 mL/min infusion rate.
b 2 mL/min infusion rate.
c 0.9% sodium chloride infused at 2 mL/min.

Systemic reactions, such as chills, muscle cramps, back pain, fever, nausea, vomiting, and wheezing, were the most frequent adverse reactions observed during the clinical trials of other similarly prepared human intravenous immunoglobulins (IGIVs). The incidence of these reactions was less than 5% of all infusions, most often related to infusion rates greater than those recommended for VIG-IV. If a patient develops any infusion-related adverse reaction, slow the rate of infusion immediately or temporarily interrupt the infusion.

Infectious: VIG-IV is derived from human plasma. Few experimental or epidemiological studies of variant Creutzfeldt-Jacob disease (vCJD) transmissibility by blood components or plasma derivatives have been published. It is not known whether plasma-derived products can transmit the vCJD agent. No such transmissions have been reported to date. Source plasma donors for VIG-IV may have lived in areas where there is a known risk of exposure to the vCJD agent (eg, American military bases in northern Europe for 6 months or more between 1980 and 1990 or at bases elsewhere in Europe for 6 months between 1980 and 1996). To date, no donors of any source plasma have been diagnosed with vCJD. The risk of transmission of recognized blood-borne viruses has been reduced by the viral inactivation and/or removal properties of the procedures used in the manufacturing of VIG-IV, including cold ethanol precipitation, nanofiltration, and solvent/detergent treatment with C18 column chromatography. The ability of these procedures to reduce infectivity of the causative agent of vCJD has not been evaluated for VIG-IV. Prions associated with VCJD have low solubility below a pH of 9, a high tendency to form aggregates, and adhere to surfaces readily; therefore, prions have the potential to be removed by the precipitation and adsorption technologies used in the plasma fractionation for VIG-IV. Despite these measures, some still unrecognized blood-borne viruses or other infectious agents may not be inactivated or removed by the manufacturing process. Therefore, give VIG-IV only if a benefit is expected.

CNS: Aseptic meningitis syndrome (AMS) has been reported infrequently in association with IGIV administration. The syndrome usually begins within several hours to 2 days after IGIV treatment. It is characterized by symptoms and signs such as severe headache, nuchal rigidity, drowsiness, fever, photophobia, painful eye movements, and nausea and vomiting. Cerebrospinal fluid studies are frequently positive, with pleocytosis up to several thousand cells/mm^3, predominately from the granulocytic series, and with elevated protein concentrations up to several hundred mg/dL. Give patients exhibiting such symptoms and signs a thorough neurological examination to rule out other causes of meningitis. AMS may occur more frequently in association with high total doses (2 g/kg) of IGIV treatment. Discontinuing IGIV treatment resulted in remission of AMS within several days without sequelae.

Hematologic: IGIV products may contain blood-group antibodies that may act as hemolysins and induce in vivo coating of red blood cells (RBCs) with immunoglobulin, causing a positive direct antiglobulin reaction and, rarely, hemolysis. Hemolytic anemia may develop after IGIV therapy because of enhanced RBC sequestration. Monitor VIG-IV recipients for signs and symptoms of hemolysis. Thrombotic events have been reported in association with IGIV. Patients at risk may include those with histories of atherosclerosis, multiple cardiovascular risk factors, advanced age, impaired cardiac output, or hyperviscosity. Weigh the risks and benefits of VIG-IV against those of alternative therapies. Consider baseline assessment of blood viscosity in patients at risk for hyperviscosity, including those with cryoglobulins, fasting chylomicronemia/markedly high triacylglycerols (triglycerides), or monoclonal gammopathies.

Pulmonary: There have been reports of noncardiogenic pulmonary edema (transfusion-related acute lung injury [TRALI]) in patients given IGIV. TRALI is characterized by severe respiratory distress, pulmonary edema, hypoxemia, normal left ventricular function, and fever and typically occurs within 1 to 6 hours after transfusion. Manage patients with TRALI using oxygen therapy with adequate ventilatory support. Monitor VIG-IV recipients for pulmonary adverse reactions. If TRALI is suspected, perform appropriate tests for the presence of antineutrophil antibodies in the product and patient serum.

Renal: Increases in serum creatinine and serum urea nitrogen occur as soon as 1 to 2 days after treatment with other IGIVs. IGIV products have been reported to be associated with renal dysfunction, acute renal failure, osmotic nephrosis, proximal tubular nephropathy, and death. Although these reports of renal dysfunction and acute renal failure have been associated with many licensed IGIV products, those that contained sucrose as a stabilizer administered at daily doses of 400 mg/kg or greater accounted for a disproportionate share of the reports. Doses of VIG-IV higher than 400 mg/kg will exceed this level of sucrose and are not recommended in patients with potential renal problems. VIG-IV contains sucrose 5% as a stabilizer, and the recommended dose is 100 mg/kg. People predisposed to acute renal failure include the following: patients with any degree of preexisting renal insufficiency, diabetes mellitus, volume depletion, sepsis, or paraproteinemia, people who are 65 years of age or older, or patients who are receiving known nephrotoxic drugs. In these patients, administer VIG-IV at the minimum concentration available and at the minimum rate of infusion practical.

Consultation: Obtain advice on the diagnosis and management of vaccinia and vaccination complications from Centers for Disease Control and Prevention (CDC) or from the manufacturer.

Pharmacologic & Dosing Characteristics

Dosage: The recommended initial dosage is 6,000 units/kg.

Route: Administer directly through a dedicated IV line at 2 mL/min or less. For subjects weighing less than 50 kg, infuse the product at 0.04 mL/kg/min (133.3 units/kg/min) or less. The maximum assessed rate of infusion has been 4 mL/min.

Overdosage: Although limited data are available, clinical experience with other IG preparations suggests that the major manifestations would be those related to volume overload.

Additional Doses: This usually involves doses at intervals of 2 to 3 days, until no new lesions appear, implying the beginning of recovery.

Consider administration of higher doses (eg, 9,000 units/kg) if the patient does not respond to the initial dose.

Related Interventions: During administration, monitor the patient's vital signs continually. Observe the patient carefully for symptoms throughout the infusion. No patients should be volume depleted before starting the VIG-IV infusion. Do not exceed the recommended infusion rate, and follow the infusion schedule closely.

Laboratory Tests: Because of the potentially increased risk of thrombosis, consider baseline assessment of blood viscosity in patients at risk for hyperviscosity, including those with cryoglobulins, fasting chylomicronemia/markedly high triacylglycerols (triglycerides), or monoclonal gammopathies. If signs or symptoms of hemolysis are present after VIG-IV infusion, conduct appropriate confirmatory laboratory testing. If TRALI is suspected, conduct appropriate tests for the presence of antineutrophil antibodies in the product and patient serum.

Efficacy: The effectiveness of VIG-IV was evaluated based on serum antibody concentrations in healthy volunteers 5 days after administration and comparison with the estimated (modeled) serum antibody concentration 5 days after administration of the previously licensed product VIG-IM. There are no controlled trials demonstrating a clinical benefit, such as a reduction in mortality or in the severity of vaccinia complications.

The binding capacity and neutralizing activity of antivaccinia antibody in 60 healthy volunteers 5 days after administering VIG-IV (both 6,000 and 9,000 units/kg) were at least as high as theoretical values that would be achieved after administration of VIG-IM. Five days represents the approximate time of peak serum antibody concentrations after IM administration of other human IG products.

Data from VIG-IM administration to treat vaccinia auto-inoculation indicate that 27 of 28 VIG-IM recipients were treated successfully. Among patients with eczema vaccinatum, mortality was 7% among VIG-IM recipients compared with the 30% to 40% mortality expected with supportive care alone.

Onset: Promptly bioavailable. Clinical effect likely to be seen within 1 or 2 days.

Pharmacokinetics: Immunoglobulins are eliminated primarily by catabolism.

The circulating half-life was 30 days (range, 13 to 67 days) and the volume of distribution was 6,630 L. After IV administration of 6,000 units/kg to 31 healthy male and female volunteers, a mean peak plasma concentration of 161 units/mL was achieved within 2 hours. Five days later, the geometric mean plasma level was 60.1 units/mL (range, 36.1 to 84.6) after a 6,000 units/kg dose and 90.3 units/mL (range, 63.4 to 133.8) after a 9,000 units/kg dose.

Mechanism: Neutralization of vaccinia viruses.

Drug Interactions: VIG is effective and indicated as an antidote to certain AEs of vaccinia (smallpox) vaccine through specific antagonism of viral replication.

Inactivated vaccines generally are not affected by circulating antibodies or administration of exogenous antibodies. Immunization with such vaccines may occur at any time before or after antibody administration.

Antibodies present in IG preparations may interfere with the immune response to live-virus vaccines such as polio, measles, mumps, rubella, and varicella. Therefore, defer live-virus vaccination for 3 months after administering VIG-IV. If such vaccinations were given within 14 to 30 days before or after VIG-IV, revaccination may be necessary. Alternatively, test for corresponding antibody titers to determine need for repeat vaccination.

Lab Interference: After administration of VIG-IV, a transitory increase of passively transferred antibodies in the patient's blood may result in misleading positive results in serological testing (eg, anti-HBs).

Pharmaceutical Characteristics

Concentration: Each mL contains 2.67 to 4.67 mg/mL total protein and more than 50,000 arbitrary units of vaccinia antibody-neutralizing activity, compared with the FDA reference standard.

Vaccinia Immune Globulin Intravenous (Human)

Quality Assay: Contains IgG representative of the immunized donors who contributed to the plasma pool from which the product is derived. The IgG contains a relatively high concentration of antibodies directed against vaccinia virus.

Potency is based on ELISA assay. Each plasma donation was tested for presence of hepatitis B surface antigen and antibodies to HIV-1, HIV-2, and hepatitis C virus. Mini-pools of plasma passed nucleic-acid tests for HIV-1, hepatitis C, and hepatitis B viruses.

Packaging: 3,333 units/mL or more, or greater than or equal to 50,000 units/15 mL vial (single vial: NDC#: 60492-0173-01; 24 vials: 60492-0173-02).

NDC Number: 60492-0173-01

Doseform: Liquid

Appearance: Colorless, free of particulate matter, not turbid

Diluent:

For infusion: If a preexisting catheter must be used, flush the line with 0.9% sodium chloride for injection before administering VIG-IV. Compatibility was assessed only with 0.9% sodium chloride, not with other solutions such as dextrose in water.

Adjuvant: None

Preservative: None

Allergens: Less than 40 mcg/mL IgA.

Excipients: Stabilized with 10% maltose and 0.03% polysorbate 80.

pH: 5.0 to 6.5

Shelf Life: Expires within 24 months.

Storage/Stability: Store at 2° to 8°C (36° to 46°F). Protect vials from light. Contact the manufacturer regarding exposure to freezing or elevated temperatures. Shipped in insulated containers with coolant packs.

If product is received frozen, use within 60 days of thawing to 2° to 8°C (36° to 46°F). Begin IV infusion within 4 hours after entering the vial.

Handling: Do not shake vial. Avoid foaming.

If a preexisting catheter must be used, flush the line with 0.9% sodium chloride for injection before administering VIG-IV.

Production Process: Derived from pooled human plasma collected from donors who received booster immunizations with *Dryvax* smallpox vaccine. Pooled plasma was fractionated by cold-ethanol precipitation according to the Cohn-Oncley method, modified to yield a product suitable for IV administration.

Purified by anion-exchange column chromatography. The viral-reduction steps (ie, *Planova* 35N filtration, solvent-detergent treatment with tri-n-butylphosphate and *Triton X-100*) have been validated for ability to remove or inactivate lipid-enveloped and nonenveloped viruses that may not have been detected in source plasma. Validation involved HIV-1, bovine viral diarrhea virus, pseudorabies virus murine minute virus, and poliovirus, which are models for HIV-2, parvovirus B-19, hepatitis A, B, and C viruses, herpes virus, West Nile virus, and vaccinia virus.

Based on the size of vaccinia virus (350 × 270 nm), it is likely removed by nanofiltration and inactivated by the presence of antivaccinia antibodies. In addition, solvent/detergent treatment of bulk VIG-IV material is capable of reducing vaccinia virus to undetectable levels.

Media: Human plasma

Vaccinia Immune Globulin Intravenous (Human)

Disease Epidemiology

Incidence: Adverse events to smallpox vaccine that warrant VIG-IV treatment are very rare. With screening programs in outbreak settings to exclude people with atopic dermatitis and immune deficiency from smallpox vaccination, VIG-IV may be needed once per approximately 250,000 vaccinations. In a smallpox outbreak setting, where fewer people would be exempted from vaccination, VIG-IV may be needed once per approximately 10,000 vaccinations.

Other Information

Perspective: See also the Smallpox Vaccinia Vaccine, Live monograph.

1895: Immune calf serum used for protection against vaccinia.
1950: MacCallum and colleagues describe vaccinia immune globulin derived from human plasma.
1968: Hyland's VIG-IM licensed on December 31.
1991: VIG-IM reverts to IND status, related to color change.
2005: VIG-IV licensed to DynPort on February 18.

First Licensed:
Cangene: May 3, 2005

Discontinued Products: Dynport (licensed February 18, 2005)

National Policy: Centers for Disease Control and Prevention. Smallpox vaccination and adverse events: guidance for clinicians. *MMWR.* 2003;52(RR-4):1-30. http://www.cdc.gov/mmwr/PDF/rr/rr5204.pdf.

Centers for Disease Control and Prevention. Recommendations for using smallpox vaccine in pre-event vaccination program: supplemental recommendations of the Advisory Committee on Immunization Practices (ACIP) and the Healthcare Infection Control Practices Advisory Committee (HICPAC). *MMWR.* 2003;52(RR-7):1-16. http://www.cdc.gov/mmwr/PDF/rr/rr5207.pdf.

References: Espmark JA, Kempe CH, Neff JM, Netter R, Stickl H, Wehle PF. Which is the factual basis, in theory and general practice, for the use of vaccinia immune globulin for the prevention or attenuation of complications of smallpox vaccination. *Vox Sang.* 1979;36:121-128.

Fenner F, Henderson DA, Arita I, Jezek Z, Ladnyi ID. *Smallpox and its Eradication.* Geneva: World Health Organization; 1988. http://whqlibdoc.who.int/Smallpox/9241561106.pdf.

Fulginiti VA, Winograd LA, Jackson M, Ellis P. Therapy of experimental vaccinal keratitis. Effect of idox-uridine and VIG. *Arch Ophthalmol.* 1965;74:539-544.

Kempe CH. Studies on smallpox and complications of smallpox vaccination. *Pediatrics.* 1960;26:176-189.

Marennikova SS. The use of hyperimmune antivaccinia gamma-globulin for the prevention and treatment of smallpox. *Bull World Health Organ.* 1962;27:325-330.

Botulism Immune Globulin Intravenous (Human)

Immunoantidotes

Name:
  BabyBIG

Manufacturer:
  Manufactured by Cangene Corporation, distributed by FFF Enterprises and California Department of Health Services

Synonyms: BIG-IV

Comparison: Prepared from human plasma, unlike botulinum antitoxin (equine), which is prepared from suitable horse plasma. Antibodies derived from human sources typically have more favorable pharmacokinetic and adverse-event profiles compared with equine-source antibodies.

Immunologic Characteristics

Microorganism: Bacterial exotoxin, *Clostridium botulinum*, anaerobic endospore-forming gram-positive rod

Viability: Inactive, passive, transient

Antigenic Form: Human immunoglobulin, unmodified (antitoxin)

Antigenic Type: Protein, IgG antibody, polyclonal, polymeric. One mcg of toxin is equivalent to 200,000 median lethal doses for a mouse and close to the median lethal dose in humans.

Strains: Activity against toxin types A and B confirmed. Activity against toxins C, D, and E not evaluated.

Use Characteristics

Indications: To treat patients younger than 1 year of age diagnosed with infant botulism caused by toxin type A or B.

Limitations: BIG-IV has not been tested for safety and efficacy in adults.

Antitoxin does not prevent microbial spread of the toxigenic organism. Conversely, antibiotics have no effect on the toxin. Botulinum toxoid is needed to confer long-lasting immunity. Select appropriate antibiotics to treat the active infection (eg, a penicillin or tetracycline).

Contraindications:

Absolute: Essentially none.

Relative: Do not use BIG-IV in people with a history of severe reaction to other human Ig preparations. People with selective immunoglobulin A (IgA) deficiency may develop antibodies to IgA and could have anaphylactic reactions to subsequent administration of blood products containing IgA. BIG-IV contains only trace amounts of IgA.

Immunodeficiency: No impairment of effect is likely. People with selective immunoglobulin A deficiency may develop antibodies to IgA and could have anaphylactic reactions to subsequent administration of blood products containing IgA. BIG-IV contains trace amounts of immunoglobulin A.

Elderly: BIG-IV has not been tested for safety and efficacy in adults.

Carcinogenicity: BIG-IV has not been evaluated for carcinogenic potential.

Mutagenicity: BIG-IV has not been evaluated for mutagenic potential.

Fertility Impairment: BIG-IV has not been evaluated for impairment of fertility.

Pregnancy: Category C. Use only if clearly needed. It is not known if BIG-IV crosses the placenta. Generally, most IgG passage across the placenta occurs during the third trimester. Animal reproduction studies have not been conducted with BIG-IV. Problems in humans have not been documented and are unlikely.

Lactation: It is not known if BIG-IV crosses into human breast milk. Problems in humans have not been documented and are unlikely.

Children: Safety and efficacy in children older than 1 year of age have not been established.

Adverse Reactions: Different methods were used to collect adverse events in the controlled study and open-label study. Minor clinical events not recorded as adverse events in the controlled study were recorded as adverse events in the open-label study. As a result, a larger number of adverse events were recorded in the open-label study. The only adverse event possibly related to BIG-IV administration was a mild, transient erythematous rash of the face or trunk. When only treatment emergent events are considered, 14% of BIG-treated patients experienced erythematous rash during or after study infusion in the controlled study. Eight percent of placebo-treated patients also experienced erythematous rash in the controlled study. A similar rash is known to occur both in infant botulism patients who have not received any IGIV products, and in patients treated with other IGIVs, making it difficult to ascertain the causality of the rash.

In the controlled study, the following adverse events occurred in at least 5% of patients:

Adverse Reactions Occurring in ≥ 5% of Patients		
	BIG-IV (N = 65)	Placebo (N = 64)
Adverse event	n (%)	
Patients with any adverse event	20 (31)	29 (45)
Rash, erythematous	9 (14)	5 (8)
Otitis media	7 (11)	5 (8)
Pneumonia	7 (11)	9 (14)
Anemia	3 (5)	9 (14)
Hyponatremia	3 (5)	9 (14)
Hypertension	1 (2)	3 (5)
Respiratory arrest	1 (2)	6 (9)
Urinary tract infection	1 (2)	8 (13)
Convulsions	0 (0)	3 (5)

In the open-label study, the following adverse events occurred in at least 5% of 293 patients: patients with any adverse event (97%), increased blood pressure (75%), dysphagia (65%), irritability (41%), atelectasis (39%), rhonchi (34%), pallor (28%), loose stools (25%), contact dermatitis (24%), erythematous rash (22%), vomiting (20%), nasal congestion (18%), edema (18%), decreased oxygen saturation, pyrexia (17%), decreased body temperature, decreased blood pressure (16%), cardiac murmur (15%), cough, rales (13%), abdominal distension (11%), decreased breath sounds, dehydration, agitation (10%), decreased hemoglobin, stridor (9%), lower respiratory tract infection, oral candidiasis (8%), injection-site reaction, tachycardia, peripheral coldness (7%), dyspnea, hyponatremia (6%), injection-site erythema, intubation, metabolic acidosis, neurogenic bladder, anemia, and tachypnea (5%).

Many adverse events observed in the clinical studies are part of the known pathophysiology of infant botulism. Minor reactions, such as chills, muscle cramps, back pain, fever, nausea, vomiting, and wheezing, were the most frequent adverse reactions observed during the clinical trials of other human IGIVs. The incidence of these reactions was less than 5% of all infusions, most often related to infusion rates. If a patient develops a minor side effect, slow the rate of infusion immediately or temporarily interrupt the infusion.

Severe reactions, such as angioneurotic edema and anaphylactic shock (although not observed during clinical trials with BIG-IV) are a possibility. Clinical anaphylaxis may occur even when the patient is not known to be sensitive to Ig products. A reaction may be related to the rate of infusion. Carefully adhere to recommended infusion rates. If anaphylaxis or a drop in blood pressure occurs, discontinue the infusion and administer epinephrine.

Infection: BIG-IV is made from human plasma and, like other plasma products, carries the possibility for transmission of blood-borne viral agents and, theoretically, the Creutzfeldt-Jakob disease agent. The risk of transmission of blood-borne viruses has been reduced by screening plasma donors for prior exposure to certain viruses and for the current presence of certain viral infections, and by the viral inactivation and/or removal properties of the precipitation procedures used to purify BIG-IV. Despite these measures, some unrecognized blood-borne viruses may not be inactivated by the manufacturing process.

Meningitis: An aseptic meningitis syndrome (AMS) has been reported infrequently in association with IGIV administration. The syndrome usually begins within several hours to 2 days after IGIV treatment. It is characterized by severe headache, nuchal rigidity, drowsiness, fever, photophobia, painful eye movements, and nausea and vomiting. Cerebrospinal fluid studies are frequently positive with pleocytosis up to several thousand cells per mm^3, predominately granulocytes, and with elevated protein levels up to several hundred mg/dL. Give patients exhibiting such symptoms and signs a thorough neurological examination to rule out other causes of meningitis. AMS may occur more frequently in association with high total doses (2 g/kg) of IGIV. Discontinuation of IGIV treatment resulted in remission of AMS within several days without sequelae.

Renal: Use BIG-IV with caution in patients with preexisting renal insufficiency and in patients judged to be at increased risk of developing renal insufficiency (eg, those with diabetes mellitus, volume depletion, paraproteinemia, or sepsis, those receiving known nephrotoxic drugs). Increases in serum creatinine and BUN have been observed as soon as 1 to 2 days after treatment with other IGIVs. In the absence of prospective data allowing identification of the maximum safe dose, concentration, and rate of infusion in these patients, do not exceed the dose, concentration, and rate of infusion recommended (see Dosage section).

Consultation: For information about treating infant botulism, contact Infant Botulism Treatment and Prevention Program, California Department of Health Services, 850 Marina Bay Parkway, Room E-361, Richmond, CA 94804; 510-231-7600.

See also http://www.infantbotulism.org.

Pharmacologic & Dosing Characteristics

Dosage: The recommended total dosage of BIG-IV is 1 mL/kg (50 mg/kg), given as a single IV infusion as soon as the clinical diagnosis of infant botulism is made.

Begin the infusion slowly. Administer IV at 0.5 mL/kg/h (25 mg/kg/h). If no untoward reactions occur after 15 minutes, the rate may be increased to 1 mL/kg/h (50 mg/kg/h). Do not exceed this rate of administration. Monitor the patient closely during and after each rate change. At the recommended rates, infusion of the indicated dose should take 67.5 minutes total elapsed time.

Minor adverse reactions experienced by patients treated with IGIV products have been related to the infusion rate. Continuously monitor vital signs during infusion. If the patient develops a minor side effect (ie, flushing), slow the rate of infusion or temporarily interrupt the infusion. If anaphylaxis or a significant drop in blood pressure occurs, stop the infusion and administer epinephrine.

Route: IV infusion only.

Overdosage: Although limited data are available, clinical experience with other Ig preparations suggests that the major manifestations would be related to volume overload.

Additional Doses: Not recommended.

Laboratory Tests: Assess renal function, including blood urea nitrogen or serum creatinine, before initial infusion. No patient should be volume-depleted. Periodically monitor renal function tests and urine output in patients at risk for developing acute renal failure.

Efficacy: Two clinical studies evaluated BIG-IV: a placebo-controlled trial (N = 129) and an open-label study to collect additional safety data and confirm efficacy (N = 293). In the placebo-controlled trial, BIG-IV given within the first 3 days of hospital admission to 59 patients with laboratory-confirmed infant botulism reduced the following:

(a) the average length of hospital stay, from 5.7 weeks (placebo group) to 2.6 weeks (BIG-treated group; $P < 0.0001$);

(b) the average length of stay in ICU, from 3.6 weeks to 1.3 weeks ($P < 0.01$);

(c) the average length of time on a mechanical ventilator, from 2.4 weeks to 0.7 weeks ($P < 0.05$); and

(d) the average number of weeks the patients had to be tube-fed, from 10 weeks to 3.6 weeks ($P < 0.01$).

Length of hospital stay also was analyzed by patient age in both the placebo-controlled trial and open-label study, as shown in the following table. The observed reduction in length of hospital stay was statistically significant ($P < 0.01$), except for the 0- to 60-day age stratum, where the small study population limited the statistical power.

Mean Length of Hospital Stay in Weeks			
	Randomized trial		Open-label study
Age (days)	BIG-IV	Placebo	BIG-IV
0 to 60	2.8	3.8	2
61 to 120	1.9	5.6	2
> 120	3	6.6	1.8

Length of hospital stay was analyzed in the adequate and well-controlled study by race (white versus nonwhite), as shown in the following table. Length of hospital stay was reduced significantly in both white and nonwhite patients ($P = 0.002$).

Mean Length of Hospital Stay in Weeks		
Race	Placebo	BIG-IV
White	6.3	2.8
Nonwhite	4.6	2.4

Onset: Prompt.

Duration: A single IV infusion of BIG-IV is expected to provide a protective level (more than 0.1 milliunits/mL) of neutralizing antibodies for 6 months.

Pharmacokinetics: Immunoglobulins are primarily eliminated by catabolism. The half-life of BIG-IV is approximately 28 days in infants, similar to data for other IgG preparations. Immunoglobulins are eliminated primarily by catabolism.

For infants who may be exposed to botulinum toxin types A or B, this product is expected to provide relevant antibodies at levels sufficient to neutralize the expected levels of circulating neurotoxin. Traditional pharmacokinetic studies of BIG-IV have not been performed; however, the following table summarizes the mean serum titer of the anti-A component of BIG-IV after IV administration.

Botulism Immune Globulin Intravenous (Human)

	Mean Serum Titer of Anti-A Component of BIG-IV After IV Administration	
Time	BIG-IV Lot 1 anti-A titer (mean ± SD)	BIG-IV Lot 2 anti-A titer (mean ± SD)
	milliunits/mL	
Day 1	not done	537.1 ± 213.4
Week 2	106.7 ± 44.6	192.2 ± 71.2
Week 4	90.0 ± 39.2	155.5 ± 56.7
Week 8	54.9 ± 22.8	96.0 ± 33.2
Week 12	26.0 ± 20.5	61.4 ± 32.3
Week 16	15.6 ± 10.4	33.0 ± 22.3
Week 20	7.6 ± 6.6	19.3 ± 14.1

Protective Level: More than 0.1 milliunits per mL.

Mechanism: Antitoxin does not reverse symptoms of botulism, but it does prevent disease progression by binding circulating toxin.

Drug Interactions: Antibodies present in IgG preparations may interfere with immune response to live virus vaccines. Defer live-virus vaccinations until approximately 5 months after administering BIG-IV. If such vaccinations were given shortly before or after BIG-IV administration, revaccination may be necessary.

Hypothetically, botulinum antitoxin might interfere with the ability of botulinum toxoid to induce active immunity, but this effect has not been studied in any systematic fashion.

Pharmaceutical Characteristics

Concentration: 50 ± 10 mg immunoglobulin per mL, primarily IgG.

Quality Assay: Contains IgG antibodies from the immunized donors who contributed to the plasma pool from which the product was derived. The titer of antibodies against type A botulinum toxin is at least 15 units/mL and against type B toxin is at least 4 units/mL. For toxin types A and B, by definition, 1 unit of botulinum antitoxin neutralizes 10,000 intraperitoneal mouse LD_{50} of botulinum toxin. The titers of antibody against botulinum neurotoxins C, D, and E have not been determined.

Packaging: Single-dose vial containing 100 mg ± 20 mg immunoglobulin for reconstitution with 2 mL sterile water for injection.

NDC Number: 68403-1100-06

Doseform: Powder for solution

Appearance: White powder yielding a colorless and translucent solution. Do not use if turbid.

Diluent:

For reconstitution: Sterile water for injection

For infusion: Administer BIG-IV using low-volume tubing and a constant infusion pump (ie, IVAC pump). Predilution of BIG-IV before infusion is not recommended. Administer BIG-IV through a separate IV line. If this is not possible, it may be piggybacked into a preexisting line if that line contains either 0.9% sodium chloride injection or one of the following dextrose solutions (with or without sodium chloride added): 2.5% dextrose in water, 5% dextrose in water, 10% dextrose in water, or 20% dextrose in water. If a preexisting line must be used, do not dilute BIG-IV more than 1:2 with any of the above-named solutions. Admixtures of BIG-IV with any other solutions have not been evaluated. Use of an in-line or syringe-tip sterile, disposable filter (18 mcm) is recommended for the administration of BIG-IV.

Adjuvant: None

Preservative: None

Allergens: Trace amounts of human IgA and IgM.

Excipients: Stabilized with 50 mg/mL sucrose and 10 mg/mL albumin (human); 20×10^{-3} mEq/mL sodium.

pH: 5.42

Shelf Life: Expires within 24 months, unless extended by FDA based on stability and potency tests.

Storage/Stability: Store at 2° to 8°C (36° to 46°F). Do not freeze. Contact the manufacturer regarding exposure to elevated temperatures. Shipped after consultation with receiving physician, in insulated container with coolant packs on next-available airplane, with door-to-door ground courier support at destination.

Begin infusion within 2 hours after complete reconstitution. Conclude infusion within 4 hours of reconstitution. Do not store BIG-IV in the reconstituted state. Admixtures of BIG-IV with other drugs have not been evaluated. Administer BIG-IV separately from other drugs or medications.

Handling: Reconstitute the powder with 2 mL of sterile water for injection to obtain a 50 mg/mL BIG-IV solution. A double-ended transfer needle or large syringe is suitable for adding the water for reconstitution. When using a double-ended transfer needle, insert one end first into the vial of water. The lyophilized powder is supplied in an evacuated vial; therefore, the water should transfer by suction. Aim the jet of water to the side of the vial, to avoid foaming. After the water is transferred into the evacuated vial, release the residual vacuum to hasten dissolution. Rotate the container gently to wet all the powder. Allow approximately 30 minutes for dissolving the powder. To avoid foaming, do not shake the vial.

Production Process: Purified immunoglobulin is derived from pooled adult plasma from people immunized with pentavalent botulinum toxoid, who were selected for high titers of neutralizing antibody against botulinum neurotoxins type A and B. All donors were tested and found negative for antibodies against HIV and the hepatitis B and hepatitis C viruses. The pooled plasma was fractionated by cold-ethanol precipitation of proteins according to the Cohn-Oncley method, modified to yield a product suitable for IV administration.

Several manufacturing steps have been validated for the ability to inactivate or remove viruses that may not have been detected in source plasma. These include Cohn-Oncley fractionation (Fraction I through Supernatant III Filtrate); nanofiltration through one 75 nm and two 35 nm filters; and solvent/detergent viral inactivation. These viral-reduction steps have been validated in in vitro experiments for the capacity to inactivate and/or remove HIV-1 and the following model viruses: bovine viral diarrhea virus (BVDV) as a model for hepatitis C virus; mouse encephalomyelitis virus (MEMV) as a model for hepatitis A virus; and pseudorabies virus (PRV), feline calicivirus (FCV), and Sindbis virus to cover a range of physicochemical properties in model viruses studied. Total mean $\log_{10}$ reductions range from 6.07 to greater than 16 $\log_{10}$.

Additional testing performed with bovine parvovirus (to model parvovirus B19) showed a mean cumulative reduction factor more than 7.34 $\log_{10}$ for Cohn-Oncley fractionation and solvent/detergent treatment followed by hydrophobic chromatography. A mean cumulative reduction factor of 2.55 $\log_{10}$ was observed for removal of porcine parvovirus by nanofiltration.

Media: Human plasma.

Botulism Immune Globulin Intravenous (Human)

Disease Epidemiology

Incidence: The mortality rate from botulism was highest in the first quarter of the 20th century. From 1981 through 1991, the total number of reported cases of botulism ranged from 82 to 133 per year. Roughly two thirds of these cases are infant botulism, and 25% to 30% are food-borne.

Susceptible Pools: Essentially, the entire population is susceptible to the neurotoxic effects of botulinum toxin poisoning.

Transmission: Infant botulism results from ingestion of spores rather than preformed toxin. Honey, a food item that should not be fed to infants, often contains botulinum spores.

Ingestion of food in which toxin has been formed causes classical botulism, mostly after inadequate heating during canning and with subsequent inadequate cooking. Improperly preserved meat and other improperly processed, canned, low-acid, or alkaline foods are the usual sources of type A or B intoxication. Most type E intoxications result from ingestion of fish, seafood, and meat from marine animals.

Most cases of wound botulism are secondary to contamination of the wound by ground-in soil or gravel. Cases have been reported among chronic IV drug users. Spread of botulinum toxin is considered a biological-warfare threat.

Incubation: Neurologic symptoms usually appear within 12 to 36 hours, sometimes several days, after ingestion. The shorter the incubation period, the more severe the disease and the higher the case-fatality rate. The incubation period of infant botulism is unknown.

Communicability: No instances of secondary person-to-person transmission have been documented.

Other Information

Perspective:

1817 to 1822: Kerner describes disease now known as food borne botulism and extracts botulinum toxin from sausages.

1870: Müller names sausage poisoning with the word botulism (from the Latin *botulus*, meaning "sausage").

1896: van Ermengem discovers causative microorganism, initially called *Bacillus botulinus*.

1897: Kempner prepares botulinum antitoxin from goat plasma.

1947: Nigg, Reames, and colleagues develop polyvalent botulinum toxoids.

1992: Clinical trials of human botulinum immune globulin (BIG) begin in California. Designated an orphan drug on January 31, 1989.

First Licensed: October 23, 2003.

Discontinued Products: None

National Policy: CDC. New telephone number to report botulism cases and request antitoxin. *MMWR*. 2003;52:774. http://www.cdc.gov/mmwr/preview/mmwrhtml/mm5232a8.htm.

References: Arnon SS, Schechter R, Inglesby TV, et al, for Working Group on Civilian Biodefense. Botulinum toxin as a biological weapon: medical and public health management. *JAMA*. 2001;285:1059-1070.

Arnon SS, Schechter R, Maslanka SE, Jewell NP, Hatheway CL. Human botulism immune globulin for the treatment of infant botulism. *N Engl J Med*. 2006;354(5):462-471.

Shapiro RL, Hatheway C, Becher J, Swerdlow DL. Botulism surveillance and emergency response: a public health strategy for a global challenge. *JAMA*. 1997;278:433-435.

Wang YC, et al. Acute toxicity of aminoglycoside antibiotics as an aid in detecting botulism. *Appl Environ Microbiol*. 1984;48:951-955.

Arnon SS. Creation and development of the public service orphan drug human botulism immune globulin. *Pediatrics*. 2007;119(Apr):785-789.

CDC. Investigational heptavalent botulinum antitoxin (HBAT) to replace licensed botulinum antitoxin AB and investigational botulinum antitoxin E. *MMWR*. 2010;59:299.

Immunoantidotes

Name:
Generic

Manufacturer:
Manufactured by Instituto Butantan (São Paulo, Brazil); distributed by the Centers for Disease Control and Prevention.
Investigational new drug (IND)

Immunologic Characteristics

Microorganism: Bacterial exotoxin, *Corynebacterium diphtheriae*, facultative anaerobic gram-positive rod

Viability: Inactive, passive, transient

Antigenic Form: Equine immunoglobulin, unmodified (antitoxin)

Antigenic Type: Protein, IgG antibody, polyclonal, polymeric. Skin tests assess immediate (type I) hypersensitivity.

Strains: Data not provided

Use Characteristics

Indications: For passive, transient protection against or for treatment of diphtheria infections.

Limitations: Antitoxin does nothing to prevent microbial spread of the toxigenic organism. Conversely, antibiotics have no effect on the toxin. A drug containing diphtheria toxoid is needed to confer long-lasting immunity. Select appropriate antibiotics to treat the active infection (eg, erythromycin, penicillin G).

Contraindications:

Absolute: Essentially none

Relative: Patients with a history of a severe hypersensitivity reaction to this drug or any of its components. Use desensitization protocol if the patient is hypersensitive and this drug is urgently needed. If diphtheria is present, antitoxin must be given.

Immunodeficiency: No impairment of effect is likely.

Elderly: No specific information is available about geriatric use of diphtheria antitoxin.

Pregnancy: Category C. Use only if clearly needed. Intact IgG crosses the placenta from the maternal circulation increasingly after 30 weeks gestation.

Lactation: It is not known if antitoxin antibodies are excreted into breast milk. Problems in humans have not been documented.

Children: Give children the same antitoxin dose as adults. At the same time, but in a different extremity and with a separate syringe, continue or complete the child's basic immunizing series with DTP or DT, as appropriate.

Adverse Reactions: Fever, arthralgia, skin rash, or lymphadenopathy may occur and are dose-related. Anaphylaxis with urticaria, respiratory distress, and vascular collapse occurred after administration of diphtheria antitoxin.

The incidence of serum sickness with contemporary enzyme-refined serum is approximately 10%. Serum sickness may appear 7 to 12 days after administration of equine serum.

Diphtheria Antitoxin (Equine)

Pharmacologic & Dosing Characteristics

Dosage: Perform hypersensitivity tests before administering therapeutic doses of antitoxin. If hypersensitivity tests are positive, perform desensitization before giving therapeutic dose.

Sensitivity test: Whenever possible, perform both the conjunctival test and the ID (also called intracutaneous) or scratch tests. The ID test is the most sensitive test of these, yielding the fewest false-negative results.

For the conjunctival test, place 1 drop of a freshly compounded 1:10 v/v dilution of diphtheria antitoxin in 0.9% sodium chloride in the lower conjunctival sac of 1 eye. Instill 1 drop of 0.9% sodium chloride ophthalmic solution in the other eye to serve as a negative control. A positive reaction indicating hypersensitivity consists of itching, burning, redness, and lacrimation appearing within 15 minutes. These symptoms can be relieved by instilling a drop of epinephrine ophthalmic solution. The control eye should remain normal. If both eyes remain normal, the conjunctival test is negative.

For the ID test, inject 0.1 mL of a 1:100 v/v dilution of diphtheria antitoxin freshly compounded in 0.9% sodium chloride. For allergic individuals, a preliminary test with 0.05 mL of a 1:1,000 v/v dilution may be advisable. Inject a separate but comparable skin site with 0.1 mL of 0.9% sodium chloride ID as a negative control. Compare the results of the 2 doses 20 minutes after injection. A positive hypersensitivity test to diphtheria antitoxin consists of an urticarial wheal with or without pseudopods, surrounded by a halo of erythema. This is in contradistinction to a negative or minimal reaction, with no wheal or pseudopods, at the saline injection site.

For a scratch test, make a ¼-inch skin scratch through a freshly compounded 1:100 v/v dilution of diphtheria antitoxin. For a negative control, make a similar scratch through a drop of 0.9% sodium chloride placed on a different but comparable skin site. Evaluate the test after 20 minutes by comparing the 2 sites. A positive hypersensitivity test consists of an urticarial wheal, with or without pseudopods, surrounded by a halo of erythema. This is in contradistinction to a negative or minimal reaction, with no wheal or pseudopods, at the saline scratch site.

If the patient exhibits a positive hypersensitivity test or a doubtful reaction, conduct careful desensitization of the patient.

Desensitization protocol: Serial. Give escalating injections of diluted diphtheria antitoxin at intervals of 15 minutes, as described below, provided no reaction occurs following any of the doses. If a reaction occurs after an injection, allow 60 minutes to elapse before repeating the last dose that failed to cause a reaction.

Dose 1: 0.05 mL of a 1:20 v/v dilution subcutaneously.
Dose 2: 0.1 mL of a 1:10 v/v dilution subcutaneously.
Dose 3: 0.3 mL of a 1:10 v/v dilution subcutaneously.
Dose 4: 0.1 mL of undiluted antitoxin subcutaneously.
Dose 5: 0.2 mL of undiluted antitoxin subcutaneously.
Dose 6: 0.5 mL of undiluted antitoxin subcutaneously.
Dose 7: Inject remaining therapeutic dose IM.
Alternatively, omit dose 7 and give the remaining amount of antitoxin cautiously by IV infusion. Do not exceed 1 mL of antitoxin per minute, in the proportion of 1 mL antitoxin per 20 mL of 0.9% sodium chloride or 5% dextrose.

Therapeutic dose: For pharyngeal or laryngeal disease evident for 48 hours, give 20,000 to 40,000 units. In the case of nasopharyngeal lesions, give 40,000 to 60,000 units. For extensive disease lasting 3 days or longer or for any patient with brawny swelling of the neck, give 80,000 to 120,000 units. Give children the same dose as adults. In addition, give appropriate antimicrobial agents at a therapeutic dose. Warm diphtheria antitoxin before injection but not greater than 32° to 34°C (90° to 93°F).

Route: Conjunctival, ID, or scratch hypersensitivity tests. Subcutaneous and IM injections for desensitization. IM or slow IV infusion for therapy, not to exceed 1 mL antitoxin per minute. In severe cases, the preferred route of administration is IV to neutralize toxin most rapidly.

Overdosage: Although few data are available, clinical experience with other immune globulin preparations suggests that the major manifestations of overdosage would be related to fluid volume overload. Severity of serum sickness may be dose-related.

Additional Doses: Additional antitoxin doses may be warranted by the patient's symptoms and response. A complete immunizing series of a product containing diphtheria toxoid is needed for long-lasting immunity.

Missed Doses: Each hour of delay in administration increases the dosage required and decreases beneficial effects.

Efficacy: The efficacy of diphtheria antitoxin decreases as the duration of pharyngeal diphtheria increases. The risk/benefit ratio appears to be better for diphtheria antitoxin use in pharyngeal disease, compared with cutaneous diphtheria.

Onset: IV effect is rapid; concentrations peak several hours after IM injection.

Duration: Mean half-life is shorter than 15 days, as with any equine immunoglobulin.

Pharmacokinetics: Immunoglobulins are primarily eliminated by catabolism.

Protective Level: Antidiphtheria levels of 0.01 or higher antitoxin units/mL.

Mechanism: Antitoxin neutralizes circulating toxin. Toxin produced by *Corynebacterium diphtheriae* already fixed to tissue is unaffected. Antitoxin does not reverse symptoms, but it does prevent progression of the disease by binding circulating toxin.

Drug Interactions: Delay administration of products containing diphtheria toxoid (eg, DTP, Td) for 3 to 4 weeks after diphtheria antitoxin administration to minimize the possibility of antigen-antibody antagonism.

Pharmaceutical Characteristics

Concentration: Lots contain 20,000 units in 1 to 10 mL containers. The exact concentration is marked on individual containers. Contains excess potency, 20% greater than labeled potency.

Quality Assay: Contains 500 or more antitoxin units/mL.

Packaging: 20,000 unit vial

Doseform: Solution

Appearance: Practically colorless, transparent, or slightly opalescent liquid. Contains not less than 20% solids.

Solvent: Equine serum

Diluent:
> *For infusion:* Dilute each mL of antitoxin in 20 mL 0.9% sodium chloride or 5% dextrose for IV infusion.

Adjuvant: None

Allergens: Equine serum

Excipients: None

pH: 6 to 7

Diphtheria Antitoxin (Equine)

Storage/Stability: Store at 2° to 8°C (36° to 46°F). Potency is not affected by freezing. Contact manufacturer regarding prolonged exposure to room temperature or elevated temperatures. Shipped in insulated containers with coolant packs.

Production Process: Immunization of horses with diphtheria toxoid alone or in combination with diphtheria toxin. Antitoxin is harvested by precipitation and dialysis of equine plasma then refined by pepsin digestion and microfiltration.

Media: Equine plasma

Disease Epidemiology

See the Diphtheria Toxoid monograph in the Vaccines/Toxoids section.

Other Information

Perspective: See also the Diphtheria Toxoid monograph in the Vaccines/Toxoids section.

1890: Behring and Kitasato describe treatment of sheep with diphtheria antitoxin.

1891: A young girl in Berlin is the first human patient successfully treated with diphtheria antitoxin. Behring earns the 1901 Nobel Prize for this and related work.

1897: Ehrlich standardizes antitoxin. Ehrlich earns the 1908 Nobel Prize for this and related work.

1901: Antitoxin produced by St. Louis Health Department contaminated with tetanus spores causes death of 14 children.

1902: Congress enacts "An act to regulate the sale of viruses, serums, toxins, and analogous products" (subsequently called the Biologics Control Act), the first modern federal legislation to control the quality of pharmaceutical products. Diphtheria antitoxin is the first drug licensed under the act in the following year.

1911: Von Pirquet and Schick describe serum sickness following equine diphtheria antitoxin.

1920: Anchorage to Iditarod, Alaska, dog-sled run against a blizzard to deliver diphtheria antitoxin. Similar crisis in 1925 involved race from Anchorage to Nome.

Discontinued Products: Generic bovine antitoxin

National Policy: CDC. Availability of diphtheria antitoxin through an investigational new drug protocol. *MMWR.* 2004;53:413. http://www.cdc.gov/mmwr/preview/mmwrhtml/mm5319a3.htm.

CDC. Diphtheria, tetanus and pertussis: recommendations for vaccine use and other preventive measures. Recommendations of the Immunization Practices Advisory Committee (ACIP). *MMWR.* 1991;40(RR-10):1-28.

WHO. Diphtheria vaccine. *Wkly Epidemiol Rec.* 2006;81:24-32. www.who.int/wer/2006/wer8103.pdf.

Tetanus Immune Globulin (Human)

Immunoantidotes

Name:
HyperTet S/D

Manufacturer:
Talecris Biotherapeutics

Synonyms: TIG. The disease is also known as lockjaw. The neurotoxin associated with tetanus is called tetanospasmin.

Immunologic Characteristics

Microorganism: Bacterial exotoxin, *Clostridium tetani*, aerobic endospore-forming gram-positive rod

Viability: Inactive, passive, transient

Antigenic Form: Human immunoglobulin, unmodified (antitoxin)

Antigenic Type: Protein, IgG antibody, polyclonal, polymeric

Strains: Harvested without regard to strain

Use Characteristics

Indications: For passive, transient protection against tetanus in any person with a wound that may be contaminated with tetanus spores when:

(1) The patient's personal history of active immunization with tetanus toxoid is unknown or uncertain, or

(2) The person has received less than 3 prior doses of tetanus toxoid, or

(3) The person has received 3 prior doses of tetanus toxoid, but a delay of 24 hours or longer has occurred between the time of injury and initiation of tetanus prophylaxis.

Use TIG as soon as possible following tetanus-prone injuries. TIG has been used in treating clinical tetanus, but its use for this purpose is less clearly defined.

A history of having received tetanus "shots" is not reliable, unless it can be confirmed that such prior "shots" were tetanus toxoid and not tetanus antitoxin (TAT) or TIG. However, a history of service in the US Armed Forces for 3 months or longer since 1940 suggests that the person has received at least 1 dose and probably a complete immunizing series.

Unlabeled Uses: If hyperimmune TIG is unavailable, IGIV may be used to provide prompt passive immunity against tetanus. Among 29 lots tested, antitetanus IgG level varied from 4 to 90 units/mL (geometric mean: 18.6). A dose of 6 g (at 4 units/mL) is likely to provide an equivalent quantity of antitetanus IgG antibodies as a 500 unit dose of TIG, although the actual dose varies between lots. Just 1.6 g of lots with antibody levels greater than 15 units/mL would be needed.

Limitations: Provides only short-term passive immunity. A product containing tetanus toxoid adsorbed is needed to induce long-lasting active immunity. TIG does nothing to prevent microbial spread of the toxigenic organism. Conversely, antibiotics have no effect on the toxin. Select appropriate antibiotics to treat active infections (eg, penicillin G, a tetracycline). Further, adequate debridement and removal of all foreign materials and devitalized tissue is very important.

Outmoded Practices: Unlike immunoglobulin products harvested from animals, do not perform skin tests prior to administration of TIG. In most humans, intradermal injection of concentrated immune globulin with its buffers causes a localized area of inflammation that can be misinterpreted as a positive allergic reaction. This reaction is caused by localized tissue irritation of a chemical nature. Misinterpretation of such a test may cause urgently needed immunoglobulin to be withheld from a patient not actually allergic to it. True allergic responses to TIG IM are rare.

Contraindications:

Absolute: None

Relative: Patients with a history of systemic hypersensitivity reactions following administration of human immune globulin products. Persons with selective immunoglobulin A (IgA) deficiency have the potential for developing anti-IgA antibodies and could have anaphylactic reactions to subsequent administration of blood products (including immune globulin preparations) that contain IgA.

Immunodeficiency: In patients with impaired immunological response, as in agammaglobulinemia or during immunosuppressive therapy, consider the use of TIG in all tetanus-prone injuries.

Elderly: No specific information is available about geriatric use of TIG.

Pregnancy: Category C. Use only if clearly needed. Intact IgG crosses the placenta from the maternal circulation increasingly after 30 weeks gestation. Problems in humans have not been documented and are unlikely.

Lactation: It is not known if TIG antibodies are excreted into breast milk. Problems in humans have not been documented and are unlikely.

Children: Safe and effective in children. The pediatric dose is the same as for adults because, theoretically, the same amount of toxin will be produced in the child's body by the infective tetanus organism as it will in an adult's body. Alternatively, give 4 units/kg. At the same time, but in a different extremity and with a separate syringe, continue or complete the child's basic immunizing series with diphtheria and tetanus toxoids with pertussis vaccine (DTP) or pediatric strength diphtheria and tetanus toxoids (DT), as appropriate.

Adverse Reactions: Local and systemic reactions following TIG are infrequent and usually mild. Expect some pain, tenderness, and muscle stiffness at the injection site, persisting for several hours. Hives, angioedema, nephrotic syndrome, and local inflammation occur occasionally. Anaphylactic reactions are very infrequent.

Pharmacologic & Dosing Characteristics

Dosage: The Centers for Disease Control and Preventions (CDC) wound management guidelines appear in the DTP Overview in the Vaccines/Toxoids section.

Usual prophylactic TIG dose is 250 units. Give 500 units if wounds are severe or if treatment is delayed. Dosage may be increased to 1,000 to 2,000 units.

For therapy of tetanus, give 500 to 3,000 or 6,000 units.

See also the CDC's wound management guidelines at the end of this monograph.

Route & Site: Deep IM, preferably in the buttock, usually the upper, outer quadrant of the gluteal muscle. A meta-analysis of intrathecal therapy of tetanus with TIG or tetanus antitoxin found no conclusive evidence of efficacy by that route of administration.

Overdosage: Although few data are available, clinical experience with other immune globulin preparations suggests that the major manifestations of overdose would be pain and tenderness at the injection site.

Additional Doses: If wound contamination persists after 3 weeks, give second dose of TIG. Give repeat dose at time of any secondary surgery required 30 to 60 days following initial treatment.

Related Interventions: If needed, give a product containing tetanus toxoid adsorbed (eg, DTP, adult strength diphtheria and tetanus toxoids [Td] bivalent or with acellular pertussis vaccine [Tdap]) at the same time but in a different extremity and with a separate syringe.

Efficacy: High

Onset: Rapid, peak serum titer occurs within 2 to 3 days after IM injection.

Duration: Mean half-life is 3.5 to 4.5 weeks. An adequate antibody titer persists approximately 4 weeks.

Pharmacokinetics: Immunoglobulins are primarily eliminated by catabolism.

Protective Level: 0.01 antitoxin units/mL; 250 units yield at least 0.01 units/mL of tetanus antitoxin in serum for 4 weeks, which is an adequate response.

Mechanism: TIG is an antibody preparation containing antitoxin that neutralizes the free form of the powerful tetanus exotoxin. TIG does not affect toxin fixed to nerve tissue.

Drug Interactions: Concurrent administration of tetanus toxoid and TIG may delay development of active immunity by several days through partial antigen-antibody antagonism. However, this interaction is not considered clinically significant and does not preclude concurrent administration of both drugs if both are needed. Nonetheless, follow the CDC's wound management guidelines closely (see DTP Overview in the Vaccines/Toxoids section).

TIG may diminish the antibody response to attenuated measles, mumps, and rubella vaccines through antigen-antibody antagonism. As a general rule, administer live virus vaccines 14 to 30 days before or 6 to 12 weeks after immune globulin administration. Alternatively, administer live virus vaccines during this interval if corresponding antibody titers are measured 3 months after TIG administration. Base the interval on the dose of IgG administered. For varicella or a measles-containing vaccine, wait 3 months after standard TIG doses before giving the vaccine. Wait longer after high doses of TIG.

Inactivated vaccines generally are not affected by circulating antibodies or administration of exogenous antibodies. Immunization with such vaccines may occur at any time before or after antibody administration.

IGIM does not appear to interfere with development of immunity following oral poliovirus (OPV) or yellow fever vaccination. However, it may be prudent not to administer these vaccines shortly after IG administration. Exceptions include unexpected travel to or contact with epidemic or endemic areas or persons. If OPV is given with or shortly after TIG, repeat the OPV dose 3 months later if immunization is still indicated.

It is not know if TIG interferes with the efficacy of other attenuated vaccines (eg, adenovirus, Bacillus Calmette-Guérin, typhoid, vaccinia). It may be prudent not to administer these vaccines shortly after TIG administration unless unavoidable.

As with other drugs administered by IM injection, give TIG with caution to persons receiving anticoagulant therapy.

Pharmaceutical Characteristics

Concentration: 15% to 18% protein, not less than 90% IgG and not less than 250 antitoxin units per container.

Quality Assay:
  USP requirement: Standardized against US Reference Standard Tetanus Antitoxin and US Control Tetanus Toxin, using a guinea pig potency test.

Packaging: 250 units occupy approximately 1 mL. Contains excess potency, 10% greater than labeled potency. 250 unit single-dose prefilled syringe with 22-gauge, 1¼-inch needle (NDC#: 13533-0634-02).

Doseform: Solution

Tetanus Immune Globulin (Human)

Appearance: Transparent to slightly opalescent; essentially colorless. May develop slight granular deposit during storage.

Solvent: Sterile water for injection

Adjuvant: None

Preservative: None

Allergens: 0.2 to 0.8 mg/mL IgA, a trace amount of IgM

Excipients: 0.21 to 0.32 molar glycine, sodium carbonate or acetic acid to adjust pH

pH: 6.4 to 7.2

Shelf Life: Expires within 36 months

Storage/Stability: Store at 2° to 8°C (36° to 46°F). Product can tolerate 30 days at 30°C (86°F). Discard if frozen. Contact manufacturer regarding prolonged exposure to room temperature or elevated temperatures. Shipping data not provided.

Production Process: Cohn-Oncley methods 6 & 9 cold-ethanol fractionation process of plasma of people hyperimmunized with tetanus toxoid. A virucidal solvent-detergent treatment step using 0.3% tri-n-butylphosphate and 0.2% sodium cholate at 30°C (86°F) for at least 6 hours is performed. It is incubated in the final container for 21 to 28 days at 20° to 27°C (68° to 81°F).

Media: Human plasma, at least 10 units per lot

Disease Epidemiology

See the Tetanus Toxoid Adsorbed monograph in the Vaccines/Toxoids section.

Other Information

Perspective: See also the Tetanus Toxoid Adsorbed monograph in the Vaccines/Toxoids section.

1890: Behring and Kitisato use tetanus antitoxin in animals. Humans are treated beginning a year later.

1903: Tetanus antitoxin used in humans in the United States, contributing to decline in tetanus cases resulting from fireworks on Independence Day.

1950s: Rubbo and Suri develop human tetanus immune globulin. Human tetanus immune globulin supercedes equine tetanus antitoxin (antiserum).

First Licensed:
Cutter (now Talecris): October 17, 1957
Massachusetts: May 1968

Discontinued Products:
Equine antitoxin: Tet-GG Antitoxin (Lilly)
Human TIG: AR-Tet (Armour); *BayTet* (Bayer), *Gamatet, Homo-Tet, Gamulin-T* (Dow); *Hu-Tet* (Hyland); *HyperTet* (Miles, Bayer); *Immu-Tetanus* (Parke-Davis); *Pro-Tet* (Lederle); *T-I-Gammagee* (Merck).

National Policy: CDC. Diphtheria, tetanus and pertussis: recommendations for vaccine use and other preventive measures. Recommendations of the Immunization Practices Advisory Committee (ACIP). *MMWR.* 1991;40(RR-10):1-28.

CDC Wound Management Guidelines				
	Clean, minor wounds		All other wounds[a]	
History of adsorbed tetanus toxoid	Td or Tdap[b]	TIG	Td or Tdap[b]	TIG
Unknown or less than 3 doses	Yes	No	Yes	Yes
3 or more doses[c]	No[d]	No	No[e]	No

a Including, but not limited to, wounds contaminated with dirt, feces, soil, or saliva; puncture wounds; avulsions; or wounds resulting from missiles, crushing, burns, or frostbite.

b For children younger than 7 years of age, trivalent DTP is preferred to tetanus toxoid alone. Use DT if pertussis vaccine is validly contraindicated. For people 7 years of age and older, Td bivalent or with acellular pertussis vaccine (Tdap) is preferred.

c If the patient has received only 3 doses of fluid toxoid, give a fourth dose of toxoid, preferably an adsorbed toxoid.

d Yes, if more than 10 years have elapsed since the last dose of tetanus toxoid.

e Yes, if more than 5 years have elapsed since the last dose of tetanus toxoid.

Antivenin Summary

Immunoantidotes

Obscure & Exotic Antivenins: To manage bites of exotic animals, contact the nearest drug information center or large zoological park.

The American Zoo and Aquarium Association coordinates publication of the Antivenom Index. This inventory lists information on venomous snakes and sources of antivenom. At this time, the Antivenom Index is maintained through voluntary contribution and covers only those venomous snakes held in zoos. For more information, contact the publications department at (301) 562-0777 ext. 253 or http://www.aza.org.

Antivenin Comparison

	Crotalid snakes	Coral snakes	Widow spiders	Scorpion
Manufacturer	Protherics, BTG	Pfizer	Merck	Accredo Health Group for Rare Diseases Therapeutics, Instituto Bioclon
Species contents	*Crotalus, Agkistrodon*	*Micrurus fulvius fulvius*	*Latrodectus mactans*	*Centruroides noxius, Centruroides limpidus limpidus, Centruroides limpidus tecomanus, Centruroides staffusus staffusus*
Cross-efficacy	Some related species	*Micrurus fulvius tenere*	Other *Latrodectus* species	*Centruroides sculpturatis* (also called *Centruroides exilicauda*)
Limitations	Other crotalids, vipers	*Micruroides euryxanthus*	—	Other scorpion genera
Treatment threshold	Prompt administration if symptoms progressing	Consider prompt administration	Primarily for children and elderly patients	Prompt administration if symptoms progressing
Dosage range	4 to 6 vials or more	3 to 15 vials	1 to 2 vials	3 vials or more
Route:				
Sensitivity test	Not required	ID	ID, conjunctival	Not required
Therapy	IV infusion	IV infusion	IV infusion, IM	IV infusion
Source	Ovine (Fab)	Equine (intact IgG)	Equine (intact IgG)	Equine, F(ab')$_2$
Routine storage	Refrigerate	Refrigerate	Refrigerate	Room temperature (up to 25°C [77°F])
Diluent:				
For reconstitution	0.9% NaCl	Sterile water	Sterile water	0.9% NaCl
For injection	0.9% NaCl	0.9% NaCl	0.9% NaCl	0.9% NaCl

References: Allen C. Arachnid envenomations. *Emerg Med Clin North Am.* 1992;10:269-298.

Auerbach PS. Marine envenomations. *N Engl J Med.* 1991;325:486-493.

Chippaux JP, et al. Production and use of snake antivenin. In: Tu AT, ed. *Handbook of Natural Toxins, Volume 5: Reptile Venoms & Toxins.* New York, NY: Marcel Dekker; 1991:529-555.

Chippaux JP, Goyffon M. Venoms, antivenoms and immunotherapy. *Toxicon.* 1998;36(6):823-846.

Russell FE. Snake venom immunology: historical and practical considerations. *J Toxicol Toxin Rev.* 1988;7:1-82.

Theakston RD, Warrell DA. Antivenoms: a list of hyperimmune sera currently available for the treatment of envenoming by bites and stings. *Toxicon.* 1991;29:1419-1470.

WHO. *Progress in the Characterization of Venoms and Standardization of Antivenoms.* Geneva, Switzerland: WHO Offset Publication #58; 1981.

Crotalidae Polyvalent Immune Fab (Ovine)

Immunoantidotes

Name:
  CroFab

Manufacturer:
  Manufactured by Protherics, distributed by BTG International

Synonyms: Early in its development, this product was known as *CroTab*.

Comparison: No clinical studies have been conducted comparing *CroFab* with other antivenins, therefore, no objective comparisons can be made. Theoretically, Fab fragments should induce serum sickness less often than intact equine IgG products.

Immunologic Characteristics

Antigen Source: Venoms of pit viper (crotalid) snakes. Family Crotalidae (but not the Old World vipers, family Viperidae).

Viability: Inactive, passive, transient

Antigenic Form: Ovine (sheep) immunoglobulin, fragmented (antivenin)

Antigenic Type: Protein, IgG antibody fragments, polyclonal, antigen-binding (Fab) fragments

Strains: *Crotalus atrox* (western diamondback rattlesnake), *Crotalus adamanteus* (eastern diamondback rattlesnake), *Crotalus scutulatus* (Mojave rattlesnake), and *Agkistrodon piscivorus* (cottonmouth or water moccasin)

Use Characteristics

Indications: For clinical management of patients with minimal or moderate North American rattlesnake envenomation. Administer within 6 hours of snakebite to prevent clinical deterioration and systemic coagulation abnormalities.

Definition of Minimal, Moderate, and Severe Envenomation in Clinical Studies of *CroFab*	
Envenomation category	Definition
Minimal	Swelling, pain, and ecchymosis limited to immediate bite site; systemic signs and symptoms absent; coagulation parameters normal with no evidence of bleeding.
Moderate	Swelling, pain, and ecchymosis involving less than a full extremity or, if bite sustained on the trunk, head, or neck, extending < 50 cm; systemic signs and symptoms may be present but not life-threatening (eg, nausea, vomiting, oral paresthesia or unusual tastes, systolic blood pressure < 90 mm Hg, heart rate < 150, tachypnea); coagulation parameters may be abnormal, but no evidence of bleeding present. Minor hematuria, gum bleeding, and nosebleeds allowed if not considered clinically severe.
Severe	Swelling, pain, and ecchymosis involving more than an entire extremity or threatening the airway; systemic signs and symptoms markedly abnormal, including severe alteration of mental status, severe hypotension, severe tachycardia, tachypnea, or respiratory insufficiency; coagulation parameters are abnormal, with serious bleeding or severe threat of bleeding.

Unlabeled Uses: Preliminary data from experiments in mice using whole IgG from the sheep immunized for *CroFab* production suggest that *CroFab* might possess antigenic cross-reactivity against the venoms of some Middle Eastern and North African snakes, however, there are no human clinical data available to confirm these findings. In these experiments, separate groups of mice were injected with increasing doses of *CroFab* premixed with two LD$_{50}$ of each venom tested. Based on the data from this study in mice, *CroFab* has relatively good cross-protection against venoms not used in the immunization of flocks used to produce it (eg, *C. h. atricaudatus*, *A. c. contortrix*, *S. m. barbouri*, *C. h. horridus*), except for *C. v. helleri*, where a very high dose is required, and for *C. m. molossus*, where a moderately high dose is required.

Contraindications:

Absolute: Essentially none

Relative: People with a known history of hypersensitivity to papaya or papain, unless the benefits outweigh the risks.

Immunodeficiency: Impairment of effect is unlikely.

Elderly: No specific information is available about geriatric use of *CroFab*.

Carcinogenicity: Animal carcinogenicity studies have not been conducted with *CroFab*.

Mutagenicity: Animal mutagenicity studies have not been conducted with *CroFab*.

Fertility Impairment: Animal reproduction studies have not been conducted with *CroFab*.

Pregnancy: Category C. Use if clearly needed. It is not known if antivenin antibody fragments cross the placenta. Intact IgG increasingly crosses the placenta from the maternal circulation during the third trimester. Problems in humans have not been documented.

Lactation: It is not known if antivenin antibody fragments cross into human breast milk. Problems in humans have not been documented.

Children: Safety and efficacy of antivenin antibody fragments in children younger than 11 years of age have not been established. The absolute venom dose following snakebite is expected to be the same in children and adults. Therefore, no dosage adjustment for age should be made.

Adverse Reactions: Most adverse reactions to *CroFab* reported in clinical studies were mild or moderate in severity. The most common adverse events reported in the clinical studies were urticaria and rash. Adverse events involving the skin and appendages (primarily rash, urticaria, and pruritus) were reported in 14 of the 42 patients. An allergic reaction with urticaria, dyspnea, and wheezing occurred in one patient.

Of the 25 patients who experienced adverse reactions, 3 experienced severe or serious adverse reactions. The patient who experienced a serious adverse event had a recurrent coagulopathy caused by envenomation, which required rehospitalization and additional antivenin administration. This patient eventually made a complete recovery. The other 2 patients had severe adverse reactions consisting of severe hives following treatment in 1 case and a severe rash and pruritus several days after treatment in the other. Both patients recovered after treatment with antihistamines and prednisone. One patient discontinued *CroFab* therapy because of a recurrent coagulation abnormality.

In the 42 patients treated with *CroFab* for minimal or moderate crotalid envenomations, there were 7 events classified as early serum reactions and 5 events classified as late serum reactions, and none were serious. In the clinical studies, serum reactions consisted mainly of urticaria and rash, and all patients recovered without sequelae. Serum sickness consisting of severe rash and pruritus developed in 1 patient.

Hematology: Coagulopathy arises in many victims of viper envenomation, as the venom interferes with the blood coagulation cascade. In clinical trials with *CroFab*, recurrent coagulopathy (return of a coagulation abnormality after successful treatment with antivenin), characterized by decreased fibrinogen, decreased platelets, and elevated prothrom-

Crotalidae Polyvalent Immune Fab (Ovine)

bin time, occurred in about half of patients studied. The clinical significance of these recurrent abnormalities is not known. Recurrent coagulation abnormalities were observed only in patients who experienced coagulation abnormalities during their initial hospitalization. Optimal dosing to completely prevent recurrent coagulopathy has not been determined. Because crotalid venoms can leak from depot sites and persist in the blood longer than *CroFab*, repeat dosing to prevent or treat such recurrence may be necessary. Recurrent coagulopathy may persist for 1 to 2 weeks or more. Monitor patients who experience coagulopathy caused by snakebite during initial hospitalization for signs and symptoms of recurrent coagulopathy for 1 week or longer at the physician's discretion. During this period, carefully assess the need for retreatment with *CroFab* and use of any type of anticoagulant or antiplatelet drug.

Hypersensitivity: The possible risks and side effects that attend the administration of heterologous animal proteins in humans include anaphylactic and anaphylactoid reactions, delayed allergic reactions (late serum reaction or serum sickness), and a possible febrile response to immune complexes formed by animal antibodies and neutralized venom components. Although no patient in the clinical studies of *CroFab* experienced a severe anaphylactic reaction, consider and inform the patient of the possibility of an anaphylactic reaction. If an anaphylactic reaction occurs during the infusion, cease *CroFab* administration at once and administer appropriate treatment (eg, epinephrine). Patients with known allergies to sheep protein would be particularly at risk for an anaphylactic reaction. Trace amounts of papain or inactivated papain residues may be present. Patients with allergies to papain, chymopapain, other papaya extracts, or the pineapple enzyme bromelain also may be at risk for an allergic reaction to *CroFab*. In addition, some dust mite allergens and some latex allergens share antigenic structures with papain; patients with these allergies may be allergic to papain. Monitor all patients treated with antivenin carefully for signs and symptoms of an acute allergic reaction (eg, urticaria, pruritus, erythema, angioedema, bronchospasm with wheezing or cough, stridor, laryngeal edema, hypotension, tachycardia). Follow up all patients for signs and symptoms of delayed allergic reactions or serum sickness (eg, rash, fever, myalgia, arthralgia) and treat appropriately if necessary.

Consultation: Poison control centers are helpful resources for individual treatment advice.

Pharmacologic & Dosing Characteristics

Dosage: Initiate antivenin administration as soon as possible after crotalid snakebite in patients who develop signs of progressive envenomation (eg, worsening local injury, coagulation abnormality, systemic signs of envenomation). Antivenin dosage requirements depend upon an individual patient's response. The recommended initial dose is 4 to 6 vials. Infuse the initial dose of *CroFab* diluted in 250 mL of 0.9% sodium chloride over 60 minutes.

Route: IV infusion. Administer the infusion slowly over the first 10 minutes at a 25 to 50 mL/h rate, with careful observation for any allergic reaction. If no such reaction occurs, the infusion rate may be increased to the full 250 mL/h rate until completion. Close patient monitoring is necessary.

Special Handling: With other antibody therapies, reactions during the infusion such as fever, low back pain, wheezing, and nausea are often related to the rate of infusion and can be controlled by decreasing the rate of administration of the solution.

Overdosage: The maximum amount that can safely be administered in single or multiple doses has not been determined. Doses of up to 18 vials (approximately 13.5 g of protein) have been administered without any observed direct toxic effect.

Additional Doses: Observe the patient for up to 1 hour after completing this first dose to determine if initial control of the envenomation has been achieved (defined as complete arrest of local manifestations, and return of coagulation tests and systemic signs to normal). If initial control is not achieved by the first dose, give an additional dose of 4 to 6 vials until initial control of the envenomation syndrome has been achieved. After initial control has been established, additional 2-vial doses of *CroFab* every 6 hours for up to 18 hours (3 doses) is recommended. Optimal dosing following the 18-hour scheduled regimen of *CroFab* has not been determined. Additional 2-vial doses may be administered as deemed necessary by the treating physician, based on the patient's clinical course.

Related Interventions: Supportive measures are often used to treat certain manifestations of crotalid snake envenomation, such as pain, swelling, hypotension, and wound infection.

Laboratory Tests: None known

Efficacy: In animal studies, *CroFab* neutralized the venoms of 10 clinically important North American crotalid snakes in a murine lethality model.

Two open-label, multicenter clinical trials using *CroFab* were conducted in otherwise healthy patients 11 years of age and older who had suffered from minimal or moderate North American crotalid envenomation that showed evidence of progression. Progression was defined as the worsening of any evaluation parameter used in the grading of an envenomation: local injury, laboratory abnormality, or symptoms and signs attributable to crotalid snake venom poisoning. To date, there are no clinical data supporting the efficacy of *CroFab* in patients presenting with severe envenomation. In both clinical studies, efficacy was determined using a Snakebite Severity Score (SSS) and an investigator's clinical assessment (ICA) of efficacy. The SSS measures the severity of envenomation based on 6 body categories: local wound (eg, pain, swelling, ecchymosis), pulmonary, cardiovascular, gastrointestinal, hematological, and nervous system effects. A higher score indicates worse symptoms. The ICA was based on the investigator's clinical judgment as to whether the patient had a clinical response (pretreatment signs and symptoms of envenomation arrested or improved after treatment), partial response (signs and symptoms worsened, but at a slower rate than expected after treatment), or nonresponse (patient's condition not favorably affected by the treatment).

In the first study (TAb001), 11 patients received an IV dose of 4 vials over 60 minutes. An additional 4-vial dose was administered after the first *CroFab* infusion, if deemed necessary by the investigator. At the 1-hour assessment, 10 of 11 patients had no change or a decrease in SSS. Ten of 11 patients also were judged to have a clinical response by the ICA. Several patients, after initial clinical response, subsequently required additional vials of *CroFab* to stem progressive or recurrent symptoms and signs. No patient in this first study experienced an anaphylactic or anaphylactoid response or evidence of an early or late serum reaction as a result of administration of *CroFab*.

Based on observations from the first study, the second study (TAb002) compared 2 different dosage schedules. Patients were given an initial IV dose of 6 vials with an option to retreat with an additional 6 vials, if needed, to achieve initial control of the envenomation syndrome. Initial control was defined as complete arrest of local manifestations, and return of coagulation tests and systemic signs to normal. Once initial control was achieved, patients were randomized to receive additional *CroFab* either every 6 hours for 18 hours (scheduled group) or as needed (PRN group). In this trial, *CroFab* was administered safely to 31 patients with minimal or moderate crotalid envenomation. All 31 patients enrolled in the study achieved initial control of their envenomation with *CroFab*, and 30, 25, and 26 of the 31 patients achieved a clinical response based on the ICA at 1, 6, and 12 hours, respectively, following initial control. Additionally, the mean SSS was significantly decreased across the patient groups by the 12-hour evaluation time point ($P = 0.05$ for the scheduled group; $P = 0.05$ for the PRN group). There was no statistically significant difference between the scheduled group and the PRN group with regard to the decrease in SSS.

In published accounts of rattlesnake bites, a decrease in platelets accompanied moderately severe envenomation, which whole blood transfusions could not correct. These platelet count decreases can last for many hours and often several days following the venomous bite. In this clinical study, 6 patients had predosing platelet counts below 100,000 cells/mm^3 (baseline average, 44,000 cells/mm^3). Of note, the platelet counts for all 6 patients increased to normal levels (average, 209,000 cells/mm^3) at 1 hour following initial control dosing with *CroFab*.

Although there was no significant difference in the decrease in SSS between the scheduled and PRN treatment groups, data suggest that scheduled dosing may provide better control of envenomation symptoms caused by the continued leaking of venom from depot sites. Scheduled patients experienced a lower incidence of coagulation abnormalities at follow-up compared with PRN patients (14% vs 44% to 56%). In addition, the need to administer additional *CroFab* to patients in the PRN group after initial control suggests that there is a continued need for antivenin for adequate treatment.

Sensitization: Skin testing has not been used in clinical trials of *CroFab* and is not required. Patients who receive a course of treatment with a foreign protein such as *CroFab* may become sensitized to it. Therefore, caution should be used when administering a repeat course of treatment with *CroFab* for a subsequent envenomation episode.

Onset: Prompt, minutes

Duration: Hours

Pharmacokinetics: Based on data from 3 patients, the elimination half-life for total Fab ranged from approximately 12 to 23 hours. These limited pharmacokinetic estimates of half-life are augmented by data obtained with an analogous ovine Fab product produced by Protherics using a similar production process. In that study, 8 healthy subjects were given 1 mg IV digoxin followed by an approximately equimolar neutralizing dose of 76 mg digoxin immune Fab (ovine). Total Fab was shown to have a volume of distribution of 0.3 L/kg, a systemic clearance of 32 mL/min (approximately 0.4 mL/min/kg) and an elimination half-life of approximately 15 hours.

Mechanism: Venom-specific Fab fragment of IgG bind and neutralize venom toxins, facilitating their redistribution away from target tissues and their elimination from the body.

Drug Interactions: No specific drug interactions with *CroFab* are known.

Patient Information: Advise the patient to contact the physician immediately if any signs and symptoms of delayed allergic reactions or serum sickness (eg, rash, pruritus, urticaria) develop after hospital discharge. Advise the patient to contact the physician immediately if unusual bruising or bleeding (eg, nosebleeds, excessive bleeding after brushing teeth, appearance of blood in stools or urine, excessive menstrual bleeding, petechiae, excessive bruising, persistent oozing from superficial injuries) develop after hospital discharge, to see if additional antivenin treatment is needed. Such bruising or bleeding may occur for up to 1 week or longer after initial treatment. Advise patients to follow up with the physician for monitoring.

Pharmaceutical Characteristics

Concentration: Each vial contains 1 g or less of total protein and not less than the indicated number of mouse LD$_{50}$ neutralizing units: *C. atrox* (western diamondback rattlesnake): 1,270; *C. adamanteus* (eastern diamondback rattlesnake): 420; *C. scutulatus* (Mojave rattlesnake): 5,570; *A. piscivorus* (cottonmouth or water moccasin): 780.

Quality Assay: Each monospecific antivenin is isolated on ion-exchange and affinity-chromatography columns. *CroFab* is standardized by its ability to neutralize the lethal action of each of 4 venom immunogens after IV injection in mice. Potency varies from batch to batch; however, a minimum number of mouse LD$_{50}$ neutralizing units against each of the 4 venoms is included in every vial of final product. One neutralizing unit is determined as the amount of the mixed monospecific Fab proteins necessary to neutralize one LD$_{50}$ of each of the four venoms, where the LD$_{50}$ is the amount of venom that would be lethal in 50% of mice.

Packaging: Box containing 2 vials of *CroFab*, diluent not included

NDC Number: 50633-0110-12

Doseform: Lyophilized powder for solution

Appearance: White lyophilized powder

Diluent:

For reconstitution: 10 mL of sterile water for injection per vial

For infusion: Reconstituted vials should be further diluted in 250 mL of sodium chloride 0.9%.

Preservative: Residual thimerosal from the manufacturing process (representing 104.5 mcg or less elemental mercury per vial)

Allergens: Trace amounts of papain or inactivated papain residues may be present.

Excipients: Sodium phosphate buffer, consisting of dibasic sodium phosphate and sodium chloride. The final product contains up to 30 mcg of mercury per vial, which amounts to no more than 0.6 mg of mercury per dose (based on the maximum dose of 18 vials studied in clinical trials).

pH: 7 to 8

Shelf Life: Expires within 30 months

Storage/Stability: Store at 2° to 8°C (36° to 46°F). Do not freeze. Contact the manufacturer regarding exposure to extreme temperatures. Shipped in insulated containers with coolant packs, usually by second-day courier.

Use the product within 4 hours after reconstitution.

Handling: Reconstitute each vial of *CroFab* with 18 mL sterile water, mixing by continuous gentle swirling. Further dilute the contents of reconstituted vials in 250 mL of sodium chloride 0.9%, mixing gently. Use both the reconstituted and diluted product within 4 hours.

Production Process: Fab (monovalent) immunoglobulin fragments are obtained from the blood of healthy sheep flocks immunized with one of several North American snake venoms. To obtain the final antivenin product, the 4 different monospecific antivenins are mixed. Each monospecific antivenin is prepared by separating the immunoglobulin from the ovine serum, using papain to cleave whole antibody into Fab and Fc fragments, and isolating the venom-specific Fab fragments on ion exchange and affinity chromatography columns.

Other Information

Perspective:

1887: Sewall shows that repeated administration of small doses of snake venom to pigeons leads to resistance.

1894: Calmette prepares antivenene, an equine preparation against mixed cobra and viperine venoms.

1895: Fraser develops cobra antivenom.

1898: Brazil demonstrates specificity of antivenoms.

1938: Mulford produces Antivenin Nearctic Cotalidae. Nearctic refers to the geographic region of North America north of Mexico. A separate bothrops antitoxin was also produced.

1947: Wyeth refines Antivenin Nearctic Crotalidae, yielding Antivenin Crotalidae (Equine) in 1956. Product distributed until approximately 2001.

First Licensed: October 2, 2000

References: Consroe P, et al. Comparison of a new ovine antigen binding fragment (Fab) antivenin for United States Crotalidae with the commercial antivenin for protection against venom-induced lethality in mice. *Am J Trop Med Hyg.* 1995;53:507-510.

Antivenin *Micrurus fulvius* (Equine)

Immunoantidotes

Name:
Generic

Manufacturer:
Pfizer

Synonyms: North American coral snake antivenin

Immunologic Characteristics

Antigen Source: Venom of coral snakes, family Elapidae

Viability: Inactive, passive, transient

Antigenic Form: Equine immunoglobulin, unmodified (antivenin)

Antigenic Type: Protein, IgG antibody, polyclonal, polymeric. Skin tests assess immediate (type I) hypersensitivity.

Strains: *Micrurus fulvius fulvius*

Use Characteristics

Indications: For passive, transient protection from the toxic effects of venoms of *Micrurus fulvius fulvius* (Eastern coral snake). Also neutralizes the venom of *Micrurus fulvius tenere* (Texas coral snake). If indicated, the best effect results if antivenin administration begins within 4 hours after envenomation.

This antivenin partially neutralizes the venom of *Micrurus dumerilii carinicauda* and minimally neutralizes the venom of *Micrurus spixii*. It also may provide some protection against the venom of *Micrurus nigrocinctus.*

Limitations: Not effective against the venom of *Micruroides euryxanthus* (Arizonan or Sonoran coral snake), found only in southeastern Arizona, southwestern New Mexico, and portions of Mexico, or other snakes not described above.

Contraindications:

Absolute: Essentially none

Relative: Patients with a history of severe hypersensitivity reactions to products containing equine serum or similar proteins. Even in the case of horse-serum hypersensitivity in a severely envenomed patient, cautious antivenin administration with concurrent titrated epinephrine and antihistamine may be attempted.

Immunodeficiency: No impairment of effect is likely.

Elderly: No specific information is available about geriatric use of coral snake antivenin.

Pregnancy: Category C. Use only if clearly needed, with appropriate consideration of the risk-benefit ratio. It is not known if antivenom antibodies cross the placenta. Intact IgG crosses the placenta from the maternal circulation increasingly after 30 weeks gestation.

Lactation: It is not known if antivenom antibodies are excreted into breast milk. Problems in humans have not been documented.

Children: The pediatric dose is equivalent to the adult dose. Pediatric doses are not adjusted by the weight of the patient.

Adverse Reactions: Immediate reactions (eg, shock, anaphylaxis) usually occur within 30 minutes of administration. Should any systemic reaction occur during antivenin administration, discontinue antivenin and initiate appropriate treatment. The following signs and symptoms may develop before withdrawing the administration needle: apprehension, flushing, itching, urticaria, edema of the face, tongue, and throat, cough, dyspnea, cyanosis, vomiting, and collapse. Defibrination and disseminated intravascular coagulation syndromes may occur.

Serum sickness may occur 5 to 24 days after administration. The interval may be shorter than 5 days, especially in those who have received preparations containing horse serum in the past. The usual signs and symptoms are malaise, fever, urticaria, lymphadenopathy, edema, arthralgia, nausea, and vomiting. Occasionally, neurological manifestations develop, such as meningismus or peripheral neuritis. Peripheral neuritis usually involves the shoulders and arms. Pain and weakness are frequently present, and permanent atrophy may result.

Habitat: Two genera of coral snakes inhabit the United States: *Micrurus* (including the eastern and Texas varieties), and *Micruroides* (the Arizonan or Sonoran variety). *Micrurus fulvius fulvius* inhabits an area from North Carolina south to Florida and west to the Mississippi River. *Micrurus fulvius tenere* inhabits an area including Louisiana, Arkansas, central Texas, and northern Mexico. Several other species of coral snake inhabit much of Central and South America, including 3 genera, *Leptomicrurus*, *Micrurus*, and *Micruroides*.

Identification: These subspecies can be differentiated by experts but are very similar in appearance. The adult coral snake (*Micrurus fulvius*) may vary between 20 to 44 inches in length, has a black snout, and yellow, black, and red bands encircling the body. The red and black rings are wider than the interposed yellow rings. However, melanistic (all black), albino (all white), and partially pigmented snakes are seen rarely. Coral snakes are secretive and rarely bite unless disturbed or handled. The fangs are short, erect, and fixed to the maxilla. Venom flows through the fang from a duct at its base. In contrast to pit vipers (eg, rattlesnakes, copperheads, cottonmouths), coral snakes have round pupils and lack facial pits.

Snake Bite Information: Unlike pit vipers that strike and rapidly withdraw after insertion of the fangs, coral snakes may strike, hold on, and "chew," presumably so their less efficient biting mechanism can introduce a sufficient amount of venom to immobilize prey. This chewing may result in 1 or more bites. Permitted to bite under laboratory conditions, *Micrurus fulvius fulvius* snakes have yielded 1 to 28 mg of venom per envenomation.

There is a direct, linear relationship between length of the snake and venom yield. The adult human LD_{50} may be 4 to 5 mg of venom.

Signs & Symptoms of Envenomation: Coral snake venom is chiefly paralytic (neurotoxic) in action, although it may have other systemic effects. Envenomation usually produces only minimal to moderate tissue reaction and pain at the site of the bite. Although patients who exhibit 1 or more fang punctures are most likely to be victims of envenomation, there is no way to predict if any given victim has been envenomed by a coral snake bite. Similar to crotalid bites, only 40% to 50% of coral snake bites involve envenomation.

Most coral snake bites are inflicted upon the upper extremities, especially the hands and fingers. The limited size of the biting apparatus makes it difficult for the coral snake to penetrate clothing or to successfully grasp any part of the body except hands and feet. Never picking up colorful snakes, never putting hands where they cannot be seen (eg, reaching behind rocks, logs, flowers), and always wearing leather shoes will substantially reduce the chances of a bite.

Unlike crotalid bites, severe and even fatal envenomation from a coral snake bite can be present without any significant local tissue reaction.

Local: Scratch marks or fang puncture wounds, no edema to moderate edema, erythema, pain or discoloration at the bite, and paresthesia in the bitten extremity.

Systemic: Euphoria, lethargy, weakness, nausea, vomiting, excessive salivation, ptosis of the eyelids, dyspnea, abnormal reflexes, convulsions, and motor weakness or paralysis, including complete respiratory paralysis. Signs and symptoms of envenomation usually begin 1 to 7 hours after the bite, but may be delayed for as long as 18 hours. If envenomation occurs, the signs and symptoms may progress rapidly and precipitously. Paralysis has occurred within 2.5 hours after a bite and appears to be of a bulbar type, involving cranial motor nerves. Death from respiratory paralysis has occurred within 4 hours of envenomation.

Envenomation Management: If possible, immobilize the patient immediately and completely. Transport the patient to the nearest hospital as soon as possible. If complete immobilization is not practical, splint the bitten extremity to limit systemic spread of venom. If the biting snake was killed, bring it to the hospital. Any victim of a coral snake bite who has any evidence of a break in the skin caused by the snake's teeth or fangs should be hospitalized for observation or treatment.

Cleanse the bite area with germicidal soap and water to remove any venom remaining on the skin. If fang puncture wounds are present, application of a tourniquet and incision and suction over the fang punctures has previously been recommended, even though there is no evidence that incision and suction are of value in removing coral snake venom. Maintain close observation of the patient for 24 hours, checking the respiratory rate every 30 minutes. Perform appropriate horse-serum hypersensitivity tests ahead of time, so that if administration of antivenin is required, data on how to proceed will be available.

It has been recommended to begin IV administration of coral snake antivenin to patients with 1 or more fang puncture wounds as soon as possible and before onset of signs and symptoms of envenomation. If signs and symptoms of envenomation occur in a patient under observation or are already present at the time the patient is first seen, give antivenin promptly by the IV route. With vigorous treatment and careful observation, patients with complete respiratory paralysis have recovered, indicating that the respiratory paralysis is reversible. Hemoglobinuria has been observed in experimental animals envenomed by coral snakes. Hence, continuous bladder drainage is recommended, with careful attention to urinary output and blood-electrolyte balance.

Do not pack the bitten extremity in ice. Cryotherapy is contraindicated because of the possibility of additional tissue damage.

Pharmacologic & Dosing Characteristics

Dosage: Mix by gentle swirling. To avoid foaming and protein degradation, do not shake.

Sensitivity test: Carefully review the patient's history, including any report of asthma, hay fever, urticaria, or other allergic manifestations, allergic reactions upon exposure to horses, or prior injections of horse serum. Perform a skin test prior to any antivenin administration, regardless of clinical history, as a guide to speed of therapeutic antivenin administration. Immediate-hypersensitivity skin tests have no bearing on whether or not delayed reactions will occur after administration of the full dose.

To apply a skin test, inject 0.02 to 0.03 mL ID of a 1:10 v/v dilution of horse serum or antivenin, typically on the dorsal forearm. Use a freshly compounded 1:100 v/v or weaker dilution for preliminary skin testing if the patient's history suggests hypersensitivity. Apply a negative control test of the same volume of 0.9% sodium chloride to the comparable site on the opposite extremity. Use of larger amounts for the skin-test dose increases the likelihood of false-positive reactions, and, in an exquisitely hypersensitive patient, increases the risk of a systemic reaction from the skin-test dose.

A positive reaction to a skin test occurs within 5 to 30 minutes, manifested by a wheal with or without pseudopods and surrounding erythema. In general, the shorter the interval between injection and the beginning of the skin reaction, the greater the hypersensitivity.

If history and skin test are both negative, proceed with antivenin administration as described below, recognizing that an immediate reaction to antivenin infusion has not been ruled out.

If the history is positive and the skin test is clearly positive, administration may be dangerous. In such instances, weigh the risk of antivenin administration against the risk of withholding it, given that envenomation may be fatal. Use the desensitization protocol if antivenin administration is elected.

If the history is negative and the skin test is mildly or questionably positive, administer the antivenin according to the desensitization protocol to reduce risk of severe immediate systemic reaction.

Desensitization protocol:

(1) In separate vials or syringes, compound fresh 1:100 and 1:10 v/v dilutions of antivenin. 0.9% sodium chloride is frequently selected as the solvent for such dilutions.

(2) Inject subcutaneously 0.1, 0.2, and then 0.5 mL of the 1:100 v/v dilution at 15-minute intervals. Repeat this 3-volume sequence with the 1:10 v/v dilution, and then repeat the 3-volume sequence with undiluted antivenin.

(3) Allow 15 minutes or longer between injections and proceed with the next dose if no reaction follows the previous dose.

(4) If a systemic reaction occurs after any injection, place a tourniquet proximal to the site of injection and administer an appropriate subcutaneous dose of epinephrine 1:1,000, proximal to the tourniquet or into another extremity. Wait 30 minutes or longer before injecting another dose. For the next dose, repeat the last dose that did not evoke a reaction.

(5) If no reaction occurs after 0.5 mL of undiluted antivenin, switch to the IM route and continue doubling the dose at 15-minute intervals until the entire dose has been injected, or proceed to the IV route as described below.

(6) The preceding schedule may require 3 to 5 hours or longer to administer the initial dose, even though time is an important factor in neutralization of venom in a critically ill patient. Alternatively, give 50 to 100 mg of diphenhydramine IV, followed by slow infusion of diluted antivenin for 15 to 20 minutes while carefully observing the patient for signs and symptoms of anaphylaxis. If anaphylaxis does not occur, continue the infusion as described below. If anaphylaxis does occur during antivenin administration, discontinue antivenin and initiate appropriate treatment. If antivenin is still needed, seek expert consultation.

Antivenin therapy: Depending on the nature and severity of the signs and symptoms of envenomation, administer the contents of 3 to 5 vials as the initial dose. Observe the patient carefully and administer additional antivenin as required. Some envenomed patients may need the contents of more than 10 vials.

Route: ID skin test or conjunctival test to assess hypersensitivity. Subcutaneous and IM injection for desensitization.

Administer therapeutic doses by slow IV injection or by IV infusion. In either case, give the first 1 to 2 mL of the antivenin dilution over 3 to 5 minutes and watch the patient carefully for evidence of an allergic reaction. If no signs or symptoms of anaphylaxis appear, continue the injection or infusion.

Adjust the rate of delivery by the severity of signs and symptoms of envenomation and tolerance of antivenin. Nonetheless, until the contents of 3 to 5 vials of antivenin have been given, administer at the maximum safe rate for IV fluids, based on body weight and general condition of the patient. For example, 250 to 500 mL over 30 minutes may be appropriate in a healthy adult, while small children may receive the first 100 mL rapidly, followed by a rate not to exceed 4 mL per minute. Response to treatment may be rapid and dramatic.

Additional Doses: Observe the patient carefully and administer additional antivenin as required. Some envenomed patients may need the contents of 10 to 15 or more vials.

Antivenin *Micrurus fulvius* (Equine)

Related Interventions: Snakes' mouths do not harbor *Clostridium tetani*, but tetanus spores may be carried into the puncture wounds by dirt present on skin at the time of the bite or by non-sterile first-aid procedures. Give appropriate tetanus prophylaxis to inadequately immunized snake bite victims (eg, DTP for young children, Td or Tdap for adults).

Broad-spectrum antibiotic therapy is indicated if local tissue damage is evident. Use morphine, other narcotics that depress respiration, and sedatives with extreme caution. Corticosteroids may be needed to treat immediate allergic reactions to antivenin therapy. Corticosteroids are preferred for treating serious delayed reactions to antivenin (eg, serum sickness).

Efficacy: Good

Onset: IV effect is rapid, IM absorption may not peak until the second day.

Duration: Mean half-life is shorter than 15 days, as with any equine immunoglobulin.

Pharmacokinetics: Immunoglobulins are primarily eliminated by catabolism.

Protective Level: Unknown

Mechanism: Specific binding with circulating venom

Drug Interactions: None known

Pharmaceutical Characteristics

Concentration: Each vial contains sufficient antivenin to neutralize 250 times the median lethal mouse dose (LD_{50}), or approximately 2 mg venom per vial.

Quality Assay:
USP requirement: Standardized for potency in mice by capacity to neutralize the lethal action of standard venom.

Packaging: 250 units in a single-dose vial yielding 10 mL. Contains excess potency, 10% greater than labeled potency. Package includes a 10 mL vial of diluent plus a 1 mL vial of horse serum 1:10 v/v with 0.35% phenol, 0.005% thimerosal, and 0.85% sodium chloride for hypersensitivity testing.

NDC Number: 00008-0407-03

Doseform: Powder for solution

Appearance: Light cream-colored solid, yielding an opalescent solution. Not more than 20% solids.

Diluent:
For reconstitution: Sterile water with 0.001% phenylmercuric nitrate

Adjuvant: None

Preservative: 0.25% phenol and 0.005% thimerosal

Allergens: Equine serum

Excipients: None

pH: 6.5 to 7.5

Shelf Life: Expires within 60 months

Storage/Stability: Store at 2° to 8°C (36° to 46°F). Do not expose to temperatures above 40°C (104°F). Do not freeze diluent. Product can tolerate 10 days in solution at room temperature. Shipped by overnight courier in insulated containers with coolant packs and freeze indicators.

Use reconstituted solutions within 48 hours and dilutions within 12 hours. To avoid foaming and protein degradation, mix by gently swirling rather than shaking.

Production Process: Fractionation of plasma harvested from healthy horses immunized with eastern coral snake (*Micrurus fulvius fulvius*) venom, then lyophilized.

Antivenin *Micrurus fulvius* (Equine)

Media: Equine plasma

Dilution: 0.9% sodium chloride

Infusion: 0.9% sodium chloride for IV infusion: the contents of 3 to 5 vials diluted in 250 to 500 mL.

Threat Epidemiology

Incidence: Only approximately 15 to 25 coral snake bites occur in the United States each year. Deaths are rare.

Susceptible Pools: Entire population

Other Information

Perspective:

1887: Sewall shows that repeated administration of small doses of snake venom to pigeons leads to resistance.

1894: Calmette prepares antivenene, an equine preparation against mixed cobra and viperine venoms.

1895: Fraser develops cobra antivenom.

1898: Brazil demonstrates specificity of antivenoms.

First Licensed: August 28, 1967

References: Nelson BK. Snake envenomation: Incidence, clinical presentation, and management. *Med Toxicol Adverse Drug Exp.* 1989;4:17-31.

Smith TA II, et al. Treatment of snake-bite poisoning. *Am J Hosp Pharm.* 1991;48:2190-2196.

Antivenin *Latrodectus mactans* (Equine)

Immunoantidotes

Name:
Generic

Manufacturer:
Merck

Synonyms: Black widow spider antivenin. Antivenin Widow Spider Species is the name used by the US Adopted Names (USAN) Council to describe this drug.

Immunologic Characteristics

Antigen Source: Venoms of black widow spiders, class Arachnida, phyllum Arthropoda

Viability: Inactive, passive, transient

Antigenic Form: Equine immunoglobulin, unmodified (antivenin)

Antigenic Type: Protein, IgG antibody, polyclonal, polymeric. Skin tests assess immediate (type I) hypersensitivity.

Strains: Black widow spider (*Latrodectus mactans*). The antivenin had earlier been produced from a variety of related spiders from both North and South America, venoms with a high degree of cross-reactivity. Antivenin Widow Spider Species is the name used by the US Adopted Names (USAN) Council to describe this drug.

Use Characteristics

Indications: For passive, transient protection from toxic effects of bites by the black widow and similar spiders. Emphasize early use of this antivenin for prompt relief. The best effect occurs with antivenin administration within 4 hours after envenomation.

Limitations: The mortality rate of *Latrodectus* envenomations since 1965 is less than 1%, but drug-induced complication rates in antivenin recipients range from 9% to 80% for immediate-hypersensitivity reactions and 36% to 80% for serum sickness. In otherwise healthy individuals between 16 and 60 years of age, consider deferring use of antivenin and treating with muscle relaxants (eg, methocarbamol, benzodiazepines, analgesics). It has been recommended to reserve antivenin for life-threatening situations only.

Contraindications:

Absolute: None

Relative: Patients with a history of severe hypersensitivity reactions to equine immune globulin products. In otherwise healthy individuals between 16 and 60 years of age, consider deferring the use of antivenin and treating with muscle relaxants.

Immunodeficiency: No impairment of efficacy is likely.

Elderly: No specific information is available about geriatric use of widow spider antivenin.

Pregnancy: Category C. Use only if clearly needed, with appropriate consideration of the risk-benefit ratio. Envenomation has induced spontaneous abortion. It is not known if antivenom antibodies cross the placenta. Intact IgG crosses the placenta from the maternal circulation increasingly after 30 weeks gestation.

Lactation: It is not known if antivenin antibodies are excreted in breast milk. Problems in humans have not been documented.

Children: Give by IV infusion; 1 vial is usually sufficient. Virtually no adverse effects have been reported in children who have received this product.

Adverse Reactions: Anaphylaxis may occur with antivenin administration. Serum sickness may occur an average of 8 to 12 days following antivenin administration.

Habitat: *Latrodectus mactans* is found throughout the temperate and tropical latitudes but not in Alaska. These spiders live in crevices and under close ground cover. They may be found in stone walls, rubbish piles, barns, stables, or outhouses. Spiders are most numerous and envenomations are most common in late summer and early autumn months.

Other widow-spider species found in the United States include *Latrodectus hesperus* in western states, the brown widow spider in southern states (*Latrodectus bishopi*), and the red widow spider in Florida (*Latrodectus geometricus*).

Signs & Symptoms of Envenomation: The majority of human bites occur on the distal extremities, buttocks, or genitalia. Local muscular cramps begin from 15 minutes to several hours after the bite, which usually produces a sharp pain similar to that caused by puncture with a needle. The sequence of symptoms depends somewhat on the location of the bite. The venom acts on the myoneuronal junctions or on the nerve endings, causing an ascending motor paralysis or destruction of the peripheral nerve endings. The groups of muscles most frequently affected initially are those of the thigh, shoulder, and back.

After a varying length of time, the pain becomes more severe, spreading to the abdomen, and weakness and tremor usually develop. The abdominal muscles assume a board-like rigidity, but tenderness is slight.

Respiration is thoracic and the patient will likely be restless and anxious. Other symptoms include feeble pulse, cold, clammy skin, labored breathing and speech, light stupor, delirium, convulsions (particularly in small children), temperature normal or slightly elevated, urinary retention, shock, cyanosis, nausea and vomiting, insomnia, or cold sweats. The syndrome following bite of the black widow spider may easily be confused with conditions involving acute abdominal symptoms.

The symptoms of a black widow spider bite increase in severity for several hours to a day, then slowly become less severe, subsiding over 2 to 3 days, except in fatal cases. Residual symptoms such as general weakness, tingling, nervousness, and transient muscle spasm may persist weeks or months after recovery from the acute stage.

Envenomation Management: Local treatment at the site of the bite is of no value.

Nothing is gained by applying a tourniquet or by attempting to remove venom from the site of the bite by incision and suction.

Pharmacologic & Dosing Characteristics

Dosage: Mix by gentle swirling. To avoid foaming and protein degradation, do not shake.

Sensitivity test: Carefully review the patient's history, including any report of asthma, hay fever, urticaria, or other allergic manifestations, allergic reactions upon exposure to horses, or prior injections of horse serum. Perform a skin or conjunctival test prior to any antivenin administration, regardless of clinical history, as a guide to speed of therapeutic antivenin administration. Immediate-hypersensitivity skin tests have no bearing on whether or not delayed reactions will occur after administration of the full dose.

To apply a skin test, inject not more than 0.02 mL ID of a 1:10 v/v dilution of horse serum, typically on the dorsal forearm. Use a freshly compounded 1:100 v/v or weaker dilution for preliminary skin testing if the history suggests hypersensitivity. Apply a negative control test of the same volume of 0.9% sodium chloride at a comparable site on the opposite extremity. After 10 minutes, a positive reaction consists of an urticarial wheal surrounded by a zone of erythema. Use of larger amounts for the skin-test dose increases the likelihood of false-positive reactions, and, in an exquisitely hypersensitive patient, increases the risk of a systemic reaction from the skin-test dose. Skin testing is approximately 22% sensitive in predicting subsequent immediate-hypersensitivity reactions but 100% specific.

For a conjunctival test in adults, instill into either conjunctival sac 1 drop of a 1:10 v/v dilution of horse serum. For children, instill 1 drop of a freshly prepared 1:100 v/v dilution. Itching of the eye and reddening of the conjunctiva constitute a positive reaction, usually within 10 minutes.

If history and hypersensitivity test are both negative, proceed with antivenin administration as described below, recognizing that an immediate reaction to antivenin infusion has not been ruled out.

If the history is positive and the hypersensitivity test is clearly positive, administration may be dangerous. In such instances, weigh the risk of antivenin administration against the risk of withholding it. Use the desensitization protocol if antivenin administration is elected.

If the history is negative and the hypersensitivity test is mildly or questionably positive, administer the antivenin according to a desensitization protocol to reduce the risk of severe immediate systemic reaction.

Desensitization protocol: Attempt desensitization only when the administration of antivenin is considered necessary to save life.

(1) In separate vials or syringes, compound fresh 1:100 and 1:10 v/v dilutions of antivenin. Frequently, 0.9% sodium chloride is selected as the solvent for such dilutions.

(2) Inject subcutaneously 0.1, 0.2, and then 0.5 mL of the 1:100 v/v dilution at 15-minute intervals. Repeat this 3-volume sequence with the 1:10 v/v dilution, and then repeat the 3-volume sequence with undiluted antivenin.

(3) Allow at least 15 to 30 minutes between injections, and proceed with the next dose only if no reaction follows the previous dose.

(4) If a systemic reaction occurs after any injection, place a tourniquet proximal to the site of injection and administer an appropriate subcutaneous dose of epinephrine 1:1,000 proximal to the tourniquet or into another extremity. Wait at least 30 minutes before injecting another dose. For the next dose, repeat the last dose that did not evoke a reaction.

(5) If no reaction occurs after 0.5 mL of undiluted antivenin, switch to the IM route and continue doubling the dose at 15-minute intervals until the entire dose has been injected.

Antivenin therapy: For adults and children, give the entire contents of 1 vial. The manufacturer recommends IM administration so that a tourniquet may be applied in the event of a systemic reaction, although this route may significantly delay absorption. Symptoms usually subside within 1 to 3 hours following IV administration. Although 1 dose of antivenin usually suffices, a second dose may be necessary in some cases.

Alternately, for quickest systemic absorption, give antivenin by IV infusion, diluted in 10 to 50 mL of 0.9% sodium chloride, administered over a 15-minute period. Infusion is especially preferred in severe cases, when the patient is younger than 12 years of age, or when the patient is in shock.

Route: ID skin test or conjunctival test to assess hypersensitivity; subcutaneous and IM injection for desensitization. Although the manufacturer recommends IM administration so that a tourniquet may be applied in the event of a systemic reaction, a 1985 FDA advisory panel cautions against this practice to avoid delayed absorption and possible inadequate treatment. Antivenin may be given by IV infusion, diluted in 10 to 50 mL of 0.9% sodium chloride, over a 15-minute period. Infusion is especially preferred in severe cases, when the patient is younger than 12 years of age, or when the patient is in shock.

Additional Doses: Although 1 vial of antivenin usually suffices, a second dose may be necessary in some cases.

Related Interventions: Additional measures giving relief include prolonged warm baths and slow IV push injection of 2 to 3 mL of 10% calcium gluconate with cardiac monitoring, titrated as necessary with additional 2 mL doses to control muscle pain. Morphine also may be required to control pain. Sedation may be indicated but not in the presence of respiratory failure. Corticosteroids have been used with varying degrees of success in treating the effects of envenomation. Corticosteroids may be needed to treat allergic reactions to antivenin therapy. Corticosteroids are preferred for treating serious delayed reactions to antivenin (eg, serum sickness). Provide supportive therapy according to the patient's clinical status.

Efficacy: Moderately effective in pain relief. Can be life-saving.

Onset: IV effect is rapid; concentration peaks 2 to 3 days after IM injection.

Duration: Mean half-life is shorter than 15 days, as with other equine immunoglobulins

Pharmacokinetics: Immunoglobulins are primarily eliminated by catabolism.

Protective Level: Unknown

Mechanism: Specific binding with circulating venom

Drug Interactions: None known

Pharmaceutical Characteristics

Concentration: Each vial contains antivenin sufficient to neutralize 6,000 times the median lethal dose of venom in mice (LD_{50}). Reconstitute this quantity of antivenin to 2.5 mL according to package instructions.

Quality Assay:
USP requirement: Standardized for potency in mice by capacity to neutralize the lethal action of standard venom. The agent used to immunize the horses is not a secreted product, but an extract of the removed venom sacs of a large number of individual spiders. For this reason, materials derived from the insects' venom-producing apparati may be present in venom preparations.

Packaging: 6,000 units in a single-dose vial. Contains excess potency, 10% greater than labeled potency. Package includes a 2.5 mL vial of diluent plus a 1 mL vial of horse serum 1:10 v/v in 0.9% sodium chloride for hypersensitivity testing.

NDC Number: 00006-4084-00

Doseform: Powder for solution

Appearance: White to gray crystalline powder, yielding an opalescent solution from light straw to very dark (like iced tea) in color. The variation in color does not affect potency. Contains 20% or less solids.

Diluent:
For reconstitution: Sterile water for injection
For infusion: If given by IV infusion, dilute the contents of 1 vial in 10 to 50 mL 0.9% sodium chloride and administer over 15 minutes.

Adjuvant: None

Preservative: 0.01% thimerosal in both the diluent and the skin-test reagent

Allergens: Equine serum

Excipients: None

pH: Data unavailable

Shelf Life: Expires within 36 months

Storage/Stability: Refrigerate at 2° to 8°C (36° to 46°F) during storage and shipment. Discard if frozen. Do not expose to excessive heat. Contact manufacturer regarding prolonged exposure to room temperature or elevated temperatures.

After reconstitution, refrigerate and discard within 6 hours.

Antivenin *Latrodectus mactans* (Equine)

Production Process: Fractionation from equine plasma harvested from healthy horses immunized against venom of black widow (*Latrodectus mactans*) and similar spiders. Plasma is pooled and defibrinated, subjected to pepsin digestion and ammonium sulfate fractionation, dialyzed, and adjusted to yield a protein concentration of approximately 20%.

Media: Equine plasma

Threat Epidemiology

Incidence: *Latrodectus* envenomations are the leading cause of death from arthropod envenomations in the United States and one of the leading causes worldwide. An estimated 3,000 spider envenomations and 6 deaths occur each year in the United States.

Susceptible Pools: Entire population

Other Information

Perspective: See Antivenin Crotalidae monograph.

First Licensed: February 13, 1936.

References: Allen C. Arachnid envenomations. *Emerg Med Clin North Amer.* 1992;10:269-298.

Binder LS. Acute arthropod envenomation. Incidence, clinical features, and management. *Med Toxicol Adverse Drug Exp.* 1989;4:163-173.

Clark RF, et al. Clinical presentation and treatment of black widow spider envenomation: A review of 163 cases. *Ann Emerg Med.* 1992;21:782-787.

Immunoantidotes

Name:
Anascorp

Manufacturer:
Manufactured by Instituto Bioclon, distributed by Accredo Health Group for Rare Diseases Therapeutics

Immunologic Characteristics

Antigen Source: Venom of *Centruroides* genus scorpions, class Arachnida, phyllum Arthropoda

Viability: Inactive, passive, transient

Antigenic Form: F(ab')₂ fragments of equine immune globulin, polyvalent preparation

Antigenic Type: Protein, equine IgG F(ab')₂ fragments, polyclonal, polymeric

Strains: Derived from plasma of horses immunized with venoms of *Centruroides noxius, Centruroides limpidus limpidus, Centruroides limpidus tecomanus,* and *Centruroides suffusus suffusus.* Cross-neutralizes the venom of *Centruroides sculpturatus* (also called *Centruroides exilicauda*), the Arizona bark scorpion.

Use Characteristics

Indications: To treat clinical signs of scorpion envenomation

Contraindications: None

Immunodeficiency: No impairment of effect is expected.

Elderly: Specific studies in elderly patients have not been conducted. Centruroides immune F(ab')₂ was administered to 77 patients older than 65 years with comparable efficacy and safety in the overall patient population.

Pregnancy: Category C. Animal reproduction studies have not been conducted with Centruroides immune F(ab')₂. It is not known whether Centruroides immune F(ab')₂ can cause fetal harm when administered to a pregnant woman or can affect reproduction capacity. Centruroides immune F(ab')₂ should be given to a pregnant woman only if clearly needed.

Lactation: It is not known whether Centruroides immune F(ab')₂ crosses into human breast milk. Because many drugs are excreted in human milk, exercise caution when Centruroides immune F(ab')₂ is administered to a breast-feeding woman.

Children: Seventy-eight percent (1,204/1,534) of patients enrolled in the clinical studies were children (age range, younger than 1 month to 18.7 years). Patient age groups were as follows: younger than 2 years (29%), 2 to 5 years (37%), and 5 to 18 years (34%). The efficacy and safety of Centruroides immune F(ab')₂ is comparable in pediatric and adult patients.

Adverse Reactions: The most common adverse events observed in at least 2% of patients in clinical studies for Centruroides immune F(ab')₂ were vomiting, pyrexia, rash, nausea, and pruritus.

A total of 1,534 patients were treated with Centruroides immune F(ab')₂ (age range, younger than 1 month to 90 years). The patient population included 802 males and 732 females. Follow-up telephone interviews were conducted at 24 hours, 7 days, and 14 days after treatment to assess symptoms suggestive of ongoing venom effect, serum sickness, and any other adverse reactions. The following table shows the adverse events occurring in patients across

Centruroides (Scorpion) Immune F(ab')₂ (Equine)

all clinical trials for Centruroides immune F(ab')$_2$. Twenty-seven percent (421/1,534) of patients receiving Centruroides immune F(ab')$_2$ reported at least 1 adverse event.

Adverse Reactions Reported in ≥ 1% of Patients	
Adverse event	Centruroides Immune F(ab')$_2$ (N = 1,534)
Vomiting	72 (4.7%)
Pyrexia	63 (4.1%)
Rash	41 (2.7%)
Nausea	32 (2.1%)
Pruritus	31 (2%)
Headache	29 (1.9%)
Rhinorrhea	28 (1.8%)
Myalgia	25 (1.6%)
Fatigue	24 (1.6%)
Cough	22 (1.4%)
Diarrhea	20 (1.3%)
Lethargy	17 (1.1%)

No patients died or discontinued study participation for severe adverse events. Thirty-four patients experienced a total of 39 severe adverse events, such as respiratory distress, aspiration, hypoxia, ataxia, pneumonia, and eye swelling. It is not clear whether these adverse events were related to Centruroides immune F(ab')$_2$, envenomation, or a combination of both.

Postmarketing experience: The following adverse events have been identified during postapproval use of Centruroides immune F(ab')$_2$: chest tightness, palpitations, rash, and pruritus.

Hypersensitivity: Severe hypersensitivity reactions, including anaphylaxis, may occur with Centruroides immune F(ab')$_2$. Be prepared to monitor and manage allergic reactions, particularly in patients with a history of hypersensitivity to equine (horse) proteins or in patients who have previously received therapy with antivenoms containing equine proteins.

Localized reactions and generalized myalgias have been reported with the use of cresol as an injectable excipient.

Serum sickness: Delayed allergic reactions, such as serum sickness (eg, rash, fever, myalgia, arthralgia), may occur after treatment with Centruroides immune F(ab')$_2$. Monitor patients carefully (including a follow-up visit), and treat appropriately. Eight of 1,534 (0.5%) patients in clinical trials exhibited symptoms suggestive of serum sickness. None manifested the full serum sickness syndrome. Three patients were treated with systemic corticosteroids and 5 others received either no treatment or symptomatic therapy.

Adventitious agents: Centruroides immune F(ab')$_2$ is made from equine plasma and may contain infectious agents (eg, viruses).

Pharmacologic & Dosing Characteristics

Dosage:

Initial dose: 3 vials. Start treatment as soon as possible after scorpion sting in patients who develop clinically important signs of scorpion envenomation, including but not limited to loss of muscle control, roving or abnormal eye movements, slurred speech, respiratory distress, excessive salivation, frothing at the mouth, and vomiting.

Give additional dose(s) based on clinical situation. Administer 1 vial at a time at 30- to 60-minute intervals.

Route: Infuse each dose intravenously (IV) over 10 minutes.

Overdosage: Although few data are available, clinical experience with similar products suggests that the major manifestations of overdosage would be pain and tenderness at the injection site.

Related Interventions: Monitor patients closely, during and up to 60 minutes after completing the infusion, to determine if clinically important signs of envenomation have resolved. If an anaphylactic reaction occurs during infusion, discontinue administration at once and administer appropriate emergency medical care (eg, IV therapy using epinephrine, corticosteroids, diphenhydramine).

Efficacy: Efficacy of Centruroides immune $F(ab')_2$ was assessed in 1 prospective, double-blind, randomized, placebo-controlled study, 4 open-label studies, and 1 retrospective study in various treatment settings in the United States and Mexico, where scorpion envenomation is common.

A total of 1,534 patients (age range, younger than 1 month to 90 years) were treated. Most (78% [1,204/1,534]) were pediatric patients (age range, younger than 1 month to 18.7 years). Male (52.3%) and female (47.7%) patients were equally represented. Treatment success was determined by resolution of clinically important signs of scorpion envenomation within 4 hours of starting infusion.

The randomized study enrolled 15 subjects, 8 randomized to receive Centruroides immune $F(ab')_2$ and 7 to receive placebo. The symptom resolution success rate was 100% for the Centruroides immune $F(ab')_2$–treated group and 14.3% for the placebo group.

A retrospective hospital chart review provided historical data from envenomated patients (N = 97) who did not receive antivenom but who were treated with sedatives and supportive care for symptoms of envenomation. These data were used as a historical control for expected outcomes in the absence of antivenom treatment. Historical controls were pediatric patients admitted to 2 pediatric intensive care units between 1990 and 2003 for the treatment of scorpion envenomation with supportive care only. The proportion of patients who required intensive care support 4 hours after intensive care unit admission and the overall duration of the intensive care support requirement were calculated. Overall, 95% to 100% of patients were relieved of systemic signs associated with scorpion envenomation in less than 4 hours after initiating Centruroides immune $F(ab')_2$ treatment. In the historical control database, only 3.1% of patients experienced relief of symptoms within 4 hours of hospital admission.

In 1,396 of 1,534 patients, the mean time from start of Centruroides immune $F(ab')_2$ infusion to resolution of clinical signs and symptoms of envenomation was 1.42 hours (0.2 to 20.5 hours). Pediatric patients generally experienced a slightly faster time to resolution (1.28 ± 0.8 hours) compared with that of adult patients (1.91 ± 1.4 hours). The time to resolution of symptoms was not affected by use of sedatives (474 patients who received sedatives had resolved symptoms in 1.49 ± 1.1 hours, and 922 patients who did not receive sedatives had resolved symptoms in 1.38 ± 0.9 hours).

Onset: Within hours

Duration: Days

Pharmacokinetics: Eight clinically healthy volunteers (6 males and 2 females; age range, 17 to 26 years) received an IV bolus dose of 47.5 mg of Centruroides immune $F(ab')_2$. Blood samples were collected for 504 hours (21 days); pharmacokinetic parameters were estimated by noncompartmental analysis and are summarized in the following table.

Pharmacokinetic Parameters of Centruroides Immune $F(ab')_2$[a]	
Parameters	Mean ± SD
$AUC_{(0-\infty)}$ (mcg•h/mL)	706 ± 352
Clearance (mL/h)	84 ± 38

Centruroides (Scorpion) Immune F(ab')₂ (Equine)

Pharmacokinetic Parameters of Centruroides Immune F(ab')$_2$[a]	
Parameters	Mean ± SD
Half-life (h)	159 ± 57
Vss (L)	13.6 ± 5.4

a AUC = area under the curve; SD = standard deviation; Vss = volume of distribution at steady state.

Protective Level: Not established

Mechanism: Venom-specific F(ab')$_2$ fragments of IgG bind and neutralize venom toxins, facilitating redistribution away from target tissues and elimination from the body.

Drug Interactions: No drug interaction studies have been conducted with Centruroides immune F(ab')$_2$.

Patient Information: Advise patients to contact their physician or emergency department immediately if any signs and symptoms of delayed allergic reactions or serum sickness develop up to 14 days following hospital discharge. Symptoms include rash, pruritus, joint pain, arthralgia, fever, lymphadenopathy, and malaise.

Pharmaceutical Characteristics

Concentration: Not more than 120 mg of total protein and not less than median lethal dose (LD$_{50}$) (mouse) of 150 neutralizing units per vial

Packaging: 1 single-use vial

NDC Number: 66621-0150-01

Doseform: Lyophilized powder yielding solution

Appearance: Data not provided

Diluent:

For reconstitution: Reconstitute each vial with 5 mL of sodium chloride 0.9%. Mix by continuous gentle swirling.

For infusion: Combine contents of appropriate number of vials promptly and further dilute with sodium chloride 0.9% to a total of 50 mL.

Adjuvant: None

Preservative: None

Allergens: Equine plasma

Excipients: Each vial contains sodium chloride 45 to 80 mg, sucrose 4.3 to 38.3 mg, and glycine 6.6 to 94.9 mg as stabilizers. Trace amounts of pepsin, cresol (less than 0.41 mg/vial), borates (less than 1 mg/vial), and sulfates (less than 1.7 mg/vial) may be present from the manufacturing process.

pH: Data not provided

Shelf Life: Expires within 24 months

Storage/Stability: Store at room temperature (up to 25°C [77°F]). Temperature excursions are permitted up to 40°C (104°F). Do not freeze. Shipping data not provided.

Production Process: The product is obtained by pepsin digestion of horse plasma to remove the Fc portion of immune globulin, followed by fractionation and purification steps. The F(ab')$_2$ content is greater than or equal to 85%, F(ab') content is less than or equal to 7%, and the product contains less than 5% intact immunoglobulin. The manufacturing procedures that contribute to the reduction in risk of viral transmission include pepsin digestion, ammonium sulfate precipitation/heat treatment, and nanofiltration.

Media: Equine plasma

Centruroides (Scorpion) Immune F(ab')₂ (Equine)

Disease Epidemiology

Incidence: Between 1931 and 1940, there were at least 40 deaths attributed to envenomation by Centruroides scorpions, predominantly among infants and children. Antivenin use started in Arizona in the late 1950s, when deaths from scorpion stings outnumbered those from rattlesnake bites.

In recent years, few deaths have been reported from Centruroides stings, despite an estimated 11,000 people stung by scorpions in Arizona alone each year; 17,000 stings were reported to US poison centers nationwide in 2009. Most stings occur in young children, in whom the effects of envenomation can be life-threatening.

Habitat: Centruroides scorpions inhabit the arid southwestern United States, especially southern and central portions of Arizona. Colonies also exist in northern Arizona and in parts of Texas, New Mexico, California, Nevada, and northern Mexico.

Scorpions are typically nocturnal, hiding in damp, cool areas (eg, under rocks or the bark of logs, in cracks and crevices of homes). Most bites occur in homes or backyards during the evening or night, most commonly from May through July.

Other Information

Perspective:

1930s: Antivenin is harvested from horses and imported from Mexico into Arizona. Stahnke subsequently develops both rabbit and cat serum scorpion antivenin for human use at Arizona State University.

1965: Polyclonal Centruroides antivenin IgG is harvested from goats.

1980: The Arizona State Board of Pharmacy accepts *C. sculpturatus* (caprine) antivenin to neutralize venom of bark scorpion. The drug was provided without charge and the expenses incurred in preparation were borne by Arizona State University. The product never received a US Food and Drug Administration (FDA) license. Distribution ceased around 2006.

First Licensed: July 27, 2011

References: Boyer LV, Theodorou AA, Berg RA, Mallie J; Arizona Envenomation Investigators. Antivenom for critically ill children with neurotoxicity from scorpion stings. *N Engl J Med.* 2009;360(20):2090-2098.

Gateau T, Bloom M, Clark R. Response to specific *Centruroides sculpturatus* antivenom in 151 cases of scorpion stings. *J Toxicol Clin Toxicol.* 1994;32(2):165-171.

Digoxin Immune Fab (Ovine)

Immunoantidotes

Names:
   Digibind

   DigiFab

Manufacturers:
   GlaxoSmithKline (no longer distributed in United States; distribution in Europe continues)
   Manufactured by Protherics, distributed by BTG International

Synonyms: Digoxin Fab, digoxin antibody-binding fragments

Comparison: The comparability of digoxin-binding antibodies is currently unknown because directly comparative studies have not been published.

Immunologic Characteristics

Antigen Source: Drug-hapten complex of digoxin-dicarboxymethoxylamine (DDMA), a digoxin analog containing the functionally essential cyclopentaperhydrophenanthrene:lactone ring moiety coupled to keyhole-limpet hemocyanin (KLH)

Viability: Inactive, passive, transient

Antigenic Form: Ovine (sheep) immunoglobulin, fragmented (antitoxin)

Antigenic Type: Protein, IgG antibody, polyclonal, antigen-binding (Fab) fragments. The Fab fragments have a molecular weight of approximately 46,000 daltons each. The molecular weight of digoxin is 781 daltons.

Strains: Active against both digoxin and digitoxin.

Use Characteristics

Indications: For the passive, transient treatment of potentially life-threatening acute digoxin intoxication. Digoxin Fab also has been used to treat life-threatening digitoxin overdose. Life-threatening toxicity is manifested by severe ventricular dysrhythmias (eg, tachycardia, fibrillation) or progressive bradydysrhythmias (eg, severe sinus bradycardia, second- or third-degree heart block not responsive to atropine), serum potassium levels higher than 5.5 mEq/L in adults or 6 mEq/L in children with rapidly progressive signs and symptoms of digoxin toxicity.

Cardiac arrest often follows ingestion of digoxin 10 mg in healthy adults, 4 mg (or more than 0.1 mg/kg) in previously healthy children, or ingestion causing steady-state serum digoxin concentrations higher than 10 ng/mL. If the potassium concentration exceeds 5 mEq/L in the setting of severe digitalis intoxication, digoxin Fab therapy is indicated. Improvement in signs and symptoms usually begins within 30 minutes.

Digoxin Fab therapy also is indicated for chronic ingestion causing steady-state serum digoxin concentrations higher than 6 ng/mL in adults or 4 ng/mL in children.

Unlabeled Uses: Physical binding occurs in vitro against a variety of plant extracts containing cardiac glycosides, including pheasant's eye, oleander, yellow oleander, and rubber vine. Digoxin Fab may be expected to be effective in poisonings caused by ingestion of these plants. *Digibind* was shown effective in a canine model of oleander toxicity. One published human case of digoxin Fab administration to reverse oleander (*Nerium oleander*) toxicity was successful and 1 was unsuccessful.

Successful use of digoxin Fab to reverse lanatoside C intoxication was reported in 1 case. Because lanatoside C (ie, deslanoside, desacetyl-lanatoside C) is hydrolyzed in the intestine to digoxin and acetyldigoxin, and all 3 compounds bind to digoxin Fab, digoxin Fab would be expected to reverse toxicity secondary to lanatoside C.

Limitations: Because human experience is limited and the consequences of repeated exposures to digoxin Fab are unknown, digoxin Fab is not indicated for milder cases of digitalis toxicity.

Suicidal ingestion may involve more than one drug. Do not overlook toxic effects of other drugs or poisons, especially in cases where signs and symptoms of digitalis toxicity are not relieved by administration of digoxin Fab.

Contraindications:

Absolute: None known

Relative: Patients with known hypersensitivities to constituents of this drug may be at increased risk, as would individuals who previously received antibodies or Fab fragments raised in sheep. Patients with allergies to papain, chymopapain, other papaya extracts, or the pineapple enzyme bromelain may be particularly at risk for an allergic reaction. Some dust mite allergens and some latex allergens share antigenic structures with papain; patients with these allergies may be allergic to papain. Skin testing has not proved useful in predicting allergic response to *Digibind*. Because of this, and because it may delay urgently needed therapy, skin testing was not performed during the clinical studies of *DigiFab* and is not suggested prior to dosing.

Immunodeficiency: Impairment of effect is unlikely.

Elderly: Specific studies in elderly patients have not been conducted. Of 150 patients given *Digibind* in a open-label study, 42% were 65 years of age and older, while 21% were 75 years of age and older. During postmarketing surveillance of 717 adults, 84% were 60 years of age and older and 60% were 70 years of age and older. Of 15 patients given *DigiFab* for digoxin toxicity in 1 clinical trial, the average age of all patients was 64 years and 8 of the 15 were 65 years of age and older. The oldest patient studied was 86 years of age. There is no evidence that the efficacy of digoxin Fab would be altered because of advanced age alone; however, elderly patients have a higher chance of having impaired renal function and, therefore, should be monitored more closely for recurrent toxicity.

Carcinogenicity: Animal carcinogenicity studies have not been conducted with digoxin Fab.

Mutagenicity: Digoxin Fab has not been evaluated for mutagenic potential.

Fertility Impairment: Digoxin Fab has not been evaluated for impairment of fertility.

Pregnancy: Category C. Use only if clearly needed. It is not known if antidigoxin antibody fragments cross the placenta. Intact IgG crosses the placenta increasingly from the maternal circulation after 30 weeks gestation. Problems in humans have not been documented.

Lactation: It is not known if antidigoxin antibody fragments are excreted in breast milk. Problems in humans have not been documented.

Children: Digoxin Fab has been used successfully in infants with no apparent adverse sequelae. In considering pediatric therapy with digoxin Fab, balance the benefits of drug use against the risks involved. In infants and children weighing less than 20 kg, the contents of a single vial usually suffice. Monitor for volume overload in children.

Adverse Reactions: Allergic reactions to digoxin Fab occur rarely. Patients with a history of allergy, especially to antibiotics, appear to be at particular risk. In a few instances, low cardiac output states and congestive heart failure (CHF) could have been exacerbated by withdrawal of the inotropic effects of digitalis. Hypokalemia may occur from reactivation of sodium/potassium adenosine triphosphatase (ATPase). Patients with atrial fibrillation may develop a rapid ventricular response from withdrawal of the effects of digitalis on the atrioventricular node.

In the clinical trials of *DigiFab*, 6 of 15 digoxin overdose patients had a total of 17 adverse experiences. Most were mild to moderate in nature and all were deemed remotely associated with *DigiFab*. Three events were deemed "severe"; all occurred in 1 patient and consisted of the following: pulmonary edema, bilateral pleural effusion, and renal failure. Review of the case determined that these events were likely because of the loss of digoxin inotropic support in combination with the patient's underlying medical condition. Of 8 healthy volunteers who received *DigiFab*, only 2 experienced an adverse reaction associated with *DigiFab*. The reactions were 1 episode of phlebitis of the infusion vein and 1 episode of moderate postural hypotension that became mild prior to resolving.

Possible risks after administration of heterologous animal proteins to humans include anaphylactic and anaphylactoid reactions, delayed allergic reactions, and a possible febrile response to immune complexes formed by animal antibodies.

No toxic effects resulted after administering digoxin Fab to healthy male Sprague-Dawley rats in equimolar doses sufficient to neutralize a 1 mg/kg dose of digoxin. In these studies, administration of either *Digibind* or *DigiFab* rapidly ameliorated physiologic changes produced by toxic serum concentrations of digoxin. Statistically equivalent responses were observed with both *Digibind* and *DigiFab* to the following variables: PTQ index, heart rate, mean arterial pressure, ventilation, arterial blood gases, and serum potassium concentrations.

Pharmacologic & Dosing Characteristics

Dosage:

Sensitivity test: Because few patients respond positively to hypersensitivity skin testing and because hypersensitivity testing can delay urgently needed therapy, it is not routinely required before treatment of life-threatening digitalis toxicity with digoxin Fab. Skin testing may be appropriate for high-risk individuals, especially those with known allergies or those previously treated with digoxin Fab.

To prepare a test dose, dilute 0.1 mL of reconstituted digoxin Fab (9.5 mg/mL) in 9.9 mL of sodium chloride 0.9% (a 1:100 v/v dilution, 95 mcg/mL), or make two 10-fold serial dilutions. Then inject 0.1 mL of this solution (95 mcg intradermally). Apply a negative control test of an equal volume of sodium chloride 0.9% at the corresponding site on the opposite extremity. After 20 minutes, observe the test site for an urticarial wheal surrounded by a zone of erythema.

Alternatively, apply a scratch test by placing 1 drop of a 1:100 v/v dilution (95 mcg per 0.1 mL) of digoxin Fab on the skin and then making a ¼-inch long scratch through the drop with a sterile needle. Inspect the scratch site after 20 minutes for an urticarial wheal surrounded by erythema.

If skin testing causes a systemic reaction, use a tourniquet proximal to the test site and institute appropriate therapy. Avoid further administration of digoxin Fab unless absolutely necessary. In such a case, pretreat the patient with corticosteroids and diphenhydramine.

Therapeutic dose: The recommended dose of digoxin Fab varies according to the amount of digoxin or digitoxin to be neutralized. The average dose used during clinical trials was 10 vials. For adults, the contents of 6 vials (228 mg) are usually adequate to reverse most cases of toxicity. This dose can be used in patients in acute distress or for whom a total digoxin concentration is unavailable. In infants and children weighing less than 20 kg, the contents of a single vial usually suffice. Various methods for calculating the appropriate dose of digoxin Fab required to neutralize the known or estimated amount of digoxin or digitoxin in the body appear below. For acute ingestion of an unknown amount of digitalis, 20 vials (760 mg) of digoxin Fab is adequate to treat most life-threatening ingestions in adults and children. In children, monitor for volume overload.

In general, a large digoxin Fab dose has a faster onset of effect but may enhance the possibility of a febrile reaction. Consider administering 10 vials and observing the patient's response. Follow with an additional 10 vials if clinically indicated.

When determining the appropriate dose of digoxin Fab, consider the following guidelines:

(1) Erroneous calculations may result from inaccurate historical estimates of the amount of digitalis ingested or absorbed, non–steady-state serum digitalis concentrations, or inaccurate total concentration measurements. Most total digoxin assay kits are designed to measure values lower than 5 ng/mL. Dilution of samples is required to obtain accurate measures higher than 5 ng/mL.

(2) Base dosage calculations on a steady-state volume of distribution of approximately 5 L/kg for digoxin (0.5 L/kg for digitoxin) to convert a total digitalis concentration to the amount of digitalis in the body. These volumes are population averages and vary widely among individuals. Many patients require higher doses for complete neutralization. Round up most doses to the next whole vial. If the dose, based on the actual or presumed ingested amount, differs substantially from that calculated from the total digoxin or digitoxin concentration, it may be preferable to use the higher dose.

(3) If toxicity is not adequately reversed after several hours or appears to recur, readministration of digoxin Fab at a dose guided by clinical judgment may be required.

(4) A patient's failure to respond to digoxin Fab raises the possibility that the clinical problem is not caused by digitalis intoxication. If there is no response to an adequate dose of digoxin Fab, question the diagnosis of digitalis toxicity.

(5) If a patient needs readministration of digoxin Fab because of recurrent toxicity or to a new toxic episode soon after the first episode, consider measuring free (unbound) serum digitalis concentrations because Fab may still be present in the body.

Approximate Digoxin Fab Dose for Reversal of a Single Large Digoxin Overdose in Adults and Children[a]						
Number of digoxin tablets or capsules ingested	25	50	75	100	150	200
Number of digoxin Fab vials	10	20	30	40	60	80

a Based on Formula 1: The dose in vials is equal to the total digitalis body load in mg divided by 0.5 mg of digitalis bound per vial. Based on 80% bioavailability of 0.25 mg *Lanoxin* tablets and 100% bioavailability of 0.2 mg *Lanoxicaps* capsules.

Adult Dose Estimate of Digoxin Fab (in Number of Vials) From Steady-State Total Digoxin Concentration[a]							
	Serum digoxin concentration (ng/mL)						
Patient weight (kg)	1	2	4	8	12	16	20
40	0.5	1	2	3	5	7	8
60	0.5	1	3	5	7	10	12
70	1	2	3	6	9	11	14
80	1	2	3	7	10	13	16
100	1	2	4	8	12	16	20

a Based on Formula 2: The dose in vials is equal to the product of the serum digoxin concentration in ng/mL multiplied by the patient's body weight in kg divided by 100.

Infants and Small Children Dose Estimates of Digoxin Fab (in mg) from Steady-State Serum Digoxin Concentration[a]							
Patient weight (kg)	Serum digoxin concentration (ng/mL)						
	1	2	4	8	12	16	20
1	0.4 mg[b]	1 mg[b]	1.5 mg[b]	3 mg[b]	5 mg	6.5 mg	8 mg
3	1 mg[b]	2.5 mg[b]	5 mg	10 mg	14 mg	19 mg	24 mg
5	2 mg[b]	4 mg	8 mg	16 mg	24 mg	32 mg	40 mg
10	4 mg	8 mg	16 mg	32 mg	48 mg	64 mg	80 mg
20	8 mg	16 mg	32 mg	64 mg	96 mg	128 mg	160 mg

a Based on Formula 3: Dose of digoxin Fab to administer in mg equals the dose in number of vials (calculated from formula above) multiplied by 40 mg per vial.

If very small doses are needed, dilute as follows, then administer with a tuberculin syringe: Dilute a 40 mg per 4 mL reconstituted vial of *DigiFab* with 36 mL of sodium chloride 0.9% to yield a 1 mg/mL solution.

Formula 4: A fourth method of calculation is based on steady-state digitoxin concentration. The dose in vials is equal to the product of the serum digitoxin concentration in ng/mL multiplied by the patient's body weight in kg divided by 1,000. This differs from Formula 2 in the denominator due to a 10-fold decrease in the volume of distribution of digitoxin as compared with digoxin.

If, in any case, the dose estimated based on ingested amount (Formula 1) differs substantially from that calculated based on the serum digoxin or digitoxin concentration (Formulas 2 or 4), it may be preferable to use the higher dose estimate.
b Dilution of reconstituted vial to 1 mg/mL may be desirable.

Route & Site: Administer an IV infusion for 30 minutes or longer. If infusion rate-related reactions occur, stop the infusion and restart at a slower rate. Give as an IV bolus if cardiac arrest is imminent. With bolus injection, an increased incidence of infusion-related reactions may be expected.

Overdosage: The maximum amount of digoxin Fab that can safely be administered in single or multiple doses has not been determined.

Additional Doses: If toxicity is not adequately reversed after several hours or appears to recur, readministration of digoxin Fab at a dose guided by clinical judgment may be required. Free digoxin concentrations rebound upward within 12 to 24 hours after giving digoxin Fab; this rebound may be delayed by 12 to 130 hours in patients with renal disease. Rarely does this rebound exceed a free digoxin concentration of 1 to 1.5 mcg/L (1.28 to 1.92 nmol/L); levels higher than this may indicate need for an additional dose of digoxin Fab. If signs and symptoms of digitalis toxicity recur shortly after giving digoxin Fab (within 12 to 72 hours or within 14 days in patients with renal disease), determining the patient's free digoxin concentration can help in assessing the need for an additional dose.

Related Interventions: Closely monitor patients, including temperature, blood pressure, electrocardiogram (ECG), and potassium concentration, during and after administration of *DigiFab*. Patients with intrinsically poor cardiac function may gradually deteriorate from withdrawal of the inotropic action of digoxin. When needed, additional symptomatic support can be provided by use of dopamine, dobutamine, or vasodilators. Provide appropriate supportive therapy for electrolyte disturbances, hypoxia, acid-base disturbances, or dysrhythmias. Massive digitalis intoxication can cause hyperkalemia. Administering potassium supplements in the setting of digitalis intoxication may be hazardous. After treatment with digoxin Fab, serum potassium concentrations may drop rapidly and must be monitored frequently, especially for the first several hours after digoxin Fab administration. Treat hypokalemia cautiously.

Laboratory Tests: Obtain total digoxin concentrations before digoxin Fab administration, if possible. Interpretation may be difficult if drawn soon after the last oral dose because equilibration of digoxin between serum and tissue requires at least 6 to 8 hours. The apparent total digoxin concentration may rise precipitously following administration of digoxin Fab, but the drug will be almost entirely bound to the Fab fragments and, therefore, will not be able to react with receptors in the body. Free digoxin concentrations rebound upward within 12 to 24 hours after giving digoxin Fab, although this rebound may be delayed by 12 to 130 hours in patients with renal disease. Rarely does this rebound exceed a free digoxin concentration of 1 to 1.5 mcg/L.

In normal circumstances, free digoxin concentrations reflect 125% of total digoxin concentrations, with respect to generally accepted concentration-versus-effect relationships. This results from 20% to 25% of digoxin being normally bound to serum proteins.

Efficacy: Treatment response to *Digibind* in a multicenter, controlled clinical trial of 150 cases of life-threatening digitalis intoxication was 90%.

In the clinical trial of *DigiFab*, serum-free digoxin concentrations in all patients fell to undetectable levels after *DigiFab* administration. Independent blinded review of each patient's ECG showed that 10 of the 15 patients studied had ECG abnormalities that improved within 4 hours after *DigiFab* infusion. The remaining 5 patients had ECG abnormalities that were unchanged from baseline throughout the 24-hour assessment period, and in 1 case through the 30-day follow-up period. Although the reason for the lack of ECG resolution could not be clearly determined in all cases, it is possible that the ECG abnormalities observed in these patients were not entirely due to digoxin toxicity, but rather to another underlying cardiac problem. Assessing all manifestations of toxicity, investigators classified 7 out of the 15 patients (47%) studied as having complete resolution of digoxin toxicity within 4 hours of *DigiFab* administration, and 14 patients (93%) were classified as having resolved their digoxin toxicity by 20 hours.

Sensitization: Prior treatment with digoxin-specific ovine immune Fab carries a theoretical risk of sensitization to ovine serum protein and possible reduction in efficacy because of human antibodies against ovine Fab. Because Fab fragments lack the antigenic determinants of the Fc fragment, they should pose a reduced immunogenic threat to patients compared with intact immunoglobulin molecules. Being monovalent, digoxin Fab is also unlikely to form extended immune complexes with the antigen.

Human antibodies to ovine Fab have been reported in some patients receiving *Digibind*; however, there have been no clinical reports of human anti-ovine immunoglobulin antibodies causing a reduction in binding of ovine digoxin immune Fab or neutralization response to ovine digoxin immune Fab to date. Among 8 healthy volunteers and 2 digoxin-intoxicated patients, none developed a measurable immune response (human anti-ovine antibodies) after *DigiFab* administration.

Onset: 30 minutes or shorter

Duration: Mean half-life is 15 to 20 hours.

Pharmacokinetics: Fab fragment-digoxin complexes accumulate in the blood, from which they are excreted by the kidney and reticuloendothelial system. In humans with normal renal function, the biological half-life is 15 to 20 hours. The Fab's volume of distribution slightly exceeds extracellular volume (0.25 to 0.4 L/kg). Systemic clearance is 0.17 to 0.52 mL/min/kg in digoxin-toxic patients with normal renal function. The elimination of total digoxin is dependent on the disposition of digoxin Fab.

Pharmacokinetics of *Digibind* and *DigiFab* were assessed in a randomized and controlled study. Pharmacokinetic profiles of Fab were similar for both *DigiFab* and *Digibind* after administration to 16 healthy subjects given digoxin 1 mg IV 2 hours earlier. The similar volumes of distribution (0.3 L/kg and 0.4 L/kg for *DigiFab* and *Digibind*, respectively) indicate considerable penetration from the circulation into the extracellular space and are consistent with previous reports of ovine Fab distribution, as are the elimination half-life values (15 hours and 23 hours for *DigiFab* and *Digibind*, respectively). Cumulative urinary excretion of digoxin was comparable for both products and exceeded 40% of the administered dose by 24 hours. The elimination half-life of 15 to 20 hours in patients with normal renal function appears to be increased up to 10-fold in patients with renal impairment, although volume of distribution remains unaffected.

In patients with renal failure, excretion of Fab fragment-digoxin complexes is delayed. In a study of 5 patients with a mean serum creatinine of 5.9 ± 1.2 mg/dL, the mean Fab half-lives of the α and β disposition phases were 14 ± 4 and 123 ± 6 hours, respectively. Monitor patients with renal failure for a prolonged period for possible recurrence of digitalis toxicity. Digoxin Fab binds digoxin as long as it remains in plasma. Fab-digoxin complexes do not release free digoxin into the blood, even in severe renal failure.

Atrioventricular block caused by digoxin recurred in a functionally anephric patient 10 days after its initial reversal by ovine Fab therapy. This clinical event persisted for longer than 1 week. In functionally anephric patients, anticipate failure to clear Fab-digoxin complexes from the blood by glomerular filtration and renal excretion. Failure to eliminate Fab-digoxin complexes in severe renal impairment could lead to reintoxication with digoxin after the release of previously bound digoxin into the blood. Monitor patients with severe renal failure treated with digoxin Fab for possible recurrence of toxicity over a prolonged period. Monitoring concentrations of free (unbound) digoxin after administration may be appropriate.

Postpone redigitalization, if possible, until the Fab fragments have been eliminated from the body, which may require 48 to 72 hours. Patients with impaired renal function may require a week or longer. Standard digoxin immunoassays can be used again reliably after these intervals.

Mechanism: Digoxin Fab binds molecules of digoxin, making them unavailable for binding at their site of action on cells in the body. The net effect is to shift the equilibrium away from binding of digoxin to its receptors in the body, thereby reversing both its toxic and therapeutic effects. Within minutes of giving digoxin Fab, there is a 10- to 30-fold increase in total digoxin concentrations. The binding affinity of digoxin Fab for digoxin is 10^9 to 10^{10} M^{-1}. This is greater than the affinity of digoxin for sodium/potassium ATPase, its sodium pump receptor, the presumed receptor for digoxin's therapeutic and toxic effects. The affinity of digoxin Fab for digitoxin is 10^8 to 10^9 M^{-1}. Osmolality ranges from 349 to 359 mOsm/kg.

Drug Interactions: Digoxin Fab interacts with cardiac glycosides by design. No other drug interactions are known.

Lab Interference: Digoxin Fab also will interfere with digitalis immunoassay measurements. Thus, the standard serum (ie, total) digoxin concentration can be clinically misleading until the Fab fragments conjugated to the cardiac drug are eliminated from the body. Obtain serum digoxin concentrations before digoxin immune Fab administration, if possible. Interpretation of any digoxin assay may be difficult if drawn too soon after the last oral dose, because equilibration of digoxin between serum and tissue requires at least 6 to 8 hours. The total digoxin concentration may rise precipitously following administration of digoxin Fab, but the digoxin measured will be almost entirely bound to Fab fragments and, therefore, will not able to react with receptors in the body. Free digoxin concentrations can, at present, only be measured reliably through ultrafiltration of the serum sample, followed by fluorescence polarization immunoassay (FPIA).

In a study of 14 digoxin-intoxicated patients, total digoxin concentrations before administration of digoxin Fab ranged from 3.5 to 10.5 nmol/mL, measured by FPIA. After treatment, total digoxin increased rapidly to 51.8 ± 22.7 nmol/mL. Total digoxin was eliminated in a 2-phase manner, with half-lives of 11.6 ± 4.1 hours and 118 ± 57 hours, respectively. Free digoxin levels fell rapidly after Fab therapy, to a mean nadir of 0.6 ± 1.1 nmol/mL but rebounded to a mean maximum free digoxin concentration of 1.7 ± 1.3 nmol/mL in 77 ± 46 hours. The time to maximum rebound occurred later in patients with end-stage renal disease compared with other patients (127 ± 40 hours vs 55 ± 28 hours). Additional doses of digoxin Fab may be warranted if the rebound in free digoxin produces reintoxication. Clinically monitor patients with renal dysfunction with ECG longer than patients with normal renal function.

Digoxin causes a shift of potassium from inside to outside the cell, such that severe intoxication can cause a life-threatening elevation of serum potassium. This may lead to increased urinary excretion of potassium so that a patient may have hyperkalemia but a whole-body deficit of potassium. When the toxic effects of digoxin are reversed by digoxin Fab, potassium shifts back into the cell with a resulting decline in serum potassium concentration. This hypokalemia may develop rapidly. For these reasons, follow serum potassium concentrations closely, especially during the first several hours after digoxin Fab administration.

Patient Information: Advise patients to contact their physician immediately if they experience any signs and symptoms of delayed allergic reactions of serum sickness (eg, rash, pruritus, urticaria) after hospital discharge.

Pharmaceutical Characteristics

Concentration: Each vial binds or antagonizes approximately 500 mcg of digoxin or digitoxin.

40 mg of digoxin-specific Fab fragments per vial, providing approximately 10 mg/mL of digoxin immune Fab protein

Quality Assay: Purified by affinity chromatography

Packaging: 40 mg vial

NDC Number: 00281-0365-10

Doseform: Powder for solution

Appearance: Off-white, crystalline powder yielding a clear, colorless solution

Diluent:

For reconstitution: 4 mL/vial sterile water for injection

For infusion: Dilute with 0.9% sodium chloride to a convenient volume

Adjuvant: None

Preservative: None

Allergens: Because the Fab fragments of these antibodies lack the antigenic determinants of the Fc fragment, they pose less of an immunogenic threat than an intact immunoglobulin molecule.

Sheep proteins, residual papain

Excipients: Approximately 75 mg mannitol and approximately 2 mg sodium acetate as a buffering agent per vial

pH: 6 to 8

Shelf Life: Expires within 36 months

Storage/Stability: Store powder at 2° to 8°C (36° to 46°F). After reconstitution, refrigerate and discard within 4 hours. Contact the manufacturer regarding exposure to freezing temperatures.

Shipped in insulated containers with coolant packs, usually by second-day courier.

Production Process: The digoxin-binding fragments are obtained from the blood of healthy sheep immunized with a digoxin derivative, DDMA, a digoxin analog containing the functionally essential cyclopentaperhydrophenanthrene:lactone ring moiety coupled to KLH. The final product is prepared by isolating the immunoglobulin fraction of the ovine serum, digesting it with papain and isolating the digoxin-specific Fab fragments by affinity chromatography.

Media: Ovine (sheep) plasma

Digoxin Immune Fab (Ovine)

Threat Epidemiology

Incidence: Studies in the 1960s and 1970s found that approximately 20% of patients receiving maintenance digoxin therapy had signs or symptoms of toxicity at some point in their clinical course. Experts believe that incidence of digitalis intoxication has decreased since the 1970s, secondary to the availability and use of serum drug level monitoring and heightened awareness of drug interactions. In a retrospective epidemiologic study conducted during 1987, the prevalence of definite or possible digoxin intoxication among 556 patients receiving maintenance digoxin for CHF was 4.8%. In the same report, the authors retrospectively reviewed the medical records of patients with a discharge diagnosis of digitalis intoxication from 1980 through 1988. The mortality rate in patients with definite or possible digoxin toxicity was 4.6%. Mortality as a result of digitalis cardiac toxicity affects 3% to 21% of patients presenting with manifestations of digitalis toxicity.

Approximately 2,500 courses of digoxin Fab therapy per year were reported from July 1986 to July 1988. More than half the recipients of digoxin Fab developed toxicity during the course of routine therapy. The balance resulted from suicide attempts and accidental ingestions.

Susceptible Pools: An estimated 25.3 million ambulatory digitalis glycoside prescriptions were written in the United States in 1987. It was the ninth most common chemical entity dispensed, representing approximately 2% of all prescriptions dispensed. Digoxin, the sixteenth most commonly used drug in hospitalized patients, was used in some 2.9 million hospitalizations, predominantly among people older than 64 years of age.

Excluding generic forms of digoxin, more than 20.8 million prescriptions for GlaxoSmithKline's *Lanoxin* brand of digoxin were dispensed in 1991. This was the fourth most common prescription drug brand dispensed, representing 1% of all prescriptions dispensed.

Other Information

Perspective:
1785: Withering reports the beneficial use of the foxglove plant (*Digitalis purpurea*) for a variety of diseases.
1930: Smith isolates digoxin from *Digitalis lanata*.
1934: Digoxin licensed for distribution in the United States.
1967: Antibodies to digoxin produced, initially used for measurement of digoxin concentrations in body fluids.
1971: Efficacy of digoxin Fab demonstrated in dogs.
1976: Human patient receives digoxin Fab treatment.
1985: *Digidote* (Boehringer Mannheim Corporation) designates an orphan drug, March 11, but not yet licensed.
1986: *Digibind* licensed on April 22, 1986 (designated an orphan drug November 1, 1984).
1995: Burroughs Wellcome revises the description of the protein content and binding capacity of *Digibind*. Dosing recommendations modified. Product itself is unchanged.
2001: *DigiFab* brand licensed to Protherics, Inc. (August 31).

References: Allen NM, Dunham GD. Treatment of digitalis intoxication with emphasis on the clinical use of digoxin immune Fab. *DICP*. 1990;24(10):991-998.

Bateman DN. Digoxin-specific antibody fragments: how much and when? *Toxicol Rev*. 2004;23(3):135-143.

Ujhelyi MR, Robert S. Pharmacokinetic aspects of digoxin-specific Fab therapy in the management of digitalis toxicity. *Clin Pharmacokinet*. 1995;28(6):483-493.

Woolf AD, Wenger T, Smith TW, Lovejoy FH Jr. The use of digoxin-specific Fab fragments for severe digitalis intoxication in children. *N Engl J Med*. 1992;326(26):1739-1744.

Comparison of Digoxin Immune Fab (Ovine) Immune Globulins		
	Digibind[a]	*DigiFab*
Indication	To treat digoxin intoxication	To treat digoxin intoxication
Antigenic type	Fab fragments of IgG	Fab fragments of IgG
Generic name	Digoxin Fab (ovine)	Digoxin Fab (ovine)
Manufacturer	GlaxoSmithKline	Protherics, Inc.
Dosage	Each vial binds ≈ 500 mcg digoxin	Each vial binds ≈ 500 mcg digoxin
Route	IV infusion	IV infusion
Doseform	Powder for solution	Powder for solution
Concentration	38 mg per vial	40 mg per vial
Packaging	Vial	Vial
Diluent	Sodium chloride 0.9%	Sodium chloride 0.9%
Routine storage	2° to 8°C	2° to 8°C

a *Digibind* no longer distributed in the United States; information provided for historical comparisons.

Rh$_o$(D) Immune Globulins

Isoantibodies

Terminology of Rh$_o$(D) Status			
Person's native antigen status	Person's antibody status	Category	Effect of exogenous Rh$_o$(D) administration
positive	negative	Rh +	RhIG will bind antigen but not affect recipient or offspring. Patient does not develop own anti-Rh$_o$(D) antibodies because the Rh$_o$(D) antigen is recognized as "self."
negative	negative	Rh –, unsensitized	Appropriate use of RhIG will prevent sensitization of recipient that would otherwise result from exposure to antigen.
negative	positive	Rh –, sensitized	RhIG will have no effect, because recipient is already sensitized and has already developed own capacity to produce anti-Rh$_o$(D) antibodies.

Comparison of Rh$_o$(D) IG Products			
Generic name	Rh$_o$(D) immune globulin intramuscular	Rh$_o$(D) immune globulin intravenous	
Brand name (distributor)	*HyperRho S/D* (Talecris), *MICRhoGam* (Ortho), *RhoGam* (Ortho)	*Rhophylac* (CSL Behring)	*WinRho SDF* (Cangene)
Synonym	RhIGIM	RhIGIV	
Concentration	250 IU (50 mcg) or 1,500 IU (300 mcg) per container	1,500 IU per 2 mL syringes	600 IU (120 mcg), 1,500 IU (300 mcg), 2,500 IU (500 mcg), 5,000 IU (1,000 mcg), or 15,000 IU (3,000 mcg) per vial
Preservative	None	None	None
Production medium	Human plasma	Human plasma	Human plasma
Doseform	Solution	Solution	Powder or solution
Diluent/Solvent	Sterile water	Glycine and saline	Powder: sodium chloride 0.9% Solution: maltose 10%
Packaging	Single-use syringes	Single-use syringes	Vials
Routine storage	2° to 8°C	2° to 8°C	2° to 8°C
Dosage	Various	Various	Various
Route	IM	IV or IM (IV for ITP)[a]	IV or IM (IV for ITP)

a CSL Behring: IM or IV, IV slow push.

Rh$_o$(D) Immune Globulin (RhIG) (Human)

Isoantibodies

Names:
   HyperRho S/D
   RhoGAM, MICRhoGAM

Manufacturers:
   Talecris Biotherapeutics
   Ortho-Clinical Diagnostics

Synonyms: Rh$_o$(D)IG, Rh$_o$IG, RhIG, anti-D immunoglobulin, anti-Rh D immunoglobulin, D immunoglobulin. Simply put, the D allele genetically codes for the Rh$_o$ antigen. The designation Rh was chosen because of similarity to an antigen detected in animals immunized with rhesus monkey red blood cells.

Comparison: Traditional IM forms of RhIG are therapeutically equivalent to RhIGIV in preventing Rh isoimmunization, although IV administration may more promptly provide circulating anti-Rh$_o$(D) antibodies.

Immunologic Characteristics

Target Antigen: Human erythrocytes with the surface antigen Rh$_o$(D). Antibodies are harvested from both male and female donors.

Viability: Inactive, passive, transient

Antigenic Form: Human immunoglobulin, unmodified

Antigenic Type: Protein, IgG antibody to human red blood cell (RBC) factor Rh$_o$(D), polyclonal, substantially polymeric

Strains: Harvested without regard to strain or subtype

Use Characteristics

Indications: For passive, transient protection against development of endogenous anti-Rh$_o$ or anti-D antibodies (isoimmunization) in nonsensitized Rh$_o$ or D antigen-negative persons who receive Rh$_o$ or D antigen-positive blood. Such exposure may result from a transfusion accident or from fetomaternal hemorrhage occurring during delivery, abortion (spontaneous or induced), abdominal trauma, ectopic pregnancy, chorionic villus sampling (CVS), percutaneous umbilical-cord blood sampling (PUBS), amniocentesis, or fetal surgery or manipulation.

Used in this way, Rh$_o$(D)IG provides secondary prophylaxis of hemolytic disease of the fetus and newborn (including erythroblastosis fetalis and hydrops fetalis) in subsequent Rh$_o$(D) antigen-positive children of nonsensitized Rh$_o$(D) antigen-negative mothers. If Rh typing of the fetus is not possible, assume the fetus is Rh$_o$(D) antigen-positive. In such a case, consider the mother a candidate for Rh$_o$(D)IG administration. To warrant Rh$_o$(D)IG administration, the following are necessary:

(1) the mother must be Rh$_o$(D) antigen-negative,

(2) the mother should not have been previously sensitized to the Rh factor and, thus, have already developed anti-Rh$_o$(D) antibodies, and

(3) the infant must be Rh$_o$(D) antigen-positive and direct antiglobulin-negative.

If the father can be determined to be Rh$_o$(D) antigen-negative, Rh$_o$(D) need not be given.

Do not perform Rh$_o$(D) cross-match prior to administration.

Full-term delivery: Rh$_o$(D)IG prevents sensitization to the Rh factor and thus prevents hemolytic disease of the fetus and newborn in subsequent Rh$_o$(D) antigen-positive children.

Rh$_o$(D)IG effectively suppresses the immune response of nonsensitized Rh$_o$(D) antigen-negative mothers after delivery of an Rh$_o$(D) antigen-positive infant.

Other obstetric conditions: Administer Rh$_o$(D)IG to all nonsensitized Rh$_o$(D) antigen-negative women after spontaneous or induced abortions, ruptured tubal pregnancies, amniocentesis; other abdominal trauma, CVS, PUBS, fetal surgery, or manipulation or any occurrence of transplacental hemorrhage, unless the blood type of the fetus has been determined to be Rh$_o$(D) antigen-negative. Sensitization occurs more frequently in women undergoing induced abortions than in those aborting spontaneously.

Administer Rh$_o$(D)IG promptly following spontaneous or induced abortion. If prompt administration is not possible, give Rh$_o$(D)IG within 72 hours following termination of the pregnancy. However, even if Rh$_o$(D)IG is not given within this time period, consider administration of the drug. Rh$_o$(D)IG may be of some value 2 weeks or less after exposure.

Transfusion accidents: Rh$_o$(D)IG can be used to prevent Rh$_o$(D) sensitization in Rh$_o$(D) antigen-negative patients accidentally transfused with Rh$_o$(D) antigen-positive RBCs or blood components containing RBCs, platelets, or granulocytes prepared from Rh$_o$(D) antigen-positive blood. Administer it within 72 hours following Rh-incompatible transfusion.

Limitations: Prophylaxis is not indicated if the fetus or father can be determined to be Rh$_o$(D) antigen-negative.

There is no benefit from Rh$_o$(D)IG administration to Rh$_o$(D) antigen-positive people; to Rh$_o$(D) antigen-negative people known to have been sensitized and, thus, with circulating anti-Rh$_o$(D) antibodies; or to a Rh$_o$(D) antigen-negative woman whose fetus is known to be Rh$_o$(D) antigen-negative.

Contraindications:

Absolute: None

Relative: Exercise caution in patients with selective IgA deficiency because they may have circulating anti-IgA antibodies that may precipitate a hypersensitivity reaction in Rh$_o$(D)IG recipients. Do not administer to infants.

Immunodeficiency: Impairment of effect is unlikely.

Elderly: Not generally indicated for geriatric patients because of the low probability of pregnancy.

Pregnancy: Category C. Use when indicated. Use of Rh$_o$(D)IG during the third trimester in full doses has produced no evidence of hemolysis in the infant. Intact IgG crosses the placenta from the maternal circulation increasingly after 30 weeks gestation.

Lactation: It is not known if Rh$_o$(D)IG antibodies are excreted into breast milk. Problems in humans have not been documented.

Children: Has no value if given to infants. Use in mothers to protect subsequent infants.

Adverse Reactions: As with most IM IgG products, adverse reactions are infrequent, usually mild in nature and generally confined to the site of injection. An occasional patient may react more strongly with localized tenderness, erythema, or low-grade fever. Fever, splenomegaly, myalgia, and lethargy have occurred in some individuals receiving multiple doses of Rh$_o$(D)IG following mismatched transfusions, as have elevated bilirubin levels. This latter reaction may be caused by a relatively rapid rate of foreign red-cell destruction, not to Rh$_o$(D)IG. Hypersensitivity and systemic reactions and induced sensitization with repeated injections occur rarely.

Pharmacologic & Dosing Characteristics

Dosage:

Before administration: Immediately after delivery, determine the infant's ABO and Rh$_o$(D) blood group and perform a direct antiglobulin test. Umbilical cord, venous, or capillary blood may be used. Confirm that the mother is Rh$_o$(D) antigen-negative.

RBC volume estimation: To determine the dose of Rh$_o$(D)IG required for antigen neutralization, the volume of packed fetal RBCs must be determined by an approved laboratory assay, such as the Kleihauer-Betke Acid Elution Stain Technique or the Clayton Modification, based on rosetting. The volume of fetomaternal hemorrhage divided by 2 gives the volume of packed fetal RBCs in the maternal blood. The dose of Rh$_o$(D)IG needed is calculated by dividing the volume (measured in mL) of packed RBCs by 15. Fetomaternal hemorrhages over 15 mL occur in only approximately 0.2% of pregnancies.

Postpartum prophylaxis, miscarriage, abortion, or ectopic pregnancy: One full-dose (1,500 unit) vial or syringe of Rh$_o$(D)IG suffices to prevent maternal sensitization to the Rh factor if the fetal packed RBC volume that entered the mother's circulation because of fetomaternal hemorrhage is less than 15 mL (less than 30 mL of whole blood). When the fetomaternal hemorrhage exceeds 15 mL of packed cells or 30 mL of whole blood, administer more than 1 vial or syringe of Rh$_o$(D)IG. One mini-dose (300 unit) vial or syringe of Rh$_o$(D)IG will prevent formation of anti-Rh$_o$(D) antibodies during transplacental hemorrhage resulting from spontaneous or induced abortion 12 weeks gestation or less. After 12 weeks gestation, give a full-dose (1,500 unit) vial or syringe.

Antepartum prophylaxis: The contents of 1 full-dose (1,500 unit) vial or syringe of Rh$_o$(D)IG given at approximately 28 weeks gestation and again within 72 hours after an Rh-incompatible delivery are highly effective in preventing Rh isoimmunization during pregnancy.

Threatened abortion: Following threatened abortion at any stage of gestation with continuation of pregnancy, give 1 full-dose (1,500 unit) vial or syringe of Rh$_o$(D)IG. If more than 15 mL of packed RBCs is suspected because of fetomaternal hemorrhage, calculate the proper dose as described above.

Amniocentesis or abdominal trauma: Following amniocentesis at either 15 to 18 weeks gestation or during the third trimester, or following abdominal trauma in the second or third trimester, give 1 full-dose (1,500 unit) vial or syringe of Rh$_o$(D)IG, unless a larger dose is needed.

Transfusion accidents: The dose of Rh$_o$(D)IG is dependent on the volume of packed red cells or whole blood transfused. To determine the amount of Rh$_o$(D)IG needed, multiply the volume (measured in mL) of Rh$_o$(D) antigen-positive whole blood administered by the hematocrit of the donor unit. This value equals the volume of packed RBCs transfused. Divide the volume (measured in mL) of RBCs by 15 to obtain the dose of Rh$_o$(D)IG needed. If the dose calculation results in a fraction, administer the next higher whole number of full-dose (1,500 unit) vials or syringes of Rh$_o$(D)IG. Rh$_o$(D) antigen-negative patients transfused with Rh$_o$(D) antigen-positive blood have received as many as 15 to 33 vials of Rh$_o$(D)IG without adverse reaction.

Route & Site: IM only. Do not inject IV. The contents of the total dose may be injected as a divided dose at different injection sites at the same time, or the total dosage may be divided and injected at intervals, provided the total dosage is injected within 72 hours postpartum or after a transfusion accident.

Overdosage: Although few data are available, clinical experience with similar products suggests that the major manifestations of overdosage would be pain and tenderness at the injection site.

Additional Doses: To prevent sensitization, Rh$_o$(D)IG must be administered after each exposure to Rh$_o$(D) antigen-positive RBCs.

If any event requires administration of Rh$_o$(D)IG at 13 to 18 weeks gestation, give another full-dose (1,500 unit) vial at 26 to 28 weeks gestation. To maintain protection throughout pregnancy, do not allow the level of passively acquired anti-Rh$_o$(D) to fall below the level required to prevent an immune response (ie, titers over 1:5 by Rapid Fluorescent Focus Inhibition Test [RFFIT]). In any case, give an additional full dose (1,500 units) of Rh$_o$(D)IG within 72 hours after delivery if the baby is Rh$_o$(D) antigen-positive. If delivery occurs within 3 weeks after the last dose, the postpartum dose may be withheld unless there is a fetomaternal hemorrhage over 15 mL of packed RBC.

If more than 15 mL of Rh$_o$(D) antigen-positive RBCs are present in the mother's circulation, more than 1 full-dose (1,500 unit) vial or syringe of Rh$_o$(D)IG is required. Failure to recognize this need may result in the administration of an inadequate dose.

Efficacy: The incidence of sensitization without Rh$_o$(D)IG administration is 12% to 13%. Administration lowers the incidence to 1% to 2% when given postpartum or 0.1% to 0.7% when given antepartum at 28 weeks gestation and again immediately after delivery.

Onset: Prompt. In one study, 99% of Rh$_o$(D)-positive RBCs injected into Rh$_o$(D)-negative healthy men were cleared from circulation within 144 hours after IM administration.

Duration: Mean half-life is 23 to 26 days.

Pharmacokinetics: Immunoglobulins are primarily eliminated by catabolism. In one study, peak serum concentrations of anti-Rh$_o$(D) IgG ranged from 7 to 46 ng/mL, achieved 2 to 7 days after IM injection. The mean apparent clearance was 0.29 ± 0.12 mL/min and the mean half-life was 18 ± 5 days. Anti-D IgG titers were measurable in all subjects at least 9 weeks after administration.

Protective Level: Antibody titers 1:5 or more by RFFIT are indicative of adequate protection.

Mechanism: Passive immunization with Rh$_o$(D)IG prevents the formation of anti-Rh$_o$(D) antibodies in nonsensitized Rh$_o$(D) antigen-negative individuals who receive Rh$_o$(D) antigen-positive RBCs. Rh$_o$(D) antibody binds circulating antigen, thus preventing stimulation of antigen-sensitive lymphocytes and the resulting production of anti-Rh$_o$(D). Prevention of Rh$_o$(D) sensitization in turn prevents hemolytic disease of the fetus and newborn in subsequent Rh$_o$(D) antigen-positive children.

Drug Interactions: Other antibodies in Rh$_o$(D)IG may interfere with the response to live vaccines such as measles, mumps, polio, or rubella. Therefore, do not immunize with live vaccines within 14 to 30 days before or 3 months after Rh$_o$(D)IG administration. For varicella vaccine, wait 5 months. For a vaccine containing measles virus, wait 3 months or longer.

Nonetheless, Rh$_o$(D)IG does not appear to impair the efficacy of rubella vaccine. Rubella-susceptible postpartum women who received blood products or Rh$_o$(D)IG may receive rubella vaccine prior to discharge, provided that an HI titer for rubella antibody is drawn 6 to 8 weeks after vaccination to ensure seroconversion.

Inactivated vaccines are not generally affected by circulating antibodies or administration of exogenous antibodies. Immunization with such vaccines may occur at any time before or after antibody administration.

As with other drugs given by IM injection, give Rh$_o$(D)IG with caution to patients taking anticoagulants.

Lab Interference: Babies born of women given Rh$_o$(D)IG antepartum may have a weakly positive antiglobulin (Coombs') test at birth.

Passively acquired anti-Rh$_o$(D) may be detected in maternal serum by antibody screening tests performed within several weeks of administration of Rh$_o$(D)IG. Such a finding does not preclude further Rh$_o$(D)IG administration. However, the presence of passively administered Rh$_o$(D) antibody in a maternal blood sample can affect the interpretation of laboratory tests to identify the patient as a candidate for Rh$_o$(D)IG. In case of doubt as to the patient's Rh group or immune status, give Rh$_o$(D)IG.

A large fetomaternal hemorrhage late in pregnancy or following delivery may cause a weak, mixed field positive D$_U$ test result. If there is any doubt about the mother's Rh type, give her Rh$_o$(D)IG. A screening test for fetal RBCs may help in such cases.

Pharmaceutical Characteristics

Concentration: Contains 90% or more IgG. Each full-dose vial or syringe inhibits the immunizing potential of 30 mL of whole blood or 15 mL of Rh$_o$(D) (RH1) antigen-positive packed RBCs. Each mini-dose vial or syringe contains one-sixth the full dose and inhibits the immunizing potential of 5 mL of whole blood or 2.5 mL of Rh$_o$(D) antigen-positive packed RBCs.

A full dose of Rh$_o$(D)IG is traditionally referred to in the United States as 300 mcg of anti-Rh$_o$(D) (corresponding to a 1,500 international unit dose). In the same way, minidose preparations are labeled as 50 mcg (250 international unit) containers.

Ortho: 4% to 6%

Talecris: 15% to 18% globulin

Quality Assay: Standardized by D-antiglobulin titer. Rh$_o$(D) antibody content meets or exceeds the content of 1 mL of the US Reference Standard Rh$_o$(D) Immune Globulin.

Ortho: Contains less than 10 picokatal (pkat)/mL of plasmin and less than 40 pkat/mL of plasminogen.

Packaging: Vials and syringes generally contain 1 to 2 mL.

Ortho: Each package includes package inserts, control forms, and patient identification cards.

Full-dose (1,500 units) RhoGAM: One single-dose prefilled syringes with 22-gauge, ¾-inch needles (00562-7805-01), 5 syringes (00562-7805-05), 25 syringes (00562-7805-25)

Minidose (250 units) MICRhoGAM: One single-dose prefilled syringe with 22-gauge, ¾-inch needles (00562-7806-01), 5 syringes (00562-7806-05), 25 syringes (00562-7806-25)

Talecris: Each package or carton includes directions for use, patient identification cards, and patient information booklets.

Full-dose (1,500 units) HyperRho S/D: One single-dose prefilled syringe with 22-gauge, 1¼-inch needle (NDC#: 13533-0631-02)

Minidose (250 units) HyperRho S/D: 10 single-dose prefilled syringes with 22-gauge, 1¼-inch needles (13533-0631-06)

Doseform: Solution

Appearance: Clear, colorless solution

Solvent: Sterile water for injection

Adjuvant: None

Preservative:

Ortho: None

Talecris: None

Allergens: Check package labeling regarding the presence of latex rubber content.

Ortho: Less than 1% IgA, IgM undetectable

Talecris: IgA content not measured

Rh$_o$(D) Immune Globulin (RhIG) (Human)

Excipients:
> *Ortho:* 15 mg/mL glycine, 2.9 mg/mL sodium chloride, 0.01% polysorbate 80
> *Talecris:* 0.21 to 0.32 molar glycine, pH adjusted with sodium carbonate

pH: 6.4 to 7.2

Shelf Life: Expires within 12 to 24 months

Storage/Stability: Store at 2° to 8°C (36° to 46°F). Discard if frozen.
> *Ortho:* Contact manufacturer regarding prolonged exposure to room temperature or elevated temperatures. Shipped at ambient temperature.
> *Talecris:* Product can tolerate 30 days at 30°C (86°F). Shipping data not provided.

Production Process: Rh$_o$(D) antigen-negative men or sterile women are immunized with Rh$_o$(D) cells to produce anti-Rh$_o$(D) antibodies. The antibodies are harvested by Cohn-Oncley methods 6 & 9 cold-ethanol fractionation process of plasma collected from these donors.
> *Ortho:* After plasma fractionation, filtration and viral inactivation steps are performed. The viral filtration step removes viruses via a size-exclusion mechanism utilizing an ultrafiltration membrane with defined pore-size distribution of 12 to 18 nm to remove enveloped and nonenveloped viruses. Next, quality control tests are performed on the membrane to ensure filter integrity. The viral inactivation step uses p-isooctylphenyl ether (Triton X-100) and tri-n-butyl phosphate to inactivate enveloped viruses such as hepatitis C virus, HIV, and West Nile virus.
> *Talecris:* A virucidal solvent-detergent treatment step is performed using 0.3% tri-n-butylphosphate and 0.2% sodium cholate at 30°C (86°F) for 6 hours or longer. Next, reactants are removed by precipitation, filtration, ultrafiltration, then diafiltration. Final containers are incubated for 21 to 28 days at 20° to 27°C (68° to 80.6°F).

Media: Human plasma, 20 units or more per lot

Disease Epidemiology

Incidence: Rh-negative women carrying Rh-positive fetuses represent 9% to 10% of all pregnancies. In the absence of RhIG prophylaxis, 0.7% to 1.8% of these Rh-negative women will be isoimmunized antenatally, 8% to 15% at birth, 3% to 5% after spontaneous or induced abortion, and 2.1% to 3.4% after amniocentesis.

In 1968, 2.7 deaths from hemolytic disease of the newborn (HDN) occurred per 10,000 live births. HDN accounted for 10% or fewer of all perinatal mortality in the United States. Between 1970 and 1975, disease rates declined from 45.1 to 20.6 per 10,000 total births (live births and stillbirths).

In 1980, 14.9 cases of HDN per 10,000 total births were noted. The incidence in 1986 was 10.6 per 10,000 births, with some regional variations. This amounts to approximately 10,000 infant deaths per year. Incidence is highest among Hispanics, Caucasians, and Chinese and lowest among other Asians, African-Americans, and Native Americans. HDN incidence rates have remained relatively stable since 1979.

Susceptible Pools: In 1974, 20% of those women who needed passive Rh$_o$(D) immunization did not receive it. Based on current usage data, some 1,100 to 1,900 cases of HDN could be prevented each year if Rh$_o$(D)IG were used more extensively. Compliance rates with dosing recommendations are nearly complete postpartum but substantially less for other indications:

- abortion: 88% to 94%;
- antepartum hemorrhage: 31%;
- amniocentesis: 14%.

Rh$_o$(D) Immune Globulin (RhIG) (Human)

Other Information

Perspective:

1900: Landsteiner identifies the ABO blood-group system. He earns the 1930 Nobel Prize for this and related work.

1939: Levine and Stetson explain hemolytic disease of the fetus and newborn in terms of Rh specificity.

1940: Landsteiner and Weiner discover Rh specificity.

1945: Coombs, Race, and Mourant develop antiglobulin test for incomplete Rh antibodies.

1950: Coombs Test introduced to identify sensitized Rh-negative patients.

1960: Gorman, Freda, and Pollack in New York and Finn and Clarke in Liverpool begin research into use of Rh$_o$(D)IG to prevent Rh$_o$(D) isoimmunization of unsensitized women.

1961: US human safety studies of Rh$_o$(D)IG are conducted among male inmates at Sing Sing Prison.

1966: Gorman, Freda, and Pollack report first successful prevention of maternal sensitization to the Rh factor by the administration of anti-Rh$_o$(D) preparation following delivery.

1968: First batch of Rh$_o$(D)IG licensed and first dose administered on May 29.

1977: First minidose of Rh$_o$(D)IG licensed.

1984: Antepartum protocols recommended by the American College of Obstetricians and Gynecologists (ACOG).

First Licensed:

Cutter (now Talecris): June 11, 1971

Ortho: April 10, 1968 (1979 for *MicRhoGam* formulation

Discontinued Products: *BayRho-D* (Bayer), *D-Imune* (Lederle), *Gamulin, MicroGamulin* (Armour, later Aventis Behring, 1982 to approximately 2000), *HypRhoD* (Cutter, Bayer), *RhesoNativ* (Kabi), *Rho-Imune* (Lederle, December 6, 1972)

National Policy: ACOG. Educational Bulletin: #227. Management of isoimmunization in pregnancy. *Int J Gynaecol Obstet.* 1996;55:183-190.

ACOG. Practice Bulletin: #4. Prevention of Rh D isoimmunization. *Int J Gynaecol Obstet.* 1999;66:63-70.

References: Bowman J. Thirty-five years of Rh prophylaxis. *Transfusion.* 2003;43(12):1661-1666.

Chavez GF, et al. Epidemiology of Rh hemolytic disease of the newborn in the United States. *JAMA.* 1991;265:3270-3274.

Chilcott, J, Lloyd Jones M, Wight J, et al. A review of the clinical effectiveness and cost-effectiveness of routine anti-D prophylaxis for pregnant women who are rhesus-negative. *Health Technol Assess.* 2003;7(4):iii-62.

Greenough A. The role of immunoglobulins in neonatal Rhesus haemolyic disease. *BioDrugs.* 2001:16:533-541.

Moise KJ. Red blood cell alloimmunization in pregnancy. *Semin Hematol.* 2005;42(3):169-178.

Nakhoul IN, Kozuch P, Varma M. Management of adult idiopathic thrombocytopenic purpura. *Clin Adv Hematol Oncol.* 2006;4(2):136-144.

Sandler SG, Tutuncuoglu SO. Immune thrombocytopenic purpura-current management practices. *Expert Opin Pharmacother.* 2004;5(12):2515-2527.

Urbaniak SJ. Alloimmunity to RhD in humans. *Transfus Clin Biol.* 2006;13(1-2):19-22.

Westhoff CM. The structure and function of the Rh antigen complex. *Semin Hematol.* 2007;44(1):42-50.

Zimmerman DR. *Rh: The Intimate History of a Disease and Its Conquest.* New York, NY: MacMillan Publishing Company; 1973.

Rh$_o$(D) Immune Globulin Intravenous (RhIGIV) (Human)

Isoantibodies

Names:
WinRho SDF

Rhophylac

Manufacturers:
Manufactured by Cangene Corporation, distributed by Baxter Healthcare Corporation
CSL Behring

Synonyms: RhIGIV. Generically known as Rh$_o$(D)IG, Rh$_o$IG, RhIG, anti-D immunoglobulin, anti-Rh D immunoglobulin, D immunoglobulin. The D allele genetically codes for the Rh$_o$ antigen. The designation Rh was chosen because of similarity to an antigen detected in animals immunized with rhesus monkey red blood cells.

Comparison: Traditional IM forms of RhIG are therapeutically equivalent to RhIGIV in preventing Rh isoimmunization, although IV administration may more promptly provide circulating anti-Rh$_o$(D) antibodies.

Compared with IGIV therapy of immune thrombocytopenic purpura (ITP), RhIGIV can be administered in lower total antibody doses over shorter periods of time.

Immunologic Characteristics

Target Antigen: Human erythrocytes with the surface antigen Rh$_o$(D), harvested from both male and female donors

Viability: Inactive, passive, transient

Antigenic Form: Human immunoglobulin, unmodified

Antigenic Type: Protein, IgG antibody to human red blood cell (RBC) factor Rh$_o$(D), polyclonal, substantially monomeric

Strains: Harvested without regard to strain or subtype

Use Characteristics

Indications: For passive, transient protection against developing endogenous anti-Rh$_o$ or anti-D antibodies (isoimmunization) in nonsensitized Rh$_o$ or D antigen-negative persons who receive Rh$_o$ or D antigen-positive blood. Such exposure may result from fetomaternal hemorrhage during delivery, abortion (spontaneous or induced), abdominal trauma, ectopic pregnancy, chorionic villus sampling (CVS), amniocentesis, fetal surgery or manipulation, or as a result of a transfusion accident.

Used in this way, RhIGIV provides secondary prophylaxis of hemolytic disease of the fetus and newborn (including erythroblastosis fetalis and hydrops fetalis) in subsequent Rh$_o$(D) antigen-positive children. If Rh typing of the fetus is not possible, assume the fetus is Rh$_o$(D) antigen-positive. In such a case, consider the mother a candidate for Rh$_o$(D)IG administration.

Also used in the treatment of ITP in certain children and adults who are Rh$_o$(D) antigen-positive.

Obstetric conditions: To suppress Rh$_o$(D) sensitization (isoimmunization) in nonsensitized (Rh$_o$[D] antibody-negative) Rh$_o$(D) antigen-negative women within 72 hours after spontaneous or induced abortions, amniocentesis, CVS, ruptured tubal pregnancy, abdominal trauma, transplacental hemorrhage, or in the normal course of pregnancy, unless the blood type of the fetus or father is known to be Rh$_o$(D) antigen-negative. In maternal bleeding caused by threatened abortion, give RhIGIV as soon as possible. Suppression of Rh isoimmunization reduces the likelihood of hemolytic disease in an $Rh_o(D)$ antigen-positive fetus in present and future pregnancies.

The criteria for an Rh-incompatible pregnancy requiring administration of RhIGIV at 28 weeks gestation and within 72 hours after delivery are:

(1) The mother must be $Rh_o(D)$ antigen-negative;

(2) the mother is carrying a child whose father is either $Rh_o(D)$ antigen-positive or $Rh_o(D)$ unknown;

(3) the infant is either $Rh_o(D)$ antigen-positive or $Rh_o(D)$ unknown; and

(4) the mother must not be previously sensitized to the $Rh_o(D)$ antigen and, thus, possessing anti-$Rh_o(D)$ antibodies.

A large fetomaternal hemorrhage late in pregnancy or following delivery may cause a weak mixed field positive D_U test result. Such an individual should be assessed for a large fetomaternal hemorrhage and the dose of RhIGIV adjusted accordingly. Give RhIGIV if there is any doubt about the mother's blood type.

Transfusion accidents: RhIGIV is recommended to suppress Rh isoimmunization in $Rh_o(D)$ antigen-negative female children and adults in their childbearing years transfused with $Rh_o(D)$ antigen-positive RBCs or blood components containing $Rh_o(D)$ antigen-positive RBCs. Initiate treatment within 72 hours of exposure. Begin treatment (without preceding exchange transfusion) only if the transfused $Rh_o(D)$ antigen-positive blood represents less than 20% of the total circulating red cells. A 1,500 international unit (300 mcg) dose will suppress the immunizing potential of approximately 17 mL of $Rh_o(D)$ antigen-positive RBCs.

ITP: To increase platelets in ITP patients who have an uncommon immune bleeding disorder. Platelet counts usually rise within 1 to 2 days and peak within 7 to 14 days after initiation of therapy. The duration of response is variable; however, the average duration is approximately 30 days. RhIGIV is recommended for treatment of the following patients who are nonsplenectomized $Rh_o(D)$ antigen-positive:

(1) Children with chronic or acute ITP;

(2) adults with chronic ITP; or

(3) children and adults with ITP secondary to HIV infection in clinical situations requiring an increase in platelet count to prevent excessive hemorrhage.

Limitations:

Rh isoimmunization: Rh prophylaxis is not indicated if the fetus or father can be determined to be $Rh_o(D)$ antigen-negative. RhIGIV will not benefit patients who are both $Rh_o(D)$ antigen-negative and Rh immunized (Rh antibody-positive). This condition can be diagnosed by standard manual Rh antibody screening tests.

ITP: The efficacy of RhIGIV in ITP has not been established by the IM or subcutaneous routes. Do not give RhIGIV to $Rh_o(D)$ antigen-negative or splenectomized individuals, as its efficacy in these patients has not been demonstrated. If a patient has a lower than normal hemoglobin level (lower than 10 g/dL), give a reduced dose of 125 to 200 international units (25 to 40 mcg) per kg to minimize the risk of increasing the severity of anemia in the patient. RhIGIV must be used with extreme caution in patients with a hemoglobin level lower than 8 g/dL because of the risk of increasing the severity of the anemia.

Contraindications:

Absolute: Patients with a history of an anaphylactic or severe systemic reaction to human globulin.

RhIGIV suppresses Rh isoimmunization in the mother; do not administer to the infant.

Relative: Patients who are deficient in IgA may develop anti-IgA antibodies and have anaphylactic reactions. Weigh the potential benefit of treatment against the potential for hypersensitivity reactions.

Immunodeficiency: Impairment of effect is unlikely.

Elderly: Not generally indicated for geriatric patients because of the low probability of pregnancy. RhIGIV has not been studied in elderly patients being treated for incompatible transfusion. In treatment of ITP, no overall differences in safety or efficacy were observed between elderly subjects and younger subjects.

Pregnancy: Category C. Use when indicated. Use of IM forms of RhIG in full doses during the third trimester has produced no evidence of hemolysis in the infant. Intact IgG crosses the placenta from the maternal circulation increasingly after 30 weeks gestation. RhIGIV has not been studied in pregnant women with ITP.

Lactation: It is not known whether RhIGIV antibodies cross into human breast milk. Problems in humans have not been documented.

Children: RhIGIV suppresses Rh isoimmunization in the mother; do not administer to the infant. The safety and effectiveness of RhIGIV have not been established in pediatric patients being treated for incompatible transfusion. Weigh the potential risks and benefits, particularly in girls whose later pregnancies may be affected if Rh isoimmunization occurs.

Adverse Reactions: The most common adverse events among people treated for any indication are injection-site pain, headaches, chills, fevers, asthenia, pallor, diarrhea, nausea, vomiting, arthralgia, myalgia, dizziness, hyperkinesia, abdominal or back pain, hypotension, hypertension, increased lactate dehydrogenase (LDH) levels, somnolence, vasodilation, pruritus, rash, and sweating. Rare cases of anaphylaxis, vertigo, tachycardia, dyspnea, and erythema have been reported.

Adverse reactions to RhIGIV are infrequent in Rh$_o$(D) antigen-negative individuals. In the clinical trial of 1,186 Rh$_o$(D) antigen-negative pregnant women, no adverse events were attributed to RhIGIV. A small number of cases report discomfort and slight swelling at the site of injection and slight elevation in temperature. As is the case with all antibody products, there is a remote chance of an anaphylactic reaction with RhIGIV in patients hypersensitive to blood products. There was 1 report of an Rh$_o$(D) antigen-negative patient receiving 1 unit of Rh$_o$(D) antigen-positive blood; the patient reported chills, shaking, nausea, myalgia, vomiting, drowsiness, disorientation, and lethargy after receiving 6,000 international units (1,200 mcg) of RhIGIV.

A postmarketing survey conducted after the Canadian licensure of RhIGIV in 1980 included data obtained from 31,059 injections, including 9,905 Rh$_o$(D) antigen-negative women who delivered Rh$_o$(D) antigen-positive infants, almost all of whom had received antenatal and postnatal prophylaxis. No adverse experiences related to RhIGIV were reported in the survey.

RhIGIV is given to Rh$_o$(D) antigen-positive patients with ITP. Side effects related to the destruction of Rh$_o$(D) antigen-positive red cells, such as decreased hemoglobin, can be expected. At the recommended initial IV dose of 250 international units/kg, the mean maximum decrease in hemoglobin was 1.7 g/dL. At a reduced dose, ranging from 125 to 200 international units/kg, the mean maximum decrease in hemoglobin was 0.61 g/dL. Only 3.7% of patients had a maximum decrease in hemoglobin of higher than 4 g/dL.

Among patients treated for ITP, there have been rare reports of signs and symptoms consistent with intravascular hemolysis that included back pain, shaking chills, fever, and discolored urine occurring, in most cases, within 4 hours of administration. Reports of potentially serious complications of intravascular hemolysis included clinically compromising anemia, acute renal insufficiency, or disseminated intravascular coagulation. There were no discern-

Rh$_o$(D) Immune Globulin Intravenous (RhIGIV) (Human)

ible contributions of age, gender, pretreatment renal function, pretreatment hemoglobin, concomitantly administered blood or blood products, comorbid conditions, or previous treatment with RhIGIV.

IGIV products have been reported to produce renal dysfunction in patients predisposed to acute renal failure or those who have renal insufficiency. Most of these reports involved products containing sucrose as a stabilizer, unlike current RhIGIV products. Nonetheless, assess renal function before and after RhIGIV administration, especially for patients at risk of developing acute renal failure.

In trials of 161 subjects with various forms of ITP, 7% of infusions involved at least 1 adverse event considered to be related to RhIGIV. The most common adverse events were headache (2%), chills (less than 2%), and fever (1%). All are expected adverse events associated with immunoglobulin infusions.

One child with chronic ITP who received an initial dose of 250 international units/kg RhIGIV followed by 175 international units/kg on day 15 had a drop in hemoglobin from 12.4 to 7.6 g/dL after the second course of treatment. RhIGIV was subsequently withheld.

Monitor Rh$_o$(D)-positive patients treated with RhIGIV for signs or symptoms of intravascular hemolysis, clinically compromising anemia, disseminated intravascular coagulation, or renal insufficiency.

Pharmacologic & Dosing Characteristics

Dosage: See RhIG Intramuscular monograph for discussion of calculating RBC volume.

Pregnancy: Give 1,500 international units (300 mcg) either IV or IM at 28 to 30 weeks gestation. If given early in the pregnancy, give RhIGIV at 12-week intervals to maintain an adequate level of passively acquired anti-Rh antibodies.

Give 600 international units (120 mcg) (Cangene) or 1,500 international units (CSL) either IV or IM as soon as possible after delivery of a confirmed Rh$_o$(D) antigen-positive baby, normally 72 hours or less after delivery. If the Rh status of the baby is not known, give RhIGIV to the mother at 72 hours after delivery. If more than 72 hours have elapsed, do not withhold RhIGIV. Rather, give it as soon as possible, up to 28 days after delivery.

Other obstetric conditions: Give 600 international units (120 mcg) (Cangene) or 1,500 international units (CSL), either IV or IM immediately after abortion, amniocentesis (after 34 weeks gestation), or any other manipulation late in pregnancy (after 34 weeks gestation) associated with increased risk of Rh isoimmunization. Administer within 72 hours after the event.

Give 1,500 international units (300 mcg) either IV or IM immediately after amniocentesis performed before 34 weeks gestation or after chorionic villus sampling. Repeat this dose every 12 weeks while the woman is pregnant. In the case of threatened abortion, give RhIGIV as soon as possible.

Transfusion: Give RhIGIV within 72 hours after exposure for treatment of incompatible blood transfusions or massive fetal hemorrhage. The dose depends on route of administration.

Cangene:

IV: Give 45 international units (9 mcg)/mL Rh$_o$(D)-positive blood or 90 international units (18 mcg)/mL of Rh$_o$(D)-positive red blood cells. Give 3,000 international units (600 mcg) IV every 8 hours until total dose is given.

IM: Give 60 international units (12 mcg)/mL Rh$_o$(D)-positive blood or 120 international units (24 mcg)/mL of Rh$_o$(D)-positive red blood cells. Give 6,000 international units (1,200 mcg) IM every 12 hours until total dose is given.

CSL: For massive fetomaternal hemorrhage, give 1,500 international units (300 mcg), either IM or IV, plus 100 international units (20 mcg) per mL fetal RBCs in excess of 15 mL if excess transplacental bleeding is quantified. If bleeding cannot be quantified, give two 1,500 international unit doses. For incompatible transfusions, give 100 international units (20 mcg) per 2 mL transfused blood or per 1 mL erythrocyte concentrate within 72 hours of exposure.

ITP: An initial IV dose of 250 international units (50 mcg) per kg is recommended for the treatment of ITP. If the patient has a hemoglobin level that is lower than 10 g/dL, a reduced dose of 125 to 200 international units (25 to 40 mcg)/kg should be given to minimize the risk of increasing the severity of anemia. Use extreme caution in patients with a hemoglobin level of less than 8 g/dL, due to the risk of increasing the severity of the anemia. The initial dose may be given as a single dose or in 2 divided doses given on separate days.

Route & Site:

IV, slow push: Infuse into a suitable vein over 3 to 5 minutes (or 2 mL per 15 to 60 seconds). Administer separately from other drugs. The IV route must be used to treat ITP.

IM: Inject into the deltoid muscle of the upper arm or the anterolateral aspect of the upper thigh. To avoid sciatic nerve injury, do not use the gluteal region as a routine injection site. If the gluteal region is used, use only the upper outer quadrant.

Overdosage: There are no reports of overdose in patients treated for Rh isoimmunization. In clinical studies of 141 nonpregnant Rh$_o$(D) antigen-positive patients with ITP treated with 600 to 32,500 international units (120 to 6,500 mcg) of RhIGIV, there were no signs or symptoms that warranted medical intervention. However, these doses were associated with mild, transient hemolytic anemia. Monitor patients with incompatible transfusion or ITP who receive an overdose because of the risk of hemolysis.

Additional Doses:

Rh isoimmunization: To prevent sensitization, RhIG must be given after each exposure to Rh$_o$(D) antigen-positive red blood cells. If given early in pregnancy, administer RhIGIV at 12-week intervals during the pregnancy to maintain an adequate level of passively acquired anti-Rh antibodies.

ITP: If subsequent therapy is required to raise platelet counts, an IV dose of 125 to 300 international units (25 to 60 mcg)/kg is recommended. Determine the optimal frequency and dose for maintenance therapy from the patient's clinical response by assessing platelet counts, red cell counts, hemoglobin, and reticulocyte levels. If the patient did not respond to the initial dose with a satisfactory increase in platelets, administer a subsequent dose based on hemoglobin level. For hemoglobin between 8 and 10 g/dL, administer 125 to 200 international units (25 to 40 mcg)/kg. For hemoglobin higher than 10 g/dL, administer 250 to 300 international units (50 to 60 mcg)/kg. For hemoglobin lower than 8 g/dL, use with caution.

Laboratory Tests: Monitor all ITP patients to determine clinical response by assessing platelet counts, red cell counts, hemoglobin, and reticulocyte levels.

Efficacy:

Rh isoimmunization: RhIGIV, when administered within 72 hours of a full-term delivery of an Rh$_o$(D) antigen-positive infant by an Rh$_o$(D) antigen-negative mother, will reduce the incidence of Rh isoimmunization from 12% to 13% to 1% to 2%. The 1% to 2% incidence is, for the most part, caused by isoimmunization during the last trimester of pregnancy. When treatment is given both antenatally at 28 weeks gestation and postpartum, the Rh immunization rate drops to approximately 0.1%.

Of 1,186 women who received antenatal RhIGIV in a clinical trial, 806 also were given RhIGIV postnatally following the delivery of an Rh$_o$(D) antigen-positive infant, of which 325 women underwent testing at 6 months after delivery for evidence of Rh isoimmuni-

Rh$_o$(D) Immune Globulin Intravenous (RhIGIV) (Human)

zation. Of these 325 women, 23 would have been expected to display signs of Rh isoimmunization; however, no signs of Rh isoimmunization were observed ($P < 0.001$).

A postmarketing survey conducted after the Canadian licensure of RhIGIV in 1980 for this indication included data obtained from 31,059 injections, including 9,905 Rh$_o$(D) antigen-negative women who delivered Rh$_o$(D) antigen-positive infants, almost all of whom had received antenatal as well as postnatal prophylaxis. Of the patients followed in this survey, there were 26 reported treatment failures that resulted in the development of Rh$_o$(D) antibodies.

Childhood chronic ITP: In an open-label, single-arm, multicenter study, 24 children with ITP of longer than 6 months duration were treated initially with 250 international units/kg RhIGIV (125 international units/kg on days 1 and 2), with subsequent doses ranging from 125 to 275 international units/kg. Response was defined as a platelet increase to 50,000/mm^3 or higher and a doubling from baseline. Nineteen of 24 patients responded, for an overall mean peak platelet count of 229,400/mm^3 (range, 43,300 to 456,000), an overall response rate of 79%, and a mean duration of response of 36.5 days (range, 6 to 84).

Childhood acute ITP: A multicenter, randomized, controlled trial comparing RhIGIV with high-dose IGIV, low-dose IGIV, and prednisone was conducted in 146 children with acute ITP and platelet counts lower than 20,000/mm^3. Of 38 patients receiving RhIGIV (125 international units/kg on days 1 and 2), 32 patients (84%) responded (platelet count 50,000/mm^3 or higher), with a mean peak platelet count of 319,500/mm^3 (range, 61,000 to 892,000) and no statistically significant differences compared with other treatment arms. The mean times to achieving 20,000/mm^3 or higher or 50,000/mm^3 platelets or higher for patients receiving RhIGIV were 1.9 and 2.6 days, respectively. When comparing the different therapies for time to reach a platelet count of 20,000/mm^3 or higher or 50,000/mm^3 or higher, no statistically significant differences among treatment groups were detected, with a range of 1.3 to 1.9 days and 2 to 3.2 days, respectively.

Adult chronic ITP: Twenty-four adults with ITP of longer than 6 months duration and platelet counts lower than 30,000/mm^3 or requiring therapy were enrolled in a single-arm, open-label trial and treated with 100 to 375 international units/kg RhIGIV (mean dose, 231 international units/kg). Twenty-one of 24 patients responded (with an increase to 20,000/mm^3 or higher) during the first 2 courses of therapy, for an overall response rate of 88% and a mean peak platelet count of 92,300/mm^3 (range, 8,000 to 229,000).

ITP secondary to HIV infection: Eleven children and 52 adults in all Walter Reed categories of HIV infection progression and ITP, with initial platelet counts of 30,000/mm^3 or lower or requiring therapy, were treated with 100 to 375 international units/kg RhIGIV in an open-label trial. RhIGIV was given for an average of 7.3 courses (range, 1 to 57) over a mean period of 407 days. Fifty-seven of 63 patients responded (with an increase to 20,000 cells/mm^3 or higher) during the first 6 courses of therapy, for an overall response rate of 90%. The overall mean change in platelet count for 6 courses was 60,900 cells/mm^3, and the mean peak platelet count was 81,700 cells/mm^3.

Onset: In a clinical study of 10 Rh$_o$(D) antigen-negative volunteers (9 men, 1 woman), Rh$_o$(D) antigen-positive red cells were completely cleared from the circulation within 8 hours of IV administration of RhIGIV. There was no indication of Rh isoimmunization of these subjects at 6 months after the clearance of the Rh$_o$(D) antigen-positive red cells.

Duration: When 600 international units (120 mcg) of RhIGIV is administered to a pregnant woman, passive anti-Rh$_o$(D) antibodies are not detectable in the circulation for more than 6 weeks; therefore, a dose of 1,500 international units (300 mcg) should be used for antenatal administration.

Pharmacokinetics: Immunoglobulins are primarily eliminated by catabolism. RhIG binds rapidly to Rho(D) antigen-positive erythrocytes. Pharmacokinetic studies were not performed in Rho(D) antigen-positive subjects with ITP.

Rh$_o$(D) Immune Globulin Intravenous (RhIGIV) (Human)

Cangene: In a study involving Rh$_o$(D) antigen-negative volunteers, 2 subjects were administered 600 international units (120 mcg) RhIGIV IM, and 2 subjects were administered the same dose IV. Peak levels (36 to 48 ng/mL) were reached within 2 hours of IV administration, and peak levels (18 to 19 ng/mL) were reached at 5 to 10 days after IM administration. The calculated areas under the curve (AUC) were the same for both routes of administration. The half-life for anti-Rh$_o$(D) was approximately 24 days after IV administration and approximately 30 days after IM administration.

CSL: 15 Rh$_o$(D)-negative pregnant women received a single 1,500 international unit dose at week 28 gestation. After IV administration, peak serum levels of RhIGIV ranged from 62 to 84 ng/mL after 1 day. Mean systemic clearance was 0.2 ± 0.03 mL/min, with a half-life of 16 ± 4 days. After IM administration, peak serum levels ranged from 7 to 46 ng/mL, achieved between 2 and 7 days after injection. Mean apparent clearance was 0.29 ± 0.12 mL/min, with a half-life of 18 ± 5 days. The absolute bioavailability was 69%. Regardless of route of administration, RhIGIV titers were detected in all women 9 weeks or more after administration.

Immunoglobulins are primarily eliminated by catabolism.

Protective Level: Antibody titers 1:5 or more by RFFIT indicate adequate protection.

Mechanism: Passive immunization with RhIG prevents the formation of anti-Rh$_o$(D) antibodies in nonsensitized Rh$_o$(D) antigen-negative individuals who receive Rh$_o$(D) antigen-positive RBCs. Rh$_o$(D) antibody binds circulating antigen, thus preventing stimulation of antigen-sensitive lymphocytes and the resulting production of anti-Rh$_o$(D). Prevention of Rh$_o$(D) sensitization in turn prevents hemolytic disease of the fetus and newborn in subsequent Rh$_o$(D) antigen-positive children.

The mechanism of action in ITP is not fully understood, but may involve RhIGIV/RBC complexes blocking the destruction of antibody/platelet complexes of ITP by the immune system. This mode of action is supported by the fact that RhIGIV is not effective against ITP in Rh$_o$(D) antigen-negative patients.

Drug Interactions: Other antibodies in RhIG may interfere with the response to live vaccines (eg, measles, mumps, rubella). Therefore, do not give live vaccines within 30 to 14 days before or 3 months after RhIG administration. However, RhIG does not appear to impair the efficacy of rubella vaccine. Rubella-susceptible postpartum women who received blood products or RhIG may receive rubella vaccine before discharge, provided that an HI titer for rubella antibody is drawn 6 to 8 weeks after vaccination to ensure seroconversion.

As with other drugs administered by IM injection, give RhIG with caution to patients on anticoagulant therapy.

Lab Interference: Passively acquired anti-A, anti-B, anti-C, and anti-E blood group antibodies may be detectable in direct and indirect antiglobulin (Coombs') tests after RhIGIV administration. Passively administered anti-Rh$_o$(D) antibodies in maternal or fetal blood can lead to a false-positive direct antiglobulin (Coombs') test. If there is an uncertainty about the mother's Rh group or immune status, give RhIGIV to the mother. IGIV products containing maltose may cause misinterpretation of glucose concentrations by certain blood-glucose testing systems (eg, those based on the glucose dehydrogenase pyrroloquinolinequinone [GDH-PQQ] method).

Pharmaceutical Characteristics

Concentration:

Cangene: Each 1,500 international unit vial or syringe (corresponding to a nominal 300 mcg dose) inhibits the immunizing potential of approximately 34 mL of whole blood or 17 mL of Rh$_o$(D) antigen-positive packed red RBCs. Each 600 international unit vial inhibits the immunizing potential of 6 mL of whole blood or 3 mL of Rh$_o$(D) antigen-positive packed RBCs.

CSL: Human plasma proteins of 3% or less, including human albumin 10 mg/mL added as a stabilizer

Quality Assay:

Cangene: Traditionally, a full dose of RhIG has been referred to as a "300 mcg" dose. Potency and dosing recommendations are now expressed in units by comparison to the WHO Anti-D standard. The conversion of "mcg" to "units" is 1 mcg = 5 units. The product potency is expressed in international units by comparison to the WHO standard.

CSL: Protein is more than 95% IgG.

Packaging:

Cangene: Solution: Single-dose vial of 600 international units (120 mcg) anti-Rh$_o$(D)IGIV (53270-3120-01), single-dose vial of 1,500 international units (300 mcg) anti-Rh$_o$(D)IGIV (53270-3300-01), single-dose vial of 2,500 international units (500 mcg) anti-Rh$_o$(D)IGIV (53270-3500-01), single-dose vial of 5,000 international units (1,000 mcg) anti-Rh$_o$(D)IGIV (53270-3100-01), single-dose vial of 15,000 international units (3,000 mcg) anti-Rh$_o$(D)IGIV (53270-3000-01).

CSL: Full-dose *Rhophylac*: One single-dose prefilled 1,500 international unit/2 mL syringe with 21-gauge, 1½-inch needle (44206-0300-01); ten 1,500 international unit/2 mL syringes with 21-gauge, 1½-inch needles (44206-0300-10).

Doseform:

Cangene: Solution

CSL: Solution

Appearance:

Cangene: White, freeze-dried powder yielding an undescribed solution

CSL: Clear or slightly opalescent, colorless to pale yellow solution

Solvent:

Cangene: Maltose 10%

CSL: Glycine and saline solution

Diluent:

For reconstitution: Cangene: Aseptically reconstitute the product shortly before use with the appropriate volume of 0.9% sodium chloride injection (see table). Inject the diluent slowly onto the inside wall of the vial and wet the pellet by gently swirling until dissolved. To avoid denaturing the antibody proteins, do not shake.

Reconstitution of *WinRho SDF*			
Vial size	Volume of diluent added to vial	Approximate available volume	Nominal concentration per mL
IV injection			
600 IU (120 mcg)	2.5 mL	2.4 mL	240 IU (48 mcg)/mL
1,500 IU (300 mcg)	2.5 mL	2.4 mL	600 IU (120 mcg)/mL
5,000 IU (1,000 mcg)	8.5 mL	8.4 mL	588 IU (118 mcg)/mL

Rh$_o$(D) Immune Globulin Intravenous (RhIGIV) (Human)

Reconstitution of *WinRho SDF*			
Vial size	Volume of diluent added to vial	Approximate available volume	Nominal concentration per mL
IM injection			
600 IU (120 mcg)	1.25 mL	1.2 mL	480 IU (96 mcg)/mL
1,500 IU (300 mcg)	1.25 mL	1.2 mL	1,200 IU (240 mcg)/mL
5,000 IU (1,000 mcg)	8.5 mL	8.4 mL	588 IU (118 mcg)/mL

For infusion: Do not combine RhIGIV with other products.

Adjuvant: None

Preservative: None

Allergens: IgA of 5 mcg or less per mL

Excipients:

Cangene: Powder: Glycine 0.1 M, sodium chloride 0.04 M, polysorbate 80 0.01%

  Solution: Maltose 10%, polysorbate 80 0.01%

CSL: Human albumin 10 mg/mL, glycine 20 mg/mL, sodium chloride less than or equal to 0.25 M

pH: 6.4 to 7.6

Shelf Life:

Cangene: Expires within 24 months

CSL: Expires within 36 months

Storage/Stability: Store at 2° to 8°C (35° to 46°F). Do not freeze. Contact the manufacturer regarding exposure to extreme temperatures. Shipped in insulated containers with coolant packs by overnight courier.

Reconstituted vials will tolerate up to 12 hours at room temperature. Do not freeze the reconstituted product. Discard any portion not used within 12 hours.

Production Process:

Cangene: Rh$_o$(D) antigen-negative men or sterile women are immunized with Rh$_o$(D) cells to produce anti-Rh$_o$(D) antibodies. The antibodies are harvested by Cohn-Oncley methods 6 & 9 cold-ethanol fractionation process of plasma collected from these donors. RhIGIV is prepared from human plasma by an anion-exchange column chromatography method. The manufacturing process includes a solvent-detergent treatment step (using tri-n-butyl phosphate and *Triton X-100*) that is effective in inactivating lipid-enveloped viruses such as hepatitis B, hepatitis C, and HIV. The product is then filtered through a *Planova* 20N microfilter, known to remove some nonlipid enveloped viruses. These processes are designed to increase product safety by reducing the risk of virus transmission.

CSL: Produced by an ion-exchange chromatography isolation procedure, using pooled plasma obtained by plasmapheresis of immunized Rho(D)-negative US donors. The manufacturing process includes a solvent-detergent treatment step using tri-n-butyl phosphate and *Triton X-100* that inactivates enveloped viruses such as HBV, HCV, and HIV. The product is nanofiltered using a *Planova* 15 nm virus filter, effective in removing enveloped and nonenveloped viruses.

Media: Human plasma

Rh₀(D) Immune Globulin Intravenous (RhIGIV) (Human)

Disease Epidemiology

Syndrome:

Rh sensitization: For information on Rh sensitization, see the Rh$_o$(D) Immune Globulin (RhIG) monograph.

ITP: ITP is a blood disorder that results in the destruction of platelets. Because platelets have an essential role in blood clotting, ITP can lead to uncontrolled bleeding and excessive bruising. ITP may occur as a primary disease or in association with an underlying condition such as HIV infection. Although the exact cause of ITP is unknown, it is believed to be an autoimmune condition in which circulating antibodies bind to platelets and mediate their destruction by the immune system.

A platelet count higher than 150,000 cells/mm^3 is considered normal. Any patient with a platelet count lower than 150,000 is considered thrombocytopenic. Most ITP patients are not treated unless their platelet count falls below 50,000. Depending on individual circumstances, patients with platelet counts between 20,000 and 50,000 may receive treatment, while patients with counts lower than 20,000 often require aggressive therapy. At these low platelet levels, the patient can experience frequent bleeding episodes, including potentially fatal central nervous system or gastrointestinal hemorrhages.

Prevalence: In the United States, approximately 100,000 patients suffer from ITP each year, including 18,000 cases of primary ITP, 50,000 cases of ITP secondary to HIV infection, and approximately 30,000 cases arising from other conditions. In the non-HIV-infected population, approximately 4,000 children have acute ITP, which generally resolves within 6 months. In contrast, most adults afflicted with ITP, either with or without concomitant HIV infection, have a chronic, refractory condition characterized by an insidious onset and long duration. In the non-HIV-infected population, the disease disproportionately affects females.

Other Information

Perspective: Also see the Rh$_o$(D) Immune Globulin (RhIG) and Immune Globulin Intravenous (IGIV) monographs.

1993: WinRho SD granted orphan drug status for treatment of ITP on November 9, conferring 7 years of market exclusivity for that indication upon licensing.

1994: Recommended for licensing by FDA advisory panel in March.

First Licensed:

Cangene: March 24, 1995

ZLB (now CSL Behring): February 12, 2004

National Policy: ACOG. Educational bulletin # 227: management of isoimmunization in pregnancy. *Int J Gynaecol Obstet.* 1996;55:183-190.

ACOG. Practice bulletin # 4: prevention of Rh D isoimmunization. *Int J Gynaecol Obstet.* 1999;66:63-70.

References: Andrew M, Blanchette VS, Adams M, et al. A multicenter study of the treatment of childhood chronic idiopathic thrombocytopenic purpura with anti-D. *J Pediatr.* 1992;120(4 pt 1):522-527.

Chavez GF, Mulinare J, Edmonds LD. Epidemiology of Rh hemolytic disease of the newborn in the United States. *JAMA.* 1991;265:3270-3274.

Greenough A. The role of immunoglobulins in neonatal Rhesus haemolytic disease. *BioDrugs.* 2001;15:533-541.

Nakhoul IN, Kozuch P, Varma M. Management of adult idiopathic thrombocytopenic purpura. *Clin Adv Hematol Oncol.* 2006;4(2):136-144, 153.

Sandler SG, Tutuncuoglu SO. Immune thrombocytopenic purpura-current management practices. *Expert Opin Pharmacother.* 2004;5(12):2515-2527.

Westhoff CM. The structure and function of the Rh antigen complex. *Semin Hematol.* 2007;44(1):42-50.

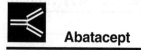
Abatacept

Isoantibodies

Name:
Orencia

Manufacturer:
Bristol-Myers Squibb Company

Comparison: Compared to abatacept, 2 amino acid substitutions (L104 to E; A29 to Y) were made in the ligand binding region of CTLA-4 to create belatacept. As a result of these modifications, belatacept binds CD80 and CD86 more avidly than abatacept, the parent CTLA-4–immunoglobulin (CTLA4-Ig) molecule from which it is derived.

Immunologic Characteristics

Target Antigen: Human cytotoxic T-lymphocyte–associated antigen 4 (CTLA-4) linked to Fc portion of immunoglobulin G1 (IgG1)

Viability: Not viable, but immunologically active

Antigenic Form: Soluble fusion protein of antigen and Fc portion of IgG1

Antigenic Type: Extracellular domain of human cytotoxic T-lymphocyte-associated antigen 4 (CTLA-4) linked to modified Fc portion of human IgG1. The Fc portion contains the hinge, CH2, and CH3 domains of IgG1. The apparent molecular weight of abatacept is 92 kilodaltons.

Use Characteristics

Indications: To reduce signs and symptoms (eg, major clinical response, slowing progression of structural damage, improving physical function) in adult patients with moderately to severely active rheumatoid arthritis (RA) who had an inadequate response to 1 or more disease-modifying antirheumatic drugs (DMARDs), such as methotrexate or tumor necrosis factor (TNF) antagonists. Abatacept may be used as monotherapy or concomitantly with DMARDs other than TNF antagonists.

Juvenile idiopathic arthritis: To reduce signs and symptoms in pediatric patients 6 years and older with moderately to severely active polyarticular juvenile idiopathic arthritis (JIA). Abatacept may be used as monotherapy or concomitantly with methotrexate.

Contraindications:

Absolute: People with known hypersensitivity to abatacept or any of its components.

Relative: Abatacept should not be administered concomitantly with TNF antagonists. Abatacept is not recommended for concomitant use with anakinra.

Immunodeficiency: Drugs inhibiting T-lymphocyte activation, including abatacept, may affect host defenses against infections and malignancies because T-cells mediate cellular immune responses. The safety and efficacy of abatacept in immunodeficient patients are not fully understood. In clinical trials, a higher rate of infections was seen in abatacept-treated patients than in placebo-treated patients.

Elderly: In clinical studies, 323 patients 65 years of age and older, including 53 patients 75 years of age and older, received abatacept. No overall differences in safety or effectiveness were observed between these patients and younger patients, but these numbers are too low to rule out differences. The frequency of serious infection and malignancy among abatacept-treated patients older than 65 years of age was higher than for those younger than 65 years of age. Because there is a higher incidence of infections and malignancies in the elderly population in general, use caution when treating elderly patients.

Carcinogenicity: In a mouse carcinogenicity study, weekly subcutaneous injections of abatacept 20, 65, or 200 mg/kg for up to 84 weeks in males and 88 weeks in females were associated with increases in the incidence of malignant lymphomas (all doses) and mammary gland tumors (intermediate and high doses in females). These mice were infected with murine leukemia virus and mouse mammary tumor virus. These viruses are associated with an increased incidence of lymphomas and mammary gland tumors, respectively, in immunosuppressed mice. The doses in these studies were 0.8, 2, and 3 times the human exposure at 10 mg/kg, respectively, based on area under the curve (AUC). The relevance of these findings to the clinical use of abatacept is unknown.

Mutagenicity: No mutagenic potential of abatacept was observed in the in vitro reverse Ames or Chinese hamster ovary/hypoxanthine guanine phosphoribosyl-transferase (CHO/HGPRT) forward-point mutation (with or without metabolic activation) assays, and no chromosomal aberrations were observed in human lymphocytes (with or without metabolic activation) treated with abatacept.

Fertility Impairment: In rats, abatacept had no adverse effects on male or female fertility at dosages up to 200 mg/kg every 3 days (11 times the human dose based on AUC).

Pregnancy: Category C. Use only if clearly needed. Abatacept crosses the placenta. Abatacept was found not to be teratogenic in mice at daily doses up to 300 mg/kg and in rats and rabbits at doses up to 200 mg/kg (29 times the human 10 mg/kg dose based on AUC in rats and rabbits). Rats treated with abatacept every 3 days during early gestation throughout lactation showed no adverse effects in offspring at doses up to 45 mg/kg (3 times the human dose). At a dose of 200 mg/kg (11 times the human dose), alterations of immune function consisted of a 9-fold increase in T-cell–dependent antibody response in female pups and inflammation of the thyroid in 1 female pup out of 10 males and 10 females evaluated. Whether these findings indicate a risk for development of autoimmune diseases in humans exposed in utero to abatacept has not been determined. Because animal reproduction studies are not always predictive of human response, use abatacept during pregnancy only if clearly needed. There are no adequate and well-controlled studies in pregnant women.

Lactation: Abatacept has been shown to be present in rat milk. It is not known whether abatacept is excreted in human milk or absorbed systemically after ingestion. Because many drugs are excreted in human milk, and because of the potential for serious adverse reactions in breast-feeding infants from abatacept, possibly including effects on the developing immune system, decide whether to discontinue breast-feeding or the drug, taking into account the importance of the drug to the mother.

Children: Safety and effectiveness in pediatric patients younger than 6 years of age have not been established. Safety and efficacy in pediatric patients for uses other than JIA have not been established.

Studies in juvenile rats exposed to abatacept before immune system maturity showed immune system abnormalities, including increased incidence of infections leading to death, as well as inflammation of the thyroid and pancreas. Studies in adult mice and monkeys have not demonstrated similar findings. As the immune system of the rat is undeveloped in the first few weeks after birth, the relevance of these results to humans older than 6 years of age (when the immune system is largely developed) is unknown.

Adverse Reactions: The most serious adverse reactions were serious infections and malignancies. The most commonly reported adverse events (at least 10% of patients treated with abatacept) were headache, upper respiratory tract infection, nasopharyngitis, and nausea. The adverse events most frequently resulting in clinical intervention (eg, interruption or discontinuation of abatacept) were due to infection. The most frequently reported infections resulting in dose interruption were upper respiratory tract infection (1%), bronchitis (0.7%), and herpes zoster (0.7%). The most frequent infections resulting in discontinuation were pneumonia (0.2%), localized infection (0.2%), and bronchitis (0.1%).

The following data reflect exposure to abatacept in patients with active RA in placebo-controlled studies (1,955 patients with abatacept, 989 with placebo). The studies had a double-blind, placebo-controlled period of either 6 months (258 patients with abatacept, 133 with placebo) or 1 year (1,697 patients with abatacept, 856 with placebo). A subset of these patients received concomitant biologic DMARD therapy, such as a TNF-blocking agent (204 patients with abatacept, 134 with placebo).

Adverse Events Occurring in ≥ 3% of Patients and ≥ 1% More Frequently in Abatacept-Treated Patients During Placebo-Controlled RA Studies		
Adverse event	Abatacept (n = 1,955)[a]	Placebo (n = 989)[b]
Headache	18%	13%
Nasopharyngitis	12%	9%
Dizziness	9%	7%
Cough	8%	7%
Back pain	7%	6%
Hypertension	7%	4%
Dyspepsia	6%	4%
Urinary tract infection	6%	5%
Rash	4%	3%
Pain in extremity	3%	2%

a Includes 204 patients on concomitant biologic DMARDs (ie, adalimumab, anakinra, etanercept, infliximab).
b Includes 134 patients on concomitant biologic DMARDs (ie, adalimumab, anakinra, etanercept, infliximab).

Infusion-related reactions: Acute infusion-related reactions (within 1 hour of start of infusion) in studies 3, 4, and 5 were more common in the abatacept-treated patients than in placebo-treated patients (9% vs 6%). The most frequently reported events (1% to 2%) were dizziness, headache, and hypertension. Acute infusion-related events reported in 0.1% to 1% of patients treated with abatacept included cardiopulmonary symptoms, such as hypotension, increased blood pressure, and dyspnea; other symptoms included nausea, flushing, urticaria, cough, hypersensitivity, pruritus, rash, and wheezing. Most of these reactions were mild to moderate. Fewer than 1% of abatacept-treated patients discontinued because of an acute infusion-related event. In controlled trials, 6 abatacept-treated patients compared with 2 placebo-treated patients discontinued study treatment because of acute infusion-related events.

Infections: Exercise caution when considering the use of abatacept in patients with a history of recurrent infections, underlying conditions that may predispose them to infections, or chronic, latent, or localized infections. Closely monitor patients who develop a new infection while undergoing treatment with abatacept. Discontinue administration of abatacept if a patient develops a serious infection. A higher rate of serious infections has been observed in patients treated with concurrent TNF antagonists and abatacept. Before starting immunomodulatory therapies, including abatacept, screen patients for latent tuberculosis infection with a tuberculin skin test. Abatacept has not been studied in patients with a positive tuberculosis screen, and the safety of abatacept in people with latent tuberculosis infection is unknown. Treat patients testing positive in tuberculosis screening using standard medical practice before therapy with abatacept. In placebo-controlled trials, infections of any type were reported in 54% of abatacept-treated patients and 48% of placebo-treated patients. The most commonly reported infections (reported in 5% to 13% of patients) were upper respiratory tract infection, nasopharyngitis, sinusitis, urinary tract infection, influenza, and bronchitis. Other infections reported in less than 5% of patients at a higher frequency (greater than 0.5%) with abatacept compared with placebo were rhinitis, herpes simplex, and pneumonia. Serious infections were reported in 3% of patients treated with abatacept and 1.9% of patients treated with placebo. The most common (0.2% to 0.5%) serious infections reported with abatacept were pneumonia, cellulitis, urinary tract infection, bronchitis, diverticulitis, and acute pyelonephritis.

Malignancies: In placebo-controlled portions of clinical trials (1,955 patients for a median of 12 months), the overall frequencies of malignancies were similar in the abatacept- and placebo-treated patients (1.3% and 1.1%, respectively). However, more cases of lung cancer were observed in abatacept-treated patients (4 [0.2%]) than in placebo-treated patients (0). In the cumulative abatacept clinical trials (placebo-controlled and uncontrolled, open-label), a total of 8 cases of lung cancer (0.21 cases per 100 patient-years) and 4 lymphomas (0.1 cases per 100 patient-years) were observed in 2,688 patients (3,827 patient-years). The rate observed for lymphoma is approximately 3.5-fold higher than that expected in an age- and gender-matched general population based on the Surveillance, Epidemiology, and End Results (SEER) Program database. Patients with RA, particularly those with highly active disease, are at a higher risk for the development of lymphoma. Other malignancies included skin, breast, bile duct, bladder, cervical, endometrial, ovarian, prostate, renal, thyroid, and uterine cancers; lymphoma, melanoma, and myelodysplastic syndrome. The potential role of abatacept in the development of malignancies in humans is unknown.

Immunogenicity: Antibodies directed against the entire abatacept molecule or to the CTLA-4 portion of abatacept were assessed by enzyme-linked immunosorbent assay (ELISA) in RA patients for up to 2 years following repeated treatment with abatacept. Thirty-four of 1,993 (1.7%) patients developed binding antibodies to the entire abatacept molecule or to the CTLA-4 portion of abatacept. Because trough levels of abatacept can interfere with assay results, a subset analysis was performed. In this analysis, 9 of 154 (5.8%) patients who discontinued treatment with abatacept for more than 56 days developed antibodies. Samples with confirmed binding activity to CTLA-4 were assessed for neutralizing antibodies in a cell-based luciferase reporter assay. Six of 9 (67%) evaluable patients possessed neutralizing antibodies. No correlation of antibody development with clinical response or adverse events was observed. The data reflect the percentage of patients whose test results were positive for antibodies to abatacept in specific assays, and are highly dependent on the sensitivity and specificity of the assays.

General toxicity: In a 1-year toxicity study in cynomolgus monkeys, abatacept was administered intravenously (IV) weekly at doses up to 50 mg/kg (9 times the human exposure at 10 mg/kg dose based on AUC). Abatacept was not associated with any significant drug-related toxicity. Reversible pharmacological effects consisted of minimal transient decreases in serum IgG and minimal to severe lymphoid depletion of germinal centers in the spleen and/or lymph nodes. No evidence of lymphomas or preneoplastic morphologic changes was observed within the time frame of this study, despite the presence of a virus (lymphocryptovirus) known to cause these lesions in immunosuppressed monkeys. The relevance of these findings to the clinical use of abatacept is unknown.

Hypersensitivity: Of 2,688 patients treated with abatacept in clinical trials, 2 cases of anaphylaxis or anaphylactoid reactions occurred. Other events potentially associated with drug hypersensitivity, such as hypotension, urticaria, and dyspnea, each occurred in less than 0.9% of abatacept-treated patients. These generally occurred within 24 hours of abatacept infusion.

Pulmonary: Thirty-seven patients with chronic obstructive pulmonary disease (COPD) treated with abatacept developed respiratory disorder adverse events more frequently than 17 COPD patients treated with placebo (43% vs 24%), including COPD exacerbations, cough, rhonchi, and dyspnea. A greater percentage of abatacept-treated patients developed a serious adverse event than placebo-treated patients (27% vs 6%), including COPD exacerbation (8%) and pneumonia (3%). Use abatacept in patients with RA and COPD with caution; monitor such patients for worsening of their respiratory status.

Pharmacologic & Dosing Characteristics

Dosage: Based on the patient's body weight.

Adults: For body weight less than 60 kg, 500 mg (2 vials). For body weight 60 to 100 kg, 750 mg (3 vials). For body weight greater than 100 kg, 1 g (4 vials). Use abatacept as monotherapy or concomitantly with DMARDs other than TNF antagonists.

Subcutaneous dosing for adult rheumatoid arthritis: After a single IV infusion as a loading dose, give 125 mg as a subcutaneous injection within 1 day, followed by 125 mg subcutaneously once a week. Patients unable to receive an infusion may start weekly injections without an IV loading dose. Patients transitioning from IV therapy to subcutaneous therapy should administer the first subcutaneous dose instead of the next scheduled IV dose.

Children: For patients 6 to 17 years of age with JIA who weigh less than 75 kg, administer 10 mg/kg based on body weight at each administration. For patients weighing 75 kg or more, administer according to the adult dosing regimen, up to a maximum dose of 1,000 mg.

Route: 30-minute IV infusion. For adults, subcutaneous injection.

Overdosage: Doses up to 50 mg/kg IV have been administered without apparent toxic effect. In case of overdosage, monitor the patient for signs or symptoms of adverse reactions and start symptomatic treatment.

Additional Doses: Give abatacept 2 and 4 weeks after the first infusion, then every 4 weeks thereafter.

Missed Doses: Interrupting the recommended schedule or delaying subsequent doses does not require restarting the series.

Efficacy: The efficacy and safety of abatacept were assessed in 5 randomized, double-blind, placebo-controlled studies in patients 18 years of age and older with active RA diagnosed according to American College of Rheumatology (ACR) criteria. Studies 1, 2, 3, and 4 required patients to have at least 12 tender and 10 swollen joints at randomization. Study 5 did not require any specific number of tender or swollen joints. Abatacept or placebo treatment was given IV at weeks 0, 2, and 4 and then every 4 weeks thereafter.

Study 1 evaluated abatacept as monotherapy in 122 patients with active RA who had failed at least 1 nonbiologic DMARD or etanercept. In study 2 and study 3, the efficacy and safety of abatacept were assessed in patients with an inadequate response to methotrexate and who were continued on their stable dose of methotrexate. In study 4, the efficacy and safety of abatacept were assessed in patients with an inadequate response to a TNF-blocking agent, with the TNF-blocking agent discontinued prior to randomization; other DMARDs were permitted. Study 5 primarily assessed safety in patients with active RA requiring additional intervention despite of current therapy with DMARDs; all DMARDs used at enrollment were continued. Patients in study 5 were not excluded for comorbid medical conditions.

Study 1 patients were randomized to receive abatacept 0.5, 2, or 10 mg/kg or placebo, ending at week 8. Study 2 patients were randomized to receive abatacept 2 or 10 mg/kg or placebo for 12 months. Study 3, 4, and 5 patients were randomized to receive a dose of abatacept based on weight range or placebo for 12 months (studies 3 and 5) or 6 months (study 4). The dose of abatacept was 500 mg for patients weighing less than 60 kg, 750 mg for patients weighing 60 to 100 kg, and 1 g for patients weighing more than 100 kg.

The percent of abatacept-treated patients achieving ACR 20, 50, and 70 responses and major clinical response in studies 1, 3, and 4 are shown in the following table. Abatacept-treated patients had higher ACR 20, 50, and 70 response rates at 6 months compared with placebo-treated patients. Month 6 ACR response rates in study 2 for the 10 mg/kg group were similar to rates in the abatacept group in study 3.

ACR Responses in Placebo-Controlled Trials						
		Inadequate response to DMARDs (Study 1)		Inadequate response to methotrexate (Study 3)		Inadequate response to TNF-blocking agent (Study 4)	
Response rate		Abatacept 10 mg/kg (n = 32)	Placebo (n = 32)	Abatacept[a] + methotrexate (n = 424)	Placebo + methotrexate (n = 214)	Abatacept[a] + DMARDs (n = 256)	Placebo + DMARDs (n = 133)
ACR 20	Month 3	53%	31%	62%[b]	37%	46%[b]	18%
	Month 6	NA	NA	68%[b]	40%	50%[b]	20%
	Month 12	NA	NA	73%[b]	40%	NA	NA
ACR 50	Month 3	16%	6%	32%[b]	8%	18%[c]	6%
	Month 6	NA	NA	40%[b]	17%	20%[b]	4%
	Month 12	NA	NA	48%[b]	18%	NA	NA
ACR 70	Month 3	6%	0	13%[b]	3%	6%[d]	1%
	Month 6	NA	NA	20%[b]	7%	10%[c]	2%
	Month 12	NA	NA	29%[b]	6%	NA	NA
Major clinical response[e]		NA	NA	14%[b]	2%	NA	NA

a Dosing based on weight range.
b $P < 0.001$.
c $P < 0.01$.
d $P < 0.05$.
e Major clinical response is defined as achieving ACR 70 response for a continuous 6-month period.

The results of the components of the ACR response criteria for studies 3 and 4 are shown in the following table. In abatacept-treated patients, greater improvement was seen in all ACR response criteria components through 6 and 12 months than in placebo-treated patients. Abatacept-treated patients experienced greater improvement than placebo-treated patients in morning stiffness.

Components of ACR Response at 6 Months								
	Inadequate response to methotrexate (Study 3)				Inadequate response to TNF-blocking agent (Study 4)			
	Abatacept + methotrexate (n = 424)		Placebo + methotrexate (n = 214)		Abatacept + DMARDs (n = 256)		Placebo + DMARDs (n = 133)	
Component (median)	Baseline	Month 6	Baseline	Month 6	Baseline	Month 6	Baseline	Month 6
Number of tender joints	28	7[a]	31	14	30	13[a]	31	24
Number of swollen joints	19	5[a]	20	11	21	10[a]	20	14
Pain[b]	67	27[a]	70	50	73	43[c]	74	64
Patient global assessment[b]	66	29[a]	64	48	71	44[a]	73	63
Disability index[d]	1.75	1.13[a]	1.75	1.38	1.88	1.38[a]	2	1.75
Physician global assessment[b]	69	21[a]	68	40	71	32[a]	69	54
CRP[e] (mg/dL)	2.2	0.9[a]	2.1	1.8	3.4	1.3[a]	2.8	2.3

a $P < 0.001$.
b Visual analog scale: 0 = best, 100 = worst.
c $P < 0.01$.
d Health Assessment Questionnaire: 0 = best, 3 = worst; based on dressing and grooming, arising, eating, walking, hygiene, reach, grip, and activities.
e CRP = C-reactive protein.

Radiographic response: Structural damage was assessed radiographically and expressed as change in Genant-modified Total Sharp Score (TSS) and its components, the erosion score and Joint Space Narrowing (JSN) score, at month 12 compared with baseline. In study 3, the baseline median TSS was 31.7 in abatacept-treated patients and 33.4 in placebo-treated patients. Abatacept-methotrexate slowed the progression of structural damage more than placebo-methotrexate alone.

Mean Radiographic Changes Over 12 Months in Study 3				
Parameter	Abatacept/Methotrexate (n = 391)	Placebo/Methotrexate (n = 195)	Difference (95% CI)	P value[a]
TSS	1.21	2.32	1.11 (0.35, 1.88)	0.012
Erosion score	0.63	1.14	0.51 (0.08, 0.94)	0.029
JSN score	0.58	1.18	0.6 (0.21, 0.99)	0.009

a Based on nonparametric analysis.

Physical function response: Improvement in physical function was measured by the Health Assessment Questionnaire Disability Index (HAQ-DI). In studies 2 to 5, abatacept demonstrated greater improvement from baseline than placebo in the HAQ-DI. The results from studies 2 and 3 are shown in the following table. Similar results were observed in study 5. During the open-label period of study 2, the improvement in physical function had been maintained for up to 3 years.

Mean Improvement from Baseline in Health Assessment Questionnaire Disability Index (HAQ-DI)				
	Inadequate response to methotrexate			
	Study 2		Study 3	
HAQ-DI	Abatacept[a] + methotrexate (n = 115)	Placebo + methotrexate (n = 119)	Abatacept[b] + methotrexate (n = 422)	Placebo + methotrexate (n = 212)
Baseline (mean)	0.98[c]	0.97[c]	169[d]	169[d]
Mean improvement year 1	0.4[c,e]	0.15[c]	0.66[d,e]	0.37[d]

a 10 mg/kg.
b Dosing based on weight range.
c Modified Health Assessment Questionnaire: 0 = best, 3 = worst; based on dressing and grooming, arising, eating, walking, hygiene, reach, grip, and activities.
d Health Assessment Questionnaire: 0 = best, 3 = worst; based on dressing and grooming, arising, eating, walking, hygiene, reach, grip, and activities.
e $P < 0.001$.

Health-related quality of life was assessed by the SF-36 questionnaire at 6 months in studies 2, 3, and 4 and at 12 months in studies 2 and 3. In these studies, improvement was observed in the abatacept group as compared with the placebo group in all 8 domains of the SF-36 as well as the Physical Component Summary (PCS) and the Mental Component Summary (MCS).

Juvenile idiopathic arthritis: Safety and efficacy were assessed in a 3-part study, including an open-label extension in children with polyarticular JIA. Patients 6 to 17 years of age (n = 190) with moderately to severely active polyarticular JIA who had an inadequate response to 1 or more DMARDs, such as methotrexate or TNF antagonists, were treated. Patients had disease duration of approximately 4 years, with moderately to severely active disease at study entry, as determined by baseline counts of active joints (mean, 16) and joints with loss of motion (mean, 16); patients had elevated CRP levels (mean, 3.2 mg/dL) and erythrocyte sedimentation rates (ESR) (mean, 32 mm/h). At study entry, 74% of patients were receiving methotrexate (mean dose, 13.2 mg/m² per week) and remained on a stable dose of methotrexate (those not receiving methotrexate did not initiate methotrexate treatment during the study). In period A (open-label, lead-in), patients received 10 mg/kg (maximum, 1,000 mg per dose) IV on days 1, 15, and 29, and monthly thereafter. Response was assessed utilizing the ACR Pediatric 30 definition of improvement, defined as 30% or greater improvement in 3 or more of 6 JIA core set variables and 30% or more worsening in 1 or less of 6 JIA core set variables. Patients demonstrating an ACR Pedi 30 response at the end of period A were randomized into the double-blind phase (period B) and received either abatacept or placebo for 6 months or until disease flare. At the end of period A, pediatric ACR 30/50/70 responses were 65%, 50%, and 28%, respectively. Pediatric ACR 30 responses were similar in all subtypes of JIA studied. During the double-blind, randomized withdrawal phase (period B), abatacept-treated patients experienced significantly fewer disease flares compared with placebo-treated patients (20% vs 53%). The risk of disease flare among patients continuing on abatacept was less than one-third of that for patients withdrawn from abatacept treatment (hazard ratio = 0.31; 95% CI, 0.16-0.59). Among patients who received abatacept throughout the study (period A, period B, and the open-label extension period C), the proportion of pediatric ACR 30/50/70 responders remained consistent for 1 year.

Onset: In studies 3 and 4, improvement in the ACR 20 response rate versus placebo was observed within 15 days in some patients.

Duration: In abatacept-treated patients, greater improvement was seen in all ACR response criteria components through 6 and 12 months than in placebo-treated patients. In studies 2 and 3, ACR response rates were maintained to 12 months in abatacept-treated patients. ACR responses were maintained up to 3 years in the open-label extension of study 2.

Pharmacokinetics: Abatacept pharmacokinetics were studied in healthy adult subjects after a single 10 mg/kg IV infusion and in RA patients after multiple 10 mg/kg IV infusions.

Pharmacokinetic Parameters in Healthy Subjects and RA Patients		
Parameter	Healthy subjects after 10 mg/kg single dose (n = 13)	RA patients after 10 mg/kg multiple doses[a] (n = 14)
Peak concentration (C_{max}) (mcg/mL)	292 (175 to 427)	295 (171 to 398)
Terminal half-life ($t_{1/2}$) (days)	16.7 (12 to 23)	13.1 (8 to 25)
Systemic clearance (CL) (mL/h/kg)	0.23 (0.16 to 0.3)	0.22 (0.13 to 0.47)
Volume of distribution (Vss) (L/kg)	0.09 (0.06 to 0.13)	0.07 (0.02 to 0.13)

a Multiple IV infusions administered at days 1, 15, 30, and monthly thereafter.

Abatacept pharmacokinetics in RA patients and healthy subjects appeared comparable. In RA patients, after multiple IV infusions, pharmacokinetics showed proportional increases of C_{max} and AUC over the dose range of 2 to 10 mg/kg. At 10 mg/kg, serum concentration appeared to reach a steady state by day 60 with a mean (range) trough concentration of 24 (1 to 66) mcg/mL. No systemic accumulation of abatacept occurred upon continued repeated treatment with 10 mg/kg at monthly intervals in RA patients.

Population pharmacokinetic analyses in RA patients revealed that there was a trend toward higher clearance of abatacept with increasing body weight. Age and gender (adjusted for body weight) did not affect clearance. Concomitant methotrexate, nonsteroidal anti-inflammatory drugs (NSAIDs), corticosteroids, and TNF-blocking agents did not influence abatacept clearance.

Pharmacokinetics have not been studied in children and adolescents. No formal studies were conducted to examine the effects of either renal or hepatic impairment on pharmacokinetics.

Juvenile idiopathic arthritis: In patients 6 to 17 years of age, the mean (range) steady-state serum peak and trough concentrations of abatacept were 217 (57 to 700) and 11.9 (0.15 to

44.6) mcg/mL, respectively. Population pharmacokinetic analyses of the serum concentration data showed that clearance of abatacept increased with baseline body weight. The estimated mean (range) clearance of abatacept in patients with JIA was 0.4 (0.2 to 1.12) mL/h/kg. After accounting for body weight, the clearance of abatacept was not related to age and gender. Concomitant methotrexate, corticosteroids, and NSAIDs were also shown not to influence abatacept clearance.

Subcutaneous dosing: Abatacept exhibited linear pharmacokinetics after subcutaneous administration. The mean (range) for C_{min} and C_{max} at steady state observed after 85 days of treatment was 32.5 mcg/mL (6.6 to 113.8 mcg/mL) and 48.1 mcg/mL (9.8 to 132.4 mcg/mL), respectively. Bioavailability after subcutaneous dosing relative to IV infusion is 78.6%. Mean estimates for systemic clearance (0.28 mL/h/kg), volume of distribution (0.11 L/kg), and terminal half-life (14.3 days) were comparable between subcutaneous and IV administration.

Study SC-II was conducted to determine the effect of abatacept monotherapy on immunogenicity after subcutaneous dosing without an IV loading dose. When the IV loading dose was not administered, a mean trough concentration of 12.6 mcg/mL was achieved after 2 weeks of dosing. Consistent with the IV data, population pharmacokinetic analyses for subcutaneous abatacept in RA patients revealed that there was a trend toward higher clearance of abatacept with increasing body weight. Age and gender (when corrected for body weight) did not affect apparent clearance. Concomitant medication, such as methotrexate, corticosteroids, and NSAIDs, did not influence abatacept apparent clearance.

Mechanism: Abatacept, a selective costimulation modulator, inhibits T-lymphocyte activation by binding to CD80 and CD86, thereby blocking interaction with CD28. This interaction provides a costimulatory signal necessary for full activation of T-lymphocytes, implicated in the pathogenesis of RA. Activated T-lymphocytes are found in the synovium of patients with RA.

In vitro, abatacept decreases T-cell proliferation and inhibits the production of the cytokines TNF-α, interferon-gamma, and interleukin-2. In a rat collagen-induced arthritis model, abatacept suppresses inflammation, decreases anticollagen antibody production, and reduces antigen-specific production of interferon-gamma. The relationship of these biological response markers to the mechanisms by which abatacept exerts its effects in RA is unknown.

In clinical trials with abatacept dosed at approximately 10 mg/kg, decreases were observed in serum levels of soluble interleukin-2 receptor (sIL-2r), interleukin-6 (IL-6), rheumatoid factor (RF), CRP, matrix metalloproteinase-3 (MMP3), and TNF-α. The relationship of these biological response markers to the mechanisms by which abatacept exerts its effects in RA is unknown.

Drug Interactions: Population pharmacokinetic analyses revealed that methotrexate, NSAIDs, corticosteroids, and TNF-blocking agents did not influence abatacept clearance. The majority of patients in RA clinical studies received one or more of the following concomitant medications with abatacept: methotrexate, NSAIDs, corticosteroids, TNF-blocking agents, azathioprine, chloroquine, gold, hydroxychloroquine, leflunomide, sulfasalazine, and anakinra.

Do not administer abatacept concomitantly with TNF antagonists. In controlled clinical trials, patients receiving concomitant abatacept and TNF-antagonist therapy experienced more infections (63% vs 43%) and serious infections (4.4% vs 0.8%) than patients treated with only TNF antagonists. These trials failed to demonstrate an important enhancement of efficacy with coadministration of abatacept with TNF antagonists; therefore, concurrent therapy with abatacept and a TNF antagonist is not recommended. While transitioning from TNF-antagonist therapy to abatacept therapy, monitor patients for signs of infection.

Abatacept is not recommended for use concomitantly with anakinra because of insufficient clinical experience.

Do not give live vaccines concurrently with abatacept or within 3 months of its discontinuation. No data are available on secondary transmission of infection from people receiving live vaccines to patients receiving abatacept. The efficacy of immunization in patients receiving abatacept is not known. Based on its mechanism of action, abatacept may blunt the effectiveness of some immunizations.

Lab Interference: Parenteral drug products containing maltose may interfere with blood glucose monitors that use test strips with glucose dehydrogenase pyrroloquinolinequinone (GDH-PQQ). GDH-PQQ–based glucose monitoring systems may react with the maltose present in this product, resulting in falsely elevated blood glucose readings on the day of infusion. Advise patients who require blood glucose monitoring to consider alternative monitoring methods, such as those based on glucose dehydrogenase nicotine adenine dinucleotide (GDH-NAD), glucose oxidase, or glucose hexokinase test methods.

Pharmaceutical Characteristics

Concentration:

IV: Abatacept 250 mg per 10 mL, after reconstitution

Subcutaneous: Abatacept 125 mg per 1 mL

Packaging:

IV: Abatacept 250 mg per vial, with a silicone-free disposable syringe (NDC#: 00003-2187-10)

Subcutaneous: Pack of 4 abatacept 125 mg per 1 mL prefilled syringes with 29-gauge, ½-inch needles (00003-2188-31)

Doseform:

IV: Powder for solution

Subcutaneous: Solution

Appearance: White freeze-dried powder, yielding clear, colorless to pale yellow solution.

Diluent:

For reconstitution: Sterile water for injection, 10 mL per 250 mg vial

For infusion: Dilute the reconstituted abatacept solution to 100 mL as follows: From a 100 mL infusion bag or bottle of sodium chloride 0.9% injection, withdraw the volume of the reconstituted abatacept vials (ie, for 2 vials remove 20 mL, for 3 vials remove 30 mL, for 4 vials remove 40 mL). Slowly add the reconstituted abatacept solution from each vial into the infusion bag or bottle using the same silicone-free disposable syringe provided with each vial. Gently mix. The concentration of the diluted abatacept solution in the infusion container will be approximately 5, 7.5, or 10 mg of abatacept per mL, depending on whether 2, 3, or 4 vials of abatacept were added. Discard any unused portion.

Adjuvant: None

Preservative: None

Allergens: None

Excipients:

IV: Maltose 500 mg, monobasic sodium phosphate 17.2 mg, and sodium chloride 14.6 mg per vial

Subcutaneous: Dibasic sodium phosphate anhydrous 0.838 mg, monobasic sodium phosphate monohydrate 0.286 mg, poloxamer-188 8 mg, and sucrose 170 mg, each per 1 mL in water for injection. Contains no maltose.

pH:
IV: 7 to 8 after reconstitution
Subcutaneous: 6.8 to 7.4

Shelf Life: Data not provided.

Storage/Stability: Store abatacept powder and abatacept syringes at 2° to 8°C (36° to 46°F). Protect vials from light by storing in the original package until time of use. Contact the manufacturer regarding exposure to freezing or elevated temperatures. Shipping data not provided.

Handling: Use only the silicone-free disposable syringe provided with each vial. Use an 18- to 21-gauge needle. If the abatacept powder is accidentally reconstituted using a siliconized syringe, the solution may develop a few translucent particles. Discard any solutions prepared using siliconized syringes. To obtain additional silicone-free disposable syringes, contact the manufacturer at 1-800-ORENCIA.

During reconstitution, to minimize foam formation in solutions of abatacept, rotate the vial with gentle swirling until the contents are completely dissolved. Avoid prolonged or vigorous agitation. Do not shake. Upon complete dissolution of the lyophilized powder, vent the vial with a needle to dissipate any foam that may be present. The solution should be clear and colorless to pale yellow. Do not use if opaque particles, discoloration, or other foreign particles are present.

Administer the diluted abatacept solution over 30 minutes, using an infusion set and a nonpyrogenic, low-protein–binding filter (pore size of 0.2 to 1.2 mcm). Complete the infusion of the diluted abatacept solution within 24 hours of reconstitution of the abatacept vials. Store the fully diluted abatacept solution at room temperature or refrigerated at 2° to 8°C (36° to 46°F) before use. Do not infuse abatacept concomitantly in the same IV line with other agents. No physical or biochemical compatibility studies have been conducted to evaluate the coadministration of abatacept with other agents.

Production Process: Abatacept is produced by recombinant DNA technology in a mammalian cell-expression system.

Media: Chinese hamster ovary cell-expression system

Other Information

First Licensed: December 23, 2005

References: Dumont FJ. Technology evaluation: abatacept, Bristol-Myers Squibb. *Curr Opin Mol Ther.* 2004;6(3):318-330.

Ruderman EM, Pope RM. The evolving clinical profile of abatacept (CTLA4-Ig): a novel co-stimulatory modulator for the treatment of rheumatoid arthritis. *Arthritis Res Ther.* 2005;7(suppl 2):S21-S25.

Isoantibodies

Name:
  ReoPro

Manufacturer:
  Manufactured by Centocor N.V. in Leiden, the
  Netherlands; distributed by Eli Lilly & Co.

Synonyms: c7E3, 7E3, initially called *CentoRx*, abcirximab, CAS 143653-53-6

Immunologic Characteristics

Target Antigen: Glycoprotein IIb/IIIa (GPIIb/IIIa) receptor of human platelets

Viability: Inactive, passive, transient

Antigenic Form: Chimeric, human-murine immunoglobulin, fragmented

Antigenic Type: Protein, IgG antibody, monoclonal, antigen-binding (Fab) fragments. The Fab fragments have an average molecular weight of 47,615 daltons. The fragments contain murine variable heavy- and light-chain regions and human constant heavy- and light-chain regions.

Use Characteristics

Indications: As an adjunct to percutaneous coronary intervention (PCI) for the prevention of acute cardiac ischemic complications in patients undergoing PCI and in patients with unstable angina not responding to conventional medical therapy when PCI is planned within 24 hours.

Patients at high risk for abrupt closure include those undergoing PCI with 1 or more of the following conditions:

(1) Unstable angina or a non-Q-wave myocardial infarction (MI)

(2) An acute Q-wave MI within 12 hours of the onset of symptoms

(3) Other high-risk clinical or morphologic characteristics (as adapted from the classification of the ACC/AHA):

  (a) two type B lesions in the artery to be dilated,

  (b) one type B lesion in the artery to be dilated in a woman of 65 years of age or older,

  (c) one type B lesion in the artery to be dilated in a patient with diabetes mellitus,

  (d) one type C lesion in the artery to be dilated.

Limitations: Therapy with abciximab requires careful attention to all potential bleeding sites (including catheter insertion sites, arterial and venous puncture sites, cutdown sites, needle puncture sites, and gastrointestinal [GI], genitourinary [GU], and retroperitoneal sites).

Abciximab is associated with an increase in bleeding rate, particularly at the site of arterial access for femoral sheath placement. Take care when attempting vascular access so that only the anterior wall of the femoral artery is punctured, avoiding a Seldinger (through-and-through) technique for obtaining sheath access. Avoid femoral vein sheath placement unless needed. While the vascular sheath is in place, maintain patients on complete bed rest with the head of the bed 30° or lower and the affected limb restrained in a straight position. Discontinue heparin 4 hours or longer prior to arterial sheath removal. Following sheath removal, apply pressure to the femoral artery for 30 minutes or longer using either manual compression or a mechanical device for hemostasis. Apply a pressure dressing following hemostasis. Maintain the patient on bed rest for 6 to 8 hours following sheath removal or discontinuation of abciximab, whichever is later.

Frequently check the sheath insertion site and distal pulses of affected leg(s) while the femoral artery sheath is in place and for 6 hours after femoral artery sheath removal. Measure any hematoma and monitor for enlargement.

Contraindications:

Absolute: Because abciximab increases the risks of bleeding, it is contraindicated in the following clinical situations:

- Active internal bleeding
- Recent (within 6 weeks) GI or GU bleeding of clinical significance
- History of cerebrovascular accident (CVA) within 2 years, or CVA with a significant residual neurological deficit
- Bleeding diathesis
- Administration of oral anticoagulants within 7 days unless prothrombin time is 1.2 or less times control
- Thrombocytopenia (less than 100,000 cells/mcL)
- Recent (within 6 weeks) major surgery or trauma
- Intracranial neoplasm, arteriovenous malformation, or aneurysm
- Severe, uncontrolled hypertension
- Presumed or documented history of vasculitis
- Use of IV dextran before PCI, or intent to use it during PCI
- Patients with known hypersensitivity to any component of this product or to murine proteins.

Immunodeficiency: Impairment of effect is unlikely.

Elderly: Of 7,860 patients in four phase III trials, 37% were 65 years of age and older, with 8% 75 years of age and older. No overall differences in safety or efficacy were observed between patients of 65 to 74 years of age compared with younger patients. The clinical experience is not adequate to determine whether patients 75 years of age and older respond differently than younger patients.

Carcinogenicity: Long-term studies in animals have not been performed to evaluate carcinogenic potential.

Mutagenicity: In vitro and in vivo mutagenicity studies have not demonstrated any mutagenic effect.

Fertility Impairment: Long-term studies in animals have not been performed to evaluate effects on fertility in male or female animals.

Pregnancy: Category C. Use only if clearly needed. It is not known if abciximab crosses the placenta. Generally, most IgG passage across the placenta occurs during the third trimester. Give abciximab to a pregnant woman only if clearly needed.

Lactation: It is not known if abciximab crosses into breast milk or is absorbed systemically after ingestion. Problems in humans have not been documented.

Children: Safety and efficacy of abciximab in children have not been studied.

Adverse Reactions: The most common complication encountered during abciximab therapy is bleeding. Major bleeding events occurred most commonly in patients treated with the bolus-plus-infusion regimen. If serious bleeding occurs that is not controllable with pressure, stop the infusion of abciximab and any concomitant heparin. The types of bleeding associated with abciximab therapy fall into 2 broad categories: (1) Bleeding observed at the arterial access site for cardiac catheterization; and (2) internal bleeding involving the GI or GU tract or retroperitoneal sites.

In the following conditions, clinical data suggest that the risks of major bleeds caused by abciximab therapy may be increased and should be weighed against the anticipated benefits:

- Patients who weigh less than 75 kg
- Patients older than 65 years of age

- Patients with a history of prior GI disease
- Patients receiving thrombolytic therapy

The following conditions also are associated with an increased risk of bleeding in the angioplasty setting, which may be additive to that of abciximab:

- PCI within 12 hours of the onset of symptoms of acute MI
- Prolonged PCI (lasting longer than 70 minutes)
- Pain, involving primarily the extremities (3.4%); peripheral edema (1.6%); abnormal vision (0.7%).

The manufacturer is gathering data on the effects of modifications to the therapeutic regimen on efficacy and bleeding risk, including intracranial hemorrhage and stroke. It also is seeking information about the effects of platelet transfusions.

The following additional adverse events from the EPIC, EPILOG, and CAPTURE trials were reported by investigators for patients treated with a bolus plus infusion of abciximab at incidences which were less than 0.5% higher than for patients in the placebo arm:

Cardiovascular: Ventricular tachycardia (1.4%); pseudoaneurysm (0.8%); palpitation (0.5%); arteriovenous fistula (0.4%); incomplete AV block (0.3%); nodal arrhythmia (0.2%); complete AV block (0.1%); embolism (limb) (0.1%); thrombophlebitis (0.1%).

CNS: Dizziness (2.9%); anxiety (1.7%); abnormal thinking (1.3%); agitation (0.7%); hypesthesia (0.6%); confusion (0.5%); muscle contractions (0.4%); coma (0.2%); hypertonia (0.2%); diplopia (0.1%).

GI: Dyspepsia (2.1%); diarrhea (1.1%); ileus (0.1%); gastroesophageal reflux (0.1%).

GU: Urinary retention (0.7%); dysuria (0.4%); abnormal renal function (0.4%); frequent micturition (0.1%); cystalgia (0.1%); urinary incontinence (0.1%); prostatitis (0.1%).

Hematologic/Lymphatic: Anemia (1.3%); leukocytosis (0.5%); petechiae (0.2%).

Miscellaneous: Pain (5.4%); increased sweating (1%); asthenia (0.7%); incisional pain (0.6%); pruritus (0.5%); abnormal vision (0.3%); edema (0.3%); wound (0.2%); abscess (0.2%); cellulitis (0.2%); peripheral coldness (0.2%); injection-site pain (0.1%); dry mouth (0.1%); pallor (0.1%); diabetes mellitus (0.1%); hyperkalemia (0.1%); enlarged abdomen (0.1%); bullous eruption (0.1%); inflammation (0.1%); drug toxicity (0.1%).

Musculoskeletal: Myalgia (0.2%).

Respiratory: Pneumonia (0.4%); rales (0.4%); pleural effusion (0.3%); bronchitis (0.3%); bronchospasm (0.3%); pleurisy (0.2%); pulmonary embolism (0.2%); rhonchi (0.1%).

Pharmacologic & Dosing Characteristics

Dosage: The safety and efficacy of abciximab have only been investigated with concomitant administration of heparin and aspirin. In patients with failed PCIs, the continuous infusion of abciximab should be stopped because there is no evidence for abciximab efficacy in that setting. In the event of serious bleeding that cannot be controlled by compression, immediately discontinue abciximab and heparin.

The recommended dosage of abciximab is an IV bolus of 0.25 mg/kg administered 10 to 60 minutes before the start of PCI, followed by a continuous IV infusion of 0.125 mcg/kg/min (to a maximum of 10 mcg/min) for 12 hours.

Patients with unstable angina not responding to conventional medical therapy and who are planned to undergo PCI within 24 hours may be treated with 0.25 mg/kg abciximab IV bolus, followed by an 18- to 24-hour IV infusion of 10 mcg/min, concluding 1 hour after PCI.

In patients with failed PCIs, stop the continuous infusion of abciximab because there is no evidence for abciximab efficacy in that setting. In case of serious bleeding that cannot be controlled by compression, discontinue abciximab and heparin immediately.

Route: IV bolus and infusion

Handling: Do not shake. Withdraw the necessary amount of abciximab (2 mg/mL) for bolus injection through a sterile, nonpyrogenic, low protein-binding 0.2- or 0.22-micron filter (eg, Millipore SLGV025LS) into a syringe. Give the bolus 10 to 60 minutes before the procedure.

Withdraw 4.5 mL of abciximab for the continuous infusion through a sterile, nonpyrogenic, low protein-binding 0.2 or 0.22-micron filter (eg, Millipore SLGV025LS) into a syringe. Inject into 250 mL 0.9% sodium chloride or 5% dextrose and infuse at a rate of 17 mL/h (10 mcg/min) for 12 hours via a continuous infusion pump equipped with an in-line sterile, nonpyrogenic, low protein-binding 0.2 or 0.22-micron filter (eg, Abbott # 4524). Discard the unused portion at the end of the 12-hour infusion.

Overdosage: There has been no experience of overdosage in human clinical trials. It is recommended that infusion be discontinued after 12 hours to avoid the effects of prolonged platelet receptor blockade.

Additional Doses: Human antichimeric antibodies (HACAs) can appear in response to the administration of abciximab. In the EPIC, EPILOG, and CAPTURE trials, positive responses occurred in approximately 5.8% of treated patients. There was no excess of hypersensitivity or allergic reactions related to abciximab treatment compared with placebo treatment. Giving abciximab again to a patient with HACAs could theoretically cause an allergic or hypersensitivity reaction (including anaphylaxis), thrombocytopenia, or diminished benefit upon readministration of abciximab.

Readministration of abciximab to 29 healthy volunteers who had not developed a HACA response after first administration did not lead to any change in abciximab pharmacokinetics or to reduced antiplatelet potency. However, results in this small group suggest that the incidence of HACA response may be increased after readministration. Readministration to patients who developed a positive HACA response after the first administration has not been evaluated in clinical trials.

Related Interventions: Abciximab is intended for use with aspirin and heparin and has been studied only in that setting.

Minimize arterial and venous punctures, IM injections, and use of urinary catheters, nasotracheal intubation, nasogastric tubes, and automatic blood pressure cuffs. When obtaining IV access, avoid noncompressible sites (eg, subclavian or jugular veins). Consider saline or heparin locks for blood drawing. Document and monitor vascular puncture sites. Provide gentle care when removing dressings.

In the EPILOG and EPISTENT studies, careful vascular access site management and discontinuation of heparin after the procedure with early removal (within 6 hours) of the femoral arterial sheath were used. The initial heparin bolus was based on the baseline ACT (less than 150 seconds: 70 mcg/kg heparin; 150 to 199 seconds: 50 mcg/kg heparin; 200 or more seconds: no heparin). Additional 20 mcg/kg heparin boluses were given to achieve and maintain ACT 200 or more seconds during the procedure. If prolonged heparin therapy or delayed sheath removal were clinically indicated, heparin was adjusted to keep the activated partial thromboplastin time (APTT) between 60 and 85 seconds (EPILOG) or 55 to 75 seconds (EPISTENT).

In the CAPTURE trail, anticoagulation was initiated before administration of abciximab, with heparin IV infusion to achieve a target APTT of 60 to 85 seconds. The heparin infusion was maintained during the abciximab infusion and adjusted to achieve an ACT of 300 seconds or an APTT of 70 seconds during the PCI. After the intervention, heparin management corresponded with EPILOG guidelines.

Laboratory Tests: Before infusion of abciximab, measure platelet count, prothrombin time, and APTT to identify preexisting hemostatic abnormalities. During and after abciximab treatment, closely monitor platelet counts and extent of heparin anticoagulation, as assessed by activated clotting time or APTT.

Monitor platelet counts prior to treatment, 2 to 4 hours following the bolus dose of abciximab, and at 24 hours or before discharge, whichever is first. If a patient experiences an acute platelet decrease (eg, a platelet decrease to lower than 100,000 cells/mcL or a decrease of 25% or more from pretreatment value), determine additional platelet counts. These platelet counts should be drawn in separate tubes containing ethylenediaminetetraacetic acid (EDTA), citrate, or heparin to exclude pseudothrombocytopenia due to in vitro anticoagulant interaction. If true thrombocytopenia is verified, immediately discontinue abciximab and appropriately monitor and treat the condition. For patients with thrombocytopenia in the EPIC trial, a daily platelet count was obtained until it returned to normal. If a patient's platelet count dropped to 60,000 cells/mcL, heparin and aspirin were discontinued. If a patient's platelet count dropped below 50,000 cells/mcL, platelets were transfused.

In the event of serious uncontrolled bleeding or the need for surgery (especially major procedures within 48 to 72 hours of treatment with abciximab), determine an Ivy bleeding time. Preliminary evidence suggests that platelet function may be restored, at least in part, with platelet transfusions.

Efficacy: The Evaluation of c7E3 to Prevent Ischemic Complications (EPIC) trial was a multicenter, double-blind, placebo-controlled trial of abciximab in patients undergoing percutaneous transluminal coronary angioplasty (PTCA) or atherectomy. In the EPIC trial, 2,099 patients between 26 and 83 years of age who were at high risk for abrupt closure of the treated coronary vessel were randomly allocated to 1 of 3 treatments: 1) An abciximab bolus (0.25 mg/kg) followed by an abciximab infusion (10 mcg/min) for 12 hours (bolus plus infusion group); 2) an abciximab bolus (0.25 mg/kg) followed by a placebo infusion (bolus group); or 3) a placebo bolus followed by a placebo infusion (placebo group). Treatment with a study agent in each of the 3 arms was initiated 10 to 60 minutes before the onset of PCI. All patients initially received an IV heparin bolus (10,000 to 12,000 units) and boluses of up to 3,000 units thereafter to a maximum of 20,000 units during PCI. Heparin infusion was continued for 12 hours to maintain a therapeutic elevation of APTT (1.5 to 2.5 times normal). Unless contraindicated, aspirin (325 mg) was administered orally 2 hours before the planned procedure and then once daily.

The primary endpoint was the occurrence of any of the following events within 30 days of PCI: death, MI, or the need for urgent intervention for recurrent ischemia (ie, urgent PCI, urgent coronary artery bypass graft [CABG] surgery, a coronary stent, or an intra-aortic balloon pump). The incidence of the primary endpoint in the bolus-plus-infusion treatment group (8.3%), compared with the placebo group (12.8%), was statistically significant ($P = 0.008$), but the lower incidence in the bolus treatment group (11.5%) was not. A lower incidence of the primary endpoint was observed in the bolus-plus-infusion treatment arm for all 3 high-risk subgroups: patients with unstable angina, patients presenting within 12 hours of the onset of symptoms of an acute MI, and patients with other high-risk characteristics.

Mortality was uncommon and similar rates were observed in all arms. The rate of acute MI was significantly lower in the groups treated with abciximab. While 80% of MIs in the study were non-Q-wave infarctions, patients in the bolus-plus-infusion arm experienced a lower incidence of both Q-wave and non-Q-wave infarctions. Urgent intervention rates were lower in the groups treated with abciximab, mostly because of lower rates of emergency PCI, and, to a lesser extent, emergency CABG surgery. The primary endpoint events in the bolus-plus-infusion treatment group were reduced mostly in the first 48 hours and this benefit was sustained through 30 days and 6 months. At the 6-month follow-up visit, this event rate remained lower in the bolus-plus-infusion arm (12.3%) than in the placebo arm (17.6%).

EPILOG was a randomized, double-blind, placebo-controlled trial to evaluate abciximab in a broad population of patients undergoing PCI (excluding patients with MI or unstable angina meeting the EPID high-risk criteria). EPILOG was a 3-arm trial, comparing abciximab plus standard-dose heparin, abciximab plus low-dose heparin, and placebo plus standard-dose heparin. The abciximab regimen was 0.25 mg/kg bolus followed by 0.125 mcg/kg/min (maximum, 10 mcg/min) infusion for 12 hours. The primary endpoint of the EPILOG trial was the composite of death or MI occurring within 30 days of PCI. The composite of death, MI, or urgent intervention was an important secondary endpoint. The endpoint values in both abciximab treatment groups were reduced mostly in the first 48 hours and this benefit was sustained through 30 days, 6 months, and 1 year. The proportionate reductions in endpoint event rates were similar regardless of type of coronary intervention used (eg, balloon angioplasty, atherectomy, or stent placement).

EPISTENT was a randomized trial evaluating 3 treatment strategies in patients undergoing PCI: conventional PTCA with abciximab plus low-dose heparin, primary intracoronary stent implantation with abciximab plus low-dose heparin, and primary intracoronary stent implantation with placebo plus standard-dose heparin. The results demonstrated benefit in both abciximab arms (ie, with and without stents), compared with stenting alone, on the composite of death, MI, or urgent intervention within 30 days of PCI. This benefit was maintained at 6 months.

CAPTURE was a randomized, double-blind, placebo-controlled trial to evaluate abciximab in unstable angina patients not responding to conventional medical therapy for whom PCI was planned, but not immediately performed. The CAPTURE trial administered either placebo or abciximab starting 18 to 24 hours before PCI and continuing until 1 hour after completion of intervention. The 30-day results are consistent with the results of the other 3 trials, with the greatest effects on the MI and urgent intervention components of the composite endpoint. The greatest difference in MI rates occurred in the post-intervention period. No effect on mortality was seen. After 6 months of follow-up, the composite endpoint of death, MI, or repeat intervention was not different between abciximab and placebo groups.

Onset: Drug effect begins within 10 to 60 minutes after administration.

Duration: Platelet function recovers over the course of 48 hours, but abciximab remains in the circulation up to 10 days in a platelet-bound state.

Pharmacokinetics: Immunoglobulins are primarily eliminated by catabolism. After IV bolus administration, free plasma concentrations of abciximab decrease rapidly, with an initial half-life of shorter than 10 minutes. The second phase half-life of approximately 30 minutes is probably related to rapid binding to the platelet GPIIb/IIIa receptors. Platelet function recovers over the course of 48 hours, but abciximab remains in the circulation for 15 days or longer in a platelet-bound state. IV 0.25 mg/kg bolus doses of abciximab followed by infusion of 10 mcg/min produces level-free plasma concentrations throughout the infusion. At the end of the infusion period, free plasma concentrations fall rapidly for approximately 6 hours, then decline at a slower rate.

IV administration in humans of single bolus doses of abciximab from 0.15 to 0.30 mg/kg produced rapid dose-dependent inhibition of platelet function as measured by ex vivo platelet aggregation in response to adenosine diphosphate (ADP) or by prolongation of bleeding time. At the 2 highest doses (0.25 and 0.30 mg/kg) at 2 hours after injection, 80% or more of the GPIIb/IIIa receptors were blocked, and platelet aggregation in response to 20 micromolar ADP was almost abolished. The median bleeding time increased to longer than 30 minutes at both doses compared with a baseline value of approximately 5 minutes.

IV administration in humans of a single bolus dose of 0.25 mg/kg followed by a continuous IV of 10 mcg/min for periods of 12 to 96 hours produced sustained high-grade GPIIb/IIIa receptor blockade (80% or more) and inhibition of platelet function (ex vivo platelet aggregation in response to 5 micromolar or 20 micromolar ADP less than 20% of baseline and bleeding time longer than 30 minutes) for the duration of the infusion in most patients. Similar results were obtained when a weight-adjusted infusion dose (0.125 mcg/kg/min to a maximum of 10 mcg/min) was given to patients weighing 80 kg or less. Results in patients who received the 0.25 mg/kg bolus followed by a 5 mcg/min infusion for 24 hours showed a similar initial receptor blockade and inhibition of platelet aggregation, but the response was not maintained throughout the infusion period.

Low levels of GPIIb/IIIa receptor blockade were present for longer than 10 days after ending the infusion. Bleeding time returned to 12 minutes or shorter within 12 hours after stopping the infusion in 15 of 20 patients (75%) and within 24 hours in 18 of 20 patients (90%). Ex vivo platelet aggregation in response to 5 micromolar ADP returned to 50% or more of baseline within 24 hours following the end of infusion in 11 of 32 patients (34%) and within 48 hours in 23 of 32 patients (72%). In response to 20 micromolar ADP, ex vivo platelet aggregation returned to 50% or more of baseline within 24 hours in 20 of 32 patients (62%) and within 48 hours in 28 of 32 patients (88%).

Mechanism: Abciximab binds to the intact GPIIb/IIIa receptor, which is a member of the integrin family of adhesion receptors and the major platelet surface receptor involved in platelet aggregation. Abciximab inhibits platelet aggregation by preventing the binding of fibrinogen, von Willebrand factor, and other adhesive molecules to GPIIb/IIIa receptor sites on activated platelets. The mechanism of action is thought to involve steric hindrance or conformational effects to block access of large molecules to the receptor rather than interacting directly with the arginine-glycine-aspartic acid (RGD) binding site of GPIIb/IIIa.

Abciximab also binds to the vitronectin ($\alpha_v\beta_3$) receptor found on platelets and vessel wall endothelial and smooth muscle cells. The vitronectin receptor mediates the procoagulant properties of platelets and the proliferative properties of vascular endothelial and smooth muscle cells. In vitro studies show that abciximab blocked $\alpha_v\beta_3$-mediated effects, including cell adhesion. At concentrations that, in vitro, provide more than 80% GPIIb/IIIa receptor blockade, but above the in vivo therapeutic range, abciximab more effectively blocked the burst of thrombin generation that followed platelet activation than select comparator antibodies that inhibit GPIIb/IIIa alone. The clinical significance of these findings is unknown.

Abciximab also binds to the activated Mac-1 receptor on monocytes and neutrophils. In vitro studies show that abciximab and 7E3-IgG block Mac-1 receptor function, based on inhibition of monocyte adhesion. In addition, the degree of activated Mac-1 expression on circulating leukocytes and number of circulating leukocyte-platelet complexes is reduced in people treated with abciximab compared with control patients. The clinical significance of these findings is unknown.

Drug Interactions: Although drug interactions with abciximab have not been studied systematically, abciximab has been given to patients with ischemic heart disease treated with a broad range of medications used in the treatment of angina, MI, and hypertension. These medications have included heparin, warfarin, beta-adrenergic receptor blockers, calcium-channel antagonists, angiotensin-converting enzyme (ACE) inhibitors, IV and oral nitrates, ticlopidine, and aspirin. Heparin, other anticoagulants, thrombolytics, and antiplatelet agents may be associated with an increase in bleeding.

In the EPIC, EPILOG, CAPTURE, and EPISTENT trials, abciximab was used concomitantly with heparin and aspirin. Because abciximab inhibits platelet aggregation, use caution when it is used with other drugs that affect hemostasis, including thrombolytics, oral anticoagulants, nonsteroidal anti-inflammatory drugs, dipyridamole, and ticlopidine. Use of oral anticoagulants is contraindicated within 7 days of abciximab administration unless prothrombin time is 1.2 times control or less. There are limited data on the use of abciximab in patients receiving thrombolytic agents. Because of concern about synergistic effects on bleeding, use systemic thrombolytic therapy judiciously.

Abciximab (Chimeric)

In the EPIC trial, there was limited experience with the administration of abciximab with low molecular weight dextran. Low molecular weight dextran was usually given for the deployment of a coronary stent, for which oral anticoagulants were also given. In the 11 patients who received low molecular weight dextran with abciximab, 5 had major bleeding events and 4 had minor bleeding events. None of the 5 placebo patients treated with low molecular weight dextran had a major bleeding event. Administration of abciximab is contraindicated with use of IV dextran before PCI or intent to use it during PCI.

Patients with HACA titers theoretically may have allergic or hypersensitivity reactions when treated with other diagnostic or therapeutic monoclonal antibodies.

Patient Information: Inform patients that receipt of abciximab may affect the future use of other murine-based products. They should discuss prior use of murine-antibody based products with their clinicians.

Pharmaceutical Characteristics

Concentration: 10 mg per 5 mL

Quality Assay: Sterile, pyrogen-free

Packaging: 5 mL single-use vial

NDC Number: 00002-7140-01

Doseform: Solution

Appearance: Clear, colorless. Inspect parenteral drug products visually for particulate matter before use. Do not use preparations of abciximab containing visibly opaque particles.

Solvent: Water for injection

Diluent:

For infusion: 0.9% sodium chloride or 5% dextrose

Adjuvant: None

Preservative: None

Allergens: None

Excipients: Buffered solution of 0.01 M sodium phosphate, 0.15 M sodium chloride, and 0.001% polysorbate 80 in water for injection

pH: 7.2

Shelf Life: Expires within 30 months

Storage/Stability: Store at 2° to 8°C (36° to 46°F). Discard if frozen, because freezing can denature the product. No information is presently available about stability at elevated temperatures. Give the drug within 72 hours after removal from refrigeration. Contact the manufacturer for future data. Shipped by overnight courier in insulated containers.

Production Process: Prepared by immunizing mice with whole human platelets. Murine monoclonal IgG antibody m7E3 was harvested and cloned in a mouse myeloma cell line. The immunoglobulin gene sequence was altered to resemble human IgG, yet the antigen recognition region remained unchanged. The hybrid molecule is called chimeric or murine-human c7E3 IgG. The chimeric 7E3 antibody is produced by continuous perfusion in mammalian cell culture. The Fab fragment is purified from cell culture supernatant by a series of steps involving specific viral inactivation and removal procedures, digestion with papain, and column chromatography.

Media: Murine myeloma cell line

Compatibility: Administer abciximab in a separate IV line; add no other medication to the infusion solutions. No incompatibilities have been observed with glass bottles or polyvinyl chloride bags and administration sets.

Abciximab (Chimeric)

Disease Epidemiology

Incidence: Angioplasty is performed on more than 400,000 heart patients each year in the United States to restore blood flow to narrowed coronary arteries. Of these, 30% (120,000) are at high risk for complications. More than 1 million people each year arrive at health care centers complaining of chest pain. About 800,000 to 1 million people in the United States have unstable angina.

Other Information

Perspective:
1984: First animal trials with abciximab.
1994: Publication of the 2,100-patient EPIC (Evaluation of c7E3 to Prevent Ischemic Complications) clinical trial.

First Licensed: December 22, 1994

References: EPIC Investigators. Use of a monoclonal antibody directed against the platelet glycoprotein IIb/IIIa receptor in high-risk coronary angioplasty. *N Engl J Med.* 1994;330:956-961.

Faulds D, et al. Abciximab (c7E3 Fab): a review of its pharmacology and therapeutic potential in ischaemic heart disease. *Drugs.* 1994;48:583-598.

Foster, RH, Wiseman LR. Abciximab: an updated review of its use in ischaemic heart disease. *Drugs.* 1998;56:629-665.

Gabriel HM, Oliveira EI. Role of abciximab in the treatment of coronary artery disease. *Expert Opin Biol Ther.* 2006;6(9):935-942.

Topol EJ, et al. Randomized trial of coronary intervention with antibody against platelet IIb/IIIa integrin for reduction of clinical restenosis: results at six months. *Lancet.* 1994;343:881-886.

Adalimumab (Recombinant)

Isoantibodies

Name:
Humira
Synonyms: D2E7, LU200134

Manufacturer:
Abbott Laboratories

Immunologic Characteristics

Target Antigen: Human tumor necrosis factor-alpha (TNF-α)

Viability: Inactive, passive, transient

Antigenic Form: Human immunoglobulin, created using phage-display technology resulting in antibody with human-derived heavy- and light-chain variable regions and human IgG1κ constant regions, D2E7 heavy chain with disulfide bond to D2E7 light chain, dimer.

Antigenic Type: Protein, IgG1 antibody, monoclonal, 1,330 amino acids, molecular weight approximately 148 kilodaltons

Use Characteristics

Indications: To reduce signs and symptoms, inhibit progression of structural damage, and improve physical function in adult patients with moderately to severely active rheumatoid arthritis (RA). Adalimumab can be used alone or in combination with disease-modifying antirheumatic drugs (DMARDs).

To reduce signs and symptoms of moderately to severely active polyarticular juvenile idiopathic arthritis in pediatric patients 4 years of age and older.

To reduce signs and symptoms of active arthritis, inhibit the progression of structural damage, and improve physical function in patients with psoriatic arthritis. Adalimumab can be used alone or in combination with DMARDs.

To reduce signs and symptoms in patients with active ankylosing spondylitis.

To reduce signs and symptoms and to induce and maintain clinical remission in adults with moderately to severely active Crohn disease who responded inadequately to conventional therapy. This includes patients who lost response or are intolerant to infliximab.

To treat adults with moderate to severe chronic plaque psoriasis who are candidates for systemic therapy or phototherapy, and when other systemic therapies are medically less appropriate.

Contraindications:

Absolute: None

Relative: People with known hypersensitivity to adalimumab or any of its components.

Immunodeficiency: TNF-α mediates inflammation and modulates cellular immune function. Therefore, it is possible for anti-TNF therapies, including adalimumab, to affect normal immune responses. The safety and efficacy of adalimumab in patients with immunosuppression have not been evaluated.

Elderly: Pharmacokinetic analyses revealed that there was a trend toward lower clearance with increasing age in patients aged 40 years of age and older. A total of 519 patients 65 years of age and older, including 107 patients 75 years of age and older, received adalimumab in clinical studies. No overall difference in effectiveness was observed between these subjects and younger subjects. The frequency of serious infection and malignancy among adalimumab-treated subjects older than 65 years of age was higher than for those younger than 65 years of age. Because there is a higher incidence of infections and malignancies in the elderly population in general, use caution when treating the elderly.

Carcinogenicity: Long-term animal studies of adalimumab have not been conducted to evaluate the carcinogenic potential.

Mutagenicity: No clastogenic or mutagenic effects of adalimumab were observed in the in vivo mouse micronucleus test or the *Salmonella-Escherichia coli* (Ames) assay, respectively.

Fertility Impairment: Long-term animal studies of adalimumab have not been conducted to evaluate its effect on fertility.

Pregnancy: Category B. An embryo-fetal, perinatal-developmental toxicity study was performed in cynomolgus monkeys at dosages up to 100 mg/kg (266 times human area-under-concentration curve [AUC], when given 40 mg subcutaneously with methotrexate every week or 373 times human AUC when given 40 mg subcutaneously without methotrexate) and revealed no evidence of harm to the fetuses because of adalimumab. There are, however, no adequate and well-controlled studies in pregnant women. Because animal reproduction and developmental studies are not always predictive of human response, use adalimumab during pregnancy only if clearly needed.

Lactation: It is not known if adalimumab crosses into human breast milk or is absorbed systemically after ingestion. Because many drugs and immunoglobulins are excreted in human milk and because of the potential for serious adverse reactions in nursing infants from adalimumab, decide whether to discontinue nursing or to discontinue the drug, taking into account the importance of the drug to the mother.

Children: Safety and efficacy of adalimumab in children younger than 18 years of age for uses other than juvenile idiopathic arthritis have not been established. In the juvenile idiopathic arthritis study, adalimumab reduced signs and symptoms of active polyarticular juvenile idiopathic arthritis in patients 4 to 17 years of age. Adalimumab has not been studied in children younger than 4 years of age, and there are limited data on treatment in children weighing less than 15 kg.

Safety of adalimumab in pediatric patients was generally similar to that observed in adults, with certain exceptions. At the start of treatment, the most common adverse reactions in the pediatric population were injection-site pain (19%) and injection-site reaction (16%). A less commonly reported adverse event was granuloma annulare, which did not lead to discontinuation of treatment. In the first 48 weeks of treatment, nonserious hypersensitivity reactions were seen in approximately 6% of children and included primarily localized allergic hypersensitivity reactions and allergic rash.

Adverse Reactions: The most serious adverse reactions were serious infections, neurologic events, and malignancies. The most common adverse reaction with adalimumab was injection-site reactions. In placebo-controlled trials, 20% of patients treated with adalimumab developed injection-site reactions (erythema and/or itching, hemorrhage, pain, or swelling), compared with 14% of patients receiving placebo. Most injection-site reactions were described as mild and generally did not require drug discontinuation.

The proportion of patients who discontinued treatment because of adverse events during the double-blind, placebo-controlled portion of clinical trials was 7% for adalimumab-treated patients and 4% for placebo-treated patients. The most common adverse events leading to stopping adalimumab treatment were clinical flare reaction (0.7%), rash (0.3%), and pneumonia (0.3%).

Allergic: Allergic reactions developed in approximately 1% of patients receiving adalimumab. If an anaphylactic reaction or other serious allergic reaction occurs, discontinue adalimumab immediately and initiate appropriate therapy.

Autoimmunity: In controlled trials, 12% of patients treated with adalimumab and 7% of placebo-treated patients who had negative baseline ANA titers developed positive titers at week 24. One patient out of 2,334 treated with adalimumab developed clinical signs suggestive of new-onset lupus-like syndrome. The patient improved after stopping therapy. No patients developed lupus nephritis or CNS symptoms. The impact of long-term treatment with adalimumab on the development of autoimmune diseases is unknown. If a patient develops symptoms suggestive of a lupus-like syndrome following treatment with adalimumab, discontinue treatment.

Immunogenicity: Patients in clinical trials were tested at multiple time points for antibodies to adalimumab during a 6- to 12-month period. Approximately 5% (58 of 1,062) of adult RA patients receiving adalimumab developed low-titer antibodies to adalimumab at least once during treatment, which were neutralizing in vitro. Patients treated with concomitant methotrexate had a lower rate of antibody development than patients on adalimumab monotherapy (1% vs 12%). No apparent correlation of antibody development to adverse events was observed. With monotherapy, patients receiving every-other-week dosing may develop antibodies more frequently than those receiving weekly dosing. In patients receiving the recommended dosage of 40 mg every other week as monotherapy, the American College of Rheumatology (ACR) 20 response was lower among antibody-positive patients than among antibody-negative patients. In patients with juvenile idiopathic arthritis, adalimumab antibodies were identified in 16% of treated patients. In adult patients receiving concomitant methotrexate, the incidence was 6% compared with 26% with adalimumab monotherapy. The long-term immunogenicity of adalimumab is unknown. The data reflect the percentage of patients whose test results were considered positive for antibodies to adalimumab in an ELISA assay, and are highly dependent on the sensitivity and specificity of the assay. Comparison of the incidence of antibodies to adalimumab with the incidence of antibodies to other products may be misleading.

Immunosuppression: TNF-blocking agents, including adalimumab, may affect host defenses against infections and malignancies, because TNF mediates inflammation and modulates cellular immune responses. In a study of 64 patients with RA treated with adalimumab, there was no evidence of depression of delayed-type hypersensitivity, depression of immunoglobulin levels, or change in enumeration of effector T- and B-cells and NK-cells, monocyte/macrophages, and neutrophils. The impact of treatment with adalimumab on the development and course of malignancies, as well as active and/or chronic infections is not fully understood. The safety and efficacy of adalimumab in patients with immunosuppression have not been evaluated.

Infections: In placebo-controlled trials, the rate of infection was 1 per patient-year in adalimumab-treated patients and 0.9 per patient-year in placebo-treated patients. Most patients continued on adalimumab after the infection resolved. The incidence of serious infections was 0.04 per patient-year in adalimumab-treated patients and 0.02 per patient-year in placebo-treated patients. Serious infections observed included pneumonia, septic arthritis, prosthetic and postsurgical infections, erysipelas, cellulitis, diverticulitis, and pyelonephritis.

Thirteen cases of tuberculosis, including miliary, lymphatic, peritoneal, and pulmonary were reported in clinical trials. Most cases of tuberculosis occurred within the first 8 months after starting therapy and may have reflected recrudescence of latent disease. While cases were observed at all doses, the incidence of tuberculosis reactivations was particularly increased at adalimumab doses higher than the recommended dose. All patients recovered after standard antimicrobial therapy.

There is a risk of opportunistic fungal infections, possibly fatal. Six cases of invasive opportunistic infections caused by histoplasma, aspergillus, and the bacterium nocardia also were reported in clinical trials.

Before beginning therapy with adalimumab, evaluate patients for active or latent tuberculosis with a tuberculin skin test. Treat latent tuberculosis before adalimumab therapy according to Centers for Disease Control and Prevention guidelines. Instruct patients to seek medical advice if signs/symptoms (eg, persistent cough, wasting/weight loss, low grade fever) suggestive of tuberculosis occur.

Do not begin treatment with adalimumab in patients with active infections, including chronic or localized infections. Monitor patients who develop a new infection during adalimumab therapy closely. Discontinue adalimumab if a patient develops a serious infection. Exercise caution when considering the use of adalimumab in patients with a history of recurrent infection or underlying conditions that may predispose them to infections, or patients who resided in regions where tuberculosis or histoplasmosis is endemic. Carefully consider the benefits and risks of adalimumab before beginning adalimumab therapy.

Use of TNF-blockers, including adalimumab, may increase the risk of reactivation of hepatitis B virus in patients who are chronic carriers of this virus. In some cases, reactivation has been fatal. Most of these cases concomitantly received other immune-suppressing medications. Exercise caution in prescribing TNF-blockers for chronic HBV carriers. Monitor such patients closely for clinical and laboratory signs of active HBV infection throughout therapy and for several months after stopping therapy. In patients who develop HBV reactivation, stop adalimumab and begin effective antiviral therapy with appropriate supportive treatment. The safety of resuming TNF-blocker therapy after HBV reactivation is controlled is not known.

Malignancies: In controlled clinical trials of some TNF-blocking agents, including adalimumab, more cases of malignancies occurred among patients receiving TNF-blockers than occurred among control patients. More cases of lymphoma occurred among patients receiving TNF-blockers compared with control patients.

Among 2,468 RA patients treated in clinical trials with adalimumab for a median of 24 months, 48 malignancies of various types were observed, including 10 patients with lymphomas. The ratio of observed rate to age-adjusted expected frequency in the general population for malignancies was 1.0 (95% CI, 0.7, 1.3) and for lymphomas was 5.4 (95% CI, 2.6, 10). While patients with RA, particularly those with highly active diseases, may be several times more likely to develop lymphomas, the role of TNF-blockers in the development of malignancy is not known. The other malignancies observed during use of adalimumab were breast, colon-rectum, uterine-cervical, prostate, melanoma, gallbladder-bile ducts, and other carcinomas.

Cases of hepatosplenic T-cell lymphoma (HSTCL), a rare type of T-cell lymphoma, have occurred in adolescents and young adults with inflammatory bowel disease treated with TNF blockers, including adalimumab.

Neurologic: Use of TNF-blocking agents, including adalimumab, has been associated with rare cases of exacerbation of clinical symptoms and/or radiographic evidence of demyelinating disease. Exercise caution in considering the use of adalimumab in patients with pre-existing or recent-onset CNS-demyelinating disorders.

Data below reflect exposure to adalimumab in 2,334 patients, including 2,073 exposed for 6 months, 1,497 exposed for longer than 1 year, and 1,380 in adequate and well-controlled studies (studies I, II, III, and IV). Adalimumab was studied primarily in placebo-controlled trials and in long-term follow-up studies for up to 36 months duration. The population had a mean age of 54 years; 77% were female, 91% were white and had moderately to severely active RA. Most patients received 40 mg adalimumab every other week.

Other infrequent serious adverse events occurring at an incidence less than 5% in patients treated with adalimumab were:

Adalimumab (Recombinant)

Neoplasia: Adenoma, carcinomas such as breast, gastrointestinal, skin, urogenital, and others; lymphoma and melanoma.

Body as a whole: Fever, infection, pain in extremity, pelvic pain, sepsis, surgery, thorax pain, tuberculosis reactivated.

Cardiovascular: Arrhythmia, atrial fibrillation, cardiovascular disorder, chest pain, congestive heart failure, coronary artery disorder, heart arrest, hypertensive encephalopathy, myocardial infarction, palpitation, pericardial effusion, pericarditis, syncope, tachycardia, vascular disorder, thrombosis (leg).

CNS: Confusion, multiple sclerosis, paresthesia, subdural hematoma, tremor.

Dermatologic: Cellulitis, erysipelas, herpes zoster.

GI: Cholecystitis, cholelithiasis, esophagitis, gastroenteritis, gastrointestinal disorder, gastrointestinal hemorrhage, hepatic necrosis, vomiting.

GU: Cystitis, kidney calculus, menstrual disorder, pyelonephritis.

Endocrine: Parathyroid disorder.

Hematologic/Lymphatic: Agranulocytosis, granulocytopenia, leukopenia, lymphoma-like reaction, pancytopenia, polycythemia.

Metabolic/Nutritional: Dehydration, healing abnormal, ketosis, paraproteinemia, peripheral edema.

Miscellaneous: Lupus erythematosus syndrome.

Musculoskeletal: Arthritis, bone disorder, bone fracture (not spontaneous), bone necrosis, joint disorder, muscle cramps, myasthenia, pyogenic arthritis, synovitis, tendon disorder.

Respiratory: Asthma, bronchospasm, dyspnea, lung disorder, lung function decreased, pleural effusion, pneumonia.

Special Senses: Cataract.

Pharmacologic & Dosing Characteristics

Dosage:

For RA, psoriatic arthritis, or ankylosing spondylitis: 40 mg every other week. Methotrexate, glucocorticoids, salicylates, nonsteroidal anti-inflammatory drugs (NSAIDs), analgesics, or other DMARDs may be continued during treatment with adalimumab. Some patients not taking concomitant methotrexate may derive additional benefit from increasing the dosing frequency of adalimumab to 40 mg every week.

For Crohn disease: 160 mg initially at week 0, 80 mg at week 2, then a maintenance dose of 40 mg every other week beginning at week 4. The initial dose may be given as 4 injections on 1 day or divided over 2 days.

For plaque psoriasis: 80 mg initially, then 40 mg every other week starting 1 week after initial dose.

For juvenile idiopathic arthritis:
- 15 kg to less than 30 kg: 20 mg every other week.
- More than 30 kg: 40 mg every other week.

Route: Subcutaneous

Overdosage: The maximum tolerated dose of adalimumab has not been established in humans. Multiple doses up to 10 mg/kg have been administered to patients in clinical trials without evidence of dose-limiting toxicities. In case of overdosage, monitor the patient for signs or symptoms of adverse reactions or effects. Institute appropriate symptomatic treatment immediately.

Missed Doses: If a dose of adalimumab is missed, inject the next dose right away. Then take the next dose when next scheduled. This will put the patient back on schedule.

Efficacy: The efficacy and safety of adalimumab were assessed in 4 randomized, double-blind studies in patients 18 years of age and older with active RA diagnosed according to ACR criteria. Patients had at least 6 swollen and 9 tender joints. Adalimumab was administered subcutaneously in combination with methotrexate (12.5 to 25 mg, studies I and III) or as monotherapy (study II), or with other DMARDs (study IV).

Study I evaluated 271 patients who had failed therapy with 1 to 4 DMARDs and had inadequate response to methotrexate. Doses of 20, 40, or 80 mg adalimumab or placebo were given every other week for 24 weeks.

Study II evaluated 544 patients who had failed therapy with 1 or more DMARD. Doses of placebo or 20 or 40 mg adalimumab were given as monotherapy every other week or weekly for 26 weeks.

Study III evaluated 619 patients who had an inadequate response to methotrexate. Patients received placebo, 40 mg adalimumab every other week with placebo injections on alternate weeks, or 20 mg of adalimumab weekly for up to 52 weeks. Study III had an additional primary endpoint at 52 weeks of inhibition of disease progression (as detected by x-ray results).

Study IV assessed safety in 636 patients who were either DMARD-naïve or were permitted to remain on their preexisting rheumatologic therapy, provided that therapy was stable for at least 28 days. Patients were randomized to 40 mg adalimumab or placebo every other week for 24 weeks.

The percent of adalimumab-treated patients achieving ACR 20, 50, and 70 responses in studies II and III are shown in the following table.

ACR Responses in Placebo-Controlled Trials (Percent of Patients)					
	Study II, monotherapy (26 weeks)			Study III, methotrexate combination (24 and 52 weeks)	
Response	Placebo (N = 110)	Humira 40 mg every other week (N = 113)	Humira 40 mg weekly (N = 103)	Placebo with Methotrexate (N = 200)	Humira with Methotrexate 40 mg every other week (N = 207)
ACR 20					
Month 6	19%	46%[a]	53%[a]	30%	63%[a]
Month 12	NA	NA	NA	24%	59%[a]
ACR 50					
Month 6	8%	22%[a]	35%[a]	10%	39%[a]
Month 12	NA	NA	NA	10%	42%[a]
ACR 70					
Month 6	2%	12%[a]	18%[a]	3%	21%[a]
Month 12	NA	NA	NA	5%	23%[a]

a $P < 0.01$, adalimumab vs placebo.

The results of study I were similar to study III; patients receiving 40 mg adalimumab every other week in study I also achieved ACR 20, 50, and 70 response rates of 65%, 52%, and 24%, respectively, compared with placebo responses of 13%, 7%, and 3%, respectively, at 6 months ($P < 0.01$).

Improvement was seen in all components of the ACR response criteria for studies II and III components and was maintained to week 52.

In study III, 85% of patients with ACR 20 responses at week 24 maintained the response at 52 weeks. The time course of ACR 20 response for study I and study II were similar. In study

IV, 53% of patients treated with adalimumab 40 mg every other week plus standard of care had an ACR 20 response at week 24, compared with 35% on placebo plus standard of care ($P < 0.001$). No unique adverse reactions related to the combination of adalimumab and other DMARDs were observed.

In all 4 studies, adalimumab showed significantly greater improvement than placebo in the disability index of Health Assessment Questionnaire (HAQ) from baseline to the end of study, and significantly greater improvement than placebo in the health outcomes as assessed by The Short Form Health Survey (SF 36). Improvement was seen in both the Physical Component Summary (PCS) and the Mental Component Summary (MCS).

In study III, structural joint damage was assessed radiographically and expressed as change in Total Sharp Score (TSS) and its components, the erosion score, and Joint Space Narrowing (JSN) score at month 12 compared with baseline. At baseline, the median TSS was approximately 55 in the placebo and 40 mg every other week groups. Adalimumab-methotrexate treated patients demonstrated less radiographic progression than patients receiving methotrexate alone.

Onset: Adalimumab begins to outperform placebo about 4 weeks into therapy, based on results from study III.

Pharmacokinetics: Immunoglobulins are primarily eliminated by catabolism. After treatment with adalimumab, a rapid decrease in levels of acute phase reactants of inflammation (C-reactive protein [CRP] and erythrocyte sedimentation rate [ESR]) and serum cytokines (IL-6) was observed compared with baseline in patients with RA. Serum levels of matrix metalloproteinases (MMP-1 and MMP-3) that produce tissue remodeling responsible for cartilage destruction were also decreased after adalimumab administration.

The maximum serum concentration (C_{max}) and the time to reach the maximum concentration (T_{max}) were 4.7 ± 1.6 mcg/mL and 131 ± 56 hours respectively, following a single 40 mg subcutaneous administration of adalimumab to healthy adult subjects. The average absolute bioavailability of adalimumab estimated from 3 studies following a single 40 mg subcutaneous dose was 64%. The pharmacokinetics of adalimumab were linear over the dose range of 0.5 to 10 mg/kg following a single IV dose. The single-dose pharmacokinetics of adalimumab were determined in several studies with IV doses ranging from 0.25 to 10 mg/kg. The distribution volume ranged from 4.7 to 6.0 L. The systemic clearance of adalimumab was approximately 12 mL/h. The mean terminal half-life was approximately 2 weeks, ranging from 10 to 20 days across studies. Adalimumab concentrations in the synovial fluid from 5 RA patients ranged from 31% to 96% of those in serum.

Adalimumab mean steady-state trough concentrations of approximately 5 mcg/mL and 8 to 9 mcg/mL were observed without and with methotrexate, respectively. The serum adalimumab trough levels at steady state increased proportionally with dose, following 20, 40, and 80 mg every other week and every week subcutaneous dosing. In long-term studies with dosing longer than 2 years, there was no evidence of changes in clearance over time.

Population pharmacokinetic analyses revealed that there was a trend toward higher apparent clearance of adalimumab in the presence of anti-adalimumab antibodies, and lower clearance with increasing age in patients aged 40 to 75 years and older.

Minor increases in apparent clearance were also predicted in patients receiving doses lower than the recommended dose and in patients with high rheumatoid factor or CRP concentrations. These increases are not likely to be clinically important.

No gender-related pharmacokinetic differences were observed after correction for a patient's body weight. Healthy volunteers and patients with RA displayed similar adalimumab pharmacokinetics.

No pharmacokinetic data are available in patients with hepatic or renal impairment.

Adalimumab (Recombinant)

In subjects with juvenile idiopathic arthritis (4 to 17 years of age), the mean steady-state trough serum concentrations for subjects weighing less than 30 kg receiving adalimumab 20 mg subcutaneously every other week as monotherapy or with concomitant methotrexate were 6.8 mcg/mL and 10.9 mcg/mL, respectively. The mean steady-state trough serum concentrations for subjects weighing 30 kg or more receiving adalimumab 40 mg subcutaneously every other week as monotherapy or with concomitant methotrexate were 6.6 and 8.1 mcg/mL, respectively.

Mechanism: Adalimumab binds specifically to TNF-α and blocks its interaction with the p55 and p75 cell-surface TNF receptors. Adalimumab also lyses surface TNF-expressing cells in vitro in the presence of complement. Adalimumab does not bind or inactivate lymphotoxin (TNF-β). TNF is a naturally occurring cytokine involved in normal inflammatory and immune responses. Elevated levels of TNF are found in the synovial fluid of RA patients and play an important role in pathologic inflammation and joint destruction, both which are hallmarks of RA. Adalimumab also modulates biological responses induced or regulated by TNF, including changes in levels of adhesion molecules responsible for leukocyte migration (ELAM-1, VCAM-1, and ICAM-1 with an IC_{50} of 1-2 $\times$ 10^{-10} M).

Drug Interactions: Methotrexate reduced adalimumab-apparent clearance after single and multiple dosing by 29% and 44%, respectively. In RA patients taking methotrexate and adalimumab concomitantly, data do not suggest the need for dose adjustment of either adalimumab or methotrexate.

Serious infections were seen in clinical studies with concurrent use of anakinra and another TNF-blocking agent, with no added benefit. Similar toxicities may also result from combination of anakinra and other TNF-blocking agents. Therefore, the combination of adalimumab and anakinra is not recommended.

Limited data are available on the effects of vaccination in patients receiving adalimumab. Do not give live vaccines concurrently with adalimumab therapy. No data are available on secondary transmission of infection by live vaccines in patients receiving adalimumab. In a placebo-controlled trial of patients with RA, no difference was detected in antipneumococcal antibody response between adalimumab and placebo arms. Similar proportions of patients developed protective levels of anti-influenza antibodies, but mean anti-influenza antibody concentrations were moderately lower in the adalimumab-treated group. The clinical significance of this finding is unknown. Bring patients with juvenile idiopathic arthritis up to date with current vaccination guidelines before starting adalimumab therapy. Patients receiving adalimumab may receive concurrent vaccinations, except for live vaccines.

In a study of 64 patients with RA treated with adalimumab, there was no evidence of depression of delayed-type hypersensitivity.

Patient Information: If skin around the injection area still hurts or is swollen, try using a towel soaked with cold water on the injection site. Instruct patients to seek medical advice if signs/symptoms (eg, persistent cough, wasting/weight loss, low-grade fever) suggestive of tuberculosis occur.

Pharmaceutical Characteristics

Concentration: 40 mg per 0.8 mL

Quality Assay: Purified by a process that includes specific viral inactivation and removal steps.

Packaging:

Pen cartons: Carton containing 2 alcohol pads and 2 dose trays, each containing a single-use pen with a fixed 27-gauge, ½-inch needle delivering 40 mg/0.8 mL (00074-4339-02). The Crohn disease starter packaging contains 6 alcohol pads and 6 dose trays, each containing a single-use pen with a fixed 27-gauge, ½-inch needle delivering 40 mg/0.8 mL

Adalimumab (Recombinant)

(00074-4339-06). The psoriasis starter packaging contains 4 alcohol pads and 4 dose trays, each containing a single-use pen with a fixed 27-gauge, ½-inch needle delivering 40 mg/ 0.8 mL (00074-4339-07).

Syringes: Patient-use carton containing 2 alcohol prep pads and 2 dose trays; each dose tray includes a single-use 1 mL prefilled glass syringe with a fixed 27-gauge ½-inch needle, providing 40 mg (0.8 mL) of adalimumab (NDC#: 00074-3799-02). Institutional-use carton containing 2 alcohol prep pads and 1 dose tray; each dose tray includes a single use, 1 mL prefilled glass syringe with a fixed 27-gauge ½-inch needle (with needle-stick protection device) providing 40 mg (0.8 mL) adalimumab (00074-3799-01).

For pediatric use, a carton containing 2 alcohol preps and 2 dose trays; each dose tray includes a single-use, 1 mL prefilled glass syringe with a fixed 27-gauge ½-inch needle, providing adalimumab 20 mg (0.4 mL) (00074-9374-02).

Doseform: Solution

Appearance: Clear and colorless

Solvent: Buffered saline

Adjuvant: None

Preservative: None

Allergens: The needle cover on the prefilled syringe contains dry natural rubber.

Excipients: Each 0.8 mL contains sodium chloride 4.93 mg, monobasic sodium phosphate dihydrate 0.69 mg, dibasic sodium phosphate dihydrate 1.22 mg, sodium citrate 0.24 mg, citric acid monohydrate 1.04 mg, mannitol 9.6 mg, polysorbate 80 0.8 mg, and water for injection. Sodium hydroxide added as necessary to adjust pH.

pH: about 5.2

Shelf Life: Not longer than 18 months

Storage/Stability: Store at 2° to 8°C (36° to 46°F). Do not freeze. Contact the manufacturer regarding exposure to extreme temperatures. Shipped by overnight courier in insulated containers with refrigerated and frozen coolant packs and fill void space in the shipping container with paper.

Handling: Protect the vial and prefilled syringe from exposure to light. To avoid degrading the product, do not shake the vial. When traveling, store in a cool carrier with a coolant pack and protect from light.

Production Process: Adalimumab is produced by recombinant DNA technology in a mammalian cell-expression system and is purified by a process that includes specific viral inactivation and removal steps.

Media: Transfected Chinese hamster ovary (CHO) cells

Other Information

First Licensed: December 31, 2002

References: Mease PJ, Gladman DD, Ritchlin CT, et al; Adalimumab Effectiveness in Psoriatic Arthritis Trial Study Group. Adalimumab for the treatment of patients with moderately to severely active psoriatic arthritis: results of a double-blind, randomized, placebo-controlled trial. *Arthritis Rheum.* 2005;52:3279-3289.

Voulgari PV, Drosos AA. Adalimumab for rheumatoid arthritis. *Expert Opin Biol Ther.* 2006;6(12):1349-1360.

Isoantibodies

Names: *Manufacturers:*
Eylea   Regeneron Pharmaceuticals

Immunologic Characteristics

Antigen Source: Human vascular endothelial growth factor (VEGF)

Viability: Not viable, but immunologically active

Antigenic Form: Soluble VEGF receptor domains linked to Fc portion of IgG1

Antigenic Type: Fusion protein containing portions of human VEGF receptors 1 and 2 extracellular domains fused to the Fc portion of human IgG1. Aflibercept has a protein molecular weight of 97 kDa in addition to glycosylation, constituting an additional 15% of the total molecular mass, resulting in a total molecular weight of 115 kDa.

Use Characteristics

Indications: To treat patients with neovascular (wet) age-related macular degeneration (AMD)

Contraindications: Patients with ocular or periocular infections, with active intraocular inflammation, or with known hypersensitivity to aflibercept or any excipient

Immunodeficiency: No impairment of effect is expected.

Elderly: In clinical studies, 89% (1,616/1,817) of patients randomized to treatment with aflibercept were 65 years of age and older, and 63% (1,139/1,817) were 75 years of age and older. No significant differences in efficacy or safety were seen with increasing age in these studies.

Carcinogenicity: Aflibercept has not been evaluated for carcinogenic potential.

Mutagenicity: Aflibercept has not been evaluated for mutagenic potential.

Fertility Impairment: Effects on male and female fertility were assessed as part of a 6-month study in monkeys with aflibercept at doses ranging from 3 to 30 mg/kg intravenously (IV). Absent or irregular menses associated with alterations in female reproductive hormone levels and changes in sperm morphology and motility were observed at all dose levels. In addition, females showed decreased ovarian and uterine weight accompanied by compromised luteal development and reduction of maturing follicles. These changes correlated with uterine and vaginal atrophy. A no observed adverse effect level (NOAEL) was not identified. Based on maximum plasma concentration (C_{max}) and area under the curve (AUC) for free aflibercept observed at the 3 mg/kg dose, the systemic exposures were approximately 4,900 times and 1,500 times higher, respectively, than the exposure observed in humans after an intravitreal dose of 2 mg. All changes were reversible.

Pregnancy: Category C. There are no adequate and well-controlled studies in pregnant women. Use aflibercept during pregnancy only if the potential benefit justifies the potential risk to the fetus. Aflibercept produced embryofetal toxicity when administered during organogenesis in pregnant rabbits at IV doses of 3 to 60 mg/kg. A series of external, visceral, and skeletal malformations were observed in the fetuses. The maternal NOAEL was 3 mg/kg, whereas the fetal NOAEL was below 3 mg/kg. At this dose, the systemic exposures based on C_{max} and AUC for free aflibercept were approximately 2,900 times and 600 times higher, respectively, compared with corresponding values observed in humans after an intravitreal dose of 2 mg.

Lactation: It is not known if aflibercept crosses into human breast milk. Aflibercept is not recommended during breast-feeding. Decide whether to discontinue breast-feeding or treatment with aflibercept, taking into account the importance of the drug to the mother.

Children: Safety and efficacy of aflibercept in children younger than 18 years have not been established.

Adverse Reactions: The most common adverse reactions (incidence of at least 5%) reported in patients receiving aflibercept were conjunctival hemorrhage, eye pain, cataract, vitreous detachment, vitreous floaters, and increased intraocular pressure (IOP).

The data in the following table reflect exposure to aflibercept in 1,824 patients with wet AMD, including 1,223 patients treated with the 2 mg dose, in 2 double-masked, active-controlled clinical studies (VIEW1 and VIEW2) for 12 months.

Most Common Adverse Events (≥ 1%) in Phase 3 Wet AMD Studies		
Adverse events	Aflibercept (n = 1,824)	Ranibizumab (n = 595)
Conjunctival hemorrhage	25%	28%
Eye pain	9%	9%
Cataract	7%	7%
Vitreous detachment	6%	6%
Vitreous floaters	6%	7%
IOP increased	5%	7%
Conjunctival hyperemia	4%	8%
Corneal erosion	4%	5%
Detachment of the retinal pigment epithelium	3%	3%
Injection-site pain	3%	3%
Foreign body sensation in eyes	3%	4%
Lacrimation increased	3%	1%
Vision blurred	2%	2%
Retinal pigment epithelium tear	2%	1%
Injection-site hemorrhage	1%	2%
Eyelid edema	1%	2%
Corneal edema	1%	1%

Hypersensitivity was reported in less than 1% of the patients treated with aflibercept.

Injection procedure: Serious adverse reactions related to the injection procedure have occurred in less than 0.1% of intravitreal injections with aflibercept and included endophthalmitis, retinal tear, traumatic cataract, and increased IOP.

Endophthalmitis and retinal detachments: Use proper aseptic technique when administering aflibercept. Instruct patients to report any symptoms suggestive of endophthalmitis or retinal detachment without delay, and manage appropriately.

Intraocular pressure: Acute increases in IOP have been seen within 60 minutes of intravitreal injection, including with aflibercept. Sustained increases in IOP have also been reported after repeated intravitreal dosing with VEGF inhibitors. Monitor IOP and perfusion of the optic nerve head and manage appropriately.

Immunogenicity: As with all therapeutic proteins, there is the potential for an immune response in patients treated with aflibercept. The immunogenicity of aflibercept was evaluated in serum samples. The immunogenicity data reflect the percentage of patients whose test results were considered positive for antibodies to aflibercept in immunoassays. In the phase 3 studies, the pretreatment incidence of immunoreactivity to aflibercept was 1% to 3% across treatment groups. After dosing with aflibercept for 52 weeks, antibodies to aflibercept were detected in a similar percentage range of patients. There were no differences in efficacy or safety between patients with or without immunoreactivity.

Thromboembolic events: There is a potential risk of arterial thromboembolic events after intravitreal use of VEGF inhibitors, including aflibercept. Arterial thromboembolic events are defined as nonfatal stroke, nonfatal myocardial infarction, or vascular death (including deaths of unknown cause). The incidence in the VIEW1 and VIEW2 wet AMD studies during the first year was 1.8% (32/1,824) in the combined group of patients treated with aflibercept.

Pharmacologic & Dosing Characteristics

Dosage: 2 mg (0.05 mL or 50 mcL) administered by intravitreal injection every 4 weeks for the first 12 weeks, followed by 2 mg (0.05 mL) once every 8 weeks. Although aflibercept may be dosed as frequently as 2 mg every 4 weeks, additional efficacy was not demonstrated when aflibercept was dosed every 4 weeks compared with every 8 weeks.

No special dosage modification is required for any of the populations studied (eg, gender, elderly).

Route & Site: Intravitreal injection with 30-gauge, ½-inch needle

Special Handling: Use the 19-gauge, 1½-inch, 5-micron filter needle and 1 mL syringe to withdraw aflibercept from the vial. Draw back the plunger rod to completely empty the filter needle. Remove the filter needle from the syringe and replace it with the 30-gauge, ½-inch injection needle. Slowly depress the plunger so that the plunger tip aligns with the line that marks 0.05 mL on the syringe. Conduct intravitreal injection under controlled aseptic conditions. Give adequate anesthesia and a topical broad-spectrum microbicide before injection. Immediately after injection, monitor patients for elevation in IOP. Use each vial to treat only a single eye. If the contralateral eye requires treatment, use a new vial and change the sterile field, syringe, gloves, drapes, eyelid speculum, filter, and injection needles.

Overdosage: Although few data are available, clinical experience with similar products suggests that the major manifestations of overdosage would be pain and tenderness at the injection site.

Efficacy: The safety and efficacy of aflibercept were assessed in 2 randomized, multicenter, double-masked, active-controlled studies in patients with wet AMD. A total of 2,412 patients were treated and evaluable for efficacy (1,817 treated with aflibercept) in the VIEW1 and VIEW2 studies. In each study, patients were randomly assigned in a 1:1:1:1 ratio to 1 of 4 dosing regimens: aflibercept 2 mg every 8 weeks after 3 initial monthly doses, aflibercept 2 mg every 4 weeks, aflibercept 0.5 mg every 4 weeks, or ranibizumab 0.5 mg administered every 4 weeks. Patient ages ranged from 49 to 99 years (mean age, 76 years).

In both studies, the primary efficacy end point was the proportion of patients who maintained vision, defined as losing fewer than 15 letters of visual acuity at week 52 compared with baseline. Data are available through week 52. The groups that received aflibercept 2 mg every 8 weeks and aflibercept 2 mg every 4 weeks were shown to have efficacy clinically equivalent to the group that received ranibizumab 0.5 mg every 4 weeks. Results are shown in the following table.

In the phase 3 studies, anatomic measures of disease activity improved similarly in all treatment groups from baseline to week 52. Anatomic data were not used to influence treatment decisions.

Efficacy at Week 52 (Full Analysis Set With LOCF) in VIEW1 and VIEW2 Studies[a]					
	VIEW1			VIEW2		
	Aflibercept 2 mg every 8 weeks[b]	Aflibercept 2 mg every 4 weeks	Ranibizumab 0.5 mg every 4 weeks	Aflibercept 2 mg every 8 weeks[b]	Aflibercept 2 mg every 4 weeks	Ranibizumab 0.5 mg every 4 weeks
Full analysis set	n = 301	n = 304	n = 304	n = 306	n = 309	n = 291
Efficacy outcomes						
Proportion of patients who maintained visual acuity (< 15 letters of BCVA loss)	94%	95%	94%	95%	95%	95%
Difference[c] (95% CI)	0.6% (−3.2, 4.4)	1.3% (−2.4, 5)		0.6% (−2.9, 4)	−0.3% (−4, 3.3)	
Mean change in BCVA as measured by ETDRS letter score from baseline	7.9	10.9	8.1	8.9	7.6	9.4
Difference[c] in LS mean (95% CI)	0.3 (−2, 2.5)	3.2 (0.9, 5.4)		−0.9 (−3.1, 1.3)	−2 (−4.1, 0.2)	
Number of patients who gained ≥ 15 letters of vision from baseline	92 (31%)	114 (38%)	94 (31%)	96 (31%)	91 (29%)	99 (34%)
Difference[c] (95% CI)	−0.4% (−7.7, 7)	6.6% (−1, 14.1)		−2.6% (−10.2, 4.9)	−4.6% (−12.1, 2.9)	

a BCVA = best corrected visual acuity; CI = confidence interval; ETDRS = early treatment diabetic retinopathy study; LOCF = last observation carried forward (baseline values are not carried forward); CI = confidence interval (95% CIs were presented to adjust for safety assessment conducted during the study).
b After treatment initiation with 3 monthly doses.
c Aflibercept group minus the ranibizumab group.

Pharmacokinetics:

Absorption: Aflibercept is administered intravitreally to exert local effects in the eye. In patients with wet AMD, following intravitreal administration of aflibercept, a fraction of the administered dose is expected to bind with endogenous VEGF in the eye to form an inactive aflibercept-VEGF complex. Once absorbed into the systemic circulation, aflibercept presents in the plasma as free aflibercept (unbound to VEGF) and a more predominant stable inactive form with circulating endogenous VEGF (ie, aflibercept-VEGF complex).

Distribution: After intravitreal administration of 2 mg per eye to patients with wet AMD, the mean C_{max} of free aflibercept in the plasma was 0.02 mcg/mL (range, 0 to 0.054 mcg/mL), attained in 1 to 3 days. The free aflibercept plasma concentrations were undetectable 2 weeks postdosing in all patients. Aflibercept did not accumulate in plasma when administered as repeated doses intravitreally every 4 weeks. After intravitreal administration of 2 mg, the mean maximum plasma concentration of free aflibercept is greater than 100-fold lower than the concentration required to half-maximally bind systemic VEGF. The volume of distribution of free aflibercept after IV administration is approximately 6 L.

Elimination: Aflibercept is a therapeutic protein and no drug metabolism studies have been conducted. Aflibercept is expected to undergo elimination through both target-mediated disposition via binding to free endogenous VEGF and metabolism via proteolysis. The terminal elimination half-life ($t_{1/2}$) of free aflibercept in plasma was approximately 5 to 6 days after IV administration of 2 to 4 mg/kg.

Renal impairment: Pharmacokinetic analysis of a subgroup of patients (n = 492) in 1 phase 3 study, of whom 43% had renal impairment (mild, n = 120; moderate, n = 74; severe, n = 16), revealed no differences with respect to plasma concentrations of free aflibercept after intravitreal administration every 4 or 8 weeks. No dose adjustment based on renal impairment status is needed.

Animal toxicology: Erosions and ulcerations of the respiratory epithelium in nasal turbinates in monkeys treated with aflibercept intravitreally were observed at intravitreal doses of 2 or 4 mg per eye. At the NOAEL of 0.5 mg per eye in monkeys, the systemic exposure was 42 times and 56 times higher based on C_{max} and AUC, respectively, than the exposure observed in humans after an intravitreal dose of 2 mg. Similar effects were not seen in clinical studies.

Mechanism: Vascular endothelial growth factor A (VEGF-A) and placental growth factor (PGF) are members of the VEGF family of angiogenic factors that can act as mitogenic, chemotactic, and vascular permeability factors for endothelial cells. VEGF acts via 2 receptor tyrosine kinases, VEGFR-1 and VEGFR-2, present on the surface of endothelial cells. PGF binds only to VEGFR-1, which is also present on the surface of leukocytes. Activation of these receptors by VEGF-A can result in neovascularization and vascular permeability.

Aflibercept acts as a soluble decoy receptor that binds VEGF-A and PGF, thereby inhibiting the binding and activation of these cognate VEGF receptors.

Drug Interactions: No drug interaction studies with aflibercept have been reported.

Patient Information: Instruct patients to report any symptoms suggestive of endophthalmitis or retinal detachment (eg, eye pain, redness, photophobia, blurred vision) without delay. Patients may experience temporary visual disturbances after an intravitreal injection with aflibercept and the associated eye examinations. Advise patients not to drive or use machinery until visual function has recovered sufficiently.

Pharmaceutical Characteristics

Concentration: 40 mg/mL

Packaging: Carton contains 1 single-use, 3 mL glass vial containing a 0.278 mL fill of aflibercept 40 mg/mL; one 19-gauge, 1½-inch, 5-micron filter needle; one 30-gauge, ½-inch injection needle; one 1 mL syringe for administration

NDC Number: 61755-0005-02

Doseform: Iso-osmotic saline-sucrose solution

Appearance: Clear, colorless to pale yellow solution

Solvent: None

Adjuvant: None

Preservative: None

Allergens: None

Excipients: Iso-osmotic solution containing sodium phosphate 10 mM, sodium chloride 40 mM, 0.03% of polysorbate 20, and sucrose 5%

pH: 6.2

Shelf Life: Data not provided

Storage/Stability: Store at 2° to 8°C (36° to 46°F). Protect vial from light. Do not freeze. Contact the manufacturer regarding exposure to freezing or elevated temperatures. Shipping data not provided.

Media: Aflibercept is produced in recombinant Chinese hamster ovary (CHO) cells.

Aflibercept

Other Information

First Licensed: November 18, 2011

Alefacept (Recombinant)

Isoantibodies

Name:
Amevive

Manufacturer:
Astellas

Synonyms: LFA-3/IgG1 fusion protein, BG9712, BG9273, LFA3TIP

Comparison: Alefacept acts as a soluble receptor for the CD2 antigen.

Immunologic Characteristics

Target Antigen: Human CD2 antigen

Viability: Not viable, but immunologically active

Antigenic Form: Soluble receptor linked to Fc antibody fragments, 1-92-antigen LFA-3 fusion protein with IgG1 (hinge-CH2-CH3 γ1-chain), dimer

Antigenic Type: Dimeric fusion protein consisting of the extracellular CD2-binding portion of the human leukocyte function antigen-3 (LFA-3) linked to the Fc (hinge, CH2, and CH3 domains) portion of human IgG1. The molecular weight of alefacept is 91.4 kilodaltons.

Use Characteristics

Indications: To treat adult patients with moderate to severe chronic plaque psoriasis who are candidates for systemic therapy or phototherapy.

Contraindications: Do not administer alefacept to patients infected with HIV. Alefacept reduces CD4+ T-lymphocyte counts, which may accelerate disease progression or increase complications of disease in these patients.

People with known hypersensitivity to alefacept or any of its components.

Immunodeficiency: Alefacept is an immunosuppressive agent and, therefore, may increase the risk of infection and reactivate latent, chronic infections.

Elderly: Of 1,357 patients who received alefacept in clinical trials, 100 were 65 years of age and older and 13 were 75 years of age and older. No differences in safety or efficacy were observed between older and younger patients, but there were not sufficient data to exclude important differences. Because the incidence of infections and certain malignancies is higher in the elderly population, use caution in treating elderly patients.

Carcinogenicity: In a chronic toxicity study, cynomolgus monkeys were dosed weekly for 52 weeks with intravenous (IV) alefacept at 1 mg/kg/dose or 20 mg/kg/dose. One animal in the high-dose group developed a B-cell lymphoma detected after 28 weeks of dosing. Additional animals in both dose groups developed B-cell hyperplasia of the spleen and lymph nodes. All animals in the study were positive for an endemic primate gammaherpes virus, also known as lymphocryptovirus. Latent lymphocryptovirus infection is generally asymptomatic, but can lead to B-cell lymphomas when animals are immune suppressed.

In a separate study, baboons given 3 doses of alefacept at 1 mg/kg every 8 weeks were found to have centroblast proliferation in B-cell–dependent areas in the germinal centers of the spleen after a 116-day washout period.

The role of alefacept in the development of the lymphoid malignancy and the hyperplasia observed in nonhuman primates and the relevance to humans is unknown. Immunodeficiency-associated lymphocyte disorders (plasmacytic hyperplasia, polymorphic proliferation, and B-cell lymphomas) occur in patients who have congenital or acquired immunodeficiencies, including those resulting from immunosuppressive therapy.

Alefacept (Recombinant)

Mutagenicity: Mutagenicity studies were conducted in vitro and in vivo; no evidence of mutagenicity was observed.

Fertility Impairment: Alefacept has not been evaluated for impairment of fertility.

Pregnancy: Category B. Women of childbearing potential make up a considerable segment of patients affected by psoriasis. Because the effect of alefacept on pregnancy and fetal development, including immune system development, is not known, health care providers should enroll patients currently taking alefacept who become pregnant into the Biogen Idec Pregnancy Registry by calling (866) AME-VIVE ([866] 263-8483). It is not known if alefacept crosses the human placenta.

Reproductive toxicology studies have been performed in cynomolgus monkeys at doses up to 5 mg/kg/week (approximately 62 times the human dose based on body weight) and revealed no evidence of impaired fertility or harm to the fetus caused by alefacept. No abortifacient or teratogenic effects were observed in cynomolgus monkeys after weekly IV bolus injections of alefacept during the period of organogenesis to gestation. Alefacept underwent transplacental passage and produced in utero exposure in the developing monkeys. In utero, serum levels of exposure in these monkeys were 23% of maternal serum levels. No evidence of fetal toxicity, including adverse effects on immune system development, was observed in any of these animals.

Animal reproduction studies, however, are not always predictive of human response and there are no adequate and well-controlled studies in pregnant women. Because the risk to the development of the fetal immune system and postnatal immune function in humans is unknown, use alefacept during pregnancy only if clearly needed. If pregnancy occurs while taking alefacept, continued use of the drug should be assessed.

Lactation: It is not known if alefacept crosses into human breast milk. Decide whether to discontinue breast-feeding or the drug, taking into account the importance of the drug to the mother.

Children: Safety and efficacy of alefacept in children younger than 18 years of age have not been established. Alefacept is not indicated for pediatric patients.

Adverse Reactions: The most serious adverse reactions were lymphopenia, malignancies, serious infections requiring hospitalization, and hypersensitivity reactions.

Commonly observed adverse events seen in the first course of clinical trials with at least 2% higher incidence in alefacept-treated patients compared with placebo-treated patients were pharyngitis, dizziness, increased cough, nausea, pruritus, myalgia, chills, injection-site pain, injection-site inflammation, and accidental injury. The only adverse event that occurred at an incidence of 5% or more among alefacept-treated patients compared with placebo-treated patients was chills (1% in those receiving placebo vs 6% in those receiving alefacept), predominantly with IV dosing.

Adverse reactions most commonly resulting in clinical intervention were cardiovascular events, including coronary artery disorder (less than 1%) and myocardial infarction (less than 1%). These events were not observed in any of the 413 placebo-treated patients. The number of patients hospitalized for cardiovascular events in the alefacept-treated group was 1.2%.

The most common events resulting in discontinuation of alefacept were CD4+ T-lymphocyte levels less than 250 cells/mcL, headache (0.2%), and nausea (0.2%).

The following data reflect exposure to alefacept in 1,357 psoriasis patients, 85% of whom received 1 to 2 courses of therapy and the rest of whom received 3 to 6 courses and were followed for up to 3 years. Of 1,357 patients, 876 received their first course in placebo-controlled studies. The population studied ranged from 16 to 84 years of age and included 69% men and 31% women. The patients were mostly white (89%), reflecting the general psoriatic population. Disease severity at baseline was moderate to severe psoriasis.

576

Hematologic: Alefacept induces dose-dependent reductions in circulating CD4+ and CD8+ T-lymphocyte counts. Do not start a course of alefacept therapy in patients with a CD4+ T-lymphocyte count below normal. Monitor CD4+ T-lymphocyte counts weekly throughout the course of the 12-week dosing regimen. Withhold dosing if CD4+ T-lymphocyte counts fall below 250 cells/mcL. Discontinue the drug if the counts remain less than 250 cells/mcL for 1 month.

In the intramuscular (IM) study (study 2), 4% of patients temporarily discontinued treatment and no patients permanently discontinued treatment due to CD4+ T-lymphocyte counts below the specified threshold of 250 cells/mcL. In study 2, 10%, 28%, and 42% of patients had total lymphocyte, CD4+, and CD8+ T-lymphocyte counts below normal, respectively. Twelve weeks after a course of therapy (12 weekly doses), 2%, 8%, and 21% of patients had total lymphocyte, CD4+, and CD8+ T-cell counts below normal.

In the first course of the IV study (study 1), 10% of patients temporarily discontinued treatment and 2% permanently discontinued treatment due to CD4+ T-lymphocyte counts below the specified threshold of 250 cells/mcL. During the first course of study 1, 22% of patients had total lymphocyte counts below normal, 48% had CD4+ T-lymphocyte counts below normal, and 59% had CD8+ T-lymphocyte counts below normal. The maximal effect on lymphocytes was observed within 6 to 8 weeks of initiation of treatment. Twelve weeks after a course of therapy (12 weekly doses), 4% of patients had total lymphocyte counts below normal, 19% had CD4+ T-lymphocyte counts below normal, and 36% had CD8+ T-lymphocyte counts below normal.

For patients receiving a second course of alefacept in study 1, 17% of patients had total lymphocyte counts below normal, 44% had CD4+ T-lymphocyte counts below normal, and 56% had CD8+ T-lymphocyte counts below normal. Twelve weeks after completing dosing, 3% of patients had total lymphocyte counts below normal, 17% had CD4+ T-lymphocyte counts below normal, and 35% had CD8+ T-lymphocyte counts below normal.

Hepatic: Rare cases of transaminase elevations 5 to 10 times the upper limit of normal occurred during alefacept therapy.

Hypersensitivity: In clinical studies, 2 patients experienced angioedema; 1 was hospitalized. In the 24-week period constituting the first course of placebo-controlled studies, urticaria was reported in 6 (less than 1%) alefacept-treated patients versus 1 patient in the control group. Urticaria resulted in discontinuation of therapy in 1 of the alefacept-treated patients. Hypersensitivity reactions (eg, urticaria, angioedema) were associated with alefacept. If an anaphylactic reaction or other serious allergic reaction occurs, discontinue alefacept immediately and start appropriate therapy.

Immunogenicity: Approximately 3% (35/1,306) of patients receiving alefacept developed low-titer antibodies to alefacept. No apparent correlation of antibody development and clinical response or adverse events was observed. The long-term immunogenicity of alefacept is unknown. The data reflect the percentage of patients whose test results were considered positive for antibodies to alefacept in an enzyme-linked immunosorbent assay (ELISA) and are highly dependent on the sensitivity and specificity of the assay.

Infections: Alefacept is an immunosuppressive agent and, therefore, may increase the risk of infection and reactivate latent, chronic infections. Do not administer alefacept to patients with a clinically important infection. Exercise caution in patients with chronic infections or a history of recurrent infection. Monitor patients for signs and symptoms of infection during or after a course of alefacept. Closely monitor new infections. If a patient develops a serious infection, discontinue alefacept.

In the 24-week period constituting the first course of placebo-controlled studies, serious infections (infections requiring hospitalization) occurred at a rate of 0.9% (8/876) in alefacept-treated patients and 0.2% (1/413) in the placebo group. In patients receiving repeated courses of alefacept therapy, the rates were 0.7% (5/756) and 11% (3/199) in the second and third course of therapy, respectively. Serious infections among 1,357 alefacept-treated patients included necrotizing cellulitis, peritonsillar abscess, postoperative and burn-wound infection, toxic shock, pneumonia, appendicitis, preseptal cellulitis, cholecystitis, gastroenteritis, and herpes simplex infection.

Injection-site reactions: In the IM study (study 2), 16% of alefacept-treated patients and 8% of placebo-treated patients reported injection-site reactions. These reactions were generally mild, typically occurred on single occasions, and included either pain (7%), inflammation (4%), bleeding (4%), edema (2%), nonspecific reaction (2%), mass (1%), or skin hypersensitivity (less than 1%). In clinical trials, 1 injection-site reaction led to discontinuation of alefacept.

Malignancies: Alefacept may increase the risk of malignancies. Some patients who received alefacept in clinical studies developed malignancies. In preclinical studies, animals developed B-cell hyperplasia, and 1 animal developed a lymphoma. Do not administer alefacept to patients with a history of systemic malignancy. Exercise caution when considering alefacept in patients at a high risk for malignancy. If a patient develops a malignancy, discontinue alefacept. In the 24-week period constituting the first course of placebo-controlled studies, the incidence of malignancies was 1.3% (11/876) for alefacept-treated patients compared with 0.5% (2/413) in the placebo group.

Among 1,357 patients who received alefacept, 25 patients were diagnosed with 35 treatment-emergent malignancies. Most of these malignancies (23) were basal (6) or squamous-cell cancers (17) of the skin. Three cases of lymphoma were observed; 1 non-Hodgkin follicle-center cell lymphoma and 2 cases of Hodgkin disease.

Pharmacologic & Dosing Characteristics

Dosage: 15 mg given once weekly as an IM injection. The recommended regimen is a course of 12 weekly injections. Retreatment with an additional 12-week course may be given, if CD4+ T-lymphocyte counts are within the normal range and at least 12 weeks pass after the previous course of treatment. Data on retreatment beyond 2 cycles are limited.

Route & Site: IM. Rotate injection sites. Do not inject into skin that is tender, bruised, red, or hard.

Overdosage: The highest dose tested in humans (0.75 mg/kg IV) was associated with chills, headache, arthralgia, and sinusitis within 1 day of dosing. Closely monitor patients who have been inadvertently administered an excess dose for effects on total lymphocyte count and CD4+ T-lymphocyte count.

Missed Doses: Interrupting the recommended schedule or delaying subsequent doses does not require restarting the series.

Laboratory Tests: Monitor CD4+ T-lymphocyte counts weekly during the 12-week dosing period to guide dosing. Patients should have normal CD4+ T-lymphocyte counts before an initial or a subsequent course of treatment with alefacept. Withhold dosing if CD4+ T-lymphocyte counts fall below 250 cells/mcL. Discontinue alefacept if CD4+ T-lymphocyte counts remain less than 250 cells/mcL for 1 month.

Efficacy: Two randomized, double-blind, placebo-controlled studies evaluated alefacept in adults with chronic (1 year or more) plaque psoriasis and at least 10% body surface area involvement who were candidates for or previously received systemic therapy or phototherapy. Each course consisted of 1 weekly dose for 12 weeks (IV for study 1, IM for study 2) of placebo or alefacept. Patients could receive concomitant low-potency topical steroids. Concomitant phototherapy or systemic therapy was not allowed.

In study 1, patients randomly received 1 or 2 courses of alefacept 7.5 mg by IV bolus. The first and second courses in the 2-course cohort were separated by at least 12 weeks. Study 2 compared patients treated with either 10 mg or 15 mg of alefacept IM.

In studies 1 and 2, 77% of patients had previously received systemic therapy and/or photo-therapy for psoriasis. Of these, 23% and 19%, respectively, had failed to respond to 1 or more of these previous therapies.

The table below shows treatment response in the first course of study 1 and study 2. Response to treatment was defined as the proportion of patients with a reduction in score on the Psoriasis Area Sensitivity Index (PASI) of 75% or more from baseline at 2 weeks after the 12-week treatment period. Other treatment responses included the proportion of patients who achieved a scoring of "almost clear" or "clear" by physician global assessment (PGA) and the proportion of patients with a reduction in PASI of 50% or more from baseline 2 weeks after the 12-week treatment period.

Percentage of Patients Responding to the First Course of Treatment in Study 1 (IV Study) and Study 2 (IM Study)						
	Alefacept study 1			Alefacept study 2		
Treatment response	Placebo (n = 186)	7.5 mg IV (n = 367)[a]	Difference (95% CI)	Placebo (n = 168)	15 mg IM (n = 166)	Difference (95% CI)
≥ 75% reduction PASI	4%	14%	10[b] (6, 15)	5%	21%	16[b] (9, 23)
≥ 50% reduction PASI	10%	38%	28[b] (22, 35)	18%	42%	24[b] (14, 33)
PGA "almost clear" or "clear"	4%	11%	7[c] (3, 12)	5%	14%	9[d](3, 15)

a Cohorts 1 and 2 combined.
b P values < 0.001.
c P value = 0.004.
d P value = 0.006.

In study 2, the proportion of responders to 10 mg IM was higher than placebo, but the difference was not statistically significant.

Onset: In both studies, onset of response to alefacept treatment (50% or more reduction in PASI) began 60 days after the start of therapy. Some patients achieved their maximal response beyond 2 weeks postdosing. In studies 1 and 2, an additional 11% (42/367) and 7% (12/166) of patients treated with alefacept, respectively, achieved a 75% reduction from baseline PASI score at 1 or more visits after the first 2 weeks of the follow-up period.

Duration: With 1 course of therapy in study I (IV route), the median duration of response (75% or more reduction in PASI) was 3.5 months for alefacept-treated patients and 1 month for placebo-treated patients. In study 2 (IM route), the median duration of response was approximately 2 months for both alefacept-treated patients and placebo-treated patients. Most patients who responded to either alefacept or placebo maintained a 50% or more reduction in PASI through the 3-month observation period. The responders (n = 52) in a subset of patients in study 1 who crossed over to placebo for course 2 (Cohort 2) maintained a 50% or more reduction in PASI for a median of 7 months.

Pharmacokinetics: Immunoglobulins are primarily eliminated by catabolism. In patients with moderate to severe plaque psoriasis, after a 7.5 mg IV administration, the mean volume of distribution of alefacept was 94 mL/kg, the mean clearance was 0.25 mL/h/kg, and the mean elimination half-life was approximately 270 hours. After IM injection, bioavailability was 63%.

In healthy male volunteers administered a 0.15 mg/kg IV bolus, 0.04 mg/kg IM injection, or 0.04 mg/kg 30-minute IV infusion, IV infusion produced a higher maximal drug concentration (C_{max}) (0.96 ± 0.26 mcg/mL vs 0.36 ± 0.19 mcg/mL) and a shorter time to maximal drug concentration (T_{max}) (2.8 ± 1.9 h vs 86 ± 60 h) compared with IM injection. Based on area under the curve, the relative bioavailability of IM to IV infusion was approximately 60%. After absorption from IM injection was complete, the rate of alefacept elimination from serum appeared consistent with IV infusion half-life (approximately 12 days). Biologic activity was demonstrated by transient reductions in CD2-positive lymphocytes, with notable specificity for memory T-cell subsets.

The pharmacokinetics of alefacept in pediatric patients have not been studied. The effects of renal or hepatic impairment on the pharmacokinetics of alefacept have not been studied.

At doses tested in clinical trials, alefacept therapy resulted in a dose-dependent decrease in circulating total lymphocytes. This reduction predominantly affected the memory-effector subset of the CD4+ and CD8+ T-lymphocyte compartments (CD4+CD45RO+ and CD8+CD45RO+), the predominant phenotype in psoriatic lesions. Circulating naive T-lymphocyte and natural killer cell counts appeared to be only minimally susceptible to alefacept treatment, while circulating B-lymphocyte counts appeared not to be affected by alefacept.

Mechanism: Alefacept interferes with lymphocyte activation by specifically binding to lymphocyte antigen CD2 and inhibiting LFA-3/CD2 interaction. Activation of T-lymphocytes involving the interaction between LFA-3 on antigen-presenting cells and CD2 on T-lymphocytes plays a role in the pathophysiology of chronic plaque psoriasis. Most T-lymphocytes in psoriatic lesions are of the memory effector phenotype characterized by the presence of the CD45RO marker, express activation markers (eg, CD25, CD69), and release inflammatory cytokines, such as interferon gamma.

Alefacept also reduces subsets of CD2+ T-lymphocytes (primarily CD45RO+), presumably by bridging between CD2 on target lymphocytes and immunoglobulin Fc receptors on cytotoxic cells, such as natural killer cells. Alefacept reduces total CD4+ and CD8+ T-lymphocyte counts. CD2 is also expressed at low levels on the surface of natural killer cells and certain bone marrow B-lymphocytes. Therefore, the potential exists for alefacept to affect the activation and numbers of cells other than T-lymphocytes. In clinical studies, minor changes in the numbers of circulating cells other than T-lymphocytes have been observed.

Drug Interactions: No formal drug-interaction studies have been performed. Patients receiving other immunosuppressive agents or phototherapy should not receive concurrent therapy with alefacept because of the possibility of excessive immunosuppression. The duration of the period after treatment with alefacept before starting other immunosuppressive therapy has not been evaluated.

The safety and efficacy of vaccines, especially live or live-attenuated vaccines, administered to patients treated with alefacept have not been studied. Among 46 patients with chronic plaque psoriasis, the ability to mount immunity to tetanus toxoid (recall antigen) and an experimental neoantigen was preserved in those patients undergoing alefacept therapy.

Patient Information: Inform patients of the need for regular monitoring of lymphocyte counts during therapy. Inform patients that alefacept reduces lymphocyte counts, which could increase their chances of developing an infection or a malignancy. Advise patients to inform their physicians promptly if they develop any signs of an infection or malignancy while undergoing a course of treatment with alefacept. Advise female patients to notify their physicians if they become pregnant while taking alefacept (or within 8 weeks after discontinuing alefacept). In such cases, encourage enrollment in the pregnancy registry (call [866] AMEVIVE for information).

Pharmaceutical Characteristics

Packaging: Carton containing 1 alefacept 15 mg vial, one 10 mL single-use vial of sterile water, one 1 mL syringe, and two 23-gauge 1¼-inch needles (NDC#: 00469-0021-04); or carton containing 4 alefacept 15 mg vials, four 10 mL single-use vials of sterile water, four 1 mL syringes, and eight 23-gauge 1¼-inch needles (00469-0021-03)

Doseform: Powder for solution

Appearance: White-to-off-white powder. After reconstitution, the solution is clear and colorless to slightly yellow.

Diluent:

For reconstitution: 0.6 mL of sterile water. When adding diluent, keep the needle pointed at the side wall of the vial and slowly inject the diluent into the vial. Some foaming will occur, which is normal. To avoid excessive foaming, do not shake or vigorously agitate. Swirl the contents gently during dissolution. Generally, dissolution of alefacept takes less than 2 minutes. After withdrawing reconstituted alefacept solution from vial into syringe, some foam or bubbles may remain in the vial.

Adjuvant: None

Preservative: None

Allergens: None

Excipients: Both the IV and the IM formulations contain sucrose 12.5 mg, glycine 5 mg, sodium citrate dihydrate 3.6 mg, and citric acid monohydrate 0.06 mg per 0.5 mL.

pH: 6.9 after reconstitution

Shelf Life: Expires within 24 months

Storage/Stability: Store dose trays of alefacept powder at controlled room temperature (15° to 30°C [59° to 86°F]). Contact the manufacturer regarding exposure to extreme temperatures. Shipped by overnight courier in insulated container with coolant packs to maintain temperature between 2° and 25°C (36° to 77°F).

After reconstitution, use the product within 4 hours if stored in the vial at 2° to 8°C (36° to 46°F). Discard unused alefacept after 4 hours.

Handling: Protect from light. Retain in carton until time of use. Do not add other medications to solutions containing alefacept. Do not reconstitute alefacept with other diluents. Do not filter reconstituted solution during preparation or administration.

Production Process: Produced by recombinant-DNA technology using a Chinese hamster ovary (CHO) mammalian cell expression system.

Media: CHO cells

Other Information

First Licensed: January 30, 2003

References: Kyle S, Chandler D, Griffiths CE, et al; British Society for Rheumatology Standards Guidelines Audit Working Group (SGAWG). Guideline for anti-TNF-alpha therapy in psoriatic arthritis [published corrections appear in *Rheumatology (Oxford)*. 2005;44(4):569; *Rheumatology (Oxford)*. 2005;44(5):701]. *Rheumatology (Oxford)*. 2005;44(3):390-397.

Langley RG, Cherman AM, Gupta AK. Alefacept: an expert review concerning the treatment of psoriasis. *Expert Opin Pharmacother*. 2005;6(13):2327-2333.

Scheinfeld N. Alefacept: a safety profile. *Expert Opin Drug Saf*. 2005;4(6):975-985.

Alemtuzumab (Humanized)

Isoantibodies

Name:
CamPath

Manufacturer:
Genzyme

Synonyms: CamPath-1H, anti-CD52 antibody

Immunologic Characteristics

Target Antigen: 21-28 kD cell surface glycoprotein, CD52. CD52 is expressed on the surface of normal and malignant B and T lymphocytes, natural killer (NK) cells, monocytes, macrophages, and tissues of the male reproductive system.

Viability: Inactive, passive, transient

Antigenic Form: Humanized (human/murine) monoclonal IgG1 antibody

Antigenic Type: Protein, IgG1κ with human variable framework and constant regions and complementarity-determining regions from a murine (rat) monoclonal antibody (CamPath-1G). Molecular weight of approximately 150 kilodaltons.

Use Characteristics

Indications: To treat B-cell chronic lymphocytic leukemia (B-CLL) in patients who have been treated with alkylating agents and who have failed fludarabine therapy. Determination of the effectiveness of alemtuzumab is based on overall response rates.

Unlabeled Uses: Alemtuzumab is being investigated in the treatment of solid organ-transplant rejection, multiple sclerosis, and non-Hodgkin lymphoma.

Limitations: Comparative, randomized trials demonstrating increased survival or clinical benefits, such as improvement in disease-related symptoms, have not yet been conducted.

Contraindications:

Absolute: None

Relative: People who have active systemic infections, underlying immunodeficiency (eg, seropositive for HIV), or known type I hypersensitivity or anaphylactic reactions to alemtuzumab or any of its components.

Immunodeficiency: Alemtuzumab is contraindicated in immunocompromised patients because the medication induces profound lymphopenia.

Elderly: Of the 149 patients with B-CLL enrolled in the 3 clinical studies, 66 (44%) were 65 years of age and older, while 15 (10%) were 75 years of age and older. Substantial differences in safety and efficacy related to age were not observed; however, the size of the database is not sufficient to exclude important differences.

Carcinogenicity: No long-term studies in animals have been performed to establish the carcinogenic potential of alemtuzumab.

Mutagenicity: No long-term studies in animals have been performed to establish the mutagenic potential of alemtuzumab.

Fertility Impairment: Alemtuzumab has not been evaluated for fertility impairment in males or females. Women and men of reproductive potential should use effective contraceptive methods during treatment and for 6 months or longer following alemtuzumab therapy.

Pregnancy: Category C. Animal reproduction studies have not been conducted with alemtuzumab. It is not known whether alemtuzumab can cause fetal harm when administered to a pregnant woman. However, human IgG is known to cross the placental barrier and, therefore, alemtuzumab may cross the placental barrier and cause fetal B- and T-lymphocyte depletion. Alemtuzumab should be given to a pregnant woman only if clearly needed.

Lactation: Excretion of alemtuzumab in human breast milk has not been studied. Because many drugs, including human IgG, are excreted in human breast milk, breastfeeding should be discontinued during treatment and for 3 months or longer following the last dose of alemtuzumab.

Children: Safety and efficacy of alemtuzumab in children have not been established.

Adverse Reactions: Safety data, except where indicated, are based on 149 patients with B-CLL enrolled in studies of alemtuzumab administered at a maintenance dose of 30 mg IV 3 times weekly for 4 to 12 weeks as a single agent. More detailed information and follow-up were available for study 1 (93 patients); therefore, the narrative description of certain events, noted below, is based on this study.

Infusion-related adverse events resulted in discontinuation of alemtuzumab therapy in 6% of the patients enrolled in study 1. The most commonly reported infusion-related adverse events in this study included rigors (89%), drug-related fever (83%), nausea (47%), vomiting (33%), and hypotension (15%). Other frequently reported infusion-related events included rash (30%), fatigue (22%), urticaria (22%), dyspnea (17%), pruritus (14%), headache (13%), and diarrhea (13%). Similar types of adverse events were reported on the supporting studies. Acute infusion-related events were most common during the first week of therapy. Antihistamines, acetaminophen, antiemetics, meperidine, and corticosteroids, as well as incremental dose escalation were used to prevent or ameliorate infusion-related events.

Infection: During study 1, all patients were required to receive antiherpes and anti-*Pneumocystis carinii* pneumonia (PCP) prophylaxis and were followed for infections for 6 months. Forty (43%) of 93 patients experienced 59 infections (1 or more infections per patient) related to alemtuzumab during treatment or within 6 months of the last dose. Of these, 34 (37%) patients experienced 42 infections that were of NCI-CTC grade 3 or 4 severity; 11 (18%) were fatal. Fifty-five percent of the grade 3 or 4 infections occurred during treatment or within 30 days of the last dose. In addition 1 or more episodes of febrile neutropenia (absolute neutrophil count [ANC] 500 cells/mcL or fewer) were reported in 10% of patients.

The following types of infections were reported in study 1: grade 3 or 4 sepsis in 12% of patients with 1 fatality, grade 3 or 4 pneumonia in 15% with 5 fatalities, and opportunistic infections in 17% with 4 fatalities. *Candida* infections were reported in 5% of patients; cytomegalovirus infections in 8% (4% of grade 3 or 4 severity); aspergillosis in 2% with fatal aspergillosis in 1%; fatal mucormycosis in 2%; fatal cryptococcal pneumonia in 1%; *Listeria monocytogenes* meningitis in 1%; disseminated herpes zoster in 1%; grade 3 herpes simplex in 2%; and *Torulopsis* pneumonia in 1%. PCP occurred in 1 (1%) patient who discontinued PCP prophylaxis.

In studies 2 and 3 in which antiherpes and anti-PCP prophylaxis were optional, 37 (66%) patients had 47 infections while or after receiving alemtuzumab therapy. In addition to the opportunistic infections reported above, the following types of related events were observed on these studies: interstitial pneumonitis of unknown etiology and progressive multifocal leukoencephalopathy.

Hematologic: Severe, prolonged, and in rare instances, fatal myelosuppression has occurred in patients with leukemia and lymphoma receiving alemtuzumab. Bone marrow aplasia and hypoplasia were observed in the clinical studies at the recommended dose. The incidence of these complications increased with doses above the recommended dose. In addition, severe and fatal autoimmune anemia and thrombocytopenia were observed in patients with CLL. Discontinue alemtuzumab for severe hematologic toxicity or in any patient with evidence of autoimmune hematologic toxicity. Following resolution of transient, non-immune myelosuppression, alemtuzumab may be reinitiated with caution. There is no information on the safety of resumption of alemtuzumab in patients with autoimmune cytopenias or marrow aplasia.

Anemia: Forty-four (47%) patients had 1 or more episodes of new onset NCI-CTC grade 3 or 4 anemia. Sixty-two (67%) patients required red blood cell (RBC) transfusions. In addition, erythropoietin use was reported in 19 (20%) patients. Autoimmune hemolytic anemia secondary to alemtuzumab therapy was reported in 1% of patients. Positive Coombs test without hemolysis was reported in 2%.

Lymphopenia: The median CD4$^+$ count at 4 weeks after initiation of alemtuzumab therapy was 2 cells/mcL; 207 cells/mcL at 2 months after discontinuation of alemtuzumab therapy, and 470 cells/mcL at 6 months after discontinuation. The pattern of change in median CD8$^+$ lymphocyte counts was similar to that of CD4$^+$ cells. In some patients treated with alemtuzumab, CD4$^+$ and CD8$^+$ lymphocyte counts had not returned to baseline levels more than 1 year posttherapy.

Neutropenia: Sixty-five (70%) patients had 1 or more episodes of NCI-CTC grade 3 or 4 neutropenia. Median duration of grade 3 or 4 neutropenia was 28 days (range, 2 to 165 days).

Pancytopenia/Marrow hypoplasia: Alemtuzumab therapy was permanently discontinued in 6 (6%) patients because of pancytopenia/marrow hypoplasia. Two (2%) cases were fatal.

Thrombocytopenia: Forty-eight (52%) patients had one or more episodes of new onset grade 3 or 4 thrombocytopenia. Median duration of thrombocytopenia was 21 days (range, 2 to 165 days). Thirty-five (38%) patients required platelet transfusions for management of thrombocytopenia. Autoimmune thrombocytopenia was reported in 2% of patients with 1 fatal case of alemtuzumab-related autoimmune thrombocytopenia.

Immunosuppression: Alemtuzumab induces profound lymphopenia. A variety of opportunistic infections have been reported in patients receiving alemtuzumab therapy. If a serious infection occurs, interrupt alemtuzumab therapy. It may be reinitiated following resolution of the infection.

Infections: Serious, sometimes fatal bacterial, viral, fungal, and protozoan infections have been reported in patients receiving alemtuzumab therapy. Prophylaxis directed against PCP and herpes virus infections decreased, but did not eliminate, the occurrence of these infections.

Immunogenicity: Four (1.9%) of 211 patients evaluated for development of an immune response were found to have antibodies to alemtuzumab. The data reflect the percentage of patients whose test results were considered positive for antibody to alemtuzumab in a kinetic enzyme immunoassay, and are highly dependent on the sensitivity and specificity of the assay. The observed incidence of antibody positivity may be influenced by several additional factors, including sample handling, concomitant medications, and underlying disease. For these reasons, comparison of the incidence of antibodies to alemtuzumab with the incidence of antibodies to other products may be misleading. Patients who develop hypersensitivity to alemtuzumab may have allergic or hypersensitivity reactions to other monoclonal antibodies.

Serious adverse events: The following serious adverse events, defined as events that result in death, require or prolong hospitalization, or require medical intervention to prevent hospitalization or malignancy, were reported in at least 1 patient treated in studies where alemtuzumab was used as a single agent. These studies were conducted in patients with lymphocytic leukemia and lymphoma (n = 745) and in patients with nonmalignant diseases (n = 152), such as rheumatoid arthritis, solid organ transplant, or multiple sclerosis.

Body as a whole: Allergic reactions, anaphylactoid reaction, ascites, hypovolemia, influenza-like syndrome, mouth edema, neutropenic fever, syncope.

Cardiovascular: Cardiac failure, cyanosis, atrial fibrillation, cardiac arrest, ventricular arrhythmia, ventricular tachycardia, angina pectoris, coronary artery disorder, myocardial infarction, pericarditis.

Central/Peripheral nervous system: Abnormal gait, aphasia, coma, grand mal convulsions, paralysis, meningitis.

Endocrine: Hyperthyroidism.

Gastrointestinal (GI): Duodenal ulcer, esophagitis, gingivitis, gastroenteritis, GI hemorrhage, hematemesis, hemorrhoids, intestinal obstruction, intestinal perforation, melena, paralytic ileus, peptic ulcer, pseudomembranous colitis, colitis, pancreatitis, peritonitis, hyperbilirubinemia, hepatic failure, hepatocellular damage, hypoalbuminemia, biliary pain.

Hearing/Vestibular: Decreased hearing.

Metabolic/Nutritional: Acidosis, aggravated diabetes mellitus, dehydration, fluid overload, hyperglycemia, hyperkalemia, hypokalemia, hypoglycemia, hyponatremia, increased alkaline phosphatase, respiratory alkalosis.

Musculoskeletal: Arthritis or worsening arthritis, arthropathy, bone fracture, myositis, muscle atrophy, muscle weakness, osteomyelitis, polymyositis.

Neoplasms: Malignant lymphoma, malignant testicular neoplasm, prostatic cancer, plasma cell dyscrasia, secondary leukemia, squamous cell carcinoma, transformation to aggressive lymphoma, transformation to prolymphocytic leukemia.

Platelet/Bleeding/Clotting disorders: Coagulation disorder, disseminated intravascular coagulation, hematoma, pulmonary embolism, thrombocythemia.

Psychiatric: Confusion, hallucinations, nervousness, abnormal thinking, apathy.

RBC disorder: Hemolysis, hemolytic anemia, splenic infarction, splenomegaly.

Reproductive system: Cervical dysplasia.

Resistance mechanism: Abscess, bacterial infection, herpes zoster infection, *Pneumocystis carinii* infection, otitis media, tuberculosis infection, viral infection.

Respiratory: Asthma, bronchitis, chronic obstructive pulmonary disease, hemoptysis, hypoxia, pleural effusion, pleurisy, pneumothorax, pulmonary edema, pulmonary fibrosis, pulmonary infiltration, respiratory depression, respiratory insufficiency, sinusitis, stridor, throat tightness.

Skin/Appendages: Angioedema, bullous eruption, cellulitis, purpuric rash.

Special senses: Taste loss.

Urinary: Abnormal renal function, acute renal failure, anuria, facial edema, hematuria, toxic nephropathy, ureteric obstruction, urinary retention, urinary tract infection.

Vascular (extracardiac): Cerebral hemorrhage, cerebrovascular disorder, deep vein thrombosis, increased capillary fragility, intracranial hemorrhage, phlebitis, subarachnoid hemorrhage, thrombophlebitis.

Vision: Endophthalmitis.

White cell and reticuloendothelial: Agranulocytosis, aplasia, decreased haptoglobin, lymphadenopathy, marrow depression.

Other adverse events: The following adverse events occurred in more than 5% of the B-CLL study population during treatment or within 30 days (n = 149). The percentages reflect occurrences in any grade, followed by the frequency of severity grade 3 or 4.

Body as a whole: Rigors (86%, 16%), fever (85%, 19%), fatigue (34%, 5%), pain or skeletal pain (24%, 2%), anorexia (20%, 3%), asthenia (13%, 4%), edema or peripheral edema (13%, 1%), back pain (10%, 3%), chest pain (10%, 1%), malaise (9%, 1%), temperature change sensation (5%, 0%).

Cardiovascular: Hypotension (32%, 5%), hypertension (11%, 2%).

Central nervous system: Headache (24%, 1%), dysthesia (15%, 0%), dizziness (12%, 1%), tremor (7%, 0%).

Alemtuzumab (Humanized)

GI: Nausea (54%, 2%), vomiting (41%, 4%), diarrhea (22%, 1%), stomatitis, ulcerative stomatitis, or mucositis (14%, 1%), abdominal pain (11%, 2%), dyspepsia (10%, 0%), constipation (9%, 1%).

Heart rate and rhythm: Tachycardia (11%, 3%).

Hematologic: Neutropenia (85%, 64%), anemia (80%, 38%), pancytopenia (5%, 3%), thrombocytopenia (72%, 50%), purpura (8%, 0%), epistaxis (7%, 1%).

Musculoskeletal: Myalgia (11%, 0%).

Psychiatric: Insomnia (10%, 0%), depression (7%, 1%), somnolence (5%, 1%).

Resistance mechanism: Sepsis (15%, 10%), herpes simplex (11%, 1%), moniliasis (8%, 1%), other viral or unidentified infection (7%, 1%).

Respiratory: Dyspnea (26%, 9%), cough (25%, 2%), bronchitis or pneumonitis (21%, 13%), pneumonia (16%, 10%), pharyngitis (12%, 0%), bronchospasm (9%, 2%), rhinitis (7%, 0%).

Skin and appendage: Rash, maculopapular rash, or erythematous rash (40%, 3%), urticaria (30%, 5%), pruritus (24%, 1%), increased sweating (19%, 1%).

Pharmacologic & Dosing Characteristics

Dosage: Initiate alemtuzumab therapy at a 3 mg dose administered as a 2-hour IV infusion daily. When the alemtuzumab 3 mg daily dose is tolerated (eg, infusion-related toxicities are grade 2), escalate the daily dose to 10 mg and continue as tolerated. After the 10 mg dose is tolerated, the maintenance dose of alemtuzumab 30 mg may be initiated. The maintenance dose of alemtuzumab is 30 mg/day administered 3 times per week on alternate days (ie, Monday, Wednesday, and Friday) for up to 12 weeks. In most patients, escalation to 30 mg can be accomplished in 3 to 7 days. Dose escalation to the recommended maintenance dose of 30 mg administered 3 times per week is required.

Route: IV only. Administer the infusion over a 2-hour period. Do not administer as an IV push or bolus.

Special Handling: Alemtuzumab has been associated with infusion-related events, including: Hypotension, rigors, fever, shortness of breath, bronchospasm, chills, or rash. To ameliorate or avoid infusion-related events, premedicate patients with an oral antihistamine (eg, diphenhydramine 50 mg) and acetaminophen (eg, 650 mg) 30 minutes before the first dose, at dose escalations, and as clinically indicated. In cases where severe infusion-related events occur, treatment with hydrocortisone 200 mg was used during clinical trials to decrease infusion-related events. Monitor patients closely. In addition, initiate alemtuzumab at a low dose with gradual escalation to the effective dose. Carefully monitor blood pressure and hypotensive symptoms, especially in patients with ischemic heart disease and in patients on antihypertensive medications.

Discontinue alemtuzumab therapy during serious infection, serious hematologic toxicity, or other serious toxicity until the event resolves. Permanently discontinue alemtuzumab therapy if evidence of autoimmune anemia or thrombocytopenia appears. Consider the following recommendations for dose modification for severe neutropenia or thrombocytopenia:

- For first occurrence of ANC lower than 250 cells/mcL or platelet count 25,000 cells/mcL or lower: Withhold alemtuzumab therapy. When ANC is 500 cells/mcL or higher and platelet count is 50,000 cells/mcL or higher, resume alemtuzumab therapy at same dose. If delay between dosing is 7 days or longer, initiate therapy at alemtuzumab 3 mg, and escalate to 10 mg and then to 30 mg as tolerated.

- For second occurrence of ANC lower than 250 cells/mcL or platelet count 25,000 cells/mcL or lower: Withhold alemtuzumab therapy. When ANC is 500 cells/mcL or higher and platelet count is 50,000 cells/mcL or higher, resume alemtuzumab therapy at 10 mg. If delay between dosing is 7 days or longer, initiate therapy at alemtuzumab 3 mg and escalate to 10 mg only.

- For third occurrence of ANC lower than 250 cells/mcL or platelet count 25,000 cells/mcL or lower: Discontinue alemtuzumab therapy permanently.
- For a decrease of ANC or platelet count to 50% or less of the baseline value in patients initiating therapy with a baseline ANC 500 cells/mcL or lower or a baseline platelet count 25,000 cells/mcL or lower: Withhold alemtuzumab therapy. When ANC or platelet count return to baseline value(s), resume alemtuzumab therapy. If the delay between dosing 7 days or longer, initiate therapy at alemtuzumab 3 mg, escalate to 10 mg, and then to 30 mg as tolerated.

Overdosage: Do not administer single doses of alemtuzumab larger than 30 mg nor cumulative doses higher than 90 mg per week because these doses are associated with a higher incidence of pancytopenia. Initial doses of alemtuzumab higher than 3 mg are not well-tolerated. One patient who received 80 mg as an initial dose by IV infusion experienced acute bronchospasm, cough, and shortness of breath, followed by anuria and death. A review of the case suggested that tumor lysis syndrome may have played a role. There is no known specific antidote for alemtuzumab overdosage. Treatment consists of drug discontinuation and supportive therapy.

Missed Doses: If therapy is interrupted for 7 days or longer, reinstitute alemtuzumab with gradual dose escalation.

Related Interventions: Anti-infective prophylaxis is recommended upon initiation of therapy and for 2 months or longer following the last dose of alemtuzumab or until $CD4^+$ counts reaches 200 cells/mcL or higher. The anti-infective regimen used in study 1 consisted of trimethoprim/sulfamethoxazole double-strength twice daily 3 times per week and famciclovir or equivalent 250 mg twice a day upon initiation of alemtuzumab therapy. The median time to recovery of $CD4^+$ counts to 200 cells/mcL or higher was 2 months; however, full recovery (to baseline) of $CD4^+$ and $CD8^+$ counts may take longer than 12 months. Because of the potential for graft-versus-host disease (GVHD) in severely lymphopenic patients, irradiation of any blood products administered prior to recovery from lymphopenia is recommended.

Laboratory Tests: Obtain complete blood counts (CBC) and platelet counts at weekly intervals during alemtuzumab therapy and more frequently if worsening anemia, neutropenia, or thrombocytopenia is observed on therapy. Assess $CD4^+$ counts after treatment until recovery to 200 cells/mcL or higher.

Efficacy: Alemtuzumab was evaluated in an open-label, noncomparative study (study 1) of 93 patients with B-CLL previously treated with alkylating agents and who had failed treatment with fludarabine. Patients were gradually escalated to a maintenance dose of alemtuzumab 30 mg IV 3 times per week for 4 to 12 weeks.

Two supportive, open-label, noncomparative studies of alemtuzumab enrolled 56 patients with B-CLL (studies 2 and 3). These patients had been previously treated with fludarabine or other chemotherapies. In studies 2 and 3, the maintenance dose of alemtuzumab was 30 mg 3 times per week with treatment cycles of 8 and 6 weeks, respectively. A slightly different dose escalation scheme was used in these trials.

Objective tumor response rates and duration of response were determined using the NCI Working Group Response Criteria. A comparison of patient characteristics and the results for each of these studies appears in the following table. Time-to-event parameters, except for duration of response, are calculated from initiation of alemtuzumab therapy. Duration of response is calculated from the onset of the response.

Alemtuzumab (Humanized)

Summary of Patient Populations and Outcomes			
	Study 1 (n = 93)	Study 2 (n = 32)	Study 3 (n = 24)
Median age in years (range)	66 (32 to 68)	57 (46 to 75)	62 (44 to 77)
Median number of prior regimens (range)	3 (2 to 7)	3 (1 to 10)	3 (1 to 8)
Prior therapies			
Alkylating agents	100%	100%	92%
Fludarabine	100%	34%	100%
Disease characteristics			
Rai stage III/IV disease	76%	72%	71%
B-symptoms	42%	31%	21%
Overall response rate (95% CI)	33% (23%, 43%)	21% (8%, 33%)	29% (11%, 47%)
Complete response	2%	0%	0%
Partial response	31%	21%	29%
Median duration of response (months) (95% CI)	7 (5, 8)	7 (5, 23)	11 (6, 19)
Median time to response (months) (95% CI)	2 (1, 2)	4 (1, 5)	4 (2, 4)
Progression-free survival (months) (95% CI)	4 (3, 5)	5 (3, 7)	7 (3, 9)

Pharmacokinetics: Immunoglobulins are primarily eliminated by catabolism. The pharmacokinetic profile of alemtuzumab was studied in a rising-dose trial in non-Hodgkin lymphoma and CLL. Alemtuzumab was administered once weekly for 12 weeks or less. Following IV infusions over a range of doses, the maximum serum concentration (C_{max}) and the area under the curve (AUC) showed relative dose proportionality. The overall average half-life ($t_{\frac{1}{2}}$) over the dosing interval was approximately 12 days. The pharmacokinetic profile as a 30 mg IV infusion 3 times per week was evaluated in CLL patients. Peak and trough levels of alemtuzumab rose during the first few weeks of treatment and appeared to approach steady state by approximately week 6, although there was marked inter-patient variability. The rise in serum alemtuzumab concentration corresponded with the reduction in malignant lymphocytosis.

Mechanism: Alemtuzumab binds to CD52, a nonmodulating antigen that is present on the surface of essentially all B and T lymphocytes, a majority of monocytes, macrophages, NK cells, and a subpopulation of granulocytes. Analysis of samples collected from multiple volunteers did not identify CD52 expression on erythrocytes or hematopoetic stem cells. The proposed mechanism of action is antibody-dependent lysis of leukemic cells following cell surface binding. CamPath-1H Fab binding was observed in lymphoid tissues and the mononuclear phagocyte system. A proportion of bone marrow cells, including some CD34$^+$ cells, express variable levels of CD52. Significant binding was also observed in the skin and male reproductive tract (epididymis, sperm, seminal vesicle). Mature spermatozoa stain for CD52, but neither spermatogenic cells nor immature spermatozoa show evidence of staining.

Drug Interactions: No formal drug interaction studies have been performed with alemtuzumab. Patients who have recently received alemtuzumab should not be immunized with live viral vaccines due to immunosuppression. The safety of immunization with live viral vaccines following alemtuzumab therapy has not been studied. The ability to generate a primary or anamnestic humoral response to any vaccine following alemtuzumab therapy has not been studied.

Lab Interference: An immune response to alemtuzumab may interfere with subsequent diagnostic serum tests that utilize antibodies.

Patient Information:

Consultation: Alemtuzumab should be administered under the supervision of a physician experienced in the use of antineoplastic therapy. Serious hematologic toxicity has occurred in patients treated with alemtuzumab. Alemtuzumab can result in serious infusion reactions. Gradual escalation to the maintenance dose is required when beginning therapy and after interruption for 7 days or longer.

Pharmaceutical Characteristics

Concentration: 30 mg per 1 mL vial

Packaging: Single-use 30 mg per 1 mL clear glass vial (NDC#: 50419-0357-01, 50419-0355-10, 58468-0357-01), carton of 3 vials (58468-0357-03)

Doseform: Solution

Appearance: Clear, colorless solution

Solvent: Phosphate-buffered sodium chloride

Diluent:

For infusion: Withdraw desired quantity of alemtuzumab from the vial into a syringe. Inject alemtuzumab into 100 mL sodium chloride 0.9% or dextrose 5%. Gently invert the bag to mix the solution. Discard syringe and any unused drug product.

Adjuvant: None

Preservative: None

Allergens: Neomycin, used in manufacturing, is not detectable in the final product.

Excipients: Each 1 mL vial contains 8 mg sodium chloride, 1.44 mg dibasic sodium phosphate, 0.2 mg potassium chloride, 0.2 mg monobasic potassium phosphate, 0.1 mg polysorbate 80, and 0.0187 mg disodium edetate.

pH: 6.8 to 7.4

Shelf Life: Expires within 24 months

Storage/Stability: Store at 2° to 8°C (36° to 46°F). Discard frozen product. Contact the manufacturer regarding exposure to extreme temperatures. Shipping data not provided.

Use solution within 8 hours after dilution. Alemtuzumab solutions may be stored at room temperature (15° to 30°C, 59° to 86°F) or refrigerated. Protect alemtuzumab solutions from light.

No incompatibilities between alemtuzumab and polyvinylchloride (PVC) bags, PVC or polyethylene-lined PVC administration sets, or low-protein binding filters have been observed. No data are available concerning the incompatibility of alemtuzumab with other drug substances. Do not add or simultaneously infuse other drug substances through the same IV line.

Handling: Do not shake ampule before use. Protect from direct sunlight.

Production Process: Produced in mammalian cell (Chinese hamster ovary) suspension culture in a medium containing neomycin.

Media: Recombinant DNA Chinese hamster ovary cells

Disease Epidemiology

Prevalence: CLL is the most prevalent form of adult leukemia, affecting approximately 120,000 patients in the United States and Europe.

Alemtuzumab (Humanized)

Other Information

First Licensed: May 7, 2001

References: Dearden C. The role of alemtuzumab in the management of T-cell malignancies. *Semin Oncol.* 2006;33(2 Suppl 5):S44-S52.

Magliocca JF, Knechtle SJ. The evolving role of alemtuzumab (*Campath-1H*) for immunosuppressive therapy in organ transplantation. *Transpl Int.* 2006;19(9):705-714.

Morris PJ, Russell NK. Alemtuzumab (*Campath-1H*): a systematic review in organ transplantation. *Transplantation.* 2006;81(10):1361-1367.

Isoantibodies

Name:
  Benlysta

Manufacturer:
  Manufactured by Human Genome Sciences,
  distributed by GlaxoSmithKline

Synonyms: The target antigen is known as B-cell activating factor (BAFF)

Immunologic Characteristics

Target Antigen: Soluble human B lymphocyte stimulator (BLyS) protein (also referred to as BAFF and TNFSF13B)

Viability: Inactive, passive, transient

Antigenic Form: Human monoclonal IgG1λ antibody

Antigenic Type: Protein, human IgG1λ, anti-human cytokine BAFF (human monoclonal heavy chain) with disulfide bond to human BAFF lambda chain. Molecular weight approximately 147,000 daltons.

Use Characteristics

Indications: To treat adult patients with active, autoantibody-positive, systemic lupus erythematosus (SLE) who are receiving standard therapy.

Limitations: The efficacy of belimumab has not been evaluated in patients with severe active lupus nephritis or severe active CNS lupus. Belimumab has not been studied in combination with other biologics or intravenous (IV) cyclophosphamide and is not recommended in these situations.

Contraindications: People with a history of anaphylaxis with belimumab.

Immunodeficiency: No safety or efficacy data are available for immunodeficient patients.

Elderly: Clinical studies of belimumab did not include a sufficient number of subjects 65 years or older to determine if they respond differently from younger subjects. Use with caution in elderly patients.

Carcinogenicity: The effect of belimumab on the development of malignancies is not known. In controlled clinical trials, malignancies (including nonmelanoma skin cancers) were reported in 0.4% of patients receiving belimumab and 0.4% of patients receiving placebo. In controlled clinical trials, malignancies (excluding nonmelanoma skin cancers) were observed in 0.2% (3/1458) and 0.3% (2/675) of patients receiving belimumab and placebo, respectively. As with other immunomodulating agents, the mechanism of action of belimumab could increase the risk for the development of malignancies.

Mutagenicity: Belimumab has not been evaluated for mutagenic potential.

Fertility Impairment: Belimumab has not been evaluated for impairment of fertility.

Pregnancy: Category C. There are no adequate and well-controlled clinical studies using belimumab in pregnant women. Immunoglobulin G (IgG) antibodies, including belimumab, can cross the placenta. Because animal reproduction studies are not always predictive of human response, use belimumab during pregnancy only if the potential benefit to the mother justifies the potential risk to the fetus. Women of childbearing potential should use adequate contraception during treatment with belimumab and for at least 4 months after the final treatment. To monitor maternal-fetal outcomes of pregnant women exposed to belimumab, enroll these women in the belimumab pregnancy registry by calling 1-877-681-6296.

Nonclinical reproductive studies have been performed in pregnant cynomolgus monkeys receiving belimumab at doses of 0, 5, and 150 mg/kg by IV infusion (the high dose was approximately 9 times the anticipated maximum human exposure) every 2 weeks from gestation day 20 to 150. Belimumab was shown to cross the monkey placenta. Belimumab was not associated with direct or indirect teratogenicity under the conditions tested. Fetal deaths were observed in 14%, 24%, and 15% of pregnant females in the 0, 5, and 150 mg/kg groups, respectively. Infant deaths occurred at an incidence of 0%, 8%, and 5%. The cause of fetal and infant deaths is not known. The relevance of these findings to humans is not known. Other treatment-related findings were limited to the expected reversible reduction of B cells in both dams and infants and reversible reduction of immunoglobulin M (IgM) in infant monkeys. B cell numbers recovered after cessation of belimumab treatment by about 1 year postpartum in adult monkeys and by 3 months of age in infant monkeys. In infants exposed to belimumab in utero, IgM levels recovered by 6 months of age.

Lactation: It is not known whether belimumab is excreted in human milk or absorbed systemically after ingestion. However, belimumab was excreted into the milk of cynomolgus monkeys. Because maternal antibodies are excreted in human breast milk, decide whether to discontinue breast-feeding or the drug, taking into account the importance of breast-feeding to the infant and the importance of the drug to the mother.

Children: Safety and effectiveness of belimumab have not been established in children.

Adverse Reactions: The following data reflect exposure to belimumab plus standard of care compared with placebo plus standard of care in 2,133 patients in 3 controlled studies. Patients received belimumab at doses of 1 mg/kg (n = 673), 4 mg/kg (n = 111, trial 1 only), or 10 mg/kg (n = 674), or placebo (n = 675) IV over a 1-hour period on days 0, 14, and 28, and then every 28 days. In 2 of the studies (trials 1 and 3), treatment was given for 48 weeks, whereas in the other study (trial 2), treatment was given for 72 weeks. Because there was no apparent dose-related increase in most adverse events observed with belimumab, the safety data summarized below are presented for the 3 doses pooled unless otherwise indicated. The table displays the results for the recommended dose of 10 mg/kg compared with placebo. Treated patients had a mean age of 39 years (range, 18 to 75 years), 94% were women, and 52% were white. In these trials, 93% of patients treated with belimumab reported an adverse event compared with 92% treated with placebo.

The most common serious adverse events were serious infections (6% and 5.2% in the groups receiving belimumab and placebo, respectively). The most commonly reported adverse events occurring in at least 5% of patients in clinical trials were nausea, diarrhea, pyrexia, nasopharyngitis, bronchitis, insomnia, pain in extremity, depression, migraine, and pharyngitis. The proportion of patients who discontinued treatment because of any adverse reaction during the controlled clinical trials was 6.2% for patients receiving belimumab and 7.1% for patients receiving placebo. The most common adverse reactions resulting in discontinuation of treatment (at least 1% of patients receiving belimumab or placebo) were infusion reactions (1.6% belimumab vs 0.9% placebo), lupus nephritis (0.7% belimumab vs 1.2% placebo), and infections (0.7% belimumab vs 1% placebo).

The following table lists adverse events, regardless of causality, occurring in at least 3% of patients with SLE who received belimumab 10 mg/kg and at an incidence of at least 1% greater than that observed with placebo in the 3 controlled studies.

	Incidence of Adverse Events Occurring in ≥ 3% of Patients Treated With Belimumab 10 mg/kg Plus Standard of Care and ≥ 1% More Frequently Than in Patients Receiving Placebo plus Standard of Care	
Preferred term	Belimumab 10 mg/kg + standard of care (n = 674)	Placebo + standard of care (n = 675)
Nausea	15%	12%
Diarrhea	12%	9%
Pyrexia	10%	8%
Nasopharyngitis	9%	7%
Bronchitis	9%	5%
Insomnia	7%	5%
Pain in extremity	6%	4%
Depression	5%	4%
Migraine	5%	4%
Pharyngitis	5%	3%
Cystitis	4%	3%
Leukopenia	4%	2%
Gastroenteritis viral	35%	1%

Mortality: There were more deaths reported with belimumab than with placebo during the controlled period of the clinical trials. Of 2,133 patients in 3 clinical trials, 14 deaths occurred during the placebo-controlled, double-blind treatment periods: 3/675 (0.4%), 5/673 (0.7%), 0/111 (0%), and 6/674 (0.9%) deaths in the placebo, belimumab 1, 4, and 10 mg/kg groups, respectively. No single cause of death predominated. Etiologies included infection, cardiovascular disease, and suicide.

Serious infections: Serious and sometimes fatal infections have been reported in patients receiving immunosuppressive agents, including belimumab. Exercise caution when considering belimumab for patients with chronic infections. Patients receiving any therapy for chronic infection should not begin therapy with belimumab. Consider interrupting belimumab therapy in patients who develop a new infection while undergoing treatment with belimumab and monitor these patients closely. In controlled clinical trials, the overall incidence of infections was 71% in patients treated with belimumab compared with 67% in patients who received placebo. The most frequent infections (more than 5% of patients receiving belimumab) were upper respiratory tract infection, urinary tract infection, nasopharyngitis, sinusitis, bronchitis, and influenza. Serious infections occurred in 6% of patients treated with belimumab and in 5.2% of patients who received placebo. The most frequent serious infections included pneumonia, urinary tract infection, cellulitis, and bronchitis. Infections leading to discontinuation of treatment occurred in 0.7% of patients receiving belimumab and 1% of patients receiving placebo. Infections resulting in death occurred in 0.3% (4/1,458) of patients treated with belimumab and in 0.1% (1/675) of patients receiving placebo.

Hypersensitivity reactions: In controlled clinical trials, hypersensitivity reactions on the day of infusion were reported in 13% (191/1,458) of patients receiving belimumab and 11% (76/675) of patients receiving placebo. Anaphylaxis was observed in 0.6% (9/1,458) of patients receiving belimumab and 0.4% (3/675) of patients receiving placebo. Manifestations included hypotension, angioedema, urticaria or other rash, pruritus, and dyspnea. Because of overlap in signs and symptoms, it was not possible to distinguish between hypersensitivity reactions and infusion reactions in all cases. Some patients (13%) received premedication, which may have mitigated or masked a hypersensitivity response; however, there is insufficient evidence to determine whether premedication diminishes the frequency or severity of hypersensitivity reactions.

Infusion reactions: In controlled clinical trials, adverse events associated with infusion were reported in 17% (251/1,458) of patients receiving belimumab and 15% (99/675) of patients receiving placebo. Serious infusion reactions (excluding hypersensitivity reactions) were reported in 0.5% of patients receiving belimumab and 0.4% of patients receiving placebo, and included bradycardia, myalgia, headache, rash, urticaria, and hypotension. The most common infusion reactions (at least 3% of patients receiving belimumab) were headache, nausea, and skin reactions. Because of overlap in signs and symptoms, it was not possible to distinguish between hypersensitivity reactions and infusion reactions in all cases. Some patients (13%) received premedication, which may have mitigated or masked an infusion reaction; however, there is insufficient evidence to determine whether premedication diminishes the frequency or severity of infusion reactions.

Depression: In controlled clinical trials, psychiatric events were reported more frequently with belimumab (16%) than with placebo (12%), related primarily to depression-related events (6.3% belimumab vs 4.7% placebo), insomnia (6% belimumab vs 5.3% placebo), and anxiety (3.9% belimumab vs 2.8% placebo). Serious psychiatric events were reported in 0.8% of patients receiving belimumab (0.6% and 1.2% with 1 and 10 mg/kg, respectively) and 0.4% of patients receiving placebo. Serious depression was reported in 0.4% (6/1,458) of patients receiving belimumab and 0.1% (1/675) of patients receiving placebo. Two suicides (0.1%) were reported in patients receiving belimumab. Most patients who reported serious depression or suicidal behavior had a history of depression or other serious psychiatric disorders, and most were receiving psychoactive medications. It is unknown if belimumab treatment is associated with an increased risk of these events. Instruct patients receiving belimumab to contact their health care provider if they experience new or worsening depression, suicidal thoughts, or other mood changes.

Immunogenicity: In trials 2 and 3, antibelimumab antibodies were detected in 4 (0.7%) of 563 patients receiving belimumab 10 mg/kg and in 27 (4.8%) of 559 patients receiving belimumab 1 mg/kg. The reported frequency for the group receiving 10 mg/kg may underestimate the actual frequency because of lower assay sensitivity in the presence of high drug concentrations. Neutralizing antibodies were detected in 3 patients receiving belimumab 1 mg/kg. Three patients with antibelimumab antibodies experienced mild infusion reactions of nausea, erythematous rash, pruritus, eyelid edema, headache, and dyspnea; none of the reactions were life-threatening. The clinical relevance of the presence of antibelimumab antibodies is not known.

Pharmacologic & Dosing Characteristics

Dosage: 10 mg/kg at 2-week intervals for the first 3 doses and at 4-week intervals thereafter. Before dosing with belimumab, consider administering premedication for prophylaxis against infusion reactions and hypersensitivity reactions.

Route: IV infusion over 1 hour. Do not administer as an IV push or bolus. Slow or interrupt the infusion rate if the patient develops an infusion reaction. Discontinue infusion if the patient experiences a serious hypersensitivity reaction.

Overdosage: There is no clinical experience with overdosage of belimumab. Two doses of up to 20 mg/kg have been given by IV infusion to humans with no increase in incidence or severity of adverse events compared with doses of 1, 4, or 10 mg/kg.

Efficacy: The safety and effectiveness of belimumab were evaluated in 3 randomized, double-blind, placebo-controlled studies involving 2,133 patients with SLE according to American College of Rheumatology criteria (trials 1, 2, and 3). Patients with severe active lupus nephritis and severe active CNS lupus were excluded. Patients were on a stable standard of care SLE treatment regimen comprising any of the following (alone or in combination): corticosteroids, antimalarials, nonsteroidal anti-inflammatory drugs (NSAIDs), and immunosuppressives. Use of other biologics and IV cyclophosphamide were not permitted.

Trial 1 enrolled 449 patients and evaluated doses of 1, 4, and 10 mg/kg belimumab plus standard of care compared with placebo plus standard of care over 52 weeks in patients with SLE. The coprimary end points were percent change in Safety of Estrogens in Lupus Erythematous - National Assessment (SELENA)–Systemic Lupus Erythematosus Disease Activity Index (SLEDAI) score at week 24 and time to first flare over 52 weeks. No significant differences between any of the belimumab groups and the placebo group were observed. Exploratory analysis of this study identified a subgroup of patients (72%) who were autoantibody positive in whom belimumab appeared to offer benefit. The results of this study informed the design of trials 2 and 3 and led to the selection of a target population and indication that is limited to autoantibody-positive SLE patients.

Trials 2 and 3, which assessed patients with SLE, were similar in design except duration (76 and 52 weeks' duration, respectively). Eligible patients had active SLE disease and positive autoantibody test results at screening. Patients were excluded if they had ever received treatment with a B cell–targeted agent or if they were currently receiving other biologic agents. IV cyclophosphamide was not permitted within the previous 6 months or during study. Baseline concomitant medications included corticosteroids, immunosuppressives (eg, azathioprine, methotrexate, mycophenolate), and antimalarials.

At screening, patients were stratified by disease severity and race, and then randomly assigned to receive belimumab 1 or 10 mg/kg or placebo in addition to standard of care. The patients were administered study medication IV over a 1-hour period on days 0, 14, and 28, and then every 28 days for 48 weeks in trial 3 and for 72 weeks in trial 2. The primary efficacy end point was a composite end point (SLE responder index) that defined response as meeting each of the following criteria at week 52 compared with baseline:

- at least 4-point reduction in the SELENA-SLEDAI score, and
- no new British Isles Lupus Assessment Group (BILAG) A organ domain score or 2 new BILAG B organ domain scores, and
- no worsening (less than 0.3-point increase) in physician global assessment score.

In trials 2 and 3, the proportion of SLE patients achieving an SLE responder index response, as defined for the primary end point, was significantly higher in the belimumab 10 mg/kg group than in the placebo group. The effect on the SLE responder index was not consistently significantly different for the belimumab 1 mg/kg group relative to placebo in both trials. The 1 mg/kg dose is not recommended. The trends in comparisons between the treatment groups for the rates of response for the individual components of the end point were generally consistent with that of the SLE responder index. At week 76 in trial 2, the SLE responder index response rate with belimumab 10 mg/kg was not significantly different from that of placebo (39% and 32%, respectively).

Clinical Response Rate in Patients With SLE After 52 Weeks of Treatment						
	Trial 2			Trial 3		
Response[a]	Placebo + standard of care (n = 275)	Belimumab 1 mg/kg + standard of care[b] (n = 271)	Belimumab 10 mg/kg + standard of care (n = 273)	Placebo + standard of care (n = 287)	Belimumab 1 mg/kg + standard of care[b] (n = 288)	Belimumab 10 mg/kg + standard of care (n = 290)
SLE Responder Index	34%	41% (P = 0.104)	43% (P = 0.021)	44%	51% (P = 0.013)	58% (P < 0.001)
Odds ratio (95% confidence interval) vs placebo		1.3 (0.9, 1.9)	1.5 (1.1, 2.2)		1.6 (1.1, 2.2)	1.8 (1.3, 2.6)
Components of SLE responder index						
% of patients with reduced SELENA-SLEDAI ≥ 4	36%	43%	47%	46%	53%	58%
% of patients with no worsening by BILAG index	65%	75%	69%	73%	79%	81%
% of patients with no worsening by Physicians Global Assessment	63%	73%	69%	69%	79%	80%

a Patients dropping out of the study early or experiencing certain increases in background medication were considered patients in whom treatment failed in these analyses. In both studies, the placebo groups had a higher proportion of patients in whom treatment failed for this reason, compared with the belimumab groups.

b The 1 mg/kg dose is not recommended.

The reduction in disease activity seen in the SLE responder index was related primarily to improvement in the most commonly involved organ systems, namely, mucocutaneous, musculoskeletal, and immunology.

Effect in black patients: Exploratory subgroup analyses of SLE responder index response rate in black patients were performed. In trials 2 and 3 combined, the SRI response rate in black patients (n = 148) in the belimumab groups was less than that in the placebo group (22/50 or 44% for placebo, 15/48 or 31% for belimumab 1 mg/kg, and 18/50 or 36% for belimumab 10 mg/kg). In trial 1, black patients (n = 106) in the belimumab groups did not appear to have a different response than the rest of the study population. Although no definitive conclusions can be drawn from these subgroup analyses, use caution when considering belimumab treatment in black SLE patients.

Effect on concomitant steroid treatment: In trials 2 and 3, 46% and 69% of patients, respectively, were receiving prednisone at doses greater than 7.5 mg/day at baseline. The proportion of patients able to reduce their average prednisone dose by at least 25% to 7.5 mg/day or less during weeks 40 through 52 was not consistently significantly different for belimumab relative to placebo in both trials. In trial 2, 17% of patients receiving belimumab 10 mg/kg and 19% of patients receiving belimumab 1 mg/kg achieved this level of steroid reduction compared with 13% of patients receiving placebo. In trial 3, 19%, 21%, and 12% of patients receiving belimumab 10 or 1 mg/kg, and placebo, respectively, achieved this level of steroid reduction.

Effect on severe SLE flares: The probability of experiencing a severe SLE flare, as defined by a modification of the SELENA trial flare criteria that excluded severe flares triggered only by an increase of the SELENA-SLEDAI score to more than 12, was calculated for trials 2 and 3. The proportion of patients having at least 1 severe flare over 52 weeks was not consistently significantly different for belimumab relative to placebo in both trials. In trial 2, 18% of patients receiving belimumab 10 mg/kg and 16% of patients receiving belimumab 1 mg/kg had a severe flare compared with 24% of patients receiving placebo. In trial 3, 14%, 18%, and 23% of patients receiving belimumab 10 and 1 mg/kg and placebo, respectively, had a severe flare.

Onset: Some effects are apparent as early as week 8. See Pharmacokinetics.

Duration: Effects apparent at week 52. See Pharmacokinetics.

Pharmacokinetics: In trials 1 and 2 in which B cells were measured, treatment with belimumab significantly reduced circulating CD19+, CD2+, naive, and activated B cells; plasmacytoid cells; and the SLE B-cell subset at week 52. Reductions in naive and the SLE B-cell subset were observed as early as week 8 and were sustained to week 52. Memory cells increased initially and slowly declined toward baseline levels by week 52. The clinical relevance of these effects on B cells has not been established.

Treatment with belimumab led to reductions in IgG and anti-dsDNA and increases in complement (C3 and C4). These changes were observed as early as week 8 and were sustained through week 52. The clinical relevance of normalizing these biomarkers has not been definitively established.

Pharmacokinetic parameters in the following table are based on population parameter estimates specific to 563 patients who received belimumab 10 mg/kg in trials 2 and 3. Limited data suggest that age, gender, and race have no known effect on pharmacokinetics.

Pharmacokinetic Parameters in Patients With SLE After IV Infusion of Belimumab 10 mg/kg[a]	
Pharmacokinetic parameter	Population estimates (n = 563)
Peak concentration	313 mcg/mL
Area under the curve	3,083 day•mcg/mL
Distribution half-life	1.75 days
Terminal half-life	19.4 days
Systemic clearance	215 mL/day
Volume of distribution	5.29 L

a IV infusions of 10 mg/kg were administered at 2-week intervals for the first 3 doses and at 4-week intervals thereafter.

Renal impairment: Belimumab has been studied in a limited number of patients with SLE and renal impairment (261 subjects with moderate renal impairment, creatinine clearance [CrCl] ≥ 30 and < 60 mL/min; 14 subjects with severe renal impairment, CrCl ≥ 15 and < 30 mL/min). Although increases in CrCl and proteinuria (> 2 g/day) increased belimumab clearance, these effects were within the expected range of variability. Therefore, dosage adjustment in patients with renal impairment is not recommended.

Hepatic impairment: Belimumab has not been studied in patients with severe hepatic impairment. Baseline ALT and AST levels did not significantly influence belimumab pharmacokinetics.

Mechanism: Belimumab is a BLyS-specific inhibitor that blocks the binding of soluble BLyS, a B-cell survival factor, to its receptors on B cells. Belimumab does not bind B cells directly. By binding BLyS, belimumab inhibits the survival of B cells, including autoreactive B cells, and reduces the differentiation of B cells into immunoglobulin-producing plasma cells.

Belimumab

Drug Interactions: Do not give live vaccines for 30 days before or concurrently with belimumab because clinical safety has not been established. No data are available on secondary transmission of infection from persons receiving live vaccines to patients receiving belimumab or the effect of belimumab on new immunizations. Because of its mechanism of action, belimumab may interfere with the response to immunization.

In clinical trials of patients with SLE, belimumab was coadministered with other drugs, including corticosteroids, antimalarials, immunomodulatory and immunosuppressive agents (eg, azathioprine, methotrexate, mycophenolate), angiotensin-pathway antihypertensives, 3-hydroxy-3-methylglutaryl coenzyme A reductase inhibitors (statins), and NSAIDs without evidence of a clinically significant effect of these concomitant medications on belimumab pharmacokinetics. The effect of belimumab on the pharmacokinetics of other drugs has not been evaluated.

Because belimumab has not been studied in combination with other biologic therapies, including B cell–targeted therapies, or IV cyclophosphamide, it is not recommended in combination with such agents.

Pharmaceutical Characteristics

Concentration: 80 mg per mL after proper reconstitution

Packaging: 120 mg powder in a single-use 5 mL glass vial (NDC # 49401-0101-01), 400 mg powder in a single-use 20 mL glass vial (NDC # 49401-0102-01)

Doseform: Powder for solution

Appearance: White to off-white powder. After reconstitution, the solution should be opalescent, colorless to pale yellow, without particles. However, small air bubbles are expected and acceptable.

Diluent:

For reconstitution: Allow 10 to 15 minutes for belimumab to reach room temperature. Reconstitute the 120 mg vial with 1.5 mL sterile water. Reconstitute the 400 mg vial with 4.8 mL sterile water. Direct the stream of sterile water toward the side of the vial to minimize foaming. Gently swirl the vial for 60 seconds. Allow the vial to sit at room temperature during reconstitution, gently swirling the vial for 60 seconds every 5 minutes until the powder is dissolved. Do not shake. Reconstitution is typically complete within 10 to 15 minutes, but may take up to 30 minutes. Protect the reconstituted solution from sunlight. If a mechanical reconstitution device (swirler) is used, it should not exceed 500 rpm and the vial should not be swirled for longer than 30 minutes.

For infusion: Belimumab is incompatible with IV dextrose solutions. Dilute belimumab only with sodium chloride 0.9%. Dilute the reconstituted product to 250 mL in sodium chloride 0.9%. From a 250 mL infusion bag or bottle, withdraw and discard a volume equal to the volume of the reconstituted solution of belimumab required for the patient's dose. Then add the required volume of the reconstituted solution of belimumab into the infusion bag or bottle. Gently invert the bag or bottle to mix the solution. Discard any unused solution in the vials.

Adjuvant: None

Preservative: None

Allergens: None

Excipients: Upon reconstitution, each single-use vial contains citric acid 0.16 mg/mL, polysorbate 80 0.4 mg/mL, sodium citrate 2.7 mg/mL, and sucrose 80 mg/mL

pH: 6.5

Shelf Life: Data not provided.

Storage/Stability: Store at 2° to 8°C (36° to 46°F). Protect vials from light. Do not freeze. Contact the manufacturer regarding exposure to freezing or elevated temperatures. Shipping data not provided.

If not used immediately, refrigerate the reconstituted belimumab solution at 2° to 8°C (36° to 46°F). Solutions of belimumab diluted in sodium chloride 0.9% may be stored at 2° to 8°C (36° to 46°F) or room temperature. The total time from reconstitution of belimumab to completion of infusion should not exceed 8 hours.

Production Process: Belimumab is produced by recombinant DNA technology in a mammalian cell expression system and manufactured using standard bioreactor and purification methods.

Media: NS0 mouse myeloma cell line

Other Information

First Licensed: March 10, 2011

References: Ding C, Jones G. Belimumab: Human Genome Sciences/Cambridge Antibody Technology/ GlaxoSmithKline. *Curr Opin Investig Drugs.* 2006;7(5):464-472.

Bevacizumab (Humanized)

Isoantibodies

Name:
  Avastin
Synonyms: CAS 216974-75-3

Manufacturer:
  Genentech

Immunologic Characteristics

Target Antigen: Human vascular endothelial growth factor (VEGF) in in vitro and in vivo assay systems.

Viability: Inactive, passive, transient

Antigenic Form: Humanized (human/murine) monoclonal IgG1 antibody

Antigenic Type: Protein, IgG1 molecule composed of human framework regions and the complementarity-determining regions of a murine antibody that binds to VEGF. Molecular weight approximately 149 kilodaltons.

Use Characteristics

Indications: As first- or second-line treatment of patients with metastatic carcinoma of the colon or rectum, in combination with IV 5-fluorouracil (FU)–based chemotherapy.

As first-line treatment of patients with unresectable, locally advanced, recurrent or metastatic nonsquamous, non–small cell lung cancer (NSCLC) in combination with carboplatin and paclitaxel.

As a single agent for patients with glioblastoma with progressive disease following prior therapy.

With interferon alfa for treatment of metastatic renal cell carcinoma.

Unlabeled Uses: Research in progress is assessing the role of bevacizumab in the treatment of other forms of cancer.

In November 2011, the Food and Drug Administration (FDA) withdrew its accelerated approval of the indication for use with paclitaxel in treating patients who have not received chemotherapy for metastatic HER2-negative breast cancer. The FDA concluded that bevacizumab used for metastatic breast cancer has not been shown to provide a benefit, in terms of delay in tumor growth, that would justify its serious and potentially life-threatening risks. There is also no evidence that its use will help women with breast cancer live longer or improve their quality of life.

Limitations: Efficacy of bevacizumab alone in colorectal cancer has not been established. In an ongoing, randomized study of patients with metastatic colorectal cancer that had progressed after a 5-FU and irinotecan-based regimen, the arm in which patients were treated with single-agent bevacizumab was closed early because of evidence of an inferior survival in that arm compared with patients treated with the FOLFOX regimen of 5-FU, leucovorin, and oxaliplatin.

Effectiveness in metastatic breast cancer is based on improvement in progression-free survival. No data are available demonstrating improvement in disease-related symptoms or survival. Bevacizumab is not indicated for disease progression following anthracycline and taxane chemotherapy administered for metastatic disease.

Effectiveness in glioblastoma with progressive disease is based on improvement in objective response rate. Currently, no data are available from randomized, controlled trials demonstrating an improvement in disease-related symptoms or increased survival with bevacizumab in glioblastoma.

Contraindications:

Absolute: Patients who developed GI perforation, serious bleeding, severe arterial thromboembolic event, nephrotic syndrome, hypertensive crisis, or other serious events during bevacizumab therapy.

Relative: None. Use bevacizumab with caution in patients with known hypersensitivity to bevacizumab or any component of this drug product.

Immunodeficiency: No impairment of effect expected.

Elderly: There were insufficient patients 65 years of age and older in which grade 1 to 4 adverse events were collected to determine whether the overall adverse event profile was different in elderly compared with younger patients. Among 392 patients receiving bolus-IFL (IFL refers to a regimen containing irinotecan, fluorouracil, and leucovorin) plus bevacizumab, 126 patients were 65 years of age and older. Severe adverse events that occurred at a higher incidence (at least 2%) in the elderly compared with those younger than 65 years of age were asthenia, sepsis, deep thrombophlebitis, hypertension, hypotension, myocardial infarction, congestive heart failure (CHF), diarrhea, constipation, anorexia, leukopenia, anemia, dehydration, hypokalemia, and hyponatremia. The effect of bevacizumab on overall survival was similar in elderly patients compared with younger patients.

Of 742 patients enrolled in clinical studies in which all adverse events were captured, 212 (29%) were 65 years of age and older and 43 (6%) were 75 years of age and older. Adverse events of any severity that occurred at a higher incidence in elderly patients compared with younger patients, in addition to those previously described, were dyspepsia, GI hemorrhage, edema, epistaxis, increased cough, and voice alteration.

Carcinogenicity: Bevacizumab has not been evaluated for carcinogenic potential in animals or humans.

Mutagenicity: Bevacizumab has not been evaluated for mutagenic potential.

Fertility Impairment: Bevacizumab may impair fertility. The incidence of ovarian failure was higher (34% vs 2%) in premenopausal women receiving bevacizumab in combination with mFOLFOX chemotherapy compared with those receiving mFOLFOX chemotherapy alone for adjuvant treatment for colorectal cancer, a use for which bevacizumab is not approved. Inform women of reproductive potential of the risk of ovarian failure before starting treatment with bevacizumab. Dose-related decreases in ovarian and uterine weights, endometrial proliferation, number of menstrual cycles, and arrested follicular development or absent corpora lutea were observed in female cynomolgus monkeys treated with bevacizumab 10 or 50 mg/kg for 13 or 26 weeks. After a 4- or 12-week recovery period, in which only the high-dose group was examined, trends suggestive of reversibility were noted in the 2 females for each regimen that were assigned to recover. After the 12-week recovery period, follicular maturation arrest was no longer observed, but ovarian weights were still moderately decreased. Reduced endometrial proliferation was no longer observed at the 12-week recovery time point, but uterine weight decreases were still notable, corpora lutea were absent in 1 of 2 animals, and the number of menstrual cycles remained reduced (67%).

Pregnancy: Category C. It is not known if bevacizumab crosses the placenta. Generally, most IgG passage across the placenta occurs during the third trimester. Bevacizumab is teratogenic in rabbits when administered at doses 2-fold greater than recommended for humans on a mg/kg basis. Observed effects included decreases in maternal and fetal body weights, an increased number of fetal resorptions, and an increased incidence of specific gross and skeletal fetal alterations. Adverse fetal outcomes were observed at all doses tested.

Angiogenesis is critical to fetal development. Inhibition of angiogenesis after administration of bevacizumab is likely to result in adverse effects on pregnancy. There are no adequate and well-controlled studies in pregnant women. Use bevacizumab during pregnancy or in any woman not employing adequate contraception only if the potential benefit justifies the potential risk to the fetus. Before starting therapy, counsel all patients regarding the potential risk of bevacizumab to the developing fetus. If the patient becomes pregnant while receiving bevacizumab, inform her of the potential hazard to the fetus and/or the risk of loss of pregnancy. Counsel patients who discontinue bevacizumab concerning prolonged exposure after discontinuing therapy (half-life approximately 20 days) and possible effects of bevacizumab on fetal development.

Lactation: It is not known if bevacizumab crosses into human breast milk. Because human IgG1 is secreted into human milk, the potential for absorption and harm to the infant after ingestion is unknown. Advise women to discontinue breast-feeding during treatment with bevacizumab and for a prolonged period after use of bevacizumab, taking into account the half-life of the product (approximately 20 days [range, 11 to 50 days]).

Children: Safety and efficacy of bevacizumab in children younger than 18 years have not been established. However, physeal dysplasia was observed in juvenile cynomolgus monkeys with open growth plates treated for 4 weeks with doses less than recommended for humans based on mg/kg and exposure. The incidence and severity of physeal dysplasia were dose-related and were at least partially reversible upon cessation of treatment.

Adverse Reactions: The most serious adverse events associated with bevacizumab were GI perforations and wound healing complications, hemorrhage, and hypertensive crises. The most common severe (grade 3 to 4) adverse events were asthenia, pain, hypertension, diarrhea, and leukopenia. The risk of arterial thromboembolic events, including cerebral infarction, transient ischemic attacks, myocardial infarction, and angina are increased in patients receiving bevacizumab in combination with chemotherapy.

The most common adverse reactions observed in bevacizumab patients at a rate greater than 10% and at least twice the control arm rate are epistaxis, headache, hypertension, rhinitis, proteinuria, taste alteration, dry skin, rectal hemorrhage, lacrimation disorder, back pain, and exfoliative dermatitis.

Comparative data on adverse experiences, except where indicated, are limited to study 1, a randomized, active-controlled study in 897 patients receiving initial treatment for metastatic colorectal cancer. All grade 3 and 4 adverse events and selected grade 1 and 2 adverse events (hypertension, proteinuria, thromboembolic events) were reported for the overall study population. In study 1, the median age was 60 years of age, 60% were male, 78% had colon-primary lesion, and 29% had prior adjuvant or neoadjuvant chemotherapy. The median duration of exposure to bevacizumab in study 1 was 8 months in arm 2 and 7 months in arm 3. All adverse events, including all grade 1 and 2 events, were reported in a subset of 309 patients. The baseline entry characteristics in the 309 patient safety subset were similar to the overall study population and well balanced across the 3 study arms.

The following other serious adverse events are considered unusual in cancer patients receiving cytotoxic chemotherapy and occurred in at least 1 subject treated with bevacizumab in clinical studies: polyserositis, intestinal obstruction, intestinal necrosis, mesenteric venous occlusion, anastomotic ulceration, pancytopenia, hyponatremia, ureteral stricture.

Severe and life-threatening (grade 3 and 4) adverse events, which occurred at a higher incidence (at least 2%) in patients receiving bolus-IFL plus bevacizumab compared with bolus-IFL plus placebo, are presented in the following table.

Grade 3 and 4 Adverse Events in Study 1 Occurring at Higher Incidence (≥ 2%) in Bevacizumab vs Control		
	Arm 1 IFL + placebo (n = 396)	Arm 2 IFL + bevacizumab (n = 392)
Grade 3 to 4 events	74%	87%
Body as a whole		
Asthenia	7%	10%
Abdominal pain	5%	8%
Pain	5%	8%
Cardiovascular		
Deep vein thrombosis	5%	9%
Hypertension	2%	12%
Intra-abdominal thrombosis	1%	3%
Syncope	1%	3%
GI		
Diarrhea	25%	34%
Constipation	2%	4%
Hematologic/Lymphatic		
Leukopenia	31%	37%
Neutropenia	14%	21%

Adverse events of any severity, which occurred at a higher incidence (at least 5%) in the initial phase of the study in patients receiving bevacizumab (bolus-IFL plus bevacizumab or 5-FU/LV plus bevacizumab) compared with the bolus-IFL plus placebo arm, are presented in the following table.

Grade 1 to 4 Adverse Events in Study 1 Occurring at Higher Incidence (≥ 5%) in Bevacizumab vs Control			
Adverse event	Arm 1 IFL + placebo (n = 98)	Arm 2 IFL + bevacizumab (n = 102)	Arm 3 5-FU/LV + bevacizumab (n = 109)
Body as a whole			
Pain	55%	61%	62%
Abdominal pain	55%	61%	50%
Headache	19%	26%	26%
Cardiovascular			
Hypertension	14%	23%	34%
Hypotension	7%	15%	7%
Deep vein thrombosis	3%	9%	6%
CNS			
Dizziness	20%	26%	19%
Dermatologic			
Alopecia	26%	32%	6%
Skin ulcer	1%	6%	6%

Grade 1 to 4 Adverse Events in Study 1 Occurring at Higher Incidence (≥ 5%) in Bevacizumab vs Control			
Adverse event	Arm 1 IFL + placebo (n = 98)	Arm 2 IFL + bevacizumab (n = 102)	Arm 3 5-FU/LV + bevacizumab (n = 109)
GI			
Vomiting	47%	52%	47%
Anorexia	30%	43%	35%
Constipation	29%	40%	29%
Stomatitis	18%	32%	30%
Dyspepsia	15%	24%	17%
Hemorrhage	6%	24%	19%
Weight loss	10%	15%	16%
Dry mouth	2%	7%	4%
Colitis	1%	6%	1%
Hemic/Lymphatic			
Thrombocytopenia	0%	5%	5%
Respiratory			
Upper respiratory infection	39%	47%	40%
Dyspnea	15%	26%	25%
Epistaxis	10%	35%	32%
Voice alteration	2%	9%	6%
Special senses			
Taste disorder	9%	14%	21%
Urogenital			
Proteinuria	24%	36%	36%

GI: Bevacizumab can result in GI perforation and wound dehiscence, in some cases resulting in death. GI perforation, sometimes associated with intra-abdominal abscess, occurred throughout treatment with bevacizumab (ie, not correlated to duration of exposure). The incidence of GI perforation in patients receiving bolus-IFL with bevacizumab was 2%. These episodes occurred with or without intra-abdominal abscesses and at various time points during treatment. The typical presentation was reported as abdominal pain associated with symptoms such as constipation and vomiting. One of 501 patients receiving bevacizumab on study 1 developed an anastomotic dehiscence when bevacizumab was initiated per protocol more than 2 months after surgery. Bevacizumab also has been shown to impair wound healing in preclinical animal models. Include GI perforation in the differential diagnosis of patients on bevacizumab presenting with abdominal pain. Permanently discontinue bevacizumab therapy in patients with GI perforation or wound dehiscence requiring medical intervention. The appropriate interval between termination of bevacizumab and subsequent elective surgery required to avoid the risks of impaired wound healing/wound dehiscence has not been determined. Similarly, the appropriate interval between termination of bevacizumab and subsequent elective surgery required to avoid the risks of impaired wound healing has not been determined. In study 1, 6 of 39 (15%) patients receiving bolus-IFL plus bevacizumab who underwent surgery after bevacizumab therapy had wound healing/bleeding complications, compared with 1 of 25 (4%) patients in the bolus-IFL arm. The longest interval between last dose of study drug and dehiscence was 56 days in a patient on the bolus-IFL plus bevacizumab arm. The interval between termination of bevacizumab and subsequent elective surgery should take into consideration the calculated half-life of bevacizumab (approximately 20 days). Tracheoesophageal fistulas have formed in patients with limited stage small cell lung cancer treated with bevacizumab. Other types of GI tract fistulas have been reported in patients treated for colorectal or other types of cancer.

Hemorrhage: Two distinct patterns of bleeding have occurred in patients receiving bevacizumab. The first is minor hemorrhage, most commonly grade 1 epistaxis. Serious, sometimes fatal, hemoptysis has occurred in patients with NSCLC treated with chemotherapy and bevacizumab. In a small study, the incidence of life-threatening or fatal hemoptysis was 4 of 13 (31%) patients with squamous histology and 2 of 53 (4%) patients with adenocarcinoma receiving bevacizumab compared with 0 of 32 (0%) patients treated with chemotherapy alone. Of patients experiencing events of pulmonary hemorrhage, many had cavitation and/or necrosis of the tumor, either preexisting or developing during bevacizumab therapy. These serious hemorrhagic events occurred suddenly and presented as major or massive hemoptysis. Discontinue bevacizumab treatment in patients with serious hemorrhage (ie, requiring medical intervention), and provide aggressive medical management. Patients with recent hemoptysis should not receive bevacizumab. The risk of CNS bleeding in patients with CNS metastases receiving bevacizumab has not been evaluated because these patients were excluded from Genentech-sponsored studies after CNS hemorrhage developed in a patient with a CNS metastasis in phase 1 studies. Other serious bleeding events reported in patients receiving bevacizumab were uncommon and included GI hemorrhage, subarachnoid hemorrhage, and hemorrhagic stroke.

Hypertension: The incidence of hypertension and severe hypertension on 1 or more occasions was increased in patients receiving bevacizumab in study 1. In patients treated with IFL plus placebo, the rate of hypertension (higher than 150/100 mm Hg) was 43%, and the rate of severe hypertension (higher than 200/110 mm Hg) was 2%. For patients treated with IFL plus bevacizumab, the rates were 60% and 7%. For patients treated with 5-FU/LV plus bevacizumab, the rates were 67% and 10%. Among patients with severe hypertension in the bevacizumab arms, 51% had a diastolic reading higher than 110 associated with a systolic reading below 200. Medication classes used to manage patients with grade 3 hypertension receiving bevacizumab included angiotensin-converting enzyme inhibitors, beta-adrenergic blockers, diuretics, and calcium-channel blockers. Four months after discontinuing therapy, persistent hypertension was present in 18 of 26 (69%) patients who received bolus-IFL plus bevacizumab and 8 of 10 (80%) patients who received bolus-IFL plus placebo. Across all clinical studies (N = 1,032), development or worsening of hypertension resulted in hospitalization or discontinuation of bevacizumab in 17 patients (2%). Four of these 17 patients (24%) developed hypertensive encephalopathy. Severe hypertension was complicated by subarachnoid hemorrhage in 1 patient. Permanently discontinue bevacizumab in patients with hypertensive crisis. Temporary suspension is recommended in patients with severe hypertension not controlled with medical management.

Mucocutaneous hemorrhage: In study 1, both serious and nonserious hemorrhagic events occurred at a higher incidence in patients receiving bevacizumab. In the 309 patients in which grade 1 to 4 events were collected, epistaxis was common and reported in 35% of patients receiving bolus-IFL plus bevacizumab compared with 10% of patients receiving bolus-IFL plus placebo. These events were generally mild in severity (grade 1) and resolved without medical intervention. Other mild to moderate hemorrhagic events reported more frequently in patients receiving bolus-IFL plus bevacizumab when compared with those receiving bolus-IFL plus placebo included GI hemorrhage (24% vs 6%), minor gum bleeding (2% vs 0%), and vaginal hemorrhage (4% vs 2%).

Proteinuria: Monitor urine protein and discontinue if nephrotic syndrome occurs; temporarily suspend if moderate proteinuria develops. In study 1, both the incidence and severity of proteinuria (defined as a urine dipstick reading of 1+ or greater) was increased in patients receiving bevacizumab compared with those receiving bolus-IFL plus placebo. Urinary dipstick readings of 2+ or greater occurred in 14% of patients receiving bolus-IFL plus placebo, 17% receiving bolus-IFL plus bevacizumab, and 28% of patients receiving 5-FU/LV plus bevacizumab. In patients with new-onset or worsening proteinuria, 24-hour urine collections were obtained. None of the 118 patients (0%) receiving bolus-IFL plus placebo, 3 of 158 patients (2%) receiving bolus-IFL plus bevacizumab, and 2 of 50 (4%) patients receiving 5-FU/LV plus bevacizumab who had a 24-hour collection experienced grade 3 proteinuria (more than 3.5 g of protein per 24 hours). In a dose-ranging, placebo-controlled, randomized study of bevacizumab in patients with metastatic renal cell carcinoma, 24-hour urine collections were obtained in approximately half of the patients enrolled. Among patients in whom 24-hour urine collections were obtained, 4 of 19 patients (21%) receiving bevacizumab at 10 mg/kg every 2 weeks, 2 of 14 (14%) receiving bevacizumab at 3 mg/kg every 2 weeks, and 0 of the 15 placebo patients experienced grade 3 proteinuria (more than 3.5 g of protein per 24 hours).

Renal: Nephrotic syndrome occurred in 5 of 1,032 (0.5%) patients receiving bevacizumab. One patient died and 1 required dialysis. In 3 patients, proteinuria decreased in severity several months after stopping bevacizumab. No patient had normalization of urinary protein levels (by 24-hour urine) after discontinuing bevacizumab. Discontinue bevacizumab in patients with nephrotic syndrome. The safety of continued bevacizumab treatment in patients with moderate to severe proteinuria has not been evaluated. In most clinical studies, bevacizumab was interrupted for at least 2 g of proteinuria per 24 hours and resumed when proteinuria was less than 2 g per 24 hours. Monitor patients with moderate to severe proteinuria based on 24-hour collections regularly until improvement and/or resolution is observed.

Thromboembolism: Discontinue if severe thromboembolic events occur. In study 1, 18% of patients receiving bolus-IFL plus bevacizumab and 15% of patients receiving bolus-IFL plus placebo experienced a grade 3 to 4 thromboembolic event. The incidence of the following grade 3 and 4 thromboembolic events were higher in patients receiving bolus-IFL plus bevacizumab, compared with patients receiving bolus-IFL plus placebo: cerebrovascular events (4 vs 0 patients), myocardial infarction (6 vs 3), deep venous thrombosis (34 vs 19), and intra-abdominal thrombosis (13 vs 5). In contrast, the incidence of pulmonary embolism was higher in patients receiving bolus-IFL plus placebo (16 vs 20). In study 1, 53 of 392 (14%) patients who received bolus-IFL plus bevacizumab and 30 of 396 (8%) patients who received bolus-IFL plus placebo had a thromboembolic event and received full-dose warfarin. Two patients in each treatment arm (4 total) developed bleeding complications. In the 2 patients treated with full-dose warfarin and bevacizumab, these events were associated with marked elevations in their INR. Eleven of 53 (21%) patients receiving bolus-IFL plus bevacizumab and 1 of 30 (3%) patients receiving bolus-IFL developed an additional thromboembolic event.

Cardiac: CHF, defined as grade 2 to 4 left ventricular dysfunction, was reported in 22 of 1,032 (2%) patients receiving bevacizumab. CHF occurred in 6 of 44 (14%) patients receiving bevacizumab and concurrent anthracyclines. CHF occurred in 13 of 299 (4%) patients who received prior anthracyclines and/or left chest wall irradiation. In a controlled study, the incidence was higher in patients receiving bevacizumab plus chemotherapy compared with patients receiving chemotherapy alone. The safety of continuation or resumption of bevacizumab in patients with cardiac dysfunction has not been studied. Patients were excluded from participation in bevacizumab clinical trials if, in the previous year, they had experienced clinically significant cardiovascular disease. Thus, the safety of bevacizumab in patients with clinically significant cardiovascular disease has not been adequately evaluated.

Infusion: Infusion reactions with the first dose of bevacizumab were uncommon (less than 3%). Severe reactions during the infusion of bevacizumab occurred in 2 patients. One patient developed stridor and wheezing during the first dose. A second patient, receiving paclitaxel followed by bevacizumab, developed a grade 3 hypersensitivity reaction requiring hospitalization during the third infusion of bevacizumab. Both patients responded to medical management. Information on rechallenge is not available. There are no data regarding the most appropriate method of identifying patients who may safely be retreated with bevacizumab after experiencing a severe infusion reaction.

Surgery: Do not begin bevacizumab therapy for at least 28 days after major surgery. The surgical incision should heal fully before starting bevacizumab. Because of the potential for impaired wound healing, suspend bevacizumab before elective surgery. The appropriate interval between the last dose of bevacizumab and elective surgery is unknown. The half-life of bevacizumab is approximately 20 days and the interval chosen should take into consideration the half-life of the drug.

Immunogenicity: As with all therapeutic proteins, there is a potential for immunogenicity. The incidence of antibody development in patients receiving bevacizumab has not been adequately determined because the assay sensitivity was inadequate to reliably detect lower titers. Enzyme-linked immunosorbent assays (ELISAs) were performed on sera from approximately 500 patients treated with bevacizumab, primarily in combination with chemotherapy; high-titer human antibevacizumab antibodies were not detected.

Hematologic: Microangiopathic hemolytic anemia has been reported in patients with solid tumors receiving both bevacizumab and sunitinib maleate.

Fistulas: Serious and sometimes fatal non-GI fistula formation involving tracheoesophageal, bronchopleural, biliary, vaginal, and bladder sites occurs at a higher incidence in bevacizumab-treated patients compared with controls. The incidence of non-GI perforation was less than 0.3% in clinical studies. Most events occurred within the first 6 months of therapy. Discontinue bevacizumab in patients with fistula formation involving an internal organ.

Leukoencephalopathy: Reversible posterior leukoencephalopathy syndrome (RPLS) has been reported, with an incidence of less than 0.1% in clinical studies. The onset of symptoms occurred from 16 hours to 1 year after starting bevacizumab. RPLS is a neurological disorder that can present with headache, seizure, lethargy, confusion, blindness, and other visual and neurologic disturbances. Mild to severe hypertension may be present. Magnetic resonance imaging (MRI) is necessary to confirm the diagnosis of RPLS. Discontinue bevacizumab in patients who develop RPLS. Symptoms usually resolve or improve within days, although some patients have experienced ongoing neurologic sequelae. The safety of restarting bevacizumab in patients previously experiencing RPLS is not known.

Pharmacologic & Dosing Characteristics

Dosage: Do not start bevacizumab therapy for at least 28 days after major surgery. The surgical incision should heal fully before starting bevacizumab. Administer until disease progression or unacceptable toxicity.

For colorectal cancer: 5 mg/kg with bolus IFL or 10 mg/kg with FOLFOX4 given once every 14 days.

For NSCLC: 15 mg/kg as IV infusion every 3 weeks.

For glioblastoma: 10 mg/kg every 2 weeks.

For metastatic renal cell carcinoma: 10 mg/kg every 2 weeks with interferon alfa.

Route & Site: Deliver initial bevacizumab dose over 90 minutes as an IV infusion after chemotherapy. If the first infusion is well tolerated, the second infusion may be administered over

60 minutes. If the 60-minute infusion is well tolerated, all subsequent infusions may be administered over 30 minutes. Do not administer as an IV push or bolus.

Overdosage: The maximum tolerated dose of bevacizumab has not been determined. The highest dose tested in humans (20 mg/kg IV) was associated with headache in 9 of 16 patients, and with severe headache in 3 of 16 patients.

Additional Doses: Permanently discontinue bevacizumab in patients who develop GI perforation, wound dehiscence requiring medical intervention, serious bleeding, nephrotic syndrome, or hypertensive crisis.

Suspend bevacizumab temporarily in patients with evidence of moderate to severe proteinuria, pending further evaluation, and in patients with severe hypertension not controlled with medical management. The risk of continuation or temporary suspension of bevacizumab in patients with moderate to severe proteinuria is unknown.

Suspend bevacizumab at least several weeks before elective surgery. Do not resume bevacizumab until the surgical incision heals fully.

Missed Doses: Interrupting the recommended schedule or delaying subsequent doses does not require restarting the series.

Laboratory Tests: Monitor blood pressure every 2 to 3 weeks during treatment with bevacizumab. Patients who develop hypertension on bevacizumab may require blood pressure monitoring at more frequent intervals. Patients with bevacizumab-induced or -exacerbated hypertension who discontinue bevacizumab should continue to have their blood pressure monitored at regular intervals.

Monitor patients receiving bevacizumab for development or worsening of proteinuria with serial urinalyses. Patients with a 2+ or greater urine dipstick reading should undergo further assessment (eg, a 24-hour urine collection).

Efficacy: The safety and efficacy of bevacizumab in the initial treatment of patients with metastatic carcinoma of the colon and rectum were studied in 2 randomized, controlled clinical trials in combination with IV 5-FU–based chemotherapy.

Bevacizumab with bolus-IFL: Study 1 was a double-blind trial evaluating bevacizumab as first-line treatment of metastatic carcinoma of the colon or rectum. Patients were randomized to bolus-IFL (irinotecan 125 mg/m^2 IV, 5-FU 500 mg/m^2 IV, and leucovorin 20 mg/m^2 IV given once weekly for 4 weeks every 6 weeks) plus placebo (arm 1), bolus-IFL plus bevacizumab (5 mg/kg every 2 weeks) (arm 2), or 5-FU/LV plus bevacizumab (5 mg/kg every 2 weeks) (arm 3). Enrollment in arm 3 was discontinued when the toxicity of bevacizumab in combination with the bolus-IFL regimen was deemed acceptable. Of the 813 patients randomized to arms 1 and 2, the median age was 60 years, 40% were female, and 79% were white. Fifty-seven percent had an Eastern Cooperative Oncology Group (ECOG) performance status of 0. Twenty-one percent had a rectal primary and 28% received prior adjuvant chemotherapy. In most patients (56%) the dominant site of disease was extra-abdominal, while the liver was the dominant site in 38% of patients. The patient characteristics were similar across the study arms. The primary end point of this trial was overall survival. The clinical benefit of bevacizumab, as measured by survival in the 2 principal arms, was seen in all subgroups tested. The subgroups examined were based on age, sex, race, ECOG performance status, location of primary tumor, prior adjuvant therapy, number of metastatic sites, and tumor burden. Among 110 patients enrolled in arm 3, median overall survival was 18.3 months, median progression-free survival was 8.8 months, overall response rate was 39%, and median duration of response was 8.5 months. Results of study 1 appear in the following table.

Study 1 Efficacy Results		
	IFL + placebo	IFL + bevacizumab 5 mg/kg every 2 weeks
Number of patients	411	402
Overall survival[a]		
Median (months)	15.6	20.3
Hazard ratio	—	0.66
Progression-free survival[a]		
Median (months)	6.2	10.6
Hazard ratio	—	0.54
Overall response rate[b]		
Rate (percent)	35%	45%
Duration of response	—	—
Median (months)	7.1	10.4

a $P < 0.001$ by stratified log-rank test.
b $P < 0.001$ by x^2 test.

Bevacizumab with 5-FU/LV chemotherapy: Study 2 tested bevacizumab with 5-FU/LV as first-line treatment of metastatic colorectal cancer. Patients were randomized to receive 5-FU/LV (5-fluorouracil 500 mg/m^2 and leucovorin 500 mg/m^2 weekly for 6 weeks every 8 weeks) or 5-FU/LV plus bevacizumab (5 mg/kg every 2 weeks) or 5-FU/LV plus bevacizumab (10 mg/kg every 2 weeks). Patients were treated until disease progression. The primary end points of the trial were objective response rate and progression-free survival. Progression-free survival was significantly better in patients receiving 5-FU/LV plus bevacizumab at 5 mg/kg when compared to those not receiving bevacizumab. However, overall survival and overall response rate were not significantly different. Outcomes for patients receiving 5-FU/LV plus bevacizumab at 10 mg/kg were not significantly different than for patients who did not receive bevacizumab. Results appear in the following table.

Study 2 Efficacy Results			
	5-FU/LV	5-FU/LV + bevacizumab 5 mg/kg	5-FU/LV + bevacizumab 10 mg/kg
Number of patients	36	35	33
Overall survival			
Median (months)	13.6	17.7	15.2
Progression-free survival			
Median (months)	5.2	9.0	7.2
Overall response rate			
Rate (%)	17	40	24

Onset: Prompt

Duration: With a mean half-life of approximately 20 days, an anti-VEGF effect may persist for several months.

Pharmacokinetics: Immunoglobulins are primarily eliminated by catabolism. The pharmacokinetic profile of bevacizumab was assessed using an assay for total serum bevacizumab concentrations, not distinguishing free bevacizumab and bevacizumab bound to VEGF ligand. Based on a population pharmacokinetic analysis of 491 patients who received 1 to 20 mg/kg of bevacizumab weekly, every 2 weeks, or every 3 weeks, the estimated half-life of bevaci-

Bevacizumab (Humanized)

zumab was approximately 20 days (range, 11 to 50 days). The predicted time to reach steady state was 100 days. The accumulation ratio after a 10 mg/kg dose of bevacizumab every 2 weeks was 2.8.

The clearance of bevacizumab varied by body weight, gender, and tumor burden. After correcting for body weight, males had a higher bevacizumab clearance (0.262 L/day vs 0.207 L/day) and a larger Vc (3.25 L vs 2.66 L) than females. Patients with higher tumor burden (at or above median value of tumor surface area) had a higher bevacizumab clearance (0.249 L/day vs 0.199 L/day) than patients with tumor burdens below the median. In a randomized study of 813 patients (study 1), there was no evidence of lesser efficacy (hazard ratio for overall survival) in males or patients with higher tumor burden treated with bevacizumab compared with females and patients with low tumor burden. The relationship between bevacizumab exposure and clinical outcomes has not been explored.

Analyses of demographic data suggest that no dose adjustments are necessary for age or gender. No studies have been conducted to examine the pharmacokinetics of bevacizumab in patients with renal impairment, nor in patients with hepatic impairment.

Mechanism: Bevacizumab binds VEGF and prevents the interaction of VEGF to its receptors (Flt-1 and KDR) on the surface of endothelial cells. The interaction of VEGF with its receptors leads to endothelial cell proliferation and new blood vessel formation in in vitro models of angiogenesis. Administration of bevacizumab to xenotransplant models of colon cancer in nude (athymic) mice caused reduction of microvascular growth and inhibition of metastatic disease progression.

Drug Interactions: No formal drug interaction studies with antineoplastic agents have been conducted. In clinical trials, patients with colorectal cancer were given irinotecan/5-FU/leucovorin (bolus-IFL) with or without bevacizumab. Irinotecan concentrations were similar in patients receiving bolus-IFL alone and in combination with bevacizumab. The concentrations of SN38, the active metabolite of irinotecan, were on average 33% higher in patients receiving bolus-IFL in combination with bevacizumab, compared to bolus-IFL alone. Patients receiving bolus-IFL plus bevacizumab had a higher incidence of grade 3 to 4 diarrhea and neutropenia. Due to high interpatient variability and limited sampling, the extent of the increase in SN38 levels in patients receiving concurrent irinotecan and bevacizumab is uncertain.

Concurrent therapy with bevacizumab and sunitinib maleate has resulted in microangiopathic hemolytic anemia in some patients with solid tumors.

In a limited number of NSCLC patients, there did not appear to be a difference in the mean exposure of either carboplatin or paclitaxel when each was administered alone or in combination with bevacizumab. However, 3 of 8 patients receiving bevacizumab plus paclitaxel/carboplatin had substantially lower paclitaxel exposure after 4 cycles of treatment at day 63 than those at day 0, while patients receiving paclitaxel/carboplatin without bevacizumab had a greater paclitaxel exposure at day 63 than those at day 0.

Pharmaceutical Characteristics

Concentration: Bevacizumab 25 mg per mL
Packaging: 100 mg per 4 mL glass vial (NDC#: 50242-0060-01); 400 mg per 16 mL glass vial (50242-0061-01)
Doseform: Solution
Appearance: Clear to slightly opalescent, colorless to pale brown
Solvent: Phosphate-buffered saline

Diluent:

For infusion: Dilute the bevacizumab dose of 5 mg/kg in a total volume of 100 mL of sodium chloride 0.9% injection. Do not administer or mix bevacizumab infusions with dextrose solutions.

Adjuvant: None

Preservative: None

Allergens: None

Excipients: α, α-trehalose dihydrate 60 mg/mL, sodium phosphate (monobasic, monohydrate) 5.8 mg/mL, sodium phosphate (dibasic, anhydrous) 1.2 mg/mL, polysorbate 20 0.5 mL/mL, and sterile water for injection

pH: 6.2

Shelf Life: The 100 mg package expires within 24 months. The 400 mg package expires within 18 months.

Storage/Stability: Store at 2° to 8°C (36° to 46°F). Protect vials from light. Do not freeze. Contact the manufacturer regarding exposure to freezing or elevated temperatures. Shipped in insulated containers with coolant packs by second-day courier.

Diluted bevacizumab solutions for infusion may be stored at 2° to 8°C (36° to 46°F) for up to 8 hours and can also tolerate up to 8 hours at temperatures up to 25°C (86°F). No incompatibilities between bevacizumab and polyvinyl chloride or polyolefin bags have been observed.

Handling: Do not shake.

Production Process: Bevacizumab is produced in a Chinese hamster ovary (CHO) mammalian cell expression system in a nutrient medium containing the antibiotic gentamicin.

Media: CHO cell expression system

Disease Epidemiology

Incidence: Colorectal cancer is the second leading cause of cancer death among men and women in the United States. In 2011, an estimated 140,000 new cases of colorectal cancer will be diagnosed in the United States. In 2011, an estimated 50,000 deaths from colon and rectal cancers will occur in the United States. Colorectal cancers are rare in young people. They usually occur in men and women older than 50 years of age.

Other Information

Perspective:

1989: Key growth factor influencing angiogenesis process (VEGF) discovered and cloned by Napoleone Ferrara at Genentech.

1993: Ferrara and colleagues develop mouse antibody to VEGF and demonstrate that the antibody could suppress angiogenesis and tumor growth in preclinical models.

1997: Clinical studies with bevacizumab begin.

First Licensed: February 26, 2004

References: Hochster HS. Bevacizumab in combination with chemotherapy: first-line treatment of patients with metastatic colorectal cancer. *Semin Oncol.* 2006;33(5)(suppl 10):S8-S14.

Hurwitz H, Saini S. Bevacizumab in the treatment of metastatic colorectal cancer: safety profile and management of adverse events. *Semin Oncol.* 2006;33(5)(suppl 10):S26-S34.

Presta LG, Chen H, O'Connor SJ, et al. Humanization of an anti-vascular endothelial growth factor monoclonal antibody for the therapy of solid tumors and other disorders. *Cancer Res.* 1997;57(20):4593-4599.

Brentuximab Vedotin

Isoantibodies

Names: Manufacturers:
  Adcetris   Seattle Genetics

Immunologic Characteristics

Antigen Source: Human CD30
Viability: Not viable, but immunologically active
Antigenic Form: Humanized IgG1
Antigenic Type: Protein-drug conjugate, IgG1. Composed of the chimeric IgG1 antibody
    cAC10 (specific for human CD30), the microtubule disrupting agent monomethyl auristatin
    E (MMAE), and a protease-cleavable linker that covalently attaches MMAE to cAC10. Bren-
    tuximab vedotin has a molecular weight of approximately 153 kDa. Approximately 4 mol-
    ecules of MMAE are attached to each antibody molecule.

Use Characteristics

Indications: To treat patients with Hodgkin lymphoma after failure of autologous stem cell
    transplant (ASCT) or after failure of 2 or more prior multiagent chemotherapy regimens in
    patients who are not ASCT candidates.

   To treat patients with systemic anaplastic large cell lymphoma (sALCL) after failure of at least
    1 prior multiagent chemotherapy regimen.
Limitations: Brentuximab vedotin indications are based on response rates. There are no data
    available demonstrating improvement in patient-reported outcomes or survival with brentux-
    imab vedotin.
Contraindications: None
Immunodeficiency: No impairment of effect is expected.
Elderly: Clinical trials of brentuximab vedotin did not include sufficient numbers of patients
    65 years of age and older to determine whether they respond differently from younger patients.
    Safety and efficacy have not been established.
Carcinogenicity: Brentuximab vedotin has not been evaluated for carcinogenic potential. Car-
    cinogenicity studies with brentuximab vedotin or the small molecule (MMAE) have not been
    conducted.
Mutagenicity: Brentuximab vedotin has not been evaluated for mutagenic potential. MMAE
    was genotoxic in the rat bone marrow micronucleus study through an aneugenic mechanism.
    This effect is consistent with the pharmacological effect of MMAE as a microtubule disrupt-
    ing agent. MMAE was not mutagenic in the bacterial reverse mutation assay (Ames test) or the
    L5178Y mouse lymphoma forward mutation assay.
Fertility Impairment: Fertility studies with brentuximab vedotin or MMAE have not been
    conducted. However, results of repeat-dose toxicity studies in rats indicate the potential for
    brentuximab vedotin to impair male reproductive function and fertility. In a 4-week, repeat-
    dose toxicity study in rats with weekly dosing of brentuximab vedotin 0.5, 5, or 10 mg/kg,
    seminiferous tubule degeneration, Sertoli cell vacuolation, reduced spermatogenesis, and
    aspermia were observed. Effects in animals were seen mainly with brentuximab vedotin 5 and
    10 mg/kg. These doses are approximately 3- and 6-fold the human recommended dose of
    1.8 mg/kg, respectively, based on body weight.

Pregnancy: Category D. There are no adequate and well-controlled studies with brentuximab vedotin in pregnant women. However, based on its mechanism of action and findings in animals, brentuximab vedotin can cause fetal harm when administered to a pregnant woman. Brentuximab vedotin caused embryofetal toxicities in animals at maternal exposures that were similar to human exposures at the recommended doses for patients with Hodgkin lymphoma and sALCL. If this drug is used during pregnancy, or if the patient becomes pregnant while receiving this drug, advise the patient of the potential hazard to the fetus.

In an embryofetal developmental study, pregnant rats received 2 intravenous (IV) doses of brentuximab vedotin 0.3, 1, 3, or 10 mg/kg during the period of organogenesis (once each on pregnancy days 6 and 13). Drug-induced embryofetal toxicities were seen mainly in animals treated with brentuximab vedotin 3 and 10 mg/kg and included increased early resorption (greater than or equal to 99%), postimplantation loss (greater than or equal to 99%), decreased numbers of live fetuses, and external malformations (ie, umbilical hernias and malrotated hindlimbs). Systemic exposure in animals at the brentuximab vedotin dose of 3 mg/kg is approximately the same exposure in patients with Hodgkin lymphoma or sALCL who received the recommended dose of 1.8 mg/kg every 3 weeks.

Lactation: It is not known if brentuximab vedotin crosses into human breast milk. Because many drugs are excreted in human milk and because of the potential for serious adverse events in breast-feeding infants from brentuximab vedotin, decide whether to discontinue breast-feeding or the drug, taking into account the importance of the drug to the mother.

Children: Safety and efficacy of brentuximab vedotin in children younger than 18 years have not been established. Clinical trials included only 9 pediatric patients, which was insufficient to determine whether children respond differently than adults.

Adverse Reactions: Brentuximab vedotin was studied as monotherapy in 160 patients in 2 phase 2 trials. Across both trials, the most common adverse events (incidence of at least 20%), regardless of causality, were neutropenia, peripheral sensory neuropathy, fatigue, nausea, anemia, upper respiratory tract infection, diarrhea, pyrexia, rash, thrombocytopenia, cough, and vomiting.

Hodgkin lymphoma: Brentuximab vedotin was studied in 102 patients in a single-arm trial with a recommended starting dose and schedule of 1.8 mg/kg IV every 3 weeks. Median duration of treatment was 27 weeks (range, 3 to 56 weeks). The most common adverse events (at least 20%), regardless of causality, were neutropenia, peripheral sensory neuropathy, fatigue, upper respiratory tract infection, nausea, diarrhea, anemia, pyrexia, thrombocytopenia, rash, abdominal pain, cough, and vomiting.

Systemic anaplastic large cell lymphoma: Brentuximab vedotin was studied in 58 patients in a single-arm trial with a recommended starting dose and schedule of 1.8 mg/kg IV every 3 weeks. Median duration of treatment was 24 weeks (range, 3 to 56 weeks). The most common adverse events (at least 20%), regardless of causality, were neutropenia, anemia, peripheral sensory neuropathy, fatigue, nausea, pyrexia, rash, diarrhea, and pain.

Two cases of anaphylaxis were reported in phase 1 trials. No grade 3 or 4 infusion-related reactions were reported in phase 2 trials; however, grade 1 or 2 infusion-related reactions were reported for 19 (12%) patients. The most common adverse events (at least 2%) associated with infusion-related reactions were chills (4%), nausea (3%), dyspnea (3%), pruritus (3%), pyrexia (2%), and cough (2%).

Serious adverse events: In phase 2 trials, serious adverse events, regardless of causality, were reported in 31% of patients receiving brentuximab vedotin. The most common serious adverse events experienced by patients with Hodgkin lymphoma include peripheral motor neuropathy (4%), abdominal pain (3%), pulmonary embolism (2%), pneumonitis (2%), pneumothorax (2%), pyelonephritis (2%), and pyrexia (2%). The most common serious adverse events experienced by patients with sALCL were septic shock (3%), supraventricular arrhythmia (3%), pain in extremity (3%), and urinary tract infection (3%). Other important serious adverse events reported included 1 case each of progressive multifocal leukoencephalopathy (PML), Stevens-Johnson syndrome, and tumor lysis syndrome.

Dose modifications: Adverse events that led to dose delays in more than 5% of patients were neutropenia (14%) and peripheral sensory neuropathy (11%).

Discontinuations: Adverse events led to treatment discontinuation in 21% of patients. Adverse events that led to treatment discontinuation in 2 or more patients with Hodgkin lymphoma or sALCL were peripheral sensory neuropathy (8%) and peripheral motor neuropathy (3%).

Peripheral neuropathy: Brentuximab vedotin treatment causes peripheral neuropathy that is predominantly sensory. Cases of peripheral motor neuropathy have also been reported. Brentuximab vedotin–induced peripheral neuropathy is cumulative. In the Hodgkin lymphoma and sALCL clinical trials, 54% of patients experienced any grade of neuropathy. Of these patients, 49% had complete resolution, 31% had partial improvement, and 20% had no improvement. Of the patients who reported neuropathy, 51% had residual neuropathy at the time of their last evaluation. Monitor patients for symptoms of neuropathy, such as hypoesthesia, hyperesthesia, paresthesia, discomfort, burning sensation, neuropathic pain, or weakness. Patients experiencing new or worsening peripheral neuropathy may require a delay, change in dose, or discontinuation of brentuximab vedotin.

Infusion reactions: Infusion-related reactions, including anaphylaxis, have occurred with brentuximab vedotin. Monitor patients during infusion. If anaphylaxis occurs, immediately and permanently discontinue brentuximab vedotin and administer appropriate medical therapy. If an infusion-related reaction occurs, interrupt the infusion and provide appropriate medical management. Premedicate patients who experienced a prior infusion-related reaction before subsequent infusions. Premedication may include acetaminophen, an antihistamine, and a corticosteroid.

Neutropenia: Monitor complete blood cell counts before each dose of brentuximab vedotin. Consider more frequent monitoring for patients with grade 3 or 4 neutropenia. Prolonged (1 week or longer) severe neutropenia can occur with brentuximab vedotin. If grade 3 or 4 neutropenia develops, manage by dose delays, reductions, or discontinuations.

Tumor lysis syndrome: Tumor lysis syndrome may occur. Patients with rapidly proliferating tumor and high tumor burden may be at increased risk. Monitor closely and take appropriate measures.

Stevens-Johnson syndrome: Stevens-Johnson syndrome has been reported with brentuximab vedotin. If Stevens-Johnson syndrome occurs, discontinue brentuximab vedotin and administer appropriate medical therapy.

Progressive multifocal leukoencephalopathy: A fatal case of PML was reported in a patient who received 4 chemotherapy regimens before receiving brentuximab vedotin.

Immunogenicity: Patients with Hodgkin lymphoma and sALCL in phase 2 trials were tested for antibodies to brentuximab vedotin every 3 weeks using a sensitive electrochemiluminescent immunoassay. Approximately 7% of patients in these trials developed persistently positive antibodies (positive test at more than 2 time points) and 30% developed transiently positive antibodies (positive in 1 or 2 postbaseline time points). Anti-brentuximab antibodies were directed against the antibody component of brentuximab vedotin in all patients with transiently or persistently positive antibodies. Two (1%) of the patients with persistently positive antibodies experienced adverse events consistent with infusion reactions that led to discontinuation of treatment. Overall, a higher incidence of infusion-related reactions was observed in patients who developed persistently positive antibodies. A total of 58 patient samples that were either transiently or persistently positive for anti-brentuximab vedotin antibodies were tested for the presence of neutralizing antibodies. Sixty-two percent of these patients had at least 1 sample that was positive for the presence of neutralizing antibodies. The effect of anti-brentuximab vedotin antibodies on safety and efficacy is not known.

Pharmacologic & Dosing Characteristics

Dosage: 1.8 mg/kg as an IV infusion over 30 minutes every 3 weeks. Continue treatment until a maximum of 16 cycles, disease progression, or unacceptable toxicity. The dose for patients weighing more than 100 kg should be calculated for 100 kg.

Dose modification:

Peripheral neuropathy: Use a combination of dose delay and reduction to 1.2 mg/kg. For new or worsening grade 2 or 3 neuropathy, hold dosing until neuropathy improves to grade 1 or baseline and then restart at 1.2 mg/kg. For grade 4 peripheral neuropathy, discontinue brentuximab vedotin.

Neutropenia: Use a combination of dose delays and reductions. For grade 3 or 4 neutropenia, hold the brentuximab vedotin dose until resolution to baseline or grade 2 or lower. Consider growth factor support for subsequent cycles in patients who experience grade 3 or 4 neutropenia. In patients with recurrent grade 4 neutropenia despite use of growth factors, consider discontinuation or dose reduction of brentuximab vedotin to 1.2 mg/kg.

Route: IV infusion. Do not administer as an IV push or bolus.

Overdosage: There is no known antidote for overdosage of brentuximab vedotin. In case of overdosage, closely monitor the patient for adverse events, particularly neutropenia, and administer supportive treatment.

Efficacy:

Hodgkin lymphoma: The efficacy of brentuximab vedotin in patients with Hodgkin lymphoma who relapsed after ASCT was evaluated in 1 open-label, single-arm, multicenter trial. Patients were treated with 1.8 mg/kg of brentuximab vedotin IV over 30 minutes every 3 weeks. Efficacy evaluations were based on overall response rate (ORR = complete remission + partial remission) and duration of response (defined by clinical and radiographic measures, including computed tomography [CT] and positron emission tomography [PET]), as defined in the 2007 Revised Response Criteria for Malignant Lymphoma (modified). The 102 patients ranged in age from 15 to 77 years (median age, 31 years), and most were female (53%) and white (87%). Patients had received a median of 5 prior therapies, including ASCT. The efficacy results are summarized in the following table. Duration of response is calculated from date of first response to date of progression or data cutoff date.

Efficacy Results in Patients With Hodgkin Lymphoma (N = 102)[a]			
		Duration of response (months)	
	Percent (95% CI)	Median (95% CI)	Range
Complete remission	32 (23, 42)	20.5 (12, NE)	1.4 to 21.9[b]
Partial remission	40 (32, 49)	3.5 (2.2, 4.1)	1.3 to 18.7
ORR	73 (65, 83)	6.7 (4, 14.8)	1.3 to 21.9[b]

a CI = confidence interval; NE = not estimable.
b Follow-up was ongoing at time of data submission.

Systemic anaplastic large cell lymphoma: The efficacy of brentuximab vedotin in patients with relapsed sALCL was evaluated in 1 phase 2, open-label, single-arm, multicenter trial. This trial included patients who had sALCL relapse after prior therapy. Fifty-eight patients were treated with brentuximab vedotin 1.8 mg/kg administered IV over 30 minutes every 3 weeks. Efficacy evaluations were based on ORR (complete remission + partial remission) and duration of response (defined by clinical and radiographic measures, including CT and PET), as defined in the 2007 Revised Response Criteria for Malignant Lymphoma (modified).

The 58 patients ranged in age from 14 to 76 years (median age, 52 years), and most were male (57%) and white (83%). Patients had received a median of 2 prior therapies; 26% of patients had received prior ASCT. Fifty percent of patients had relapsed and 50% of patients were refractory to their most recent therapy. Seventy-two percent were anaplastic lymphoma kinase (ALK) negative. Efficacy results are summarized in the following table. Duration of response is calculated from date of first response to date of progression or data cutoff date.

Efficacy Results in Patients With Systemic Anaplastic Large Cell Lymphoma (N = 58)			
		Duration of response (months)	
	Percent (95% CI)	Median (95% CI)	Range
Complete remission	57 (44, 70)	13.2 (10.8, NE)	0.7 to 15.9[a]
Partial remission	29 (18, 41)	2.1 (1.3, 5.7)	0.1 to 15.8[a]
ORR	86 (77, 95)	12.6 (5.7, NE)	0.1 to 15.9[a]

a Follow-up was ongoing at time of data submission.

Pharmacokinetics: The pharmacokinetics of brentuximab vedotin were evaluated in phase 1 trials and in a population pharmacokinetic analysis of data from 314 patients. The pharmacokinetics of 3 analytes were determined: the antibody-drug conjugate, MMAE, and total antibody. Total antibody had the greatest exposure and had a similar pharmacokinetic profile as the antibody-drug conjugate. Therefore, data on the pharmacokinetics of the antibody-drug conjugate and MMAE have been summarized.

Absorption: Maximum concentrations of antibody-drug conjugate were typically observed near the end of infusion. A multiexponential decline in antibody-drug conjugate serum concentrations was observed with a terminal half-life of approximately 4 to 6 days. Exposures were approximately dose proportional from 1.2 to 2.7 mg/kg. Steady state of the antibody-drug conjugate was achieved within 21 days with every-3-week dosing of brentuximab vedotin, consistent with the terminal half-life estimate. Minimal to no accumulation of antibody-drug conjugate was observed with multiple doses at the every-3-week schedule.

The time to maximum concentration for MMAE ranged from approximately 1 to 3 days. Similar to the antibody-drug conjugate, steady state of MMAE was achieved within 21 days with every-3-week dosing of brentuximab vedotin. MMAE exposures decreased with continued administration of brentuximab vedotin, with approximately 50% to 80% of the exposure of the first dose being observed at subsequent doses.

Distribution: In vitro, the binding of MMAE to human plasma proteins ranged from 68% to 82%. MMAE is not likely to displace or to be displaced by highly protein-bound drugs. In vitro, MMAE was a substrate of P-glycoprotein (P-gp) and was not a potent inhibitor of P-gp. In humans, the mean steady-state volume of distribution was approximately 6 to 10 L for antibody-drug conjugate.

Elimination: In vivo data in animals and humans suggest that only a small fraction of MMAE released from brentuximab vedotin is metabolized. In vitro data indicate that the MMAE metabolism that occurs is primarily via oxidation by CYP3A4/5. In vitro studies using human liver microsomes indicate that MMAE inhibits CYP3A4/5, but not other CYP isoforms. MMAE did not induce any major cytochrome P450 (CYP-450) enzymes in primary cultures of human hepatocytes.

MMAE appeared to follow metabolite kinetics, with the elimination of MMAE appearing to be limited by its rate of release from antibody-drug conjugate. An excretion study was undertaken in patients who received a dose of brentuximab vedotin 1.8 mg/kg. Approximately 24% of the total MMAE administered as part of the antibody-drug conjugate during a brentuximab vedotin infusion was recovered in both urine and feces over a 1-week period. Of the recovered MMAE, approximately 72% was recovered in the feces, and the majority of the excreted MMAE was unchanged. The kidney and liver are routes of excretion for MMAE. Neither the influence of renal impairment nor hepatic impairment on the pharmacokinetics of MMAE has been determined.

QT/QTc prolongation potential: The effect of brentuximab vedotin (1.8 mg/kg) on the QTc interval was evaluated in an open-label, single-arm study in 46 evaluable patients with CD30-expressing hematologic malignancies. Administration of brentuximab vedotin did not prolong the mean QTc interval more than 10 msec from baseline. Small increases in the mean QTc interval (less than 10 msec) cannot be excluded because this study did not include a placebo arm and a positive control arm.

Effects of gender, age, and race: Based on the population pharmacokinetic analysis, gender, age, and race do not have a meaningful effect on the pharmacokinetics of brentuximab vedotin.

Mechanism: Brentuximab vedotin is an antibody-drug conjugate. The antibody is a chimeric IgG1 directed against CD30. The small molecule, MMAE, is a microtubule disrupting agent. MMAE is covalently attached to the antibody via a linker. Nonclinical data suggest that the anticancer activity of brentuximab vedotin is due to the binding of the antibody-drug conjugant to CD30-expressing cells, followed by internalization of the antibody-drug conjugate–CD30 complex, and the release of MMAE via proteolytic cleavage. Binding of MMAE to tubulin disrupts the microtubule network within the cell, subsequently inducing cell cycle arrest and apoptotic death of the cells.

Drug Interactions: In vitro data indicate that MMAE is a substrate and an inhibitor of CYP3A4/5. MMAE is primarily metabolized by CYP3A. Coadministration of brentuximab vedotin with ketoconazole, a potent CYP3A4 inhibitor, increased exposure to MMAE by approximately 34%. Closely monitor patients receiving strong CYP3A4 inhibitors concomitantly with brentuximab vedotin for adverse events. Coadministration of brentuximab vedotin with rifampin, a potent CYP3A4 inducer, reduced exposure to MMAE by approximately 46%.

Coadministration of brentuximab vedotin did not affect exposure to midazolam, a CYP3A4 substrate. MMAE does not inhibit other CYP enzymes at relevant clinical concentrations. Brentuximab vedotin is not expected to alter the exposure to drugs that are metabolized by CYP3A4 enzymes.

Patient Information: Advise patients that brentuximab vedotin can cause peripheral neuropathy. Patients should report any numbness or tingling of the hands or feet or any muscle weakness. Advise patients to contact their health care provider if a fever of 100.5°F or greater or other evidence of potential infection (eg, chills, cough, pain on urination) develops. Advise patients to contact their health care provider if they experience signs and symptoms of infusion reactions, including fever, chills, rash, or breathing problems, within 24 hours of infusion. Advise women receiving brentuximab vedotin to avoid pregnancy and breast-feeding while receiving brentuximab vedotin.

Pharmaceutical Characteristics

Concentration: Brentuximab vedotin 5 mg/mL after proper reconstitution
Packaging: Single-use 50 mg vial
NDC Number: 51144-0050-01
Doseform: Lyophilized powder for solution

Brentuximab Vedotin

Appearance: White to off-white cake or powder, yielding a clear to slightly opalescent, colorless solution

Diluent:

For reconstitution: Reconstitute each 50 mg vial with 10.5 mL of sterile water to yield a single-use solution containing 5 mg/mL. Direct the stream toward the wall of the vial to avoid foaming. Gently swirl the vial to aid dissolution. Do not shake.

For infusion: After reconstitution, dilute immediately into an infusion bag (minimum, 100 mL) to achieve a final concentration of 0.4 to 1.8 mg/mL, or store the solution at 2° to 8°C (36° to 46°F) and use within 24 h. Brentuximab vedotin can be diluted into sodium chloride 0.9%, dextrose 5%, or Ringer's lactate injection. Gently invert the bag to mix the solution. Do not freeze. Discard any unused portion.

Do not mix brentuximab vedotin with, or administer as an infusion with, other medicinal products.

Adjuvant: None

Preservative: None

Allergens: None

Excipients: The reconstituted product contains trehalose dihydrate 70 mg/mL, sodium citrate dehydrate 5.6 mg/mL, citric acid monohydrate 0.21 mg/mL, and 0.2 mg/mL of polysorbate 80.

pH: Approximately 6.6

Shelf Life: Data not provided

Storage/Stability: Store vials at 2° to 8°C (36° to 46°F). Protect vials from light. Do not freeze. Contact the manufacturer regarding exposure to freezing or elevated temperatures. Shipping data not provided.

Production Process: Brentuximab vedotin is produced by chemical conjugation of the antibody and small molecule components. The antibody is produced by mammalian (Chinese hamster ovary) cells, and the small molecule components are produced by chemical synthesis.

Other Information

First Licensed: August 19, 2011

Canakinumab (Humanized)

Isoantibodies

Name
Ilaris

Manufacturer
Novartis Pharmaceuticals Corporation

Synonyms: ACZ885

Immunologic Characteristics

Target Antigen: Human interleukin-1β

Viability: Inactive, passive, transient

Antigenic Form: Humanized immunoglobulin G1κ

Antigenic Type: Protein, immunoglobulin G1κ, with high affinity for human interleukin-1β. It is comprised of two 447- (or 448-) residue heavy chains and two 214-residue light chains, with a molecular mass of 145,157 daltons when deglycosylated. Both heavy chains of canakinumab contain oligosaccharide chains linked to the protein backbone at asparagine 298 (Asn 298).

Use Characteristics

Indications: To treat cryopyrin-associated periodic syndromes (CAPS) in adults and children 4 years of age or older, including familial cold auto-inflammatory syndrome (FCAS) and Muckle-Wells syndrome (MWS).

Contraindications: None

Immunodeficiency: The effect of anti-interleukin-1 (IL-1) therapy on the development of malignancies is not known. However, treatment with immunosuppressants, including canakinumab, may result in an increase in the risk of malignancies.

Elderly: Clinical studies of canakinumab did not include sufficient numbers of subjects 65 years of age and older to determine whether they respond differently from younger subjects.

Carcinogenicity: Long-term animal studies to evaluate the carcinogenic potential of canakinumab have not been performed.

Mutagenicity: Canakinumab has not been evaluated for mutagenic potential.

Fertility Impairment: Because canakinumab does not cross-react with rodent IL-1β, male and female fertility was evaluated in a mouse model using a murine analog of canakinumab. Male mice were treated weekly beginning 4 weeks before mating and continuing through 3 weeks after mating. Female mice were treated weekly for 2 weeks before mating through gestation day 3 or 4. The murine analog of canakinumab did not alter male or female fertility parameters at subcutaneous doses of up to 150 mg/kg.

Pregnancy: Category C. Use only if clearly needed. It is not known if canakinumab crosses the placenta. Generally, most IgG passage across the placenta occurs during the third trimester. Canakinumab has been shown to produce delays in fetal skeletal development when evaluated in marmoset monkeys using doses 23-fold the maximum recommended human dose (MRHD) and greater (based on a plasma area under the curve [AUC] comparison). Doses producing exposures within the clinical-exposure range at the MRHD were not evaluated. Similar delays in fetal skeletal development were observed in mice administered a murine analog of canakinumab. There are no adequate and well-controlled studies of canakinumab in pregnant women. Because animal reproduction studies are not always predictive of human response, this drug should be used during pregnancy only if clearly needed.

Embryofetal developmental toxicity studies were performed in marmoset monkeys and mice. Pregnant marmoset monkeys were given canakinumab subcutaneously twice weekly at doses of 15, 50, or 150 mg/kg (representing 23- to 230-fold the human dose) from gestation days 25 to 109, with no evidence of embryotoxicity or fetal malformations. There were increases in the incidence of incomplete ossification of the terminal caudal vertebra and misaligned and/or bipartite vertebra in fetuses at all dose levels compared with concurrent controls, suggesting delay in skeletal development in the marmoset. Because canakinumab does not cross-react with mouse or rat IL-1, pregnant mice were subcutaneously administered a murine analog of canakinumab at doses of 15, 50, or 150 mg/kg on gestation days 6, 11, and 17. The incidence of incomplete ossification of the parietal and frontal skull bones of fetuses was increased in a dose-dependent manner at all dose levels tested.

Lactation: It is not known if canakinumab crosses into human breast milk. Problems in humans have not been documented. Use caution when canakinumab is administered to a breast-feeding woman.

Children: The CAPS trials with canakinumab included 23 patients 4 to 17 years of age (11 adolescents were treated with 150 mg subcutaneously, and 12 children were treated with 2 mg/kg based on body mass between 15 and 40 kg). Clinical symptoms and objective markers of inflammation (eg, serum amyloid A [SAA], C-reactive protein [CRP]) improved in most patients. Overall, the efficacy and safety of canakinumab in pediatric and adult patients were comparable. Upper respiratory infections were the most frequently reported infection. The safety and effectiveness of canakinumab in patients younger than 4 years of age have not been established.

Adverse Reactions: The most common adverse reactions reported by patients with CAPS treated with canakinumab were nasopharyngitis, diarrhea, influenza-like illness, headache, and nausea. The following data reflect exposure to canakinumab in 104 adult and pediatric patients with CAPS (including 20 patients with FCAS, 72 with MWS, 10 with neonatal-onset multisystem inflammatory disorder (MWS/NOMID) overlap, 1 without FCAS or MWS, and 1 who was misdiagnosed in placebo-controlled (35 patients) and noncontrolled trials. Sixty-two patients received canakinumab for at least 6 months, 56 for at least 1 year, and 4 for at least 3 years. Nine serious adverse reactions were reported for patients with CAPS. Among these were vertigo (2 patients), infections (3 patients), including intraabdominal abscess after appendectomy (1 patient). The most commonly reported adverse reactions associated with canakinumab in CAPS patients were nasopharyngitis, diarrhea, influenza-like illness, headache, and nausea. No effect on type or frequency of adverse events was seen with longer-term treatment. One patient discontinued treatment because of potential infection.

Approximately 833 subjects have been treated with canakinumab in blinded and open-label clinical trials in patients with CAPS and other diseases, and healthy volunteers. Fifteen patients reported serious adverse reactions during the clinical program. Study 1 investigated canakinumab in an 8-week, open-label period (part 1), followed by a 24-week, randomized withdrawal period (part 2), followed by a 16-week, open-label period (part 3). All patients were treated with canakinumab 150 mg subcutaneously or 2 mg/kg if body mass was between 15 and 40 kg. All patients with CAPS received canakinumab in part 1, so there are no controlled data on adverse events. Data in the following table are for all adverse events for all patients with CAPS receiving canakinumab. In study 1, no pattern was observed for any type or frequency of adverse events throughout the 3 study periods.

Number (%) of Patients with Adverse Events by Preferred Terms in > 10% of Patients in Parts 1 to 3 of the Phase 3 Trial for CAPS Patients	
Adverse event	Canakinumab (Humanized) N = 35 n (%)
Patients with adverse events	35 (100%)
Nasopharyngitis	12 (34%)
Diarrhea	7 (20%)
Influenza	6 (17%)
Rhinitis	6 (17%)
Nausea	5 (14%)
Headache	5 (14%)
Bronchitis	4 (11%)
Gastroenteritis	4 (11%)
Pharyngitis	4 (11%)
Weight increased	4 (11%)
Musculoskeletal pain	4 (11%)
Vertigo	4 (11%)

Infections: IL-1 blockade may interfere with immune response to infections and increase the risk of serious infections. Use caution when administering canakinumab to patients with infections, a history of recurring infections, or underlying conditions that may predispose them to infections. Discontinue treatment with canakinumab if a patient develops a serious infection. Do not initiate treatment in patients with active infection requiring medical intervention. Infections, predominantly of the upper respiratory tract, in some instances serious, have been reported with canakinumab. The observed infections responded to standard therapy. No unusual or opportunistic infections were reported. In clinical trials, canakinumab was not administered concomitantly with tumor necrosis factor (TNF) inhibitors. An increased incidence of serious infections has been associated with administration of another IL-1 blocker in combination with TNF inhibitors. Taking canakinumab with TNF inhibitors is not recommended, because this may increase the risk of serious infections.

Vertigo: Vertigo has been reported in 9% to 14% of patients in CAPS studies, exclusively in patients with MWS, and as a serious adverse event in 2 cases. All events resolved with continued treatment with canakinumab.

Injection-site reactions: In study 1, subcutaneous injection-site reactions were observed in 9% of patients in part 1 with mild tolerability reactions; in part 2, 1 (7%) patient each had a mild or moderate tolerability reaction and, in part 3, 1 patient had a mild local tolerability reaction. No severe injection-site reactions were reported and none led to discontinuation of treatment. Avoid injecting into an area that is already swollen or red.

Immunogenicity: A specific biosensor binding assay was used to detect antibodies directed against canakinumab in patients who received canakinumab. None of the 60 patients with CAPS tested positive for treatment-emergent binding antibodies at the time points tested. Thirty-one of 60 patients with CAPS were treated longer than 48 weeks.

Pharmacologic & Dosing Characteristics

Dosage: 150 mg for patients with CAPS and body mass greater than 40 kg. For patients with CAPS and body mass between 15 and 40 kg, the recommended dose is 2 mg/kg. For children 15 to 40 kg with an inadequate response, the dose can be increased to 3 mg/kg.

Canakinumab (Humanized)

Route: Subcutaneous

Overdosage: No case of overdose has been reported. In case of overdose, monitor the subject for signs and symptoms of adverse events, and promptly start symptomatic treatment.

Additional Doses: Give canakinumab every 8 weeks.

Related Interventions: Drugs that affect the immune system by blocking TNF have been associated with an increased risk of reactivation of latent tuberculosis (TB). It is possible that taking drugs such as canakinumab that block IL-1 increases the risk of TB or other atypical or opportunistic infections. Before starting immunomodulatory therapies, including canakinumab, test patients for latent TB infection. Canakinumab has not been studied in patients with a positive TB screen, and safety in this setting is unknown. Treat patients testing positive in TB screening according to standard medical practice before therapy with canakinumab.

Efficacy: The efficacy and safety of canakinumab to treat patients with CAPS were demonstrated in study 1, a 3-part trial in patients 9 to 74 years of age with the MWS phenotype of CAPS. Throughout the trial, patients weighing more than 40 kg received canakinumab 150 mg and patients weighing 15 to 40 kg received 2 mg/kg. Part 1 was an 8-week, open-label, single-dose period during which all patients received canakinumab. Patients who achieved a complete clinical response and did not relapse by week 8 were randomized into part 2, a 24-week, randomized, double-blind, placebo-controlled withdrawal period. Patients who completed part 2 or experienced a disease flare entered part 3, a 16-week, open-label, active-treatment phase. A complete response was defined as ratings of minimal or better for physician's assessment of disease activity and assessment of skin disease and serum levels of CRP and SAA less than 10 mg/L. A disease flare was defined as CRP and/or SAA values greater than 30 mg/L and either a score of mild or worse for physician's assessment or a score of minimal or worse for physician's assessment of disease activity and skin disease. In part 1, a complete clinical response was observed in 71% of patients 1 week after starting treatment and in 97% of patients by week 8. In the randomized withdrawal period, 81% of patients randomized to placebo flared compared with none (0%) of the patients randomized to canakinumab. The 95% confidence interval (CI) for treatment difference in the proportion of flares was 53% to 96%. At the end of part 2, all 15 patients treated with canakinumab had absent or minimal disease activity and skin disease.

In a second trial, patients 4 to 74 years of age with both MWS and FCAS phenotypes of CAPS were treated in an open-label manner. Treatment with canakinumab resulted in clinically significant improvement of signs and symptoms and in normalization of high CRP and SAA in a majority of patients within 1 week.

Physician's Global Assessment of Auto-Inflammatory Disease Activity and Assessment of Skin Disease: Frequency Table and Treatment Comparison in Part 2					
		Canakinumab (Humanized) N = 15		Placebo N = 16	
	Baseline	Start of part 2 (Week 8)	End of part 2	Start of part 2 (Week 8)	End of part 2
Physician's global assessment of auto-inflammatory disease activity - n (%)					
Absent	0/31 (0)	9/15 (60)	8/15 (53)	8/16 (50)	0/16 (0)
Minimal	1/31 (3)	4/15 (27)	7/15 (47)	8/16 (50)	4/16 (25)
Mild	7/31 (23)	2/15 (13)	0/15 (0)	0/16 (0)	8/16 (50)
Moderate	19/31 (61)	0/15 (0)	0/15 (0)	0/16 (0)	4/16 (25)
Severe	4/31 (13)	0/15 (0)	0/15 (0)	0/16 (0)	0/16 (0)

Physician's Global Assessment of Auto-Inflammatory Disease Activity and Assessment of Skin Disease: Frequency Table and Treatment Comparison in Part 2					
		Canakinumab (Humanized) N = 15		Placebo N = 16	
	Baseline	Start of part 2 (Week 8)	End of part 2	Start of part 2 (Week 8)	End of part 2
Assessment of skin disease - n (%)					
Absent	3/31 (10)	13/15 (87)	14/15 (93)	13/16 (81)	5/16 (31)
Minimal	6/31 (19)	2/15 (13)	1/15 (7)	3/16 (19)	3/16 (19)
Mild	9/31 (29)	0/15 (0)	0/15 (0)	0/16 (0)	5/16 (31)
Moderate	12/31 (39)	0/15 (0)	0/15 (0)	0/16 (0)	3/16 (19)
Severe	1/32 (3)	0/15 (0)	0/15 (0)	0/16 (0)	0/16 (0)

Markers of inflammation CRP and SAA normalized within 8 days of treatment in the majority of patients. Normal mean CRP and SAA values were sustained throughout study 1 in patients continuously treated with canakinumab. After withdrawal of canakinumab in part 2, CRP and SAA values again returned to abnormal values and subsequently normalized after reintroduction of canakinumab in part 3. The pattern of normalization of CRP and SAA was similar.

Onset: CRP and SAA are indicators of inflammatory disease activity that are elevated in patients with CAPS. Elevated SAA has been associated with the development of systemic amyloidosis in patients with CAPS. Following canakinumab treatment, CRP and SAA levels normalize within 8 days.

Pharmacokinetics:

Absorption: Peak serum canakinumab concentration (C_{max}) of 16 ± 3.5 mcg/mL occurred approximately 7 days after subcutaneous administration of a single 150 mg dose to adult patients with CAPS. The mean terminal half-life was 26 days. The absolute bioavailability of subcutaneous canakinumab was approximately 70%. Exposure parameters (such as AUC and C_{max}) increased in proportion to dose over the dose range of 0.3 to 10 mg/kg given as an IV infusion or from 150 to 300 mg as a subcutaneous injection. In children, peak concentrations of canakinumab occurred between 2 and 7 days following single subcutaneous administration of canakinumab 150 mg or 2 mg/kg in pediatric patients. The terminal half-life ranged from 22.9 to 25.7 days, similar to the pharmacokinetic properties observed in adults.

Distribution: Canakinumab binds to serum IL-1β. Canakinumab volume of distribution (at steady-state) varied according to body mass and was estimated to be 6.01 L in a typical patient with CAPS weighing 70 kg. The expected accumulation ratio was 1.3-fold following 6 months of canakinumab 150 mg subcutaneously every 8 weeks.

Elimination: Clearance of canakinumab varied according to body mass and was estimated to be 0.174 L/day in a typical patient with CAPS weighing 70 kg. There was no indication of accelerated clearance or time-dependent change in the pharmacokinetic properties of canakinumab following repeated administration. No gender- or age-related pharmacokinetic differences were observed after correction for body mass.

Mechanism: Canakinumab binds to human IL-1β and neutralizes its activity by blocking its interaction with IL-1 receptors, but it does not bind IL-1α or IL-1 receptor antagonist (IL-1ra).

Drug Interactions: No formal drug interaction studies have been conducted with canakinumab.

IL-1 inhibitors: The concomitant administration of canakinumab with other drugs (eg, rilonacept, anakinra) that block IL-1 has not been studied. Based on the potential for pharmaco-

Canakinumab (Humanized)

logical interactions between canakinumab and a recombinant IL-1ra, concomitant administration of canakinumab and other agents that block IL-1 or its receptors is not recommended.

TNF inhibitors: An increased incidence of serious infections and an increased risk of neutropenia have been associated with administration of another IL-1 blocker in combination with TNF inhibitors in another patient population. Use of canakinumab with TNF inhibitors may also result in similar toxicities and is not recommended because this may increase the risk of serious infections.

Cytochrome P450 substrates: The formation of cytochrome P450 enzymes is suppressed by increased levels of cytokines (eg, IL-1) during chronic inflammation. Thus, it is expected that for a molecule that binds to IL-1, such as canakinumab, the formation of cytochrome P450 enzymes could be normalized. This is clinically relevant for cytochrome P450 substrates with a narrow therapeutic index, where the dose is individually adjusted (eg, warfarin). Upon initiation of canakinumab in patients being treated with these types of medicinal products, perform therapeutic monitoring of the effect or drug concentration and adjust dosages as needed.

Vaccines: No data are available on either the effects of live vaccination or the secondary transmission of infection by live vaccines in patients receiving canakinumab. Therefore, do not give live vaccines concurrently with canakinumab. In addition, because canakinumab may interfere with normal immune response to new antigens, vaccinations may not be effective in patients receiving canakinumab. No data are available on the effectiveness of vaccinations with inactivated (killed) antigens in patients receiving canakinumab. Complete all recommended immunizations in accordance with current guidelines before starting canakinumab therapy.

Pharmaceutical Characteristics

Concentration: After reconstituting the 180 mg powder with 1 mL of sterile water, it yields 180 mg per 1.2 mL or 150 mg/mL solution.

Quality Assay: Biological activity of canakinumab is measured by comparing its inhibition of IL-1β–dependent expression of the reporter gene luciferase to that of a canakinumab internal reference standard, using a stably transfected cell line.

Packaging: Single-use canakinumab 180 mg powder in 6 mL glass vial

NDC Number: 00078-0582-61

Doseform: Powder for solution

Appearance: White powder yielding clear to opalescent solution, essentially free of particulates. The solution may have a slight brownish-yellow tint. Do not use if the solution has a distinctly brown discoloration.

Diluent:
For reconstitution: Preservative-free sterile water

Adjuvant: None

Preservative: None

Allergens: None

Excipients: Sucrose, L-histidine, L-histidine HCL monohydrate, polysorbate 80

pH: Data not provided

Shelf Life: Data not provided

Storage/Stability: Store at 2° to 8°C (36° to 46°F). Protect vials from light. Do not freeze. Contact the manufacturer regarding exposure to freezing or elevated temperatures. Shipping data not provided.

After reconstitution, protect from light and store at room temperature for up to 60 minutes. Otherwise, refrigerate at 2° to 8°C (36° to 46°F) and use within 4 hours.

Handling: To reconstitute, slowly inject 1 mL of preservative-free sterile water. Swirl the vial slowly at a 45° angle for approximately 1 minute and allow to stand for 5 minutes. Then gently turn the vial upside down and back again 10 times. Do not shake. Avoid touching the rubber stopper with fingers. Allow to stand for approximately 15 minutes at room temperature to obtain a clear solution. Tap the vial to remove any residual liquid from stopper. Slight foaming of the product upon reconstitution is not unusual.

Inject using a 27-gauge, ½-inch needle. Avoid injecting into scar tissue, as this may result in insufficient dosing.

Production Process: Expressed in a murine Sp2/0-Ag14 cell line.

Media: Murine Sp2/0-Ag14 cell line

Disease Epidemiology

CAPS refers to rare genetic syndromes generally caused by mutations in the nucleotide-binding domain, leucine-rich family (NLR), pyrin domain containing 3 (NLRP-3) gene (also known as cold-induced auto-inflammatory syndrome-1). CAPS disorders are inherited in an autosomal dominant pattern with male and female offspring equally affected. Features common to all disorders include fever, urticaria-like rash, arthralgia, myalgia, fatigue, and conjunctivitis. The NLRP-3 gene encodes the protein cryopyrin, an important component of the inflammasome. Cryopyrin regulates the protease caspase-1 and controls activation of IL-1β. Mutations in NLRP-3 result in an overactive inflammasome, resulting in excessive release of activated IL-1β that drives inflammation.

Prevalence: There are believed to be approximately 300 cases in the United States, but many patients may remain undiagnosed because of poor disease recognition.

Other Information

First Licensed: June 18, 2009

References: Lachmann HJ, Kone-Paut I, Kuemmerle-Deschner JB, et al; Canakinumab in CAPS Study Group. Use of canakinumab in the cryopyrin-associated periodic syndrome. *N Engl J Med.* 2009;360(23):2416-2425.

Church LD, McDermott MF. Canakinumab, a fully-human mAb against IL-1beta for the potential treatment of inflammatory disorders. *Curr Opin Mol Ther.* 2009;11(1):81-89.

Certolizumab Pegol (Humanized)

Isoantibodies

Name:
  Cimzia
Synonyms: CDP-870

Manufacturers:
  Nektar Therapeutics and UCB Pharmaceuticals

Immunologic Characteristics

Target Antigen: Human tumor necrosis factor-alpha (TNF-α)

Viability: Inactive, passive, transient

Antigenic Form: Humanized immunoglobulin fragment Fab', conjugated to approximately 40 kDa polyethylene glycol (PEG2MAL40K)

Antigenic Type: Protein, immunoglobulin G (IgG) Fab' fragment of humanized anti–TNF-α monoclonal antibody linked to PEG (pegylated), with high affinity for soluble and membrane-bound TNF-α. The Fab' fragment is composed of a light chain with 214 amino acids and a heavy chain with 229 amino acids. The molecular weight of certolizumab pegol is approximately 91 kDa.

Use Characteristics

Indications: To reduce signs and symptoms of Crohn disease and maintain clinical response in adult patients with moderately to severely active disease who have had an inadequate response to conventional therapy

To treat moderately to severely active rheumatoid arthritis

Contraindications: None

Immunodeficiency: TNF mediates inflammation and modulates cellular immune responses, so TNF blockers may affect host defenses against infections and malignancies. The effect of certolizumab pegol on the development and course of malignancies, as well as active and/or chronic infections, is not fully understood. Safety and efficacy of certolizumab pegol in patients with immunosuppression have not been formally evaluated.

Elderly: Studies of certolizumab pegol did not include a sufficient number of subjects 65 years of age and older to determine whether they respond differently from younger volunteers. Other clinical experience has not identified differences in responses between elderly and younger patients. A population pharmacokinetic analysis of all patients enrolled in certolizumab pegol studies concluded that there was no apparent difference in drug concentration by age. Because there is generally a higher incidence of infections in the elderly population, use caution when treating elderly patients.

Carcinogenicity: Long-term animal studies with certolizumab pegol have not been conducted to assess its carcinogenic potential.

Mutagenicity: Certolizumab pegol was not genotoxic in the Ames test, the human peripheral blood lymphocytes chromosomal aberration assay, or the mouse bone marrow micronucleus assay.

Fertility Impairment: Because certolizumab pegol does not cross-react with mouse or rat TNF-α, reproduction studies were performed in rats using a rodent anti-murine TNF-α pegylated Fab fragment (cTNF PF) that is similar to certolizumab pegol. cTNF PF had no effects on the fertility and general reproductive performance of male and female rats at intravenous (IV) doses of up to 100 mg/kg administered twice weekly.

Pregnancy: Category B. Because certolizumab pegol does not cross-react with mouse or rat TNF-α, reproduction studies were performed in rats using a rodent anti-murine TNF-α

pegylated Fab' fragment (cTN3 PF) that is similar to certolizumab pegol. Reproduction studies have been performed in rats at doses of up to 100 mg/kg and revealed no evidence of impaired fertility or harm to the fetus caused by cTN3 PF. There are, however, no adequate and well-controlled studies of certolizumab pegol in pregnant women. Because animal reproduction studies are not always predictive of human response, use this drug during pregnancy only if clearly needed. It is not known if certolizumab pegol crosses the placenta.

Lactation: It is not known if this drug is excreted in human milk. Because many drugs are excreted in human milk and because of the potential for serious adverse reactions in breast-feeding infants from certolizumab pegol, decide whether to discontinue breast-feeding or the drug, taking into account the importance of the drug to the mother.

Children: The safety and efficacy of certolizumab pegol in children have not been established.

Adverse Reactions: The following data reflect certolizumab pegol 400 mg subcutaneous dosing in studies of patients with Crohn disease. In the safety population in controlled studies, 620 subjects with Crohn disease received certolizumab pegol and 614 subjects received placebo. In controlled and uncontrolled studies, 1,564 subjects received certolizumab pegol at some dose level; of these, 1,350 received certolizumab pegol 400 mg. Approximately 55% were women, 45% were men, and 94% were white. Most patients in the active group were 18 to 64 years of age.

During controlled studies, the portion of patients with serious adverse reactions was 10% for certolizumab pegol and 9% for placebo. The most common adverse reactions (more than 5% of certolizumab pegol-treated patients, with a higher incidence compared with placebo) in controlled studies were upper respiratory tract infection (20% vs 13%), urinary tract infection (7% vs 6%), and arthralgia (6% vs 4%).

The portion of patients who discontinued treatment because of adverse reactions in controlled studies was 8% for certolizumab pegol and 7% for placebo. The most common adverse reactions leading to discontinuation of certolizumab pegol (for 2 or more patients, with a higher incidence than placebo) were abdominal pain (0.4% vs 0.2%), diarrhea (0.4% vs 0%), and intestinal obstruction (0.4% vs 0%).

Autoimmunity: Patients were tested at multiple time points for antibodies to certolizumab pegol during studies CD1 and CD2. The percentage of antibody-positive patients was 8% in patients continuously exposed to certolizumab pegol, of which approximately 80% were neutralizing in vitro. No apparent correlation of antibody development with adverse events or efficacy was observed. Patients treated with concomitant immunosuppressants had a lower rate of antibody development than patients not taking immunosuppressants at baseline (3% vs 11%). The following adverse events were reported in antibody-positive patients (N = 100) at an incidence of at least 3% higher than antibody-negative patients (N = 1,242): abdominal pain, arthralgia, peripheral edema, erythema nodosum, injection-site erythema, injection-site pain, pain in extremity, and upper respiratory tract infection. In studies of Crohn disease, 4% of patients treated with certolizumab pegol and 2% of patients treated with placebo who had negative baseline antinuclear antibody (ANA) titers developed positive titers during the studies. One of the 1,564 patients with Crohn disease treated with certolizumab pegol developed symptoms of a lupus-like syndrome. The impact of long-term certolizumab pegol treatment on the development of autoimmune diseases is not known. If a patient develops symptoms suggestive of a lupus-like syndrome with certolizumab pegol treatment, discontinue treatment.

Infections: The incidence of infections in controlled studies was 38% for certolizumab pegol-treated patients and 30% for placebo-treated patients. The infections primarily consisted of upper respiratory tract infection (20% vs 13%, respectively). The incidence of serious infections during controlled studies was 3% for certolizumab pegol and 1% for placebo. Serious infections, sepsis, and cases of opportunistic infections, including fatalities, have been reported in patients receiving TNF blockers. Many occurred in patients on concomitant immunosuppressive therapy that, in addition to their Crohn disease, could predispose them to infections. In postapproval experience with TNF blockers, infections have been observed with various pathogens, including viral, bacterial, fungal, and protozoal organisms, involving all organ systems. These infections occurred in patients receiving certolizumab pegol alone or in conjunction with immunosuppressive agents. Do not start treatment with certolizumab pegol in patients with active infections, including chronic or localized infections. Monitor patients for signs and symptoms of infection during and after treatment. If an infection develops, monitor the patient carefully, and stop certolizumab pegol if the infection becomes serious. Exercise caution in patients with a history of recurrent infection, concomitant immunosuppressive therapy, or underlying conditions that may predispose them to infections, or in patients who have resided in regions where tuberculosis and histoplasmosis are endemic. Carefully assess the benefits and risks of certolizumab pegol treatment before starting therapy.

Opportunistic infection: In studies that included more than 4,650 patients, the overall rate of tuberculosis was approximately 0.5 per 100 patient-years. The rate in Crohn disease studies was 0.3 cases per 100 patient-years. Tuberculosis, invasive fungal, and other opportunistic infections, some fatal, have occurred. Test for latent tuberculosis using purified protein derivative; consider an induration of 5 mm or greater to be positive, even if previously vaccinated with Bacillus Calmette-Guérin. Consider the possibility of a false-negative test result. If latent infection is diagnosed, start appropriate prophylaxis in accordance with current Centers for Disease Control and Prevention guidelines. Monitor all patients for active tuberculosis during certolizumab pegol treatment, even if the initial tuberculin skin test is negative.

Hepatitis B: Evaluate patients at risk for hepatitis B virus (HBV) infection for prior evidence of HBV infection before starting certolizumab pegol therapy. Monitor HBV carriers for reactivation during and several months after therapy. Most reported cases of reactivation with anti-TNF therapy occurred in patients concomitantly receiving other medications that suppress the immune system. If reactivation occurs, stop certolizumab pegol and begin antiviral therapy. The safety of resuming TNF-blocker therapy after HBV reactivation is controlled is not known.

Malignancies: For some TNF blockers, more cases of malignancies have been observed among patients receiving those TNF blockers compared with control patients. During controlled and open-label portions of certolizumab pegol studies of Crohn disease and other investigational uses, malignancies (excluding nonmelanoma skin cancer) were observed at a rate (95% confidence interval [CI]) of 0.6% (0.4% to 0.8%) per 100 patient-years among 4,650 certolizumab pegol-treated patients compared with a rate of 0.6% (0.2% to 1.7%) per 100 patient-years among 1,319 placebo-treated patients. In clinical trials of all TNF blockers, more cases of lymphoma occurred among patients receiving TNF blockers than occurred in control patients. In controlled studies of certolizumab pegol for Crohn disease and other investigational uses, there was one case of lymphoma among 2,657 certolizumab pegol-treated patients and one case of Hodgkin lymphoma among 1,319 placebo-treated patients. Patients with Crohn disease or other diseases that require long-term exposure to immunosuppressant therapies may be at higher risk than the general population for the development of lymphoma, even in the absence of anti-TNF therapy. The potential role of anti-TNF therapy in the development of malignancies is not known.

CNS: Use of TNF blockers has been associated with rare cases of new-onset or exacerbation of clinical symptoms and/or radiographic evidence of demyelinating disease. Use caution with certolizumab pegol in patients with preexisting or recent-onset CNS demyelinating disorders. Rare cases of neurological disorders, including seizure disorder, optic neuritis, and peripheral neuropathy, have been reported in patients treated with certolizumab pegol; the causal relationship to certolizumab pegol remains unclear.

Hematologic: Rare reports of pancytopenia, including aplastic anemia, have been reported with TNF blockers. Adverse reactions of the hematologic system, including medically significant cytopenia (eg, leukopenia, pancytopenia, thrombocytopenia), have infrequently been reported. A causal relationship remains unclear. Use caution in patients who have ongoing or prior significant hematologic abnormalities. Advise all patients to seek immediate medical attention if they develop signs or symptoms suggestive of blood dyscrasias or infection (eg, persistent fever, bruising, bleeding, pallor) while on certolizumab pegol. Consider discontinuation of certolizumab pegol therapy in patients with confirmed significant hematologic abnormalities. Other serious or significant adverse reactions reported include anemia, lymphadenopathy, and thrombophilia.

Cardiovascular: Cases of worsening congestive heart failure (CHF) and new-onset CHF have been reported with TNF blockers. Certolizumab pegol has not been formally studied in patients with CHF; however, in clinical studies of another TNF blocker in CHF, a higher rate of serious CHF-related adverse reactions was observed. Use caution with certolizumab pegol in patients who have heart failure. Other serious or significant adverse reactions reported include angina pectoris, arrhythmias, hypertensive heart disease, myocardial infarction, myocardial ischemia, pericardial effusion, and pericarditis.

Hypersensitivity: Symptoms compatible with hypersensitivity reactions have rarely been reported after certolizumab pegol treatment (eg, angioedema, dyspnea, hypotension, rash, serum sickness, urticaria). If such reactions occur, stop further administration and institute appropriate therapy.

Miscellaneous: Other serious or significant adverse reactions reported in controlled and uncontrolled studies in Crohn disease and other diseases under investigation occurring in patients receiving certolizumab pegol 400 mg or other doses include the following:

General: Bleeding and injection-site reactions.

Hepatobiliary: Elevated liver enzymes and hepatitis.

Immunologic: Alopecia totalis.

Ophthalmic: Optic neuritis, retinal hemorrhage, and uveitis.

Psychiatric: Anxiety, bipolar disorder, and suicide attempt.

Renal: Nephrotic syndrome and renal failure.

Reproductive: Menstrual disorder.

Skin and soft tissue: Dermatitis, erythema nodosum, and urticaria. Severe skin reactions, including Stevens-Johnson syndrome, toxic epidermal necrolysis, and erythema multiforme, have been identified during postapproval use of other TNF blockers. Because these reactions are voluntarily reported from a population of uncertain size, it is not always possible to reliably estimate their frequency or establish a causal relationship to drug exposure.

Vascular: Vasculitis.

Pharmacologic & Dosing Characteristics

Dosage:

Crohn disease: 400 mg subcutaneously initially and at weeks 2 and 4. If response occurs, follow with 400 mg subcutaneously every 4 weeks.

Rheumatoid arthritis: 400 mg subcutaneously initially and at weeks 2 and 4, followed by 200 mg every other week. For maintenance dosing, consider 400 mg every 4 weeks.

Route & Site: Subcutaneously into separate sites on the abdomen or thigh

Overdosage: The maximum tolerated dose of certolizumab pegol has not been established. Doses of up to 800 mg subcutaneously and 20 mg/kg IV have been administered without serious adverse reactions. In cases of overdosage, closely monitor patients for adverse effects and immediately start appropriate symptomatic treatment.

Certolizumab Pegol (Humanized)

Efficacy: Efficacy and safety of certolizumab pegol were assessed in 2 double-blind, randomized, placebo-controlled studies in patients 18 years of age and older with moderately to severely active Crohn disease, as defined by a Crohn Disease Activity Index (CDAI) of 220 to 450 points. Certolizumab pegol 400 mg was administered subcutaneously in each study. Stable concomitant medications for Crohn disease were permitted.

Study CD1, a randomized, placebo-controlled study of 662 patients with active Crohn disease: Certolizumab pegol or placebo was administered at weeks 0, 2, and 4, then every 4 weeks until week 24. Clinical response was defined as a 100-point or more reduction in CDAI score compared with baseline, and clinical remission was defined as an absolute CDAI score of 150 points or less. Results appear in the following table. At week 6, the proportion of clinical responders was significantly greater for treated patients than for controls. The difference in clinical remission rates was not statistically significant at week 6. The difference in the portion of patients in clinical response at weeks 6 and 26 was significant and demonstrated a maintenance of clinical response.

Study CD1: Clinical Response and Remission, Overall Study Population		
	% Response or remission (95% CI)	
Time point	Placebo (n = 328)	Certolizumab pegol 400 mg (n = 331)
Week 6		
Clinical response	27% (22% to 32%)	35% (30% to 40%)[a]
Clinical remission	17% (13% to 22%)	22% (17% to 26%)
Week 26		
Clinical response	27% (22% to 31%)	37% (32% to 42%)[a]
Clinical remission	18% (14% to 22%)	29% (25% to 34%)[a]
Both weeks 6 and 26		
Clinical response	16% (12% to 20%)	23% (18% to 28%)[a]
Clinical remission	10% (7% to 13%)	14% (11% to 18%)

a $P < 0.05$.

Study CD2, a randomized, treatment-withdrawal study of patients with active Crohn disease: All patients who entered the study were dosed initially with certolizumab pegol 400 mg at weeks 0, 2, and 4, then assessed for clinical response (as previously defined) at week 6. At week 6, a group of 428 clinical responders was randomized to receive certolizumab pegol 400 mg or placebo as maintenance therapy every 4 weeks, starting at week 8 and continuing through week 24. Nonresponders at week 6 were withdrawn from the study. Final evaluation was based on the CDAI score at week 26. Patients who withdrew or received rescue therapy were not considered in clinical response. The results are shown in the following table. At week 26, significantly more week-6 responders were in clinical response and clinical remission in the certolizumab pegol group than in the placebo group.

Study CD2: Clinical Response and Clinical Remission		
	% Response or remission (95% CI)	
	Certolizumab pegol 400 mg × 3 + placebo (n = 210)	Certolizumab pegol 400 mg (n = 215)
Week 26		
Clinical response	36% (30% to 43%)	63% (56% to 69%)[a]
Clinical remission	29% (22% to 35%)	48% (41% to 55%)[a]

a $P < 0.05$.

Baseline use of immunosuppressants or corticosteroids had no effect on clinical response to certolizumab pegol.

Pharmacokinetics: Seventy-eight healthy subjects received doses of up to certolizumab pegol 800 mg subcutaneously and up to 10 mg/kg IV in 3 pharmacokinetic studies. Single IV and subcutaneous doses of certolizumab pegol had predictable dose-related plasma concentrations, with a linear relationship between dose administered and maximum serum concentration (C_{max}) and the area under the certolizumab pegol plasma concentration vs time curve (AUC). Patients with Crohn disease were dosed subcutaneously every 4 weeks with certolizumab pegol at 100, 200, or 400 mg and at 400 mg every 2 weeks for 3 doses, followed by a maintenance dose of 400 mg every 4 weeks. Certolizumab pegol plasma concentrations were broadly dose proportional, and pharmacokinetics observed in patients with Crohn disease were consistent with those seen in healthy subjects.

The pharmacokinetics of certolizumab pegol were evaluated in a cross-study population pharmacokinetic analysis of data from 1,580 subjects, of whom 1,268 were patients with Crohn disease. The population pharmacokinetic analysis concluded that age, gender, creatinine clearance, and white blood cell count did not influence the pharmacokinetics of certolizumab pegol. The population pharmacokinetic analysis was unable to draw any conclusion on the effect of hepatic impairment.

Anticertolizumab pegol antibodies, repeated administration, weight, and immunosuppressant use were covariates that had a statistically significant effect on the pharmacokinetics of certolizumab pegol. Only the presence of antibodies had more than a 30% effect on C_{max} and/or AUC. None of the subject-dependent covariates identified in the population pharmacokinetic analysis had an effect that would require dose adjustment.

Pharmacokinetic parameters in Japanese subjects were similar to those in white subjects following subcutaneous dosing at 3 dose levels in a biocomparability study.

Absorption: Following subcutaneous administration, peak plasma concentrations of certolizumab pegol were attained between 54 and 171 hours postinjection. Certolizumab pegol has bioavailability of approximately 80% (range, 76% to 88%) after subcutaneous administration compared with IV administration. Steady state concentrations range from 0.5 to 90 mcg/mL for a fixed dose of certolizumab pegol 400 mg. For patients developing anticertolizumab pegol antibodies, the steady state concentrations range from 0.5 to 75 mcg/mL.

Distribution: The steady state volume of distribution was estimated as 6.4 L in the population pharmacokinetic analysis.

Metabolism & Elimination: Pegylation, the covalent attachment of PEG polymers to peptides, delays the elimination of these entities from the circulation by a variety of mechanisms, including decreased renal clearance, proteolysis, and immunogenicity. Accordingly, certolizumab pegol is an antibody Fab' fragment conjugated with PEG to extend the terminal plasma elimination half-life of the Fab' to a value comparable with a whole antibody product. The terminal elimination phase half-life was approximately 14 days for all doses tested. The clearance following subcutaneous dosing was estimated as 17 mL/hour in the population pharmacokinetic analysis, with an intersubject variability of 38% (coefficient of variation) and an interoccasion variability of 16%. The route of elimination of certolizumab pegol has not been studied in human subjects.

Mechanism: Certolizumab pegol binds to human TNF-α with a partition coefficient of 90 pM. TNF-α is a key proinflammatory cytokine with a central role in inflammatory processes. Certolizumab pegol selectively neutralizes TNF-α (concentration that inhibits 90% [IC_{90}] of 0.4 ng/mL for inhibition of human TNF-α by in vitro L929 murine fibrosarcoma cytotoxicity assay), but it does not neutralize lymphotoxin-α (TNF-β). Certolizumab pegol cross-reacts poorly with TNF from rodents and rabbits; therefore, in vivo efficacy was evaluated using animal models in which human TNF-α was the physiologically active molecule. Certolizumab pegol neutralizes membrane-associated and soluble human TNF-α in a dose-dependent manner. Incubation of monocytes with certolizumab pegol resulted in a dose-dependent inhibition of lipopolysaccharide-induced TNF-α and interleukin (IL)-1β production in human monocytes. Certolizumab pegol does not contain a fragment crystallizable region, normally present in a complete antibody, and, therefore, does not fix complement or cause antibody-dependent, cell-mediated cytotoxicity in vitro. Certolizumab pegol does not induce apoptosis in vitro in human peripheral blood-derived monocytes or lymphocytes, nor does it induce neutrophil degranulation.

A tissue reactivity study was carried out ex vivo to evaluate potential cross-reactivity of certolizumab pegol with cryosections of normal human tissues. Certolizumab pegol showed no reactivity with a designated standard panel of healthy human tissues.

Biological activities ascribed to TNF-α include the upregulation of cellular adhesion molecules and chemokines, upregulation of major histocompatibility complex class I and class II molecules, and direct leukocyte activation. TNF-α stimulates the production of downstream inflammatory mediators, including IL-1, prostaglandins, platelet activating factor, and nitric oxide. Elevated levels of TNF-α have been implicated in the pathology of Crohn disease. TNF-α is strongly expressed in the bowel wall in areas involved by Crohn disease, and fecal concentrations of TNF-α in patients with Crohn disease have been shown to reflect clinical severity of the disease. After treatment with certolizumab pegol, patients with Crohn disease demonstrated a decrease in the levels of C-reactive protein.

Drug Interactions: Baseline use of immunosuppressants or corticosteroids had no effect on clinical response to certolizumab pegol. Formal drug-drug interaction studies have not been conducted with certolizumab pegol.

Anakinra: Serious infections were seen in clinical studies with concurrent use of anakinra (an IL-1 antagonist) and another TNF blocker, with no added benefit. Because of the nature of adverse reactions seen with this combination therapy, similar toxicities may also result from combination of anakinra and other TNF blockers. Therefore, concurrent use of certolizumab pegol with anakinra is not recommended.

Immunization: No data are available on the response to vaccination or the secondary transmission of infection by live vaccines in patients receiving certolizumab pegol. Do not coadminister live or attenuated vaccines and certolizumab pegol.

Lab Interference: Interference with certain coagulation assays has been detected in patients treated with certolizumab pegol. Certolizumab pegol may cause false-positive elevated activated partial thromboplastin time (aPTT) results in patients without coagulation abnormalities. This effect has been observed with the PTT-LA test from Diagnostica Stago and the *HemosIL* APTT-SP (liquid) and *HemosIL* lyophilized silica tests from Instrumentation Laboratories. Other aPTT assays may be affected as well. Interference with thrombin time and prothrombin time assays has not been observed. There is no evidence that certolizumab pegol therapy has an effect on in vivo coagulation.

Patient Information: Advise patients to inform their health care providers if they develop any signs or symptoms of severe allergic reactions, infection (eg, tuberculosis, reactivation of hepatitis B), new or worsening medical conditions (eg, heart, neurologic, autoimmune), or cytopenia (eg, bruising, bleeding, persistent fever). Counsel patients about the possible risk of lymphoma and other malignancies while receiving certolizumab pegol.

Pharmaceutical Characteristics

Concentration: 200 mg per 1 mL after reconstitution

Packaging:

Powder: Each pack contains 2 glass vials with rubber stoppers, each containing certolizumab pegol 200 mg powder; two 2 mL glass vials containing 1 mL sterile water; two

3 mL plastic syringes; four 20-gauge, 1 inch needles; two 23-gauge, 1 inch needles; 8 alcohol swabs (NDC #: 50474-0700-62)

Solution: Package with 2 alcohol swabs and 2 single-use prefilled glass syringes with a fixed 25 ½-gauge thin-wall needle, each containing 200 mg (1 mL) of certolizumab pegol (50474-0710-79). Starter package with 6 alcohol swabs and 6 single-use prefilled glass syringes with a fixed 25 ½-gauge thin-wall needle, each containing 200 mg (1 mL) of certolizumab pegol (50474-0710-81).

Doseform: Either solution or lyophilized powder for solution

Appearance: White, lyophilized powder yielding a clear to opalescent, colorless to pale-yellow liquid, with no visible particulates or gels in solution

Solvent: Isotonic saline solution

Diluent:
For reconstitution: 1 mL sterile water per 200 mg vial

Adjuvant: None

Preservative: None

Allergens: None

Excipients:
Powder: Sucrose 100 mg, lactic acid 0.9 mg, and polysorbate 0.1 mg per 200 mg vial
Syringe: Each 1 mL syringe contains sodium acetate 1.36 mg, sodium chloride 7.31 mg.

pH:
Powder: Approximately 5.2 after reconstitution
Syringe: Approximately 4.7

Shelf Life: Data not provided.

Storage/Stability: Store at 2° to 8°C (36° to 46°F). Protect vials from light. Do not freeze. Reconstituted product in vial can tolerate 2 hours at room temperature or 24 hours at 2° to 8°C (36° to 46°F). Contact the manufacturer regarding exposure to freezing or elevated temperatures. Shipping data not provided.

Bring the drug to room temperature before reconstituting to facilitate dissolution. Gently swirl each vial without shaking so the powder comes into contact with the sterile water. Leave vials undisturbed to fully reconstitute (may take up to 30 minutes).

Handling: Do not separate the contents of the carton prior to use. Before injection, allow reconstituted certolizumab pegol to reach room temperature. Using a new 20-gauge needle for each vial, withdraw the reconstituted solution into a separate syringe for each vial. Switch each needle to a 23-gauge needle and inject the full contents of each syringe subcutaneously into separate sites on the abdomen or thigh.

Production Process: Fab′ fragment is manufactured in *Escherichia coli* and subsequently purified, then conjugated to PEG2MAL40K to generate certolizumab pegol.

Media: *E. coli*

Other Information

First Licensed: April 22, 2008

References: Kaushik VV, Moots RJ. CDP-870 (certolizumab) in rheumatoid arthritis. *Expert Opin Biol Ther.* 2005;5(4):601-606.

Schreiber S, Rutgeerts P, Fedorak RN, et al; CDP870 Crohn Disease Study Group. A randomized, placebo-controlled trial of certolizumab pegol (CDP870) for treatment of Crohn disease. *Gastroenterology.* 2005;129(3):807-818. Erratum 1808.

Cetuximab (Chimeric)

Isoantibodies

Name:
  Erbitux

Manufacturer:
  Manufactured by ImClone System, distributed
  by Bristol-Myers Squibb Company

Synonyms: IMC-C225

Immunologic Characteristics

Target Antigen: Extracellular domain of the human epidermal growth factor receptor (EGFR).

Viability: Inactive, passive transient

Antigenic Form: Chimeric (murine/human) monoclonal IgG1 antibody

Antigenic Type: Protein, IgG1 molecule composed of Fv regions of a murine anti-EGFR antibody with human IgG1 heavy and kappa light chain constant regions. Molecular weight approximately 152 kilodaltons.

Use Characteristics

Indications: Cetuximab, used in combination with irinotecan, is indicated for the treatment of EGFR-expressing, metastatic colorectal carcinoma in patients who are refractory to irinotecan-based chemotherapy.

Cetuximab administered as a single agent is indicated for the treatment of EGFR-expressing, metastatic colorectal carcinoma in patients who are intolerant to irinotecan-based chemotherapy.

For treatment of certain head and neck cancers: locally or regionally advanced squamous cell carcinoma of the head and neck (SCCHN) in combination with radiation therapy; recurrent locoregional disease or metastatic SCCHN in combination with platinum-based therapy with 5-FU; or recurrent or metastatic SCCHN progressing after platinum-based therapy.

In combination with radiation therapy to treat patients with SCCHN that cannot be removed by surgery (unresectable SCCHN). Also approved as monotherapy to treat patients whose head and neck cancer has metastasized despite use of standard chemotherapy.

Limitations: The effectiveness of cetuximab is based on objective response rates. Currently, no data are available that demonstrate an improvement in disease-related symptoms or increased survival with cetuximab.

Contraindications:
  Absolute: None.
  Relative: Use with caution in patients with known hypersensitivity to cetuximab, murine proteins, or any component of this product.

Immunodeficiency: No impairment of effect expected.

Elderly: Of 633 patients who received cetuximab with irinotecan or cetuximab alone in 4 advanced colorectal cancer studies, 206 patients (33%) were 65 years of age and older. No overall differences in safety or efficacy were observed between these patients and younger patients.

Carcinogenicity: Long-term animal studies have not been performed to test cetuximab for carcinogenic potential.

Mutagenicity: No mutagenic or clastogenic potential of cetuximab was observed in the *Salmonella-Escherichia coli* (Ames) assay or in the in vivo rat micronucleus test.

Fertility Impairment: A 39-week toxicity study in cynomolgus monkeys receiving 0.4 to 4 times the human dose of cetuximab (based on total body surface area) revealed a tendency to impair menstrual cycling in female monkeys, including increased incidences of irregularity or absence of cycles, when compared with control animals beginning from week 25 of treatment and continuing through the 6-week recovery period. Serum testosterone levels and analysis of sperm counts, viability, and motility were not remarkably different between cetuximab-treated and control male monkeys. It is not known if cetuximab can impair fertility in humans.

Pregnancy: Category C. Animal reproduction studies have not been conducted with cetuximab. However, the EGFR has been implicated in the control of prenatal development and may be essential for normal organogenesis, proliferation, and differentiation in the developing embryo. In addition, human IgG1 is known to cross the placental barrier. Therefore, cetuximab has the potential to be transmitted from the mother to the developing fetus. It is not known whether cetuximab can cause fetal harm when administered to a pregnant woman or whether cetuximab can affect reproductive capacity. There are no adequate and well-controlled studies in pregnant women. Only give cetuximab to a pregnant woman or any woman not employing adequate contraception if the potential benefit justifies the potential risk to the fetus. Counsel all patients regarding the potential risk of cetuximab treatment to the developing fetus before beginning therapy. If the patient becomes pregnant while receiving this drug, inform her of the potential hazard to the fetus and/or the potential risk for loss of the pregnancy.

Lactation: It is not known if cetuximab crosses into human breast milk. Because human IgG1 is secreted in human milk, the potential for absorption and harm to the infant after ingestion is unknown. Based on the mean half-life of cetuximab after multiple dosing of 114 hours (range, 75 to 188 hours), advise women to discontinue breast-feeding during treatment with cetuximab and for 60 days after the last dose of cetuximab.

Children: Safety and efficacy of cetuximab in children have not been established.

Adverse Reactions: Most data described below reflect exposure to cetuximab in 633 patients with advanced metastatic colorectal cancer. Cetuximab was studied in combination with irinotecan (n = 354) or alone (n = 279). Patients receiving cetuximab plus irinotecan received a median of 12 doses (with 88/354 [25%] treated for longer than 6 months) and patients receiving cetuximab alone received a median of 7 doses (with 26/279 [9%] treated for longer than 6 months). The group had a median age of 59 years and was 60% male and 91% white. The range of dosing for patients receiving cetuximab plus irinotecan was 1 to 84 infusions, and the range of dosing for patients receiving cetuximab alone was 1 to 63 infusions.

The most serious adverse reactions associated with cetuximab were diarrhea (6% in patients receiving cetuximab plus irinotecan, 0% in patients receiving cetuximab alone); fever (5%); dehydration (5% in patients receiving cetuximab plus irinotecan, 2% in patients receiving cetuximab alone); infusion reaction, sepsis (3%); kidney failure (2%); dermatologic toxicity, pulmonary embolus (1%); and interstitial lung disease (0.5%). Thirty-seven (10%) patients receiving cetuximab plus irinotecan and 14 (5%) patients receiving cetuximab alone discontinued treatment primarily because of adverse events.

The most common adverse events seen in 354 patients receiving cetuximab plus irinotecan were acneform rash (88%), asthenia/malaise (73%), diarrhea (72%), nausea (55%), abdominal pain (45%), and vomiting (41%).

The most common adverse events seen in 279 patients receiving cetuximab alone were acneform rash (90%), asthenia/malaise (49%), fever (33%), nausea (29%), constipation (28%), and diarrhea (28%).

Data in patients with advanced colorectal carcinoma in the following table are based on the experience of 354 patients treated with cetuximab plus irinotecan and 279 patients treated with cetuximab alone.

Incidence of Adverse Events in ≥ 10% of Treated Patients With Advanced Colorectal Carcinoma (%)				
	Cetuximab plus irinotecan (n = 354)		Cetuximab alone (n = 279)	
Body system	Grades 1 to 4	Grades 3 and 4	Grades 1 to 4	Grades 3 and 4
Body as a Whole				
Asthenia/malaise[a]	73	16	49	10
Abdominal pain	45	8	25	7
Fever[b]	34	4	33	0
Pain	23	6	19	5
Infusion reaction[c]	19	3	25	2
Infection	16	1	11	1
Back pain	16	3	11	3
Headache	14	2	25	3
CNS				
Insomnia	12	0	10	< 1
Depression	10	0	9	0
Dermatologic				
Acneform rash[d]	88	14	90	10
Alopecia	21	0	5	0
Skin disorder	15	1	5	0
Nail disorder	12	< 1	16	< 1
Pruritus	10	1	10	< 1
Conjunctivitis	14	1	7	< 1
GI				
Diarrhea	72	22	28	2
Nausea	55	6	29	2
Vomiting	41	7	25	3
Anorexia	36	4	25	3
Constipation	30	2	28	1
Stomatitis	26	2	11	< 1
Dyspepsia	14	0	7	0
Hematic/Lymphatic				
Leukopenia	25	17	1	0
Anemia	16	5	10	4
Metabolic/Nutritional				
Weight loss	21	0	9	1
Peripheral edema	16	1	10	< 1
Dehydration	15	6	9	2

Incidence of Adverse Events in ≥ 10% of Treated Patients With Advanced Colorectal Carcinoma (%)				
	Cetuximab plus irinotecan (n = 354)		Cetuximab alone (n = 279)	
Body system	Grades 1 to 4	Grades 3 and 4	Grades 1 to 4	Grades 3 and 4
Respiratory				
Dyspnea[b]	23	2	20	7
Cough increased	20	0	10	1

a Asthenia/malaise is defined as any event described as asthenia, malaise, or somnolence.
b Includes cases reported as infusion reaction.
c Infusion reaction is defined as any event described at any time during the clinical study as allergic reaction or anaphylactoid reaction, or any event occurring on the first day of dosing described as allergic reaction, anaphylactoid reaction, fever, chills, chills and fever, or dyspnea.
d Acneform rash is defined as any event described as acne, rash, maculopapular rash, pustular rash, dry skin, or exfoliative dermatitis.

Dermatologic: In human studies of cetuximab, dermatologic toxicities, including acneform rash, skin drying and fissuring, and inflammatory and infectious sequelae (eg, blepharitis, cheilitis, cellulitis, cyst) were reported. In patients with advanced colorectal cancer, acneform rash was reported in 88% (560/633) of all treated patients and was severe (grade 3 or 4) in 12% (79/633) of these patients. Acneform rash most commonly occurred on the face, upper chest, and back, but could extend to the extremities and was characterized by multiple follicular- or pustular-appearing lesions. Skin drying and fissuring were common and were associated with inflammatory and infectious sequelae (eg, blepharitis, cellulitis, cyst). The onset of acneform rash was generally within the first 2 weeks of therapy. Although the event resolved following stopping treatment in most patients, in nearly half of the cases, the event continued beyond 28 days. After severe dermatologic toxicities appeared, complications including *Staphylococcus aureus* sepsis and abscesses requiring incision and drainage were reported. Monitor patients developing dermatologic toxicities while receiving cetuximab for inflammatory or infectious sequelae, and start appropriate treatment of these conditions. Modify the dose of any future cetuximab infusions in case of severe acneform rash. Consider treatment with topical and/or oral antibiotics; topical corticosteroids are not recommended.

A related nail disorder, occurring in 14% of patients (0.3% grade 3), was characterized as a paronychial inflammation with associated swelling of the lateral nail folds of the toes and fingers, with the great toes and thumbs as the most commonly affected digits.

In cynomolgus monkeys, cetuximab administered at doses approximately 0.4 to 4 times the weekly human exposure (based on total body surface area) resulted in dermatologic findings, including inflammation at the injection site and desquamation of the external integument. At the highest dose level, the epithelial mucosa of the nasal passage, esophagus, and tongue were similarly affected, and degenerative changes in the renal tubular epithelium occurred. Deaths caused by sepsis were observed in 5 of 10 animals at the highest dose level, beginning after approximately 13 weeks of treatment.

Immunogenicity: As with all therapeutic proteins, there is potential for immunogenicity. Potential immunogenic responses to cetuximab were assessed using either a double-antigen radiometric assay or enzyme-linked immunosorbent assay (ELISA). Because of limitations in assay performance and sample timing, the incidence of antibody development in patients receiving cetuximab has not been adequately determined. The incidence of antibodies to cetuximab was measured by collecting and analyzing serum prestudy, before selected infusions, and during treatment follow-up. Patients were considered evaluable if they had a negative pretreatment sample and a posttreatment sample. Nonneutralizing anti-cetuximab antibodies were detected in 5% (28/530) of evaluable patients. In patients positive for anti-cetuximab antibody, the median time to onset was 44 days (range, 8 to 281 days). Although the number of seropositive patients is limited, there does not appear to be any relationship between the appearance of antibodies to cetuximab and the safety or antitumor activity of the molecule. The observed incidence of anti-cetuximab antibody responses may be influenced by the low sensitivity of available assays, inadequate to reliably detect lower antibody titers.

Infusion reactions: In clinical trials, severe, potentially fatal infusion reactions were reported. These events included the rapid onset of airway obstruction (eg, bronchospasm, stridor, hoarseness), urticaria, and/or hypotension. In studies in advanced colorectal cancer, severe infusion reactions were observed in 3% of patients receiving cetuximab plus irinotecan and in 2% of patients receiving cetuximab alone (17 of 633 patients, rarely with fatal outcome, less than 1 in 1,000). Grade 1 and 2 infusion reactions, including chills, fever, and dyspnea usually occurring on the first day of initial dosing, were observed in 16% of patients receiving cetuximab plus irinotecan and 23% of patients receiving cetuximab alone. In the clinical studies described above, a 20 mg test dose was administered IV over 10 minutes before the loading dose to all patients. The test dose did not reliably identify patients at risk for severe allergic reactions. Approximately 90% of severe infusion reactions were associated with the first infusion of cetuximab, despite the use of prophylactic antihistamines. Caution must be exercised with every cetuximab infusion, as there were patients who experienced their first severe infusion reaction during later infusions.

Pulmonary: Interstitial lung disease (ILD) was reported in 3 of 633 (less than 0.5%) patients with advanced colorectal cancer receiving cetuximab. One case of interstitial pneumonitis with noncardiogenic pulmonary edema resulting in death was reported. Two patients had preexisting fibrotic lung disease and experienced an acute exacerbation while receiving cetuximab plus irinotecan. In the clinical investigational program, an additional case of interstitial pneumonitis was reported in a patient with head and neck cancer treated with cetuximab plus cisplatin. The onset of symptoms occurred between doses 4 and 11 in all reported cases. In the event of acute onset or worsening pulmonary symptoms, interrupt cetuximab therapy and promptly investigate these symptoms. If ILD is confirmed, discontinue cetuximab and treat the patient appropriately.

With radiation therapy: In a study of 21 patients with locally advanced SCCHN, patients treated with cetuximab, cisplatin, and radiation had a 95% incidence of rash (19% grade 3). The incidence and severity of cutaneous reactions with combined modality therapy appears to be additive, particularly within the radiation port. Use caution in adding radiation to cetuximab therapy in patients with colorectal cancer.

Pharmacologic & Dosing Characteristics

Dosage: Cetuximab 400 mg/m^2 as an initial loading dose given as a 120-minute IV infusion, as monotherapy or in combination with irinotecan. The recommended weekly maintenance dose is 250 mg/m^2 infused over 60 minutes.

Infusion reactions: If the patient experiences a mild or moderate infusion reaction, permanently reduce the infusion rate by 50%. Immediately and permanently discontinue cetuximab in patients who experience severe infusion reactions.

Dermatologic toxicity: If a patient experiences severe acneform rash, adjust cetuximab treatment according to the following table. In patients with mild and moderate skin toxicity, continue treatment without dose modification.

Cetuximab Dose Modification Guidelines			
Severe acneform rash	Cetuximab	Outcome	Cetuximab dose modification
1st occurrence	Delay infusion 1 to 2 weeks	Improvement	Continue at 250 mg/m^2
		No improvement	Discontinue cetuximab
2nd occurrence	Delay infusion 1 to 2 weeks	Improvement	Reduce dose to 200 mg/m^2
		No improvement	Discontinue cetuximab
3rd occurrence	Delay infusion 1 to 2 weeks	Improvement	Reduce dose to 150 mg/m^2
		No improvement	Discontinue cetuximab
4th occurrence	Discontinue cetuximab	—	—

Route: For IV infusion via infusion pump or syringe pump. Do not administer as IV push or bolus. Piggyback the cetuximab solution to the patient's infusion line. After the cetuximab infusion, observe the patient for 1 hour.

Infusion pump: Draw up the volume of a vial using a sterile syringe and appropriate needle (eg, vented spike, transfer device). Fill cetuximab into a sterile evacuated container or bag such as glass containers, polyolefin bags (eg, *Intravia* [Baxter]), ethylene vinyl acetate bags (eg, Baxter, Clintec), diethylhexyl phthalate (DEHP)-plasticized polyvinyl chloride (PVC) bags (eg, *Lifecare* [Abbott]), or PVC bags. Repeat until the calculated volume has been put into the container. Use a new needle for each vial. Administer through a low–protein-binding 0.22-micrometer in-line filter, placed proximal to the patient. Affix the infusion line and prime it with cetuximab before starting the infusion. Do not exceed 5 mL/min maximum infusion rate. Use sodium chloride 0.9% to flush line at the end of infusion.

Syringe pump: Draw up the volume of a vial using a sterile syringe and appropriate needle (eg, vented spike). Place the syringe into the syringe driver of a syringe pump and set the rate. Administer through a low–protein-binding 0.22-micrometer in-line filter rated for syringe-pump use, placed proximal to the patient. Connect the infusion line and start the infusion after priming the line with cetuximab. Repeat procedure until the calculated dose has been infused. Use a new needle and filter for each vial. Do not exceed 5 mL/min maximum infusion rate. Use sodium chloride 0.9% to flush line at the end of infusion.

Overdosage: Single doses of cetuximab greater than 500 mg/m^2 have not been tested. There is no experience with overdosage in human clinical trials.

Missed Doses: Interrupting the recommended schedule or delaying subsequent doses does not require restarting the series.

Related Interventions: Premedication with an H$_1$ antagonist (eg, diphenhydramine 50 mg IV) is recommended.

Laboratory Tests:

EGFR testing: Patients enrolled in clinical studies were required to have immunohistochemical evidence of positive EGFR expression using *DakoCytomation's EGFR pharmDx* test kit. Assessment for EGFR expression should be performed by laboratories with demonstrated proficiency in the specific technology being utilized. Improper assay performance, including use of suboptimally fixed tissue, failure to utilize specified reagents, deviation from specific assay instructions, and failure to include appropriate controls for assay validation, can lead to unreliable results. Refer to the *DakoCytomation* test kit package insert for full instructions on assay performance.

Efficacy: A controlled clinical trial was conducted in 329 patients randomized to receive either cetuximab plus irinotecan (218 patients) or cetuximab alone (111 patients). In both arms of the study, cetuximab was administered as a 400 mg/m^2 initial dose, followed by 250 mg/m^2 weekly until disease progression or unacceptable toxicity. All patients received a 20 mg test dose on day 1. In the cetuximab-plus-irinotecan arm, irinotecan was added to cetuximab using the same dose and schedule for irinotecan as the patient had previously failed. Acceptable irinotecan schedules were 350 mg/m^2 every 3 weeks, 180 mg/m^2 every 2 weeks, or 125 mg/m^2 weekly times 4 doses every 6 weeks. An Independent Radiographic Review Committee (IRC), blinded to the treatment arms, assessed both the progression on prior irinotecan and the response to protocol treatment for all patients.

Of the 329 randomized patients, 206 (63%) were male. The median age was 59 years (range, 26 to 84 years), and the majority was white (323, 98%). Eighty-eight percent of patients had baseline Karnofsky Performance Status greater than 80. Fifty-eight percent of patients had colon cancer and 40% had rectal cancer. Approximately two-thirds (63%) of patients previously had failed oxaliplatin treatment.

The efficacy of cetuximab plus irinotecan or cetuximab alone was evaluated in all randomized patients. Analyses also were conducted in 2 prespecified subgroups: irinotecan refractory and irinotecan and oxaliplatin failures. The irinotecan-refractory group included patients who had received at least 2 cycles of irinotecan-based chemotherapy before treatment with cetuximab and had independent confirmation of disease progression within 30 days of completion of the last cycle of irinotecan-based chemotherapy. The irinotecan and oxaliplatin failure group was defined as irinotecan-refractory patients who had previously been treated with and failed an oxaliplatin-containing regimen. The objective response rates (ORR) in these groups are presented in the following table.

Objective Response Rates per Independent Review						
	Cetuximab + irinotecan		Cetuximab monotherapy		Difference (95% CI[a])	
Groups	n	ORR (%)	n	ORR (%)	%	P value[b]
All patients	218	22.9	111	10.8	12.1 (4.1 to 20.2)	0.007
Irinotecan-oxaliplatin failure	80	23.8	44	11.4	12.4 (-0.8 to 25.6)	0.09
Irinotecan refractory	132	25.8	69	14.5	11.3 (0.1 to 22.4)	0.07

a 95% confidence interval for the difference in objective response rates.
b Cochran-Mantel-Haenszel test.

The median duration of response in the overall group was 5.7 months in the combination arm and 4.2 months in the monotherapy arm. Compared with patients randomized to cetuximab alone, patients randomized to cetuximab and irinotecan experienced a significantly longer median time to disease progression.

Time to Progression per Independent Review				
Groups	Cetuximab + irinotecan (median)	Cetuximab monotherapy (median)	Hazard ratio (95% CI[a])	Log-rank P value
All patients	4.1 mo	1.5 mo	0.54 (0.42 to 0.71)	< 0.001
Irinotecan-oxaliplatin failure	2.9 mo	1.5 mo	0.48 (0.31 to 0.72)	< 0.001
Irinotecan refractory	4 mo	1.5 mo	0.52 (0.37 to 0.73)	< 0.001

a Hazard ratio of cetuximab plus irinotecan: cetuximab monotherapy with 95% CI.

Single-arm trials: Cetuximab combined with irinotecan was studied in a single-arm, openlabel clinical trial in 138 patients with EGFR-expressing metastatic colorectal cancer who had progressed following an irinotecan-containing regimen. Patients received a 20 mg test dose of cetuximab on day 1, followed by a 400 mg/m^2 initial dose, and 250 mg/m^2 weekly until disease progression or unacceptable toxicity. Patients received the same dose and schedule for irinotecan as the patient had previously failed. Acceptable irinotecan schedules were 350 mg/m^2 every 3 weeks, or 125 mg/m^2 weekly times 4 doses every 6 weeks. Of 138 patients enrolled, 74 patients had documented progression to irinotecan as determined by an IRC. The overall response rate was 15% for the overall group and 12% for the irinotecan failure group. The median durations of response were 6.5 and 6.7 months, respectively.

Cetuximab was studied as a single agent in a multicenter, open-label, single-arm clinical trial in patients with EGFR-expressing metastatic colorectal cancer who progressed following an irinotecan-containing regimen. Of 57 patients enrolled, 28 patients had documented progression to irinotecan. The overall response rate was 9% for the treated group and 14% for the irinotecan failure group. The median times to progression were 1.4 and 1.3 months, respectively. The median duration of response was 4.2 months for both groups.

Pharmacokinetics: Immunoglobulins are primarily eliminated by catabolism. Cetuximab administered alone or in combination with concomitant chemotherapy or radiotherapy exhibits nonlinear pharmacokinetics. The area under the concentration-time curve (AUC) increased in a greater than dose-proportional manner as the dose increased from 20 to 400 mg/m^2. Cetuximab clearance decreased from 0.08 to 0.02 L/h/m^2 as the dose increased from 20 to 200 mg/m^2, and at doses greater than 200 mg/m^2, it appeared to plateau. The volume of distribution for cetuximab appeared to be independent of dose and approximated the vascular space of 2 to 3 L/m^2.

After a 2-hour infusion of 400 mg/m^2 cetuximab, the maximum mean serum concentration (C_{max}) was 184 mcg/mL (range, 92 to 327 mcg/mL), and the mean elimination half-life was 97 hours (range, 41 to 213 hours). A 1-hour infusion of 250 mg/m^2 produced a mean C_{max} of 140 mcg/mL (range, 120 to 170 mcg/mL). Following the recommended dose regimen (400 mg/m^2 initial dose, 250 mg/m^2 weekly dose), cetuximab concentrations reached steady-state levels by the third weekly infusion, with mean peak and trough concentrations across studies ranging from 168 to 235 mcg/mL and 41 to 85 mcg/mL, respectively. The mean half-life was 114 hours (range, 75 to 188 hours).

A group pharmacokinetic analysis was performed to explore the potential effects of selected covariates, including race, gender, age, and hepatic and renal function, on cetuximab pharmacokinetics. Female patients had a 25% lower intrinsic cetuximab clearance than male patients. Similar efficacy and safety were observed for female and male patients in the clinical trials; therefore, dose modification based on gender is not necessary. None of the other covariates explored appeared to have an impact on cetuximab pharmacokinetics.

Mechanism: Cetuximab binds specifically to the EGFR (HER1, c-ErbB-1) on normal and tumor cells, and competitively inhibits the binding of epidermal growth factor (EGF) and other ligands, such as transforming growth factor-alpha. Binding of cetuximab to the EGFR blocks phosphorylation and activation of receptor-associated kinases, resulting in inhibition of cell growth, induction of apoptosis, and decreased matrix metalloproteinase and vascular endothelial growth factor production. The EGFR is a transmembrane glycoprotein that is a member of a subfamily of type I receptor tyrosine kinases including EGFR (HER1), HER2, HER3, and HER4. The EGFR is expressed constitutively in many normal epithelial tissues, including the skin and hair follicle. Overexpression of EGFR also is detected in many human cancers including those of the colon and rectum.

In vitro assays and in vivo animal studies have shown that cetuximab inhibits the growth and survival of tumor cells that overexpress the EGFR. No antitumor effects of cetuximab were observed in human tumor xenografts lacking EGFR expression. The addition of cetuximab to irinotecan or irinotecan plus 5-fluorouracil in animal studies resulted in an increase in antitumor effects compared with chemotherapy alone.

Patients enrolled in the clinical studies were required to have immunohistochemical evidence of positive EGFR expression. Primary tumor or tumor from a metastatic site was tested with *DakoCytomation's EGFR pharmDx* test kit. Specimens were scored based on the percentage of cells expressing EGFR and intensity (ie, barely/faint, weak to moderate, strong). Response rate did not correlate with either the percentage of positive cells or the intensity of EGFR expression.

Drug Interactions: A drug interaction study was performed in which cetuximab was administered in combination with irinotecan. There was no evidence of any pharmacokinetic interactions between cetuximab and irinotecan.

Patient Information: Patients should wear sunscreen and hats and limit sun exposure while receiving cetuximab, as sunlight can exacerbate any skin reactions that may occur.

Pharmaceutical Characteristics

Concentration: 2 mg/mL

Packaging: 100 mg per 50 mL single-use vial (NDC#: 66733-0948-23) or 200 mg per 100 mL single-use vial (66733-0958-23)

Doseform: Solution

Appearance: Clear and colorless liquid that may contain a small amount of easily visible white amorphous cetuximab particulates.

Solvent: Phosphate-buffered saline

Diluent:

For infusion: Do not dilute. Piggyback into infusion line.

Adjuvant: None

Preservative: None

Allergens: None

Excipients: Sodium chloride 8.48 mg/mL, sodium phosphate dibasic heptahydrate 1.88 mg/mL, sodium phosphate monobasic monohydrate 0.42 mg/mL, water for injection.

pH: 7 to 7.4

Shelf Life: Expires within an unspecified period of time.

Storage/Stability: Store at 2° to 8°C (36° to 46°F). Discard if frozen. Increased particulate formation may occur at temperatures at or below 0°C. Contact the manufacturer regarding exposure to freezing temperatures. Shipping data not provided.

Preparations of cetuximab in infusion containers are chemically and physically stable for up to 12 hours at 2° to 8°C (36° to 46°F) and up to 8 hours at controlled room temperature (20° to 25°C [68° to 77°F]). Discard any remaining solution in the infusion container after that interval. Discard any unused portion of the vial.

Handling: Do not shake or dilute.

Media: Cetuximab is produced in a mammalian (ie, murine myeloma) cell culture.

Disease Epidemiology

Incidence: In the United States, approximately 148,000 people are diagnosed with cancer of the colon or rectum every year. Half of these patients have metastatic disease, or cancer that has spread to other organs, at the time of diagnosis. EGFR is expressed in up to 77% of colorectal cancer tumors. Colorectal cancer is the third leading cause of cancer death in the United States.

Other Information

First Licensed: February 12, 2004

References: Bernier J. Cetuximab in the treatment of head and neck cancer. *Expert Rev Anticancer Ther.* 2006;6(11):1539-1552.

Hitt R, Martín P, Hidalgo M. Cetuximab in squamous cel l carcinoma of the head and neck. *Future Oncol.* 2006;2(4):449-457.

Denosumab (Humanized)

Isoantibodies

Name:
   Prolia
   Xgeva

Manufacturer:
   Amgen
   Amgen

Synonyms: AMG162

Immunologic Characteristics

Target Antigen: Human receptor activator of nuclear factor kappa-B (RANK) ligand.

Viability: Inactive, passive transient

Antigenic Form: Humanized immunoglobulin.

Antigenic Type: Protein, IgG2, antihuman osteoclast differentiation factor, with affinity and specificity for human RANK ligand (RANKL), dimer. Molecular weight approximately 147 kilodaltons.

Use Characteristics

Indications:

> *Prolia*: To treat postmenopausal women with osteoporosis at high risk for fracture, defined as a history of osteoporotic fracture, or multiple risk factors for fracture; or patients who have failed or are intolerant to other available osteoporosis therapy. In postmenopausal women with osteoporosis, denosumab reduces the incidence of vertebral, nonvertebral, and hip fractures.

> As a treatment to increase bone mass in women at high risk for fracture receiving adjuvant aromatase inhibitor therapy for breast cancer.

> As a treatment to increase bone mass in men at high risk for fracture receiving androgen deprivation therapy for nonmetastatic prostate cancer. In these patients, denosumab reduces the incidence of vertebral fractures.

> *Xgeva*: To prevent skeletal-related events in patients with bone metastases from solid tumors. Not indicated for preventing skeletal-related events in patients with multiple myeloma.

Contraindications: Correct preexisting hypocalcemia before starting denosumab therapy.

Immunodeficiency: No impairment of effect is expected.

Elderly:

> *Prolia*: In clinical studies, 9,943 patients (76%) were 65 years and older, with 3,576 (27%) 75 years and older. No overall differences in safety or efficacy were observed between these patients and younger patients. Other reported clinical experience has not identified differences in responses between elderly and younger patients.

> *Xgeva*: In clinical trials, 1,260 (44%) were 65 years or older. No overall differences in safety or efficacy were observed between these patients and younger patients.

Carcinogenicity: Denosumab has not been evaluated for carcinogenic potential in long-term animal studies.

Mutagenicity: Denosumab has not been evaluated for mutagenic potential.

Fertility Impairment: Denosumab had no effect on female fertility or male reproductive organs in monkeys at doses 13- to 50-fold more than the recommended human dose, based on body weight (mg/kg).

Pregnancy: Category C. It is not known if denosumab crosses the placenta. There are no adequate and well-controlled studies of denosumab in pregnant women. Enroll women who become pregnant during denosumab treatment in Amgen's pregnancy surveillance program (800–772–6436). In genetically engineered mice in which RANKL was turned off by gene removal, absence of RANKL (the denosumab [humanized] target) caused fetal lymph node agenesis and postnatal impairment of dentition and bone growth. These pregnant mice also showed altered maturation of the maternal mammary gland, leading to impaired lactation postpartum. In an embryofetal developmental study, cynomolgus monkeys received denosumab subcutaneously weekly during organogenesis at doses up to 13-fold more than the recommended human dose based on body weight. No evidence of maternal toxicity or fetal harm was observed. This study only assessed fetal toxicity during a period equivalent to the first trimester; fetal lymph nodes were not examined. Monoclonal antibodies are transported across the placenta in a linearly increasing fashion as pregnancy progresses, with the largest amount transferred during the third trimester. Potential adverse developmental effects resulting from exposures during the second and third trimesters have not been assessed in animals.

Lactation: It is not known whether denosumab crosses into human milk. Because many drugs are excreted in human milk and because of the potential for serious adverse reactions in breast-feeding infants from denosumab, decide whether to discontinue breast-feeding or the drug, taking into account the importance of the drug to the mother. Maternal exposure to denosumab during pregnancy may impair mammary gland development and lactation based on animal studies in pregnant mice lacking the RANK/RANKL signaling pathway (ie, OPG-Fc), leading to impaired lactation postpartum.

Children: Denosumab is not recommended in pediatric patients. The safety and effectiveness of denosumab in pediatric patients have not been established. Denosumab may impair bone growth in children with open growth plates and may inhibit eruption of dentition. In neonatal rats, inhibition of RANKL with a construct of osteoprotegerin bound to Fc (OPG-Fc) at doses less than or equal to 10 mg/kg was associated with inhibition of bone growth and tooth eruption. Adolescent primates dosed with denosumab at 10 and 50 times (10 and 50 mg/kg dose) more than the recommended human dose based on the body weight had abnormal growth plates.

Adverse Reactions: Denosumab safety in postmenopausal osteoporosis was assessed in a 3-year, randomized, double-blind, placebo-controlled study of 7,808 postmenopausal women aged 60 to 91 years (placebo, n = 3,876; denosumab, n = 3,886). All women were instructed to take at least 1,000 mg of calcium and 400 international units of vitamin D per day. All-cause mortality was 2.3% (n = 90) for placebo and 1.8% (n = 70) for denosumab. Incidence of nonfatal serious adverse events was 24% for placebo and 25% for denosumab. The percentage of patients who withdrew due to adverse events was 2.1% and 2.4% for placebo and denosumab, respectively.

The most common adverse reactions reported with denosumab are back pain, pain in extremity, musculoskeletal pain, hypercholesterolemia, and cystitis. The most common adverse reactions leading to discontinuation of denosumab are breast cancer, back pain, and constipation.

Adverse reactions reported in at least 2% of postmenopausal women with osteoporosis and more frequently in the denosumab-treated women than in the placebo-treated women included anemia (3.3%), angina pectoris (2.6%), atrial fibrillation (2%), vertigo (5%), upper abdominal pain (3.3%), flatulence (2.2%), gastroesophageal reflux disease (2.1%), peripheral edema (4.9%), asthenia (2.3%), cystitis (5.9%), upper respiratory tract infection (4.9%), pneumonia (3.9%), pharyngitis (2.3%), herpes zoster (2%), hypercholesterolemia (7.2%), back pain (34.7%), pain in extremity (11.7%), musculoskeletal pain (7.6%), bone pain (3.7%), myalgia (2.9%), spinal osteoarthritis (2.1%), sciatica (4.6%), insomnia (3.2%), rash (2.5%), and pruritus (2.2%).

Denosumab (Humanized)

Denosumab safety in bone metastasis was assessed in participants who received at least 1 dose of *Xgeva*. In clinical trials, patients were randomized to receive either 120 mg of *Xgeva* every 4 weeks as a subcutaneous injection or 4 mg (dose adjusted for reduced renal function) of zoledronic acid every 4 weeks by IV infusion. Entry criteria included serum calcium (corrected) from 8 to 11.5 mg/dL (2 to 2.9 mmol/L) and creatinine clearance (CrCl) 30 mL/min or higher. Patients who had received IV bisphosphonates were excluded, as were patients with a history of osteonecrosis of the jaw or osteomyelitis of the jaw, an active dental or jaw condition requiring oral surgery, nonhealed dental/oral surgery, or any planned invasive dental procedure. During the study, serum chemistries, including calcium and phosphorus were monitored every 4 weeks. The most common adverse reactions in patients receiving *Xgeva* (per-patient incidence of at least 25%) were fatigue/asthenia, hypophosphatemia, and nausea. The most common serious adverse reaction in patients receiving *Xgeva* was dyspnea. The most common adverse reactions resulting in discontinuation of *Xgeva* were osteonecrosis and hypocalcemia.

Mineral metabolism: Hypocalcemia may be exacerbated by denosumab. Correct preexisting hypocalcemia before starting denosumab therapy. Hypocalcemia after denosumab administration is a significant risk in patients with severe renal impairment or receiving dialysis. Instruct all such patients about symptoms of hypocalcemia and the importance of maintaining calcium levels with adequate calcium and vitamin D supplementation. Adequately supplement all patients with calcium and vitamin D.

Hypocalcemia: Decreases in serum calcium levels to less than 8.5 mg/dL were reported in 0.4% of women in the placebo group and 1.7% of women in the denosumab group at the 1-month visit. The nadir in serum calcium level occurs at approximately day 10 after denosumab dosing in subjects with healthy renal function. In clinical studies, subjects with impaired renal function were more likely to have greater reductions in serum calcium levels compared to those with healthy renal function. In 55 patients with varying degrees of renal function, serum calcium levels less than 7.5 mg/dL or symptomatic hypocalcemia were observed in 5 subjects. These included no subjects with healthy renal function, 10% of those with CrCl 50 to 80 mL/min, 29% of those with CrCl less than 30 mL/min, and 29% of those undergoing hemodialysis. These subjects did not receive calcium and vitamin D supplementation. In a study of 4,550 postmenopausal women with osteoporosis, the mean change from baseline in serum calcium level 10 days after denosumab dosing was −5.5% in subjects with CrCl less than 30 mL/min versus −3.1% in those with CrCl greater than or equal to 30 mL/min.

Infections: RANKL is expressed on activated T- and B-lymphocytes and in lymph nodes. Therefore, a RANKL inhibitor like denosumab may increase the risk of infection. The incidence of infections resulting in death was 0.2% in both placebo and denosumab groups. However, the incidence of nonfatal serious infections was 3.3% in the placebo group and 4% in the denosumab group. Hospitalizations due to serious infections in the abdomen (0.7% for placebo vs 0.9% for denosumab), urinary tract (0.5% for placebo vs 0.7% for denosumab), and ear (0% for placebo vs 0.1% for denosumab) were reported. Endocarditis was reported in no placebo patients and 3 denosumab patients. Skin infections, including erysipelas and cellulitis, leading to hospitalization were more frequent with denosumab (less than 0.1% for placebo vs 0.4% for denosumab). The incidence of opportunistic infections was balanced between placebo and denosumab groups, and the overall incidence of infections was similar between the groups. Advise patients to seek prompt medical attention if they develop signs or symptoms of severe infection, including cellulitis. Patients receiving concomitant immunosuppressant agents or with impaired immune systems may be at increased risk for serious infections. Consider the benefit-risk profile in such patients before treating with denosumab.

Dermatologic: Significantly more patients treated with denosumab developed epidermal and dermal adverse events (eg, dermatitis, eczema, rashes): 8.2% of the placebo and 10.8% of the denosumab group ($P < 0.0001$). Most events were not specific to the injection site. Consider discontinuing denosumab if severe symptoms develop.

Osteonecrosis of the jaw: Osteonecrosis of the jaw can occur spontaneously and is generally associated with tooth extraction and/or local infection with delayed healing. Osteonecrosis of the jaw has been reported in patients receiving denosumab. Perform a routine oral exam before starting denosumab treatment. Consider a dental examination with appropriate preventative dentistry before denosumab in patients with risk factors for osteonecrosis of the jaw, such as invasive dental procedures (eg, tooth extraction, dental implants, oral surgery), diagnosis of cancer, concomitant therapies (eg, chemotherapy, corticosteroids), poor oral hygiene, and comorbid disorders (eg, periodontal or other preexisting dental disease, anemia, coagulopathy, infection, ill-fitting dentures). Encourage good oral hygiene practices during denosumab treatment. Patients suspected of having or who develop osteonecrosis of the jaw while taking denosumab should receive care by a dentist or an oral surgeon. In these patients, extensive dental surgery to treat osteonecrosis of the jaw may exacerbate the condition. Consider stopping denosumab therapy.

Bone turnover: In clinical trials in women with postmenopausal osteoporosis, denosumab resulted in significant suppression of bone remodeling, as evidenced by markers of bone turnover and bone histomorphometry. The significance of these findings and the effect of long-term treatment with denosumab are unknown. The long-term consequences of the degree of suppression of bone remodeling observed with denosumab may contribute to adverse outcomes such as osteonecrosis of the jaw, atypical fractures, and delayed fracture healing.

Pancreatitis: Reported in 4 patients (0.1%) with placebo and 8 patients (0.2%) with denosumab. One placebo recipient and all 8 denosumab recipients had serious events, including 1 death.

Malignancies: The incidence of new malignancies was 4.3% with placebo and 4.8% with denosumab. New malignancies related to breast (0.7% for placebo vs 0.9% for denosumab), reproductive (0.2% for placebo vs 0.5% for denosumab), and GI systems (0.6% for placebo vs 0.9% for denosumab) were reported. A causal relationship has not been established.

Animal toxicology: In ovariectomized monkeys, once-monthly treatment with denosumab suppressed bone turnover and increased bone mineral density (BMD) and strength of cancellous and cortical bone at doses 50-fold more than the recommended human dose, based on body weight (mg/kg). Bone tissue was normal with no evidence of mineralization defects, accumulation of osteoid, or woven bone. Adolescent primates treated with denosumab at doses greater than 10 times (10 and 50 mg/kg dose) more than the recommended human dose, based on mg/kg, had abnormal growth plates, considered to be consistent with the pharmacological activity of denosumab.

Immunologic: Using an electrochemiluminescent bridging immunoassay, 1% (55/8,113) or less of osteoporosis patients and less than 1% (7/2,758) of patients with osseous metastases for up to 5 years tested positive for binding antibodies (including preexisting, transient, and developing antibodies). No patients tested positive for neutralizing antibodies. No evidence of altered pharmacokinetic profile, toxicity profile, or clinical response was associated with binding antibody development.

Pharmacologic & Dosing Characteristics

Dosage:
Prolia: 60 mg every 6 months.
Xgeva: 120 mg every 4 weeks.
Route & Site: Subcutaneous in upper arm, upper thigh, or abdomen.

Overdosage: There is no experience with overdosage with denosumab.

Missed Doses: Give the dose as soon as the patient is available.

Related Interventions: Calcium 1,000 mg daily and vitamin D at least 400 international units daily.

Laboratory Tests: In patients predisposed to hypocalcemia or disturbances of mineral metabolism (eg, history of hypoparathyroidism, thyroid surgery, parathyroid surgery, malabsorption syndromes, excision of small intestine, severe renal impairment [CrCl less than 30 mL/min] or dialysis), monitor calcium and mineral levels (eg, phosphorus, magnesium).

Efficacy:

Prolia: Efficacy and safety in treating postmenopausal osteoporosis were demonstrated in a 3-year, double-blind, placebo-controlled trial. Enrolled women had a baseline BMD T-score between -2.5 and -4 at either lumbar spine or total hip. Women with other diseases (eg, rheumatoid arthritis, osteogenesis imperfecta, Paget disease) or on therapies that affect bone were excluded. The 7,808 enrolled women were 60 to 91 years of age (mean, 72 years). Overall, the mean baseline lumbar spine BMD T-score was -2.8, and 23% of women had a vertebral fracture at baseline. Women were randomized to receive subcutaneous injections of either placebo (n = 3,906) or denosumab 60 mg (n = 3,902) once every 6 months. All women received at least 1,000 mg of calcium and 400 international units of vitamin D supplementation daily. Denosumab significantly reduced incidence of new morphometric vertebral fractures at 1, 2, and 3 years ($P < 0.0001$). Incidence of new vertebral fractures at year 3 was 7.2% in placebo-treated women, compared to 2.3% for denosumab-treated women. Absolute risk reduction was 4.8% and relative risk reduction was 68% for new morphometric vertebral fractures at year 3. Denosumab reduced the risk for new morphometric vertebral fractures regardless of age, baseline rate of bone turnover, baseline BMD, baseline history of fracture, or prior use of a drug for osteoporosis.

Xgeva: In trial 1 of patients with metastatic breast cancer, the hazard ratio for SRE was 0.82 (95% confidence interval [CI], 0.71 to 0.95). In trial 2 of patients with metastatic solid tumors or multiple myeloma, the hazard ratio for SRE was 0.84 (95% CI, 0.71 to 0.98). In trial 3 of patients with metastatic castrate-resistant prostate cancer, the hazard ratio for SRE was 0.82 (95% CI, 0.71 to 0.95).

Incidence of New Vertebral Fractures				
	Proportion of women with fractures (%)[a]			
	Placebo (n = 3,691) (%)	Denosumab (n = 3,702) (%)	Absolute risk reduction (%)[b] (95% CI)	Relative risk reduction (%)[b] (95% CI)
0 to 1 year	2.2	0.9	1.4 (0.8, 1.9)	61 (42, 74)
0 to 2 years	5	1.4	3.5 (2.7, 4.3)	71 (61, 79)
0 to 3 years	7.2	2.3	4.8 (3.9, 5.8)	68 (59, 74)

a Event rates based on crude rates in each interval.

b Absolute risk reduction and relative risk reduction based on Mantel-Haenszel method adjusting for age group variable.

Hip fractures: Incidence of hip fracture was 1.2% for placebo-treated women, compared to 0.7% for denosumab-treated women at year 3. The age-adjusted absolute risk reduction of hip fractures was 0.3%, with a relative risk reduction of 40% at 3 years ($P = 0.04$).

Nonvertebral fractures: Denosumab reduced the incidence of nonvertebral fractures from 8% among placebo recipients to 6.5% among the denosumab group. The absolute risk reduction was 1.5% (95% CI, 0.3% to 2.7%). The relative risk reduction was 20% (95% CI, 5% to 33%). This analysis excluded fractures of the vertebrae (cervical, thoracic, and lumbar), skull, facial, mandible, metacarpus, and finger and toe phalanges.

Bone mineral density: Denosumab significantly increased BMD at all anatomic sites measured at 3 years. The treatment differences in BMD at 3 years were 8.8% at the lumbar spine, 6.4% at the total hip, and 5.2% at the femoral neck. Consistent effects on BMD were observed at the lumbar spine, regardless of baseline age, race, weight/body mass index (BMI), baseline BMD, and level of bone turnover. After stopping denosumab, BMD returned to near baseline levels within 12 months.

Bone: 115 transiliac-crest bone biopsy specimens were obtained from 92 postmenopausal women with osteoporosis at either month 24 and/or month 36. Qualitative histology assessments showed normal architecture and quality with no evidence of mineralization defects, woven bone, or marrow fibrosis in patients treated with denosumab. The presence of double tetracycline labeling in a biopsy specimen indicates active bone remodeling, whereas the absence of tetracycline label suggests suppressed bone formation. In denosumab subjects, 35% had no tetracycline label present at the month 24 biopsy, and 38% had no tetracycline label present at the month 36 biopsy, whereas 100% of placebo patients had double label present at both time points. When compared to placebo, denosumab resulted in virtually absent activation frequency and markedly reduced bone formation rates. However, long-term consequences of this degree of suppression of bone remodeling are unknown.

Onset: The cumulative incidence of hip fractures for denosumab-treated women began to diverge from the placebo group around the 12-month point.

Duration: Not established.

Pharmacokinetics: In clinical studies of osteoporosis, denosumab reduced bone resorption marker serum type 1 C-telopeptide (CTX) by approximately 85% within 3 days, with maximal reductions occurring within 1 month. CTX levels were below the limit of assay quantitation (0.049 ng/mL) in 39% to 68% of subjects 1 to 3 months after dosing denosumab. After each dosing interval, CTX reductions were partially attenuated from a maximal reduction of greater than or equal to 87% to greater than or equal to 45% (range, 45% to 80%) as serum denosumab levels diminished, reflecting the reversibility of the effects of denosumab on bone remodeling. These effects were sustained with continued treatment. Upon reinitiation, the degree of inhibition of CTX by denosumab was similar to that observed in patients starting denosumab. Consistent with the physiological coupling of bone formation and resorption in skeletal remodeling, subsequent reductions in bone-formation markers (ie, osteocalcin and procollagen type 1 N-terminal peptide [PINP]) were observed starting 1 month after the first dose of denosumab. After stopping denosumab therapy, markers of bone resorption increased to levels 40% to 60% above pretreatment values, but returned to baseline levels within 12 months.

In a study in healthy male and female volunteers (n = 73; age range, 18 to 64 years) after a single denosumab 60 mg subcutaneous dose after fasting (12 hours or longer), the mean maximum denosumab concentration (C_{max}) was 6.75 mcg/mL ($\pm$ 1.89 mcg/mL). The median time to maximum denosumab concentration (T_{max}) was 10 days (range, 3 to 21 days). After C_{max}, serum denosumab concentrations declined over 4 to 5 months, with a mean half-life of 25.4 days ($\pm$ 8.5 days; n = 46). The mean area under the curve up to 16 weeks (AUC_{0-16} weeks) of denosumab was 316 mcg•day/mL ($\pm$ 101 mcg•day/mL). No accumulation or change in denosumab pharmacokinetics with time was observed upon multiple dosing of 60 mg subcutaneously once every 6 months. A population pharmacokinetic analysis was performed to evaluate the effects of demographic characteristics. This analysis showed no notable differences in pharmacokinetics with age (in postmenopausal women), race, or body weight (36 to 140 kg).

Bone cancer: In patients with breast cancer and bone metastases, the median reduction in urinary N-terminal telopeptide corrected for creatinine (uNTx/Cr) was 82% within 1 week after starting *Xgeva* 120 mg subcutaneously. In trials, the median reduction in uNTx/Cr from baseline to month 3 was approximately 80% in 2,075 *Xgeva*-treated patients. After subcutaneous administration, bioavailability was 62%. Denosumab displayed nonlinear pharmacokinetics at doses below 60 mg, but approximately dose-proportional increases in exposure at higher doses. With multiple 120 mg subcutaneous doses every 4 weeks in patients with metastatic cancer to the bone, up to 2.8-fold accumulation in serum denosumab concentrations was observed, and steady state was achieved by 6 months. At steady state, the mean ± standard deviation (SD) serum trough concentration was 20.5 ± 13.5 mcg/mL at the recommended *Xgeva* dose, and the mean elimination half-life was 28 days. A population pharmacokinetic analysis was performed to evaluate the effects of demographic characteristics. Denosumab clearance and volume of distribution were proportional to body weight. The steady-state exposure after repeat 120 mg subcutaneous doses every 4 weeks to subjects weighing 45 kg and 120 kg were, respectively, 48% higher and 46% lower than an exposure of the typical 66 kg subject.

Gender: Mean serum concentration-time profiles observed in a study conducted in healthy men 50 years and older were similar to those observed in a study conducted in postmenopausal women using the same dose regimen.

Age: Pharmacokinetics were not affected by age across all populations studied whose ages ranged from 28 to 87 years.

Race: The pharmacokinetics of denosumab were not affected by race.

Renal: In 55 patients with varying degrees of renal function, including patients on dialysis, the degree of renal impairment had no effect on pharmacokinetics; thus, dose adjustment for renal impairment is not necessary. Adequate intake of calcium and vitamin D is important in patients with severe renal impairment or receiving dialysis.

Hepatic: No clinical studies have been conducted to evaluate the effect of hepatic impairment on pharmacokinetics of denosumab.

Mechanism: Binds to RANKL, a transmembrane or soluble protein essential for formation, function, and survival of osteoclasts, cells responsible for bone resorption. Denosumab prevents RANKL from activating its receptor, RANK, on the surface of osteoclasts and their precursors. Preventing RANKL/RANK interaction inhibits osteoclast formation, function, and survival, thereby decreasing bone resorption and increasing bone mass and strength in both cortical and trabecular bone. Increased osteoclast activity, stimulated by RANKL, is a mediator of bone pathology in solid tumors with osseous metastases.

Drug Interactions: No specific drug-drug interaction studies have been conducted with denosumab.

Pharmaceutical Characteristics

Concentration:
Prolia: 60 mg per mL
Xgeva: 70 mg per mL

Packaging:
Prolia: One single-use 60 mg per 1 mL syringe (NDC#: 55513-0710-01), 1 single-use 60 mg per 1 mL vial (55513-0720-01)
Xgeva: One single-use 120 mg per 1.7 mL vial (55513-0730-01)

Doseform: Solution

Appearance: Clear, colorless to pale yellow solution, that may contain trace amounts of translucent to white proteinaceous particles. Do not use if discolored or cloudy.

Solvent: Water for injection with sorbitol.

Adjuvant: None

Preservative: None

Allergens: Grey needle cap on prefilled syringe contains dry natural rubber (a derivative of latex).

Excipients:

Prolia: Sorbitol 4.7%, acetate 17 mM, polysorbate-20 0.01%, and sodium hydroxide to adjust pH

Xgeva: Sorbitol 4.7%, acetate 18 mM, and sodium hydroxide

pH: 5.2

Shelf Life: Data not provided.

Storage/Stability: Store at 2° to 8°C (36° to 46°F). Do not freeze. Once removed from refrigerator, do not expose denosumab to temperatures greater than 25°C (77°F). Discard if not used within 14 days. Protect denosumab from direct light and heat. Avoid vigorous shaking. Contact the manufacturer regarding exposure to freezing or elevated temperatures. Shipping data not provided.

Handling: Before administration, remove denosumab from refrigerator and bring to room temperature (up to 25°C, 77°F) by standing in the original container. This generally takes 15 to 30 minutes. Do not warm denosumab in any other way.

Production Process: Antibody harvested from genetically engineered Chinese hamster ovary cells.

Media: Genetically engineered Chinese hamster ovary cells.

Other Information

First Licensed: June 1, 2010

References: Lewiecki EM. RANK ligand inhibition with denosumab for the management of osteoporosis. *Expert Opin Biol Ther*. 2006;6(10):1041-1050.

McClung MR, Lewiecki EM, Cohen SB, et al; AMG 162 Bone Loss Study Group. Denosumab in postmenopausal women with low bone mineral density. *N Engl J Med*. 2006;354(8):821-831.

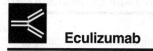

Eculizumab

Isoantibodies

Name:
 Soliris
Synonyms: 5G1.1, h5G1.1

Manufacturer:
 Alexion Pharmaceuticals

Immunologic Characteristics

Target Antigen: Human complement protein C5

Viability: Not viable, but immunologically active

Antigenic Form: Recombinant humanized monoclonal $IgG_{2/4k}$ antibody containing human constant regions from human IgG2 sequences and human IgG4 sequences and murine complementarity-determining regions grafted onto the human framework light- and heavy-chain variable regions.

Antigenic Type: Protein, two 448 amino acid heavy chains and two 214 amino acid light chains and has a molecular weight of approximately 148 kDa.

Use Characteristics

Indications: To reduce hemolysis caused by paroxysmal nocturnal hemoglobinuria (PNH).

To treat patients with atypical hemolytic uremic syndrome (HUS) to inhibit complement-mediated thrombotic microangiopathy.

Contraindications:
 Absolute: People with unresolved serious *Neisseria meningitidis* infection. People not currently vaccinated against *N. meningitidis.*
 Relative: Use caution when administering eculizumab to patients with any systemic infection.

Elderly: In PNH studies, 15 patients 65 years of age and older received eculizumab. Although no apparent age-related differences occurred, the number of patients 65 years of age and older is not sufficient to determine whether they respond differently than younger patients.

Carcinogenicity: Eculizumab has not been evaluated for carcinogenic potential.

Mutagenicity: Eculizumab has not been evaluated for mutagenic potential.

Fertility Impairment: Effects of eculizumab upon fertility have not been studied in animals. Intravenous (IV) injections of male and female mice with a murine anti-C5 antibody at up to 4 to 8 times the human equivalent dose of eculizumab had no adverse effects on mating or fertility.

Pregnancy: Category C. PNH is a serious illness. Pregnant women with PNH and their fetuses have high rates of morbidity and mortality during pregnancy and the postpartum period. There are no adequate and well-controlled studies of eculizumab in pregnant women. Eculizumab is expected to cross the placenta. Animal studies using a mouse analog of eculizumab (murine anti-C5 antibody) showed increased rates of developmental abnormalities and an increased rate of dead and moribund offspring at doses 2 to 8 times the human dose. Use eculizumab during pregnancy only if the potential benefit justifies the potential risk to the fetus. Animal reproduction studies were conducted in mice using doses of a murine anti-C5 antibody at approximately 2 to 4 times (low dose) and 4 to 8 times (high dose) the recommended human eculizumab dose, based on body mass. When animal exposure to the antibody occurred from before mating until early gestation, no decrease in fertility or reproductive performance was observed. When maternal exposure to the antibody occurred during organogenesis, 2 cases of retinal dysplasia and 1 case of umbilical hernia were observed among 230 offspring born to mothers exposed to the higher antibody dose; however, the exposure did not increase fetal loss or neonatal death. When maternal exposure to the antibody occurred from implantation through weaning, a higher number of male offspring became moribund or died (1 of 25 controls, 2 of 25 in the low-dose group, 5 of 25 in the high-dose group). Surviving offspring had normal development and reproductive performance. No information is available on the effects of eculizumab during labor and delivery.

Lactation: It is not known whether eculizumab crosses into human breast milk. Because IgG is excreted in human milk, eculizumab may also be secreted. Published data suggest that breast milk antibodies do not enter the neonatal and infant circulation in substantial amounts. Exercise caution when eculizumab is administered to a breast-feeding woman. Weigh the unknown risks to the infant from GI or limited systemic exposure to eculizumab against the known benefits of breast-feeding.

Children: Safety and efficacy of eculizumab in children younger than 18 years have not been established for PNH. For atypical HUS, safety and effectiveness in children are similar to adult patients.

Adverse Reactions: The following data reflect exposure to eculizumab in 196 adult patients 18 to 85 years of age with PNH (55% were women). All had signs or symptoms of intravascular hemolysis. Eculizumab was studied in a placebo-controlled clinical study, a single-arm clinical study, and a long-term extension study; 182 patients were exposed for 1 year or more. All patients received the recommended eculizumab dose regimen.

The most frequently reported adverse reactions in atypical HUS single-arm prospective trials (at least 15% combined per-patient incidence) were hypertension, upper respiratory tract infection, diarrhea, headache, anemia, vomiting, nausea, urinary tract infection, and leukopenia.

Adverse events that occurred at a higher rate in the eculizumab group than the placebo group and at a rate of 5% or more in the eculizumab include the following:

Adverse Events in the Controlled Clinical Study		
Reaction	Eculizumab (n = 43)	Placebo (n = 44)
Headache	19 (44%)	12 (27%)
Nasopharyngitis	10 (23%)	8 (18%)
Back pain	8 (19%)	4 (9%)
Nausea	7 (16%)	5 (11%)
Fatigue	5 (12%)	1 (2%)
Cough	5 (12%)	4 (9%)
Herpes simplex infections	3 (7%)	0 (0%)
Sinusitis	3 (7%)	0 (0%)
Respiratory tract infection	3 (7%)	1 (2%)
Constipation	3 (7%)	2 (5%)
Myalgia	3 (7%)	1 (2%)
Pain in extremity	3 (7%)	1 (2%)
Influenza-like illness	2 (5%)	1 (2%)

In the placebo-controlled clinical study, serious adverse events, including infections and progression of PNH, occurred in 4 patients (9%) receiving eculizumab and in 9 patients (21%) receiving placebo. No deaths occurred in the study and no patients receiving eculizumab experienced a thrombotic event; 1 thrombotic event occurred in a patient receiving placebo.

Among 193 patients with PNH treated with eculizumab in the single-arm study or the follow-up study, adverse events were similar to those reported in the placebo-controlled clinical study. Serious adverse events occurred among 16% of patients. The most common serious adverse events were viral infection (2%), headache (2%), anemia (2%), and pyrexia (2%).

Infections: Eculizumab increases a patient's susceptibility to serious meningococcal infections (ie, septicemia, meningitis). In clinical studies, 2 of 196 patients with PNH developed serious meningococcal infections while receiving eculizumab treatment; both had been vaccinated. In clinical studies among patients without PNH, meningococcal meningitis occurred in an unvaccinated patient. Vaccinate all patients against meningococci at least 2 weeks before the first dose of eculizumab. However, vaccination may not always prevent meningococcal infections.

Eculizumab blocks terminal complement; therefore, patients may have increased susceptibility to infections, especially with encapsulated bacteria. Use caution when administering eculizumab to patients with any systemic infection.

Hematologic: Eculizumab therapy increases the number of PNH cells; patients who discontinue eculizumab treatment may be at increased risk for serious hemolysis. Serious hemolysis is identified by serum lactate dehydrogenase (LDH) levels higher than the pretreatment level, along with any of the following: at least 25% absolute decrease in PNH clone size (in the absence of dilution due to transfusion) in 1 week or less; a hemoglobin level of less than 5 g/dL or a decrease of more than 4 g/dL in 1 week or less; angina; change in mental status; a 50% increase in serum creatinine level; and thrombosis. Monitor any patient who discontinues eculizumab for at least 8 weeks to detect serious hemolysis and other reactions. If serious hemolysis occurs after discontinuing eculizumab, consider the following procedures or treatments: blood transfusion (packed red blood cells [RBCs]), or exchange transfusion if the PNH RBCs are more than 50% of the total RBCs by flow cytometry; anticoagulation; corticosteroids; or reinstitution of eculizumab. In clinical studies, 16 of 196 patients with PNH discontinued treatment with eculizumab. Patients were followed for evidence of worsening hemolysis and no serious hemolysis was observed.

Immunologic: As with all proteins, there is a potential for immunogenicity. Low titers of antibodies to eculizumab were detected in 3 of 196 (2%) of all PNH patients treated with eculizumab. No apparent correlation of antibody development to clinical response was observed. Immunogenicity data reflect the percentage of patients whose test results were considered positive for antibodies to eculizumab in an enzyme-linked immunosorbent assay (ELISA) and are highly dependent on the sensitivity and specificity of the assay.

Pharmacologic & Dosing Characteristics

Dosage: Administer eculizumab at the recommended dosage regimen time points, or within 2 days of these time points.

Paroxysmal nocturnal hemoglobinuria: 600 mg via 35-minute IV infusion every 7 days for the first 4 weeks, followed by 900 mg for the fifth dose 7 days later, then 900 mg every 14 days thereafter.

Atypical hemolytic uremic syndrome: For patients 18 years of age and older: 900 mg weekly for 4 weeks, then 1,200 mg 1 week later, then 1,200 mg every 2 weeks thereafter.

For patients younger than 18 years, calculate dose based on body weight:
- 40 kg or more: 900 mg weekly for 4 doses, then 1,200 mg at week 5, then 1,200 mg every 2 weeks
- 30 to 39 kg: 600 mg weekly for 2 doses, then 900 mg at week 3, then 900 mg every 2 weeks
- 20 to 29 kg: 600 mg weekly for 2 doses, then 600 mg at week 3, then 600 mg every 2 weeks
- 10 to 19 kg: 600 mg weekly for 1 dose, then 300 mg at week 2, then 300 mg every 2 weeks
- 5 to 9 kg: 300 mg weekly for 1 dose, then 300 mg at week 2, then 300 mg every 3 weeks

Supplemental dosing is needed in the setting of concomitant support with plasmapheresis/ plasma exchange or fresh frozen plasma infusion, according to the following schedule.

Supplemental Dosing for Eculizumab Based on Concomitant Interventions			
Type of intervention	Most recent eculizumab dose	Supplemental eculizumab dose with each plasmapheresis/ plasma exchange or fresh frozen plasma infusion intervention	Timing of supplemental eculizumab dose
Plasmapheresis or plasma exchange	300 mg	300 mg per each plasmapheresis or plasma exchange session	Within 60 minutes after each plasmapheresis or plasma exchange session
	600 mg or more	600 mg per each plasmapheresis or plasma exchange session	
Fresh frozen plasma infusion	300 mg or more	300 mg per each unit of fresh frozen plasma	60 minutes before each 1 unit of fresh frozen plasma infusion

Route: IV infusion, via gravity feed, a syringe-type pump, or an infusion pump. Do not administer as an IV push or bolus.

If an adverse reaction occurs during administration of eculizumab, slow or stop the infusion. If the infusion is slowed, the total infusion time should not exceed 2 hours. Monitor the patient for at least 1 hour after completing the infusion for signs or symptoms of an infusion reaction.

After Discontinuation: Eculizumab increases the number of PNH RBCs. Monitor all patients who discontinue eculizumab therapy for signs and symptoms of intravascular hemolysis, including evaluation of serum LDH levels.

The effect of withdrawal of anticoagulant therapy during eculizumab treatment has not been established. Therefore, treatment with eculizumab should not alter anticoagulant management.

Monitor patients with atypical HUS for signs and symptoms of thrombotic microangiopathy (TMA) complications for at least 12 weeks. In atypical HUS clinical studies, 18 patients (5 in the prospective studies) discontinued eculizumab treatment. TMA complications occurred following a missed dose in 5 patients, and eculizumab was reinitiated in 4 of these 5 patients. Clinical signs and symptoms of TMA include changes in mental status, seizures, angina, dyspnea, or thrombosis. In addition, the following changes in laboratory parameters may identify a TMA complication: occurrence of 2, or repeated measurement of any one, of the following: a decrease in platelet count by 25% or more compared with baseline or the peak platelet count during eculizumab treatment; an increase in serum creatinine by 25% or more compared with baseline or nadir during eculizumab treatment; or an increase in serum LDH by 25% or more compared with baseline or nadir during eculizumab treatment. If TMA complications occur, consider reinstitution of eculizumab treatment, plasma therapy (plasmapheresis, plasma exchange, or fresh frozen plasma infusion), or appropriate organ-specific supportive measures.

Overdosage: No specific data are available.

Missed Doses: Interrupting the recommended schedule or delaying subsequent doses does not require restarting the series.

Related Interventions: Eculizumab increases the risk of meningococcal infections. Vaccinate patients with a meningococcal vaccine at least 2 weeks before the first dose of eculizumab; revaccinate according to current standard of care. Quadrivalent meningococcal conjugate vaccines are preferred. Monitor patients for early signs of meningococcal infections; evaluate immediately if infection is suspected, and treat with antibiotics if necessary.

Laboratory Tests: Serum LDH levels increase during hemolysis and may assist in monitoring eculizumab effects, including response to discontinuing therapy. In clinical studies, 6 patients achieved a reduction in serum LDH levels only after a decrease in the eculizumab dosing interval from 14 to 12 days. All other patients achieved a reduction in serum LDH levels with the 14-day dosing interval.

Efficacy: The safety and efficacy of eculizumab in PNH patients with hemolysis were assessed in a randomized, double-blind, placebo-controlled, 26-week study (study 1). PNH patients were also treated with eculizumab in a single-arm, 52-week study (study 2) and in a long-term extension study.

Study 1: PNH patients with 4 or more transfusions in the prior 12 months, flow cytometric confirmation of at least 10% PNH cells, and platelet counts of at least 100,000 cells/mcL were randomized to eculizumab (n = 43) or placebo (n = 44). Before randomization, all patients were observed to confirm the need for RBC transfusion and to identify the hemoglobin concentration (the "set point") that would define each patient's hemoglobin stabilization and transfusion outcome. The hemoglobin set point was 9 g/dL or less in patients with symptoms and 7 g/dL or less in patients without symptoms. End points related to hemolysis included the numbers of patients achieving hemoglobin stabilization, the number of RBC units transfused, fatigue, and health-related quality of life. Hemoglobin stabilization was defined as maintaining a hemoglobin concentration above the hemoglobin set point and avoiding RBC transfusion for the entire 26-week period. Hemolysis was monitored mainly through serum LDH levels. The proportion of PNH RBCs was monitored by flow cytometry. Patients receiving anticoagulants and systemic corticosteroids at baseline continued these medications. Major baseline characteristics were balanced.

Patients treated with eculizumab had less hemolysis ($P < 0.001$), with improved anemia based on hemoglobin stabilization and a reduced need for RBC transfusions than patients treated with placebo. These effects were seen regardless of prestudy RBC transfusion strata. After 3 weeks of eculizumab treatment, patients reported less fatigue and improved health-related quality of life. Because of study sample size and duration, effects of eculizumab on thrombotic events could not be determined.

Study 1 Results		
	Placebo (n = 44)	Eculizumab (n = 43)
Percentage of patients with stabilized hemoglobin levels	0%	49%
Packed RBC units transfused per patient (median) (range)	10 (2 to 21)	0 (0 to 16)
Transfusion avoidance (%)	0%	51%
LDH levels at end of study (median, units/L)	2,167	239
Free hemoglobin at end of study (median, mg/dL)	62	5

Study 2 and extension study: PNH patients with 1 transfusion or more in the prior 24 months and at least 30,000 platelets/mcL received eculizumab over a 52-week period. Concomitant medications included antithrombotic agents in 63% of patients and systemic corticosteroids in 40% of patients. Overall, 96 of the 97 enrolled patients completed the study (1 patient died following a thrombotic event). A reduction in intravascular hemolysis as measured by serum LDH levels was sustained for the treatment period and resulted in a reduced need for RBC transfusion and less fatigue; 187 eculizumab-treated PNH patients were enrolled in a long-term extension study. All patients sustained a reduction in intravascular hemolysis during eculizumab treatment ranging from 10 to 54 months. Fewer thrombotic events occurred with eculizumab treatment than during the same period of time before treatment. However, the majority of patients received concomitant anticoagulants; the effect of anticoagulant withdrawal during eculizumab therapy was not studied.

Pharmacokinetics: In the placebo-controlled clinical study, eculizumab reduced hemolysis, manifested as lowered serum LDH levels from 2,200 ± 1,034 units/L (mean ± SD) at baseline to 700 ± 388 units/L by week 1 and maintained the effect through the end of the study at week 26 (327 ± 433 units/L). In the single-arm clinical study, eculizumab maintained this effect through 52 weeks.

A pharmacokinetic analysis with a standard 1-compartmental model was conducted with 40 PNH patients who received the recommended multidose eculizumab regimen. Eculizumab clearance for a typical PNH patient weighing 70 kg was 22 mL/h, with a volume of distribution of 7.7 L. The half-life was 272 ± 82 hours (mean ± SD). The mean observed peak and trough serum concentrations of eculizumab by week 26 were 194 ± 76 mcg/mL and 97 ± 60 mcg/mL, respectively.

Studies have not been conducted to evaluate the pharmacokinetics of eculizumab in special patient populations identified by gender, race, age (pediatric or geriatric), or the presence of renal or hepatic impairment.

Mechanism: Eculizumab specifically binds to the complement protein C5 with high affinity, thereby inhibiting its cleavage to C5a and C5b and preventing the generation of the terminal complement complex C5b-9. Eculizumab inhibits terminal complement-mediated intravascular hemolysis in PNH patients and complement-mediated TMA in atypical HUS patients.

A genetic mutation in PNH patients leads to the generation of populations of abnormal RBCs (known as PNH cells) that are deficient in terminal-complement inhibitors, rendering PNH RBCs sensitive to persistent terminal complement-mediated destruction. The destruction and loss of these PNH cells (intravascular hemolysis) results in low RBC counts (anemia), and fatigue, difficulty in functioning, pain, dark urine, shortness of breath, and blood clots. In atypical HUS, impairment in the regulation of complement activity leads to uncontrolled terminal complement activation, resulting in platelet activation, endothelial cell damage, and TMA.

Because eculizumab blocks terminal complement, patients may have increased susceptibility to infections, especially with encapsulated bacteria (eg, meningococci).

Drug Interactions: Drug interaction studies have not been performed with eculizumab.

Patient Information: Give patient a safety card that lists symptoms warranting immediate medical attention (eg, signs and symptoms of meningococcal infection). Signs and symptoms of meningococcal infection include moderate to severe headache with nausea or vomiting, fever (often as high as 39.4°C [103°F]), or stiff neck or stiff back; rash; confusion; severe muscle aches with influenza-like symptoms; and eye sensitivity to light. Patients should carry this card at all times and show the card to health care providers who treat them. Advise patients to be monitored for hemolysis (breakdown of RBCs) at least 8 weeks after stopping eculizumab.

Pharmaceutical Characteristics

Concentration: 10 mg/mL

Quality Assay: Purified by standard bioprocess technology

Packaging: Single 300 mg per 30 mL vial

NDC Number: 25682-0001-01

Doseform: Solution

Appearance: Clear, colorless solution

Solvent: Phosphate-buffered saline solution

Eculizumab

Diluent:
> *For infusion:* Dilute to a final concentration of 5 mg/mL before administration by adding an equal volume of diluent (ie, sodium chloride 0.9%, sodium chloride 0.45%, dextrose 5%, or Ringer's lactate injection, USP, to the infusion bag).

Adjuvant: None

Preservative: None

Allergens: None

Excipients: Each vial contains sodium phosphate monobasic 13.8 mg, sodium phosphate dibasic 53.4 mg, sodium chloride 263.1 mg, and polysorbate 80 (vegetable origin) 6.6 mg.

pH: 7

Shelf Life: Data not provided.

Storage/Stability: Store at 2° to 8°C (36° to 46°F). Protect vials from light. Do not shake. Discard if frozen. Contact the manufacturer regarding exposure to freezing or elevated temperatures. Shipping data not provided.

Diluted solutions of eculizumab are stable for 24 hours at 2° to 8°C (36° to 46°F) and at room temperature.

Handling: The final admixed eculizumab 5 mg/mL infusion volume is 60 mL for 300 mg doses, 120 mL for 600 mg doses, 180 mL for 900 mg doses, or 240 mL for 1,200 mg doses. Gently invert the infusion bag to ensure thorough mixing. Discard any unused portion left in a vial. Before administration, allow the admixture to adjust to room temperature (18° to 25°C [64° to 77°F]). Do not heat the admixture in a microwave or with any heat source other than ambient air temperature.

Media: Murine myeloma cell culture

Disease Epidemiology

Prevalence: PNH affects 1 to 2 people per million population. PNH is primarily a disease of adults (median age of diagnosis, 35 to 40 years of age) with occasional cases diagnosed in children or adolescents.

Other Information

Perspective:
> *1852:* Strübing describes paroxysmal hemoglobinuria.

First Licensed: March 16, 2007.

References: Hill A, Hillmen P, Richards SJ, et al. Sustained response and long-term safety of eculizumab in paroxysmal nocturnal hemoglobinuria. *Blood.* 2005;106(7):2559-2565.

Isoantibodies

Name:
  Enbrel

Manufacturer:
  Manufactured by Immunex Corporation,
  distributed by Amgen

Synonyms: Tumor necrosis factor receptor-p75 fusion protein, TNFR:Fc

Comparison: Etanercept is a molecule that acts as a soluble receptor for tumor necrosis factor (TNF). Etanercept is categorically and structurally different from antibodies that neutralize TNF (eg, infliximab).

Immunologic Characteristics

Target Antigen: Human tissue necrosis factor receptor fused to Fc antibody fragments

Viability: Not viable, but immunologically active

Antigenic Form: Soluble receptors linked to Fc fragments of IgG1 antibody

Antigenic Type: Dimeric fusion protein consisting of the extracellular ligand-binding portion of the human 75-kilodalton (p75) tumor necrosis factor receptor (TNFR) linked to the Fc portion of human IgG1. The Fc component of etanercept contains the C_H2 domain, the C_H3 domain and hinge region, but not the C_H1 domain of IgG1. Etanercept consists of 934 amino acids and has an apparent molecular weight of approximately 150 kilodaltons.

Use Characteristics

Indications: To reduce signs and symptoms, delay progression of structural damage, and improve physical function in patients with moderately to severely active rheumatoid arthritis (RA), including patients who have or have not had an inadequate response to 1 or more disease-modifying antirheumatic drugs (DMARDs) (eg, hydroxychloroquine, oral or injectable gold, methotrexate, azathioprine, D-penicillamine, sulfasalazine). Etanercept can be used in combination with methotrexate in patients who do not respond adequately to methotrexate alone.

To reduce the signs and symptoms of moderately to severely active polyarticular-course juvenile rheumatoid arthritis (JRA) in children who have had an inadequate response to one or more DMARDs.

To reduce signs and symptoms of active arthritis, delay progression of structural damage in patients with psoriatic arthritis, and improve physical function in patients with psoriatic arthritis. Etanercept can be used in combination with methotrexate in patients who do not respond adequately to methotrexate alone.

To reduce signs and symptoms in patients with active ankylosing spondylitis.

To treat adult patients with chronic moderate to severe plaque psoriasis who are candidates for systemic therapy or phototherapy.

Unlabeled Uses: Research in progress is assessing the value of etanercept in treating congestive heart failure, septic shock, and other disorders.

Contraindications:

Absolute: Patients with sepsis.

Relative: Patients with known severe hypersensitivity to etanercept or any of its components.

Etanercept (Recombinant)

Immunodeficiency: The possibility exists that anti-TNF therapies, including etanercept, may affect host defenses against infections and malignancies because TNF mediates inflammation and modulates cellular immune responses. The safety and efficacy of etanercept in immunodeficient patients is not fully known.

Elderly: At least 197 RA and 89 plaque psoriasis patients 65 years of age and older were studied in clinical trials. No overall differences in safety or efficacy were observed between these patients and younger patients. Greater sensitivity of some older individuals cannot be ruled out. Because the incidence of infections is higher among the elderly in general, use caution in treating this population.

Carcinogenicity: Long-term animal studies have not been conducted to evaluate the carcinogenic potential of etanercept.

Mutagenicity: Mutagenesis studies were conducted in vitro and in vivo. No evidence of mutagenic activity was observed.

Fertility Impairment: Long-term animal studies have not been conducted to evaluate the effect of etanercept on fertility.

Pregnancy: Category B. Developmental toxicity studies were performed in rats and rabbits at doses 60- to 100-fold greater than the human dose, and revealed no evidence of harm to the fetus caused by etanercept. However, there are no studies in pregnant women. Because animal reproduction studies are not always predictive of human response, use etanercept during pregnancy only if clearly needed.

Lactation: It is not known if etanercept crosses into human breast milk or is absorbed systemically after ingestion. Because many drugs and immunoglobulins are excreted in human milk, and because of the potential for serious adverse reactions in nursing infants, decide whether to discontinue nursing or discontinue etanercept.

Children: In an open-label study, 69 children (4 to 17 years of age) were given etanercept 0.4 mg/kg (maximum: 25 mg) subcutaneously twice weekly for 3 months. These children had moderately to severely active polyarticular-course JRA, refractory to or intolerant of methotrexate. Of 54 patients for whom 3-month treatment data were available, 76% demonstrated a clinical response measured by the JRA definition of improvement. The JRA definition of improvement involves 30% or greater improvement in 3 or more of 6 criteria and 30% or greater worsening in no more than 1 of 6 JRA core set criteria, which include physician and patient global assessments, active joint count, limitation of motion, functional assessment, and erythrocyte sedimentation rate (ESR).

Of 69 JRA patients for whom safety data were available, the safety profile was similar to that seen in adult RA patients treated with etanercept. However, the fraction of JRA patients reporting abdominal pain (17%) and vomiting (14.5%) was higher than in adult RA patients. While receiving etanercept, 2 JRA patients developed varicella infection associated with signs and symptoms of aseptic meningitis; the infections resolved without sequelae. In patients with a significant exposure to varicella virus, temporarily discontinue etanercept therapy and consider treatment with varicella-zoster immune globulin (VZIG). Etanercept has not been studied in children under 4 years of age.

Adverse Reactions: Etanercept has been studied in approximately 1,200 patients with RA, followed for up to 36 months, and in 157 patients with psoriatic arthritis, followed for 6 months. The proportion of patients who discontinued treatment because of adverse events was the same in both the etanercept and placebo treatment groups (4%).

Allergic reactions: Allergic reactions associated with etanercept were reported rarely (less than 2%). Anaphylaxis has not yet been observed. If an anaphylactic reaction or another serious allergic reaction occurs, discontinue etanercept immediately and initiate appropriate therapy.

Auto-antibodies: Patients had serum samples tested for auto-antibodies at multiple time-points. Of patients evaluated for antinuclear antibodies (ANA), the fraction who developed new positive ANA (greater than or equal to 1:40) was higher in people treated with etanercept (11%) than in placebo-treated patients (5%). The fraction who developed new positive anti-double-stranded DNA antibodies was also higher by radioimmunoassay (15% for etanercept compared with 4% for placebo) and by crithidia lucilae assay (3% for etanercept, none for placebo). The fraction of patients treated with etanercept who developed anticardiolipin antibodies was similarly increased compared with placebo-treated patients. No patients developed clinical signs suggesting a lupus-like syndrome or other new autoimmune disease. The effect of long-term treatment with etanercept on developing autoimmune diseases is unknown.

Hematologic: Several cases of blood dyscrasias during etanercept therapy have been reported, between 2 weeks and 5 months after initiation of treatment. Some of these cases had fatal outcomes related to sepsis. The blood dyscrasias included pancytopenia (less than 1 case per 1,000 treated patients) and aplastic anemia (less than 1 case per 10,000 treated patients). Discontinue etanercept if blood dyscrasias are confirmed.

Immunogenicity: Patients were tested at multiple time-points for antibodies to etanercept. Antibodies to etanercept, all nonneutralizing, were detected at least once in sera of up to 5% of adult patients with RA or psoriatic arthritis. No apparent correlation of antibody development to clinical response or adverse events was observed. The immunogenicity of long-term therapy with etanercept is unknown.

Immunosuppression: The possibility exists that anti-TNF therapies, including etanercept, may affect host defenses against infections and malignancies because TNF mediates inflammation and modulates cellular immune responses. In a study of 49 patients with RA treated with etanercept, there was no evidence of depression of delayed-type hypersensitivity, depression of immunoglobulin levels, or change in enumeration of effector cell populations. The impact of etanercept on the development and course of malignancies and infections is not fully understood. The safety and efficacy of etanercept in patients with immunosuppression or chronic infections have not been evaluated.

Infections: Serious infections, including sepsis and fatal infections, have been reported in patients receiving TNF-blocking agents. Do not give etanercept to patients with any infection, including chronic or localized infections. Exercise caution when considering etanercept for patients with a chronic infection or a history of recurrent infection. Do not give etanercept to patients with clinically important, active infections. Rare cases of tuberculosis occurred in patients treated with TNF-antagonists. Closely monitor patients who develop a new infection during treatment. If a patient develops a serious infection or sepsis, discontinue therapy. Upper respiratory tract infections (URIs; colds) and sinusitis were the most frequently reported infections in patients receiving etanercept or placebo. In placebo-controlled trials, the incidence of URIs was 16% in the placebo group and 29% in the etanercept group. Accounting for the longer observation period among patients taking etanercept, 0.68 events per patient-year occurred in the placebo group and 0.82 events per patient-year occurred in the etanercept group. No increase in the incidence of serious infections was observed (1.3% for placebo, 0.9% for etanercept). In open-label and placebo-controlled trials, 22 serious infections were observed among 745 subjects exposed to etanercept, including pyelonephritis, bronchitis, septic arthritis, abdominal abscess, cellulitis, osteomyelitis, wound infection, pneumonia, foot abscess, leg ulcer, diarrhea, sinusitis, and sepsis. Data from a sepsis clinical trial not specifically involving patients with RA suggest that etanercept treatment may increase mortality in patients with established sepsis.

Injection-site reactions: In controlled trials, 37% of patients treated with etanercept developed injection-site reactions. All injection-site reactions were described as mild to moderate (eg, erythema, itching, pain, swelling) and generally did not require stopping therapy.

Etanercept (Recombinant)

Injection-site reactions generally occurred in the first month of therapy and subsequently decreased in frequency. The mean duration of injection-site reactions was 3 to 5 days. Seven percent of patients experienced redness at a previous injection site when subsequent injections were given.

Malignancies: Seventeen new malignancies of various types were observed in 1,197 RA patients treated with etanercept for up to 36 months. The observed rates and incidences were similar to those expected for the population studied.

Nervous system: Rare cases of CNS demyelinating disorders have been reported, although a causal relationship to etanercept therapy is unclear. Cases of transverse myelitis, optic neuritis, multiple sclerosis, and new onset or exacerbation of seizure disorders have been observed in association with etanercept therapy. While no clinical trials have been performed evaluating etanercept in people with multiple sclerosis, administering other TNF antagonists to people with multiple sclerosis resulted in increases in disease activity. Carefully consider the risk/benefit ratio in patients with preexisting or recent onset CNS-demyelinating disorders.

Other adverse reactions: Events reported in 3% or more of patients, with higher incidence in patients treated with etanercept compared with controls in placebo-controlled RA trials (including the combination methotrexate trial), were as follows:

Adverse Events in Placebo-Controlled Clinical Trials[a]			
	Percent of patients		Events per patient-year
Event	Placebo (n = 152)	Etanercept (n = 349)	Placebo (40 pt-y)	Etanercept (117 pt-y)
Injection-site reaction	10	37	0.62	7.73
Infection	32	35	1.86	1.82
Nonupper respiratory infection[b]	32	38	1.54	1.5
Upper respiratory tract infection[b]	16	29	0.68	0.82
Headache	13	17	0.62	0.68
Rhinitis	8	12	0.35	0.45
Dizziness	5	7	0.25	0.21
Pharyngitis	5	7	0.17	0.24
Cough	3	6	0.17	0.18
Asthenia	3	5	0.1	0.16
Pain, abdominal	3	5	0.12	0.17
Rash	3	5	0.12	0.21
Respiratory disorder	1	5	0.05	0.17
Dyspepsia	1	4	0.05	0.12
Sinusitis	2	3	0.07	0.12

a Includes data from the 6-month study in which patients received concurrent methotrexate therapy.
b Includes data from 2 of the 3 controlled trials.

Among RA patients treated in controlled trials, serious adverse events occurred in 4% of patients treated with etanercept compared with 5% of placebo-treated patients. Among RA patients in controlled and open-label trials of etanercept, malignancies and infections were the most common serious adverse events observed. Other infrequent serious adverse events included: Heart failure, MI, myocardial ischemia, cerebral ischemia, hypertension, hypotension, cholecystitis, pancreatitis, GI hemorrhage, bursitis, depression, and dyspnea.

Pediatric patients: In general, adverse events in pediatric patients are similar in frequency and type to those seen in adults. Severe adverse reactions reported in 69 JRA patients 4 to

17 years of age included varicella, gastroenteritis, depression/personality disorder, cutaneous ulcer, and esophagitis/gastritis. Of the 69 patients, 43 (62%) experienced an infection while receiving etanercept during 3 months of observation. The types of infections reported were generally mild and consistent with those commonly seen in outpatient pediatric populations. Several adverse events were reported more commonly in JRA patients compared with adult RA patients. These included headache (19%, 1.7 events per patient-year), nausea (9%, 1 event per patient-year), abdominal pain (19%, 0.74 events per patient-year), and vomiting (13%, 0.74 per patient-year).

Pharmacologic & Dosing Characteristics

Dosage: For adult patients with RA, psoriatic arthritis, or ankylosing spondylitis, 50 mg/week given as two 25 mg injections at separate sites. The two injections may be given on the same day or 3 to 4 days apart. Methotrexate, glucocorticoids, salicylates, nonsteroidal anti-inflammatory drugs (NSAIDs), or analgesics may be continued during treatment with etanercept. A dose of 50 mg twice weekly suggested a higher incidence of adverse events, but similar ACR response rates to doses higher than 50 mg per week are not recommended.

For adult plaque psoriasis patients, the recommended starting dose is 50 mg twice weekly for 3 months, followed by reduction to a maintenance dose of 50 mg per week. Starting doses of 25 mg or 50 mg per week have also been shown to be effective. The proportion of responders is related to etanercept dose.

For pediatric patients 4 to 17 years of age, 0.8 mg/kg/week (maximum, 50 mg per dose and 25 mg per injection), either on the same day or as two doses 3 to 4 days apart. The dose for children 31 kg (68 pounds) or less should be given as a single injection once weekly. Glucocorticoids, NSAIDs, or analgesics may be continued during treatment with etanercept. Neither higher doses of etanercept nor concurrent use with methotrexate has been studied.

Give doses at least 72 to 96 hours apart.

Route: Subcutaneous injection

Overdosage: The maximum tolerated dose of etanercept has not been established in humans. Toxicology studies in monkeys at doses up to 30 times the human dose showed no evidence of dose-limiting toxicities. No dose-limiting toxicities were observed during clinical trials of etanercept. Single IV doses up to 60 mg/m^2 were administered to healthy volunteers in an endotoxemia study, without evidence of dose-limiting toxicities. The highest dose level evaluated in RA patients has been a single IV loading dose of 32 mg/m^2, followed by subcutaneous doses of 16 mg/m^2 (approximately 25 mg) administered twice weekly. In an RA trial, 1 patient mistakenly self-administered 62 mg etanercept subcutaneously twice weekly for 3 weeks without experiencing adverse effects.

Efficacy: Safety and efficacy of etanercept were assessed in several randomized, double-blind, placebo-controlled studies. Study I evaluated 234 adults with active RA who had failed therapy with at least 1 but no more than 4 DMARDs, and had 12 or more tender joints, 10 or more swollen joints, and either erythrocyte sedimentation rate greater than or equal to 28 mm/h, C-reactive protein (CRP) over 2 mg/dL, or morning stiffness for 45 minutes or longer. Doses of 10 or 25 mg etanercept or placebo were administered subcutaneously twice a week for 6 consecutive months. Study II evaluated 89 patients with similar inclusion criteria, except that these subjects had additionally received methotrexate for 6 months or longer, with a stable dose (12.5 to 25 mg/wk) for 4 weeks or longer, and they had 6 or more tender or painful joints. Subjects in study II received a dose of 25 mg etanercept or placebo subcutaneously twice a week for 6 months in addition to their stable methotrexate dose.

The results of the controlled trials were expressed in percentage improvements in RA using American College of Rheumatology (ACR) response criteria. The primary endpoint of study I was achievement of an ACR 20 response at month 3. Subjects who failed to respond based on prespecified criteria for lack of efficacy before month 3 were allowed to drop out early and were considered treatment failures. For study II, the primary endpoint was achievement of an ACR 20 response at month 6. By definition, an ACR 20 response is achieved if patients experience a 20% improvement in their tender joint count and swollen joint count plus 20% or greater improvement in 3 or more of the following 5 criteria: Patient pain assessment, patient global assessment, physician global assessment, patient self-assessed disability, and acute-phase reactant (ESR or CRP). ACR 50 and 70 responses are defined using the same criteria as a 50% improvement or a 70% improvement, respectively.

Responses were higher in people treated with etanercept at 3 and 6 months in both trials. The results of the 2 trials are summarized in the table below:

ACR Responses (% of patients)				
	Study I		Study II	
Response	Placebo (n = 80)	Etanercept[a] (n = 78)	Placebo and Methotrexate (n = 30)	Etanercept[a] and Methotrexate (n = 59)
ACR 20				
Month 3	23	62[b]	33	66[b]
Month 6	11	59[b]	27	71[b]
ACR 50				
Month 3	8	41[b]	0	42[b]
Month 6	5	40[b]	3	39[b]

a 25 mg etanercept subcutaneously twice weekly.
b $P \leq 0.01$, etanercept vs placebo.

In both studies, approximately 15% of subjects who received etanercept achieved an ACR 70 response at month 3 and month 6, compared with less than 5% of subjects in the placebo groups.

A dose-response relationship was observed in study I. Results with 10 mg were intermediate between placebo and 25 mg. Etanercept performed significantly better than placebo in all components of the ACR criteria, as well as other measures of RA disease activity not included in the ACR response criteria, such as morning stiffness. A health assessment questionnaire (HAQ), which included disability, vitality, mental health, general health status, and arthritis-associated health status subdomains, was administered every 3 months during the trial. All subdomains of the HAQ improved in patients treated with etanercept, compared with controls, at 3 and 6 months. The table below shows the results of the components of the ACR response criteria for study I. Findings were similar in study II.

Components of ACR Response in Study I				
	Placebo (n = 80)		Etanercept[a] (n = 78)	
Parameter (median)	Baseline	3 months	Baseline	3 months[b]
Number of tender joints[c]	34	29.5	31.2	10[d]
Number of swollen joints[e]	24	22	23.5	12.6[d]
Physician global assessment[f]	7	6.5	7	3[d]
Patient global assessment[f]	7	7	7	3[d]
Pain[f]	6.9	6.6	6.9	2.4[d]
Disability index[g]	1.7	1.8	1.6	1[d]

Components of ACR Response in Study I				
	Placebo (n = 80)		Etanercept[a] (n = 78)	
Parameter (median)	Baseline	3 months	Baseline	3 months[b]
ESR (mm/h)	31	32	28	15.5[d]
CRP (mg/dL)	2.8	3.9	3.5	0.9[d]

a 25 mg etanercept subcutaneously twice weekly.
b Results at 6 months showed similar improvement.
c Scale 0 to 71.
d $P < 0.01$, etanercept vs placebo, based on mean percent changes from baseline.
e Scale 0 to 68.
f Visual analog scale; 0 = best, 10 = worst.
g Health assessment questionnaire; 0 = best, 3 = worst; includes 8 categories: dressing and grooming, arising, eating, walking, hygiene, reach, grip, and activities.

An additional randomized, controlled, double-blind trial evaluated 180 patients with similar criteria to study I. Doses of 0.25, 2, and 16 mg/m^2 etanercept were administered subcutaneously twice a week for 3 consecutive months. A dose-dependent increase in the fraction of subjects achieving an ACR 20 response was seen, with 75% of subjects responding in the highest dose group (16 mg/m^2 etanercept).

Ankylosing spondylitis: Etanercept was assessed in 277 patients with active ankylosing spondylitis, 18 to 70 years of age. Compared with placebo, treatment with etanercept resulted in improvements in the Assessment in Ankylosing Spondylitis (ASAS) response criteria and other measures of disease activity. After 12 weeks, the ASAS 20/50/70 responses were achieved by 60%, 45%, and 29% of patients receiving etanercept, compared to 27%, 13%, and 7% of patients receiving placebo. Similar responses were seen at week 24. Responses were similar between patients receiving or not receiving concomitant therapies at baseline.

Plaque psoriasis: Etanercept was assessed in adults with chronic stable plaque psoriasis involving at least 10% of body surface area, a Psoriasis Area and Severity Index (PASI) score of at least 10, and who had received or were candidates for systemic antipsoriatic therapy or phototherapy. More patients randomized to etanercept than placebo achieved at least 75% reduction from baseline PASI score (PASI 75), with a dose-response relationship across doses of 25 mg once a week, 25 mg twice a week, and 50 mg twice a week. The individual components of the PASI (induration, erythema, scaling) contributed comparably to the overall improvement in PASI. Among responders, the median time to PASI 50 and PASI 75 was approximately 1 and approximately 2 months, respectively, after start of therapy with either 25 or 50 mg twice a week. Patients who achieved PASI 75 at month 6 were entered into a study drug withdrawal and retreatment period. After withdrawal of study drug, these patients had a median duration of PASI 75 between 1 and 2 months. In patients who were PASI 75 responders at 3 months, retreatment with open-label etanercept after discontinuation of up to 5 months resulted in a similar proportion of responders as seen during the initial double-blind portion of the study. Most patients initially randomized to 50 mg twice a week continued after month 3 and had their dose reduced to 25 mg twice a week. Of 91 patients who were PASI 75 responders at month 3, 77% maintained their PASI 75 response at month 6.

Polyarticular-course JRA: Etanercept was assessed in 69 children 4 to 17 years of age with moderately to severely active polyarticular-course JRA refractory to or intolerant of methotrexate. In the first part of the study, all patients received 0.4 mg/kg etanercept subcutaneously twice weekly. Clinical response was seen in 51 of 69 patients (74%).

In part 2, patients with a clinical response at day 90 were randomized to remain on etanercept or receive placebo for 4 months. From the start of part 2, the median time to disease flare was 116 days or longer for etanercept-treated patients and 28 days for placebo-treated patients. The data suggested the possibility of a higher flare rate among patients with a higher baseline erythrocyte sedimentation rate. Some of the etanercept-treated patients continued to improve from month 3 through month 7, while placebo-treated patients did not improve.

Psoriatic arthritis: The efficacy of etanercept was assessed in a randomized, double-blind, placebo-controlled study of 205 patients 18 to 70 years of age with psoriatic arthritis. Patients had active psoriatic arthritis (3 or more swollen joints and 3 or more tender joints) in 1 or more of the following forms: distal interphalangeal involvement, polyarticular arthritis (absence of rheumatoid nodules and presence of psoriasis), arthritis mutilans, asymmetric psoriatic arthritis, or ankylosing spondylitis-like. Patients also had plaque psoriasis with a qualifying target lesion 2 cm or more in diameter. Patients currently on stable methotrexate therapy could continue at a stable dose of up to 25 mg/week. These patients received 25 mg etanercept or placebo subcutaneously twice a week for 6 months. Compared with placebo recipients, etanercept-treated patients had fewer tender joints, fewer swollen joints, superior assessment scores and disability index, less morning stiffness, less pain, and lower C-reactive protein concentrations. Clinical responses were apparent at 4 weeks and persisted through 6 months of therapy. Responses were similar in patients who were or were not receiving concomitant methotrexate therapy at baseline. Improvements in physical function and disability measures were maintained for up to 2 years through the open-label portion of the study.

Onset: Among patients receiving etanercept, the clinical responses generally appeared within 1 to 2 weeks after the start of therapy and nearly always occurred by 3 months.

Duration: After discontinuing etanercept, symptoms of arthritis generally returned within a month. Reintroduction of treatment with etanercept after discontinuations of up to 18 months resulted in the same magnitudes of response as in patients who received etanercept without interrupting therapy, based on results of open-label studies. Continued durable responses were seen for up to 18 months in open-label extension treatment trials when patients received etanercept without interruption.

Pharmacokinetics: Immunoglobulins are primarily eliminated by catabolism. After administration of 25 mg etanercept by a single subcutaneous injection to 25 patients with RA, a median half-life of 102 ± 30 hours was observed, with a clearance of 160 ± 80 mL/h. A maximum serum concentration (C_{max}) of 1.1 ± 0.6 mcg/mL and time to C_{max} of 69 ± 34 hours was observed after a single 25 mg dose. After continued dosing with etanercept for 6 months at 25 mg twice weekly, the mean C_{max} was 2.4 ± 1 mcg/mL. Based on available data, individual patients may undergo a 2- to 5-fold increase in serum levels with repeated dosing. Serum concentrations in people with RA have not been measured for dosing intervals longer than 6 months.

Pharmacokinetic parameters do not differ between men and women or vary with age in adult or pediatric patients. No formal pharmacokinetic studies have been conducted to examine the effects of renal or hepatic impairment on etanercept pharmacokinetics or drug interactions with methotrexate.

Pediatric patients with JRA, 4 to 17 years of age, were administered 0.4 mg/kg of etanercept for up to 18 weeks. The average serum concentration after repeated dosing was 2.1 mcg/mL, with a range of 0.7 to 4.3 mcg/mL. Clearance of etanercept was 45.9 mL/h/m^2. Limited data suggests that the clearance of etanercept is reduced slightly in children 4 to 8 years of age. Population pharmacokinetic analyses predict that administration of 0.8 mg/kg once weekly will result in C_{max} 11% higher and C_{min} 20% lower at steady state compared with 0.4 mg/kg twice weekly. The predicted pharmacokinetic differences between regiments in JRA patients are of the same magnitude as differences observed between twice weekly and weekly regimens in adult RA patients. Pharmacokinetics in children younger than 4 years of age have not been studied.

Etanercept (Recombinant)

Mechanism: Etanercept binds specifically to TNF and blocks its interaction with cell-surface TNF receptors. TNF is a naturally occurring cytokine involved in normal inflammatory and immune responses. TNF plays an important role in the inflammatory processes of RA and resulting joint pathology. Elevated levels of TNF are found in the synovial fluid of RA patients.

Two distinct TNF receptors (TNFRs), a 55-kilodalton protein (p55) and a 75-kilodalton protein (p75), exist naturally as monomeric molecules on cell surfaces and in soluble forms. The biological activity of TNF depends upon binding to either cell surface TNFR.

Etanercept is a dimeric soluble form of the p75 TNF receptor that can bind to 2 TNF molecules. It inhibits the activity of TNF in vitro and has been shown to affect several animal models of inflammation, including murine collagen-induced arthritis. Etanercept inhibits binding of both TNF-α and TNF-β (lymphotoxin alpha [LT-α]) to cell surface TNFRs, rendering TNF biologically inactive. Cells expressing transmembrane TNF that bind etanercept are not lysed in vitro in the presence or absence of complement. Etanercept can also modulate biological responses that are induced or regulated by TNF, including expression of adhesion molecules responsible for leukocyte migration (ie, E-selectin and to a lesser extent intercellular adhesion molecule-1 [ICAM-1]), serum levels of cytokines (eg, IL-6), and serum levels of matrix metalloproteinase-3 (MMP-3 or stromelysin).

Drug Interactions: Specific drug interaction studies have not been conducted with etanercept.

Little data are available on the effects of vaccinating patients (either children or adults) receiving etanercept. But based on known effects of etanercept, there is a risk that etanercept could impair patient responses to live and inactivated vaccines. Most psoriatic arthritis patients receiving etanercept mounted an effective B-cell immune response to pneumococcal 23-valent polysaccharide vaccine, but titers in aggregate were moderately lower and fewer patients had 2-fold rises in titers, compared with patients not receiving etanercept. The clinical significance of this finding is unknown.

Some live, attenuated vaccines pose safety risks to immunosuppressed people. Do not give live vaccines concurrently with anti-TNF. No data are available on the secondary transmission of attenuated microbes contained in live vaccines among patients receiving etanercept. Ensure that patients with JRA are up-to-date with current immunization guidelines before beginning etanercept therapy.

Two etanercept-treated patients developed varicella infection and signs and symptoms of aseptic meningitis, which resolved without sequelae. Patients with a significant exposure to varicella should temporarily discontinue etanercept therapy and be considered for prophylactic treatment with varicella-zoster immune globulin.

In a 24-week study of concurrent etanercept and anakinra therapy, the rate of serious infections in the combination arm (7%) was higher than with etanercept alone (0%). Combination therapy did not result in higher ACR response rates compared with etanercept alone.

Patient Information: Sites for self-injection include the thigh, abdomen, or upper arm. Rotate injection sites. Give new injections 1 inch or further from an old site, but not into areas where the skin is tender, bruised, red, or hard.

Pharmaceutical Characteristics

Concentration:
Syringes: Etanercept 50 mg/mL
Vials: Etanercept 25 mg per vial

Quality Assay: Polyacrylimide gel electrophoresis and other methods.

Etanercept (Recombinant)

Packaging:

Prefilled syringes: Carton of four 25 mcg single-use prefilled syringes with ½-inch, 27-guage needles (58406-0455-04). Carton of four 50 mcg single-use prefilled syringes (58406-0435-04).

Autoinjectors: Carton of four 50 mg single-use prefilled *SureClick* autoinjectors with ½-inch, 27-guage needles (58406-0445-04).

Multidose vials: Carton of 4 trays. Each tray contains one 25 mg single-use vial of lyophilized powder, 1 prefilled glass syringe of diluent with ½-inch, 27-gauge needle, 1 vial adapter, 1 plunger, and 2 alcohol swabs (58406-0425-34).

Doseform: Either solution or powder for reconstitution as a solution

Appearance:

Syringes: Clear, colorless solution

Vials: White lyophilized powder, yielding a clear and colorless solution after reconstitution.

Solvent: For ready-to-use syringes, phosphate-buffered saline

Diluent:

For reconstitution: 1 mL bacteriostatic water for injection. Do not reconstitute etanercept with other diluents.

Preservative:

Syringes: None

Vials: Powder contains no preservative. Bacteriostatic diluent contains 0.9% benzyl alcohol.

Allergens: The needle cover of the diluent syringe contains dry natural rubber (latex).

Excipients:

Syringes: Sucrose 10 mg/mL, sodium chloride 5.8 mg/mL, L-arginine hydrochloride 5.3 mg/mL, sodium phosphate monobasic monohydrate 2.6 mg/mL, sodium phosphate dibasic anhydrous 0.9 mg/mL

Vials: Mannitol 40 mg, sucrose 10 mg, and tromethamine 1.2 mg, each per vial

pH:

Syringes: 6.1 to 6.5

Vials: 7.1 to 7.7, after reconstitution

Shelf Life: Expires within 12 months

Storage/Stability: Store at 2° to 8°C (36° to 46°F). Do not freeze. Contact the manufacturer regarding exposure to extreme temperatures. Shipped in insulated containers with coolant packs via overnight courier.

Administer reconstituted solutions of etanercept as soon as possible after reconstitution. If not administered immediately, etanercept may be stored in the vial at 2° to 8°C (36° to 46°F) for up to 14 days, if the supplied diluent was used.

Do not add any other medications to solutions containing etanercept.

Handling: To reconstitute, slowly inject diluent into the vial. Some foaming will occur. To avoid excessive foaming, do not shake or agitate vigorously. Gently swirl contents during dissolution. Generally, dissolution takes less than 10 minutes. Do not filter reconstituted solutions during preparation or administration.

Production Process: Etanercept is produced by recombinant DNA technology in a Chinese hamster ovary (CHO) mammalian cell expression system.

Media: Chinese hamster ovary (CHO) cell culture

Disease Epidemiology

Prevalence: Rheumatoid arthritis is a painful, potentially debilitating disease characterized by chronic inflammation of joint linings. In severe cases, this inflammation extends to other joint tissues and surrounding cartilage, where it may erode bone and cartilage and lead to joint deformities. Symptoms include stiffness, pain, and swelling of multiple joints. Approximately 2.2 million Americans have rheumatoid arthritis, and approximately 84,000 new cases are diagnosed each year. Two to 3 times more women than men are affected.

Other Information

First Licensed: November 2, 1998

References: Kyle S, Chandler D, Griffiths CE, et al; British Society for Rheumatology Standards Guidelines Audit Working Group (SGAWG). Guideline for anti-TNF-alpha therapy in psoriatic arthritis. *Rheumatology (Oxford)*. 2005;44:390-397. Erratum in: *Rheumatology (Oxford)*. 2005;44:569. *Rheumatology (Oxford)*. 2005;44:701.

Moreland LW, Baumgartner SW, Schiff MH, et al. Treatment of rheumatoid arthritis with a recombinant human tumor necrosis factor receptor (p75)-Fc fusion protein. *N Engl J Med*. 1997;337:141-147.

Sun YN, Lu JF, Joshi A, Compton P, Kwon P, Bruno RA. Population pharmacokinetics of efalizumab (humanized monoclonal anti-CD11a antibody) following long-term subcutaneous weekly dosing in psoriasis subjects. *J Clin Pharmacol*. 2005;45:468-476.

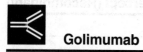 **Golimumab**

Isoantibodies

Name:
   Simponi
Synonyms: CNTO 148

Manufacturer:
   Janssen Biotech

Immunologic Characteristics

Target Antigen: Human tumor necrosis factor alpha (TNF-α)
Viability: Inactive, passive, transient
Antigenic Form: Human IgG-1κ monoclonal antibody
Antigenic Type: Protein, IgG1κ antibody, monoclonal, with multiple glycoforms with molecular masses of approximately 150 to 151 kilodaltons

Use Characteristics

Indications:

To treat: Moderately to severely active rheumatoid arthritis (RA) in adults, in combination with methotrexate.

Active psoriatic arthritis (PsA) in adults, alone or in combination with methotrexate.

Active ankylosing spondylitis (AS) in adults.

Contraindications: None

Immunodeficiency: No impairment of effect expected.

Elderly: In phase 3 trials, there were no overall differences in serious adverse events, serious infections, and adverse events in golimumab-treated patients 65 years and older (N = 155) compared with younger golimumab-treated patients. Because there is a higher incidence of infections in the elderly population in general, use caution in treating elderly patients with golimumab.

Carcinogenicity: Golimumab has not been evaluated for carcinogenic potential.

Mutagenicity: Golimumab has not been evaluated for mutagenic potential.

Fertility Impairment: A fertility study conducted in mice using an analogous antimouse TNF-α antibody showed no impairment of fertility.

Pregnancy: Category B. There are no adequate and well-controlled studies of golimumab in pregnant women. Because animal reproduction and developmental studies are not always predictive of human response, it is not known whether golimumab can affect reproduction capacity or cause fetal harm when administered to a pregnant woman. Use golimumab during pregnancy only if clearly needed.

An embryo-fetal developmental toxicology study was performed in pregnant cynomolgus monkeys treated with golimumab during the first trimester with doses of up to 50 mg/kg subcutaneously twice weekly (360 times greater than the maximum recommended human dose) and revealed no evidence of harm to maternal animals or fetuses. Umbilical cord blood samples collected at the end of the second trimester showed that fetuses were exposed to golimumab during gestation. In this study, in utero exposure to golimumab produced no developmental defects in the fetus.

A pre- and postnatal developmental study was performed in which pregnant cynomolgus monkeys were treated with golimumab during the second and third trimesters and during lactation at doses of up to 50 mg/kg twice weekly (860 and 310 times greater than the maximal steady-state human blood levels for maternal animals and neonates, respectively) and revealed no evidence of harm to maternal animals or neonates. Golimumab was present in the neonatal serum from the time of birth and for up to 6 months postpartum. Exposure to golimumab during gestation and during the postnatal period caused no developmental defects in the infants.

Lactation: It is not known whether golimumab is excreted in human milk or absorbed systemically after ingestion. Because many drugs and immune globulins are excreted in human milk, and because of the potential for adverse reactions in breast-feeding infants from golimumab, decide whether to discontinue breast-feeding or to discontinue the drug, taking into account the importance of the drug to the mother.

In the pre- and postnatal developmental study in cynomolgus monkeys in which golimumab was administered subcutaneously during pregnancy and lactation, golimumab was detected in the breast milk at concentrations approximately 400-fold lower than the maternal serum concentrations.

Children: Safety and effectiveness of golimumab in pediatric patients younger than 18 years of age have not been established.

Adverse Reactions: The following safety data are based on 5 pooled, randomized, double-blind, controlled phase 3 trials in patients with RA, psoriatic arthritis, and ankylosing spondylitis (studies RA-1, RA-2, RA-3, PsA, and AS). These trials included 639 control-treated patients and 1,659 golimumab-treated patients, including 1,089 with RA, 292 with psoriatic arthritis, and 278 with ankylosing spondylitis. The proportion of patients who discontinued treatment because of adverse reactions in the controlled phase 3 trials through week 16 in RA, psoriatic arthritis, and ankylosing spondylitis was 2% for golimumab-treated patients and 3% for placebo-treated patients. The most common adverse reactions leading to discontinuation of golimumab in the controlled phase 3 trials through week 16 were sepsis (0.2%), alanine aminotransferase increase (0.2%), and aspartate aminotransferase increase (0.2%). Upper respiratory tract infection and nasopharyngitis were the most common adverse reactions reported in the combined phase 3 RA, psoriatic arthritis, and ankylosing spondylitis trials through week 16, occurring in 7% and 6% of golimumab-treated patients compared with 6% and 5% of control-treated patients, respectively.

Serious infections: Patients treated with golimumab are at increased risk for developing serious infections that may lead to hospitalization or death. Most patients who developed these infections were taking concomitant immunosuppressants such as methotrexate or corticosteroids. Concomitant use of a TNF-blocker and abatacept or anakinra was associated with a higher risk of serious infections; therefore, concomitant use of these products is not recommended. Do not start golimumab during an active infection, including clinically important localized infections. If an infection develops, monitor carefully and stop golimumab if infection becomes serious. Discontinue golimumab if a patient develops a serious infection. Carefully consider the risks and benefits of treatment with golimumab before starting therapy in patients with chronic or recurrent infections. In controlled trials through week 16 in patients with RA, psoriatic arthritis, and ankylosing spondylitis, serious infections were observed in 1.4% of golimumab-treated patients and 1.3% of control-treated patients. In the controlled trials through week 16 in patients with RA, psoriatic arthritis, and ankylosing spondylitis, the incidence of serious infections per 100 patient-years of follow-up was 5.4 (95% confidence interval [CI], 4-7.2) for the golimumab group and 5.3 (95% CI, 3.1-8.7) for the placebo group. Serious infections observed in golimumab-treated patients included sepsis, pneumonia, cellulitis, abscess, tuberculosis (TB), invasive fungal infections, and hepatitis B virus (HBV) infection. Reported infections include:

- Active TB, including reactivation of latent TB. Patients with TB have frequently presented with disseminated or extrapulmonary diseases. Test patients for latent TB before golimumab use and during therapy. Start treatment for latent infection before using golimumab. In the controlled and noncontrolled portions of RA, psoriatic arthritis, and ankylosing spondylitis trials, the incidence of active TB was 0.23 and 0 per 100 patient-years in 2,347 golimumab-treated patients and 674 placebo-treated patients, respectively. Cases of TB included pulmonary and extrapulmonary TB. Most TB cases occurred in countries with a high incidence rate of TB.

- Invasive fungal infections, including histoplasmosis, coccidioidomycosis, and pneumocystosis. Patients with histoplasmosis or other invasive fungal infections may present with disseminated, rather than localized, disease. Antigen and antibody testing for histoplasmosis may be negative in some patients with active infection. Consider empiric antifungal therapy in patients at risk for invasive fungal infections who develop severe systemic illness. Consider empiric antifungal therapy for those who reside in or travel to regions where mycoses are endemic (eg, histoplasmosis, coccidioidomycosis, blastomycosis).
- Bacterial, viral, protozoal, and other infections caused by opportunistic pathogens.
- Hepatitis B reactivation. Evaluate patients at risk for HBV infection for prior evidence of HBV infection before starting TNF-blocker therapy. Monitor HBV carriers (ie, HBsAg+) during and several months after therapy. In some instances, HBV reactivation occurring in conjunction with TNF-blocker therapy has been fatal. Adequate data are not available on whether antiviral therapy can reduce the risk of HBV reactivation in HBV carriers who are treated with TNF-blockers. If reactivation occurs, stop golimumab and begin antiviral therapy. The safety of resuming TNF-blockers after HBV reactivation has been controlled is not known.

Malignancies: The incidence of lymphoma in clinical trials was higher in TNF-blocker recipients than in control groups and in the general US population. Cases of other malignancies have been observed among patients receiving TNF-blockers. Consider the risks and benefits of TNF-blocker treatment before starting therapy in patients with a known malignancy other than a successfully treated nonmelanoma skin cancer (NMSC) or when considering continuing a TNF-blocker in patients who develop a malignancy. During the controlled portions of trials with golimumab in RA, psoriatic arthritis, and ankylosing spondylitis, the incidence of lymphoma per 100 patient-years of follow-up was 0.21 (95% CI, 0.03-0.77) in the golimumab groups compared with 0 (95% CI, 0-0.96) in the placebo group. In the controlled and noncontrolled portions of these clinical trials in 2,347 golimumab-treated patients with a median follow-up of 1.4 years, the incidence of lymphoma was 3.8-fold higher than expected in the general US population (adjusted for age, gender, and race). Patients with RA and other chronic inflammatory diseases, particularly patients with highly active disease and/or chronic exposure to immunosuppressant therapies, may be at several-fold higher risk than the general population for developing lymphoma, even in the absence of TNF-blocking therapy. During controlled portions of trials in RA, psoriatic arthritis, and ankylosing spondylitis, the incidence of malignancies other than lymphoma per 100 patient-years of follow-up was not elevated in the golimumab groups compared with the placebo group. In the controlled and noncontrolled portions of these trials, the incidence of malignancies other than lymphoma in golimumab-treated patients was similar to that expected in the general US population (adjusted for age, gender, and race). In controlled trials of other TNF-blockers in patients at higher risk for malignancies (eg, patients with chronic obstructive pulmonary disease [COPD], patients with Wegener granulomatosis treated with concomitant cyclophosphamide), a greater portion of malignancies occurred in the TNF-blocker group compared with the controlled group. In an exploratory 1-year clinical trial evaluating the use of golimumab 50, 100, and 200 mg in 309 patients with severe persistent asthma, 6 patients developed malignancies other than NMSC in the golimumab groups compared with none in the control group. Three of the 6 patients were in the golimumab 200 mg group.

Heart failure: Cases of worsening congestive heart failure (CHF) and new-onset CHF have been reported with TNF-blockers. In several exploratory trials of other TNF-blockers in treating CHF, there were greater proportions of TNF-blocker–treated patients who had CHF exacerbations requiring hospitalization or increased mortality. Golimumab has not been studied in patients with a history of CHF; use golimumab with caution in patients with CHF. If a decision is made to administer golimumab to patients with CHF, monitor these patients closely during therapy, and discontinue golimumab if new or worsening symptoms of CHF appear.

Demyelinating disorders: Use of TNF-blockers has been associated with cases of new-onset or exacerbation of CNS demyelinating disorders, including multiple sclerosis (MS). While no trials have been performed evaluating golimumab in treating patients with MS, another TNF-blocker was associated with increased disease activity in patients with MS. Therefore, use caution in considering TNF-blockers in patients with CNS demyelinating disorders, including MS.

Hematologic: There have been postlicensing reports of pancytopenia, leukopenia, neutropenia, aplastic anemia, and thrombocytopenia in patients receiving TNF-blockers. Although there were no cases of severe cytopenias seen in golimumab clinical trials, use caution when using TNF-blockers in patients who have significant cytopenias.

Hepatic: There have been reports of severe hepatic reactions, including acute liver failure, in patients receiving TNF-blockers. In controlled phase 3 trials of golimumab in patients with RA, psoriatic arthritis, and ankylosing spondylitis through week 16, ALT elevations 5 or more times the upper limit of normal (ULN) occurred in 0.2% of control-treated patients and 0.7% of golimumab-treated patients, and ALT elevations 3 or more times ULN occurred in 2% of control-treated patients and 2% of golimumab-treated patients. Because many of the patients in phase 3 trials were also taking medications that cause liver enzyme elevations (eg, nonsteroidal anti-inflammatory agents [NSAIDs], methotrexate), the relationship between golimumab and liver elevation is not clear.

Autoimmunity: Use of TNF-blockers has been associated with formation of autoantibodies and, rarely, with developing a lupus-like syndrome. In controlled phase 3 trials in patients with RA, psoriatic arthritis, and ankylosing spondylitis through week 14, there was no association of golimumab treatment and development of newly positive anti-dsDNA antibodies.

Injection-site reactions: In controlled phase 3 trials through week 16 in RA, psoriatic arthritis, and ankylosing spondylitis, 6% of golimumab-treated patients had injection-site reactions compared with 2% of control-treated patients. Most injection-site reactions were mild, and the most frequent manifestation was erythema. In controlled trials in RA, psoriatic arthritis, and ankylosing spondylitis, no patients treated with golimumab developed anaphylactic reactions.

Psoriasis: Cases of new-onset psoriasis, including pustular psoriasis and palmoplantar psoriasis, have been reported with TNF-blockers. Exacerbation of preexisting psoriasis has been reported with TNF-blockers. Many of these patients were taking concomitant immunosuppressants (eg, methotrexate, corticosteroids). Some patients required hospitalization. Psoriasis improved in most patients after discontinuing their TNF-blocker. Some patients had psoriasis recur when they were rechallenged with a different TNF-blocker. Consider discontinuing golimumab for severe cases and for those who do not improve or who worsen despite topical treatments.

Immunogenicity: Antibodies to golimumab were detected in 57 (4%) golimumab-treated patients across the phase 3 RA, psoriatic arthritis, and ankylosing spondylitis trials through week 24. Similar rates occurred in each of the 3 indications. Patients who received golimumab with concomitant methotrexate had a lower proportion of antibodies to golimumab than patients who received golimumab without methotrexate (approximately 2% vs 7%

respectively). Of patients with a positive antibody response to golimumab in trials, most had neutralizing antibodies to golimumab as measured by a cell-based functional assay. The small number of patients positive for antibodies to golimumab limits the ability to draw definitive conclusions regarding the relationship between antibodies to golimumab and clinical efficacy or safety measures. The previously described data reflect the percentage of patients whose test results were considered positive for antibodies to golimumab in an ELISA assay and are highly dependent on the sensitivity and specificity of the assay.

The following table summarizes the adverse events that occurred in 1% or more in the combined golimumab groups during 5 pooled trials through week 16 in patients with RA, psoriatic arthritis, and ankylosing spondylitis.

Adverse Events Reported by ≥ 1% of Patients in RA, Psoriatic Arthritis, and Ankylosing Spondylitis Trials Through Week 16ᵃ		
Adverse reaction	Placebo ± DMARDsᵇ (n = 639)	Golimumab ± DMARDs (n = 1,659)
Upper respiratory tract infection	37 (6%)	120 (7%)
Nasopharyngitis	31 (5%)	91 (6%)
Alanine aminotransferase increased	18 (3%)	58 (4%)
Injection-site erythema	6 (1%)	56 (3%)
Hypertension	9 (1%)	48 (3%)
Aspartate aminotransferase increased	10 (2%)	44 (3%)
Bronchitis	9 (1%)	31 (2%)
Dizziness	7 (1%)	32 (2%)
Sinusitis	7 (1%)	27 (2%)
Influenza	7 (1%)	25 (2%)
Pharyngitis	8 (1%)	22 (1%)
Rhinitis	4 (< 1%)	20 (1%)
Pyrexia	4 (< 1%)	20 (1%)
Oral herpes	2 (< 1%)	16 (1%)
Paresthesia	2 (< 1%)	16 (1%)

a Patients may have taken concomitant methotrexate, sulfasalazine, hydroxychloroquine, low-dose corticosteroids (prednisone ≤ 10 mg/day or equivalent), and/or NSAIDs during trials.
b DMARDs = disease-modifying antirheumatic drugs.

Consultation: Consult specialists in diagnosis and treatment of TB, invasive fungal infections, and other serious infections.

Pharmacologic & Dosing Characteristics

Dosage: 50 mg once a month

Route: Subcutaneous

Overdosage: In a clinical study, 5 patients received protocol-directed single infusions of golimumab 10 mg/kg intravenously (IV) without serious adverse reactions or other significant reactions. The highest patient weight was 100 kg, and therefore that patient received a single IV infusion of 1,000 mg of golimumab. There were no golimumab overdoses in the clinical studies.

Related Interventions: Test for latent TB; if positive (induration 5 mm and larger, even for patients previously vaccinated with BCG), start treatment for TB before starting golimumab. Monitor all patients for active TB during treatment, even if initial latent TB test is negative.

For patients with RA, golimumab should be given in combination with methotrexate. For patients with psoriatic arthritis or ankylosing spondylitis, golimumab may be given with or without methotrexate or other nonbiologic DMARDs. For patients with RA, psoriatic arthritis, or ankylosing spondylitis, corticosteroids, nonbiologic DMARDs, and/or NSAIDs may be continued during treatment with golimumab.

Efficacy:

Rheumatoid arthritis: Efficacy and safety of golimumab were evaluated in 3 multicenter, randomized, double-blind, controlled trials (studies RA-1, RA-2, and RA-3) in 1,542 patients 18 years of age and older with moderately to severely active RA, diagnosed according to American College of Rheumatology (ACR) criteria, for at least 3 months before administration of study agent. Patients were required to have at least 4 swollen and 4 tender joints. Golimumab was administered at doses of 50 or 100 mg subcutaneously every 4 weeks. Double-blind, controlled efficacy data were collected and analyzed through week 24. Patients were allowed to continue stable doses of concomitant low-dose corticosteroids (prednisone 10 mg/day or less) and/or NSAIDs, and patients may have received oral methotrexate during the trials.

Study RA-1 evaluated 461 patients previously treated (at least 8 to 12 weeks before administration of study agent) with 1 or more doses of a TNF-blocker without a serious adverse reaction. Patients may have discontinued the biologic TNF-blocker for a variety of reasons. Patients were randomized to receive placebo (n = 155), golimumab 50 mg (n = 153), or golimumab 100 mg (n = 153). Patients were allowed to continue stable doses of concomitant methotrexate, sulfasalazine, and/or hydroxychloroquine during the trial. The use of other DMARDs, including cytotoxic agents or other biologics, was prohibited.

Study RA-2 evaluated 444 patients who had active RA despite a stable dose of at least 15 mg/wk of methotrexate and who had not been previously treated with a TNF-blocker. Patients were randomized to receive methotrexate (n = 133), golimumab 50 mg plus methotrexate (n = 89), golimumab 100 mg plus methotrexate (n = 89), or golimumab 100 mg as monotherapy (n = 133). The use of other DMARDs (eg, sulfasalazine, hydroxychloroquine, cytotoxic agents, other biologics) was prohibited.

Study RA-3 evaluated 637 patients with active RA who were methotrexate naive and had not previously been treated with a TNF-blocker. Patients were randomized to receive methotrexate (n = 160), golimumab 50 mg plus methotrexate (n = 159), golimumab 100 mg plus methotrexate (n = 159), or golimumab 100 mg monotherapy (n = 159). For patients receiving methotrexate, methotrexate was administered at a dose of 10 mg/wk beginning at week 0 and increased to 20 mg/wk by week 8. Use of other DMARDs, including sulfasalazine, hydroxychloroquine, cytotoxic agents, or other biologics, was prohibited.

The primary end point in studies RA-1 and RA-2 was the proportion of patients achieving an ACR 20 response at week 14. The primary end point in study RA-3 was the proportion of patients achieving an ACR 50 response at week 24.

In studies RA-1, RA-2, and RA-3, the median duration of RA disease was 9.4, 5.7, and 1.2 years; and 99%, 75%, and 54% of patients used at least 1 DMARD in the past, respectively. Approximately 77% and 57% of patients received concomitant NSAIDs and low-dose corticosteroids, respectively, in the 3 pooled RA trials.

In the 3 RA trials, a greater percentage of patients treated with a combination of golimumab and methotrexate achieved ACR responses at week 14 (studies RA-1 and RA-2) and week 24 (studies RA-1, RA-2, and RA-3) versus patients treated with methotrexate alone. There was no clear evidence of improved ACR response with the golimumab 100 mg group compared with the golimumab 50 mg group. In studies RA-2 and RA-3, the golimumab monotherapy groups were not statistically different from the methotrexate monotherapy groups in ACR responses. The following table shows the proportion of patients with the ACR response for the golimumab 50 mg and control groups in studies RA-1, RA-2, and RA-3. In the subset of patients who received golimumab in combination with methotrexate in study RA-1, the proportion of patients achieving ACR 20, 50, and 70 responses at week 14 were 40%, 18%, and 13%, respectively, in the golimumab 50 mg plus methotrexate group (n = 103) compared with 17%, 6%, and 2%, respectively, in the placebo plus methotrexate group (n = 107). The following table shows the percent improvement in components of the ACR response criteria for the golimumab 50 mg plus methotrexate and methotrexate groups in study RA-2. ACR 20 responses were observed in 38% of patients in the golimumab 50 mg plus methotrexate group at the first assessment (week 4) after the initial golimumab administration.

Studies RA-1, RA-2, and RA-3 Proportion of Patients With an ACR Response[a]						
	Study RA-1 Active RA previously treated with 1 or more doses of TNF-blockers		Study RA-2 Active RA, despite methotrexate		Study RA-3 Active RA, methotrexate naive	
	Placebo ± DMARDs[b]	Golimumab 50 mg ± DMARDs[b]	Background methotrexate	Golimumab 50 mg + background methotrexate	Methotrexate	Golimumab 50 mg + methotrexate
N[c]	155	153	133	89	160	159
ACR 20						
Week 14	18%	35%	33%	55%	NA[d]	NA
Week 24	17%	34%	28%	60%	49%	62%
ACR 50						
Week 14	6%	16%	10%	35%	NA	NA
Week 24	5%	18%	14%	37%	29%	40%
ACR 70						
Week 14	2%	10%	4%	13%	NA	NA
Week 24	3%	12%	5%	20%	16%	24%[e]

a Approximately 78% and 58% of patients received concomitant low-dose corticosteroids (prednisone 10 mg/day or less) and NSAIDs, respectively, during the 3 pooled RA trials.
b DMARDs in study RA-1 included methotrexate, hydroxychloroquine, and/or sulfasalazine (approximately 68%, 8%, and 5% of patients received methotrexate, hydroxychloroquine, and sulfasalazine, respectively).
c N reflects randomized patients.
d NA = Not applicable, because data were not collected at week 14 in study RA-3.
e Not significantly different from methotrexate monotherapy.

Study RA-2: Median Percent Improvement From Baseline in Individual ACR Components at Week 14[a]		
	Background methotrexate (N[b] = 133)	Golimumab 50 mg + background methotrexate (N[b] = 89)
Number of swollen joints (0 to 66)		
Baseline	12	13
Week 14	38%	62%

Study RA-2: Median Percent Improvement From Baseline in Individual ACR Components at Week 14[a]		
	Background methotrexate (N^b = 133)	Golimumab 50 mg + background methotrexate (N^b = 89)
Number of tender joints (0 to 68)		
Baseline	21	26
Week 14	30%	60%
Patient's assessment of pain (0 to 10)		
Baseline	5.7	6.1
Week 14	18%	55%
Patient's global assessment of disease activity (0 to 10)		
Baseline	5.3	6
Week 14	15%	45%
Physician's global assessment of disease activity (0 to 10)		
Baseline	5.7	6.1
Week 14	35%	55%
HAQ[c] score (0 to 3)		
Baseline	1.25	1.38
Week 14	10%	29%
CRP[c] (mg/dL)		
Baseline	0.8	1
Week 14	2%	44%

a In study RA-2, approximately 70% and 85% of patients received concomitant low-dose corticosteroids (prednisone 10 mg/day or less) and/or NSAIDs during the trials, respectively.

b N reflects randomized patients; actual number of patients evaluable for each end point may vary.

c HAQ = Health Assessment Questionnaire; CRP = C-reactive protein.

Note: Baseline values are medians.

Physical function: In studies RA-1 and RA-2, the golimumab 50 mg groups demonstrated a greater improvement compared with control groups in change in mean Health Assessment Questionnaire Disability Index (HAQ-DI) score from baseline to week 24 (0.25 vs 0.05 in RA-1, 0.47 vs 0.13 in RA-2). Also in studies RA-1 and RA-2, the golimumab 50 mg groups had a greater proportion of HAQ responders compared with control groups (change from baseline greater than 0.22) at week 24 (44% vs 28%, 65% vs 35%, respectively).

Psoriatic arthritis: Safety and efficacy of golimumab were evaluated in a multicenter, randomized, double-blind, placebo-controlled trial in 405 adult patients with moderately to severely active psoriatic arthritis (at least 3 swollen joints and at least 3 tender joints) despite NSAID or DMARD therapy (study PsA). Patients in this study had a diagnosis of psoriatic arthritis for at least 6 months with a qualifying psoriatic skin lesion of at least 2 cm in diameter. Previous treatment with a TNF-blocker was not allowed. Patients were randomly assigned to placebo (n = 113), golimumab 50 mg (n = 146), or golimumab 100 mg (n = 146) given subcutaneously every 4 weeks. Patients were allowed to receive stable doses of concomitant methotrexate (25 mg/wk or less), low-dose oral corticosteroids (prednisone 10 mg/day or less), and/or NSAIDs during the trial. The use of other DMARDs, including sulfasalazine, hydroxychloroquine, cytotoxic agents, or other biologics, was prohibited. The primary end point was the proportion of patients achieving ACR 20 response at week 14. Placebo-controlled efficacy data were collected and analyzed through week 24. Patients with each subtype of psoriatic arthritis were enrolled, including polyarticular arthritis with no rheumatoid nodules (43%), asymmetric peripheral arthritis (30%), distal interphalangeal joint arthritis (15%), spondylitis with peripheral arthritis (11%), and arthritis mutilans (1%). The median duration of psoriatic arthritis disease was 5.1 years; 78% of patients received at least 1 DMARD in the past, approximately 48% of patients received methotrexate, and 16% received low-dose oral steroids.

Clinical response: Golimumab with or without methotrexate, compared with placebo with or without methotrexate, resulted in significant improvement in signs and symptoms, as demonstrated by the proportion of patients with an ACR 20 response at week 14 in study PsA. There was no clear evidence of improved ACR response with the golimumab 100 mg dose group compared with the golimumab 50 mg group. ACR responses observed in the golimumab-treated groups were similar in patients receiving and not receiving concomitant methotrexate. Similar ACR 20 responses at week 14 were observed in patients with different psoriatic arthritis subtypes. However, the number of patients with arthritis mutilans was too small to allow meaningful assessment. Golimumab 50 mg treatment also resulted in significantly greater improvement compared with placebo for each ACR component in study PsA. Treatment with golimumab resulted in improvement in enthesitis and skin manifestations in patients with psoriatic arthritis. However, the safety and efficacy of golimumab in the treatment of patients with plaque psoriasis have not been established.

ACR 20 responses were observed in 31% of patients in the golimumab 50 mg plus methotrexate group at the first assessment (week 4) after the initial golimumab administration.

Study PsA: Proportion of Patients with ACR Responses		
	Placebo $\pm$ methotrexate[a] (N^b = 113)	Golimumab 50 mg $\pm$ methotrexate[a] (N^b = 146)
ACR 20		
Week 14	9%	51%
Week 24	12%	52%
ACR 50		
Week 14	2%	30%
Week 24	4%	32%
ACR 70		
Week 14	1%	12%
Week 24	1%	19%

a In study PsA, approximately 48%, 16%, and 72% of patients received stable doses of methotrexate ($\leq$ 25 mg/day), low-dose corticosteroids (prednisone $\leq$ 10 mg/day), and NSAIDs, respectively.
b N reflects randomized patients.

Study PsA: Percent Improvement in ACR Components at Week 14		
	Placebo $\pm$ methotrexate[a] (N^b = 113)	Golimumab 50 mg $\pm$ methotrexate[a] (N^b = 146)
Number of swollen joints (0 to 66)		
Baseline	10	11
Week 14	8%	60%
Number of tender joints (0 to 68)		
Baseline	18	19
Week 14	0%	54%
Patient's assessment of pain (0 to 10)		
Baseline	5.4	5.8
Week 14	−1%	48%

Study PsA: Percent Improvement in ACR Components at Week 14		
	Placebo ± methotrexate[a] (N[b] = 113)	Golimumab 50 mg ± methotrexate[a] (N[b] = 146)
Patient's global assessment of disease activity (0 to 10)		
Baseline	5.2	5.2
Week 14	2%	49%
Physician's global assessment of disease activity (0 to 10)		
Baseline	5.2	5.4
Week 14	7%	59%
HAQ score (0 to 10)		
Baseline	1	1
Week 14	0%	28%
CRP (mg/dL) (0 to 10)		
Baseline	0.6	0.6
Week 14	0%	40%

Note: Baseline are median values.

a In study PsA, approximately 48%, 16%, and 78% of patients received stable doses of methotrexate (≤ 25 mg/day), low-dose corticosteroids (prednisone ≤ 10 mg/day), and NSAIDs, respectively.

b N reflects randomized patients; actual number of patients evaluable for each end point may vary by time point.

Physical function: In Study PsA, golimumab 50 mg demonstrated a greater improvement compared with placebo in change in mean HAQ-DI score from baseline to week 24 (0.33 and −0.01, respectively). In addition, the golimumab 50 mg group had a greater proportion of HAQ responders compared with the placebo group (0.3 or more change from baseline) at week 24 (43% vs 22%, respectively).

Ankylosing spondylitis: Safety and efficacy of golimumab were evaluated in a multicenter, randomized, double-blind, placebo-controlled trial in 356 adult patients with active ankylosing spondylitis according to modified New York criteria for at least 3 months (study AS). Patients had symptoms of active disease (defined as a Bath Ankylosing Spondylitis Disease Activity Index [BASDAI] of at least 4 and visual analog scale for total back pain of at least 4 on scales of 0 to 10 cm) despite current or previous NSAID therapy. Patients were excluded if they were previously treated with a TNF-blocker or if they had complete ankylosis of the spine. Patients were randomly assigned to placebo (n = 78), golimumab 50 mg (n = 138), or golimumab 100 mg (n = 140) administered subcutaneously every 4 weeks. Patients were allowed to continue stable doses of concomitant methotrexate, sulfasalazine, hydroxychloroquine, low-dose corticosteroids (prednisone 10 mg/day or less), and/or NSAIDs during the trial. Use of other DMARDs, including cytotoxic agents or other biologics, was prohibited. The primary end point was the percentage of patients achieving an Assessment in Ankylosing Spondylitis (ASAS) 20 response at week 14. Placebo-controlled efficacy data were collected and analyzed through week 24.

In study AS, the median duration of ankylosing spondylitis disease was 5.6 years, median duration of inflammatory back pain was 12 years, 83% were HLA-B27 positive, 24% had prior joint surgery or procedure, and 55% received at least 1 DMARD in the past. During the clinical trial, the use of concomitant DMARDs and/or NSAIDs was as follows: methotrexate (20%), sulfasalazine (26%), hydroxychloroquine (1%), low-dose oral steroids (16%), and NSAIDs (90%). Golimumab with or without DMARDs compared with placebo with or without DMARDs resulted in a significant improvement in signs and symptoms as demonstrated by the proportion of patients with an ASAS 20 response at week 14. There was no clear evidence of improved ASAS response with the golimumab 100 mg group compared with the golimumab 50 mg group. The following table shows the percent improvement in the components of the ASAS response criteria for the golimumab 50 mg with or without DMARDs and placebo with or without DMARDs groups in study AS. ASAS 20 responses were observed in 48% of patients in the golimumab 50 mg plus methotrexate group at the first assessment (week 4) after the initial golimumab administration.

Study AS: Proportion of ASAS Responders at Weeks 14 and 24		
	Placebo ± DMARDs[a] (N[b] = 78)	Golimumab 50 mg ± DMARDs[a] (N[b] = 138)
Responders, % of patients		
ASAS 20		
Week 14	22%	59%
Week 24	23%	56%
ASAS 40		
Week 14	15%	45%
Week 24	15%	44%

a During the trial, concomitant use of stable doses of DMARDS was as follows: methotrexate (21%), sulfasalazine (25%), and hydroxychloroquine (1%). Approximately 16% and 89% of patients received stable doses of low-dose oral steroids and NSAIDs during the trial, respectively.
b N reflects randomized patients.

Study AS: Median Percent Improvement in ASAS Components at Week 14		
	Placebo ± DMARDs[a] (N[b] = 78)	Golimumab 50 mg ± DMARDs[a] (N[b] = 138)
ASAS components		
Patient global assessment (0 to 10)		
Baseline	7.2	7
Week 14	13%	47%
Total back pain (0 to 10)		
Baseline	7.6	7.5
Week 14	9%	50%
BASFI[c] (0 to 10)		
Baseline	4.9	5
Week 14	−3%	37%
Inflammation (0 to 10)[d]		
Baseline	7.1	7.1
Week 14	6%	59%

a During the trial, concomitant use of stable doses of DMARDs was as follows: methotrexate (21%), sulfasalazine (25%), and hydroxychloroquine (1%). Approximately 16% and 89% of patients received stable doses of low-dose oral steroids and NSAIDs during the trial, respectively.
b N reflects randomized patients.
c BASFI = Bath Ankylosing Spondylitis Functional Index.
d Inflammation is the mean of 2 patient-reported stiffness self-assessments in the BASDAI.

Pharmacokinetics: In clinical studies, decreases in CRP, interleukin-6 (IL-6), matrix metalloproteinase 3, intercellular adhesion molecule-1 [ICAM-1]) and vascular endothelial growth factor were observed after golimumab administration in patients with RA, psoriatic arthritis, and ankylosing spondylitis.

After subcutaneous administration of golimumab to healthy subjects and patients with active RA, the median time to reach maximum serum concentrations (T_{max}) ranged from 2 to 6 days. Subcutaneous injection of golimumab 50 mg to healthy subjects produced a mean maximum serum concentration (C_{max}) of approximately 2.5 mcg/mL. Golimumab exhibited dose-proportional pharmacokinetics (PK) in patients with active RA over the dose range of 0.1 to 10 mg/kg after a single IV dose. After a single IV administration over the same dose range in patients with active RA, mean systemic clearance of golimumab was 4.9 to 6.7 mL/day/kg, and mean volume of distribution ranged from 58 to 126 mL/kg. The volume of distribution for golimumab indicates that golimumab is distributed primarily in the circulatory system with limited extravascular distribution. Median terminal half-life values were estimated to be approximately 2 weeks in healthy subjects and patients with active RA, psoriatic arthritis, or ankylosing spondylitis. By cross-study comparisons of mean area under the curve (AUC_{∞}) values after IV or subcutaneous administration of golimumab, the absolute bioavailability of subcutaneous golimumab was estimated to be approximately 53%.

When golimumab 50 mg was administered subcutaneously to patients with RA, psoriatic arthritis, or ankylosing spondylitis every 4 weeks, serum concentrations appeared to reach steady state by week 12. With concomitant use of methotrexate, treatment with golimumab 50 mg subcutaneously every 4 weeks resulted in a mean steady-state trough serum concentration of approximately 0.4 to 0.6 mcg/mL in patients with active RA, approximately 0.5 mcg/mL in patients with active psoriatic arthritis, and approximately 0.8 mcg/mL in patients with active ankylosing spondylitis. Patients with RA, psoriatic arthritis, and ankylosing spondylitis treated with golimumab 50 mg and methotrexate had approximately 52%, 36%, and 21% higher mean steady-state trough concentrations of golimumab, respectively, compared with those treated with golimumab 50 mg without methotrexate. The presence of methotrexate also decreased antigolimumab antibody incidence from 7% to 2%. For RA, golimumab should be used with methotrexate. In the psoriatic arthritis and ankylosing spondylitis trials, the presence or absence of concomitant methotrexate did not appear to influence clinical efficacy and safety parameters.

Population PK analyses indicated that concomitant use of NSAIDs, oral corticosteroids, or sulfasalazine did not influence the apparent clearance of golimumab.

Population PK analyses showed there was a trend toward higher apparent clearance of golimumab with increasing weight. However, across the psoriatic arthritis and ankylosing spondylitis populations, no meaningful differences in clinical efficacy were observed among the subgroups by weight quartile. The RA trial in methotrexate-experienced and TNF-blocker–naive patients (study RA-2) did show evidence of a reduction in clinical efficacy with increasing body weight, but this effect was observed for both tested doses of golimumab (50 and 100 mg). Therefore, there is no need to adjust the dosage of golimumab based on a patient's weight.

Population PK analyses suggested no PK differences between male and female patients after body weight adjustment in the RA and psoriatic arthritis trials. In the AS trial, female patients showed 13% higher apparent clearance than male patients after body weight adjustment. Subgroup analysis based on gender showed that both female and male patients achieved clinically significant response at the proposed clinical dose. Dosage adjustment based on gender is not needed.

Population PK analyses indicated that PK parameters of golimumab were not influenced by age in adult patients. Patients 65 years and older had apparent clearance of golimumab similar to patients younger than 65 years of age. No ethnicity-related PK differences were observed between white patients and Asian patients, and there were too few patients of other races to assess for PK differences.

Patients who developed antigolimumab antibodies generally had lower steady-state serum trough concentrations of golimumab.

No formal study of the effect of renal or hepatic impairment on the PK of golimumab was conducted.

Golimumab

Mechanism: Golimumab is a human monoclonal antibody that binds to both the soluble and transmembrane bioactive forms of human TNF-α. This interaction prevents the binding of TNF-α to its receptors, thereby inhibiting the biological activity of TNF-α (a cytokine protein). There was no evidence of golimumab binding to other TNF superfamily ligands; in particular, the golimumab antibody did not bind or neutralize human lymphotoxin. Golimumab did not lyse human monocytes expressing transmembrane TNF in the presence of complement or effector cells.

Elevated TNF-α levels in the blood, synovium, and joints have been implicated in the pathophysiology of several chronic inflammatory diseases such as RA, psoriatic arthritis, and ankylosing spondylitis. TNF-α is an important mediator of the articular inflammation characteristic of these diseases. Golimumab modulated the in vitro biological effects mediated by TNF in several bioassays, including the expression of adhesion proteins responsible for leukocyte infiltration (E-selectin, ICAM-1 and vascular cell adhesion molecule-1 [VCAM-1]) and the secretion of proinflammatory cytokines (IL-6, IL-8, G-CSF, and GM-CSF).

Drug Interactions:

Abatacept: In controlled trials, the concurrent administration of another TNF-blocker and abatacept was associated with a greater proportion of serious infections than the use of a TNF-blocker alone; combination therapy has not demonstrated improved clinical benefit in treating RA. Therefore, combining TNF-blockers and abatacept is not recommended.

Anakinra: Concurrent administration of anakinra (an IL-1 antagonist) and another TNF-blocker was associated with a greater portion of serious infections and neutropenia and no additional benefits, compared with the TNF-blocker alone. Therefore, combining anakinra with TNF-blockers is not recommended.

Methotrexate: In treating RA, use golimumab with methotrexate. Because using or not using methotrexate did not appear to influence the efficacy or safety of golimumab in treating psoriatic arthritis or ankylosing spondylitis, golimumab can be used with or without methotrexate in treating psoriatic arthritis and ankylosing spondylitis.

Cytochrome P450 substrates: Formation of cytochrome P450 enzymes may be suppressed by increased levels of cytokines (eg, TNF-α) during chronic inflammation. Therefore, a molecule that antagonizes cytokine activity, such as golimumab, could normalize formation of cytochrome P450 enzymes. Upon starting or stopping golimumab in patients being treated with cytochrome P450 substrates with a narrow therapeutic index, monitor the effect (eg, warfarin) or drug concentration (eg, cyclosporine, theophylline) and adjust the individual dose of the drug as needed.

Live vaccines: Patients treated with golimumab may receive vaccinations, except for live vaccines. No data are available on the response to live vaccines or the risk of disseminated infection, or transmission of infection after administering live vaccines to patients receiving golimumab. In the phase 3 psoriatic arthritis study, after pneumococcal vaccination, a similar proportion of golimumab- and placebo-treated patients were able to mount an adequate immune response of at least a 2-fold increase in antibody titers to pneumococcal polysaccharide vaccine (*Pneumovax 23*, Merck). In both golimumab- and placebo-treated patients, the proportions of patients who responded to pneumococcal vaccine were lower among patients receiving methotrexate compared with patients not receiving methotrexate. The data suggest that golimumab does not suppress the humoral immune response to pneumococcal 23-valent vaccine.

Patient Information: For patients using the autoinjector, advise them not to pull the autoinjector away from the skin until they hear a first click sound and then a second click sound (the injection is finished and the needle is pulled back). It usually takes approximately 3 to 6 seconds, but it may take up to 15 seconds to hear the second click after the first click. If the autoinjector is pulled away from the skin before the injection is completed, a full dose of golimumab may not be administered.

Pharmaceutical Characteristics

Concentration: 50 mg per 0.5 mL

Packaging:

Autoinjector: Single-dose 50 mg per 0.5 mL glass autoinjector with stainless steel, 5-bevel, 27-gauge, ½-inch needle (NDC #: 57894-0070-02)

Syringe: Single-dose 50 mg per 0.5 mL glass syringe with stainless steel, 5-bevel, 27-gauge, ½-inch needle with a passive needle safety guard (57894-0070-01)

Doseform: Solution

Appearance: Clear to slightly opalescent and colorless to light yellow.

Solvent: L-histidine 0.44 mg per 0.5 mL, L-histidine monohydrochloride monohydrate 0.44 mg per 0.5 mL, sorbitol 20.5 mg per 0.5 mL, 0.08 mg of polysorbate 80 per 0.5 mL

Adjuvant: None

Preservative: None

Allergens: The needle cover on the prefilled syringe, as well as the prefilled syringe in the auto-injector, contain dry natural rubber (a derivative of latex).

Excipients: None

pH: Approximately 5.5

Shelf Life: Expires within an unspecified period of time.

Storage/Stability: Store at 2° to 8°C (36° to 46°F). Protect vials from light. Do not freeze. Contact the manufacturer regarding exposure to freezing or elevated temperatures. Shipping data not provided.

Handling: To ensure proper use, allow the prefilled syringe or autoinjector to sit at room temperature outside the carton for 30 minutes before injection. Do not warm golimumab in any other way.

Production Process: Golimumab was created using genetically engineered mice immunized with human TNF, resulting in an antibody with human-derived antibody variable and constant regions. Golimumab is produced by a recombinant cell line cultured by continuous perfusion and is purified by a series of steps that includes measures to inactivate and remove viruses.

Media: Data not provided.

Other Information

First Licensed: April 24, 2009

References: Hutas G. Golimumab, a fully human monoclonal antibody against TNF-alpha. *Curr Opin Mol Ther.* 2008;10(4):393-406.

Inman RD, Davis JC Jr, Heijde D, et al. Efficacy and safety of golimumab in patients with ankylosing spondylitis: results of a randomized, double-blind, placebo-controlled, phase III trial. *Arthritis Rheum.* 2008;58(11):3402-3412.

Kavanaugh A, McInnes I, Mease P, et al. Golimumab, a new human tumor necrosis factor alpha antibody, administered every four weeks as a subcutaneous injection in psoriatic arthritis: twenty-four-week efficacy and safety results of a randomized, placebo-controlled study. *Arthritis Rheum.* 2009;60(4):976-986.

Kay J, Matteson EL, Dasgupta B, et al. Golimumab in patients with active rheumatoid arthritis despite treatment with methotrexate: a randomized, double-blind, placebo-controlled, dose-ranging study. *Arthritis Rheum.* 2008;58(4):964-975.

Golimumab

Keystone EC, Genovese MC, Klareskog L, et al; GO-FORWARD Study. Golimumab, a human antibody to tumour necrosis factor α given by monthly subcutaneous injections, in active rheumatoid arthritis despite methotrexate therapy: the GO-FORWARD Study. *Ann Rheum Dis.* 2009;68(6):789-796.

Zhou H, Jang H, Fleischmann RM, et al. Pharmacokinetics and safety of golimumab, a fully human anti-TNF-alpha monoclonal antibody, in subjects with rheumatoid arthritis. *J Clin Pharmacol.* 2007;47(3):383-396.

Isoantibodies

Name:
Remicade

Manufacturer:
Janssen Biotech

Synonyms: cA2, antitumor necrosis factor-alpha (TNF-α), *CenTNF*. Initially known as *Avakine*, a name unintentionally suggestive of a cytokine.

Immunologic Characteristics

Target Antigen: Human tumor necrosis factor-alpha (TNF-α).

Viability: Inactive, passive, transient

Antigenic Form: Chimeric, human-murine immunoglobulin. Contains human constant regions and murine variable regions.

Antigenic Type: Protein, IgG1κ antibody, monoclonal, with a molecular weight of approximately 149,100 daltons.

Use Characteristics

Indications:

Ankylosing spondylitis: To reduce signs and symptoms in patients with active ankylosing spondylitis.

Crohn disease: To reduce signs and symptoms and induce and maintain clinical remission in adult and pediatric patients with moderately to severely active Crohn disease who had inadequate response to conventional therapy. Also to reduce the number of draining enterocutaneous and rectovaginal fistulas and maintaining fistula closure in people with fistulizing Crohn disease. Safety and efficacy in fistulizing Crohn disease beyond 3 doses have not been studied.

To induce and maintain clinical remission in patients with moderately to severely active Crohn disease.

Plaque psoriasis: To treat adult patients with chronic severe (ie, extensive and/or disabling) plaque psoriasis who are candidates for systemic therapy and when other systemic therapies are medically less appropriate.

Psoriatic arthritis: To reduce signs and symptoms of active arthritis in patients with psoriatic arthritis.

Rheumatoid arthritis: In combination with methotrexate, to reduce signs and symptoms, inhibiting progression of structural damage and improving physical function in people with moderately to severely active rheumatoid arthritis (RA) who had inadequate response to methotrexate alone.

Ulcerative colitis: To reduce signs and symptoms, achieve clinical remission and mucosal healing, and eliminate corticosteroid use in adult patients with moderately to severely active ulcerative colitis who have had an inadequate response to conventional therapy.

Pediatric ulcerative colitis: For reducing signs and symptoms and inducing and maintaining clinical remission in pediatric patients with moderately to severely active disease who have had an inadequate response to conventional therapy.

Limitations: Studies at other doses or regimens have not been completed. Studies have not been conducted to assess the effects of infliximab on healing of the internal fistular canal, on closure of noncutaneously draining fistulas (eg, entero-entero), or on cutaneously draining fistulas in locations other than perianal and periabdominal.

Infliximab (Chimeric)

Contraindications:

Absolute: None

Relative: Patients with known hypersensitivity to murine proteins or other components of the product

Immunodeficiency: TNF-α mediates inflammation and modulates cellular immune function. Therefore, it is possible for anti-TNF therapies, including infliximab, to affect normal immune responses.

Elderly: In RA, no overall differences were observed in effectiveness or safety in 72 patients 65 years of age and older, compared with younger patients.

In Crohn disease studies, clinical studies of infliximab did not include sufficient patients 65 years of age and older to determine if their responses differ from those of younger adults. No overall differences were observed in safety or efficacy in 72 patients 65 years of age and older with RA compared with younger patients. Because of the effect of infliximab on the risk of infections and the higher risk of infections among the elderly in general, use caution in treating the elderly with infliximab.

Carcinogenicity: Long-term animal studies have not been performed to assess the carcinogenic potential of infliximab. Patients with long duration of Crohn disease, RA, or chronic exposure to immunosuppressant therapies are more prone to develop lymphomas. The effect of infliximab on these phenomena is unknown.

Mutagenicity: No clastogenic or mutagenic effects of infliximab were observed in the in vivo mouse micronucleus test or the *Salmonella-Escherichia coli* (Ames) assay, respectively.

Fertility Impairment: No impairment of fertility was observed in a fertility and general reproduction toxicity study with the analogous mouse antibody used in the 6-month chronic toxicity study. It is not known whether infliximab can impair fertility in humans.

Pregnancy: Category B. Give infliximab to a pregnant woman only if clearly needed. Use caution in administering live vaccines to infants born to female patients treated with infliximab during pregnancy because infliximab is known to cross the placenta and has been detected in the serum of infants up to 6 months of age born to female patients treated during pregnancy.

Because infliximab does not cross-react with TNF-α in species other than humans and chimpanzees, animal reproduction studies have not been conducted. No evidence of maternal toxicity, embryotoxicity, or terotogenicity was observed in a developmental toxicity study conducted in mice using an analogous antibody that selectively inhibits the functional activity of mouse TNF-α. Doses of 10 to 15 mg/kg in pharmacodynamic animal models with the anti-TNF analogous antibody produced maximal pharmacologic effectiveness. Doses up to 40 mg/kg were shown to produce no adverse effects in animal reproduction studies. It is not known whether infliximab can cause fetal harm when administered to a pregnant woman or can affect reproduction capacity.

Lactation: It is not known if infliximab crosses into human breast milk or is absorbed systemically after ingestion. Because of the potential for serious adverse reactions in breast-feeding infants, decide whether to discontinue breast-feeding or infliximab, taking into account the importance of the drug to the mother.

Children: Safety and efficacy of infliximab in children younger than 6 years of age have not been established.

Adverse Reactions: In clinical trials of RA, Crohn disease, and other diseases, 771 patients were treated with infliximab doses up to 20 mg/kg. Approximately 33% of the patients received a single infusion of infliximab, while the others received up to 5 infusions. In studies of both Crohn disease and RA, approximately 5% of patients discontinued scheduled infliximab infusions because of an adverse experience. The most common reasons for discontinuation of treatment were dyspnea, urticaria, and headache. Adverse events have been reported in a higher proportion of patients receiving the 10 mg/kg dose than the 3 mg/kg dose.

Antichimeric antibodies: Of 134 Crohn disease patients treated with infliximab and evaluated for human antichimeric antibody (HACA) development, 18 (13%) were HACA positive, the majority at low titer (less than or equal to 1:20). Patients who were HACA positive were more likely to experience an infusion reaction than HACA-negative patients (36% vs 11%, respectively). The incidence of positive HACA responses was lower among Crohn disease patients receiving immunosuppressant therapies such as mercaptopurine (6-MP), azathioprine, or corticosteroids than among those not receiving these agents (10% vs 23%, respectively). With repeated dosing of infliximab, serum concentrations of infliximab were higher in RA patients who received concomitant methotrexate. There are limited data available on development of anti-infliximab antibodies in patients receiving long-term treatment with infliximab. Because immunogenicity analyses are product specific, comparison of antibody rates with those from other products is not appropriate.

Autoimmunity: Anti-TNF therapy may result in formation of autoimmune antibodies and, rarely, in development of a lupus-like syndrome. Among RA patients treated with infliximab, 62% developed antinuclear antibodies (ANAs) between screening and last evaluation, compared with 27% of placebo-treated patients. Anti–double-strand DNA (dsDNA) antibodies developed in 15% of infliximab-treated patients, compared with 0% for placebo. Three patients treated with infliximab developed clinical signs consistent with a lupus-like syndrome. All 3 improved after discontinuation of infliximab and initiation of appropriate medical treatment. No other autoimmune disorders were reported in patients followed for 6 months to 3 years after the last infusion.

If a patient develops symptoms suggestive of a lupus-like syndrome after treatment with infliximab and is positive for antibodies against dsDNA, discontinue treatment. In clinical trials, discontinuing infliximab led to disappearance of anti-dsDNA antibodies or resolution of symptoms of a lupus-like syndrome.

Of infliximab-treated patients with Crohn disease evaluated for ANA, 34% developed ANA between screening and final evaluation. Anti-dsDNA antibodies developed in approximately 9% of patients treated with infliximab. No association of total infliximab exposure with development of anti-dsDNA antibodies was noted. Baseline therapy with an immunosuppressant at any time reduced development of anti-dsDNA antibodies from 21% among patients not receiving immunosuppressants to 3% among those receiving immunosuppressants. This effect was noted particularly among Crohn disease patients. Crohn disease patients were approximately 2 times more likely to develop anti-dsDNA antibodies if they were ANA positive at study entry.

Of the infliximab-treated RA patients tested, 23% developed ANA between screening and last evaluation, compared with 6% of placebo-treated patients. Anti-dsDNA antibodies developed in approximately 4% of infliximab-treated patients, compared with 1 of the placebo-treated patients. No association was seen between infliximab dose or schedule and development of ANA or anti-dsDNA.

Hepatic: Severe hepatic reactions, including acute liver failure, jaundice, hepatitis, and cholestasis have been reported rarely in patients receiving infliximab.

Hypersensitivity: Infliximab has been associated with hypersensitivity reactions, including urticaria, dyspnea, and hypotension, typically during or within 2 hours after infusion. Discontinue infliximab if severe reactions occur.

In some cases, serum sickness–like reactions occurred in Crohn disease patients 3 to 12 days after infliximab therapy was restarted after an extended period without infliximab treatment. Symptoms included fever, rash, headache, sore throat, myalgias, polyarthralgias, hand and facial edema, or dysphagia. These reactions were associated with marked increase in anti-infliximab antibodies, loss of detectable serum concentrations of infliximab, and possible loss of drug efficacy.

Immune response: TNF-α mediates inflammation and modulates cellular immune function. Therefore, it is possible for anti-TNF therapies, including infliximab, to affect normal immune responses.

Infections: Patients with chronic exposure to immunosuppressant therapies are more prone to develop infections. The effect of infliximab treatment on these phenomena is unknown. Serious infections, including pneumonia, sepsis, and fatal infections, have been reported in patients receiving TNF-blocking agents. Many of these serious infections in patients treated with infliximab occurred in patients on concomitant immunosuppressive therapy that, in addition to their Crohn disease or RA, could predispose them to infection. Exercise caution when considering infliximab for patients with a chronic infection (eg, tuberculosis, coccidioidomycosis) or a history of recurrent infection. Do not give infliximab to patients with clinically important, active infections. Closely monitor patients who develop new infection during treatment. If a patient develops a serious infection or sepsis, discontinue infliximab therapy. Rare cases of tuberculosis, invasive fungal infections, and other opportunistic infections occurred in patients treated with TNF-antagonists.

In placebo-controlled trials evaluating infliximab, infections were reported in 26% of infliximab-treated patients (followed an average of 27 weeks) compared with 16% of placebo recipients (followed an average of 20 weeks). The infections most frequently reported were upper respiratory tract infections (eg, sinusitis, pharyngitis, bronchitis) and urinary tract infections. No increased risk of serious infections or sepsis was observed with infliximab compared with placebo. Among infliximab-treated patients, these serious infections included pneumonia, cellulitis, pyelonephritis, and sepsis. In patients with fistulizing Crohn disease, 12% developed a new abscess 8 to 16 weeks after the last infusion with infliximab.

Infusion reactions: An infusion reaction was defined as any adverse event occurring during the infusion or within 2 hours after the infusion; 20% of infliximab-treated patients in clinical trials experienced an infusion reaction compared with 9% of placebo-treated subjects. Among the 3284 infliximab infusions, 3% were accompanied by nonspecific symptoms (eg, fever, chills), 1% were accompanied by pruritus or urticaria, 1% involved cardiopulmonary reactions (primarily chest pain, hypotension, hypertension, or dyspnea), and 0.1% were accompanied by combined symptoms of pruritus/urticaria and cardiopulmonary reactions. Two percent of patients discontinued infliximab because of infusion reactions. All patients recovered following treatment or discontinuation of infusion. In patients with Crohn disease, an infusion reaction affected 7% of patients during the initial infusion and 10% during the second infliximab infusion. Subsequent infliximab infusions beyond the second were not associated with a higher incidence of reactions. In people with RA, infusions after the initial infusion were not associated with a higher incidence of reactions.

Malignancies or lymphoproliferative disorders: Patients with Crohn disease, RA, or chronic exposure to immunosuppressant therapies are more prone to develop lymphomas. The effect of infliximab treatment on these phenomena is unknown. Five new and 2 recurrent malignancies were observed in 6 of 771 patients treated with infliximab for up to 36 weeks in clinical trials. These were non-Hodgkin B-cell lymphoma, breast cancer, melanoma, squamous cell cancer of the skin, and basal cell cancer. There are insufficient data to determine whether infliximab contributed to the development of these malignancies. The observed incidence rates were similar to those expected for the populations studied.

Nervous system: TNF inhibitors have been associated with rare cases of optic neuritis, seizure, and new-onset or exacerbation of clinical symptoms or radiographic evidence of CNS demyelinating disorders, including multiple sclerosis. Exercise caution before using infliximab in patients with preexisting or recent onset CNS demyelinating or seizure disorders.

Serious events: Among infliximab-treated patients, serious adverse events occurred in up to 2%, with most occurring in up to 0.5%. These included the following: abdominal pain, abdominal hernia, abscess, adult respiratory distress syndrome, anxiety, arthralgia, arthropathy, azotemia, back pain, bacterial infection, bone fracture, brain infarction, bronchitis, cardiac failure, cellulitis, chest pain, cholecystitis, confusion, coughing, dehydration, delirium, depression, diarrhea, dizziness, dyspnea, dysuria, endophthalmitis, erythematous rash, falling, fever, furunculosis, gastric ulcer, headache, hydronephrosis, hypertension, hypotension, injection-site inflammation, intestinal obstruction, intestinal perforation, intestinal stenosis, kidney infarction, leukopenia, liver function elevations (transient), lymphadenopathy, lymphoma, lupus erythematosus syndrome, malignant breast neoplasm, myalgia, myocardial ischemia, nausea, palpitation, pancreatic insufficiency, pleurisy, pneumonia, proctalgia, pulmonary embolus, pulmonary infiltration, renal calculus, renal failure, respiratory insufficiency, rheumatoid nodules, sepsis, somnolence, splenic infarction, splenomegaly, suicide attempt, increased sweating, syncope, tachycardia, tendon injury, thrombocytopenia, thrombophlebitis, upper motor neuron lesion, ureteral obstruction, vomiting, and weight decrease.

At least 1 adverse event occurred in 63% of placebo-treated patients compared with 84% of infliximab-treated patients. Among people treated with infliximab, those with Crohn disease were more likely than those with RA to report adverse events associated with GI symptoms. Adverse events occurring in 1% or more of patients are listed below.

Cardiovascular: Hypertension, hypotension, ecchymosis, flushing, hematoma (1% to 5%).

CNS: Fever (6% to 10%); involuntary muscle contractions, paresthesia, vertigo (1% to 5%).

Dermatologic: Rash, pruritus, moniliasis (5%); acne, alopecia, fungal dermatitis, eczema, erythema, erythematous rash, maculopapular rash, papular rash, dry skin, increased sweating, urticaria (1% to 5%).

GI: Nausea (14% to 17%); abdominal pain (8% to 12%); vomiting (5% to 9%); diarrhea, constipation, dyspepsia, flatulence, intestinal obstruction, oral pain, ulcerative stomatitis, toothache (1% to 5%).

GU: Urinary tract infection (3% to 6%); dysuria, micturition frequency (1% to 5%).

Immunologic: Abscess, herpes simplex, herpes zoster (1% to 5%).

Miscellaneous: Headache (20% to 23%); fatigue (6% to 11%); pain (6% to 9%); flu-like syndrome, chest pain, chills, peripheral edema, fall, hot flushes, malaise, anemia, increased hepatic enzymes, conjunctivitis, tachycardia (1% to 5%).

Musculoskeletal: Back pain (5%); arthralgia, arthritis, myalgia (1% to 5%).

Psychiatric: Anxiety, depression, insomnia (1% to 5%).

Respiratory: Upper respiratory tract infection (16% to 20%); pharyngitis (8% to 9%); bronchitis (4% to 7%); rhinitis (6% to 8%); sinusitis (5% to 9%); coughing (5% to 10%); dyspnea, laryngitis, respiratory tract allergic reaction (1% to 5%).

Pharmacologic & Dosing Characteristics

Dosage:

Ankylosing spondylitis: 5 mg/kg by IV infusion, with additional doses 2 and 6 weeks after the first infusion and every 6 weeks thereafter.

Crohn disease: 5 mg/kg as a single IV infusion to treat moderately to severely active Crohn disease in patients who respond inadequately to conventional therapy. In patients with fistulizing disease, follow an initial 5 mg/kg dose with additional 5 mg/kg doses 2 and 6 weeks after the initial infusion. The average patient will require 3 to 4 vials of infliximab per infusion.

Plaque psoriasis: 5 mg/kg at 0, 2 and 6 weeks, then every 8 weeks.

Psoriatic arthritis: 5 mg/kg by IV infusion, with additional doses 2 and 6 weeks after the first infusion and every 8 weeks thereafter. Infliximab may be used in combination with methotrexate.

Rheumatoid arthritis: 3 mg/kg by IV infusion, followed by additional similar doses 2 and 6 weeks after first infusion, and then every 8 weeks thereafter. Give infliximab in combination with methotrexate therapy. For patients who have an incomplete response to infliximab, consider adjusting the infliximab dose up to 10 mg/kg or treating as often as every 4 weeks.

Ulcerative colitis: The recommended dose of infliximab is 5 mg/kg given as an induction regimen at 0, 2, and 6 weeks, followed by a maintenance regimen of 5 mg/kg every 8 weeks thereafter for the treatment of moderately to severely active ulcerative colitis.

Route: IV infusion over 2 or more hours.

Overdosage: Single doses up to 20 mg/kg have been administered without any direct toxic effect. Monitor patients for signs or symptoms of adverse effects and institute appropriate symptomatic treatment immediately.

Additional Doses: Among 40 patients with Crohn disease retreated with infliximab after a 2- to 4-year interval without infliximab treatment, 10 patients experienced adverse events manifesting 3 to 12 days after infusion. Six events were considered serious. Signs and symptoms included myalgia or arthralgia with fever or rash. Some patients also experienced pruritus; facial, hand, or lip edema; dysphagia; urticaria; sore throat; and headache. These patients had not experienced infusion-related adverse events with their initial infliximab therapy. Of the 40 patients, these adverse events occurred in 9 of 23 (39%) who received infliximab from a liquid formulation no longer in use and in 1 of 17 (6%) who received a lyophilized formulation. Signs and symptoms resolved in all cases.

Missed Doses: Interrupting the recommended schedule or delaying subsequent doses does not require restarting the series.

Related Interventions: Evaluate patients for latent tuberculosis infection with a tuberculin skin test before therapy with infliximab.

Efficacy:

Ankylosing spondylitis: The primary end point was the proportion of patients demonstrating 20% or greater improvement in signs and symptoms at 24 weeks, as measured by Assessment in Ankylosing Spondylitis Response Criteria. Improvement in signs and symptoms of ankylosing spondylitis was seen in 60% of the patients in the infliximab group, compared with 18% of the placebo group. Improvement was observed at week 2 and maintained through week 24. At 24 weeks, the proportions of patients achieving 50% and 70% improvement were 44% and 28%, respectively, for the infliximab group, compared with 9% and 4% of the placebo group. In the infliximab group, 22% achieved a low level of disease activity, compared with 1% of the placebo group.

Active Crohn disease: In a study of 108 patients with moderately to severely active Crohn disease (Crohn disease activity index [CDAI] of more than or equal to 200 but 400 or less) who did not respond adequately to conventional therapies, 82% of patients treated with infliximab at 5 mg/kg achieved a clinical response (decrease in CDAI by 70 points or more from baseline) at week 4 compared with 16% of placebo recipients. In this study, 48% of infliximab recipients went into clinical remission at week 4 compared with 4% of placebo recipients. Overall, 92% of patients in the trial continued to receive stable doses of corticosteroids, antibiotics, aminosalicylates, or other immunomodulators. Patients treated with infliximab had higher scores on a quality-of-life scale than did placebo recipients.

When patients who had not responded to infliximab received a single 10 mg/kg dose of infliximab 4 weeks after the first dose, 34% experienced a response 4 weeks after the second dose.

Patients who remained in clinical response at week 8 were eligible for the retreatment phase. Patients were rerandomized at week 12 to receive 4 infusions of placebo or 10 mg/kg of infliximab at 8-week intervals (weeks 12, 20, 28, 36) and were followed to week 48. In the limited data set available, no significant differences were observed between the infliximab and placebo groups.

Fistulizing Crohn disease: Infliximab was also effective in reducing the number of open, draining fistulas that were of 3 or more months' duration. In a clinical study of 94 patients, 68% of infliximab recipients experienced closure of 50% or more of fistulas for 4 weeks or longer, compared with 26% of placebo recipients. The primary end point was based on drainage upon gentle compression on 2 or more consecutive visits, without an increase in medication or surgery for Crohn disease. Approximately 55% of patients with infliximab-treated fistulas experienced closure of their fistulas compared with 13% of placebo recipients. Six patients with a demonstrated clinical response to treatment with infliximab developed an abscess in the area of the fistula between 8 and 16 weeks after the last infusion. New fistulas developed in approximately 15% of both infliximab- and placebo-treated patients.

Plaque psoriasis: Safety and efficacy of infliximab were assessed in 3 randomized, double-blind, placebo-controlled studies in patients 18 years of age and older with chronic, stable plaque psoriasis involving 10% body surface area, a minimum Psoriasis Area Sensitivity Index (PASI) score of 12, and who were candidates for systemic therapy or phototherapy. In study I, in patients with more extensive psoriasis who previously received phototherapy, 85% of patients on infliximab 5 mg/kg achieved a PASI 75 at week 10, compared with 4% on placebo. In study II, in patients with more extensive psoriasis who previously received phototherapy, 72% and 77% of patients on infliximab 3 mg/kg and 5 mg/kg achieved a PASI 75 at week 10 respectively, compared with 1% on placebo. In study II, among patients with more extensive psoriasis who failed or were intolerant to phototherapy, 70% and 78% of patients on infliximab 3 mg/kg and 5 mg/kg achieved a PASI 75 at week 10 respectively, compared with 2% on placebo. Maintenance of response was studied in infliximab-treated patients in the 3 mg/kg and 5 mg/kg groups. The groups that received a maintenance dose every 8 weeks appear to have a greater percentage of patients maintaining a PASI 75 through week 50, compared with patients who received as-needed (or PRN) doses. The best response was maintained with the 5 mg/kg every-8-week dose. At week 46, when infliximab serum concentrations were at trough level in the every-8-week dose group, 54% of patients in the 5 mg/kg group, compared with 36% in the 3 mg/kg group, achieved PASI 75. The lower percentage of PASI 75 responders in the 3 mg/kg every-8-week dose group compared with the 5 mg/kg group was associated with a lower percentage of patients with detectable trough serum infliximab levels. Regardless of whether the maintenance doses are PRN or every 8 weeks, there is a decline in response in a subpopulation of patients in each group over time. The results of study I through week 50 in the 5 mg/kg every 8 weeks maintenance dose group were similar to the results from study II. Efficacy and safety of infliximab beyond 50 weeks have not been evaluated in patients with plaque psoriasis.

Psoriatic arthritis: In a study of 200 patients with active psoriatic arthritis, treatment with infliximab 5 mg/kg resulted in improvements in American College of Rheumatology (ACR) response criteria, dactylitis, and enthesopathy.

Rheumatoid arthritis: Efficacy of infliximab in conjunction with methotrexate was assessed in a randomized, double-blind, placebo-controlled study of 428 patients with active RA despite treatment with methotrexate. Patients enrolled had a median age of 54 years, median disease duration of 8.4 years, median swollen and tender joint count of 20 and 31 respectively, and were on a median dose of 15 mg/wk of methotrexate. Patients received either placebo plus methotrexate or 1 of 4 doses of infliximab plus methotrexate. All doses and schedules of infliximab with methotrexate resulted in improved signs and symptoms. This improvement was observed at week 2 and maintained through week 102. Approximately 10% of patients treated with infliximab achieved a major clinical response, defined as maintenance of an ACR response level 20 over one 6-month period, compared with 0% of placebo-treated patients. Compared with placebo recipients, infliximab-treated patients had fewer tender joints, fewer swollen joints, superior assessment scores and disability index, less pain, and lower C-reactive protein concentrations. Inhibition of progression of structural damage by radiograph was observed at week 54 and maintained through week 102. All doses and schedules of infliximab showed significantly greater improvement from baseline in physical function, disability, and quality of life through week 54, compared with placebo.

Ulcerative colitis: The safety and efficacy of infliximab were assessed in 2 randomized, double-blind, placebo-controlled studies enrolling 728 patients with moderately to severely active ulcerative colitis. In both studies, greater percentages of patients in the infliximab groups achieved a clinical response, a sustained clinical response, clinical remission, and other assessed clinical outcomes than in the placebo groups. Of patients on corticosteroids, greater proportions of patients in the infliximab groups were in clinical remission and able to discontinue corticosteroids at week 30, compared with patients in the placebo groups.

Onset: Efficacy was demonstrated in moderately to severely active Crohn disease when measured 4 weeks after a single infusion of infliximab. The median time to onset of response in patients with fistulizing disease was 2 weeks. In RA, differences between infliximab and placebo treatment groups were apparent within the first 2 to 6 weeks of therapy.

Duration: The proportion of patients with moderately to severely active Crohn disease in remission gradually diminished over the 12-week observation period after the single dose. The median duration of response after 3 doses in patients with fistulizing disease was 12 weeks; after 22 weeks, there was no difference between infliximab-treated patients and placebo recipients. In RA, differences between infliximab and placebo treatment groups were sustained throughout the 30-week observation interval.

Pharmacokinetics: Immunoglobulins are primarily eliminated by catabolism. Elevated concentrations of TNF-α are found in the stools of Crohn disease patients and in the joints of RA patients, and correlate with elevated disease activity.

In Crohn disease, treatment with infliximab reduced infiltration of inflammatory cells and TNF-α production in inflamed areas of the intestine and reduced the proportion of mononuclear cells from the lamina propria able to express TNF-α and interferon-gamma.

In RA, treatment with infliximab reduced infiltration of inflammatory cells into inflamed areas of the joint, expression of molecules mediating cellular adhesion, chemoattraction, and tissue degradation.

After treatment with infliximab, patients with Crohn disease or RA have decreased levels of serum IL-6 and C-reactive protein compared with baseline. However, peripheral blood lymphocytes from infliximab-treated patients showed no decrease in proliferative responses to in vitro mitogenic stimulation when compared with cells from untreated patients.

Data from single IV infusions of 1 to 20 mg/kg showed a direct and linear relationship between the dose administered and the maximum serum concentration (C_{max}) and area under the plasma concentration-time curve (AUC). The volume of distribution at steady state (Vd), clearance, and mean residence time were independent of the dose. Infliximab has a prolonged terminal half-life and is predominantly distributed within the vascular compartment. Median pharmacokinetic results for doses of 3 to 10 mg/kg in RA and 5 mg/kg in Crohn disease indicate that the terminal half-life of infliximab is 8 to 9.5 days. No systematic accumulation of infliximab occurred upon continued repeated treatment with 3 or 10 mg/kg at 4- or 8-week intervals. No major differences in clearance or volume of distribution were observed in subgroups defined by age or weight. It is not known if there are differences in patients with marked impairment of hepatic or renal function. Corticosteroid use significantly increased the Vd of infliximab from 2.8 to 3.3 L (a 17% increase, possibly secondary to corticosteroid-mediated changes in electrolyte balance and fluid retention). A single infusion of 3 mg/kg in patients with RA resulted in a terminal half-life of 8 days.

No major differences in clearance or volume of distribution were observed in patient subgroups defined by age or weight. It is not known whether there are differences in clearance or volume of distribution between gender subgroups or in patients with marked impairment of hepatic or renal function.

After an initial dose of infliximab, repeated infusions at 2 and 6 weeks in fistulizing Crohn disease and RA patients resulted in predictable concentration-time profiles following each treatment. No systemic accumulation of infliximab occurred upon continued repeated treatment with 3 or 10 mg/kg at 4- or 8-week intervals. In RA patients or patients with moderate or severe Crohn disease who were retreated with 4 infusions of infliximab 10 mg/kg at 8-week intervals, no systemic accumulation of infliximab occurred.

Mechanism: Infliximab binds specifically with TNF-α, with an association constant of 10^{10} M^{-1}. Infliximab neutralizes the biological activity of TNF-α by binding with high affinity to the soluble and transmembrane forms of TNF-α. Infliximab destroys TNF-α–producing cells. Infliximab also binds TNF-α with its receptors. Infliximab does not neutralize TNF-β (lymphotoxin-α), a related cytokine that uses the same receptors as TNF-α.

Biological activities attributed to TNF-α include induction of proinflammatory cytokines, such as IL-1 and IL-6, enhancement of leukocyte migration by increasing endothelial layer permeability and expression of adhesion molecules by endothelial cells and leukocytes, activation of neutrophil and eosinophil functional activity, and induction of acute phase and other liver proteins as well as tissue-degrading enzymes produced by synoviocytes and/or chondrocytes. Cells expressing transmembrane TNF-α bound by infliximab can be lysed in vitro by complement or effector cells. Anti–TNF-α antibodies reduce disease activity in a cotton-top tamarind colitis model and decrease synovitis and joint erosions in a murine model of collagen-induced arthritis. Infliximab prevents disease in transgenic mice that develop polyarthritis as a result of constitutive expression of human TNF-α and, when administered after disease onset, allows eroded joints to heal. Infliximab inhibits the functional activity of TNF-α in a variety of in vitro bioassays using human fibroblasts, endothelial cells, neutrophils, B- and T-lymphocytes, and epithelial cells.

Drug Interactions: In RA, concomitant medications besides methotrexate were nonsteroidal anti-inflammatory drugs (NSAIDs), folic acid, corticosteroids, and narcotics. Most patients in clinical trials received 1 or more of the following concomitant medications: antibiotics, antivirals, corticosteroids, folic acid, mercaptopurine-azathioprine, NSAIDs, and aminosalicylates. Patients with Crohn disease receiving immunosuppressants tended to experience fewer infusion reactions compared with patients not receiving immunosuppressants.

Based on the known effects of infliximab, there is a theoretical risk that infliximab could impair patient responsiveness to live and inactivated vaccines. Live vaccines should not be given concurrently with infliximab therapy.

Infliximab (Chimeric)

Pharmaceutical Characteristics

Concentration: 100 mg/vial

Packaging: Single-use 20 mL vial

NDC Number: 57894-0030-01

Doseform: Lyophilized powder for solution

Appearance: White, lyophilized powder, yielding a colorless to light yellow and opalescent solution. Foaming of the solution on reconstitution is not unusual. Because infliximab is a protein, the solution may develop a few translucent particles. Do not use if opaque particles, discoloration, or other foreign particles are present.

Diluent:

For reconstitution: 10 mL of sterile water for injection per vial. Direct the diluent against the glass wall of the vial. Gently swirl the solution by rotating the vial to dissolve the powder. Avoid prolonged or vigorous agitation. Do not shake. Allow the reconstituted solution to stand for 5 minutes.

For infusion: Further dilute the reconstituted infliximab in 250 mL of sodium chloride 0.9%. The infusion concentration should range between 0.4 and 4 mg/mL (100 mg per 250 mL = 0.4 mg/mL; 1,000 mg per 250 mL = 4 mg/mL). Add the reconstituted infliximab solution to the infusion container slowly. Mix gently. Infuse over 2 or more hours.

Adjuvant: None

Preservative: None

Allergens: None

Excipients: Each 100 mg vial contains sucrose 500 mg, 0.5 mg of polysorbate 80, monobasic sodium phosphate 2.2 mg, and dibasic sodium phosphate 6.1 mg.

pH: 7.2 after reconstitution with 10 mL of sterile water

Shelf Life: Expires within 18 months.

Storage/Stability: Store powder at 2° to 8°C (36° to 46°F). Discard frozen infliximab. Contact the manufacturer regarding exposure to extreme temperatures. Shipped by overnight courier in insulated containers with refrigerated and frozen coolant packs and fill void space in the shipping container with paper.

Discard if not used within 3 hours after reconstitution. Discard unused portions.

Do not infuse infliximab concomitantly in the same IV line with other agents.

Handling: Reconstituted infliximab and diluted infliximab are incompatible with plasticized polyvinylchloride (PVC) equipment and devices. Prepare diluted infliximab solutions only in glass infusion bottles or polypropylene or polyolefin infusion bags. Administer infliximab solutions through polyethylene-lined administration sets, using an in-line, low–protein-binding filter (pore size, 1.2 micron or smaller).

Production Process: Infliximab is produced by a recombinant cell line cultured by continuous perfusion and is purified by a series of steps that includes measures to inactivate and remove viruses.

Media: Recombinant cell line

Disease Epidemiology

Prevalence:

Crohn disease: Crohn disease is a chronic and debilitating disorder of the GI tract. Crohn disease causes fever, diarrhea, abdominal pain, weight loss, and general fatigue. In severe cases, it causes blockage of the intestines and creates painful fistulas, deep openings that drain mucus or fecal material from the bowel wall through the skin, bladder, vagina, and rectum. Crohn disease most often begins in young adults 20 to 35 years of age. Approximately 250,000 people with Crohn disease live in the United States.

Rheumatoid arthritis: RA is a painful, potentially debilitating disease characterized by chronic inflammation of joint linings. In severe cases, this inflammation extends to other joint tissues and surrounding cartilage, where it may erode bone and cartilage and lead to joint deformities. Symptoms include stiffness, pain, and swelling of multiple joints. Approximately 2.1 million Americans have RA. Two to 3 times more women than men are affected.

Other Information

Perspective:

1932: Burrill Crohn describes a serious inflammatory disease of the GI tract at Mount Sinai Medical Center in New York City.

1993: Infliximab initially constructed and characterized.

First Licensed: August 24, 1998

References: Bodger K. Economic implications of biological therapies for Crohn's disease: review of infliximab. *Pharmacoeconomics.* 2005;23(9):875-888.

Siddiqui MA, Scott LJ. Infliximab: a review of its use in Crohn's disease and rheumatoid arthritis. *Drugs.* 2005;65(15):2179-2208.

Targan SR, Hanauer SB, van Deventer SJ, et al. A short-term study of chimeric monoclonal antibody cA2 to tumor necrosis factor alpha for Crohn's disease. *N Engl J Med.* 1997;337(15):1029-1035.

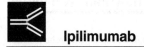
Ipilimumab

Isoantibodies

Name:
Yervoy
Synonyms: MDX-010, MDX-CTLA-4

Manufacturer:
Bristol-Myers Squibb Company

Immunologic Characteristics

Target Antigen: Cytotoxic T-lymphocyte antigen 4 (CTLA-4)

Viability: Inactive, passive, transient

Antigenic Form: Human monoclonal IgG1κ antibody

Antigenic Type: Protein, IgG1κ, anti-human cytotoxic T-lymphocyte antigen 4 (CTLA-4) antigen. Molecular weight approximately 148,000 daltons.

Use Characteristics

Indications: To treat unresectable or metastatic melanoma.

Contraindications: None

Elderly: Of the 511 patients treated with ipilimumab at 3 mg/kg, 28% were 65 years and older. No overall differences in safety or efficacy were reported between elderly patients (≥ 65 years) and younger patients (< 65 years).

Carcinogenicity: The carcinogenic potential of ipilimumab has not been evaluated in long-term animal studies.

Mutagenicity: The genotoxic potential of ipilimumab has not been evaluated.

Fertility Impairment: Human fertility studies have not been performed with ipilimumab. The effects of ipilimumab on prenatal and postnatal development in monkeys have not been fully investigated. Preliminary results are available from an ongoing study in which pregnant cynomolgus monkeys received ipilimumab every 21 days from the onset of organogenesis in the first trimester through delivery, at dose levels either 2.6 or 7.2 times higher than the clinical dose of 3 mg/kg of ipilimumab (by area under the curve [AUC]). No treatment-related adverse effects on reproduction were detected during the first 2 trimesters of pregnancy. Beginning in the third trimester, the ipilimumab groups experienced higher incidences of abortion, stillbirth, premature delivery (with corresponding lower birth weight), and higher incidences of infant mortality in a dose-related manner compared with controls. Genetically engineered mice heterozygous for CTLA-4 (CTLA-4±), the target for ipilimumab, appeared healthy and gave birth to healthy CTLA-4± heterozygous offspring. Mated CTLA-4± heterozygous mice also produced offspring deficient in CTLA-4 (homozygous negative, CTLA-4−/−). The CTLA-4−/− homozygous-negative offspring appeared healthy at birth, exhibited signs of multiorgan lymphoproliferative disease by 2 weeks of age, and all died by 34 weeks of age with massive lymphoproliferation and multiorgan tissue destruction.

Pregnancy: Category C. There are no adequate and well-controlled studies of ipilimumab in pregnant women. Because ipilimumab is an IgG1-type antibody, it has the potential to cross the placenta and reach the developing fetus. Use ipilimumab during pregnancy only if the potential benefit justifies the potential risk to the fetus. In a combined study of embryo-fetal and peri- and postnatal development, severe toxicities, including increased incidences of third-trimester abortion, stillbirth, premature delivery, low birth weight, and infant mortality occurred following intravenous (IV) administration of ipilimumab to pregnant cynomolgus monkeys every 21 days from the onset of organogenesis through parturition at doses of 2.6 or

7.2 times the recommended human dose of 3 mg/kg (by AUC). In genetically engineered mice in which the gene for CTLA-4 has been deleted, offspring lacking CTLA-4 were born apparently healthy, but died within 34 weeks due to multi-organ infiltration and damage by lymphocytes. Human IgG1 (such as ipilimumab) is known to cross the placental barrier; therefore, ipilimumab has the potential to be transmitted from the mother to the developing fetus.

Lactation: It is not known whether ipilimumab is secreted in human milk. Because many drugs are secreted in human milk and because of the potential for serious adverse reactions in breast-feeding infants from ipilimumab, decide whether to discontinue breast-feeding or ipilimumab, taking into account the importance of ipilimumab to the mother.

Children: Safety and effectiveness of ipilimumab have not been established in pediatric patients.

Adverse Reactions: The clinical development program excluded patients with active autoimmune diseases or those receiving systemic immunosuppression for organ transplantations. Exposure to ipilimumab 3 mg/kg for 4 doses given by IV infusion in previously treated patients with unresectable or metastatic melanoma was assessed in a randomized, double-blind clinical study (study 1); 131 patients (median age, 57 years; 60% men) received ipilimumab as a single agent, 380 patients (median age, 56 years; 61% men) received ipilimumab with an investigational gp100 peptide vaccine (gp100), and 132 patients (median age, 57 years; 54% men) received gp100 peptide vaccine alone. Patients in the study received a median of 4 doses (range, 1 to 4 doses). Ipilimumab was discontinued because of adverse reactions in 10% of patients.

The most common adverse reactions ($\geq$ 5%) in patients who received ipilimumab at 3 mg/kg were fatigue, diarrhea, pruritus, rash, and colitis. The following table presents selected adverse reactions from study 1, which occurred in 5% or more of patients in the ipilimumab-containing arms, with 5% or greater increased incidence over the control gp100 arm for all-grade events, and with 1% or more incidence over the control group for grade 3 to 5 events.

Ipilimumab Adverse Reactions (5% or more)[a]						
	Ipilimumab 3 mg/kg (n = 131)		Ipilimumab 3 mg/kg + gp100 (n = 380)		gp100 (n = 132)	
System Organ Class	Any grade	Grade 3-5	Any grade	Grade 3-5	Any grade	Grade 3-5
GI Disorders						
Diarrhea	32%	5%	37%	4%	20%	1%
Colitis	8%	5%	5%	3%	2%	0%
Skin and SC Tissue Disorders						
Pruritus	31%	0%	21%	< 1%	11%	0%
Rash	29%	2%	25%	2%	8%	0%
Fatigue	41%	7%	34%	5%	31%	3%

a Percentage (%) of patients.

The following table presents the per-patient incidence of severe, life-threatening, or fatal immune-mediated adverse reactions from study 1.

Severe to Fatal Immune-Mediated Adverse Reactions in Study 1		
	Percentage of Patients	
	Ipilimumab 3 mg/kg (n = 131)	Ipilimumab 3 mg/kg + gp100 (n = 380)
Any immune-mediated adverse event	15%	12%
Enterocolitis[a,b]	7%	7%
Hepatotoxicity[a]	1%	2%
Dermatitis	2%	3%
Neuropathy[a]	1%	< 1%
Endocrinopathy	4%	1%
Hypopituitarism	4%	1%
Adrenal insufficiency	0%	1%
Other		
Pneumonitis	0%	< 1%
Meningitis	0%	< 1%
Nephritis	1%	0%
Eosinophilia[c]	1%	0%
Pericarditis[a,c]	0%	< 1%

a Including fatal outcome.
b Including intestinal perforation.
c Underlying etiology not established.

Across clinical studies that utilized ipilimumab doses ranging from 0.3 to 10 mg/kg, the following adverse reactions were also reported (incidence less than 1% unless otherwise noted): urticaria (2%), large intestinal ulcer, esophagitis, acute respiratory distress syndrome, renal failure, and infusion reaction. Based on the experience in the entire clinical program for melanoma, the incidence and severity of enterocolitis and hepatitis appear to be dose-dependent.

Immune-mediated events: Ipilimumab can result in severe and fatal immune-mediated adverse reactions due to T-cell activation and proliferation. These immune-mediated reactions may involve any organ system; the most common severe immune-mediated adverse reactions are enterocolitis, hepatitis, dermatitis (including toxic epidermal necrolysis [TEN]), neuropathy, and endocrinopathy. Most of these immune-mediated reactions initially manifested during treatment; however, a minority occurred weeks to months after discontinuing ipilimumab.

Permanently discontinue ipilimumab and initiate systemic high-dose corticosteroid therapy for severe immune-mediated reactions. Withhold dose for moderate immune-mediated adverse reactions until return to baseline, improvement to mild severity, or complete resolution, and patient is receiving < 7.5 mg of prednisone or equivalent per day. Administer systemic high-dose corticosteroids for severe, persistent, or recurring immune-mediated reactions.

Assess patients for signs and symptoms of enterocolitis, dermatitis, neuropathy, and endocrinopathy, and evaluate clinical chemistries, including liver function tests and thyroid function tests, at baseline and before each dose.

Enterocolitis: In study 1, severe, life-threatening, or fatal (diarrhea of 7 or more stools above baseline, fever, ileus, peritoneal signs; grade 3 to 5) immune-mediated enterocolitis occurred in 34 (7%) ipilimumab-treated patients, and moderate (diarrhea with up to 6 stools above baseline, abdominal pain, mucus or blood in stool; grade 2) enterocolitis occurred in 28 (5%) ipilimumab-treated patients. Across all ipilimumab-treated patients (n = 511),

5 (1%) patients developed intestinal perforation, 4 (0.8%) patients died as a result of complications, and 26 (5%) patients were hospitalized for severe enterocolitis. The median time to onset was 7.4 weeks (range, 1.6 to 13.4) and 6.3 weeks (range, 0.3 to 18.9) after starting ipilimumab in patients with grade 3 to 5 enterocolitis and with grade 2 enterocolitis, respectively. Twenty-nine patients (85%) with grade 3 to 5 enterocolitis were treated with high-dose (≥ 40 mg of prednisone equivalent per day) corticosteroids; the median duration of treatment was 2.3 weeks (ranging up to 13.9 weeks) followed by corticosteroid taper. Of 28 patients with moderate enterocolitis, 46% were not treated with systemic corticosteroids, 29% were treated with < 40 mg of prednisone or equivalent per day for a median 5.1 weeks, and 25% were treated with high-dose corticosteroids for a median 10 days prior to corticosteroid taper. Infliximab was administered to 5 of the 62 patients (8%) with moderate, severe, or life-threatening immune-mediated enterocolitis after inadequate response to corticosteroids. Of the 34 patients with grade 3 to 5 enterocolitis, 74% experienced complete resolution, 3% experienced improvement to grade 2 severity, and 24% did not improve. Among the 28 patients with grade 2 enterocolitis, 79% experienced complete resolution, 11% improved, and 11% did not improve. Monitor patients for signs and symptoms of enterocolitis (eg, diarrhea, abdominal pain, mucus or blood in stool, with or without fever) and bowel perforation (eg, peritoneal signs, ileus). In symptomatic patients, rule out infectious etiologies and consider endoscopic evaluation for persistent or severe symptoms. Permanently discontinue ipilimumab in patients with severe enterocolitis and initiate systemic prednisone 1 to 2 mg/kg/day or equivalent. Upon improvement to grade 1 or less, initiate corticosteroid taper and continue to taper over 1 month or longer. In clinical trials, rapid corticosteroid tapering resulted in recurrence or worsening symptoms of enterocolitis in some patients. Withhold ipilimumab dosing for moderate enterocolitis; administer antidiarrheal treatment and, if persistent for more than 1 week, initiate systemic prednisone 0.5 mg/kg/day or equivalent.

Immune-mediated hepatitis: In study 1, severe, life-threatening, or fatal hepatotoxicity occurred in 8 (2%) ipilimumab-treated patients, with fatal hepatic failure in 0.2% and hospitalization in 0.4% of ipilimumab-treated patients. An additional 13 (2.5%) patients experienced moderate hepatotoxicity manifested by liver function test abnormalities. The underlying pathology was not ascertained in all patients, but in some instances, included immune-mediated hepatitis. There were insufficient numbers of patients with biopsy-proven hepatitis to characterize the clinical course of this event. Monitor liver function tests (hepatic transaminase and bilirubin levels) and assess patients for signs and symptoms of hepatotoxicity before each dose of ipilimumab. In patients with hepatotoxicity, rule out infectious or malignant causes and increase frequency of liver function test monitoring until resolution. Permanently discontinue ipilimumab in patients with grade 3 to 5 hepatotoxicity and administer systemic prednisone 1 to 2 mg/kg/day or equivalent. When liver function tests show sustained improvement or return to baseline, start corticosteroid tapering and continue to taper over 1 month. Across the clinical development program for ipilimumab, mycophenolate treatment has been administered in patients who have persistent severe hepatitis despite high-dose corticosteroids. Withhold ipilimumab in patients with grade 2 hepatotoxicity.

Immune-mediated dermatitis: In study 1, severe, life-threatening, or fatal immune-mediated dermatitis (eg, Stevens-Johnson syndrome, TEN, or rash complicated by full thickness dermal ulceration; or necrotic, bullous, or hemorrhagic manifestations; grade 3 to 5) occurred in 13 (2.5%) ipilimumab-treated patients. One (0.2%) patient died as a result of TEN and 1 additional patient required hospitalization for severe dermatitis. There were 63 (12%) patients with moderate (grade 2) dermatitis. The median time to onset of moderate, severe, or life-threatening immune-mediated dermatitis was 3.1 weeks, and ranged up to 17.3 weeks from start of ipilimumab. Seven (54%) ipilimumab-treated patients with severe dermatitis received high-dose corticosteroids (median dose, 60 mg prednisone/day or equivalent) for up to 14.9 weeks followed by corticosteroid taper. Of these 7 patients, 6 had complete resolution; time to resolution ranged up to 15.6 weeks. Of the 63 patients with moderate dermatitis, 25 (40%) were treated with systemic corticosteroids (median, 60 mg/day of prednisone or equivalent) for a median of 2.1 weeks, 7 (11%) were treated with only topical corticosteroids, and 31 (49%) did not receive systemic or topical corticosteroids. Forty-four (70%) patients with moderate dermatitis were reported to have complete resolution, 7 (11%) improved to mild (grade 1) severity, and 12 (19%) had no reported improvement. Monitor patients for signs and symptoms of dermatitis, such as rash and pruritus. Unless an alternate etiology has been identified, signs or symptoms of dermatitis should be considered immune-mediated. Permanently discontinue ipilimumab in patients with Stevens-Johnson syndrome, TEN, or rash complicated by full thickness dermal ulceration; or necrotic, bullous, or hemorrhagic manifestations. Administer systemic prednisone 1 to 2 mg/kg/day or equivalent. When dermatitis is controlled, taper corticosteroids over 1 month or longer. Withhold ipilimumab dosing in patients with moderate to severe signs and symptoms. For mild to moderate dermatitis, such as localized rash and pruritus, treat symptomatically. Administer topical or systemic corticosteroids if there is no improvement of symptoms within 1 week.

Immune-mediated neuropathies: In study 1, one case of fatal Guillain-Barré syndrome and 1 case of severe (grade 3) peripheral motor neuropathy were reported. Across the clinical development program of ipilimumab, myasthenia gravis and additional cases of Guillain-Barré syndrome have been reported. Monitor for symptoms of motor or sensory neuropathy, such as unilateral or bilateral weakness, sensory alterations, or paresthesia. Permanently discontinue ipilimumab in patients with severe neuropathy (interfering with daily activities) such as Guillain-Barré–like syndromes. Institute medical intervention as appropriate to manage severe neuropathy. Consider systemic prednisone 1 to 2 mg/kg/day or equivalent for severe neuropathies. Withhold ipilimumab dosing in patients with moderate neuropathy (not interfering with daily activities).

Immune-mediated endocrinopathies: In study 1, severe to life-threatening immune-mediated endocrinopathies (requiring hospitalization, urgent medical intervention, or interfering with activities of daily living; grade 3 to 4) occurred in 9 (1.8%) ipilimumab-treated patients. All patients had hypopituitarism and some had additional concomitant endocrinopathies, such as adrenal insufficiency, hypogonadism, and hypothyroidism. Six of the 9 patients were hospitalized for severe endocrinopathies. Moderate endocrinopathy (requiring hormone replacement or medical intervention; grade 2) occurred in 12 (2.3%) patients, and consisted of hypothyroidism, adrenal insufficiency, hypopituitarism, and 1 case each of hyperthyroidism and Cushing syndrome. The median time to onset of moderate to severe immune-mediated endocrinopathy was 11 weeks and ranged up to 19.3 weeks after the initiation of ipilimumab. Of the 21 patients with moderate to life-threatening endocrinopathy, 17 patients required long-term hormone replacement therapy including, most commonly, adrenal hormones (n = 10) and thyroid hormones (n = 13). Monitor patients for clinical signs and symptoms of hypophysitis, adrenal insufficiency (including adrenal crisis), and hyper or hypothyroidism. Patients may experience fatigue, headache, mental status changes, abdominal pain, unusual bowel habits, and hypotension, or nonspecific symptoms that may resemble other causes, such as brain metastasis or underlying disease. Unless an alternate etiology has been identified, consider signs or symptoms of endocrinopathies immune-mediated. Monitor thyroid function tests and clinical chemistries at the start of treatment, before each dose, and as clinically indicated, based on symptoms. In a limited number of patients, hypophysitis was diagnosed by imaging studies through enlargement of the pituitary gland. Withhold ipilimumab dosing in symptomatic patients. Initiate systemic prednisone 1 to 2 mg/kg/day or equivalent, and initiate appropriate hormone replacement therapy.

Other immune-mediated adverse reactions: The following clinically significant immune-mediated adverse reactions were seen in 1% or fewer of ipilimumab-treated patients in study 1: nephritis, pneumonitis, meningitis, pericarditis, uveitis, iritis, and hemolytic anemia. Across the clinical development program for ipilimumab, the following likely immune-mediated adverse reactions were also reported with an incidence of 1% or less: myocarditis, angiopathy, temporal arteritis, vasculitis, polymyalgia rheumatica, conjunctivitis, blepharitis, episcleritis, scleritis, leukocytoclastic vasculitis, erythema multiforme, psoriasis, pancreatitis, arthritis, and autoimmune thyroiditis. Permanently discontinue ipilimumab for clinically significant or severe immune-mediated adverse reactions. Initiate systemic prednisone 1 to 2 mg/kg/day or equivalent for severe immune-mediated adverse reactions. Administer corticosteroid eye drops to patients who develop uveitis, iritis, or episcleritis. Permanently discontinue ipilimumab for immune-mediated ocular disease that is unresponsive to local immunosuppressive therapy.

Immunogenicity: In clinical studies, 1.1% of 1,024 evaluable patients tested positive for binding antibodies against ipilimumab in an electrochemiluminescent (ECL)–based assay. This assay has substantial limitations in detecting anti-ipilimumab antibodies in the presence of ipilimumab. Infusion-related or peri-infusional reactions consistent with hypersensitivity or anaphylaxis were not reported in these 11 patients, nor were neutralizing antibodies against ipilimumab detected. Because trough levels of ipilimumab interfere with the ECL assay results, a subset analysis was performed in the dose cohort with the lowest trough levels. In this analysis, 6.9% of 58 evaluable patients treated with 0.3 mg/kg dose tested positive for binding antibodies against ipilimumab.

Pharmacologic & Dosing Characteristics

Dosage: 3 mg/kg given IV over 90 minutes every 3 weeks for a total of 4 doses. Withhold the scheduled dose of ipilimumab for any moderate immune-mediated adverse reactions or for symptomatic endocrinopathy. For patients with complete or partial resolution of adverse reactions (grade 0 to 1) who are receiving less than 7.5 mg of prednisone or equivalent per day, resume ipilimumab at 3 mg/kg every 3 weeks until administration of all 4 planned doses or 16 weeks from first dose, whichever occurs earlier. Permanently discontinue ipilimumab for any of the following:

- Persistent moderate adverse reactions or inability to reduce corticosteroid dose to prednisone 7.5 mg or equivalent per day.
- Failure to complete full treatment course within 16 weeks from administration of first dose.
- Severe or life-threatening adverse reactions, including any of the following:
  - Colitis with abdominal pain, fever, ileus, or peritoneal signs; increase in stool frequency (7 or more over baseline), stool incontinence; need for IV hydration for longer than 24 hours; GI hemorrhage; and GI perforation
  - AST or ALT over 5 times the upper limit of normal (ULN) or total bilirubin over 3 times the ULN
  - Stevens-Johnson syndrome, TEN, or rash complicated by full-thickness dermal ulceration, or necrotic, bullous, or hemorrhagic manifestations
  - Severe motor or sensory neuropathy, Guillain-Barré syndrome, or myasthenia gravis
  - Severe immune-mediated reactions involving any organ system (eg, nephritis, pneumonitis, pancreatitis, non-infectious myocarditis)
  - Immune-mediated ocular disease that is unresponsive to topical immunosuppressive therapy

Route: IV infusion

Overdosage: There is no information on overdosage with ipilimumab.

Ipilimumab

Efficacy: The safety and efficacy of ipilimumab were investigated in a randomized (3:1:1), double-blind, double-dummy study (study 1) that included 676 randomized patients with unresectable or metastatic melanoma previously treated with 1 or more of the following: aldesleukin, dacarbazine, temozolomide, fotemustine, or carboplatin. Of these 676 patients, 403 were randomized to receive ipilimumab at 3 mg/kg in combination with an investigational peptide vaccine with incomplete Freund adjuvant (gp100), 137 were randomized to receive ipilimumab at 3 mg/kg, and 136 were randomized to receive gp100 alone. The study enrolled only patients with HLA-A2*0201 genotype; this HLA genotype facilitates the immune presentation of the investigational peptide vaccine. The study excluded patients with active autoimmune disease or those receiving systemic immunosuppression for organ transplantation. Ipilimumab/placebo was administered at 3 mg/kg as an IV infusion every 3 weeks for 4 doses. Gp100/placebo was administered at a dose of 2 mg peptide by deep subcutaneous injection every 3 weeks for 4 doses. Assessment of tumor response was conducted at weeks 12 and 24, and every 3 months thereafter. Patients with evidence of objective tumor response at 12 or 24 weeks had assessment for confirmation of durability of response at 16 or 28 weeks, respectively. The major efficacy outcome measure was overall survival (OS) in the ipilimumab+gp100 arm compared with that in the gp100 arm. Secondary efficacy outcome measures were OS in the ipilimumab+gp100 arm compared with that in the ipilimumab arm, OS in the ipilimumab arm compared with that in the gp100 arm, best overall response rates (BORR) at week 24 among each of the study arms, and duration of responses. Of the randomized patients, 61%, 59%, and 54% in the ipilimumab+gp100, ipilimumab, and gp100 arms, respectively, were men. Twenty-nine percent were 65 years or older; the median age was 57 years; 71% had M1c stage; 12% had a history of previously treated brain metastasis; 98% had Eastern Cooperative Oncology Group performance status of 0 and 1; 23% had received aldesleukin; and 38% had elevated lactate dehydrogenase (LDH) levels. Sixty-one percent of patients randomized to either ipilimumab-containing arms received all 4 planned doses. The median duration of follow-up was 8.9 months. The OS results are shown below.

Ipilimumab Overall Survival Results			
	Ipilimumab (n = 137)	Ipilimumab + gp100 (n = 403)	gp100 (n = 136)
Hazard ratio (vs. gp100) (95% CI[a])	0.66 (0.51, 0.87)	0.68 (0.55, 0.85)	
P value	P = 0.0026	P = 0.0004	
Hazard ratio (vs. ipilimumab) (95% CI)		1.04 (0.83, 1.3)	
Median (months) (95% CI)	10 (8, 13.8)	10 (8.5, 11.5)	6 (5.5, 8.7)

a CI = confidence interval.

The BORR, as assessed by the investigator, was 5.7% (95% CI, 3.7%-8.4%) in the ipilimumab+gp100 arm, 10.9% (95% CI, 6.3%-17.4%) in the ipilimumab arm, and 1.5% (95% CI, 0.2%-5.2%) in the gp100 arm. The median duration of response was 11.5 months in the ipilimumab+gp100 arm and was not reached in the ipilimumab or gp100 arm.

Onset: Within approximately 4 to 8 months

Duration: Not established

Pharmacokinetics: The pharmacokinetics of ipilimumab were studied in 499 patients with unresectable or metastatic melanoma who received doses of 0.3, 3, or 10 mg/kg administered once every 3 weeks for 4 doses. Peak concentration (C_{max}), trough concentration (C_{min}), and AUC of ipilimumab were found to be dose-proportional within the dose range examined. Upon repeated dosing of ipilimumab administered every 3 weeks, ipilimumab clearance (Cl) was time-invariant. Minimal systemic accumulation was observed as evident by an accumulation index of 1.5-fold or less. Ipilimumab steady-state concentration was reached by the third dose. The following mean (percent coefficient of variation) parameters were generated through population pharmacokinetic analysis: terminal half-life of 14.7 days (30.1%);

systemic Cl of 15.3 mL/h (38.5%); and volume of distribution at steady-state (V_{ss}) of 7.21 L (10.5%). The mean ($\pm$ standard deviation [SD]) ipilimumab C_{min} achieved at steady-state with the 3-mg/kg regimen was 21.8 mcg/mL (± 11.2).

Specific populations: Cross-study analyses were performed on data from patients with a variety of conditions, including 420 patients with melanoma who received single or multiple infusions of ipilimumab at doses of 0.3, 3, or 10 mg/kg. The effects of various covariates on ipilimumab pharmacokinetics were assessed in population pharmacokinetic analyses. Ipilimumab Cl increased with increasing body weight; however, no dose adjustment of ipilimumab is required for body weight after administration on a mg/kg basis. The following factors had no clinically significant effect on the Cl of ipilimumab: age (range, 26 to 86 years), gender, concomitant use of budesonide, performance status, HLA-A2*0201 status, positive anti-ipilimumab antibody status, prior use of systemic anticancer therapy, or baseline LDH levels. The effect of race was not examined because there were insufficient numbers of patients in nonwhite ethnic groups.

Renal impairment: Creatinine clearance (CrCl) at baseline did not have a clinically important effect on ipilimumab pharmacokinetics in patients with calculated CrCl values 29 mL/min or more.

Hepatic impairment: Baseline AST, total bilirubin, and ALT levels did not have a clinically important effect on ipilimumab pharmacokinetics in patients with various degrees of hepatic impairment.

Mechanism: CTLA-4 is a negative regulator of T-cell activation. Ipilimumab binds to CTLA-4 and blocks the interaction of CTLA-4 with its ligands, CD80/CD86. Blockade of CTLA-4 augments T-cell activation and proliferation. Ipilimumab's effect in patients with melanoma is indirect, possibly through T-cell–mediated antitumor immune responses.

Drug Interactions: No formal drug-drug interaction studies have been conducted with ipilimumab.

Pharmaceutical Characteristics

Concentration: 5 mg per mL

Packaging: One single-use 50 mg/10 mL vial (NDC #: 00003-2327-11). One single-use 200 mg/40 mL vial (00003-2328-22)

Doseform: Solution

Appearance: Clear to slightly opalescent, colorless to pale yellow solution. May contain a small amount of visible translucent to white, amorphous ipilimumab particulates.

Solvent: Sterile water

Diluent:

For infusion: Allow vials to stand at room temperature for approximately 5 minutes before preparing infusion. Withdraw the required volume of ipilimumab and transfer into an IV bag. Dilute with sodium chloride 0.9% injection or dextrose 5% injection to prepare a diluted solution with a final concentration ranging from 1 to 2 mg/mL. Mix diluted solution by gentle inversion. Store the diluted solution for 24 hours or less under refrigeration (2° to 8°C, 36° to 46°F) or at room temperature (20° to 25°C, 68° to 77°F). Discard partially used vials of ipilimumab.

Adjuvant: None

Preservative: None

Allergens: None

Excipients: Diethylene triamine pentaacetic acid (DTPA) (0.04 mg/mL), mannitol (10 mg/mL), polysorbate 80 (vegetable origin) (0.1 mg/mL), sodium chloride (5.85 mg/mL), tris hydrochloride (3.15 mg/mL)

Ipilimumab

pH: 7

Shelf Life: Data not provided.

Storage/Stability: Store between 2° and 8°C (36° and 46°F). Protect vials from light. Do not freeze. Contact the manufacturer regarding exposure to freezing or elevated temperatures. Shipping data not provided.

Handling: Do not shake product. Discard vial if solution is cloudy, there is pronounced discoloration (solution may have pale yellow color), or there is foreign particulate matter other than translucent to white, amorphous particles.

Administer diluted solution over 90 minutes through an IV line containing a sterile, nonpyrogenic, low-protein–binding in-line filter. Do not mix ipilimumab with, or administer as an infusion with, other medicinal products. Flush the IV line with sodium chloride 0.9% or dextrose 5% after each dose.

Media: Chinese hamster ovary cell culture

Other Information

First Licensed: March 25, 2011

References: Weber J, Thompson JA, Hamid O, et al. A randomized, double-blind, placebo-controlled, phase II study comparing the tolerability and efficacy of ipilimumab administered with or without prophylactic budesonide in patients with unresectable stage III or IV melanoma. *Clin Cancer Res.* 2009;15(17):5591-5598.

Isoantibodies

Name:
   Tysabri

Manufacturer:
   Biogen Idec

Synonyms: Antegren (an early brand name), AN 100226

Immunologic Characteristics

Target Antigen: α_4-integrin. Integrins are receptor proteins involved in cell-cell and other cellular interactions.

Viability: Inactive, passive, transient

Antigenic Form: Humanized immunoglobulin produced in murine myeloma cells. Contains human framework regions and the complementarity-determining regions of a murine antibody that binds to α_4-integrin.

Antigenic Type: Protein, IgG4κ antibody, monoclonal. Molecular weight approximately 149 kilodaltons.

Use Characteristics

Indications:

Multiple sclerosis: As monotherapy for treating patients with relapsing forms of multiple sclerosis (MS), to delay the accumulation of physical disability and reduce the frequency of clinical exacerbations.

Natalizumab is generally recommended for patients who have had an inadequate response to or are unable to tolerate alternative MS therapies.

Crohn disease: For inducing and maintaining clinical response and remission in adult patients with moderately to severely active Crohn disease with evidence of inflammation who have had an inadequate response to or are unable to tolerate conventional Crohn disease therapies and inhibitors of TNF-α.

Unlabeled Uses: Research in progress is assessing the role of natalizumab in the treatment of Crohn disease and ulcerative colitis.

Limitations: Because natalizumab increases the risk of progressive multifocal leukoencephalopathy (PML), an opportunistic viral infection of the brain that usually leads to death or severe disability, natalizumab is generally recommended for patients who have had an inadequate response to, or are unable to tolerate, alternative MS therapies.

The safety and efficacy of natalizumab beyond 2 years are unknown. Safety and efficacy in patients with chronic progressive MS have not been established.

In Crohn disease, do not use natalizumab in combination with immunosuppressants or inhibitors of TNF-α.

Contraindications:

Absolute: Do not treat patients who have or have had PML. Do not re-treat patients who experienced hypersensitivity reactions with natalizumab.

Relative: People with known hypersensitivity to natalizumab or any of its components.

Immunodeficiency: No impairment of effect expected, but safety concerns apply. PML, an opportunistic infection of the brain caused by the JC virus that typically occurs in patients who are immunocompromised, occurred in 3 patients who received natalizumab in clinical trials, and several dozen additional patients since then. Cases of PML have been reported in patients taking natalizumab who were recently or concomitantly treated with immunomodulators or immunosuppressants, as well as in patients receiving natalizumab as monotherapy. Ordinarily, patients receiving chronic immunosuppressant or immunomodulatory therapy or who have systemic medical conditions resulting in significantly compromised immune system function should not be treated with natalizumab.

Elderly: Clinical studies of natalizumab did not include sufficient numbers of patients 65 years of age and older to determine whether they respond differently than younger patients.

Carcinogenicity: No clastogenic effects of natalizumab were observed in the Ames or human chromosomal aberration assays. Xenograft transplantation models in severe combined immunodeficient (SCID) and nude mice with two α_4-integrin-positive tumor lines (ie, leukemia, melanoma) demonstrated no increase in tumor growth rates or metastasis resulting from natalizumab treatment.

Mutagenicity: No mutagenic effects of natalizumab were observed in the Ames or human chromosomal aberration assays. Natalizumab showed no effects on in vitro assays of α_4-integrin-positive tumor line proliferation or cytotoxicity.

Fertility Impairment: Reductions in female guinea pig fertility were observed at dose levels of 30 mg/kg, but not at 10 mg/kg (2.3-fold the clinical dose). A 47% reduction in pregnancy rate was observed in guinea pigs receiving 30 mg/kg compared with controls. Implantations were seen in only 36% of animals having corpora lutea in the 30 mg/kg group vs 66% to 72% in the other groups. Natalizumab did not affect male fertility at doses up to 7-fold the clinical dose.

Pregnancy: Category C. In reproductive studies in monkeys and guinea pigs, there was no evidence of teratogenic effects at doses up to 30 mg/kg (7 times the human clinical dose based on body weight). When female guinea pigs were exposed to natalizumab during the second half of pregnancy, a small reduction in pup survival was noted at postnatal day 14 with respect to control (3 pups/litter for the natalizumab group, 4.3 pups/litter for the control group). In 1 of 5 studies that exposed monkeys or guinea pigs during pregnancy, the number of abortions in treated monkeys was 33% vs 17% in controls. No effects on abortion rates were noted in any other study. Natalizumab underwent transplacental transfer and produced in utero exposure in developing guinea pigs and cynomolgus monkeys. When pregnant dams were exposed to natalizumab at approximately 7-fold the clinical dose, serum levels in fetal animals at delivery were approximately 35% of maternal serum natalizumab levels. A study in pregnant cynomolgus monkeys treated at 2.3-fold the clinical dose demonstrated natalizumab-related changes in the fetus. These changes included mild anemia, reduced platelet count, increased spleen weights, and reduced liver and thymus weights associated with increased splenic extramedullary hematopoiesis, thymic atrophy, and decreased hepatic hematopoiesis. In offspring born to mothers treated with natalizumab at 7-fold the clinical dose, platelet counts were also reduced. This effect was reversed upon clearance of natalizumab. There was no evidence of anemia in these offspring. There are no adequate and well-controlled studies of natalizumab therapy in pregnant women. Because animal reproduction studies are not always predictive of human response, use natalizumab during pregnancy only if clearly needed. Consider discontinuing natalizumab in a woman who becomes pregnant. Generally, most IgG passage across the placenta occurs during the third trimester.

Lactation: It is not known if natalizumab crosses into human breast milk. Because many drugs and immunoglobulins are excreted in human milk, and because the potential for serious adverse reactions is unknown, decide whether to discontinue nursing or natalizumab, taking into account the importance of therapy to the mother.

Children: Safety and efficacy of natalizumab in children with MS younger than 18 years of age have not been established.

Adverse Reactions:

Leukoencephalopathy: Progressive multifocal leukoencephalopathy (PML), an opportunistic infection caused by the JC virus that typically only occurs in patients who are immunocompromised, developed in 3 patients who received natalizumab in clinical trials. Two cases of PML were observed among 1,869 patients with MS treated for a median of 120 weeks. The third case occurred among 1,043 patients with Crohn disease after the patient received 8 doses. Both MS patients were receiving concomitant immunomodulatory therapy, and the patient with Crohn disease had been treated in the past with immunosuppressive therapy. In the postmarketing setting, additional cases of PML have been reported in patients with MS who were receiving no concomitant immunomodulatory therapy. The absolute risk for PML in patients treated with natalizumab cannot be precisely estimated. There are no known interventions that can reliably prevent PML or adequately treat PML if it occurs. It is not known whether early detection of PML and discontinuation of natalizumab will mitigate the disease. In patients treated with natalizumab, the risk of developing PML increases with longer treatment duration. The estimated incidence of PML since licensing based on duration of therapy is as follows: up to 24 infusions, 0.3 cases per 1,000 patients; 25 to 36 infusions, 1.5 cases per 1,000 patients; 37 to 48 infusions, 0.9 cases per 1,000 patients. There is limited experience beyond 4 years of treatment. The risk of PML is also increased in patients who have been treated with an immunosuppressant before receiving natalizumab; this increased risk appears to be independent of natalizumab treatment duration. Ordinarily, patients receiving chronic immunosuppressant or immunomodulatory therapy or who have systemic medical conditions resulting in significantly compromised immune system function should not be treated with natalizumab. The incidence of PML appears to be lower in patients receiving natalizumab as monotherapy; however, the number of cases is too few and the number of patients treated too small to reliably conclude that the true risk of PML is lower in patients treated with natalizumab alone than in patients who are receiving other drugs that decrease immune function or who are otherwise immunocompromised.

Because of the risk of PML, natalizumab is available only under a special restricted distribution program, the TOUCH Prescribing Program. In patients with MS, obtain a magnetic resonance imaging (MRI) scan before starting therapy with natalizumab. This scan may be helpful in differentiating subsequent MS symptoms from those of PML. In patients with Crohn disease, a baseline brain MRI may also be helpful to distinguish preexistent lesions from newly developed lesions, but brain lesions at baseline that could cause diagnostic difficulty while on natalizumab therapy are uncommon. Monitor patients on natalizumab for any new sign or symptom suggestive of PML. For diagnosis, an evaluation, including a gadolinium-enhanced MRI scan of the brain and, when indicated, CSF analysis for JC viral DNA, are recommended. Typical symptoms associated with PML are diverse, progress over days to weeks, and include progressive weakness on one side of the body or clumsiness of limbs, disturbance of vision, and changes in thinking, memory, and orientation leading to confusion and personality changes. The progression of deficits usually leads to death or severe disability over weeks or months.

Withhold natalizumab dosing immediately at the first sign or symptom suggestive of PML. Three sessions of plasma exchange over 5 to 8 days were shown to accelerate natalizumab clearance in a study of 12 patients, although in the majority of patients, alpha-4 integrin receptor binding remained high. Adverse events that may occur during plasma exchange include clearance of other medications and volume shifts, which have the potential to lead to hypotension or pulmonary edema. There is no evidence that plasma exchange has any benefit in the treatment of opportunistic infections such as PML.

During study 1, the most frequently reported serious adverse reactions with natalizumab were infections (3.2% vs 2.6% in placebo), acute hypersensitivity reactions (1.1%, including anaphylaxis or anaphylactoid reaction [0.8%]), depression (1%, including suicidal ideation [0.6%]), and cholelithiasis (1%).

The most frequently reported adverse reactions resulting in clinical intervention (ie, discontinuation of natalizumab) were urticaria and other hypersensitivity reactions (1%).

The following table lists adverse events and selected laboratory abnormalities occurring at an incidence of 1% or higher in natalizumab-treated patients than in the placebo control group during study 1. The adverse event profile in study 2 was similar.

Adverse Events in Study 1		
Adverse events	Natalizumab (n = 627)	Control (n = 312)
General		
Headache	38%	33%
Fatigue	27%	21%
Arthralgia	19%	14%
Chest discomfort	5%	3%
Acute hypersensitivity reaction	4%	< 1%
Other hypersensitivity reaction	5%	2%
Seasonal allergy	3%	2%
Rigors	3%	< 1%
Weight increased	2%	< 1%
Weight decreased	2%	< 1%
Infection		
Urinary tract infection	21%	17%
Lower respiratory tract infection	17%	16%
Gastroenteritis	11%	9%
Vaginitis[a]	10%	6%
Tooth infections	9%	7%
Herpes	8%	7%
Tonsillitis	7%	5%
Psychiatric		
Depression	19%	16%
Musculoskeletal/Connective tissue disorders		
Pain in extremity	16%	14%
Muscle cramp	5%	3%
Joint swelling	2%	1%
Gastrointestinal		
Abdominal discomfort	11%	10%
Diarrhea	10%	9%
Abnormal liver function test	5%	4%
Skin		
Rash	12%	9%
Dermatitis	7%	4%
Pruritus	4%	2%
Night sweats	1%	0%

Adverse Events in Study 1		
Adverse events	Natalizumab (n = 627)	Control (n = 312)
Menstrual disorders[a]		
Irregular menstruation	5%	4%
Dysmenorrhea	3%	< 1%
Amenorrhea	2%	1%
Ovarian cyst	2%	< 1%
Neurologic		
Somnolence	2%	< 1%
Vertigo	6%	5%
Renal and urinary disorders		
Urinary incontinence	4%	3%
Urinary urgency/frequency	9%	7%
Injury		
Limb injury	3%	2%
Skin laceration	2%	< 1%
Thermal burn	1%	< 1%

a Percentage among females.

Consult manufacturer's prescribing information for most recent clinical management information.

Immunosuppression: Concomitant treatment of relapses with a short course of corticosteroids was not associated with an increased rate of infection. The safety and efficacy of natalizumab with other immunosuppressive agents have not been evaluated. Do not give patients receiving these agents concurrent therapy with natalizumab because of the possibility of an increased risk of infections.

Infections: The rate of infection was approximately 1.5 per patient-year in both natalizumab-treated patients and placebo recipients. The infections were predominately upper respiratory tract infections, influenza, and urinary tract infections. Most patients did not interrupt treatment with natalizumab during the infection. In study 1, the incidence of serious infection was 3.2% for natalizumab vs 2.6% for placebo. Rates of urinary tract infections (0.8% vs 0.3%) and pneumonia (0.6% vs 0%) were higher in the natalizumab group compared with the placebo group. In study 2, appendicitis was more common in the natalizumab group (0.8% vs 0.2%).

A cryptosporidial gastroenteritis with a prolonged course occurred in one patient. In clinical studies for indications other than MS, opportunistic infections (eg, *Pneumocystis jiroveci* pneumonia, pulmonary *Mycobacterium avium intracellulare*, bronchopulmonary aspergillosis, *Burkholderia cepacia*) have occurred uncommonly in natalizumab-treated patients, some of whom were receiving concurrent immunosuppressants. Two serious nonbacterial meningitides occurred in natalizumab-treated patients (but none in placebo-treated patients). In postmarketing experience, one natalizumab-treated patient developed herpes encephalitis and died; a second patient developed herpes meningitis and recovered after appropriate treatment.

Infusion reactions: An infusion-related reaction included any adverse event within 2 hours of starting an infusion. Approximately 24% of natalizumab patients experienced an infusion-related reaction, compared with 18% of placebo recipients. Events more common in natalizumab patients included headache, dizziness, fatigue, hypersensitivity reactions, urticaria, pruritus, and rigors. Acute urticaria occurred in approximately 2% of patients. Other hypersensitivity reactions occurred in 1% of patients receiving natalizumab.

Serious systemic hypersensitivity infusion reactions occurred in less than 1% of patients. All patients recovered with treatment and/or discontinuation of the infusion. Patients who became persistently positive for antibodies to natalizumab were more likely to have an infusion-related reaction than those who were antibody negative.

Immunogenicity: Patients in study 1 and study 2 were tested for antibodies to natalizumab every 12 weeks. The assays used were unable to detect low to moderate levels of antibodies to natalizumab. Antibodies were detected in approximately 9% of MS patients receiving natalizumab at least once during treatment, with persistent antibody positivity in 6% of patients. Approximately 82% of patients who became persistently antibody-positive by this assay had developed detectable antibodies by 12 weeks. Antinatalizumab antibodies were neutralizing in vitro. The presence of antinatalizumab antibodies correlated with a reduction in serum natalizumab levels. Across studies, the week-12 preinfusion mean natalizumab serum concentrations in antibody-negative patients were 14.9 mcg/mL, compared with 1.3 mcg/mL in antibody-positive patients. Persistent antibody-positivity to natalizumab was associated with a substantial decrease in the effectiveness of natalizumab, based on increased disability and annualized relapse rates. Adverse events more common in patients with persistent antibody-positivity included infusion-related reactions, myalgia, hypertension, dyspnea, anxiety, and tachycardia. If the presence of persistent antibodies is suspected, perform an antibody test. Antibodies may be detected and confirmed with sequential serum antibody tests. Antibodies detected early in treatment (eg, within the first 6 months) may be transient and disappear with continued dosing. Repeat testing 3 months after the initial positive result helps assess persistence of these antibodies. Consider the overall benefits and risks of natalizumab in a patient with persistent antibodies. The long-term immunogenicity of natalizumab and the effects of low to moderate levels of antibody to natalizumab are unknown.

Hepatic: Clinically significant liver injury was reported after natalizumab was marketed. Signs of liver injury, including markedly elevated serum hepatic enzymes and elevated total bilirubin, occurred as early as 6 days after the first dose. Signs of liver injury also were first reported after multiple doses. In some patients, liver injury recurred upon rechallenge, providing evidence that natalizumab caused the injury. The combination of transaminase elevations and elevated bilirubin without evidence of obstruction is generally recognized as an important predictor of severe liver injury that may lead to death or the need for a liver transplant in some patients. Discontinue natalizumab in patients with jaundice or other evidence of significant liver injury (eg, laboratory evidence).

Hypersensitivity: Natalizumab has been associated with hypersensitivity reactions, including serious systemic reactions (eg, anaphylaxis) at an incidence of less than 1%. These reactions usually occur within 2 hours of starting infusion. Associated symptoms can include chest pain, dizziness, dyspnea, fever, flushing, hypotension, nausea, pruritus, rash, rigors, and urticaria. Generally, these reactions are associated with antibodies to natalizumab. If a hypersensitivity reaction occurs, discontinue administration of natalizumab and initiate appropriate therapy.

Pharmacologic & Dosing Characteristics

Dosage: 300 mg IV infusion every 4 weeks.

If a patient with Crohn disease has not experienced therapeutic benefit by 12 weeks of induction therapy, discontinue natalizumab. For patients with Crohn disease who start natalizumab while taking chronic oral corticosteroids, begin tapering the steroid dose as soon as a therapeutic benefit of natalizumab has occurred. If the patient cannot be tapered off of oral corticosteroids within 6 months of starting natalizumab, discontinue natalizumab. Other than the initial 6-month taper, consider discontinuing natalizumab in patients who require additional steroid use that exceeds 3 months in a calendar year to control their Crohn disease.

Route: IV infusion. Do not administer natalizumab as an IV push or bolus injection. Dilute natalizumab concentrate 300 mg/15 mL in 100 mL 0.9% sodium chloride injection, and infuse over approximately 1 hour. After the infusion is complete, flush the line with 0.9% sodium chloride. Observe patients during the infusion and for 1 hour after the infusion is complete. Promptly discontinue the infusion upon the first observation of any signs or symptoms consistent with a hypersensitivity-type reaction.

Overdosage: Safety of doses higher than 300 mg has not been adequately evaluated. The maximum amount of natalizumab that can be safely administered has not been determined.

Related Interventions: Obtain an MRI scan before beginning natalizumab therapy to help differentiate active or progressing MS from PML. Monitor patients receiving natalizumab for any new sign or symptom suggestive of PML. Withhold natalizumab immediately at the first sign or symptom suggestive of PML. For diagnosis, an evaluation that includes a gadolinium-enhanced MRI scan of the brain and, when indicated, CSF analysis for JC viral DNA are recommended. The patient should be evaluated 3 and 6 months after the first infusion and every 6 months thereafter.

Laboratory Tests: Natalizumab increases circulating lymphocytes, monocytes, eosinophils, basophils, and nucleated red blood cells. These increases persist during natalizumab exposure, but are reversible, returning to baseline levels usually within 16 weeks of the last dose. Elevations of neutrophils have not been observed. Natalizumab induces mild decreases in hemoglobin levels that are frequently transient.

Efficacy: Natalizumab was evaluated in 2 randomized, double-blind, placebo-controlled trials in patients with MS. Both studies enrolled patients who had experienced 1 or more clinical relapses during the prior year and had Kurtzke Expanded Disability Status Scale (EDSS) scores between 0 and 5. In both studies, neurological evaluations were performed every 12 weeks and at times of suspected relapse. MRI evaluations for T1-weighted gadolinium (Gd)-enhancing lesions and T2-hyperintense lesions were performed annually.

Study 1 enrolled patients who had not received any interferon-beta or glatiramer acetate for at least 6 months; approximately 94% had never been treated with these agents. Median age was 37 years, with a median disease duration of 5 years. Patients were randomized to receive natalizumab 300 mg IV infusion (n = 627) or placebo (n = 315) every 4 weeks for up to 28 months.

Study 2 enrolled patients who had experienced 1 or more relapses while being treated with interferon beta-1a 30 mcg IM once weekly during the prior year. Median age was 39 years, with a median disease duration of 7 years. Patients were randomized to receive natalizumab 300 mg (n = 589) or placebo (n = 582) every 4 weeks for up to 28 months. All patients continued to receive interferon beta-1a 30 mcg IM once weekly.

Study results appear below. The primary end point after 2 years was time to onset of sustained increase in disability, defined as an increase of 1 point or more on the EDSS from baseline EDSS of 1 point or more that was sustained for 12 weeks, or at least a 1.5 point increase on the EDSS from baseline EDSS equal to 0 that was sustained for 12 weeks. Time to onset of sustained increase in disability was longer in natalizumab-treated patients than in the placebo group in both studies 1 and 2. The proportion of patients with increased disability and the annualized relapse rate were also lower in natalizumab-treated patients in both studies. Changes in MRI findings often do not correlate with changes in the clinical status of disabled patients (eg, disability progression). The prognostic significance of the MRI findings in these studies has not been evaluated.

Natalizumab (Humanized)

Study 1 (Monotherapy) Results: Clinical and MRI End Points at 2 Years[a]		
	Natalizumab (n = 627)	Placebo (n = 315)
Clinical end points		
Percentage with sustained increase in disability	17%	29%
Relative risk reduction	42% (95% CI; 23%, 57%)	
Annualized relapse rate	0.22	0.67
Relative reduction	67%	
Percentage of patients remaining relapse free	67%	41%
MRI end points		
New or newly enlarging T2–hyperintense lesions		
Median	0	5
Percentage of patients with:		
0 lesions	57%	15%
1 lesion	17%	10%
2 lesions	8%	8%
3 or more lesions	18%	68%
Gd-enhancing lesions		
Median	0	0
Percentage of patients with:		
0 lesions	97%	72%
1 lesion	2%	12%
2 or more lesions	1%	16%

a All analyses based on intent to treat. For each end point, $P < 0.001$.

Study 2 (Add-On Study) Results: Clinical and MRI End Points at 2 Years[a]		
	Natalizumab plus *Avonex* (n = 589)	Placebo plus *Avonex* (n = 582)
Clinical end points		
Percentage with sustained increase in disability	23%	29%
Relative risk reduction	24% (95% CI; 4%, 39%)	
Annualized relapse rate	0.33	0.75
Relative reduction	56%	
Percentage of patients remaining relapse free	54%	32%
MRI end points		
New or newly enlarging T2–hyperintense lesions		
Median	0	3
Percentage of patients with:		
0 lesions	67%	30%
1 lesion	13%	9%
2 lesions	7%	10%
3 or more lesions	14%	50%
Gd-enhancing lesions		
Median	0	0
Percentage of patients with:		
0 lesions	96%	75%
1 lesion	2%	12%
2 or more lesions	1%	14%

a All analyses based on intent to treat. For each end point, $P < 0.001$.

Onset: Not described.

Duration: Not determined.

Pharmacokinetics: After repeated IV administration of 300 mg doses to MS patients, the mean maximum serum concentration was 110 ± 52 mcg/mL. Mean average steady-state concentrations over the dosing period were 23 to 29 mcg/mL. The observed time to steady state was approximately 24 weeks after every 4 weeks of dosing. The mean half-life was 11 ± 4 days with a clearance of 16 ± 5 mL/h. The distribution volume of 5.7 ± 1.9 L was consistent with plasma volume. Pharmacokinetics of natalizumab in pediatric MS patients or patients with renal or hepatic insufficiency have not been studied.

The effects of covariates, such as body mass, age, gender, and presence of anti-natalizumab antibodies on natalizumab pharmacokinetics were investigated. Natalizumab clearance increased with body mass in a less-than-proportional manner, with a 43% increase in body mass resulting in a 32% increase in clearance. The presence of persistent anti-natalizumab antibodies increased natalizumab clearance approximately 3-fold. Age (18 to 62 years) and gender did not influence natalizumab pharmacokinetics.

Natalizumab administration increases the number of circulating leukocytes, (including lymphocytes, monocytes, basophils, and eosinophils) due to inhibition of transmigration out of the vascular space. Natalizumab does not affect the number of circulating neutrophils.

Mechanism: Natalizumab binds to the α_4-subunit of $\alpha_4\beta_1$ and $\alpha_4\beta_7$ integrins expressed on the surface of all leukocytes except neutrophils. Natalizumab inhibits the α_4-mediated adhesion of leukocytes to their counter-receptor(s). The receptors for the α_4 family of integrins include vascular cell adhesion molecule-1 (VCAM-1), which is expressed on activated vascular endothelium, and mucosal addressin cell adhesion molecule-1 (MadCAM-1) present on vascular endothelial cells of the GI tract. Disruption of these molecular interactions prevents transmigration of leukocytes across the endothelium into inflamed parenchymal tissue. In vitro, anti-α_4-integrin antibodies also block α_4-mediated cell binding to ligands such as osteopontin and an alternatively spliced domain of fibronectin, connecting segment-1 (CS-1). In vivo, natalizumab may further act to inhibit the interaction of α_4-expressing leukocytes with their ligand(s) in the extracellular matrix and on parenchymal cells, thereby inhibiting further recruitment and inflammatory activity of activated immune cells.

The specific mechanism(s) by which natalizumab exerts its effects in MS have not been fully defined. In MS, lesions are believed to occur when activated inflammatory cells, including T-lymphocytes, cross the blood-brain barrier (BBB). Leukocyte migration across the BBB involves interaction between adhesion molecules on inflammatory cells and their counter-receptors present on endothelial cells of the vessel wall. The clinical effect of natalizumab in MS may be secondary to blockade of the molecular interaction of $\alpha_4\beta_1$-integrin expressed by inflammatory cells with VCAM-1 on vascular endothelial cells, and with CS-1 and/or osteopontin expressed by parenchymal cells in the brain. Data from an experimental autoimmune encephalitis animal model of MS demonstrate reduction of leukocyte migration into brain parenchyma and reduction of plaque formation detected by MRI after repeated administration of natalizumab. The clinical significance of these animal data is unknown.

Drug Interactions: Concurrent use of antineoplastic, immunosuppressant, or immunomodulating agents may further increase the risk of infections, including PML and other opportunistic infections, over risk observed with natalizumab alone. All 3 cases of PML during clinical trials occurred in patients concomitantly exposed to immunomodulators (interferon-beta in patients with MS) or were immunocompromised due to recent treatment with immunosuppressants (eg, azathioprine). Ordinarily, patients receiving chronic immunosuppressant or immunomodulatory therapy or who have systemic medical conditions resulting in significantly compromised immune function should not receive natalizumab.

713

Natalizumab (Humanized)

Concurrent use of short courses of corticosteroids was associated with an increase in infections in studies 1 and 2. However, the increase in infections in natalizumab-treated patients who received steroids was similar to the increase in placebo-treated patients who received steroids.

After multiple dosing, interferon beta-1a 30 mcg IM weekly reduced natalizumab clearance by approximately 30% The similarity of the natalizumab-associated adverse event profile with or without coadministered interferon beta-1a indicates that this alteration in clearance does not require reduction of the natalizumab dose to maintain safety. Results of studies in MS patients taking natalizumab and concomitant interferon beta-1a 30 mcg IM once weekly or glatiramer acetate were inconclusive regarding need for dose adjustment of interferon or glatiramer.

No data are available on the effects of vaccination in patients receiving natalizumab. No data are available on the secondary transmission of infection by live vaccines in patients receiving natalizumab.

Patient Information: Counsel patients fully about the risks and benefits of natalizumab. Patients should report any continually worsening symptoms that persist over several days to their physician. If symptoms consistent with a hypersensitivity reaction (eg, urticaria) occur during or after a natalizumab infusion, these should be reported to a physician immediately.

Pharmaceutical Characteristics

Concentration: 300 mg per 15 mL or 20 mg/mL

Packaging: 300 mg per 10 mL single-use vial

NDC Number: 59075-0730-15

Doseform: Solution for further dilution

Appearance: Colorless and clear to slightly opalescent solution

Solvent: Phosphate-buffered saline for injection

Diluent:
> *For infusion:* Add natalizumab concentrate 300 mg/15 mL to 100 mL 0.9% sodium chloride injection. Use no other IV diluents to prepare the natalizumab solution. Gently invert the natalizumab solution to mix completely. Do not inject other medications into infusion set side ports.

Adjuvant: None

Preservative: None

Allergens: None

Excipients: Each 15 mL dose contains sodium chloride 123 mg, sodium phosphate monobasic monohydrate 17 mg, sodium phosphate dibasic heptahydrate 7.24 mg, and 3 mg polysorbate 80.

pH: 6.1

Shelf Life: No data from manufacturer.

Storage/Stability: Store at 2° to 8°C (36° to 46°F). Protect vials from light. Discard if frozen. Contact the manufacturer regarding exposure to freezing or elevated temperatures. Shipped in insulated containers with coolant packs.

> After dilution, infuse natalizumab solution immediately, or refrigerate solution at 2° to 8°C and use within 8 hours. If stored at 2° to 8°C, allow the solution to warm to room temperature before infusion.

Handling: Use of filtration devices during administration has not been evaluated.

Media: Produced in murine myeloma cells.

Other Information

First Licensed: November 23, 2004

References: Anonymous. Natalizumab: AN 100226, anti-4α integrin monoclonal antibody. *Drugs R&D.* 2004;5:102-107.

Sanborn WJ, Colombel JF, Enns R, et al; International Efficacy of Natalizumab as Active Crohn's Therapy (ENACT-1) Trial Group; Evaluation of Natalizumab as Continuous Therapy (ENACT-2) Trial Group. Natalizumab induction and maintenance therapy for Crohn's disease. *N Engl J Med.* 2005;353:1912-1925.

Clifford DB, et al. Natalizumab-associated progressive multifocal leukoencephalopathy in patients with multiple sclerosis: Lessons from 28 cases. *Lancet Neurol.* 2010;9:438-46, erratum: 463.

Iaffaldano P, et al. Safety profile of Tysabri: International risk management plan. *Neurol Sci.* 2009;30(Suppl 2):S159-S162.

Tan CS, Koralnik IJ. Progressive multifocal leukoencephalopathy and other disorders caused by JC virus: Clinical features and pathogenesis. *Lancet Neurol.* 2010;9:425-437.

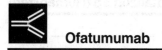 **Ofatumumab**

Isoantibodies

Name:
Arzerra
Synonyms: HuMax-CD20

Manufacturer:
GlaxoSmithKline

Immunologic Characteristics

Target Antigen: CD20 antigen

Viability: Inactive, passive, transient

Antigenic Form: Human IgG1κ monoclonal antibody

Antigenic Type: Protein, IgG1κ antibody, monoclonal, with molecular weight of approximately 149 kilodaltons

Use Characteristics

Indications: To treat patients with chronic lymphocytic leukemia (CLL) refractory to fludarabine and alemtuzumab. The effectiveness of ofatumumab is based on the demonstration of durable objective responses. No data demonstrate improvement in disease-related symptoms or increased survival with ofatumumab.

Contraindications: None

Elderly: Clinical studies of ofatumumab did not include sufficient numbers of subjects 65 years of age and older to determine whether they respond differently from younger subjects.

Carcinogenicity: Ofatumumab has not been evaluated for carcinogenic potential.

Mutagenicity: Ofatumumab has not been evaluated for mutagenic potential. In a repeat-dose toxicity study, no tumorigenic or unexpected mitogenic responses were noted in cynomolgus monkeys treated for 7 months with up to 3.5 times the human dose of ofatumumab.

Fertility Impairment: Effects on male and female fertility have not been evaluated in animal studies.

Pregnancy: Category C. There are no adequate or well-controlled studies of ofatumumab in pregnant women. Pregnant cynomolgus monkeys dosed with 0.7 or 3.5 times the human dose of ofatumumab weekly during organogenesis (gestation days 20 to 50) had no maternal toxicity or teratogenicity. Both dose levels of ofatumumab depleted circulating B cells in the dams, with signs of initial B-cell recovery 50 days after the final dose. Ofatumumab crossed the placental barrier. Following cesarean delivery at gestational day 100, fetuses from ofatumumab-treated dams exhibited decreases in mean peripheral B-cell counts (decreased to approximately 10% of control values), splenic B-cell counts (decreased to approximately 15% to 20% of control values), and spleen weight (decreased by 15% for the low-dose and by 30% for the high-dose group, compared with control values). Fetuses from treated dams exhibiting antiofatumumab antibody responses had higher B-cell counts and higher spleen weight compared with the fetuses from other treated dams, indicating partial recovery in those animals developing antiofatumumab antibodies. When compared with control animals, fetuses from treated dams in both dose groups had a 10% decrease in mean placental weight. A 15% decrease in mean thymus weight compared with the controls was also observed in fetuses from dams treated with 3.5 times the human dose of ofatumumab. The biological significance of decreased placental and thymic weight is unknown.

Ofatumumab should be used during pregnancy only if the potential benefit to the mother justifies the potential risk to the fetus. There are no human or animal data on the potential short-

716

and long-term effects of perinatal B-cell depletion in offspring following in utero exposure to ofatumumab. Ofatumumab does not bind normal human tissues other than B-lymphocytes. It is not known if binding occurs to unique embryonic or fetal tissue targets. In addition, the kinetics of B-lymphocyte recovery are unknown in offspring with B-cell depletion.

Lactation: It is not known whether ofatumumab crosses into human milk; however, human IgG is secreted in human milk. Published data suggest that neonatal and infant consumption of breast milk does not result in substantial absorption of these maternal antibodies into circulation. Because the effects of local GI and limited systemic exposure to ofatumumab are unknown, use caution when ofatumumab is administered to a breast-feeding woman.

Children: Safety and effectiveness of ofatumumab have not been established in children.

Adverse Reactions: Most common adverse reactions (10% or more) were neutropenia, pneumonia, pyrexia, cough, diarrhea, anemia, fatigue, dyspnea, rash, nausea, bronchitis, and upper respiratory tract infections.

The most common serious adverse reactions in study 1 were infections (including pneumonia and sepsis), neutropenia, and pyrexia. Infections were the most common adverse reactions leading to drug discontinuation in study 1.

The safety of ofatumumab monotherapy was evaluated in 181 patients with relapsed or refractory CLL in 2 open-label, nonrandomized, single-arm studies. In these studies, ofatumumab was administered at 2,000 mg beginning with the second dose for 11 doses (study 1, N = 154) or 3 doses (study 2, N = 27).

The data described in the following table and other sections are derived from 154 patients in study 1. All patients received 2,000 mg weekly from the second dose onward. Ninety percent of patients received at least 8 infusions of ofatumumab and 55% received all 12 infusions. The median age was 63 years (range, 41 to 86 years of age); 72% were men; 97% were white.

Incidence of All Adverse Reactions Occurring in ≥ 5% of Patients in Study 1 and in the Fludarabine- and Alemtuzumab-Refractory Subset of Study 1				
	Total population (N = 154)		Fludarabine- and alemtuzumab-refractory (n = 59)	
Adverse event	All grades	Grade ≥ 3	All grades	Grade ≥ 3
Blood and lymphatic system				
Anemia	16%	5%	17%	8%
Cardiovascular				
Hypertension	5%	0%	8%	0%
Hypotension	5%	0%	3%	0%
Tachycardia	5%	< 1%	7%	2%
GI				
Diarrhea	18%	0%	19%	0%
Nausea	11%	0%	12%	5%
Infections and infestations				
Pneumonia[a]	23%	14%	25%	15%
Upper respiratory tract infection	11%	0%	3%	0%
Bronchitis	11%	< 1%	19%	2%
Sepsis[b]	8%	8%	10%	10%
Nasopharyngitis	8%	0%	8%	0%

Incidence of All Adverse Reactions Occurring in ≥ 5% of Patients in Study 1 and in the Fludarabine- and Alemtuzumab-Refractory Subset of Study 1				
	Total population (N = 154)		Fludarabine- and alemtuzumab-refractory (n = 59)	
Adverse event	All grades	Grade ≥ 3	All grades	Grade ≥ 3
Infections and infestations (cont.)				
Herpes zoster	6%	1%	7%	2%
Sinusitis	5%	2%	3%	2%
Musculoskeletal and connective tissue				
Back pain	8%	1%	12%	2%
Muscle spasms	5%	0%	3%	0%
Nervous system				
Headache	6%	0%	7%	0%
Psychiatric				
Insomnia	7%	0%	10%	0%
Respiratory, thoracic, and mediastinal				
Cough	19%	0%	19%	0%
Dyspnea	14%	2%	19%	5%
Skin and subcutaneous tissue				
Rash^c	14%	< 1%	17%	2%
Urticaria	8%	0%	5%	0%
Hyperhidrosis	5%	0%	5%	0%
General disorders and administration-site conditions				
Pyrexia	20%	3%	25%	5%
Fatigue	15%	0%	15%	0%
Edema peripheral	9%	< 1%	8%	2%
Chills	8%	0%	10%	0%

a Pneumonia includes pneumonia, lung infection, lobar pneumonia, and bronchopneumonia.
b Sepsis includes sepsis, neutropenic sepsis, bacteremia, and septic shock.
c Includes rash, rash macular, and rash vesicular.

Infusion reactions: Ofatumumab can cause serious infusion reactions manifesting as bronchospasm, dyspnea, laryngeal edema, pulmonary edema, flushing, hypertension, hypotension, syncope, cardiac ischemia/infarction, back pain, abdominal pain, pyrexia, rash, urticaria, and angioedema. Infusion reactions occurred in 44% of patients on the day of the first infusion (300 mg), 29% on the day of the second infusion (2,000 mg), and less frequently during subsequent infusions. Institute medical management for severe infusion reactions, including angina or other signs and symptoms of myocardial ischemia. In a study of patients with moderate to severe chronic obstructive pulmonary disease, an indication for which ofatumumab is not approved, 2 of 5 patients developed grade 3 bronchospasm during infusion.

Cytopenias: Prolonged (1 week or longer) severe neutropenia and thrombocytopenia can occur with ofatumumab. Of 108 patients with healthy neutrophil counts at baseline, 45 (42%) developed grade 3 or higher neutropenia. Nineteen (18%) developed grade 4 neutropenia. Some patients experienced new-onset grade 4 neutropenia longer than 2 weeks in duration. Monitor complete blood cell counts (CBCs) and platelet counts at regular intervals during therapy, and increase the frequency of monitoring in patients who develop grade 3 or 4 cytopenias.

Progressive multifocal leukoencephalopathy: Consider progressive multifocal leukoencephalopathy (PML) in any patient with new onset of or changes in preexisting neurological signs or symptoms. If PML is suspected, discontinue ofatumumab and evaluate for PML, including consultation with a neurologist, brain magnetic resonance imaging (MRI), and lumbar puncture.

Infections: A total of 108 patients (70%) experienced bacterial, viral, or fungal infections. A total of 45 patients (29%) experienced grade 3 or higher infections, of which 19 (12%) were fatal. The proportion of fatal infections in the fludarabine- and alemtuzumab-refractory group was 17%.

Immunogenicity: Serum samples from patients with CLL in study 1 were tested by enzyme-linked immunosorbent assay (ELISA) for antiofatumumab antibodies during and after the 24-week treatment period. Results were negative in 46 patients after the eighth infusion and in 33 patients after the twelfth infusion.

Hepatitis B: Reactivation, including fulminant hepatitis and death, occurs with other monoclonal antibodies directed against CD20. Screen patients at high risk of hepatitis B virus (HBV) infection before starting ofatumumab. Closely monitor carriers of HBV for clinical and laboratory signs of active HBV infection during treatment with ofatumumab and for 6 to 12 months after last infusion of ofatumumab. Discontinue ofatumumab in patients who develop viral hepatitis or reactivation of viral hepatitis, and institute appropriate treatment. Insufficient data exist regarding the safety of ofatumumab in patients with active hepatitis.

GI: Obstruction of the small intestine can occur in patients receiving ofatumumab. Perform a diagnostic evaluation if obstruction is suspected.

Pharmacologic & Dosing Characteristics

Dosage: 12 doses administered as follows:
- 300 mg initial dose, followed 1 week later by
- 2,000 mg weekly for 7 doses, followed 4 weeks later by
- 2,000 mg every 4 weeks for 4 doses.

Route & Site: IV infusion. Do not administer as an IV push or bolus. Prepare all doses in 1,000 mL of sodium chloride 0.9%.
- Dose 1: Start infusion at 3.6 mg/h (12 mL/h).
- Dose 2: Start infusion at 24 mg/h (12 mL/h).
- Doses 3 through 12: Start infusion at 50 mg/h (25 mL/h).

In the absence of infusional toxicity, the rate of infusion may be increased every 30 minutes. Do not exceed the infusion rates in the following table.

Infusion Rates for Ofatumumab			
Interval after start of infusion (min)	Dose 1[a] (mL/h)	Dose 2[b] (mL/h)	Doses 3 to 12[b] (mL/h)
0-30	12	12	25
31-60	25	25	50
61-90	50	50	100
91-120	100	100	200
>120	200	200	400

a Dose 1 = 300 mg in 1,000 mL of sodium chloride 0.9% (0.3 mg/mL).
b Doses 2 and 3 to 12 = 2,000 mg in 1,000 mL of sodium chloride 0.9% (2 mg/mL).

Interrupt infusion for infusion reactions of any severity. For grade 4 infusion reactions, do not resume infusion. If grade 1, 2, or 3 infusion reaction resolves or remains less than or equal to grade 2, resume infusion with modifications according to initial grade of infusion reaction. For grade 1 or 2, infuse at one-half of the previous infusion rate. For grade 3, infuse at a rate of 12 mL/h. After resuming infusion, rate may be increased according to the table, based on patient tolerance.

Overdosage: No data are available regarding overdosage with ofatumumab.

Related Interventions: Premedicate patients 30 minutes to 2 hours before each dose with oral acetaminophen 1,000 mg (or equivalent), oral or IV antihistamine (cetirizine 10 mg or equivalent), and IV corticosteroid (prednisolone 100 mg or equivalent). Monitor patients closely during infusions. Interrupt infusion if reactions occur. Do not reduce corticosteroid dose for doses 1, 2, and 9. Corticosteroid may be reduced as follows: for doses 3 through 8, gradually reduce with successive infusions if a grade 3 or higher infusion reaction did not occur with the preceding dose; for doses 10 through 12, administer prednisolone 50 to 100 mg or equivalent if a grade 3 or higher infusion reaction did not occur with dose 9.

Efficacy: Study 1 was a single-group, multicenter study in 154 patients with relapsed or refractory CLL. Ofatumumab was administered by IV infusion as follows: 300 mg (week 0), 2,000 mg weekly for 7 infusions (weeks 1 through 7), and 2,000 mg every 4 weeks for 4 infusions (weeks 12 through 24). Patients with CLL refractory to fludarabine and alemtuzumab (n = 59) comprised the efficacy population. Drug refractoriness was defined as failure to achieve at least a partial response to, or disease progression within 6 months of, the last dose of fludarabine or alemtuzumab. The main efficacy outcome was durable objective tumor response rate. Objective tumor responses were determined using the 1996 National Cancer Institute Working Group (NCIWG) Guidelines for CLL.

In patients with CLL refractory to fludarabine and alemtuzumab, the median age was 64 years (range, 41 to 86 years of age), 75% were men, and 95% were white. The median number of prior therapies was 5; 93% received prior alkylating agents, 59% received prior rituximab, and all received prior fludarabine and alemtuzumab. Eighty-eight percent of patients received at least 8 infusions of ofatumumab and 54% received 12 infusions. The investigator-determined overall response rate in patients with CLL refractory to fludarabine and alemtuzumab was 42% (99% confidence interval [CI], 26% to 60%) with a median duration of response of 6.5 months (95% CI, 5.8 to 8.3). There were no complete responses. Antitumor activity was also observed in additional patients in study 1 and in a multicenter, open-label, dose-escalation study (study 2) conducted in patients with relapsed or refractory CLL.

Pharmacokinetics: In patients with CLL refractory to fludarabine and alemtuzumab, the median decrease in circulating CD19-positive B cells was 91% (n = 50) with the eighth infusion and 85% (n = 32) with the twelfth infusion. The time to recovery of lymphocytes, including CD19-positive B cells, to normal levels was not determined.

Pharmacokinetic data were obtained from 146 patients with refractory CLL who received a 300 mg initial dose followed by 7 weekly and 4 monthly infusions of 2,000 mg. The maximum concentration (C_{max}) and area under the curve ($AUC_{0-\infty}$) after the eighth infusion in study 1 were approximately 40% and 60% higher than after the fourth infusion in study 2. The mean volume of distribution at steady-state (Vss) ranged from 1.7 to 5.1 L. Ofatumumab is eliminated through both a target-independent and a B cell–mediated route. Ofatumumab exhibited dose-dependent clearance in the dose range of 100 to 2,000 mg. Because of the depletion of B cells, the clearance of ofatumumab decreased substantially after subsequent infusions, compared with the first infusion. The mean clearance between the fourth and twelfth infusions was approximately 0.01 L/h and exhibited large intersubject variability, with a coefficient of variation of 50%. The mean half-life between the fourth and twelfth infusions was approximately 14 days (range, 2.3 to 61.5 days).

Cross-study analyses were performed on data from patients with a variety of conditions, including 162 patients with CLL, who received multiple infusions of ofatumumab as a single agent at doses ranging from 100 to 2,000 mg. The effects of various covariates (eg, body size [weight, height, body surface area], age, gender, baseline creatinine clearance [CrCl]) on ofatumumab pharmacokinetics were assessed in a population pharmacokinetic analysis.

Body mass: Volume of distribution and clearance increased with body mass; however, this increase was not clinically significant. No dosage adjustment is recommended based on body mass.

Age: Age did not significantly influence ofatumumab pharmacokinetics in patients ranging from 21 to 86 years of age. No pharmacokinetic data are available in children.

Gender: Gender had a modest effect on ofatumumab pharmacokinetics (14% to 25% lower clearance and volume of distribution in women compared with men) in a cross-study population analysis (41% men; 59% women). These effects are not considered clinically important, and no dosage adjustment is recommended.

Renal Impairment: CrCl at baseline did not have a clinically important effect on ofatumumab pharmacokinetics in patients with calculated CrCl values ranging from 33 to 287 mL/min.

Mechanism: Ofatumumab binds specifically to both the small and large extracellular loops of the CD20 molecule. The CD20 molecule is expressed on normal B-lymphocytes (pre–B- to mature B-lymphocytes) and on B-cell CLL. The CD20 molecule is not shed from the cell surface and is not internalized after antibody binding. The Fab domain of ofatumumab binds to the CD20 molecule and the Fc domain mediates immune effector functions to result in B-cell lysis in vitro. Possible mechanisms of cell lysis include complement-dependent cytotoxicity and antibody-dependent, cell-mediated cytotoxicity.

Drug Interactions: No formal drug-drug interaction studies have been conducted with ofatumumab.

The safety of immunization with live viral vaccines during or after administration of ofatumumab has not been studied. Do not administer live viral vaccines to patients who recently received ofatumumab. The ability to generate an immune response to any vaccine following administration of ofatumumab has not been studied.

Patient Information: Advise patients to contact a health care provider for any of the following:

- signs and symptoms of infusion reactions, including fever, chills, rash, or breathing problems, within 24 hours of infusion
- bleeding, easy bruising, petechiae, pallor, worsening weakness, or fatigue
- signs of infection, including fever and cough
- new neurological symptoms, such as confusion, dizziness or loss of balance, difficulty talking or walking, or vision problems
- symptoms of hepatitis, including worsening fatigue or yellow discoloration of skin or eyes
- new or worsening abdominal pain or nausea
- pregnancy or breast-feeding

Advise patients of the need for periodic monitoring of CBCs and to avoid vaccination with live viral vaccines.

Pharmaceutical Characteristics

Concentration: 20 mg/mL

Packaging: 100 mg per 5 mL single-use glass vials with a latex-free rubber stopper and an aluminum overseal.

NDC Number: Carton of 3 single-use vials with 2 filters (00173-0808-02). Carton of 10 single-use vials with 2 filters (00173-0808-05).

Ofatumumab

Doseform: Solution

Appearance: Clear to opalescent, colorless solution; may contain a small amount of visible, translucent to white, amorphous ofatumumab particles

Solvent: Buffered saline

Diluent:

For infusion: 300 mg dose: Withdraw and discard 15 mL from a 1,000 mL bag of sodium chloride 0.9%. Withdraw 5 mL from each of 3 vials of ofatumumab and add to the bag. Mix diluted solution by gentle inversion.

> *2,000 mg dose:* Withdraw and discard 100 mL from a 1,000 mL bag of sodium chloride 0.9%. Withdraw 5 mL from each of 20 vials of ofatumumab and add to the bag. Mix diluted solution by gentle inversion.

Adjuvant: None

Preservative: None

Allergens: None

Excipients: Sodium citrate 8.55 mg/mL, citric acid monohydrate 0.195 mg/mL as buffering agents, sodium chloride 5.85 mg/mL as an isotonic agent

pH: 6.5

Shelf Life: Expires within 24 months.

Storage/Stability: Store vials at 2° to 8°C (36° to 46°F). Protect vials from light. Do not freeze. Contact the manufacturer regarding exposure to freezing or elevated temperatures. Shipping data not provided. Store diluted solution between 2° to 8°C (36° to 46°F).

Handling: Administer using an infusion pump, the in-line filter provided with the product, and polyvinyl chloride administration sets. Flush the IV line with sodium chloride 0.9% before and after each dose. Start infusion within 12 hours of preparation.

Production Process: Generated via transgenic mouse and hybridoma technology.

Media: Produced in a recombinant murine cell line (NS0) using standard mammalian cell cultivation and purification technologies.

Other Information

First Licensed: October 26, 2009

Omalizumab (Humanized)

Isoantibodies

Name:
  Xolair

Manufacturer:
  Manufactured by Genentech, distributed by
  Genentech and Novartis

Synonyms: CAS # 242138-07-4, rhuMab-E25

Immunologic Characteristics

Target Antigen: Fc region of human immunoglobulin E (IgE).

Viability: Inactive, passive, transient

Antigenic Form: Humanized monoclonal IgG1κ antibody, anti-(human IgE Fc region) human-mouse E25 clone PSVIE 26 γ1-chain with disulfide bond to human-mouse E25 clone PSVIE26 κ-chain, dimer

Antigenic Type: Protein, IgG1κ immunoglobulin. Molecular weight of approximately 149 kilodaltons.

Use Characteristics

Indications: For treating adults and adolescents (12 years of age and older) with moderate to severe persistent asthma who have a positive skin test or in vitro reactivity to a perennial aeroallergen and whose symptoms are inadequately controlled with inhaled corticosteroids. Omalizumab decreases the incidence of asthma exacerbations in these patients.

Limitations: Safety and efficacy have not been established in other allergic conditions. Omalizumab has not been shown to alleviate asthma exacerbations acutely and should not be used to treat acute bronchospasm or status asthmaticus.

Contraindications:

Absolute: None.

Relative: People who experienced a severe hypersensitivity reaction to omalizumab.

Immunodeficiency: No differential effect of omalizumab in immunodeficient patients has been identified.

Elderly: In clinical trials, 134 patients 65 years of age and older were treated with omalizumab. Although there were no apparent age-related differences observed in these studies, the number of patients 65 years of age and older is not sufficient to determine whether they respond differently from younger patients.

Carcinogenicity: Omalizumab has not been evaluated for carcinogenic potential.

Mutagenicity: No evidence of mutagenic activity was observed in Ames tests using 6 different strains of bacteria with and without metabolic activation at omalizumab concentrations up to 5,000 mcg/mL.

Fertility Impairment: The effects of omalizumab on male and female fertility have been assessed in cynomolgus monkeys. Omalizumab doses less than or equal to 75 mg/kg/week did not elicit reproductive toxicity in male cynomolgus monkeys and did not inhibit reproductive capability, including implantation, in female cynomolgus monkeys. These doses provide a 2- to 16-fold safety factor based on total dose and 2- to 5-fold safety factor based on AUC over the range of adult clinical doses.

Pregnancy: Category B. Reproduction studies in cynomolgus monkeys have been conducted with omalizumab. Subcutaneous doses up to 75 mg/kg (12 times the maximum clinical dose)

of omalizumab did not elicit maternal toxicity, embryotoxicity, or teratogenicity when administered throughout organogenesis and did not elicit adverse effects on fetal or neonatal growth when administered throughout late gestation, delivery, and nursing. IgG molecules are known to cross the placental barrier, especially during the third trimester. There are no adequate and well-controlled studies of omalizumab in pregnant women. Because animal reproduction studies are not always predictive of human response, omalizumab should be used during pregnancy only if clearly needed.

Lactation: Excretion of omalizumab in milk was evaluated in female cynomolgus monkeys receiving subcutaneous doses of 75 mg/kg/week. Neonatal plasma levels of omalizumab after in utero exposure and 28 days of nursing were between 11% and 94% of the maternal plasma level. Milk levels of omalizumab were 1.5% of maternal blood concentration. While omalizumab presence in human milk has not been studied, IgG is excreted in human milk and therefore it is expected that omalizumab will be present in human milk. The potential for omalizumab absorption or harm to the infant are unknown. Exercise caution when administering omalizumab to a breastfeeding woman.

Children: Safety and efficacy of omalizumab in children younger than 12 years of age have not been established. Safety and effectiveness of omalizumab were evaluated in 2 studies in 926 asthma patients 6 to younger than 12 years of age (624 omalizumab, 302 placebo). One study was a pivotal study of similar design and conduct to that of adult and adolescent studies 1 and 2. The other study was primarily a safety study and included evaluation of efficacy as a secondary outcome. In the pivotal study, omalizumab-treated patients had a statistically significant reduction in the rate of exacerbations (worsening of asthma that required systemic corticosteroids or a doubling of the baseline ICS dose), but other efficacy variables, such as nocturnal symptom scores, beta-agonist use, and measures of airflow (FEV1), were not significantly different in treated patients compared with placebo. Considering the risk of anaphylaxis and malignancy seen in omalizumab-treated patients older than 12 years of age and the modest efficacy of omalizumab in the pivotal pediatric study, the risk-benefit assessment does not support the use of omalizumab in patients 6 to younger than 12 years of age. There is no reason to expect that children would not be at risk for anaphylaxis and malignancy as seen in adults and adolescents receiving omalizumab.

Adverse Reactions: The most serious adverse reactions occurring in clinical studies with omalizumab were malignancies and anaphylaxis. The adverse reactions most commonly observed among patients treated with omalizumab included injection-site reaction (45%), viral infections (23%), upper respiratory tract infection (20%), sinusitis (16%), headache (15%), and pharyngitis (11%). These events were observed at similar rates in omalizumab-treated patients and control patients. These were also the most frequently reported adverse reactions resulting in clinical intervention (eg, discontinuing therapy, adding a medication to treat an adverse reaction).

The data described above reflect omalizumab exposure for 2,076 adult and adolescent patients 12 years of age and older, including 1,687 patients exposed for 6 months and 555 exposed for at least 1 year, in either placebo-controlled or other controlled asthma studies. The mean age of patients receiving omalizumab was 42 years, with 134 patients 65 years of age and older; 60% were women, and 85% were white. Patients received omalizumab 150 to 375 mg every 2 or 4 weeks or, for patients assigned to control groups, standard therapy with or without a placebo.

Adverse events that occurred at least 1% more often in patients receiving omalizumab, compared with placebo, appear below. Age (among patients younger than 65 years of age), race, and gender did not affect the between-group differences in the rates of adverse events.

Malignancy: Malignant neoplasms were observed in 20 of 4,127 (0.5%) omalizumab-treated patients, compared with 5 of 2,236 (0.2%) control patients in clinical studies of asthma and other allergic disorders. The observed malignancies in omalizumab-treated patients were a variety of types, principally breast, nonmelanoma skin, prostate, melanoma, and parotid. Most patients were observed for less than 1 year. The impact of longer exposure to omalizumab or use in patients at higher risk for malignancy (eg, elderly, current smokers) is not known.

Anaphylaxis: Anaphylaxis occurred within 2 hours of the first or subsequent administration of omalizumab in 3 (less than 0.1%) patients without other identifiable allergic triggers. These events included urticaria and throat and/or tongue edema. Observe patients after injection of omalizumab. Have medications for the treatment of severe hypersensitivity reactions readily available. If a severe hypersensitivity reaction occurs, discontinue therapy.

Injection-site reactions: Severe injection-site reactions occurred more frequently in omalizumab-treated patients compared with patients in the placebo group (12% vs 9%). Injection-site reactions of any severity occurred in 45% of omalizumab-treated patients, compared with 43% in placebo-treated patients. The types of injection-site reactions included: bruising, redness, warmth, burning, stinging, itching, hive formation, pain, indurations, mass, and inflammation. Most injection-site reactions occurred within 1 after injection, lasted less than 8 days, and generally decreased in frequency at subsequent dosing visits.

Neutralizing antibodies: Low titers of antibodies to omalizumab were detected in approximately 1/1,723 (less than 0.1%) of patients treated with omalizumab. The data reflect the percentage of patients whose test results were considered positive for antibodies to omalizumab in an ELISA assay and are highly dependent on the sensitivity and specificity of the assay.

Allergy: Allergic symptoms, including urticaria, dermatitis, and pruritus were observed in patients treated with omalizumab. There were also 3 cases of anaphylaxis observed within 2 hours of omalizumab administration in which there were no other identifiable allergic triggers.

Pharmacologic & Dosing Characteristics

Dosage: 150 to 375 mg injected subcutaneously every 2 or 4 weeks. Because the solution is slightly viscous, the injection may take 5 to 10 seconds to administer. Doses (mg) and dosing frequency are determined by serum total IgE level (units/mL), measured before the start of treatment, and body weight (kg). Doses of more than 150 mg are divided among more than 1 injection site to limit injections to no greater than 150 mg per site.

Dose (mg) for Administration Every 4 Weeks				
Pretreatment serum IgE (units/mL)	Body weight (kg)			
	30-60	> 60-70	> 70-90	> 90-150
≥ 30-100	150	150	150	300
> 100-200	300	300	300	
> 200-300	300			
> 300-400	See Every-2-Week table			
> 400-500				
> 500-600				

Omalizumab (Humanized)

Dose (mg) for Administration Every 2 Weeks				
Pretreatment serum IgE (units/mL)	Body weight (kg)			
	30-60	> 60-70	> 70-90	> 90-150
≥ 30-100				
> 100-200	See Every-4-Week table			225
> 200-300		225	225	300
> 300-400	225	225	300	
> 400-500	300	300	375	
> 500-600	300	375		
> 600-700	375	Do not dose		

Number of Injections and Total Injection Volumes for Asthma		
Dose (mg)	Number of injections	Total volume injected[a]
150	1	1.2 mL
225	2	1.8 mL
300	2	2.4 mL
375	3	3.0 mL

a 1.2 mL maximum delivered volume per vial.

Dosing adjustments: Adjust doses for significant changes in body weight. Total IgE levels are elevated during treatment and remain elevated up to 1 year after ceasing treatment. Therefore, retesting of IgE levels during omalizumab treatment cannot be used as a guide for dose determination. Base dose determinations after treatment interruptions lasting less than 1 year on serum IgE levels obtained at the initial dose determination. Total serum IgE levels may be retested for dose determination if treatment with omalizumab has been interrupted for at least 1 year.

Route: Subcutaneous

Overdosage: The maximum tolerated dose of omalizumab has not been determined. Single IV doses up to 4,000 mg have been administered to patients without evidence of dose-limiting toxicities. The highest cumulative dose administered to patients was 44,000 mg over a 20-week period, which was not associated with toxicities.

Related Interventions: Do not abruptly discontinue systemic or inhaled corticosteroids upon initiation of omalizumab therapy. Decrease corticosteroids under the direct supervision of a physician, at a clinically appropriate pace.

Efficacy: The safety and efficacy of omalizumab were evaluated in 3 placebo-controlled trials. The trials enrolled patients 12 to 76 years of age, with moderate to severe persistent asthma for at least 1 year, and a positive skin-test reaction to a perennial aeroallergen. At screening, patients in studies 1 and 2 had a forced expiratory volume in 1 second (FEV_1) between 40% and 80% predicted, while in study 3 there was no restriction on screening FEV_1. All patients had FEV_1 improvement of at least 12% following beta-agonist administration. All patients were symptomatic and treated with inhaled corticosteroids (ICS) and short-acting beta-agonists. In study 3, long-acting beta-agonists were allowed. Study 3 patients were receiving at least 1,000 mcg/day fluticasone propionate and a subset was also receiving oral cortico-steroids. Patients receiving other concomitant controller medications were excluded, and initiation of additional controller medications while on study was prohibited. Patients currently smoking were excluded. In study 3, patients were stratified by use of ICS-only or ICS with concomitant use of oral steroids. Patients received omalizumab for 16 weeks with an unchanged corticosteroid dose unless an acute exacerbation necessitated an increase. Patients then entered an ICS reduction phase of 12 weeks (studies 1 and 2) or 16 weeks (study 3) during which ICS (or oral steroid in study 3 subset) dose reduction was attempted in a step-wise manner.

Omalizumab dosing was based on body weight and baseline serum total IgE concentration. All patients were required to have a baseline IgE between 30 and 700 units/mL and body weight no greater than 150 kg. Patients were treated according to a dosing table to administer at least 0.016 mg/kg/unit (IgE/mL) of omalizumab or a matching volume of placebo over each 4-week period. The maximum omalizumab dose per 4 weeks was 750 mg; patients who had a weight-IgE combination that yielded a dose greater than 750 mg were excluded from the studies. Patients who were to receive more than 300 mg within the 4-week period were administered half the total dose every 2 weeks.

The distribution of the number of asthma exacerbations per patient in each group during a study was analyzed separately for the stable steroid and steroid-reduction periods. In all 3 studies, exacerbation was defined as worsening of asthma that required treatment with systemic corticosteroids or a doubling of the baseline ICS dose.

In both studies 1 and 2, the number of exacerbations per patient was reduced in patients treated with omalizumab compared with placebo. In study 3, the number of exacerbations in patients treated with omalizumab was similar to that in placebo-treated patients. The absence of an observed treatment effect in study 3 may be related to differences in the patient population or other factors. In all 3 studies, most exacerbations were managed in the outpatient setting and most were treated with systemic steroids. Hospitalization rates were not significantly different between omalizumab and placebo-treated patients; however, the overall hospitalization rate was small. Among those patients who experienced an exacerbation, the distribution of exacerbation severity was similar between treatment groups.

Frequency of Asthma Exacerbations per Patient by Phase in Studies 1 and 2				
Stable Steroid Phase (16 wks)				
	Study 1		Study 2	
Exacerbations per patient	Omalizumab (N = 268)	Placebo (N = 257)	Omalizumab (N = 274)	Placebo (N = 272)
0	85.8%	76.7%	87.6%	69.9%
1	11.9%	16.7%	11.3%	25.0%
≥ 2	2.2%	6.6%	1.1%	5.1%
P value	0.005		< 0.001	
Mean exacerbations/patient	0.2	0.3	0.1	0.4
Steroid Reduction Phase (12 wks)				
Exacerbations per patient	Omalizumab (N = 268)	Placebo (N = 257)	Omalizumab (N = 274)	Placebo (N = 272)
0	78.7%	67.7%	83.9%	70.2%
1	19.0%	28.4%	14.2%	26.1%
≥ 2	2.2%	3.9%	1.8%	3.7%
P value	0.004		< 0.001	
Mean exacerbations/patient	0.2	0.4	0.2	0.3

Omalizumab (Humanized)

Percentage of Patients with Asthma Exacerbations by Subgroup and Phase in Study 3				
Stable Steroid Phase (16 wks)				
	Inhaled only		Oral + inhaled	
	Omalizumab (N = 126)	Placebo (N = 120)	Omalizumab (N = 50)	Placebo (N = 45)
% Patients with ≥ 1 exacerbations	15.9	15	32	22.2
Difference (95% CI)	0.9% (−9.7%, 13.7%)		9.8% (−10.5%, 31.4%)	
Steroid Reduction Phase (12 wks)				
	Omalizumab (N = 126)	Placebo (N = 120)	Omalizumab (N = 50)	Placebo (N = 45)
% Patients with ≥ 1 exacerbations	22.2	26.7	42	42.2
Difference (95% CI)	−4.4% (−17.6%, 7.4%)		−0.2% (−22.4%, 20.1%)	

In all 3 studies, a reduction of asthma exacerbations was not observed in omalizumab-treated patients who had FEV$_1$ more than 80% at time of randomization. Reductions in exacerbations were not seen in patients who required oral steroids as maintenance therapy. In studies 1 and 2, measures of airflow (FEV$_1$) and asthma symptoms were evaluated. The clinical relevance of the treatment-associated differences is unknown.

Asthma Symptoms and Pulmonary Function During Stable Steroid Phase of Study 1[a]				
	Omalizumab (n = 268)[b]		Placebo (n = 257)[b]	
Endpoint	Mean baseline	Median change (baseline to week 16)	Mean baseline	Median change (baseline to week 16)
Total asthma symptom score	4.3	−1.5[c]	4.2	−1.1[c]
Nocturnal asthma score	1.2	−0.4[c]	1.1	−0.2[c]
Daytime asthma score	2.3	−0.9[c]	2.3	−0.6[c]
FEV$_1$ % predicted	68	3[c]	68	0[c]

a Asthma symptom scale = total score from 0 (least) to 9 (most); nocturnal and daytime scores from 0 (least) to 4 (most) symptoms.
b Number of patients available for analysis ranges 255 to 258 in the omalizumab group and 238 to 239 in the placebo group.
c Comparison of omalizumab versus placebo ($P < 0.05$).

Onset: Within weeks

Duration: Not established

Pharmacokinetics:

Absorption: After subcutaneous administration, omalizumab is absorbed with an average absolute bioavailability of 62%. After a single subcutaneous dose in adult and adolescent patients with asthma, omalizumab was absorbed slowly, reaching peak serum concentrations after an average of 7 to 8 days. The pharmacokinetics of omalizumab are linear at doses greater than 0.5 mg/kg. After multiple doses of omalizumab, areas under the serum concentration-time curve from day 0 to day 14 at steady state were up to 6 times those after the first dose.

Distribution: In vitro, omalizumab forms complexes of limited size with IgE. Precipitating complexes and complexes more than 1 million daltons in molecular weight are not observed in vitro or in vivo. Tissue distribution studies in cynomolgus monkeys showed no specific uptake of ^{125}I-omalizumab by any organ or tissue. The apparent volume of distribution in patients following subcutaneous administration was 78 ± 32 mL/kg.

Elimination: Immunoglobulins are primarily eliminated by catabolism. Clearance of omalizumab involves IgG clearance processes as well as clearance via specific binding and complex formation with its target ligand, IgE. Liver elimination of IgG includes degradation in the liver reticuloendothelial system (RES) and endothelial cells. Intact IgG is also excreted in bile. In studies with mice and monkeys, omalizumab:IgE complexes were eliminated by interactions with Fc-gamma receptors within the RES at rates that were generally faster than IgG clearance. In asthma patients, omalizumab serum elimination half-life averaged 26 days, with apparent clearance averaging 2.4 ± 1.1 mL/kg/day. In addition, doubling body weight approximately doubled apparent clearance.

Pharmacodynamics: In clinical studies, serum free IgE levels were reduced in a dose-dependent manner within 1 hour after the first dose and maintained between doses. Mean serum free IgE decrease was more than 96% using recommended doses. Serum total IgE levels (ie, bound and unbound) increased after the first dose due to formation of omalizumab:IgE complexes, which have a slower elimination rate compared with free IgE. At 16 weeks after the first dose, average serum total IgE levels were 5-fold higher compared with pretreatment when using standard assays. After discontinuation of omalizumab dosing, the omalizumab-induced increase in total IgE and decrease in free IgE were reversible, with no observed rebound in IgE levels after drug washout. Total IgE levels did not return to pretreatment levels for up to 1 year after discontinuing omalizumab.

Special populations: The population pharmacokinetics of omalizumab were analyzed to evaluate the effects of demographic characteristics. Analyses of these limited data suggest that no dose adjustments are necessary for age (12 to 76 years of age), race, ethnicity, or gender.

Mechanism: Omalizumab inhibits the binding of IgE to the high-affinity IgE receptor (FcεRI) on the surface of mast cells and basophils. Reduction in surface-bound IgE on FcεRI-bearing cells limits the degree of release of mediators of the allergic response. Treatment with omalizumab also reduces the number of FcεRI receptors on basophils in atopic patients.

Drug Interactions: No formal drug interaction studies have been performed with omalizumab. The concomitant use of omalizumab and allergen immunotherapy has not been evaluated.

Lab Interference: Serum total IgE levels increase after administration of omalizumab due to formation of omalizumab:IgE complexes. Elevated serum total IgE levels may persist up to 1 year after discontinuing omalizumab. Serum total IgE levels obtained less than 1 year following discontinuation may not reflect steady state free IgE levels and should not be used to reassess the dosing regimen.

Patient Information: Advise patients receiving omalizumab not to decrease the dose or stop taking any other asthma medications unless otherwise instructed by a physician. Advise patients that they may not see immediate improvement in their asthma after beginning omalizumab therapy.

Pharmaceutical Characteristics

Concentration: 150 mg of omalizumab per 1.2 mL after reconstitution with 1.4 mL sterile water

Packaging: Single-use vial containing 202.5 mg of omalizumab (NDC#: 50242-0040-62)

Doseform: Powder for solution

Appearance: White lyophilized powder. The fully reconstituted product will appear clear or slightly opalescent and may have a few small bubbles or foam around the edge of the vial. The reconstituted product is somewhat viscous.

Omalizumab (Humanized)

Diluent:
> *For reconstitution:* Sterile water for injection. The lyophilized product typically takes 15 to 20 minutes to dissolve.

Adjuvant: None

Preservative: None

Allergens: Gentamicin is added during manufacturing, but is not detectable in the final product.

Excipients: 145.5 mg sucrose, 2.8 mg L-histidine hydrochloride monohydrate, 1.8 mg L-histidine, and 0.5 mg polysorbate 20 per vial

pH: 5.8 to 6.5

Shelf Life: Expires within 12 months

Storage/Stability: Store at 2° to 8°C (36° to 46°F). Contact the manufacturer regarding exposure to extreme temperatures. Shipped at controlled ambient temperature (30°C or below, 86°F or below).

The solution may be used within 8 hours after reconstitution if refrigerated, or within 4 hours if stored at room temperature.

Handling: After adding the diluent, gently swirl the upright vial for approximately 1 minute to evenly wet the powder. Do not shake.

Gently swirl the vial for 5 to 10 seconds every 5 minutes to dissolve any remaining solids. There should be no visible gel-like particles in the solution. Do not use if foreign particles are present. For vials that take longer than 20 minutes to dissolve completely, continue gently swirling the vial every 5 minutes, until there are no visible gel-like particles in the solution. It is acceptable to have small bubbles or foam around the edge of the vial. Do not use if the contents of the vial do not dissolve completely by 40 minutes.

Invert the vial for 15 seconds to allow the solution to drain toward the stopper. Using a new 3 mL syringe with a 1-inch, 18-gauge needle, insert the needle into the inverted vial. Position the needle tip at the very bottom of the solution in the vial stopper when drawing the solution into the syringe. Before removing the needle from the vial, pull the plunger all the way back to the end of the syringe barrel to remove all of the solution from the inverted vial.

Replace the 18-gauge needle with a 25-gauge needle for subcutaneous injection.

Expel air, large bubbles, and any excess solution to obtain the required 1.2 mL dose.

Each vial delivers 150 mg omalizumab per 1.2 mL. For a 75 mg dose, draw up 0.6 mL into the syringe and discard the remaining product. A thin layer of small bubbles may remain at the top of the solution in the syringe. Because the solution is slightly viscous, the injection may take 5 to 10 seconds to administer. Protect reconstituted omalizumab vials from direct sunlight.

Production Process: Produced by a Chinese hamster ovary (CHO) cell suspension culture in a nutrient medium containing the antibiotic gentamicin.

Media: Chinese hamster ovary (CHO) cell suspension

Other Information

First Licensed: June 20, 2003

References: Chang TW, Shiung YY. Anti-IgE as a mast cell-stabilizing therapeutic agent. *J Allergy Clin Immunol*. 2006;117(6):1203-1212.

Nowak D. Management of asthma with anti-immunoglobulin E: a review of clinical trials of omalizumab. *Respir Med*. 2006;100(11):1907-1917.

Name: *Manufacturer:*
Vectibix   Amgen
Synonyms: ABX-EGF

Immunologic Characteristics

Target Antigen: Human epidermal growth factor receptor (EGFR).

Viability: Inactive, passive, transient

Antigenic Form: Human monoclonal IgG2-κ antibody

Antigenic Type: Protein, IgG2 kappa molecule composed of human monoclonal ABX-EGF heavy chain with disulfide bond to human ABX-EGF light chain, a dimer. Molecular weight approximately 147 kilodaltons.

Use Characteristics

Indications: To treat EGFR-expressing, metastatic colorectal carcinoma with disease progression on or after fluoropyrimidine-, oxaliplatin-, and irinotecan-containing chemotherapy regimens.

Limitations: The efficacy of panitumumab in treating EGFR-expressing, metastatic colorectal carcinoma is based on progression-free survival. Currently no data are available that demonstrate an improvement in disease-related symptoms or increased survival with panitumumab.

Detection of EGFR protein expression is necessary to select patients appropriate for panitumumab therapy; these are the only patients studied and for whom benefit has been shown. Patients enrolled in the colorectal cancer clinical studies were required to have immunohistochemical evidence of EGFR expression using the Dako *EGFR pharmDx* test kit. Assess EGFR expression in laboratories with demonstrated proficiency in the specific technology used. Improper assay performance, including use of suboptimally fixed tissue, failure to utilize specific reagents, deviation from specific assay instructions, and failure to include appropriate controls for assay validation can lead to unreliable results. Refer to the Dako *EGFR pharmDx* test kit or other test kits approved by FDA to identify patients eligible for treatment with panitumumab and instructions on assay performance.

Contraindications:
Absolute: None.
Relative: People with known hypersensitivity to panitumumab or any component of the drug product.

Elderly: Of 229 patients with metastatic colorectal carcinoma who received panitumumab in the controlled study, 96 (42%) were 65 years of age and older. Although the clinical study did not include a sufficient number of elderly patients to determine whether they respond differently from younger patients, there were no apparent differences in safety and efficacy of panitumumab between these patients and younger patients.

Carcinogenicity: Panitumumab has not been evaluated for carcinogenic potential in animals or humans.

Mutagenicity: Panitumumab has not been evaluated for mutagenic potential in vitro or in vivo.

Fertility Impairment: Panitumumab may impair fertility in women of childbearing potential. Prolonged menstrual cycles and/or amenorrhea were observed in normally cycling, female cynomolgus monkeys after weekly doses of panitumumab 1.25- to 5-fold greater than the recommended human dose (based on body weight). Menstrual cycle irregularities in panitumumab-treated, female cynomolgus monkeys were accompanied by both a decrease and a delay in peak progesterone and 17β-estradiol levels. Normal menstrual cycling resumed in most animals after discontinuing panitumumab treatment. A no-effect level for menstrual cycle irregularities and serum hormone levels was not identified.

The effects of panitumumab on male fertility have not been studied. However, no adverse effects were observed microscopically in reproductive organs from male cynomolgus monkeys treated for 26 weeks with panitumumab at doses of up to 5-fold the recommended human dose (based on body weight).

Pregnancy: Category C. There are no adequate and well-controlled studies in pregnant women. However, EGFR has been implicated in the control of prenatal development and may be essential for normal organogenesis, proliferation, and differentiation in the developing embryo. Panitumumab treatment was associated with significant increases in embryolethal or abortifacient effects in pregnant cynomolgus monkeys when administered weekly during the period of organogenesis (gestation day 20 to 50), at doses approximately 1.25- to 5-fold greater than the recommended human dose (based on body weight). There were no fetal malformations or other evidence of teratogenesis noted in the offspring. While no panitumumab was detected in serum of neonates from panitumumab-treated dams, antipanitumumab antibody titers were present in 14 of 27 offspring delivered at gestation day 100. Therefore, while no teratogenic effects were observed in panitumumab-treated monkeys, panitumumab has the potential to cause fetal harm when administered to pregnant women. Human IgG is known to cross the placental barrier; therefore, panitumumab may be transmitted from the mother to the developing fetus. In women of childbearing potential, appropriate contraceptive measures must be used during treatment with panitumumab and for 6 months after the last dose of panitumumab. If panitumumab is used during pregnancy or if the patient becomes pregnant while receiving this drug, inform her of the potential risk for loss of the pregnancy or potential hazard to the fetus.

Lactation: It is not known if panitumumab crosses into human breast milk. Because human IgG is secreted into human milk, panitumumab might also be secreted. The potential for absorption and harm to the infant after ingestion is unknown. Advise women to discontinue breast-feeding during treatment with panitumumab and for 2 months after the last dose of panitumumab.

Children: Safety and efficacy of panitumumab in children younger than 18 years of age have not been studied.

Adverse Reactions: Safety data are available from 15 clinical trials in which 1,467 patients received panitumumab. Of these, 1,293 received panitumumab monotherapy and 174 received panitumumab in combination with chemotherapy. The most common adverse events observed were skin rash with variable presentations, hypomagnesemia, paronychia, fatigue, abdominal pain, nausea, and diarrhea. The most serious adverse events observed were pulmonary fibrosis, severe dermatologic toxicity complicated by infectious sequelae and septic death, infusion reactions, abdominal pain, hypomagnesemia, nausea, vomiting, and constipation. Severe toxicity necessitated dose interruption in 11% of panitumumab-treated patients. Adverse events requiring discontinuation of panitumumab were infusion reactions, severe skin toxicity, paronychia, and pulmonary fibrosis.

The following data, except where noted, reflect exposure to panitumumab administered as a single agent at the recommended dose and schedule (6 mg/kg every 2 weeks) in 229 patients with metastatic carcinoma of the colon or rectum in the controlled trial. The median number of doses was 5 (range, 1 to 26 doses), and 71% of patients received 8 or fewer doses. The population had a median age of 62 years (range, 27 to 82 years); 63% were men; and 99% were white, with less than 1% black, less than 1% Hispanic, and 0% other.

Per-Patient Incidence of Adverse Events Occurring in ≥ 5% of Patients with a Between-Group Difference of ≥ 5%				
	Patients treated with panitumumab plus BSC[a] (n = 229)		BSC[a] alone (n = 234)	
Adverse reaction	All grades[b]	Grade 3 to 4[b]	All grades[b]	Grade 3 to 4[b]
Body as a whole				
Fatigue	26%	4%	15%	3%
General deterioration	11%	8%	4%	3%
Digestive				
Abdominal pain	25%	7%	17%	5%
Nausea	23%	1%	16%	< 1%
Diarrhea	21%	2%	11%	0%
Constipation	21%	3%	9%	1%
Vomiting	19%	2%	12%	1%
Stomatitis	7%	0%	1%	0%
Mucosal inflammation	6%	< 1%	1%	0%
Metabolic/Nutritional				
Peripheral edema	12%	1%	6%	< 1%
Hypomagnesemia (laboratory)	39%	4%	2%	0%
Respiratory				
Cough	14%	< 1%	7%	0%
Skin/Appendages				
All skin/integument toxicity	90%	16%	9%	0%
Skin	90%	14%	6%	0%
Erythema	65%	5%	1%	0%
Acneiform dermatitis	57%	7%	1%	0%
Pruritus	57%	2%	2%	0%
Exfoliation	25%	2%	0%	0%
Rash	22%	1%	1%	0%
Skin fissures	20%	1%	< 1%	0%
Dry skin	10%	0%	0%	0%
Acne	13%	1%	0%	0%
Nail	29%	2%	0%	0%
Paronychia	25%	2%	0%	0%
Other nail disorder	9%	0%	0%	0%
Hair	9%	0%	1%	0%
Growth of eyelashes	6%	0%	0%	0%
Eye	15%	< 1%	2%	0%

a Best supportive care.
b Version 2.0 of the NCI-Common Toxicity Criteria (CTC) was used to grade toxicities. Skin toxicity was coded based on a modification of version 3.0.

Infusion reactions: In clinical trials of panitumumab, 4% of patients experienced infusion reactions, and in 1% reactions were graded as severe (grade 3 to 4). Severe infusion reactions were identified by reports of anaphylactic reaction, bronchospasm, fever, chills, and hypotension. Although fatal infusion reactions have not been reported with panitumumab, fatalities have occurred with other monoclonal antibodies. Stop infusion if a severe infusion reaction occurs. Depending on the severity and/or persistence of the reaction, permanently discontinue panitumumab. The use of premedication was not standardized in clinical trials. Thus, the utility of premedication in preventing the first or subsequent episodes of infusional toxicity is unknown.

Immunogenicity: Immunogenicity has been evaluated using 2 screening immunoassays to detect antipanitumumab antibodies: an acid dissociation-bridging enzyme-linked immunosorbent assay (ELISA) (detecting high-affinity antibodies) and a *Biacore* biosensor immunoassay (detecting high- and low-affinity antibodies). The incidence of binding antibodies to panitumumab (excluding predose and transient positive patients) detected by the ELISA assay, was 2 of 612 (less than 1%). The incidence detected by the *Biacore* assay was 25 of 610 (4.1%). For patients whose sera tested positive in screening immunoassays, an in vitro biological assay was performed to detect neutralizing antibodies. Excluding predose and transient positive patients, 8 of the 604 patients (1.3%) with postdose samples and 1 of 350 (less than 1%) of the patients with follow-up samples tested positive for neutralizing antibodies. There was no evidence of altered pharmacokinetic profile or toxicity profile between patients who developed antibodies to panitumumab as detected by screening immunoassays and those who did not.

Dermatologic: Dermatologic toxicities related to panitumumab blockade of EGF binding and subsequent inhibition of EGFR-mediated signaling pathways were reported in 89% of patients and were severe (grade 3 and higher) in 12% to 16% of patients receiving monotherapy. The clinical manifestations included acneiform dermatitis, pruritus, erythema, rash, skin exfoliation, paronychia, dry skin, and skin fissures. Severe dermatologic toxicities were complicated by infection including sepsis, septic death, and abscesses requiring incisions and drainage. Median time to development of skin/eye-related toxicity was 14 days; time to most severe skin/eye-related toxicity was 15 days after the first dose of panitumumab, and median time to resolution after the last dose of panitumumab was 84 days. Withhold or discontinue panitumumab and monitor for inflammatory or infectious sequelae in patients with severe dermatologic toxicities. Weekly administration of panitumumab to cynomolgus monkeys for 4 to 26 weeks resulted in dermatologic findings, including dermatitis, pustule formation and exfoliative rash, and deaths secondary to bacterial infection and sepsis at doses of 1.25- to 5-fold higher (on a mg/kg basis) than the recommended human dose.

Ophthalmic: Eye-related toxicities occurred in 15% of patients and included conjunctivitis (4%), ocular hyperemia (3%), increased lacrimation (2%), and eye/eyelid irritation (1%).

Pulmonary: Pulmonary fibrosis occurred in less than 1% (2 of 1,467) of patients enrolled in clinical studies of panitumumab. A case in a patient with underlying idiopathic pulmonary fibrosis who received panitumumab combined with chemotherapy resulted in death from worsening pulmonary fibrosis after 4 doses of panitumumab. The second case was characterized by cough and wheezing 8 days after the initial dose, exertional dyspnea on the day of the seventh dose, and persistent symptoms and computed tomography evidence of pulmonary fibrosis after the eleventh dose of panitumumab as monotherapy. An additional patient died with bilateral pulmonary infiltrates of uncertain etiology with hypoxia, after 23 doses of panitumumab combined with chemotherapy. After the initial fatality, patients with a history of interstitial pneumonitis, pulmonary fibrosis, evidence of interstitial pneumonitis, or pulmonary fibrosis were excluded from clinical studies. Therefore, the estimated risk in a general population that may include such patients is uncertain. Permanently discontinue panitumumab therapy in patients developing interstitial lung disease, pneumonitis, or lung infiltrates.

GI: Panitumumab treatment can cause diarrhea, and, when used in combination with irinotecan, appears to increase the incidence and severity of chemotherapy-induced diarrhea. In a study of 19 patients receiving panitumumab in combination with irinotecan, bolus 5-fluorouracil, and leucovorin (IFL), the incidence of grade 3 to 4 diarrhea was 58% and was fatal in 1 patient. In a study of 24 patients receiving panitumumab plus IFL, the incidence of grade 3 diarrhea was 25%. The combination of panitumumab with IFL is not recommended.

Electrolyte Disturbance: In the clinical trial of panitumumab, median magnesium levels decreased by 0.1 mMol/L in the panitumumab arm. Hypomagnesemia (grade 3 or 4) requiring oral or IV electrolyte repletion occurred in 2% of patients. Hypomagnesemia occurred 6 weeks or longer after initiation of panitumumab. In some patients, hypomagnesemia was associated with hypocalcemia. Monitor electrolytes during and for 8 weeks after completion of panitumumab therapy. Provide appropriate treatment (eg, oral or IV electrolyte repletion), as needed.

Pharmacologic & Dosing Characteristics

Dosage: 6 mg/kg every 14 days.

Route: By IV infusion, using an infusion pump with a low protein-binding 0.2- or 0.22-micron in-line filter. Infuse over 60 minutes through a peripheral line or indwelling catheter. Infuse doses of more than 1,000 mg over 90 minutes. Do not administer by IV push or as a bolus.

Overdosage: The highest per-infusion dose administered in clinical studies was 9 mg/kg administered every 3 weeks. There is no experience with overdosage in human clinical trials.

Related Interventions:

Infusion reactions: Reduce infusion rate by 50% in patients experiencing a mild or moderate (grade 1 or 2) infusion reaction for the duration of that infusion. Immediately and permanently discontinue infusion in patients experiencing severe (grade 3 or 4) infusion reactions.

Withhold panitumumab for dermatologic toxicities that are grade 3 or higher or are considered intolerable. If toxicity does not improve to grade 2 or less within 1 month, permanently discontinue this therapy. If dermatologic toxicity improves to grade 2 or less, and the patient is symptomatically improved after withholding no more than 2 doses, treatment may be resumed at 50% of the original dose. If toxicities recur, permanently discontinue panitumumab. If toxicities do not recur, subsequent doses may be increased by increments of 25% of the original dose until the recommended dose of 6 mg/kg is reached.

Efficacy: Panitumumab was studied in an open-label, multinational, randomized, controlled trial of 463 patients with EGFR-expressing, metastatic carcinoma of the colon or rectum. Patients were required to have progressed on or after treatment with a regimen(s) containing a fluoropyrimidine, oxaliplatin, and irinotecan. All patients were required to have EGFR expression defined as at least 1+ membrane staining in 1% or more of tumor cells by the Dako *EGFR pharmDx* test kit. Patients were randomized to receive panitumumab 6 mg/kg once every 2 weeks plus best supportive care (n = 231) or best supportive care alone (n = 232) until investigator-determined disease progression. Upon investigator-determined disease progression, patients in the best supportive care-alone arm were eligible to receive panitumumab and were followed until disease progression was independently confirmed. The analyses of progression-free survival, objective response, and response duration were based on events confirmed by reviewers masked to treatment assignment. Among the 463 patients, 63% were men, median age was 62 years, 40% were 65 years or older, 99% were white, 86% had a baseline Eastern Cooperative Oncology Group (ECOG) performance status of 0 or 1, and 67% had colon cancer. The median number of prior therapies for metastatic disease was 2.4. The membrane-staining intensity for EGFR was 3+ in 19%, 2+ in 51%, and 1+ in 30% of patients' tumors.

A statistically significant prolongation in progression-free survival was observed in patients receiving panitumumab, compared with those receiving best supportive care alone. The mean progression-free survival was 96 days in the panitumumab arm and 60 days in the best supportive care-alone arm. In a series of sensitivity analyses, including one adjusting for potential ascertainment bias, progression-free survival was still significantly prolonged among patients receiving panitumumab compared with best supportive care alone. Of the 232 patients randomized to best supportive care alone, 75% crossed over to receive panitumumab after investigator determination of disease progression; the median time to crossover was 8.4 weeks (0.3 to 26.4 weeks).

There were 19 partial responses in patients randomized to panitumumab, for an overall response of 8% (95% CI, 5% to 12.6%). No patient in the control arm had an objective response. The median duration of response was 17 weeks (95% CI, 16 to 25 weeks). There was no difference in overall survival observed between the study arms.

EGFR expression and response: Patients enrolled in the colorectal cancer clinical studies were required to have immunohistochemical evidence of EGFR expression; these were the only patients studied and for whom benefit was shown. EGFR tumor expression was determined using the Dako *EGFR pharmDx* test kit. Specimens were scored based on the percentage of cells expressing EGFR and staining intensity (3+, 2+, and 1+). Exploratory univariate analyses assessing the relationship between EGFR expression and progression-free survival did not suggest that the progression-free survival benefit differed as a function of EGFR staining intensity or percentage of EGFR-expressing tumor cells.

Pharmacokinetics: Panitumumab administered as a single agent exhibits nonlinear pharmacokinetics. After a single 1-hour infusion, the area under the curve (AUC) increased in a greater than dose-proportional manner, and the clearance of panitumumab decreased from 30.6 to 4.6 mL/day/kg as the dose increased from 0.75 to 9 mg/kg. However, at doses above 2 mg/kg, the AUC of panitumumab increases in a dose-proportional manner.

With the recommended 6 mg/kg every-2-week regimen, panitumumab concentrations reached steady-state levels by the third infusion with mean ($\pm$ SD) peak and trough concentrations of 213 $\pm$ 59 and 39 $\pm$ 14 mcg/mL, respectively. The mean ($\pm$ SD) AUC_{0-tau} and clearance were 1,306 $\pm$ 374 mcg•day/mL and 4.9 $\pm$ 1.4 mL/kg/day, respectively. The elimination half-life was approximately 7.5 days (range, 3.6 to 10.9 days). A population pharmacokinetic analysis was performed to explore the potential effects of covariates on panitumumab pharmacokinetics. Results suggest that age (21 to 88 years), gender, race (15% nonwhite), mild to moderate renal dysfunction, mild to moderate hepatic dysfunction, and EGFR membrane-staining intensity (1+, 2+, 3+) in tumor cells had no apparent impact on the pharmacokinetics of panitumumab. No formal pharmacokinetic studies of panitumumab have been conducted in patients with renal or hepatic impairment.

Mechanism: EGFR is a member of a subfamily of type 1 receptor tyrosine kinases, including EGFR (HER1, c-ErbB-1), HER2/neu, HER3, and HER4. EGFR is a transmembrane glycoprotein expressed in many normal epithelial tissues, including skin and hair follicle. Overexpression of EGFR is also detected in many human cancers, including those of the colon and rectum. Interaction of EGFR with its normal ligands (eg, EGF, transforming growth factor-alpha) leads to phosphorylation and activation of a series of intracellular tyrosine kinases, which in turn regulate transcription of molecules involved with cellular growth and survival, motility, proliferation, and transformation. Panitumumab binds specifically to EGFR on both normal and tumor cells and competitively inhibits the binding of ligands for EGFR. In nonclinical studies, binding of panitumumab to EGFR prevents ligand-induced receptor autophosphorylation and activation of receptor-associated kinases, resulting in inhibition of cell growth, induction of apoptosis, decreased proinflammatory cytokine and vascular growth factor production, and internalization of EGFR. In vitro assays and in vivo animal studies show that panitumumab inhibits growth and survival of selected human tumor cell lines expressing EGFR.

Drug Interactions: No formal drug-drug interaction studies have been conducted with panitumumab.

Patient Information: Inform patients about possible adverse effects of panitumumab, including dermatologic toxicity, infusion reactions, pulmonary fibrosis, and potential embryofetal lethality. Instruct patients to report skin and ocular changes, and dyspnea to a health care professional. Advise patients that periodic monitoring of electrolyte levels is required. Encourage patients to wear sunscreen and hats and limit sun exposure while receiving panitumumab, because sunlight can exacerbate any skin reactions that may occur.

Pharmaceutical Characteristics

Concentration: 20 mg/mL

Packaging: 100 mg per 5 mL single-use vial (NDC#: 55513-954-01), 200 mg per 10 mL single-use vial (55513-955-01), 400 mg per 20 mL single-use vial (55513-956-01).

Doseform: Solution

Appearance: Colorless solution. The solution may contain a small amount of visible translucent-to-white, amorphous, proteinaceous panitumumab particulates, to be removed by filtration.

Diluent: Aqueous.

For infusion: Withdraw the necessary amount for a dose of 6 mg/kg. Dilute to a total volume of 100 mL with 0.9% sodium chloride injection. Dilute doses of more than 1,000 mg to 150 mL with 0.9% sodium chloride injection. Do not exceed 10 mg/mL final concentration. Mix diluted solution by gentle inversion; do not shake. Administer using a low-protein-binding 0.2-micron or 0.22-micron in-line filter. Flush the line before and after administration with 0.9% sodium chloride injection, to avoid mixing with other drug products or IV solutions.

Adjuvant: None

Preservative: None

Allergens: None

Excipients: Sodium chloride 5.8 mg/mL, sodium acetate 6.8 mg/mL, and water for injection

pH: 5.6 to 6

Shelf Life: Data not provided.

Storage/Stability: Store at 2° to 8°C (36° to 46°F). Protect vials from direct sunlight. Discard if frozen. Contact the manufacturer regarding exposure to freezing or elevated temperatures. Shipping data not provided.

Use the diluted infusion solution within 6 hours if stored at room temperature or within 24 hours of dilution if stored at 2° to 8°C (36° to 46°F).

Handling: Do not mix panitumumab with, or administer it as an infusion with, other medicinal products. Do not add other medications to solutions containing panitumumab.

Media: Produced in genetically engineered Chinese hamster ovary cells.

Disease Epidemiology

Incidence: An estimated 150,000 new cases of colon cancer were diagnosed, and 55,000 deaths occurred from colon and rectal cancer in the United States in 2006. Approximately 70% of colorectal carcinomas test positive for EGFR. Colorectal cancer is the third most common cancer and the third leading cause of cancer mortality in the United States.

Panitumumab

Other Information

First Licensed: September 27, 2006.

References: McIntyre JA, Martin L. Panitumumab. *Drugs Future*. 2004;29:793-797.

Wainberg Z, Hecht JR. A phase III randomized, open-label, controlled trial of chemotherapy and bevacizumab with or without panitumumab in the first-line treatment of patients with metastatic colorectal cancer. *Clin Colorectal Cancer*. 2006;5(5):363-367.

Isoantibodies

Name:
Perjeta

Manufacturer:
Genentech

Synonyms: 2C4, *Omnitarg*

Immunologic Characteristics

Target Antigen: Extracellular dimerization domain (subdomain II) of the human epidermal growth factor receptor 2 (HER2) protein

Viability: Inactive, passive, transient

Antigenic Form: Humanized IgG1, antihuman neu (receptor) (human-mouse monoclonal 2C4 heavy chain) with disulfide bond to human-mouse 2C4 κ-chain, dimer

Antigenic Type: Protein, approximate molecular weight of 148 kDa.

Use Characteristics

Indications: In combination with trastuzumab and docetaxel to treat patients with HER2-positive metastatic breast cancer who have not received prior anti-HER2 therapy or chemotherapy for metastatic disease.

Limitations: Detection of HER2 protein overexpression is necessary for selection of patients appropriate for pertuzumab therapy because these are the only patients studied and for whom benefit has been shown. In the randomized trial, patients with breast cancer were required to have evidence of HER2 overexpression, defined as 3+ immunohistochemistry (IHC) by *Dako Herceptest* or fluorescent in situ hybridization (FISH) amplification ratio of 2 or more by *Dako HER2 FISH PharmDx* test kit. Only limited data were available for patients whose breast cancer was positive according to FISH but did not demonstrate protein overexpression by IHC. Assess HER2 status via laboratories with demonstrated proficiency in the specific technology being used. Improper assay performance, including use of suboptimally fixed tissue, failure to utilize specified reagents, deviation from specific assay instructions, and failure to include appropriate controls for assay validation, can lead to unreliable results.

Contraindications: None

Elderly: Of 402 patients who received pertuzumab in the randomized trial, 60 (15%) patients were 65 years and older, and 5 (1%) patients were 75 years and older. No overall differences in efficacy and safety of pertuzumab were observed between these patients and younger patients. Based on a population pharmacokinetic analysis, no significant difference was observed in the pharmacokinetics of pertuzumab between patients younger than 65 years (n = 306) and patients 65 years of age and older (n = 175).

Carcinogenicity: Pertuzumab has not been evaluated for carcinogenic potential.

Mutagenicity: Pertuzumab has not been evaluated for mutagenic potential.

Pregnancy: Category D: There are no adequate and well-controlled studies of pertuzumab in pregnant women. Based on findings in animal studies, pertuzumab can cause fetal harm when administered to a pregnant woman. The effects of pertuzumab are likely to be present during all trimesters of pregnancy. Pertuzumab administered to pregnant cynomolgus monkeys resulted in oligohydramnios, delayed fetal kidney development, and embryofetal deaths at clinically relevant exposures 2.5- to 20-fold greater than the recommended human dose, based on maximal drug concentration (C_{max}). If pertuzumab is administered during pregnancy, or if the patient becomes pregnant while receiving this drug, inform the patient of the potential hazard to the fetus. Verify pregnancy status before starting pertuzumab. Advise patients of the risks of embryofetal death and birth defects and the need for contraception during and after treatment. Advise patients to contact their health care provider immediately if they suspect they might be pregnant. If pertuzumab is administered during pregnancy or if a patient becomes pregnant while receiving pertuzumab, immediately report exposure to the Genentech Adverse Event Line at 1-888-835-2555. Encourage women who may be exposed during pregnancy to enroll in the MotHER Pregnancy Registry by contacting 1-800-690-6720. Monitor women who become pregnant during pertuzumab therapy for oligohydramnios. If oligohydramnios occurs, perform fetal testing appropriate for gestational age and consistent with community standards of care. The efficacy of intravenous (IV) hydration in managing oligohydramnios due to pertuzumab exposure is not known.

Lactation: It is not known if pertuzumab crosses into human breast milk, but human IgG is excreted in human milk. Discontinue breast-feeding or discontinue pertuzumab, taking into consideration the elimination half-life of pertuzumab and the importance of the drug to the mother.

Children: Safety and efficacy of pertuzumab in children younger than 18 years have not been established.

Adverse Reactions: The most common adverse events (incidence greater than 30%) with pertuzumab in combination with trastuzumab and docetaxel were diarrhea, alopecia, neutropenia, nausea, fatigue, rash, and peripheral neuropathy. The most common grade 3 to 4 adverse reactions (greater than 2%) were neutropenia, febrile neutropenia, leukopenia, diarrhea, peripheral neuropathy, anemia, asthenia, and fatigue. An increased incidence of febrile neutropenia was observed for Asian patients in both treatment arms compared with patients of other races and from other geographic regions. Among Asian patients, the incidence of febrile neutropenia was higher in the pertuzumab-treated group (26%) compared with the placebo-treated group (12%).

In clinical trials, pertuzumab was evaluated (predominantly in combination with other antineoplastic agents) in more than 1,400 patients with various malignancies. The adverse reactions described in the following table were identified in 804 patients with HER2-positive metastatic breast cancer treated in a randomized trial. Patients were randomized to receive pertuzumab in combination with trastuzumab and docetaxel or placebo in combination with trastuzumab and docetaxel. The median duration of study treatment was 18 months for patients in the pertuzumab-treated group and 12 months for patients in the placebo-treated group. No dose adjustment was permitted for pertuzumab or trastuzumab. The rates of adverse events resulting in permanent discontinuation of all study therapy were 6.1% for patients in the pertuzumab-treated group and 5.3% for patients in the placebo-treated group. Adverse events led to discontinuation of docetaxel alone in 24% of patients in the pertuzumab-treated group and 23% of patients in the placebo-treated group.

Adverse Reactions Occurring in ≥ 10% of Patients in the Pertuzumab Treatment Arm of the Randomized Trial				
	Pertuzumab + trastuzumab + docetaxel (n = 407)		Placebo + trastuzumab + docetaxel (n = 397)	
Body system/ adverse reactions	All grades	Grades 3 to 4	All grades	Grades 3 to 4
General disorders and administration-site conditions				
Fatigue	37.6%	2.2%	36.8%	3.3%
Asthenia	26%	2.5%	30.2%	1.5%
Edema, peripheral	23.1%	0.5%	30%	0.8%

Adverse Reactions Occurring in ≥ 10% of Patients in the Pertuzumab Treatment Arm of the Randomized Trial				
	Pertuzumab + trastuzumab + docetaxel (n = 407)		Placebo + trastuzumab + docetaxel (n = 397)	
Body system/ adverse reactions	All grades	Grades 3 to 4	All grades	Grades 3 to 4
Mucosal inflammation	27.8%	1.5%	19.9%	1%
Pyrexia	18.7%	1.2%	17.9%	0.5%
Skin and subcutaneous tissue disorders				
Alopecia	60.9%	0%	60.5%	0.3%
Rash	33.7%	0.7%	24.2%	0.8%
Nail disorder	22.9%	1.2%	22.9%	0.3%
Pruritus	14%	0%	10.1%	0%
Dry skin	10.6%	0%	4.3%	0%
GI disorders				
Diarrhea	66.8%	7.9%	46.3%	5%
Nausea	42.3%	1.2%	41.6%	0.5%
Vomiting	24.1%	1.5%	23.9%	1.5%
Constipation	15%	0%	24.9%	1%
Stomatitis	18.9%	0.5%	15.4%	0.3%
Blood and lymphatic system disorders				
Neutropenia	52.8%	48.9%	49.6%	45.8%
Anemia	23.1%	2.5%	18.9%	3.5%
Leukopenia	18.2%	12.3%	20.4%	14.6%
Febrile neutropenia[a]	13.8%	13%	7.6%	7.3%
Nervous system disorders				
Neuropathy, peripheral	32.4%	3.2%	33.8%	2%
Headache	20.9%	1.2%	16.9%	0.5%
Dysgeusia	18.4%	0%	15.6%	0%
Dizziness	12.5%	0.5%	12.1%	0%
Musculoskeletal and connective tissue disorders				
Myalgia	22.9%	1%	23.9%	0.8%
Arthralgia	15.5%	0.2%	16.1%	0.8%
Infections and infestations				
Upper respiratory tract infection	16.7%	0.7%	13.4%	0%
Nasopharyngitis	11.8%	0%	12.8%	0.3%
Respiratory, thoracic, and mediastinal disorders				
Dyspnea	14%	1%	15.6%	2%
Metabolism and nutrition disorders				
Decreased appetite	29.2%	1.7%	26.4%	1.5%
Eye disorders				
Lacrimation increased	14%	0%	13.9%	0%
Psychiatric disorders				
Insomnia	13.3%	0%	13.4%	0%

a Denotes an adverse reaction reported in association with a fatal outcome.

The following clinically relevant adverse reaction was reported in less than 10% of patients in the pertuzumab-treated group and more often than in the placebo-treated group: paronychia (7.1% in the pertuzumab-treated group vs 3.5% in the placebo group).

Left ventricular dysfunction: Decreases in left ventricular ejection fraction (LVEF) have been reported with drugs that block HER2 activity, including pertuzumab. In the randomized trial, pertuzumab in combination with trastuzumab and docetaxel was not associated with increases in the incidence of symptomatic left ventricular systolic dysfunction (LVSD) or decreases in LVEF compared with placebo in combination with trastuzumab and docetaxel. Left ventricular dysfunction occurred in 4.4% of patients in the pertuzumab-treated group and 8.3% of patients in the placebo-treated group. Symptomatic LVSD (congestive heart failure [CHF]) occurred in 1% of patients in the pertuzumab-treated group and 1.8% of patients in the placebo-treated group. Patients who have received prior anthracyclines or prior radiotherapy to the chest area may be at higher risk of decreased LVEF. Pertuzumab has not been studied in patients with a pretreatment LVEF value of 50% or less, a history of CHF, decreases in LVEF to less than 50% during prior trastuzumab therapy, or conditions that could impair left ventricular function, such as uncontrolled hypertension, recent myocardial infarction, serious cardiac arrhythmia requiring treatment, or a cumulative prior anthracycline exposure to more than 360 mg/m^2 of doxorubicin or its equivalent. Assess LVEF before starting pertuzumab and at regular intervals (eg, every 3 months) during treatment to ensure that LVEF is within the institution's normal limits. If LVEF is less than 40%, or is 40% to 45% with a 10% or greater absolute decrease below the pretreatment value, withhold pertuzumab and trastuzumab and repeat LVEF assessment within approximately 3 weeks. Discontinue pertuzumab and trastuzumab if LVEF does not improve or declines further, unless the benefits for the individual patient outweigh the risks.

Patients receiving pertuzumab and trastuzumab after discontinuation of docetaxel: In the randomized trial, adverse reactions were reported less frequently after discontinuation of docetaxel treatment. All adverse reactions in the pertuzumab plus trastuzumab treatment group occurred in less than 10% of patients, except for diarrhea (19%), upper respiratory tract infection (13%), rash (12%), headache (11%), and fatigue (11%).

Infusion-associated reactions, hypersensitivity: Pertuzumab has been associated with infusion and hypersensitivity reactions. An infusion reaction was defined as any event described as a hypersensitivity reaction, an anaphylactic reaction, an acute infusion reaction, or cytokine-release syndrome during an infusion or on the same day as the infusion. The initial dose of pertuzumab was given the day before trastuzumab and docetaxel to allow assessment of pertuzumab-associated reactions. On the first day, when only pertuzumab was administered, the overall frequency of infusion reactions was 13% in the pertuzumab-treated group and 9.8% in the placebo-treated group; less than 1% were grade 3 or 4. The most common infusion reactions (1% or more) were pyrexia, chills, fatigue, headache, asthenia, hypersensitivity, and vomiting. During the second cycle, when all drugs were administered on the same day, the most common infusion reactions in the pertuzumab-treated group (1% or more) were fatigue, dysgeusia, hypersensitivity, myalgia, and vomiting.

In the randomized trial, the overall frequency of hypersensitivity or anaphylaxis reactions was 10.8% in the pertuzumab-treated group and 9.1% in the placebo-treated group. The incidence of grade 3 to 4 hypersensitivity or anaphylaxis reactions was 2% in the pertuzumab-treated group and 2.5% in the placebo-treated group.

Cardiac electrophysiology: The effect of an initial pertuzumab dose of 840 mg followed by a maintenance dose of 420 mg every 3 weeks on QTc interval was evaluated in a subgroup of 20 patients with HER2-positive breast cancer in the randomized trial. No significant changes in the mean QT interval (ie, greater than 20 msec) due to placebo, based on

Fridericia correction method, were detected in the trial. A small increase in the mean QTc interval (ie, less than 10 msec) cannot be excluded because of the limitations of the trial design.

Immunogenicity: As with all therapeutic proteins, there is the potential for an immune response to pertuzumab. Patients in the randomized trial were tested at multiple time-points for antibodies to pertuzumab. Approximately 2.8% (11/386) of patients in the pertuzumab-treated group and 6.2% (23/372) of patients in the placebo-treated group tested positive for anti-pertuzumab antibodies. Of these 34 patients, none experienced anaphylactic/hypersensitivity reactions that were clearly related to the antitherapeutic antibodies. The presence of pertuzumab in patient serum at the levels expected at the time of antitherapeutic antibodies sampling can interfere with the ability of this assay to detect anti-pertuzumab antibodies. In addition, the assay might be detecting antibodies to trastuzumab. As a result, data may not accurately reflect the true incidence of anti-pertuzumab antibody development.

Pharmacologic & Dosing Characteristics

Dosage: 840 mg administered as a 60-minute IV infusion, followed every 3 weeks thereafter by 420 mg administered as a 30- to 60-minute IV infusion. If a significant infusion-associated reaction occurs, slow or interrupt the infusion and administer appropriate medical therapy. Monitor patients carefully until complete resolution of signs and symptoms. Consider permanent discontinuation in patients with severe infusion reactions.

Left-ventricular ejection fraction: Monitor LVEF. Withhold pertuzumab and trastuzumab dosing for at least 3 weeks for either a drop in LVEF to less than 40%, or for LVEF of 40% to 45% with a 10% or greater absolute decrease below pretreatment values. Pertuzumab may be resumed if LVEF has recovered to greater than 45% or to 40% to 45% associated with a less than 10% absolute decrease below pretreatment values. If after a repeat assessment within approximately 3 weeks LVEF has not improved or has declined further, consider discontinuation of pertuzumab and trastuzumab, unless the benefits for the individual patient outweigh the risks. Withhold or discontinue pertuzumab if trastuzumab treatment is withheld or discontinued. If docetaxel is discontinued, treatment with pertuzumab and trastuzumab may continue.

Dose reductions are not recommended for pertuzumab. For docetaxel dose modifications, see the docetaxel prescribing information.

Route: IV infusion only. Do not administer as an IV push or bolus.

Overdosage: No drug overdoses have been reported with pertuzumab to date.

Missed Doses: For delayed or missed doses, if the time between 2 sequential infusions is less than 6 weeks, administer the pertuzumab 420 mg dose. Do not wait until the next planned dose.

If the time between 2 sequential infusions is 6 weeks or longer, readminister the initial dose of pertuzumab 840 mg followed every 3 weeks thereafter by a dose of 420 mg.

Related Interventions:

Trastuzumab: When administered with pertuzumab, the recommended initial dose of trastuzumab is 8 mg/kg administered as a 90-minute IV infusion, followed every 3 weeks thereafter by a dose of 6 mg/kg administered as an IV infusion over 30 to 90 minutes.

Docetaxel: When administered with pertuzumab, the recommended initial dose of docetaxel is 75 mg/m^2 administered as an IV infusion. The dose may be escalated to 100 mg/m^2 administered every 3 weeks if the initial dose is well tolerated.

Laboratory Tests:

HER2 testing: Perform HER2 testing using US Food and Drug Administration (FDA)-approved tests by laboratories with demonstrated proficiency.

Efficacy: The randomized trial was a multicenter, double-blind, placebo-controlled trial of 808 patients with HER2-positive metastatic breast cancer. Breast tumor specimens were required to show HER2 overexpression, defined as 3+ IHC or FISH amplification ratio of 2 or more determined at a central laboratory. Patients were randomized 1:1 to receive placebo plus trastuzumab and docetaxel or pertuzumab plus trastuzumab and docetaxel. Randomization was stratified by prior treatment (prior or no prior adjuvant/neoadjuvant anti-HER2 therapy or chemotherapy) and geographic region (Europe, North America, South America, and Asia). Patients with prior adjuvant or neoadjuvant therapy were required to have a disease-free interval of more than 12 months before trial enrollment. Pertuzumab was given IV at an initial dose of 840 mg, followed by 420 mg every 3 weeks thereafter. Trastuzumab was given IV at an initial dose of 8 mg/kg, followed by 6 mg/kg every 3 weeks thereafter. Patients were treated with pertuzumab and trastuzumab until progression of disease, withdrawal of consent, or unacceptable toxicity. Docetaxel was given as an initial dose of 75 mg/m^2 by IV infusion every 3 weeks for at least 6 cycles. The docetaxel dose could be escalated to 100 mg/m^2 at the investigator's discretion if the initial dose was well tolerated. At the time of the primary analysis, the mean number of cycles of study treatment administered was 16.2 in the placebo-treated group and 19.9 in the pertuzumab-treated group.

The primary end point of the randomized trial was progression-free survival (PFS), as assessed by an independent review facility. PFS was defined as the time from the date of randomization to the date of disease progression or death (from any cause) if the death occurred within 18 weeks of the last tumor assessment. Additional end points included overall survival (OS), PFS (investigator-assessed), objective response rate, and duration of response.

The median age of patients was 54 years (range, 22 to 89 years), 59% were white, 32% were Asian, and 4% were black. All were women, with the exception of 2 patients. Seventeen percent of the patients were enrolled in North America, 14% in South America, 38% in Europe, and 31% in Asia. Tumor prognostic characteristics, including hormone receptor status (positive 48%, negative 50%) and presence of visceral disease (78%) and nonvisceral disease only (22%), were similar in the study arms. Approximately half of the patients received prior adjuvant or neoadjuvant anti-HER2 therapy or chemotherapy (47% in the placebo group, 46% in the pertuzumab group). Among patients with hormone receptor–positive tumors, 45% received prior adjuvant hormonal therapy and 11% received hormonal therapy for metastatic disease. Eleven percent of patients received prior adjuvant or neoadjuvant trastuzumab.

The randomized trial demonstrated a statistically significant improvement in independent review facility–assessed PFS in the pertuzumab-treated group compared with the placebo-treated group (hazard ratio, 0.62; 95% confidence interval [CI], 0.51-0.75; $P < 0.0001$) and an increase in median PFS of 6.1 months (median PFS of 18.5 months in the pertuzumab-treated group vs 12.4 months in the placebo-treated group). The results for investigator-assessed PFS were comparable with those observed for independent review facility–assessed PFS.

Consistent results were observed across several patient subgroups, including age (younger than 65 years or 65 years and older), race, geographic region, prior adjuvant/neoadjuvant anti-HER2 therapy or chemotherapy (yes or no), and prior adjuvant/neoadjuvant trastuzumab therapy (yes or no). In the subgroup of patients with hormone receptor–negative disease (n = 408), the hazard ratio was 0.55 (95% CI, 0.42-0.72). In the subgroup of patients with hormone receptor–positive disease (n = 388), the hazard ratio was 0.72 (95% CI, 0.55-0.95). In the subgroup of patients with disease limited to nonvisceral metastasis (n = 178), the hazard ratio was 0.96 (95% CI, 0.61-1.52).

At the time of the PFS analysis, 165 patients had died. More deaths occurred in the placebo-treated group (23.6%) compared with the pertuzumab-treated group (17.2%). At the interim OS analysis, the results were not mature and did not meet the prespecified stopping boundary for statistical significance.

Pharmacokinetics: Pertuzumab demonstrated linear pharmacokinetics at a dose range of 2 to 25 mg/kg. Based on a population pharmacokinetic analysis that included 481 patients, the median clearance of pertuzumab was 0.24 L/day, and the median half-life was 18 days. With an initial dose of 840 mg followed by a maintenance dose of 420 mg every 3 weeks thereafter, the steady-state concentration of pertuzumab was reached after the first maintenance dose. The population pharmacokinetic analysis suggested no pharmacokinetic differences based on age, gender, and ethnicity (Japanese vs non-Japanese). Baseline serum albumin level and lean body weight as covariates only exerted a minor influence on pharmacokinetic parameters. Therefore, no dose adjustments based on body weight or baseline albumin level are needed.

Renal impairment: No dedicated renal impairment trial for pertuzumab has been conducted. No relationship between creatinine clearance (CrCl) and pertuzumab exposure was observed over the range of observed CrCl (27 to 244 mL/min). Based on the results of the population pharmacokinetic analysis, pertuzumab exposure in patients with mild (CrCl 60 to 90 mL/min, n = 200) and moderate (CrCl 30 to 60 mL/min, n = 71) renal impairment was similar to that in patients with healthy renal function (CrCl greater than 90 mL/min, n = 200). Dose adjustments of pertuzumab are not needed in patients with mild or moderate renal impairment. No dose adjustment can be recommended for patients with severe renal impairment (CrCl less than 30 mL/min) because of the limited pharmacokinetic data available.

Hepatic impairment: No clinical studies have been conducted to evaluate the effect of hepatic impairment on the pharmacokinetics of pertuzumab.

Mechanism: Pertuzumab is an HER2/neu receptor antagonist. Pertuzumab targets the extracellular dimerization domain (subdomain II) of the HER2 protein and, thereby, blocks ligand-dependent heterodimerization of HER2 with other HER family members, including epidermal growth factor receptor (EGFR), HER3, and HER4. As a result, pertuzumab inhibits ligand-initiated intracellular signaling through 2 major signal pathways, mitogen-activated protein (MAP) kinase and phosphoinositide 3-kinase (PI3K). Inhibition of these signaling pathways can result in cell growth arrest and apoptosis, respectively. In addition, pertuzumab mediates antibody-dependent cell-mediated cytotoxicity. While pertuzumab alone inhibited the proliferation of human tumor cells, the combination of pertuzumab and trastuzumab significantly augmented antitumor activity in HER2-overexpressing xenograft models.

Drug Interactions: No drug-drug interactions were observed between pertuzumab and trastuzumab, or between pertuzumab and docetaxel in a substudy of 37 patients in the randomized trial.

Pharmaceutical Characteristics

Concentration: Pertuzumab 420 mg per 14 mL vial, or 30 mg/mL

Packaging: 420 mg per 14 mL (30 mg/mL) single-use vial (NDC#: 50242-0145-01)

Doseform: Solution for further dilution

Appearance: Clear to slightly opalescent, colorless to pale brown liquid

Solvent: Sucrose-histidine solution

Diluent:
For infusion: Withdraw the appropriate volume of pertuzumab solution from the vial(s). Dilute into a 250 mL sodium chloride 0.9% polyvinyl chloride (PVC) or non-PVC polyolefin infusion bag. Do not use dextrose solutions. Mix diluted solution by gentle inversion. Do not shake.

Adjuvant: None

Preservative: None

Pertuzumab

Allergens: Gentamicin used in processing is not detectable in the final product.

Excipients: Each single-use vial contains L-histidine acetate 20 mM, sucrose 120 mM, and 0.02% of polysorbate 20.

pH: 6

Shelf Life: Data not provided

Storage/Stability: Store at 2° to 8°C (36° to 46°F). Protect vials from light. Do not freeze. Contact the manufacturer regarding exposure to freezing or elevated temperatures. Shipping data not provided.

If the diluted infusion solution is not used immediately, it can be stored at 2°C to 8°C (36° to 46°F) for up to 24 hours.

Handling: Do not shake. Do not mix pertuzumab with other drugs.

Production Process: Pertuzumab is produced by recombinant DNA technology in a mammalian (Chinese hamster ovary) cell culture containing the antibiotic gentamicin.

Media: Chinese hamster ovary cell culture

Other Information

First Licensed: June 8, 2012

746

Ranibizumab (Humanized)

Isoantibodies

Name:
Lucentis
Synonyms: RhuFab V2

Manufacturer:
Genentech

Immunologic Characteristics

Target Antigen: Human vascular endothelial growth factor A (VEGF-A).

Viability: Inactive, passive, transient

Antigenic Form: Humanized (human/murine) IgG1-κ antibody fragment

Antigenic Type: Protein, IgG1 anti-(human vascular endothelial growth factor (VEGF)) Fab fragment (human-mouse monoclonal rhuFAB V2γ1-chain) with disulfide bond to human-mouse rhuFAB V2 light chain. Molecular weight approximately 48,000 daltons.

Use Characteristics

Indications: To treat patients with neovascular (wet) age-related macular degeneration.

Contraindications:

Absolute: People with ocular or periocular infections.

Relative: People with known hypersensitivity to ranibizumab or any of the excipients.

Elderly: In clinical studies, approximately 94% (822 of 879) of ranibizumab-treated patients were 65 years of age or older and approximately 68% (601 of 879) were 75 years of age or older. No notable difference in treatment effect was seen with increasing age in any study. Age did not have a significant effect on systemic exposure in a population pharmacokinetic analysis after correcting for creatinine clearance.

Carcinogenicity: Ranibizumab has not been evaluated for carcinogenic potential.

Mutagenicity: Ranibizumab has not been evaluated for mutagenic potential.

Fertility Impairment: Ranibizumab has not been evaluated for impairment of fertility.

Pregnancy: Category C. Use only if clearly needed. It is not known if ranibizumab crosses the placenta. Generally, most IgG passage across the placenta occurs during the third trimester. Animal reproduction studies have not been conducted with ranibizumab.

Lactation: It is not known if ranibizumab crosses into human breast milk. Because many drugs are excreted in human milk and because the potential for absorption and harm to infant growth and development exists, exercise caution when ranibizumab is administered to a breast-feeding woman.

Children: Safety and efficacy of ranibizumab in children younger than 18 years of age have not been established.

Adverse Reactions:

Safety data: In 3 double-masked, controlled studies, 874 patients treated with ranibizumab for neovascular age-related macular degeneration with dosage regimens of 0.3 mg (375 patients) or 0.5 mg (379 patients) administered monthly by intravitreal injection (studies 1 and 2), and dosage regimens of 0.3 mg (59 patients) or 0.5 mg (61 patients) administered once a month for 3 consecutive doses followed by a dose administered once every 3 months (study 3).

The most frequently reported ocular adverse events with ranibizumab treatment that occurred at a higher incidence in the ranibizumab group appear in the following table. The ranges represent the minimum and maximum rates across all 3 studies for control patients, and across all 3 studies and both dose groups for ranibizumab.

Most Frequently Reported Ocular Adverse Events Reported With Ranibizumab (Humanized)		
Adverse Event	Ranibizumab (Humanized)	Control
Conjunctival hemorrhage	43% to 77%	29% to 66%
Eye pain	17% to 37%	11% to 33%
Vitreous floaters	3% to 32%	3% to 10%
Intraocular pressure increased	8% to 24%	3% to 7%
Foreign body sensation in eyes	6% to 19%	6% to 14%
Eye irritation	4% to 19%	6% to 20%
Intraocular inflammation	5% to 18%	3% to 11%
Lacrimation increased	3% to 17%	0% to 16%
Cataract	5% to 16%	6% to 16%
Visual disturbance	0% to 14%	2% to 9%
Blepharitis	3% to 13%	4% to 9%
Eye pruritus	0% to 13%	3% to 12%
Retinal disorder	0% to 13%	0% to 9%
Retinal degeneration	1% to 11%	1% to 7%
Ocular hyperemia	5% to 10%	1% to 10%
Maculopathy	3% to 10%	3% to 11%
Dry eye	3% to 10%	5% to 8%
Conjunctival hyperemia	0% to 9%	0% to 7%
Ocular discomfort	0% to 8%	0% to 5%
Posterior capsule opacification	0% to 8%	0% to 5%
Injection-site hemorrhage	0% to 5%	0% to 2%
Vitreous hemorrhage	0% to 4%	1% to 3%

The most frequently reported nonocular adverse events with ranibizumab treatment that occurred at a higher incidence in the ranibizumab group appear in the following table. The ranges represent the minimum and maximum rates across all 3 studies for control patients, and across all 3 studies and both dose groups for ranibizumab.

Most Frequently Reported Nonocular Adverse Events With Ranibizumab (Humanized)		
Adverse Event	Ranibizumab	Control
Hypertension/elevated blood pressure	5% to 23%	8% to 23%
Nasopharyngitis	5% to 16%	5% to 13%
Headache	2% to 15%	3% to 10%
Arthralgia	3% to 11%	0% to 9%
Bronchitis	3% to 10%	2% to 8%
Cough	3% to 10%	2% to 7%
Influenza	2% to 10%	1% to 5%
Nausea	2% to 9%	4% to 6%
Anemia	3% to 8%	0% to 8%
Sinusitis	2% to 8%	4% to 6%
Hypercholesterolemia	1% to 8%	2% to 5%
Insomnia	1% to 6%	1% to 6%
Atrial fibrillation	0% to 5%	2% to 4%

Most Frequently Reported Nonocular Adverse Events With Ranibizumab (Humanized)		
Adverse Event	Ranibizumab	Control
Dyspnea	0% to 5%	1% to 3%
Chronic obstructive pulmonary disease	0% to 5%	0% to 2%
Herpes zoster	0% to 5%	0% to 2%
Diabetes mellitus	0% to 5%	0% to 1%
Fall	1% to 4%	1% to 4%
Gastroenteritis, viral	0% to 4%	0% to 2%

Ophthalmic: Intravitreal injections, including those with ranibizumab, have been associated with endophthalmitis and retinal detachments. Increases in intraocular pressure have occurred within 60 minutes of intravitreal ranibizumab injection. Monitor intraocular pressure and perfusion of the optic nerve head.

Serious adverse events related to injection, including endophthalmitis, rhegmatogenous retinal detachments, and iatrogenic traumatic cataracts occurred in less than 0.1% of intravitreal injections.

Cardiovascular: The rate of arterial thromboembolic events in the 3 studies in the first year was 2.1% (18 out of 874) of patients treated with ranibizumab, compared with 1.1% (5 out of 441) of patients in the control arms. In the second year of study 1, the rate of arterial thromboembolic events was 3% (14 out of 466) of patients in the combined group of patients treated with ranibizumab, compared with 3.2% (7 out of 216) of patients in the control arm. There is a theoretical risk of arterial thromboembolic events after intravitreal use of VEGF inhibitors.

Immunologic: The pretreatment rate of immunoreactivity to ranibizumab was 0% to 3% across treatment groups. After monthly dosing with ranibizumab for 12 to 24 months, low titers of anti-ranibizumab antibodies were detected in 1% to 6% of patients. Immunogenicity data reflect an electrochemiluminescence assay, highly dependent on the sensitivity and specificity of the assay. The clinical significance of immunoreactivity to ranibizumab is unclear, although some patients with the highest levels of immunoreactivity were noted to have iritis or vitreitis.

Pharmacologic & Dosing Characteristics

Dosage: 0.5 mg per 0.05 mL, administered by intravitreal injection once a month. Withdraw entire vial contents through the filter needle attached to a 1 mL syringe. Then discard the filter needle and replace it with a 30-gauge, ½-inch needle for intravitreal injection.

Although less effective, treatment may be reduced to 1 injection every 3 months after the first 4 injections if monthly injections are not feasible. Compared with continued monthly dosing, dosing every 3 months will lead to approximately 5-letter (1-line) loss of visual acuity benefit, on average, over the following 9 months.

Route & Site: For ophthalmic intravitreal injection only.

Overdosage: Initial single doses of ranibizumab injection 1 mg were associated with intraocular inflammation in 2 of 2 patients injected. With an escalating regimen of doses beginning with initial 0.3 mg ranibizumab doses, doses as high as 2 mg were tolerated in 15 of 20 patients.

Dose Preparation:

Special handling: Conduct intravitreal injection under controlled aseptic conditions, using sterile gloves, a sterile drape, and a sterile eyelid speculum (or equivalent). Provide adequate anesthesia and a broad-spectrum microbicide before injection.

Monitor: After intravitreal injection, monitor patients for elevation in intraocular pressure and for endophthalmitis (eg, red eye, sensitivity to light, pain, change in vision). Monitoring may consist of a check for perfusion of the optic nerve head immediately after the injection, tonometry within 30 minutes after injection, and biomicroscopy between 2 and 7 days after injection. Instruct patients to report any symptoms suggestive of endophthalmitis without delay. Evaluate patients regularly during therapy. Use each vial to treat only a single eye. If the contralateral eye requires treatment, use a new vial and change the sterile field, syringe, gloves, drapes, eyelid speculum, filter, and injection needles.

Missed Doses: Interrupting the recommended schedule or delaying subsequent doses does not require restarting the series.

Related Interventions: Ranibizumab intravitreal injection has been used adjunctively with verteporfin photodynamic therapy. Twelve of 105 (11%) patients developed serious intraocular inflammation; in 10 of the 12 patients, this occurred when ranibizumab was administered 7 days (± 2 days) after verteporfin photodynamic therapy.

Efficacy: The safety and efficacy of ranibizumab were assessed in 3 randomized, double-masked, sham- or active-controlled studies in patients with neovascular age-related macular degeneration. A total of 1,323 patients (879 ranibizumab, 444 control) were enrolled in the 3 studies. In study 1, patients with minimally classic or occult (without classic) choroidal neovascularization lesions received monthly ranibizumab 0.3 or 0.5 mg intravitreal injections or monthly sham injections. Data are available through month 24. Patients treated with ranibizumab in study 1 received a mean of 22 total treatments out of a possible 24 from day 0 to month 24.

In study 2, patients with predominantly classic choroidal neovascularization lesions received: 1) monthly ranibizumab 0.3 mg and sham photodynamic therapy; 2) monthly ranibizumab 0.5 mg and sham photodynamic therapy; or 3) sham intravitreal injections and active verteporfin photodynamic therapy. Sham photodynamic therapy (or active verteporfin photodynamic therapy) was given with the initial ranibizumab (or sham) injection and every 3 months thereafter if fluorescein angiography showed persistence or recurrence of leakage. Data are available through month 12. Patients treated with ranibizumab in study 2 received a mean of 12 total treatments out of a possible 13 from day 0 through month 12. In both studies, the primary efficacy end point was the proportion of patients who maintained vision, defined as losing fewer than 15 letters of visual acuity at 12 months compared with baseline. Almost 95% of ranibizumab-treated patients maintained their visual acuity; 34% to 40% of ranibizumab-treated patients experienced a clinically significant improvement in vision, defined as gaining 15 or more letters at 12 months. The size of the lesion did not significantly affect the results. Detailed results appear in the following table.

Outcomes at Month 12 and Month 24 in Study 1				
Outcome measure	Month	Sham (n = 238)	Ranibizumab 0.5 mg (n = 240)	Estimated difference (95% CI)[a]
Loss of < 15 letters in visual acuity (%)[b]	Month 12	62%	95%	32% (26%, 39%)
	Month 24	53%	90%	37% (29%, 44%)
Gain of ≥ 15 letters in visual acuity (%)[b]	Month 12	5%	34%	29% (22%, 35%)
	Month 24	4%	33%	29% (23%, 35%)

Outcomes at Month 12 and Month 24 in Study 1				
Outcome measure	Month	Sham (n = 238)	Ranibizumab 0.5 mg (n = 240)	Estimated difference (95% CI)[a]
Mean change in visual acuity (letters) (SD)[b]	Month 12	−10.5 (16.6)	+7.2 (14.4)	17.5 (14.8, 20.2)
	Month 24	−14.9 (18.7)	+6.6 (16.5)	21.1 (18.1, 24.2)

a Adjusted estimate based on the stratified model.
b P < 0.01.

Outcomes at Month 12 in Study 2			
Outcome measure	Verteporfin PDT[a] (n = 143)	Ranibizumab 0.5 mg (n =140)	Estimated difference (95% CI)[b]
Loss of < 15 letters in visual acuity (%)[c]	64%	96%	33% (25%, 41%)
Gain of ≥ 15 letters in visual acuity (%)[c]	6%	40%	35% (26%, 44%)
Mean change in visual acuity (letters) (SD)[c]	−9.5 (16.4)	+11.3 (14.6)	21.1 (17.5, 24.6)

a Photodynamic therapy.
b Adjusted estimate based on the stratified model.
c P < 0.01.

Ranibizumab-treated patients had minimal observable choroidal neovascularization lesion growth. At month 12, the mean change in the total area of the choroidal neovascularization lesion was 0.1 to 0.3 DA for ranibizumab versus 2.3 to 2.6 DA for the control arms.

The use of ranibizumab beyond 24 months has not been studied.

Study 3 was a randomized, double-masked, sham-controlled, 2-year study assessing ranibizumab in patients with neovascular age-related macular degeneration (with or without a classic choroidal neovascularization component). Data are available through month 12. Patients received ranibizumab 0.3 or 0.5 mg or sham injections once a month for 3 consecutive doses, followed by a dose administered once every 3 months. One hundred eighty-four patients were enrolled in this study (ranibizumab 0.3 mg, 60; ranibizumab 0.5 mg, 61; sham, 63); 171 (93%) completed 12 months of this study. Ranibizumab-treated patients in study 3 received a mean of 6 total treatments out of a possible 6 from day 0 through month 12.

In study 3, the primary efficacy end point was mean change in visual acuity at 12 months compared with baseline. After an initial increase in visual acuity (following monthly dosing), on average, patients dosed once every 3 months with ranibizumab lost visual acuity, returning to baseline at month 12. In study 3, 90% of ranibizumab-treated patients maintained visual acuity at month 12.

Onset: Improved visual acuity with monthly dosing is evident within approximately 2 months of ranibizumab therapy (studies 1 and 2).

Pharmacokinetics: In animal studies, after intravitreal injection, ranibizumab was cleared from the vitreous with a half-life of approximately 3 days. After reaching a maximum at approximately 1 day, the serum concentration of ranibizumab declined in parallel with the vitreous concentration. In these animal studies, systemic exposure of ranibizumab was more than 2,000-fold lower than in the vitreous. In patients with neovascular age-related macular degeneration following monthly intravitreal administration, maximum ranibizumab serum concentrations were low (0.3 to 2.36 ng/mL). These levels were less than the concentration of

Ranibizumab (Humanized)

ranibizumab (11 to 27 ng/mL) thought necessary to inhibit VEGF-A by 50%, as measured in an in vitro cellular proliferation assay. The maximum serum concentration was dose-proportional over the dose range of 0.05 to 1 mg per eye. Based on a population pharmacokinetic analysis, maximum serum concentrations of 1.5 ng/mL are predicted to be reached at approximately 1 day after monthly intravitreal administration of ranibizumab 0.5 mg per eye. Based on the disappearance of ranibizumab from serum, the estimated average vitreous elimination half-life was approximately 9 days. Steady-state minimum concentration is predicted to be 0.22 ng/mL with a monthly dosing regimen. In humans, serum ranibizumab concentrations are predicted to be approximately 90,000-fold lower than vitreal concentrations.

Renal: No formal studies have been conducted to examine the pharmacokinetics of ranibizumab in patients with renal impairment. Sixty-eight percent of (136 of 200) patients in the population pharmacokinetic analysis had renal impairment (46.5% mild, 20% moderate, and 1.5% severe). Reduction in ranibizumab clearance is minimal in patients with renal impairment and is considered clinically insignificant. Dose adjustment is not expected to be needed for patients with renal impairment.

Hepatic: No formal studies have been conducted to examine the pharmacokinetics of ranibizumab in patients with hepatic impairment. Dose adjustment is not expected to be needed for patients with hepatic dysfunction.

Pharmacodynamics: Neovascular age-related macular degeneration is associated with foveal retinal thickening, as assessed by optical coherence tomography and leakage from choroidal neovascularization as assessed by fluorescein angiography. In study 3, foveal retinal thickness was assessed by optical coherence tomography in 118 of 184 patients. Optical coherence tomography measurements were collected at baseline, months 1, 2, 3, 5, 8, and 12. In ranibizumab-treated patients, foveal retinal thickness decreased, on average, more than the sham group from baseline through month 12. Retinal thickness decreased by month 1 and decreased further at month 3. Foveal retinal thickness data did not provide information useful in influencing treatment decisions. In ranibizumab-treated patients, the area of vascular leakage, on average, decreased by month 3, as assessed by fluorescein angiography. The area of vascular leakage for an individual patient was not correlated with visual acuity.

Mechanism: Ranibizumab binds to the receptor binding site of active forms of VEGF-A, including the cleaved form of this molecule, VEGF110. VEGF-A causes neovascularization and leakage in models of ocular angiogenesis and is thought to contribute to progression of neovascular age-related macular degeneration. Binding of ranibizumab to VEGF-A prevents the interaction of VEGF-A with its receptors (VEGFR1 and VEGFR2) on the surface of endothelial cells, reducing endothelial cell proliferation, vascular leakage, and new blood vessel formation.

Drug Interactions: Drug interaction studies have not been conducted with ranibizumab.

Pharmaceutical Characteristics

Concentration: 0.5 mg per 0.05 mL (ie, 10 mg/mL)

Packaging: Carton containing 1 single-use glass vial of ranibizumab, one 5-micron, 19-gauge, 1½-inch filter needle to withdraw vial contents, and one 30-gauge, ½-inch injection needle.

NDC Number: 50242-080-01

Doseform: Solution

Appearance: Colorless to pale yellow solution

Solvent: Water with 10 mM histidine hydrochloride, 10% α,α-trehalose dihydrate, and 0.01% polysorbate 20 per 0.05 mL vial

Adjuvant: None

Preservative: None

Ranibizumab (Humanized)

Allergens: None

Excipients: The nutrient system contains the antibiotic tetracycline. Tetracycline is not detectable in the final product.

pH: 5.5

Shelf Life: Data not provided.

Storage/Stability: Store at 2° to 8°C (36° to 46°F). Protect vials from light. Do not freeze. Contact the manufacturer regarding exposure to freezing or elevated temperatures. Shipping data not provided.

Handling: Withdraw entire contents (0.2 mL) of the vial through a 5-micron, 19-gauge filter needle attached to a 1 mL tuberculin syringe; then discard the filter needle and replace it with a 30-gauge, ½-inch needle for intravitreal injection. Expel contents until the plunger tip is aligned with the line that marks 0.05 mL on the syringe.

Production Process: Produced by an *Escherichia coli* expression system in a nutrient medium.

Media: *E. coli* expression system

Disease Epidemiology

Incidence: 155,000 Americans are diagnosed each year with age-related macular degeneration. Wet age-related macular degeneration, which accounts for 10% of all age-related macular degeneration, is responsible for 80% of the associated vision loss. Vision loss in wet age-related macular degeneration is caused by the growth of abnormal leaky blood vessels that eventually damage the area of the eye responsible for central vision.

Other Information

First Licensed: June 30, 2006.

References: Dugel PU. Ranibizumab treatment of patients with ocular diseases. *Int Ophthalmol Clin.* 2006;46(4):131-140.

Ferrara N, Damico L, Shams N, Lowman H, Kim R. Development of ranibizumab, an anti-vascular endothelial growth factor antigen binding fragment, as therapy for neovascular age-related macular degeneration. *Retina.* 2006;26(8):859-870.

Rosenfeld PJ, Rich RM, Lalwani GA. Ranibizumab: Phase III clinical trial results. *Ophthalmol Clin North Am.* 2006;19(3):361-372.

Comparison of Agents Used to Treat Macular Degeneration		
	Bevacizumab	Ranibizumab
Brand name	*Avastin*	*Lucentis*
Manufacturer	Genentech	Genentech
Antibody type	Humanized IgG1, 149 kilodaltons	Humanized IgG1-κ Fab, 48 kilodaltons
Activity	Binds VEGF	Binds VEGF-α
Labeled indication	Metastatic carcinoma of colon or rectum; non-small cell lung cancer	Age-related macular degeneration
Dosage, Route	5 to 15 mg/kg IV every 14 days	0.5 mg per 0.05 mL intravitreous monthly
Doseform	Solution	Solution
Concentration	25 mg/mL	10 mg/mL
Packaging	100 mg per 4 mL vial; 400 mg per 16 mL vial	2 mg per 0.2 mL vial
Solvent	Phosphate-buffered saline with trehalose	Sterile water with histidine and trehalose
Preservative	None	None
Routine storage	2° to 8°C	2° to 8°C

Rituximab (Chimeric)

Isoantibodies

Name:
   Rituxan

Manufacturer:
   Manufactured jointly by Biogen Idec and
   Genentech, Inc.

Synonyms: Anti-CD20 pan-B-cell monoclonal antibody, C2B8, IDEC-102, CAS 174722-31-7

Immunologic Characteristics

Target Antigen: CD20 antigen found on the surface of normal and malignant B lymphocytes. The antibody is produced by mammalian cell (Chinese hamster ovary) suspension culture.

Viability: Inactive, passive, transient

Antigenic Form: Chimeric (murine/human) monoclonal IgG1 antibody

Antigenic Type: Protein, IgG1κ immunoglobulin containing murine light- and heavy-chain variable region sequences and human constant region sequences, with a weight of 144,187 daltons. It consists of 2 heavy chains of 451 amino acids and 2 light chains of 213 amino acids, with a binding affinity for the CD20 antigen of approximately 8 nM.

Use Characteristics

Indications:

Non-Hodgkin's Lymphoma (NHL): To treat patients with relapsed or refractory, low-grade or follicular, CD20-positive, B-cell NHL as a single agent; previously untreated follicular, CD20-positive, B-cell NHL combined with first-line chemotherapy and, in patients achieving a complete or partial response to rituximab combined with chemotherapy, as single-agent maintenance therapy; non-progressing (including stable disease), low-grade, CD20-positive, B-cell NHL as a single agent after first-line CVP chemotherapy; and previously untreated diffuse large B-cell, CD20-positive NHL combined with CHOP or other anthracycline-based chemotherapy regimens.

Chronic Lymphocytic Leukemia (CLL): Combined with fludarabine and cyclophosphamide (FC), to treat patients with previously untreated and previously treated CD20-positive CLL.

Rheumatoid Arthritis (RA): Combined with methotrexate, to treat adult patients with moderately- to severely- active rheumatoid arthritis who had an inadequate response to one or more TNF-antagonist therapies.

Wegener's Granulomatosis (WG) and Microscopic Polyangiitis (MPA): Combined with glucocorticoids, to treat adult patients.

Unlabeled Uses: Research in progress is assessing the role of rituximab in the treatment of HIV-associated lymphomas.

Contraindications:

Absolute: Patients with known type I (immediate) hypersensitivity or anaphylactic reactions to murine proteins or to any component of this product.

Relative: None known

Elderly: Among 331 patients enrolled in clinical studies of rituximab, 24% were 65 to 75 years of age and 5% were 75 years of age or older. The overall response rates were higher in patients 65 years of age or older, compared with younger patients (52% vs 44%). However, the median duration of response was shorter in older patients (10.1 vs 11.4 months). This shorter duration was not statistically significant. Adverse reactions, including incidence, severity, and type of adverse reaction, were similar in both groups.

Fertility Impairment: Advise patients of childbearing potential to use effective contraceptive methods during treatment and for up to 12 months after therapy.

Pregnancy: Category C. It is not known whether rituximab can cause fetal harm or affect reproductive capacity. Human IgG can cross the placenta, especially in the third trimester. It may potentially cause fetal B-cell depletion. Therefore, give rituximab to a pregnant woman only if clearly needed.

Lactation: It is not known whether rituximab is excreted in breast milk. Because human IgG is excreted in breast milk and the potential for absorption and immunosuppression in the infant is unknown, advise women to discontinue nursing until circulating drug levels are no longer detectable.

Children: The safety and efficacy of rituximab in children have not been established.

Adverse Reactions: Safety data are based on 315 patients treated in 5 studies. This includes patients with bulky disease (lesions larger than 10 cm), patients who have received more than 1 course of rituximab, and patients who were receiving 375 mg/m^2 for 8 doses.

Deaths within 24 hours of rituximab infusion have been reported. These fatal reactions followed reactions that included hypoxia, pulmonary infiltrates, acute respiratory distress syndrome, myocardial infarction, ventricular fibrillation, or cardiogenic shock. About 80% of fatal infusion reactions occurred in association with the first infusion.

Severe and life-threatening events (grade 3 or 4) were reported in 10% of patients. The following adverse events were reported: Neutropenia (1.9%); chills (1.6%); leukopenia, thrombocytopenia (1.3% for each); hypotension, anemia, bronchospasm, urticaria (1% for each); headache, abdominal pain, arrhythmia (0.6% for each); asthenia, hypertension, nausea, vomiting, coagulation disorder, angioedema, arthralgia, pain, rhinitis, increased cough, dyspnea, bronchiolitis obliterans, hypoxia, asthma, pruritus, rash (each occurring in 1 patient; 0.3% each).

The following adverse events occurred in at least 1% but no more than 5% of patients, in order of decreasing incidence: Flushing, arthralgia, diarrhea, anemia, cough, hypertension, lacrimation disorder, pain, hyperglycemia, back pain, peripheral edema, paresthesia, dyspepsia, chest pain, anorexia, anxiety, malaise, tachycardia, agitation, insomnia, sinusitis, conjunctivitis, abdominal enlargement, postural hypotension, LDH increase, hypocalcemia, hypesthesia, respiratory disorder, tumor pain, pain at injection site, bradycardia, hypertonia, nervousness, bronchitis, and taste perversion.

Bulky disease: The proportion of patients reporting any adverse event was similar in patients with bulky disease and those with lesions smaller than 10 cm in diameter. However, the rate of dizziness, neutropenia, thrombocytopenia, myalgia, anemia, and chest pain was higher in patients with lesions larger than 10 cm. The incidence of any grade 3 and 4 event was higher (31% vs 13%), and the incidence of grade 3 or 4 neutropenia, anemia, hypotension, and dyspnea was also higher in patients with bulky disease, compared with patients with lesions smaller than 10 cm.

Infection: Serious, including fatal, bacterial, fungal, and new or reactivated viral infections can occur during and up to 1 year after completing rituximab-based therapy. New or reactivated viral infections included cytomegalovirus, herpes simplex virus, parvovirus B19, varicella zoster virus, West Nile virus, hepatitis B, and hepatitis C. Discontinue rituximab for serious infections and institute appropriate anti-infective therapy. Hepatitis B virus (HBV) reactivation with fulminant hepatitis, hepatic failure, and death can occur in patients with hematologic malignancies treated with rituximab. The median time to the diagnosis of hepatitis was about 4 months after starting rituximab and about 1 month after the last dose. Screen patients at high risk of HBV infection before initiation of rituximab. Closely monitor carriers of hepatitis B for clinical and laboratory signs of active HBV infection for several months after rituximab therapy. Discontinue rituximab and any concomitant chemotherapy in patients who develop viral hepatitis, and institute appropriate treatment including antiviral therapy. Insufficient data exist regarding the safety of resuming rituximab in patients who develop hepatitis subsequent to HBV reactivation.

Leukoencephalopathy: JC virus infection resulting in progressive multifocal leukoencephalopathy (PML) and death can occur in rituximab-treated patients with hematologic malignancies or with autoimmune diseases. Most patients with hematologic malignancies diagnosed with PML received rituximab in combination with chemotherapy or as part of a hematopoietic stem cell transplant. The patients with autoimmune diseases had prior or concurrent immunosuppressive therapy. Most cases of PML were diagnosed within 12 months of their last infusion of rituximab. Consider a PML diagnosis in any patient presenting with new-onset neurologic manifestations. Evaluation of PML includes consultation with a neurologist, brain MRI, and lumbar puncture. Discontinue rituximab and consider discontinuation or reduction of any concomitant chemotherapy or immunosuppressive therapy in patients who develop PML.

Body as a whole: An infusion-related symptom complex consisting of fever and chills/rigors occurred in the majority of patients during the first rituximab infusion. Other frequent infusion-related symptoms included nausea, urticaria, fatigue, headache, pruritus, bronchospasm, dyspnea, sensation of tongue or throat swelling (angioedema), rhinitis, vomiting, hypotension, flushing, and pain at disease sites. These reactions generally occurred within 30 minutes to 2 hours of beginning the first infusion and resolved with slowing or interrupting the infusion and with supportive care (eg, IV saline, diphenhydramine, acetaminophen).

The incidence of infusion-related events decreased from 80% (7%, grade 3/4) during the first infusion to approximately 40% (5% to 10%, grade 3/4) with later infusions. Mild to moderate hypotension requiring interruption of infusion with or without giving IV saline occurred in 32 (10%) patients. Isolated severe reactions requiring epinephrine have been reported in patients receiving rituximab for other indications. Angioedema was reported in 41 (13%) patients and was serious in 1 patient. Bronchospasm occurred in 25 (8%) patients; 25% of these patients were treated with bronchodilators. A single report of bronchiolitis obliterans was noted.

Interrupt rituximab infusion if severe reactions occur. Infusions can be resumed at a 50% reduction in rate (eg, from 100 to 50 mg/h) when symptoms completely resolve. These symptoms can be treated with diphenhydramine and acetaminophen; bronchodilators or IV saline may be needed. In most cases, patients who have experienced non-life-threatening reactions have been able to complete the full course of therapy.

Discontinue infusions if serious or life-threatening cardiac arrhythmias occur. Patients who develop clinically significant arrhythmias need cardiac monitoring during and after subsequent infusions of rituximab. Patients with preexisting cardiac conditions, including arrhythmias and angina, have had recurrences of these events during rituximab therapy. Monitor these patients throughout and immediately after infusion.

Cardiovascular: Four patients developed arrhythmias during rituximab infusion. One discontinued treatment because of ventricular tachycardia and supraventricular tachycardia. The other 3 experienced trigeminy or irregular pulse and did not require discontinuation. Angina was reported during infusion, and MI occurred 4 days after infusion in 1 subject with a history of MI.

Dermatologic: Severe mucocutaneous reactions, some fatal, have been reported in association with rituximab treatment. These reports include paraneoplastic pemphigus, Stevens-Johnson syndrome, lichenoid dermatitis, vesiculobullous dermatitis, and toxic epidermal necrolysis. The onset of the reaction varied from 1 to 13 weeks after rituximab exposure.

Do not administer further infusions to patients experiencing a severe mucocutaneous reaction. Seek prompt medical evaluation. Skin biopsy may help distinguish among different mucocutaneous reactions and guide subsequent treatment. Safety of readministration of rituximab to patients with any of these reactions has not been determined.

Hematologic: Severe thrombocytopenia occurred in 1.3% of patients treated with rituximab, severe neutropenia occurred in 1.9%, and severe anemia occurred in 1%. A single case of transient aplastic anemia (pure red cell aplasia) and 2 cases of hemolytic anemia after therapy were reported.

Immunologic: Rituximab induced B-cell depletion in 70% to 80% of patients and was associated with decreased serum immunoglobulins in a minority of patients. The lymphopenia persisted a median of 14 days. Infectious events occurred in 31% of patients. Serious infectious events, including sepsis, occurred in 2% of patients. Of the serious infectious events, none were associated with neutropenia. The serious bacterial events included sepsis due to *Listeria*, staphylococcal bacteremia, or polymicrobial sepsis. Significant viral infections included herpes simplex infections (n = 2) and herpes zoster (n = 3).

Miscellaneous: Among 21 patients who received more than 1 course of rituximab, the fraction of patients reporting any adverse event upon re-treatment was similar to the percentage of patients reporting adverse events upon initial exposure. The following events were reported more frequently in retreated subjects: asthenia, throat irritation, flushing, tachycardia, anorexia, leukopenia, thrombocytopenia, anemia, peripheral edema, dizziness, depression, respiratory symptoms, night sweats, and pruritus.

Renal: Acute renal failure, sometimes fatal, that requires dialysis has been reported in the setting of tumor lysis syndrome (TLS) within 12 to 24 hours after first treatment with rituximab. Other features included hypocalcemia, hyperuricemia, or hyperphosphatemia. The risk of TLS appears to be greater in patients with 25,000 or more circulating malignant cells/mm^3 or high tumor burden. Consider prophylaxis for TLS in patients at high risk. Correct electrolyte abnormalities, monitor renal function and fluid balance, and administer supportive care as indicated. After complete resolution of the complications of TLS, rituximab has been tolerated when readministered with prophylactic therapy for TLS in a limited number of cases.

Pharmacologic & Dosing Characteristics

Dosage:

Non-Hodgkin lymphoma: The recommended dosage of rituximab is 375 mg/m^2 given as an IV infusion once weekly for 4 or 8 doses.

Re-treatment therapy: Patients who subsequently develop progressive disease may be safely retreated with rituximab 375 mg/m^2 IV infusion once weekly for 4 doses. Currently, there are limited data on administering more than 2 courses.

Diffuse large B-cell NHL: The recommended dosage is 375 mg/m^2 IV preinfusion, given on day 1 of each cycle of chemotherapy for up to 8 infusions.

Chronic lymphocytic leukemia: 375 mg/m^2 the day before starting FC chemotherapy, then 500 mg/m^2 on day 1 of cycles 2 through 6 (every 28 days).

Rheumatoid arthritis: Two, 1,000 mg IV infusions separated by 2 weeks. Glucocorticoids administered as methylprednisolone 100 mg IV or its equivalent 30 minutes before each infusion are recommended to reduce incidence and severity of infusion reactions. Administer subsequent courses every 24 weeks or based on clinical evaluation, but not sooner than every 16 weeks. Rituximab is given in combination with methotrexate.

Route: IV infusion. Rituximab may be administered in an outpatient setting. Do not administer as an IV push or bolus. Do not mix or dilute rituximab with other drugs.

First infusion: Administer the solution for infusion at an initial rate of 50 mg/h. If hypersensitivity or infusion-related events do not occur, increase the rate in 50 mg/h increments every 30 minutes, to a maximum of 400 mg/h. If an adverse event develops, temporarily slow or interrupt the infusion. The infusion can continue at half the previous rate upon improvement of symptoms.

Subsequent infusions: Subsequent doses can be started at an initial rate of 100 mg/h and increased by 100 mg/h increments at 30-minute intervals, to a maximum of 400 mg/h, as tolerated.

Overdosage: There has been no experience with overdosage in human clinical trials. Single doses over 500 mg/m^2 have not been tested.

Monitor: Obtain complete blood counts (CBC) and platelet counts at regular intervals during rituximab therapy and more frequently in patients who develop cytopenias.

Related Interventions: Consider premedication with acetaminophen and diphenhydramine before each infusion of rituximab. Premedication may attenuate infusion-related events. Because transient hypotension may occur during rituximab infusion, consider withholding antihypertensive medications 12 hours before rituximab infusion.

CLL: Pneumocystis jiroveci pneumonia (PCP) and anti-herpetic viral prophylaxis is recommended for patients with CLL during treatment and for up to 12 months after treatment as appropriate.

Efficacy: A study was conducted in 166 patients with relapsed or refractory low-grade or follicular B-cell non-Hodgkin lymphoma (NHL) who received 375 mg/m^2 of rituximab weekly for 4 doses. Patients with tumor masses larger than 10 cm or with more than 5,000 lymphocytes/mcL in peripheral blood were excluded. The overall response rate (ORR) was 48%, with a 6% complete response (CR) and a 42% partial response rate (PRR). Disease-related signs and symptoms were present in 23% of patients at study entry and resolved in 64% of those patients. The median time to onset of response was 50 days, and the median duration of response was projected to be 10 to 12 months. The ORR was higher in patients with International Working Formulation (IWF) B, C, and D histologic subtypes, in contrast to IWF A subtype (58% vs 12%), higher in patients whose largest lesion was smaller than 5 cm vs larger than 7 cm in greatest diameter (55% vs 38%), and higher in patients with chemosensitive relapse within 3 months as compared with chemoresistant (53% vs 36%). ORR in patients previously treated with autologous bone marrow transplant was 78%. The following factors were not associated with a lower response rate: older than 60 years of age, extranodal disease, prior anthracycline therapy, and bone marrow involvement.

In a second study, 37 patients with relapsed or refractory B-cell NHL received 375 mg/m^2 of rituximab weekly for 4 doses. The ORR was 46% with a median duration of response of 8.6 months (range, 2.6 to 26.2).

Thirty-seven patients with relapsed or refractory low-grade NHL received 375 mg/m^2 rituximab weekly for 8 doses. The overall response rate was 57% (14% complete response, 43% partial response) with a median duration of response of 13.4 months (range, 2.5 to 36 or more).

Thirty-nine patients with relapsed or refractory bulky disease (single lesion larger than 10 cm diameter) low-grade NHL received 375 mg/m^2 rituximab weekly for 4 doses. The overall response rate was 36% (3% complete response, 33% partial response) with a median duration of response of 6.9 months (range, 2.8 to 25 or more).

Sixty patients received 375 mg/m^2 rituximab weekly for 4 doses. All patients had relapsed or refractory low-grade or follicular B-cell NHL and achieved an objective clinical response to a prior course of rituximab. Of the 60 patients, 55 received their second course of rituximab, 3 patients received a third course, and 2 patients received their second and third courses in this study. The overall response rate was 38% (10% complete response, 28% partial response) with a median duration of response of 15 months (range, 3 to 25 or more).

Rheumatoid arthritis: Efficacy was evaluated in 517 adult patients with active disease (at least 8 swollen and 8 tender joints) receiving methotrexate who had inadequate response to at least 1 TNF inhibitor. Patients received two 1,000 mg doses or placebo as an IV infusion on days 1 and 15, in combination with continued methotrexate 10 to 25 mg weekly. Efficacy was assessed at 24 weeks: 51% in the rituximab-methotrexate arm versus 18% in the placebo-methotrexate arm achieved an ACR-20 response; 27% in the rituximab-methotrexate arm versus 5% in the placebo-methotrexate arm achieved an ACR-50 response; 12% in the rituximab-methotrexate arm versus 1% in the placebo-methotrexate arm achieved an ACR-70 response. Improvement was also noted for number of tender or swollen joints, physician global assessment, patient global assessment, pain, disability index, and C-reactive protein concentration.

Onset: Rituximab resulted in a rapid and sustained depletion of circulating and tissue-based B cells. Lymph node biopsies performed 14 days after therapy showed a decrease in the percentage of B cells in 7 of 8 patients who received single doses of rituximab larger than 100 mg/m^2. Among the 166 patients in the pivotal study, circulating B cells (measured as CD19-positive cells) were depleted within the first 3 doses, with sustained depletion for up to 9 months posttreatment in 83% of patients. One of the responding patients (1%) failed to show significant depletion of CD19-positive cells after the third infusion of rituximab, in contrast to 19% of the nonresponding patients.

Rheumatoid arthritis: Higher ACR-20 responses were observed by week 8 after a single course of treatment (ie, 2 infusions). Similar patterns were seen for ACR-50 and ACR-70 responses.

Duration: B-cell recovery began at approximately 6 months after completing treatment. Median B-cell levels returned to normal by 12 months after completing treatment. There were sustained and statistically significant reductions in IgM and IgG serum levels from 5 to 11 months after rituximab therapy. Only 14% of patients had reductions in IgG or IgM serum levels, resulting in values below normal.

Rheumatoid arthritis: Higher ACR-20 responses were maintained through week 24 after a single course of treatment (ie, 2 infusions). Similar patterns were seen for ACR-50 and ACR-70 responses. About 4% of RA patients had prolonged peripheral B-cell depletion lasting longer than 3 years after a single treatment.

Pharmacokinetics: Immunoglobulins are primarily eliminated by catabolism. In patients given single doses of 10, 50, 100, 250, or 500 mg/m^2 as an IV infusion, serum levels and the half-life of rituximab were proportional to dose. In 14 patients given 375 mg/m^2 as an IV infusion for 4 weekly doses, the mean serum half-life was 76 hours (range, 32 to 153 hours) after the first infusion and 206 hours (range, 84 to 407 hours) after the fourth infusion. The wide range of half-lives may reflect variable tumor burden among patients and changes in CD20-positive (normal and malignant) B-cell populations upon repeated administrations.

Rituximab 375 mg/m^2 was given as an IV infusion weekly for 4 doses to 203 patients naive to rituximab. The mean C_{max} after the fourth infusion was 486 mcg/mL (range, 78 to 997 mcg/mL). The peak and trough serum levels of rituximab were inversely correlated with baseline values for the number of circulating CD20-positive B cells and measures of disease burden. Median steady-state serum levels were higher for responders, compared with nonresponders. However, no difference was found in rate of elimination measured by serum half-life. Serum levels were higher in patients with IWF subtypes B, C, and D, compared with those with subtype A. Rituximab was detectable in serum of patients 3 to 6 months after completing treatment.

Rituximab at a dose of 375 mg/m^2 was administered as an IV infusion weekly for 8 doses to 37 patients. The mean C_{max} after 8 infusions was 550 mcg/mL (range, 171 to 1,177 mcg/mL). The mean C_{max} increased with each successive infusion through the eighth infusion (from 243 to 550 mcg/mL).

The pharmacokinetic profile of rituximab, when administered as 6 infusions of 375 mg/m² in combination with 6 cycles of CHOP chemotherapy, was similar to that seen with rituximab alone.

Rheumatoid arthritis: After administration of 2 doses of rituximab in patients with RA, the mean C_{max} values were 183 mcg/mL (CV = 24%) for the 2 × 500 mg dose and 370 mcg/mL (CV = 25%) for the 2 × 1,000 mg dose, respectively. Following the 2 × 1,000 mg dose, mean volume of distribution at steady state was 4.3 L (CV = 28%). Mean systemic serum clearance of rituximab was 0.01 L/h (CV = 38%) and mean terminal elimination half-life after the second dose was 19 days (CV = 32%). Female patients (n = 86) had a 37% lower clearance of rituximab than male RA patients (n = 25). This gender difference does not necessitate dose adjustment, because safety and efficacy do not appear to be influenced by gender.

Serum neutralizing activity: Human antimurine antibody (HAMA) was not detected in 67 patients evaluated. Four of 356 patients evaluated for human antichimeric antibody (HACA) were positive, and 3 had an objective clinical response. Patients who develop HAMA or HACA titers may have allergic or hypersensitivity reactions when treated with this or other murine or chimeric monoclonal antibodies.

Mechanism: Rituximab binds specifically to the antigen CD20 (human B-lymphocyte-restricted differentiation antigen, Bp35), a hydrophobic transmembrane protein on premature and mature B lymphocytes. The antigen is also expressed on more than 90% of B-cell non-Hodgkin lymphomas (NHL) but is not found on hematopoietic stem cells, pro-B cells, normal plasma cells, or other normal tissues. CD20 regulates early steps in the activation process for cell-cycle initiation and differentiation and possibly functions as a calcium ion channel. CD20 is not shed from the cell surface and does not internalize upon antibody binding. Free CD20 antigen is not found in the circulation.

The Fab domain of rituximab binds to the CD20 antigen on B lymphocytes. The Fc domain recruits immune effector functions to mediate B-cell lysis in vitro. Possible mechanisms of cell lysis include complement-dependent cytotoxicity and antibody-dependent cellular cytotoxicity. Rituximab can induce apoptosis in the DHL-4 human B-cell lymphoma line. Rituximab binding was observed on lymphoid cells in the thymus, the white pulp of the spleen, and a majority of B lymphocytes in peripheral blood and lymph nodes. Little or no binding was observed in nonlymphoid tissues.

Drug Interactions: No formal drug interaction studies have been performed with rituximab.

The safety of immunization with any vaccine, particularly live viral vaccines, following rituximab therapy has not been studied. The ability of rituximab recipients to generate a primary or anamnestic humoral response to any vaccine has also not been studied. For RA patients, follow current immunization guidelines and administer non-live vaccines at least 4 weeks before a course of rituximab. A response to pneumococcal polysaccharide vaccination (a T-cell independent antigen) as measured by an increase in antibody titers to at least 6 of 12 serotypes was lower in patients treated with rituximab plus methotrexate (MTX), compared to patients treated with MTX alone (19% vs. 61%). A lower proportion of patients in the rituximab plus MTX group developed detectable levels of anti-keyhole limpet hemocyanin antibodies (a novel protein antigen) after vaccination compared to patients on MTX alone (47% vs. 93%). A positive response to tetanus toxoid vaccine (a T-cell dependent antigen with existing immunity) was similar in patients treated with rituximab plus MTX compared to patients on MTX alone (39% vs. 42%). The proportion of patients maintaining a positive Candida skin test (to evaluate delayed-type hypersensitivity) was also similar (77% of patients on rituximab plus MTX vs. 70% of patients on MTX alone). Most patients in the rituximab-treated group had B-cell counts below the lower limit of normal at the time of immunization. The clinical implications of these findings are not known.

The effect of rituximab on immune responses was assessed in a randomized, controlled study in patients with RA treated with rituximab and MTX) compared to patients treated with MTX alone.

Most patients with hematologic malignancies diagnosed with PML received rituximab in combination with chemotherapy or as part of a hematopoietic stem cell transplant.

Pharmaceutical Characteristics

Concentration: 10 mg/mL

Packaging: Single-use 100 mg/10 mL vial (NDC#: 50242-051-21); single-use 500 mg/50 mL vial (50242-053-06)

Doseform: Solution for further dilution

Appearance: Clear, colorless liquid

Solvent: Buffered sodium chloride solution

Diluent:

For infusion: Dilute to a final concentration of 1 to 4 mg/mL in an infusion bag containing either 0.9% sodium chloride or 5% dextrose in water. Gently invert the bag to mix the solution.

Adjuvant: None

Preservative: None

Allergens: Gentamicin, used in the production process, is not detectable in the final product.

Excipients: 9 mg/mL sodium chloride, 7.35 mg/mL sodium citrate dihydrate, 0.7 mg/mL polysorbate 80

pH: 6.5

Shelf Life: Expires within 24 months

Storage/Stability: Store at 2° to 8°C (36° to 46°F). Discard frozen rituximab. Contact the manufacturer regarding exposure to extreme temperatures. Shipped at ambient temperatures via overnight courier. Protect rituximab vials from direct sunlight. Discard any unused portion.

Rituximab solutions for infusion are stable at 2° to 8°C (36° to 46°F) for 24 hours and at room temperature for an additional 24 hours. No incompatibilities between rituximab and polyvinylchloride or polyethylene bags have been observed.

Production Process: The chimeric (murine/human) anti-CD20 antibody is produced by mammalian cell (Chinese hamster ovary) suspension culture in a nutrient medium containing the antibiotic gentamicin, which is not detectable in the final product. The anti-CD20 antibody is purified by affinity and ion-exchange chromatography. Purification includes specific viral inactivation and removal.

Media: Chinese hamster ovary cell culture

Disease Epidemiology

Incidence: Most cases of non-Hodgkin lymphoma (NHL) are B-cell malignancies composed of clonal proliferations of B lymphocytes arrested at specific stages in the normal differentiation pathway. NHL is the sixth most common cause of cancer-related deaths in the United States. In 1997, approximately 53,600 cases of NHL were diagnosed in the United States. Approximately 23,000 people died of NHL in this country in 1997. Low-grade or follicular lymphomas account for approximately 43% of new cases of malignant B-cell lymphomas in North America and more than 65% of the prevalence. A variety of congenital and acquired immunodeficiency states, autoimmune disorders, infectious organisms, and physical or chemical agents have been associated with an increased risk of developing NHL.

Rituximab (Chimeric)

Prevalence: Approximately 240,000 Americans have B-cell NHL. Approximately 50% of these cases are of the low-grade or follicular subgroup. Patients with this type of NHL may remain in remission for years, but eventually have multiple recurrences of symptoms or relapses that occur with increasing frequency over the course of the disease.

Other Information

Perspective:
1994: Rituximab designated an orphan drug.

First Licensed: November 26, 1997

References: Demidem A, Lam T, Alas S, Hariharan K, Hanna N, Bonavida B. Chimeric anti-CD20 (IDEC-C2B8) monoclonal antibody sensitizes a B cell lymphoma cell line to cell killing by cytotoxic drugs. *Cancer Biother Radiopharm.* 1997;12:177-186.

Maloney DG, Grillo-Lopez AJ, White CA, et al. IDEC-C2B8 (Rituximab) anti-CD20 monoclonal antibody therapy in patients with relapsed low-grade non-Hodgkin's lymphoma. *Blood.* 1997;90:2188-2195.

Summers KM, Kockler DR. Rituximab treatment of refractory rheumatoid arthritis. *Ann Pharmacother.* 2005;39:2091-2095.

Tocilizumab (Humanized)

Name:
Actemra

Manufacturer:
Genentech

Synonyms: *RoActemra* (within the European Union)

Immunologic Characteristics

Target Antigen: Human interleukin 6 (IL-6)

Viability: Inactive, passive, transient

Antigenic Form: Humanized immunoglobulin

Antigenic Type: Protein, IgG-1κ antibody, monoclonal with typical H2L2 polypeptide structure. Each light chain and heavy chain consists of 214 and 448 amino acids, respectively, with a molecular weight of approximately 148 kilodaltons.

Use Characteristics

Indications: To treat adults with moderately to severely active rheumatoid arthritis (RA) who had an inadequate response to one or more tumor necrosis factor (TNF) antagonist therapies.

Limitations: Avoid using tocilizumab in combination with biological disease modifying antirheumatic drugs (DMARDs), such as TNF antagonists, interleukin-1 receptor (IL-1R) antagonists, anti-CD20 monoclonal antibodies, and selective costimulation modulators, because of the possibility of increased immunosuppression and increased risk of infection.

Do not start tocilizumab in patients with an absolute neutrophil count (ANC) less than 2,000 cells/mm^3, a platelet count less than 100,000 cells/mm^3, or in those who have ALT or AST greater than 1.5 times the upper limit of normal (ULN).

Contraindications: None

Elderly: Of 2,644 patients who received tocilizumab in studies 1 to 5, 435 patients with RA were older than 65 years of age, including 50 patients at least 75 years of age. The frequency of serious infection among subjects 65 years of age and older was higher than in those younger than 65 years of age. As there is a higher incidence of infection in the elderly population in general, use caution when treating these patients.

Carcinogenicity: No long-term animal studies have been performed to establish the carcinogenic potential of tocilizumab.

Mutagenicity: Tocilizumab was negative in the in vitro Ames bacterial reverse mutation assay and the in vitro chromosomal aberrations assay using human peripheral blood lymphocytes.

Fertility Impairment: Fertility studies conducted in male and female mice using a murine analog of tocilizumab showed no impairment of fertility.

Pregnancy: Category C. There are no adequate and well-controlled studies in pregnant women. Use tocilizumab during pregnancy only if the potential benefit justifies the potential risk to the fetus. In an embryo-fetal development toxicity study, pregnant cynomolgus monkeys were treated with intravenous (IV) tocilizumab (daily doses of 2, 10, or 50 mg/kg from gestation day 20 to 50) during organogenesis. Although there was no evidence for a teratogenic or dysmorphogenic effect at any dose, tocilizumab produced an increase in the incidence of abortion/embryo-fetal death at 10 and 50 mg/kg doses (1.25 and 6.25 times the human dose of 8 mg/kg every 4 weeks based on a mg/kg comparison).

Testing of a murine analog of tocilizumab in mice did not yield any evidence of harm to offspring during the pre- and postnatal development phase when dosed at 50 mg/kg IV, with treatment every 3 days from implantation until day 21 after delivery (weaning). There was no evidence for any functional impairment of the development and behavior, learning ability, immune competence, and fertility of the offspring.

To monitor the outcomes of pregnant women exposed to tocilizumab, a pregnancy registry has been established. To register, call 877-311-8972.

Lactation: It is not known whether tocilizumab crosses into human milk or is absorbed systemically after ingestion. Because many drugs are excreted in human milk, and because of the potential for serious adverse reactions in breast-feeding infants from tocilizumab, decide whether to discontinue breast-feeding or the drug, taking into account the importance of the drug to the mother.

Children: Safety and effectiveness of tocilizumab in pediatric patients have not been established.

Adverse Reactions: The following adverse reactions include data from 5 double-blind, controlled, multicenter studies. In these studies, patients received tocilizumab 8 mg/kg monotherapy (288 patients), tocilizumab 8 mg/kg in combination with DMARDs (including methotrexate) (1,582 patients), or tocilizumab 4 mg/kg in combination with methotrexate (774 patients).

The all-exposure population includes all patients in registration studies who received at least 1 dose of tocilizumab. Of these 4,009 patients, 3,577 received treatment for at least 6 months, 3,296 for at least 1 year, 2,806 for at least 2 years, and 1,222 for 3 years. All patients had moderately to severely active RA. The study population had a mean age of 52 years, 82% were female, and 74% were white.

The most common serious adverse reactions were infections. The most commonly reported adverse reactions in controlled studies up to 6 months' duration (occurring in at least 5% of patients treated with tocilizumab monotherapy or in combination with DMARDs) were upper respiratory tract infections, nasopharyngitis, headache, hypertension, and increased ALT. The proportion of patients who discontinued treatment because of any adverse reactions during the double-blind, placebo-controlled studies was 5% for patients taking tocilizumab and 3% for placebo-treated patients. The most common adverse reactions that required discontinuation of tocilizumab were increased hepatic transaminase values (per protocol requirement) and serious infections.

Infections: In the 6-month, controlled clinical studies, the rate of infections in the tocilizumab monotherapy group was 119 events per 100 patient-years, similar to the methotrexate monotherapy group. The rate of infections in the tocilizumab 4 and 8 mg/kg plus DMARD groups was 133 and 127 events per 100 patient-years, respectively, compared with 112 events per 100 patient-years in the placebo plus DMARD group. The most commonly reported infections (5% to 8% of patients) were upper respiratory tract infections and nasopharyngitis. The overall rate of infections with tocilizumab in the all-exposure population was 108 events per 100 patient-years.

Serious and sometimes fatal infections caused by bacterial, mycobacterial, invasive fungal, viral, protozoal, or other opportunistic pathogens have been reported in patients receiving immunosuppressive agents, including tocilizumab, for RA. The most common serious infections included pneumonia, urinary tract infection, cellulitis, herpes zoster, gastroenteritis, diverticulitis, sepsis, and bacterial arthritis. Among opportunistic infections, tuberculosis (TB), cryptococcosis, aspergillosis, candidiasis, and pneumocystosis were reported with tocilizumab. Other serious infections, not reported in clinical studies, may also occur (eg, histoplasmosis, coccidioidomycosis, listeriosis). Patients with disseminated rather than localized disease were often taking concomitant immunosuppressants, such as methotrexate or corticosteroids, which, in addition to RA, may predispose them to infections. In the 6-month, controlled clinical studies, the rate of serious infections in the tocilizumab monotherapy group was 3.6 per 100 patient-years compared with 1.5 per 100 patient-years in the methotrexate group. The rate of serious infections in the tocilizumab 4 and 8 mg/kg plus DMARD groups was 4.4 and 5.3 events per 100 patient-years, respectively, compared with 3.9 events per 100 patient-years in the placebo plus DMARD group. In the all-exposure population, the overall rate of serious infections was 4.7 events per 100 patient-years. The overall rate of fatal serious infections was 0.13 per 100 patient-years. Cases of opportunistic infections have been reported. If a serious infection develops, interrupt tocilizumab until the infection is controlled. Perform test for latent TB; if positive, start treatment for TB prior to starting tocilizumab. Monitor all patients for the development of signs and symptoms of infection during and after treatment with tocilizumab, as signs and symptoms of acute inflammation may be lessened because of suppression of the acute phase reactants. Viral reactivation has been reported with immunosuppressive biologic therapies, and cases of herpes zoster exacerbation were observed in clinical studies with tocilizumab. No cases of hepatitis B reactivation were observed in the trials; however, patients who screened positive for hepatitis were excluded.

GI: During the 6-month, controlled clinical trials, the overall rate of GI perforation was 0.26 events per 100 patient-years with tocilizumab therapy. In the all-exposure population, the overall rate of GI perforation was 0.28 events per 100 patient-years. GI perforation was primarily reported as complications of diverticulitis, including generalized purulent peritonitis, lower GI perforation, fistula, and abscess. Most patients who developed GI perforations were taking concomitant nonsteroidal anti-inflammatory drugs (NSAIDs), corticosteroids, or methotrexate. The relative contribution of these concomitant medications versus tocilizumab to the development of GI perforations is not known. Evaluate patients presenting with new-onset abdominal symptoms promptly for early identification of GI perforation.

Infusion: In the 6-month, controlled clinical studies, adverse events associated with the infusion (occurring during or within 24 hours of the start of infusion) were reported in 8% and 7% of patients in the tocilizumab 4 and 8 mg/kg plus DMARD groups, respectively, compared with 5% of patients in the placebo plus DMARD group. The most frequently reported event with the 4 and 8 mg/kg doses during the infusion was hypertension (1% for both doses), whereas the most frequently reported event occurring within 24 hours of finishing an infusion were headache (1% for both doses) and skin reactions (1% for both doses), including rash, pruritus, and urticaria. These events were not treatment limiting. Clinically significant hypersensitivity reactions (eg, anaphylactoid and anaphylactic reactions) associated with tocilizumab and requiring treatment discontinuation were reported in 0.1% (3/2,644) patients in the 6-month, controlled trials and in 0.2% (9/4,009) patients in the all-exposure population. These reactions were generally observed during the second to fourth infusion of tocilizumab.

Laboratory:

Neutrophils: Treatment with tocilizumab was associated with a higher incidence of neutropenia than with placebo. In the 6-month, controlled clinical studies, decreases in neutrophil counts less than 1,000 cells/mm^3 occurred in 1.8% and 3.4% of patients in the tocilizumab 4 and 8 mg/kg plus DMARD groups, respectively, compared with 0.1% of patients in the placebo plus DMARD group. Approximately half of the instances of ANC less than 1,000 cells/mm^3 occurred within 8 weeks of starting therapy. Decreases in neutrophil counts to less than 500 cells/mm^3 occurred in 0.4% and 0.3% of patients in the tocilizumab 4 and 8 mg/kg plus DMARD groups, respectively, compared with 0.1% of patients in the placebo plus DMARD group. There was no clear relationship between decreases in neutrophils to less than 1,000 cells/mm^3 and the occurrence of serious infections. In the all-exposure population, the pattern and incidence of decreases in neutrophil counts remained consistent with that seen in the 6-month, controlled clinical studies. Tocilizumab treatment should not be started in patients with a low neutrophil count (ie, ANC less than 2,000 cells/mm^3). In patients who develop an ANC less than 500 cells/mm^3, treatment is not recommended.

Platelets: Treatment with tocilizumab was associated with a reduction in platelet counts. In the 6-month, controlled clinical studies, decreases in platelet counts to less than 100,000 cells/mm^3 occurred in 1.3% and 1.7% of patients in the tocilizumab 4 and 8 mg/kg plus DMARD groups, respectively, compared with 0.5% of patients taking placebo plus DMARD, without associated bleeding events. In the all-exposure population, the pattern and incidence of decreases in platelet counts remained consistent with that seen in the 6-month, controlled clinical studies. Tocilizumab treatment should not be started in patients with platelet counts less than 100,000 cells/mm^3. In patients who develop platelet counts less than 50,000 cells/mm^3, treatment is not recommended.

Liver function tests: Treatment with tocilizumab was associated with a higher incidence of transaminase elevations than with placebo. Increased frequency and magnitude of these elevations were observed when potentially hepatotoxic drugs (eg, methotrexate) were used in combination with tocilizumab. Transaminases normalized when both treatments were withheld, but elevations recurred when methotrexate and tocilizumab were restarted at lower doses. Elevations resolved when methotrexate and tocilizumab were discontinued. In patients experiencing liver enzyme elevation, modification of treatment regimen, such as reduction in the dose of concomitant DMARD, interruption of tocilizumab, or reduction in tocilizumab dose, resulted in decrease or normalization of liver enzymes. These elevations were not associated with clinically relevant increases in direct bilirubin, nor were they associated with clinical evidence of hepatitis or hepatic insufficiency. Tocilizumab treatment should not be started in patients with elevated transaminases ALT or AST higher than 1.5 times ULN. In patients who develop elevated ALT or AST higher than 5 times ULN, treatment is not recommended.

	Incidence of Liver Enzyme Abnormalities in the 6-Month, Controlled Period of Studies 1 through 5				
	Tocilizumab 8 mg/kg monotherapy (n = 288)	Methotrexate (n = 284)	Tocilizumab 4 mg/kg + DMARDs (n = 774)	Tocilizumab 8 mg/kg + DMARDs (n = 1,582)	Placebo + DMARDs (n = 1,170)
AST (unit/liter)					
> ULN to 3 × ULN	22%	26%	34%	41%	17%
> 3 × ULN to 5 × ULN	0.3%	2%	1%	2%	0.3%
> 5 × ULN	0.7%	0.4%	0.1%	0.2%	< 0.1%
ALT (unit/liter)					
> ULN to 3 × ULN	36%	33%	45%	48%	23%
> 3 × ULN to 5 × ULN	1%	4%	5%	5%	1%
> 5 × ULN	0.7%	1%	1.3%	1.5%	0.3%

Lipids: Treatment with tocilizumab was associated with increases in lipid parameters, such as total cholesterol, triglycerides, low-density lipoprotein (LDL) cholesterol, and/or high-density lipoprotein (HDL) cholesterol. Elevations in lipid parameters (total cholesterol, LDL, HDL, triglycerides) were first assessed at 6 weeks after starting tocilizumab in 6-month, controlled clinical trials. Increases were observed at the 6-week assessment and remained stable thereafter. Increases in triglycerides levels to greater than 500 mg/dL were rarely observed. Changes in other lipid parameters from baseline to week 24 were evaluated. Mean LDL increased by 13 mg/dL in the tocilizumab

4 mg/kg plus DMARD group, 20 mg/dL in the tocilizumab 8 mg/kg plus DMARD group, and 25 mg/dL in tocilizumab 8 mg/kg monotherapy group. Mean HDL increased by 3 mg/dL in the tocilizumab 4 mg/kg plus DMARD group, 5 mg/dL in the tocilizumab 8 mg/kg plus DMARD group, and 4 mg/dL in tocilizumab 8 mg/kg monotherapy group. Mean LDL/HDL ratio increased by an average of 0.14 in the tocilizumab 4 mg/kg plus DMARD group, 0.15 in the tocilizumab 8 mg/kg plus DMARD group, and 0.26 in the tocilizumab 8 mg/kg monotherapy. Apolipoprotein (Apo) B/ApoA1 ratios were essentially unchanged in tocilizumab-treated patients. Elevated lipids responded to lipid-lowering agents.

Immunogenicity: In the 6-month, controlled clinical studies, 2,876 patients were tested for antitocilizumab antibodies. Forty-six (2%) patients developed antitocilizumab antibodies, of whom 5 had an associated, medically significant hypersensitivity reaction leading to withdrawal. Thirty (1%) patients developed neutralizing antibodies.

Malignancies: During the 6-month, controlled period of the studies, exposure-adjusted incidence was similar in the tocilizumab groups (1.32 events per 100 patient-years) and in the placebo plus DMARD group (1.37 events per 100 patient-years). In the all-exposure population, the rate of malignancies remained consistent (1.1 events per 100 patient-years) with the rate observed in the 6-month, controlled period.

Demyelinating disorders: The impact of treatment with tocilizumab on demyelinating disorders is not known, but multiple sclerosis and chronic inflammatory demyelinating polyneuropathy were reported rarely in clinical studies. Patients should be monitored closely for signs and symptoms potentially indicative of demyelinating disorders. Use caution in considering the use of tocilizumab in patients with preexisting or recent-onset demyelinating disorders.

Hepatic: Treatment with tocilizumab is not recommended in patients with active hepatic disease or hepatic impairment.

Other events: Adverse reactions occurring in at least 2% of patients on tocilizumab 4 or 8 mg/kg plus DMARD and at least 1% more than that observed in patients on placebo plus DMARD are summarized in this table.

Adverse Reactions Occurring in at Least 2% of Patients on Tocilizumab (Humanized) 4 or 8 mg/kg Plus DMARD[a]				
Preferred term	Tocilizumab 8 mg/kg monotherapy (n = 288)	Methotrexate (n = 284)	Tocilizumab 4 mg/kg + DMARDs (n = 774)	Tocilizumab 8 mg/kg + DMARDs (n = 1,582)	Placebo + DMARDs (n = 1,170)
Upper espiratory tract infection	7%	5%	6%	8%	6%
Nasopharyngitis	7%	6%	4%	6%	4%
Headache	7%	2%	6%	5%	3%
Hypertension	6%	2%	4%	4%	3%
ALT increased	6%	4%	3%	3%	1%
Dizziness	3%	1%	2%	3%	2%
Bronchitis	3%	2%	4%	3%	3%
Rash	2%	1%	4%	3%	1%
Mouth ulceration	2%	2%	1%	2%	1%
Abdominal pain, upper	2%	2%	3%	3%	2%
Gastritis	1%	2%	1%	2%	1%
Transaminase increased	1%	5%	2%	2%	1%

a Reactions listed also occurred ≥ 1% more in patients receiving tocilizumab than in patients receiving placebo plus DMARD.

Tocilizumab (Humanized)

Pharmacologic & Dosing Characteristics

Dosage: For adults who have had an inadequate response to 1 or more TNF antagonist, when used in combination with DMARDs or as monotherapy, the recommended starting dosage is 4 mg/kg followed by an increase to 8 mg/kg based on clinical response every 4 weeks. Reduce dose from 8 to 4 mg/kg to manage certain dose-related laboratory changes, including elevated liver enzymes, neutropenia, and thrombocytopenia. Do not exceed 800 mg per infusion. If a serious infection develops, interrupt tocilizumab treatment until infection is controlled.

Liver enzyme abnormalities
- For greater than 1 to 3 times ULN, modify dose of concomitant DMARDs, if appropriate. For persistent increases in this range, reduce tocilizumab dose to 4 mg/kg or interrupt tocilizumab until ALT/AST have normalized.
- For greater than 3 to 5 times ULN (confirmed by repeat testing), interrupt tocilizumab dosing until less than 3 times ULN and follow the previous recommendations for greater than 1 to 3 times ULN. For persistent increases greater than 3 times ULN, discontinue tocilizumab.
- For greater than 5 times ULN, discontinue tocilizumab.

Low ANC
- ANC greater than 1,000 cells/mm^3, maintain dose.
- ANC 500 to 1,000 cells/mm^3, interrupt tocilizumab dosing. When ANC is greater than 1,000 cells/mm^3, resume tocilizumab at 4 mg/kg and increase to 8 mg/kg as clinically appropriate.
- ANC less than 500 cells/mm^3, discontinue tocilizumab.

Low platelet count
- 50,000 to 100,000 cells/mm^3, interrupt tocilizumab dosing. When platelet count is greater than 100,000 cells/mm^3, resume tocilizumab at 4 mg/kg and increase to 8 mg/kg as clinically appropriate.
- Less than 50,000 cells/mm^3, discontinue tocilizumab.

No dose adjustment is required in patients with mild renal impairment. Tocilizumab has not been studied in patients with moderate to severe renal impairment.

Route: IV infusion over 60 minutes. Do not infuse concomitantly in the same IV line with other drugs. No physical or biochemical compatibility studies have been conducted to evaluate the coadministration of tocilizumab with other drugs.

Overdosage: There are limited data available on overdoses with tocilizumab. One case of accidental overdose was reported in which a patient with multiple myeloma received a dose of 40 mg/kg. No adverse reactions were observed. No serious adverse reactions were observed in healthy volunteers who received single doses of up to 28 mg/kg, although all 5 patients at the highest dose of 28 mg/kg developed dose-limiting neutropenia.

Laboratory Tests: Monitor neutrophils, platelets, and ALT and AST levels every 4 to 8 weeks. When clinically indicated, consider other liver function tests, such as bilirubin. Assess lipid parameters approximately 4 to 8 weeks after starting tocilizumab therapy, then at approximately 6-month intervals.

Efficacy: The efficacy of tocilizumab was assessed in 5 randomized, double-blind, multicenter studies in patients older than 18 years of age with active RA diagnosed according to American College of Rheumatology (ACR) criteria. Patients had at least 8 tender and 6 swollen joints at baseline. Tocilizumab was given IV every 4 weeks as monotherapy (study 1), in combination with methotrexate (studies 2 and 3) or other DMARDs (study 4) in patients with an inadequate response to those drugs, or in combination with methotrexate in patients with an inadequate response to TNF antagonists (study 5).

Study 1 evaluated patients with moderately to severely active RA who had not been treated with methotrexate within 6 months prior to randomization or who had not discontinued previous methotrexate treatment as a result of clinically important toxic effects or lack of response. In this study, 67% of patients were methotrexate-naive, and more than 40% of patients had RA for less than 2 years. Patients received tocilizumab 8 mg/kg monotherapy or methotrexate alone (dose titrated over 8 weeks from 7.5 mg to a maximum of 20 mg weekly). The primary end point was the number of tocilizumab patients who achieved an ACR20 response at week 24. Tocilizumab recipients achieved 70% response for ACR20, 44% for ACR50, and 28% for ACR70. The weighted difference beyond the response of the methotrexate-treated control group ranged from 12% to 19%.

Study 2 is an ongoing, 2-year study with a planned interim analysis at week 24 that evaluated patients with moderately to severely active RA who had an inadequate clinical response to methotrexate. Patients received tocilizumab 8 mg/kg, tocilizumab 4 mg/kg, or placebo every 4 weeks in combination with methotrexate 10 to 25 mg weekly. The primary end point at week 24 was the number of patients who achieved an ACR20 response. Tocilizumab recipients achieved 51% to 56% response for ACR20, 25% to 32% for ACR50, and 11% to 13% for ACR70. The weighted difference beyond the response of the methotrexate-treated control group ranged from 8% to 29%.

Study 3 evaluated patients with moderately to severely active RA who had an inadequate clinical response to methotrexate. Patients received tocilizumab 8 mg/kg, tocilizumab 4 mg/kg, or placebo every 4 weeks in combination with methotrexate 10 to 25 mg weekly. The primary end point was the number of patients who achieved an ACR20 response at week 24. Tocilizumab recipients achieved 48% to 59% response for ACR20, 32% to 44% for ACR50, and 12% to 22% for ACR70. The weighted difference beyond the response of the methotrexate-treated control group ranged from 11% to 33%.

Study 4 evaluated patients who had an inadequate response to their existing therapy, including 1 or more DMARD. Patients received tocilizumab 8 mg/kg or placebo every 4 weeks in combination with the stable DMARDs. The primary end point was the number of patients who achieved an ACR20 response at week 24. Tocilizumab recipients achieved 61% response for ACR20, 38% for ACR50, and 21% for ACR70. The weighted difference beyond the response of the DMARD-treated control group ranged from 17% to 35%.

Study 5 evaluated patients with moderately to severely active RA who had an inadequate clinical response or were intolerant to 1 or more TNF antagonist therapies. The TNF antagonist therapy was discontinued prior to randomization. Patients received tocilizumab 8 mg/kg, tocilizumab 4 mg/kg, or placebo every 4 weeks in combination with methotrexate 10 to 25 mg weekly. The primary end point was the number of patients who achieved an ACR20 response at week 24. Tocilizumab recipients achieved 30% to 50% response for ACR20, 17% to 29% for ACR50, and 5% to 12% for ACR70. The weighted difference beyond the response of the methotrexate-treated control group ranged from 4% to 46%.

In all studies, patients treated with tocilizumab 8 mg/kg had statistically significant ACR20, ACR50, and ACR70 response rates versus methotrexate- or placebo-treated patients at week 24. Patients with inadequate response to DMARDs or TNF antagonist therapy treated with tocilizumab 4 mg/kg had lower response rates compared with patients treated with tocilizumab 8 mg/kg.

Onset: In clinical studies with tocilizumab 4 and 8 mg/kg, decreases in levels of C-reactive protein to within normal ranges were seen as early as week 2. Changes in pharmacodynamic parameters were observed (ie, decreases in rheumatoid factor, erythrocyte sedimentation rate, serum amyloid A; increases in hemoglobin) with both doses; however, the greatest improvements were observed with tocilizumab 8 mg/kg. In healthy subjects administered tocilizumab doses ranging from 2 to 28 mg/kg, ANCs decreased to their nadirs 3 to 5 days following tocilizumab administration. Thereafter, neutrophils recovered toward baseline in a dose-dependent manner. RA patients demonstrated a similar pattern of ANCs following tocilizumab administration.

Pharmacokinetics: Pharmacokinetics in healthy subjects and patients with RA were similar. The clearance of tocilizumab decreased with increased doses. At the 10 mg/kg single dose in RA patients, mean clearance was 0.29 ± 0.1 mL/h/kg and mean apparent terminal half-life was 151 ± 59 hours (6.3 days). The pharmacokinetics of tocilizumab were determined using a population pharmacokinetic analysis of 1,793 RA patients treated with tocilizumab 4 and 8 mg/kg every 4 weeks for 24 weeks. The pharmacokinetic parameters of tocilizumab did not change with time. A more than dose-proportional increase in area under the curve (AUC) and trough concentration (C_{min}) was observed for doses of 4 and 8 mg/kg every 4 weeks. Maximum concentration (C_{max}) increased dose proportionally. At steady state, predicted AUC and C_{min} were 2.7 and 6.5-fold higher with 8 mg/kg compared with 4 mg/kg, respectively.

For doses of tocilizumab 4 mg/kg given every 4 weeks, the predicted mean ($\pm$ standard deviation [SD]) steady-state AUC, C_{min}, and C_{max} of tocilizumab were $13{,}000 \pm 5{,}800$ mcg•h/mL, 1.49 ± 2.13 mcg/mL, and 88.3 ± 41.4 mcg/mL, respectively. The accumulation ratios for AUC and C_{max} were 1.11 and 1.02, respectively. The accumulation ratio was higher for C_{min} (1.96). Steady state was reached following the first administration for C_{max} and AUC, respectively, and after 16 weeks for C_{min}.

For doses of tocilizumab 8 mg/kg given every 4 weeks, the predicted mean ($\pm$ SD) steady-state AUC, C_{min}, and C_{max} of tocilizumab were $35{,}000 \pm 15{,}500$ mcg•h/mL, 9.74 ± 10.5 mcg/mL, and 183 ± 85.6 mcg/mL, respectively. The accumulation ratios for AUC and C_{max} were 1.22 and 1.06, respectively. The accumulation ratio was higher for C_{min} (2.35). Steady state was reached following the first administration and after 8 and 20 weeks for C_{max}, AUC, and C_{min}, respectively. Tocilizumab AUC, C_{min}, and C_{max} increased with increase of body weight. At body weight of at least 100 kg, the predicted mean ($\pm$ SD) steady-state AUC, C_{min}, and C_{max} of tocilizumab were $55{,}500 \pm 14{,}100$ mcg•h/mL, 19 ± 12 mcg/mL, and 269 ± 57 mcg/mL, respectively, which are higher than mean exposure values for the patient population. Therefore, tocilizumab doses exceeding 800 mg per infusion are not recommended.

Distribution: Following IV dosing, tocilizumab undergoes biphasic elimination from the circulation. In patients with RA, the central volume of distribution (Vd) was 3.5 L and the peripheral Vd was 2.9 L, resulting in a Vd at steady state of 6.4 L.

Elimination: The total clearance of tocilizumab is concentration dependent and is the sum of the linear clearance and the nonlinear clearance. The linear clearance was estimated to be 12.5 mL/h in the population pharmacokinetic analysis. The concentration-dependent nonlinear clearance plays a major role at low tocilizumab concentrations. Once the nonlinear clearance pathway is saturated at higher tocilizumab concentrations, clearance is mainly determined by the linear clearance.

The half-life of tocilizumab is concentration dependent. The concentration-dependent apparent half-life is up to 11 days for 4 mg/kg and up to 13 days for 8 mg/kg every 4 weeks at steady-state.

Special populations: Population pharmacokinetic analyses in adults with RA showed that age, gender, and race did not affect the pharmacokinetics of tocilizumab. Linear clearance was found to increase with body size. The body weight–based dose (8 mg/kg) resulted in approximately 86% higher exposure in patients weighing more than 100 kg compared with patients weighing less than 60 kg. No formal study of the effect of hepatic or renal impairment on the pharmacokinetics of tocilizumab was conducted. Most patients in the population pharmacokinetic analysis had normal renal function or mild renal impairment.

Mild renal impairment (creatinine clearance less than 80 mL/min and at least 50 mL/min based on Cockcroft-Gault) did not impact the pharmacokinetics of tocilizumab; no dose adjustment is required.

Mechanism: Tocilizumab binds specifically to both soluble and membrane-bound IL-6 receptors (sIL-6R and mIL-6R) and inhibits IL-6-mediated signaling through these receptors. IL-6 is a pleiotropic proinflammatory cytokine produced by a variety of cell types, including T- and B-cells, lymphocytes, monocytes, and fibroblasts. IL-6 is involved in diverse physiological processes, such as T-cell activation, induction of immunoglobulin secretion, initiation of hepatic acute phase protein synthesis, and stimulation of hematopoietic precursor cell proliferation and differentiation. IL-6 is also produced by synovial and endothelial cells, leading to its local production in joints affected by inflammatory processes, such as RA.

Drug Interactions: Population pharmacokinetic analyses did not detect any effect of methotrexate, NSAIDs, or corticosteroids on tocilizumab clearance. Coadministration of a single dose of tocilizumab 10 mg/kg with methotrexate 10 to 25 mg once weekly had no clinically significant effect on methotrexate exposure. Tocilizumab has not been studied in combination with biological DMARDs, such as TNF antagonists.

Cytochrome P450s (CYP-450) in the liver are down-regulated by infection and inflammation stimuli, including cytokines such as IL-6. Inhibition of IL-6 signaling in RA patients treated with tocilizumab may restore CYP-450 activities to levels higher than those in the absence of tocilizumab, leading to increased metabolism of drugs that are CYP-450 substrates. In vitro studies showed that tocilizumab has the potential to affect expression of multiple CYP enzymes, including CYP1A2, 2B6, 2C9, 2C19, 2D6, and 3A4. Its effects on CYP2C8 or transporters is unknown. In vivo studies with omeprazole (metabolized by CYP2C19 and CYP3A4) and simvastatin (metabolized by CYP3A4) showed up to a 28% and 57% decrease in exposure 1 week following a single dose of tocilizumab, respectively. The effect of tocilizumab on CYP enzymes may be clinically relevant for CYP-450 substrates with narrow therapeutic index in which the dose is individually adjusted. Therapeutic monitoring of effect (eg, warfarin) or drug concentration (eg, cyclosporine, theophylline) and any necessary adjustment of the individual dosages should be performed when starting or discontinuing tocilizumab with these drugs. Use caution when tocilizumab is coadministered with CYP3A4 substrate drugs in which decrease in effectiveness is undesirable (eg, oral contraceptives, lovastatin, atorvastatin). The effect of tocilizumab on CYP-450 enzyme activity may persist for several weeks after therapy.

Do not give live vaccines concurrently with tocilizumab. No data are available on the secondary transmission of infection from persons receiving live vaccines to patients receiving tocilizumab. No data are available on the effectiveness of vaccination in patients receiving tocilizumab. Because IL-6 inhibition may interfere with the normal immune response to new antigens, give patients all recommended vaccinations before starting therapy with tocilizumab.

Patient Information:

Infections: Inform patients that tocilizumab may lower their resistance to infections. Instruct patients to contact their doctor immediately when symptoms suggesting infection appear.

GI perforation: Inform patients that some patients treated with tocilizumab had serious adverse effects in the stomach and intestines. Instruct patients to contact their doctor immediately when symptoms of severe, persistent abdominal pain appear.

Tocilizumab (Humanized)

Pharmaceutical Characteristics

Concentration: 20 mg per mL

Packaging: Single-use vial of 80 mg per 4 mL (NDC#: 50242-0135-01), box of four 80 mg per 4 mL vials (50242-0135-04); single-use vial of 200 mg per 10 mL (50242-0136-01), box of four 200 mg per 10 mL vials (50242-0136-04); single-use vial of 400 mg per 20 mL (50242-0137-01), box of four 400 mg per 20 mL vials (50242-0137-04)

Doseform: Solution

Appearance: Colorless to pale yellow liquid

Solvent: Phosphate-buffered aqueous solution

Diluent:

For infusion: Dilute tocilizumab to 100 mL. From a 100 mL infusion bag or bottle, withdraw a volume of sodium chloride 0.9% equal to the volume of tocilizumab solution required.

Adjuvant: None

Preservative: None

Allergens: None

Excipients: Disodium phosphate dodecahydrate and sodium dihydrogen phosphate dehydrate (as a 15 mmol/L phosphate buffer), polysorbate 80 (0.5 mg/mL), sucrose (50 mg/mL)

pH: Approximately 6.5

Shelf Life: Data not provided.

Storage/Stability: Store at 2° to 8°C (36° to 46°F). Protect vials from light by storage in original packages until time of use. Do not freeze. Contact the manufacturer regarding exposure to freezing or elevated temperatures. Shipping data not provided.

Store the fully diluted tocilizumab solution for infusion at 2° to 8°C (36° to 46°F) or room temperature for up to 24 hours. Protect from light. Allow fully diluted tocilizumab solution to reach room temperature before infusion.

Production Process: Data not provided.

Media: Data not provided.

Other Information

First Licensed: January 8, 2010

References: Oldfield V, Dhillon S, Plosker GL. Tocilizumab: a review of its use in the management of rheumatoid arthritis. *Drugs.* 2009;69(5):609-632.

Trastuzumab (Humanized)

Isoantibodies

Name: *Manufacturer:*
Herceptin   Genentech

Synonyms: MDX-210, 520C9x22, anti-p185HER2, *Metavert*

Immunologic Characteristics

Target Antigen: Human epidermal growth factor receptor 2 (HER2) protein

Viability: Inactive, passive, transient

Antigenic Form: Chimeric, human-murine immunoglobulin. Contains human framework regions with the complementarity-determining regions of a murine antibody (4D5) that binds to HER2.

Antigenic Type: Protein, IgG1κ antibody, monoclonal. Inhibits the proliferation of human tumor cells that overexpress HER2.

Use Characteristics

Indications: As a single agent, for the adjuvant treatment of HER2-overexpressing node-negative (ER/PR negative or with one high-risk feature) or node-positive breast cancer, following multimodality anthracycline-based therapy.

As part of a treatment regimen containing doxorubicin, cyclophosphamide, and either paclitaxel or docetaxel for the adjuvant treatment of HER2-overexpressing breast cancer, or as part of a regimen with docetaxel and carboplatin.

Combined with cisplatin and capecitabine or 5-fluorouracil, to treat patients with HER2 over-expressing metastatic gastric or gastroesophageal junction adenocarcinoma, who have not received prior treatment for metastatic disease.

Unlabeled Uses: Research in progress is assessing the role of trastuzumab in the treatment of prostate, non-small cell lung, pancreatic, and ovarian cancers.

Limitations: Only use trastuzumab in patients whose tumors have HER2 protein overexpression.

Contraindications:

Absolute: None

Relative: Patients with a prior severe hypersensitivity reaction to trastuzumab, Chinese hamster ovary cell proteins, or any component of this product. For patients with a known hypersensitivity to benzyl alcohol (the preservative in bacteriostatic water for injection), reconstitute trastuzumab with sterile water for injection, USP, and discard the reconstituted vial after a single use.

Immunodeficiency: Specific data on the use of trastuzumab in immunodeficient people is not available, although impairment of effect is unlikely.

Elderly: Trastuzumab was administered to 133 patients 65 years of age or older. The risk of cardiac dysfunction may be increased in geriatric patients. The reported clinical experience is not adequate to determine whether older patients respond differently than younger patients.

Pregnancy: Category D. Trastuzumab can cause fetal harm when administered to a pregnant woman. Postmarketing case reports suggest that trastuzumab use during pregnancy increases the risk of oligohydramnios during the second and third trimesters. If trastuzumab is used during pregnancy or if a woman becomes pregnant while taking trastuzumab, inform her of the potential hazard to a fetus. HER2 protein expression is high in many embryonic tissues, including cardiac and neural tissues. In mutant mice lacking HER2, embryos died in early gestation. Placental transfer of trastuzumab during the early (days 20 to 50 of gestation) and late (days 120 to 150 of gestation) fetal development period was observed.

Lactation: A study conducted in lactating cynomolgus monkeys at doses 25 times the weekly human maintenance dose of 2 mg/kg trastuzumab demonstrated that trastuzumab is secreted in breast milk. The presence of trastuzumab in the serum of infant monkeys was not associated with any adverse effects on their growth or development from birth to 3 months of age. It is not known whether trastuzumab is excreted in human breast milk. Because human IgG is excreted in human breast milk and the potential for absorption and harm to the infant is unknown, advise women to discontinue nursing during trastuzumab therapy and for 6 months after the last dose of trastuzumab.

Children: Safety and efficacy have not been established.

Adverse Reactions: In clinical trials, 958 patients received trastuzumab alone or in combination with chemotherapy. Data below are based on the randomized, controlled clinical trial in 234 patients who received recommended doses of trastuzumab in combination with chemotherapy and 4 open-label studies of trastuzumab as a single agent in 352 patients at doses of 10 to 500 mg administered weekly.

Adverse Events Occurring in ≥ 5% of Patients or at Increased Incidence in the Trastuzumab Arm of the Randomized Study (%)					
Adverse event	Single agent (n = 352)	Trastuzumab + paclitaxel (n = 91)	Paclitaxel alone (n = 95)	Trastuzumab + AC[a] (n = 143)	AC[a] alone (n = 135)
Cardiovascular					
Tachycardia	5	12	4	10	5
CHF	7	11	1	28	7
CNS					
Insomnia	14	25	13	29	15
Dizziness	13	22	24	24	18
Paresthesia	9	48	39	17	11
Depression	6	12	13	20	12
Peripheral neuritis	2	23	16	2	2
Neuropathy	1	13	5	4	4
Dermatologic					
Rash	18	38	18	27	17
Herpes simplex	2	12	3	7	9
Acne	2	11	3	3	< 1
GI					
Nausea	33	51	9	76	77
Diarrhea	25	45	29	45	26
Vomiting	23	37	28	53	49
Nausea and vomiting	8	14	11	18	9
Anorexia	14	24	16	31	26
Hematologic/Lymphatic					
Anemia	4	14	9	36	26
Leukopenia	3	24	17	52	34
Metabolic					
Peripheral edema	10	22	20	20	17
Edema	8	10	8	11	5

Adverse event	Single agent (n = 352)	Trastuzumab + paclitaxel (n = 91)	Paclitaxel alone (n = 95)	Trastuzumab + AC[a] (n = 143)	AC[a] alone (n = 135)
Musculoskeletal					
Bone pain	7	24	18	7	7
Arthralgia	6	37	21	8	9
Respiratory					
Cough increased	26	41	22	43	29
Dyspnea	22	27	26	42	25
Rhinitis	14	22	5	22	16
Pharyngitis	12	22	14	30	18
Sinusitis	9	21	7	13	6
Body as a whole					
Pain	47	61	62	57	42
Asthenia	42	62	57	54	55
Fever	36	49	23	56	34
Chills	32	41	4	35	11
Headache	26	36	28	44	31
Abdominal pain	22	34	22	23	18
Back pain	22	34	30	27	15
Infection	20	47	27	47	31
Viral-like syndrome	10	12	5	12	6
Accidental injury	6	13	3	9	4
Allergic reaction	3	8	2	4	2
UTI	5	18	14	13	7

Table title: Adverse Events Occurring in ≥ 5% of Patients or at Increased Incidence in the Trastuzumab Arm of the Randomized Study (%)

a AC = Anthracycline (doxorubicin or epirubicin) and cyclophosphamide.

Infection: An increased incidence of infections, primarily mild upper respiratory tract infections or catheter infections, was observed in patients receiving trastuzumab in combination with chemotherapy.

Infusion-associated symptoms: During the first infusion with trastuzumab, a symptom complex most commonly consisting of chills or fever was observed in approximately 40% of patients. The symptoms were usually mild to moderate in severity and were treated with acetaminophen, diphenhydramine, and meperidine (with or without reduction in the rate of trastuzumab infusion). Trastuzumab discontinuation was infrequent. Other signs or symptoms may include nausea, vomiting, pain (in some cases at tumor sites), rigors, headache, dizziness, dyspnea, hypotension, rash, and asthenia. The symptoms occurred infrequently with subsequent trastuzumab infusions.

Body as a whole: Trastuzumab can result in severe hypersensitivity reactions, including anaphylaxis, infusion reactions, and pulmonary events. Rarely, these have been fatal. Strongly consider discontinuing trastuzumab therapy in patients who develop anaphylaxis, angioedema, or acute respiratory distress. Cellulitis, anaphylactoid reaction, ascites, hydrocephalus, radiation injury, deafness, hypothyroidism, and amblyopia have occurred in patients treated with trastuzumab.

Cardiovascular: Vascular thrombosis; pericardial effusion; heart arrest; hypotension; syncope; hemorrhage; shock; arrhythmia. Signs and symptoms of cardiac dysfunction, such as dyspnea, increased cough, paroxysmal nocturnal dyspnea, peripheral edema, S3 gallop, or reduced ejection fraction, have been observed in patients treated with trastuzumab. Use of trastuzumab can result in ventricular dysfunction and congestive heart failure. Con-

Trastuzumab (Humanized)

gestive heart failure associated with trastuzumab therapy may be severe and has been associated with disabling cardiac failure, death, and mural thrombosis leading to stroke. Perform baseline cardiac assessment on candidates for treatment with trastuzumab, including history and physical exam and 1 or more of the following: EKG, echocardiogram, MUGA scan. Evaluate left ventricular function in all patients before and during treatment with trastuzumab. Exercise extreme caution in treating patients with preexisting cardiac dysfunction. Conduct frequent monitoring for deteriorating cardiac function. Consider discontinuing trastuzumab in patients who develop clinically significant congestive heart failure or decrease in left ventricular function. Most patients with cardiac dysfunction responded to appropriate medical therapy. There is a 4- to 6-fold increase in the incidence of symptomatic myocardial dysfunction among patients receiving trastuzumab as a single agent or in combination therapy compared with those not receiving trastuzumab. The highest absolute incidence occurs when trastuzumab is administered with an anthracycline. The safety of continuation or resumption of trastuzumab in patients who have previously experienced cardiac toxicity has not been studied.

The incidence and severity of cardiac dysfunction was particularly high in patients who received trastuzumab in combination with anthracyclines and cyclophosphamide. The probability of cardiac dysfunction was highest in patients who received trastuzumab concurrently with anthracyclines. The data suggest that advanced age may increase the probability of cardiac dysfunction. Preexisting cardiac disease or prior cardiotoxic therapy (eg, anthracycline or radiation therapy to the chest) may decrease the ability to tolerate trastuzumab therapy; however, the data are not adequate to evaluate the correlation between trastuzumab-induced cardiotoxicity and these factors.

The clinical status of patients in the trials who developed congestive heart failure were classified for severity using the New York Heart Association functional classification system (I through IV, IV being the most severe level of cardiac failure).

Incidence and Severity of Cardiac Dysfunction with Trastuzumab (%)				
	Trastuzumab[a] alone (n = 213)	Trastuzumab + Paclitaxel[b] (n = 91)	Paclitaxel[b] (n = 95)	Trastuzumab + AC[b,c] (n = 143)	AC[b,c] (n = 135)
Any cardiac dysfunction	7	11	1	28	7
Class III to IV	5	4	1	19	3

a Open-label, single-agent phase 2 study (94% received prior anthracyclines).
b Randomized phase 3 study comparing chemotherapy plus trastuzumab with chemotherapy alone, where chemotherapy is either AC or paclitaxel.
c AC = Anthracycline (doxorubicin or epirubicin) and cyclophosphamide.

CNS: Convulsion; ataxia; confusion; manic reaction.

Dermatologic: Herpes zoster; skin ulceration.

GI: Hepatic failure; gastroenteritis; hematemesis; ileus; intestinal obstruction; colitis; esophageal ulcer; stomatitis; pancreatitis; hepatitis.

Of patients treated with trastuzumab as a single agent, 25% experienced diarrhea. An increased incidence of diarrhea, primarily mild to moderate in severity, was observed in patients receiving trastuzumab in combination with chemotherapy.

GU: Hydronephrosis; kidney failure; cervical cancer; hematuria; hemorrhagic cystitis; pyelonephritis.

Hematologic: Pancytopenia; acute leukemia; coagulation disorder; lymphangitis.

An increased incidence of anemia and leukopenia was observed in the treatment group receiving trastuzumab and chemotherapy, especially in the trastuzumab and anthracycline-cyclophosphamide (AC) subgroup, compared with the treatment group receiving chemotherapy alone. The majority of these cytopenic events were mild or moderate in intensity and reversible, and none resulted in discontinuation of therapy with trastuzumab. Hematologic toxicity is infrequent following the administration of trastuzumab as a single agent, with an incidence of grade III toxicities for white blood cells, platelets, and hemoglobin at less than 1%. No grade IV toxicities were observed.

Immunologic: Of 903 patients, human anti-human antibodies (HAHA) to trastuzumab were detected in 1 patient, who had no allergic manifestations.

Metabolic: Hypercalcemia; hypomagnesemia; hyponatremia; hypoglycemia; growth retardation; weight loss.

Musculoskeletal: Pathological fractures; bone necrosis; myopathy.

Respiratory: Apnea; pneumothorax; asthma; hypoxia; laryngitis; pneumonitis; pulmonary fibrosis. Severe pulmonary events leading to death occur rarely with the use of trastuzumab. Clinical findings include dyspnea, pulmonary infiltrates, pleural effusions, noncardiogenic pulmonary edema, pulmonary insufficiency and hypoxia, and acute respiratory distress syndrome. Patients with symptomatic intrinsic lung disease or with extensive tumor involvement of the lungs, resulting in dyspnea at rest, may be at greater risk of severe reactions.

Pharmacologic & Dosing Characteristics

Dosage:

Breast cancer: The recommended initial loading dose is 4 mg/kg. The recommended weekly maintenance dose is 2 mg/kg.

Adjuvant treatment of breast cancer: Administer according to one of the following dosing schedules for a total of 52 weeks of trastuzumab therapy:

- During and following paclitaxel, docetaxel, or docetaxel/carboplatin: Administer trastuzumab at an initial dose of 4 mg/kg as a 90-minute IV infusion, followed by weekly doses of 2 mg/kg as 30-minute IV infusions, as tolerated, during chemotherapy for the first 12 weeks (paclitaxel or docetaxel) or 18 weeks (docetaxel/carboplatin). One week following the last weekly dose of trastuzumab, administer trastuzumab at 6 mg/kg as a 30- to 90-minute IV infusion every 3 weeks.
- Initiate trastuzumab after completing all chemotherapy. Administer trastuzumab at an initial dose of 8 mg/kg, followed by doses of 6 mg/kg every 3 weeks for a total of 17 doses (52 weeks of therapy). Administer all doses of more than 4 mg/kg as 90-minute IV infusions.
- As a single agent within 3 weeks after completing multimodality, anthracycline-based chemotherapy regimens: Initial dose at 8 mg/kg as a 90-minute IV infusion, with subsequent doses at 6 mg/kg as a 30- to 90-minute IV infusion every 3 weeks.

Metastatic treatment of breast cancer: Administer trastuzumab, alone or in combination with paclitaxel, at an initial dose of 4 mg/kg as a 90-minute IV infusion, followed by subsequent weekly doses of 2 mg/kg as 30-minute IV infusions until disease progression.

If needed, modify the dose.

Gastric cancer: Initial dose of 8 mg/kg, followed by subsequent doses of 6 mg/kg as IV infusion over 30 to 90 min every 3 weeks until disease progression occurs.

Infusion reactions: To manage mild or moderate infusion reactions, decrease the rate of infusion. Interrupt the infusion in patients with dyspnea or clinically significant hypotension. Discontinue trastuzumab in case of severe or life-threatening infusion reactions.

Cardiomyopathy: Assess left ventricular ejection fraction (LVEF) before starting trastuzumab and at regular intervals during treatment. Withhold trastuzumab doses for at least 4 weeks for either a 16% or more absolute decrease in LVEF from pretreatment values or LVEF below institutional limits of normal and 10% or more absolute decrease in LVEF from pretreatment values. Trastuzumab may be resumed if, within 4 to 8 weeks, the LVEF returns to normal values and the absolute decrease from baseline is 15% or less. Permanently discontinue trastuzumab for a persistent (more than 8 weeks) LVEF decline or for suspension of dosing on more than 3 occasions related to cardiomyopathy.

Route: IV infusion. Administer the initial loading dose as a 90-minute IV infusion. The recommended weekly maintenance dose can be administered as a 30-minute infusion if the initial loading dose was well tolerated. Trastuzumab may be administered in an outpatient setting. Do not administer as an IV push or bolus dose. Observe patients for fever and chills or other infusion-associated symptoms.

Overdosage: There is no experience with overdosage of trastuzumab in human clinical trials. Single doses over 500 mg have not been tested.

Laboratory Tests: In clinical trials, the Clinical Trial Assay (CTA) was used for immunohistochemical detection of HER2 protein overexpression. The DAKO *HercepTest*, another immunohistochemical test for HER2 protein overexpression, has not been directly studied for its ability to predict trastuzumab treatment effect, but it has been compared with the CTA on more than 500 breast cancer histology specimens obtained from the National Cancer Institute Cooperative Breast Cancer Tissue Resource. Based upon these results and an expected incidence of 33% of 2+ or 3+ HER2 overexpression in tumors from women with metastatic breast cancer, one can estimate the correlation of the *HercepTest* results with CTA results. Of specimens testing 3+ (strongly positive) on the *HercepTest*, 94% would be expected to test at least 2+ on the CTA (ie, meeting the study entry criterion), including 82% that would be expected to test 3+ on the CTA (ie, the reading most associated with clinical benefit). Of specimens testing 2+ (weakly positive) on the *HercepTest*, only 34% would be expected to test at least 2+ on the CTA, including 14% that would be expected to test 3+ on the CTA.

Efficacy: The safety and efficacy of trastuzumab were studied in a randomized, controlled clinical trial in combination with chemotherapy (469 patients) and an open-label single-agent clinical trial (222 patients). Both trials studied patients with metastatic breast cancer whose tumors overexpress the HER2 protein. Patients were eligible if they had 2+ or 3+ levels of overexpression (based on a 0 to 3+ scale) by immunohistochemical assessment of tumor tissue performed by a central testing lab.

A multicenter, randomized, controlled clinical trial was conducted in 469 patients with metastatic breast cancer who had not been previously treated with chemotherapy for metastatic disease. Patients were randomized to receive chemotherapy alone or in combination with trastuzumab. For those who had received prior anthracycline therapy in the adjuvant setting, chemotherapy consisted of paclitaxel (175 mg/m^2 over 3 hours every 21 days for at least 6 cycles); for all other patients, chemotherapy consisted of anthracycline plus cyclophosphamide (AC: doxorubicin 60 mg/m^2 or epirubicin 75 mg/m^2 plus 600 mg/m^2 cyclophosphamide every 21 days for 6 cycles). Compared with patients in the AC subgroups, patients in the paclitaxel subgroups were more likely to have had the following: Poor prognostic factors (eg, premenopausal status, estrogen or progesterone receptor negative tumors, positive lymph nodes), prior therapy (eg, adjuvant chemotherapy, myeloablative chemotherapy, radiotherapy), and a shorter disease-free interval.

Compared with patients randomized to chemotherapy alone, the patients randomized to trastuzumab and chemotherapy experienced a significantly longer time to disease progression, a higher overall response rate (ORR), a longer median duration of response, and a higher 1-year survival rate. These treatment effects were observed both in patients who received trastuzumab plus paclitaxel and in those who received trastuzumab plus AC. But the magnitude of the effects was greater in the paclitaxel subgroup. The degree of HER2 overexpression was a predictor of treatment effect.

Clinical Efficacy of Trastuzumab in First-Line Treatment					
	Combined results		Paclitaxel subgroup		AC subgroup	
	Trastuzumab + all chemotherapy (n = 235)	All chemotherapy (n = 234)	Trastuzumab + paclitaxel (n = 92)	Paclitaxel (n = 96)	Trastuzumab + AC[a] (n = 143)	AC[a] (n = 138)
Time to progression[b,c]						
Median (months)	7.2	4.5	6.7	2.5	7.6	5.7
Overall response rate[b]						
Rate (%)	45	29	38	15	50	38
Duration of response[b,c]						
Median (months)	9.1	5.8	8.3	4.3	9.1	6.4
25%, 75% quantile	5.5, 14.9	3.9, 8.5	4.9, 11	3.7, 7.4	5.8, 14.9	4.5, 8.5
1-year survival[c]						
% alive	79	68	73	61	83	73

a AC = Anthracycline (doxorubicin or epirubicin) and cyclophosphamide.
b Assessed by an independent Response Evaluation Committee.
c Kaplan-Meier Estimate.

Trastuzumab was studied as a single agent in a multicenter, open-label, single-arm clinical trial in patients with HER2-overexpressing metastatic breast cancer who had relapsed following 1 or 2 prior chemotherapy regimens for metastatic disease. Of 222 patients enrolled, 66% had received prior adjuvant chemotherapy, 68% had received 2 prior chemotherapy regimens for metastatic disease, and 25% had received prior myeloablative treatment with hematopoietic rescue. The ORR (complete response + partial response) was 14%, with a 2% complete response rate and a 12% partial response rate. Complete responses were observed only in patients with disease limited to skin and lymph nodes. The degree of HER2 overexpression was a predictor of treatment effect.

HER2 protein overexpression: In the clinical studies described, patient eligibility was determined by testing tumor specimens for overexpression of HER2 protein. Specimens were tested with the CTA and scored as 0, 1+, 2+, or 3+, with 3+ indicating the strongest positivity. Only patients with 2+ or 3+ positive tumors were eligible (approximately 33% of those screened). Data from both efficacy trials suggest that the beneficial treatment effects were largely limited to patients with the highest level of HER2 protein overexpression (3+).

Treatment Effect of Trastuzumab vs Level of HER2 Expression					
	Single-arm trial	Treatment subgroups in randomized trial			
	Trastuzumab	Trastuzumab + paclitaxel	Paclitaxel	Trastuzumab + AC[a]	AC[a]
Overall response rate					
2+ overexpression	4%	21%	16%	40%	43%
3+ overexpression	17%	44%	14%	53%	36%
Median time to progression (months)					
2+ overexpression	N/A[b]	4.4	3.2	7.6	7.1
3+ overexpression	N/A	7.1	2.2	7.3	4.9

a AC = Anthracycline (doxorubicin or epirubicin) and cyclophosphamide.
b N/A = Not assessed.

Trastuzumab (Humanized)

Pharmacokinetics: Immunoglobulins are primarily eliminated by catabolism. Data are based on breast cancer patients with metastatic disease. Short-duration IV infusions of 10 to 500 mg once weekly demonstrated dose-dependent pharmacokinetics. Mean half-life increased and clearance decreased with increasing dose level. The half-life averaged 1.7 and 12 days at the 10 and 500 mg dose levels, respectively. The volume of distribution was approximately that of serum volume (44 mL/kg). At the highest weekly dose studied (500 mg), mean peak serum concentrations were 377 mcg/mL.

In studies using a loading dose of 4 mg/kg followed by a weekly maintenance dose of 2 mg/kg, a mean half-life of 5.8 days (range, 1 to 32 days) was observed. Between weeks 16 and 32, trastuzumab serum concentrations reached a steady-state with mean trough and peak concentrations of approximately 79 and 123 mcg/mL, respectively.

Preliminary data from Europe suggest that the mean half-life may be closer to 25 days. These data are being evaluated further. If confirmed, a longer half-life could warrant avoiding anthracycline-based therapy for up to 22 weeks after stopping trastuzumab therapy.

Detectable concentrations of the circulating extracellular domain of the HER2 receptor (shed antigen) are found in the serum of some patients with HER2-overexpressing tumors. Determination of shed antigen in baseline serum samples revealed that 64% (286/447) of patients had detectable shed antigen, which ranged as high as 1880 ng/mL (median, 11 ng/mL). Patients with higher baseline shed antigen levels were more likely to have lower serum trough concentrations. However, with weekly dosing, most patients with elevated shed antigen levels achieved target serum concentrations of trastuzumab by week 6.

Data suggest that the disposition of trastuzumab is not altered based on age or serum creatinine (up to 2 mg/dL). No formal interaction studies have been performed.

Mean serum trough concentrations of trastuzumab, when administered in combination with paclitaxel, were consistently elevated approximately 1.5-fold, compared with serum concentrations of trastuzumab used in combination with anthracycline plus cyclophosphamide. In primate studies, administration of trastuzumab with paclitaxel resulted in a reduction in trastuzumab clearance. Serum levels of trastuzumab in combination with cisplatin or in combination with doxorubicin or epirubicin plus cyclophosphamide did not suggest any interactions; no formal drug interaction studies were performed.

Mechanism: The HER2 (or c-erbB2) proto-oncogene encodes a transmembrane receptor protein of 185 kDa, which is structurally related to the epidermal growth factor receptor. HER2 protein overexpression is observed in 25% to 30% of primary breast cancers. HER2 protein overexpression can be determined using an immunohistochemistry-based assessment of fixed tumor blocks. Trastuzumab binds with high affinity in a cell-based assay (Kd = 5 nM) to the extracellular domain of the human epidermal growth factor receptor 2 (HER2) protein. Trastuzumab has been shown, in both in vitro assays and in animals, to inhibit the proliferation of human tumor cells that overexpress HER2. Trastuzumab is a mediator of antibody-dependent cellular cytotoxicity (ADCC). In vitro, trastuzumab-mediated ADCC has been shown to be preferentially exerted on HER2-overexpressing cancer cells compared with cancer cells that do not overexpress HER2.

Drug Interactions: There have been no formal drug interaction studies performed with trastuzumab in humans. Administration of paclitaxel in combination with trastuzumab resulted in a 2-fold decrease in trastuzumab clearance in a nonhuman primate study and in a 1.5-fold increase in trastuzumab serum levels in clinical studies. Do not mix or dilute trastuzumab with other drugs. Do not administer or mix trastuzumab infusions with dextrose solutions.

Trastuzumab (Humanized)

Pharmaceutical Characteristics

Concentration: 440 mg per vial, yielding trastuzumab 21 mg/mL

Packaging: Lyophilized, sterile powder containing 440 mg trastuzumab per vial under vacuum. Each carton contains 1 vial of 440 mg trastuzumab and one 20 mL vial of bacteriostatic water for injection containing 1.1% benzyl alcohol.

NDC Number: 50242-0134-68

Doseform: Lyophilized powder for reconstitution

Appearance: White to pale yellow powder, yielding a colorless to pale yellow transparent solution.

Diluent:

For reconstitution: 20 mL bacteriostatic water for injection, containing 1.1% benzyl alcohol, yielding 21 mL of a multidose solution containing trastuzumab 21 mg/mL. Use only 20 mL of fluid from the 30 mL vial. Do not dilute with volumes other than 20 mL. Shaking or causing excessive foaming during addition of diluent may cause problems with dissolution or the amount of trastuzumab that can be withdrawn from the vial. For patients hypersensitive to benzyl alcohol, sterile water for injection without preservatives may be used, but trastuzumab vials reconstituted in this way must be discarded after a single use.

For infusion: Add reconstituted trastuzumab solution to an infusion bag containing 250 mL of 0.9% sodium chloride. Do not use dextrose 5%. Gently invert the bag to mix the solution. No incompatibilities between trastuzumab and polyvinylchloride or polyethylene bags have been observed.

Adjuvant: None

Preservative: None in powder. Standard diluent contains benzyl alcohol.

Allergens: Gentamicin is added to mammalian cell cultures during manufacture, but it is undetectable in the final product. For patients hypersensitive to benzyl alcohol, sterile water for injection without preservatives may be used, but trastuzumab vials reconstituted in this way must be discarded after a single use.

Excipients: Each vial contains 9.9 mg L-histidine hydrochloride, 6.4 mg L-histidine, 400 mg α,α-trehalose dihydrate, and 1.8 mg polysorbate 20.

pH: 6 after reconstitution

Shelf Life: Expires within 30 months

Storage/Stability: Store powder at 2° to 8°C (36° to 46°F) before reconstitution. After reconstitution with bacteriostatic water, as supplied, trastuzumab is stable for 28 days when stored refrigerated at 2° to 8°C (36° to 46°F), and the solution is preserved for multiple use. Discard any remaining multidose reconstituted solution after 28 days. If unpreserved sterile water (not supplied) is used, use the reconstituted trastuzumab solution immediately and discard any unused portion. If reconstituted trastuzumab is inadvertently frozen, discard it. Contact the manufacturer regarding exposure to elevated temperatures. Shipping data not provided.

Store solutions of trastuzumab for infusion diluted in polyvinylchloride or polyethylene bags containing 0.9% sodium chloride for injection at 2° to 8°C (36° to 46°F) for up to 24 hours before administration. Diluted trastuzumab has been shown to be stable for up to 24 hours at room temperature (2° to 25°C [36° to 77°F]). However, because diluted trastuzumab contains no effective preservative, refrigerate the reconstituted and diluted solution.

Handling: Reconstitution with bacteriostatic water according to package directions yields a multidose solution containing 21 mg/mL trastuzumab. Label such vials with an expiration date 28 days from the date of reconstitution. If sterile water is used as the diluent, use the product immediately and discard unused portions.

781

Trastuzumab (Humanized)

Based on the patient's body weight, determine the dose of trastuzumab needed. Calculate the volume of 21 mg/mL trastuzumab solution needed. Withdraw this volume from the vial and add it to an infusion bag containing 250 mL of 0.9% sodium chloride, USP. Do not use dextrose 5%. Gently invert the bag to mix the solution. Incompatibilities between trastuzumab and polyvinylchloride or polyethylene bags have not been observed.

Production Process: Produced by mammalian cell (Chinese hamster ovary) suspension culture in a nutrient medium-containing gentamicin. Gentamicin is undetectable in the final product.

Media: Chinese hamster ovary (CHO) suspension culture in a nutrient medium

Disease Epidemiology

Incidence: The HER2/neu antigen is present in approximately 33% of breast cancer and 20% of ovarian cancer cases diagnosed each year.

Breast cancer: Worldwide, more than 300,000 cases of breast cancer are diagnosed annually, with 180,000 new cases and 46,300 deaths in the United States each year. The 5-year survival rate for localized breast cancer rose from 78% in the 1940s to 92% currently. If the cancer is not invasive, survival approaches 100%. If spread regionally, the survival rate is 71%. With distant metastases, the rate is 18%.

Other Information

Perspective:

1979: Weinberg identifies HER2/neu gene. This gene was first detected in neurologic tumors of rats, evoking the "neu" notation. HER2 refers to the second known human epidermal growth factor receptor. The gene is sometimes called erbB2, referring to its origin in the erbB oncogene.

1983: Ullrich identifies protein produced by HER2/neu gene.

1985: HER2/neu gene discovered in cancerous breast cells.

1993: Trastuzumab designated an orphan drug, October 5.

First Licensed: September 24, 1998

References: Baselga J, et al. Receptor blockade with monoclonal antibodies as anti-cancer therapy. *Pharmacol Ther.* 1994;64:127-154.

Baselga J, et al. Recombinant humanized anti-HER2 antibody (*Herceptin*) enhances the antitumor activity of paclitaxel and doxorubicin against HER2/neu overexpressing human breast cancer xenografts. *Cancer Res.* 1998;58:2825-2831.

Bazell R. *HER-2: The Making of Herceptin, a Revolutionary Treatment for Breast Cancer.* New York, NY: Random House; 1998.

Kabe KL, Kolesar JM. Role of trastuzumab in adjuvant therapy for locally invasive breast cancer. *Am J Health Syst Pharm.* 2006;63:527-533.

Ustekinumab

Name:
Stelara
Synonyms: CNTO 1275

Manufacturer:
Janssen Biotech

Immunologic Characteristics

Target Antigen: p40 subunit of the IL-12 and IL-23 cytokines
Viability: Inactive, passive, transient
Antigenic Form: Human IgG1κ monoclonal antibody
Antigenic Type: Protein, IgG1κ antibody, monoclonal, comprised of 1,326 amino acids, with estimated molecular mass ranging from 148,079 to 149,690 daltons.

Use Characteristics

Indications: To treat adults (18 years of age and older) with moderate to severe plaque psoriasis who are candidates for phototherapy or systemic therapy.

Contraindications: None.

Elderly: Of the 2,266 patients with psoriasis given ustekinumab, 131 were 65 years of age and older and 14 patients were 75 years of age and older. Although no differences in safety or efficacy were observed between older and younger patients, the number of patients 65 years of age and older is not sufficient to determine whether they respond differently from younger patients.

Carcinogenicity: Ustekinumab has not been evaluated for carcinogenic potential. Published literature showed that administration of murine IL-12 caused an antitumor effect in mice with transplanted tumors and IL-12/IL-23p40 knockout mice or mice treated with anti-IL-12/IL-23p40 antibody had decreased host defense to tumors. Mice genetically manipulated to be deficient in both IL-12 and IL-23 or IL-12 alone developed UV-induced skin cancers earlier and more frequently compared with wild-type mice. The relevance of these experimental findings in mouse models for malignancy risk in humans is unknown.

Mutagenicity: Ustekinumab has not been evaluated for mutagenic potential.

Fertility Impairment: Ustekinumab has not been evaluated for impairment of fertility. A male fertility study was conducted with only 6 male monkeys per group given subcutaneous doses of ustekinumab 0, 22.5, or 45 mg/kg twice weekly before mating and during the mating period for 13 weeks, followed by a 13-week, treatment-free period. Although fertility and pregnancy outcomes were not evaluated in mated females, there were no treatment-related effects on parental toxicity or male fertility parameters.

A female fertility study was conducted in mice using an analogous IL-12/IL-23p40 antibody administered subcutaneously at doses of up to 50 mg/kg twice weekly, beginning 15 days before cohabitation and continuing through gestational day 7. There were no treatment-related effects on maternal toxicity or female fertility parameters.

Pregnancy: Category B. There are no studies of ustekinumab in pregnant women. Use ustekinumab during pregnancy only if the potential benefit justifies the potential risk to the fetus. No teratogenic effects were observed in developmental and reproductive toxicology studies performed in cynomolgus monkeys at doses of up to ustekinumab 45 mg/kg, which is 45 times (based on mg/kg) the highest intended clinical dose in psoriasis patients (approximately 1 mg/kg based on a 90 mg dose given to a 90 kg patient with psoriasis).

Ustekinumab was tested in 2 embryo-fetal development toxicity studies. Pregnant cynomolgus monkeys were administered ustekinumab at doses of up to 45 mg/kg during organogenesis either twice weekly via subcutaneous injections or weekly by IV injections. No significant adverse developmental effects were noted in either study.

In an embryo-fetal development and pre- and postnatal development toxicity study, 3 groups of 20 pregnant cynomolgus monkeys were administered subcutaneous doses of ustekinumab 0, 22.5, or 45 mg/kg twice weekly from the beginning of organogenesis in cynomolgus monkeys to day 33 after delivery. There were no treatment-related effects on mortality, clinical signs, body weight, food consumption, hematology, or serum biochemistry in dams. Fetal losses occurred in 6 control monkeys, 6 monkeys treated with 22.5 mg/kg, and 5 monkeys treated with 45 mg/kg. Neonatal deaths occurred in 1 monkey treated with 22.5 mg/kg and in 1 monkey treated with 45 mg/kg. No ustekinumab-related abnormalities were observed in the neonates from birth through 6 months of age in clinical signs, body mass, hematology, or serum biochemistry. There were no treatment-related effects on functional development until weaning, functional development after weaning, morphological development, immunological development, and gross and histopathological examinations of offspring by the age of 6 months.

Lactation: Use caution when ustekinumab is administered to a breast-feeding woman. Weigh the unknown risks to the infant from GI or systemic exposure to ustekinumab against the known benefits of breast-feeding. Ustekinumab is excreted in the milk of lactating monkeys administered ustekinumab. Because IgG is excreted in human milk, it is expected that ustekinumab will be present as well. It is not known if ustekinumab is absorbed systemically after ingestion; however, published data suggest that antibodies in breast milk do not enter the neonatal and infant circulation in substantial amounts.

Children: Safety and efficacy of ustekinumab in children younger than 18 years of age have not been established.

Adverse Reactions: Most common adverse reactions (incidence greater than 3% and greater than with placebo): nasopharyngitis, upper respiratory tract infection, headache, and fatigue.

The safety data reflect exposure to ustekinumab in 2,266 psoriasis patients, including 1,970 patients exposed for at least 6 months, 1,285 patients exposed for at least 1 year, and 373 patients exposed for at least 18 months.

The following table summarizes the adverse reactions that occurred at a rate of at least 1% and at a higher rate in the ustekinumab groups than in the placebo group during the placebo-controlled period of study 1 and study 2.

Adverse Reactions Reported by ≥ 1% of Patients Through Week 12 in Study 1 and Study 2			
		Ustekinumab	
	Placebo	45 mg	90 mg
Patients treated	665	664	666
Nasopharyngitis	51 (8%)	56 (8%)	49 (7%)
Upper respiratory tract infection	30 (5%)	36 (5%)	28 (4%)
Headache	23 (3%)	33 (5%)	32 (5%)
Fatigue	14 (2%)	18 (3%)	17 (3%)
Diarrhea	12 (2%)	13 (2%)	13 (2%)
Back pain	8 (1%)	9 (1%)	14 (2%)
Dizziness	8 (1%)	8 (1%)	14 (2%)
Pharyngolaryngeal pain	7 (1%)	9 (1%)	12 (2%)
Pruritus	9 (1%)	10 (2%)	9 (1%)
Injection-site erythema	3 (< 1%)	6 (1%)	13 (2%)
Myalgia	4 (1%)	7 (1%)	8 (1%)
Depression	3 (< 1%)	8 (1%)	4 (1%)

Adverse drug reactions that occurred at rates of at least 1% included: cellulitis and certain injection-site reactions (pain, swelling, pruritus, induration, hemorrhage, bruising, and irritation).

Infections: In the placebo-controlled period of clinical studies of psoriasis patients (average follow-up of 12.6 weeks for placebo-treated patients and 13.4 weeks for ustekinumab-treated patients), 27% of ustekinumab-treated patients reported infections (1.39 per patient-year of follow-up) compared with 24% of placebo-treated patients (1.21 per patient-year of follow-up). Serious infections occurred in 0.3% of ustekinumab-treated patients (0.01 per patient-year of follow-up) and in 0.4% of placebo-treated patients (0.02 per patient-year of follow-up). In the controlled and noncontrolled portions of psoriasis clinical trials, 61% of ustekinumab-treated patients reported infections (1.24 per patient-year of follow-up). Serious infections were reported in 0.9% of patients (0.01 per patient-year of follow-up). Do not start ustekinumab during any clinically important active infection. If a serious infection develops, stop ustekinumab until infection resolves. Use caution when considering the use of ustekinumab in patients with a chronic infection or a history of recurrent infection. Serious infections requiring hospitalization included cellulitis, diverticulitis, osteomyelitis, viral infections, gastroenteritis, pneumonia, and urinary tract infections. Individuals genetically deficient in IL-12/IL-23 are particularly vulnerable to disseminated infections from mycobacteria (including nontuberculous, environmental mycobacteria), salmonella (including nontyphi strains), and bacillus Calmette-Guérin (BCG) vaccinations, with serious infections and fatal outcomes reported. Because it is not known whether patients with pharmacologic blockade of IL-12/IL-23 from treatment with ustekinumab will be susceptible to these infections, diagnostic tests should be considered according to clinical circumstances. Evaluate patients for tuberculosis (TB) before starting treatment with ustekinumab, starting treatment of latent TB before administering ustekinumab.

Malignancies: Ustekinumab may increase the risk of malignancy. In the controlled and non-controlled portions of psoriasis clinical trials, 0.4% of ustekinumab-treated patients reported malignancies, excluding nonmelanoma skin cancers (0.36 per 100 patient-years of follow-up). Nonmelanoma skin cancer was reported in 0.8% of ustekinumab-treated patients (0.8 per 100 patient-years of follow-up). Serious malignancies included breast, colon, head and neck, kidney, prostate, and thyroid cancers. The safety of ustekinumab in patients with a history of or a known malignancy has not been evaluated. In rodent models, inhibition of IL-12/IL-23p40 increased the risk of malignancy.

Reversible posterior leukoencephalopathy syndrome: One case was reported among 3,523 ustekinumab-treated patients. The patient, who received 12 doses of ustekinumab over approximately 2 years, experienced headache, seizures, and confusion. No additional ustekinumab injections were administered, and the patient fully recovered with appropriate treatment. Treat reversible posterior leukoencephalopathy syndrome (RPLS) promptly and discontinue ustekinumab.

Immunogenicity: The presence of ustekinumab in the serum can interfere with the detection of antiustekinumab antibodies, resulting in inconclusive results because of assay interference. In studies 1 and 2, antibody testing was done when ustekinumab may have been present in the serum. The following table summarizes the antibody results from studies 1 and 2. In study 1, the last ustekinumab injection was between weeks 28 and 48, with the last test for antiustekinumab antibodies at week 52. In study 2, the last ustekinumab injection was at week 16 and the last test for antiustekinumab antibodies was at week 24.

Ustekinumab

Antiustekinumab Immunogenicity		
Antibody Results	Study 1 (n = 743)	Study 2 (n = 1,198)
Positive	38 (5%)	33 (3%)
Negative	351 (47%)	90 (8%)
Inconclusive	354 (48%)	1,075 (90%)

The data reflect the percentage of patients whose test results were positive for antibodies to ustekinumab in a bridging immunoassay and are highly dependent on the sensitivity and specificity of the assay.

Pharmacologic & Dosing Characteristics

Dosage: The safety and efficacy of ustekinumab have not been evaluated beyond 2 years.

For patients weighing less than 100 kg, the recommended dose is 45 mg initially and 4 weeks later, followed by 45 mg every 12 weeks.

For patients weighing more than 100 kg, the recommended dose is 90 mg initially and 4 weeks later, followed by 90 mg every 12 weeks. In patients weighing more than 100 kg, 45 mg was also efficacious; however, 90 mg resulted in greater efficacy in these patients.

Route: Subcutaneous

Overdosage: Single doses of up to 4.5 mg/kg IV have been administered in clinical studies without dose-limiting toxicity. In case of overdosage, monitor the patient for any signs or symptoms of adverse reactions or effects and start appropriate symptomatic treatment immediately.

Efficacy: Two multicenter, randomized, double-blind, placebo-controlled studies (study 1 and study 2) enrolled a total of 1,996 patients at least 18 years of age with plaque psoriasis who had a minimum body surface area involvement of 10%, Psoriasis Area and Severity Index (PASI) score greater than 12, and who were candidates for phototherapy or systemic therapy. Patients with guttate, erythrodermic, or pustular psoriasis were excluded from the studies.

Study 1 enrolled 766 patients and study 2 enrolled 1,230 patients. The studies had the same design through week 28. In both studies, patients were randomized in equal proportion to placebo or ustekinumab 45 or 90 mg. Patients randomized to ustekinumab received 45 or 90 mg doses, regardless of weight, at weeks 0, 4, and 16. Patients randomized to receive placebo at weeks 0 and 4 crossed over to receive ustekinumab (either 45 or 90 mg) at weeks 12 and 16.

In both studies, the end points were the proportion of patients who achieved 75% or greater reduction in PASI score (PASI 75) from baseline to week 12 and treatment success (cleared or minimal) on the Physician's Global Assessment (PGA). The PGA is a 6-category scale ranging from 0 (cleared) to 5 (severe) that indicates the physician's overall assessment of psoriasis, focusing on plaque thickness/induration, erythema, and scaling.

In both studies, patients in all treatment groups had a median baseline PASI score ranging from approximately 17 to 18. Baseline PGA score was marked or severe in 44% of patients in study 1 and 40% of patients in study 2. Approximately two-thirds of all patients had received prior phototherapy; 69% had received either prior conventional systemic or biologic therapy for the treatment of psoriasis, with 56% receiving prior conventional systemic therapy and 43% receiving prior biologic therapy. A total of 28% of study patients had a history of psoriatic arthritis.

The results are presented in the following table.

Clinical Outcomes of Study 1 and Study 2 Week 12						
	Study 1			Study 2		
		Ustekinumab			Ustekinumab	
	Placebo	45 mg	90 mg	Placebo	45 mg	90 mg
Patients randomized	255	255	256	410	409	411
PASI 75 response	8 (3%)	171 (67%)	170 (66%)	15 (4%)	273 (67%)	311 (76%)
PGA of cleared or minimal	10 (4%)	151 (59%)	156 (61%)	18 (4%)	277 (68%)	300 (73%)

Examination of age, gender, and race subgroups did not identify differences in response to ustekinumab among these subgroups. In patients who weighed less than 100 kg, response rates were similar with the 45 and 90 mg doses; however, in patients who weighed more than 100 kg, higher response rates were seen with 90 mg dosing compared with 45 mg dosing.

Clinical Outcomes by Weight, Study 1 and Study 2						
	Study 1			Study 2		
		Ustekinumab			Ustekinumab	
	Placebo	45 mg	90 mg	Placebo	45 mg	90 mg
Patients randomized	255	255	256	410	409	411
Week 12 PASI 75 response						
< 100 kg	4% 6/166	74% 124/168	65% 107/164	4% 12/290	73% 218/297	78% 225/289
> 100 kg	2% 2/89	54% 47/87	68% 63/92	3% 3/120	49% 55/112	71% 86/121
PGA of cleared or minimal						
< 100 kg	4% 7/166	64% 108/168	63% 103/164	5% 14/290	74% 220/297	75% 216/289
> 100 kg	3% 3/89	49% 43/87	58% 53/92	3% 4/120	51% 57/112	69% 84/121

Patients in study 1 were evaluated through week 52. At week 40, those who were PASI 75 responders at both weeks 28 and 40 were rerandomized to either continued dosing of ustekinumab at week 40 or withdrawal of therapy (placebo at week 40). At week 52, 89% (144/162) of patients rerandomized to ustekinumab treatment were PASI 75 responders, compared with 63% (100/159) of patients rerandomized to placebo (treatment withdrawal after week 28 dose).

Pharmacokinetics: In a small exploratory study, a decrease was observed in the expression of mRNA of its molecular targets IL-12 and IL-23 in lesional skin biopsies measured at baseline and up to 2 weeks posttreatment in psoriatic patients.

Absorption: In psoriasis patients, the median time to reach the maximum serum concentration (T_{max}) was 13.5 and 7 days, respectively, after a single subcutaneous ustekinumab dose of 45 mg (n = 22) and 90 mg (n = 24). In healthy patients (n = 30), the median T_{max} value (8.5 days) following a single subcutaneous 90 mg dose was comparable with that observed in psoriasis patients. After multiple subcutaneous doses, steady-state serum concentrations were achieved by week 28. The mean (± standard deviation [SD]) steady-state trough serum concentration ranged from 0.31 ± 0.33 mcg/mL (45 mg) to 0.64 ± 0.64 mcg/mL (90 mg). There was no apparent accumulation in serum ustekinumab concentration over time when given subcutaneously every 12 weeks.

Distribution: After subcutaneous administration of ustekinumab 45 mg (n = 18) and 90 mg (n = 21) to patients with psoriasis, the mean (± SD) apparent volume of distribution during the terminal phase (Vz/F) was 161 ± 65 mL/kg and 179 ± 85 mL/kg, respectively. The mean (± SD) volume of distribution during the terminal phase (Vz) following a single

IV dose to patients with psoriasis ranged from 56.1 ± 6.5 to 82.1 ± 23.6 mL/kg.

Weight: When given the same dose, patients weighing more than 100 kg had lower median serum ustekinumab concentrations, compared with those patients weighing 100 kg or less.

Hepatic and renal impairment: No pharmacokinetic data are available in patients with hepatic or renal impairment.

Elderly: A population pharmacokinetic analysis (n = 106/1,937 patients 65 years of age and older) was performed to evaluate the effect of age on the pharmacokinetics of ustekinumab. There were no apparent changes in pharmacokinetic parameters (clearance and volume of distribution) in patients older than 65 years of age.

Elimination: The metabolic pathway of ustekinumab has not been characterized. As a human IgG1κ monoclonal antibody, ustekinumab is expected to be degraded into small peptides and amino acids via catabolic pathways in the same manner as endogenous IgG. The mean (± SD) systemic clearance (CL) following a single IV dose of ustekinumab to administered psoriasis patients ranged from 1.9 ± 0.28 to 2.22 ± 0.63 mL/day/kg. The mean (± SD) half-life ranged from 14.9 ± 4.6 to 45.6 ± 80.2 days across all psoriasis studies following IV and subcutaneous administration.

Mechanism: Ustekinumab is a human interleukin-12 and -23 antagonist. Ustekinumab is a human IgG1κ monoclonal antibody that binds with high affinity and specificity to the p40 protein subunit used by both the IL-12 and IL-23 cytokines. IL-12 and IL-23 are naturally occurring cytokines involved in inflammatory and immune responses, such as natural killer cell activation and CD4+ T-cell differentiation and activation. In in vitro models, ustekinumab was shown to disrupt IL-12 and IL-23 mediated signaling and cytokine cascades by disrupting the interaction of these cytokines with a shared cell-surface receptor chain, IL-12 β1.

Drug Interactions: The safety of ustekinumab in combination with other immunosuppressive agents or phototherapy has not been evaluated. Ultraviolet-induced skin cancers developed earlier and more frequently in mice genetically manipulated to be deficient in both IL-12 and IL-23 or IL-12 alone.

Before starting ustekinumab therapy, give patients all vaccinations appropriate for age or other risk factors. Nonlive vaccinations received during a course of ustekinumab may not elicit an immune response sufficient to prevent disease. Do not give live vaccines to patients being treated with ustekinumab. Do not give BCG vaccines during ustekinumab treatment or for 1 year before starting treatment or 1 year after discontinuing treatment. Use caution when administering live vaccines to household contacts of patients receiving ustekinumab, because of the potential risk for transmission to patient.

CYP450 substrates: Formation of CYP450 enzymes can be altered by increased levels of certain cytokines (eg, IL-1, IL-6, IL-10, TNFα, IFN) during chronic inflammation. Thus, ustekinumab could normalize the formation of CYP450 enzymes. A role for IL-12 or IL-23 in the regulation of CYP450 enzymes has not been reported. However, upon starting ustekinumab in patients who are receiving concomitant CYP450 substrates, particularly those with a narrow therapeutic index, consider monitoring for therapeutic effect (eg, for warfarin) or drug concentration (eg, for cyclosporine) and adjust the individual dose of the drug needed.

Patient Information:

Infections: Inform patients that ustekinumab may lower the ability of their immune system to fight infections. Instruct patients to describe any history of infections to the health care provider, and to contact their health care provider if they develop any symptoms of infection.

Malignancies: Counsel patients about the risk of malignancies while receiving ustekinumab.

Ustekinumab

Pharmaceutical Characteristics

Concentration: Ustekinumab 90 mg/mL

Packaging: Each prefilled syringe is equipped with a needle safety guard. Single-use 45 mg/0.5 mL prefilled syringe with a 27-gauge, ½-inch needle (NDC #: 57894-0060-03). Single-use 90 mg/1 mL prefilled syringe with a 27-gauge, ½-inch needle (57894-0061-03). Single-use 45 mg/0.5 mL vial (57894-0060-02). Single-use 90 mg/1 mL vial (57894-0061-02).

Doseform: Solution

Appearance: Colorless to light yellow; may contain a few small translucent or white particles.

Solvent: Histidine-sucrose solution

Adjuvant: None

Preservative: None

Allergens: The needle cover on the prefilled syringe contains dry natural rubber (a derivative of latex).

Excipients: L-histidine and L-histidine monohydrochloride monohydrate 1 mg/mL, polysorbate-80 0.04 mg/mL, and sucrose 76 mg/mL.

pH: 5.7 to 6.3

Shelf Life: Data not provided.

Storage/Stability: Store upright at 2° to 8°C (36° to 46°F). Keep the product in the original carton to protect from light until the time of use. Do not freeze. Do not shake. Contact the manufacturer regarding exposure to freezing or elevated temperatures. Shipping data are not provided.

Handling: When using the single-use vial, a 27-gauge, ½-inch needle is recommended.

Production Process: Using DNA recombinant technology, ustekinumab is produced in a well-characterized recombinant cell line and is purified using standard bioprocessing technology. The manufacturing process contains steps for the clearance of viruses.

Media: Data are not provided.

Other Information

First Licensed: September 25, 2009

References: Chien AL, Elder JT, Ellis CN. Ustekinumab: a new option in psoriasis therapy. *Drugs.* 2009;69(9):1141-1152.

Ziv-aflibercept

Isoantibodies

Name:
Zaltrap

Manufacturer:
Sanofi-Aventis and Regeneron Pharmaceuticals

Immunologic Characteristics

Target Antigen: Vascular endothelial growth factor (VEGF) receptors 1 and 2

Viability: Not viable, but immunologically active

Antigenic Form: VEGF-binding portions from extracellular domains of human VEGF receptors 1 and 2 fused to Fc portion of human IgG1

Antigenic Type: Dimeric glycoprotein with molecular weight of 97 kDa, with glycosylation constituting an additional 15% of the total molecular mass, resulting in a total molecular weight of 115 kDa.

Use Characteristics

Indications: In combination with 5-fluorouracil-leucovorin-irinotecan (FOLFIRI) to treat patients with metastatic colorectal cancer (MCRC) that is resistant to or has progressed following an oxaliplatin-containing regimen.

Contraindications: None

Immunodeficiency: No impairment of effect has been noted.

Elderly: Of 611 MCRC patients treated with ziv-aflibercept/FOLFIRI, 205 (34%) were 65 years or older, and 33 (5%) were 75 years or older. Elderly patients (65 years and older) experienced higher incidences (5% or more) of diarrhea, dizziness, asthenia, weight decrease, and dehydration compared with younger patients. Monitor elderly patients more closely for diarrhea and dehydration.

The effect of ziv-aflibercept on overall survival was similar in patients younger than 65 years and patients 65 years and older who received ziv-aflibercept/FOLFIRI. No dose adjustment is recommended for patients 65 years of age and older.

Carcinogenicity: Ziv-aflibercept has not been evaluated for carcinogenic potential.

Mutagenicity: Ziv-aflibercept has not been evaluated for mutagenic potential.

Fertility Impairment: Male and female reproductive function and fertility may be compromised during treatment with ziv-aflibercept, based on findings in sexually mature monkeys. In a 6-month repeat-dose toxicology study, ziv-aflibercept inhibited ovarian function and follicular development, as evidenced by decreased ovary weight, decreased amount of luteal tissue, decreased number of maturing follicles, atrophy of uterine endometrium and myometrium, vaginal atrophy, and abrogation of progesterone peaks and menstrual bleeding. Alterations in sperm morphology and decreased sperm motility were noted in male monkeys. These effects were observed at all doses tested, including the lowest dose tested (3 mg/kg). These animal findings were reversible within 18 weeks after cessation of treatment.

Weekly/every 2 weeks intravenous (IV) administration of ziv-aflibercept to growing young adult (sexually mature) cynomolgus monkeys for up to 6 months resulted in changes in bone (effects on growth plate and the axial and appendicular skeleton), nasal cavity (atrophy/loss of the septum and/or turbinates), kidney (glomerulopathy with inflammation), ovary (decreased number of maturing follicles, granulosa cells, and/or theca cells), and adrenal gland (decreased vacuolation with inflammation). Most ziv-aflibercept–related findings were noted from the lowest dose tested (3 mg/kg per dose), correlating to 60% of area under the curve

(AUC) at the human recommended dose. In another study in sexually immature cynomolgus monkeys (treated IV for 3 months), similar effects were observed. The skeletal and nasal cavity effects were not reversible after a postdosing recovery period.

Females and males of reproductive potential should use highly effective contraception during and up to a minimum of 3 months after the last dose of treatment.

Pregnancy: Category C. It is not known if ziv-aflibercept crosses the placenta. There are no adequate and well-controlled studies in pregnant women. Ziv-aflibercept was embryotoxic and teratogenic in rabbits at exposure levels lower than human exposures at the recommended dose, with increased incidences of external, visceral, and skeletal fetal malformations. Use during pregnancy only if the potential benefit justifies the potential risk to the fetus.

Lactation: It is not known if ziv-aflibercept crosses into human breast milk. Because of the potential for serious adverse reactions in breast-feeding infants, decide whether to discontinue breast-feeding or the drug, taking into account the importance of the drug to the mother.

Children: Safety and efficacy of ziv-aflibercept in children younger than 18 years have not been established.

Adverse Reactions: The safety of ziv-aflibercept in combination with FOLFIRI was evaluated in 1,216 previously treated patients with MCRC (study 1). Patients were treated with ziv-aflibercept 4 mg/kg IV (n = 611) or placebo (n = 605) every 2 weeks (one cycle) in a randomized (1:1), double-blind, placebo-controlled phase 3 study. Patients received a median of 9 cycles of ziv-aflibercept/FOLFIRI or 8 cycles of placebo/FOLFIRI.

The most common adverse events (all grades, 20% or greater incidence and at least 2% greater incidence for the ziv-aflibercept/FOLFIRI regimen) were leukopenia, diarrhea, neutropenia, proteinuria, AST increased, stomatitis, fatigue, thrombocytopenia, ALT increased, hypertension, weight decreased, decreased appetite, epistaxis, abdominal pain, dysphonia, serum creatinine increased, and headache.

The most common grade 3 to 4 adverse events (at least 5%) reported at a higher incidence (at least 2% between-arm difference) in the ziv-aflibercept/FOLFIRI arm (in order of decreasing frequency) were neutropenia, diarrhea, hypertension, leukopenia, stomatitis, fatigue, proteinuria, and asthenia. The most frequent adverse events leading to permanent discontinuation in at least 1% of patients treated with the ziv-aflibercept/FOLFIRI regimen were asthenia/fatigue, infections, diarrhea, dehydration, hypertension, stomatitis, venous thromboembolic events, neutropenia, and proteinuria. The ziv-aflibercept dose was reduced and/or omitted in 17% of patients compared with a placebo dose modification in 5% of patients. Cycle delays of more than 7 days occurred in 60% of patients treated with ziv-aflibercept/FOLFIRI compared with 43% of patients treated with placebo/FOLFIRI.

Hemorrhage: Severe and sometimes fatal hemorrhage, including GI hemorrhage, has been reported in patients who received ziv-aflibercept. In patients with MCRC, bleeding/hemorrhage (all grades) was reported in 38% of patients treated with ziv-aflibercept/FOLFIRI compared with 19% of patients treated with placebo/FOLFIRI. Grade 3 to 4 hemorrhagic events, including GI hemorrhage, hematuria, and postprocedural hemorrhage, were reported in 3% of patients receiving ziv-aflibercept/FOLFIRI compared with 1% of patients receiving placebo/FOLFIRI. Severe intracranial hemorrhage and pulmonary hemorrhage/hemoptysis, including fatal events, have also occurred in patients receiving ziv-aflibercept. Do not administer to patients with severe hemorrhage.

GI: Discontinue ziv-aflibercept therapy in patients who experience GI perforation. Incidence of severe diarrhea and dehydration is increased; monitor elderly patients more closely.

Compromised wound healing: Repeated administration of ziv-aflibercept resulted in a delay in wound healing in rabbits. In full-thickness excisional and incisional skin wound models, ziv-aflibercept administration reduced fibrous response, neovascularization, epidermal hyperplasia/reepithelialization, and tensile strength. Discontinue ziv-aflibercept in patients with compromised wound healing. Suspend for at least 4 weeks before elective surgery, and do not resume for at least 4 weeks following major surgery and until the surgical wound is fully healed.

Fistula formation: Fistula formation involving GI and non-GI sites occurs at a higher incidence in patients treated with ziv-aflibercept. Discontinue ziv-aflibercept if fistula occurs.

Hypertension: Ziv-aflibercept increases the risk of grade 3 to 4 hypertension. Monitor blood pressure and treat hypertension. Temporarily suspend ziv-aflibercept if hypertension is not controlled. Discontinue if hypertensive crisis develops.

Arterial thromboembolic events: Arterial thromboembolic events (eg, transient ischemic attacks, cerebrovascular accident, angina pectoris) have occurred. Discontinue ziv-aflibercept if arterial thromboembolic events develop.

Proteinuria: Severe proteinuria, nephrotic syndrome, and thrombotic microangiopathy (TMA) occurred more frequently in patients treated with ziv-aflibercept. Monitor urine protein. Suspend ziv-aflibercept for proteinuria of 2 g per 24 hours. Discontinue if nephrotic syndrome or TMA develops.

Hematology: A higher incidence of neutropenic complications (febrile neutropenia and neutropenic infection) occurred in patients receiving ziv-aflibercept. Delay administration of ziv-aflibercept/FOLFIRI until neutrophil count is at least 1.5×10^9/L.

Reversible posterior leukoencephalopathy syndrome: Discontinue ziv-aflibercept.

Infection: Infections occurred at a higher frequency in patients receiving ziv-aflibercept/FOLFIRI (all grades, 46%; grades 3 to 4, 12%) than in patients receiving placebo/FOLFIRI (all grades, 33%; grades 3 to 4, 7%), including urinary tract infection, nasopharyngitis, upper respiratory tract infection, pneumonia, catheter-site infection, and tooth infection.

Cardiac electrophysiology: The effect of ziv-aflibercept 6 mg/kg IV every 3 weeks on QTc interval was evaluated in 87 patients with solid tumors in a randomized, placebo-controlled study. No large changes in the mean QT interval from baseline (ie, more than 20 ms as corrected for placebo) based on Fridericia correction method were detected in the study. However, a small increase in the mean QTc interval (ie, less than 10 ms) cannot be excluded due to limitations of the study design.

Immunogenicity: In patients with various cancers across 15 studies, 1.4% (41/2,862) of patients tested positive for antiproduct antibody at baseline. The incidence of antiproduct antibody development was 3.1% (53/1,687) in patients receiving IV ziv-aflibercept and 1.7% (19/1,134) in patients receiving placebo. Among patients who tested positive for antiproduct antibody and had sufficient samples for further testing, neutralizing antibodies were detected in 17 of 48 ziv-aflibercept–treated patients and in 2 of 40 patients receiving placebo. Mean free ziv-aflibercept trough concentrations were lower in patients with positive neutralizing antibodies than in the overall population. The effect of neutralizing antibodies on efficacy and safety could not be assessed based on limited available data.

Pharmacologic & Dosing Characteristics

Dosage: 4 mg/kg every 2 weeks. Administer ziv-aflibercept before any component of the FOLFIRI regimen on the day of treatment.

Discontinue ziv-aflibercept in the event of severe hemorrhage, GI perforation, compromised wound healing, fistula formation, hypertensive crisis or hypertensive encephalopathy, arterial thromboembolic events, nephrotic syndrome or TMA, or reversible posterior leukoencephalopathy syndrome (RPLS).

Temporarily suspend ziv-aflibercept
- at least 4 weeks before elective surgery.
- for recurrent or severe hypertension, until controlled. Upon resumption, permanently reduce the ziv-aflibercept dose to 2 mg/kg.
- for proteinuria of 2 g per 24 hours. Resume when proteinuria is less than 2 g per 24 hours. For recurrent proteinuria, suspend ziv-aflibercept until proteinuria is less than 2 g per 24 hours and then permanently reduce to 2 mg/kg.

For toxicities related to irinotecan, 5-fluorouracil (5-FU), or leucovorin, refer to the current respective prescribing information.

Route: IV infusion over 1 hour. Do not administer as an IV push or bolus.

Overdosage: There is no information on the safety of ziv-aflibercept given at doses above 7 mg/kg every 2 weeks or 9 mg/kg every 3 weeks.

Additional Doses: Continue ziv-aflibercept until disease progression or unacceptable toxicity.

Duration: Study 1 was a randomized, double-blind, placebo-controlled study in patients with MCRC who were resistant to or who progressed during or within 6 months of receiving oxaliplatin-based combination chemotherapy, with or without prior bevacizumab. A total of 1,226 patients were randomized (1:1) to receive either ziv-aflibercept (4 mg/kg IV infusion on day 1, n = 612) or placebo (n = 614) in combination with 5-fluorouracil plus irinotecan (FOL-FIRI: irinotecan 180 mg/m^2 IV infusion and leucovorin (dl-racemic) 400 mg/m^2 IV infusion at the same time on day 1, followed by 5-FU 400 mg/m^2 IV bolus, followed by 5-FU 2,400 mg/m^2 IV infusion). The treatment cycles for both arms were repeated every 2 weeks. Patients were treated until disease progression or unacceptable toxicity. The primary efficacy end point was overall survival. Treatment assignment was stratified by electrocochleography (ECOG) performance status (0 versus 1 versus 2) and according to prior therapy with bevacizumab (yes or no).

Demographics characteristics were similar between treatment arms. Of the 1,226 patients randomized, the median age was 61 years, 59% were men, 87% were white, 7% were Asian, 3.5% were black, and 98% had a baseline ECOG performance status of 0 or 1. Among the 1,226 randomized patients, 89% and 90% of patients treated with placebo/FOLFIRI and ziv-aflibercept/FOLFIRI, respectively, had received prior oxaliplatin-based combination chemotherapy in the metastatic/advanced setting. A total of 346 (28%) patients received bevacizumab in combination with prior oxaliplatin-based treatment.

Overall efficacy results for the ziv-aflibercept/FOLFIRI regimen versus the placebo/FOL-FIRI regimen are summarized in the following table. Planned subgroup analyses for overall survival based on stratification factors at randomization yielded a hazard ratio (HR) of 0.86 (95% confidence interval [CI], 0.68 to 1.1) in patients who received prior bevacizumab and an HR of 0.79 (95% CI, 0.67 to 0.93) in patients without prior bevacizumab exposure.

Efficacy Outcome Measures for Ziv-Aflibercept		
	Placebo/FOLFIRI (n = 614)	Ziv-aflibercept/FOLFIRI (n = 612)
Overall survival		
Number of deaths, n (%)	460 (75%)	403 (66%)
Median overall survival (95% CI) (months)	12.1 (11.1 to 13.1)	13.5 (12.5 to 15)
Stratified HR (95% CI)	0.82 (0.71 to 0.94)	
Stratified log-rank test *P* value	0.0032	

Ziv-aflibercept

Efficacy Outcome Measures for Ziv-Aflibercept		
	Placebo/FOLFIRI (n = 614)	Ziv-aflibercept/FOLFIRI (n = 612)
Progression-free Survival (PFS)[a]		
Number of events, n (%)	454 (74%)	393 (64%)
Median PFS (95% CI) (months)	4.7 (4.2 to 5.4)	6.9 (6.5 to 7.2)
Stratified HR (95% CI)	0.76 (0.66 to 0.87)	
Stratified log-rank test *P* value[b]	0.00007	
Overall response rate (95% CI) (%)[c]	11.1 (8.5 to 13.8)	19.8 (16.4 to 23.2)
Stratified Cochran-Mantel-Haenszel test *P* value	0.0001	

a PFS (based on tumor assessment): Significance threshold is set to 0.0001.
b Stratified on ECOG performance status (0 vs 1 vs 2) and prior bevacizumab (yes vs no).
c Overall objective response rate.

Pharmacokinetics: Plasma concentrations of free and VEGF-bound ziv-aflibercept were measured using specific enzyme-linked immunosorbent assays (ELISAs). Free ziv-aflibercept concentrations appear to exhibit linear pharmacokinetics in the dose range of 2 to 9 mg/kg. Following IV administration of 4 mg/kg every 2 weeks, the elimination half-life of free ziv-aflibercept was approximately 6 days (range, 4 to 7 days). Steady-state concentrations of free ziv-aflibercept were reached by the second dose. The accumulation ratio for free ziv-aflibercept was approximately 1.2 after 4 mg/kg every 2 weeks.

Specific populations: Based on a population pharmacokinetic analysis, age, race, and gender did not have a clinically important effect on the exposure of free ziv-aflibercept. Patients weighing 100 kg or more had a 29% increase in systemic exposure compared with patients weighing 50 to 100 kg.

Hepatic impairment: Based on a population pharmacokinetic analysis that included patients with mild (total bilirubin greater than 1 to 1.5 times the upper limit of normal [ULN] and any AST, n = 63) and moderate (total bilirubin greater than 1.5 to 3 times the ULN and any AST, n = 5) hepatic impairment, there was no effect of total bilirubin, AST, and ALT on the clearance of free ziv-aflibercept. There are no data available for patients with severe hepatic impairment (total bilirubin greater than 3 times the ULN and any AST).

Renal impairment: Based on a population pharmacokinetic analysis that included patients with mild (creatinine clearance [CrCl] 50 to 80 mL/min, n = 549), moderate (CrCl, 30 to 50 mL/min, n = 96), and severe renal impairment (CrCl, less than 30 mL/min, n = 5), there was no clinically important effect of CrCl on the clearance of free ziv-aflibercept.

Mechanism: Ziv-aflibercept acts as a soluble receptor that binds to human VEGF-A (equilibrium dissociation constant KD of 0.5 pM for VEGF-A165 and 0.36 pM for VEGF-A121), to human VEGF-B (KD of 1.92 pM), and to human PlGF (KD of 39 pM for PlGF-2). By binding to these endogenous ligands, ziv-aflibercept can inhibit the binding and activation of their cognate receptors. This inhibition can result in decreased neovascularization and decreased vascular permeability. In animals, ziv-aflibercept inhibits proliferation of endothelial cells, thereby inhibiting growth of new blood vessels. Ziv-aflibercept inhibited the growth of xenotransplanted colon tumors in mice.

Drug Interactions: No dedicated drug-drug interaction studies have been conducted for ziv-aflibercept. No clinically important pharmacokinetic drug-drug interactions were found between ziv-aflibercept and irinotecan/SN-38 or 5-FU, based on cross-study comparisons and population pharmacokinetic analyses.

Pharmaceutical Characteristics

Concentration: 25 mg/mL

Packaging: One single-use 100 mg per 4 mL vial (NDC#: 00024-5840-01), 3 single-use 100 mg per 4 mL vials (00024-5840-03); 1 single-use 200 mg per 8 mL vial (00024-5841-01)

Doseform: Solution

Appearance: Clear, colorless to pale yellow solution. Do not use if solution is discolored or cloudy or contains particles.

Solvent: Buffered saline solution

Diluent:

For infusion: Withdraw the dose of ziv-aflibercept and dilute in sodium chloride 0.9% or dextrose 5% sufficient to achieve a final concentration of 0.6 to 8 mg/mL. Use polyvinyl chloride (PVC) infusion bags containing bis(2-ethylhexyl) phthalate (DEHP) or polyolefin infusion bags.

Adjuvant: None

Preservative: None

Allergens: None

Excipients: Polysorbate-20 0.1%, sodium chloride 100 mM, sodium citrate 5 mM, sodium phosphate 5 mM, and sucrose 20% in water for injection

pH: 6.2

Shelf Life: Data not provided

Storage/Stability: Store at 2° to 8°C (36° to 46°F). Keep the vials in the original outer carton to protect from light. Do not freeze. Contact the manufacturer regarding exposure to freezing or elevated temperatures. Shipping data not provided.

Store diluted ziv-aflibercept at 2° to 8°C (36° to 46°F) for up to 4 hours. Discard any unused portion left in the infusion bag.

Handling: Administer the diluted ziv-aflibercept solution through a 0.2-micron polyethersulfone filter. Do not use filters made of polyvinylidene fluoride (PVDF) or nylon. Administer ziv-aflibercept using an infusion set made of one of the following materials: PVC containing DEHP, DEHP-free PVC containing trioctyl-trimellitate (TOTM), polypropylene, polyethylene-lined PVC, or polyurethane. Do not combine ziv-aflibercept with other drugs in the same infusion bag or IV line.

Production Process: Ziv-aflibercept is produced by recombinant DNA technology in a Chinese hamster ovary (CHO) K-1 mammalian expression system.

Media: CHO K-1 cells

Other Information

First Licensed: August 3, 2012

Transplantation General Statement: Antilymphocyte Antibody Summary

Isoantibodies

Antilymphocyte Antibody Comparisons

	Lymphocyte Immune Globulin	Antithymocyte Globulin	Muromonab-CD3	Daclizumab	Basiliximab	Belatacept
Manufacturer/distributor	Pfizer	Genzyme	Ortho Biotech	Hoffman-LaRoche	Novartis	Bristol-Myers Squibb
Proprietary name	Atgam	Thymoglobulin	Orthoclone OKT3	Zenapax	Simulect	Nulojix
Abbreviation	ATG	ATG	OKT3			
Protein concentration	50 mg/mL	5 mg/mL	1 mg/mL	5 mg/mL	20 mg/5 mL	25 mg/mL
Doseform	Solution	Powder for reconstitution	Solution	Solution	Powder for reconstitution	Powder for reconstitution
Packaging	5 mL ampule	25 mg vial plus 5 mL diluent	5 mL ampule	25 mg/5 mL vial	Box of 10 or 20 mg vials	250 mg vial of powder
Route & Rate	IV infusion over 4 to 6 hours	IV infusion over 4 to 6 hours	IV bolus over ≤ 60 seconds	IV bolus over 1 minute	IV infusion over 20 to 30 minutes	IV infusion over 30 min
Source	Equine	Rabbit	Murine	Chimeric (90% human, 10% murine)	Chimeric (human/murine)	Human fusion protein
Antigenic type	Polyclonal	Polyclonal	Monoclonal	Monoclonal	Monoclonal	CTLA-4 fused to Fc of IgG1
Antigenic targets (specificity)	Multiple (broad-spectrum)	Multiple (broad-spectrum)	CD3 receptors on T-cells (broad-spectrum)	CD25 subunit of IL-2 receptors on T-cells (selective)	CD25 subunit of IL-2 receptors on T-cells (selective)	Binds to CD80 and CD86
Indications	Prevention or treatment of allograft rejection; aplastic anemia	Treatment of acute allograft rejection	Treatment of acute allograft rejection	Prevention of acute allograft rejection	Prevention of acute allograft rejection	Prevention of acute allograft rejection (kidney) in seropositive patients

Antilymphocyte Antibody Comparisons						
	Lymphocyte Immune Globulin	Antithymocyte Globulin	Muromonab-CD3	Daclizumab	Basiliximab	Belatacept
Lot-to-lot potency variation	Yes	No	No	No	No	No
Sensitivity test suggested	Yes	No	No	No	No	No
Human neutralizing antibodies develop	Yes, antihorse ("minimal")	Yes, antirabbit	Yes, antimouse (80% after 2 weeks)	Yes, anti-daclizumab (8.4%)	Yes, anti-basiliximab (0.4% to 1.4%)	Yes, anti-belatacept
Regimen	21 doses in 28 days	Daily for 7 to 14 days	Daily for 10 to 14 days	5 doses, each 14 days apart	2 doses, day of transplant (within 2 hours before surgery) and on day 4	Initial, then maintenance
Typical dose	10-30 mg/kg/day	1.5 mg/kg	5 mg/day	1 mg/kg	20 mg per dose; pediatric dose: 12 mg/m^2	10 mg/kg, then 5 mg/kg

Transplantation General Statement: Antilymphocyte Antibody Summary

Disease Epidemiology

Incidence: By the mid-1990s, the number of organ transplants had increased to more than 11,000 kidneys, 1,000 livers, and thousands of other organs annually in more than 200 centers in the United States. The 1-year graft survival for recipients of first cadaveric kidneys is approximately 90%. The expected half-life of a cadaveric allograft that remained functional for 1 year is an additional 8.5 years. Of the 12,000 US kidney transplants each year, 20% to 60% develop acute rejection within the first year after surgery.

Other Information

Perspective:

1899: Metchnikoff demonstrates ability of a guinea pig antilymphoid serum to destroy white blood cells.

1908: Ottenberg performs pretransfusion tests in vitro to determine compatability of blood.

1940s: Interest in skin grafts, evident in 1924, rekindles in care of World War II burn patients.

1954: Murray and colleagues transplant a human kidney with recipient surviving longer than 1 year. The operation exchanged a kidney between a living pair of identical twins in Boston, because antirejection drugs had not yet been developed.

1960s: Various researchers experiment with polyclonal antilymphocyte sera (ALS).

1966: First successful pancreas transplant (success defined as recipient survival 1 year or longer), led by Kelly and Lillehie in Minneapolis.

Starzl, Iwasaki, and colleagues use refined antilymphocyte globulin (ALG) IM for prevention and treatment of human kidney allograph rejection.

1967: First successful liver transplant, led by Starzl in Denver.

Human heart transplanted by South Africa's Christiaan Barnard, and human liver transplanted by Starzl in Denver. Patient survival is measured in weeks.

1968: First successful heart transplant, led by Shumway in Stanford.

1970: Initial use of antilymphoblast globulin (MALG) by the University of Minnesota.

1975: Köhler and Milstein develop techniques for mass-producing monoclonal antibodies by fusing mouse splenocytes with myeloma cells. They earn the 1984 Nobel Prize in Medicine for this and related work.

1979: OKT monoclonal antibodies developed that detect distinct types of circulating human lymphocytes.

1981: First successful heart-lung transplant, led by Reitz at Stanford. *ATGAM* licensed on November 17, the first antibody product licensed for lymphoid depletion.

1983: First successful lung transplant, led by Cooper in Toronto.

1986: Muromonab-CD3, the first monoclonal antibody for human therapy, licensed in the United States on June 19.

1994: Antilymphoblast globulin (equine and caprine, MALG) produced by the University of Minnesota Department of Surgery recalled amid controversy over alleged commercial distribution without confirmation of safety and efficacy by the FDA.

1997: Daclizumab licensed in the United States on December 10.

1998: Basiliximab licensed on May 12. *Thymoglobulin* licensed on December 28.

References: Turka LA. What's new in transplant immunology: problems and prospects. *Ann Intern Med.* 1998;128:946-948.

Lymphocyte Immune Globulin, Antithymocyte Globulin (Equine)

Isoantibodies

Name:
 Atgam

Manufacturer:
 Pfizer

Synonyms: LIG, ATG, horse antihuman thymocyte gamma globulin, HAHTGG

Comparison: Several antibody products (eg, basiliximab, daclizumab, antithymocyte globulin) are licensed for prevention of allograft rejection. Some of these and some other antibody products (eg, antithymocyte globulin, muromonab-CD3) are licensed for treatment of acute allograft rejection. These drugs vary in their efficacy, adverse event profile, and use characteristics.

Immunologic Characteristics

Target Antigen: Human thymus lymphocytes

Viability: Inactive, passive, transient

Antigenic Form: Equine immunoglobulin, unmodified

Antigenic Type: Protein, IgG antibody, polyclonal, primarily monomeric. The molecular weight of this type of IgG ranges from 150,000 to 160,000 daltons. Skin tests assess immediate (type I) hypersensitivity.

Strains: The horses are immunized with thymocytes routinely removed from children undergoing thoracic surgery, harvested without regard to HLA specificity.

Use Characteristics

Indications: For prevention or treatment of allograft rejection in renal transplant patients. ATG may be used with conventional chemotherapy at time of rejection to increase the frequency of resolution of acute rejection episodes. ATG may be used as an adjunct to other immunosuppressive therapy to delay the onset of the first rejection episode, although data for this use are inconsistent. Most patients who received ATG for the treatment of acute rejection had not received it starting at the time of transplantation.

ATG is also indicated for treatment of moderate to severe aplastic anemia in patients unsuited for bone marrow transplantation. When administered with a regimen of supportive care, ATG may induce partial or complete hematologic remission.

Caution: Only physicians experienced in immunosuppressive therapy in the management of renal transplant or aplastic anemia patients should use ATG.

Unlabeled Uses: ATG has also been used as an immunosuppressant in the course of liver, bone marrow, heart, and other organ transplants. ATG has been used in the treatment of multiple sclerosis, myasthenia gravis, pure red-cell aplasia, and for scleroderma, although efficacy has not been definitively established.

Limitations: ATG is of no proven value in patients with aplastic anemia who are candidates for bone marrow transplantation or in patients with aplastic anemia secondary to neoplastic disease, storage disease, myelofibrosis, Fanconi syndrome, or in patients known to have been exposed to myelotoxic agents or radiation.

Contraindications:

Absolute: Do not give patients with a history of a systemic reaction (eg, generalized rash, tachycardia, dyspnea, hypotension, or anaphylaxis) any additional doses of ATG or any other equine IgG preparation. Discontinue treatment with ATG in case of anaphylaxis, severe and unremitting thrombocytopenia, or severe unremitting leukopenia.

Lymphocyte Immune Globulin, Antithymocyte Globulin (Equine)

Relative: Consider the risk-benefit ratio before administering ATG to a patient who has had severe systemic reaction during prior administration of any other equine IgG preparation.

Immunodeficiency: Because ATG is an immunosuppressive agent, carefully monitor recipients for signs of leukopenia, thrombocytopenia, or concurrent infection. Studies suggest an increase in the incidence of cytomegalovirus infection in recipients of ATG. Reducing the dose of other adjunctive immunosuppressive agents may reduce this risk. If infection occurs, start appropriate adjunctive therapy promptly.

Elderly: No specific information is available about geriatric use of ATG.

Pregnancy: Category C. ATG administration to pregnant women is not recommended; consider it only under exceptional circumstances. It is not known if ATG antibodies cross the placenta. Intact IgG crosses the placenta from the maternal circulation increasingly after 30 weeks gestation.

Lactation: It is not known if ATG antibodies are excreted into breast milk. Problems in humans have not been documented.

Children: Experience in children is limited. ATG has been administered safely to a small number of pediatric renal allograft recipients and pediatric aplastic anemia patients at dosages comparable with those used in adults.

Adverse Reactions:

Renal transplantation: The primary clinical experience with ATG has been in renal allograft patients who were also receiving concurrent standard immunosuppressive therapy (eg, azathioprine, corticosteroids): Fever (33%), chills (14%), leukopenia (14%), thrombocytopenia (11%), and dermatological reactions (eg, rash, pruritus, urticaria, wheal, flare; 13%). Reactions reported in 1% to 5% of recipients: Arthralgia, chest or back pain, clotted arterial-venous fistula, diarrhea, dyspnea, headache, hypotension, nausea or vomiting, night sweats, pain at the infusion site, peripheral thrombophlebitis, stomatitis. Reactions reported in less than 1% of recipients: Anaphylaxis, dizziness, weakness or faintness, edema, herpes simplex reactivation, hiccoughs or epigastric pain, hyperglycemia, hypertension, iliac vein obstruction, laryngospasm, localized infection, lymphadenopathy, malaise, myalgia, paresthesia, possible serum sickness, pulmonary edema, renal artery thrombosis, seizures, systemic infection, tachycardia, toxic epidermal necrosis, wound dehiscence.

Aplastic anemia: In trials with ATG in the treatment of aplastic anemia, patients were also being concurrently managed with supportive therapy (eg, transfusions, corticosteroids, antibiotics, antihistamines). In these trials, most patients experienced fever and skin reactions. Frequently reported reactions: Chills (50%), arthralgia (50%), headache (17%), myalgia (10%), nausea (7%), chest pain (7%), phlebitis (5%). Reactions reported in less than 5% of recipients: Diaphoresis, joint stiffness, periorbital edema, aches, edema, muscle ache, vomiting, agitation/lethargy, listlessness, light-headedness, seizures, diarrhea, bradycardia, myocarditis, cardiac irregularity, hepatosplenomegaly, possible encephalitis or postviral encephalopathy, hypotension, CHF, hypertension, burning soles or palms, foot sole pain, lymphadenopathy, postcervical lymphadenopathy, tender lymph nodes, bilateral pleural effusion, respiratory distress, anaphylaxis, proteinuria. In other studies of patients with aplastic anemia and other hematological abnormalities who received ATG, abnormal tests of liver function (eg, AST, ALT, alkaline phosphatase) and renal function (eg, serum creatinine) have been observed. In some trials, clinical and laboratory findings of serum sickness were seen in a majority of patients.

Postmarketing experience: Fever (51%), thrombocytopenia (30%), rashes (27%), chills (16%), leukopenia (14%), systemic infection (13%). Events reported in 5% to 10% of recipients: Abnormal renal function tests; serum sickness-like symptoms; dyspnea or apnea; arthralgia; chest, back, or flank pain; diarrhea; nausea; vomiting. Events reported in less than 5% of recipients: Hypertension; herpes simplex infection; pain; swelling or redness at the infusion site; eosinophilia; headache; myalgia or leg pains; hypotension; anaphylaxis; tachycardia; edema; localized infection; malaise; seizures; GI bleeding or perforation; deep vein thrombosis; sour mouth or throat; hyperglycemia; acute renal failure; abnormal liver function tests; confusion or disorientation; cough; neutropenia or granulocytopenia; anemia; thrombophlebitis; dizziness; epigastric or stomach pain; lymphadenopathy; pulmonary edema or CHF; abdominal pain; nosebleed, vasculitis; aplasia or pancytopenia; abnormal involuntary movement or tremor; rigidity; sweating; laryngospasm or edema; hemolysis or hemolytic anemia; viral hepatitis; faintness; enlarged or ruptured kidney; paresthesia; renal artery thrombosis.

A cause-effect relationship between some side effects and ATG administration is not established. In some cases, the side effects may merely be temporally associated, but not causally associated, with ATG.

Pharmacologic & Dosing Characteristics

Dosage:

Sensitivity test: Apply an intradermal skin test starting with 0.1 mL of a freshly compounded 1:1,000 v/v dilution (5 mcg IgG/mL) in 0.9% sodium chloride on 1 arm, with a contralateral injection of an equal volume of 0.9% sodium chloride as a negative-control reagent. Observe the patient and skin-test site at least every 15 to 20 minutes over the first hour after the intradermal injection. Other volumes and concentrations have also been used by the epicutaneous route.

A local reaction of 10 mm or greater with wheal, erythema, or both, with or without pseudopod formation and itching or a marked local swelling, constitute a positive test. The predictive value of this test has not been proven clinically. Allergic reactions, such as anaphylaxis, have occurred in patients whose skin test is negative. In the presence of a positive skin test to ATG, consider alternative forms of immunotherapy. A systemic reaction, such as generalized rash, tachycardia, dyspnea, hypotension, or anaphylaxis, precludes any additional administration of ATG.

If therapy with ATG is conducted despite a positive skin test, administer the drug in a setting where intensive life-support facilities for potentially life-threatening allergic reactions are available.

Therapeutic dose for renal allograft recipients: Usual dose is 10 to 30 mg/kg daily. The few children studied received 5 to 25 mg/kg daily. ATG is usually given concomitantly with azathioprine and corticosteroids. To delay the onset of allograft rejection, a fixed dose is often given: 15 mg/kg daily for 14 days, followed by 15 mg every other day for the next 14 days (ie, 21 doses over 28 days). Give the first dose within 24 hours before or after the transplant.

To treat rejection, the first dose of ATG can be delayed until diagnosis of the first rejection episode. Give 10 to 15 mg/kg daily for 14 days. Additional alternate-day therapy up to a total of 21 doses can be given.

Therapeutic dose for aplastic anemia: Give 10 to 20 mg/kg daily for 8 to 14 days. Additional alternate-day therapy up to a total of 21 doses can be given. Because thrombocytopenia can be associated with ATG administration, patients receiving it may need prophylactic platelet transfusions to maintain platelets at clinically acceptable levels.

Route & Site: Skin test by ID injection. Therapy by IV infusion, frequently into a vascular shunt, arterial-venous fistula or a high-flow central vein through an in-line filter with a pore diameter of 0.2- to 5-micron. Using high-flow veins will minimize the occurrence of phlebitis and thrombosis. Use the in-line filter to prevent inadvertent administration of insoluble material that may develop in the product during storage. Infuse the daily dose over at least 4 hours.

Lymphocyte Immune Globulin, Antithymocyte Globulin (Equine)

Overdosage: The maximal tolerated dose of ATG varies from patient to patient. The largest single dose to date was 7,000 mg in a renal-transplant recipient, at a concentration of approximately 10 mg/mL. This was about 7 times the recommended total dose and infusion concentration. No signs of acute intoxication developed in this patient. Some patients have received up to 50 doses in 4 months. Others have received 28-day courses of 21 doses, followed by as many as 3 more courses for the treatment of acute rejection, without increasing the incidence of toxic manifestations.

Additional Doses: Exercise caution during repeat courses of ATG. Carefully observe patients for signs of allergic reactions.

Efficacy: In general, ATG enables a 1-year graft survival rate of 80% or higher. Graft and patient survival are dependent on whether the transplanted organ is harvested from a living or deceased host, the degree of antigenic matching, the combination of immunosuppressive drugs delivered, and other factors.

Onset: Rapid

Duration: Mean half-life: 5.7 ± 3 days (range: 1.5 to 13 days).

Pharmacokinetics: Immunoglobulins are primarily eliminated by catabolism. The peak plasma level of equine IgG occurs after 5 days of infusion at 10 mg/kg/day. Peak values vary depending on the recipient's ability to catabolize equine IgG. In a small study, the mean peak plasma value was 727 ± 310 mcg/mL. Rosette-forming cells decrease immediately after beginning ATG therapy. Recovery to normal values after cessation of therapy is dependent upon the recipient's catabolic rate and, in some cases, upon the length of therapy. About 1% of equine IgG is excreted in the urine, mostly intact. Mean urine levels (over 21 doses in 28 days) are 4,061 ± 2,429 ng/mL. Human antibody responses against the equine IgG are generally minimal.

Mechanism: ATG is a lymphocyte-selective immunosuppressant, as demonstrated by its ability to reduce the number of circulating thymus-dependent lymphocytes that form rosettes with sheep erythrocytes. This antilymphocytic effect probably reflects an alteration of the function of T-lymphocytes, responsible in part for cell-mediated immunity and involved in humoral immunity.

ATG also contains low concentrations of antibodies against other formed elements of the blood. ATG has specific binding activity against surface antigens of granulocytes, platelets, B- and T-lymphocytes, and other nuclear and cytoplasmic components. In monkeys, ATG reduces the number of thymus-dependent areas of the spleen and lymph nodes. It also decreases circulating sheep-erythrocyte-rosetting lymphocytes that can be detected, but, ordinarily, ATG does not cause severe lymphopenia. It tends to spare natural killer cells.

Drug Interactions: Combined therapy with antilymphocytic antibodies and other immunosuppressant drugs may increase the recipient's risk of infection and neoplasm. Use the lowest effective dose of each agent. When ATG is given with other immunosuppressive therapy, such as antimetabolites and corticosteroids, the patient's own antibody response to horse IgG is minimal. As other immunosuppressive drugs are withdrawn or reduced in dosage, some previously masked reactions to ATG may become apparent.

Minnesota antilymphoblast globulin can suppress delayed-hypersensitivity responses. It is likely that ATG would have similar effects.

Pharmaceutical Characteristics

Concentration: 50 mg/mL equine protein, primarily monomeric IgG. Precise methods of determining the potency of ATG have not been established; thus, activity may potentially vary from lot to lot.

Quality Assay: Each lot is tested to assure ability to inhibit rosette formation between human peripheral lymphocytes and sheep red blood cells in vitro. In vitro tests of potency are not always indicative of clinical immunosuppression. Antibody activity against human red blood cells and platelets is also measured to assure acceptably low activity. Only lots that test negative for antihuman serum protein antibody, antiglomerular basement membrane antibody, pyrogens, and HBsAg are released.

Packaging: Box of 5 ampules, containing 5 mL each

NDC Number: 00009-7224-02

Doseform: Solution

Appearance: Colorless to faintly pink or brown; nearly odorless. May develop a granular or flaky deposit during storage.

Solvent: Sterile water for injection

Diluent:

For testing: Use 0.9% sodium chloride for dilution of ID hypersensitivity tests.

For infusion: Do not exceed a 4 mg/mL concentration, using a suitable IV fluid containing 0.225% to 0.9% sodium chloride. Do not use dextrose injection because the low salt concentration may cause precipitation. Highly acidic pH can also contribute to physical instability over time.

Invert IV containers during admixture to prevent foaming if the undiluted ATG contacts the air inside. To avoid foaming and protein denaturation, do not shake. Gently rotate or swirl to achieve thorough mixing. Use a 0.2- to 1-micron low protein-binding filter (eg, *Millex* GV).

Adjuvant: None

Preservative: None

Allergens: Equine serum

Excipients: Glycine 0.3 molar

pH: Approximately 6.8

Shelf Life: Expires within 24 months

Storage/Stability: Store at 2° to 8°C (36° to 46°F). Discard if frozen because freeze/thaw cycles may fracture ampules and compromise sterility. When ATG is stored at 25°C (77°F), it shows a significant decline in rosette-inhibiting activity by the end of 6 months. Storage at 40°C (104°F) causes formation of an insoluble material. Shipped in insulated containers with coolant packs. Transport should not take longer than 3 days, although 1 to 2 days is more common.

Diluted ATG is physically and chemically stable for up to 24 hours in concentrations of up to 4 mg/mL in 0.9% sodium chloride, 5% dextrose with 0.225% sodium chloride, and 5% dextrose with 0.45% sodium chloride. Store diluted ATG in a refrigerator if prepared prior to the time of infusion. Even if stored in a refrigerator, the total time in dilution should not exceed 24 hours, including infusion time.

Handling: Invert the infusion container to avoid foaming that would occur if the undiluted ATG were to contact the air inside. Do not shake, to avoid foaming and protein denaturation. Gently rotate or swirl to achieve thorough mixing. Use a 0.2- to 1-micron low protein-binding filter (eg, *Millex* GV). Allow diluted ATG to reach room temperature before infusion.

Production Process: Harvested from the hyperimmune plasma of horses immunized with human thymus lymphocytes and Freund's complete adjuvant. The plasma is precipitated from solution with acrinol. Then, it is adsorbed with human erythrocyte stroma to reduce the hemagglutinin titer and with precipitated human plasma to remove antibodies to circulat-

Lymphocyte Immune Globulin, Antithymocyte Globulin (Equine)

ing plasma proteins. The resulting plasma is subsequently processed by Cohn-Oncley methods 6 & 9 to increase the concentration. DEAE-ion exchange chromatography is performed for purification.

Media: Equine plasma

Disease Epidemiology

Incidence: See the Transplantation General Statement in the Antilymphocyte Antibody Summary monograph.

Other Information

Perspective: See the Transplantation General Statement in the Antilymphocyte Antibody Summary monograph.

1981: Atgam licensed November 17.

References: Chan GLC, et al. Principles of immunosuppression. *Crit Care Clinics.* 1990;6:841-892.

Wechter WJ, et al. Manufacture of antithymocyte globulin (*Atgam*) for clinical trials. *Transplantation.* 1979;28:303-307.

Lymphocyte Immune Globulin, Antithymocyte Globulin (Rabbit)

Isoantibodies

Name:
Thymoglobulin

Manufacturer:
Genzyme

Synonyms: ATG (caution: Note distinctions between *Thymoglobulin* and *Atgam* [antithymocyte globulin equine])

Comparison: Several antibody products (eg, basiliximab, daclizumab, antithymocyte globulin) are licensed for prevention of allograft rejection. Some of these and some other antibody products (eg, antithymocyte globulin, muromonab-CD3) are licensed for treatment of acute allograft rejection. These drugs vary in their efficacy, adverse event profile, and use characteristics.

Immunologic Characteristics

Target Antigen: Human thymus lymphocytes

Viability: Inactive, passive, transient

Antigenic Form: Rabbit immunoglobulin, unmodified

Antigenic Type: Protein, more than 90% rabbit IgG antibody, polyclonal, primarily monomeric

Strains: The rabbits are immunized with thymocytes harvested without regard to HLA specificity. Includes antibodies against T-cell markers such as CD2, CD3, CD4, CD8, CD11a, CD18, CD25, CD44, CD45, HLA-DR, HLA Class I heavy chains, and β_2 microglobulin.

Use Characteristics

Indications: For the treatment of renal transplant acute rejection in conjunction with concomitant immunosuppression.

Limitations: This agent has not been shown to be effective for treating antibody- (humoral) mediated rejections.

Contraindications:

Absolute: Patients with a history of a severe systemic reaction to this drug or other products containing rabbit proteins.

Relative: Patients with an acute viral illness.

Immunodeficiency: Because this is an immunosuppressive agent, carefully monitor recipients for signs of leukopenia, thrombocytopenia, or concurrent infection. If infection occurs, start appropriate adjunctive therapy promptly.

Elderly: No specific information is available about geriatric use.

Pregnancy: Category C. Animal reproduction studies have not been conducted. Give to a pregnant woman only if clearly needed. It is not known if antibodies cross the placenta or if ATG can cause fetal harm or affect reproduction capacity. Intact human IgG crosses the placenta from the maternal circulation increasingly after 30 weeks gestation.

Lactation: It is not known if ATG antibodies cross into human breast milk. Problems in humans have not been documented. Exercise caution when administering to a nursing woman.

Children: Safety and efficacy in pediatric patients have not been established in controlled trials. However, the dose, efficacy, and adverse event profile are not thought to be different from adults based on limited European and US studies.

Lymphocyte Immune Globulin, Antithymocyte Globulin (Rabbit)

Adverse Reactions: Adverse events are generally manageable or reversible. In the phase III trial of 163 kidney transplant patients comparing the safety and efficacy of *Thymoglobulin* and *Atgam*, there were no significant differences in clinically significant adverse events between the 2 treatment groups.

Infusion may produce fever and chills. To minimize these reactions, infuse the first dose over 6 hours or less into a high-flow vein. Premedication with corticosteroids, acetaminophen, or an antihistamine, or slowing the infusion rate, may reduce reaction incidence and intensity.

Malignancies were reported in 3 patients who received *Thymoglobulin* and in 3 patients who received *Atgam* during the 1-year follow-up period. Prolonged use or overdosage of *Thymoglobulin* with other immunosuppressive agents may cause over-immunosuppression resulting in severe infections and may increase the incidence of lymphoma or posttransplant lymphoproliferative disease (PTLD) or other malignancies.

No significant differences were observed between the *Thymoglobulin* and *Atgam* groups for infections overall, and the incidence of cytomegalovirus (CMV) infection was equivalent in both groups. Viral prophylaxis was at the center's discretion during antibody treatment, but all centers used gancyclovir infusion during treatment. Appropriate antiviral, antibacterial, antiprotozoal, or antifungal prophylaxis is recommended.

In rare instances, anaphylaxis has been reported with use. In such cases, stop the infusion immediately. Treat the patient as clinically indicated. Thrombocytopenia or neutropenia may result from cross-reactive antibodies and is reversible following dose adjustments.

Adverse events reported by more than 25% of patients in a treatment group included the following: Fever (63%); chills, leukopenia (57%); pain (46%); headache (40%); abdominal pain (38%); diarrhea, hypertension, nausea, thrombocytopenia (37%); peripheral edema (34%); dyspnea (28%); asthenia, hyperkalemia, tachycardia (27%). Malaise was reported more often among *Thymoglobulin* recipients (13%) than among *Atgam* recipients (4%). Dizziness was reported more often among *Atgam* recipients (25%) than among *Thymoglobulin* recipients (9%).

Anti-rabbit antibodies developed in 68% of patients treated with *Thymoglobulin* in the phase III randomized trial. No controlled studies have been conducted to study the effect of anti-rabbit antibodies on repeat use. However, the manufacturer recommends monitoring the lymphocyte count to ensure that T-cell depletion is achieved upon retreatment.

Pharmacologic & Dosing Characteristics

Dosage: The recommended dosage for treatment of acute renal graft rejection is 1.5 mg/kg of body weight administered daily for 7 to 14 days.

Route: IV infusion into a high-flow vein. Infuse over 6 hours or longer for the first infusion and over 4 hours or longer on subsequent days of therapy.

Overdosage: Overdosage may result in leukopenia or thrombocytopenia, which can be managed with dose reduction. Reduce the dose by one-half if the WBC count is between 2,000 and 3,000 cells/mm^3 or if the platelet count is between 50,000 and 75,000 cells/mm^3. Consider stopping treatment if the WBC count falls below 2,000 cells/mm^3 or platelets below 50,000 cells/mm^3.

Additional Doses: Exercise caution during repeat courses.

Carefully observe patients for signs of allergic reactions.

Missed Doses: Interrupting the recommended schedule or delaying subsequent doses does not require restarting the series.

Related Interventions: Administration of antiviral prophylactic therapy is recommended. Premedication with corticosteroids, acetaminophen, or an antihistamine 1 hour before infusion may reduce the incidence and intensity of side effects during infusion. Monitor patients for adverse events during and after infusion. Monitor T-cell counts (absolute or subsets) to assess the level of T-cell depletion, as well as total WBC and platelet counts.

Laboratory Tests: During therapy, monitoring the lymphocyte count (ie, total lymphocyte or T-cell subset) may help assess the degree of T-cell depletion. For safety, also monitor WBC and platelet counts.

Efficacy: A controlled, double-blind, multicenter, randomized clinical trial comparing *Thymoglobulin* 1.5 mg/kg/day and *Atgam* 15 mg/kg/day was conducted in 163 renal transplant patients with biopsy-proven Banff Grade II (moderate), Grade III (severe), or steroid-resistant Grade I (mild) acute graft rejection. *Thymoglobulin* was at least as effective as *Atgam* in reversing acute rejection episodes in this setting. During the trial, the FDA approved new maintenance immunosuppressive agents (tacrolimus and mycophenolate). Off-protocol use of these agents occurred during the second half of the study in some patients without affecting the overall conclusions.

Successful treatment was defined as a serum creatinine level (14 days from diagnosis of rejection) returned to baseline and a functioning graft on day 30 after the end of therapy. There were no significant differences between the 2 treatments with respect to: (1) day 30 serum creatinine levels relative to baseline; (2) improvement rate in posttreatment histology; (3) 1-year post-rejection Kaplan-Meier patient survival (*Thymoglobulin* 93%, [n = 82] and *Atgam* 96%, [n = 80]); (4) day 30, and (5) 1-year post-rejection graft survival (*Thymoglobulin* 83%, [n = 82]; *Atgam* 75%, [n = 80]).

Onset: T-cell depletion is usually observed within a day of initiating therapy.

Duration: Not described

Pharmacokinetics: Immunoglobulins are primarily eliminated by catabolism. After an initial IV dose of 1.25 to 1.5 mg/kg, mean levels 4 to 8 hours after a 4-hour infusion were 21.5 mcg/mL with a half-life of 2 to 3 days. After 7 to 11 daily doses, the mean concentration was 87 mcg/mL.

Mechanism: This immunosuppressive product contains cytotoxic antibodies directed against antigens expressed on human T-lymphocytes. The mechanism by which polyclonal antilymphocyte preparations suppress immune responses is not fully understood. Possible mechanisms include T-cell clearance from the circulation and modulation of T-cell activation, homing, and cytotoxic activities. This agent includes antibodies against T-cell markers such as CD2, CD3, CD4, CD8, CD11a, CD18, CD25, CD44, CD45, HLA-DR, HLA Class I heavy chains, and β_2 microglobulin. In vitro, at concentrations higher than 0.1 mg/mL, it mediates T-cell suppressive effects via inhibition of proliferative responses to several mitogens.

Drug Interactions: Combined therapy with antithymocytic antibodies and other immunosuppressant drugs may increase the recipient's risk of infection and neoplasm. Use the lowest effective dose of each agent. Many transplant centers decrease maintenance immunosuppression therapy during the period of antibody therapy.

Minnesota antilymphoblast globulin was known to suppress delayed-hypersensitivity responses. It is likely that this agent would have similar effects.

It is a common practice to wait several months after discontinuation of immunosuppressive therapy before immunizing patients with inactivated or attenuated vaccines. Active immunization of immunosuppressed patients may result in an inadequate response to immunization. They may remain susceptible despite immunization. Some live, attenuated vaccines pose safety risks to immunosuppressed patients.

Lab Interference: This agent has not been shown to interfere with any routine clinical laboratory tests that do not use immunoglobulins, but it may interfere with rabbit antibody-based immunoassays and with cross-match or panel-reactive antibody cytotoxicity assays.

Lymphocyte Immune Globulin, Antithymocyte Globulin (Rabbit)

Pharmaceutical Characteristics

Concentration: After reconstitution, 25 mg antithymocyte globulin (rabbit) per 5 mL (5 mg/mL)

Quality Assay: Each lot is released following potency testing (lymphocytotoxicity and E-rosette inhibition assays) and cross-reactive antibody testing (hemagglutination, platelet agglutination, antihuman serum protein antibody, antiglomerular basement membrane antibody, and fibroblast toxicity assays on every fifth lot).

Packaging: Package containing 10 mL vial with 25 mg powder (NDC#: 58468-0080-01)

Doseform: Powder for solution

Appearance: White lyophilized powder. Colorless, slightly opalescent solution.

Diluent:

For reconstitution: Sterile water for injection.

For infusion: Sodium chloride 0.9% or dextrose 5%. Dilute each vial in 50 mL of infusion solution (total volume usually between 50 to 500 mL). Mix the solution by inverting the bag gently once or twice. Infuse through a 0.22-micron filter into a high-flow vein.

Adjuvant: None

Preservative: None

Allergens: Rabbit serum proteins

Excipients: Glycine (50 mg/5 mL), mannitol (50 mg/5 mL), sodium chloride (10 mg/5 mL)

pH: 6.6 to 7.4

Shelf Life: Expires within 24 months

Storage/Stability: Store at 2° to 8°C (36° to 46°F). Do not freeze. Protect from light. Contact the manufacturer regarding exposure to extreme temperatures. Shipping data not provided.

Administer drug in reconstituted vials within 4 hours. Infuse solutions immediately after dilution. Protect from light.

Handling: Allow powder and diluent vials to reach room temperature before reconstituting the lyophilized product. Rotate vial gently until powder is completely dissolved. If any particulate matter is visible, continue to gently rotate the vial until no particulate matter is visible. If particulate matter persists, discard the vial. Administer through an in-line 0.22-micron filter.

Production Process: Harvested from the plasma of rabbits immunized with human thymocytes. Human RBC are used in the manufacturing process to deplete cross-reactive antibodies to non-T-cell antigens. The manufacturing process is validated to remove or inactivate potential exogenous viruses. All human RBC are from US-registered or FDA-licensed blood banks. A viral inactivation step (pasteurization; ie, heat treatment of active ingredient at 60°C [140°F] for 10 hours) is performed for each lot. Processing steps include purification using ion-exchange chromatography.

Media: Rabbit plasma

Disease Epidemiology

Incidence: See the Transplantation General Statement.

Other Information

Perspective: See the Transplantation General Statement.

First Licensed: December 30, 1998

References: Hardinger KL. Rabbit antithymocyte globulin induction therapy in adult renal transplantation. *Pharmacotherapy.* 2006;26(12):1771-1783.

Name:
Simulect

Manufacturer:
Novartis Pharmaceuticals Corporation

Comparison: Several antibody products (eg, basiliximab, daclizumab, antithymocyte globulin) are licensed for the prevention of allograft rejection. Some of these and some other antibody products (eg, antithymocyte globulin, muromonab-CD3) are licensed for treatment of acute allograft rejection. These drugs vary in their efficacy, adverse event profile, and use characteristics.

Immunologic Characteristics

Target Antigen: Interleukin-2 receptor α-chain (IL-2Ra, also known as CD25 antigen) on the surface of activated T-lymphocytes.

Viability: Inactive, passive, transient

Antigenic Form: Chimeric (murine/human) monoclonal IgG1κ antibody, a glycoprotein

Antigenic Type: Protein, IgG1κ antibody that specifically binds to and blocks the interleukin-2 receptor α-chain (IL-2Ra, also known as CD25 antigen) on the surface of activated T-lymphocytes. The calculated molecular weight of basiliximab is 144 kilodaltons.

Use Characteristics

Indications: Basiliximab is indicated for the prophylaxis of acute organ rejection in patients receiving renal transplantation when used as part of an immunosuppressive regimen that includes cyclosporine and corticosteroids. Basiliximab is also indicated in renal transplantation in combination with triple immunosuppressive therapy and in pediatric renal transplantation. Basiliximab should only be used by clinicians experienced in immunosuppression therapy and management of organ transplantation patients.

Limitations: The efficacy of basiliximab in preventing acute rejection in recipients of other solid organ allografts has not been demonstrated.

Contraindications:

Absolute: Patients with a history of a severe acute hypersensitivity reaction after basiliximab therapy.

Relative: Patients with known hypersensitivity to basiliximab or any other component of the formulation (other than severe).

Immunodeficiency: While in the circulation, basiliximab impairs the response of the immune system to antigenic challenges. Whether the ability to respond to repeated or ongoing challenges with those antigens returns to normal after basiliximab is cleared is unknown.

Elderly: Clinical studies of basiliximab included a small number of patients 65 years of age or older (15 patients received basiliximab; 19 received placebo). From the data, the adverse event profile in patients 65 years of age or older is similar to that of patients younger than 65 years of age, and no age-related dosage adjustment is required. Use caution in giving immunosuppressive drugs to elderly patients.

Carcinogenicity: No long-term studies in laboratory animals have been performed to evaluate basiliximab's potential to produce carcinogenicity.

Mutagenicity: No mutagenic potential was observed in the in vitro assays with *Salmonella* (Ames) and V79 Chinese hamster cells.

Fertility Impairment: No fertility studies in laboratory animals have been performed to evaluate the potential to impair fertility.

Pregnancy: Category B. There are no adequate and well-controlled studies in pregnant women. No maternal toxicity, embryotoxicity, or teratogenicity was observed in cynomolgus monkeys 100 days postcoitum following dosing with basiliximab during the organogenesis period; blood levels in pregnant monkeys were 13-fold higher than those seen in human patients. Immunotoxicology studies have not been performed in the offspring. Because IgG molecules are known to cross the placental barrier (especially during the third trimester), the IL-2 receptor may play an important role in development of the immune system, and animal reproduction studies are not always predictive of human response, use basiliximab in pregnant women only when the potential benefit justifies the potential risk to the fetus. Women of child-bearing potential should use effective contraception before beginning basiliximab therapy, during therapy, and for 4 months after completion of basiliximab therapy.

Lactation: It is not known if basiliximab crosses into human breast milk. Because many drugs (including human antibodies) are excreted in breast milk, and because of the potential for adverse reactions, decide whether to discontinue nursing or to discontinue the drug, taking into account the importance of the drug to the mother.

Children: No adequate and well-controlled studies of basiliximab have been completed in pediatric patients. In an ongoing safety and pharmacokinetic study, pediatric patients (2 to 11 years of age [n = 8], 12 to 15 years of age [n = 4], median age 9.5 years of age) were treated with basiliximab, in addition to standard immunosuppressive agents including cyclosporine, corticosteroids, azathioprine, and mycophenolate mofetil. Preliminary results indicate that 2 of 12 patients (16.7%) experienced an acute rejection episode within 3 months of transplantation. The most frequently reported adverse events were fever and urinary tract infections (41.7% each). Overall, the adverse event profile was consistent with general clinical experience in the pediatric renal transplantation population and with the profile in the controlled adult renal transplantation studies.

Adverse Reactions: The incidence of adverse events from basiliximab was determined in 2 randomized, double-masked trials for the prevention of renal allograft rejection. All patients received concomitant cyclosporine for microemulsion and corticosteroids. Basiliximab did not appear to add to the background of adverse events seen in organ transplantation patients as a consequence of their underlying disease and the concurrent administration of immunosuppressants and other medications. Adverse events were reported by 99% of the patients in the placebo-treated group and 99% of the patients in the basiliximab-treated group. Basiliximab did not increase the incidence of serious adverse events observed, compared with placebo. The most frequently reported adverse events were GI disorders, reported in 75% of basiliximab-treated patients and 73% of placebo-treated patients.

The incidence and types of adverse events were similar in basiliximab-treated and placebo-treated patients.

Body as a whole: Pain, peripheral edema, edema, fever, viral infection, leg edema, asthenia (10% or more), accidental trauma, chest pain, increased drug level, face edema, fatigue, infection, malaise, generalized edema, rigors, sepsis (3% to 10%).

Cardiovascular: Hypertension (10% or more), angina pectoris, cardiac failure, chest pain, abnormal heart sounds, aggravated hypertension, hypotension, arrhythmia, atrial fibrillation, tachycardia, vascular disorder (3% to 10%).

CNS: Headache, tremor, dizziness (10% or more), hypoesthesia, neuropathy, paresthesia (3% to 10%).

Dermatologic: Surgical wound complications, acne (10% or more), cyst, herpes simplex, herpes zoster, hypertrichosis, pruritus, rash, skin disorder, skin ulceration (3% to 10%).

Endocrine: Increased glucocorticoids (3% to 10%).

Basiliximab (Chimeric)

GI: Constipation, nausea, diarrhea, abdominal pain, vomiting, dyspepsia, moniliasis (10% or more), enlarged abdomen, flatulence, GI disorder, gastroenteritis, GI hemorrhage, gum hyperplasia, melena, esophagitis, ulcerative stomatitis (3% to less than 10%).

GU: Dysuria, increased nonprotein nitrogen, urinary tract infection (10% or more), impotence, genital edema, albuminuria, bladder disorder, hematuria, frequent micturition, oliguria, abnormal renal function, renal tubular necrosis, surgery, ureteral disorder, urinary retention (3% to 10%).

Hematologic: Anemia (10% or more), hematoma, hemorrhage, purpura, thrombocytopenia, thrombosis, polycythemia (3% to 10%).

Hypersensitivity: At least 17 cases of severe acute hypersensitivity (eg, anaphylaxis, tachycardia, dyspnea, bronchospasm, pulmonary edema, respiratory failure, capillary leak syndrome, cytokine release syndrome) have occurred after basiliximab administration, both initial doses and re-exposures.

Metabolic/Nutritional: Hyperkalemia, hypokalemia, hyperglycemia, hyperuricemia, hypophosphatemia, hypocalcemia, weight increase, hypercholesterolemia, acidosis (10% or more), dehydration, diabetes mellitus, fluid overload, hypercalcemia, hyperlipemia, hypoglycemia, hypoproteinemia, hypomagnesemia (3% to 10%).

Miscellaneous: The incidence of malignancies among all patients in the two 12-month trials was not significantly different between the basiliximab and placebo groups. Lymphoma or lymphoproliferative disease occurred in 1 patient (0.3%) in the basiliximab group compared with 2 patients (0.6%) in the placebo group. Other malignancies were reported among 5 patients (1.4%) in the basiliximab group, compared with 7 patients (1.9%) in patients treated with placebo. Patients on immunosuppressive therapy are known to be at increased risk for developing these complications; monitor patients accordingly.

Cytomegalovirus infection was reported in 14% of basiliximab-treated patients and 18% of placebo-treated patients. The rates of infections, serious infections, and infectious organisms were similar in the basiliximab and placebo treatment groups.

Musculoskeletal: Leg pain, back pain (10% or more), arthralgia, arthropathy, bone fracture, cramps, hernia, myalgia (3% to 10%).

Respiratory: Dyspnea, upper respiratory tract infection, coughing, rhinitis, pharyngitis (10% or more), bronchitis, bronchospasm, abnormal chest sounds, pneumonia, pulmonary disorder, pulmonary edema, sinusitis (3% to less than 10%).

Psychiatric: Insomnia (10% or more), agitation, anxiety, depression (3% to 10%).

Special Senses: Cataract, conjunctivitis, abnormal vision (3% to 10%).

Pharmacologic & Dosing Characteristics

Dosage: Basiliximab is used as part of an immunosuppressive regimen that includes cyclosporine and corticosteroids.

Adult: In adult patients, the recommended regimen is 2 doses of 20 mg each. Give the first 20 mg dose within 2 hours before transplantation surgery. Give the second 20 mg dose 4 days after transplantation.

Pediatric: In pediatric patients weighing less than 35 kg, the recommended regimen is 2 doses of 10 mg each. In pediatric patients weighing 35 kg or more, the recommended regimen is 2 doses of 20 mg each. Give the first dose within 2 hours before transplantation surgery. Give the second dose 4 days after transplantation.

Route: For central or peripheral IV administration only. Administer as a bolus injection or diluted to a volume of 50 mL with sodium chloride 0.9% or dextrose 5% administered over 20 to 30 minutes. Bolus administration may be associated with nausea, vomiting, and local reactions, including pain.

Basiliximab (Chimeric)

Overdosage: A maximum tolerated dose has not been determined. In clinical studies, basiliximab has been administered to renal transplantation patients in single doses of 60 mg or lower, or in divided doses over 3 to 5 days of 120 mg or lower, without any associated serious adverse events. There has been 1 report of a pediatric renal transplantation patient receiving a single 20 mg dose (2.3 mg/kg) without adverse effect.

Additional Doses: Readministration of basiliximab after an initial course of therapy has not been formally studied in humans. Severe acute hypersensitivity reactions have been reported after re-exposures to basiliximab after intervals of several months. The potential risks of such readministration, specifically those associated with immunosuppression or the occurrence of anaphylactoid reactions, are not fully understood.

Missed Doses: Interrupting the recommended schedule or delaying subsequent doses does not require restarting the series.

Efficacy: Basiliximab in the prophylaxis of acute organ rejection in adults following first cadaveric- or living-donor renal transplantation was assessed in 2 randomized, double-masked, placebo-controlled trials. The studies compared two 20 mg doses of basiliximab with placebo, as part of a standard immunosuppressive regimen including cyclosporine for micro-emulsion and corticosteroids, administered starting on day 0. The first dose of basiliximab or placebo was administered within 2 hours before transplantation surgery (day 0), with the second dose on day 4 posttransplantation. A total of 729 patients 18 to 75 years of age undergoing first cadaveric or living donor renal transplantation with HLA mismatch were enrolled.

Patients receiving basiliximab experienced a significantly lower incidence of biopsy-confirmed rejection episodes at 6 and 12 months posttransplantation. There was no difference in the rate of delayed graft function, patient survival, or graft survival between basiliximab-treated patients and placebo-treated patients. There was no evidence that the clinical benefit of basiliximab was limited to specific subpopulations based on age, gender, race, donor type (cadaveric- or living-donor allograft), or a history of diabetes mellitus.

Efficacy Parameters (% of Patients)						
	European/Canadian study			US study		
	Placebo (n = 185)	Basiliximab (n = 190)	P value	Placebo (n = 173)	Basiliximab (n = 173)	P value
Primary endpoint						
Death, graft loss, or acute rejection episode (0 to 6 months)	57%	42%	0.003	55%	38%	0.002
Secondary endpoints						
Death, graft loss, or acute rejection episode (0 to 12 months)	60%	46%	0.007	58%	41%	0.001
Biopsy-confirmed rejection episode (0 to 6 months)	44%	30%	0.007	46%	33%	0.015
Biopsy-confirmed rejection episode (0 to 12 months)	46%	32%	0.005	49%	35%	0.009
Patient survival (12 months)	97%	95%	0.29	96%	97%	0.56
Patients with functioning graft (12 months)	87%	88%	0.7	93%	95%	0.5

Sensitization: Among renal transplantation patients (n = 246) treated with basiliximab and tested for anti-idiotype antibodies, 1 developed an anti-idiotype antibody response with no deleterious clinical effect. The incidence of human antimurine antibody (HAMA) in renal transplantation patients treated with basiliximab was 2 of 138 patients not exposed to muromonab-CD3 and 4 of 34 patients who subsequently received muromonab-CD3. The available clinical data on the use of muromonab-CD3 in patients previously treated with basiliximab suggest that subsequent use of muromonab-CD3 or other murine antilymphocytic antibody preparations is not precluded.

Onset: Prompt

Duration: At the recommended dosing regimen, the mean ± SD duration of basiliximab saturation of IL-2Ra was 36 ± 14 days. The duration of clinically significant IL-2 receptor blockade after the recommended course of basiliximab is not known. No significant changes to circulating lymphocyte numbers or cell phenotypes were observed by flow cytometry. Whether the ability to respond to repeated or ongoing antigenic challenges returns to normal after basiliximab is cleared is unknown.

Pharmacokinetics: Complete and consistent binding to IL-2Ra in adults is maintained as long as serum basiliximab levels exceed 0.2 mcg/mL. As concentrations fall below this threshold, the IL-2Ra sites are no longer fully bound, and the number of T-cells expressing unbound IL-2Ra returns to pretherapy values within 1 to 2 weeks. The relationship between serum concentration and receptor saturation was assessed in 2 pediatric patients (2 and 12 years of age) and was similar to that seen in adult renal transplantation patients. In vitro studies using human tissues indicate that basiliximab binds only to lymphocytes.

Absorption: Adults: Single-dose and multiple-dose pharmacokinetic studies have been conducted in patients undergoing first kidney transplantation. Cumulative doses ranged from 15 to 150 mg. Peak serum concentration (mean ± standard deviation) following IV infusion of 20 mg over 30 minutes is 7.1 ± 5.1 mg/L. There is a dose-proportional increase in maximal concentration (C_{max}) and area under the curve (AUC) up to the highest tested single dose of 60 mg.

Children: The pharmacokinetics of basiliximab were assessed in 12 pediatric renal transplantation patients, 8 children 2 to 11 years of age and 4 adolescents 12 to 15 years of age.

Distribution: Adults: The volume of distribution at steady state is 8.6 ± 4.1 L. The extent and degree of distribution to various body compartments have not been fully studied.

Children: These data indicate that the volume of distribution at steady state in children was 4.8 ± 2.1 L. Distribution volume was reduced by approximately 50% compared with adult renal transplantation patients. Disposition parameters were not influenced to a clinically relevant extent by age, body weight (9 to 37 kg), or body surface area (0.44 to 1.2 m^2) in this age group. In adolescents, the volume of distribution at steady state was 7.8 ± 5.1 L. Disposition in adolescents was similar to that seen in adult renal transplantation patients.

Elimination: Immunoglobulins are primarily eliminated by catabolism.

Adults: The terminal half-life is 7.2 ± 3.2 days. Total body clearance is 41 ± 19 mL/h. No clinically relevant influence of body weight or gender on distribution volume or clearance has been observed in adults. Elimination half-life was not influenced by age (20 to 69 years), gender, or race.

Children: The half-life for children 1 to 11 years of age was 9.5 ± 4.5 days and clearance was 17 ± 6 mL/h. Clearance was reduced by approximately 50% compared with adult renal transplantation patients. Disposition parameters were not influenced to a clinically relevant extent by age, body mass, or body surface area. In adolescents, the half-life was 9.1 ± 3.9 days and clearance was 31 ± 19 mL/h.

Mechanism: Specifically binds to and blocks the interleukin-2 receptor α-chain (IL-2Ra, also known as CD25 antigen) selectively expressed on the surface of activated T-lymphocytes, acting as a receptor antagonist with high affinity (Ka = 1 × 10^{10} M^{-1}). This specific high-affinity binding of basiliximab to IL-2Ra competitively inhibits IL-2-mediated activation of lymphocytes, a critical pathway in the cellular immune response involved in allograft rejection.

While in the circulation, basiliximab impairs the response of the immune system to antigenic challenges. Whether the ability to respond to repeated or ongoing challenges with antigens first encountered during basiliximab-induced immunosuppression returns to normal after basiliximab is cleared is unknown.

Drug Interactions: No formal drug interaction studies have been conducted. The following medications have been administered in clinical trials with basiliximab with no incremental increase in adverse reactions: Antilymphocyte globulin, antithymocyte globulin, azathioprine, corticosteroids, cyclosporine, mycophenolate mofetil, and muromonab-CD3. The available clinical data on the use of muromonab-CD3 in patients previously treated with basiliximab suggest that subsequent use of muromonab-CD3 or other murine antilymphocytic antibody preparations is not precluded.

It is not known whether the immune response to vaccines, infection, and other antigenic stimuli administered or encountered during basiliximab therapy is impaired or whether such response will remain impaired after basiliximab therapy.

It is a common practice to wait several months after discontinuation of immunosuppressive therapy before immunizing patients with inactivated or attenuated vaccines. Active immunization of immunosuppressed patients may result in an inadequate response to immunization. They may remain susceptible despite immunization. Some live, attenuated vaccines pose safety risks to immunosuppressed patients.

Pharmaceutical Characteristics

Concentration: Each vial contains 20 mg basiliximab for reconstitution.

Quality Assay: Data not provided

Packaging: Single-use glass vial containing either 10 mg basiliximab (NDC#: 00078-0393-61) or 20 mg basiliximab (00078-0331-84).

Doseform: Lyophilized powder for reconstitution in 6 mL colorless glass vials. Basiliximab is water-soluble.

Appearance: White, lyophilized powder. After reconstitution, a clear-to-opalescent, colorless solution.

Diluent:

For reconstitution: Reconstitute each 10 mg vial of basiliximab powder with 2.5 mL of sterile water for injection and each 20 mg vial with 5 mL of sterile water. Shake the vial gently to dissolve the powder. The reconstituted solution is isotonic.

For infusion: Dilute reconstituted basiliximab to a volume of 25 mL (children) or 50 mL (adolescents and adults) with sodium chloride 0.9% or dextrose 5% for infusion. When mixing the solution, gently invert the bag to avoid foaming. Do not shake.

Adjuvant: None

Preservative: None

Allergens: None

Excipients: Each 20 mg vial contains 7.21 mg monobasic potassium phosphate, 0.99 mg disodium hydrogen phosphate (anhydrous), 1.61 mg sodium chloride, 20 mg sucrose, 80 mg mannitol, and 40 mg glycine. Each 10 mg vial contains half this quantity.

pH: 6 after reconstitution

Shelf Life: Expires within 24 months.

Storage/Stability: Store powder at 2° to 8°C (36° to 46°F). Discard if frozen. Contact the manufacturer regarding exposure to extreme temperatures. Shipped with temperature monitors to identify conditions hotter than 41°C (105°F).

Use promptly after reconstituting the solution. If not used immediately, solution can be stored at 2° to 8°C (36° to 46°F) for 24 hours or at room temperature for 4 hours. Discard the reconstituted solution if not used within 24 hours.

No incompatibility between basiliximab and polyvinyl chloride bags or infusion sets has been observed. No data are available on the compatibility of basiliximab with other IV substances. Do not add or simultaneously infuse other drug substances through the same IV line.

Production Process: Basiliximab is produced by recombinant DNA technology, with the glycoprotein obtained from fermentation of an established mouse myeloma cell line genetically engineered to express plasmids containing the human heavy and light chain constant region genes and mouse heavy and light chain variable region genes encoding the RFT5 antibody that binds selectively to the IL-2Ra.

Media: Mouse myeloma cell line

Other Information

First Licensed: May 12, 1998

References: Nashan B, et al. Randomised trial of basiliximab versus placebo for control of acute cellular rejection in renal allograft recipients. *Lancet*. 1997;350:1193-1198. Errata 1484.

Ramirez CB, Marino IR. The role of basiliximab induction therapy in organ transplantation. *Expert Opin Biol Ther*. 2007;7(1):137-148.

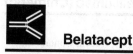

Belatacept

Isoantibodies

Name:
Nulojix

Manufacturer:
Bristol-Myers Squibb

Synonyms: BMS-224818

Comparison: Compared with abatacept, 2 amino acid substitutions (L104 to E; A29 to Y) were made in the ligand binding region of CTLA-4 to create belatacept. As a result of these modifications, belatacept binds CD80 and CD86 more avidly than abatacept, the parent CTLA4-immunoglobulin (CTLA4-Ig) molecule from which it is derived.

Immunologic Characteristics

Target Antigen: Human cytotoxic T-lymphocyte-associated antigen 4 (CTLA-4) linked to a portion of Fc domain of human IgG1

Viability: Not viable, but immunologically active

Antigenic Form: Soluble fusion protein of antigen and Fc portion of IgG1

Antigenic Type: Extracellular domain of human cytotoxic T-lymphocyte-associated antigen 4 (CTLA-4) fused to a portion (hinge-CH2-CH3 domains) of the Fc domain of a human IgG1. The apparent molecular weight of belatacept is approximately 90 kilodaltons.

Use Characteristics

Indications: To prevent organ rejection in adult patients receiving a kidney transplant. Use belatacept in combination with basiliximab induction, mycophenolate mofetil, and corticosteroids, and only in patients who are Epstein-Barr virus (EBV)–seropositive.

Limitations: Use of belatacept to prevent rejection in transplanted organs other than kidney has not been established. In a clinical trial of liver transplant patients, use of belatacept regimens with more frequent administration of belatacept than any of those studied in kidney transplant, along with mycophenolate mofetil and corticosteroids, was associated with a higher rate of graft loss and death compared to the tacrolimus control arms. In addition, 2 cases of posttransplant lymphoproliferative disorder (PTLD) involving the liver allograft (1 fatal) and 1 fatal case of progressive multifocal leukoencephalopathy (PML) were observed among the 147 patients randomized to belatacept. The 2 cases of PTLD were reported among the 140 EBV seropositive patients (1.4%). The fatal case of PML was reported in a patient receiving higher than recommended doses of belatacept and mycophenolate.

Contraindications: Transplant recipients who are Epstein-Barr virus (EBV) seronegative (based on IgG antibodies to viral capsid antigen [VCA] and EBV nuclear antigen [EBNA]) or with unknown EBV serostatus, due to the risk of PTLD.

Immunodeficiency: Because this is an immunosuppressive agent, carefully monitor recipients for signs of leukopenia or concurrent infection. If infection occurs, start appropriate adjunctive therapy promptly.

Elderly: Of 401 patients treated with the recommended dosage regimen of belatacept, 15% were 65 years of age or older, while 3% were 75 years of age or older. No overall differences in safety or effectiveness were observed between these subjects and younger subjects, but greater sensitivity or less efficacy in older individuals cannot be ruled out.

Carcinogenicity: Belatacept has not been evaluated for carcinogenic potential. However, a murine carcinogenicity study was conducted with abatacept (a more active analog in rodents) to determine the carcinogenic potential of CD28 blockade. Weekly SC injections of 20, 65, or 200 mg/kg of abatacept were associated with increases in the incidence of malignant lymphomas (all doses) and mammary gland tumors (intermediate- and high-dose in females) at clinically relevant exposures. The mice in this study were infected with endogenous murine leukemia and mouse mammary tumor viruses that are associated with an increased incidence of lymphomas and mammary gland tumors, respectively, in immunosuppressed mice. Although the precise relevance of these findings to the clinical use of belatacept is unknown, cases of PTLD (a premalignant or malignant proliferation of B lymphocytes) were reported in clinical trials.

Mutagenicity: Belatacept has not been evaluated for mutagenic potential.

Fertility Impairment: Belatacept had no adverse effects on male or female fertility in rats at doses up to 200 mg/kg daily (25 times the maximum recommended human dose).

Pregnancy: Category C. Use only if clearly needed. There are no studies of belatacept treatment in pregnant women. To monitor maternal-fetal outcomes, pregnant women exposed to belatacept or whose partners have received belatacept should be enrolled in the National Transplant Pregnancy Registry (NTPR) by calling 1-877-955-6877. Belatacept is known to cross the placenta of animals. Belatacept was not teratogenic in pregnant rats and rabbits at doses approximately 16 and 19 times greater than the exposure associated with the maximum recommended human dose of 10 mg/kg administered over the first month of treatment, based on area under the concentration-time curve (AUC). Belatacept administered to female rats daily during gestation and throughout the lactation period was associated with maternal toxicity (infections) in a small percentage of dams at doses of at least 20 mg/kg (at least 3 times the maximum recommended human dose, based on AUC) resulting in increased pup mortality (up to 100% pup mortality in some dams). In pups that survived, there were no abnormalities or malformations at doses up to 200 mg/kg (19 times the maximum recommended human dose). In vitro data indicate that belatacept has lower binding affinity to CD80/CD86 and lower potency in rodents than in humans. Although the rat toxicity studies with belatacept were done at pharmacologically saturating doses, the in vivo difference in potency between rats and humans is unknown. Therefore, the relevance of the rat toxicities to humans and the significance of the magnitude of the relative exposures are unknown. Abatacept, a fusion protein that differs from belatacept by 2 amino acids, binds to the same ligands (CD80/CD86) and blocks T-cell costimulation like belatacept, but is more active than belatacept in rodents. Therefore, toxicities identified with abatacept in rodents, including infections and autoimmunity, may be predictive of adverse effects in humans treated with belatacept. Autoimmunity was observed in one rat offspring exposed to abatacept in utero and/or during lactation and in juvenile rats after treatment with abatacept. However, the clinical relevance of autoimmunity in rats to patients or a fetus exposed in utero is unknown.

Lactation: It is not known if belatacept crosses into human breast milk. However, belatacept is excreted in rat milk. Because many drugs are excreted in human milk and because of the potential for serious adverse reactions from belatacept in breast-feeding infants, decide whether to discontinue breast-feeding or to discontinue the drug, taking into account the importance of the drug to the mother.

Children: The safety and efficacy of belatacept in patients younger than 18 years of age have not been established. Because T-cell development continues into the teenage years, the potential concern for autoimmunity in neonates applies to pediatric use as well.

Adverse Reactions: The data described below primarily derive from 2 randomized, active-controlled 3-year trials of belatacept in de novo kidney transplant patients. In study 1 and study 2, belatacept was studied at the recommended dose and frequency in 401 patients, compared with a cyclosporine control regimen in 405 patients. These 2 trials also included 403 patients treated with a belatacept regimen of higher cumulative dose and more frequent dosing than recommended. All patients also received basiliximab induction, mycophenolate mofetil, and corticosteroids. Patients were treated and followed for 3 years.

Most common adverse reactions (20% or more on belatacept treatment): Anemia, diarrhea, urinary tract infection, peripheral edema, constipation, hypertension, pyrexia, graft dysfunction, cough, nausea, vomiting, headache, hypokalemia, hyperkalemia, and leukopenia. The proportion of patients who discontinued treatment due to adverse reactions was 13% for the recommended belatacept regimen and 19% for the cyclosporine control arm through 3 years of treatment. The most common adverse reactions leading to discontinuation in belatacept-treated patients were cytomegalovirus (CMV) infection (1.5%) and complications of transplanted kidney (1.5%).

Posttransplant Lymphoproliferative Disorder (PTLD): Increased risk, predominantly involving the CNS, compared to patients on a cyclosporine-based regimen. Monitor recipients for new or worsening neurological, cognitive, or behavioral signs and symptoms. Other known risk factors for PTLD include CMV infection and T-cell-depleting therapy. Use T-cell–depleting therapies to treat acute rejection cautiously.

Malignancies: Patients receiving immunosuppressants, including belatacept, are at increased risk of developing malignancies, in addition to PTLD, including those of the skin. Limit exposure to sunlight and UV light by wearing protective clothing and using a sunscreen with a high protection factor.

Progressive Multifocal Leukoencephalopathy (PML): PML is an often rapidly progressive and fatal opportunistic CNS infection caused by the JC virus, a human polyoma virus. In clinical trials with belatacept, two cases of PML were reported in patients receiving belatacept at higher cumulative doses and more frequently than the recommended regimen, along with mycophenolate mofetil and corticosteroids; one case occurred in a kidney transplant recipient and the second case occurred in a liver transplant recipient. As PML has been associated with high levels of overall immunosuppression, do not exceed the recommended doses and frequency of belatacept and concomitant immunosuppressives, including mycophenolate. Consider PML in the differential diagnosis in patients with new or worsening neurological, cognitive, or behavioral signs or symptoms. If PML is diagnosed, consider reducing or withdrawing immunosuppression, taking into account the risk to the allograft.

Infections: Patients receiving immunosuppressants, including belatacept, are at increased risk of developing bacterial, viral (eg, CMV and herpes), fungal, and protozoal infections. These infections may lead to serious, including fatal, outcomes. Prophylaxis for CMV is recommended for at least 3 months after transplantation. Prophylaxis for *Pneumocystis jiroveci* is recommended after transplantation. Tuberculosis (TB) was more frequently observed in patients receiving belatacept than in those receiving cyclosporine in clinical trials. Evaluate patients for TB before starting belatacept. Treat latent TB infection before starting belatacept. In addition to cases of JC virus–associated PML, cases of polyoma virus–associated nephropathy (PVAN), mostly due to BK virus infection, have been reported. PVAN is associated with serious outcomes; including deteriorating renal function and kidney graft loss. Patient monitoring may help detect patients at risk for PVAN. Consider reducing immunosuppression for patients who develop evidence of PVAN, taking into account the risk to the allograft.

Infusion Reactions: There were no reports of anaphylaxis or drug hypersensitivity in patients treated with belatacept in studies 1 and 2 through 3 years. Infusion-related reactions within 1 hour of infusion were reported in 5% of patients treated with the recommended dose of belatacept, similar to the placebo rate. No serious events were reported through year 3. The most frequent reactions were hypotension and hypertension.

Proteinuria: At month 1 after transplantation in studies 1 and 2, the frequency of 2+ proteinuria on urine dipstick in patients treated with the belatacept recommended regimen was 33% (130/390) and 28% (107/384) in patients treated with the cyclosporine control regimen. The frequency of 2+ proteinuria was similar between the 2 treatment groups between 1 and 3 years after transplantation (less than 10% in both studies). There were no differences in the occurrence of 3+ proteinuria (less than 4% in both studies) at any time point, and no patient experienced 4+ proteinuria. The clinical significance of this increase in early proteinuria is unknown.

Immunogenicity: Antibodies directed against the belatacept molecule were assessed in 398 patients treated with the belatacept recommended regimen in studies 1 and 2 (212 of these patients were treated for at least 2 years). Of the 372 patients with immunogenicity assessment at baseline (before receiving belatacept), 29 patients tested positive for antibelatacept antibodies; 13 of these patients had antibodies to the modified cytotoxic T-lymphocyte–associated antigen 4 (CTLA-4). Antibelatacept antibody titers did not increase during treatment in these 29 patients. Eight (2%) patients developed antibodies during treatment with the belatacept recommended regimen. In the patients who developed antibodies during treatment, the median titer (by dilution method) was 8, with a range of 5 to 80. Of 56 patients who tested negative for antibodies during treatment and reassessed approximately 7 half-lives after discontinuation of belatacept, one tested antibody positive. Antibelatacept antibody development was not associated with altered clearance of belatacept. Samples from 6 patients with confirmed binding activity to the modified cytotoxic T-lymphocyte–associated antigen 4 (CTLA-4) region of the belatacept molecule were assessed by an in vitro bioassay for the presence of neutralizing antibodies. Three of these 6 patients tested positive for neutralizing antibodies. However, the development of neutralizing antibodies may be underreported due to lack of assay sensitivity. The clinical impact of anti-belatacept antibodies (including neutralizing antibelatacept antibodies) could not be determined in the studies.

New-Onset Diabetes After Transplantation (NODAT): The incidence of NODAT was defined in studies 1 and 2 as use of an antidiabetic agent for at least 30 days or at least 2 fasting plasma glucose values of 126 mg/dL (7 mmol/L) or more posttransplantation. Of the patients treated with the belatacept recommended regimen, 5% (14/304) developed NODAT by the end of 1 year, compared to 10% (27/280) of patients on the cyclosporine control regimen. However, by the end of year 3, the cumulative incidence of NODAT was 8% (24/304) in patients treated with the belatacept recommended regimen and 10% (29/280) in patients treated with cyclosporine.

Hypertension: Blood pressure and use of antihypertensive medications were reported in studies 1 and 2. By year 3, one or more antihypertensive medications were used in 85% of belatacept-treated patients and 92% of cyclosporine-treated patients. At 1 year after transplantation, systolic blood pressures were 8 mm Hg lower and diastolic blood pressures were 3 mm Hg lower in patients treated with the belatacept recommended regimen, compared to the cyclosporine control regimen. At 3 years after transplantation, systolic blood pressures were 6 mm Hg lower and diastolic blood pressures were 3 mm Hg lower in belatacept-treated patients, compared to cyclosporine-treated patients. Hypertension was reported as an adverse reaction in 32% of belatacept-treated patients and 37% of cyclosporine-treated patients.

Dyslipidemia: Mean values of total cholesterol, HDL, LDL, and triglycerides were reported in studies 1 and 2. At 1 year after transplantation, these values were 183 mg/dL, 50 mg/dL, 102 mg/dL, and 151 mg/dL, respectively, in 401 patients treated with the belatacept recommended regimen and 196 mg/dL, 48 mg/dL, 108 mg/dL, and 195 mg/dL, respectively, in 405 patients treated with the cyclosporine control regimen. At 3 years after transplantation, the total cholesterol, HDL, LDL, and triglycerides were 176 mg/dL, 49 mg/dL, 100 mg/dL, and 141 mg/dL, respectively, in belatacept-treated patients compared to 193 mg/dL, 48 mg/dL, 106 mg/dL, and 180 mg/dL in cyclosporine-treated patients. The clinical significance of the lower mean triglyceride values in belatacept-treated patients at 1 and 3 years is unknown.

Pharmacologic & Dosing Characteristics

Dosage: Base the total infusion dose of belatacept on the actual body weight of the patient at time of transplantation. Do not modify the dose during therapy, unless body weight changes more than 10%. The prescribed dose of belatacept must be evenly divisible by 12.5 mg for the dose to be prepared accurately using the reconstituted solution and the silicone-free disposable syringe provided. Evenly divisible increments are 0, 12.5, 25, 37.5, 50, 62.5, 75, 87.5, and 100.

Administration of higher than the recommended doses or more frequent dosing of belatacept is not recommended, due to an increased risk of PTLD predominantly involving the CNS, PML, and serious CNS infections.

Initial-Phase Dose: Day 1 (day of transplantation, before implantation) and day 5 (approximately 96 hours after day-1 dose): 10 mg/kg.

>*End of week 2 and week 4 after transplantation:* 10 mg/kg.

>*End of week 8 and week 12 after transplantation:* 10 mg/kg.

Maintenance-Phase Dose: End of week 16 after transplantation and every 4 weeks (± 3 d) thereafter: 5 mg/kg.

>Use of higher than recommended or more frequent dosing is not recommended, due to increased risk of serious infections and malignancy.

Route & Site: For IV infusion only; administer over 30 minutes.

Overdosage: Single doses up to 20 mg/kg have been administered to healthy subjects without apparent toxic effect. Administration of belatacept of higher cumulative dose and more frequent dosing than recommended in kidney transplant patients resulted in a higher frequency of CNS-related adverse events. In case of overdosage, monitor the patient for signs or symptoms of adverse reactions and provide appropriate symptomatic treatment.

Related Interventions: Patients do not require premedication before administering belatacept.

CMV prophylaxis is recommended for at least 3 months after transplantation.

Laboratory Tests: Determine EBV serology before administering belatacept; give belatacept only to patients who are EBV seropositive.

Efficacy: The efficacy and safety of belatacept in de novo kidney transplantation were assessed in 2 open-label, randomized, multicenter, active-controlled trials (study 1 and study 2). These trials evaluated two dose regimens of belatacept, the recommended dosage regimen and a regimen with higher cumulative doses and more frequent dosing than the recommended dosage regimen, compared to a cyclosporine control regimen. All treatment groups also received basiliximab induction, mycophenolate mofetil (MMF), and corticosteroids. Study 1 enrolled recipients of living donor and standard criteria deceased donor organs and Study 2 enrolled recipients of extended criteria donor organs. Standard criteria donor organs were defined as organs from a deceased donor with anticipated cold ischemia time of less than 24 hours and not meeting the definition of extended criteria donor organs. Extended criteria donors were defined as deceased donors with at least one of the following: (1) donor age 60 years or older; (2) donor age 50 years or older and other donor comorbidities (at least 2 of the following: stroke, hypertension, serum creatinine more than 1.5 mg/dL); (3) donation of organ after cardiac death; or (4) anticipated cold ischemia time of the organ of 24 hours or longer. The belatacept regimen with higher cumulative doses and more frequent dosing was associated with more efficacy failures. Higher doses and/or more frequent dosing of belatacept are not recommended.

Belatacept is recommended for use only in EBV seropositive patients. In study 1, approximately 87% of patients were EBV seropositive before transplant. Efficacy results in the EBV seropositive subpopulation were consistent with those in the total population studied. By 1 year, the efficacy failure rate in the EBV seropositive population was 21% (42/202) in patients treated with the belatacept recommended regimen and 17% (31/184) in patients treated with cyclosporine (difference, 4%; 97.3% CI, −4.8 to 12.8). Patient and graft survival was 98% (198/202) in belatacept-treated patients and 92% (170/184) in cyclosporine-treated patients (difference, 5.6%; 97.3% CI, 0.8 to 10.4). By 3 years, efficacy failure was 25% in both treatment groups and patient and graft survival was 94% (187/202) in belatacept-treated patients compared with 88% (162/184) in cyclosporine-treated patients (difference, 4.6%; 97.3% CI, −2.1 to 11.3).

In study 2, approximately 91% of patients were EBV seropositive before transplant. Efficacy results in the EBV seropositive subpopulation were consistent with those in the total population studied. By 1 year, the efficacy failure rate in the EBV seropositive population was 29% (45/156) in patients treated with the belatacept recommended regimen and 28% (47/168) in patients treated with cyclosporine (difference, 0.8%; 97.3% CI, −10.3 to 11.9). Patient and graft survival rate in the EBV seropositive population was 89% (139/156) in belatacept-treated patients and 86% (144/168) in cyclosporine-treated patients (difference, 3.4; 97.3% CI, −4.7 to 11.5). By 3 years, efficacy failure was 35% (54/156) in belatacept-treated patients and 36% (61/168) in cyclosporine-treated patients. Patient and graft survival was 83% (130/156) in belatacept-treated patients compared with 77% (130/168) in cyclosporine-treated patients (difference, 5.9%; 97.3% CI, −3.8 to 15.6).

Pharmacokinetics: Belatacept-mediated costimulation blockade results in the inhibition of cytokine production by T-cells required for antigen-specific antibody production by B-cells. In clinical trials, greater reductions in mean IgG, IgM, and IgA concentrations were observed from baseline to month 6 and month 12 posttransplant in belatacept-treated patients compared to cyclosporine-treated patients. In an exploratory subset analysis, a trend of decreasing IgG concentrations with increasing belatacept trough concentrations was observed at month 6. Also in this exploratory subset analysis, belatacept-treated patients with CNS PTLD, CNS infections including PML, other serious infections, and malignancies were observed to have a higher incidence of IgG concentrations below the lower limit of the normal range (less than 694 mg/dL) at month 6 than those patients who did not experience these adverse events. This observation was more pronounced with the higher than recommended dose of belatacept. A similar trend was also observed for cyclosporine-treated patients with serious infections and malignancies. However, it is unclear whether any causal relationship between an IgG concentration below the lower level of normal and these adverse events exists, as the analysis may have been confounded by other factors (eg, age older than 60 years, receipt of an extended criteria donor kidney, exposure to lymphocyte depleting agents) which were also associated with IgG below the lower level of normal at month 6 in these trials. The following table summarizes the pharmacokinetic parameters of belatacept in healthy adult and in kidney transplant patients after the 10 mg/kg IV infusion at week 12, and after 5 mg/kg IV infusion every 4 weeks at month 12 posttransplant or later.

Pharmacokinetic Parameters of Belatacept in Healthy Subjects and Kidney Transplant Patients			
Pharmacokinetic Parameter (Mean ± SD [Range])	Healthy Subjects (After 10 mg/kg Single Dose) n = 15	Kidney Transplant Patients (After 10 mg/kg Multiple Doses) n = 10	Kidney Transplant Patients (After 5 mg/kg Multiple Doses) n = 14
Peak concentration (C_{max}) (mcg/mL)	300 ± 77 (190 to 492)	247 ± 68 (161 to 340)	139 ± 28 (80 to 176)
AUC[a] (mcg•h/mL)	26,398 ± 5,175 (18,964 to 40,684)	22,252 ± 7,868 (13,575 to 42,144)	14,090 ± 3,860 (7,906 to 20,510)
Terminal half-life ($t_{1/2}$) (days)	9.8 ± 2.8 (6.4 to 15.6)	9.8 ± 3.2 (6.1 to 15.1)	8.2 ± 2.4 (3.1 to 11.9)
Systemic clearance (CL) (mL/h/kg)	0.39 ± 0.07 (0.25 to 0.53)	0.49 ± 0.13 (0.23 to 0.7)	0.51 ± 0.14 (0.33 to 0.75)

Belatacept

Pharmacokinetic Parameters of Belatacept in Healthy Subjects and Kidney Transplant Patients			
Pharmacokinetic Parameter (Mean ± SD [Range])	Healthy Subjects (After 10 mg/kg Single Dose) n = 15	Kidney Transplant Patients (After 10 mg/kg Multiple Doses) n = 10	Kidney Transplant Patients (After 5 mg/kg Multiple Doses) n = 14
Volume of distribution (V_{ss}) (L/kg)	0.09 ± 0.02 (0.07 to 0.15)	0.11 ± 0.03 (0.067 to 0.17)	0.12 ± 0.03 (0.09 to 0.17)

a AUC = AUC_{inf} after single dose and AUC_{tau} after multiple doses, where tau = 4 weeks.

In healthy subjects, the pharmacokinetics of belatacept was linear and exposure to belatacept increased proportionally after a single IV infusion dose of 1 to 20 mg/kg. The pharmacokinetics of belatacept in de novo kidney transplant patients and healthy subjects were comparable. Following the recommended regimen, the mean belatacept serum concentration reached steady-state by week 8 in the initial phase after transplantation and by month 6 during the maintenance phase. Following once monthly IV infusion of 10 mg/kg and 5 mg/kg, there was about 20% and 10% systemic accumulation of belatacept in kidney transplant patients, respectively.

Based on population pharmacokinetic analysis of 924 kidney transplant patients up to 1 year posttransplant, the pharmacokinetics of belatacept were similar at different time periods posttransplant. In clinical trials, trough concentrations of belatacept were consistently maintained from month 6 up to 3 years posttransplant. Population pharmacokinetic analyses in kidney transplant patients revealed that there was a trend toward higher clearance of belatacept with increasing body weight. Age, gender, race, renal function (measured by calculated glomerular filtration rate [GFR]), hepatic function (measured by albumin), diabetes, and concomitant dialysis did not affect the clearance of belatacept.

Mechanism: Belatacept is a selective T-cell costimulation blocker that binds to CD80 and CD86 on antigen-presenting cells, thereby blocking CD28-mediated costimulation of T lymphocytes. In vitro, belatacept inhibits T-lymphocyte proliferation and the production of the cytokines interleukin-2, interferon-gamma, interleukin-4, and TNF-alfa. Activated T-lymphocytes are the predominant mediators of immunologic rejection. In nonhuman primate models of renal transplantation, belatacept monotherapy prolonged graft survival and decreased the production of antidonor antibodies, compared with vehicle.

Drug Interactions: Avoid the use of live vaccines during treatment with belatacept, including but not limited to the following: intranasal influenza, measles, mumps, rubella, oral polio, BCG, yellow fever, varicella, and Ty21a typhoid vaccines.

Cytochrome P450 Substrates: No formal drug interaction studies have been conducted with belatacept. Other biologic therapies that are cytokines or cytokine modulators have been shown to affect the expression and/or functional activities of cytochrome P450 (CYP-450) enzymes in vitro and/or in vivo. In vitro studies have shown that belatacept inhibits the production of certain cytokines during an alloimmune response. No studies in kidney transplant patients have been conducted to assess if belatacept inhibits cytokine production in vivo. The potential for belatacept to alter the systemic concentrations of drugs that are CYP-450 substrates has not been studied. Consider potentially altered CYP-450 metabolism in kidney transplant patients receiving belatacept who exhibit signs and symptoms of altered efficacy or adverse events associated with coadministered drugs known to be metabolized by CYP-450.

Mycophenolate Mofetil: In a pharmacokinetic substudy of studies 1 and 2, plasma concentrations of mycophenolic acid (MPA) were measured in 41 patients who received fixed MMF doses of 500 mg to 1500 mg twice daily with either 5 mg/kg of belatacept or cyclosporine. The mean dose-normalized MPA C_{max} and AUC_{0-12} were approximately 20% and 40% higher, respectively, with belatacept coadministration than with cyclosporine coadministration. Consider the potential for a change of MPA exposure after crossover from cyclosporine to belatacept or from belatacept to cyclosporine in patients concomitantly receiving MMF.

Patient Information: Counsel potential recipients regarding the elevated risk of posttransplant lymphoproliferative disorders, malignancies, and serious infections. Instruct patients to immediately report neurological, cognitive, or behavioral signs and symptoms during and after therapy with belatacept. Instruct patients to limit exposure to sunlight and UV light by wearing protective clothing and using a sunscreen with a high protection factor. Instruct patients to look for any signs and symptoms of skin cancer, such as suspicious moles or lesions.

Pharmaceutical Characteristics

Concentration: 250 mg belatacept powder per vial, 25 mg/ml after reconstitution as instructed

Packaging: Carton with one 250 mg single-use vial with a 12 mL silicone-free disposable syringe

NDC Number: 00003-0371-13

Doseform: Lyophilized powder for injection

Appearance: White or off-white powder, yielding a clear to slightly opalescent and colorless to pale yellow solution. Do not use if opaque particles, discoloration, or other foreign particles are present.

Diluent:

For reconstitution: Reconstitute contents of each vial with 10.5 mL of a suitable diluent. Suitable diluents include: sterile water for injection, sodium chloride 0.9%, or dextrose 5%. To minimize foam formation, rotate the vial and invert with gentle swirling until the contents are completely dissolved. Avoid prolonged or vigorous agitation. Do not shake.

For infusion: Dilute the required volume of reconstituted belatacept solution diluted with sodium chloride 0.9% or dextrose 5%. Belatacept reconstituted with sterile water should be further diluted with either sodium chloride 0.9% or dextrose 5% in water. If reconstituted with sodium chloride 0.9%, further dilute with sodium chloride 0.9% before infusion. If reconstituted with dextrose 5% in water, further dilute with dextrose 5% in water before infusion. From an appropriate infusion container, withdraw a volume of infusion fluid equal to the volume of the reconstituted belatacept solution required to provide the prescribed dose. With the same silicone-free disposable syringe used for reconstitution, withdraw the required amount of belatacept solution from the vial, inject it into the infusion container, and gently rotate the infusion container to ensure mixing. The final belatacept concentration in the infusion container should range from 2 to 10 mg/mL. Typically, an infusion volume of 100 mL will be appropriate for most patients and doses, but total infusion volumes ranging from 50 to 250 mL may be used. Administer over 30 minutes, using an infusion set and a low–protein-binding filter with pore size of 0.2 to 1.2 mcm.

Adjuvant: None

Preservative: None

Allergens: None

Excipients: Each 250 mg vial of belatacept also contains monobasic sodium phosphate 34.5 mg, sodium chloride 5.8 mg, and sucrose 500 mg

pH: 7.2 to 7.8

Shelf Life: Data not provided.

Storage/Stability: Store between 2° and 8°C (36° and 46°F). Protect vials from light by storing in the original package. Contact the manufacturer regarding exposure to freezing or elevated temperatures. Shipping data not provided.

Belatacept

Transfer the reconstituted solution from the vial to the infusion container immediately. Complete the belatacept infusion within 24 hours of reconstitution. If not used immediately, infusion solution may be stored between 2° and 8°C (36° and 46°F) and protected from light for up to 24 hours (a maximum of 4 hours of those 24 hours can be at room temperature (20° to 25°C [68° to 77°F]) with room lighting. Infuse belatacept in a separate line from other concomitantly infused agents. Do not infuse belatacept in the same IV line with other agents. No physical or biochemical compatibility studies have been conducted to evaluate the administration of belatacept with other agents.

Handling: Only use the enclosed silicone-free disposable syringe to prepare each dose. If the silicone-free disposable syringe is dropped or becomes contaminated, use a new silicone-free disposable syringe from inventory. To obtain additional silicone-free disposable syringes, contact Bristol-Myers Squibb at 1-888-NULOJIX. If belatacept is accidentally reconstituted using a different syringe, the solution may develop a few translucent particles. Discard any solutions prepared using siliconized syringes.

Production Process: Produced by recombinant DNA technology in a mammalian cell expression system.

Media: Chinese hamster ovary cell-expression system

Other Information

First Licensed: June 15, 2011

References: Gupta G, Womer KL. Profile of belatacept and its potential role in prevention of graft rejection following renal transplantation. *Drug Des Devel Ther*. 2010;4:375-382.

Daclizumab (Chimeric)

Isoantibodies

Name:
Zenapax

Manufacturer:
Roche Laboratories, under license from Protein Design Laboratories

Synonyms: Anti-interleukin-2 receptor monoclonal antibody, SMART Anti-Tac (anti-T-cell activation) antibodies. Initially known as dacliximab.

Comparison: Several antibody products (eg, basiliximab, daclizumab, antithymocyte globulin) are licensed for prevention of allograft rejection. Some of these and some other antibody products (eg, antithymocyte globulin, muromunab-CD3) are licensed for treatment of acute allograft rejection. These drugs vary in their efficacy, adverse event profile, and use characteristics.

Immunologic Characteristics

Target Antigen: Alpha subunit (p55 alpha, CD25, or Tac subunit) of the human high-affinity interleukin-2 (IL-2) receptor expressed on the surface of activated lymphocytes.

Viability: Inactive, passive, transient

Antigenic Form: Chimeric (90% human, 10% murine) IgG1

Antigenic Type: Protein, IgG1, monoclonal, targeting only recently activated T-cells. The human amino acid sequences derive from constant domains of human IgG1 and the variable framework regions of the Eu myeloma antibody. The murine sequences derive from complementarily determining regions of a murine anti-Tac antibody. The molecular weight is 144 kilodaltons.

Use Characteristics

Indications: For prophylaxis of acute organ rejection in patients receiving renal transplants, as part of an immunosuppressive regimen that includes cyclosporine and corticosteroids.

Unlabeled Uses: Daclizumab is being investigated for efficacy in preventing acute rejection in organ transplants other than renal transplants.

Contraindications:

Absolute: Patients with known hypersensitivity to daclizumab or to any components of this product.

Relative: None

Elderly: Clinical studies of daclizumab did not include enough subjects 65 years of age or older to determine whether they differ from younger subjects. Use caution in giving immunosuppressive drugs to elderly patients.

Fertility Impairment: The effect of daclizumab on fertility is not known.

Pregnancy: Category C. It is not known whether daclizumab can cause fetal harm or affect reproductive capacity. In general, IgG can cross the placental barrier, especially during the third trimester. Do not use daclizumab in pregnant women unless the potential benefit justifies the potential risk to the fetus. Advise women of childbearing potential to use effective contraception before beginning daclizumab therapy, during therapy, and for 4 months after completing therapy.

Lactation: It is not known whether daclizumab is excreted in breast milk. Many drugs are excreted in breast milk, including human IgG antibodies. Because of potential adverse reactions, decide whether to discontinue nursing or to discontinue the drug, taking into account the importance of the drug to the mother.

Children: No adequate studies have been completed in children. Initial results of an ongoing study among 25 children 11 months to 17 years of age (median, 12 years) treated with daclizumab plus standard immunosuppressive agents (eg, mycophenolate, cyclosporine, tacrolimus, azathioprine, corticosteroids) indicate the most frequent adverse events were hypertension (48%), postoperative (posttraumatic) pain (44%), diarrhea (36%), and vomiting (32%). Reported rates of hypertension and dehydration were higher for pediatric patients than for adult patients.

It is not known whether the immune response to vaccines, infection, and other antigenic stimuli administered or encountered during daclizumab therapy is impaired or whether such response will remain impaired after daclizumab therapy.

Preliminary results among 6 children suggest serum daclizumab levels are somewhat lower in pediatric renal-transplant patients than in adult transplant patients given the same dosage. However, daclizumab levels in these pediatric patients were sufficient to saturate the Tac subunit of the IL-2 receptor on lymphocytes measured by flow cytometry. The Tac subunit was saturated immediately after the first dose of 1 mg/kg of daclizumab and remained saturated for at least the first 3 months posttransplant. Saturation of the Tac subunit of the IL-2 receptor was similar to that observed in adult patients receiving the same dosage.

Adverse Reactions: The safety of daclizumab was determined in 4 studies among 629 patients receiving renal allografts, of whom 336 received daclizumab and 293 received placebo. All patients received concomitant cyclosporine and corticosteroids. Daclizumab did not alter the pattern, frequency, or severity of known major toxicities associated with the use of immunosuppressive drugs.

Adverse events were reported by 95% of the placebo-treated group and 96% of the daclizumab-treated group. The proportion of patients prematurely withdrawn from the studies because of adverse events was 8.5% in the placebo-treated group and 8.6% in the daclizumab-treated group.

Daclizumab did not increase the number of serious adverse events observed, compared with placebo. The most frequently reported adverse events were GI disorders, reported with equal frequency in daclizumab- (67%) and placebo-treated (68%) patients. The incidence and types of adverse events were similar in both groups.

Carcinogenesis: One year after treatment, the incidence of malignancies was 2.7% in the placebo group, compared with 1.5% in the daclizumab group. Daclizumab did not increase the number of posttransplant lymphomas, which occurred with a frequency of less than 1% in both groups. The following events occurred in daclizumab-treated patients:

Body as a whole: Posttraumatic pain, chest pain, fever, pain, fatigue (more than 5%); shivering, generalized weakness (between 2% and 5%).

Cardiovascular: Hypertension, hypotension, tachycardia, thrombosis, bleeding (more than 5%).

CNS: Tremor, headache, dizziness (more than 5%); urinary retention, leg cramps, prickly sensation (between 2% and 5%).

Dermatologic: Impaired wound healing without infection, acne (more than 5%); pruritus, hirsutism, rash, night sweats, increased sweating (between 2% and 5%).

GI: Constipation, nausea, diarrhea, vomiting, abdominal pain, pyrosis, dyspepsia, abdominal distention, epigastric pain (not food-related) (more than 5%); flatulence, gastritis, hemorrhoids (between 2% and 5%).

GU: Oliguria, dysuria, renal tubular necrosis (more than 5%).

Hematologic: Lymphocele.

Local: Injection-site reaction (between 2% and 5%).

Daclizumab (Chimeric)

Metabolic/Nutritional: Edema of extremities, edema (more than 5%); fluid overload, diabetes mellitus, dehydration (between 2% and 5%).

Musculoskeletal: Musculoskeletal pain, back pain (more than 5%); arthralgia, myalgia (between 2% and 5%).

Ophthalmic: Blurred vision (between 2% and 5%).

Psychiatric: Insomnia (more than 5%); depression, anxiety (between 2% and 5%).

Renal: Renal damage, hydronephrosis, urinary tract bleeding, urinary tract disorder, renal insufficiency (between 2% and 5%).

Respiratory: Dyspnea, pulmonary edema, coughing (more than 5%); atelectasis, congestion, pharyngitis, rhinitis, hypoxia, rales, abnormal breath sounds, pleural effusion (between 2% and 5%).

Hypersensitivity: Anaphylactoid reactions after daclizumab have not been reported, but can occur after administration of proteins.

Lab test abnormalities: No differences in abnormal hematologic or chemical laboratory test results were seen between groups, except for fasting blood glucose. Approximately 16% (10/64) of placebo-treated and 32% (28/88) of daclizumab-treated patients had high-fasting blood glucose values. Most of these high values occurred either on the first day post-transplant, when patients received high doses of corticosteroids, or in patients with diabetes.

Miscellaneous: Incidence and types of infectious episodes, including viral infections, fungal infections, bacteremia and septicemia, and pneumonia did not vary between groups. Cytomegalovirus infection occurred in 16% of the placebo group and 13% of the daclizumab group. One exception was cellulitis and wound infections, which occurred in 4.1% of placebo-treated patients and 8.4% of daclizumab-treated patients. One year after transplant, 7 placebo-treated patients and only 1 daclizumab-treated patient had died of an infection.

Pharmacologic & Dosing Characteristics

Dosage: Daclizumab is used as part of an immunosuppressive regimen that includes cyclosporine and corticosteroids. The recommended dose for daclizumab is 1 mg/kg. The standard course of daclizumab therapy is 5 doses. Give the first dose less than 24 hours before transplantation. Give the 4 remaining doses at intervals of 14 days.

No dosage adjustment is necessary for patients with severe renal impairment. No dosage adjustments based on other identified covariates (eg, age, gender, proteinuria, race) are required for renal allograft patients. No data are available for administration to patients with severe hepatic impairment. The influence of body weight on systemic clearance supports dosing daclizumab on a mg/kg basis. This dosing maintained drug exposure within 30% of the reference exposure.

Route: IV. Mix the proper dose of daclizumab with 50 mL of 0.9% sodium chloride and administer via a peripheral or central vein over 1 minute. Do not inject undiluted.

Overdosage: No overdoses with daclizumab have been reported. A maximum tolerated dose has not been determined. A dose of 1.5 mg/kg has been administered to bone-marrow transplant recipients without associated adverse events.

Additional Doses: Readministration of daclizumab after an initial course of therapy has not been studied in humans. The potential risks of such readministration (eg, immunosuppression, anaphylactoid reactions) are not known.

Efficacy: Two trials assessed daclizumab for prophylaxis of acute organ rejection in adult patients receiving their first cadaveric kidney transplant. These trials compared daclizumab 1 mg/kg with placebo, in the course of standard immunosuppressive regimens containing either cyclosporine and corticosteroids (double-therapy trial) or cyclosporine, corticosteroids and azathioprine (triple-therapy trial). Daclizumab dosing was initiated within 24 hours before transplant, with subsequent doses given every 14 days for 5 doses. The proportion of patients who developed a biopsy-proven acute rejection episode within the first 6 months following transplantation was significantly lower in the daclizumab-treated group in both the double-therapy and triple-therapy trials. No difference in patient survival was observed in the triple-therapy study between daclizumab- and placebo-treated patients. Treatment with daclizumab was associated with better patient survival at 1 year posttransplant in the double-therapy study. The incidence of delayed graft function was no different between groups in either study. No difference in graft function was observed 1 year posttransplant in either study between groups.

In another study, daclizumab or placebo was added to a regimen of cyclosporine, mycophenolate, and steroids. Daclizumab did not affect the incidence or types of adverse events reported. The incidence of the combined endpoint of biopsy-proven or clinically presumptive acute rejection was 20% (5 of 25) in the placebo group and 12% (6 of 50) in the daclizumab group. Although numerically lower, the difference in acute rejection was not statistically significant.

Efficacy Parameters						
	Triple-therapy regimen (cyclosporine, corticosteroids, and azathioprine)			Double-therapy regimen (cyclosporine and corticosteroids)		
	Placebo (n = 134)	Daclizumab (n = 126)	P value	Placebo (n = 134)	Daclizumab (n = 141)	P value
Primary endpoint (incidence of biopsy-proven acute rejection at 6 months)						
No. of patients	47 (35%)	28 (22%)	0.03	63 (47%)	39 (28%)	0.001
Secondary endpoints (incidence of biopsy-proven acute rejection at 1 year)						
No. of patients	51 (38%)	35 (28%)	0.09	65 (49%)	39 (28%)	< 0.001
Patient survival at 1 year posttransplant						
No. of patients	129 (96%)	123 (98%)	0.51	126 (94%)	140 (99%)	0.01
Graft survival at 1 year posttransplant						
No. of patients with functioning graft	121 (90%)	120 (95%)	0.08	111 (83%)	124 (88%)	0.3

Onset: Rapid

Duration: At the recommended dose, daclizumab saturates the Tac subunit of the IL-2 receptor for approximately 120 days posttransplant. The duration of clinically significant IL-2 receptor blockade after the recommended course of daclizumab is unknown. Whether the ability to respond to repeated or ongoing challenges with antigens returns to normal after daclizumab is cleared is unknown. No significant changes to circulating lymphocyte numbers or cell phenotypes were observed by flow cytometry. Cytokine-release syndrome has not been observed after daclizumab administration.

Pharmacokinetics: Immunoglobulins are primarily eliminated by catabolism. In clinical trials involving renal allograft patients treated with a 1 mg/kg IV dose of daclizumab every 14 days for 5 doses, peak serum concentration (mean $\pm$ SD) rose between the first dose (21 $\pm$ 14 mcg/mL) and the fifth (32 $\pm$ 22 mcg/mL). The mean trough serum concentration before the fifth dose was 7.6 $\pm$ 4 mcg/mL. In vitro and in vivo data suggest that serum levels of 5 to 10 mcg/mL are necessary for saturation of the Tac subunit of the IL-2 receptors to block the responses of activated T-lymphocytes.

Analysis of the data using a two-compartment open model gave the following values for a reference patient (a 45-year-old white male with a body weight of 80 kg and no proteinuria): Systemic clearance, 15 mL/h; volume of central compartment, 2.5 L; volume of peripheral compartment, 3.4 L. The estimated terminal elimination half-life for the reference patient was 20 days (480 hours), similar to the terminal elimination half-life for human IgG (18 to 23 days). Bayesian estimates of terminal elimination half-life ranged from 11 to 38 days for the 123 patients included in the population analysis. Estimated interpatient variability in systemic clearance and central volume of distribution were 15% and 27%, respectively.

Serum neutralizing activity: Low titers of anti-idiotype antibodies to daclizumab were detected among 8.4% of daclizumab-treated patients. No antibodies that affected efficacy, safety, serum daclizumab tests, or any other clinically relevant parameters examined were detected.

Mechanism: Daclizumab functions as an IL-2 receptor antagonist that binds with high affinity to the Tac subunit of the high-affinity IL-2 receptor complex and inhibits IL-2 binding. Daclizumab binding is highly specific for Tac, which is expressed on activated but not resting lymphocytes. Daclizumab inhibits IL-2-mediated activation of lymphocytes, a critical pathway in the cellular immune response involved in allograft rejection.

While circulating, daclizumab impairs the response of the immune system to antigenic challenges. Whether the ability to respond to repeated or ongoing challenges with those antigens returns to normal after daclizumab is cleared is unknown.

Drug Interactions: It is not known whether daclizumab use will have a long-term effect on the ability of the immune system to respond to antigens first encountered (eg, via immunization) during daclizumab-induced immunosuppression.

The following medications have been administered in clinical trials with daclizumab with no incremental increase in adverse reactions: Cyclosporine, mycophenolate, ganciclovir, acyclovir, azathioprine, and corticosteroids. Very limited experience exists with the use of daclizumab concomitantly with tacrolimus, muromonab-CD3, antithymocyte globulin, and antilymphocyte globulin.

In renal allograft recipients treated with daclizumab and mycophenolate mofetil, no pharmacokinetic interaction between daclizumab and mycophenolic acid, the active metabolite of mycophenolate mofetil, was observed.

A common rule of thumb is to wait several months after discontinuation of immunosuppressive therapy before immunizing people with inactivated or attenuated vaccines. Active immunization of immunosuppressed people may result in an inadequate response to immunization. They may remain susceptible despite immunization. Some live, attenuated vaccines pose safety risks to immunosuppressed people.

Patient Information: Inform patients of the risks and potential benefits associated with immunosuppressive therapy. While the incidence of lymphoproliferative disorders and opportunistic infections in the limited clinical trial experience was no higher in daclizumab-treated patients compared with placebo-treated patients, patients on immunosuppressive therapy are at increased risk for developing lymphoproliferative disorders and opportunistic infections.

Pharmaceutical Characteristics

Concentration: 5 mg/mL

Packaging: Single-use 25 mg/5 mL vial

NDC Number: 00004-0501-09

Doseform: Solution for further dilution

Appearance: Clear, colorless fluid

Solvent: Phosphate-buffered saline

Daclizumab (Chimeric)

Diluent:
For infusion: 0.9% sodium chloride

Adjuvant: None

Preservative: None

Allergens: None

Excipients: 3.6 mg/mL sodium phosphate monobasic monohydrate, 11 mg/mL sodium phosphate dibasic heptahydrate, 4.6 mg/mL sodium chloride, 0.2 mg/mL polysorbate 80; may contain hydrochloric acid or sodium hydroxide to adjust the pH.

pH: 6.9

Shelf Life: Expires within 12 months

Storage/Stability: Store at 2° to 8°C (36° to 46°F). Do not freeze. Discard frozen product. Contact the manufacturer regarding exposure to extreme temperatures. Shipping data not provided. Do not shake. Protect undiluted solution from direct light.

Diluted medication is stable for 24 hours at 4°C (39°F) or for 4 hours at room temperature. After this time, discard the prepared solution. No incompatibility between daclizumab and polyvinyl chloride or polyethylene bags or infusion sets has been observed. No data are available concerning the incompatibility of daclizumab with other drug substances. Do not add or infuse other drug substances simultaneously through the same IV line.

Handling: When mixing the solution, gently invert the bag to avoid foaming. Do not shake. Discard any unused portion.

Production Process: Data not provided

Media: Data not provided

Disease Epidemiology

Incidence: In 1996, approximately 11,100 people received kidney transplants. In approximately 40% of these surgeries, signs of organ rejection appeared, requiring additional intervention to preclude rejection.

Other Information

First Licensed: December 10, 1997

References: Vincenti F, et al. Interleukin-2-receptor blockade with daclizumab to prevent acute rejection in renal transplantation. *N Engl J Med.* 1998;338:161-165.

Wiland AM, Philosophe B. Daclizumab induction in solid organ transplantation. *Expert Opin Biol Ther.* 2004;4(5):729-740.

Isoantibodies

Name:
Orthoclone OKT3

Manufacturer:
Janssen Biotech

Synonyms: OKT-3, anti-CD3. OKT is an abbreviation for Ortho Kung T-cell; Kung is the name of an Ortho researcher who developed monoclonal antibodies against human T-cell surface antigens. CD3 identifies the specificity of the antibody as cell differentiation cluster 3.

Comparison: Several antibody products (eg, basiliximab, daclizumab, antithymocyte globulin) are licensed for prevention of allograft rejection. Some of these and some other antibody products (eg, antithymocyte globulin, muromonab-CD3) are licensed for treatment of acute allograft rejection. These drugs vary in their efficacy, adverse event profile, and use characteristics.

Immunologic Characteristics

Target Antigen: Human T-cell T3 (CD3) antigen. The T3 complex consists of 3 glycoprotein subunits positioned adjacent to the T-cell receptor (Ti) complex involved in recognition of nonself antigens.

Viability: Inactive, passive, transient

Antigenic Form: Murine immunoglobulin, unmodified

Antigenic Type: Protein, IgG2a antibody, monoclonal, polymeric. Consists of 2 heavy chains of approximately 50,000 daltons each and 2 light chains of approximately 25,000 daltons each, for a total weight of 150,000 daltons. The antibody binds a glycoprotein with a molecular weight of 20,000 daltons on the surface of mature human T-lymphocytes.

Strains: T3 (CD3) antigen-receptor complex of human peripheral T-lymphocytes.

Use Characteristics

Indications: For the treatment of acute allograft rejection in renal transplant patients. For the treatment of acute allograft rejection in heart and liver transplant recipients resistant to standard steroid therapy.

Unlabeled Uses: Muromonab-CD3 has also been used with success in reversing acute and resistant rejection in liver- and cardiac-transplant recipients. It has also been used prophylactically in various solid organ transplantations. The drug has been used for both ex vivo and in vivo treatment of donor bone marrow to prevent or reverse graft-vs-host disease (GVHD). The commercial product cannot be used for ex vivo treatment because it contains polysorbate 80.

Limitations: Contains polysorbate 80; do not use for in vitro treatment of bone marrow.
Caution: Only physicians experienced in immunosuppressive therapy in the management of renal transplant patients should use muromonab-CD3.

Contraindications:
Absolute: Patients with a history of a serious hypersensitivity reaction to this or any other product of murine (mouse) origin, patients with a history of seizures or predisposed to seizures, patients known or suspected to be pregnant or breastfeeding.
Relative: Patients in uncompensated heart failure or fluid overload as evidenced by chest radiograph or a weight gain over 3% during the week preceding planned muromonab-CD3 administration. If the patient's temperature is higher than 37.8°C (100°F) at the time of first muromonab-CD3 administration, withhold the drug. Antipyretic drugs may be

used to lower the temperature. A human antimouse antibody titer more than 1:1,000 is a contraindication to further use.

Immunodeficiency: Muromonab-CD3 therapy can lead to increased susceptibility to infection. Further, lymphomas have been reported following immunosuppressive therapy, perhaps related to the intensity and duration of therapy.

Elderly: No specific information is available about geriatric use of muromonab-CD3.

Pregnancy: Category C. It is not known whether muromonab-CD3 can cause fetal harm when administered to a pregnant woman or can affect reproduction capacity. If this drug is used during pregnancy or the patient becomes pregnant while taking this drug, advise the patient of the potential hazard to the fetus. Intact IgG crosses the placenta from the maternal circulation increasingly after 30 weeks gestation.

Lactation: It is not known if muromonab-CD3 antibodies are excreted into breast milk. Because of the potential for serious adverse reactions or oncogenesis shown for muromonab-CD3 in human studies, make a decision to discontinue nursing or to discontinue the drug, taking into account the importance of the drug to the mother.

Children: Safety and efficacy in children have not been established. No controlled clinical studies have been conducted in children. Published literature has reported the use of muromonab-CD3 in infants and children beginning with a dose of 0.1 mg/kg. Based on immunologic monitoring, the dosage has been adjusted accordingly. Pediatric recipients are significantly immunosuppressed for a prolonged period of time and therefore require close monitoring after therapy for opportunistic infections, particularly varicella, which poses an infectious complication unique to that population.

GI fluid loss secondary to diarrhea or vomiting resulting from the cytokine-release syndrome (CRS) may be significant when treating small children and may require parenteral hydration. It is unknown whether there may be significant long-term sequelae (eg, neurodevelopmental language difficulties in infants younger than 1 year old) related to the occurrence of seizures, high fever, CNS infections, or aseptic meningitis following muromonab-CD3 treatment. If administration of muromonab-CD3 is deemed medically appropriate, children require more vigilant and frequent monitoring than adults.

Adverse Reactions: Severe pulmonary edema has occurred in patients with fluid overload prior to treatment with muromonab-CD3. Significant fever, chills, dyspnea, and malaise may occur 30 minutes to 6 hours after the first dose of muromonab-CD3. First-dose reactions may be minimized by using a regimen of corticosteroids. If the patient's temperature exceeds 37.8°C (100°F), lower it with antipyretics before muromonab-CD3 administration.

Compared with conventional treatment (azathioprine and corticosteroids), patients treated with muromonab-CD3 experienced increased adverse reactions during the first 2 days of therapy: Fever (90%); chills (59%); headache (11%, but 44% of patients experiencing aseptic-meningitis syndrome); dyspnea (21%); chest pain, neck stiffness (14%); vomiting (13%); wheezing, nausea (11%); diarrhea, tremor, photophobia (10%).

The most common infections observed during the first 45 days following start of muromonab-CD3 therapy were due to herpes simplex (27%) and cytomegalovirus (19%). Other severe and life-threatening infections included *Staphylococcus epidermidis, Pneumocystis carinii, Legionella, Cryptococcus, Serratia,* and gram-negative bacteria. The incidence of infections was not statistically different with muromonab-CD3 than with high-dose corticosteroids.

Anaphylaxis, aseptic-meningitis syndrome, serum sickness, lymphoma, neuropsychiatric events, encephalopathy, cerebral edema, intravascular thrombosis, and seizures have occurred. In patients treated with muromonab-CD3, posttransplant lymphoproliferative disorders reported have ranged from lymphadenopathy or benign polyclonal B-cell hyperplasia to malignant and often fatal monoclonal B-cell lymphomas. In postmarketing experience, approximately one-third of the lymphoproliferations reported were benign and two-thirds were malignant.

Muromonab-CD3 is a mouse protein that can induce human antimouse antibody (HAMA) production in patients following exposure. Antibodies against muromonab-CD3 develop in 80% of patients during or after the second week of treatment. These neutralizing antibodies are primarily IgG, with titers of 1:100 to 1:1000 by ELISA. A titer more than 1:1,000 is a contraindication to further use.

Temporally associated with administration of the first few doses of muromonab-CD3 (particularly the first 2 to 3 doses), most patients have developed an acute clinical syndrome, labeled the cytokine-release syndrome (CRS), that has been attributed to the release of cytokines by activated lymphocytes or monocytes. The clinical syndrome has ranged from a more frequently reported mild, self-limited, flu-like illness to a less frequently reported severe, life-threatening shock-like reaction which may include serious cardiovascular and CNS manifestations. The syndrome typically begins 30 to 60 minutes after administration of a dose of muromonab-CD3 (but may occur later) and may persist for several hours. The frequency and severity of this symptom complex is usually greatest with the first dose. With each successive dose, both the frequency and severity of the cytokine-release syndrome tends to diminish. Increasing the amount of a dose or resuming treatment after a hiatus may preclude the syndrome.

Pharmacologic & Dosing Characteristics

Dosage:
> *Adults and adolescents:* 5 mg daily for 10 to 14 days. Begin treatment once acute renal rejection is diagnosed. Monitor patients closely for 48 hours after the first dose.
> *Children:* 0.1 mg/kg for 10 to 14 days

Route & Site: IV bolus injection. Draw solution from ampule into syringe through a low protein-binding 0.2- or 0.22-micron filter (eg, *Millex* GV) to prepare injections. Then discard the filter and attach needle to be used for IV bolus injection.

Inject quickly, over 60 seconds or less. Do not administer by IV infusion or in conjunction with other drug solutions. To avoid foaming and protein degradation, do not shake.

Laboratory Data: Monitor various tests prior to and during muromonab-CD3 therapy, including:
- Renal—BUN, serum creatinine;
- Hepatic—transaminases, alkaline phosphatase, bilirubin;
- Hematology—WBC with differential cell counts.

Additional Doses: Only limited data are available about re-treatment with muromonab-CD3. The presence of anti-muromonab-CD3 antibodies may limit the efficacy of subsequent administration and possibly cause serious adverse reactions. Use caution.

Related Interventions: IV methylprednisolone sodium succinate 8 mg/kg given 1 to 4 hours prior to the first muromonab-CD3 dose can decrease the incidence and severity of reactions to the first dose.

Oral acetaminophen and antihistamines can be given concomitantly with muromonab-CD3 to reduce early reactions.

Reduce conventional concomitant immunosuppressive chemotherapy to the lowest dose compatible with an effective therapeutic response in order to reduce the potential for malignant transformations and the incidence or severity of infections. Discontinue cyclosporine during muromonab-CD3 therapy. Resume maintenance immunosuppression, including cyclosporine if indicated, about 3 days prior to cessation of muromonab-CD3 therapy.

Muromonab-CD3 (Murine)

Efficacy: In a randomized trial of 123 patients with acute rejection of cadaveric renal transplants, muromonab-CD3 reversed 94% of the rejections, compared to 75% with conventional corticosteroid treatment.

Muromonab-CD3 may be more effective in cardiac allograft rejection prophylaxis than antithymocyte globulin, as indicated by shorter hospitalizations, better biopsy scores, decreased incidence and severity of rejection, and longer time to the first rejection episode.

Onset: Rapid, 10 to 15 minutes

Duration: Mean half-life: 18 hours

Pharmacokinetics: Immunoglobulins are primarily eliminated by catabolism. During treatment with 5 mg daily for 14 days, mean serum trough levels of muromonab-CD3, measured by ELISA, rose over the first 3 days and then averaged 0.9 mcg/mL on days 3 through 14.

A rapid and concomitant decrease in the number of circulating CD3-positive, CD4-positive (T-helper cells), and CD8-positive (T-suppressor cells) T-cells has been observed within minutes after administration of muromonab-CD3. Between the second and seventh day, increasing numbers of circulating CD4- and CD8-positive cells have been observed in patients, although CD3-positive cells remain undetectable. The presence of these CD4- and CD8-positive cells has not been found to affect the clinical course of the patient. CD3-positive cells reappear rapidly and reach pretreatment levels within a week after termination of muromonab-CD3 therapy.

Increasing numbers of CD3-positive cells have been observed in some patients during the second week of therapy, possibly as a result of development of antibodies that neutralize muromonab-CD3. The distribution of anti-muromonab-CD3 antibodies include 86% IgG, 29% IgE, and 21% IgM. The mean time of appearance of anti-muromonab-CD3 IgG was 18 to 22 days. IgG antibodies appeared by the end of the second week of treatment in 80% of patients.

Muromonab-CD3 administered after development of neutralizing antibodies may be consumed and rendered unavailable for binding to the T3 antigen-receptor complex on T-cells.

Anti-muromonab-CD3 antibodies may be of 2 types: (1) Anti-isotypic antibodies that bind to the Fc region of muromonab-CD3 and do not inhibit its immunosuppressive activity, and (2) anti-idiotypic antibodies that bind to the variable portion of muromonab-CD3, where it attaches to the T3 antigen, reducing efficacy.

Muromonab-CD3's route of metabolism is unclear. Bound to T-lymphocytes, it may be opsonized by the reticuloendothelial system or be neutralized by human antimurine antibodies. The specific route of elimination of unbound murine immunoglobulin is unknown, but may be eliminated by catabolism.

Muromonab-CD3 is unlikely to be dialyzed by either hemodialysis or peritoneal dialysis, but may be dialyzed by high-flux dialysis. Daily dosing is recommended after dialysis.

Effective level: Assay plasma muromonab-CD3 levels by ELISA, using a target level after the third day of therapy more than 800 ng/mL. Another option is to measure quantitative T-lymphocyte surface phenotyping (eg, CD3, CD4, CD8), with a target of CD3-positive T-cells less than 25 cells/mm^3.

Mechanism: Muromonab-CD3 probably blocks the function of all T-cells that play a role in acute renal rejection. Specifically, it blocks the function of a 20,000 dalton subunit (CD3) on the surface membrane of human T-cells associated in vitro with the antigen recognition structure of T-cells, essential for signal transduction. During in vitro cytolytic assays, muromonab-CD3 blocks both the generation and function of effecter cells. In vivo, muromonab-CD3 reacts with most peripheral blood T-cells and T-cells in body tissues, but not with other hematopoietic elements or other tissues of the body.

Muromonab-CD3 opsonizes circulating T-lymphocytes that are then removed by reticuloendothelial cells, modulating (ie, removing) the T3-antigen recognition complex from the surface of T-cells, thus rendering the T-cells immunologically unable to function. Muromonab-CD3 may also inhibit functions of sessile killer cells in transplanted organ.

Leukocytes have been observed in cerebrospinal and peritoneal fluids, although the mechanism of this effect is not understood.

Drug Interactions: Combined therapy with antilymphocytic antibodies and other immunosuppressant drugs may increase the recipient's risk of infection and neoplasm. Use the lowest effective dose of each agent.

Minnesota antilymphoblast globulin can suppress delayed-hypersensitivity responses. It is possible, but not established, that muromonab-CD3 would have similar effects, although suppression may not persist as long as that associated with other lymphocyte immune globulins.

It is a common practice to wait several months after discontinuation of immunosuppressive therapy before immunizing people with inactivated or attenuated vaccines. Active immunization of immunosuppressed people may result in an inadequate response to immunization. They remain susceptible despite immunization. Some live, attenuated vaccines pose safety risks to immunosuppressed people.

Lab Interference: Patients who develop human antimouse antibodies (HAMAs) may show either falsely elevated or depressed values when tested with assay kits that employ mouse monoclonal antibodies (eg, some serum pregnancy tests). Consider alternate diagnostic procedures.

Pharmaceutical Characteristics

Concentration: 5 mg/5 mL

Quality Assay: Monoclonal nature provides reproducible antibody product with consistent, measurable reactivity to human T-cells.

Packaging: Package of five 5 mL ampules

NDC Number: 59676-0101-01

Doseform: Solution

Appearance: Clear, colorless solution with a few fine translucent protein particles.

Solvent: Phosphate-buffered saline: 2.25 mg monobasic sodium phosphate, 9 mg dibasic sodium phosphate, and 43 mg sodium chloride, each per 5 mL

Adjuvant: None

Preservative: None

Allergens: Murine IgG

Excipients: 1 mg per ampule polysorbate 80

pH: 6.5 to 7.5

Shelf Life: Expires within 9 months

Storage/Stability: Store at 2° to 8°C (36° to 46°F). Discard if frozen. Do not store at room temperature longer than 4 hours. Shipped in insulated containers with coolant packs and temperature-monitoring strips. Reportedly stable for 16 hours in plastic syringes.

Production Process: Murine monoclonal antibodies are produced using seed lots of the parent hybridoma. The immunoglobulin is purified from murine ascites fluid by fractionation followed by ion-exchange chromatography. The purified bulk is formulated to final dose strength, filter-sterilized, and aseptically filled into ampules.

Media: Mouse ascites fluid

Muromonab-CD3 (Murine)

Disease Epidemiology

Incidence: See the Transplantation General Statement in the Antilymphocyte Antibody summary-monograph.

Other Information

Perspective: See the Transplantation General Statement in the Antilymphocyte Antibody summary monograph.

References: Chan GLC, Gruber SA, Skjei KL, et al. Principles of immunosuppression. *Crit Care Clinics*. 1990;6:841-892.

Hooks MA, Wade CS, Millikan WJ Jr. Muromonab CD-3: A review of its pharmacology, pharmacokinetics and clinical use in transplantation. *Pharmacotherapy*. 1991;11:26-37.

Todd PA, Brogden RN. Muromonab CD-3: A review of its pharmacology and therapeutic potential. *Drugs*. 1989;37:871-899.

Smith SL. Ten years of Orthoclone OKT3 (muromonab-CD3): A review. *J Transpl Coord*. 1996;6(Sep):109-121.

Isoantibodies

Most antibodies conjugated to radioisotopes are used as immunoimaging agents for radioimmunoscintigraphy. This process uses the specificity of antibodies and the imaging potential of radioisotopes to aid in the diagnosis of a wide variety of diseases. Other radiolabeled antibodies will carry therapeutic doses of alpha, beta, or gamma radiation to specific sites in the body. This combined use of antibodies and radiation may be humanity's closest step yet to Paul Ehrlich's ideal "magic bullet" that targets diseased tissue without harming healthy tissue.

This section begins with a table describing isotope-conjugated antibodies licensed for use in the United States. The table is followed by another table identifying the chemical and physical characteristics of radioisotopes considered for radiolabeling antibodies. The choice of a radioisotope is based largely on the time required for the antibody to diffuse to the tissue to be imaged or irradiated. While indium-111 may be preferred with intact antibodies, 99m-technetium may be more likely to be conjugated to antibody fragments (eg, Fab).

Products currently in clinical trials are listed in the Investigational Immunologic Drugs section. A wide variety of immunoimaging agents are in advanced clinical trials, have achieved orphan drug status, or are undergoing safety and efficacy review by the FDA.

Advantages and Disadvantages of Selected Isotopes for Radioimmunoscintigraphy		
Isotope	Advantages	Disadvantages
^{67}Cu, Copper	Image quality	Availability
^{99m}Tc, Technetium	Decay energy Availability Cost	Labeling chemistry Kidney uptake Limited follow-up imaging (short half-life)
^{111}In, Indium	Decay energy Labeling chemistry	Cost Uptake by reticuloendothelial system
^{123}I, Iodine	Decay energy Chelation chemistry	Availability Cost In vivo dehalogenation Decreased immunoreactivity
^{125}I, Iodine	Short range	Poor images
^{131}I, Iodine	Labeling chemistry Availability	Decay energy In vivo dehalogenation Decreased immunoreactivity
^{188}Re, Rhenium	Generator-produced Technetium chemistry Image quality	Availability
^{211}At, Astatine	Iodine chemistry Short range	Not suitable for imaging

Isotope-Conjugated Antibodies

Isotopes for Diagnostic and Therapeutic Radiology				
Isotope symbol[a]	Element	Physical half-life[b]	Main photon energies (keV)	Decay type[c]
$^{32}_{15}$ P	Phosphorus	14.3 days	1,710	Beta –, gamma
$^{51}_{24}$ Cr	Chromium	27.8 days	320	Electron capture, gamma
$^{67}_{29}$ Cu	Copper	2.6 days	93, 185	Beta –
$^{90}_{39}$ Y	Yttrium	64.2 hours	2,260 (B)	Beta –
$^{99m}_{43}$ Tc	Technetium	6.02 hours	2, 140, 142	Isomeric transition, gamma
$^{111}_{49}$ In	Indium	2.83 days	173, 247	Electron capture, gamma
$^{123}_{53}$ I	Iodine	13.3 hours	159	Electron capture, gamma
$^{125}_{53}$ I	Iodine	60.1 days	35	Electron capture
$^{131}_{53}$ I	Iodine	8.06 days	284, 364, 637	Beta –, gamma
$^{186}_{75}$ Re	Rhenium	3.7 days	123 to 774, 137	Beta –, electron capture, gamma
$^{188}_{75}$ Re	Rhenium	17 hours	155 to 2,021	Beta –
$^{211}_{85}$ At	Astatine	7.2 hours	96 to 1,067	Alpha, electron capture

a In the nomenclature of radioisotopes, the superscript refers to the combined number of protons and neutrons in the atom (the mass number), while the subscript denotes the number of protons. The difference between these 2 integers is the number of neutrons.

b The physical half-life is the amount of time for a quantity of an isotope to decay to the point where only half the original quantity remains. This value does not take into account the biological properties and biological half-life of an isotopic drug.

c Several types of radioactive decay may occur. Each isotope has at least 1 characteristic mode of decay:

Alpha decay involves the emission of a helium atom.

Beta – ("beta minus") decay involves the emission of an electron, also called a negatron.

Electron capture involves the capture of an orbital electron by a nucleus to achieve a more stable neutron-proton ratio.

Gamma rays are a form of electromagnetic radiation emitted with varying energy.

Isometric transition releases gamma radiation as the atom changes from the metastable to stable state.

Other Information

Perspective:

1896: Becquerel observes natural radioactivity from uranium fogging his photographic plates.

1899: Rutherford differentiates alpha and beta radiation.

1900: Pierre Curie and Villard observe gamma radiation.

1903: Rutherford and Soddy propose theory of radioactive disintegration.

1919: Rutherford observes first artificial transmutation. This first successful act of alchemy bombarded nitrogen with alpha particles, converting it to oxygen-17.

1949: Pressman and Keighley demonstrate that rabbit antibodies to rat kidney labeled with iodine-131 will localize in the kidneys of living rats.

1965: Carcinoembryonic antigen (CEA) discovered.

1975: Köhler and Milstein develop techniques for mass-producing monoclonal antibodies by fusing mouse splenocytes with myeloma cells. They earn the 1984 Nobel Prize in Medicine.

1978: Goldenberg and colleagues report use of ^{131}I-labeled antibodies that target CEA to detect and localize cancers in humans by external photoscanning.

References: Bogard WC Jr, et al. Practical considerations in the production, purification, and formulation of monoclonal antibodies for immunoscintigraphy and immunotherapy. *Semin Nucl Med.* 1989;19:202-220.

Kassis AI. Optimizing antibodies for use in nuclear medicine. *J Nucl Med.* 1991;32:1751-1753.

Kenanova V, Wu AM. Tailoring antibodies for radionuclide delivery. *Expert Opin Drug Deliv.* 2006;3(1):53-70.

McKearn TJ. Future directions in tumor radioimmunodetection. In: Maguire RT, Van Nostrand D, eds. *Diagnosis of Colorectal and Ovarian Carcinoma: Application of Immunoscintigraphic Technology.* New York, NY: Marcel Dekker; 1992:211-232.

Pangalis GA, Kyrtsonis MC, Vassilakopoulos TP, et al. Immunotherapeutic and immunoregulatory drugs in haematologic malignancies. *Curr Top Med Chem.* 2006;6(16):1657-1686.

Pohlman B, Sweetenham J, Macklis RM. Review of clinical radioimmunotherapy. *Expert Rev Anticancer Ther.* 2006;6(3):445-461.

Reilly RM. Radioimmunotherapy of malignancies. *Clin Pharmacol Ther.* 1991;10:359-375.

Reilly RM, et al. Problems of delivery of monoclonal antibodies: pharmaceutical and pharmacokinetic solutions. *Clin Pharmacokinet.* 1995;28:126-142.

Wong JY. Systemic targeted radionuclide therapy: potential new areas. *Int J Radiat Oncol Biol Phys.* 2006;66(2 Suppl):S74-S82.

Isoantibodies

Yttrium Y 90:

Radioisotope: The source of yttrium-90 (Y-90) is strontium-90 (Sr-90). Yttrium-90 (Y-90) decays by emission of beta particles, with a physical half-life of 64.1 hours (2.67 days). The product of radioactive decay is nonradioactive zirconium-90. The range of beta particles in soft tissue is 5 mm. Radiation emission data for Y-90 appear below.

Radiation	Mean % of Disintegration	Mean Energy (keV)
Beta minus	100	750 to 935

External Radiation: The exposure rate for 37 MBq (1 mCi) of Y-90 is 8.3×10^{-3} Ci/kg/h (32 R/h) at the mouth of an open Y-90 vial. Use adequate shielding with this beta-emitter, in accordance with institutional good radiation safety practices. Beta particles have low penetrating capacity. The maximum range of beta minus from Y-90 in tissue is approximately 11 mm.

Physical Decay: To allow correction for physical decay of Y-90, the fractions that remain at selected intervals before and after the time of calibration appear below.

Yttrium Y 90 Fractions Remaining at Selected Intervals			
Time elapsed (h)	Fraction remaining	Time elapsed (h)	Fraction remaining
−36	1.48	1	0.99
−24	1.30	2	0.98
−12	1.14	3	0.97
−8	1.09	4	0.96
−7	1.08	5	0.95
−6	1.07	6	0.94
−5	1.06	7	0.93
−4	1.04	8	0.92
−3	1.03	12	0.88
−2	1.02	24	0.77
−1	1.01	36	0.68
0	1.00		

Technetium Tc 99m:

Radioisotope: This radioisotope is extracted from a generator (or "cow") containing molybdenum-99, which decays to produce technetium-99m. Technetium-99m (Tc-99m or ^{99m}Tc), which decays by isometric transition with a physical half-life of 6.02 hours. The product of radioactive decay is technetium-99, sometimes called "Tc-99g." The principal photon that is useful for detection and imaging is Gamma-2, with a mean proportion per disintegration of 89.07% and an energy of 140.5 keV. Other gamma particles are emitted with energy of 18 keV and mean proportion per disintegration of 6.2%.

External Radiation: The specific gamma ray constant for Tc-99m is 5.4 microcoulombs/kg-MBq-h (0.78 R/mCi-h) at 1 cm. The first half-value thickness of lead for Tc-99m is 0.017 cm. A range of values for the relative attenuation of the radiation emitted by this radionuclide from various thicknesses of lead appears below. For example, the use of 0.25 cm of lead will decrease the external radiation exposure by a factor of approximately 1,000.

Shield Thickness (Lead, cm)	Coefficient of Attenuation
0.017	1/2
0.08	1/10
0.16	1/100
0.25	1/1,000
0.33	1/10,000

Physical Decay: To correct for physical decay of Tc-99m, the fractions that remain at selected intervals after dose calibration appear below.

Technetium Tc 99m Fractions Remaining at Selected Intervals			
Time elapsed after calibration (h)	Fraction remaining	Time elapsed after calibration (h)	Fraction remaining
0	1	8	0.398
1	0.891	9	0.355
2	0.794	10	0.316
3	0.708	11	0.282
4	0.631	12	0.251
5	0.562	18	0.13
6	0.501	24	0.06
7	0.447		

Indium In 111:

Radioisotope: The principal source of indium-111 (In-111) is tin-111 (Sn-111). Indium-111 (In-111) decays by electron capture with a physical half-life of 67.2 hours. The product of radioactive decay is cadmium-111 (Cd-111). The energies of the photons useful for detection and imaging studies appear below.

Radiation	Mean % of Disintegration	Mean Energy (keV)
Gamma-2	90.2	171.3
Gamma-3	94	245.4

External Radiation: The exposure rate constant for 37 MBq (1 mCi) of In-111 is 8.3×10^{-4} Ci/kg/h (3.21 R/h). The first half-value thickness of lead for In-111 is 0.023 cm. A range of values for the relative attenuation of radiation emitted by this radionuclide for various thicknesses of lead appears below. For example, 0.834 cm of lead will decrease the external radiation exposure by a factor of approximately 1,000. These estimates of attenuation do not take into consideration the presence of longer-lived contaminants with higher energy photons, namely In-114m/114.

Shield Thickness (Lead, cm)	Coefficient of Attenuation
0.023	1/2
0.203	1/10
0.513	1/100
0.834	1/1,000
1.12	1/10,000

Physical Decay: To allow correction for physical decay of In-111, fractions remaining at selected intervals before and after dose calibration ([a]) appear below.

Indium In 111 Fractions Remaining at Selected Intervals			
Time elapsed (h)	Fraction remaining	Time elapsed (h)	Fraction remaining
−48	1.64	+36	0.69
−42	1.54	+42	0.65
−36	1.44	+48	0.61
−30	1.35	+54	0.58
−24	1.28	+60	0.54
−18	1.2	+66	0.51
−12	1.13	+72	0.48
−6	1.06	+84	0.42
0[a]	1	+96	0.37
+6	0.94	+108	0.33
+12	0.88	+120	0.29
+18	0.83	+132	0.26
+24	0.78	+144	0.23
+30	0.74		

a Dose calibration.

Radiologic Characteristics of Isotopes

Iodine I 131:

Radioisotope: The source of iodine-131 (I-131) is tellurium-131 (Te-131). Iodine-131 (I-131) decays with beta and gamma emissions with a physical half-life of 8.04 days. The product of radioactive decay is xenon-131 (Xe-131). The principal beta emission has a mean energy of 191.6 keV and the principal gamma emission has an energy of 364.5 keV.

External Radiation: The specific gamma ray constant for I-131 is 2.2 R/mCi-h at 1 cm. The first half-value layer is 0.24 cm lead shielding. A range of values for the relative attenuation of the radiation emitted by this radionuclide that results from interposition of various thicknesses of lead appears below. To facilitate control of the radiation exposure from this radionuclide, the use of a 2.55 cm thickness of lead will attenuate the radiation emitted by a factor of about 1,000.

Shield Thickness (Lead, cm)	Coefficient of Attenuation
0.24	1/2
0.89	1/10
1.60	1/100
2.55	1/1,000
3.7	1/10,000

Physical Decay: To allow correction for physical decay of I-131, the fraction of I-131 radioactivity that remains in the vial after the date of calibration is calculated as follows: fraction of remaining radioactivity of I-131 after $\times$ days = $2^{-(\times/804)}$. Physical decay calculations appear below.

Iodine I 131 Fractions Remaining at Selected Intervals	
Time elapsed after calibration (d)	Fraction remaining
0[a]	1.000
1	0.917
2	0.842
3	0.772
4	0.708
5	0.650
6	0.596
7	0.547
8	0.502
9	0.460
10	0.422
11	0.387
12	0.355
13	0.326
14	0.299[a]

a Calibration day.

Capromab Pendetide (Murine)

Isoantibodies

Name:
ProstaScint Kit for the Preparation of
Indium-111 Capromab Pendetide

Manufacturer:
Manufactured by Laureate Pharma for EUSA
Pharma (USA)

Synonyms: *OncoScint* PR356, CYT-356-In-111, 7E11-C5.3, CAS 145464-28-4

Immunologic Characteristics

Target Antigen: A glycoprotein expressed by prostate epithelium known as prostate specific membrane antigen (PSMA). The PSMA epitope recognized by monoclonal antibody 7E11-C5.3 is located in the cytoplasmic domain. Expression of this glycoprotein has not been demonstrated on any other adenocarcinomas or transitional cell cancers tested.

Viability: Inactive, passive, transient

Antigenic Form: Murine immunoglobulin

Antigenic Type: IgG1, kappa subclass, monoclonal, 150,000 daltons, recognizing a cytoplasmic membrane-specific epitope. Conjugated to the linker-chelator glycyltyrosyl-(N,E-diethylenetriamine pentaacetic acid)-lysine hydrochloride (GYK-DTPA-HCl).

Strains: Recognizes prostate specific membrane antigen (PSMA), a glycoprotein found on adenocarcinomas of the prostate.

Use Characteristics

Indications: For use as a diagnostic imaging agent in newly diagnosed patients with biopsy-proven prostate cancer thought to be clinically localized after standard diagnostic evaluation (eg, chest x-ray, bone scan, CT scan, MRI) who are at high risk for pelvic lymph node metastases. It is not indicated in patients who are not at high risk.

Indium-111 capromab is also indicated as a diagnostic imaging agent in post-prostatectomy patients with a rising prostate-specific antigen (PSA) and a negative or equivocal standard metastatic evaluation in whom there is a high clinical suspicion of occult metastatic disease. The imaging performance of indium-111 capromab following radiation therapy has not been studied.

Limitations: Do not base patient management on indium-111 capromab scan results without appropriate confirmatory studies. In clinical trials, there was a high rate of false-positive and false-negative image interpretations. False-positive scan interpretations may result in:
(1) Inappropriate surgical intervention to confirm scan results; (2) inappropriate denial of curative therapy if results are not confirmed; or (3) inadequate surgical staging if only areas of uptake are sampled. Do not limit surgical sampling to the areas of positive uptake unless histologic examination of these areas is diagnostic. Because of the potential for false-negative scan interpretations, do not use negative images in lieu of histologic confirmation.

Capromab is not indicated as a screening tool for carcinoma of the prostate nor for readministration for the purpose of assessment of response to treatment. Indium-111 capromab images should be interpreted only by physicians who have had specific training in indium-111 capromab image interpretation. Proper patient preparation is mandatory to obtain optimal images for interpretation.

Bone scans are more sensitive than capromab for the detection of metastases to bone. Indium-111 capromab should not replace bone scans for the evaluation of skeletal metastases.

Contraindications:

Absolute: Patients who are hypersensitive to this or any other product of murine origin or to indium-111 chloride

Relative: None

Immunodeficiency: No impairment of effect is likely.

Elderly: No specific information is available about geriatric use of capromab. Older patients were entered into clinical trials.

Carcinogenicity: Long-term animal studies have not been performed to evaluate the carcinogenic potential of indium-111 capromab.

Mutagenicity: Long-term animal studies have not been performed to evaluate the mutagenic potential of indium-111 capromab.

Fertility Impairment: Long-term animal studies have not been performed to evaluate the effect of indium-111 capromab on fertility.

Pregnancy: Capromab is not indicated for use in women. It is not known if capromab crosses the placenta nor whether capromab can cause fetal harm if administered to a pregnant woman or affect reproductive capacity.

Lactation: Capromab is not indicated for use in women.

Children: The safety and efficacy of indium-111 capromab in children have not been established. Capromab is not indicated for use in children.

Adverse Reactions: Capromab was generally well tolerated in clinical trials. After administration of 529 single doses of indium-111 capromab, adverse reactions were observed in 4% of patients. The most commonly reported adverse reactions were: Increases in bilirubin, hypotension, and hypertension occurring in 1% of patients. Elevated liver enzymes and injection-site reactions occurred in slightly less than 1% of patients. Other adverse reactions, in order of decreasing frequency, were: Pruritus, fever, rash, headache, myalgia, asthenia, burning sensation in thigh, shortness of breath, and taste alteration. Most adverse reactions were mild and readily reversible. Data from repeat administration in 61 patients revealed a similar incidence of adverse reactions (5%). No deaths were attributable to indium-111 capromab.

Indium-111 capromab can induce human antimouse antibody (HAMA) responses to murine IgG infrequently and with low peak levels after single administration. HAMA levels were detected (at higher than 8 ng/mL) by radioimmune assay (RIA) after single infusion in 8% (20/239) of patients, while 1% of patients had levels higher than 100 ng/mL. In addition, serum HAMA levels were detected by RIA after repeat infusion in 19% (5/27) of the patients. While limited data exist concerning the clinical significance of HAMA, detectable serum levels can alter the clearance and tissue biodistribution of MAbs. The development of persistently elevated serum HAMA levels could compromise the efficacy of diagnostic or therapeutic murine antibody-based agents. In repeat administration trials, 93% (65/70) of the evaluable repeat infusions were associated with normal tissue distribution of the monoclonal antibodies conjugate. Pre-infusion serum HAMA levels were generally not predictive of altered distribution.

When considering the administration of indium-111 capromab to patients who have previously received other murine antibody-based products, be aware of the potential for assay interference and increased clearance and altered biodistribution. This may interfere with the quality or sensitivity of the imaging study. Before administration of murine antibodies, including indium-111 capromab, review the patient's history to determine whether the patient has previously received such products.

Caution: Only clinicians experienced in the safe handling of radionuclides should use radiopharmaceuticals.

Capromab Pendetide (Murine)

Pharmacologic & Dosing Characteristics

Dosage: Do not inject capromab directly into a patient. Use the indium-111 chloride only to radiolabel capromab. Do not inject it directly into the patient. The imaging agent, indium-111 capromab, is formed by combining capromab with indium-111 as described below. Reducing the dose of indium-111, unlabeled capromab, or indium-111 capromab may adversely impact imaging results and is not recommended.

The recommended dose of capromab is 0.5 mg radiolabeled with 5 mCi of indium-111 chloride. Each dose is administered IV over 5 minutes. Do not mix it with any other medication during its administration. Indium-111 capromab may be readministered after infiltration or a technically inadequate scan; however, it is not indicated for readministration to assess response to treatment.

Route & Site: IV

Overdosage: The maximum amount of indium-111 capromab that can be safely administered has not been determined. In clinical studies, single doses of 10 mg of indium-111 capromab were administered to 20 patients with prostate cancer. The type and frequency of adverse reactions at this dose were similar to those observed with lower doses. The maximum indium-111 dose administered with capromab in a clinical study was 6.5 mCi.

Dose Preparation: Read complete directions before starting the preparation procedure. Conduct all procedures using aseptic technique and standard precautions for handling radionuclides. Prepare indium-111 capromab using waterproof gloves, adequate shielding of radioactivity, and aseptic techniques. Before radiolabeling, allow the 2 vials to reach room temperature.

The following materials are required but not supplied with the drug kit: Indium-111 chloride, sterile syringes, vial shield, dose calibrator, ITLC-GC strips, chromatography chamber, sterile needles, syringe shield, waterproof gloves, alcohol wipe, water-soluble marker, 0.9% sodium chloride solution, diethylenetriamine pentaacetic acid solution, and gamma-ray detector.

Before radiolabeling, bring the refrigerated capromab to room temperature. Capromab is a protein solution that may develop translucent particulates. These particulates will be removed by filtration. Clean the rubber stopper of each vial with an alcohol wipe. With a sterile 1 mL syringe, add 0.1 mL of sodium acetate solution to the shielded vial of indium-111 chloride and mix. Retain remaining sodium acetate for use later. With the same 1 mL syringe, withdraw 6 to 7 mCi of the buffered indium-111 chloride and add to the capromab vial. Flush the syringe to mix the preparation. To normalize pressure, withdraw an equal volume of air. Swirl gently to mix and assay contents in a dose calibrator. On 1 of the labels, record the patient's identification and the date, time of preparation, and activity in the vial. Affix the label to the vial shield. Allow the labeling reaction to proceed at room temperature for 30 minutes.

With a syringe, add the remaining sodium acetate to the capromab reaction vial. To normalize pressure, withdraw an equal volume of air. Aseptically attach the 0.22-micrometer Millex-GV sterile filter and a sterile needle to a 10 mL sterile disposable syringe, and withdraw the contents of the reaction vial through the filter into the syringe. Keep the needle immersed in the solution to avoid creating an air lock in the filter. Remove the filter and needle. Aseptically attach a new sterile needle to the syringe. Assay syringe and contents in a dose calibrator. The syringe should contain 4 mCi (148 MBq) or more of indium-111. Determine radiochemical purity by instant thin-layer chromatography (ITLC). If the radiochemical purity is less than 90%, repeat the ITLC procedure. If repeat testing remains less than 90%, properly discard the preparation and do not administer it.

On the second label provided in the kit, record the patient's identification and the date, time of assay, and activity in the syringe. Affix this label to the syringe shield. Use the indium-111 capromab within 8 hours of radiolabeling.

Related Interventions: There may be indium-111 capromab clearance and imaging localization observed in the bowel, blood pool, kidneys, and urinary bladder. When obtaining all 72- to 120-hour planar and SPECT images, catheterize and irrigate the bladder. Administer a cathartic the evening before imaging the patient and give a cleansing enema within an hour before each 72- to 120-hour imaging session.

Waste Disposal: Discard vials, needles, and syringes according to local, state, and federal regulations governing radioactive and biohazardous waste.

Radiation Protection: After the indium-111 is added to the capromab, shield the drug appropriately to minimize radiation exposure to patients, family, and medical personnel, consistent with proper hospital and patient-management procedures.

Image Acquisition: Acquire images using a large field-of-view gamma camera equipped with a parallel-hole medium-energy collimator. Calibrate the gamma camera using the 172 and 247 keV photopeaks for indium-111 with a 20% symmetric window. Perform whole body or spot planar views of the pelvis, abdomen, and thorax between 72 and 120 hours after indium-111 capromab infusion.

Conduct whole-body acquisition from skull through mid-femur. The total scan time over this area should be 35 minutes or longer using a 128×512 or $256 \times 1,024$ matrix.

Acquire planar images in anterior and posterior views for 7.5 minutes per view using a 128×128 or 256×256 matrix. Because of uptake of indium-111 capromab by the liver, planar images obtained with the liver in the field of view must be acquired with adequate counts to allow the detection of lesions in the adjacent extrahepatic abdomen and pelvis. This may result in pixel overflow with image degradation in the region of the liver.

Two single-photon emission computed tomography (SPECT) imaging sessions are necessary. The first SPECT session should be of the pelvis and be performed approximately 30 minutes after infusion to obtain a blood pool image. The second SPECT session includes the pelvis and abdomen, including the lower liver margin through the prostatic fossa, and should be performed between 72 and 120 hours after infusion for detection of benign and malignant prostate tissue sites. Depending upon the capability of the camera's field-of-view to include both pelvis and abdomen, either 1 or 2 separate acquisitions may be necessary during the second session.

To resolve imaging ambiguities possibly resulting from activity in blood pool, stool, or urinary bladder, perform follow-up imaging sessions with full patient preparation.

Acquire the SPECT images using a 64×64 or 128×128 matrix for a minimum of 60 to 120 stops, respectively, over 360° rotation for approximately 25 seconds per view at the first session and 50 seconds per view at the second session. Perform reconstruction using a Butterworth filter or equivalent in the transverse, coronal, and sagittal views. An order of 5 and cut-off of 0.5 may be used as a starting point. Slice thickness should be in the range of 6 to 12 mm.

Efficacy: Indium-111 capromab has been administered in single doses to more than 600 patients in clinical studies and in repeat administrations (2 to 4 infusions) to 61 patients. A 0.5 mg dose was determined to be the lowest effective dose. The imaging performance of indium-111 capromab was evaluated in a phase 2 and a phase 3 trial in each of 2 clinical settings: (1) Patients with clinically localized prostate cancer who were at high risk for metastases, and (2) patients with a high clinical suspicion for occult recurrent or residual prostate cancer.

Newly diagnosed patients: In 1 of 2 open-label, uncontrolled phase 3 trials, 160 patients with a tissue diagnosis of prostate cancer who were considered at high risk for lymph node metastases underwent indium-111 capromab immunoscintigraphy before scheduled staging pelvic lymphadenectomy. High risk was defined as 1 or more of the following:

(1) PSA 10 or more times the upper limit of normal and a Gleason score of 7 or more; (2) prostatic acid phosphatase above the upper limit of normal; (3) equivocal evidence of lymph node metastases on CT or ultrasound and PSA 8 or more times the upper limit of normal; (4) Gleason score of 8 or more; or (5) clinical stage C and Gleason score of 6 or more. All patients had been evaluated for metastatic disease using standard noninvasive imaging techniques and were considered to have clinically localized prostate cancer. The indium-111 capromab uptake to specific sites of tumor involvement was not performed.

One hundred fifty-two patients had an interpretable scan and surgical staging. Forty scans were classified as true-positive, 25 as false-positive, 63 as true-negative, and 24 as false-negative. Thus, the test yielded a sensitivity of 62%, specificity of 72%, positive-predictive value of 62%, negative-predictive value of 72%, and an overall accuracy of 68%.

A retrospective subset analysis suggested that a positive indium-111 capromab scan in patients with a Gleason score of 7 or more and a PSA of 40 or higher contained additional information regarding the likelihood that tumor metastases would be found at the scheduled staging pelvic lymphadenectomy.

Patients with occult recurrent or residual disease: In the second open-label, uncontrolled phase 3 trial, 183 patients with a high clinical suspicion of residual or recurrent prostate cancer following radical prostatectomy were evaluated. Patients with a rising PSA, a negative bone scan, and negative or equivocal standard diagnostic techniques (eg, transrectal ultrasound, CT scan, MRI) underwent indium-111 capromab immunoscintigraphy before biopsy of the prostatic fossa. The interpretations were correlated with the results of histopathologic analysis of the prostatic fossa biopsy specimens.

One hundred fifty-eight patients had an interpretable scan and prostatic fossa biopsy. Twenty-nine scans were classified as true-positive, 29 as false-positive, 70 as true-negative, and 30 as false-negative. This test yielded a sensitivity of 49%, specificity of 71%, positive-predictive value of 50%, negative-predictive value of 70%, and an overall accuracy of 63%.

Indium-111 capromab localized to only the prostatic fossa in 29 (18%) patients, to prostatic fossa and extrafossa sites in 29 (18%) patients, and to only extrafossa sites in 39 (25%) patients. The study was not designed to evaluate extrafossa sites of uptake. Three extrafossa sites of uptake were biopsied, 1 of which was positive for metastatic prostate cancer.

Patients with distant metastases: Clinical trials have not specifically studied the ability of indium-111 capromab to image distant (extrapelvic) metastases, and a limited number of patients with distant (primarily bone) metastases were enrolled. Thirteen patients out of 16 (81%) with CT evidence of distant soft tissue disease had positive extrafossa indium-111 capromab scans. Thirty-five out of 61 patients (57%) with bone-scan evidence of disease had positive indium-111 capromab skeletal uptake; however, indium-111 capromab imaging did not identify most sites of abnormal bone uptake on bone scan. Nor did it demonstrate any new sites of metastasis that were not seen on bone scan. However, the indium-111 capromab scan did demonstrate sites of bone-marrow metastases that were not seen on bone scan in 2 of 43 patients in the phase 1 study.

Time of Reading: Conduct the first SPECT session approximately 30 minutes after infusion to obtain a blood pool image. Perform planar views between 72 and 120 hours after indium-111 capromab infusion. The second SPECT session is performed between 72 and 120 hours after infusion to detect benign and malignant prostate tissue sites.

Interpretation: Interpret diagnostic images acquired with indium-111 capromab in conjunction with other appropriate diagnostic tests.

Following indium-111 capromab administration, some of the radiolabel localizes in normal liver, spleen, bone marrow, and genitalia. Indium-111-labeled antibodies may localize nonspecifically in colostomy sites, degenerative joint disease, abdominal aneurysms, postoperative bowel adhesions, and local inflammatory lesions, including those typically associated with inflammatory bowel disease or secondary to surgery or radiation. Indium-111 capromab can demonstrate apparent localization to sites of tortuous blood vessels. Careful review of the patient's medical history and other diagnostic information will aid in the interpretation of the images.

Subsequent Tests: Sixty-one patients received a total of 74 repeat infusions of indium-111 capromab. The incidence of adverse reactions upon repeat infusion (5%) was comparable with that observed after single infusion (4%). Human antimouse antibody (HAMA) levels were detected (at levels higher than 8 ng/mL) by RIA after single infusion in 8% (20/239) of patients, while 1% of patients had levels higher than 100 ng/mL. Serum HAMA levels were detected by RIA after repeat infusion in 19% (5/27) of patients. Biodistribution was unaltered on 65 of 70 (93%) evaluable repeat scans. The efficacy of repeat indium-111 capromab imaging was not evaluated.

Onset: Sufficient antibodies have localized so that optimal images are routinely obtained between 72 and 120 hours after injection.

Duration: Interpretable images may be obtained as late as 120 hours after injection.

Pharmacokinetics: Immunoglobulins are primarily eliminated by catabolism. Based on data from clinical studies, indium-111 capromab demonstrated a monoexponential elimination pattern with a terminal-phase half-life of 67 $\pm$ 11 hours (mean $\pm$ SD). Approximately 10% of the administered radioisotope dose is excreted in the urine during the 72 hours after IV infusion. The pharmacokinetics of indium-111 capromab are characterized by slow serum clearance (42 $\pm$ 22 mL/h) and small volume of distribution (4 $\pm$ 2.1 L).

Mechanism: PSMA is expressed in many primary and metastatic prostate cancer lesions, and in vitro immunohistologic studies have shown 7E11-C5.3 to be reactive to more than 95% of the prostate adenocarcinomas evaluated. In general, PSMA expression by prostate cancer cells is either unchanged or increased in patients treated with hormonal therapy. The 7E11-C5.3 antibody is immunoreactive with normal and hypertrophic adult prostate tissue. In clinical studies of patients with prostate cancer, indium-111 capromab localized in the prostate and some known primary and metastatic tumor sites.

Non-antigen-dependent localization, suspected to be secondary to catabolism, has been observed in the liver, spleen, and bone marrow. Although there is variation among individuals, there may also be localization and imaging activity in the bowel, blood pool, kidneys, urinary bladder, and genitalia. Intracellular localization of 7E11-C5.3 has been observed in histochemically prepared tissue sections from normal adult skeletal and cardiac muscle, although primate studies revealed no specific localization to these tissues.

Drug Interactions: The effect of surgical or medical androgen ablation on the imaging performance of indium-111 capromab has not been studied. Preliminary data suggest hormone ablation may increase PSMA expression with concurrent decrease in tumor expression of PSA. The use of capromab in this patient population cannot be recommended at this time.

Lab Interference: The presence of HAMA in serum as a result of capromab may interfere with some antibody-based immunoassays (eg, PSA, digoxin). When present, this interference generally results in falsely high values. When following PSA levels, use assay methods resistant to HAMA interference. PSA assays resistant to HAMA interference include *Hybritech Tandem-R* and *Abbott IMX*.

When patients receive indium-111 capromab, notify the clinical laboratory to take appropriate measures to avoid interference by HAMA with clinical laboratory testing procedures.

These methods include the use of non-murine-based immunoassays, HAMA removal by adsorption, or sample pre-treatment to block HAMA activity.

Patient Information: Murine antibodies are foreign proteins and they can induce HAMAs. While limited data exist about the clinical significance of HAMAs, HAMAs may interfere with murine antibody-based immunoassays. They can compromise the efficacy of in vitro or in vivo diagnostic or therapeutic murine antibody-based drugs and may increase the risk of adverse reactions. Inform patients that use of this product could adversely affect the future ability to diagnose recurrence of their tumor, the ability to perform certain other laboratory tests, or to use other murine-based products. Advise patients to discuss prior use of murine-antibody-based products with their clinicians.

Pharmaceutical Characteristics

Concentration: The capromab vial contains 0.5 mg/mL of capromab pendetide.

Quality Assay: Sterile, pyrogen-free. Immediately before administration, measure the patient dose in a dose calibrator. Radiochemical purity must be more than 90% by instant thin-layer chromatography. Inspect the solution visually; if there is particulate matter or discoloration, discard the preparation and notify the manufacturer.

Packaging: Single-dose kit containing 2 vials. The capromab vial contains 0.5 mg/mL capromab pendetide. The buffer vial contains sodium acetate solution. Each kit also includes 1 sterile 0.22 micrometer Millex-GV filter, prescribing information, and 2 identification labels.

NDC Number: 57902-0817-01

Doseform: Solution for further processing

Appearance:
Buffer vial: Clear, colorless solution
Capromab vial: Clear, colorless solution that may contain some translucent particles

Solvent: Capromab pentetate is initially provided in sodium phosphate-buffered saline solution.

Adjuvant: None

Preservative: None

Allergens: None

Excipients:
Buffer vial: 82 mg of sodium acetate (0.5 M) in 2 mL of water for injection, pH adjusted with glacial acetic acid.

pH:
Buffer vial: pH 5 to 7
Capromab vial: pH 6

Shelf Life: Expires within an unspecified period of time

Storage/Stability: Store at 2° to 8°C (36° to 46°F). Discard frozen product. Contact the manufacturer regarding exposure to elevated or prolonged room temperature. Shipping data not provided. Store upright.

Administer indium-111 capromab within 8 hours of formulation.

Production Process: The antibody is produced by serum-free in vitro cultivation of cells and purified by sequential protein isolation and chromatographic separation procedures.

Media: Data not provided

Radiologic Characteristics

Radiation Dosimetry: The estimated absorbed radiation dose to an average adult patient from an IV injection of capromab labeled with 5 mCi of indium-111 are shown below. Total dose estimates include absorbed radiation doses from indium-111 and the indium-114m radiocontaminant. A level of 0.06% of indium-114m was used for the dose estimates presented.

Average Absorbed Radiation Doses in Adult Patients from IV Capromab Labeled with 5 mCi (185 MBq) Indium-111		
Organ	Average dose (rad/5 mCi)	Average dose (mGy/185 MBq)
Total body	2.7	27
Brain	1.1	11
Liver	18.5	185
Spleen	16.3	163
Kidney	12.4	124
Lungs	5.6	56
Heart wall	7.8	78
Red marrow	4.3	43
Adrenals	5.2	52
Urine bladder wall	2.2	22
Bone surfaces	4.0	40
Stomach	3.1	31
Gall bladder wall	7.3	73
Small intestine	3.3	33
Upper large intestine wall	5.0	50
Lower large intestine wall	7.6	76
Pancreas	5.1	51
Skin	1.1	11
Testes	5.6	56
Prostate	8.2	82
Thymus	2.6	26
Thyroid	1.4	14
Other tissues	2.0	20

Disease Epidemiology

Incidence: An estimated 165,000 cases of prostate cancer, the second leading cause of cancer death in men, are diagnosed annually in the United States, resulting in approximately 35,000 deaths per year. One in every 10 men will develop prostate cancer by 85 years of age.

Other Information

First Licensed: October 28, 1996

References: Wright GL Jr, et al. Expression of prostate-specific membrane antigen in normal, benign and malignant prostate tissues. *Urol Oncol.* 1995;1:18-28.

Sodee DB, Nelson AD, Faulhaber PF, Maclennan GT, Resnick MI, Bakale G. Update on fused capromab pendetide imaging of prostate cancer. *Clin Prostate Cancer.* 2005;3(4):230-238.

Isoantibodies for Non-Hodgkin Lymphoma

Isoantibodies

Comparison of Therapies for Non-Hodgkin Lymphoma		
Brand names	*Zevalin*	*Bexxar*
Generic names	Ibritumomab tiuxetan	Tositumomab
Manufacturer	Cell Therapeutics	Corixa Corporation, with GlaxoSmithKline
Indication	Low-grade, follicular, or transformed B-cell NHL, including patients with rituximab-refractory follicular non-Hodgkin lymphoma	CD20-positive, follicular, NHL, with and without transformation, refractory to rituximab and relapsed after chemotherapy
Antigenic type	IgG1κ monoclonal antibody against CD20 antigen	IgG2aλ monoclonal antibody against CD20 antigen
Source	Murine	Murine
Isotope	In-111 for dosimetry, Y-90 for therapy	I-131 for dosimetry and therapy
Dose	*Step 1, day 0, dosimetry:* Rituximab 250 mg/m^2, then 5 mCi (1.6 mg antibody) of In-111 *Zevalin*. *Step 2, days 7 to 9, therapy:* Rituximab 250 mg/m^2, then 0.4 mCi/kg Y-90 *Zevalin*. If platelets 100,000 to 149,000 cells/mm^3, 0.3 mCi/kg.	*Step 1, day 0, dosimetry:* Tositumomab 450 mg, then 5 mCi I-131 tositumomab (35 mg). *Step 2, days 7 to 14, therapy:* Tositumomab 450 mg, then 75 cGy I-131 tositumomab (35 mg). If platelets 100,000 to 150,000 cells/mm^3, 65 cGy.
Route	IV push	IV infusion
Doseform	Solution	Solution
Concentration	3.2 mg ibritumomab tiuxetan per 2 mL	*Tositumomab*: 14 mg/mL *I-131 tositumomab*: 0.1 mg protein/mL and 0.61 mCi/mL (at calibration).
Packaging	2 kits	2 kits
Solvent	Buffered sodium chloride 0.9%	Buffered water
Routine storage	2° to 8°C. Administer *Zevalin* within 12 h of In-111 labeling or 8 h of Y-90 labeling.	*Tositumomab*: 2° to 8°C; after dilution, stable 24 h at 2° to 8°C or 8 h at room temperature. *I-131 tositumomab*: Freeze in lead pots -20°C or below, until thawed before administration. Thawed doses stable 8 h at 2° to 8°C or room temperature.
Media	Chinese hamster ovary cells	Murine cell culture

Isoantibodies

Name:
Zevalin Kits to Prepare In-111 *Zevalin* and Y-90 *Zevalin*

Manufacturer:
Spectrum Pharmaceuticals

Synonyms: Indium-111 ibritumomab tiuxetan and Yttrium-90 ibritumomab tiuxetan are components of the *Zevalin* therapeutic regimen.

Immunologic Characteristics

Target Antigen: CD20 antigen is found on the surface of normal and malignant B-lymphocytes.

Viability: Inactive, passive, transient

Antigenic Form: Murine IgG1κ immunoglobulin, composed of 2 murine gamma-1 heavy chains of 445 amino acids each and 2 kappa light chains of 213 amino acids each.

Antigenic Type: Protein, IgG1κ monoclonal antibody directed against CD20 antigen. The tiuxetan linker-chelator provides a high-affinity, conformation-restricted chelation site for In-111 or Y-90. The molecular weight of ibritumomab tiuxetan is approximately 148 kilodaltons.

Use Characteristics

Indications: In a multistage regimen, to treat patients with relapsed or refractory low-grade, follicular, or transformed B-cell non-Hodgkin lymphoma, including patients with rituximab refractory follicular non-Hodgkin lymphoma. Effectiveness of the regimen in a relapsed or refractory patient population is based on overall response rates.

To treat previously untreated follicular non-Hodgkin lymphoma in patients who achieve a partial or complete response to first-line chemotherapy.

Caution: Only clinicians experienced in the safe handling of radionuclides should use radiopharmaceuticals.

Limitations: The effects of the *Zevalin* regimen on survival are not known.

Contraindications:

Absolute: Do not administer Y-90 *Zevalin* to patients with altered biodistribution, as determined by imaging with In-111 *Zevalin*. Do not treat patients with fewer than 100,000 platelets/mm^3.

Relative: Zevalin regimen is contraindicated in patients with known immediate hypersensitivity or anaphylactic reactions to murine proteins or to any component of this product, including rituximab, yttrium chloride, and indium chloride.

Immunodeficiency: No impairment of effect is expected.

Elderly: Of 349 patients treated with the *Zevalin* regimen in clinical studies, 38% (132 patients) were 65 years of age or older, while 12% (41 patients) were 75 years of age or older. No overall differences in safety or effectiveness were observed between these subjects and younger subjects, but greater sensitivity of some older individuals cannot be ruled out.

Carcinogenicity: No long-term animal studies have been performed to establish the carcinogenic potential of the *Zevalin* regimen. However, radiation is a potential carcinogen.

Mutagenicity: No long-term animal studies have been performed to establish the mutagenic potential of the *Zevalin* regimen. However, radiation is a potential mutagen. There have been no studies to evaluate whether the *Zevalin* regimen causes mutagenic alterations to germ cells.

Fertility Impairment: No long-term animal studies have evaluated the effect of the *Zevalin* regimen on fertility in males or females. The *Zevalin* regimen results in a significant radiation dose to the testes. The radiation dose to the ovaries has not been established. There have been no studies to evaluate whether the *Zevalin* regimen causes hypogonadism, premature menopause, or azoospermia.

Pregnancy: Category D. Y-90 *Zevalin* can cause fetal harm when administered to a pregnant woman. There are no adequate and well-controlled studies in pregnant women. There is a potential risk that the *Zevalin* regimen could cause toxic effects on the male and female gonads. If this drug is used during pregnancy, or if the patient becomes pregnant while receiving this drug, inform the woman of the potential hazard to the fetus. Advise women of childbearing potential to avoid becoming pregnant for up to 12 months after the *Zevalin* regimen.

Lactation: It is not known whether *Zevalin* is excreted in human milk. Because human IgG is excreted in human milk and the potential for *Zevalin* exposure in the infant is unknown, advise women to discontinue nursing and substitute formula feeding for breast feedings.

Children: Safety and effectiveness of the *Zevalin* regimen in children have not been established.

Adverse Reactions: Safety data are based on 349 patients treated in 5 clinical studies with the *Zevalin* regimen. The most serious adverse reactions caused by the *Zevalin* regimen include infections (predominantly bacterial), allergic reactions (eg, bronchospasm and angioedema), and hemorrhage while thrombocytopenic (resulting in deaths). Patients who received the *Zevalin* regimen have developed myeloid malignancies and dysplasias. Fatal infusion reactions have occurred after the infusion of rituximab.

The most common toxicities reported were neutropenia, thrombocytopenia, anemia, gastrointestinal symptoms (eg, nausea, vomiting, abdominal pain, and diarrhea), increased cough, dyspnea, dizziness, arthralgia, anorexia, anxiety, and ecchymosis. Hematologic toxicity was often severe and prolonged, whereas most nonhematologic toxicity was mild.

Severe or life-threatening adverse events occurring in 1% to 5% of patients not already mentioned include: Pancytopenia (2%), allergic reaction (1%), gastrointestinal hemorrhage (1%), melena (1%), tumor pain (1%), and apnea (1%). The following severe or life-threatening events occurred in less than 1% of patients: Angioedema, tachycardia, urticaria, arthritis, lung edema, pulmonary embolus, encephalopathy, hematemesis, subdural hematoma, and vaginal hemorrhage.

Severe infusion reactions: The *Zevalin* regimen may cause severe, sometimes fatal, infusion reactions. These severe reactions typically occur within 30 to 120 minutes of the first rituximab infusion. Signs and symptoms of severe infusion reaction may include: Hypotension, angioedema, hypoxia, or bronchospasm, and may require interruption of rituximab, In-111 *Zevalin*, or Y-90 *Zevalin* administration. The most severe manifestations and sequelae may include: Pulmonary infiltrates, acute respiratory distress syndrome, myocardial infarction, ventricular fibrillation, and cardiogenic shock.

At least 1 adverse event occurred in 99% of participants. Adverse events scored as grade 3 or 4 occurred in 89% of participants. Adverse events occurring in 5% or more of the 349 patients included:

Body as a whole: 80% overall, 12% in grade 3 or 4. Asthenia (43%, 3%); infection (29%, 5%); chills (24%, less than 1%); fever (17%, 1%); abdominal pain (16%, 3%); pain (13%, 1%); headache (12%, 1%); throat irritation (10%, 0%); back pain (8%, 1%); flushing (6%, 0%).

Cardiovascular: 17% overall, 3% in grade 3 or 4. Hypotension (6%, 1%).

Hemorrhage, including fatal cerebral hemorrhage, and severe infections occurred in a minority of patients in clinical studies. Carefully monitor and manage cytopenias and their complications (eg, febrile neutropenia, hemorrhage) for up to 3 months after use of the *Zevalin* regimen. Exercise caution in treating patients with drugs that interfere with platelet function or coagulation after the *Zevalin* regimen.

CNS: 27% overall, 2% in grade 3 or 4. Dizziness (10%, less than 1%); insomnia (5%, 0%).

Dermatologic: 28% overall, 1% in grade 3 or 4. Pruritus (9%, less than 1%); rash (8%, less than 1%).

GI: 48% overall, 3% in grade 3 or 4. Nausea (31%, 1%); vomiting (12%, 0%); diarrhea (9%, less than 1%); anorexia (8%, 0%); abdominal enlargement (5%, 0%); constipation (5%, 0%).

GU: 6% overall, less than 1% in grade 3 or 4.

Hematologic/Lymphatic: 98% overall, 86% in grade 3 or 4. Thrombocytopenia (95%, 63%); neutropenia (77%, 60%); anemia (61%, 17%); ecchymosis (7%, less than 1%).

The most common severe adverse events reported with the *Zevalin* regimen were thrombocytopenia and neutropenia. In less than 5% of cases, severe cytopenia extended more than 12 weeks after the *Zevalin* regimen. Some of these patients eventually recovered from cytopenia, while others experienced progressive disease, received further anticancer therapy, or died of their lymphoma without having recovered from cytopenia. The cytopenias may have influenced subsequent treatment decisions. Do not administer the *Zevalin* regimen to patients with 25% or greater lymphoma marrow involvement and/or impaired bone-marrow reserve (eg, prior myeloablative therapies); platelet count less than 100,000 cells/mm^3; neutrophil count less than 1,500 cells/mm^3; hypocellular bone marrow (up to 15% cellularity or marked reduction in bone marrow precursors); or to patients with a history of failed stem-cell collection.

Incidence and Duration of Severe Hematologic Toxicity		
	Zevalin regimen using 0.4 mCi/kg Y-90 dose (14.8 MBq/kg)	Modified *Zevalin* regimen using 0.3 mCi/kg Y-90 dose (11.1 MBq/kg)
ANC		
Median nadir (cells/mm^3)	800	600
Among patients with ANC < 1,000 cells/mm^3	57%	74%
Among patients with ANC < 500 cells/mm^3	30%	35%
Median duration of ANC < 1,000 cells/mm^3	22 d	29 d
Platelets		
Median nadir (cells/mm^3)	41,000	24,000
Among patients with platelets < 50,000 cells/mm^3	61%	78%
Among patients with platelets < 10,000 cells/mm^3	10%	14%
Median duration of platelets < 50,000 cells/mm^3	24 d	35 d

Median time to ANC nadir was 62 days, to platelet nadir was 53 days, and to hemoglobin nadir was 68 days. Information on growth factor use and platelet transfusions is based on 211 patients for whom data were collected. Filgrastim was given to 13% of patients and erythropoietin to 8%. Platelet transfusions were given to 22% of patients and red blood cell transfusions to 20%.

Immunologic: Of 211 patients who received the *Zevalin* regimen in clinical trials and were followed for 90 days, there were 8 (3.8%) patients with evidence of human anti-mouse antibody (HAMA) (n = 5) or human anti-chimeric antibody (HACA) (n = 4) at any time during the course of the study. Two patients had low titers of HAMA before starting the *Zevalin* regimen; 1 remained positive without an increase in titer, while the other had a negative titer posttreatment. Three patients had evidence of HACA responses before initiation of the *Zevalin* regimen; 1 had a marked increase in HACA titer while the others had negative titers posttreatment. Of the 3 patients who had negative HAMA or HACA titers before the *Zevalin* regimen, 2 developed HAMA in absence of HACA titers, and 1 had both HAMA and HACA positive titers posttreatment. There has not been adequate evaluation of HAMA and HACA at delayed time-points, concurrent with recovery from lymphopenia at 6 to 12 months, to establish whether masking of immunogenicity at early time-points occurs. Patients who received murine proteins previously should be screened for HAMA. Patients with evidence of HAMA have not been studied and may be at increased risk of allergic or serious hypersensitivity reactions during *Zevalin* regimen administrations.

Metabolic/Nutritional: 23% overall, 3% in grade 3 or 4. Peripheral edema (8%, 1%); angioedema (5%, less than 1%).

Miscellaneous:

Leukemia & Myelodysplastia: Myelodysplastic syndrome (MDS) and/or acute myelogenous leukemia (AML) were reported in 5.2% (11/211) of patients with relapsed or refractory NHL enrolled in clinical studies and 1.5% (8/535) of patients included in the expanded-access trial, with median follow-up of 6.5 and 4.4 y, respectively. Among the 19 reported cases, the median time to the diagnosis of MDS or AML was 1.9 y after treatment with the *Zevalin* therapeutic regimen; however, the cumulative incidence continues to increase. Among 204 patients receiving Y-90 *Zevalin* following first-line chemotherapy, two patients (1%) were diagnosed with AML within 3 y of receiving *Zevalin*.

Cutaneous: Erythema multiforme, Stevens-Johnson syndrome, toxic epidermal necrolysis, bullous dermatitis, and exfoliative dermatitis, some fatal, were reported in post-marketing experience. The time to onset of these reactions was variable, ranging from a few days to 4 months after *Zevalin* therapeutic regimen. Discontinue the regimen in patients experiencing a severe cutaneous or mucocutaneous reaction.

Musculoskeletal: 18% overall, 1% in grade 3 or 4. Arthralgia (7%, 1%); myalgia (7%, less than 1%).

Respiratory: 36% overall, 3% in grade 3 or 4. Dyspnea (14%, 2%); increased cough (10%, 0%); rhinitis (6%, 0%); bronchospasm (5%, 0%).

Special Senses: 7% overall, less than 1% in grade 3 or 4.

Systemic: During the first 3 months after initiating the *Zevalin* regimen, 29% of patients developed infections. Three percent developed serious infections comprising urinary tract infection, febrile neutropenia, sepsis, pneumonia, cellulitis, colitis, diarrhea, osteomyelitis, and upper respiratory tract infection. Life-threatening infections were reported for 2%, including sepsis, empyema, pneumonia, febrile neutropenia, fever, and biliary stent-associated cholangitis. Between 3 months and 4 years after starting the *Zevalin* regimen, 6% of patients developed infections. Two percent had serious infections comprising urinary tract infection, bacterial or viral pneumonia, febrile neutropenia, perihilar infiltrate, pericarditis, and IV drug-associated viral hepatitis. One percent had life-threatening infections that included bacterial pneumonia, respiratory disease, and sepsis.

Pharmacologic & Dosing Characteristics

Dosage: Initiate the *Zevalin* therapeutic regimen following recovery of platelet counts to $\geq 150,000$ cells/mm^3 at least 6 weeks, but no more than 12 weeks, after the last dose of first-line chemotherapy. The *Zevalin* regimen is administered in 2 steps: Step 1 begins with 1 IV infusion of rituximab 250 mg/m^2 at an initial rate of 50 mg/h. Do not mix or dilute rituximab with other drugs. If hypersensitivity or infusion-related events do not occur, escalate the infusion rate in 50 mg/h increments every 30 minutes, to a maximum of 400 mg/h. If hypersensitivity or an infusion-related event develops, temporarily slow or interrupt the infusion. The infusion can continue at one half the previous rate upon improvement of patient symptoms. Within 4 hours of completing the rituximab infusion, administer a fixed dose of 5 mCi (1.6 mg total antibody dose) of In-111 *Zevalin* as a 10-minute IV push. Note that the rituximab dose is less when used as part of the *Zevalin* regimen, compared to rituximab used alone.

Next, assess biodistribution with a series of images. Capture the first image 2 to 24 hours after In-111 *Zevalin* administration, with the second image 48 to 72 hours after In-111 *Zevalin*. An optional third image 90 to 120 hours after In-111 *Zevalin* may be useful. If biodistribution is acceptable, proceed to step 2. If not acceptable, do not proceed with *Zevalin* regimen.

Step 2 follows 7 to 9 days after In-111 *Zevalin*, with a second IV infusion of rituximab 250 mg/m^2 at an initial rate of 100 mg/h (50 mg/h if infusion-related events were documented during the first rituximab administration). Increase by 100 mg/h increments at 30-minute intervals, to a maximum of 400 mg/h, as tolerated. Within 4 hours after completing the rituximab administration, administer 0.4 mCi/kg actual body weight of Y-90 *Zevalin* as a 10-minute IV push for patients with normal platelet count. For patients with mild thrombocytopenia (ie, baseline platelet count between 100,000 and 149,000 cells/mm^3), reduce the Y-90 *Zevalin* dose to 0.3 mCi/kg (11.1 MBq/kg).

Do not treat patients with fewer than 100,000 platelets/mm^3.

Do not allow the prescribed, measured, and administered dose of Y-90 *Zevalin* to exceed the absolute maximum allowable dose of 32 mCi (1184 MBq), regardless of the patient's body weight. Do not administer Y-90 *Zevalin* to patients with altered biodistribution, as determined by imaging with In-111 *Zevalin*.

Do not use In-111 *Zevalin* and Y-90 *Zevalin* in the absence of the rituximab pre-dose.

Route: Administer rituximab as an IV infusion, not by IV push or bolus. Administer In-111 and Y-90 *Zevalin* by 10-minute IV push.

Overdosage: Doses as high as 0.52 mCi/kg (19.2 MBq/kg) of Y-90 *Zevalin* were administered in clinical trials, with severe hematological toxicities. No fatalities or second organ injury resulting from overdosage were documented. However, single doses up to 50 mCi (1,850 MBq) of Y-90 *Zevalin*, and multiple doses of 20 mCi (740 MBq) followed by 40 mCi (1,480 MBq) of Y-90 *Zevalin*, were studied in a limited number of subjects. In these trials, some patients required autologous stem cell support to manage hematologic toxicity.

Dose Preparation: Changing the ratio of any of the reactants in the radiolabeling process may adversely impact therapeutic results. Significant differences exist in the preparation of the In-111 *Zevalin* dose and the Y-90 *Zevalin* dose. Read all directions thoroughly and assemble all materials before starting. Required materials not supplied in the kit: In-111 chloride solution, three 1 mL syringes, one 3 mL syringe, two 10 mL syringes with 18- to 20-gauge needles, instant thin-layer chromatographic silica gel (ITLC-SG) strips, sodium chloride 0.9% for the chromatography solvent, developing chamber for chromatography, suitable radioactivity counting apparatus, 0.22 micrometer low-protein-binding filter, vial, and syringe shield. Measure the patient dose by a suitable radioactivity calibration system immediately before administration. Use proper aseptic technique and precautions for handling radioactive materials. Use waterproof gloves in the preparation and during the determination of radiochemical purity of radiolabeled *Zevalin*. Use appropriate shielding during radiolabeling. Use a syringe shield during administration to the patient.

Preparing the In-111 Zevalin dose: Use sterile, pyrogen-free In-111 chloride to prepare In-111 *Zevalin*. Before radiolabeling, allow contents of the refrigerated carton to reach room temperature. Clean the rubber stoppers of all vials in the kit and the In-111 chloride vial with a suitable alcohol swab and allow to air dry. Place the empty reaction vial in a suitable dispensing shield (prewarmed to room temperature). To avoid the buildup of excessive pressure during the procedure, use a 10 mL syringe to withdraw 10 mL of air from the reaction vial. Before initiating the radiolabeling reaction, determine the amount of each component needed. Calculate the volume of In-111 chloride equivalent to 5.5 mCi, based on the activity concentration of the In-111 chloride stock. The volume of 50 mM sodium acetate solution needed to adjust the pH for the radiolabeling reaction is 1.2 times the volume of In-111 chloride solution determined above. Calculate the volume of formulation buffer needed to bring the reaction vial contents to a final volume of 10 mL. This is the volume of formulation buffer needed to protect the labeled product from radiolysis and to terminate the labeling reaction. For example, if volumes of 0.5 mL of In-111 chloride, 0.6 mL of sodium acetate, and 1 mL of *Zevalin* were used, then the amount of formulation buffer would be: $10 - (0.5 + 0.6 + 1.0) = 7.9$ mL. With a 1 mL syringe, transfer the calculated volume of 50 mM of sodium acetate to the empty reaction vial. Coat the entire liner surface of the reaction vial by gentle inversion or rolling. Transfer 5.5 mCi of In-111 chloride to the reaction vial with a 1 mL syringe. Mix the 2 solutions and coat the entire liner surface of the reaction vial by gentle inversion or rolling. With a 3 mL syringe, transfer 1 mL of *Zevalin* to the reaction vial. Coat the entire surface of the reaction vial by gentle inversion or rolling. Do not shake or agitate the vial contents, to avoid foaming and protein denaturation. Allow the labeling reaction to proceed at room temperature for 30 minutes. Allowing the labeling reaction to proceed for a longer or shorter time may result in inadequate labeling. Immediately after the 30-minute incubation period, using a 10 mL syringe with a large-bore, 18- to 20-gauge needle, transfer the calculated volume of formulation buffer to the reaction vial. Gently add the formulation buffer down the side of the reaction vial. If necessary, to normalize air pressure, withdraw an equal volume of air. Coat the entire liner surface of the reaction vial by gentle inversion or rolling. Do not shake or agitate the vial contents. Avoid foaming. Record patient identification, date and time of preparation, total activity and volume, and date and time of expiration on the supplied labels. Affix these labels to the reaction vial and shielded reaction-vial container. Calculate the volume required for an In-111 *Zevalin* dose of 5 mCi. Withdraw the required volume from the reaction vial contents into a 10 mL syringe with a large-bore, 18- to 20-gauge needle. Assay the syringe and contents in a dose calibrator. The syringe should contain the dose of In-111 *Zevalin* to be administered to the patient. Record patient identification, date and time of preparation, total activity and volume added, and date and time of expiration on the supplied labels. Affix these labels to the syringe and shielded unit-dose container. Determine radiochemical purity. Store In-111 *Zevalin* at 2° to 8°C (36° to 46°F) until use. Administer within 12 hours of radiolabeling.

Preparing the Y-90 Zevalin dose: Use sterile, pyrogen-free Y-90 chloride to prepare Y-90 *Zevalin*. Before radiolabeling, allow the contents of the refrigerated carton to reach room temperature. Clean the rubber stoppers of all vials in the kit and the Y-90 chloride vial with a suitable alcohol swab and allow to air dry. Place the empty reaction vial in a suitable dispensing shield (prewarmed to room temperature). To avoid the buildup of excessive pressure during the procedure, use a 10 mL syringe to withdraw 10 mL of air from the reaction vial. Before initiating the radiolabeling reaction, determine the amount of each component needed. Calculate the volume of Y-90 chloride equivalent to 40 mCi, based on the activity concentration of the Y-90 chloride stock. The volume of 50 mM sodium acetate solution needed to adjust the pH for the radiolabeling reaction is 1.2 times the volume of Y-90 chloride solution determined above. Calculate the volume of formulation buffer needed to bring the reaction vial contents to a final volume of 10 mL. This is the volume of formulation buffer needed to protect the labeled product from radiolysis and to terminate the labeling reaction. For example if the volumes were 0.5 mL of Y-90 chloride, 0.6 mL of sodium acetate, and 1.3 mL of *Zevalin*, then the amount of formulation buffer would be: $10 - (0.5 + 0.6 + 1.3) = 7.6$ mL. With a 1 mL syringe, transfer the calculated volume 50 mM of sodium acetate to the empty reaction vial. Coat the entire liner surface of the reaction vial by gentle inversion or rolling. Transfer 40 mCi of Y-90 chloride to the reaction vial with a 1 mL syringe. Mix the 2 solutions and coat the entire liner surface of the reaction vial by gentle inversion or rolling. With a 3 mL syringe, transfer 1.3 mL of *Zevalin* to the reaction vial. Coat the entire surface of the reaction vial by gentle inversion or rolling. Do not shake or agitate the vial contents. Allow the labeling reaction to proceed at room temperature for 5 minutes. Allowing the labeling reaction to proceed for a longer or shorter time may result in inadequate labeling. Immediately after the 5-minute incubation period, use a 10 mL syringe with a large-bore, 18- to 20-gauge needle to transfer the calculated volume of formulation buffer to the reaction vial, which terminates incubation. Gently add the formulation buffer down the side of the reaction vial. If necessary to normalize air pressure, withdraw an equal volume of air. Coat the entire liner surface of the reaction vial by gentle inversion or rolling. Do not shake or agitate the vial contents. Avoid foaming. Record patient identification, date and time of preparation, total activity and volume, and date and time of expiration on the supplied labels. Affix these labels to the reaction vial and shielded reaction-vial container. Calculate the volume required for a Y-90 *Zevalin* dose of 0.4 mCi/kg (14.8 MBq/kg) actual body weight for patients with normal platelet count, and 0.3 mCi/kg (11.1 MBq/kg) actual body weight for patients with platelet count of 100,000 to 149,000 cells/mm^3. Do not exceed the absolute maximum allowable dose of 32 mCi (1184 MBq). Withdraw the required volume from the reaction vial contents into a 10 mL syringe with a large-bore 18- to 20-gauge needle. Assay the syringe and contents in a dose calibrator. The syringe should contain the dose of Y-90 *Zevalin* to be administered to the patient, within 10% of the actual prescribed dose of Y-90 *Zevalin*, not to exceed a maximum dose of 32 mCi. Do not under administer or exceed the prescribed dose by more than 10%. Record patient identification, date and time of preparation, total activity and volume added, and date and time of expiration on the supplied labels. Affix these labels to the syringe and shielded unit-dose container. Determine radiochemical purity. Store Y-90 *Zevalin* at 2° to 8°C (36° to 46°F) until use. Administer within 8 hours of radiolabeling.

Determining radiochemical purity for both In-111 Zevalin and Y-90 Zevalin: At room temperature, place a small drop of either In-111 *Zevalin* or Y-90 *Zevalin* at the origin of an ILTC-SG strip. Place the ITLC-SG strip into a chromatography chamber with the origin at the bottom and the solvent front at the top. Allow the 0.9% NaCl solvent to migrate 5 cm or more from the bottom of the strip. Remove the strip from the chamber and cut the strip in half. Count each half of the ITLC-SG strip for 1 minute (CPM) with a suitable counting apparatus. Calculate the percent RCP as follows: % RCP = [CPM bottom half] / [CPM bottom half + CPM top half] × 100. If the radiochemical purity is less than 95%, repeat the ITLC procedure. If repeat testing confirms that radiochemical purity is less than 95%, do not administer the preparation.

Additional Doses: The *Zevalin* regimen is intended as a single treatment. The safety and toxicity profile from multiple courses of the *Zevalin* regimen or other forms of therapeutic irradiation preceding, after, or in combination with the *Zevalin* regimen have not been established.

Related Interventions: Take precautions to avoid extravasations. Establish a free-flowing IV line before Y-90 *Zevalin* injection. Closely monitor for evidence of extravasations during Y-90 *Zevalin* injection. If any signs or symptoms of extravasation occur, immediately terminate and restart the infusion in another vein. Hypersensitivity reactions may occur. Consider premedication with acetaminophen and diphenhydramine before each infusion of rituximab.

Ibritumomab Tiuxetan (Murine)

Laboratory Tests: Obtain complete blood counts (CBC) and platelet counts weekly after the *Zevalin* regimen and continue until levels recover. Monitor CBC and platelet counts more frequently in patients who develop severe cytopenia, or as clinically indicated.

Waste Disposal: After performing *Zevalin* regimen administration steps 1 or 2, discard vials, needles, and syringes in accordance with regulations governing radioactive and biohazardous waste.

Radiation Protection: After the isotope is added to the *Zevalin*, shield the drug appropriately to minimize radiation exposure to patients, family, and medical personnel. Y-90 *Zevalin* is suitable for administration on an outpatient basis. Beyond the use of vial and syringe shields for preparation and injection, no special shielding is necessary.

Image Acquisition: Assess the biodistribution of In-111 *Zevalin* by a visual evaluation of whole-body, planar-view anterior and posterior gamma images at 2 to 24 hours and 48 to 72 hours after injection. To resolve ambiguities, a third image at 90 to 120 hours may be necessary. Acquire images using a large field-of-view gamma camera equipped with a medium-energy collimator. Calibrate the gamma camera using the 171 and 245 keV photopeaks for In-111 with a 15% to 20% symmetric window. Using a $256 \times 1,024$ computer acquisition matrix, set the scan speed at 10 cm/min for the first scan, 7 cm/min for the second scan, and 5 cm/min for the optional third scan.

Efficacy: Safety and efficacy of the *Zevalin* regimen were evaluated in 2 multicenter trials with 197 subjects. The *Zevalin* regimen was administered in 2 steps. The activity and toxicity of a variation of the *Zevalin* regimen employing a reduced dose of Y-90 *Zevalin* was further defined in a third study enrolling 30 patients with mild thrombocytopenia (platelet count 100,000 to 149,000 cells/mm^3).

Study 1 assessed 54 patients with relapsed follicular lymphoma refractory to rituximab treatment. The primary efficacy endpoint was the overall response rate (ORR) using International Workshop Response Criteria (IWRC). Secondary efficacy endpoints included time to disease progression (TTP) and duration of response (DR). In a secondary analysis comparing objective response to the *Zevalin* regimen with that observed with the most recent treatment with rituximab, the median duration of response after the *Zevalin* regimen was 6 vs 4 months.

Study 2 compared the *Zevalin* regimen to rituximab therapy (4 weekly doses of 375 mg/m^2 IV) in a randomized study of 143 patients with relapsed or refractory low-grade or follicular non-Hodgkin lymphoma (NHL), or transformed B-cell NHL. The primary efficacy endpoint of the study was to determine the ORR using the IWRC. The ORR was significantly higher (80% vs 56%, $P = 0.002$) for patients treated with the *Zevalin* regimen, as was the complete response rate (30% vs 16%). The secondary endpoints, duration of response and time to progression, were not significantly different between the 2 treatment arms.

Study 3 assessed 30 patients with relapsed or refractory low-grade, follicular, or transformed B-cell NHL who had mild thrombocytopenia (platelet count 100,000 to 149,000 cells/mm^3). Excluded from the study were patients with 25% lymphoma marrow involvement and/or impaired bone marrow reserve. Investigators defined impaired bone marrow reserve as any of the following: Prior myeloablative therapy with stem-cell support; prior external beam radiation to more than 25% of active marrow; a platelet count less than 100,000 cells/mm^3 or neutrophil count less than 1,500 cells/mm^3. In this study, a modification of the *Zevalin* regimen with a lower specific activity Y-90 *Zevalin* dose (Y-90 *Zevalin* at 0.3 mCi/kg [11.1 MBq/kg]) was used. Objective, durable clinical responses were observed (67% ORR [95% CI: 48% to 85%], 11.8 months median DR [range: 4 to 17 months]) and resulted in a greater incidence of hematologic toxicity than studies 1 and 2.

Interpretation: The radiopharmaceutical is expected to be easily detectable in the blood-pool areas at the first time-point, with less activity in the blood pool on later images. Moder-

860

ately high to high uptake is seen in the normal liver and spleen, with moderately low or very low uptake in normal kidneys, urinary bladder, and normal bowel on the first-day image and the second- or third-day image. Localization to lymphoid aggregates in the bowel wall has been reported. Tumor uptake may be visualized in soft tissue as areas of increased intensity. Tumor-bearing areas in normal organs may be seen as areas of increased or decreased intensity.

If a visual inspection of the gamma images reveals an altered biodistribution, do not proceed to the Y-90 *Zevalin* dose. The patient may be considered to have an altered biodistribution if the blood pool is not visualized on the first image, indicating rapid clearance of the radiopharmaceutical by the reticuloendothelial system to the liver, spleen, and/or marrow. Other potential examples of altered biodistribution may include: Diffuse uptake in the normal lungs more intense than the cardiac blood pool on the first-day image; kidney uptake more intense than the liver on the posterior view on the second- or third-day image; or intense areas of uptake throughout the normal bowel comparable to uptake by the liver on the second- or third-day images.

During *Zevalin* clinical development, individual tumor radiation-absorbed dose estimates as high as 778 cGy/mCi were reported. Although solid-organ toxicity has not been directly attributed to radiation from adjacent tumors, apply careful consideration before proceeding with treatment in patients with very high tumor uptake next to critical organs or structures.

Pharmacokinetics: Immunoglobulins are primarily eliminated by catabolism. Pharmacokinetic and biodistribution studies were performed using In-111 *Zevalin* (5 mCi [185 MBq] In-111, 1.6 mg ibritumomab tiuxetan). In a study designed to assess the need for preadministration of unlabeled antibody, only 18% of known sites of disease were imaged when In-111 *Zevalin* was administered without unlabeled ibritumomab. When preceded by unlabeled ibritumomab (1 mg/kg or 2.5 mg/kg), In-111 *Zevalin* detected 56% and 92% of known disease sites, respectively.

In pharmacokinetic studies of patients receiving the Zevalin regimen, the mean effective half-life for Y-90 activity in blood was 30 hours, and the mean area under the fraction of injected activity (FIA) vs time-curve in blood was 39 hours. Over 7 days, a median of 7.2% of the injected activity was excreted in urine.

In clinical studies, administration of the *Zevalin* regimen resulted in sustained depletion of circulating B cells. At 4 weeks, the median number of circulating B cells was zero (range, 0 to 1,084 cells/mm^3). B-cell recovery began at approximately 12 weeks after treatment, and the median level of B cells was within the normal range (32 to 341 cells/mm^3) by 9 months after treatment. Median serum levels of IgG and IgA remained within the normal range throughout the period of B-cell depletion. Median IgM serum levels dropped below normal (median 49 mg/dL, range 13 to 3,990 mg/dL) after treatment and recovered to normal values by 6 months post-therapy.

Mechanism: Ibritumomab tiuxetan binds specifically to the CD20 antigen (human B-lymphocyte-restricted differentiation antigen, Bp35). The apparent affinity (KD) of ibritumomab tiuxetan for the CD20 antigen ranges between 14 to 18 nM. The CD20 antigen is expressed on pre-B and mature B lymphocytes and on greater than 90% of B-cell non-Hodgkin lymphomas (NHL). The CD20 antigen is not shed from the cell surface and does not internalize upon antibody binding.

The complementarity-determining regions of ibritumomab bind to the CD20 antigen on B-lymphocytes. Ibritumomab, like rituximab, induces apoptosis in CD20+ B-cell lines in vitro. The chelate tiuxetan, which tightly binds In-111 or Y-90, is covalently linked to the amino groups of exposed lysines and arginines contained within the antibody. The beta emission from Y-90 induces cellular damage by forming free radicals in the target and neighboring cells.

Ibritumomab Tiuxetan (Murine)

Normal human tissue cross-reactivity: Ibritumomab-tiuxetan binding was observed in vitro on lymphoid cells of the bone marrow, lymph node, thymus, red and white pulp of the spleen, and lymphoid follicles of the tonsil, as well as lymphoid nodules of other organs such as the large and small intestines. Binding was not observed on the nonlymphoid tissues or gonadal tissues.

Drug Interactions: No formal drug interaction studies have been performed with *Zevalin*. Due to the frequent occurrence of severe and prolonged thrombocytopenia, weigh the potential benefits of medications that interfere with platelet function and/or anticoagulation against the risks of bleeding and hemorrhage. Patients receiving medications that interfere with platelet function or coagulation should have more frequent laboratory monitoring for thrombocytopenia. In addition, modify transfusion practices for such patients, given the increased risk of bleeding.

The safety of immunization with live vaccines after the *Zevalin* regimen has not been studied. Also, the ability of patients who received the *Zevalin* regimen to generate a primary or anamnestic humoral response to any vaccine has not been studied.

Pharmaceutical Characteristics

Concentration: 3.2 mg ibritumomab tiuxetan per 2 mL

Quality Assay: Perform radiochemical purity tests before administration.

Packaging: Supplied as 2 separate, distinctly labeled kits containing the nonradioactive ingredients needed for a single dose of In-111 *Zevalin* and a single dose of Y-90 *Zevalin*, both essential components of the *Zevalin* regimen. Order In-111 chloride and rituximab separately. MDS Nordion supplies Y-90 chloride solution upon ordering the Y-90 *Zevalin* kit. Each of the 2 *Zevalin* kits contains 4 vials used to produce a single dose of either In-111 *Zevalin* or Y-90 *Zevalin*: (1) One *Zevalin* vial containing 3.2 mg of ibritumomab tiuxetan in 2 mL sodium chloride 0.9%; (2) one 50 mM sodium acetate vial containing 13.6 mg sodium acetate trihydrate in 2 mL water; (3) one formulation buffer vial containing 750 mg albumin human, 76 mg sodium chloride, 21 mg sodium phosphate dibasic heptahydrate, 4 mg pentetic acid, 2 mg potassium phosphate monobasic, and 2 mg potassium chloride in 10 mL of water adjusted to pH 7.1 with either sodium hydroxide or hydrochloric acid; and (4) one empty reaction vial and 4 identification labels.

NDC Number:
In-111 Zevalin kit: 68152-104-04
Y-90 Zevalin kit: 68152-103-03

Appearance: Ibritumomab tiuxetan is a clear, colorless solution that may contain translucent particles; these particulates will be removed by filtration before administration. The formulation buffer solution is clear yellow to amber colored.

Solvent: Sodium chloride 0.9%

Adjuvant: None

Preservative: None

Allergens: None

Excipients: Sodium acetate trihydrate 50 mM for the radiolabeling reaction, with 750 mg albumin human, 76 mg sodium chloride, 21 mg sodium phosphate dibasic heptahydrate, 4 mg pentetic acid, 2 mg potassium phosphate monobasic, and 2 mg potassium chloride in the formulation buffer vial.

pH: 7.1

Shelf Life: Expires within 12 months.

Storage/Stability: Store at 2° to 8°C (36° to 46°F). Do not freeze. Store radiolabeled *Zevalin* at 2° to 8°C (36° to 46°F) until use. Administer In-111 *Zevalin* within 12 hours of radiolabeling. Administer Y-90 *Zevalin* within 8 hours of radiolabeling. Contact the manufacturer regarding exposure to extreme temperatures. Shipped by overnight courier in insulated container with coolant packs to maintain temperature between 1° and 25°C.

Production Process: Ibritumomab is produced in Chinese hamster ovary cells. Ibritumomab tiuxetan results from a stable thiourea covalent bond between ibritumomab and the linker-chelator tiuxetan (N-[2-bis(carboxymethyl)amino]-3-[p-isothiocyanatophenyl]propyl)-(N-[2-bis(carboxymethyl)amino]-2-[methyl]-ethyl)glycine.

Media: Chinese hamster ovary cells

Radiologic Characteristics

Radiation Dosimetry: Radiation-absorbed doses for In-111 *Zevalin* and Y-90 *Zevalin* were estimated using sequential whole-body images and Miridose-3 software. The estimated radiation absorbed doses to organs and marrow from a course of the *Zevalin* regimen appear below. Absorbed dose estimates for the lower large intestine, upper large intestine, and small intestine have been modified from the standard Miridose-3 output, under the assumption that activity is within the intestine wall rather than the intestine contents.

Estimated Absorbed Radiation Doses from Y-90 *Zevalin* and In-111 *Zevalin*				
	Y-90 *Zevalin* mGy/MBq		In-111 *Zevalin* mGy/MBq	
Organ	Median	Range	Median	Range
Spleen[a]	9.4	1.8 to 14.4	0.9	0.2 to 1.2
Testes [a]	9.1	5.4 to 11.4	0.6	0.4 to 0.8
Liver [a]	4.8	2.3 to 8.1	0.7	0.3 to 1.1
Lower large intestinal wall [a]	4.8	3.1 to 8.2	0.4	0.2 to 0.6
Upper large intestinal wall [a]	3.6	2.0 to 6.7	0.3	0.2 to 0.6
Heart wall [a]	2.8	1.5 to 3.2	0.4	0.2 to 0.5
Lungs [a]	2.0	1.2 to 3.4	0.2	0.1 to 0.4
Small intestine [a]	1.4	0.8 to 2.1	0.2	0.1 to 0.3
Red marrow [b]	1.3	0.7 to 1.8	0.2	0.1 to 0.2
Urinary bladder wall [c]	0.9	0.7 to 2.1	0.2	0.1 to 0.2
Bone surfaces [b]	0.9	0.5 to 1.2	0.2	0.1 to 0.2
Ovaries [c]	0.4	0.3 to 0.5	0.2	0.2 to 0.2
Uterus [c]	0.4	0.3 to 0.5	0.2	0.1 to 0.2
Adrenals [c]	0.3	0.0 to 0.5	0.2	0.1 to 0.3
Brain [c]	0.3	0.0 to 0.5	0.1	0.0 to 0.1
Breasts [c]	0.3	0.0 to 0.5	0.1	0.0 to 0.1
Gallbladder wall [c]	0.3	0.0 to 0.5	0.3	0.1 to 0.4
Muscle [c]	0.3	0.0 to 0.5	0.1	0.0 to 0.1
Pancreas [c]	0.3	0.0 to 0.5	0.2	0.1 to 0.3
Skin [c]	0.3	0.0 to 0.5	0.1	0.0 to 0.1
Stomach [c]	0.3	0.0 to 0.5	0.1	0.1 to 0.2
Thymus [c]	0.3	0.0 to 0.5	0.1	0.1 to 0.2
Thyroid [c]	0.3	0.0 to 0.5	0.1	0.0 to 0.1
Kidneys [a]	0.1	0.0 to 0.2	0.2	0.1 to 0.2
Total Body [c]	0.5	0.2 to 0.7	0.1	0.1 to 0.2

a Organ region of interest.
b Sacrum region of interest.
c Whole body region of interest.

Ibritumomab Tiuxetan (Murine)

Disease Epidemiology

Incidence: Of the estimated 61,000 new cases of lymphoma in 2003, 7,600 were Hodgkin disease and 53,400 were non-Hodgkin lymphoma (NHL). Since the early 1970s, incidence rates for NHL have nearly doubled, but those rates stabilized in the 1990s, primarily because of the decline in AIDS-related NHL.

Other Information

First Licensed: February 19, 2002

References: Cheson BD. The role of radioimmunotherapy with yttrium-90 ibritumomab tiuxetan in the treatment of non-Hodgkin lymphoma. *BioDrugs.* 2005;19(5):309-322.

Johnston PB, Bondly C, Micallef IN. Ibritumomab tiuxetan for non-Hodgkin's lymphoma. *Expert Rev Anticancer Ther.* 2006;6(6):861-869.

Isoantibodies

Name:
  Bexxar Kits

Manufacturer:
  GlaxoSmithKline

Immunologic Characteristics

Target Antigen: CD20 antigen is found on the surface of normal and malignant B-lymphocytes.

Viability: Inactive, passive, transient

Antigenic Form: Murine IgG2a lambda immunoglobulin, comprised of 2 murine gamma 2a heavy chains of 451 amino acids each and 2 lambda light chains of 220 amino acids each. The molecular weight of tositumomab is approximately 150 kilodaltons.

Antigenic Type: Protein, IgG2a lambda monoclonal antibody directed against CD20 antigen. The *Bexxar* therapeutic regimen consists of tositumomab and Iodine I-131 tositumomab.

Use Characteristics

Indications: To treat patients with CD20 antigen-expressing relapsed or refractory, low-grade, follicular, or transformed non-Hodgkin lymphoma, including patients with rituximab-refractory non-Hodgkin lymphoma.

Limitations: The *Bexxar* regimen is not indicated for the initial treatment of patients with CD20-positive NHL. The *Bexxar* regimen is intended as a single course of treatment. The safety of multiple courses of the *Bexxar* regimen or combination of this regimen with other forms of irradiation or chemotherapy has not been evaluated.

Contraindications:

Absolute: Do not administer the *Bexxar* regimen to patients with more than 25% lymphoma marrow involvement and/or impaired bone marrow reserve.

Any patient unable to tolerate thyroid-blocking agents should not receive the *Bexxar* regimen.

Relative: The safety of the *Bexxar* regimen has not been established in patients with more than 25% lymphoma marrow involvement, platelet count less than 100,000 cells/mm^3, or neutrophil count less than 1,500 cells/mm^3.

The *Bexxar* therapeutic regimen is contraindicated in patients with known hypersensitivity to murine proteins or any other component of the *Bexxar* therapeutic regimen. Patients who are human antimouse antibody (HAMA) positive may be at increased risk for serious allergic reactions and other side effects if they undergo in vivo diagnostic testing or treatment with murine monoclonal antibodies.

Immunodeficiency: No impairment of effect is expected.

Elderly: Clinical studies of the *Bexxar* regimen did not include enough people 65 years of age or older to determine whether they respond differently from younger patients. Of 230 patients who received the *Bexxar* regimen at the recommended dose, 27% were 65 years of age or older and 4% were 75 years of age or older. Across all studies, the overall response rate was lower in patients 65 years of age and older (41% vs 61%), and the duration of responses were shorter (10 months vs 16 months); however, these findings are primarily derived from 2 of the 5 studies. While the incidence of severe hematologic toxicity was lower, the duration of severe hematologic toxicity was longer in those 65 years of age or older compared with patients younger than 65 years of age. Because of limited experience, greater sensitivity of some older individuals cannot be ruled out.

Tositumomab (Murine)

Carcinogenicity: Radiation is a potential carcinogen. No long-term animal studies have been performed to establish the carcinogenic potential of the *Bexxar* regimen.

Mutagenicity: Radiation is a potential mutagen. No long-term animal studies have been performed to establish the mutagenic potential of the *Bexxar* regimen.

Fertility Impairment: The *Bexxar* regimen delivers a significant radiation dose to the testes. The radiation dose to the ovaries has not been established. No studies have evaluated whether administration of the *Bexxar* therapeutic regimen causes hypogonadism, premature menopause, azoospermia, and/or mutagenic alterations to germ cells. There is a potential risk the *Bexxar* regimen may cause toxic effects on the male and female gonads. Use effective contraceptive methods during treatment and for 12 months after the *Bexxar* regimen. No long-term animal studies have been performed to establish the effect on fertility of the *Bexxar* regimen.

Pregnancy:

Category X: I-131 tositumomab is contraindicated for use in women who are pregnant. I-131 may cause harm to the fetal thyroid gland when administered to pregnant women. Transplacental passage of radioiodine may cause severe, and possibly irreversible, hypothyroidism in neonates. While there are no adequate and well-controlled studies of the *Bexxar* regimen in pregnant animals or humans, defer use of the *Bexxar* regimen in women of childbearing age until the possibility of pregnancy has been ruled out. If the patient becomes pregnant while being treated with the *Bexxar* regimen, inform the woman of the potential hazard to the fetus. It is not known if tositumomab crosses the placenta. Generally, most IgG passage across the placenta occurs during the third trimester.

Lactation: Radioiodine is excreted in breast milk and may reach concentrations equal to or greater than maternal plasma concentrations. Immunoglobulins are excreted in breast milk. The absorption potential and potential for adverse effects of tositumomab in infants are not known. Therefore, substitute formula feedings for breastfeedings before starting treatment. Advise women to discontinue nursing.

Children: Safety and efficacy of the *Bexxar* regimen in children younger than 18 years of age have not been established.

Adverse Reactions: The most serious adverse reactions observed in the clinical trials were severe and prolonged cytopenias and the sequelae of cytopenias (eg, infections, sepsis, hemorrhage), allergic reactions (eg, bronchospasm, angioedema), secondary leukemia, and myelodysplasia.

The most common adverse reactions in the clinical trials included neutropenia, thrombocytopenia, and anemia that were prolonged and severe. Less common but severe adverse reactions included pneumonia, pleural effusion, and dehydration. Data regarding adverse events were primarily obtained in 230 patients with NHL enrolled in 5 clinical trials using the recommended dose and schedule. Patients had a median follow-up of 35 months, and 79% of the patients were followed at least 12 months for survival and selected adverse events. Patients had a median of 3 prior chemotherapy regimens, a median of 55 years of age, 60% were male, 27% had transformation to a higher grade histology, 29% were intermediate grade and 2% high grade histology (IWF), and 68% had Ann Arbor stage IV disease. Patients enrolled in these studies were not permitted to have prior hematopoietic stem cell transplantation or irradiation to more than 25% of the red marrow. In the expanded access program, which included 765 patients, data regarding clinical serious adverse events and HAMA and thyroid stimulating hormone (TSH) levels were used to supplement the characterization of delayed adverse events.

Immunogenicity: Two percent of chemotherapy-relapsed or refractory patients in clinical studies had a positive serology for HAMA before treatment. With a median observation period for HAMA seroconversion of 6 months, 11% seroconverted to HAMA positivity. The median time to development of HAMA was 6 months. In a study of 77 chemotherapy-naive patients, the incidence of conversion to HAMA seropositivity was 70%, with a median time to development of HAMA of 27 days. With a median observation period of 6 months, a total of 76 patients (10%) in clinical trials and the expanded access programs became seropositive for HAMA posttreatment. The median time of HAMA development was 148 days, with 45 (59%) patients seropositive for HAMA by 6 months. No patient became seropositive for HAMA more than 30 months after the *Bexxar* regimen.

Infections: Of 230 patients, 45% patients experienced 1 or more adverse event possibly related to infection. Most were viral (eg, rhinitis, pharyngitis, viral-like symptoms, herpes) or other minor infections. Eight percent experienced serious infections involving hospitalization. Documented infections included pneumonia, bacteremia, septicemia, bronchitis, and skin infections.

Infusional toxicity: A constellation of symptoms, including fever, rigors or chills, sweating, hypotension, dyspnea, bronchospasm, and nausea, were reported during or within 48 hours of infusion. Sixty-seven patients (29%) reported fever, rigors/chills, or sweating within 14 days after the dosimetric dose. Although all patients in the clinical studies received pretreatment with acetaminophen and an antihistamine, the value of premedication in preventing infusion-related toxicity was not evaluated in any of the clinical studies. Infusional toxicities were managed by slowing and/or temporarily interrupting the infusion. Symptomatic management was required in more severe cases. Adjustment of the rate of infusion to control adverse reactions occurred in 16 patients (7%); 7 patients required adjustments for only the dosimetric infusion, 2 required adjustments for only the therapeutic infusion, and 7 required adjustments for the dosimetric and therapeutic infusions. Adjustments included 50% reduction in the rate of infusion, temporary interruption, and, in 2 patients, permanent discontinuation of infusion.

Malignancies: Myelodysplastic syndrome (MDS) and/or acute leukemia were reported in 8% (19/230) of patients enrolled in clinical studies and 2% (13/765) of patients included in expanded access programs, with median follow-up of 35 and 20 months, respectively. Among 32 reported new cases, the median time to development of MDS/leukemia was 27 months after treatment, but the cumulative rate continues to increase. The pretreatment characteristics (eg, median age, number of prior chemotherapy regimens) were similar in patients developing MDS/secondary leukemias compared with those who did not. Additional malignancies also were reported in 5% (52/995) of patients enrolled in clinical studies or included in the expanded access program. Approximately half of these were nonmelanomatous skin cancers. The remainder, which occurred in 2 or more patients, included breast cancer, lung cancer, bladder cancer, head and neck cancer, colon cancer, and melanoma, in order of decreasing incidence. The relative risk of developing secondary malignancies in patients receiving the *Bexxar* regimen over the background rate in this population cannot be determined because of the absence of controlled studies.

Adverse events that occurred in at least 5% of patients appear in the following table.

Adverse Experiences in ≥ 5% of Patients Treated with *Bexxar* Regimen[a] (n = 230)		
Adverse reactions	All grades (%)	Grade 3 or 4 (%)
Total	96	48
Body as a Whole	81	12
Asthenia	46	2
Fever	37	2
Infection[b]	21	< 1
Pain	19	1
Chills	18	1
Headache	16	0
Abdominal pain	15	3
Back pain	8	1
Chest pain	7	0
Neck pain	6	1
Cardiovascular	26	3
Hypotension	7	1
Vasodilatation	5	0
CNS	26	3
Dizziness	5	0
Somnolence	5	0
Dermatologic	44	5
Rash	17	< 1
Pruritus	10	0
Sweating	8	< 1
Endocrine	7	0
Hypothyroidism	7	0
Metabolic/Nutritional	21	3
Peripheral edema	9	0
Weight loss	6	< 1
GI	56	9
Nausea	36	3
Vomiting	15	1
Anorexia	14	0
Diarrhea	12	0
Constipation	6	1
Dyspepsia	6	< 1
Musculoskeletal	23	3
Myalgia	13	< 1
Arthralgia	10	1

Adverse Experiences in ≥ 5% of Patients Treated with *Bexxar* Regimen[a] (n = 230)		
Adverse reactions	All grades (%)	Grade 3 or 4 (%)
Respiratory	44	8
Cough increased	21	1
Pharyngitis	12	0
Dyspnea	11	3
Rhinitis	10	0
Pneumonia	6	0

a Excludes laboratory derived hematologic adverse events.
b The COSTART term for infection includes a subset of infections (eg, upper respiratory infection). Other terms are mapped to preferred terms (eg, pneumonia, sepsis).

Endocrine: Administration of the *Bexxar* regimen may result in hypothyroidism. Start thyroid-blocking medications at least 24 hours before receiving the dosimetric dose and continue until 14 days after the therapeutic dose. All patients must receive thyroid-blocking agents. Any patient unable to tolerate thyroid-blocking agents should not receive the *Bexxar* regimen. Evaluate patients for signs and symptoms of hypothyroidism and annually screen for biochemical evidence of hypothyroidism. The overall incidence of hypothyroidism in clinical study patients was 14%, with cumulative incidences of 4.2% at 6 months and 8.1%, 12.6%, and 15% at 1, 2, and 4 years, respectively. Twelve percent (117/990) of patients in clinical studies or expanded access programs had an elevated TSH level (8%) or a history of hypothyroidism (4%) before treatment, and 5 patients had no baseline information. With a median observation period of 18 months, 9% became hypothyroid as determined by elevated TSH. The cumulative incidence of hypothyroidism in the combined populations was 9.1% and 17.4% at 2 and 4 years, respectively.

GI: Eighty-seven patients (38%) experienced 1 or more GI adverse events, including nausea, emesis, abdominal pain, and diarrhea. These events were temporally related to antibody infusion. Nausea, vomiting, and abdominal pain were often reported within days of infusion, whereas diarrhea was generally reported days to weeks after infusion.

Hematologic: Most patients who received the *Bexxar* therapeutic regimen experienced severe thrombocytopenia and neutropenia. The most common adverse reactions associated with the *Bexxar* regimen were severe or life-threatening cytopenias, with 71% of 230 patients enrolled in clinical studies experiencing grade 3 or 4 cytopenias. These consisted primarily of grade 3 or 4 thrombocytopenia (53%) and grade 3 or 4 neutropenia (63%). The time to nadir was 4 to 7 weeks and the duration of cytopenias was approximately 30 days. Thrombocytopenia, neutropenia, and anemia persisted for more than 90 days after the *Bexxar* regimen in 7%, 7%, and 5% of patients respectively (this includes patients with transient recovery followed by recurrent cytopenia).

Because of the variable nature in the onset of cytopenias, obtain complete blood counts weekly for 10 to 12 weeks. The sequelae of severe cytopenias were commonly observed in the clinical studies and included infections (45% of patients), hemorrhage (12%), a requirement for growth factors (12% G- or GM-CSF; 7% epoetin alfa), and blood product support (15% platelet transfusions; 16% red blood cell transfusions). Prolonged cytopenias also may influence subsequent treatment decisions.

The following table provides a detailed description of the hematologic toxicity.

Tositumomab (Murine)

Hematologic Toxicity[a] (N = 230)	
Endpoint	Values
Median nadir (cells/mm^3)	43,000
Per patient incidence[a] platelets < 50,000/mm^3	53% (n = 123)
Median[b] duration of platelets < 50,000/mm^3 (days)	32
Grade 3/4 without recovery to grade 2, N (%)	16 (7%)
Per patient incidence[c] platelets < 25,000/mm^3	21% (n = 47)
Absolute neutrophil count (ANC)	
Median nadir (cells/mm^3)	690
Per patient incidence[a] ANC < 1,000 cells/mm^3 (%)	63% (n = 145)
Median[b] duration of ANC < 1,000 cells/mm^3 (days)	31
Grade 3/4 without recovery to grade 2, N (%)	15 (7%)
Per patient incidence[c] ANC < 500 cells/mm^3, N (%)	25% (n = 57)
Hemoglobin	
Median nadir (g/dL)	10
Per patient incidence[a] < 8 g/dL	29% (n = 66)
Median[b] duration of hemoglobin < 8 g/dL (days)	23
Grade 3/4 without recovery to grade 2, N (%)	12 (5%)
Per patient incidence[c] hemoglobin < 6.5 g/dL, N (%)	5% (n = 11)

a Grade 3/4 toxicity was assumed if patient was missing 2 of more weeks of hematology data between week 5 and week 9.
b Duration of grade 3/4 of 1,000+ days (censored) was assumed for those patients with undocumented grade 3/4 and no hematologic data on or after week 9.
c Grade 4 toxicity was assumed if patient had documented grade 3 toxicity and was missing 2 or more weeks of hematology data between week 5 and week 9.

Hypersensitivity: Hypersensitivity reactions, including anaphylaxis, were reported during and after the *Bexxar* regimen. Fourteen patients (6%) experienced 1 or more of the following adverse events: allergic reaction, face edema, injection-site hypersensitivity, anaphylactoid reaction, laryngismus, and serum sickness. Screen patients who have received murine proteins for HAMA. Patients who are positive for HAMA may be at increased risk of anaphylaxis and serious hypersensitivity reactions during administration of the *Bexxar* regimen.

Immunologic: There was no consistent effect of the *Bexxar* therapeutic regimen on posttreatment serum IgG, IgA, or IgM levels.

Renal: I-131 tositumomab and I-131 are excreted primarily by the kidneys. Impaired renal function may decrease the rate of excretion of the radiolabeled iodine and increase patient exposure to the radioactive component of the *Bexxar* regimen. There are no data regarding the safety of the *Bexxar* regimen in patients with impaired renal function.

Pharmacologic & Dosing Characteristics

Dosage: The *Bexxar* therapeutic regimen is administered in 2 discrete steps: the dosimetric and therapeutic steps. Each step consists of a sequential infusion of tositumomab followed by I-131 tositumomab. The therapeutic step is administered 7 to 14 days after the dosimetric step. The dosing steps can be summarized as follows:

Day 1: Patient begins thyro-protective regimen. This regimen continues through 14 days after the therapeutic dose.

870

Day 0: Premedication with acetaminophen and diphenhydramine. Dosimetric step: IV infusion of 450 mg tositumomab in 50 mL sodium chloride (NaCl) 0.9% over 60 minutes followed by IV infusion of 5 mCi I-131 tositumomab (35 mg) over 20 minutes. Whole-body dosimetry and biodistribution.

Day 2, 3, or 4: Whole-body dosimetry and biodistribution.

Day 6 or 7: Whole-body dosimetry and biodistribution. If biodistribution is unacceptable, do not administer therapeutic dose. Calculation of patient-specific activity of I-131 tositumomab to deliver 75 cGy total-body dose (in mCi), or 65 cGy for patients with 100,000 to 150,000 platelets/mm^3.

Day 7 (up to day 14): Premedication with acetaminophen and diphenhydramine.

Therapeutic step: IV infusion of 450 mg tositumomab in 50 mL sodium chloride 0.9% over 60 minutes, followed by prescribed therapeutic dose of I-131 tositumomab (35 mg) in 30 mL sodium chloride 0.9% over 20 minutes. Calculate I-131 activity for therapeutic dose as per the following instructions:
- Patients with at least 150,000 platelets/mm^3: sufficient I-131 to deliver 75 cGy total body irradiation and 35 mg tositumomab, administered IV over 20 minutes.
- Patients with NCI Grade 1 thrombocytopenia (100,000 to 150,000 platelets/mm^3): sufficient I-131 to deliver 65 cGy total body irradiation and 35 mg tositumomab, administered IV over 20 minutes.

Route: IV infusion. The *Bexxar* regimen is administered via an IV tubing set with an inline 0.22 micron filter. Use the same IV tubing set and filter throughout the entire dosimetric or therapeutic step. A change in filter can result in loss of drug. During infusions, reduce the rate of infusion 50% for mild to moderate infusional toxicity; interrupt infusion for severe infusional toxicity. After complete resolution of severe infusional toxicity, resume infusion with a 50% reduction in the rate of infusion.

Overdosage: The maximum dose administered in clinical trials was 88 cGy. Three patients were treated with a total body dose of 85 cGy of I-131 tositumomab in a dose-escalation study. Two of the 3 patients developed grade 4 toxicity lasting 5 weeks with subsequent recovery. In addition, accidental overdose occurred in 1 patient at total body doses of 88 cGy. The patient developed grade 3 hematologic toxicity lasting 18 days. Monitor patients who receive an accidental overdose of I-131 tositumomab closely for cytopenias and radiation-related toxicity. The effectiveness of hematopoietic stem cell transplantation as a supportive care measure for marrow injury has not been studied; however, the timing of such support should take into account the pharmacokinetics of the *Bexxar* regimen and decay rate of I-131 to minimize the irradiation of infused hematopoietic stem cells.

Dose Preparation: Read all directions thoroughly and assemble all materials before preparing the dose for administration. Measure the I-131 tositumomab dosimetric and therapeutic doses by a suitable radioactivity calibration system immediately before administration. Use waterproof gloves in preparing and administrating the product.

Preparation for dosimetric step:

Tositumomab dose: Withdraw and dispose of 32 mL from a 50 mL bag of NaCl 0.9%. Withdraw entire contents from each of two 225 mg vials (450 mg tositumomab in 32 mL) and transfer to infusion bag containing 18 mL of NaCl 0.9% to yield a final volume of 50 mL. Gently mix the solution by inverting/rotating the bag. Do not shake.

I-131 Tositumomab dosimetric dose: Allow approximately 60 minutes for thawing (at ambient temperature) of the I-131 tositumomab dosimetric vial with appropriate lead shielding. Based on activity concentration of the vial, calculate volume required for an I-131 tositumomab activity of 5 mCi. Withdraw calculated volume from I-131 tositumomab vial and transfer to shielded preparation vial. Assay the dose to ensure the mCi has been prepared.
- If the assayed dose is 4.5 to 5.5 mCi, proceed.

- If the assayed dose does not contain 4.5 to 5.5 mCi, recalculate the activity concentration of I-131 tositumomab at this time, based on volume and activity in preparation vial. Recalculate volume required for 5 mCi of I-131 tositumomab activity. Using the same 30 mL syringe, add or subtract the appropriate volume from the I-131 tositumomab vial so the preparation vial contains the volume required for I-131 tositumomab activity of 4.5 to 5.5 mCi. Re-assay the preparation vial and proceed.

Calculate amount of tositumomab contained in the solution of I-131 tositumomab in the shielded preparation vial, based on volume and protein concentration. If the shielded preparation vial contains less than 35 mg, calculate the amount of additional tositumomab needed to yield a total of 35 mg protein. Calculate the volume needed from the 35 mg vial of tositumomab, based on protein concentration. Withdraw the calculated volume of tositumomab from the 35 mg vial of tositumomab and transfer to the shielded preparation vial. The preparation vial should now contain 35 mg tositumomab. Using the 20 mL syringe containing NaCl 0.9%, add a sufficient quantity to the shielded preparation vial to yield a final volume of 30 mL. Gently mix the solutions. Withdraw the entire contents from the preparation vial into a 30 mL syringe using a large-bore needle (eg, 18 gauge). Assay and record the activity.

Administration of dosimetric step:

Tositumomab infusion: Attach a primary IV infusion set to the 0.22 micron inline filter set and the 100 mL bag of NaCl 0.9%. After priming the primary IV infusion set and filter, connect the infusion bag containing 450 mg tositumomab/50 mL via a secondary IV infusion set to primary IV set at a port distal to the filter. Infuse tositumomab over 60 minutes, then disconnect the secondary set and flush the primary set and the filter with NaCl 0.9%. Discard the tositumomab bag and secondary IV set.

I-131 tositumomab dosimetric infusion: Use appropriate shielding when administering the dosimetric dose. Deliver the dosimetric dose in a 30 mL syringe. Connect the extension set to the 3-way stopcock. Connect the 50 mL bag of NaCl 0.9% to a secondary IV set and connect the set to the 3-way stopcock. Prime the secondary IV set and the extension set. Connect the extension set to a port in the primary IV set, distal to the filter. Use the same primary set and pre-wetted filter used for the tositumomab infusion. A change in filter can result in loss of up to 7% of the I-131 tositumomab dose. Attach the syringe filled with I-131 tositumomab to the 3-way stopcock. Set syringe pump to deliver the entire 5 mCi (35 mg) dose of I-131 tositumomab over 20 minutes. After infusion, close the stopcock to the syringe. Flush the extension set and the secondary IV set with NaCl 0.9% from the 50 mL bag. After the flush, disconnect the extension set, 3-way stopcock, and syringe. Disconnect the primary IV set and filter. Determine the combined residual activity of the syringe and infusion set components (eg, stopcock, sets) by assaying in a suitable radioactivity calibration system immediately after completion of administration of the dosimetric step. Calculate and record the dose delivered to the patient by subtracting the residual activity in the syringe and infusion set components from the activity of I-131 tositumomab in the syringe before infusion.

Determination of dose for therapeutic step: After infusion of the I-131 tositumomab dosimetric dose, obtain total body gamma camera counts and whole body images:

- Within 1 hour of infusion and before urination.
- 2 to 4 days after infusion of the dosimetric dose, after urination.
- 6 to 7 days after infusion of the dosimetric dose, after urination.

Assess biodistribution. If biodistribution is altered, do not administer the therapeutic step. Determine total body residence time. Determine activity hours, according to gender. Use actual patient mass (in kg) or maximum effective mass (in kg), whichever is lower. Determine whether to reduce the desired total body dose (to 65 cGy) due to platelet count of 100,000 to less than 150,000 cells/mm^3. Based on the total body residence time and activity-hours, calculate the I-131 activity (mCi) to be administered to deliver the therapeutic dose of 65 or 75 cGy. Use the following equation to calculate the activity of I-131 required for the desired total body dose of radiation.

$$\text{I-131 Activity (mCi)} = \frac{\text{Activity-Hours (mCi-h)}}{\text{Residence Time (h)}} \times \frac{\text{Desired Total Body Dose (cGy)}}{75 \text{ cGy}}$$

Preparation for therapeutic step:

Tositumomab dose: Withdraw and dispose of 32 mL of saline from a 50 mL bag of NaCl 0.9%. Withdraw contents from each of two 225 mg tositumomab vials (450 mg/ 32 mL) and transfer to infusion bag containing 18 mL NaCl 0.9%. Gently mix the solutions by inverting or rotating the bag. Do not shake.

I-131 tositumomab therapeutic dose: Allow approximately 60 minutes for the I-131 tositumomab therapeutic vial to thaw at ambient temperature with appropriate shielding. Calculate the dose of I-131 tositumomab required. Based on the activity concentration of the vial, calculate volume required for I-131 tositumomab activity required for the therapeutic dose. Using 1 or more 30 mL syringes with 18-gauge needles, withdraw calculated volume from I-131 tositumomab vial. Transfer this volume to the shielded preparation vial. Assay the dose to ensure the appropriate activity (mCi). If the assayed dose is within ± 10% of the dose calculated for the therapeutic step, proceed. If not, recalculate the activity concentration of the I-131 tositumomab at this time, based on volume and activity in preparation vial. Recalculate the volume required for I-131 tositumomab activity for therapeutic dose. Using the same 30 mL syringe, add or subtract the appropriate volume from the I-131 tositumomab vial, so the preparation vial contains volume required for I-131 tositumomab activity required for therapeutic dose. Re-assay preparation vial. When activity is correct, calculate amount of tositumomab protein contained in solution of I-131 tositumomab in shielded preparation vial, based on volume and protein concentration. If the shielded preparation vial contains less than 35 mg, calculate the amount of additional tositumomab needed to yield 35 mg protein. Calculate volume needed from 35 mg vial of tositumomab, based on protein concentration. Withdraw calculated volume of tositumomab from 35 mg vial of tositumomab, and transfer to shielded preparation vial. The preparation vial should now contain 35 mg of tositumomab. If the dose of I-131 tositumomab requires the use of 2 vials of I-131 tositumomab or the entire contents of a single vial of I-131 tositumomab, there may be no need to add protein from the 35 mg vial of tositumomab. Using the 20 mL syringe containing NaCl 0.9%, add a sufficient volume (if needed) to shielded preparation vial to yield a final volume of 30 mL. Gently mix the solution. Withdraw entire volume from preparation vial into 1 or more sterile 30 mL syringes using a large-bore needle (eg, 18 gauge). Assay and record the activity.

Administration of therapeutic step:

Tositumomab infusion: Attach a primary IV infusion set to the 0.22 micron inline filter set and a 100 mL bag of NaCl 0.9%. After priming the primary IV set and filter set, connect infusion bag containing 450 mg tositumomab/50 mL via a secondary IV set to the primary IV set at a port distal to the filter. Infuse tositumomab over 60 minutes, then disconnect the secondary IV set and flush the primary IV set and filter set with NaCl 0.9%. Discard the tositumomab bag and secondary IV infusion set.

I-131 tositumomab therapeutic infusion: Use appropriate shielding when administering the therapeutic dose. Deliver the therapeutic dose in 1 or more 30 mL syringes. Connect the extension set to the 3-way stopcock. Connect the 50 mL bag of NaCl 0.9% to a secondary IV set and connect the infusion set to the 3-way stopcock. Prime the secondary IV set and extension set. Connect the extension set to a port in the primary IV set, distal to the filter. Use the same primary set and pre-wetted filter used for the tositumomab infusion. A change in filter can result in loss of up to 7% of the I-131 tositumomab dose.

Attach the syringe filled with I-131 tositumomab to the 3-way stopcock. Set syringe pump to deliver the entire therapeutic dose of I-131 tositumomab over 20 minutes. If more than 1 syringe is required, remove the syringe and repeat previous steps. After completely infusing the I-131 tositumomab, close the stopcock to the syringe. Flush the secondary IV set and the extension set with NaCl 0.9% from the 50 mL bag of NaCl 0.9%. After flushing, disconnect the extension set, 3-way stopcock, and syringe. Disconnect the primary IV set and filter. Determine the combined residual activity of the syringe(s) and infusion set components (eg, stopcock, sets) by assaying in a suitable radioactivity calibration system immediately after completing administration of the therapeutic step. Calculate and record the dose delivered to the patient by subtracting the residual activity from the activity of I-131 tositumomab in the syringe before infusion.

Additional Doses: The *Bexxar* regimen is intended as a single course of treatment. The safety of multiple courses of the *Bexxar* regimen or combination of this regimen with other forms of irradiation or chemotherapy has not been evaluated.

Related Interventions:

Thyroid-protective agents:

- Saturated solution of potassium iodide (SSKI) 4 drops orally 3 times/day;
- Lugol's solution 20 drops orally 3 times/day;
- or potassium iodide tablets 130 mg/day

Start thyroid-protective agents at least 24 hours before the I-131 tositumomab dosimetric dose, continuing until 2 weeks after administration of the I-131 tositumomab therapeutic dose. Do not administer the dosimetric dose of I-131 tositumomab if patient has not yet received at least 3 doses of SSKI, 3 doses of *Lugol's* solution, or one 130 mg potassium iodide tablet at least 24 hours earlier.

Acetaminophen 650 mg orally and diphenhydramine 50 mg orally 30 minutes before administration of tositumomab in the dosimetric and therapeutic steps.

Laboratory Tests: Obtain a complete blood count (CBC) with differential and platelet count before, and at least weekly after administration of the *Bexxar* regimen. Continue weekly monitoring of blood counts for at least 10 weeks or, if persistent, until severe cytopenias completely resolve. More frequent monitoring is indicated in patients with evidence of moderate or more severe cytopenias. Monitor TSH level before treatment and annually thereafter. Measure serum creatinine levels immediately before the *Bexxar* regimen.

Waste Disposal: Discard all materials used to deliver I-131 tositumomab (eg, syringes, vials, sets) according to regulations governing radioactive and biohazardous waste.

Radiation Protection: Minimize exposure of medical personnel and other patients to I-131. Shield the drug appropriately during preparation and administration to minimize radiation exposure to patients, family, and medical personnel. Beyond the use of vial and syringe shields for preparation and injection, no special shielding is necessary.

Image Acquisition:

Gamma camera and dose calibrator procedures: Follow manufacturer-specific quality-control procedures for the gamma camera/computer system, the collimator, and the dose calibrator. Less than 20% variance between maximum and minimum pixel-count values in the useful field of view is acceptable on I-131 intrinsic flood fields and variability less than 10% is preferable. I-131-specific camera uniformity corrections are strongly recommended, rather than applying lower energy correction to the I-131 window. Assess camera extrinsic uniformity at least monthly using 99m-Tc or 57-Co as a source with imaging at the appropriate window. Additional (nonroutine) quality-control procedures are required. To assure the accuracy and precision of the patient total body counts, the gamma camera must undergo validation and daily quality control on each day it is used to collect patient images. Use the same setup and region of interest (ROI) for calibration, determination of background, and whole-body patient studies.

Gamma camera setup: Use the same camera, collimator, ROI, scanning speed, energy window, and setup for all studies. The gamma camera must be capable of whole body imaging and have a large or extra large field of view with a digital interface. It must be equipped with a parallel-hole collimator rated to at least 364 keV by the manufacturer with a septal penetration for I-131 of less than 7%. The camera and computer must be set up for scanning as follows: Parallel-hole collimator rated to at least 364 keV with a septal penetration for I-131 of less than 7%. Symmetric window (20% to 25%) centered on the 364 keV photo peak of I-131 (314 to 414 keV). Matrix: minimum 128 × 128. Scanning speed: 10 to 30 cm/min.

Counts from calibrated source for quality control: Determine camera sensitivity for I-131 each day. Determine the gamma camera's sensitivity by scanning a calibrated activity of I-131 (eg, 200 to 250 microCi in at least 20 mL of saline within a sealed pharmaceutical vial). First, determine the radioactivity of the I-131 source using a NIST-traceable-calibrated clinical dose calibrator at the I-131 setting.

Background counts: Obtain the background count from a scan with no radioactive source, after the count of the calibrated source and just before obtaining the patient count. If abnormally high background counts are measured, identify the source and, if possible, remove it. If abnormally low background counts are measured, verify the camera energy window setting and collimator before repeating the background counts. Obtain the counts per microCi by dividing the background-corrected source count by the calibrated activity for that day. For a specific camera and collimator, the counts per microCi should be relatively constant. When values vary more than 10% from the established ratio, ascertain and correct the reason for the discrepancy and repeat the source count.

Patient total body counts: Obtain the source and background counts first and establish the camera sensitivity (constant counting efficiency) before obtaining the patient count. Use the same ROI for the whole body counts, the quality-control counts of the radioactive source, and the background counts. Acquire anterior and posterior whole body images for gamma camera counts. For any particular patient, use the same gamma camera for all scans. To obtain proper counts, include extremities in the images, with arms not crossing over the body. Center the scans on the midline of the patient. Record the time of the start of the radiolabeled dosimetric infusion and the time of the start of each count acquisition. Obtain gamma camera counts at the 3 imaging time points:

Count 1: Within an hour of end of the infusion of the I-131 tositumomab dosimetric dose before patient urinates.

Count 2: Two to 4 days after administration of the I-131 tositumomab dosimetric dose and immediately after patient urinates.

Count 3: Six to 7 days after the administration of the I-131 tositumomab dosimetric dose and immediately after patient urinates.

Biodistribution of I-131 tositumomab: Assess the biodistribution of I-131 tositumomab by determining total body residence time and by visual examination of whole body camera images from the image taken at Count 1 (within an hour of end of infusion) and from the image taken at Count 2 (2 to 4 days after administration). To resolve ambiguities, evaluation of the image at Count 3 (6 to 7 days after administration) may be necessary. If either of these methods indicates that biodistribution is altered, do not administer the I-131 tositumomab therapeutic dose.

Expected biodistribution: Within an hour of end of infusion, before urination, most of the activity is in the blood pool (heart and major blood vessels), and the uptake in normal liver and spleen is less than in the heart. At the second and third time points, the activity in the blood pool decreases significantly, with decreased accumulation of activity in normal liver and spleen. Images may show uptake by thyroid, kidney, and urinary bladder and minimal uptake in the lungs. Tumor uptake in soft tissues and in normal organs is seen as areas of increased intensity.

Results indicating altered biodistribution: At the first imaging time point, if the blood pool is not visualized or if there is diffuse, intense tracer uptake in the liver and/or spleen or uptake suggestive of urinary obstruction the biodistribution is altered. Diffuse lung uptake greater than that of blood pool on the first day represents altered biodistribution. At the second and third imaging time points, uptake suggestive of urinary obstruction and diffuse lung uptake greater than that of the blood pool represent altered biodistribution. Or total body residence times of less than 50 hours and more than 150 hours.

Calculation of I-131 activity for therapeutic dose:

Residence time (h): For each time point, calculate the background corrected total body count at each time point (defined as the geometric mean), using this equation: Geometric mean of counts = square root of $[(CA - CBA)(CP - CBP)]$. In this equation, CA = the anterior counts, CBA = the anterior background counts, CP = the posterior counts, and CBP = the posterior background counts. Once the geometric mean of the counts has been calculated for each of the time points, the percent injected activity remaining for each time point is calculated by dividing the geometric mean of the counts from that time point by the geometric mean of the counts from Day 0 and multiplying by 100. The residence time (h) is then determined by plotting the time from the start of infusion and the percent injected activity values for the imaging time points on Graph 1 (provided by manufacturer). A best-fit line is then drawn from 100% (the pre-plotted Day 0 value) through the other 2 plotted points (if the line does not intersect the 2 points, 1 point must lie above the best-fit line and 1 point must lie below the best-fit line). The residence time (h) is read from the x-axis of the graph at the point where the fitted line intersects with the horizontal 37% injected activity line.

Activity hours (mCi-h): To determine the activity hours (mCi-h), determine the patient's maximum effective mass derived from the patient's sex and height. If patient's actual weight is less than the maximum effective mass, use the actual weight in the activity hours table. If the patient's actual weight is greater than the maximum effective mass, use the mass from the worksheet for "Determination of Maximum Effective Mass."

Calculation of I-131 activity for therapeutic dose: Use the following equation to calculate the activity of I-131 required for the desired total body dose of radiation:

$$\text{I-131 Activity (mCi)} = \frac{\text{Activity Hours (mCi-h)}}{\text{Residence Time (h)}} \times \frac{\text{Desired Total Body Dose (cGy)}}{75 \text{ cGy}}$$

Efficacy: Efficacy was evaluated in a multicenter, single-arm study in patients with low-grade or transformed low-grade or follicular large-cell lymphoma whose disease had not responded to or had progressed after rituximab therapy. Benefit was based on durable responses without effect on survival. All patients in the study received at least 4 doses of rituximab without an objective response, or progressed after treatment. Patients also had a platelet count at least 100,000 cells/mm^3; an average of 25% or less of the intratrabecular marrow space involved by lymphoma, and no evidence of progressive disease arising in a field irradiated with more than 3,500 cGy within 1 year of completion of irradiation.

Forty patients initiated the *Bexxar* regimen. The median age was 57 (range, 35 to 78); the median time from diagnosis to protocol entry was 50 months (range, 11 to 70); and the median number of prior chemotherapy regimens was 4 (range, 1 to 11). Twenty-four patients had disease that did not respond to their last treatment with rituximab, 11 patients had disease that responded to rituximab for less than 6 months, and 5 patients had disease that responded to rituximab, with a duration of response of 6 months or greater. Overall, 35 of 40 patients met the definition of "rituximab refractory," defined as no response or a response of less than 6 months duration. The after table summarizes efficacy outcome data from this study. The median duration of follow-up was 26 months for all patients and 26 months for the rituximab-refractory subset.

Objective Responses to *Bexxar* Therapeutic Regimen			
Patients refractory to rituximab		All patients	
Response rate (95% CI) (n = 35)	Median duration of response (mo) (range)	Response rate (95% CI) (n = 40)	Median duration of response (mo) (range)
Overall response 63% (45, 79)	25 (4+, 35+)	68% (51, 81)	16 (1+, 35+)
Complete response[a] 29% (15, 46)	Not reached (4, 35+)	33% (19, 49)	Not reached (4, 35+)

a Complete response rate = pathologic and clinical complete responses.

The results of this study were supported by demonstration of durable objective responses in 4 single-arm studies enrolling 190 patients evaluable for efficacy with rituximab-naive, follicular NHL with or without transformation, who had relapsed after or were refractory to chemotherapy. In these studies, the overall response rates ranged from 47% to 64%, and the median durations of response ranged from 12 to 18 months.

Duration: The *Bexxar* therapeutic regimen results in sustained depletion of circulating CD20-positive cells. The impact of the *Bexxar* therapeutic regimen on circulating CD20-positive cells was assessed in 2 clinical studies, 1 conducted in chemotherapy-naïve patients and 1 in heavily pretreated patients. The assessment of circulating lymphocytes did not distinguish normal from malignant cells. Consequently, assessment of recovery of normal B-cell function was not directly assessed. At 7 weeks, the median number of circulating CD20-positive cells was 0 (range, 0 to 490 cells/mm^3). Lymphocyte recovery began at approximately 12 weeks after treatment. Among patients who had CD20-positive cell counts recorded at baseline and at 6 months, 8 of 58 (14%) chemotherapy-naive patients had CD20-positive cell counts below normal limits at 6 months and 6 of 19 (32%) heavily pretreated patients had CD20-positive cell counts below normal limits at 6 months.

Pharmacokinetics: Immunoglobulins are primarily eliminated by catabolism. The phase 1 study of I-131 tositumomab determined that a 475 mg predose of unlabeled antibody decreased splenic targeting and increased the terminal half-life of radiolabeled antibody. The median blood clearance after administration of 485 mg of tositumomab in 110 patients with NHL was 68.2 mg/h (range, 30.2 to 260.8 mg/h). Patients with high tumor burden, splenomegaly, or bone marrow involvement had a faster clearance, shorter terminal half-life, and larger volume of distribution. The total body clearance, as measured by total body gamma camera counts, was dependent on the same factors noted for blood clearance. Patient-specific dosing, based on total body clearance, provided a consistent radiation dose, despite variable pharmacokinetics, by allowing each patient's administered activity to be adjusted for individual patient variables

Elimination of I-131 occurs by decay and excretion in the urine. Urine was collected for 49 dosimetric doses. After 5 days, the whole body clearance was 67% of the injected dose. Urine accounts for 98% of clearance.

Mechanism: Tositumomab binds specifically to the CD20 (human B-lymphocyte-restricted differentiation antigen, Bp 35 or B1) antigen. This antigen is a transmembrane phosphoprotein expressed on pre-B lymphocytes and at higher density on mature B-lymphocytes. The antigen is also expressed on more than 90% of B-cell NHL. The recognition epitope for tositumomab is found within the extracellular domain of the CD20 antigen. CD20 does not shed from the cell surface and does not internalize after antibody binding.

Possible mechanisms of action of the *Bexxar* therapeutic regimen include induction of apoptosis, complement-dependent cytotoxicity (CDC), and antibody-dependent cellular cytotoxicity (ADCC) mediated by the antibody. Additionally, cell death is associated with ionizing radiation from the radioisotope.

Drug Interactions: The safety of immunization with live vaccines after the *Bexxar* regimen has not been studied. The ability of patients who received the *Bexxar* regimen to generate a primary or anamnestic humoral response to any vaccine has not been studied.

No formal drug interaction studies have been performed. Because of the frequent occurrence of severe and prolonged thrombocytopenia, weigh the potential benefits of medications that interfere with platelet function and/or anticoagulation against the potential increased risk of bleeding and hemorrhage.

Lab Interference: The *Bexxar* regimen may evoke HAMA. HAMA may affect the accuracy of the results of in vitro and in vivo diagnostic tests and may affect the toxicity profile and efficacy of therapeutic agents that rely on murine antibody technology.

Patient Information: Before administering the *Bexxar* regimen, inform patients that they will have a radioactive material in their body for several days upon release from the hospital or clinic. Provide patients with oral and written instructions for minimizing exposure of family members, friends, and the general public.

Advise women of the potential risks of I-131 to the fetus. Instruct women who are breastfeeding to discontinue nursing.

Advise patients of the potential risk of toxic effects on the male and female gonads from the *Bexxar* regimen. Instruct them in effective contraceptive methods during treatment and for 12 months after the *Bexxar* regimen.

Inform patients of the risks of hypothyroidism and the importance of compliance with thyroid-blocking agents and need for lifelong monitoring. Inform patients of the possibility of developing a HAMA immune response and that HAMA may affect the results of in vitro and in vivo diagnostic tests, as well as results of therapies that rely on murine antibody technology.

Inform patients of symptoms associated with cytopenia, the need for frequent monitoring for up to 12 weeks after treatment and the potential for persistent cytopenias beyond 12 weeks. Inform patients that certain antineoplastic agents used in the treatment of malignancy (eg, alkylating agents, topoisomerase II inhibitors, ionizing radiation), have been associated with the development of MDS, secondary leukemia, and solid tumors. Inform patients that MDS, secondary leukemia, and solid tumors have also been observed in patients receiving the *Bexxar* regimen.

Pharmaceutical Characteristics

Concentration: Tositumomab is provided at a nominal concentration of 14 mg/mL tositumomab in 35 and 225 mg single-use vials.

I-131 tositumomab is a radio-iodinated derivative of tositumomab covalently linked to I-131. Each single-use vial contains not less than 20 mL of I-131 tositumomab at nominal protein and activity concentrations of 0.1 mg/mL and 0.61 mCi/mL (at calibration), respectively.

Quality Assay: Unbound radio-iodine and other reactants have been removed by chromatographic purification steps. The dosimetric dosage form is supplied at nominal protein and activity concentrations of 0.1 mg/mL and 0.61 mCi/mL (at date of calibration), respectively. The therapeutic dosage form is supplied at nominal protein and activity concentrations of 1.1 mg/mL and 5.6 mCi/mL (at date of calibration), respectively.

Packaging:

Dosimetric packaging: Components are shipped from separate sites. Ensure the components are scheduled to arrive on the same day.

Tositumomab: Two single-use 225 mg/16.1 mL vials and 1 single-use 35 mg/2.5 mL vial of tositumomab supplied by McKesson Biosciences (NDC #: 00007-3260-31).

I-131 tositumomab: A single-use vial of I-131 tositumomab within a lead pot supplied by MDS Nordion (00007-3261-01). Each single-use vial contains not less than 20 mL of

I-131 tositumomab at nominal protein and activity concentrations of 0.1 mg/mL and 0.61 mCi/mL (at calibration), respectively. The product specification sheet describes the lot-specific protein concentration, activity concentration, total activity, and expiration date.

Therapeutic packaging: Components are shipped from separate sites. Ensure the components are scheduled to arrive on the same day.

Tositumomab: Two single-use 225 mg/16.1 mL vials and 1 single-use 35 mg/2.5 mL vial of tositumomab supplied by McKesson Biosciences (NDC #: 00007-3260-36).

I-131 tositumomab: One or 2 single-use vials of I-131 tositumomab within a lead pot, supplied by MDS Nordion (00007-3262-01). Each single-use vial contains not less than 20 mL of I-131 tositumomab at nominal protein and activity concentrations of 1.1 mg/mL and 5.6 mCi/mL (at calibration), respectively. The product specification sheet describes the lot-specific protein concentration, activity concentration, total activity, and expiration date.

Doseform: Liquid

Appearance: Tositumomab is a clear to opalescent, colorless to slightly yellow liquid. Diluted tositumomab may contain particulates that are generally white in nature.

Solvent: Buffered water

Diluent:
For infusion: Sodium chloride 0.9%

Adjuvant: None

Preservative: None

Allergens: None

Excipients: The tositumomab formulation contains 10% w/v maltose, 145 mM sodium chloride, and 10 mM phosphate. The I-131 tositumomab formulation for the dosimetric and the therapeutic dosage forms contains 5% to 6% (w/v) povidone, 1 to 2 mg/mL maltose (dosimetric dose) or 9 to 15 mg/mL maltose (therapeutic dose), 0.85 to 0.95 mg/mL sodium chloride, and 0.9 to 1.3 mg/mL ascorbic acid.

pH: The pH of tositumomab is approximately 7.2. The pH of I-131 tositumomab is approximately 7.

Shelf Life:
Tositumomab: Expires within 24 months.

I-131 tositumomab: Prepared shortly before shipping. Degrades according to half-life of radioisotope. Typically usable for 5 days.

Storage/Stability:
Tositumomab: Refrigerate 35 and 225 mg vials of tositumomab at 2° to 8°C (36° to 46°F) before dilution. Protect from strong light. Do not shake. Do not freeze.

Solutions of diluted tositumomab are stable for up to 24 hours if refrigerated at 2° to 8°C (36° to 46°F) or up to 8 hours at room temperature. Refrigerating the diluted solution at 2° to 8°C (36° to 46°F) before administration is preferred because it does not contain preservatives. Do not freeze solutions of diluted tositumomab.

I-131 tositumomab: Freeze in the original lead pots at -20°C or below until removed for thawing before administration. Thawed dosimetric and therapeutic doses of I-131 tositumomab are stable up to 8 hours at 2° to 8°C (36° to 46°F) or at room temperature. Solutions of I-131 tositumomab diluted for infusion contain no preservatives and should be stored refrigerated at 2° to 8°C (36° to 46°F) before administration. Do not freeze.

Contact the manufacturer regarding exposure to other temperatures. Shipping data not provided.

Production Process: Tositumomab is produced in an antibiotic-free culture of mammalian cells.

Media: Murine cell culture.

Tositumomab (Murine)

Radiation Dosimetry: Estimations of radiation-absorbed doses for I-131 tositumomab were performed using sequential whole body images and Miridose 3 software. Patients with apparent thyroid, stomach, or intestinal imaging were selected for organ-dosimetry analyses. The estimated radiation-absorbed doses to organs and marrow from a course of the *Bexxar* therapeutic regimen appear in the following table.

Estimated Radiation-Absorbed Organ Doses (*Bexxar*, mGy/MBq)		
From organ regions of interest (ROIs)	*Median*	*Range*
Thyroid	2.71	1.4 to 6.2
Kidneys	1.96	1.5 to 2.5
Intestine wall		
Upper lower	1.34	0.8 to 1.7
Lower lower	1.30	0.8 to 1.6
Heart wall	1.25	0.5 to 1.8
Spleen	1.14	0.7 to 5.4
Testes	0.83	0.3 to 1.3
Liver	0.82	0.6 to 1.3
Lungs	0.79	0.5 to 1.1
Red marrow	0.65	0.5 to 1.1
Stomach wall	0.40	0.2 to 0.8
From whole body ROIs	*Median*	*Range*
Urine bladder wall	0.64	0.6 to 0.9
Bone surfaces	0.41	0.4 to 0.6
Pancreas	0.31	0.2 to 0.4
Gall bladder wall	0.29	0.2 to 0.3
Adrenals	0.28	0.2 to 0.3
Ovaries	0.25	0.2 to 0.3
Small intestine	0.23	0.2 to 0.3
Thymus	0.22	0.1 to 0.3
Uterus	0.20	0.2 to 0.2
Muscle	0.18	0.1 to 0.2
Breasts	0.16	0.1 to 0.2
Skin	0.13	0.1 to 0.2
Brain	0.13	0.1 to 0.2
Total body	0.24	0.2 to 0.3

Other Information

First Licensed: June 27, 2003

References: Davies AJ. A review of tositumomab and I (131) tositumomab radioimmunotherapy for the treatment of follicular lymphoma. *Expert Opin Biol Ther*. 2005;5(4):577-588.

Allergen Extracts

Names:
Aquagen SQ
Immunorex
Generic

Manufacturers:
ALK-Abelló Laboratories
Antigen Laboratories
Allergy Laboratories (Oklahoma); Allermed
Laboratories; Antigen Laboratories; Greer
Laboratories; Hollister-Stier Corporation;
Nelco Laboratories

Synonyms: Allergenic extracts, desensitizing vaccines (British term). Use of these products is referred to as immunotherapy, previously described as desensitization and hyposensitization. The federal requirement for minimum antigen E (AgE) content of products containing short-ragweed extract began in January 1982. Biologically standardized products were first licensed in 1983. Potency designations for cat extracts were changed in October 1992, from 50,000 and 100,000 AU (allergy units) per mL to 5,000 and 10,000 BAU (bioequivalent allergy units) per mL, to correspond to skin-test potency of other standardized extracts.

Comparison: Theoretically, comparable extracts from the same pollen or other antigenic source are generically equivalent. However, the shortcomings of the w/v (weight-to-volume) and PNU (protein nitrogen units) measurement systems require caution and dosage reduction when changing between manufacturers and even when continuing therapy with a freshly compounded allergen-extract prescription obtained from different lots from the original manufacturer.

Immunologic Characteristics

Antigen Source: The FDA licenses over 900 distinct allergen extracts as safe and effective for immunodiagnosis. Of these, approximately 600 are also licensed as safe and effective for immunotherapy. Representative members of various allergen groups include:

Animals: eg, cat (primary allergen: Fel d 1), dog, horse, rat, guinea pig danders; chicken, duck, goose, pigeon feathers

Foods: eg, chicken egg albumin, casein, bovine alpha lactalbumin, beta lactoglobulin, almond (*Prunus amygdalus*), gum acacia (*Acacia senegal*), scallops (*Pecten irradians*)

Grasses: eg, Kentucky blue (June; *Poa pratensis*), red top (*Agrostis alba*), perennial rye (*Lolium perenne*), Bermuda (*Cynodon dactylon*), meadow fescue (*Festuca eliatior*), velvet (*Holcus lanata*)

Insects: eg, German cockroach, house-dust mite (*Dermatophagoides farinae, Dermatophagoides pteronyssinus*)

Molds: eg, various species of the following representative genera: *Alternaria, Aspergillus, Cladosporium, Fusarium, Monilia, Mucor, Helminthosporium, Penicillium, Phoma, Rhizopus, Saccharomyces, Tricophyton*

Trees: eg, white oak (*Quercus alba*), Arizona cypress (*Cupressus arizonica*), cottonwood (*Populus deltoides*), red maple (*Acer rubrum*), mountain cedar (*Juniperus sabinoides*), American elm (*Ulmus americanus*)

Weeds: eg, short ragweed (*Ambrosia artemisiifolia [elatior]*), common sagebrush (*Artemisia tridentata*), saltbush (*Atriplex wrightii*), wingscale (*Atriplex canescens*), lambs quarters (*Chenopodium album*)

Other inhalants: eg, house dust, cotton linters, gum arabic, gum karaya, green tobacco leaf, gum tragacanth, silk, castor bean

Consult the Directory of Manufacturers (in the Resources section) to obtain catalogs of specific products available from each manufacturer. The following general monograph discusses allergen extracts generically and is followed by sections on specific product types.

Viability: Not viable, but antigenically active

Antigenic Form: Allergen extract

Antigenic Type: Proteins and other constituents. Skin tests assess immediate (type I) hypersensitivity.

Strains: Multiple species, refer to container label.

Use Characteristics

Indications: For use as an aid in the diagnosis of immediate hypersensitivity through skin testing. Some extracts are indicated for induction of active immunity against subsequent hypersensitivity reactions, for the treatment of patients whose histories indicate that they experience allergic symptoms upon natural exposure to certain allergens.

Efficacy for the treatment of allergic rhinitis has been scientifically established for short ragweed, mountain cedar, birch, *Cladosporium*, timothy grass, and orchard grass extracts. Efficacy is inferred for other pollen and mold extracts.

In assessing hypersensitivity, the patient's history is the most important factor. Skin test reactions confirm or correct the clinical impression; generally, the larger the skin reaction, the more likely the response is important to the patient's illness. But even smaller reactions to prevalent potent allergens may be included in a prescription, if compatible with patient history. In assessing skin test reactions, consider symptom relationship to season, geographic location, occupation, environment, hobbies, and other special circumstances of the patient. Avoidance is the best way to control hypersensitivity responses. When avoidance is not possible, limit the number of allergens in the prescription to the smallest number possible, to avoid diluting allergens below a therapeutic concentration. Do not include allergens to which the patient is never or rarely exposed.

If the number of indicated allergens exceeds 6 to 10, the treatment may be divided among 2 or 3 separate mixtures, permitting adjustment of individual doses according to the pollination season, degree of exposure, or presence of local reactions.

Unlabeled Uses: Allergen extracts also may be used in the diagnosis and treatment of veterinary allergy. Dosage is the same for large and small animals as for human adults.

Limitations: Very young children, geriatric patients, or those suffering from autoimmune disorders or severe and unstable allergic disorders may not respond to immunotherapy.

Inappropriate Uses: Avoid several controversial practices that lack scientific evidence of efficacy: cytotoxic allergy testing, subcutaneous provocative and neutralization testing, skin titration immunotherapy (ie, Rinkel technique), urine autoinjection, remote practice of allergy, IgG to foods, Candidiasis hypersensitivity syndrome, and clinical ecology.

Alternative Tests: Radioallergosorbent test (RAST), the related fluorescent (FAST) or enzyme colorimetric (EAST) tests, and enzyme-linked immunosorbent assays (ELISA) may also be used to assess allergenic hypersensitivity, although these tests are less sensitive than intradermal skin testing with allergen extracts.

Contraindications:

Absolute: None

Relative: Do not treat patients with allergens to which they have no history of hypersensitivity nor a likelihood of exposure, regardless of skin-test results. There is inconclusive evidence that routine immunization with allergen extracts may exacerbate autoimmune diseases. Children with nephrotic syndrome probably should not receive immunotherapy. Precautions are also warranted in patients experiencing severe respiratory or cardiovascular distress and patients who have experienced an anaphylactic reaction to the offending allergen. Weigh the risks of therapy against its benefits.

Temporarily withhold allergen extracts, or reduce the dose if any of the following conditions occur:

(1) Severe symptoms of rhinitis or asthma,

(2) infection accompanied by fever, or

(3) exposure to excessive amounts of clinically relevant allergen prior to a scheduled injection.

Patient compliance is an important consideration in the decision to initiate immunotherapy with any potent allergen extract. Do not initiate therapy if the patient cannot be depended on to respond promptly and properly to an impending adverse reaction.

Patients receiving beta-adrenergic antagonists (ie, beta blockers) may be refractory to the effects of epinephrine, which may be needed to treat anaphylactic reactions.

Immunodeficiency: Immune response and resultant reduction in symptoms may be impaired in immunocompromised patients.

Elderly: Geriatric patients may not respond to immunotherapy.

Pregnancy: Category C. Use only if clearly needed. Immunotherapy has been continued during pregnancy but is not generally initiated during it. Consider the risk-benefit ratio. An anaphylactic reaction may induce a miscarriage as a result of uterine muscle contractions. It is not known if allergen extracts or corresponding antibodies cross the placenta. Generally, most IgG passage across the placenta occurs during the third trimester.

Lactation: It is not known if allergen extracts or corresponding antibodies are excreted in breast milk. Problems in humans have not been documented.

Children: Children older than 2 years of age appear to tolerate allergen-extract injections well. Adult and pediatric maintenance doses are usually equivalent. If the injection volume is too large for a small child to tolerate comfortably, split the dose among several injections.

Adverse Reactions: Allergen-extract injections may be the most common cause of systemic allergic reactions in the United States.

Anaphylaxis may occur without warning, usually within the first 20 minutes after an injection, even during the maintenance phase of therapy. Observe patients for 20 to 30 minutes after each injection and instruct them to return promptly if symptoms of an allergic reaction or shock occur. The more quickly symptoms appear, the more severe they are likely to be, and the more rapidly treatment measures should be instituted. Anaphylaxis may be a greater concern in asthmatic patients already experiencing allergic respiratory symptoms. Only conduct skin testing and immunotherapy in facilities with adequate equipment and medications and personnel trained to respond to anaphylaxis.

Immediate induration and erythema reactions are ordinarily of little consequence, but if these reactions are large (more than 3 to 5 cm in diameter) they may be the first manifestation of a systemic reaction. If large local reactions occur, observe the patient for systemic symptoms. Oral antihistamines may relieve symptoms. Reduce the next therapeutic dose by half or to the last dose that did not elicit a reaction; increase subsequent doses more slowly, through the use of intermediate dilutions if needed.

Systemic reactions: Mild exacerbation of allergic symptoms, sneezing, mild to severe generalized urticaria, angioedema, rhinitis, conjunctivitis, edema (including laryngeal edema), wheezing, asthma, dyspnea, cough, fainting, pallor, cyanosis, bradycardia, tachycardia, lacrimation, marked perspiration, hypotension, upper airway obstruction. Symptoms may progress to anaphylactic shock and death. After a systemic reaction, reduce the next therapeutic dose to the last dose that did not elicit a reaction, or lower, and increase subsequent doses more slowly, through the use of intermediate dilutions if needed. Repeated systemic reactions, even of a mild nature, may be sufficient reason for cessation of further attempts to increase the reaction-eliciting dose.

Management of systemic reactions: Apply a tourniquet above the injection site, and inject 0.3 to 0.5 mL of epinephrine 1:1,000 subcutaneously or IM into the other arm. The dose may need to be repeated every 5 to 10 minutes, since a succession of small doses is often more effective and less dangerous than a single large dose. Loosen the tourniquet at least every 10 minutes. Also inject a maximum of 0.1 mL of epinephrine 1:1,000 at the site of the allergen injection to delay allergen absorption. If more than 1 extract injection had been given, distribute the 0.1 mL evenly among the sites.

See the epinephrine monograph for a dosing chart by age and body mass. In general, the pediatric dose is 10 mcg (0.01 mL of a 1:1,000 w/v solution) per kg of body weight or 300 mcg (0.3 mL) per square meter of body surface, up to 500 mcg (0.5 mL).

Patients receiving beta-adrenergic antagonists (ie, beta blockers) may be refractory to the effects of epinephrine.

After adequate epinephrine has been given, and in cases where symptoms of angioedema, urticaria, rhinitis, or conjunctivitis are not responding rapidly, inject antihistamine (eg, 10 to 50 mg diphenhydramine [eg, *Benadryl*]) IV or IM, according to the manufacturer's direction.

Other measures may be necessary: Inhaled or parenteral bronchodilators or oxygen for cyanosis; endotracheal intubation, tracheotomy, cricothyrotomy, or transtracheal catheterization for laryngeal edema; resuscitation, defibrillation, IV sodium bicarbonate, and other proper medications for cardiac arrest; mechanical airway use if the patient becomes unconscious; and oral or IV corticosteroids if reactions are prolonged. Monitor hypotension and, if necessary, administer vasopressors along with adequate plasma volume replacement. Rarely will all the above measures be necessary. Promptness in beginning emergency treatment is important.

Pharmacologic & Dosing Characteristics

Dosage: Progressive, escalating dose, modified by patient reactions to the injections. The suggested dosages provided below are based on the concentration of the greatest single allergen present (GSAP) in the prescription formula. Adult and pediatric doses are usually equivalent. Agitate vials thoroughly but gently before withdrawing each dose.

Read vial labels carefully; selecting the wrong vial may cause a 10-fold or greater dosage error and induce a severe systemic reaction. The activity in a small volume of injected extract is absorbed more rapidly than the same activity in a larger volume.

Diagnostic tests: Single-component extracts are the optimal choice for testing because combining extracts may reduce their independent concentrations to subdiagnostic levels. Second, in the event of a positive reaction, the component of the mixture that elicited the reaction will not be known.

Skin tests are usually applied to the flexor surface of the forearm, although the back may also be used. Avoid using the spinal column, because it is not as reactive as other areas.

Prick (puncture) tests: 10,000 to 100,000 AU/mL or 1:100 to 1:10 w/v or 1,000 to 2,000 PNU/mL. Wipe prick needles used for prick tests in a suitable manner after each skin puncture to avoid cross-contamination of skin test sites.

Intradermal (ID) tests: Perform ID tests only for those allergens eliciting a negative or questionable scratch or prick test result. Inject 0.05 mL of a 1 to 10 AU/mL or 1:1,000 to 1:100 w/v or 100 to 200 PNU/mL concentration. Use separate needles and syringes for each allergen during testing, to avoid cross-contamination of stock vials. Do not use the same needle for different patients.

Administer negative- and positive-control reagents consisting of plain diluent and a dilution of histamine phosphate (prick, 2.75 mg/mL; ID, 0.275 mg/mL) to all subjects to confirm the absence of reaction-inhibiting medications.

Therapeutic dose: Warning: Dilute concentrated extracts before initiation of therapy. Use separate needles and syringes for each allergen when compounding allergen-extract prescriptions, to avoid cross-contamination of stock vials.

Therapy begins with minute, subcutaneous doses of 1 or several allergen extracts individualized to each patient. Progressively escalate the dosage to a maintenance dose. Dosage reductions 50% or more or pauses in dose escalation are warranted if the patient misses a scheduled injection, when starting therapy from a new refill prescription (especially for extracts from a different manufacturer), or during corresponding pollination seasons. All extracts lose potency over time, and a fresh extract formula could have an effective potency that is substantially greater than that of the previous prescription set. Processing and source materials may differ markedly among manufacturers, and extracts from different manufacturers may not be directly interchangeable. Inadvertently challenging a hypersensitive patient directly with a full-strength antigen may result in anaphylaxis and death.

Initial therapy: Starting with 0.05 mL of 1 to 10 AU/mL or 1:100,000 to 1:10,000 w/v or 2 to 20 PNU/mL, with escalating doses every 3 to 14 days.

Maintenance therapy: 0.1 mL to 0.3 mL of 10,000 AU/mL or 0.5 mL of 1:100 w/v or 2,000 PNU/mL, repeated every 7 to 30 days.

Transfer from nonstandardized to AU- or BAU-standardized extracts: AU- and BAU-standardized extracts may be more potent than nonstandardized w/v or PNU extracts, and are not directly interchangeable with them. Therefore, use the standardized extract for the skin test on which the initial dose will be based. For patients being switched from nonstandardized to AU- or BAU-standardized extracts, perform skin testing with dilutions of both extracts, and compare the results for a basis for adjustment of the dose.

Recommended Maintenance Doses and Major Allergen Content of Allergen Immunotherapy		
Major allergen	Dose (standard units)	Maintenance concentrate (w/v)
D. pteronyssinus (Der p 1)	600 AU	7 to 12 mcg
D. farinae (Der f 1)	2,000 AU	10 mcg
Cat (Fel d 1)	2,000 to 3,000 BAU	11 to 17 mcg
Grass (eg, timothy) (Phl p 5)	4,000 BAU	7 mcg
Short ragweed (standard) (Amb a 1)	n/a	6 to 24 mcg
Non-standard pollen	n/a	1:100 to 1:30
Non-standard fungi/mold	n/a	1:100 to 1:50

Route: Subcutaneously. Never administer IV. ID or IM injections may produce large local reactions or be excessively painful. Injections of more than 0.2 mL of a 50% glycerin product may be painful. Use a syringe graduated in units of 0.01 mL to measure each dose. A 25- to 27-gauge, 1/4- to 5/8-inch needle may be preferred.

Additional Doses: Monthly or as indicated. Because of inexact potency measurement systems, clinicians typically reduce the dose when initiating maintenance therapy from a newly compounded extract prescription set.

Missed Doses: Resume therapy as soon as possible. Large intervals since the last allergen injection may necessitate a dose reduction to reduce the likelihood of an adverse allergic reaction.

After unusually long intervals since the last dose, the patient can be assessed by ID tests to serial dilutions of the patient's allergen-extract prescription formula. Such tests have been started with 0.02 mL of a 1:100,000 w/v concentration, escalating in 10-fold steps until 10 to

15 mm induration is observed or a 1:100 concentration is reached. Allergists have then resumed therapy at the same or a weaker concentration that evoked the reaction.

Efficacy: More than 70% to 90% of patients with a proper diagnosis will demonstrate an improvement in symptoms with adequate immunotherapy.

Onset: Symptomatic improvement may occur within 12 weeks of initiation of immunotherapy and increase over a period of 1 to 2 years.

Duration: Many clinicians recommend that immunotherapy continue for 2 to 5 years after patients report few or no symptoms during seasonal exposure to corresponding allergens.

Protective Level: Not established

Mechanism: IgG ("blocking antibody") specific to each allergen appears in human serum following injection of several doses of allergen extracts. This IgG is believed to compete for specific IgE ("reagin") generated by sensitization of the patient to a specific environmental antigen, but the specific mechanism of effectiveness is not known.

IgE fixes to the target cells (eg, mast cells, basophils) with its Fc portion. This allows the Fab fraction of the IgE to be available for binding to active sites on the allergen (eg, ragweed pollen). When the allergen has bridged 2 of the IgE molecules on the surface of the target cell, adenylate cyclase activity results in a rise in cyclic AMP (adenosine 3'5' cyclic monophosphate) and culminates in the release of chemical mediators such as histamine. Action of these mediators on target organs produces the allergic response.

In patients receiving allergen-extract immunotherapy, serum IgE levels increase initially, and then gradually decrease over several years, perhaps because immunotherapy reduces IgE production. Increased T-suppressor lymphocyte effect has also been noted. The complete mechanism of action of allergen extracts has not been defined.

Drug Interactions: H_1 antihistamines (eg, chlorpheniramine, diphenhydramine, hydroxyzine, promethazine) suppress skin test reactivity to allergen extracts, although the potency and duration of skin-test suppression vary. Long-acting H_1 antihistamines, such as astemizole, may interfere for as long as 6 weeks. Other drugs with H_1 antihistaminic effects, such as tricyclic antidepressants (TCAs), may also suppress immediate hypersensitivity responses. H_2 antihistamines (eg, cimetidine, ranitidine) do not decrease skin test responsiveness alone but may increase skin test suppression synergistically in combination with H_1 antihistamines.

Topical corticosteroids suppress dermal reactivity to allergen extracts locally. Oral corticosteroids appear to have no effect on immediate hypersensitivity skin test reactivity.

Use positive-control reagents (eg, histamine, codeine) in all subjects to confirm the absence of reaction-inhibiting medications.

Drugs that appear to have no effect on immediate-hypersensitivity reagents include oral aminophylline, ephedrine, fenoterol, terbutaline, theophylline, and the latter 2 drugs combined.

Pharmaceutical Characteristics

Concentration: Weight-to-volume (w/v) ratios and protein nitrogen units (PNU) are the 2 most widely used measurement systems. The relatively new allergy unit (AU) and bioequivalent allergy unit (BAU) have certain advantages over the other systems, primarily that of biological standardization in vivo.

W/V extraction ratios indicate the relative quantities of pollen or other allergen extracted per given volume of extraction fluid (or menstruum). W/V ratios of 1:10 or 1:20 (ie, 1 g of source material, such as pollen, per 10 or 20 mL fluid) are most common, although some products are marketed as 1:50 or 1:100 w/v dilutions. These ratios describe the manufacturing process, but do not reflect the allergenicity of the resulting product. Thus, the specific antigenic proteins extracted from the raw allergenic source material are not measured, nor is potency necessarily uniform from batch to batch.

PNU standardization measures the total protein content of a finished extract, usually by the Kjeldahl or Ninhydrin methods. One PNU contains 0.01 mcg of protein nitrogen. Unfortunately, this type of assay measures protein without regard to the presence, absence, or consistency of specific allergenic components. Most commercial PNU products contain 20,000 PNU/mL, although 5,000; 10,000; and 40,000 PNU/mL concentrations are available for some extracts.

Correlation of potency between the w/v and PNU systems is incomplete and inconsistent. PNU assays for 1:10 w/v allergen-extract products generally range from 12,000 to 150,000 PNU/mL, depending on the allergen. Grass extracts typically exhibit PNU content at the top of this range, while mold extracts tend to be found near the low end. W/V products of any given allergen routinely vary in their PNU content by as much as ± 25% between batches. Even pollens taken from plants grown in the same soil in successive years yield extracts of varying potency. If the active components of allergen extracts were available in pure form, then mass alone would suffice as a standardization method, as it does for most drugs. Unfortunately, much additional work is needed to identify each active ingredient of each allergen extract.

A new composite immunologic measurement system, allergy units (AU, initially called the allergenic unit), increases qualitative and quantitative uniformity and lot-to-lot reproducibility. The FDA first licensed these products in 1983. Their standardization is analogous to that used for insulin, that is, standardization by biological activity. AU or BAU standardization is a major advance in immunotherapy, because it is the first system to assure human potency of any given extract. Extracts standardized in allergy units are typically marketed at 10,000 AU/mL and 100,000 AU/mL, although *Dermatophagoides pteronyssinus* house-dust mite extracts are marketed at 5,000, 10,000, or 30,000 AU/mL, and cat extracts are marketed at 5,000 and 10,000 BAU/mL.

The AU- or BAU-standardization methods are not perfected; they measure composite activity of a product with numerous independent active ingredients. For example, the antigen Amb a 1 (formerly called antigen E) is a good indicator for predicting the relative potency of other companion antigenic determinants in a given lot of short-ragweed extract. But Amb a 1 alone is not sufficient to relieve allergic symptoms in most short-ragweed-sensitive patients. A more complex mixture of allergens is required to treat most patients hypersensitive to this pollen.

Any empiric comparison between the various standardization systems bears risks. Use comparisons only for general guidance. Converting patients from 1 system of immunotherapy to another must be done cautiously, preferably preceded with skin tests with the new extract(s). Do not combine allergens of different standardization types. Allergists commonly reject generic substitution of w/v and PNU allergen-extract products because of the lack of potency uniformity between manufacturers and between lots of any single manufacturer.

Allergen-extract prescription formulae may include up to a dozen or more constituent allergens. Such prescriptions may be labeled on the basis of total allergen content (TAC) or according to the concentration of the greatest single allergen present (GSAP) in the formula, according to prescriber preference. Exercise caution when allergen-extract prescriptions from both labeling systems are compounded or stored in the same location to avoid dosage errors. For example, a vial containing ten 1 mL portions of 1:10 w/v concentrates may either be labeled 1:100 w/v, based on the concentration of the greatest single allergen present, or 1:10 w/v, based on the total quantity of allergens present. Vials labeled 1:100 w/v under either system would actually vary from each other by a power of 10. Since each specific allergen can be considered to interact with the human immune system independently, labeling on a GSAP basis may be preferable, and is the convention adopted for this monograph. However, it may not be the system used by most allergists.

Many manufacturers market predetermined mixes of various related allergens, usually adopting the TAC labeling method. Do not use mixes for immunodiagnosis, since unique allergens may be diluted below a reactive concentration by the presence of other allergens. Do not include mixes in allergen-extract prescriptions unless the patient is hypersensitive by testing to each of the ingredients of the mix.

Quality Assay: The following products are available in biologically standardized formulations:

> Cat hair
> Cat pelt
> Insects (whole body, mite), *Dermatophagoides farinae*
> Insects (whole body, mite), *Dermatophagoides pteronyssinus*
> Pollen, Bermuda grass, *Cynodon dactylon*
> Pollen, Kentucky bluegrass (June), *Poa pratensis*
> Pollen, meadow fescue, *Festuca elatior*
> Pollen, orchard grass, *Dactylis glomerata*
> Pollen, redtop, *Agrostis alba*
> Pollen, perennial ryegrass, *Lolium perenne*
> Pollen, sweet vernal grass, *Anthoxanthum odoratum*
> Pollen, timothy grass, *Phleum pratense*
> Pollen, short ragweed, *Ambrosia artemisiifolia*
> Pollen, short ragweed, *Ambrosia elatior*

Most w/v- and PNU-assayed allergen-extract products sold in the United States bear the proviso "No US Standard of Potency." This caution is needed because w/v and PNU assays of allergen-extract concentrations have only a limited correlation to biological and immunologic activity.

Pollen extracts may contain no more than 1% foreign pollens as determined by microscopic examination. Since January 27, 1982, extracts of short ragweed (*Ambrosia artemisiifolia* [*elatior*]) have been required to have an antigen E (Amb a 1) content of at least 135 units per mL for 1:10 w/v extracts and at least 67.5 units/mL for 1:20 w/v extracts, as measured by a radial immunodiffusion test. One antigen E unit is approximately equal to 1 mcg antigen E per mL. AU-standardized extracts at a 100,000 AU/mL concentration must contain 200 to 400 antigen E units per mL. Short-ragweed extracts are labeled with a potency declaration of the antigen E content in each vial.

Cat extracts labeled as 5,000 BAU/mL must contain 5 to 9.9 Fel d 1 units/mL. Cat extracts labeled as 10,000 BAU/mL must contain 10 to 19.9 Fel d 1 units/mL.

Mold extracts are most commonly derived from pure mold cultures obtained from the American Type Culture Collection (ATCC) and grown on synthetic, nonallergenic, nonproteinaceous liquid media.

Allergenicity, purity, and immunogenicity may be variously assessed by pH, pyrogen testing, radioallergosorbent test (RAST) inhibition, isoelectric focusing (IEF), crossed radioimmunoelectrophoresis (CRIE), quantitative immunoelectrophoresis, and quantitative skin testing.

Packaging: 1, 1.5, 5, 10, and 15 mL dropper bottles for prick-puncture skin testing; 1, 2, 5, 10, 20, 30, and 50 mL sterile vials for ID testing and compounding allergen-extract prescriptions. Various sterile diluents are packaged in vials of 1.8, 4, 4.5, 9, 30, and 100 mL and other volumes.

NDC Number: Company series: ALK—53298 or 52709; Allergy Laboratories (Oklahoma)—54575; Allermed—49643; Antigen—49288; Greer—22840; Hollister-Stier—65044; Nelco—36987.

Doseform: Suspension, solution, or powder for solution

Appearance: Clear to dark brown or black solutions. Precipitates may develop during storage, apparently without affecting potency.

Lyophilized extracts appear as a white or yellow-tinged powder or cake. Some extracts (eg, grain extracts, mushroom, avocado, privet) are normally very dark or may darken progressively in phenol-containing diluents. Do not use such extracts for immunotherapy, because they may leave residual pigmentation at injection sites.

Solvent: Allergen extracts may be manufactured in either aqueous or glycerinated form. Lyophilized and glycerinated extracts are the most stable forms. Stock containers of water-based (aqueous) allergen extracts typically contain constituents of the diluting fluid (eg, sodium chloride, sodium bicarbonate) and are usually preserved with phenol.

Diluent: Dilute aqueous extracts with a solution containing 0.03% human serum albumin (HSA) as a protein stabilizer, 0.9% sodium chloride for tonicity, and 0.4% phenol as an antimicrobial agent. Extracts in a solution with 50% glycerin offer a higher degree of protein preservation, but glycerin injections may cause local irritation or sterile abscesses. Glycerin is often used in the diluent for prick skin test dilutions, because its viscosity retards the flow of 1 prick-test reagent into neighboring reagents. However, glycerin may also increase the incidence of false-positive skin-test reactions, especially in the higher dose associated with ID injection. Label all vials with the concentration of their contents.

Suboptimal fluids for compounding dilutions of aqueous allergen extracts include phenol-saline (0.9% sodium chloride with 0.4% phenol), phosphate-buffered saline (eg, 0.5% sodium chloride with 0.08% to 0.11% sodium phosphate, 0.036% to 0.04% potassium phosphate, and 0.4% phenol), bicarbonate-saline (Coca's solution: 0.5% sodium chloride, 0.275% sodium bicarbonate, 0.4% phenol), and various glycero-saline solutions (eg, 10% glycerin with 0.5% sodium chloride and 0.4% phenol; 25% glycerin with 0.5% sodium chloride, sodium phosphate, potassium phosphate, and 0.4% phenol). Undiluted sterile parenteral glycerin, with a glycerin content of 95% or more, is available from several manufacturers.

By professional consensus, the following scheme has been adopted by allergists in the United States to designate the relative dilutions of allergen-extract prescriptions:

Color Scheme for Allergen Extract Dilutions	
Dilution strength	Cap color
Maintenance concentrate	red-capped vial
10-fold dilution	yellow-capped vial
100-fold dilution	blue-capped vial
1,000-fold dilution	green-capped vial
≥ 10,000-fold dilution	silver-capped vial

Adjuvant: None

Preservative: Usually 0.4% or 0.5% phenol; 0.01% thimerosal is used if the allergen may darken or precipitate in the presence of phenol (eg, extracts of privet pollen, mushroom, grain mill dust, white potato, avocado; food extracts of corn, barley, oat, rye, and wheat).

Allergens: Allergen extracts are allergenic by definition and intent. HSA, used in many diluents, does not sensitize recipients.

Excipients: Mannitol in some lyophilized products. Extracts may contain varying amounts of sodium chloride, sodium bicarbonate, sodium carbonate, calcium carbonate, sodium phosphate, potassium phosphate, magnesium phosphate, potassium citrate, or glycerin.

pH: 6 to 8.5

Shelf Life: Products containing 50% or more glycerin expire within 36 months, less than 50% glycerin within 18 months. Short-ragweed extracts expire within 12 months. Lyophilized products expire within 30 to 48 months.

Storage/Stability: Store at 2° to 8°C (36° to 46°F). Do not freeze.

Discard extracts after inadvertent freezing. Lyophilized extracts are variously stored at room temperature or under refrigeration; consult package labeling for details. While any elevated temperatures will speed protein degradation, allergen extracts containing 50% glycerin can typically tolerate 10 days or more at ambient room temperatures or 7 days at elevated temperatures. Typically shipped by overnight or second-day courier or first-class mail at ambient temperature.

Stability of allergen extracts is briefest at low concentrations because of protein adsorption to glass containers. Protein degradation and enzymatic autodigestion also reduce potency. Stability is favored by low temperatures; however, freezing may precipitate some proteins, especially those of high molecular weight.

Because of the intricacies of compounding and the potency variation of 1 prescription formula to the next, 12-month expiration dates for full-strength vials are frequently adopted. Shorter dating is common for more dilute concentrations. For AU-standardized products, 30 to 36 month stability is appropriate for concentrated extracts containing 50% glycerin at a concentration of 1,000 to 100,000 AU/mL, 4 months after reconstitution with an aqueous diluent at 100,000 AU/mL, 2 months at 50,000 AU/mL, and 3 weeks at 10,000 AU/mL. Concentrations up to 1,000 AU/mL demonstrate acceptable stability for 7 to 14 days, although some advocate 24-hour dating.

Extracts with high proteolytic activity (eg, molds, cockroach) may be mixed together, but should not be combined with extracts with low protease activity (eg, grasses, trees, weeds, danders).

Production Process: Preparation of an allergen extract may involve some or all of the following series of steps: 1) grinding of the source material, 2) defatting using an aromatic solvent, 3) extraction for 16 to 72 hours, 4) clarification or preliminary filtration, 5) dialysis to remove irritating substances and coloring materials (the utility of this step is controversial), 6) concentration by evaporation, 7) sterilization by filtration, 8) lyophilization, if applicable, 9) sterility testing, 10) standardization or potency measurement, and 11) general safety tests.

Media: Various biological sources

Disease Epidemiology

Prevalence: Based on skin test reactivity, allergic rhinitis affects 5% to 22% of the general population, and is the sixth most prevalent disease in the United States. It affects an estimated 22 million Americans. An estimated 5 million Americans are allergic to cat allergen. Some 1.4 million Americans receive immunotherapy, comprising some 35 million injections annually, probably the greatest single potential source of drug-induced anaphylaxis risk.

Other Information

Perspective:

1873: Blackley performs a skin test as a means to identify substances causing allergic symptoms.

1906: von Pirquet introduces the term *allergie* to describe reactions deviating from the norm.

1911: Noon and Freeman independently perform "hyposensitization" therapy for "hay fever" by injection of pollen extracts.

1915: Allergen extracts first licensed in the United States.

1935: Cooke notes that blocking antibodies (specific IgG) develop in patients treated with immunotherapy.

1941: Criep opens centralized allergen-extract laboratory at the Pittsburgh Veterans Administration Hospital.

1976: Guilbert opens US Army centralized allergen-extract pharmacy at the Walter Reed Army Medical Center.

1983: Allergy-unit (AU) standardized extracts licensed.

Specific Considerations by Type of Allergen:

Nomenclature: The nomenclature system for individual allergens was developed by the International Union of Immunological Societies. The system is based on the first 3 letters of the genus, followed by the first letter of the species, and then an Arabic number. For example, antigen E of short ragweed (*Ambrosia artemisiifolia [elatior]*) is now called Amb a 1.

Epidermal Allergens: Animal dander hypersensitivity is best treated by eliminating contact with the allergen, and hence the animal. Immunotherapy may lead to local or systemic reactions to the injections if the patient remains exposed to a constant high level of antigen.

Standardized Cat Hair Extract is not directly interchangeable with Standardized Cat Pelt Extract, nor with nonstandardized cat extracts. Cat hair and cat pelt extracts are similar in content of Fel d 1, the major allergen among cat-sensitive patients. Pelt extracts, however, contain large amounts of cat serum or albumin in addition to Fel d 1. Although approximately 97% of cat-sensitive patients respond primarily to Fel d 1, 3% also have an exquisite response to components other than Fel d 1. These latter patients may respond more to cat-pelt extracts. Given the difference in allergenic components, do not interchange these extracts during therapy. To switch patients from 1 product to the other, base the initial dose on skin tests using the new extract. Since October 1992, w/v and PNU designations are not included on cat extracts; similarly, the terms cat epithelia and cat dander are no longer used.

Bayer produced a line of acetone-precipitated epidermal allergen extracts (*Albay AP*) by reconstituting dry allergenically active concentrates precipitated from raw material extracts. For AP extracts labeled w/v, the ratio represents the dry weight of finished acetone precipitate per volume of reconstituting fluid. Hollister-Stier calls this process the Hollister-Stier AP Process.

Foods: The FDA licenses food extracts for immunodiagnosis only. There is no convincing evidence that food allergen extracts are safe and effective for immunotherapy. Foods for extracts are defatted and dehydrated before extraction. While most foods are extracted in aqueous buffered solution, some are extracted with a fluid containing 0.1% sodium formaldehyde sulfoxylate to prevent oxidation. Some food extracts are extremely potent, such as peanut extract. Egg-white extract may develop an insoluble precipitate following agitation during normal handling.

Grasses: Grass antigens may be somewhat more reactogenic than other categories of antigens. As a result, many clinicians administer them on a more conservative basis. Grasses tend to pollinate most heavily during summer months. Studies of grass allergen cross-reactivity have been published.

Insects: Extracts of common house-dust mites (*Dermatophagoides farinae* and *D. pteronyssinus*) are the only insect extracts to be standardized in allergy units (AU/mL), the modern system of biological potency measurement. Of the 2 species, *D. farinae* is found most commonly in the United States, although *D. pteronyssinus* predominates in certain coastal regions. Mites are typically grown on a yeast and pork medium under a process that limits residual medium content to less than 1%. The medium contains no material of human origin.

Harvester ants (genus *Pogonomyrmex*) rarely have been reported to cause anaphylaxis, but whole-body extracts of these insects are not readily available. Commercially available whole-body extracts of insects not members of the biological order *Hymenoptera* include black, red, and carpenter ants; American, German, and Oriental cockroaches; deer and black flies, sweat bees, mosquitoes (ie, *Aedes aegyptii, Culex pipiens*), and house-dust mites. But none of these insects is likely to evoke potentially fatal allergic reactions in its victims.

Whole-body extracts (WBE) of *Hymenoptera* insects are discussed in a separate monograph.

Molds: Mold extracts are most commonly derived from pure mold cultures obtained from the American Type Culture Collection (ATCC) and grown on synthetic, nonallergenic, protein-free liquid media.

MMP: Process mold extracts are produced by Hollister-Stier under a license from the Association of Allergists for Mycological Investigations. MMP are the initials of the 3 prime inventors of the method. Some clinicians consider MMP-process extracts to be more potent and free from nonspecific irritants than previous w/v or PNU extracts, and consequently more specific and effective, although the FDA has not accepted these claims as valid. The strongest concentrations available are 1:100 w/v in either 50% glycerin or buffered sodium chloride. PNU-standardized MMP extracts are also available. The suggested maximum maintenance dose for each MMP allergen is 0.5 mL of a 1:1,000 w/v concentration.

Allergen Extracts, Aqueous & Glycerinated

Aspergillus Skin Test Reagent: Aspergillus extracts are effective for skin test diagnosis of bronchopulmonary aspergillosis and probably effective for immunotherapy of asthma and rhinitis. They are not effective for immunotherapy of bronchopulmonary aspergillosis. Immunodeficiency increases susceptibility to infection, yet may decrease skin test responsiveness.

Aspergillus is a genus of molds. *Aspergillus fumigatus, A. niger*, and *A. flavus* are the most common causes of human disease. Extracts are manufactured by several allergen-extract producers in concentrates of 1:5, 1:10, and 1:20 w/v.

For immunodiagnosis, apply appropriate scratch or ID tests. A reaction is generally considered positive when 5 to more than 10 mm induration occurs 10 minutes after administration. If a strongly positive reaction does not occur within 15 minutes, then a second test at a higher concentration may be injected. Late reactions 4 to 6 hours after injection are considered positive if an area of redness and edema appears that is more than 15 mm in diameter.

Trees: Trees tend to pollinate most heavily during spring months. A study of tree allergen cross-reactivity has been published.

Weeds: Antigen E, a major allergen in short-ragweed extracts, is used as an indicator of the potency of extracts produced from this plant's pollen. Antigen E has a molecular weight of 38,000 daltons. Since January 27, 1982, extracts of short ragweed (*Ambrosia artemisiifolia [elatior]*) must exhibit an antigen E (Amb a 1) content of at least 135 units per mL for 1:10 or 67.5 units/mL or more for 1:20, as measured by a radial immunodiffusion test. One antigen E unit is approximately equal to 1 mcg antigen E per mL. AU-standardized extracts at a 100,000 AU/mL concentration contain 200 to 400 antigen E units per mL. Other significant allergens in short-ragweed extracts include antigen K (Amb a 2), Ra-3 (Amb a 3), Ra-5 (Amb a 5), and others.

Weeds tend to pollinate most heavily during late summer and fall months. A study of weed allergen cross-reactivity has been published.

House Dust: Allergenic constituents of house dust consist primarily of mites (*Dermatophagoides farinae* and *D. pteronyssinus*), animal danders (especially cat), hair, foods, feathers, detergents, mold spores, fibers, dust silk, pollens, and other inhalants. Nonspecific irritants and dyes may be removed during processing by dialysis. Because source material is widely inconsistent between manufacturers, but less inconsistent for any one manufacturer or production process, use the same type of dust extract for testing and for immunotherapy, if indicated.

Greer Laboratories produces a house-dust extract that is dialyzed and concentrated to 1:1 w/v. Hollister-Stier produces an acetone-precipitated (*Albay AP*) house-dust extract by reconstituting dry allergenically active concentrates precipitated from extracts of raw materials. For AP extracts labeled on a w/v basis, the ratio represents the dry weight of finished acetone precipitate per volume of reconstituting fluid.

Discontinued Products: *Panoral* (Eli Lilly); *Polligens* (Lederle)

References: Bernstein IL, Li JT, Bernstein DI, et al. Allergy diagnostic testing: An updated practice parameter. *Ann Allergy Asthma Immunol.* 2008:100(suppl):S1-S148.

Chapman JA, Bernstein IL, Lee RE, et al. Food allergy: A practice parameter. *Ann Allergy Asthma Immunol.* 2006;96(3 Suppl 2): S1-68.

Cox L, Williams B, Sicherer S, et al; American College of Allergy, Asthma and Immunology Test Task Force; American Academy of Allergy, Asthma and Immunology Specific IgE Test Task Force. Pearls and pitfalls of allergy diagnostic testing: report from the American College of Allergy, Asthma and Immunology/American Academy of Allergy, Asthma and Immunology Specific IgE Test Task Force. *Ann Allergy Asthma Immunol.* 2008;101(6):580-592.

Joint Task Force on Practice Parameters; American Academy of Allergy, Asthma and Immunology; American College of Allergy, Asthma and Immunology; Joint Council of Allergy, Asthma and Immunology. Allergen immunotherapy: a practice parameter second update [published corrections appear in *J Allergy Clin Immunol.* 2009;123(6):1421. *J Allergy Clin Immunol.* 2008;122(4):842]. *J Allergy Clin Immunol.* 2007;120(3 suppl):S25-S85.

Malling HJ. Minimizing the risks of allergen-specific injection immunotherapy. *Drug Saf.* 2000;23:323-332.

WHO/IUIS Allergen Nomenclature Subcommittee. Allergen nomenclature. *J Allergy Clin Immunol.* 1995;96:5-14.

Allergen Extracts

Standard Concentrations & Dosages of Allergen Extracts for Diagnosis & Therapy[a]

Parameter	Diagnostic tests		Immunotherapy dosage[b]		Frequency	
	Prick	Intradermal	Initial	Maintenance	Initial	Maintenance
Immunometric	10,000 to 100,000 AU/mL	1 to 10 AU/mL	0.05 mL of 1 to 10 AU/mL	0.1 to 0.3 mL of 10,000 AU/mL	3 to 14 days	7 to 30 days
Weight/volume	1/100 to 1/10 w/v	1/1,000 to 1/100 w/v	0.05 mL of 1/100,000 w/v	0.5 mL of 1/100 w/v	3 to 14 days	7 to 30 days
Protein nitrogen units	1,000 to 2,000 PNU/mL	100 to 200 PNU/mL	0.05 mL of 2 PNU/mL	0.5 mL of 2,000 PNU/mL	3 to 14 days	7 to 30 days

a Concentration comparisons are provided for general reference only. AU, w/v, and PNU systems are not directly interchangeable nor biologically equivalent in potency. Adult and pediatric doses are usually equivalent.
b Dosage based on concentration of greatest single allergen present (GSAP).

Allergen Extracts, Alum-Precipitated

Allergen Extracts

Name:
Center-Al

Manufacturer:
ALK-Abelló

Comparison: Not generically equivalent to other allergen extracts. Do not combine alum-precipitated products with other allergen extracts in the same prescription.

Immunologic Characteristics

Antigen Source: Grasses, trees, weeds, house dust

Viability: Not viable, but antigenically active

Antigenic Form: Allergen extract, adsorbed to aluminum salt

Antigenic Type: Proteins and other constituents

Strains: Multiple species, refer to container label

Use Characteristics

Indications: For induction of active immunity against subsequent hypersensitivity reactions, for the treatment of patients whose histories indicate that they experience allergic symptoms upon natural exposure to certain allergens.

Limitations: Very young children, geriatric patients, or those suffering from autoimmune disorders or severe and unstable allergic disorders may not respond to immunotherapy.

Contraindications:

Absolute: None

Relative: Do not immunize patients against a substance against which they have not demonstrated symptoms or IgE antibodies. There is inconclusive evidence that routine immunization with allergen extracts may exacerbate autoimmune diseases. Children with nephrotic syndrome probably should not receive immunotherapy. Other relative contraindications include patients experiencing severe respiratory or cardiovascular distress and patients who have experienced an anaphylactic reaction to the offending allergen. Weigh the risks of therapy against its benefits.

Patients with Alzheimer disease, Down syndrome, and renal insufficiency are theoretically at risk from aluminum intake, including alum-precipitated allergenic extracts.

Temporarily withhold allergen extracts from patients or reduce the dose if any of the following conditions occur:

(1) severe symptoms of rhinitis or asthma,

(2) infection accompanied by fever, or

(3) exposure to excessive amounts of clinically relevant allergen prior to a scheduled injection.

Patient compliance is an important consideration in the decision to initiate immunotherapy with any potent allergen extract. Do not initiate therapy if the patient cannot be depended on to respond promptly and properly to an impending adverse reaction.

Patients receiving beta-adrenergic antagonists (ie, beta-blockers) may be refractory to the effects of epinephrine, which may be needed to treat anaphylactic reactions.

Immunodeficiency: Immune response and resultant reduction in symptoms hypothetically may be impaired in immunocompromised persons.

Elderly: Geriatric patients may not respond to immunotherapy.

Pregnancy: Category C. Use only if clearly needed. Immunotherapy has been continued during pregnancy but is not generally initiated during it. Consider the risk-benefit ratio. An anaphylactic reaction may induce a miscarriage due to uterine muscle contractions. It is not known if allergen extracts or corresponding antibodies cross the placenta. Generally, most IgG passage across the placenta occurs during the third trimester.

Lactation: It is not known if allergen extracts or corresponding antibodies cross into human breast milk. Problems in humans have not been documented.

Children: Children older than 2 years of age appear to tolerate allergen-extract injections well. Adult and pediatric maintenance doses are usually equivalent. If the injection volume is too large for a small child to tolerate comfortably, split the dose among several injections.

Adverse Reactions: Anaphylaxis may occur without warning, even during the maintenance phase of therapy. Observe patients for at least 20 to 30 minutes after each allergen-extract injection and instruct them to return promptly if symptoms of an allergic reaction or shock occur. Adverse reactions that do occur may be delayed in onset by 1 hour or more, compared with minutes for nonprecipitated forms of allergen extracts. The more quickly symptoms appear, the more severe they are likely to be and the more rapidly treatment measures should be instituted. Anaphylaxis may be a greater concern in asthmatic patients already experiencing allergic respiratory symptoms. Only conduct immunotherapy in facilities with adequate equipment and medications and personnel trained to respond to anaphylaxis.

Local reactions at the site of injection may be immediate or delayed. Immediate induration and erythema reactions are ordinarily of little consequence, but if very large may be the first manifestation of a systemic reaction. If large local reactions occur, observe the patient for systemic symptoms. Delayed reactions start several hours after injection with local edema, erythema, itching, or pain. These usually peak at 24 hours and require no treatment, although oral antihistamines may be of benefit. Reduce the next therapeutic dose to the last dose that did not elicit a reaction, and increase subsequent doses more slowly through the use of intermediate dilutions if needed. Question patients before each dose regarding delayed manifestations that may have developed since the last clinic visit.

Injection site: The incidence of subcutaneous nodules increases with higher dosage of individual products and with extemporaneous mixtures at lower dosage. Do not deliver more than 5,000 PNU in any single dose, whether as a single allergen or mixture, and do not exceed 0.5 mL in volume. If nodules occur, limit the highest single dose administered to a maximum of 0.2 mL (2,000 PNU).

Systemic: Sneezing, mild to severe generalized urticaria, itching other than at the injection site, extensive or generalized edema, wheezing, asthma, dyspnea, cyanosis, tachycardia, lacrimation, marked perspiration, cough, hypotension, syncope, or upper airway obstruction. Symptoms may progress to anaphylactic shock and death. After a systemic reaction, reduce the next therapeutic dose to the last dose that did not elicit a reaction, and increase subsequent doses more slowly through the use of intermediate dilutions.

Pharmacologic & Dosing Characteristics

Dosage: Shake vial thoroughly before withdrawing each dose. Read vial labels carefully, because selecting the wrong vial may cause a 10-fold or greater dosage error and potentially cause a severe systemic reaction. The following are suggested dosages based on the concentration of the greatest single allergen present (GSAP) in the formula. Adult and pediatric doses are usually equivalent.

Diagnosis: Do not use alum-precipitated allergen extracts for diagnosis. Use aqueous allergen extracts at concentrations described in that monograph.

Therapeutic dose: Warning—Concentrated extracts must be diluted before initiation of therapy. Use separate needles and syringes for each allergen when compounding allergen-extract prescriptions to avoid cross-contamination of stock vials.

Therapy begins with minute subcutaneous doses of one or several allergen extracts individualized to each patient. Progressively escalate the dosage to a maintenance dose. Dosage reductions or pauses in dose escalation are warranted if the patient misses a scheduled injection, when starting therapy from a new refill prescription, or during corresponding pollination seasons.

Initial dose: 0.1 mL of 100 PNU/mL, with escalating doses every 7 to 14 days.

Maintenance dose: 0.5 mL of 1,000 PNU/mL, with additional doses every 2 to 6 weeks. Do not give a maintenance dose less than 3 weeks before the expected onset of the pollination season.

Transfer of therapy from aqueous allergens to alum-precipitated allergens: To avoid untoward reactions, initiate treatment as though the patient was previously untreated. In transferring from standardized extracts, consider the more rapid rate of decline in activity of aqueous extracts relative to alum-precipitated extracts in cautiously transferring patients to alum-precipitated extract. This current recommendation is more cautious than the previous, outdated guidance to make the first dose of alum-precipitated allergen equal to the last dose of PNU-standardized aqueous extract.

Transfer of therapy from alum-precipitated allergens to aqueous allergens: To avoid untoward reactions, disregard previous therapy and initiate treatment as though the patient was previously untreated. Relate the first dose of alum-precipitated extract to the patient's hypersensitivity, determined by clinical history and confirmed by skin testing. Patients who tolerate a particular dose of alum-precipitated extract may be prone to a severe constitutional reaction when injected with a lesser amount of water-soluble free antigen.

The maximum dose of Center-Al varies among available allergens: 0.6 mL for most pollens, and 0.24 mL for molds.

Route: Subcutaneously, preferably in the upper outer aspects of the arm, using a 25- or 26-gauge, ½- to ¾-inch needle. Use a syringe graduated in units of 0.01 mL to measure each dose.

Additional Doses: 0.5 mL of 1,000 PNU/mL, every 2 to 8 weeks

Missed Doses: Resume therapy as soon as possible. Large intervals since the last allergen injection (eg, longer than 6 to 8 weeks) may necessitate a dose reduction to reduce the risk of systemic reactions.

Efficacy: More than 70% to 90% of patients with a proper diagnosis will demonstrate an improvement in symptoms with adequate immunotherapy.

Onset: Symptomatic improvement may occur within 12 weeks of initiation of immunotherapy and increase over a period of 1 to 2 years.

Duration: Many clinicians recommend that immunotherapy continue for 2 to 5 years after patients report few or no symptoms during seasonal exposure to corresponding allergens.

Protective Level: Not established

Mechanism: Adsorption of the allergen onto the aluminum moiety appears to slow the biologic release of the allergen, with a consequent prolongation of the antigenic stimulus, allowing faster dosage progression to a higher maintenance dose, higher IgG responses, better relief of symptoms as related to dose, and fewer immediate adverse reactions. Nodule formation may limit therapy in some patients.

Like aqueous allergen extracts, recipients of alum-precipitated extracts develop IgG ("blocking antibody") specific to each allergen following injection of several doses. This IgG is believed to compete for specific IgE ("reagin") generated by sensitization of the patient to a specific environmental antigen.

Bound to receptors on mast cells, the IgE produces allergic reactions through the release of histamine and other mediators upon coupling with an antigen, such as ragweed pollen. In patients receiving allergen-extract immunotherapy, serum IgE levels increase initially and then gradually decrease over several years, perhaps because immunotherapy reduces IgE production. The complete mechanism of action of allergen extracts has not been defined.

Drug Interactions: Do not mix alum-precipitated allergen extracts with any non-alum containing allergens, nor mix the two forms of alum-precipitated extracts in a single prescription. Such mixing may free the alum-adsorbed allergens.

Pharmaceutical Characteristics

Concentration: 10,000 PNU per mL; some allergens are available at 20,000 PNU per mL.

Quality Assay: Most PNU-assayed allergen-extract products sold in the United States bear the proviso "No US Standard of Potency." This caution is needed because PNU assays of allergen-extract concentrations have only a limited correlation to biological and immunologic activity. Pollen extracts contain up to 1% extraneous pollens as determined by microscopic examination. For extracts of short ragweed (*Ambrosia artemisiifolia* [*elatior*]), the antigen E (Amb a I) content must be at least 135 units per mL, as measured by a radial immunodiffusion test of redissolved alum precipitate. Short-ragweed extracts are labeled with a potency declaration of the antigen E content in each vial.

Allergenicity, purity, and immunogenicity may be variously assessed by pH, pyrogen testing, radioallergosorbent test (RAST) inhibition, isoelectric focusing (IEF), crossed radioimmunoelectrophoresis (CRIE), and quantitative immunoelectrophoresis.

Packaging: 10 or 30 mL vial

NDC Number:

Company series: ALK: 53298 or 52709

Doseform: Suspension

Appearance: Off-white to light or dark brown translucent suspension

Solvent: Stock containers typically contain constituents of the diluting fluid (menstruum; eg, sodium chloride, sodium bicarbonate) and usually are preserved with phenol.

Diluent: Dilute alum-precipitated suspensions of allergen extracts with 0.9% sodium chloride with 0.4% phenol ("phenol-saline") only. Admixture of alum-precipitated allergen extracts with any diluent containing buffers will disrupt the prolonged-release character and result in resolution of some of the alum-complexed allergen, thereby producing the immediate bioavailability of the allergens. HSA may be used, but the albumin content offers no stability advantage for alum-precipitated products. Label all vials with the concentration of their contents.

Adjuvant: Each maximum recommended dose contains aluminum hydroxide not to exceed 0.85 mg aluminum per 0.5 mL.

Preservative: 0.4% phenol

Allergens: Allergen extracts are allergenic by definition and intent.

Excipients: Extracts may contain varying amounts of sodium chloride, sodium bicarbonate, sodium carbonate, calcium carbonate, sodium phosphate, potassium phosphate, magnesium phosphate, or potassium citrate.

pH: 6.3 to 7.2

Shelf Life: Expires within 18 months.

Storage/Stability: Store at 2° to 8°C (36° to 46°F). Discard if frozen, because freezing may cause agglomeration and degrade potency. Contact manufacturer regarding prolonged exposure to room temperature or elevated temperatures. Typically shipped by second-day courier or first-class mail at ambient temperature.

Stability of allergen extracts is shortest at low concentrations because of protein adsorption to the walls of glass containers. Protein degradation and enzymatic autodigestion also degrade potency. Stability is favored by low temperatures, although freezing may precipitate some proteins, especially those of high molecular weight.

Because of the intricacies of compounding and the potency variation of one prescription formula to the next, 12-month expiration dates for full-strength vials are used frequently. Use shorter dating for more dilute vials.

Production Process: Prepared from freshly extracted aqueous allergen extracts by aseptic precipitation with aluminum potassium sulfate ("alum," $AlK(SO_4)_2 \cdot 12H_2O$) at a neutral pH to preclude denaturation of the allergen fractions, creating a complex with aluminum hydroxide. Higher molecular weight antigens, such as antigen E, are adsorbed to the alum gel. Lower molecular weight materials not adsorbed are washed out by extensive treatment of the precipitate with 0.9% sodium chloride. This process removes about half the total PNU of the aqueous phase, enriching the final product with those higher molecular weight fractions adsorbed to the gel.

Media: Various biological sources

Disease Epidemiology

See Allergen Extracts, Aqueous & Glycerinated monograph.

Other Information

Perspective: See Allergen Extracts, Aqueous & Glycerinated monograph.

First Licensed:
Center Laboratories: October 19, 1971.

Discontinued Products: *Allpyral* (Hollister Stier, later Miles and Bayer)

References: Grammer LC, Shaughnessy MA. Immunotherapy with modified allergens. *Immunol Allergy Clin N Amer.* 1992;12:95-105.

Hymenoptera Venom/Venom Protein

Hymenoptera Allergens

Names:
Pharmalgen
Albay, Venomil

Manufacturers:
ALK-Abelló Laboratories
Hollister-Stier Corporation

Synonyms: Stinging insect venoms

Comparison: For honey bee, white-faced hornet, and yellow hornet venoms, the two marketed *Hymenoptera* venom sources are generically equivalent. The species mix of wasp, yellow jacket, and mixed-vespid venoms vary slightly between manufacturers; skin testing may be appropriate before interchanging the two brands.

Immunologic Characteristics

Antigen Source: Venoms of flying insects of the order *Hymenoptera*.

Five distinct venoms are marketed, along with 1 premixed combination:
Honey bee (*Apis mellifera*), family Apidae, subfamily Apinae;
Wasp (*Polistes* species), family Vespidae, subfamily Polistinae;
White-faced hornet (*Dolichovespula maculata*), family Vespidae, subfamily Vespinae;
Yellow hornet (*Dolichovespula arenaria*), family Vespidae, subfamily Vespinae; and
Yellow jacket (*Vespula* species), family Vespidae, subfamily Vespinae.
Venoms of the 2 hornets and yellow jackets are mixed in equal proportion and traditionally called mixed-vespid venom. Nonetheless, the term "vespine wasps" is taxonomically more correct for this group of insects.
Species content: The exact species content ratio of a given lot of wasp, yellow jacket, or mixed-vespid venoms is available by calling Hollister-Stier. The content ratio of these ALK venoms is fixed (although the data is proprietary) and does not vary between lots.

Viability: Not viable, but antigenically active

Antigenic Form: Purified venom

Antigenic Type: Protein. Skin tests assess immediate (type I) hypersensitivity.

Strains: Three venoms are derived from a single species of insects: Honey bee (*Apis mellifera*), white-faced hornet (*Dolichovespula maculata*), and yellow hornet (*D. arenaria*). The species mix of wasp, yellow jacket, and mixed-vespid venoms varies slightly between manufacturers.

Wasp venom marketed by ALK includes the species *Polistes annularis*, *Polistes exclamans*, *Polistes fuscatus*, *Polistes metricus*, and *Polistes apachus*. Wasp venom marketed by Hollister-Stier may include any of the following species: *Polistes annularis*, *Polistes apachus*, *Polistes canadensis*, *Polistes carolinus*, *Polistes comanchus*, *Polistes dorsalis*, *Polistes exclamans*, *Polistes flavus*, *Polistes fuscatus*, *Polistes instabilis*, *Polistes kaibabensis*, *Polistes major*, *Polistes metricus*, *Polistes pacificus*, and *Polistes perplexus*.

Yellow jacket venom produced by ALK includes the species *Vespula vulgaris*, *Vespula squamosa*, *Vespula germanica*, *Vespula pensylvanica*, *Vespula flavopilosa*, and *Vespula maculifrons*; the same venom produced by Hollister-Stier includes *Vespula vulgaris*, *Vespula squamosa*, *Vespula germanica*, and *Vespula maculifrons*.

Use Characteristics

Indications: For confirmatory diagnosis of hypersensitivity and for induction of active immunity against subsequent hypersensitivity reactions.

Skin testing with insect venoms aids in correlating the presence of IgE antibodies with the patient's symptoms. Dilutions of insect venoms help assess the hypersensitivity of the patient and whether the patient should begin immunotherapy.

Patients with a history of systemic reaction to *Hymenoptera* stings and a positive skin test to an ID venom injection of 1 mcg/mL have approximately a 60% chance of reacting again when stung by the same species of insect.

Immunotherapy is indicated for the prevention of subsequent systemic reactions to specific insect stings or a reduction in the severity of such reactions. Venom immunotherapy is indicated if the patient has a positive venom skin test and a history of generalized urticaria or angioedema, respiratory difficulty, or vascular collapse following a sting.

Limitations: Children who manifest mild, non-life-threatening systemic reactions that affect only the skin after natural stings do not benefit from venom immunotherapy and should not be treated. Similarly, do not treat adults with a positive symptomatic history but negative skin tests.

Alternative Tests: The radioallergosorbent test (RAST) is an alternative to diagnostic skin testing with purified *Hymenoptera* venom, but is less sensitive and yields more false-negative results.

Contraindications:

Absolute: None

Relative: Do not start patients with negative ID skin tests at 1 mcg/mL on immunotherapy. There is inconclusive evidence that routine immunization may exacerbate autoimmune disease; give immunotherapy cautiously to these patients and only if the risk from insect stings is greater than the risk of exacerbating an underlying disorder.

Patient compliance is an important consideration in the decision to initiate immunotherapy with any potent allergen extract. Do not initiate therapy if the patient cannot be depended on to respond promptly and properly to an impending adverse reaction.

Patients receiving beta-adrenergic antagonists (ie, beta blockers) may be refractory to the effects of epinephrine, which may be needed to treat anaphylactic reactions.

Immunodeficiency: Immune response and protection may be impaired in immunocompromised patients.

Elderly: Geriatric patients may not respond to immunotherapy.

Pregnancy: Category C. Use only if clearly needed. Given histamine's known ability to contract uterine muscle, avoid systemic reactions, whether resulting from insect sting or reaction to immunotherapy.

Consider the risk-benefit ratio of continuing an immunotherapy program during pregnancy, and especially initiation of such a program, where there is a possibility that the patient may not be able to reach the recommended maintenance dose without significant risk of a systemic reaction. It is not known if venom or corresponding antibodies cross the placenta. Generally, most IgG passage across the placenta occurs during the third trimester.

Lactation: It is not known if venom or corresponding antibodies are excreted in breast milk. Problems in humans have not been documented.

Children: The pediatric dose is the same as the adult dose.

Adverse Reactions: Anaphylaxis may occur without warning, usually within the first 20 minutes after an injection, and even during the maintenance phase of therapy. Observe patients for 20 to 30 minutes after each injection, and instruct them to return to the office promptly if symptoms of an allergic reaction or shock occur. The more quickly symptoms appear, the more severe they are likely to be, and the more rapidly treatment measures should be instituted. Only conduct skin testing and immunotherapy in facilities with adequate equipment, medications, and personnel trained to respond to anaphylaxis.

Systemic reactions may range from mild to life-threatening, and many include anaphylaxis. In 1 study, some form of systemic reaction occurred in one-third of patients treated. One systemic response occurred with the first dose given. Some systemic manifestations may have occurred because of the patient's apprehension; these did not require treatment. Approximately one-fourth of patients experiencing systemic responses were given some form of specific therapy (eg, epinephrine, theophylline, metaproterenol), some on several occasions.

Excessively large, painful, or persistent local reactions can occur from venom skin tests or from immunotherapy. Large local reactions occur in approximately 60% of patients receiving immunotherapy. Frequent application of cold packs to the area will ameliorate the discomfort. Reactions usually subside in 24 to 36 hours. Corticosteroids can be used to hasten resolution of the local reaction.

Management of systemic reaction: Apply a tourniquet above the injection site and inject 0.3 to 0.5 mL of epinephrine 1:1,000 subcutaneously or IM into the other arm. The dose may need to be repeated every 5 to 10 minutes, because a succession of small doses is often more effective and less dangerous than a single large dose.

Loosen the tourniquet at least every 10 minutes. Also, inject a maximum of 0.1 mL of epinephrine 1:1,000 at the site of the allergen injection to delay allergen absorption. If more than 1 allergen injection was given, distribute the 0.1 mL evenly among the sites.

See the epinephrine monograph for a dosing chart by age and body mass. In general, the pediatric dose is 10 mcg (0.01 mL of a 1:1,000 w/v solution) per kg body weight or 300 mcg (0.3 mL) per m^2 of body surface, up to 500 mcg (0.5 mL).

Patients receiving beta-adrenergic antagonists (ie, beta blockers) may be refractory to the effects of epinephrine.

After adequate epinephrine has been given, and in cases where symptoms of angioedema, urticaria, rhinitis, or conjunctivitis do not respond rapidly, inject antihistamine (eg, diphenhydramine [eg, *Benadryl*]) IV or IM, according to the manufacturer's direction. Other measures may be necessary: inhaled or parenteral bronchodilators or oxygen for cyanosis; endotracheal intubation, tracheotomy, cricothyrotomy, or transtracheal catheterization for laryngeal edema; resuscitation, defibrillation, IV sodium bicarbonate, and other proper medications for cardiac arrest; mechanical airway use if the patient becomes unconscious; and oral or IV corticosteroids if the reaction is prolonged. Monitor hypotension and, if necessary, administer vasopressors along with adequate plasma volume replacement. Rarely will all the above measures be necessary. Promptness in beginning emergency treatment is important.

Pharmacologic & Dosing Characteristics

Dosage: Swirl drug gently to dissolve powder. Do not shake, because foaming leads to denaturation and inactivation of venom proteins.

Diagnostic tests: Immunodiagnostic testing for *Hymenoptera* allergy is conducted to corroborate the patient's description of a previous systemic reaction suggestive of *Hymenoptera* allergy. Most allergists begin testing with a prick test using a 1 mcg/mL solution.

If these tests are negative (typically less than 5 to 10 mm induration), conduct serial ID testing, usually starting with 0.02 to 0.05 mL of a 0.001 to 1 mcg/mL solution on the flexor surface of the forearm or back, with 15- to 20-minute pauses between each 10-fold increase in concentration. A positive reaction warranting immunotherapy and cessation of testing is generally considered 5 to 10 mm induration and 11 to 20 mm erythema.

Test patients with all 5 available venoms, at least 2 to 4 weeks after any natural sting. It may be that yellow and white-faced hornet venoms are so antigenically similar that only 1 is needed for testing and therapy, although this advice is not commonly adopted.

Apply negative and positive controls consisting of plain diluent and a dilution of histamine phosphate (prick, 2.75 mg/mL, ID, 0.275 mg/mL).

Therapeutic dose: Immunotherapy starts with an initial dose of 0.02 mL of a 0.01 mcg/mL solution of each of the venoms to which the patient reacted positively. An alternate approach is to start two 10-fold dilutions below the first positive cutaneous reaction. Additional doses are given every 3 to 7 days, escalating through concentrations of 0.1 mcg/mL, 1 mcg/mL, and 10 mcg/mL.

Rush immunotherapy under controlled conditions is effective in helping patients reach maintenance doses more quickly. In either case, therapy usually plateaus at a standard maintenance dose of 1 mL of 100 mcg/mL at 30-day intervals. Alternately, for maintenance doses, reconstitute a 120 mg vial with 0.6 mL of human serum albumin (HSA) instead of the usual 1.2 mL, to yield 100 mcg/0.5 mL. Longer intervals may also be effective. Detailed recommended treatment schedules appear in each package insert.

Dosage modification is usually needed to individualize therapy to each patient's hypersensitivity, including temporary dosage plateau or reduction following large or delayed local reaction or systemic reaction to immunotherapy injections. Adjust the dose progression of immunotherapy individually in patients treated with more than 1 venom.

Maintenance doses may be increased to 200 mcg monthly if the patient manifests a systemic reaction to a natural sting while receiving 100 mcg monthly.

Route:

Testing: Prick and ID

Immunotherapy: Subcutaneous

Additional Doses: The standard maintenance dose is 100 mcg at 30-day intervals. Longer intervals may also be effective. Maintenance doses may be increased to 200 mcg monthly if the patient manifests a systemic reaction to a natural sting while receiving 100 mcg monthly.

Missed Doses: If more than 6 to 8 weeks pass without a routine immunotherapy dose, reduce the dosage by 20% or more, and then slowly escalate back up to 100 mcg/month.

Efficacy: Venom therapy is 97% effective in reducing anaphylaxis from stings in adults with previous systemic allergic reactions. Efficacy of venom immunotherapy has been confirmed in double-blind clinical trials.

Without therapy, up to 60% of these adults will react systemically again if challenged. Clinical protection has been confirmed through intentional sting challenges of hypersensitive patients in an intensive care unit.

The vespids (ie, white-faced hornet, yellow hornet, yellow jacket) are significantly cross-antigenic. Wasp venom slightly cross-reacts with the vespids. Honey bee venom is the most antigenically unique.

Purified venoms have completely replaced whole-body stinging-insect extracts for sting-induced anaphylaxis caused by honey bee, wasps, and the vespids.

Whole-body extracts of these insects contained many extraneous body proteins and only a small fraction of pure venom. They were determined to be no better than placebo in blinded trials. Do not use whole-body extracts for prophylaxis of sting-induced anaphylaxis; completely reevaluate patients on such therapy before beginning immunotherapy with *Hymenoptera* venoms.

Onset: Partial protection occurs during the escalation phase and is essentially complete when maintenance doses of 100 mcg per month are reached.

Duration: For many years after the *Hymenoptera* venoms were introduced, experts believed that immunotherapy should be continued indefinitely, given the potentially life-threatening consequences of inadequate treatment. Various parameters have been suggested to indicate when hypersensitivity is no longer present and immunotherapy may be stopped:

Suppression of previous skin test or RAST responsiveness; fall in venom-specific serum IgE levels to insignificant or undetectable levels; or an empiric length of immunotherapy such as 3 to 5 years. A 3-year policy, in consultation with the patient, has been recommended with continued availability of epinephrine for self-administration, but this cannot be considered a consensus opinion.

Protective Level: Unknown

Mechanism: As with allergen extracts, specific anti-venom IgE rises initially during immunotherapy, then declines over time. Venom immunotherapy induces specific IgG (blocking) antibody, mostly of the IgG_4 subclass, the role of which in hyposensitization is only partially known.

Drug Interactions: H_1 antihistamines (eg, chlorpheniramine, diphenhydramine, hydroxyzine, promethazine) suppress skin-test reactivity to *Hymenoptera* venoms, although the potency and duration of skin test suppression vary. Long-acting H_1 antihistamines, such as astemizole, may interfere for as long as 6 weeks. Other drugs with H_1 antihistaminic effects, such as tricyclic antidepressants (TCAs), may also suppress immediate hypersensitivity responses. H_2 antihistamines (eg, cimetidine, ranitidine) do not decrease skin test responsiveness alone, but may increase skin-test suppression synergistically in combination with H_1 antihistamines.

Topical corticosteroids suppress dermal reactivity to *Hymenoptera* venoms locally. Oral corticosteroids appear to have no effect on immediate hypersensitivity skin test reactivity.

Administer positive controls (eg, histamine, codeine) to all subjects to confirm the absence of reaction-inhibiting medications. Drugs that appear to have no effect on immediate-hypersensitivity reagents include oral aminophylline, ephedrine, fenoterol, terbutaline, theophylline, and the latter two drugs combined.

Pharmaceutical Characteristics

Concentration: After appropriate reconstitution, a full-strength concentration provides 100 mcg/mL of each venom or a total of 300 mcg/mL for mixed-vespid products.

Quality Assay: Crude venoms are separated from insect body parts, standardized by protein assay, and tested for hyaluronidase and phospholipase content, residual moisture, albumin content, and pH. Some lot-to-lot variability of potency will persist. Other active constituents of *Hymenoptera* venoms include acid phosphatase and various peptides and vasoactive amines, such as melittin, histamine, and dopamine.

Packaging:

ALK: Each of the 5 *Pharmalgen* venoms is available separately in boxes of six 120 mcg vials. The labels reflect the complete contents of the vials; adding 1.2 mL of HSA diluent yields a concentration of 100 mcg/mL.

Each venom is also available in 10-dose 1,100 mcg vials for immunotherapy, to be reconstituted with 11 mL of HSA diluent.

A mixed-vespid formulation is available in these single- and 10-dose sizes, but the quantity of venom is increased 3-fold (ie, to 360 mcg and 3,300 mcg) to account for the 3 venoms included (ie, white-faced and yellow hornets, yellow jacket).

A diagnostic kit is marketed to facilitate compounding dilutions for diagnostic skin testing, containing one 120 mcg vial of each of 5 venoms. Diluents are sold separately.

HS: Venoms for immunotherapy are packaged in boxes of 6 single-dose 120 mcg vials (*Venomil*) and one 550 mcg 5-dose (*Albay*) vial. Each container yields 100 mcg/mL when reconstituted with 1.2 or 5.5 mL of HSA diluent, respectively.

A mixed-vespid formulation is available in these single- and 5-dose sizes: 360 mcg and 1,650 mcg.

Five separate diagnostic kits are also marketed, each containing one 12 mcg vial of a single venom, using the *Venomil* name, to facilitate compounding dilutions for diagnostic skin testing after addition of 1.2 mL HSA diluent.

Each kit contains six 1.8 mL vials of HSA diluent.

NDC Number:

ALK: Single-dose 120 mcg vials: Honey bee (NDC#: 53298-0801-01), wasp (53298-1301-01), white-faced hornet (53298-1101-01), yellow hornet (53298-1001-01), yellow jacket (53298-0901-01), mixed vespids (53298-1201-01), diagnostic kit (53298-1401-01). The initial code 52709 may also be used.

10-dose 1,100 mcg vials: Honey bee (53298-0801-02), wasp (53298-1301-02), white-faced hornet (53298-1101-02), yellow hornet (53298-1001-02), yellow jacket (53298-0901-02), mixed vespids (53298-1201-02). The initial code 52709 may also be used.

HS: Single-dose 120 mcg *Venomil* vials: Honey bee (00118-6781-01), wasp (00118-6784-01), white-faced hornet (00118-6782-01), yellow hornet (00118-6783-01), yellow jacket (00118-6785-01), mixed vespids (00118-6786-01).

5-dose 550 mcg *Albay* vials: Honey bee (00118-9940-05), wasp (00118-9943-05), white-faced hornet (00118-9941-05), yellow hornet (00118-9942-05), yellow jacket (00118-9944-05), mixed vespids (00118-9945-05).

12 mcg *Venomil* vials: Honey bee (00118-6781-00), wasp (00118-6784-00), white-faced hornet (00118-6782-00), yellow hornet (00118-6783-00), yellow jacket (00118-6785-00), mixed vespids (00118-6786-00).

Doseform: Powder for solution

Appearance: White powder, yielding a opalescent solution

Diluent:

For reconstitution: 0.03% HSA in 0.9% sodium chloride with 0.4% phenol. Label all vials with the concentration of their contents.

Adjuvant: None

Preservative: The freeze-dried powder contains no preservative, but the recommended HSA diluent contains 0.4% phenol

Allergens: 0.03% HSA

Excipients: An unspecified quantity of mannitol

pH: 6.6 in HSA diluent

Shelf Life:

ALK: Expires within 30 months.

HS: Expires within 36 months.

Storage/Stability: Store at 2° to 8°C (36° to 46°F). Do not freeze.

Contact manufacturer regarding prolonged exposure to room temperature or elevated or freezing temperatures. Shipping data not provided.

Stability is briefest for dilute solutions, but quite lengthy for the 100 mcg/mL concentrate:

100 mcg/mL: 6 months (HS) or 12 months (ALK)

1 to 99 mcg/mL: 1 month

0.1 mcg/mL: 14 days

Less than 0.1 mcg/mL: Prepare fresh daily.

Handling: Do not reinsert a needle previously inserted into a venom vial into a diluent vial or a vial containing a different venom, in order to avoid contamination of either container with a different antigen.

Production Process: Most venoms are harvested by physical dissection of the insects' venom sacs. Honey bees, however, are stimulated electrically to sting; the extruded venom is then collected in a suitable receptacle.

Media: *Hymenoptera* insects

Threat Epidemiology

Incidence: At least 40 people die each year in the United States from anaphylaxis induced by stings from honey bees, wasps, or the vespids (the group of yellow jackets and hornets). Many other insect-related deaths likely are wrongly attributed to heart attacks or other causes.

Susceptible Pools: Several thousand Americans receive monthly injections of venoms as immunoprotection. Estimates of the prevalence of *Hymenoptera* hypersensitivity range from 0.15% to 4% of the American population.

Other Information

Perspective:

1930: Whole-body extracts of *Hymenoptera* insects introduced for immunotherapy.

1950s: Loveless reasons that venom proteins are the likely cause of sting-related anaphylaxis.

1970s: Researchers at Johns Hopkins University and other centers confirm that purified insect venom causes patients to develop antibodies against venom components.

1979: *Hymenoptera* venoms first licensed to Hollister-Stier (in March) and Pharmacia (now ALK).

References: Joint Council of Allergy, Asthma, & Immunology. Practice Parameters for discontinuation of *Hymenoptera* venom immunotherapy. *J Allergy Clin Immunol.* 1998;101:573-575.

Golden DB, Moffitt J, Nicklas RA, et al; Joint Task Force on Practice Parameters; American Academy of Allergy, Asthma, and Immunology (AAAAI); Americal College of Allergy, Asthma and Immunolocy (ACAAI); Joint Council of Allergy, Asthma, and Immunology. Stinging insect hypersensitivity: a practice parameter update 2011. *J Allergy Clin Immunol.* 2011;127(4):852-854. e1-e23.

Fire Ant Whole-Body Extract

Hymenoptera Allergens

Name:
Generic

Manufacturers:
Allergy Laboratories (Oklahoma); Greer Laboratories; Hollister-Stier Laboratories

Synonyms: Fire ant WBE

Comparison: Considered generically equivalent, but antigen content may vary from manufacturer to manufacturer.

Immunologic Characteristics

Antigen Source: *Solenopsis invicta* and *Solenopsis richteri*, subfamily Myrimicae, family Formicidae, order *Hymenoptera*.

Viability: Not viable, but antigenically active

Antigenic Form: Whole-body extract

Antigenic Type: Protein. Skin tests assess immediate (type I) hypersensitivity. Fire ant whole-body extracts (WBEs) contain at least 30 antigens, 5 of which may evoke IgE-mediated anaphylaxis.

Strains: *Solenopsis invicta* and *Solenopsis richteri*, known as the imported fire ants.

Use Characteristics

Indications: For confirmatory diagnosis of hypersensitivity and for induction of active immunity against subsequent hypersensitivity reactions. Skin testing with fire ant WBEs is useful to demonstrate the presence of IgE antibodies to account for the patient's symptoms.

Dilutions of fire ant WBEs help assess the hypersensitivity of the patient and whether the patient should begin immunotherapy.

While purified venoms have completely replaced WBEs for honey bees, wasps, and hornets, WBEs are still employed for certain other *Hymenoptera* insects, including the imported fire ants (*Solenopsis invicta* and *Solenopsis richteri*). Immunotherapy reduces the risk of anaphylaxis and appears to be effective in reducing mortality. Candidates for fire ant immunotherapy include patients who have had a systemic reaction correlated with positive skin tests or RAST, those who are geographically or occupationally susceptible to repeated exposure, and those who exhibit exceptional anxiety and life-style changes to avoid another exposure.

Alternative Tests: The radioallergosorbent test (RAST) is less sensitive and yields more false-negative results.

Contraindications:

Absolute: None

Relative: Do not treat patients with allergens to which they have no history of hypersensitivity, positive skin test results, or likelihood of exposure. There is inconclusive evidence that routine immunization may exacerbate autoimmune diseases. Children with nephrotic syndrome probably should not receive immunotherapy. Other relative contraindications include patients experiencing severe respiratory or cardiovascular distress and patients who have experienced an anaphylactic reaction to the offending allergen. Weigh the risks of therapy against its benefits.

Patient compliance is an important consideration in the decision to initiate immuno-therapy with any potent allergen extract. Do not initiate therapy if the patient cannot be depended on to respond promptly and properly to an impending adverse reaction.

Patients receiving beta-adrenergic antagonists (ie, beta blockers) may be refractory to the effects of epinephrine, which may be needed to treat anaphylactic reactions.

Immunodeficiency: Immune response and resultant reduction in symptoms may be impaired in immunocompromised patients.

Elderly: Geriatric patients may not respond to immunotherapy.

Pregnancy: Category C. Use only if clearly needed. Immunotherapy has been continued dur-ing pregnancy, but is not generally initiated in pregnant women. Consider the risk-benefit ratio. An anaphylactic reaction may induce a miscarriage as a result of uterine muscle contrac-tions. It is not known if fire ant WBEs or corresponding antibodies cross the placenta. Gener-ally, most IgG passage across the placenta occurs during the third trimester.

Lactation: It is not known if fire ant WBEs or corresponding antibodies are excreted in breast milk. Problems in humans have not been documented.

Children: Children younger than 2 years of age appear to tolerate allergen-extract injections well, and no special recommendations need be made for these patients. Adult and pediatric maintenance doses are usually equivalent. If the injection volume is too large for a small child to tolerate comfortably, split the dose among several injections.

Adverse Reactions: Anaphylaxis may occur without warning, usually within the first 20 min-utes after an injection, even during the maintenance phase of therapy. Observe patients for 20 to 30 minutes after each injection, and instruct them to return to the office promptly if symp-toms of an allergic reaction or shock occur. The more quickly symptoms appear, the more severe they are likely to be, and the more rapidly treatment measures should be instituted. Only conduct skin testing and immunotherapy in facilities with adequate equipment, medica-tions, and personnel trained to respond to anaphylaxis.

Immediate induration and erythema reactions are ordinarily of little consequence, but if they are large (larger than 3 to 5 cm in diameter), they may be the first manifestation of a sys-temic reaction. If large local reactions occur, observe the patient for systemic symptoms. Oral antihistamines may be of benefit in relieving symptoms. Reduce the next therapeutic dose by half or to the last dose that did not elicit a reaction. Increase subsequent doses more slowly, through the use of intermediate dilutions.

Systemic reactions: Mild exacerbation of allergic symptoms, sneezing, mild to severe gener-alized urticaria, angioedema, rhinitis, conjunctivitis, edema (including laryngeal edema), wheezing, asthma, dyspnea, cough, fainting, pallor, cyanosis, bradycardia, tachycardia, lacrimation, marked perspiration, hypotension, upper airway obstruction. Symptoms may progress to anaphylactic shock and death. After a systemic reaction, reduce the next thera-peutic dose to the last dose that did not elicit a reaction, or lower. Increase subsequent doses more slowly, through the use of intermediate dilutions.

Repeated systemic reactions, even of a mild nature, are sufficient reason for the cessation of further attempts to increase the reaction-eliciting dose.

Management of systemic reaction: Apply a tourniquet above the injection site, and inject 0.3 to 0.5 mL of epinephrine 1:1,000 subcutaneously or IM into the other arm. The dose may need to be repeated every 5 to 10 minutes, because a succession of small doses is often more effective and less dangerous than a single large dose.

Loosen the tourniquet at least every 10 minutes. Also inject a maximum of 0.1 mL of epi-nephrine 1:1,000 at the site of the allergen injection to delay allergen absorption. If more than 1 allergen injection was given, distribute the 0.1 mL evenly among the sites.

See the epinephrine monograph for a dosing chart by age and body mass. In general, the pediatric dose is 10 mcg (0.01 mL of a 1:1,000 w/v solution) per kg body weight or 300 mcg (0.3 mL) per m² of body surface, up to 500 mcg (0.5 mL).

Patients receiving beta-adrenergic antagonists (ie, beta blockers) may be refractory to the effects of epinephrine.

After adequate epinephrine has been given, and in cases where symptoms of angioedema, urticaria, rhinitis, or conjunctivitis do not respond rapidly, inject antihistamine (eg, diphenhydramine eg, [*Benadryl*]) IV or IM, according to the manufacturer's direction. Other measures may be necessary: Inhaled or parenteral bronchodilators or oxygen for cyanosis; endotracheal intubation, tracheotomy, cricothyrotomy, or transtracheal catheterization for laryngeal edema; resuscitation, defibrillation, IV sodium bicarbonate, and other proper medications for cardiac arrest; mechanical airway use if the patient becomes unconscious; and oral or IV corticosteroids if the reaction is prolonged.

Monitor hypotension and, if necessary, administer vasopressors along with adequate plasma volume replacement. Rarely will all the above measures be necessary. Promptness in beginning emergency treatment is important.

Sting information: Reactions to fire ants range from local pruritus and erythema to anaphylactic shock and death, with anaphylaxis occurring in up to 1% of stings. Hypersensitivity reactions to fire ants are more common than to other *Hymenoptera* insects. In the southeastern US, fire ants are the leading cause of insect-related anaphylactic death. Fire ant venom has a lower protein content than the venoms of other *Hymenoptera*, consisting predominantly of toxic alkaloids (primarily 2,6-disubstituted piperidines).

Pharmacologic & Dosing Characteristics

Dosage: Do not shake, because foaming leads to denaturation and inactivation of proteins.

Diagnostic tests: Whole-body fire ant extracts are used for skin-test diagnosis, beginning with 1 or an escalating series of prick tests at concentrations ranging from 1:100,000 to 1:1,000 w/v or 1 to 100 PNU/mL.

If these tests are negative (typically less than 5 to 10 mm induration), conduct serial ID testing, usually starting with 0.02 to 0.05 mL of a 1:1,000,000 w/v or 0.1 PNU/mL solution on the flexor surface of the patient's forearm or on the back, with 15- to 20-minute pauses between each 10-fold increase in concentration. Most clinically hypersensitive patients will produce a substantial induration and erythema reaction before the concentration reaches 1:500 w/v or 500 PNU/mL, with a positive reaction defined as a 5 to 10 mm induration and 11 to 20 mm erythema.

Administer negative- and positive-control reagents, consisting of plain diluent and a dilution of histamine phosphate (prick, 2.75 mg/mL; ID, 0.275 mg/mL).

Therapeutic dose: Immunotherapy begins with 0.5 mL of the first WBE dilution that produced a positive skin test (usually 1:10,000 or 1:100,000 w/v or 1 or 10 PNU/mL), although some clinicians begin 1 or two 10-fold dilutions below this point, for added safety. Dosage increases in an escalating series of injections every 3 to 7 days to a maximum tolerated dose up to 0.5 mL of a 1:100 or 1:10 w/v or 1,000 or 10,000 PNU/mL solution.

Dosage modification is usually needed to individualize therapy to each patient's hypersensitivity, including temporary dosage plateau or reduction following large or delayed local reaction or systemic reaction to immunotherapy injections.

Additional Doses: The maintenance dose may be given every 2 to 6 weeks. Continue immunotherapy against fire ants indefinitely, until data suggesting otherwise are reported.

Missed Doses: Resume therapy as soon as possible. Large intervals since the last allergen injection may necessitate a dose reduction to reduce the likelihood of an adverse allergic reaction.

Efficacy: Despite some conflicting data, purified fire ant venom appears to be no more effective than the corresponding whole-body extract, probably because fire ants lack the enzymes that biodegrade venom protein in honey bee, wasp, and vespid WBEs. Understanding of the efficacy of fire ant WBEs is based on uncontrolled studies.

Onset: Partial protection is obtained during the escalation phase and is essentially complete when maintenance doses are reached.

Duration: Many experts believe that immunotherapy should be continued indefinitely, given the potentially life-threatening consequences of inadequate treatment.

Protective Level: Unknown

Mechanism: Fire ant WBEs induce an increase in venom-specific IgG_4 (blocking antibody) that apparently protects most extract recipients. A corresponding fall in venom-specific IgE also occurs.

Drug Interactions: H_1 antihistamines (eg, chlorpheniramine, diphenhydramine, hydroxyzine, promethazine) suppress skin-test reactivity to allergens, although the potency and duration of skin-test suppression vary.

Long-acting H_1 antihistamines, such as astemizole, may interfere for as long as 6 weeks. Other drugs with H_1 antihistaminic effects, such as tricyclic antidepressants (TCAs), may also suppress immediate-hypersensitivity responses. H_2 antihistamines (eg, cimetidine, ranitidine) do not decrease skin-test responsiveness alone, but may increase skin-test suppression synergistically in combination with H_1 antihistamines.

Topical corticosteroids suppress dermal reactivity to allergens locally.

Oral corticosteroids appear to have no effect on immediate-hypersensitivity skin-test reactivity.

Administer positive controls (eg, histamine, codeine) to all subjects to confirm the absence of reaction-inhibiting medications. Drugs that appear to have no effect on immediate-hypersensitivity reagents include oral aminophylline, ephedrine, fenoterol, terbutaline, theophylline, and the latter two drugs combined.

Pharmaceutical Characteristics

Concentration:
Allergy: 5,000 and 10,000 PNU/mL
Others: 1:10 and 1:20 w/v; 10,000 and 20,000 PNU/mL

Quality Assay: Fire ant WBEs sold in the United States bear the proviso "No US Standard of Potency." This caution is needed, because w/v and PNU assays have only a limited correlation to biological and immunologic activity.

Packaging: 10, 20, 30, and 50 mL vials

NDC Number: Company series:
Greer: 22840
Hollister-Stier: 00118

Doseform: Solution

Appearance: Clear to dark brown or black solutions. Precipitates may develop during storage, apparently without affecting potency.

Solvent: Fire ant WBEs may be manufactured in either aqueous or glycerinated form. Stock containers of water-based (aqueous) allergen extracts typically contain constituents of the diluting fluid (menstruum; eg, sodium chloride, sodium bicarbonate) and are preserved with phenol.

Fire Ant Whole-Body Extract

Diluent: Dilute fire ant WBEs with a solution containing 0.03% human serum albumin (HSA) as a protein preservative, 0.9% sodium chloride for tonicity, and 0.4% phenol as an antimicrobial agent.

Adjuvant: None

Preservative: 0.4% phenol

Allergens: Fire ant WBEs are allergenic by definition and intent.

Excipients: May contain varying amounts of sodium chloride, sodium bicarbonate, sodium or potassium phosphate.

pH: 6.5 to 7.5

Shelf Life: Expires within 18 months.

Storage/Stability: Store at 2° to 8°C (36° to 46°F). Discard if frozen, because freezing may cause agglomeration and reduce potency. Contact manufacturer regarding prolonged exposure to room temperature or elevated temperatures. Typically shipped by second-day courier or first-class mail at ambient temperature.

Definitive data on fire ant extract stability are not available. Six-month expiration dates for full-strength vials are frequently adopted, with 30-day stabilities used for concentrations of 1:10,000 w/v or 20 PNU/mL or less. Shorter dates are adopted, compared with purified venoms, because no potency-measurement system based on biologic activity is available.

Stability decreases with protein adsorption to the walls of glass containers. HSA diluents reduce this effect, but protein degradation and enzymatic autodigestion also decrease potency over time. Stability is favored by low temperatures.

Production Process: Whole insects are macerated and then extracted, similar to methods used for pollen extracts and other allergen extracts.

Media: *Solenopsis* fire ants

Threat Epidemiology

Incidence: With an annual reported sting attack rate of 30% to 60% among the general population, some 12 million persons may be stung each year by fire ants in the southern US and in Puerto Rico. The prevalence of hypersensitivity to fire ant stings has not been determined.

Susceptible Pools: Hypersensitivity reactions to fire ants are likely to increase in frequency, as the habitat infested by these insects is increasing.

Other Information

Perspective: See Allergen Extract Aqueous & Glycerinated monograph.

References: Brown SG, Heddle RJ. Prevention of anaphylaxis with ant venom immunotherapy. *Curr Opin Allergy Clin Immunol.* 2003;3:511-516.

Stafford CT. Hypersensitivity to fire ant venom. *Ann Allergy Asthma Immunol.* 1996;77:87-99.

Benzylpenicilloyl Polylysine (BPL)

Immediate-Hypersensitivity Drugs, Miscellaneous

Name:
Pre-Pen Skin Test Antigen

Manufacturer:
AllerQuest

Synonyms: BPL. Older references describe it as penicilloyl polylysine (PPL).

Immunologic Characteristics

Antigen Source: Hapten-polypeptide complex

Viability: Not viable, but antigenically active

Antigenic Form: Hapten, benzylpenicilloyl moiety, $C_{16}H_{19}N_2O_5S$

Antigenic Type: Polyvalent hapten-polypeptide complex. The polylysine polymer consists of at least 40 units. Skin tests assess immediate (type I) hypersensitivity.

Strains: Chemically pure

Use Characteristics

Indications: For use as an adjunct in assessing the risk of administering benzylpenicillin (ie, penicillin G) when penicillin is the drug of choice in adult patients who have previously received penicillin and who have a history of clinical penicillin hypersensitivity.

In this situation, a negative skin test to BPL is associated with an incidence of allergic reactions less than 5% after the administration of a therapeutic dose of penicillin, whereas the incidence may be more than 20% in the presence of a positive skin test to BPL.

These allergic reactions are predominantly dermatologic. Because of the extremely low incidence of anaphylactic reactions, there are insufficient data to document that a decreased incidence of anaphylactic reactions following administration of penicillin will occur in patients with a negative skin test to BPL. Similarly, when deciding the risk of proposed penicillin treatment, there are not enough data to permit relative weighing in individual cases of a history of clinical penicillin hypersensitivity as compared with positive skin tests to BPL or minor penicillin determinants.

It has been suggested that skin testing may be appropriate when the patient's history of allergy is very weak, moderately weak, or when no details are available. If the history of allergy is strong, an alternative antibiotic may be indicated even if the skin test results are negative.

Limitations: No reagent, test, or combination of tests will completely ensure that a subsequent penicillin therapy will not induce a reaction. An allergic reaction to therapeutic penicillin may occur in patients with a negative BPL skin test. Many patients reacting positively to BPL will not develop a systemic allergic reaction on subsequent exposure to therapeutic penicillin. Thus, the BPL skin test facilitates assessing the local allergic skin reactivity of a patient to benzylpenicilloyl.

There are insufficient data to assess the potential danger of sensitization to repeated skin testing with BPL. There are also insufficient data to determine the value of BPL in: Assessing the risk of penicillin administration in adult patients who give no history of clinical penicillin hypersensitivity; assessing penicillin as a suspected cause of a drug reaction; patients undergoing routine allergy evaluation; assessing the risk of administration of semi-synthetic penicillins (eg, phenoxymethylpenicillin [penicillin V], ampicillin, carbenicillin, dicloxacillin, methicillin, nafcillin, oxacillin, phenethicillin) or cephalosporin-type antibiotics. Nonetheless, these semi-synthetic penicillins contain the same molecular nucleus as penicillin G; the nuclear configuration determines major antigenic specificity. Analogous decisions about the use of semi-synthetic penicillins based on BPL skin-test results can, with rare exception, be made.

Benzylpenicilloyl-polylysine does not contain antigens referred to as minor determinants or the minor determinant mix (MDM). MDM consists of benzylpenicillin itself and penicillin degradation products (eg, sodium benzylpenicilloate, benzylpenicilloyl n-propylamine). MDM is physically and chemically stable for only short periods of time in solution. Some clinicians compound penicillin G potassium 10,000 units/mL extemporaneously in an effort to better assess reactivity to MDM; aging the penicillin offers no advantage. Nonetheless, 5% to 10% of skin-test reactive patients may be missed.

Alternative Tests: RAST assays have been developed to detect IgE antibodies to the penicilloyl determinant, analogous to the BPL skin test. This test is positive in 60% to 95% of patients whose skin test is positive to BPL. No in vitro assay has yet been developed for minor determinant antigens.

Contraindications:

Absolute: None

Relative: Patients with a history of either a systemic or marked local reaction to a prior administration of BPL. Do not skin test patients known to be extremely hypersensitive to penicillin.

Immunodeficiency: Immunocompromised patients may be less likely to exhibit a positive skin-test response. Conversely, immunocompromised patients may also be less likely to respond antigenically with antibody production against penicillin. No specific information is available about the use of this product in immunocompromised patients.

Elderly: No specific information is available about geriatric use of BPL.

Pregnancy: Category C. Use only if clearly needed. Consider the hazards of skin testing in relation to the hazard of penicillin therapy without skin testing. It is not known if BPL or corresponding antibodies cross the placenta. Generally, most IgG passage across the placenta occurs during the third trimester.

Lactation: It is not known if BPL or corresponding antibodies are excreted in breast milk. Problems in humans have not been documented.

Children: Insufficient data exist to determine the value of performing BPL skin tests in children.

Adverse Reactions: Allergic reactions to BPL occur in less than 1% of recipients.

Occasionally, patients develop an intense local inflammatory response at the skin test site. Rarely, a systemic allergic reaction follows a BPL skin test: generalized erythema, pruritus, angioedema, urticaria, dyspnea, hypotension. Systemic allergic reactions are generally of short duration and controllable, but observe the patient for several hours.

Pharmacologic & Dosing Characteristics

Dosage: Apply a scratch or epicutaneous test first. If this test is negative or equivocal, proceed to an ID test.

Scratch or Epicutaneous Test: Apply the scratch or epicutaneous test first on the inner volar aspect of the forearm. After preparing the skin surface, make a 3 to 5 mm scratch of the epidermis using a sterile 20-gauge needle; very little pressure is needed. If bleeding occurs, prepare a second site, and scratch more lightly. Apply a small drop of BPL to the scratch, and rub gently with an applicator, toothpick, or the side of the needle. Also apply an appropriate negative (eg, 0.9% sodium chloride) control reagent at a separate but analogous site.

Time of Reading: Observe patient for induration, erythema and itching at the test site during the succeeding 15 minutes.

Interpretation: A positive reaction consists of a pale induration, usually with pseudopods, surrounding the scratch site. It may vary in diameter from 5 to 15 mm or wider, most often within 10 minutes. This induration may be surrounded by a variable diameter of erythema and accompanied by a variable degree of itching. Wipe off the solution over the scratch after 15 minutes or as soon as a positive response is evident. If the scratch test is either negative or equivocally positive (less than 5 mm induration and little or no erythema and no itching), an ID test may be performed.

ID Test: Using a syringe graduated in units of 0.01 mL, with a ⅜- to ⅝-inch, 26- to 30-gauge, short-bevel needle, withdraw the contents of the ampule.

Prepare a sterile skin-test area on the upper, outer arm, sufficiently below the deltoid muscle to permit proximal application of a tourniquet later, if needed. Eject all air from the syringe through the needle.

Insert the needle, bevel up, immediately below the skin surface. Inject an amount of BPL sufficient to raise the smallest possible perceptible bleb, between 0.01 to 0.02 mL. Using a separate syringe and needle, inject a like amount of 0.9% sodium chloride as a negative control, at least 1.5 inches from the BPL test site.

Time of Reading: Most reactions will develop within 5 to 15 minutes.

Interpretation: A positive response consists of itching and marked increase in the size of the original bleb. Induration may exceed 20 mm in diameter and exhibit pseudopods. An ambiguous response occurs when the induration is only slightly larger than the initial injection bleb, with or without accompanying erythematous flare, yet larger than the negative-control site. A negative response demonstrates no increase in size of the original bleb or no greater reaction than the negative control site.

The negative control site should be completely reactionless. If it exhibits induration more than 2 to 3 mm, repeat the test. If the same reaction occurs, consult with a specialist in allergy skin testing.

The manufacturer does not recommend skin testing with a dilution of penicillin or other penicillin-derived reagents simultaneously with BPL. Although such practices have been described in the professional literature, there is limited data on the efficacy or utility of such a procedure.

Related Interventions: If penicillin remains the drug of choice in a life-threatening situation, successful desensitization with penicillin, with appropriate precautions, may be possible regardless of a positive skin test or positive history of clinical penicillin hypersensitivity.

Efficacy: A negative skin test to BPL in patients with a clinical history of penicillin hypersensitivity is associated with an incidence of allergic reactions of less than 5% after the administration of therapeutic penicillin, whereas the incidence may be more than 20% in the presence of a positive skin test to BPL.

Predictive Capacity: Patients reporting a previous reaction to penicillin are more likely to react again than patients reporting a negative history of prior reactions.

Some 20% of positive BPL reactors will subsequently react to penicillin therapy. Positive tests develop following penicillin therapy in less than 10% of patients. A positive test does not preclude the need for desensitization prior to administration of a therapeutic dose of penicillin.

For patients with no history of clinical hypersensitivity, there are insufficient data to determine the value of a BPL test. No data are available on the value of this reagent in subsequent use of semisynthetic penicillins or cephalosporins.

This test is 89% to 96% sensitive, implying that 4% to 11% of patients who will subsequently react to a therapeutic dose of penicillin will test falsely negative to BPL on the day of penicillin therapy.

Benzylpenicilloyl Polylysine (BPL)

This test is also 89% to 96% specific, implying that 4% to 11% of patients who will not subsequently react to a therapeutic dose of penicillin will test falsely positive to BPL on the day of penicillin therapy.

Subsequent Tests: Apply the same dose. There are insufficient data to assess the potential danger of sensitization to repeated skin testing with BPL.

Sensitization: Although definitive data are unavailable, sensitization probably occurs within days or weeks after exposure to penicillin. This exposure may arise from a therapeutic course of penicillin or from other environmental exposures.

Onset: 15 minutes

Mechanism: Reacts with benzylpenicilloyl skin-sensitizing antibodies (ie, reagins, specific IgE antibodies) to initiate release of chemical mediators that produce an immediate induration and erythema reaction at a skin-test site. All individuals exhibiting a positive skin test to BPL possess IgE antibodies against the benzylpenicilloyl group, which is a hapten.

Individuals who have previously received therapeutic penicillin may have positive skin test reactions to BPL and to a number of other nonbenzylpenicilloyl haptens. The latter are described as the minor determinants, in that they are present in lesser amounts than the major determinant, benzylpenicilloyl. The minor determinants may nevertheless be associated with episodes of significant clinical hypersensitivity. A minor-determinant skin-test reagent is not licensed by the FDA, but is designated an orphan drug. Refer to the IND section.

Virtually everyone who receives penicillin develops specific antibodies to the drug, as measured by hemagglutination studies. However, positive skin tests to various penicillin and penicillin-derived reagents become positive in less than 10% of patients who have tolerated penicillin in the past.

Drug Interactions: Specific interactions have not been reported, but it is likely that immediate hypersensitivity suppressants (eg, H_1 antihistamines) will suppress reactivity to benzylpenicilloyl-polylysine.

Pharmaceutical Characteristics

Concentration: 6×10^{-5} molar benzylpenicilloyl moiety (range, 5.4 to 7×10^{-5} molar)

Quality Assay: Purity assays used to minimize the contaminants penicillanate and penamaldate

Packaging: Box of five 0.25 mL single-dose ampules

NDC Number: 49471-0001-05

Doseform: Solution

Appearance: Clear, colorless solution

Solvent: Phosphate buffer 0.01 molar with sodium chloride 0.15 molar

Adjuvant: None

Preservative: None

Allergens: None

Excipients: Phosphate buffer 0.01 molar with sodium chloride 0.15 molar

pH:
USP requirement: 6.5 to 8.5, although the product usually exhibits a pH from 7.4 to 7.6

Shelf Life: Expires within 36 months.

Storage/Stability: Store at 2° to 8°C (36° to 46°F). Discard if exposed to ambient temperatures for more than 1 day. Contact the manufacturer regarding exposure to freezing temperatures. Shipped at ambient temperature.

Production Process: Benzylpenicilloyl-polylysine is a derivative of poly-l-lysine, where 50% to 70% of the epsilon-amino groups are chemically coupled with benzylpenicilloyl groups of benzylpenicillin (penicillin G) in an alkaline medium, forming benzylpenicilloyl alpha amide.

Media: Chemically synthesized.

Threat Epidemiology

Incidence: True allergic reactions to penicillin occur in 0.7% to 8% of treatment courses. Anaphylactic reactions occur in 0.004% to 0.015% of penicillin treatment courses (4 to 15 per 100,000 courses). Among patients of sexually transmitted disease clinics, measured rates averaged 0.055% (55 per 100,000). At least 350 penicillin-induced deaths occur in the United States each year (1 death per 50,000 to 100,000 treatment courses).

From 5% to 20% of the population may claim penicillin hypersensitivity. Misdiagnosis of penicillin allergy may result from faulty recall, natural declining hypersensitivity, misattribution of symptoms to an allergic cause, and previous problems with contaminated preparations.

By contrast, ampicillin-induced rashes occur in 5.2% to 9.5% of treatment courses; 6.9% to 10% of patients given ampicillin during a viral infection may develop a rash.

Other Information

Perspective:
1928: Fleming isolates penicillin from cultures of *Penicillium notatum.*
1940: Florey, Chain & colleagues introduce penicillin into therapeutic use in humans, developing method for large-scale production.
1946: Case of penicillin-induced anaphylaxis reported.
1949: Death because of penicillin-induced anaphylaxis reported.
1950s: Parker develops BPL in St. Louis, Missouri.
1969: Levine & Zolov perform skin tests with minor determinants.
1974: *Pre-Pen* licensed on July 25.

References: Salkind AR, Cuddy PG, Foxworth JW. Is this patient allergic to penicillin? An evidence-based analysis of the likelihood of penicillin allergy. *JAMA.* 2001;285:2498-2505.

Schafer JA, Mateo N, Parlier GL, Rotschafer JC. Penicillin allergy skin testing: What do we do now? *Pharmacotherapy.* 2007;27(4):542-545.

Penicillin Desensitization: If penicillin remains the drug of choice in a life-threatening situation, desensitization to penicillin may be possible and desirable, regardless of a positive skin test or history of clinical penicillin hypersensitivity. Precautions are essential, since this procedure is nothing less than controlled anaphylaxis. Desensitization slowly and progressively antagonizes the body's pool of anti-penicillin IgE antibodies, making it safer to proceed with standard penicillin therapy.

A variety of desensitization schedules have been recommended. Typically, escalating penicillin VK or semisynthetic penicillin doses are given every 15 to 60 minutes, starting with 100 to 1,000 units or 0.05 mg orally, serially doubling the dose, progressing through 640,000 units or 400 mg. The oral route allows blood levels to rise gradually, contributing primarily univalent, inhibiting haptens into the circulation. Parenteral penicillin G or a semisynthetic penicillin follows at similar escalating doses by cautious infusion of 1 g or other appropriate dose of the desired antibiotic.

Any period of time longer than 48 hours free of penicillin may permit the patient to accumulate a substantial quantity of antipenicillin antibodies once again, making subsequent bolus doses of penicillin dangerous once more. If a substantial lapse of time ensues, apply a subsequent BPL test at the standard dose. If a desensitized patient is known to need subsequent courses of penicillin (eg, cystic fibrosis, chronic neutropenia), consider sustained oral desensitization. In such cases, chronic twice daily oral penicillin VK therapy is safe and effective.

Benzylpenicilloyl Polylysine (BPL)

Desensitization is a dangerous procedure that should be performed only in settings where emergency resuscitative equipment, supplies, and personnel are readily available, such as an intensive care unit. Fatalities have occurred during parenteral desensitization, often ascribed to higher initial doses or faster rates of escalation. Do not attempt desensitization following aberrant reactions, such as exfoliative dermatitis. Patients receiving β-adrenergic antagonists may be refractory to epinephrine given in response to anaphylaxis and may even be predisposed to anaphylaxis.

Dextran-1

Immediate-Hypersensitivity Drugs, Miscellaneous

Name:
Promit

Manufacturer:
Distributed by Amersham Biosciences, produced by Medisan Pharmaceuticals, Meda AB of Sweden

Synonyms: Promiten

Immunologic Characteristics

Antigen Source: Purified dextran-1

Viability: Not viable, but antigenically active

Antigenic Form: Hapten

Antigenic Type: Monovalent polysaccharide hapten, alpha-1,6-linked glucose polymer. The molecular weight averages 1,000 daltons. The empirical formula is $(C_6H_{10}O_5)_n$.

Strains: Chemically pure

Use Characteristics

Indications: For passive, transient prevention of serious anaphylactic reactions in connection with the IV infusion of a clinical dextran solution (eg, dextran 40; dextran 70; dextran 75; *Gentran, Macrodex, Rheomacrodex*). By means of hapten inhibition, the incidence of these reactions is significantly reduced.

Unlabeled Uses: One case report has been published of dextran-1 used to prevent anaphylactoid reactions in a patient who reacted to the test dose of an iron dextran infusion (*ImFed*). Dextran-1 was used in conjunction with diphenhydramine, methylprednisolone, and ephedrine and slowly escalating doses of iron dextran.

Limitations: Mild dextran-induced anaphylactic (allergic) reactions are not prevented by dextran-1.

Keep other means of maintaining circulation available so that dextran therapy can be stopped at the first signs of allergic reactions. Have resuscitative equipment readily available. In the event of an anaphylactoid reaction, do not administer subsequent clinical dextran infusions.

Contraindications:

Absolute: None

Relative: If the IV administration of clinical dextran solutions is contraindicated (eg, marked hemostatic defects of all types, hemorrhagic tendencies, marked cardiac decompensation, and renal disease with oliguria or anuria), do not give dextran-1. Dextran-1 may interfere with platelet function. Use dextran-1 with caution in patients with thrombocytopenia.

Immunodeficiency: No impairment of effect is likely.

Elderly: No specific information is available about geriatric use of dextran-1.

Pregnancy: Category B. In rabbits, doses 35 to 70 times the human dose resulted in increased fetal resorption, postimplantation fetal loss, retardation of long-bone ossification, and marginal retardation of growth. No evidence of impaired fertility or fetal harm was found in studies of mice. No adequate, well-controlled studies in pregnant women have been conducted. Use only if clearly needed.

Lactation: It is not known if dextran-1 is excreted in breast milk. Problems in humans have not been documented.

Dextran-1

Children: Give children a lower dose than adults.

Adverse Reactions: Among more than 70,000 recipients of dextran-1, less than 1 in 1,000 patients exhibited an adverse reaction: Cutaneous reactions, nausea, pallor, shivering, moderate hypotension, bradycardia with moderate hypotension, bradycardia alone. One patient experienced severe hypotension, and one experienced bradycardia with severe hypotension. If any reaction to dextran-1 occurs, do not give clinical dextran solutions. Another volume expander may be appropriate (eg, hetastarch).

Despite its role in hapten inhibition, dextran-1 itself may rarely induce anaphylactoid reactions. Observe patients closely during the first minutes of infusion, and make every effort to determine whether symptoms of severe hypotension result from shock initially present or from the dextran.

Pharmacologic & Dosing Characteristics

Dosage:
Adults: 20 mL of dextran-1
Children: 0.3 mL/kg of body weight

Route & Site: Administer IV, 1 to 2 minutes before IV infusion of clinical dextran solutions (eg, dextran 40, dextran 75). The full dose may be delivered rapidly, over 1 to 2 minutes, by needle and syringe or through a Y injection-site, provided there is minimal dilution of the dextran-1 dose.

Do not allow the interval between administration of dextran-1 and clinical dextran solutions to exceed 15 minutes. If a longer period has elapsed, give another dose of dextran-1. Do not administer dextran-1 through an IV set used to infuse a clinical dextran solution. Do not administer IM. To avoid decreasing efficacy, do not dilute or mix dextran-1 with clinical dextran solutions.

Overdosage: Because dextran-1 is cleared rapidly by renal excretion, any overdosage should be of short duration and minimal consequence. Dextrans with molecular weights less than 15,000 daltons are cleared similarly to creatinine.

Additional Doses: By 48 hours after the completion of infusion of 1 unit of clinical dextran solution (eg, dextran 40, dextran 75), the concentration of dextran in the serum is decreased and the concentration of free dextran-reactive antibodies may increase. In this case, the risk of formation of large anaphylactogenic immune complexes returns with any infusion of another dose of clinical dextran solution. Give an additional injection of dextran-1 if 48 hours or more have elapsed since the previous infusion of clinical dextran solution.

Efficacy: The incidence of dextran-induced anaphylactic reactions is reduced 15 to 20 times by means of hapten inhibition with dextran-1.

Onset: Within 1 to 2 minutes

Duration: Do not allow the interval between administration of dextran-1 and clinical dextran solutions to exceed 15 minutes. If a longer period has elapsed, give another dose of dextran-1. Once a clinical dextran solution has finished infusing, the protective effects persist approximately 48 hours.

Pharmacokinetics: Because of its low molecular weight, dextran-1 is rapidly and completely excreted by glomerular filtration. There is no apparent need to adjust the dextran-1 dose in patients with impaired renal function. After IV injection of a single 20 mL dose, approximately 50% of the original concentration is cleared from the blood within 30 minutes. The mean urinary elimination half-life was 41 ± 11 minutes in 12 healthy volunteers. The pharmacokinetics of dextran-1 have been described as a 2-compartment open model with elimination from the central compartment only.

920

Mechanism: Dextran-1 binds to 1 of the 2 available binding sites on dextran-reacting IgG antibodies without forming bridges between multiple IgG molecules. Therefore, there is no tendency to form large immune complexes; this prevents type III immune-complex reactions. A polyvalent hapten (eg, dextran 40, dextran 75) may form complexes with antibodies as an antigen does; a monovalent hapten can only bind to individual combining sites of antibodies, thereby eliminating the possibility of immune-complex formation.

In this way, a molar excess of monovalent hapten given just prior to the IV administration of a clinical dextran solution competitively prevents formation of immune complexes and impedes occurrence of anaphylaxis. During the later phase of the dextran infusion and on the following day, the patient is protected by the dextran molecules in the clinical dextran solutions themselves, because an antigen excess (a higher concentration of dextran, compared with dextran-reactive IgG) develops in the circulation and only small nonanaphylactogenic immune complexes can form. This effect persists approximately 48 hours.

Drug Interactions: Do not administer dextran-1 through an IV set used to infuse a clinical dextran solution.

Lab Interference: Draw blood samples for cross-matching, Rh determinations, and blood typing before injection of dextran-1, because administration of subsequent dextran infusions induce rouleaux formation. Rouleaux formation involves pseudoagglutination of erythrocytes, which can interfere with accurate blood grouping and cross matching for blood transfusions. Although the use of dextran-1 or clinical dextran infusions does not interfere with blood typing and cross matching when these tests are performed by saline agglutination and indirect antiglobulin methods, difficulties may be encountered when proteolytic-enzyme techniques are used to cross match blood.

Blood glucose determinations that involve sulfuric acid or acetic acid hydrolysis may give elevated values after any form of dextran is administered. The presence of dextran in the blood may result in turbidity that may interfere with bilirubin assays using alcohol, and in total protein assays using biuret reagent. To avoid misleading results when these tests are indicated, draw blood samples before initiating dextran therapy.

Pharmaceutical Characteristics

Concentration: 150 mg/mL

Quality Assay: Viscosity and ultraviolet absorbency tests for purity, and tests for protolytic impurities, heavy metals, and endotoxins

Packaging: 20 mL vial

NDC Number: 61569-0200-20

Doseform: Solution

Appearance: Do not administer unless clear.

Solvent: Sterile water for injection

Diluent:
For infusion: Do not dilute dextran-1 or mix it with clinical dextran solutions or any other fluid, to avoid decreasing efficacy.

Adjuvant: None

Preservative: None

Allergens: None

Excipients: Sodium chloride 6 mg/mL for tonicity, pH adjusted with hydrochloric acid

pH: 4.5

Shelf Life: Expires within 48 months.

Dextran-1

Storage/Stability: Store at room temperature, preferably 30°C (86°F) or below. Discard if frozen. Discard partially used containers. Product can tolerate 3 months at 60°C (140°F). Shipped at ambient temperature.

Production Process: Produced by action of the bacterium *Leuconostoc mesenteroides* on sucrose. The crude dextrans produced are then hydrolyzed and deferentially fractionated to obtain dextran fractions of desired molecular weight.

Threat Epidemiology

Incidence: The risk of dextran-induced anaphylactic reactions ranges from 2 to 25 per 1,000 units infused (2 to 13 per 1,000 units of dextran 40 infused, and 17 to 25 or more times per 1,000 units of dextran 60 or dextran 75 infused). An estimated 4% of the general population possesses dextran-reactive antibodies.

Other Information

Perspective:
1944: Dextran used as a plasma substitute in the United States.
1981: Human tests of dextran-1 in Germany and Scandinavia.
1984: *Promit* licensed in the United States on October 30, 1984.

References: Grabenstein JD. Dextran-1: An antibody antagonist. *Hosp Pharm.* 1993;28:140-144.

Hedin H, et al. Incidence, pathomechanism and prevention of dextran-induced anaphylactoid/anaphylactic reactions in man. *Devel Biol Stand.* 1981;48:179-189.

Ljungström KG. Dextran 40 therapy made safer by pretreatment with dextran 1. *Plast Reconstr Surg.* 2007;120(1):337-340.

Zinderman CE, Landow L, Wise RP. Anaphylactoid reactions to dextran 40 and 70: reports to the United States Food and Drug Administration, 1969 to 2004. *J Vasc Surg.* 2006;43(5):1004-1009.

Tuberculin Purified Protein Derivative Solution

Mycobacterial Antigens

Names:
    Tubersol Diagnostic Antigen
    Aplisol (Stabilized Solution)

Manufacturers:
    Sanofi Pasteur
    JHP Pharmaceuticals

Synonyms: PPD, Mantoux test, tuberculin skin test (TST)

Comparison: The various PPD solutions are generically equivalent, but differ from PPD multipuncture devices and from old tuberculin products. Intradermal PPD is more sensitive and more specific than any tuberculin delivered by multipuncture device.

Limited published data suggest that commercial brands of purified protein derivative (PPD) of tuberculin may vary in their false-positive reaction rate. Several published reports suggest that JHP's *Aplisol* may have a higher false-positive rate than Sanofi Pasteur's *Tubersol*, while *Tubersol* may produce somewhat more false-negative results than *Aplisol*. The clinical significance of these data are not yet clear.

Immunologic Characteristics

Microorganism: Bacterium, *Mycobacterium tuberculosis*, acid-fast bacillus (AFB), aerobic gram-positive rod

Viability: Inactivated

Antigenic Form: Isolate from culture filtrates

Antigenic Type: Protein. Skin tests assess delayed (type IV) hypersensitivity.

Strains:
    Sanofi Pasteur: Johnson strain of *M. tuberculosis*, derived from master batch CT68
    JHP: Human type strains, derived from master lot 154616

Use Characteristics

Indications: For detection of delayed hypersensitivity to *M. tuberculosis*. Tuberculin PPD is used as an aid in the diagnosis of infection with *M. tuberculosis*. The 5 TU/0.1 mL strength is the standard selected for the routine testing of individuals for tuberculosis, for testing of individuals suspected of having contact with active tuberculosis, and as a follow-up verification test in individuals who have had reactions to skin tests with tuberculin multiple-puncture devices, which are less sensitive diagnostic tools. Do not use multiple-puncture devices to screen high-risk populations.

Alternate concentrations: 1 TU and 250 TU/0.1 mL concentrations are no longer distributed in the United States.

The CDC Advisory Council for the Elimination of Tuberculosis recommends that the following groups be screened for tuberculosis and tuberculosis infection:

- Close contacts, those sharing the same household or other enclosed environments, of people known or suspected to have tuberculosis;
- People infected with HIV;
- People who inject illicit drugs or other locally identified high-risk substance users (eg, crack cocaine users);
- People who have medical risk factors known to increase the risk for disease if infection occurs (eg, diabetes mellitus, conditions requiring prolonged high-dose corticosteroid therapy or other immunosuppressive therapy, chronic renal failure, leukemias, lympho-

mas, carcinoma of the head or neck, weight loss to at least 10% below ideal body weight, silicosis, gastrectomy, jejunoileal bypass);
- Residents and employees of high-risk congregate settings (eg, correctional institutions, nursing homes, mental institutions, other long-term residential facilities, shelters for the homeless);
- Health care workers who serve high-risk clients;
- Foreign-born people, including children, who arrived within the last 5 years from areas that have a high tuberculosis incidence or prevalence (eg, most parts of Asia, Africa, Latin America);
- Some medically underserved, low-income populations;
- High-risk racial or ethnic minority populations, defined locally;
- Infants, children, and adolescents exposed to adults in the high-risk categories listed above.

High-risk categories will change over time as the epidemiology of tuberculosis infection changes. Screening people not members of high-risk groups is not recommended, because it diverts resources from other, more important activities.

The purpose for screening is to identify infected people who are at high risk for disease and who would benefit from preventive therapy or to find people who have clinical disease and need treatment. Screening programs can also provide epidemiologic data for assessing tuberculosis trends in a community, assessing the value of continued screening, and compiling baseline data to assess if subsequent exposure occurs (eg, for nursing-home residents and employees in some occupations). Do not undertake screening programs if necessary facilities for patient evaluation and treatment are unavailable or if patients found to be positive are unlikely to complete preventive therapy.

The American Academy of Pediatrics (AAP) recommends the following criteria for tuberculin skin testing of children:

Children for whom imminent skin testing is indicated:
- Contacts of people with confirmed or suspected infectious tuberculosis (contact investigation), including children in contact with family members or associates who spent time in jail or prison in the last 5 years.
- Children with radiographic or clinical findings suggesting tuberculosis.
- Children immigrating from endemic areas (eg, Asia, Middle East, Africa, Latin America).
- Children with travel histories to endemic countries or significant contact with indigenous persons from such countries.

Test these children annually for tuberculosis:
- Children infected with HIV.
- Incarcerated adolescents.

Test these children every 2 to 3 years (apply initial test upon diagnosis or circumstance):
- Children exposed to the following people: HIV-infected people, homeless people, residents of nursing homes, institutionalized adolescents or adults, users of illicit drugs, incarcerated adolescents or adults, and migrant farm workers. This includes foster children exposed to adults in these high-risk groups.

Consider testing these children at 4, 6, and 11 to 16 years of age:
- Children whose parents immigrated (with unknown tuberculin skin test status) from regions of the world with high prevalence of tuberculosis. Continued potential exposure by travel to the endemic areas or household contact with people from endemic areas (with unknown tuberculin skin test status) is an indication for repeat tuberculin skin testing.
- Children without specific risk factors who reside in high-prevalence areas. In general, a high-risk neighborhood or community does not mean an entire city is at high risk; rates in any city vary by neighborhood, or even from block to block. Be aware of these patterns in

determining the likelihood of exposure; public health officials or local tuberculosis experts can help clinicians identify areas that have appreciable tuberculosis rates.

AAP notes the following medical factors increase a child's risk for progression to disease: diabetes mellitus, chronic renal failure, malnutrition, and congenital or acquired immunodeficiencies. Without recent exposure, these people are not at increased risk of acquiring tuberculous infection. Underlying immune deficiencies theoretically enhance the possibility for progression to severe disease. Ask all these patients about potential exposure to tuberculosis. If exposure is possible, consider immediate and periodic tuberculin skin testing. Perform an initial intradermal tuberculin skin test before beginning immunosuppressive therapy in any child.

Limitations: A small percentage of responders may be infected with some mycobacterium other than *M. tuberculosis* (eg, *M. avium*, *M. intracellulare*). Not all patients suffering from tuberculosis will have a delayed-hypersensitivity reaction to a tuberculin test, including individuals who acquired the disease within the previous 2 to 5 weeks.

In some populations with high turnover rates (eg, some jails, prisons, homeless shelters), chest radiographs may be preferred as screening tools to PPD testing if the primary objective is to identify people with current pulmonary tuberculosis.

Contraindications:

Absolute: None

Relative: Do not administer tuberculin to known tuberculin-positive reactors because of the severity of reactions (eg, vesiculation, ulceration, necrosis) that may occur at the test site in very highly hypersensitive individuals. Rarely, tuberculin testing may activate quiescent tuberculous lesions in individuals with active tuberculosis.

Immunodeficiency: Skin-test responsiveness may be suppressed during or for as much as 6 weeks following viral infection, live viral vaccination, miliary or pulmonary tuberculosis infection, bacterial infection, severe febrile illness, malnutrition, sarcoidosis, malignancy, or immunosuppression (eg, corticosteroids or other immunosuppressive pharmacotherapy). In most patients who are very sick with tuberculosis, a previously negative tuberculin test becomes positive after a few weeks of chemotherapy. When of diagnostic importance, accept a negative test as proof that hypersensitivity is absent only after normal reactivity to common antigens has been demonstrated, such as with an anergy-test panel.

Elderly: Skin-test responsiveness may be delayed or reduced in magnitude among older patients. Two-step testing is important, especially in patients 35 years of age or older.

Once acquired, tuberculin sensitivity tends to persist, although it often wanes with time and advancing age. In older patients or in patients receiving a PPD test for the first time, the reaction may develop more slowly and may not be maximal until after 72 hours. Not all infected persons will have a delayed hypersensitivity reaction to PPD. A number of factors decrease the ability to respond to PPD, such as elderly patients with waned sensitivity. Any condition that impairs or attenuates CMI can cause a false-negative reaction, including aging

Pregnancy: Category C. The risk of unrecognized tuberculosis and the close postpartum contact between a mother with active disease and her infant leaves the infant in grave danger of tuberculosis and complications such as tuberculous meningitis. No adverse effects upon the fetus recognized as being due to tuberculosis skin testing have been reported. The state of pregnancy does not interfere with PPD test results. Test women with PPD if they have any substantial risk of disease.

Lactation: It is not likely that tuberculin is excreted in breast milk. Problems in humans have not been documented and are unlikely.

Children: A child known to have been exposed to a tuberculous adult must not be considered free of infection until the child demonstrates a negative tuberculin reaction at least 10 weeks after contact with the tuberculous person(s) has ceased.

Tuberculin Purified Protein Derivative Solution

Because their immune systems are immature, many neonates and infants younger than 6 weeks of age who are infected with *M. tuberculosis* may not have a delayed hypersensitivity reaction to a tuberculin test. Older infants and children develop tuberculin sensitivity 3 to 6 weeks and up to 3 months after initial infection.

Adverse Reactions: Immediate erythematous or other reactions may occur at the injection site. In highly hypersensitive individuals, strongly positive reactions including vesiculation, ulceration, or necrosis occur at the test site. The reasons for these infrequent occurrences are unknown. Cold packs or topical corticosteroid preparations can be used for symptomatic relief of the associated pain, pruritus, and discomfort.

Pharmacologic & Dosing Characteristics

Dosage: 0.1 mL of the appropriate concentration. The 5 TU/0.1 mL strength is the standard concentration.

Alternate concentrations: 1 TU and 250 TU/0.1 mL concentrations are no longer distributed in the United States.

Route & Site: Intradermal, also described as intracutaneous or the Mantoux method. A ½-inch, 26- or 27-gauge needle is recommended. Do not use syringes that have previously been used for another purpose or another patient.

Insert the point of the needle into the most superficial layers of the skin with the bevel pointing upward. As the tuberculin solution is injected, a pale bleb 6 to 10 mm in diameter rises over the point of the needle. This is quickly absorbed and no dressing is required. If no bleb forms (suggesting the fluid has been injected subcutaneously) or if a significant part of the dose leaks from the injection site, reapply the test at another site more than 5 cm away from the first site.

Avoid injecting subcutaneously. In such cases where no bleb forms, no local reaction develops, but a general febrile reaction or acute inflammation around old tuberculous lesions may occur in highly hypersensitive individuals.

The flexor (volar) or dorsal surface of the forearm approximately 4 inches below the elbow is preferred, although other sites may be used. Cleanse the site with 70% isopropyl alcohol and allow to dry before test injection. In patients with severe skin rashes, do not administer the test in areas where the rash occurs. Similarly, avoid hairy areas, scars, pimples, moles, and other marks.

Diagnostic Accuracy: The selection of 5 TU as the test dose is based on data indicating that:

(1) The 5 TU dose gives measurable reactions in more than 95% of the known tuberculous-infected patients tested;

(2) doses more than 5 TU may elicit reactions not caused by tuberculosis infection;

(3) nonreactors to doses considerably less than 5 TU are not accepted as negative but are retested with a stronger dose. In geographical regions with a high incidence of atypical (nontuberculous) mycobacterial infections, a threshold for positivity more than 10 mm of induration may be more accurate in delineating tuberculosis from nontuberculous mycobacterial hypersensitivity.

Time of Reading: Read test 48 to 72 hours after injection. Delayed-hypersensitivity reactions begin in 5 to 6 hours and peak after 48 to 72 hours. Reactions in elderly patients and those never before tested may peak sometime after 72 hours.

Interpretation: Consider only induration in interpreting a tuberculin test. Measure induration along the transverse diameter at a right angle to the long axis of the forearm. Detect induration by gently palpating the double skin fold between the thumb and forefinger, starting in a normal area around the test site and moving toward the test until a thickening is felt. Also record the presence of edema and necrosis. If erythema more than 10 mm in diameter occurs in the absence of induration, the injection may have been made too deeply; retest these patients.

Skin-test responsiveness may be suppressed during or for as much as 4 to 6 weeks following viral infection, live viral vaccination, miliary or pulmonary tuberculosis infection, bacterial infection, severe febrile illness, malnutrition, sarcoidosis, malignancy, or immunosuppression. In most patients who are very sick with tuberculosis, a previously negative tuberculin test becomes positive after a few weeks of treatment.

Reactions with induration of 5 mm or more diameter are classified as positive in:

(1) Patients of any age who have had recent close contact with people with active tuberculosis,

(2) patients with HIV infection or risk factors for HIV infection but unknown HIV status,

(3) patients who have fibrotic chest radiographs consistent with healed tuberculosis, and

(4) patients with organ transplants and other immune-suppressed patients (eg, those receiving prednisone 15 mg/day or more for 1 month or longer).

Reactions with induration of 10 mm or more diameter are classified as positive in patients not described above, but who belong to 1 or more of the following groups:

(1) Recent immigrants (within previous 5 years) from high-prevalence countries (eg, much of Asia, Africa, Latin America);

(2) injection-drug users;

(3) residents and employees of high-risk congregate settings, such as prisons and jails, nursing homes and other long-term facilities for the elderly, hospitals and other healthcare facilities, residential facilities for people with AIDS, and homeless shelters;

(4) mycobacteriology laboratory personnel;

(5) people with clinical conditions that place them at high risk, such as silicosis, diabetes mellitus, chronic renal failure, some hematological disorders (eg, leukemias, lymphomas), other specific malignancies (eg, carcinoma of head or neck and lung), weight loss at least 10% of ideal body weight, gastrectomy, and jejunoileal bypass;

(6) children younger than 4 years of age;

(7) infants, children, and adolescents exposed to adults in high-risk categories.

Reactions with induration at least 15 mm diameter are classified as positive in all other patients not listed above.

Skin test conversions

- For people with negative reactions who undergo repeat skin testing (eg, health care workers), consider an increase in reaction size more than 10 mm within a period of 2 years a skin-test conversion indicative of recent infection with *M. tuberculosis*.

- In some individuals who have been infected with nontuberculous mycobacteria or have undergone BCG vaccination, the skin test may show some degree of induration. For them, conversion to "positive" is defined as an increase in induration by 10 mm on subsequent tests.

Health care facilities and other high-risk settings

- For health care workers and employees in other high-risk settings with no other risk factors for TB, use a cut-off of 15 mm induration (rather than 10 mm) with PPD to define a positive baseline test at time of initial employment.

- An increase of more than 10 mm in reaction size is generally accepted as a positive result on subsequent testing, unless the worker is a contact of a TB case or has HIV infection or is otherwise immunocompromised, in which case more than 5 mm is considered positive.

Such a response indicates hypersensitivity to tuberculin and implies past or present infection with *M. tuberculosis*. A positive tuberculin reaction does not necessarily signify the presence of active disease. Conduct further diagnostic procedures before making a diagnosis of tuberculosis (eg, chest radiograph, microbiological examination of sputum). A small percentage of responders may be infected with some mycobacterium other than *M. tuberculosis* (eg, *M. avium, M. intracellulare*) or been sensitized through BCG vaccination. Tuberculin reactivity in BCG vaccinees does not reliably predict protection against *M. tuberculosis*.

Negative reactions involve induration less than 5 mm in diameter. This indicates lack of hypersensitivity to tuberculin and implies that tuberculous infection is highly unlikely.

Predictive Capacity: PPD tests are 95% sensitive, implying that 5% of infected test recipients will test falsely negative.

PPD tests are 98% specific, implying that 2% of uninfected test recipients will test falsely positive. Skin reactions may occur in individuals infected by nontuberculous mycobacteria (eg, *M. avium, M. intracellulare*). Specificity is highest among people living in Arctic areas or at high elevations and lowest in the tropics or at low elevations.

Subsequent Tests: Repeated testing of uninfected patients does not sensitize them to tuberculin. In patients with waning hypersensitivity to mycobacterial antigens, however, the stimulus of a tuberculin test may "boost" or increase the size of the reaction to a subsequent test from a week to a year later. This subsequent test may be misinterpreted as recent development of hypersensitivity in some instances. When conducting routine, periodic tuberculin testing of adults, use 2-stage testing to minimize the likelihood of interpreting a boosted reaction as a skin-test conversion from uninfected to infected. An interval of 1 to 3 weeks between tests is appropriate. A change from negative to positive results in that short interval probably indicates boosting. Classify these patients as reactors, not converters (see Interpretation of Serial Tuberculin Tests at the end of this section). The frequency of boosting is highest among people older than 55 years of age and among patients previously vaccinated with BCG.

Base the need for repeat skin testing on the degree of risk for exposure, derived from locally generated data. Base the interval for repeat testing, in part, on local rates of disease and skin-test conversion.

Sensitization: Sensitization to tuberculin occurs 2 to 10 weeks after mycobacterial infection. Negative PPD reactions 3 months after exposure imply the person was not infected.

Mechanism: Tuberculin deposited in the skin of tuberculin-reactive individuals reacts with sensitized lymphocytes to cause the release of mediators of cellular hypersensitivity. Some of these mediators (eg, skin reactive factor) induce an inflammatory response to the skin, causing the induration characteristic of a positive reaction.

The sensitization following infection with mycobacteria occurs primarily in the regional lymph nodes. Small T-lymphocytes proliferate in response to the antigenic stimulus to give rise to specifically sensitized lymphocytes. After several weeks, these lymphocytes enter the blood stream and circulate for long periods of time. Subsequent restimulation of these sensitized lymphocytes with the same or a similar antigen, such as intradermal injection of tuberculin, evokes a local reaction mediated by these cells. The tuberculin reaction is characterized by the early predominance of mononuclear cells (small- and medium-sized lymphocytes and monocytes). Only a small proportion of these cells appear to be lymphocytes sensitized to tuberculin. Most cells become involved in the reaction through the release of biologically active substances by sensitized lymphocytes. An increase in vascular permeability leading to erythema and edema also occurs in tuberculin reactions.

Drug Interactions: Reactivity to any tuberculin test may be suppressed in patients receiving high doses of corticosteroids or other immunosuppressive drugs, or in patients who were recently immunized with live virus vaccines (eg, measles, mumps, rubella). If tuberculin skin testing is indicated, perform it either preceding or simultaneous with immunization or 4 to 6 weeks after immunization.

Patients previously immunized with BCG vaccine may test positive to a tuberculin skin test. Tuberculin reactions caused by BCG cannot reliably be distinguished from reactions caused by natural mycobacterial infections. Test conversion rates after vaccination may be much less than 100%. The mean reaction size among vaccinees is often less than 10 mm, and tuberculin hypersensitivity tends to wane after vaccination. The ATS suggests it is appropriate to consider any significant reaction to 5 TU of PPD tuberculin in BCG-vaccinated patients as indicating infection with *M. tuberculosis*, especially among patients from countries with a high prevalence of tuberculosis. A compilation of global BCG vaccination policies appears at www.bcgatlas.org. Tuberculin reactivity in BCG vaccinees does not reliably predict protection against *M. tuberculosis*.

Several weeks of cimetidine therapy may augment or enhance delayed hypersensitivity responses to skin-test antigens, although this effect has not been consistently observed. The effect may be mediated through cimetidine binding to suppressor T-lymphocytes. It is presently unknown if other H_2 antagonists possess similar activity.

In a study of 24 BCG-vaccinated volunteers given 10 TU of PPD on each forearm, with one forearm randomly pretreated with a lidocaine-prilocaine mixture (EMLA cream), the treated forearm experienced less pain, but the tuberculin reaction was not affected.

Patient Information: It has been reported reported that only 37.2% of patients with more than 10 mm induration following 5 tuberculin units (TU) of tuberculin purified protein derivative (PPD) thought any induration was present. Do not rely on patients to read their own tests.

Pharmaceutical Characteristics

Concentration: 5 TU/0.1 mL, comparable to the US Reference Standard, PPD-S.

Alternate concentrations: The formerly available 1 TU/0.1 mL concentration was referred to as the "first strength" of PPD, 5 TU/0.1 mL as the "intermediate strength," and the formerly available 250 TU/0.1 mL as the "second strength." To avoid misinterpretation and dosage errors, do not use these designations.

Quality Assay: 5 TU/0.1 mL products must be clinically equivalent to the US Reference Standard, PPD-S. Other concentrations are not directly standardized; their potency is calculated based on dilution of standardized products. Produced in conformance with USP monograph, including guinea pig safety tests. The US tuberculin unit is equivalent to the international unit; 5 TU PPD-S is equivalent to 0.1 mcg/0.1 mL.

Packaging:

Sanofi Pasteur: 5 TU/0.1 mL, 10 tests per 1 mL vial (NDC #: 49281-0752-21), 50 tests per 5 mL vial (49281-0752-22)

JHP: 5 TU/0.1 mL, 10 tests per 1 mL vial (42023-0104-01), 50 tests per 5 mL vial (42023-0104-05)

Doseform: Solution

Appearance: Slightly opalescent, colorless solution

Solvent:

Sanofi Pasteur: Phosphate-buffered saline

JHP: Potassium and sodium phosphate buffers

Adjuvant: None

Preservative:

Sanofi Pasteur: 0.28% phenol

JHP: 0.35% phenol

Tuberculin Purified Protein Derivative Solution

Allergens: None

Excipients: 0.0005% to 0.0006% polysorbate 80, a stabilizer that prevents loss of potency due to adsorption to glass.

pH: 7.3 to 7.5

Shelf Life: Expires within 12 months.

Storage/Stability: Store at 2° to 8°C (36° to 46°F). Discard if frozen. PPD is light sensitive; expose to light only while measuring doses. Discard vials 1 month after first entry, because air introduced into the vial permits oxidation that reduces potency.

Prefilling syringes: PPD solution is stable when prefilled into syringes, individually labeled, and stored in a refrigerator for 30 days or less. Manipulation during prefilling increases the risk of microbial contamination. Aseptic technique in laminar-flow hoods will minimize this risk.

Sanofi Pasteur: Product can tolerate 24 hours at room temperature 24°C (75°F) or less. Vials that have not yet been entered can tolerate 24°C (75°F) for 72 hours. Use such products promptly. Shipped in insulated containers with coolant properties. Contact manufacturer regarding stability at elevated temperatures.

JHP: Product can tolerate at least 2 to 3 weeks at room temperature or 1 week at elevated temperature. Stability data suggest that frozen *Aplisol* is stable for 24 hours at −16°C (3°F). Shipped at ambient temperature.

Production Process: PPD is a precipitate of old tuberculin by ammonium sulfate or trichloroacetic acid by the method of Florence Seibert (1934). Evaporated to 10% of original volume.

Media: Protein-free synthetic medium

Disease Epidemiology

Incidence: In the middle of the 19th century, tuberculosis was the leading cause of death worldwide. An estimated 25% of the adult population of Europe in the mid-19th century died of pulmonary tuberculosis.

Disease incidence has been declining in industrialized nations since late in the 19th century. Only a limited amount of the decline in tuberculosis can be attributed to chemotherapy and BCG vaccination; most of the decline resulted from improved sanitation, less crowded urban living and working areas, improved nutrition, and other social conditions. In 1944, 126,000 cases were reported in the United States, a case rate of 95 per 100,000 population.

In 1992, approximately 26,673 cases were reported in the United States (10.5 cases per 100,000 population), continuing a pattern of increasing disease incidence since 1985. Of these cases, 2,500 were estimated to have resulted from recent infection and 23,000 from an infection in the more distant past. The incidence reported in 1990 was 9.4% greater than in 1989, the largest annual increase since 1953. Disease incidence reported in the general population was approximately 10.2 cases per 100,000 people. Disproportionately greater increases in tuberculosis occurred among Hispanics, non-Hispanic blacks, Asians, and Pacific Islanders. In contrast, decreases in tuberculosis incidence were reported among non-Hispanic whites, American Indians, and Alaskan natives. The 1995 rate for the general population, 8.7 cases per 100,000 people, is the lowest level reported since national surveillance began in 1953. The proportion of cases among foreign-born people has continued to rise, as has the incidence among people infected with HIV.

Approximately 10 to 15 million Americans have a latent tuberculosis infection (1995 CDC estimate). In the adult population of the United States, approximately 5% to 10% will react positively to a 5 TU tuberculin PPD test. Higher proportions are likely to test positive among high-risk populations.

Of patients newly infected with tuberculosis who react positively to a 5 TU tuberculin PPD test, approximately 12% can be expected to progress to active tuberculosis disease during their lifetime; this risk may be 4% for each of the first 2 years, with diminishing risk thereafter. Among patients with a positive PPD reaction from infection in the more distant past, an estimated 0.2% can be expected to progress to active tuberculosis.

Half of the world's population is infected with *M. tuberculosis*. As many as 10 million new cases of active tuberculosis occur throughout the world each year, with 2 to 3 million deaths. More than 3 billion doses of BCG vaccine have been administered worldwide, and more than 70% of the world's children receive BCG vaccination. A compilation of global BCG vaccination policies appears at www.bcgatlas.org.

Susceptible Pools: People infected with HIV comprise the largest pool of people in the United States susceptible to tuberculosis. Medically underserved populations, including racial and ethnic minorities and foreign-born people, are also at increased risk.

Transmission: Exposure to bacilli in airborne droplet nuclei produced by people with pulmonary or laryngeal tuberculosis during expiratory efforts (eg, coughing, singing, sneezing). Bovine tuberculosis in humans most often results from ingestion of unpasteurized dairy products.

Incubation: The incubation period from infection to primary lesion or significant tuberculin reaction is approximately 4 to 12 weeks. While the risk of tuberculosis peaks within the first 1 to 2 years after infection, the risk of activation persists throughout life. Among immunocompetent adults, active tuberculosis disease will develop in 5% to 15% during their lifetimes. The risk is greatest in the first 2 years, then decreases markedly. The likelihood that latent infection will progress to active disease in infants and children is substantially greater than for most other age groups. The risk for active tuberculosis disease among HIV-infected people may remain high for an indefinite period of time or may even increase as immunosuppression progresses.

Active tuberculosis disease is fatal in 50% or fewer of people who have not been treated. Chemotherapy has helped reduce the fatality rate 94%, to a mortality rate of 0.6 deaths per 100,000 population in 1993. The rate in 1954 was 12.4 deaths per 100,000 population.

Communicability: Prolonged close contact to an infectious person can lead to infection of contacts. Communicability persists as long as viable tubercle bacilli are discharged in the sputum. The status of the acid-fast bacillus smear of the source case may be the strongest predictor of which patients are most contagious.

Other Information

Perspective: Also see the BCG vaccine monograph in the Vaccines/Toxoids section.

1890: Koch discovers tuberculin, a glycerinated extract of soluble products of the tubercle bacillus. He earns the 1905 Nobel Prize in Medicine for this and related work. Koch initially thought tuberculin cured early cases of tuberculosis.

1907: Calmette introduces conjunctival tuberculin test. Pirquet develops tuberculin test in which test material is applied to a superficial abrasion of the skin.

1908: Mantoux introduces ID test for tuberculosis.

Early 20th century: Koch introduces "new" tuberculin, an emulsion of dried pulverized organisms in 50% glycerin, resulting in adoption of the term "old" tuberculin for the original product. At various times, a wide variety of tuberculin doseforms were available, including ointments, patch tests, tablets of PPD for reconstitution, and products for subcutaneous or conjunctival tests. In 1927, 65 forms of tuberculin and 36 vaccines were reportedly available in the United States.

1931: Siebert develops purified protein derivative (PPD) of tuberculin.

1939: Siebert's PPD lot 49608 prepared, the US Reference Standard. In 1952, this lot becomes the international standard, called PPD-S.

1951: Heaf describes a multiple-puncture tuberculin test using a mechanical punch device with 6 needles.

1965: Institut Mérieux develops plastic-tine multipuncture device in France.

1970: Polysorbate 80 added to PPD to prevent protein adsorption to glass walls of vials. Earlier products were unstable, with inconsistent potency.

1985: Incidence of tuberculosis begins to rise again in the United States, after declining for decades, including the threat of multiple drug-resistant strains.

Over the years, various names were used to describe tuberculin tests. A summary of names for various routes of administration follows:

Calmette test—a conjunctival test

Heaf test—a mechanical multipuncture device

Mantoux test—intradermal injection

Moro test—lanolin-based topical application

Pirquet's test—scarification

Rosenthal test—a tine test with a multipuncture device

Vollmer test—a patch test

First Licensed:
Connaught: September 26, 1969 (now Sanofi Pasteur)
Parke-Davis: 1973 (sold to Parkedale in 1998 and to JHP in 2007)

National Policy: American Thoracic Society, Centers for Disease Control and Prevention, Infectious Diseases Society of America. Controlling tuberculosis in the United States. *MMWR.* 2005;54(RR-12):1-81. Erratum in *MMWR.* 2005;54(45):1161.http://www.cdc.gov/mmwr/PDF/rr/rr5412.pdf.

CDC. Targeted tuberculin testing and treatment of latent tuberculosis infection. *MMWR.* 2000;49(RR-6):1-51. ftp.cdc.gov/pub/Publications/mmwr/rr/rr4906.pdf.

References: American Thoracic Society, CDC, Infectious Disease Society of America. Treatment of tuberculosis. *MMWR.* 2003;S2(RR-11):1-77.

Sepkowitz KA. How contagious is tuberculosis? *Clin Infect Dis.* 1996;23:954-962.

Snider DE Jr. Bacille Calmette-Guérin vaccinations and tuberculin skin tests. *JAMA.* 1985;253:3438-3439.

Zwerling A, Behr MA, Verma A, Brewer TF, Menzies D, Pai M. The BCG World Atlas: a database of global BCG vaccination policies and practices. *PLoS Med.* 2011;8(3):e1001012.

Interpretation of Serial Tuberculin Tests			
Initial reaction	Subsequent reaction	Time interval	Interpretation
Positive to any multiple-puncture device[a] (OT or PPD)	Positive to intradermal PPD	A few days	Infected
Positive to any multiple-puncture device[a] (OT or PPD)	Negative to any tuberculin test (OT or PPD)	A few days	Not infected (the initial reaction represents a false-positive reaction to the multiple-puncture device)
Negative to any tuberculin test (OT or PPD)	Positive to any tuberculin test (OT or PPD)	A few days, weeks, or a month	Infected during the entire period (the second reaction represents a "booster" reaction induced by the first test)
Negative to any tuberculin test (OT or PPD)	Positive to intradermal PPD	Months or years	Newly infected (a "converter")
Positive to intradermal PPD (negative history of BCG vaccination)	Negative to intradermal PPD	At any time in the future	Immunosuppressed (anergic, perhaps from tuberculosis itself)
Positive to intradermal PPD (positive history of BCG vaccination)	Negative to intradermal PPD	At any time in the future	Either immunosuppressed (anergic, perhaps from tuberculosis itself) or waning immunity to BCG
Negative to any tuberculin test (OT or PPD)	Negative to any tuberculin test (OT or PPD)	Weeks, months, or years	Not infected (assumes anergy is not a factor)

a Multipuncture devices (eg, OT) are no longer distributed in the United States.

Ubiquitous Delayed Antigens

Name:
Candin

Manufacturer:
Allermed Laboratories

Synonyms: Candidin is an obsolete term. The *Candida* genus of fungi was formerly called *Oidium* and later *Monilia*.

Comparison: Unlike the now-obsolete oidiomycin and other unstandardized *Candida albicans* allergen extracts, *Candin* is standardized in vivo against an internal reference product to ensure potency and reproducibility of cutaneous test results.

In the literature, the incidence of delayed-hypersensitivity reactions to unstandardized *Candida* antigens has been reported to vary from 52% to 89%, depending upon the strength of the antigen and the induration size defined as a positive test. In contrast, when healthy subjects were tested with 2 reagents, *Candin* and mumps skin test antigen, 92% were positive to at least 1 antigen, a higher response rate than to either antigen used alone.

Immunologic Characteristics

Microorganism: Fungus, *Candida albicans*. Subdivision Deuteromycotina (formerly called Fungi imperfecti), class *Blastomyces*

Viability: Inactivated

Antigenic Form: Fungal culture filtrate

Antigenic Type: Presumably polysaccharides and proteins, representing fungal cell-wall antigens. Skin tests assess delayed (type IV) hypersensitivity.

Strains: 2 proprietary strains of *Candida albicans*

Use Characteristics

Indications: For use as a recall antigen for detecting delayed hypersensitivity by intracutaneous (ID) testing. The product may be useful in evaluating the cellular immune response in patients suspected of having reduced cell-mediated immunity.

Published studies confirm that antigens of *Candida albicans* are useful in the assessment of diminished cellular immunity in patients infected with human immunodeficiency virus. Responses to delayed-hypersensitivity antigens have been reported to have prognostic value in patients with cancer.

Because HIV infection can modify the delayed-hypersensitivity response to tuberculin, it is advisable to skin test HIV-infected patients at high risk of tuberculosis with antigens in addition to tuberculin, to assess their competency to react to tuberculin.

Limitations: Because some people with normal cellular immunity are not hypersensitive to *Candida*, a response rate less than 100% to the antigen is to be expected in normal individuals. Therefore, the concurrent use of other licensed delayed-hypersensitivity skin test antigens is recommended. Do not use this product to diagnose or treat type I allergy to *Candida albicans*.

Contraindications:
Absolute: Patients who had a previous unacceptable adverse reaction to this antigen or to a similar product (ie, extreme hypersensitivity or allergy). As has been observed with other, unstandardized antigens used for delayed-hypersensitivity skin testing, it is possible that some patients may have exquisite immediate hypersensitivity to *Candin*.

Relative: Patients with bleeding tendency; bruising and nonspecific induration may occur because of the trauma of the skin test.

Immunodeficiency: Because immunodeficiencies of various types can modify the delayed-hypersensitivity response to *Candida albicans* and similar skin test antigens, negative results to panels of delayed-hypersensitivity antigens may indicate a loss or reduction of cell-mediated immunity.

Elderly: No specific information is available about geriatric use of *Candin*. The delayed-hypersensitivity response to *Candin* may be diminished in geriatric patients, because the aging process is known to alter cell-mediated immunity.

Carcinogenicity: Long-term studies in animals have not been conducted with *Candin* to determine its potential for carcinogenicity.

Mutagenicity: Long-term studies in animals have not been conducted with *Candin* to determine its potential for mutagenicity.

Fertility Impairment: Long-term studies in animals have not been conducted with *Candin* to determine its potential for impairing fertility.

Pregnancy: Category C. Animal reproduction studies have not been conducted with *Candin*. It is not known whether *Candin* can cause fetal harm when administered to a pregnant woman. Use *Candin* in pregnant women only if clearly needed. Considering the safety record of tuberculin in pregnant women, problems are unlikely.

Lactation: It is not known if *Candin* crosses into human breast milk. Problems in humans have not been documented and are unlikely.

Children: Safety and efficacy of *Candin* in children less than 18 years old have not been established.

Adverse Reactions:

Systemic: Systemic reactions to *Candin* have not been observed. However, all foreign antigens have the remote possibility of causing anaphylaxis and even death when injected intradermally. Systemic reactions usually occur within 30 minutes after the injection of antigen and may include the following symptoms: sneezing, coughing, itching, shortness of breath, abdominal cramps, vomiting, diarrhea, tachycardia, hypotension, and respiratory failure in severe cases. Progression of the delayed reaction to vesiculation, necrosis and ulceration is possible. Systemic allergic reactions including anaphylaxis must be immediately treated with epinephrine hydrochloride 1:1,000. Additional measures may be required depending upon the severity of the reaction.

Immediate hypersensitivity reactions: Immediate hypersensitivity reactions to *Candin* occur in some individuals. These reactions are characterized by the presence of an edematous hive surrounded by a zone of erythema. They occur approximately 15 to 20 minutes after the ID injection of the antigen. The size of the immediate reaction varies depending upon the sensitivity of the individual. Immediate hypersensitivity reactions have been reported in 17% to 22% of patients, with erythema of 10 to 24 mm in diameter, and in another 5% to 13% of patients, with erythema of 5 to 9 mm.

Local: Local reactions to *Candin* can include redness, swelling, pruritus, excoriation, and discoloration of the skin. These reactions usually subside within hours or days after administration of the skin test. In some patients, skin discoloration may persist for several weeks. Local reactions may be treated with a cold compress and topical steroids. Severe local reactions may require additional measures as appropriate.

In a published study of 479 HIV-positive adults tested with *Candin*, adverse local reactions were observed in six subjects as follows: pruritus (n = 3), swelling at the test site (n = 1), vesiculation (n = 1) and vesiculation with weeping edema (n = 1). Pruritus and swelling cleared within 48 hours; vesiculation with edema required about 1 week to resolve. In 2 studies involving 171 people, 1 adverse reaction was observed. This reaction consisted of induration 22 × 55 mm at 48 hours, which resolved within 1 week.

Severe local reactions including rash, vesiculation, bullae, dermal exfoliation, and cellulitis have been reported to MedWatch for unstandardized allergenic extracts of *Candida albicans* used for anergy testing.

Pharmacologic & Dosing Characteristics

Dosage: The test dose is 0.1 mL.

Route & Site: Inject *Candin* ID on the volar surface of the forearm or on the outer aspect of the upper arm. Cleanse the skin with 70% alcohol before applying the skin test. The ID injection must be given as superficially as possible, causing a distinct, sharply defined bleb. An unreliable reaction may result if the product is injected subcutaneously. Do not inject into a blood vessel.

Efficacy: In 1 group of 18 healthy adults, 14 (78%) of the individuals reacted to *Candin* with an induration response of 5 mm or more at 48 hours. In a second study of 35 subjects, 21 (60%) had induration reactions 5 mm or more at 48 hours. In this study, 65% of males tested positive compared with 53% of females; the mean induration in responding males was 12.8 mm and in responding females was 13 mm. When subjects in these studies were tested with 2 reagents, *Candin* and mumps skin test antigen, 92% were positive to at least 1 antigen, a higher response rate than to either antigen used alone.

In another study, the skin test responses of adults with HIV infection were compared with those of healthy control subjects. The responses in HIV-infected patients who did not meet the definition of AIDS were less than those in uninfected subjects, but the differences were not statistically significant. A significant difference was found between AIDS patients and uninfected controls in both mean induration ($P < 0.01$) and proportion with 5 mm or more response ($P < 0.01$).

In a related study involving 20 male patients diagnosed with AIDS, 1 subject responded to *Candin*. In this study, 65% of the male control subjects had delayed-hypersensitivity reactions of 5 mm or more to *Candin*. The mean induration response at 48 hours for control subjects was 8.33 mm, compared with 1.78 mm for the AIDS subjects. AIDS vs control *P*-values were < 0.01 for mean induration and < 0.01 for induration 5 mm or more.

In a published study of delayed-hypersensitivity anergy, 479 subjects (334 males and 145 females) infected with HIV and being screened for tuberculosis were skin tested with several additional antigens, including *Candin*. Only 12% reacted to tuberculin (5 mm or more), 57% reacted to *Candin* (3 mm or more), and 60% reacted to either tuberculin or *Candin* or both. In this study, a 3 mm induration response to *Candin* was considered positive. The authors concluded that in HIV-infected subjects, testing with other delayed-hypersensitivity antigens increases the accuracy of interpretation of negative tuberculin reactions.

In another study of 18 patients with lung cancer, *Candin* elicited a positive induration response in 5 patients (28%). In a second series of 20 patients with metastatic cancer, no reactions more than 5 mm were observed.

Time of Reading: The time required for the induration response to reach maximum intensity varies with the individual. The reaction usually begins within 24 hours and peaks between 24 and 48 hours. Read the skin test after 48 hours by visually inspecting the test site and palpating the indurated area. Measure across 2 diameters. Report the mean of the longest and midpoint diameters of the indurated area as the delayed-hypersensitivity response. For example, a reaction that is 10 mm (longest diameter) by 8 mm (midpoint orthogonal diameter) has a sum of 18 mm and a mean of 9 mm. The delayed-hypersensitivity response is therefore 9 mm.

Interpretation: Induration 5 mm or more is classified as a positive delayed-hypersensitivity reaction to *Candin*.

Predictive Capacity: Except for mumps skin test antigen and *Candin*, most commonly used recall antigens were developed for other purposes, and the size of the reaction elicited may not be directly related to cellular immunity because of variability in antigen source and dose and skin test administration and measurement techniques. Useful antigens are those which elicit a reaction size 5 mm or more in greater than 50% of normal individuals. The combination of results from skin testing with more than 1 antigen should result in detection of delayed hypersensitivity in 95% or more of healthy subjects.

Mechanism: Cellular or delayed-type hypersensitivity (delayed hypersensitivity) can be assessed by ID testing with bacterial, viral, and fungal antigens to which most healthy people are sensitized. A positive skin test denotes prior antigenic exposure, T-cell competency, and an intact inflammatory response. The reaction usually peaks 48 hours after antigen is introduced into the skin and is manifest as induration at the test site.

The inflammatory response associated with the delayed-hypersensitivity reaction is characterized by an infiltration of lymphocytes and macrophages at the site of antigen deposition. Specific cell types that appear to play a major role in the delayed-hypersensitivity response include CD4+ and CD8+ T-lymphocytes that leave the recirculating lymphocyte pool in response to exogenous antigen. Both CD4+ and CD8+ lymphocytes have been recovered from delayed-hypersensitivity reactions elicited by *Candida* antigen.

Drug Interactions: Pharmacologic doses of corticosteroids may variably suppress the delayed-hypersensitivity skin test response after 2 weeks of therapy. The mechanism of suppression is believed to involve a decrease in monocytes and lymphocytes, particularly T-cells. The skin test response usually returns to the pretreatment level within several weeks after steroid therapy is discontinued.

Pharmaceutical Characteristics

Concentration: *Candin* is not explicitly labeled in potency units.

Quality Assay: The skin-test potency of *Candin* is measured in cutaneous dose-response studies in healthy adults. The product is intended to elicit an induration response of at least 5 mm in immunologically competent people with cellular hypersensitivity to the antigen. The procedure involves concurrent (side-by-side) testing of production lots with an Internal Reference (IR), using sensitive adults who have been previously screened and qualified to serve as test subjects. The induration response at 48 hours elicited by 0.1 mL of a production lot is measured and compared with the response elicited by 0.1 mL of the IR. The test is satisfactory if the potency of the production lot does not differ more than ± 20% from the potency of the IR, when analyzed by the paired t-test (2-tailed) at a P value of 0.05.

People included in the potency assay are qualified as test subjects by receiving 4 skin tests with the IR from which a mean induration response is calculated. Current skin tests with the IR must show that the potency of the IR has not changed more than ± 20% from the mean qualifying response in the same test subjects, when analyzed by the paired t-test (2-tailed) at a P value of 0.05. The required induration response at 48 hours to the IR is 15 mm ± 20%.

Packaging: 1 mL multidose vials containing ten 0.1 mL doses

NDC Number: 49643-0138-01

Doseform: Solution

Appearance: Clear, colorless

Solvent: 0.5% sodium chloride, 0.25% sodium bicarbonate

Adjuvant: None

Preservative: 0.4% phenol

Allergens: 0.03% human serum albumin

Excipients: 0.0008% polysorbate 80

pH: 8 to 8.5

Shelf Life: Expires in 18 months or less.

Storage/Stability: Store at 2° to 8°C (36° to 46°F). Discard frozen product. Product can tolerate up to 7 days at 40°C (104°F). Shipped under ambient conditions in uninsulated containers for second-day delivery.

Production Process: *Candin* is made from the culture filtrate and cells of 2 strains of *Candida albicans*. The fungi are propagated in a chemically defined medium consisting of inorganic salts, biotin, and sucrose. Lyophilized source material is extracted with a solution of 0.25% NaCl, 0.125% NaHCO$_3$ and 50% v/v glycerol. The concentrated extract is diluted with a solution of 0.5% NaCl, 0.25% NaHCO$_3$, 0.03% albumin (human) USP, 8 ppm polysorbate 80, and 0.4% phenol.

Media: A chemically defined medium consisting of inorganic salts, biotin, and sucrose

---

Other Information

Perspective:
1839: von Langenbeck discovers *Candida albicans*.

First Licensed: November 27, 1995

Discontinued Products: *Dermatophytin "O"* (variously from Hollister-Stier, Miles and Bayer)

References: Ohri LK, Manley JM, Chatterjee A, Cornish NE. Pediatric case series evaluating a standardized *Candida albicans* skin test product. *Ann Pharmacother*. 2004;38(6):973-977.

Delayed-Hypersensitivity Antigens, Miscellaneous

Comparative Table of Contact Dermatitis Allergens		
Manufacturer	Hermal Kurt Hermann	Mekos Laboratories
Distributor	Hermal Laboratories	Allerderm Laboratories
Proprietary Name	generic	*T.R.U.E. Test*
Doseform	syringes of allergen pastes and solutions	Unit-dose prefilled allergen patches
Shelf Life	24 months	12 months
Packaging	kit of 20 reclosable syringes suitable for testing 150 patients	package of 5 pairs of patches
Route of administration	topical, preferably to upper back	topical, preferably to upper back
Contents	balsam of Peru	balsam of Peru
	benzocaine	caine mix (benzocaine, tetracaine, dibucaine)
	black rubber mix	black rubber mix
	p-tert-butylphenol formaldehyde resin	p-tert-butylphenol formaldehyde resin
	carba mix	carba mix
	cinnamic aldehyde	fragrance mix (geraniol, cinnamaldehyde, hydroxycitronellal, eugenol, isoeugenol, -amyl-cinnaldehyde, oak moss)
	—	chloromethylisothiazolione
	—	cobalt dichloride hexahydrate
	colophony	colophony
	epoxy resin	epoxy resin
	ethylenediamine dihydrochloride	ethylenediamine dihydrochloride
	formaldehyde	formaldehyde
	imidazolidinyl urea (Germall 115)	
	lanolin alcohol (wool wax alcohols)	wool alcohols (lanolin)
	mercaptobenzothiazole	mercaptobenzothiazole
	mercapto mix	mercapto mix
	neomycin sulfate	neomycin sulfate
	nickel sulfate anhydrous	nickel sulfate hexahydrate
	—	paraben mix (methyl-, ethyl-, propyl-, butyl-, and benzyl-parahydroxybenzoate)
	p-phenylenediamine	p-phenylenediamine
	potassium dichromate	potassium dichromate
	Quaternium-15	Quaternium-15
	—	quinoline mix (clioquinol and chlorquinaldol)
	—	thimerosal
	thiuram mix	thiuram mix

Allergen Reaction Frequencies & Locations	
Allergen (frequency of reaction among people with suspected contact dermatitis)	Where allergen is typically encountered
balsam of Peru (3.3% to 5.1%)	This resin is found in many cosmetics and perfumes and is also used as a flavoring agent in cough syrups, lozenges, chewing gum, and candies.
benzocaine, tetracaine, dibucaine (2% to 3.5%)	Benzocaine, tetracaine, and dibucaine are found in many topical anesthetic medications.
black rubber mix (1.4% to 2.1%)	The components of black rubber mix are antioxidant and antiozonate chemicals, found in almost all black rubber products, eg, tires, handles, hoses.
p-tert-butylphenol formaldehyde resin (0.9% to 3.1%)	This resin is found in many waterproof glues used in the leather goods, furniture, and shoe industries.
carba mix (2% to 3.3%)	These chemicals are used to stabilize rubber products. These chemical stabilizers are found in almost all rubber products, many pesticides, and some glues.
cinnamic aldehyde and other fragrances (3.1% to 7%)	The components of fragrance mix are commonly used in toiletries, fragrances, and flavorings.
chloromethylisothiazolinone (2.7%)	This antibacterial preservative is found in many shampoos, creams, lotions, and other skin care products.
chromium (potassium dichromate) (1.7% to 5.2%)	Chromium is found in cement, and in many industrial chemicals.
cobalt dichloride hexahydrate (7.3%)	Cobalt is found in metal-plated objects and costume jewelry.
colophony (1.9% to 2.7%)	Colophony, also called rosin, is found in adhesives, sealants, and pine oil cleaners.
epoxy resin (1.3% to 2.1%)	This resin is found in adhesives, surface coatings, and paints.
ethylenediamine dihydrochloride (2.3% to 5.9%)	Ethylenediamine is used as a stabilizer, emulsifier, and preservative in topical fungicides, antibiotic creams, eye drops, and nose drops
formaldehyde (5.8% to 6.8%)	Formaldehyde is found in many building materials and plastic industries.
imidazolidinyl urea (Germall 115) (1.5%)	This preservative is commonly found in cosmetics and topical nonprescription drugs.
lanolin (wood alcohols) (1.2% to 1.5%)	Wool alcohols (lanolin) is a common constituent of many ointments, creams, lotions, and soaps.
mercaptobenzothiazole (2.1% to 2.7%)	This chemical, a vulcanization accelerator, is found in most rubber products, some adhesives, and is used as an industrial anticorrosive agent.
mercapto mix (2.5% to 3.1%)	This group of chemical accelerators is found in many rubber products, eg, shoes, gloves, elastic.
neomycin sulfate (4.3% to 7.2%)	Neomycin is a common antibiotic and is found in topical antibiotic creams, lotions, ointments, eye drops, and ear drops.
nickel sulfate (10% to 20%)	Nickel is one of the most common metals in the environment and is found in most metal and metal-plated objects.

Allergen Summary

Allergen Reaction Frequencies & Locations	
Allergen (frequency of reaction among people with suspected contact dermatitis)	Where allergen is typically encountered
parabens (1.7%)	The components of paraben mix can be found in cosmetics, dermatological creams, and paste bandages.
p-phenylenediamine (4% to 6.9%)	This blue-black aniline dye is found most often in permanent and semipermanent hair dyes.
Quaternium-15 (6.2% to 6.8%)	This preservative is found in creams, lotions, shampoos, soaps, and other cosmetics and skin-care products.
quinolines (0.7%)	The components of quinoline mix are found mostly in veterinary products, in certain types of paste bandages, and in some medicated creams and ointments.
rosin	See colophony.
thimerosal (8.7% to 10.5%)	Thimerosal is a preservative that contains mercury. Thimerosal is found in some medications, cosmetics, nose drops, and ear drops.
thiuram mix (3.9% to 5.5%)	These antimicrobial and antioxidant substances are found in almost all rubber products.

Delayed-Hypersensitivity Antigens, Miscellaneous

Name:
Generic

Manufacturer:
Almirall Hermal, distributed by Hermal
Laboratories

Comparison: Hermal's allergens are provided in reclosable syringes for application to a holding device; *T.R.U.E. Test* is a unit-dose pair of patches for direct application to the skin. Available allergens vary (see table). Concordance of skin reactions with the two products will range from 60% to 80% because of variability of individual patient response.

Immunologic Characteristics

Antigen Source: 21 distinct allergens: Balsam of Peru, benzocaine, black rubber mix, p-tert-butylphenol formaldehyde, carba mix, cinnamic aldehyde, colophony, epoxy resin, ethylenediamine, formaldehyde, imidazolidinyl urea (Germall 115), lanolin alcohol (wool wax alcohols), mercaptobenzothiazole, mercapto mix, neomycin sulfate, nickel sulfate, p-phenylenediamine, potassium dichromate (chromium), Quaternium 15, thiuram mix. For details, see Pharmaceutical Characteristics.

Viability: Inactive

Antigenic Form: Chemical allergens

Antigenic Type: Various chemicals, see Pharmaceutical Characteristics. Skin tests assess delayed (type IV) hypersensitivity. Contact allergens are generally low molecular weight substances, usually less than 500 daltons, that can easily penetrate the horny layer of the epidermis.

Strains: Chemically pure

Use Characteristics

Indications: For assessment of contact dermatitis. This test kit includes a group of substances associated with contact dermatitis. The kit may be used as an aid in diagnosing contact dermatitis or as a diagnostic screen. A thorough patient history is essential in evaluating the significance of a positive reaction. These allergens may be used individually or as a battery.

Limitations: The failure of a patient to react to the allergen patch test does not rule out possible allergic-contact hypersensitivity. Active sensitization to test allergens has resulted from the testing process. Therefore, weigh clinical benefits anticipated from repetitive testing against possible increased risks of adverse reactions with repetitive use (eg, active sensitization or increased reactivity).

Contraindications:

Absolute: None

Relative: Evaluate the use of this product in patients with known severe systemic or local reactions to 1 of the allergens in this kit carefully before application.

Immunodeficiency: Patients receiving immunosuppressive therapy or with other immunodeficiencies (especially those involving cell-mediated immunity) may have a diminished skin-test response to this and other diagnostic antigens.

Elderly: No specific information is available about geriatric use of the allergen patch test kit.

Carcinogenicity: Repeated exposure to nickel refinery dust and nickel subsulfite are known to be carcinogenic in humans. Formaldehyde is a possible human carcinogen. The relevance of these findings to a single application of a nickel or formaldehyde allergen patch test is unknown.

Pregnancy: Category C. Use only if clearly needed. It is unlikely that patch test allergens cross the placenta.

Lactation: No studies have been performed to date to assess the systemic absorption of the allergen patch test reagents in nursing mothers. Problems in humans have not been reported.

Children: The safety and efficacy of the allergen patch test in children have not been established.

Adverse Reactions: Reactions associated with topical application of allergen patch test reagents are generally mild and limited to the test site. Adverse reactions that persisted more than 7 days after patch testing were generally mild:

Pruritus, erythema, hyperpigmentation, edema, hypopigmentation, irritation. One patient reported oozing skin at a nickel patch test site that remained pruritic and irritated for 3 weeks after testing. Another nickel-sensitive patient reported a subsequent flare of dermatitis of the arms and legs that did not fully resolve for several months. Cellulitis and local lymphadenitis involving the left ear lobe were observed 7 days after application of the allergen patch test in a woman with a history of contact hypersensitivity to jewelry who tested positive at the nickel patch site. Possible adverse reactions may include reactions in old areas of eczema distal to the test site. Koebner-phenomenon (isomorphic) reactions in patients with psoriasis may occur. Very rarely, anaphylactic reactions may occur, most often associated with test antibiotics (eg, neomycin).

Consultation: Advise patients to avoid extreme physical activity or mechanical action that may result in reduced adhesion, perspiration, or actual loss of the patch test material. Avoid showering or otherwise wetting the test sites while patch tests are in place. Advise patients to consult the prescriber concerning possible removal of the offending test strip(s) if they experience intense discomfort from itching, burning, erythema, or vesiculation.

Pharmacologic & Dosing Characteristics

Dosage: Apply 1, several, or all 20 allergens as a test battery. In patch testing, apply the allergen dose to a holding device. Occlusion is essential for reliable patch testing. This can be provided by using *Finn Chambers* on *Scanpor* tape. Apply a 5 mm ribbon of each petrolatum-based allergen directly into separate *Finn Chambers*. For water-based allergens, use 1 drop of each allergen solution to saturate individual 3 mm diameter paper discs in separate chambers. Do not overfill the chambers.

Apply patch tests in multiple columns, labeled with letters (eg, A, B, C, D) in indelible ink, generally as viewed from left to right. Number the individual tests in each column from top to bottom. The preferred sequence of application is the order listed under Pharmaceutical Characteristics.

Affix the lower portion of the test strip first. Then affix the chambers at the lower end of the tape by pressing them from below to let air escape from the chambers. Next, press the top of each chamber gently to obtain an even distribution of the allergen against the skin. Then press the surrounding tape against the skin. Repeat this process with each chamber, working from bottom to top.

Route & Site: Topical, to normal-appearing skin free of dermatitis. Mark test sites adequately (eg, with an indelible marker) to allow identification of individual test sites when the occlusive tape is removed 48 hours later. All controlled clinical trials were performed using *Finn Chambers* on *Scanpor* tape. The efficacy of other test modalities has not been established.

The upper back is the preferred test site, avoiding the vertebrae, although other areas may be used. In some cases, it may be necessary to shave the site prior to application of the tests. During application to the upper back, the patient should stand erect with shoulders dorsi-flexed, as in a military position of attention. This will allow the tape to fit tightly against the back when the patient assumes normal standing, sitting, and reclining postures.

Scoring: Use patch-test record sheets provided in the test kit to record the allergens tested, their position, and test results. At each test reading, score responses using the following scale (or symbol):

1 = weak, nonvesicular reaction: erythema, infiltration, possibly papules (+)
2 = strong, edematous, or vesicular reaction (++)
3 = extreme, spreading, bullous, ulcerative reaction (+++)
4 = doubtful reaction, macular erythema only (?)
5 = irritant reaction (IR)
6 = negative reaction (−)
7 = excited skin
8 = not tested

Time of Reading: Remove tests 48 hours after application. Read the skin-test sites 30 to 60 minutes after tape removal, to allow the erythema associated with tape removal to sub-side and to permit some positive patch tests to manifest. Also, delayed readings are essential because some tests may turn positive after an additional period, yielding as many as 34% more positive reactions. Generally, a delayed reading 3 to 5 days after test removal suffices.

Interpretation: Avoid allergens to which the patient tests positive, to preclude future epi-sodes of contact dermatitis. Various summaries of products to avoid for each chemical have been published. The threshold at which to begin counseling avoidance varies among clini-cians.

Predictive Capacity: When 40 patients with suspected contact dermatitis to at least 1 of the 20 allergens contained in this kit were tested to each of the 20 allergens, 21 had a positive response when read within 7 days. False-negative reactions may complicate interpretation of patch tests and most frequently result from failure of the patch test to duplicate the condi-tions of natural allergen exposure, failure to perform delayed readings, concomitant adminis-tration of corticosteroids, and miscellaneous technical failures including premature intentional or unintentional removal of test patches.

Irritant reactions, also known as false-positive reactions, are one of the most troublesome aspects of patch testing. They are most frequently seen during the first reading, or after 48 to 72 hours, and are not normally observed at later readings. As many as 22% of initially posi-tive sites become negative at the second reading. Patch test allergens with a tendency to pro-duce minor irritant reactions include carba mix, potassium dichromate, formaldehyde, and cinnamic aldehyde.

Strongly positive patch test reactions, most frequently due to nickel, may induce nonspecific reactions in adjacent test areas ("excited skin") that may be confused with an allergic reac-tion. When the clinical history of a patient strongly suggests that an allergen may produce a positive reaction, the suspect allergen may be patch tested at a site other than the back to minimize the excited-skin phenomenon.

Subsequent Tests: The safety and efficacy of this product following repetitive use is unknown. Active sensitization resulting from application of test allergens has been observed. There-fore, weigh any clinical benefits anticipated from repetitive testing against possible increased risks of adverse reactions with repetitive use (eg, active sensitization, increased reactivity).

Mechanism: In patients who have previously been sensitized to a particular allergen, reexpo-sure to the allergen by topical application normally will elicit an allergic contact-dermatitis response after 12 to 72 hours. The topical application of a low molecular weight allergen (less than 500 daltons) at an appropriate concentration and under occlusion usually results in sufficient penetration of the allergen to begin initiation of a cell-mediated immune response.

Once penetration has occurred, the allergen may associate either by covalent or noncovalent bonds with cell-surface antigens of Langerhans (dendritic) cells. It is possible that these cells can present the allergen to allergen-specific effecter helper T-lymphocytes that produce lymphokines. These inflammatory mediators include interleukin-2 (which causes proliferation of the allergen-specific T-cells), chemotactic factors (which recruit various inflammatory cells, including nonspecific T-cells, macrophages, basophils, and eosinophils), and migration inhibitory factor (which causes macrophages to remain at the reaction site).

The destructive activity of these cells leads to lysis of allergen-associated cells, probably contributing to the characteristic spongiosis found histologically in allergic contact dermatitis. These responses are observed after patch testing as erythematous, edematous, vesicular, or bullous reactions at the application site.

Drug Interactions: In general, reactivity to delayed-hypersensitivity tests (eg, PPD) may be suppressed in patients receiving corticosteroids or other immunosuppressive drugs, or in patients recently immunized with live virus vaccines (eg, measles, mumps, rubella, varicella). If delayed-hypersensitivity skin testing is indicated, perform it either preceding or simultaneously with immunization or 4 to 6 weeks after immunization.

Several weeks of cimetidine therapy may augment or enhance delayed-hypersensitivity responses to skin-test antigens, although this effect has not been consistently observed. The effect may be mediated through cimetidine binding to suppressor T-lymphocytes. It is presently unknown if other H_2 antagonists possess similar activity.

Pharmaceutical Characteristics

Concentration: The estimated application dose for each allergen patch test is based on a 5 mm ribbon of petrolatum-based allergen or 1 drop of water-based allergen. The concentration of each allergen patch test is intended to elicit an immune response in patients already hypersensitive to the allergen, while simultaneously minimizing the incidence of both irritant and false-negative reactions. The concentrations of specific allergens are provided below:

(a) 5% benzocaine in petrolatum (0.68 mg per application),

(b) 1% mercaptobenzothiazole in petrolatum (0.14 mg per application),

(c) 20% colophony in petrolatum (2.7 mg per application, 70% or more of which [1.9 mg] is abietic acid),

(d) 1% p-phenylenediamine in petrolatum (0.14 mg per application),

(e) 2% imidazolidinyl urea (*Germall* 115) in water (0.95 mg per application),

(f) 1% cinnamic aldehyde in petrolatum (0.14 mg per application),

(g) 30% lanolin alcohol (wool wax alcohols) in petrolatum (4.1 mg per application, 30% or more of which [1.2 mg] is cholesterol),

(h) 3% carba mix (carba rubber mix) in petrolatum (0.41 mg per application; including 1% 1,3-diphenylguanidine, 1% zinc diethyldithiocarbamate, and 1% zinc dibutyldithiocarbamate, 0.14 mg each per application),

(i) 20% neomycin sulfate in petrolatum (2.7 mg per application),

(j) 1% thiuram mix (thiuram rubber mix) in petrolatum (0.14 mg per application, including 0.25% tetramethylthiuram disulfide, 0.25% tetramethylthiuram monosulfide, 0.25% tetraethylthiuram disulfide, and 0.25% dipentamethylenethiuram disulfide, 0.034 mg each per application),

(k) 1% formaldehyde (contains methanol) in water (0.47 mg per application),

(l) 1% ethylenediamine dihydrochloride in petrolatum (0.14 mg per application),

(m) 1% epoxy resin in petrolatum (0.14 mg per application),

(n) 2% quaternium 15(N-(3-chlorallyl)-hexaminium chloride) in petrolatum (0.27 mg per application),

(o) 1% p-tert-butylphenol formaldehyde resin in petrolatum (0.14 mg per application),

(p) 1% mercapto mix (mercapto rubber mix) in petrolatum (0.14 mg per application, including 0.333 N-cyclohexyl-2-benzothiazole-sulfenamide, 0.333% 2,2′-benzothiazyl disulfide, and 0.333% morpholinylmercaptobenzothiazole, 0.045 mg each per application),

(q) 0.6% black rubber p-phenylenediamine mix (PPD) in petrolatum (0.081 mg per application, including 0.25% N-phenyl-N′-cyclohexyl-p-phenylenediamine [0.034 mg per application], 0.1% N-isopropyl-N′-phenyl-p-phenylenediamine [0.014 mg per application], and 0.25% N,N′-dipheny-p-phenylenediamine [0.034 mg per application]),

(r) 0.25% potassium dichromate in petrolatum (equivalent to 0.088% chromium or 0.012 mg chromium per application),

(s) 25% balsam Peru in petrolatum (3.4 mg per application, 1.2 mg benzylbenzoate or more and 0.34 mg benzylcinnamate or more),

(t) 2.5% nickel sulfate anhydrous in petrolatum (equivalent to 0.95% nickel, 0.13 mg nickel per application).

Quality Assay: Contents are provided within ± 20% of each labeled concentration. The components of some allergen patch test mixtures (eg, thiuram mix) can chemically interact to form new substances. Microbial analysis reveals fewer than 100 microorganisms per mL, with the absence of *Salmonella, Shigella, Escherichia coli, Staphylococcus aureus*, and *Pseudomonas aeruginosa*. The allergen patch test is not certified as sterile.

Packaging: 20 reclosable syringes for topical use only (not for injection), each exuding sufficient allergen to test 150 patients, housed in a plastic case with 2 drawers.

NDC Number: 48018-1056-01

Doseform: Semi-solid paste or solution. Allergens are either suspended in 4.5 g petrolatum, USP, or dissolved in 5.5 g water.

Appearance: Test allergens are generally white, off-white, cream, or light yellow in color. p-Phenylenediamine appears milk-chocolate brown. Black rubber p-phenylenediamine mix is grayish brown in color. Potassium dichromate appears medium yellow. Balsam Peru is dark brown in color. Nickel sulfate anhydrous appears light aqua.

Diluent: Petrolatum, USP, or sterile water for injection

Adjuvant: None

Preservative: None

Allergens: Allergenic by definition and intent

Excipients: None

pH: Not described

Shelf Life: Expires within 24 months.

Storage/Stability: Store at 2° to 8°C (36° to 46°F). Freezing is not known to cause harm to the product. Product can apparently tolerate repeated exposure to room temperature during office hours. Shipped by surface courier at ambient temperature.

Production Process: Prepared from the purest grade of source materials available.

Disease Epidemiology

Prevalence: At least 35 million Americans are affected by contact dermatitis. Up to 3% of the American population may be affected by hand eczema alone. Contact dermatitis accounts for as much as 40% of occupationally acquired illnesses, with at least 70,000 new cases each year in the United States.

The substances in these test panels were selected by the North American Contact Dermatitis Group of the American Academy of Dermatology, based on data developed through an ongoing program of allergen and patient screening.

Information regarding common sources of exposure to these allergens can be found in other references.

Other Information

Perspective:

1896: Jadassohn describes epicutanous testing for detection of allergic contact dermatitis.

1970s: American Academy of Dermatology works with Johnson & Johnson to standardize a patch test tray for dermatologists.

1980: Hermal assumes responsibility for continuity of supply from Johnson & Johnson.

1985: Allergen patch test kit available without FDA licensure until 1985. FDA requires withdrawal of product until safety and efficacy studies completed.

1988: Hermal's patch test kit licensed on April 20, 1988.

References: Adams RM. Recent advances in contact dermatitis. *Ann Allergy.* 1991;67:552-567.

American Academy of Allergy, Asthma and Immunology; American College of Allergy, Asthma and Immunology. Contact dermatitis: a practice parameter. *Ann Allergy Asthma Immunol.* 2006;97(3)(suppl 2): S1-S38.

Cohen DE, Brancaccio RR, Soter NA. Diagnostic tests for type IV or delayed hypersensitivity reactions. *Clin Allergy Immunol.* 2000;15:287-305.

Fischer T, et al. Easier patch testing with T.R.U.E. Test. *J Am Acad Dermatol.* 1989;20:447-453.

Fischer T, et al. Improved, but not perfect, patch testing. *Am J Contact Derm.* 1990;1:73-90.

Grabenstein JD. Allergen patches: Testing for contact dermatitis. *Hosp Pharm.* 1996;31:419-429.

Koch P. Occupational contact dermatitis. Recognition and management. *Am J Clin Dermatol.* 2001;2:353-365.

Mark BJ, Slavin RG. Allergic contact dermatitis. *Med Clin North Am.* 2006;90(1):169-185.

Nedorost ST, Cooper KD. The role of patch testing for chemical and protein allergens in atopic dermatitis. *Curr Allergy Asthma Rep.* 2001;1:323-328.

Turjanmaa K. The role of atopy patch tests in the diagnosis of allergy in atopic dermatitis. *Curr Opin Allergy Clin Immunol.* 2005;5(5):425-428.

Delayed-Hypersensitivity Antigens, Miscellaneous

Name:
T.R.U.E. Test

Manufacturer:
Manufactured by Mekos Laboratories,
distributed by Smart Practice

Synonyms: *T.R.U.E. Test* stands for thin-layer rapid use epicutaneous test.

Comparison: Hermal's allergens are provided in reclosable syringes for application to a holding device; *T.R.U.E. Test* is a unit-dose set of patches for direct application to the skin. Available allergens vary (see table). Concordance of skin reactions with the 2 products will range from 60% to 80% because of variability of individual patient response.

Immunologic Characteristics

Antigen Source: 35 distinct allergens: Nickel sulfate, wool alcohols (lanolin), neomycin sulfate, potassium dichromate (chromium), caine mix (benzocaine, dibucaine, tetracaine), fragrance mix, colophony, epoxy resin, quinoline mix, balsam of Peru, ethylenediamine, cobalt, p-tert-butylphenol formaldehyde, paraben mix, carba mix, black rubber mix, chloromethyl isothiazolinone, Quaternium-15, mercaptobenzothiazole, p-phenylenediamine, formaldehyde, mercapto mix, thimerosal, and thiuram mix. For details, see Pharmaceutical Characteristics.

Viability: Inactive

Antigenic Form: Chemical allergens

Antigenic Type: Various chemicals, see Pharmaceutical Characteristics. Skin tests assess delayed (type IV) hypersensitivity. Contact allergens are generally low molecular weight substances, usually less than 500 daltons, that can easily penetrate the horny layer of the epidermis.

Strains: Chemically pure

Use Characteristics

Indications: An aid in the diagnosis of allergic contact dermatitis in adult patients whose histories suggest sensitivity to 1 or more of the substances included on the *T.R.U.E. Test* panels. These patches include a group of substances associated with contact dermatitis. They may be used as an aid in diagnosing contact dermatitis or as a diagnostic screen. A thorough patient history is essential in evaluating the significance of a positive reaction.

To determine whether sensitization to an allergen may be etiologically important, *T.R.U.E. Test* may also be used adjunctively to evaluate other eczemas (atopic, seborrheic, venous, palmar and plantar hyperkeratotic eczema, vesiculosis, or neurodermatitis) and other dermatologic diseases that do not heal, such as leg ulcers and psoriasis, to determine whether there may be a contact hypersensitivity component.

Limitations: Failure of a patient to react to the allergen patch test does not rule out possible allergic-contact sensitivity. Active sensitization to test allergens has resulted from similar testing processes. Therefore, weigh clinical benefits anticipated from repetitive testing against possible increased risks of adverse reactions with repetitive use (eg, active sensitization or increased reactivity).

Contraindications:

Absolute: None

Relative: Carefully evaluate the use of this product in patients with known severe systemic or local reactions to 1 of the allergens on these patches before application. Do not apply during extensive, ongoing contact dermatitis. It may provoke an intensified reaction on both the present and previously affected sites and may also cause a false-positive test result.

Immunodeficiency: Patients receiving immunosuppressive therapy or having other immunodeficiencies (especially those involving cell-mediated immunity) may have a diminished skin-test response to this and other diagnostic antigens.

Elderly: More frequent patch test responses can be expected in elderly patients. While no conclusive explanation is available, older patients may exhibit an increased frequency of cutaneous allergies.

Carcinogenicity: Studies of *T.R.U.E. Test* to evaluate carcinogenic potential or mutagenesis have not been performed. Nickel refinery dust, nickel sulfite, and formaldehyde are known carcinogens. Nickel sulfate, potassium dichromate, cobalt dichloride, epoxy resin, and thiuram mix are suspected carcinogens. The potential effects of using very low concentrations of these substances for single or multiple applications are currently unknown. Some components of *T.R.U.E. Test* have been reviewed as part of the Cosmetic Ingredient Review and found to be safe or safe with qualifications. Those found to be safe are hydroxypropylcellulose, methylcellulose, wool alcohols, paraben mix, Quaternium-15, and p-phenylenediamine. Those found to be safe with qualifications are N-phenyl-p-phenylenediamine, chloromethylisothiazolinone, and formaldehyde.

Pregnancy: Category C. Use only if clearly needed. It is unlikely that patch test allergens cross the placenta.

Lactation: It is unlikely that patch test allergens cross into human breast milk. Problems in humans have not been documented.

Children: The safety and efficacy of the allergen patch test in children have not been established.

Adverse Reactions: Adverse reactions reported with the use of *T.R.U.E. Test* and patch testing in general are normally mild and usually occur only at the site of the test application. The most common adverse reactions (1% or more) were burning (25%), tape irritation (16%), persistent reactions (7%), erythema (6%), and hyper/hypopigmentation (5%). There are reports of other adverse reactions associated with patch testing. These include keloids, sarcoid infiltrates, vitiligo spots, edema, crusting, scarring, ectopic flare, and sensitization.

Extremely sensitive patients may exhibit extreme (+ + +) reactions that may be bullous or ulcerative with pronounced erythema, infiltration, and coalescing vesicles.

Excited skin syndrome ("angry back") is a state of hyperreactivity induced by a dermatitis on other parts of the body or by a strong positive skin-test reaction. Therefore, test results should be evaluated carefully in patients with multiple, positive, concomitant patch test results. To determine which reactions are false positives, retesting at a later date may be considered.

On rare occasions, it may be necessary to remove the test strip from the patient because of severe itching or burning sensations. One patient taking part in the clinical studies removed the test tape after 24 hours because of severe itching.

Occasionally, hyperpigmentation of the test site occurs during healing. Healing with or without medication normally takes place within 5 days to 2 weeks, although reactions in some individuals may persist longer. Although there are no specific data, in general, more severe positive reactions can be expected to require longer healing times. Of course, healing time can be influenced by many factors, especially the general health of the patient.

The minor amount of allergen on each *T.R.U.E. Test* patch that penetrates the skin will rarely induce a flare-up of dermatitis. In the case of extensive ongoing contact dermatitis, how-

948

ever, the test should not be applied because it may provoke an intensified reaction on both the present and previously affected sites and may also cause a false-positive test result.

In some cases, allergenic responses may be delayed in onset. One type of delayed reaction is a sensitization, which is not well defined in the literature but is described as a positive reaction observed at 10 to 14 days or later after application and at 2 to 4 days after the test is repeated. The positive reaction should meet the criteria for an allergic reaction (papular or vesicular erythema and infiltration) to distinguish between a false-positive result and a sensitization.

In clinical studies conducted with *T.R.U.E. Test*, there have been reports of delayed reactions occurring at 21 days or later. None of these patients were retested to verify a sensitization reaction. There are enough data for 2 of these patients to indicate probable sensitization.

In addition, the adhesive tape may also cause an irritation at the test site. Reports of tape irritation are infrequent, usually mild in nature and self-limiting in clinical studies conducted with *T.R.U.E. Test*, although no data were collected in these studies beyond a day 21 safety visit.

P-phenylenediamine (allergen #20) will turn the patch test area black on all patients. This allergen is a dye; the response is not allergic. This discoloration may remain for up to 2 weeks.

Pharmacologic & Dosing Characteristics

Dosage: Three rectangular patches containing 35 allergens. Apply *T.R.U.E. Test* patches either directly from the refrigerator or allow them to come to room temperature (15 to 20 minutes) before application.

Route & Site: Topical, to healthy skin free of acne, scars, dermatitis, or any other condition that may interfere with interpretation of test results. The intact skin should not be cleansed with alcohol or soap. Test sites should be adequately marked to allow identification of individual test sites when the occlusive tape is removed.

The upper portion of the back is the preferred test site, avoiding the vertebrae, although other areas may be used. In some cases, it may be necessary to use an electric shaver (not razors) on the site prior to application of the tests.

Avoid application to recently tanned or sun-exposed skin, as this may increase the risk of false-negative reactions. Avoid patch testing on patients for 3 weeks after UV treatments, heavy sun, or tanning bed exposure. Avoid excessive sweating during the testing period to maintain sufficient adhesion to the skin. Avoid excessive physical activity to maintain sufficient adhesion and to prevent actual loss of patch test material. Avoid getting the panels and surrounding area wet.

Related Interventions: If a severe patch test reaction develops, the patient may be treated with a topical corticosteroid or, in rare cases, with a systemic corticosteroid.

Efficacy: Multiple North American and European studies demonstrate that *T.R.U.E. Test* is a clinically relevant method for diagnosing allergic contact dermatitis. The persistent local response and the occurrence of late reactions are within the normal range expected for patch testing.

To further demonstrate the clinical relevance of the *T.R.U.E. Test* method for diagnosing allergic contact dermatitis, a comparison was made to data in a screening tray recommended by the North American Contact Dermatology Group. These data were collected over 4 years by 14 independent investigators in North America after testing 4,055 patients with suspect contact dermatitis: 57% female; 87% Caucasian, 7% African American, 3% Asian, 2% Hispanic; average age 43.8 years. These data demonstrate that most allergens have very similar reactivities in the 2 methods. Differences noted are most likely due to patient selection in the clinical trials.

Another test (the "nickel use test") was conducted to correlate reactions to *T.R.U.E. Test* and a medallion containing 20% nickel. This test showed a sensitivity (true positive) rate of 95.2%, a specificity (true negative) rate of 62.1%, a positive predictive value of 64.5%, and a negative predictive value of 94.7%.

Time of Reading: The patient wears *T.R.U.E. Test* for at least 48 hours before it is removed. Evaluate the test sites 72 to 96 hours after application. This allows allergic reactions to fully develop and mild irritant reactions to fade. If reading at 48 hours is considered, another reading at 72 to 96 hours is recommended.

Neomycin sulfate and p-phenylenediamine sometimes cause reactions that may not appear until 4 to 5 days (or later) after the application. Late positive reactions may occur 7 to 10 days after application. Late positive reactions occurring more than 14 days after application may indicate active sensitization.

Interpretation: An interpretation method, similar to the one recommended by the International Contact Dermatitis Research Group, is recommended:

? = Doubtful reaction: faint macular erythema only

+ = Weak (nonvesicular) positive reaction: erythema, infiltration, possibly with papules

+ + = Strong (vesicular) positive reaction: erythema, infiltration, papules and vesicles

+ + + = Extreme positive reaction: bullous reaction

− = Negative reaction

IR = Irritant reaction of different types: Pustules as well as patchy follicular or homogeneous erythema without infiltrations are usually signs of irritation and do not indicate allergy.

Itching is a subjective symptom that is expected to accompany a positive reaction.

Encourage patients to avoid allergens to which they test positive, to preclude future episodes of contact dermatitis. Various summaries of products to avoid for each chemical have been published.The threshold at which to begin counseling avoidance varies among clinicians.

Predictive Capacity: It has been estimated that approximately 2 of 100 positive test reactions or 1 of 1,000 applied patches yield false-negative results.

False-positive reactions, also known as irritant reactions, are one of the most troublesome aspects of patch testing, especially with positive reactions. Allergens most likely to produce such reactions include nickel, cobalt, and balsam of Peru.

A false-positive result may occur when an irritant reaction cannot be differentiated from an allergic reaction. Pustules and patchy follicular or homogeneous erythema without infiltration are usually signs of irritation and do not indicate allergy.

A positive test reaction should meet the criteria for an allergic reaction (papular or vesicular erythema and infiltration). If an irritant reaction cannot be distinguished from a true positive reaction or if a doubtful reaction is present, a retest may be considered in a few weeks or months.

It is important when evaluating a positive test result not only to consider the intensity of the reaction but also to consider whether it is relevant to the patient's existing condition either as a primary cause or an aggravating factor.

Excited skin syndrome ("angry back") consists of a hyperreactive state of the skin in which false-positive patch test reactions concur with dermatitis at a distant body site or with adjacent strong positive skin test reactions. This rare state of hyper-reactivity is not well understood clinically. There has been only 1 reported case of suspected angry back in a patient tested with *T.R.U.E. Test*. The patient had the standard screening allergens and a special shoe series on his back and also had *T.R.U.E. Test* on his thigh. He displayed symptoms of angry back on his back, but not on his thigh. This patient was retested 1 month after complete cure, and an accurate diagnosis was made using the standard series and *T.R.U.E. Test*.

False-negative results may be due to insufficient patch contact with the skin, sensitization to a substance not present in the test panel, or premature evaluation of the test. Retesting may be indicated.

Subsequent Tests: The safety and efficacy of repetitive testing with *T.R.U.E. Test* is unknown. Sensitization or increased reactivity to 1 or more of the allergens may occur. The benefits of repeat testing should therefore be carefully evaluated against the possible risks.

Sensitization: Sensitization to a substance included on the test panel may occur with patch testing but is extremely rare. A test reaction that appears more than 14 days after application may indicate active sensitization.

Mechanism: A positive response to the patch test is a classical delayed cell-mediated hypersensitivity reaction (type IV), which normally appears within 9 to 96 hours after exposure. The topical application of a low molecular weight allergen (less than 500 daltons) at an appropriate concentration and under occlusion usually results in sufficient penetration of the allergen to begin initiation of a cell-mediated immune response.

Following primary contact, an allergen penetrates the skin and binds covalently or noncovalently to epidermal Langerhans cells. The processed allergen is presented to helper T-lymphocytes, resulting in the release of lymphokines, including interleukin 2. Interleukin 2 stimulates the production of other lymphocytes, chemotactic factors that recruit macrophages, basophils, eosinophils, and migration inhibitory factor, which all induce macrophages to remain at the reaction site. The resulting inflammation produces a papular, vesicular, or bullous response with erythema and itching at the site of application.

Signs and symptoms of allergic contact dermatitis vary in intensity. Some patients may present with mild redness while others may present with severe swelling and bullae formation. Itching and vesiculation are common. The exposed areas of the skin (eg, hands, forearm, face, neck, the dorsal surface of the feet) are primary initial sites of contact dermatitis. However, any area of the skin that comes into contact with a sensitizing allergen may also be affected.

The destructive activity of these cells leads to lysis of allergen-associated cells, probably contributing to the characteristic spongiosis found histologically in allergic contact dermatitis. These responses are observed after patch testing as erythematous, edematous, vesicular, or bullous reactions at the application site.

Drug Interactions: In general, reactivity to any delayed-hypersensitivity test may be suppressed in patients receiving corticosteroids or other immunosuppressive drugs, or in patients who were recently immunized with live virus vaccines (eg, measles, mumps, rubella). If delayed-hypersensitivity skin testing is indicated it should either be performed preceding or simultaneously with immunization or 4 to 6 weeks after immunization.

Because steroids may suppress a positive test reaction, cease use of topical steroids on the test site or oral steroids (equivalent to 15 mg of prednisolone) at least 1 to 2 weeks before testing. Topical steroids on nontest areas may be appropriate.

The effect of concomitant systemic antihistamine administration on patch test results is unknown. The effect of concomitant or prior systemic cyclosporine administration on patch test results is unknown.

Patient Information: Warn patients that itching and burning sensations are common occurrences with patch testing and may be severe in extremely sensitive patients. Erythema and vesiculation can also occur. Medication may be necessary to relieve these itching or burning sensations. Patients who experience intense discomfort should contact their physician concerning possible removal of the test.

Advise patients to avoid extreme physical activity or mechanical action that may result in reduced adhesion or actual loss of patch test material. Use appropriate measures to avoid getting the area around the patch wet.

T.R.U.E. Test may be applied throughout the year. However, during the summer months, advise patients to avoid excessive sweating to maintain sufficient adhesion to the skin. In addition, minimize exposure to the sun to prevent a sun-induced skin reaction that may interfere with interpretation of test results.

Ask patients to report reactions occurring after 7 days to detect potential sensitizations.

Pharmaceutical Characteristics

Concentration: The concentration of each allergen patch test is intended to elicit an immune response in patients already sensitive to the allergen, while minimizing the incidence of irritant and false-negative reactions. The concentrations of specific allergens are provided below:

Allergen Panel 1.2:

(Position 1) Nickel sulfate hexahydrate 0.2 mg/cm^2 or 0.036 mg of nickel per patch (purity 98.5% to 101.5%). The active allergenic component is nickel. The gel vehicle is hydroxypropylcellulose.

(Position 2) Wool alcohols (lanolin) 1 mg/cm^2 or 0.81 mg per patch. Wool alcohols (lanolin) is a natural product obtained from the fleece of sheep. This allergen is a highly complex mixture of alcohols containing cholesterol, lanosterol, agnosterol, and their dihydro derivatives plus straight- and branched-chain aliphatic alcohols. The active allergenic component has not been identified. The gel vehicle is povidone.

(Position 3) Neomycin sulfate, USP, 0.23 mg/cm^2 or 0.19 mg per patch. The gel vehicle is methylcellulose.

(Position 4) Potassium dichromate 0.023 mg/cm^2 or 0.0067 mg of chromium per patch (purity 98.5% to 101.5%). The active allergenic component is chromium. The gel vehicle is hydroxypropylcellulose.

(Position 5) Caine mix 630 mcg/cm^2 (benzocaine, USP, 0.364 mg/cm^2; dibucaine hydrochloride, USP, 0.064 mg/cm^2; tetracaine hydrochloride, USP, 0.063 mg/cm^2). The gel vehicle is povidone.

(Position 6) Fragrance mix 430 mcg/cm^2 (cinnamyl alcohol, cinnamaldehyde, α-amylcinnamaldehyde, isoeugenol, hydroxycitronellal, eugenol, geraniol, oak moss), 0.43 mg of fragrance mix per cm^2 or 0.07 mg of geraniol, 0.034 mg of cinnamaldehyde, 0.054 mg of hydroxycitronellal, 0.054 mg of cinnamyl alcohol, 0.034 mg of eugenol, 0.015 mg of isoeugenol, 0.015 mg of -amylcinnamaldehyde, and 0.07 mg of oak moss per patch. These substances are at least 95% pure, except isoeugenol is at least 88% pure and -amylcinnaldehyde is at least 90% pure. Identity of impurities is unknown, except that cinnamaldehyde contains trace amounts of cinnamyl alcohol. Oak moss, a dark green sticky paste, is a solvent extract of the lichen *Evernia prunastri*. The chemical composition is very complex. The acid fraction (95% of the extracted material) is made up of depsides including atranorin, evernic acid, usnic acid, chloratranorin, and degradation products of these depsides. Atranorin is suspected as a prime allergenic component, and its peak (measured with gas chromatography) is used to determine the amount of oak moss in the fragrance mix patch. The gel vehicle includes hydroxypropylcellulose and β-cyclodextrin.

(Position 7) Colophony 0.85 mg/cm^2 or 0.069 mg per patch. Colophony is produced from the resin of the pine trees *Pinus massoniana* and *Pinus tabuliformis*. It is translucent, pale yellow or brownish yellow, brittle and glassy in appearance. Colophony consists of 75% to 85% resin acids, 10% neutral fractions (ie, terpenes), with the remaining part oxidation products. Oxidation products of abietic acid and other resin acids have been identified as the active allergenic components. The UV-absorbance measurement of 1 of the primary components, abietic acid, is used to quantify colophony hydroxypropylcellulose. The gel vehicle is povidone.

(Position 8) Paraben mix (containing equal parts of the 5 ester derivatives of parahydroxybenzoic acid and methyl-, ethyl-, propyl-, butyl-, and benzylparahydroxybenzoate) 1 mg/cm^2 or 0.81 mg per patch (purity of each derivative 98.5% to 101.5%). The gel vehicle is povidone.

(Position 9) Negative control: An uncoated polyester patch.

(Position 10) Balsam of Peru 0.8 mg/cm^2 or 0.65 mg per patch. Balsam of Peru is a resin from a South American tree, *Myroxylon balsamum pereirae*. The resin consists of a mixture of fragrances and other substances that have not all been identified. Balsam of Peru patch content is quantitated by gas chromatography of its 2 major constituents, benzyl cinnamate and benzyl benzoate. Several components of balsam of Peru have been identified as allergens, including cinnamic acid, benzyl alcohol, and vanillin. The gel vehicle is povidone.

(Position 11) Ethylenediamine dihydrochloride 0.05 mg/cm^2 or 0.018 mg of ethylenediamine per patch (purity 98.5% to 101.5%). The active allergenic component is ethylenediamine. The gel vehicle is methylcellulose.

(Position 12) Cobalt dichloride hexahydrate 0.02 mg/cm^2 or 0.004 mg of cobalt per patch (purity 98.5% to 101.5%). The active allergenic component is cobalt. The gel vehicle is hydroxypropylcellulose.

Allergen Panel 2.2:

(Position 13) p-tert-butylphenol formaldehyde resin 45 mcg per cm^2 or 36 mcg per patch (purity 95% or more). The active allergenic components have been identified as p-tert-butylphenol formaldehyde and numerous other compounds. The gel vehicle is hydroxypropylcellulose.

(Position 14) Epoxy resin, 50 mcg/cm^2 or 32 mcg of diglycidylether of bisphenol A per patch. Epoxy resin is a clear viscous liquid consisting of 75% to 85% diglycidylether of bisphenol A, the active allergenic component, a monomer used to prepare polymer epoxy resins. The remaining part consists of the dimer and the trimer. The gel vehicle is hydroxypropylcellulose.

(Position 15) Carba mix (1,3-diphenylguanidine, zinc dibutyldithiocarbamate, zinc diethyldithiocarbamate, in equal parts) 0.25 mg per cm^2 or 0.2 mg per patch (purity 96% to 102%). The gel vehicle is hydroxypropylcellulose.

(Position 16) Black rubber mix [N-cyclohexyl-N'-phenyl-paraphenylenediamine 0.03 mg per cm^2 (purity 90% or more), N-isopropyl-N'-phenyl-paraphenylenediamine 0.03 mg per cm^2 (purity 95% to 102%), N,N'-diphenyl-paraphenylenediamine 0.012 mg per cm^2 (purity 90% or more) in the ratio 2:5:5] 0.075 mg per cm^2 or 0.061 mg per patch. The gel vehicle is povidone.

(Position 17) Chloromethyl (Cl+Me−) isothiazolinone 0.004 mg per cm² or 0.0032 mg per patch. Chloromethylisothiazolinone consists of 2 active ingredients, 5-chloro-2-methyl-4-isothiazolin-3-1 (1.05% to 1.25% w/w) and 2-methyl-4-isothiazolin-3-1 (0.25% to 0.4% w/w) in a 3:1 ratio at a concentration of 1.5% in aqueous magnesium salts. The gel vehicle is povidone.

(Position 18) Quaternium-15 (1-(3-chloroallyl)-3,5,7,-triaza-1-azonium-adamantane chloride) 0.1 mg per cm² or 0.081 mg per patch (purity 94% to 102%). The gel vehicle is hydroxypropylcellulose.

(Position 19) Methyldibromo glutaronitrile (MDBGN), or methyldibromo glutaronitrile, 1,2-dibromo-2,4-dicyanobutane (purity 95% or more), is a component of the preservative *Euxyl K400*. The patch contains MDBGN 5 mcg/cm² or 4 mcg per patch. The gel vehicle is povidone.

(Position 20) p-Phenylenediamine 0.09 mg/cm² or 0.073 mg per patch (purity 97.5% to 101.5%). The gel vehicle is povidone.

(Position 21) Formaldehyde 0.18 mg/cm² or 0.15 mg per patch. Formaldehyde is released from the proallergen N-hydroxymethyl succinimide, which is cleaved into succinimide and formaldehyde when it comes in contact with the transepidermal water on the surface of the skin. Formaldehyde is the active allergenic compound. The content of formaldehyde in the proallergen is 22.1% to 24.1%. Methylene chloride is used as a suspending medium for this proallergen but is not present in significant quantities in the finished patch. The gel vehicle is povidone with sodium bicarbonate and sodium carbonate.

(Position 22) Mercapto mix 0.075 mg/cm² or 0.061 mg per patch. Mercapto mix is composed of benzothiazole sulfenamide derivatives: N-cyclohexylbenzothiazyl-sulfenamide (purity 85% or greater), dibenzothiazyl disulfide (purity 97% to 102%), and morpholinylmercaptobenzothiazole (purity 85% or greater), present in equal parts. The gel vehicle is povidone.

(Position 23) Thimerosal 7 mcg/cm² or 6 mcg per patch (purity 97% or more). Thimerosal is a preservative that contains mercury. The gel vehicle is povidone.

(Position 24) Thiuram mix 0.025 mg/cm² or 0.0051 mg of tetramethylthiuram monosulfide, 0.0051 mg of tetramethylthiuram disulfide, 0.0051 mg of disulfiram, USP, and 0.0051 mg of dipentamethylenethiuram disulfide per patch (purity at least 95%). The components of thiuram mix can chemically interact, resulting in the formation of mixed disulfides. Thiuram monosulfides and disulfides are the active allergens. The gel vehicle is povidone.

Allergen Panel 3.2:

(Position 25) Diazolidinyl urea (*Germall II*) is a complex mixture. The product is formulated to contain 550 mcg/cm² of diazolidinyl urea or 446 mcg per patch. The gel vehicle is povidone.

(Position 26) Quinoline mix is composed of 2 chemical germicides: equal parts of clioquinol, USP, (purity 93% or more) and chlorquinaldol (purity 95% or more), 190 mcg/cm² or 154 mcg of quinoline mix per patch. The gel vehicle is povidone.

(Position 27) Tixocortol-21-pivalate (purity 95% or more) is a corticosteroid (group A). The product is formulated to contain 3 mcg/cm² or 2 mcg of tixocortol-21-pivalate per patch. The gel vehicle is povidone.

(Position 28) Gold sodium thiosulfate (purity 90% or more) containing 75 mcg/cm^2 of gold sodium thiosulfate or 23 mcg of gold per patch. The gel vehicle is hydroxypropylcellulose.

(Position 29) Imidazolidinyl urea (*Germall 115*) is a complex mixture, with 600 mcg/cm^2 or 486 mcg of imidazolidinyl urea per patch. The gel vehicle is povidone.

(Position 30) Budesonide, USP, (purity 98% or more) is a corticosteroid, with 1 mcg/cm^2 or 0.8 mcg of budesonide per patch. The gel vehicle is povidone.

(Position 31) Hydrocortisone-17-butyrate, USP, (purity 97% or more) is a midpotent (group D2) corticosteroid containing 20 mcg/cm^2 or 16 mcg of hydrocortisone-17-butyrate per patch. The gel vehicle is povidone.

(Position 32) Mercaptobenzothiazole (purity 98.5% or more) is a vulcanization accelerator used in rubber products, containing 75 mcg/cm^2 or 61 mcg of mercaptobenzothiazole per patch. The gel vehicle is povidone.

(Position 33) Bacitracin, USP, containing 600 mcg/cm^2 or 486 mcg of bacitracin per patch. The gel vehicle is hydroxypropylcellulose.

(Position 34) Parthenolide (purity 95% or more) is a sesquiterpene lactone occurring naturally in plants such as daisies, feverfew, and magnolia. Contains 3 mcg/cm^2 or 2 mcg of parthenolide per patch. The gel vehicle is povidone.

(Position 35) Disperse Blue 106 (purity 90% or more) is a commonly used thiazol-azoyl-p-phenylene diamine derivative dye used primarily in synthetic textiles. Contains 50 mcg/cm^2 or 41 mcg of Disperse Blue 106 per patch. The gel vehicle is povidone.

(Position 36) 2-bromo-2-nitropropane-1,3-diol (*Bronopol*) (purity 95% or more), containing 250 mcg/cm^2 or 203 mcg of *Bronopol* per patch. The gel vehicle is povidone.

Quality Assay: The source materials for the *T.R.U.E. Test* allergens are obtained from outside suppliers who certify that the materials meet specific standards of purity. The manufacturer then determines the purity and identity of the source materials using validated in-house chemical analyses.

Each patch is analytically tested and contains ± 20% of its labeled value at the time of batch release. These values are maintained through expiry except for colophony, which maintains ± 30% of label value under the recommended storage conditions.

The components of the patches containing mixtures (eg, thiuram mix) have the potential to chemically interact, resulting in the formation of new substances.

T.R.U.E. Test is subjected to microbial load testing to ensure that 100 microorganisms or fewer per test are present. In addition, *T.R.U.E. Test* is further analyzed to ensure the absence of *Staphylococcus aureus* and *Pseudomonas aeruginosa*. The allergen patch test is not certified as sterile.

Packaging: Each test consists of 3 pieces of surgical tape (5.2 cm × 13 cm), each with 12 polyester patches of approximately 0.81 cm^2 each, covered with a protective sheet and packed in a pouch of laminated foil. Each multipack carton contains 5 units. Each unit consists of a set of 3 adhesive panels.

An identification template is available for quick identification of any allergen that causes a reaction. To ensure correct positioning, correlate marks on the skin with the notches on the template.

NDC Number: 67334-0457-01

Allergen Patch Test

Doseform: Three pieces of surgical tape (5.2 cm × 13 cm), each with 12 polyester patches and packed in a pouch of laminated foil. The adhesive used in the panels is acrylate based. There is no natural rubber latex, rubber components, balsams, or rosins in the adhesive or tape. Acrylate adhesives are processed to remove free monomers that may be allergenic. After being taped to the skin, the film is hydrated by perspiration and is transformed into a gel 50 to 70 microns thick.

Appearance: White, rectangular patches

Adjuvant: None

Preservative: None

Allergens: Allergenic by definition and intent.

Excipients: The allergens are homogenized in 1 or more of the following materials to produce the allergen films that coat the patches: hydroxypropylcellulose, methylcellulose, povidone (polyvinylpyrrolidone), povidone with butylhydroxyanisole and butylhydroxytoluene, povidone with sodium bicarbonate and sodium carbonate, and hydroxypropylcellulose with β-cyclodextrin.

pH: Data not provided

Shelf Life: Expires within 24 months.

Storage/Stability: Store at 2° to 8°C (36° to 46°F). Do not freeze. Shipped in insulated containers with coolant packs. Contact the manufacturer regarding exposures to extreme temperatures.

Handling:

(1) Peel open the package and remove Test Panel 1.2.

(2) Remove the protective plastic covering from the test surface of the panel. Be careful not to touch the test substances.

(3) Position the test on the upper left side of the patient's back so that allergen #1 is in the upper left corner. See packaging for diagram. Avoid applying the test on the margin of the scapula. From the center of the panel, smooth outward toward the edges, making sure each allergen makes firm contact with the skin.

(4) With a medical marking pen, indicate on the skin the location of the 2 notches on the panel.

(5) Repeat the process with Test Panel 2.2 and then Panel 3.2. See packaging for diagram.

Production Process: Prepared from the purest grade of source materials available. The allergens are incorporated into a suitable vehicle. The allergen-gel preparation is printed onto an impermeable backing of plastic and dried to a thin film. The coated sheet is cut into 9 × 9 mm squares. Squares containing 12 distinct allergens are mounted on a tape, covered with a protective sheet, and packed in an airtight and light-impermeable envelope.

Disease Epidemiology

Prevalence: At least 35 million Americans are affected by contact dermatitis. Up to 3% of the American population may be affected by hand eczema alone. Contact dermatitis accounts for as much as 40% of occupationally acquired illnesses, with at least 70,000 new cases each year in the United States.

The allergens in *T.R.U.E. Test* were selected from those substances that have been widely reported to induce allergic contact dermatitis. They represent approximately 80% of the most common allergens. Nickel sulfate, thimerosal, Quaternium-15, formaldehyde, thiuram mix, and balsam of Peru are the most commonly reported reactive allergens. The frequency of positive responses to the various allergens can change depending upon the specific patient population and occupational and environmental influences. The epidemiology of allergic contact dermatitis and the frequency of positive patch test reactions to various causative allergens have been the subject of several extensive studies. Information regarding common sources of exposure to these allergens can be found in other references.

Other Information

Perspective:
1896: Jadassohn describes epicutanous testing for detection of allergic contact dermatitis.
1970s: American Academy of Dermatology works with Johnson & Johnson to standardize a patch test tray for dermatologists.

First Licensed: Panel #1 on July 12, 1990; panel #2 on November 28, 1994

References: Adams RM. Recent advances in contact dermatitis. *Ann Allergy.* 1991;67(6):552-566.

American Academy of Allergy, Asthma and Immunology; American College of Allergy, Asthma and Immunology. Contact dermatitis: a practice parameter [published correction appears in *Ann Allergy Asthma Immunol.* 2006;97(6):819]. *Ann Allergy Asthma Immunol.* 2006;97(3)(suppl 2):S1-S38.

Cohen DE, Brancaccio RR, Soter NA. Diagnostic tests for type IV or delayed hypersensitivity reactions. *Clin Allergy Immunol.* 2000;15:287-305.

Fischer T, Maibach HI. Easier patch testing with TRUE Test. *J Am Acad Dermatol.* 1989;20(3):447-453.

Fischer T, Maibach HI. Improved, but not perfect, patch testing. *Am J Contact Derm.* 1990;1:73-90.

Koch P. Occupational contact dermatitis. Recognition and management. *Am J Clin Dermatol.* 2001;2(6):353-365.

Mark BJ, Slavin RG. Allergic contact dermatitis. *Med Clin North Am.* 2006;90(1):169-185.

Nedorost ST, Cooper KD. The role of patch testing for chemical and protein allergens in atopic dermatitis. *Curr Allergy Asthma Rep.* 2001;1(4):323-328.

Turjanmaa K. The role of atopy patch tests in the diagnosis of allergy in atopic dermatitis. *Curr Opin Allergy Clin Immunol.* 2005;5(5):425-428.

Coccidioides immitis Spherule-Derived Skin Test Antigen

Fungal Antigens

Name:
Spherusol

Manufacturer:
Allermed Laboratories

Synonyms: Coccidioidomycosis is also known as San Joaquin Valley fever, valley fever, desert fever, desert rheumatism, and Posada disease.

Comparison: Previously, 2 forms of coccidioidin were marketed in the United States: a mycelial derivative (*BioCox*, Iatric Corporation) and a spherule derivative (*Spherulin*, Berkeley Biologicals [later ALK-Abelló Laboratories]). Coccidioidin derived from spherules is considered more sensitive, although possibly less specific, than coccidioidin derived from mycelia.

Immunologic Characteristics

Microorganism: Fungus, dimorphic, *Coccidioides immitis*

Viability: Inactivated

Antigenic Form: Spherule filtrate

Antigenic Type: Proteins and polysaccharides. Skin tests assess delayed (type IV) hypersensitivity.

Strains: Not specified

Use Characteristics

Indications: To detect delayed hypersensitivity to *C. immitis* in adults 18 to 64 years of age with a history of pulmonary coccidioidomycosis. The skin test is intended to help differentiate coccidioidomycosis from other viral, bacterial, or mycotic infections (eg, blastomycosis, histoplasmosis, tuberculosis, sarcoidosis).

Limitations: The use of *Spherusol* to detect delayed-type hypersensitivity response in a general population with unknown exposure to *C. immitis* has not been evaluated. Patients with acute or disseminated coccidioidomycosis may not develop a delayed-type hypersensitivity response to *Spherusol*.

Contraindications: Severe allergic reaction (eg, anaphylaxis) to *Spherusol* or any component of *Spherusol* or other coccidioidin products.

Immunodeficiency: Patients with immunodeficiency (especially those involving cell-mediated immunity) and a history of coccidioidomycosis may not develop a delayed-type hypersensitivity response. Patients receiving immunosuppressive therapy may have a false-negative skin test response to this and other diagnostic antigens.

Elderly: No specific information is available regarding the use of *Spherusol* in the elderly population.

Pregnancy: Category C. Use only if clearly needed. It is unlikely that *Spherusol* crosses the placenta.

Lactation: It is unlikely that *Spherusol* is excreted in breast milk. Problems in humans have not been documented.

Children: Safety and efficacy of *Spherusol* have not been established in children.

Adverse Reactions: The most commonly reported local adverse reactions were itching and swelling (greater than 75%) and pain (greater than 15%) within 7 days of administration. Immediate hypersensitivity, including severe systemic reactions, may occur after administration of skin test antigens.

Pharmacologic & Dosing Characteristics

Dosage: 0.1 mL (1.27 mcg)

Route & Site: Intradermal, applied to the volar surface of the forearm using a ½-inch, 26- or 27-gauge needle with bevel side up at a 15- to 20-degree angle. Proper injection will result in a bleb 5 to 10 mm in diameter at the injection site.

Additional Doses: Repeat administration of *Spherusol* has not been evaluated.

Time of Reading: Measure induration at test site 48 ($\pm$ 4) hours after application.

Interpretation: Measure response by taking the mean of the orthogonal diameters of the area of induration. A mean induration of 5 mm or greater is considered a positive delayed-type hypersensitivity response to *Spherusol*. Erythema in the absence of induration is considered negative. This implies a past or present infection with *C. immitis*. If the patient exhibits a positive reaction to both *Spherusol* and tuberculin, the diagnosis must depend on serological tests and isolation of *C. immitis* or *Mycobacterium tuberculosis* from sputum. Simultaneous infections have been reported.

A negative test (less than 5 mm induration) indicates that the patient has not been previously sensitized to *Spherusol* or that hypersensitivity to this product has not reached, or has declined below, a detectable level. The skin test may also be negative in severe forms of disease (due to anergy) or when prolonged periods of time have passed since infection. Skin tests may be negative in cases of disseminated disease.

Predictive Capacity: The delayed-type hypersensitivity response after administration of *Spherusol* was evaluated in one US study that enrolled adults with a history of coccidioidomycosis. Two other US studies enrolled subjects without a history of coccidioidomycosis; in one of these studies, subjects had a history of histoplasmosis. In each study, concomitant with *Spherusol*, 2 additional skin test extracts, *Candin* and *Trichophyton* (positive controls), were administered along with saline (negative control) and a diluent containing less than or equal to 0.0001% of thimerosal (negative control). All skin tests and controls were administered as 0.1 mL doses in a randomized pattern on the volar surface of the forearms. Investigators and subjects were blinded to identity and placement of skin test antigens and controls. Responses were read at 48 ($\pm$ 4) hours after administration. For each subject, *Spherusol* skin test results were considered valid if induration of 5 mm or greater was observed at the positive control antigen sites and if no induration 5 mm or greater was observed at the negative control sites.

A double-blind study in endemic areas (Bakersfield, California and Tucson, Arizona) enrolled 54 adults with a history of pulmonary coccidioidomycosis. Of 51 subjects with valid skin test results, 50 (98%; 2-sided 95% confidence interval [CI], 90%-100%) had a mean induration of 5 mm or greater at the *Spherusol* site. Among subjects with valid skin test results, the average size of induration at the *Spherusol* site was 17 mm (range, 5 to 39 mm).

A double-blind study conducted in an area not endemic for *C. immitis* (Spokane, Washington) enrolled 60 adults with no known exposure to *C. immitis* by travel to or residency in an endemic area. Subjects had negative serologies to *C. immitis* by complement fixation, immunodiffusion, and/or enzyme-linked immunosorbent assay (ELISA). At the 48-hour assessment, 55 subjects had valid skin test results. One subject had a 5 mm mean induration response to *Spherusol*, and 54 subjects demonstrated negative responses (less than 5 mm mean induration) to *Spherusol*.

A double-blind study conducted in an area not endemic for *C. immitis* but endemic for *Histoplasma capsulatum* (Blair, Nebraska) enrolled 12 adults with no known exposure to *C. immitis* by travel to or residency in an endemic area. All subjects had a history of pulmonary histoplasmosis. Subjects had negative serologies to *C. immitis* by complement fixation, immunodiffusion, and/or ELISA. At the 48-hour assessment, all 12 subjects reacted to at least one of the positive controls with a 5 mm or greater mean induration and demonstrated nega-

Coccidioides immitis Spherule-Derived Skin Test Antigen

tive (less than 5 mm) responses to the negative controls. No positive induration responses to *Spherusol* were observed (1-sided 97.5% CI, 0%-26.5%) among subjects who had a history of disease caused by *H. capsulatum* and no history of travel to areas endemic for *C. immitis*. These findings support the lack of cross-reaction between the cellular immune responses induced by the 2 fungal species.

Subsequent Tests: A positive test may develop within 2 days to 3 weeks after onset of symptoms of primary coccidioidomycosis.

Mechanism: In patients with a history of pulmonary coccidioidomycosis, *Spherusol* is thought to elicit a cellular immune reaction to *C. immitis*, as evidenced by a delayed hypersensitivity response. The general mechanism is based on interaction of antigen with CD4 and CD8 lymphocytes, followed by the secretion of interleukins and other lymphokines from macrophages. Release of effector molecules causes endothelial cells lining the blood vessels to become permeable and allows fibrinogen to escape into the surrounding tissue, where it is converted to fibrin. The deposition of fibrin and accumulation of T cells and monocytes within the extracellular spaces cause the tissue to swell and become indurated. This process is usually detectable in 18 hours and typically peaks at 48 hours.

Drug Interactions: Reactivity to any delayed hypersensitivity test may be suppressed in patients receiving corticosteroids or other immunosuppressive drugs, or in patients who were recently immunized with live virus vaccines (eg, measles, mumps, rubella, varicella). If indicated, perform delayed hypersensitivity skin testing preceding immunization, simultaneously with immunization, or 4 to 6 weeks after immunization. Pharmacologic doses of corticosteroids may suppress the response to skin test antigens after 2 weeks of therapy. The mechanism of suppression is thought to involve a decrease in monocytes and lymphocytes, particularly T cells. The normal delayed hypersensitivity response usually returns to pretreatment levels within several weeks after steroid therapy is discontinued. The use of *Spherusol* has not been evaluated during or following the use of corticosteroids or immunosuppressive agents.

It is not known if concurrent treatment with antifungal medications interferes with delayed-type hypersensitivity responses to *Spherusol* in patients with a history of pulmonary coccidioidomycosis. In a clinical trial, receipt of concurrent or previous antifungal therapy did not appear to interfere with or accentuate the induration response to *Spherusol*.

Several weeks of cimetidine therapy may augment or enhance delayed hypersensitivity responses to skin test antigens, although this effect was not consistently observed. The effect may be mediated through cimetidine binding to suppressor T lymphocytes. It is presently unknown if other H_2 antagonists possess similar activity.

Pharmaceutical Characteristics

Concentration: 1.27 mcg of extracts of *C. immitis* spherules per 0.1 mL dose

Quality Assay: The potency of each lot of *Spherusol* is determined in sensitized guinea pigs.

Packaging: 1 mL multidose vial

NDC Number: 49463-0140-01

Doseform: Solution

Appearance: Clear, colorless solution

Solvent: Sodium chloride 0.9%

Adjuvant: None

Preservative: Phenol 0.4%

Allergens: None

Excipients: Sodium borate 0.014%. Residual thimerosal from the manufacturing process is present at a concentration of 0.0001% or less (less than 0.05 mcg of mercury per 0.1 mL dose)

pH: Not described

Shelf Life: Expires within an unspecified period

Storage/Stability: Store at 2° to 8°C (36° to 46°F). Discard if frozen. Contact the manufacturer regarding exposure to freezing or elevated temperatures. Shipping data not provided.

Production Process: Filtrate of spherules of *C. immitis*

Media: Liquid synthetic medium

Disease Epidemiology

Incidence: Based on delayed hypersensitivity skin testing, one-third of the population of endemic areas is infected.

Susceptible Pools: Most people living in endemic areas are susceptible to infection. Immunocompromised people are at greatest risk of progressing from infection to disease.

Transmission: Airborne transmission of fungal spores. Coccidioidomycosis is confined to the southwestern United States, contiguous areas of northern Mexico, and certain regions of Central and South America (eg, Argentina). The natural reservoir of mycelia is in soil, concentrated in California, Arizona, New Mexico, Nevada, Utah, and Texas. The mycelia can be recovered at the surface after spring rains. As the weather becomes hot and dry, mycelia convert to infectious arthroconidia that become airborne. Mycelia are rarely seen in lesions of coccidioidomycosis. The predominant form in vivo is sporangium or spherule. In coccidioidal granuloma, spores disseminate throughout the body.

Incubation: 1 to 4 weeks in primary infection (usually 10 to 16 days)

Communicability: Not directly transmitted from humans or animals to humans

Other Information

Perspective:

1892: Posada discovers *C. immitis* in tissue from a fatal human case.

1915: Coccidioidin first used in humans.

1928: First substantial use of coccidioidin.

1977: A dust storm in California causes coccidiomycosis to quadruple in the state and increase 20-fold in the San Joaquin Valley.

1994: Epidemic of coccidiomycosis in southern California after a January earthquake.

First Licensed: July 29, 2011

Discontinued Products:

Mycelia-derived BioCox 1:10 and 1:100 v/v (Iatric Corporation): Licensed in 1968; withdrawn June 25, 1997

Spherule-derived Spherulin 1:10 and 1:100 v/v (Berkeley Biologicals [later ALK-Abelló Laboratories]): Licensed January 15, 1976; withdrawn circa 2006

References: Einstein HE, Johnson RH. Coccidioidomycosis: new aspects of epidemiology and therapy. *Clin Infect Dis.* 1993;16(3):349-354.

Johnson RH, Einstein HE. Coccidioidal meningitis. *Clin Infect Dis.* 2006;42(1):103-107.

Kirkland TN, Fierer J. Coccidioidomycosis: a reemerging infectious disease. *Emerg Infect Dis.* 1996;2(3):192-199.

Coccidioides immitis Spherule-Derived Skin Test Antigen

Coccidioides Skin Test Summary	
Generic name	*Coccidioides immitis* spherule-derived skin test antigen
Brand name	*Spherusol*
Synonym	Coccidioidin
Manufacturer	Allermed Laboratories
Viability	Not viable
Indication	To detect pulmonary coccidioidomycosis
Concentration	1.27 mcg per 0.1 mL
Adjuvant	None
Preservative	Phenol 0.4%
Production medium	Liquid synthetic medium
Doseform	Solution
Solvent	Sodium chloride 0.9%
Packaging	1 mL vial
Routine storage	2° to 8°C (35° to 46°F)
Dosage, route	0.1 mL intradermally

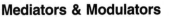

General Statement

A variety of terms is used to describe the immunologic messengers that regulate the human immune system. These messengers provide the positive and negative feedback that allow immune defenses to mobilize against an invader and also to demobilize when the acute threat has passed.

Some terms for these drugs are overly broad (overly sensitive, if you will), such as *biological response modifiers* (BRMs) or *immunomodulators*. The term *biological response modifier* does not distinguish immunologic agents from nonimmunologic agents. Based on a strict definition of the words, insulin could be categorized as a BRM, although it clearly does not act immunologically. Vaccines are immunomodulators, of course, but are adequately described in their own section.

Some of the terms used to describe these products are overly specific, such as *lymphokines* and *monokines*. *Lymphokines* refer to proteins released by immune cells, but some messengers of immunologic interest come from cells other than immune ones (eg, interferon beta from fibroblasts). *Monokines* refer just to substances secreted by monocytes and macrophages (eg, interleukin-1 and tumor necrosis factor). We could use the rubric *cytokines*, as most of the immunologic messengers currently of interest communicate between cells, but such a term is also unnecessarily restrictive.

We have chosen to use the rubric *immunologic mediators* to include both intercellular and intracellular messengers that regulate inflammation, as well as the production of antibodies, granulocytes (eg, neutrophils, eosinophils), macrophages and monocytes, hematopoietic cells and other cells.

Colony-Stimulating Factors

Colony-Stimulating Factors Comparison			
	Filgrastim	Pegfilgrastim	Sargramostim
Abbreviation	G-CSF	G-CSF pegylated	GM-CSF
Proprietary name	*Neupogen*	*Neulasta*	*Leukine*
Manufacturer	Amgen	Amgen	Berlex
Form	Nonglycosylated	Nonglycosylated	Glycosylated
Packaging	300 mcg/1 mL 480 mcg/1.6 mL	6 mg/0.6 mL	250 mcg 500 mcg
Doseform	Solution	Solution	Solution or powder
Solvent/Diluent	Buffered water	Buffered water	Sterile water
Primary indications	Following chemotherapy for nonmyeloid malignancies. In autologous stem cell transplants to aid engraftment and cell recovery. To treat chronic neutro-penia.	To prevent febrile neutropenia in patients with nonmyeloid malignancies receiving myelosuppressive anticancer drugs.	Following bone marrow transplantation for non-Hodgkin lymphoma, acute lymphocytic leukemia, or Hodgkin disease. To prevent infection after high-dose chemotherapy for AML. In allogeneic and autologous bone marrow transplants to aid engraftment and cell recovery. In autologous stem cell transplants to aid engraftment and cell recovery.
Route	Subcutaneous, IV infusion	Subcutaneous	Subcutaneous, IV infusion
IV fluid	5% dextrose	Not applicable	0.9% sodium chloride
Add albumin if final CSF concentration is:	< 15 mcg/mL	Not applicable	< 10 mcg/mL
Albumin concentration	2 mg/mL	Not applicable	1 mg/mL
Initial dose	5 mcg/kg/day for ≥ 10 days	6 mg	250 mcg/m^2/day for ≥ 21 days
Routine storage	Refrigerate	Refrigerate	Refrigerate

Cell lineages affected
  Primary
 	
  Secondary
	
	Neutrophils
		
		Neutrophils
			
			Neutrophils, monocytes, macrophages, eosinophils
			Platelets, erythrocytes (in vitro)

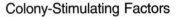

Colony-Stimulating Factors

Name:
Neupogen

Manufacturer:
Amgen

Synonyms: Granulocyte colony-stimulating factor (recombinant human), G-CSF, rG-CSF, recombinant methionyl human G-CSF (r-met-Hu-G-CSF)

Immunologic Characteristics

Source: G-CSF expressed from recombinant *Escherichia coli* bacteria

Viability: Not viable, but immunologically active

Antigenic Form: Colony-stimulating factor

Antigenic Type: Protein. Endogenous G-CSF is a glycoprotein produced by monocytes, fibroblasts and endothelial cells. Filgrastim is a protein of 175 amino acids, with a molecular weight of 18,800 daltons. Unlike native human G-CSF, filgrastim is not glycosylated. Its amino acid sequence is identical to the natural product, except for the addition of an N-terminal methionine necessary for expression in *Escherichia coli*.

Strains: r-met-Hu-G-CSF (recombinant methionyl human G-CSF)

Use Characteristics

Indications: To decrease the incidence of infection, as manifested by febrile neutropenia, in patients with nonmyeloid malignancies receiving myelosuppressive anticancer drugs associated with a significant increase of severe neutropenia with fever (eg, cyclophosphamide, doxorubicin, etoposide). Other benefits shown in clinical studies were decreased requirements for hospitalization, decreased IV antibiotic use, and decreased duration and extent of severe neutropenia.

Among cancer patients receiving bone marrow transplants, filgrastim reduces the duration of neutropenia and neutropenia-related clinical sequelae (such as febrile neutropenia) in patients with nonmyeloid malignancies undergoing myeloablative chemotherapy following marrow transplantation.

Filgrastim is effective as a chronic treatment to reduce the incidence and duration of sequelae of neutropenia (such as fever, infections, and oropharyngeal ulcers) in symptomatic patients with congenital, cyclic, or idiopathic neutropenia. Filgrastim decreases the number of infections by increasing the patient's neutrophil count and decreasing the duration of neutropenia. Rates of hospitalization and incidence of antibiotic use are also reduced.

Filgrastim mobilizes hematopoietic progenitor cells (stem cells) into the peripheral blood for collection by leukapheresis. Mobilization allows for the collection of increased numbers of progenitor cells capable of engraftment, compared with collection by leukapheresis without mobilization or bone marrow harvest. After myeloablative chemotherapy, the transplantation of an increased number of progenitor cells can lead to more rapid engraftment, which may result in decreased need for supportive care. Filgrastim in autologous peripheral blood stem (or progenitor) cell (PBPC) transplants can reduce time to engraftment and neutrophil and platelet recovery. This, in turn, can shorten hospital stays and reduce the need for transfusions.

Filgrastim is effective in reducing the time to neutrophil recovery and the duration of fever, after induction or consolidation chemotherapy in adults with acute myelogenous leukemia. Filgrastim treatment significantly reduced antibiotic use and duration of hospitalization.

Unlabeled Uses: Filgrastim is being investigated for efficacy in the treatment of myelodysplastic syndromes (orphan designation, August 3, 1990) and patients with AIDS who, in addition, are afflicted with CMV retinitis and are being treated with ganciclovir (orphan designation, September 3, 1991).

Limitations: No difference in survival or disease progression was demonstrated among cancer patients. The efficacy of filgrastim has not been evaluated in patients receiving chemotherapy associated with delayed myelosuppression (eg, nitrosoureas), with mitomycin C or with myelosuppressive doses of antimetabolites (eg, 5-fluorouracil, cytosine arabinoside). Safety and efficacy of filgrastim have not been evaluated in patients receiving concurrent radiation therapy. Avoid simultaneous use of filgrastim with chemotherapy and radiation therapy. Using filgrastim before confirming severe chronic neutropenia (SCN) may impair diagnostic efforts and thus impair or delay evaluation and treatment of an underlying condition, other than SCN, causing the neutropenia.

Contraindications:

Absolute: None

Relative: Do not administer within 24 hours before or after cytotoxic chemotherapy, because of possible sensitivity of rapidly dividing myeloid cells to chemotherapy. Do not administer to patients with known hypersensitivity to *Escherichia coli*-derived products.

Immunodeficiency: Filgrastim is being evaluated in immunocompromised patients with SCN. Preliminary data support safety and efficacy of filgrastim in these disorders.

Elderly: No specific information is available about geriatric use of filgrastim.

Carcinogenicity: The possibility that filgrastim can act as a growth factor for any tumor type, particularly myeloid malignancies, cannot be excluded. Because of the possibility of tumor growth potentiation, take care in using this drug in any malignancy with myeloid characteristics (eg, leukemias).

When filgrastim is used to mobilize peripheral blood progenitor cells, tumor cells may be released from the marrow and subsequently collected in a leukapheresis product. The effect of reinfusion of tumor cells has not been well studied. The limited data available are inconclusive.

Mutagenicity: Filgrastim failed to induce bacterial gene mutations in either the presence or absence of a drug-metabolizing enzyme system.

Fertility Impairment: Filgrastim had no observed effect on the fertility of male or female rats, or on gestation, at doses up to 500 mcg/kg.

Pregnancy: Category C. Use only if benefits exceed likely risks. It is not known if filgrastim crosses the human placenta. Filgrastim has adverse effects in pregnant rabbits at doses 2 to 10 times the human dose. But filgrastim had no lethal, teratogenic, or behavioral effects on fetuses of pregnant rats during the period of organogenesis at doses up to 575 mcg/kg/day.

Lactation: It is not known if filgrastim is excreted in breast milk. Problems in humans have not been documented.

Children: Although efficacy of filgrastim has not been demonstrated in a pediatric population, safety data indicate that filgrastim does not exhibit any greater toxicity in children than in adults. In patients receiving chronic filgrastim for the treatment of SCN, subclinical increases in spleen size were reported more often in children than in adults. The clinical significance of these findings relative to normal growth and development is not known. Limited data from patients with SCN, aged 4 months to 17 years, followed for 1.5 years do not suggest alterations in growth and development, sexual maturation, or endocrine function. Safety and efficacy in neonates and patients with autoimmune neutropenia of infancy have not been established.

Adverse Reactions: The most common adverse experience occurring with filgrastim therapy is medullary bone pain (24%). Severity ranges from mild to moderate and can be controlled in most patients with nonnarcotic analgesics; infrequently, narcotic analgesics have been required. Bone pain was reported more frequently in patients treated with higher doses (20 to 100 mcg/kg/day) administered IV than with lower or subcutaneous doses. No statistically significant increase in the incidence of fever in filgrastim-treated patients was noted. Spontaneously reversible mild to moderate elevations in uric acid, lactate dehydrogenase, and alkaline phosphatase occurred in 27% to 58% of filgrastim recipients. Transient decreases in blood pressure (less than 90/60 mm Hg), which did not require clinical treatment, were reported in 4% of recipients. Patients occasionally experience redness, swelling, or itching at the site of injection. Numerous side effects occurred more frequently among placebo recipients than those treated with filgrastim. There were no reports of viral-like symptoms, pleuritis, pericarditis, or other major systemic reactions.

Among cancer patients receiving bone marrow transplants, the most common complaints (compared with placebo recipients) were nausea (10% vs 4%), vomiting (7% vs 3%), hypertension (4% vs 0%), rash (12% vs 10%), and peritonitis (2% vs 0%). None of these events was believed by the investigator to be related to filgrastim. One episode of erythema nodosum was reported.

Among patients with SCN, the most common side effects were mild to moderate bone pain (33%), palpable splenomegaly (30%), epistaxis (15%), and anemia (10%). Thrombocytopenia (less than 50,000 cells/mm^3) occurred in 12% of those with palpable spleens, but in less than 6% overall. Infrequent events possibly related to filgrastim include injection-site reactions, rash, hepatomegaly, arthralgia, osteoporosis, cutaneous vasculitis, hematuria or proteinuria, alopecia, and exacerbations of some preexisting skin disorders, such as psoriasis.

Among cancer patients undergoing peripheral blood progenitor cell collection, the most common adverse events were mild to moderate musculoskeletal symptoms (44%), predominantly medullary bone pain (33%), transient increases in alkaline phosphatase (21%), and headache (7%). Mild to moderate anemia occurred in 65% of patients, with decreases in platelet counts in 97%.

Allergic reactions and anaphylaxis attributed to filgrastim administration have been reported at a rate less than 1 per 4,000 patients treated. There is no evidence of the development of anti-filgrastim antibodies, even among 33 patients who received filgrastim daily for almost 2 years.

Cardiac events (eg, myocardial infarctions, dysrhythmias) have affected 2.9% of cancer patients receiving filgrastim; the relationship between these events and filgrastim therapy is unknown. Monitor patients with preexisting cardiac anomalies closely.

In septic patients, be alert to the theoretical possibility of adult respiratory distress syndrome because of the possible influx of neutrophils into the lungs if this is the site of inflammation.

Because of the potential for receiving higher doses of chemotherapy (ie, full doses on the prescribed schedule), the patient may be at greater risk of thrombocytopenia, anemia and nonhematologic consequences of increased chemotherapy doses. Monitor hematocrit and platelet count regularly. Exercise caution when administering filgrastim with other drugs known to lower the platelet count.

White blood cell counts of 100,000 cells/mm^3 and above were observed in approximately 2% of patients receiving filgrastim at doses greater than 5 mcg/kg/day. To avoid the potential complications of excessive leukocytosis, check the CBC twice weekly during filgrastim therapy. One-third of patients on long-term therapy for SCN develop subclinical splenomegaly; 3% of patients were noted to have clinical splenomegaly. Less frequently observed adverse events included exacerbation of preexisting skin disorders (eg, psoriasis), alopecia, hematuria or proteinuria, thrombocytopenia (platelets less than 50,000 cells/mm^3) and osteoporosis.

Whereas 9 of 325 patients developed myelodysplasia or myeloid leukemia while receiving filgrastim during clinical trials, acute myeloid leukemia or abnormal cytogenetics are part of the natural history of SCN without cytokine therapy. The effect of filgrastim on developing abnormal cytogenetics and the effect of continued filgrastim therapy in these patients are unknown.

Cutaneous vasculitis has been reported rarely (less than 1 per 7,000 patients) after filgrastim. In most cases the severity of cutaneous vasculitis was moderate or severe. Most reports involved patients with SCN on long-term filgrastim therapy. Symptoms of vasculitis generally developed simultaneously with the increase in the absolute neutrophil count (ANC) and abated when the ANC decreased. Many patients were able to continue filgrastim at a reduced dose.

Pharmacologic & Dosing Characteristics

Dosage: Avoid shaking; a frothy appearance or the presence of bubbles does not reduce the efficacy of the drug, but may decrease the amount that can be drawn into the syringe.

Cancer patients receiving myelosuppressive chemotherapy: Initial dose: 5 mcg/kg/day, administered as a single daily injection. Give via either intermittent infusion over at least 20 to 30 minutes or continuous infusion.

Increase doses in increments of 5 mcg/kg for each chemotherapy cycle, according to the duration and severity of the nadir of the ANC. Administer filgrastim no earlier than 24 hours after administration of cytotoxic chemotherapy. Administer filgrastim daily for up to 2 weeks, until the ANC reaches 10,000 cells/mm^3 following the expected chemotherapy-induced neutrophil nadir. The duration of filgrastim therapy needed to attenuate chemotherapy-induced neutropenia may depend on the myelosuppressive potential of the chemotherapy regimen employed.

Discontinue filgrastim when the ANC exceeds 10,000 cells/mm^3 after the expected chemotherapy-induced nadir. Do not confuse this threshold with a transient increase in neutrophil counts typically seen 1 to 2 days after initiation of filgrastim therapy.

Cancer patients receiving bone marrow transplant: Give 10 mcg/kg/day as an IV infusion over 4 or 24 hours or as a continuous 24-hour subcutaneous infusion. For patients receiving bone marrow transplant, give the first dose at least 24 hours after cytotoxic chemotherapy and at least 24 hours after bone marrow infusion.

During the period of neutrophil recovery, titrate the daily dose of filgrastim against the neutrophil response. When the ANC is more than 1,000 cells/mm^3 for 3 consecutive days, reduce filgrastim to 5 mcg/kg/day. Then, if the ANC remains more than 1,000 cells/mm^3 for 3 more consecutive days, discontinue filgrastim. Then, if the ANC decreases to less than 1,000 cells/mm^3, resume filgrastim at 5 mcg/kg/day. If the ANC falls below 1,000 cells/mm^3 at any time during the 5 mcg/kg/day regimen, increase filgrastim to 10 mcg/kg/day and follow the steps above.

Patients with severe chronic neutropenia (SCN): Give filgrastim to patients in whom a diagnosis of congenital, cyclic, or idiopathic neutropenia has been definitely confirmed. Rule out other diseases associated with neutropenia. In congenital neutropenia, start at 6 mcg/kg subcutaneously twice daily. For idiopathic or cyclic neutropenia, start at 5 mcg/kg as a single subcutaneous injection daily. Chronic daily administration is required to maintain clinical benefit. Do not use ANC as the sole indication of efficacy. Individually adjust the dose based on the patient's clinical course, as well as ANC. Patients may experience clinical benefit with ANCs below a typical 1,500 to 10,000 cells/mm^3 level. Reduce the dose if the ANC is persistently more than 10,000 cells/mm^3.

Peripheral blood progenitor cell (PBPC) collection and therapy in cancer patients: Give 10 mcg/kg/day for PBPC mobilization subcutaneously, either as a bolus or as continuous infusion. Give filgrastim at least 4 days before the first leukapheresis procedure and continue until the last leukapheresis. Although the optimal duration of filgrastim administration and leukapheresis schedule have not been established, giving filgrastim for 6 to 7 days with leukapheresis on days 5, 6, and 7 was safe and effective. Filgrastim was also given after reinfusion of the collected cells.

Initial dose: 5 mcg/kg/day, administered as a single daily injection. Give via either intermittent infusion over at least 20 to 30 minutes or continuous infusion. IV infusions over 2 to 4 hours have been described.

Increase doses in increments of 5 mcg/kg for each chemotherapy cycle, according to the duration and severity of the nadir of the ANC. Administer filgrastim no earlier than 24 hours after administration of cytotoxic chemotherapy. Administer filgrastim daily for up to 2 weeks, until the ANC reaches 10,000 cells/mm^3 following the expected chemotherapy-induced neutrophil nadir. The duration of filgrastim therapy needed to attenuate chemotherapy-induced neutropenia may depend on the myelosuppressive potential of the chemotherapy regimen employed.

Discontinue filgrastim when the ANC exceeds 10,000 cells/mm^3 after the expected chemotherapy-induced nadir. Do not confuse this threshold with a transient increase in neutrophil counts typically seen 1 to 2 days after initiation of filgrastim therapy.

Another empiric method of dosing that has been employed is to give 300 mcg/day to patients weighing up to 70 kg and 480 mcg/day to patients weighing more than 70 kg. Some clinicians have chosen to stop therapy when the ANC rises to more than 1,500 to 5,000 cells/mm^3, although this method has not been scientifically evaluated.

Route: Subcutaneous injection, subcutaneous infusion, or IV infusion. Administration by IV push has not been studied.

Overdosage: Discontinue filgrastim if the ANC exceeds 10,000 cells/mm^3 to avoid the potential risks of excessive leukocytosis. The maximum tolerated dose has not been determined. Doses up to 138 mcg/kg/day have been administered without dose-limiting toxic effects attributable to filgrastim. WBC counts more than 100,000 cells/mm^3 have not been associated with any reported adverse clinical effects. A flattening of the dose-response curve above 10 mcg/kg/day has been observed.

Additional Doses: The safety and efficacy of chronic administration of filgrastim have not been established.

Missed Doses: A transient increase in neutrophil counts is typically seen 1 to 2 days after beginning filgrastim therapy. For a sustained therapeutic response, continue filgrastim until the postnadir ANC exceeds 10,000 cells/mm^3.

Laboratory Tests: Obtain a CBC prior to chemotherapy and twice per week during filgrastim therapy to avoid leukocytosis and to monitor the neutrophil count. After cytotoxic chemotherapy, the neutrophil nadir occurred earlier during cycles when filgrastim was given, and white blood cell differentials showed a left shift. The duration of severe neutropenia was reduced and was followed by accelerated recovery of WBC counts.

In cancer patients receiving bone marrow transplants, monitor CBCs and platelet counts at least 3 times per week after transplant. In patients with severe chronic neutropenia, monitor CBC with differential and platelet count twice per week during the first 4 weeks of filgrastim therapy and for 2 weeks after any dose adjustment; monitor monthly once the patient is clinically stable.

In clinical trials, cyclic fluctuations in neutrophil counts were seen frequently in patients with congenital or idiopathic neutropenia after starting filgrastim therapy. Platelet counts were generally at the upper limits of normal before starting filgrastim. After therapy began, platelet counts decreased but remained within normal limits. Early myeloid forms were noted in peripheral blood in most patients, including the appearance of metamyelocytes and myelocytes. Promyelocytes and myeloblasts were noted in some patients. Relative increases were occasionally noted in the number of circulating eosinophils and basophils. No consistent increases were observed with filgrastim therapy. As in other trials, increases were observed in serum uric acid, lactic dehydrogenase, and serum alkaline phosphatase.

Efficacy: In studies of cancer patients receiving myelosuppressive chemotherapy, filgrastim reduced the number of days during which antibiotics were used to treat fever and neutropenia, the number of days of hospitalization, and the incidence of confirmed infections by approximately 50% when G-CSF was administered, compared with placebo. At least one episode of fever with neutropenia occurred among 77% of placebo recipients and 40% of G-CSF recipients. Incidence of hospitalization fell from 69% to 52%, IV antibiotic usage fell from 60% to 38%, and the median duration of neutropenia fell from 5.6 days to 2.4 days. Over all cycles of chemotherapy, the median duration of grade IV neutropenia (ANC less than 0.5×10^9 cells/liter) was 6 days with placebo and 1 day with G-CSF.

Among cancer patients receiving bone marrow transplant, the median number of days of severe neutropenia dropped from 23 days in a control group to 11 days in the group treated with filgrastim. The median number of days of febrile neutropenia fell from 13.5 to 5.5. Reductions in numbers of days of hospitalization and antibiotic use were also seen, although these effects were not statistically significant in these trials.

In studies of patients with severe chronic neutropenia, rates of infection fell from 50% among control patients to 20% among patients treated with filgrastim. Incidence of fever fell from 25% to 20%, antibiotic use dropped from 49% to 20%, and duration of fever dropped from 0.63 days to 0.2 days. Oropharyngeal ulcer rates fell from 26% to 0%. As a result, hospitalization rates fell from 73% to 45% over a 4-month period.

In retrospective studies, patients receiving peripheral blood stem (or progenitor) cell (PBPC) transplants mobilized with filgrastim 5 to 10 mcg/kg/day showed a median time to platelet recovery of 16.5 days compared with 31 days for an untreated group. Patients treated with filgrastim had fewer platelet transfusions (10, compared with 17.5 for the untreated group), a shorter time to last red blood cell transfusion (11 vs 27 days) and a reduction in number of transfusions (8 vs 14.5). Filgrastim did not affect overall or disease-free survival.

In a randomized trial comparing filgrastim in bone marrow transplants to filgrastim in PBPC transplants, the latter therapy had shorter hospitalizations, time to neutrophil restoration (11 vs 14 days for bone-marrow transplant), time to platelet recovery (16 vs 23 days) and fewer platelet transfusion days (6 vs 10). An FDA committee did not conclude from these data that filgrastim in PBPC transplants is superior to filgrastim in bone marrow transplants.

Onset: While the net effect of filgrastim administration is a dose-dependent elevation of neutrophil counts evident 24 hours after administration, within the first 30 to 60 minutes following a dose circulating neutrophil counts in many patients drop to less than 1,000 neutrophils/mm^3. By 4 hours after administration, a rapid rise in neutrophil counts above pretreatment levels occurs. The mechanism of the early depression of circulating neutrophil counts is unknown but is consistent with neutrophil migration to endothelial cells, with the subsequent loss of detectability in peripheral blood.

Duration: When filgrastim is administered in the absence of chemotherapy, sustained elevations of the ANC occur throughout the dosing period. When administered following chemotherapy, an initial transient neutrophil increase is followed by a decrease in ANC because of the effects of cytotoxic chemotherapy. However, in patients receiving filgrastim, accelerated neutrophil recovery from the chemotherapy-induced nadir occurs with sustained neutrophil elevations throughout the remainder of the dosing period. The duration and severity of the chemotherapy-induced neutropenia are significantly decreased when filgrastim is administered.

Decreases in the ANC of 50% have occurred within 24 hours of filgrastim discontinuation. Normalization of the ANC occurs within 1 to 7 days after termination of filgrastim. There is no evidence of withdrawal effects, such as rebound neutropenia, following discontinuation of filgrastim.

Pharmacokinetics: Blood levels after subcutaneous bolus dosing increase over 2 to 8 hours with peaks 4 to 5 hours after administration. After giving 11.5 mcg/kg subcutaneously, serum levels remain greater than 10 ng/mL for 8 to 16 hours. After a single 30-minute IV infusion or subcutaneous bolus dose, a linear correlation is observed between the dose and both the serum concentration and area under the concentration-time curves (AUC).

Continuous IV infusion of 20 mcg/kg of filgrastim over 24 hours resulted in mean and median serum concentrations of 48 and 56 ng/mL, respectively. Subcutaneous administration of 3.45 mcg/kg and 11.5 mcg/kg resulted in maximum serum concentrations of 4 and 49 ng/mL, respectively, within 2 to 8 hours. The apparent volume of distribution (Vd) averaged 150 mL/kg in both normal subjects and cancer patients. Continuous IV infusions of 20 mcg/kg/day over 11 to 20 days produced steady-state serum concentrations with no evidence of drug accumulation.

IV or subcutaneous filgrastim is eliminated at a rate consistent with first-order kinetics with a clearance of 0.5 to 0.7 mL/min/kg and an average circulating elimination half-life of 3.5 hours (range, 0.77 to 8.49). Half-lives are similar for IV and subcutaneous routes, 231 and 210 minutes, respectively. The route of metabolism of filgrastim is presently unknown. Filgrastim is not dialyzed by either hemo- or peritoneal dialysis.

Protective Level: Doses of filgrastim that increase the ANC more than 10,000 cells/mm^3 may not result in any additional clinical benefit.

Mechanism: Filgrastim selectively stimulates the differentiation and proliferation of neutrophil precursors in human bone marrow, leading to the release of mature neutrophils into the circulation from the bone marrow. Filgrastim also affects the functional activities of mature neutrophils, including enhanced phagocytic ability, priming of the cellular metabolism associated with respiratory burst, antibody-dependent killing and the increased expression of some functions associated with cell-surface antigens.

The absolute monocyte count increases in a dose-dependent manner in most recipients of filgrastim, but the percentage of monocytes in the differential count remains within the normal range. In all studies to date, absolute counts of both eosinophils and basophils were within the normal range following filgrastim administration. Increases in lymphocyte counts following filgrastim administration occurred in some normal subjects and cancer patients.

White blood cell differential counts obtained during clinical trials have demonstrated a shift toward granulocyte progenitor cells (a "shift to the left"), including the appearance of promyelocytes and myeloblasts, usually during neutrophil recovery following a chemotherapy-induced nadir. Dohle bodies and increased granulocyte granulation, as well as hypersegmented neutrophils, have also been observed. Such changes were transient and were not associated with clinical sequelae, nor were they necessarily associated with infection.

Drug Interactions: Do not administer filgrastim and chemotherapy simultaneously. Use drugs that may potentiate release of neutrophils, such as lithium, with caution.

Because of the potential for receiving higher doses of chemotherapy (ie, full doses on the prescribed schedule), the patient may be at greater risk of thrombocytopenia, anemia and non-hematologic consequences of increased chemotherapy doses. Exercise care when administering filgrastim with other drugs known to lower the platelet count.

Filgrastim

Pharmaceutical Characteristics

Concentration: 300 mcg per 1 mL (vials), equivalent to activity of 0.4 to 1.6 × 10^8 units/mg

Quality Assay: Cell-mitogenesis assay

Packaging: Box of ten 300 mcg per 1 mL single-dose vials (NDC #: 55513-0530-10); box of ten 480 mcg per 1.6 mL single-dose vials (55513-0546-10)

Box of 10 single-dose 300 mcg/0.5 mL prefilled syringes with 27-gauge, ½-inch needles with needle guard (55513-924-10); box of 10 single-dose 480 mcg/0.8 mL prefilled syringes with 27 gauge, ½-inch needles with needle guard (55513-209-10)

Doseform: Solution

Appearance: Clear, colorless liquid. Do not use if discolored or cloudy, or if the vial appears to contain any precipitate.

Solvent: Sterile water for injection with buffer and excipients

Diluent:

For infusion: Dilute in 5% dextrose. Filgrastim is not physically compatible with 0.9% sodium chloride. Filgrastim is stable if the concentration after dilution is at least 15 mcg/mL in 5% dextrose. At dilutions from 2 to 15 mcg/mL, add human albumin to a final albumin concentration of 0.2% (2 mg/mL) to protect against adsorption of the filgrastim to the container walls. For example, add 2 mL of 5% albumin to each 50 mL of IV fluid. Do not dilute filgrastim to a final concentration less than 2 mcg/mL.

Compatibility: Filgrastim 30 mcg/mL combined with 75 other drugs under simulated Y-site conditions was compatible at 22°C (71.6°F) for up to 4 hours. Visual incompatibilities were noted with 22 other drugs: Amphotericin B, cefonicid, cefoperazone, cefotaxime, cefoxitin, ceftizoxime, ceftriaxone, cefuroxime, clindamycin, dactinomycin, etoposide, fluorouracil, furosemide, heparin, mannitol, metronidazole, methylprednisolone, mezlocillin, mitomycin, prochlorperazine, piperacillin, and thiotepa.

Adjuvant: None

Preservative: None

Allergens: The needle cover of prefilled syringes contains dry natural rubber (a latex derivative).

Excipients: 0.01 molar sodium acetate buffer, 5% sorbitol, and 0.004% polysorbate 80. Contains 0.035 mg/mL sodium and 0.59 mg/mL acetate.

pH: 3.8 to 4.2

Shelf Life: Expires within 24 months.

Storage/Stability: Store at 2° to 8°C (35° to 46°F). Do not freeze. If inadvertently frozen for up to 24 hours, thaw the vials and refrigerate for future use. Discard if frozen longer than 24 hours. Never expose filgrastim to dry ice. The drug cannot tolerate temperatures less than −4°C (25°F). Prior to injection, filgrastim may be allowed to reach controlled room temperature (up to 30°C or 86°F) for up to 7 days. Discard unused portions. Do not save unused drug for later administration. It is shipped in insulated containers.

If filgrastim is inadvertently left out of refrigeration for up to 7 days, it is safe to use, provided that the contents of the vial remain clear, not cloudy, and were not subjected to temperatures less than −4°C (25°F) or higher than 30°C (86°F). Filgrastim is stable for 14 days when sterilely repackaged into syringes and promptly refrigerated.

When diluted, filgrastim can remain at a neutral pH for a limited period of time. Filgrastim is stable if the concentration after dilution is at least 15 mcg/mL in 5% dextrose. At dilutions from 2 to 15 mcg/mL, add human albumin to a final albumin concentration of 0.2% (2 mg/mL) to protect against adsorption of the filgrastim to the container walls. For example, add 2 mL of 5% albumin to each 50 mL of 0.9% sodium chloride. Refrigerate diluted solutions and use within

24 hours of preparation. Sterile dilutions are stable up to 7 days at 2° to 8°C (35° to 46°F). Do not dilute to a final concentration less than 2 mcg/mL. Do not use any saline fluid as a diluent or the product may precipitate.

Handling: Avoid shaking. Filgrastim is compatible with glass bottles; polyvinylchloride and polyolefin IV bags, tubing, and related devices; and polypropylene syringes.

Production Process: Recombinant DNA technology is used to clone the gene that encodes G-CSF. That gene is introduced into *Escherichia coli* bacteria, which then produces filgrastim proteins. Prior to purification, r-met-Hu-G-CSF oxidizes to its native state. Final purity is achieved by sequential passage over a series of chromatography columns. Gene, vectors, host cells, and process were patented in March 1989 with US patent #4,810,643.

Media: *E. coli*

Disease Epidemiology

Prevalence: Severe chronic neutropenia affects 1,000 to 2,000 patients in the US. In the US, approximately 9,000 patients per year are diagnosed with acute myelogenous leukemia.

Other Information

Perspective:
1983: Nicola and colleagues identify and purify murine G-CSF.
1985: Welte and colleagues first purify human G-CSF.
1986: Nicola and colleagues isolate the gene for G-CSF and express it with *E. coli*.
1991: Filgrastim licensed on February 21, 1991 (designated an orphan drug August 30, 1990).

References: Hollingshead LM, et al. Recombinant granulocyte colony-stimulating factor (rG-CSF). A review of its pharmacological properties and prospective role in neutropenic conditions. *Drugs.* 1991;42:300-330.

Ricotta R, Cerea G, Schiavetto I, Maugeri MR, Pedrazzoli P, Siena S. Pegfilgrastim: Current and future perspectives in the treatment of chemotherapy-induced neutropenia. *Future Oncol.* 2006;2(6):667-676.

Smith TJ, Khatcheressian J, Lyman GH, et al. 2006 update of recommendations for the use of white blood cell growth factors: an evidence-based clinical practice guideline. *J Clin Oncol.* 2006;24(19):3187-3205.

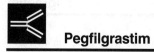

Pegfilgrastim

Colony-Stimulating Factors

Name:
Neulasta

Manufacturer:
Amgen

Synonyms: *Neulastim*

Comparison: Pegfilgrastim is a pegylated form of filgrastim, which affects dose and dosing interval.

Immunologic Characteristics

Antigen Source: Based on G-CSF expressed from recombinant *Escherichia coli* bacteria

Viability: Not viable, but immunologically active

Antigenic Form: Colony-stimulating factor

Antigenic Type: Protein covalently conjugated to monomethoxypolyethylene glycol. Endogenous G-CSF is a glycoprotein produced by monocytes, fibroblasts, and endothelial cells. Filgrastim is a water-soluble protein of 175 amino acids, with a molecular weight of 18,800 daltons. Unlike native human G-CSF, filgrastim is nonglycosylated. Its amino acid sequence is identical to the natural product, except for the addition of an N-terminal methionine necessary for expression in *E. coli*. The average molecular weight of pegfilgrastim is approximately 39 kD.

Strains: Pegylated r-met-Hu-G-CSF (recombinant methionyl human G-CSF)

Use Characteristics

Indications: To decrease the incidence of infection, as manifested by febrile neutropenia, in patients with nonmyeloid malignancies receiving myelosuppressive anticancer drugs associated with a clinically significant incidence of febrile neutropenia.

Limitations: To avoid a potential risk of splenic rupture, do not use pegfilgrastim for peripheral-blood progenitor-cell (PBPC) mobilization.

Contraindications:

Absolute: None

Relative: Pegfilgrastim is contraindicated in patients with known hypersensitivity to *E. coli*-derived proteins, pegfilgrastim, filgrastim, or any other component of the product. Do not administer pegfilgrastim in the period from 14 days before to 24 hours after administration of cytotoxic chemotherapy, because of the potential for an increase in sensitivity of rapidly dividing myeloid cells to cytotoxic chemotherapy.

Immunodeficiency: No adverse effect in immunodeficiency known. May be indicated to avert infectious complications of immunodeficiency.

Elderly: No differences were observed in clinical trials in the pharmacokinetics of geriatric patients (65 years of age and older) compared with younger patients (younger than 65 years of age). Of the subjects with cancer who received pegfilgrastim in clinical studies, 18% were 65 years of age and older, and 3% were 75 years of age and older. No overall differences in safety or effectiveness were observed between these patients and younger patients; however, because of the small number of elderly subjects, small but clinically relevant differences cannot be excluded.

Carcinogenicity: The carcinogenic potential of pegfilgrastim has not been evaluated in long-term animal studies. In a 6-month toxicity study in rats given once weekly subcutaneous injections of up to 1,000 mcg/kg of pegfilgrastim (approximately 23-fold higher than the human dose), no precancerous or cancerous lesions were noted.

Pegfilgrastim is a growth factor that primarily stimulates neutrophils and neutrophil precursors. However, the G-CSF receptor through which pegfilgrastim and filgrastim act has been found on tumor cell lines, including some myeloid, T-lymphoid, lung, head and neck, and bladder tumor cell lines. The possibility that pegfilgrastim can act as a growth factor for any tumor type cannot be excluded. Pegfilgrastim in myeloid malignancies and myelodysplasia (MDS) has not been studied. In a randomized study comparing filgrastim with placebo in patients undergoing remission induction and consolidation chemotherapy for acute myeloid leukemia, important differences in remission rate between the two arms were excluded. Disease-free survival and overall survival were comparable. However, the study was not designed to detect important differences in these endpoints.

Mutagenicity: Pegfilgrastim has not been evaluated for mutagenic potential.

Fertility Impairment: When administered once weekly via subcutaneous injections to male and female rats at doses up to 1,000 mcg/kg before and during mating, reproductive performance, fertility, and sperm assessment parameters were not affected.

Pregnancy: Category C. There are no adequate and well-controlled studies in pregnant women. Use pegfilgrastim during pregnancy only if the potential benefit to the mother justifies the potential risk to the fetus. It is not known if pegfilgrastim crosses the placenta. No gender-related differences were observed in the human pharmacokinetics of pegfilgrastim.

Pegfilgrastim has been shown to have adverse effects in pregnant rabbits when administered subcutaneously every other day during gestation at doses as low as 50 mcg/kg/dose (approximately 4-fold higher than the human dose). Decreased maternal food consumption, accompanied by decreased maternal body weight gain and decreased fetal body weights were observed at 50 to 1,000 mcg/kg/dose. Pegfilgrastim doses of 200 and 250 mcg/kg/dose resulted in an increased incidence of abortions. Increased postimplantation loss because of early resorptions was observed at doses of 200 to 1,000 mcg/kg/dose and decreased numbers of live rabbit fetuses were observed at pegfilgrastim doses of 200 to 1,000 mcg/kg/dose, given every other day.

Subcutaneous injections of pegfilgrastim of up to 1,000 mcg/kg/dose every other day during the period of organogenesis in rats were not associated with an embryotoxic or fetotoxic outcome. However, an increased incidence (compared with historical controls) of wavy ribs was observed in rat fetuses at 1,000 mcg/kg/dose every other day. Very low levels (less than 0.5%) of pegfilgrastim crossed the placenta when administered subcutaneously every other day to pregnant rats during gestation.

Once weekly subcutaneous injections of pegfilgrastim at doses up to 1,000 mcg/kg/dose to female rats from day 6 of gestation through day 18 of lactation did not result in any adverse maternal effects. There were no deleterious effects on the growth and development of the offspring, and no adverse effects were found upon assessment of fertility indices.

Lactation: It is not known if pegfilgrastim crosses into human breast milk. Problems in humans have not been documented.

Children: Safety and efficacy of pegfilgrastim in children younger than 18 years of age have not been established. The safety and pharmacokinetics of pegfilgrastim were studied in 37 children with sarcoma. The mean ($\pm$ SD) systemic exposure (AUC_{0-inf}) of pegfilgrastim 100 mcg/kg subcutaneous was 22 ($\pm$ 13.1) mcg•h/mL in the 6 to 11 years of age group (n = 10), 29.3 ($\pm$23.2) mcg•h/mL in the 12 to 21 years of age group (n = 13), and 47.9 ($\pm$ 22.5) mcg•h/mL in the youngest age group (0 to 5 years of age; n = 11). The terminal elimination half-lives of the corresponding age groups were 20.2 ($\pm$ 11.3) hours, 21.2 ($\pm$ 16) hours, and 30.1 ($\pm$ 38.2) hours, respectively. The most common adverse reaction was bone pain.

Do not use 6 mg fixed-dose, single-use syringe formulation in infants, children, and smaller adolescents weighing less than 45 kg.

Adverse Reactions: Safety data are based upon 465 subjects with lymphoma and solid tumors (breast, lung, and thoracic tumors) enrolled in 6 randomized studies. Subjects received pegfilgrastim after nonmyeloablative cytotoxic chemotherapy. Most adverse experiences were attributed by the investigators to the underlying malignancy or cytotoxic chemotherapy and occurred at similar rates in subjects who received pegfilgrastim (n = 465) or filgrastim (n = 331). These adverse experiences occurred at rates between 72% and 15% and included the following: nausea, fatigue, alopecia, diarrhea, vomiting, constipation, fever, anorexia, skeletal pain, headache, taste perversion, dyspepsia, myalgia, insomnia, abdominal pain, arthralgia, generalized weakness, peripheral edema, dizziness, granulocytopenia, stomatitis, mucositis, and neutropenic fever. In subjects receiving pegfilgrastim in clinical trials, the only serious event not deemed attributable to underlying or concurrent disease or to concurrent therapy was a case of hypoxia.

The most common adverse event attributed to pegfilgrastim in clinical trials was medullary bone pain, reported in 26% of subjects, comparable to the rate in filgrastim-treated patients. This bone pain was generally reported to be of mild to moderate severity. About 12% of all subjects used nonnarcotic analgesics and less than 6% used narcotic analgesics in association with bone pain. No patient withdrew from study because of bone pain.

Reversible elevations in LDH, alkaline phosphatase, and uric acid that did not require treatment intervention were observed. The incidences of these changes were the following: LDH (19% for pegfilgrastim vs 29% for filgrastim), alkaline phosphatase (9% vs 16%), and uric acid (8% vs 9%). For uric acid, 1% of reported cases for both treatment groups were classified as severe.

Allergic: Allergic-type reactions, including anaphylaxis, skin rash, and urticaria, occurring on initial or subsequent treatment occur with filgrastim. In some cases, symptoms have recurred with rechallenge, suggesting a causal relationship. Allergic-type reactions to pegfilgrastim were not observed in clinical trials. If a serious allergic reaction or anaphylactic reaction occurs, administer appropriate therapy and discontinue pegfilgrastim.

Hematologic: In clinical studies, leukocytosis (WBC counts greater than 100×10^9 cells/L) was observed in less than 1% of 465 subjects with nonmyeloid malignancies receiving pegfilgrastim. Leukocytosis was not associated with any adverse effects. Severe sickle-cell crises occurred in patients with sickle-cell disease (specifically homozygous sickle-cell anemia, sickle/hemoglobin C disease, and sickle/β+ thalassemia) who received filgrastim for PBPC mobilization or following chemotherapy; one of these cases was fatal. Use pegfilgrastim with caution in patients with sickle-cell disease and only after careful consideration of risks and benefits. Keep patients with sickle-cell disease who receive pegfilgrastim well hydrated and monitor for sickle-cell crises. In the event of severe sickle-cell crisis, administer supportive care and interventions to ameliorate the underlying event. Consider therapeutic red blood cell exchange transfusion.

Immunogenicity: As with all therapeutic proteins, there is a potential for immunogenicity. While available data suggest that a small proportion of patients developed binding antibodies to filgrastim or pegfilgrastim, the nature and specificity of these antibodies have not been adequately studied. No neutralizing antibodies have been detected using a cell-based bioassay in 46 patients who apparently developed binding antibodies. The detection of antibody formation is highly dependent on the sensitivity and specificity of the assay. Cytopenias resulting from an antibody response to exogenous growth factors have been reported on rare occasions in patients treated with other recombinant growth factors. There is a theoretical possibility that an antibody directed against pegfilgrastim may cross-react with endogenous G-CSF, resulting in immune-mediated neutropenia, but this has not been observed in clinical studies.

Respiratory: Adult respiratory distress syndrome (ARDS) occurred in neutropenic patients with sepsis receiving filgrastim, perhaps secondary to an influx of neutrophils to sites of inflammation in the lungs. Evaluate neutropenic patients receiving pegfilgrastim who develop fever, lung infiltrates, or respiratory distress for ARDS. If ARDS occurs, discontinue or withhold pegfilgrastim until resolution of ARDS.

Spleen: Rare cases of splenic rupture occurred after administering filgrastim for PBPC mobilization in healthy donors and patients with cancer. Some of these cases were fatal. Pegfilgrastim has not been evaluated in this setting; therefore, pegfilgrastim should not be used for PBPC mobilization. Evaluate patients receiving pegfilgrastim who report left, upper abdominal or shoulder tip pain for an enlarged spleen or splenic rupture.

Pharmacologic & Dosing Characteristics

Dosage: 6 mg administered once per chemotherapy cycle. Do not administer pegfilgrastim in the period 14 days before and 24 hours after administration of cytotoxic chemotherapy. Do not use the 6 mg fixed-dose formulation in infants, children, and smaller adolescents weighing less than 45 kg.

Route: Subcutaneous injection

Overdosage: The maximum amount of pegfilgrastim safely administered in single or multiple doses is unknown. Single doses of 300 mcg/kg administered subcutaneously to 8 normal volunteers and 3 patients with non-small cell lung cancer did not result in serious adverse effects. These subjects experienced a mean maximum ANC of 55×10^9 cells/L with a corresponding mean maximum WBC of 67×10^9 cells/L. The absolute maximum ANC observed was 96×10^9 cells/L with a corresponding observed absolute maximum WBC of 120×10^9 cells/L. The duration of leukocytosis ranged from 6 to 13 days. Consider leukapheresis to manage symptomatic patients.

Laboratory Tests: To assess a patient's hematologic status and ability to tolerate myelosuppressive chemotherapy, obtain a CBC and platelet count before administering chemotherapy. Regularly monitor hematocrit values and platelet counts.

Efficacy: Pegfilgrastim was evaluated in 2 randomized, double-blind, active-control studies employing doxorubicin 60 mg/m^2 and docetaxel 75 mg/m^2 administered every 21 days for up to 4 cycles to treat metastatic breast cancer. Study 1 investigated a fixed dose of pegfilgrastim. Study 2 employed a weight-adjusted dose. In the absence of growth factor support, similar chemotherapy regimens are expected to result in a 100% incidence of severe neutropenia (absolute neutrophil count [ANC] less than 0.5×10^9 cells/L) with a mean duration of 5 to 7 days and a 30% to 40% incidence of febrile neutropenia. Based on the correlation between duration of severe neutropenia and incidence of febrile neutropenia in studies with filgrastim, duration of severe neutropenia was chosen as the primary endpoint in both studies. The efficacy of pegfilgrastim was shown by establishing comparability to filgrastim-treated subjects in the mean number of days of severe neutropenia.

In study 1, 157 subjects randomly received either a single 6 mg subcutaneous dose of pegfilgrastim on day 2 of each chemotherapy cycle or filgrastim at 5 mcg/kg/day subcutaneously beginning on day 2 of each cycle. In study 2, 310 subjects were randomized to receive a single 100 mcg/kg subcutaneous injection of pegfilgrastim on day 2 or filgrastim at 5 mcg/kg/day subcutaneously beginning on day 2 of each chemotherapy cycle.

Both studies met the primary objective, showing that duration of severe neutropenia of pegfilgrastim-treated patients did not exceed that of filgrastim-treated patients by more than 1 day in cycle 1 of chemotherapy. The rates of febrile neutropenia in the 2 studies were comparable for pegfilgrastim and filgrastim. Other secondary endpoints included days of severe neutropenia in cycles 2 to 4, the depth of ANC nadir in cycles 1 to 4, and the time to ANC recovery after nadir. In both studies, the results for the secondary endpoints were similar between the 2 treatment groups.

Mean Days of Severe Neutropenia in Cycle 1			
	Mean duration of severe neutropenia		
Study	Pegfilgrastim[a]	Filgrastim (5 mcg/kg/day)	Difference in means (95% CI)
Study 1 (n = 157)	1.8 days	1.6 days	0.2 days (-0.2, 0.6)
Study 2 (n = 310)	1.7 days	1.6 days	0.1 days (-0.2, 0.4)

a Study 1 dose = 6 mg × 1; study 2 dose = 100 mcg/kg × 1.

Pharmacokinetics: The pharmacokinetics and pharmacodynamics of pegfilgrastim were studied in 379 patients with cancer. The pharmacokinetics of pegfilgrastim were nonlinear in cancer patients and clearance decreased with increased dose. Neutrophil receptor binding is an important factor in the clearance of pegfilgrastim. Serum clearance is directly related to the number of neutrophils. For example, the concentration of pegfilgrastim declined rapidly at the onset of neutrophil recovery following myelosuppressive chemotherapy. In addition, patients with higher body weights experienced higher systemic exposure to pegfilgrastim after receiving a dose normalized for body weight. A large variability in the pharmacokinetics of pegfilgrastim was observed in cancer patients. The half-life of pegfilgrastim ranged from 15 to 80 hours after subcutaneous injection. Pegfilgrastim has reduced renal clearance and prolonged persistence in vivo as compared with filgrastim. The pharmacokinetic profile in patients with hepatic or renal insufficiency has not been assessed.

Mechanism: Both filgrastim and pegfilgrastim are colony-stimulating factors that act on hematopoietic cells by binding to specific cell surface receptors, thereby stimulating proliferation, differentiation, commitment, and end cell functional activation. Studies on cellular proliferation, receptor binding, and neutrophil function show that filgrastim and pegfilgrastim have the same mechanism of action.

Drug Interactions: No formal drug interaction studies between pegfilgrastim and other drugs have been performed. Drugs such as lithium may potentiate the release of neutrophils; patients receiving lithium and pegfilgrastim should have more frequent monitoring of neutrophil counts.

Pegfilgrastim has not been studied in patients receiving chemotherapy associated with delayed myelosuppression (eg, nitrosoureas, mitomycin C).

Administering pegfilgrastim concomitantly with 5-fluorouracil or other antimetabolites has not been evaluated. Administration of pegfilgrastim at 0, 1, and 3 days before 5-fluorouracil resulted in increased mortality in mice; administration of pegfilgrastim 24 hours after 5-fluorouracil did not adversely affect survival.

Pegfilgrastim has not been studied in patients receiving radiation therapy.

Patient Information: Inform patients of possible side effects, instructing them to report adverse events to the prescribing physician. Inform patients of the signs and symptoms of allergic drug reactions and appropriate responses. Counsel patients on the importance of compliance with treatment, including regular monitoring of blood counts.

Pharmaceutical Characteristics

Concentration: 6 mg pegfilgrastim per 0.6 mL

Packaging: One 0.6 mL prefilled single-dose syringe with a 27-gauge, ½-inch needle and an *UltraSafe* needle guard

NDC Number: 55513-0190-01

Doseform: Solution

Appearance: Clear, colorless solution

Solvent: Sterile water

Adjuvant: None

Preservative: None

Allergens: The needle cover of prefilled syringes contains dry natural rubber (a latex derivative).

Excipients: 0.35 mg acetate, 30 mg sorbitol, 0.02 mg polysorbate 20, and 0.02 mg sodium, each per 0.6 mL syringe

pH: 4

Shelf Life: Expires within 18 months.

Storage/Stability: Store at 2° to 8°C (36° to 46°F). Avoid shaking. Before injection, pegfilgrastim may be stored at room temperature for up to 48 hours, if protected from light. Discard pegfilgrastim stored at room temperature for longer than 48 hours. Avoid freezing. If accidentally frozen, allow pegfilgrastim to thaw in the refrigerator before administration. If frozen a second time, discard pegfilgrastim. Shipping data not provided.

Handling: To activate *UltraSafe* needle guard, place hands behind the needle, grasp the guard with one hand, and slide the guard forward until the needle is completely covered and the guard audibly clicks into place.

Production Process: Filgrastim is obtained from the bacterial fermentation of a strain of *E. coli* transformed with a genetically engineered plasmid containing the human G-CSF gene. To produce pegfilgrastim, a 20 kD monomethoxypolyethylene glycol molecule is covalently bonded to the N-terminal methionyl residue of filgrastim.

Media: *E. coli*

Disease Epidemiology

See Filgrastim monograph.

Other Information

Perspective: See Filgrastim monograph.

First Licensed: January 31, 2002

References: Lyman GH. Pegfilgrastim: A granulocyte colony-stimulating factor with sustained duration of action. *Expert Opin Biol Ther.* 2005;5(12):1635-1646.

Smith TJ, Khatcheressian J, Lyman GH, et al. 2006 update of recommendations for the use of white blood cell growth factors: an evidence-based clinical practice guideline. *J Clin Oncol.* 2006;24(19):3187-3205.

Sargramostim

Colony-Stimulating Factors

Name:
 Leukine

Manufacturer:
 Genzyme Corporation

Synonyms: Granulocyte macrophage colony-stimulating factor, GM-CSF, CSF-2.

Immunologic Characteristics

Antigen Source: GM-CSF expressed from recombinant *Saccharomyces cerevisiae* yeast.

Viability: Not viable, but immunologically active.

Antigenic Form: Colony-stimulating factor.

Antigenic Type: Protein. Endogenous GM-CSF is produced by T-lymphocytes, endothelial fibroblasts, and macrophages. Sargramostim is a glycoprotein of 127 amino acids. It consists of 3 primary molecular species with weights of 19,500, 16,800, and 15,500 daltons. Sargramostim differs from natural human GM-CSF by substitution of leucine for arginine at position 23. This amino acid substitution facilitates expression of the protein in yeast. The carbohydrate moiety may differ from the natural protein.

Strains: r-Hu-GM-CSF (recombinant human GM-CSF).

Use Characteristics

Indications:

Use following induction chemotherapy in acute myelogenous leukemia (AML): Sargramostim helps prevent infection following high-dose induction chemotherapy in adult patients 55 years of age and older with AML. Sargramostim helps shorten the time to neutrophil recovery and reduces the incidence of severe and life-threatening infections. AML also is referred to as acute nonlymphocytic leukemia. It encompasses a heterogeneous group of leukemias arising from various nonlymphoid cell lines.

Use in myeloid reconstitution after autologous bone marrow transplantation (BMT): For acceleration of myeloid recovery in patients with non-Hodgkin lymphoma, acute lymphoblastic leukemia (ALL), or Hodgkin disease undergoing autologous BMT. Sargramostim accelerates neutrophil recovery and engraftment, decreases the number of days antibiotics are required in the posttransplant period, reduces the duration of infectious episodes, and shortens the duration of hospitalization. Sargramostim effectively treats neutropenia associated with BMT, treats graft failure and delay of engraftment, and promotes early engraftment.

Use in myeloid reconstitution after allogenic bone marrow transplantation: To accelerate myeloid recovery in patients undergoing allogenic BMT from HLA-matched donors. Sargramostim accelerates myeloid engraftment, reducing incidence of bacteremia and other culture-positive infections, and shortens the median duration of hospitalization.

Use in BMT failure or engraftment delay: Sargramostim helps prolong survival in patients who have undergone allogeneic or autologous BMT in whom engraftment is delayed or has failed. It is effective in the presence or absence of infection. Survival benefit may be relatively greater in those patients who demonstrate 1 or more of the following characteristics: autologous BMT failure or engraftment delay, no previous total body irradiation, malignancy other than leukemia, or a multiple organ failure score of 2 or less. Sargramostim used in allogeneic BMT in HLA-matched related donors can shorten time to white blood cell recovery, decrease length of hospital stay, reduce incidence of infection, and reduce risk of mucositis. In clinical trials, infection incidence dropped from 75% to 57% and the risk of mucositis fell from 29% to 8%.

Use in autologous peripheral blood progenitor transplantation: Use in mobilization and following transplantation of autologous peripheral blood progenitor cells (PBPC). To mobilize hematopoietic progenitor cells into peripheral blood for collection by leuokpheresis. Mobilization allows for the collection of increased numbers of progenitor cells capable of engraftment as compared with collection without mobilization. After myeloblative chemotherapy, the transplantation of an increased number of progenitor cells can lead to more rapid engraftment, which may result in a decreased need for supportive care. Myeloid reconstitution is further accelerated by administration of sargramostim after PBPC transplantation.

Unlabeled Uses: Sargramostim is being investigated for efficacy in the treatment of congenital aplastic anemia, treatment of myelodysplastic syndromes, treatment of chronic lymphocytic leukemia to increase the granulocyte count, treatment of neutropenia due to hairy-cell leukemia, treatment of patients with AIDS with neutropenia due to the disease itself or due to zidovudine or ganciclovir therapy, treatment of severe thermal injury in patients with more than 40% full or partial thickness burns, as an adjunct to chemotherapy for pediatric tumors or other neoplasms, neonatal sepsis, surgeries with high risk of infection, and to decrease transplantation-associated organ system damage, particularly in the liver and kidney.

Limitations: No significant difference in survival or rate of disease relapse was observed between sargramostim and placebo groups at 12 months after bone-marrow transplantation. Insufficient data are available to support the efficacy of sargramostim in accelerating myeloid recovery following peripheral blood stem cell transplantation.

Data obtained from uncontrolled studies suggest that if in vitro bone marrow purging with chemical agents causes a significant decrease in the number of responsive hematopoietic progenitors, the patient may not respond to sargramostim. Similarly, in patients who receive extensive radiotherapy to hematopoietic sites for the treatment of primary disease in the abdomen or chest or who have been exposed to multiple myelotoxic agents, the effect of sargramostim on myeloid reconstitution may be limited.

Contraindications:

Absolute: Sargramostim is contraindicated in patients with excessive (more than 10%) leukemic myeloid blast cells in the bone marrow or peripheral blood; for concomitant use with chemotherapy or radiotherapy; or in patients with known hypersensitivity to GM-CSF, yeast-derived products, or to any component of the formulation.

Relative: None

Immunodeficiency: May be indicated to avert infectious complications of immunodeficiency.

Elderly: In clinical trials, experience in older patients (aged 65 years and older) was limited to the acute myelogenous leukemia (AML) study. Of 52 patients treated with sargramostim, 22 patients were 65 to 70 years old and 30 patients were 55 to 64 years old. Their experience was not sufficient to reliably assess efficacy or safety. Analyses of general trends in safety and efficacy demonstrate similar patterns in older patients 65 to 70 years vs 55 to 64 years old. Greater sensitivity of some older individuals cannot be ruled out.

Carcinogenicity: The possibility that sargramostim can act as a growth factor for any tumor type, particularly myeloid malignancies, cannot be excluded. Because of the possibility of tumor growth potentiation, take precautions in using this drug in any malignancy with myeloid characteristics (eg, leukemias).

Pregnancy: Category C. Use only if clearly needed. It is not known if sargramostim crosses the placenta.

Sargramostim

Lactation: It is not known if sargramostim is excreted in breast milk. Problems in humans have not been documented.

Children: Safety and effectiveness in children have not been established. However, available safety data indicate that sargramostim does not exhibit any greater toxicity in children than in adults. A total of 124 children 4 months to 18 years old have been treated with sargramostim in clinical trials at doses ranging from 60 to 1,000 mcg/m^2/day IV and 4 to 1,500 mcg/m^2/day subcutaneously. In 53 children enrolled in controlled studies at a dose of 250 mcg/m^2/day by 2-hour IV infusion, the type and frequency of adverse events were comparable to those reported for adults. Do not give sargramostim reconstituted with any diluent containing 0.9% benzyl alcohol to neonates or infants.

Adverse Reactions: The following adverse events were reported 2% more often in treating autologous BMT transplantation in sargramostim recipients than in placebo recipients: asthenia (66%, compared with 51% in the placebo group), malaise (57% vs 51%), diarrhea (89% vs 82%), rash (44% vs 38%), and peripheral edema (11% vs 7%). In the historically controlled study, headache (26%), pericardial effusion (25%), arthralgia (21%), and myalgia (18%) were also reported among sargramostim recipients. In uncontrolled studies, the most frequent adverse events included fever, asthenia, headache, bone pain, chills, and myalgia. These systemic events were generally mild or moderate and were usually prevented or reversed by the administration of analgesics and antipyretics such as acetaminophen. Other infrequent events reported were dyspnea, peripheral edema, and rash.

No significant differences were observed between sargramostim- and placebo-treated patients in the type or of laboratory abnormalities, including renal and hepatic parameters. In some patients with preexisting renal or hepatic dysfunction enrolled in uncontrolled clinical trials, sargramostim administration induced elevation of serum creatinine or bilirubin and hepatic enzymes.

The following adverse events were reported at least 2% more often in treating acute myelogenous leukemia in sargramostim recipients than in placebo recipients: fever without infection (81%, compared with 74% in the placebo group), weight loss (37% vs 28%), nausea (58% vs 55%), vomiting (46% vs 34%), anorexia (13% vs 11%), skin disturbance (77% vs 45%), metabolic disorders (58% vs 49%), and edema (25% vs 23%). Only the difference in rates of skin-associated events was statistically significant. No significant differences were observed in laboratory results, nor in renal or hepatic toxicity. No significant differences were observed for adverse events following consolidation. There was no significant difference in response rate or relapse rate. In a study comparing sargramostim treatment with historical controls, the sargramostim group exhibited significantly increased incidence of weight gain, low serum proteins, and prolonged prothrombin time.

Fluid retention: In patients with preexisting peripheral edema, pleural or pericardial effusion, administration of sargramostim may aggravate fluid retention. In 1 patient given sargramostim despite massive weight gain and development of significant peripheral edema, a capillary leak syndrome was reported. Carefully monitor body weight and hydration status during sargramostim administration. Fluid retention associated with sargramostim has been reversible after interruption or dose reduction with or without diuretic therapy. Use caution in patients with preexisting fluid retention, pulmonary infiltrates, or CHF.

Renal and hepatic: In some patients with preexisting renal or hepatic dysfunction enrolled in uncontrolled clinical trials, sargramostim has induced elevation of serum creatinine or bilirubin and hepatic enzymes. Dose reduction or interruption of sargramostim resulted in a decrease to pretreatment values. However, in controlled clinical trials, the incidences of renal and hepatic dysfunction were comparable between sargramostim (250 mcg/m^2/day by 2-hour IV infusion) and placebo-treated patients. Monitor renal and hepatic function in patients displaying renal or hepatic dysfunction before starting treatment at least every other week during sargramostim administration.

Respiratory: Sequestration of granulocytes in the pulmonary circulation has followed sargramostim infusion; dyspnea has occurred occasionally. Give special attention to respiratory symptoms during and immediately after sargramostim infusion, especially in patients with preexisting lung disease. In patients displaying dyspnea during sargramostim administration, reduce the rate of infusion by half. Give subsequent infusions following the standard dose schedule with careful monitoring. If respiratory symptoms worsen despite infusion rate reduction, discontinue infusion. Give sargramostim with caution in patients with hypoxia.

Cardiovascular: Occasional transient supraventricular dysrhythmias have occurred during sargramostim administration in uncontrolled studies, particularly in patients with a history of cardiac dysrhythmias. These dysrhythmias reversed after discontinuing sargramostim. Use sargramostim with caution in patients with preexisting cardiac disease.

Adverse events that occurred when the WBC count reached 200,000 cells/mm^2 included dyspnea, malaise, nausea, fever, rash, sinus tachycardia, headache, and chills. Each of these effects was reversible upon discontinuation of sargramostim.

If any anaphylactoid reaction occurs, stop sargramostim immediately and initiate appropriate supportive therapy.

Anti-sargramostim antibodies have been detected in 5 of 214 patients (2.3%) who received sargramostim for 28 to 84 days in multiple courses. All 5 patients had impaired hematopoiesis before administration of sargramostim and consequently the effect of anti-GM-CSF antibodies on normal hematopoiesis could not be assessed. Drug-induced neutropenia, neutralization of endogenous GM-CSF activity, and diminution of the therapeutic effect of sargramostim secondary to formation of neutralizing antibody remain theoretical possibilities.

Pharmacologic & Dosing Characteristics

Dosage:

After autologous or allogeneic BMT: To stimulate neutrophil recovery in patients who have undergone BMT, the recommended dose of sargramostim is 250 mcg/m^2/day as a 2-hour infusion for 21 consecutive days. Begin therapy 2 to 4 hours after the autologous bone-marrow infusion, at least 24 hours after the last dose of chemotherapy or radiotherapy. Do not give sargramostim until the post-marrow infusion ANC is less than 500 cells/mm^3. Continue sargramostim until an ANC greater than 1,500 cells/mm^3 for 3 consecutive days is attained. If blast cells appear or disease progression occurs, discontinue treatment.

Following chemotherapy in AML: 250 mcg/m^2/day IV over 4 hours starting approximately on day 11 or 4 days following the completion of induction chemotherapy, if the day 10 bone marrow is hypoplastic with less than 5% blasts. If a second cycle of induction chemotherapy is necessary, give sargramostim 4 days after completing chemotherapy, if bone marrow is hypoplastic with less than 5% blasts. Continue sargramostim until an ANC greater than 1,500 cells/mm^3 for 3 consecutive days or a maximum of 42 days is reached. Discontinue immediately if leukemia regrowth occurs.

BMT failure or engraftment delay: 250 mcg/m^2/day as a 2-hour infusion for 14 consecutive days. Repeat dose after 7 days off therapy if engraftment has not occurred. If engraftment still has not occurred, a third course of 500 mcg/m^2/day for 14 days may be tried after another 7 days off therapy. If there is still no improvement, it is unlikely that further dose escalation will be beneficial. If blast cells appear or disease progression occurs, stop treatment.

Autologous PBPC transplantation (mobilization and recovery): 250 mcg/m^2/day as a continuous IV infusion or subcutaneous injection. Daily injections continue at least until sufficient mononuclear cells are harvested, usually begun by day 5. If sufficient progenitor cells are not collected, consider another mobilization therapy. If WBC is greater than 50,000 cells/mm³, reduce the sargramostim dose by 50%. In clinical trials, if sargramostim was given before and after transplant, ANC counts rose sooner. Continue sargramostim until an ANC greater than 1,500 cells/mm³ for 3 consecutive days is attained.

General principles: In case of a severe adverse reaction (eg, related to fluid retention, respiratory symptoms, cardiac dysrhythmias), reduce the dose of sargramostim by half or temporarily discontinue it until the reaction abates. If the ANC exceeds 20,000 cells/mm³ or if the platelet count is more than 500,000 cells/mm³, interrupt sargramostim administration or halve the dose. Excessive blood counts have returned to normal or baseline levels within 3 to 7 days following cessation of sargramostim therapy.

If, in the differential count, peripheral blast cells increase to 10% or more of the WBC count, discontinue sargramostim.

If underlying neoplastic disease progresses during sargramostim therapy, discontinue drug.

Another empiric method of dosing that has been employed is to give 250 mcg/day to patients weighing up to 70 kg, and 500 mcg/day to patients weighing more than 70 kg. Some clinicians have chosen to stop therapy when the ANC rises to more than 1,500 to 5,000 cells/mm³, although this method has not been scientifically evaluated.

Route & Site: IV infusion, given over 2 hours beginning 2 to 4 hours after the bone marrow transplantation. Infusions over 30 to 60 minutes, 2 to 4 hours, 5 to 12 hours, or 24 hours have also been reported. Because of potential sensitivity of rapidly dividing hematopoietic progenitor cells, do not administer sargramostim within 24 hours before or after cytotoxic chemotherapy or within 12 hours before or after radiotherapy. May also be administered by subcutaneous injection.

Overdosage: The maximum amount of sargramostim that can safely be administered has not been determined. Doses up to 100 mcg/kg/day (approximately 4,000 mcg/m²/day) have been administered by IV infusion for 7 to 18 days, yielding increases in WBC up to 200,000 cells/mm³. Adverse events at this high dose included dyspnea, malaise, nausea, fever, rash, sinus tachycardia, headache, and chills. Each of these effects was reversible upon discontinuation of sargramostim.

Laboratory Tests: To avoid potential complications of excessive leukocytosis (ie, WBC greater than 50,000 cells/mm³, ANC greater than 20,000 cells/mm³), draw a CBC twice per week during sargramostim therapy. In patients with renal or hepatic dysfunction prior to beginning treatment, monitor renal and hepatic function biweekly during sargramostim therapy.

Efficacy:

Myeloid reconstitution after autologous BMT: Placebo-controlled clinical trials in autologous bone-marrow transplant recipients demonstrated that sargramostim improved hematologic and clinical end points: Time to neutrophil engraftment (18 vs 24 days), duration of hospitalization (25 vs 31 days), infection duration (1 vs 4 days), or antibacterial utilization (21 vs 25 days of therapy).

Following chemotherapy in AML: Among patients 55 years and older, sargramostim shortened the median duration of ANC less than 500 cells/mm³ by 4 days and ANC less than 1,000 cells/mm³ by 7 days following induction; 75% of patients receiving sargramostim achieved ANC greater than 500 cells/mm³ by day 16 compared with day 25 for patients receiving placebo. Sargramostim significantly shortened the median times to neutrophil recovery whether 1 cycle or 2 cycles of induction chemotherapy was administered. During the consolidation phase of chemotherapy, sargramostim did not shorten the median time to recovery of ANC to 500 cells/mm³ compared with placebo. The incidence of severe infections and deaths associated with infections was significantly reduced in patients who received sargramostim. During induction or consolidation, 52% of patients receiving sargramostim and 74% of placebo recipients had at least 1 serious infection. The proportion of patients achieving complete remission was higher in the sargramostim group (69% compared with 55% in the placebo group). This difference was not statistically significant, nor was there a significant difference in relapse rates or median survival.

BMT failure or engraftment delay: An historically controlled study was conducted in patients experiencing graft failure following allogeneic or autologous BMT. Three categories of patients were included: Patients with a delay in engraftment (ANC up to 100 cells/mm³ by day 28 after BMT), those with a delay in engraftment (ANC up to 100 cells/mm³ by day 21 after BMT) with evidence of an active infection, and patients who lost their marrow graft after a transient engraftment (average ANC of 500 cells/mm³ or more for at least 1 week followed by loss of engraftment with ANC less than 500 cells/mm³ for at least 1 week beyond day 21 after transplant). The median survival of patients treated with sargramostim after autologous BMT failure was 474 days compared with 161 days for the historical controls. Similarly, after allogeneic BMT failure, the median survival was 97 days with sargramostim treatment or 35 days for the historical controls. Improvement in survival was considerably better in patients with fewer impaired organs. The probability of survival was relatively greater for patients with any of the following characteristics: Autologous BMT failure or delay in engraftment, exclusion of total body irradiation from the preparative regimen, a non-leukemic malignancy, or up to 2 impaired organs. Leukemic subjects derived less benefit than other subjects.

Use in autologous PBPC transplantation: Sargramostim in autologous peripheral blood stem (or progenitor) cell (PBPC) transplants can reduce time to engraftment and neutrophil and platelet recovery. In retrospective studies, patients receiving PBPC transplants mobilized with sargramostim 250 mcg/m² IV reached an ANC of more than 500 cells/mm³ in 21 days, compared with 29 days for an untreated group. Fewer apherese procedures were needed in sargramostim recipients to harvest sufficient mononuclear cells. If sargramostim was given before and after transplant, the interval fell to 12 days. The median time to last platelet transfusion following transplantation in these 3 groups was 24, 28, and 19 days, respectively. For red blood cell transfusions, the values were 19, 28, and 13.5 days, respectively. Sargramostim did not affect overall or disease-free survival.

Onset: In patients with advanced malignancy, a rise in peripheral WBC count occurs 1 to 2 days after initiation of daily sargramostim administration.

Duration: WBC counts returned to baseline levels within 1 week following cessation of sargramostim therapy. Excessive blood counts have returned to normal or baseline levels within 3 to 7 days following cessation of sargramostim.

Pharmacokinetics: Following 250 mcg/m² sargramostim by 2-hour IV infusion in 2 patients, serum concentration ranged from 22,000 to 23,000 pg/mL at the termination of the infusion. Five patients receiving 500 to 750 mcg/m² by 2-hour IV infusion demonstrated a rapid initial decline in serum concentration (half-life, 12 to 17 minutes), followed by a slower decrease (half-life, 2 hours). In 4 patients treated by subcutaneous injection at 125 mcg/m² every 12 hours, sargramostim was detected in the serum within 5 minutes of administration (range, 55 to 450 pg/mL). Peak levels were observed 2 hours after injection (range, 350 to 3,900 pg/mL), and sargramostim remained at detectable levels 6 hours following injection (range, 150 to 2,700 pg/mL).

The metabolic pathway, metabolic products, and extent of metabolism of sargramostim have not yet been determined.

Mechanism: Cellular responses (eg, division, maturation, activation) to sargramostim are induced through its binding to specific receptors on the cell surfaces of target cells. Administration of sargramostim to patients results in a dose- and schedule-related rise in the peripheral WBC count. In patients with advanced malignancy not receiving chemotherapy who received sargramostim either by daily IV bolus injections or continuous IV infusions for 14 days, the most rapid increase was in segmented neutrophils, followed by immature neutrophils, monocytes, and then eosinophils.

GM-CSF is a multilineage hematopoietic growth factor that induces partially committed progenitor cells to proliferate and differentiate along the granulocyte and macrophage pathways. It also enhances the function of mature granulocytes and macrophages/monocytes. GM-CSF increases the chemotactic, antifungal, and antiparasitic activities of granulocytes and monocytes. It increases the cytotoxicity of monocytes toward certain neoplastic cell lines and activates polymorphonuclear granulocytes to inhibit the growth of tumor cells.

GM-CSF also promotes the proliferation of megakaryocytic and erythroid progenitors. However, other factors are required to induce complete maturation of these cell lineages.

Drug Interactions: Use drugs such as lithium and corticosteroids, which may potentiate the myeloproliferative effects of sargramostim, with caution.

Because of the potential sensitivity of rapidly dividing hematopoietic progenitor cells to cytotoxic chemotherapeutic or radiologic therapies, do not give sargramostim within 24 hours before or after chemotherapy or within 12 hours before or after radiation therapy.

Because of the potential for receiving higher doses of chemotherapy (ie, full doses on the prescribed schedule), the patient may be at greater risk of thrombocytopenia, anemia, and nonhematologic consequences of increased chemotherapy doses.

Pharmaceutical Characteristics

Concentration: 5×10^7 colony-forming units per mg, comparable with 5.6×10^6 IU/mg. The liquid formulation contains 500 mg (2.8×10^6 IU) per mL.

Quality Assay: Normal human bone marrow colony-formation assay.

Packaging:
Powder: Carton of five 250 mcg (1.4×10^6 IU) single-dose vials (NDC #: 58468-0180-02)
Liquid: Carton of one 500 mcg (2.8×10^6 IU) per 1 mL multidose vial (58468-0180-01), five 500 mcg (2.8×10^6 IU) per 1 mL multidose vials (58468-0181-02)

Doseform: Solution or powder for solution

Appearance: White powder, yielding a clear, colorless solution; or a clear, colorless solution

Solvent: Sterile water for injection

Diluent:
For reconstitution: Powder: 1 mL sterile water for injection per vial. Bacteriostatic water for injection with 0.9% benzyl alcohol may also be used. Do not mix the contents of vials reconstituted with different diluents. During reconstitution, direct the diluent at the side of the vial and swirl the contents gently to avoid foaming during dissolution. Avoid excessive or vigorous agitation.

For infusion: Use only 0.9% sodium chloride for infusion. If the final concentration of sargramostim is less than 10 mcg/mL, add human albumin to a final concentration of 0.1% (1 mg/mL) to the saline solution before adding the sargramostim to prevent adsorption of the drug to the drug delivery system. For example, add 1 mL of 5% albumin to each 50 mL 0.9% sodium chloride. Addition of albumin to a sargramostim infusion may cause physical or chemical incompatibility of the solution with other drugs, such as vancomycin. Do not use an in-line membrane filter for IV infusion.

Adjuvant: None

Preservative:
Powder: None
Liquid: 1.1% benzyl alcohol

Allergens: None

Excipients: 40 mg mannitol, 10 mg sucrose, 1.2 mg tromethamine, each per vial of either powder or liquid formulation

pH:
Powder: 7.1 to 7.7, when reconstituted with sterile water
Liquid: 6.7 to 7.7

Shelf Life:
Powder: 250 mcg vials expire within 24 months and 500 mcg vials within 18 months
Liquid: Expires within 24 months

Storage/Stability: Store at 2° to 8°C (35° to 46°F). Do not freeze.

Shipped at ambient temperature via overnight courier. Any package expected to need longer than 48 hours for delivery is shipped refrigerated or chilled with coolant packs. Contact the manufacturer regarding exposure to freezing temperatures.

After reconstitution or dilution for IV infusion, store sargramostim solutions in the refrigerator. Discard unused solutions after 6 hours. Sargramostim is stable for 20 days when sterilely repackaged into syringes and promptly refrigerated.

Once the seal on a vial of the liquid formulation is pierced, that vial may be stored for up to 20 days at 2° to 8°C (35° to 46°F). Powdered sargramostim reconstituted with bacteriostatic water for injection may be retained for a like interval. Do not shake. Discard remaining solution after 20 days.

In the absence of specific compatibility information, add no other medication to infusion solutions containing sargramostim.

Production Process: Manufactured by recombinant DNA technology in a yeast expression system.

Media: *Saccharomyces cerevisiae*

Other Information

Perspective:
1991: Sargramostim licensed on March 4, 1991 (designated an orphan drug May 3, 1990).
2008: Liquid formulation revised to remove edetate disodium (EDTA).

Discontinued Products: Sargramostim was also previously marketed by Hoechst-Roussel Pharmaceuticals with the proprietary name *Prokine*.

References: Burr JM, et al. Criteria for use of sargramostim (granulocyte-macrophage colony-stimulating factor). *Clin Pharm.* 1991;10:947-949.

Lieschke GJ, et al. Granulocyte colony-stimulating factor and granulocyte-macrophage colony-stimulating factor. *N Engl J Med.* 1992;327:28-35, 99-106.

Smith TJ, Khatcheressian J, Lyman GH, et al. 2006 update of recommendations for the use of white blood cell growth factors: an evidence-based clinical practice guideline. *J Clin Oncol.* 2006;24(19):3187-3205.

Romiplostim

Colony-Stimulating Factors

Name:
Nplate

Manufacturer:
Amgen

Synonyms: Thrombopoietin mimetics

Immunologic Characteristics

Viability: Not viable, but immunologically active

Antigenic Form: Thrombopoietin receptor agonist

Antigenic Type: Protein. Fc-peptide fusion protein (peptibody) that activates intracellular transcriptional pathways leading to increased platelet production via the thrombopoietin receptor (also known as cMpl). The molecule contains 2 identical single-chain subunits, each consisting of a human immunoglobulin G1 (IgG1) Fc domain, covalently linked at the C-terminus to a peptide containing 2 thrombopoietin receptor-binding domains. Romiplostim has no amino acid sequence homology to endogenous thrombopoietin.

Use Characteristics

Indications: To treat thrombocytopenia in patients with chronic immune (idiopathic) thrombocytopenic purpura (ITP) who have had an insufficient response to corticosteroids, immunoglobulins, or splenectomy. Use romiplostim only in patients with ITP whose degree of thrombocytopenia and clinical condition increases the risk for bleeding. To minimize the risk for thrombotic-thromboembolic complications, do not use romiplostim in an attempt to normalize platelet counts.

Contraindications: None

Immunodeficiency: No impairment of effect is expected.

Elderly: Of the 271 patients who received romiplostim in ITP clinical studies, 55 (20%) were 65 years of age and older and 27 (10%) were 75 years of age and older. No overall differences in safety or efficacy have been observed between older and younger patients in placebo-controlled studies, but greater sensitivity of some older individuals cannot be ruled out. In general, be cautious with dose adjustment for elderly patients, reflecting the greater frequency of decreased hepatic, renal, or cardiac function, and of concomitant disease or other drug therapy.

Carcinogenicity: The carcinogenic potential of romiplostim has not been evaluated.

Mutagenicity: The mutagenic potential of romiplostim has not been evaluated.

Fertility Impairment: Romiplostim had no effect on the fertility of rats at doses of up to 37 times the maximum human dose based on systemic exposure.

Pregnancy: Category C. There are no adequate and well-controlled studies of romiplostim use in pregnant women. In animal reproduction and developmental toxicity studies, romiplostim crossed the placenta; adverse fetal effects included thrombocytosis, postimplantation loss, and an increase in pup mortality. Use romiplostim during pregnancy only if the potential benefit to the mother justifies the potential risk to the fetus. A pregnancy registry collects information about the effects of romiplostim use during pregnancy. Clinicians or pregnant women may enroll and contribute to the registry by calling 877-675-2831.

In rat and rabbit developmental toxicity studies, no evidence of fetal harm was observed at romiplostim doses of up to 11 times (rats) and 82 times (rabbits) the maximum human dose based on systemic exposure. In mice at doses 5 times the maximum human dose, reductions in maternal body weight and increased postimplantation loss occurred. In a prenatal and postnatal developmental study in rats at doses 11 times the maximum human dose, there was an increase in perinatal pup mortality. Romiplostim crossed the placental barrier in rats and increased fetal platelet counts at clinically equivalent and higher doses.

Lactation: It is not known if romiplostim crosses into human breast milk. Human immunoglobulin G (IgG) is excreted into human milk. Published data suggest that breast milk antibodies do not enter the neonatal and infant circulation in substantial amounts. Because many drugs are excreted into human milk and because of the potential for serious adverse reactions in breast-feeding infants from romiplostim, decide whether to discontinue breast-feeding or romiplostim, taking into account the importance of romiplostim to the mother and the known benefits of breast-feeding.

Children: Safety and efficacy in children younger than 18 years of age have not been established.

Adverse Reactions: The most common adverse reactions (at least 5% higher incidence in romiplostim vs placebo) are arthralgia, dizziness, insomnia, myalgia, pain in extremity, abdominal pain, shoulder pain, dyspepsia, and paresthesia.

Headache was the most commonly reported adverse reaction that did not occur at an incidence 5% or more higher in romiplostim versus placebo. Headache occurred in 35% of patients receiving romiplostim and 32% of patients receiving placebo. Headaches were usually of mild or moderate severity.

The following table presents adverse reactions from 2 randomized, placebo-controlled, double-blind studies (studies 1 and 2) with an incidence 5% or more higher in romiplostim versus placebo. The majority of these adverse reactions were mild to moderate in severity.

Adverse Drug Reactions Identified in 2 Placebo-Controlled Studies[a]		
Preferred term	Romiplostim (n = 84)	Placebo (n = 41)
Arthralgia	26%	20%
Dizziness	17%	0%
Insomnia	16%	7%
Myalgia	14%	2%
Pain in extremity	13%	5%
Abdominal pain	11%	0%
Shoulder pain	8%	0%
Dyspepsia	7%	0%
Paresthesia	6%	0%

a Data from romiplostim use among 271 patients 18 to 88 years of age with chronic ITP, of whom 62% were women.

Among 142 patients with chronic ITP who received romiplostim in the single-arm extension study, the incidence rates of the adverse reactions occurred in a pattern similar to those reported in the placebo-controlled clinical studies. The following data are reported from an open-label, single-arm study in which patients received romiplostim over an extended period. Overall, romiplostim was administered to 114 patients for 52 or more weeks and 53 patients for 96 or more weeks.

Hematopoietic: Romiplostim administration increases the risk for development or progression of reticulin fiber deposition within the bone marrow. In clinical studies, romiplostim was discontinued in 4 of 271 patients because of bone marrow reticulin deposition. Six additional patients had reticulin observed upon bone marrow biopsy. All 10 patients with bone marrow reticulin deposition had received romiplostim doses of at least 5 mcg/kg, and 6 received doses of at least 10 mcg/kg. Progression to marrow fibrosis with cytopenias was not reported in the controlled clinical studies. In the extension study, 1 patient with

ITP and hemolytic anemia developed marrow fibrosis with collagen during romiplostim therapy. Clinical studies have not excluded a risk of bone marrow fibrosis with cytopenias.

Hepatic: No clinical studies were conducted in patients with hepatic impairment. Use romiplostim with caution in this population.

Immunogenicity: As with all therapeutic proteins, patients may develop antibodies to romiplostim. Patients were screened for immunogenicity to romiplostim using a *BIAcore*-based biosensor immunoassay. This assay can detect both high- and low-affinity binding antibodies that bind to romiplostim and cross-react with thrombopoietin. The samples from patients that tested positive for binding antibodies were evaluated for neutralizing capacity using a cell-based bioassay. In clinical studies, the incidence of preexisting antibodies to romiplostim was 8% (17/225), and the incidence of binding antibody development during romiplostim treatment was 10% (23/225). The incidence of preexisting antibodies to endogenous thrombopoietin was 5% (12/225), and the incidence of binding antibody development to endogenous thrombopoietin during romiplostim treatment was 5% (12/225). Of the patients with positive antibodies to romiplostim or thrombopoietin, 1 (0.4%) patient had neutralizing activity to romiplostim and no patients had neutralizing activity to thrombopoietin. No correlation was observed between antibody activity and clinical effectiveness or safety.

Lack or loss of response: Hyporesponsiveness or failure to maintain a platelet response with romiplostim should prompt a search for causative factors, including neutralizing antibodies to romiplostim or bone marrow fibrosis.

Malignancies: Romiplostim stimulation of the thrombopoietin receptor on the surface of hematopoietic cells may increase the risk for hematologic malignancies. In controlled clinical studies among patients with chronic ITP, the incidence of hematologic malignancy was low and similar between romiplostim and placebo. In a separate, single-arm clinical study of 44 patients with myelodysplastic syndrome (MDS), 11 patients were reported as having possible disease progression, among whom 4 patients had confirmation of acute myelogenous leukemia (AML) during follow-up. Romiplostim is not indicated for the treatment of thrombocytopenia due to MDS or any cause of thrombocytopenia other than chronic ITP.

Renal: No clinical studies were conducted in patients with renal impairment. Use romiplostim with caution in this population.

Thrombocytopenia: Discontinuing romiplostim may result in thrombocytopenia of greater severity than was present before romiplostim therapy. This worsened thrombocytopenia may increase a patient's risk of bleeding, particularly if romiplostim is discontinued while the patient is taking anticoagulants or antiplatelet agents. In clinical studies of patients with chronic ITP who had discontinued romiplostim therapy, 4 of 57 patients (7%) developed thrombocytopenia of greater severity than was present before romiplostim therapy. This worsened thrombocytopenia resolved within 14 days.

Thrombotic/Thromboembolic: Thrombotic/thromboembolic complications may result from excessive increases in platelet counts. Excessive doses of romiplostim or medication errors that result in excessive romiplostim doses may increase platelet counts to a level that produces thrombotic/thromboembolic complications. In controlled clinical studies, the incidence of thrombotic/thromboembolic complications was similar between romiplostim and placebo. To minimize the risk for thrombotic/thromboembolic complications, do not use romiplostim in an attempt to normalize platelet counts.

Consultation: Romiplostim is available only through a restricted distribution program called the *Nplate* NEXUS (Network of Experts Understanding and Supporting *Nplate* and patients) Program. Under the NEXUS Program, only registered prescribers and patients may prescribe, administer, or receive romiplostim. To enroll, call 877-675-2831. Prescribers and patients are required to understand the risks of romiplostim therapy. Prescribers are required to understand the information in the prescribing information and be able to appropriately educate patients, document patient understanding, and report any serious adverse events.

Animal Toxicology: In a 4-week, subcutaneous, repeat-dose toxicity study in which rats were dosed 3 times per week, romiplostim caused extramedullary hematopoiesis, bone hyperostosis, and bone marrow fibrosis at clinically equivalent and higher doses. In this study, these findings were not observed in animals after a 4-week, posttreatment recovery period. Studies of long-term treatment with romiplostim in rats have not been conducted; it is not known if the fibrosis of the bone marrow is reversible in rats after long-term treatment.

Pharmacologic & Dosing Characteristics

Dosage: Give an initial dose of 1 mcg/kg once weekly, based on actual body weight.

Adjust weekly dose by increments of 1 mcg/kg to achieve and maintain a platelet count of at least 50×10^9 cells/L using the lowest doses needed to reduce the risk for bleeding. Adjust as follows:

- If platelet count is less than 50×10^9 cells/L, increase the dose by 1 mcg/kg.
- If platelet count is greater than 200×10^9 cells/L for 2 consecutive weeks, reduce the dose by 1 mcg/kg.
- If platelet count is greater than 400×10^9 cells/L, do not dose.

Continue to assess the platelet count weekly. After the platelet count has fallen to less than 200×10^9 cells/L, resume romiplostim at a dose reduced by 1 mcg/kg.

Do not exceed a maximum weekly dose of 10 mcg/kg.

Discontinue romiplostim if platelet count does not increase to a level sufficient to avoid clinically important bleeding after 4 weeks of romiplostim therapy at the maximum weekly dose of 10 mcg/kg.

In clinical studies, most patients who responded to romiplostim achieved and maintained platelet counts of at least 50×10^9 cells/L, with a median dose of 2 mcg/kg.

Route & Site: Subcutaneous

Overdosage: In the event of overdose, platelet counts may increase excessively and result in thrombotic/thromboembolic complications. In this case, discontinue romiplostim and monitor platelet counts. Reinitiate romiplostim in accordance with dosing and administration recommendations.

Laboratory Tests: Before initiating romiplostim, examine the peripheral blood differential to establish the baseline extent of red and white blood cell abnormalities. Monitor complete blood cell count (CBC), including platelet counts and peripheral blood smears, before initiating romiplostim and weekly throughout romiplostim therapy, until a stable romiplostim dose (at least 50×10^9 cells/L for 4 or more weeks without dose adjustment) has been achieved. Thereafter, monitor CBC, including platelet counts and peripheral blood smears, at least monthly. Discontinuation of romiplostim may result in worsened thrombocytopenia than was present before romiplostim therapy. Monitor CBC, including platelet counts, for 2 or more weeks after discontinuing romiplostim.

Assess patients for formation of neutralizing antibodies if platelet counts substantially decrease after an initial romiplostim response. To detect antibody formation, submit blood samples to the manufacturer (800-772-6436). The manufacturer will assay the samples for antibodies to romiplostim and thrombopoietin.

Monitor peripheral blood for signs of marrow fibrosis. Before starting romiplostim, examine the peripheral blood smear closely to establish a baseline level of cellular morphologic abnormalities. After identification of a stable romiplostim dose, examine peripheral blood

Romiplostim

smears and CBC monthly for new or worsening morphologic abnormalities (eg, teardrop and nucleated red blood cells, immature white blood cells) or cytopenia(s). If patient develops new or worsening morphologic abnormalities or cytopenia(s), discontinue treatment with romiplostim and consider a bone marrow biopsy, including staining for fibrosis.

Efficacy: The safety and efficacy of romiplostim were assessed in 2 double-blind, placebo-controlled clinical studies and in an open-label extension study. In studies 1 and 2, patients with chronic ITP who had completed at least one prior treatment and had a platelet count of 30×10^9 cells/L or lower were randomized (2:1) to 24 weeks of romiplostim (1 mcg/kg subcutaneously) or placebo. Prior ITP treatments in both study groups included corticosteroids, immunoglobulins, rituximab, cytotoxic therapies, danazol, and azathioprine. Patients already receiving ITP medical therapies at a constant dosing schedule were allowed to continue receiving these medical treatments throughout the studies. Rescue therapies (ie, corticosteroids, intravenous immunoglobulin (IVIG), platelet transfusions, and anti-D immunoglobulin) were permitted for bleeding, wet purpura, or if the patient was at immediate risk for hemorrhage. Patients received single weekly subcutaneous injections of romiplostim, with individual dose adjustments to maintain platelet counts (50 to 200×10^9 cells/L).

Study 1 evaluated patients who had not undergone splenectomy. The patients had been diagnosed with ITP for approximately 2 years and had received a median of 3 prior ITP treatments. Overall, median platelet count was 19×10^9 cells/L at study entry. During the study, median weekly romiplostim dose was 2 mcg/kg (25th to 75th percentile: 1 to 3 mcg/kg).

Study 2 evaluated patients who had undergone splenectomy. The patients had been diagnosed with ITP for approximately 8 years and had received a median of 6 prior ITP treatments. Overall, median platelet count was 14×10^9 cells/L at study entry. During the study, median weekly romiplostim dose was 3 mcg/kg (25th to 75th percentile: 2 to 7 mcg/kg).

Outcomes of studies 1 and 2 are shown in the following table. A durable platelet response was the achievement of a weekly platelet count of at least 50×10^9 cells/L for any 6 of the last 8 weeks of the 24-week treatment period in the absence of rescue medication at any time. A transient platelet response was the achievement of any weekly platelet counts of at least 50×10^9 cells/L for any 4 weeks during the treatment period without a durable platelet response. An overall platelet response was the achievement of either a durable or transient platelet response. Platelet responses were excluded for 8 weeks after receiving rescue medications.

Results From Placebo-Controlled Studies[a]				
	Study 1 nonsplenectomized patients		Study 2 splenectomized patients	
Outcomes	Romiplostim (n = 41)	Placebo (n = 21)	Romiplostim (n = 42)	Placebo (n = 21)
Platelet responses and rescue therapy				
Durable platelet response, n (%)	25 (61%)	1 (5%)	16 (38%)	0
Overall platelet response, n (%)	36 (88%)	3 (14%)	33 (79%)	0
Number of weeks with platelet counts ≥ 50 × 10⁹ cells/L, average	15	1	12	0
Requiring rescue therapy, n (%)	8 (20%)	13 (62%)	11 (26%)	12 (57%)
Reduction/discontinuation of baseline concurrent ITP medical therapy				
Receiving therapy at baseline	(n = 11)	(n = 10)	(n = 12)	(n = 6)
Patients who had > 25% dose reduction in concurrent therapy, n (%)	36%	20%	33%	17%
Patients who discontinued baseline therapy, n (%)[b]	36%	30%	67%	0%

a All P values < 0.05 for platelet response and rescue therapy comparisons between romiplostim and placebo.
b For multiple concomitant baseline therapies, all therapies were discontinued.

In studies 1 and 2, 9 patients reported a serious bleeding event (5 [6%] romiplostim, 4 [10%] placebo). Bleeding events that were grade 2 severity or higher occurred in 15% of patients treated with romiplostim and 34% of patients treated with placebo.

Extension study: Patients who participated in study 1 or 2 were withdrawn from study medications. If platelet counts subsequently decreased to 50×10^9 cells/L or less, the patients were allowed to receive romiplostim in an open-label extension study, with weekly dosing based on platelet counts. Following romiplostim discontinuation in studies 1 and 2, 7 patients maintained platelet counts of at least 50×10^9 cells/L. Among 100 patients who subsequently entered the extension study, platelet counts were increased and sustained regardless of whether they had received romiplostim or placebo in the prior placebo-controlled studies. The majority of patients reached a median platelet count of 50×10^9 cells/L after receiving 1 to 3 doses of romiplostim; these platelet counts were maintained throughout the remainder of the study, with a median duration of romiplostim treatment of 60 weeks and a maximum duration of 96 weeks.

Pharmacokinetics: In clinical studies, treatment with romiplostim resulted in dose-dependent increases in platelet counts. After a single subcutaneous dose of romiplostim 1 to 10 mcg/kg in patients with chronic ITP, the peak platelet count was 1.3 to 14.9 times higher than the baseline platelet count over a 2- to 3-week period. The platelet counts were more than 50×10^9 cells/L for 7 of 8 patients with chronic ITP who received 6 weekly doses of romiplostim at 1 mcg/kg.

In the long-term extension study in patients with ITP receiving weekly subcutaneous treatment of romiplostim, the pharmacokinetics over the dose range of 3 to 15 mcg/kg indicated that peak serum concentrations were observed approximately 7 to 50 hours after the dose (median, 14 hours), with half-life values ranging from 1 to 34 days (median, 3.5 days). The serum concentrations varied among patients and did not correlate with the dose administered. The elimination of serum romiplostim is, in part, dependent on the thrombopoietin receptor on platelets. As a result, for a given dose, patients with high platelet counts are associated with low serum concentrations and vice versa. In another ITP clinical study, no accumulation in serum concentrations was observed (n = 4) after 6 weekly doses of romiplostim (3 mcg/kg). The accumulation at higher doses of romiplostim is unknown.

Mechanism: Romiplostim increases platelet production through binding and activation of the thrombopoietin receptor, a mechanism analogous to endogenous thrombopoietin.

Drug Interactions: No formal drug interaction studies of romiplostim have been performed.

Romiplostim may be used with other medical ITP therapies, such as corticosteroids, danazol, azathioprine, IVIG, and anti-D immunoglobulin. If the patient's platelet count is at least 50×10^9 cells/L, medical ITP therapies may be reduced or discontinued.

Pharmaceutical Characteristics

Concentration: 250 or 500 mcg of deliverable romiplostim at 500 mcg/mL in single-use vials

Packaging: Single-use vials containing 250 mcg (NDC #: 55513-221-01) or 500 mcg (55513-222-01) deliverable romiplostim

Doseform: Powder for solution

Appearance: White powder yielding clear and colorless solution

Diluent:

For reconstitution: Preservative-free sterile water

    250 mcg vial: Contains romiplostim 375 mcg; add 0.72 mL of sterile water to yield a concentration of 250 mcg per 0.5 mL or 500 mcg/mL.

Romiplostim

500 mcg vial: Contains romiplostim 625 mcg; add 1.2 mL of sterile water to yield a concentration of 500 mcg/mL.

Adjuvant: None

Preservative: None

Allergens: None

Excipients:

250 mcg vial: Mannitol 30 mg, sucrose 15 mg, L-histidine 1.2 mg, polysorbate-20 0.03 mg, and hydrochloride to adjust pH.

500 mcg vial: Mannitol 50 mg, sucrose 25 mg, L-histidine 1.9 mg, polysorbate-20 0.05 mg, and hydrochloride to adjust pH.

pH: 5

Shelf Life: Data not provided.

Storage/Stability: Store at 2° to 8°C (36° to 46°F). Protect vials from light. Do not freeze. Contact the manufacturer regarding exposure to freezing or elevated temperatures. Shipping data not provided.

Gently swirl and invert the vial to reconstitute. Avoid excess or vigorous agitation. Generally, dissolution of romiplostim takes less than 2 minutes. Reconstituted romiplostim may be kept at room temperature (25°C, [77°F]) or refrigerated at 2° to 8°C (36° to 46°F) for up to 24 hours before administration.

Handling: Do not shake during reconstitution. The injection volume may be very small. Use a syringe with graduations to 0.01 mL.

Production Process: Romiplostim is produced by recombinant DNA technology in *Escherichia coli.*

Media: *E. coli*

Other Information

First Licensed: August 22, 2008

References: Stasi R, Evangelista ML, Amadori S. Novel thrombopoietic agents: A review of their use in idiopathic thrombocytopenic purpura. *Drugs.* 2008;68(7):901-912.

Interferons

Interferon was discovered in 1957 in England by Alick Isaacs and Jean Lindenmann as they investigated the phenomenon of viral interference. They discovered that embryonic chick cells exposed to inactivated influenza virus in culture secreted a substance into the culture medium that interfered with the replication of live virus in a fresh batch of cells. They named the substance "interferon." The specific product they discovered is called beta interferon in the current classification scheme.

The interferons are a family of naturally occurring small protein molecules (eg, polypeptides) or glycoproteins from 145 to 166 amino acids in length with molecular weights of approximately 15,000 to 25,000 daltons. Eukaryotic cells produce and secrete interferons in response to viral infections or various synthetic and biological inducers. Interferons are cytokines that mediate antiviral, antiproliferative, and immunomodulatory activities.

Three major classes of interferons have been identified: Alpha, beta, and gamma. Alpha interferons are proteins derived from human leukocytes. Beta interferons are glycoproteins derived from human fibroblasts. Both are acid stable and were originally referred to as type I interferon. Gamma interferons are glycoproteins derived from human T-lymphocytes. They are acid labile and previously were referred to as type II interferon. These interferons have overlapping but clearly distinct biological activities.

Comparison of Interferons	
Interferon type	Endogenous source
Alpha	Leukocytes
Beta	Fibroblasts, macrophages
Gamma	T-lymphocytes, natural killer lymphocytes

These 3 classes are not homogenous, and each may contain several different molecular species. For example, at least 18 genetically and molecularly distinct human alfa-interferons have been identified, varying slightly in amino acid sequence. Three molecules that have been isolated, purified, and undergone clinical development (eg, alfa-2a, alfa-2b, alfa-2c) differ in amino acids at the 23rd and 34th positions.

In general, specific individual forms of leukocyte interferon are spelled interferon alfa-2a, etc. The broad category that encompasses alfa-2a, alfa-2b, and alfa-n3 is generically spelled interferon alpha.

The US Adopted Names (USAN) Council uses the following style to create nonproprietary names for interferons:

The word interferon is the first element in the name. The appropriate Greek letter (spelled out) is the second word of the name: alfa, beta, gamma. An appropriate Arabic numeral and letter are appended to the Greek letter by a hyphen (no space) to delineate subcategories. The numbers conform to the recommendation of the Interferon Nomenclature Committee. The lowercase letter is assigned by the drug nomenclature agencies to differentiate one manufacturer's interferon from another's. Examples of pure interferon substances are:

- interferon alfa-2a
- interferon alfa-2b
- interferon beta-1a
- interferon beta-1b
- interferon gamma-1a

For mixtures of naturally occurring interferons, the lowercase letter "n" precedes the number. Examples of names of mixtures of interferons obtained from a natural source, whether the exact percentage of a mixture is known or not, are:

- interferon alfa-n1
- interferon alfa-n2

Alfacon refers to a "consensus" interferon that shares structural elements of both interferon-alfa and interferon-beta (eg, interferon alfacon-1).

Resources: Borden EC, Sen GC, Uze G, et al. Interferons at age 50: past, current and future impact on biomedicine. *Nat Rev Drug Discov.* 2007;6(12):975-990.

Interferon Alpha Comparison

	Alfa-2a[a]	PEG-Alfa-2a[b]	Alfa-2b	PEG-Alfa-2b	Alfa-n3	Alfacon-1
Brand name	*Roferon-A*	*Pegasys*	*Intron A*[b]	*Peg*Intron, *Sylatron*	*Alferon N*	*Infergen*
Distributor	Roche	Roche	Merck	Merck	Hemispherx Biopharma	Valeant Pharmaceuticals
Labeled indications	Hairy cell leukemia, chronic hepatitis C infection, chronic myelogenous leukemia	Chronic hepatitis C infection, chronic hepatitis B infection	Hairy cell leukemia, AIDS-related Kaposi sarcoma, chronic hepatitis C infection, condylomata acuminata, chronic hepatitis B infection, malignant melanoma, follicular lymphoma	Chronic hepatitis C infection, adjuvant treatment of metastatic melanoma	Condylomata acuminata	Chronic hepatitis C infection
Dosage	From 3 million units 3 times per week to 9 million units/day	180 mcg once/week	1 to 30 million units/day	Hepatitis C: 40 to 150 mcg once/week, Melanoma: 6 then 3 mcg/kg/week	250,000 units/wart	9 mcg 3 times/week
Routes	Subcutaneous	Subcutaneous	Subcutaneous, IM, intralesional	Subcutaneous	Intralesional	Subcutaneous
Doseform	Solution	Solution	Powder for solution	Powder for solution	Solution	Solution
Concentration	6 to 18 million units/mL	180 mcg/mL	3, 5, 10, 50 million units/mL	Various, 40 to 300 mcg/mL after reconstitution	5 million units/mL	0.03 mg/mL
Packaging	3, 6, and 9 million units in prefilled syringes	180 mcg/1 mL vial	3, 5, 10, 18, 25, 50 million units packages of various volumes	Various	5 million units/ 1 mL vial	9 mcg/0.3 mL, 15 mcg/0.5 mL vials
Solvent/ Diluent	Sodium chloride with excipients	Buffered saline	Bacteriostatic water	Sterile water	Buffered saline	Phosphate-buffered saline
Routine storage	2° to 8°C	2° to 8°C	2° to 8°C	Redipen: 2° to 8°C Vials: 25°C	2° to 8°C	2° to 8°C
Source	*Escherichia coli*	*Escherichia coli*	*Escherichia coli*	*Escherichia coli*	Human leukocytes	*Escherichia coli*
Preservative	Benzyl alcohol	Benzyl alcohol	m-cresol	None	Phenol	None
Allergens	Tetracycline not detectable	None	Tetracycline not detectable	None	Neomycin, murine IgG (egg not detectable)	None

a *Roferon-A* is no longer distributed in the United States; data provided for historical comparison reasons.
b Peginterferon alfa-2a (*Pegasys*) may be used with ribavirin (trade name *Copegus*).

Disease Epidemiology

Chronic Hepatitis B

Prevalence: Approximately 1 million to 1.25 million people in the US are carriers of hepatitis B virus; 1 in 4 will develop chronic active hepatitis B. See also Hepatitis B and HBIG monographs.

Chronic Hepatitis C

Incidence: 170,000 new cases occur each year; approximately 50% (85,000 cases) develop chronic hepatitis, and approximately 20% of chronic cases (17,000 cases) progress to cirrhosis, liver failure, or hepatocellular carcinoma, usually after 10 to 20 years or more. Approximately 4 million Americans are chronically infected with hepatitis C virus. From 50% to 80% of those infected develop chronic disease. Approximately 8,000 to 10,000 people die annually as a result of infection *sequelae*, a level likely to triple within the next 10 to 20 years without effective intervention.

Susceptible Pools: Groups at highest risk include transfusion recipients, parenteral drug users, and dialysis patients. Others include health care workers exposed to blood and household or sexual contacts of cases.

Transmission: By percutaneous exposure to contaminated blood and plasma derivatives. Contaminated needles and syringes are important vehicles of transmission, especially among parenteral drug users.

Of newly infected patients in 1 survey, 42% had a history of IV drug use, and 6% to 10% had a history of blood transfusion. The remainder became infected through other modes of transmission (hemodialysis, sexual contact with an infected partner, occupational exposure to infected blood or blood products, and unidentified sources).

In a group of 332 patients with chronic hepatitis C, 81% had a history of blood or blood-product exposure, 8% had a history of IV drug use, 2% had a history of surgery without blood products, and the remainder had other types of exposure.

Incubation: Ranges from 2 weeks to 6 months, usually 6 to 9 weeks.

Communicability: 1 or more week before onset of symptoms through the acute phase and indefinitely in chronic carriers.

Condylomata Acuminata

Incidence: Approximately 3 million new and recurrent cases of condylomata acuminata are reported annually. Genital papillomavirus infection is the most commonly diagnosed sexually transmitted viral disease.

Transmission: By direct contact, usually sexually transmitted, allowing transfer of the human papillomavirus (HPV). Papillomavirus is a double-stranded DNA virus (genus Papillomavirus, family Papovaviridae).

Incubation: Approximately 2 to 3 months (range, 1 to 20 months).

Communicability: At least as long as visible lesions persist.

Hairy Cell Leukemia

Incidence: Rare, representing only 2% of adult leukemia cases.

Kaposi Sarcoma

Incidence: Formerly a rare cancer in the US, Kaposi sarcoma (KS) is the most common malignancy associated with AIDS, affecting 14% to 31% of AIDS patients. The overall incidences of KS is 0.32 to 0.62 cases per 100,000 people per year in Europe and North America, although risk among AIDS patients may be 100-fold greater. The relative proportion of KS among AIDS patients has been declining since the early 1980s.

Perspective:
1872: Kaposi describes odd skin tumors among Mediterranean and Jewish populations.

References: Wahman A, et al. The epidemiology of classic, African, and immunosuppressed Kaposi's sarcoma. *Epidemiol Rev.* 1991;13:178–199.

Other Information

Perspective:
1957: Isaacs and Lindenmann discover interferon beta.
1979: Human gene for interferon alfa cloned.
1986: Interferon alfa licensed for therapy of hairy cell leukemia.
1989: Hepatitis C virus first cloned and characterized.
1992: Interferon alfa licensed for therapy of chronic hepatitis B.

Resources: Perry CM, Wagstaff AJ. Interferon-α-n1: A review of its pharmacological properties and therapeutic efficacy in the management of chronic viral hepatitis. *BioDrugs.* 1998;9:125-154.

Peginterferon Alfa-2a (Recombinant)

Interferons

Name:
Pegasys

Manufacturer:
Roche Pharmaceuticals

Synonyms: Pegylated interferon alfa-2a

Comparison: The various interferon alpha products are not generically interchangeable because of variations in dosage, routes of administration, and adverse events specific to different brands. Do not use different brands of interferon alpha in any single treatment regimen. For comparison of peginterferon alfa-2a and interferon alfa-2a (*Roferon-A*), see the Efficacy section of this monograph.

Immunologic Characteristics

Antigen Source: Interferon alfa expressed from recombinant *Escherichia coli* bacteria.

Viability: Not viable, but immunologically active.

Antigenic Form: Interferon, human leukocyte.

Antigenic Type: Protein, a covalent conjugate of recombinant interferon alfa-2a (approximately 20 kilodalton) with a single-branched bis-monomethoxy polyethylene glycol (PEG) chain (approximately 40 kilodalton). The PEG moiety is linked at a single site to the interferon-alfa moiety via a stable amide bond to lysine.

Strains: Interferon alfa-2a

Use Characteristics

Indications: To treat chronic hepatitis C in patients 5 years of age and older with compensated liver disease not previously treated with interferon alpha, in patients with histological evidence of cirrhosis and compensated liver disease, and in adults with chronic hepatitis C/HIV coinfection and CD4 count greater than 100 cells/mm^3.

Combination therapy with ribavirin is recommended unless patient has a contraindication to or significant intolerance of ribavirin.

As monotherapy for treatment of adult patients with HBeAg-positive and HBeAg-negative chronic hepatitis B infection who have compensated liver disease and evidence of viral replication and liver inflammation.

Limitations: The safety and efficacy of peginterferon alfa-2a have not been established in patients who have failed other alpha interferon treatments, nor in the treatment of hepatitis C in liver or other organ transplant recipients. The safety and efficacy of peginterferon alfa-2a for patients with hepatitis C virus (HCV) coinfected with HIV or hepatitis B virus (HBV) have not been established.

Contraindications:

Absolute: People with hypersensitivity to peginterferon alfa-2a or any of its components, autoimmune hepatitis, or decompensated hepatic disease (Child-Pugh class B and C) before or during treatment with peginterferon alfa-2a. Hepatic decompensation with Child-Pugh score of 6 or greater in cirrhotic chronic hepatitis C patients coinfected with HIV before treatment.

Relative: Peginterferon alfa-2a also is contraindicated in neonates and infants because it contains benzyl alcohol. Benzyl alcohol has been associated with an increased incidence of neurological and other complications in neonates and infants, which are sometimes fatal.

1002

Combination therapy with ribavirin is contraindicated in people hypersensitive to ribavirin or *Copegus*, women who are pregnant, men whose female partners are pregnant, and patients with hemoglobinopathies (eg, thalassemia major, sickle cell anemia).

Elderly: The area under the concentration curve (AUC) increased from 1,295 to 1,663 ng•h/mL in subjects older than 62 years of age taking peginterferon alfa-2a 180 mcg, but peak concentrations were similar (9 vs 10 ng/mL) in those older and younger than 62 years of age. Adverse reactions related to alpha interferons, such as CNS, cardiac, and systemic (eg, viral-like) effects, may be more severe in the elderly. Exercise caution when using peginterferon alfa-2a in this population. This drug is excreted by the kidney. The risk of toxic reactions may be greater in patients with impaired renal function. Because elderly patients are more likely to have decreased renal function, take care in dose selection, monitoring renal function as clinically appropriate.

Carcinogenicity: Peginterferon alfa-2a has not been tested for carcinogenic potential.

Mutagenicity: Peginterferon alfa-2a did not cause DNA damage when tested in the Ames bacterial mutagenicity assay and in the in vitro chromosomal aberration assay in human lymphocytes in the presence or absence of metabolic activation.

Fertility Impairment: Peginterferon alfa-2a may impair fertility. Prolonged menstrual cycles and amenorrhea were observed in female cynomolgus monkeys given subcutaneous injections of 600 mcg/kg/dose (7,200 mcg/m^2/dose) of peginterferon alfa-2a every other day for 1 month at approximately 180 times the recommended weekly human dose for a 60 kg person (based on body surface area [BSA]). Menstrual cycle irregularities were accompanied by a decrease and delay in the peak 17-beta-estradiol and progesterone levels following administration of peginterferon alfa-2a to female monkeys. A return to normal menstrual rhythm followed cessation of treatment. Every-other-day dosing with peginterferon alfa-2a 100 mcg/kg (1,200 mcg/m^2; approximately 30 times the recommended human dose) had no effects on cycle duration or reproductive hormone status.

The effects of peginterferon alfa-2a on male fertility have not been studied. However, no adverse effects on fertility were observed in male Rhesus monkeys treated with nonpegylated interferon alfa-2a for 5 months at doses up to 25×10^6 units/kg/day.

Pregnancy: Alone, Category C. Peginterferon alfa-2a has not been studied for its teratogenic effect. Nonpegylated interferon alfa-2a treatment of pregnant Rhesus monkeys at approximately 20 to 500 times the weekly human dose resulted in a statistically significant increase in abortions. No teratogenic effects were seen in the offspring delivered at term. Assume peginterferon alfa-2a has abortifacient potential. There are no adequate and well-controlled studies of peginterferon alfa-2a in pregnant women. Use peginterferon alfa-2a during pregnancy only if the potential benefit justifies the potential risk to the fetus. Peginterferon alfa-2a is recommended for use in women of childbearing potential only when they are using effective contraception during therapy.

With ribavirin, Category X. All animal species exposed to ribavirin developed significant teratogenic or embryocidal effects. Ribavirin is contraindicated in women who are pregnant and men whose female partners are pregnant.

Lactation: It is not known whether peginterferon alfa-2a or its components are excreted in human milk. The effect of orally ingested peginterferon alfa-2a from breast milk on the breast-feeding infant has not been evaluated. Because of the potential for adverse reactions from the drug in breast-feeding infants, decide whether to discontinue breast-feeding or the treatment.

Children: The safety and efficacy of peginterferon alfa-2a in children younger than 18 years of age have not been established. Peginterferon alfa-2a contains benzyl alcohol. Benzyl alcohol has been associated with an increased incidence of neurological and other complications in neonates and infants, which are sometimes fatal.

Adverse Reactions: Peginterferon alfa-2a causes a broad variety of serious adverse reactions. In all studies, one or more serious adverse reactions occurred in 9% of patients receiving peginterferon alfa-2a. Serious adverse events included the following: substance overdose, hepatic dysfunction, fatty liver, cholangitis, arrhythmia, suicidal ideation, suicide, diabetes mellitus, autoimmune phenomena, peripheral neuropathy, peptic ulcer, GI bleeding, pancreatitis, colitis, corneal ulcer, endocarditis, pneumonia, interstitial pneumonitis, pulmonary embolism, coma, myositis, cerebral hemorrhage. Each of these individual events occurred at a frequency of 1% or less. Monitor patients for serious conditions that may become life-threatening. Withdraw therapy in patients with persistently severe or worsening signs or symptoms.

Nearly all patients in clinical trials experienced one or more adverse events. The most commonly reported adverse reactions were psychiatric reactions, including depression, irritability, and anxiety, and viral-like symptoms such as fatigue, pyrexia, myalgia, headache, and rigors. The most common reason for dose modification or withdrawal from studies was hematologic abnormalities.

Because clinical trials are conducted under widely varying and controlled conditions, the adverse reaction rates of a drug cannot be directly compared with rates in the clinical trials of another drug. Also, the adverse event rates listed here may not predict the rates observed in a broader patient population in clinical practice. More than 1,000 patients have been treated with peginterferon alfa-2a in clinical trials. Adverse reactions occurring in 5% or more of patients receiving peginterferon alfa-2a 180 mcg (n = 559) in clinical trials appear below. The population encompassed an age range of 18 to 76 years. Seventy percent of the patients were male and 86% were Caucasian.

Adverse Reactions Occurring in ≥ 5% of Subjects in Chronic Hepatitis C Clinical Trials (Pooled Studies 1, 2, 3, and 4)				
	Monotherapy (studies 1, 2, and 3)		Combination therapy (study 4)	
	Peginterferon alfa-2a 180 mcg	Interferon alfa-2a 3 MIU[a] or 6/3 MIU	Peginterferon alfa-2a 180 mcg + ribavirin 1,000 mg or 1,200 mg	Interferon alfa-2a + ribavirin 1,000 mg or 1,200 mg
Body system/ adverse events	48 week[b] n = 559 %	48 week[b] n = 554 %	48 week[c] n = 451 %	48 week[c] n = 443 %
Injection-site reaction	22	18	23	16
Endocrine disorders				
Hypothyroidism	3	2	4	5
Flu-like symptoms and signs				
Fatigue/Asthenia	56	57	65	68
Pyrexia	37	41	41	55
Rigors	35	44	25	37
Pain	11	12	10	9
Gastrointestinal				
Nausea/Vomiting	24	33	25	29
Diarrhea	16	16	11	10
Abdominal pain	15	15	8	9
Dry mouth	6	3	4	7
Dyspepsia	< 1	1	6	5
Hematologic[d]				
Lymphopenia	3	5	14	12
Anemia	2	1	11	11
Neutropenia	21	8	27	8
Thrombocytopenia	5	2	5	< 1

Adverse Reactions Occurring in ≥ 5% of Subjects in Chronic Hepatitis C Clinical Trials (Pooled Studies 1, 2, 3, and 4)			
Metabolic and nutritional			
Anorexia	17	17	24	26
Weight decrease	4	3	10	10
Musculoskeletal, connective tissue and bone			
Myalgia	37	38	40	49
Arthralgia	28	29	22	23
Back pain	9	10	5	5
Neurological			
Headache	54	58	43	49
Dizziness (excluding vertigo)	16	12	14	14
Memory impairment	5	4	6	5
Resistance mechanism disorders			
Overall	10	6	12	10
Psychiatric			
Irritability/Anxiety/Nervousness	19	22	33	38
Insomnia	19	23	30	37
Depression	18	19	20	28
Concentration impairment	8	10	10	13
Mood alteration	3	3	5	6
Respiratory, thoracic, and mediastinal			
Dyspnea	4	2	13	14
Cough	4	3	10	7
Dyspnea exertional	< 1	< 1	4	7
Skin and subcutaneous			
Alopecia	23	30	28	33
Pruritus	12	8	19	18
Dermatitis	8	3	16	13
Dry skin	4	3	10	13
Rash	5	4	8	5
Sweating increased	6	7	6	5
Eczema	1	1	5	4
Visual disorders			
Vision blurred	4	2	5	2

a An induction dose of 6 million international units (MIU) 3 times a week for the first 12 weeks followed by 3 million international units 3 times a week for 36 weeks given subcutaneously.

b Pooled studies 1, 2, and 3

c Study 4

d Severe hematologic abnormalities (lymphocyte $< 0.5 \times 10^9$ cells/L; hemoglobin < 10 g/dL; neutrophil $< 0.75 \times 10^9$ cells/L; platelet $< 50 \times 10^9$ cells/L)

Autoimmune: Development or exacerbation of autoimmune disorders, including myositis, hepatitis, immune thrombocytopenic purpura, psoriasis, rheumatoid arthritis, interstitial nephritis, thyroiditis, and systemic lupus erythematosus, have been reported in patients receiving alpha interferons. Use peginterferon alfa-2a with caution in patients with autoimmune disorders.

Peginterferon Alfa-2a (Recombinant)

Pancreatitis: Pancreatitis, sometimes fatal, has occurred during alpha interferon treatment. Suspend peginterferon alfa-2a if symptoms or signs suggestive of pancreatitis are observed. Discontinue peginterferon alfa-2a in patients diagnosed with pancreatitis.

Cardiovascular: Hypertension, supraventricular arrhythmias, chest pain, and myocardial infarction have been observed in patients treated with peginterferon alfa-2a. Administer peginterferon alfa-2a with caution to patients with preexisting cardiac disease.

CNS: Life-threatening neuropsychiatric reactions may manifest in patients receiving peginterferon alfa-2a. Depression, suicidal ideation, and suicide attempt may occur in patients with and without previous psychiatric illness. Use peginterferon alfa-2a with extreme caution in patients who report a history of depression. Neuropsychiatric adverse events observed with alpha interferon treatment include relapse of drug addiction, drug overdose, aggressive behavior, psychoses, hallucinations, bipolar disorders, and mania. Monitor all patients for evidence of depression and other psychiatric symptoms. Advise patients to report any sign or symptom of depression or suicidal ideation to their physician. In severe cases, immediately stop therapy and provide psychiatric help.

Endocrine: Peginterferon alfa-2a causes or aggravates hypothyroidism and hyperthyroidism. Hyperglycemia, hypoglycemia, and diabetes mellitus have developed in patients treated with peginterferon alfa-2a. Do not begin peginterferon alfa-2a therapy in patients with these conditions at baseline who cannot be effectively treated by medication. Patients who develop these conditions during treatment and cannot be controlled with medication may require discontinuation of peginterferon alfa-2a therapy.

GI: Hemorrhagic/ischemic colitis, sometimes fatal, has been observed within 12 weeks of starting alpha interferon treatment. Abdominal pain, bloody diarrhea, and fever are typical manifestations of colitis. Discontinue peginterferon alfa-2a immediately if these symptoms develop. The colitis usually resolves within 1 to 3 weeks of stopping alpha interferon. Ulcerative colitis also has been observed in patients treated with alpha interferon.

Hematologic: Peginterferon alfa-2a suppresses bone marrow function and may result in severe cytopenias. Very rarely, alpha interferons may be associated with aplastic anemia. Obtain complete blood cell counts (CBC) before treatment and routinely during therapy. Use peginterferon alfa-2a with caution in patients with baseline neutrophil counts less than 500 cells/mm^3, baseline platelet counts less than 90,000 cells/mm^3, or baseline hemoglobin less than 10 g/dL. Discontinue peginterferon alfa-2a therapy, at least temporarily, in patients who develop severe decreases in neutrophil and platelet counts.

Hepatic: Transient elevations in ALT (2- to 5-fold above baseline) were observed in some patients receiving peginterferon alfa-2a, including patients with virologic response. Transient elevations were not associated with deterioration of other liver function tests. However, when the increase in ALT levels is progressive despite dose reduction or is accompanied by increased bilirubin, discontinue peginterferon alfa-2a.

Hypersensitivity: Severe acute hypersensitivity reactions (eg, urticaria, angioedema, bronchoconstriction, anaphylaxis) have been observed rarely during alpha interferon therapy. If such reactions occur, discontinue therapy with peginterferon alfa-2a and immediately provide appropriate therapy.

Immunologic: Two percent of patients (8/409) receiving peginterferon alfa-2a developed low-titer neutralizing antibodies (using an assay of a sensitivity of 100 interferon neutralizing units/mL). Six percent (24/409) of patients treated with peginterferon alfa-2a developed binding antibodies to interferon alfa-2a, as assessed by an ELISA assay. The clinical and pathological significance of the appearance of serum neutralizing antibodies is unknown. No apparent correlation or antibody development to clinical response or adverse events was observed. The percentage of patients whose test results were considered positive for antibodies is highly dependent on the sensitivity and specificity of the assays. Additionally, the observed incidence of antibody positivity in these assays may be influenced by several factors, including sample timing and handling, concomitant medications, and underlying disease. For these reasons, comparison of the incidence of antibodies to peginterferon alfa-2a with the incidence of antibodies to these products may be misleading.

Ophthalmic: Decrease in or loss of vision; retinopathy, including macular edema; retinal artery or vein thrombosis; retinal hemorrhages and cotton wool spots; optic neuritis; and papilledema are induced or aggravated by treatment with peginterferon alfa-2a or other alpha interferons. All patients should receive an eye examination at baseline. Patients with preexisting ophthalmologic disorders (eg, diabetic or hypertensive retinopathy) should receive periodic ophthalmologic exams during interferon alpha treatment. Any patient who develops ocular symptoms should receive a prompt and complete eye examination. Discontinue peginterferon alfa-2a treatment in patients who develop new or worsening ophthalmologic disorders.

Renal: A 25% to 45% higher exposure to peginterferon alfa-2a is seen in subjects undergoing hemodialysis. In patients with impaired renal function, closely monitor signs and symptoms of interferon toxicity. Adjust doses of peginterferon alfa-2a accordingly. Use peginterferon alfa-2a with caution in patients with creatinine clearance less than 50 mL/min.

Respiratory: Dyspnea, pulmonary infiltrates, pneumonia, bronchiolitis obliterans, interstitial pneumonitis, and sarcoidosis, some resulting in respiratory failure and/or patient deaths, may be induced or aggravated by peginterferon alfa-2a or alpha interferon therapy. Discontinue peginterferon alfa-2a treatment in patients who develop persistent or unexplained pulmonary infiltrates or pulmonary function impairment.

Pharmacologic & Dosing Characteristics

Dosage:

Adults: 180 mcg once per week for 48 weeks. There are no safety and efficacy data on treatment longer than 48 weeks. Consider discontinuing therapy after week 12 virological results are available if the patient failed to demonstrate a response.

When dose modification is required for moderate to severe adverse reactions (clinical and laboratory), initial dose reduction to 135 mcg is generally adequate. However, in some cases, dose reduction to 90 mcg may be needed. Following improvement of the adverse reaction, re-escalation of the dose may be considered.

Hematologic: Dose reduction to 135 mcg is recommended if the neutrophil count is less than 750 cells/mm^3. For patients with absolute neutrophil count (ANC) values less than 500 cells/mm^3, suspend treatment until ANC values return to more than 1,000 cells/mm^3. Resume therapy initially at 90 mcg and monitor the neutrophil count. Dose reduction to 90 mcg is recommended for platelet counts less than 50,000 cells/mm^3. Cease therapy when platelet count is less than 25,000 cells/mm^3.

Renal: In patients with end-stage renal disease requiring hemodialysis, reduce the dose to 135 mcg. Closely monitor for signs and symptoms of interferon toxicity.

Liver: In patients with progressive ALT increases above baseline values, reduce the dose to 90 mcg. If ALT increases are progressive despite dose reduction or are accompanied by increased bilirubin or evidence of hepatic decompensation, immediately discontinue therapy.

Psychiatric: Modify or discontinue therapy for patients with depression, according to the following guidelines:

Guidelines for Modification or Discontinuation of Peginterferon Alfa-2a and for Scheduling Visits for Patients With Depression					
Depression Severity	Initial management (4 to 8 weeks)		Depression		
	Dose modification	Visit schedule	Remains	Improves	Worsens
Mild	No change	Evaluate once weekly	Continue weekly schedule	Resume normal schedule	(See moderate or severe depression)
Moderate	Decrease *Pegasys* dose to 135 mcg (to 90 mcg if needed)	Evaluate once weekly	Consider psychiatric consult; continue reduced dosing	If symptoms improve and are stable for 4 weeks, may resume normal visit schedule; continue reduced dosing or return to normal dose	(See severe depression)
Severe	Discontinue *Pegasys* permanently	Obtain immediate psychiatric consultation	Psychiatric therapy necessary		

Combination therapy: In combination, the recommended dose is peginterferon alfa-2a 180 mcg once weekly. The recommended dose of ribavirin and duration of combined therapy varies on viral genotype. The daily oral dose of ribavirin is 800 mg to 1,200 mg in 2 divided doses. Individualize the ribavirin dose according to the patient's baseline disease characteristics (eg, genotype), response to therapy, and tolerance to the regimen. See preceding guidelines for modifying the peginterferon alfa-2a dose. Ribavirin absorption increases when administered with a meal, so advise patients to take ribavirin with food.

Genotype	Peginterferon alfa-2a	Ribavirin	Duration
Genotype 1, 4	180 mcg	< 75 kg = 1,000 mg	48 weeks
		≥ 75 kg = 1,200 mg	48 weeks
Genotype 2, 3	180 mcg	800 mg	24 weeks

For adults coinfected with chronic hepatitis C and HIV, the recommended dose is peginterferon alfa-2a 180 mcg once weekly and ribavirin 800 mg orally daily given in 2 divided doses for a total of 48 weeks, regardless of genotype.

For patients with no cardiac disease and hemoglobin less than 10 g/dL, reduce the ribavirin dose to 600 mg/day; discontinue ribavirin if hemoglobin less than 8.5 g/dL. For patients with a history of stable cardiac disease and a 2 g/dL or more decrease in hemoglobin during any 4-week treatment period, reduce the ribavirin dose to 600 mg/day; discontinue ribavirin if hemoglobin is less than 12 g/dL despite 4 weeks at reduced dose.

Once ribavirin has been withheld due to a laboratory abnormality or clinical manifestation, an attempt may be made to restart ribavirin at 600 mg daily and further increase the dose to 800 mg daily based on the physician's judgment, but it is not recommended to increase ribavirin to the original dose.

Pediatric patients: Peginterferon alfa-2a 180 mcg/1.73 m^2 × BSA subcutaneously once weekly, to a maximum dose of 180 mcg, given in combination with ribavirin. The recom-

mended treatment duration for patients with genotype 2 or 3 is 24 weeks and for other genotypes is 48 weeks. Ribavirin is available only as a 200 mg tablet, so determine if such a
tablet can be swallowed by the pediatric patient. Administer ribavirin with food. Patients
who start treatment before their eighteenth birthday should maintain pediatric dosing
through the completion of therapy.

Ribavirin Dosing Recommendations for Pediatric Patients		
Body weight (kg)	Ribavirin daily dose[a]	Number of tablets
23 to 33	400 mg/day	One 200 mg tablet AM
		On 200 mg tablet PM
34 to 46	600 mg/day	One 200 mg tablet AM
		One 200 mg tablet PM
47 to 59	800 mg/day	Two 200 mg tablets AM
		Two 200 mg tablets PM
60 to 74	1,000 mg/day	Two 200 mg tablets AM
		Three 200 mg tablets PM
≥ 75	1,200 mg/day	Three 200 mg tablets AM
		Three 200 mg tablets PM

a Approximately 15 mg/kg/day.

If toxicities occur that may be related to peginterferon alfa-2a or ribavirin, the dose of one
or both drugs can be modified or discontinued. Do not give ribavirin as monotherapy. Recommendations for dose modifications in pediatric patients for toxicities associated with
therapy are presented in the product's prescribing information. When dose modification is
required for moderate to severe adverse reactions (clinical or laboratory), modification
to 135 mcg/1.73 m^2 × BSA is generally adequate. However, in some cases, dose modification to 90 mcg/1.73 m^2 × BSA or 45 mcg/1.73 m^2 × BSA may be needed. Up to 3 dose
modifications for toxicity can be made before discontinuation is considered. These modifications apply to pediatric patients with depression, who can be managed similar to the
algorithm for adult patients. Upon resolution of a laboratory abnormality or clinical adverse
reaction, an increase to the original dose may be considered. If ribavirin has been withheld due to a laboratory abnormality or clinical adverse reaction, an attempt may be made
to restart it at one-half the full dose.

Route & Site: Subcutaneously in the abdomen or thigh.

Overdosage: There is limited experience with overdosage. The maximum dose received by
any patient was 7 times the intended dose of peginterferon alfa-2a (180 mcg/day for 7 days).
There were no serious reactions attributed to overdosages. Weekly doses of up to 630 mcg
have been administered to patients with cancer. Dose-limiting toxicities were fatigue, elevated
liver enzymes, neutropenia, and thrombocytopenia. There is no specific antidote for peginterferon alfa-2a. Hemodialysis and peritoneal dialysis are not effective.

Missed Doses: Missing a dose of peginterferon alfa-2a will not have immediate consequences.
If a missed dose is recognized within 2 days of when it should have been given, administer it
and give the next dose on the day it is usually given. If more than 2 days pass, administer the
missed dose as soon as possible and adjust the weekly schedule. If more than 1 dose is missed,
advise the clinician managing therapy.

Laboratory Tests: Before beginning peginterferon alfa-2a therapy, standard hematological
and biochemical laboratory tests are recommended for all patients. After beginning therapy,
perform hematological tests at 2 weeks and biochemical tests at 4 weeks. Perform additional
testing periodically during therapy. In the clinical studies, the CBC (including hemoglobin
level, white blood cell [WBC], and platelet counts) and chemistries (including liver function

Peginterferon Alfa-2a (Recombinant)

tests and uric acid) were measured at 1, 2, 4, 6, and 8 weeks, and then every 4 weeks, or more frequently if abnormalities were found. Thyroid-stimulating hormone (TSH) was measured every 12 weeks.

Entrance criteria used for the clinical studies of peginterferon alfa-2a may be considered as a guideline to acceptable baseline values for initiation of treatment:

- Platelet count 90,000 cells/mm^3 or more (as low as 75,000 cells/mm^3 in patients with cirrhosis or transition to cirrhosis)
- ANC 1,500 cells/mm^3 or more
- Serum creatinine concentration less than 1.5 times upper limit of normal
- TSH and T4 within normal limits or adequately controlled thyroid function

Treatment with peginterferon alfa-2a 180 mcg was associated with decreases in total WBC, ANC, and platelet counts, which generally improved with dosage modification and returned to pretreatment levels within 4 to 8 weeks upon cessation of therapy. Approximately 4% of patients had transient decreases in ANC to levels below 500 cells/mm^3 at some time during therapy. Peginterferon alfa-2a treatment also was associated with decreases in values for platelet counts. About 5% of patients had decreases in platelet counts to levels below 50,000 cells/mm^3.

Although treatment with peginterferon alfa-2a 180 mcg was associated with small gradual decreases in hemoglobin and hematocrit, less than 1% of all patients, including those with cirrhosis, required dose modification for anemia.

Peginterferon alfa-2a treatment was associated with the development of abnormalities in thyroid laboratory values, some with associated clinical manifestations. The rates of clinically relevant hypothyroidism or hyperthyroidism (requiring treatment dose modification or discontinuation) were 4% and 1%, respectively. Among the patients who developed new-onset thyroid abnormalities during peginterferon alfa-2a treatment, approximately half still had abnormalities during the follow-up period.

Efficacy: Peginterferon alfa-2a was studied in the treatment of hepatitis C infection in 3 randomized, open-label, active-controlled clinical studies. All patients were adults with compensated liver disease and detectable HCV who were previously untreated with interferon alfa. All patients received subcutaneous therapy for 48 weeks and were followed for 24 more weeks to assess durability of response. In studies 1 and 2, approximately 20% of subjects had cirrhosis or transition to cirrhosis. Study 3 enrolled only patients with a histological diagnosis of cirrhosis or transition to cirrhosis. The protocols defined response to treatment as 2 consecutive undetectable HCV RNA values and normalization of ALT at 24 weeks posttreatment. In all 3 studies, treatment with peginterferon alfa-2a 180 mcg resulted in significantly more patient response, compared with treatment with interferon alfa-2a. An exploratory analysis also was conducted with response to treatment defined as undetectable HCV RNA and normalization of ALT posttreatment (on or after study week 68).

In study 1 (n = 630), patients received interferon alfa-2a 3 million units 3 times per week, peginterferon alfa-2a 135 mcg once per week, or peginterferon alfa-2a 180 mcg once per week. Treatment with peginterferon alfa-2a 135 mcg was not significantly different from responses to 180 mcg.

In study 2 (n = 526), patients received either interferon alfa-2a 6 million units 3 times per week for 12 weeks followed by 3 million units 3 times per week for 36 weeks, or peginterferon alfa-2a 180 mcg once per week.

In study 3 (n = 269), patients received interferon alfa-2a 3 million units 3 times per week, peginterferon alfa-2a 90 mcg once per week, or peginterferon alfa-2a 180 mcg once per week. Treatment with peginterferon alfa-2a 90 mcg was intermediate between peginterferon alfa-2a 180 mcg and interferon alfa-2a.

Sustained Response at Week 72								
	Study 1			Study 2			Study 3 (with cirrhosis)		
	Roferon A 3 M units (n = 207)	Pegasys 180 mcg (n = 208)	Difference (95% CI)	Roferon A 6/3 M units (n = 207)	Pegasys 180 mcg (n = 208)	Difference (95% CI)	Roferon A 3 M units (n = 207)	Pegasys 180 mcg (n = 208)	Difference (95% CI)
Protocol: combined virological and biological sustained responder (week 72)	9%	20%	11% (4%, 17%)	15%	28%	13% (6%, 20%)	3%	20%	16% (7%, 25%)
Sustained virological response[a]	9%	23%	13% (7%, 20%)	17%	31%	13% (7%, 22%)	5%	28%	23% (13%, 33%)
Exploratory analysis: combined virological and biological sustained responder (week 72)	11%	24%	13% (6%, 20%)	17%	35%	18% (11%, 25%)	7%	23%	16% (6%, 26%)
Sustained virological response[a]	11%	26%	15% (8%, 23%)	19%	39%	19% (11%, 26%)	8%	30%	22% (11%, 33%)

a *Cobas Amplicor HCV* test, version 2.0.

Matched pre- and posttreatment liver biopsies obtained in approximately 70% of subjects showed similar modest reductions in inflammation and fibrosis, compared with baseline, in all treatment groups.

Of patients who did not demonstrate by 12 weeks of peginterferon alfa-2a 180 mcg therapy either undetectable HCV RNA or 2-$\log_{10}$ or more drop in HCV RNA titer from baseline, 2% (3/156) achieved a sustained virological response. Averaged over studies 1, 2, and 3, response rates to peginterferon alfa-2a were 23% among patients with viral genotype 1 and 48% in patients with other viral genotypes.

The treatment response rates were similar in men and women and in non-white compared with white patients. However, the total number of non-white patients was too small to rule out substantial differences.

Interferon alfa-2a was assessed in combination with ribavirin (trade name *Copegus*) in 2 randomized clinical trials. Combination therapy resulted in a higher sustained virologic response (undetectable HCV RNA at end of 24-week treatment-free follow-up period), compared to either interferon alfa-2a alone or the combination of interferon alfa-2a with ribavirin. In all treatment arms, patients with viral genotype 1, regardless of viral load, had a lower response rate. The HCV genotype influenced the optimal treatment duration and dose of ribavirin.

Onset: Of patients who did not demonstrate by 12 weeks of peginterferon alfa-2a 180 mcg therapy (undetectable HCV RNA or 2-$\log_{10}$ drop or more in HCV RNA titer from baseline), 2% (3/156) achieved a sustained virological response.

Duration: Proportions of subjects with sustained response through study week 72 appear in the table above.

Pharmacokinetics: Maximal serum concentrations (C_{max}) occur 72 to 96 hours after dosing and are sustained for up to 168 hours. The C_{max} and AUC measurements of peginterferon alfa-2a increase in a dose-related manner. Week 48 mean trough concentrations (16 ng/mL; range, 4 to 28) are approximately 2-fold higher than week 1 mean trough concentrations

(8 ng/mL; range, 0 to 15). Steady-state serum levels are reached within 5 to 8 weeks of once-weekly dosing. The peak-to-trough ratio at week 48 is approximately 2.

The mean systemic clearance in healthy subjects given peginterferon alfa-2a was 94 mL/h, approximately 100-fold lower than for interferon alfa-2a. The mean terminal half-life after subcutaneous dosing in patients with chronic hepatitis C infection was 80 hours (range, 50 to 140 hours), compared with 5.1 hours (range, 3.7 to 8.5 hours) for interferon alfa-2a.

Peginterferon alfa-2a administration yielded similar pharmacokinetics in healthy male and female subjects. The AUC was increased from 1,295 to 1,663 ng•h/mL in subjects older than 62 years of age taking peginterferon alfa-2a 180 mcg, but peak concentrations were similar (9 vs 10 ng/mL) in those older and younger than 62 years of age.

In patients with end-stage renal disease undergoing hemodialysis, there is a 25% to 45% reduction in clearance.

Pharmacokinetics have not been adequately studied in pediatric patients.

Mechanism: The biological activity of peginterferon alfa-2a derives from its interferon alfa-2a moiety. Interferons bind to specific membrane receptors on the cell surface and initiate a complex sequence of protein-protein interactions leading to rapid activation of gene transcription. Interferon-stimulated genes modulate many biological effects, including inhibition of virus replication in infected cells, inhibition of cell proliferation, and immunomodulation. The clinical relevance of these in vitro findings is not known.

Peginterferon alfa-2a stimulates the production of effector proteins such as serum neopterin and 2' 5' oligoadenylate synthetase, raises body temperature, and causes reversible decreases in leukocyte and platelet counts. The correlation between in vitro and in vivo pharmacologic, pharmacodynamic, and clinical effects is unknown.

Drug Interactions: Treatment with peginterferon alfa-2a once per week for 4 weeks in healthy subjects was associated with an inhibition of P-450 1A2 and a 25% increase in theophylline AUC. Monitor theophylline serum levels and consider dose adjustments for patients given theophylline and peginterferon alfa-2a. There was no effect on the pharmacokinetics of representative drugs metabolized by CYP 2C9, CYP 2C19, CYP 2D6, or CYP 3A4.

In patients with chronic hepatitis C treated with peginterferon alfa-2a in combination with ribavirin, peginterferon alfa-2a did not affect ribavirin distribution or clearance.

The pharmacokinetics of coadministration of methadone and peginterferon alfa-2a were evaluated in 24 peginterferon alfa-2a–naive chronic hepatitis C patients (15 male, 9 female) who received 180 mcg peginterferon alfa-2a subcutaneously weekly. All patients were on stable methadone maintenance therapy (median dose, 95 mg; range, 30 to 150 mcg) before receiving peginterferon alfa-2a. Mean methadone pharmacokinetic parameters were 10% to 15% higher after 4 weeks of peginterferon alfa-2a treatment, compared to baseline. Methadone did not significantly alter the pharmacokinetics of peginterferon alfa-2a, compared to 6 chronic hepatitis patients not receiving methadone.

Lab Interference: None recognized.

Patient Information: Caution patients who develop dizziness, confusion, somnolence, and fatigue to avoid driving or operating machinery. Advise patients to report any sign or symptom of depression or suicidal ideation to their prescribing physician. A patient should self-inject peginterferon alfa-2a only if the physician determines that it is appropriate, the patient agrees to medical follow-up as necessary, and training in proper injection technique has been provided in the illustrated medication guide.

Pharmaceutical Characteristics

Concentration: Either 180 or 360 mcg/mL of peginterferon alfa-2a

Packaging:

Vial: 1.2 mL per single-use clear glass vial delivering 180 mcg/mL of drug product (NDC#: 00004-0350-09)

Syringe: Four 180 mcg per 0.5 mL clear glass syringes with four 27-gauge, ½-inch needles and 4 alcohol swabs (00004-0352-39) or without alcohol swabs (00004-0357-30)

Autoinjector: One 180 mcg per 0.5 mL *ProClick* single-use autoinjector (00004-0365-09); four 180 mcg per 0.5 mL *ProClick* single-use autoinjectors (00004-0365-30). One 135 mcg per 0.5 mL *ProClick* single-use autoinjector (00004-0360-09), four 135 mcg per 0.5 mL *ProClick* single-use autoinjectors (00004-0360-30).

Pegasys can be used in combination with *Copegus* (ribavirin), 200 mg oral tablets, light pink to pink-colored, oval-shaped, film-coated, engraved with RIB 200 on 1 side and Roche on the other side. Packaged in bottles of 168 tablets (00004-0086-94). Store tablets at room temperature. Read product labeling before use.

Doseform: Solutions

Appearance: Colorless to light-yellow solution.

Solvent: Buffered saline

Adjuvant: None

Preservative: Benzyl alcohol 10 mg/mL

Allergens: None

Excipients: Sodium chloride 8 mg, 0.05 mg of polysorbate 80, sodium acetate trihydrate 2.62 mg, and acetic acid 0.05 mg per mL

pH: 5.5 to 6.5

Shelf Life: Expires within an unspecified period of time.

Storage/Stability: Store at 2° to 8°C (36° to 46°F). Discard if frozen. Product can tolerate up to 24 hours at controlled room temperature (25°C [77°F]). Contact the manufacturer regarding exposure to extreme temperatures. Shipping data not provided.

Handling: Do not shake. Protect solution from light. Discard any unused portion.

Production Process: Interferon alfa-2a is obtained from bacterial fermentation of a strain of *E. coli* bearing a genetically engineered plasmid containing an interferon gene from human leukocytes. The interferon is then conjugated to a single-branched bis-monomethoxy PEG chain.

Media: Recombinant *E. coli*

Other Information

First Licensed: October 24, 2002

References: Robins GW, Scott LJ, Keating GM. Peginterferon-alpha-2a (40kD): a review of its use in the management of patients with chronic hepatitis B. *Drugs.* 2005;65(6):809-825.

Grace MJ, Cutler DL, Bordens RW. Pegylated IFNs for chronic hepatitis C: an update. *Expert Opin Drug Deliv.* 2005;2(2):219-226.

Interferon Alfa-2b (Recombinant)

Interferons

Name:
Intron A

Manufacturer:
Merck, under license from Biogen Idec

Synonyms: IFN2αb, SCH 30500

Comparison: The various interferon alpha products are not generically interchangeable because variations in dosage, routes of administration, and adverse reactions exist among the different brands. Do not use different brands of interferon alpha in any single treatment regimen.

Immunologic Characteristics

Antigen Source: Interferon alfa expressed from recombinant *Escherichia coli* bacteria

Viability: Not viable, but immunologically active

Antigenic Form: Interferon, human leukocyte

Antigenic Type: Protein. A water-soluble protein of 165 amino acids, with an approximate molecular weight of 19,271 daltons. Possesses an arginine molecule at position 23 and a histidine molecule at position 34.

Strains: Interferon alfa-2b

Use Characteristics

Indications:

Hairy cell leukemia (HCL): For treatment of patients 18 years of age and older. Interferon alfa-2b can produce clinically meaningful regression or stabilization of this disease, both in previously splenectomized and non-splenectomized patients. Prior to initiation of therapy, and periodically during treatment, perform tests to quantify peripheral blood hemoglobin, platelets, granulocytes, hairy cells, and hairy cells in the bone marrow.

Condylomata acuminata (venereal or genital warts): For intralesional treatment of selected cases involving external surfaces of the genital and perianal areas. Therapy is particularly useful for patients who do not respond satisfactorily to other treatment methods (eg, podophyllin resin, surgery, cryotherapy, chemotherapy, laser therapy) or whose lesions are more readily treatable by interferon alfa-2b than by other treatments. The use of interferon alfa-2b in adolescents has not been studied. Consider monitoring for leukopenia and elevated serum liver enzymes (eg, AST).

AIDS-related Kaposi sarcoma: For treatment of selected patients 18 years of age and older. Studies have demonstrated a greater likelihood of response in patients without systemic symptoms, who have limited lymphadenopathy and a relatively intact immune system (as indicated by total CD4 count). Perform lesion measurements and blood counts prior to initiating therapy and periodically during treatment. Do not use interferon alfa-2b in patients with rapidly progressive visceral disease.

Chronic hepatitis B (HBV) infection: For treatment of chronic hepatitis B virus infection in adults and children 1 year of age and older with compensated liver disease and HBV replication. Patients must have been HBsAg-positive for at least 6 months and have HBV replication (serum HBeAg-positive) with elevated serum ALT levels. Prior to initiation of interferon therapy, perform a liver biopsy to establish the presence of chronic hepatitis and extent of liver damage. Consider the following criteria for interferon therapy of this infection: No history of hepatic encephalopathy, variceal bleeding, ascites or other signs of clinical decompensation, normal bilirubin levels, stable albumin levels, prothrombin time prolonged less than 3 seconds, WBC at least 4,000 cells/mm^2, and platelets at least

100,000 cells/mm^2. Evaluate CBC and platelet counts prior to initiating interferon therapy to establish baseline values for monitoring potential toxicity. Repeat these tests at treatment weeks 1, 2, 4, 8, 12, and 16. Evaluate liver function tests, including serum ALT, albumin, and bilirubin at these same times. Evaluate HBeAg, HBsAg, and ALT at the end of therapy as well as 3 and 6 months after therapy, because patients may become virologic responders during the 6-month period following the end of treatment.

Chronic hepatitis C: For treatment of patients 18 years of age and older with compensated liver disease who have a history of blood or blood-product exposure or are hepatitis C-antibody positive. Chronicity is established by elevated ALT levels for at least 6 months. Exclude patients with other causes of hepatitis, including autoimmune hepatitis.

Consider the following criteria for interferon therapy of this infection: No history of hepatic encephalopathy, variceal bleeding, ascites, or other signs of decompensation, prothrombin time prolonged less than 3 seconds, WBC at least 3,000/mm^3, and platelets at least 70,000/mm^3. Serum albumin and serum creatinine should be normal or near normal. Serum bilirubin should not exceed 2 mg/dL. Perform a liver biopsy to establish the diagnosis of chronic hepatitis. Prior to initiation of therapy, evaluate CBC and platelet counts to establish baselines for monitoring potential toxicity. Repeat these tests at weeks 1 and 2 following initiation of therapy and monthly thereafter. Evaluate ALT levels after 2, 16, and 24 weeks of therapy to assess response to therapy. Do not give interferon alfa-2b for treatment of patients with decompensated liver disease or immune-suppressed transplant recipients, because safety and efficacy studies have not been conducted in such patients.

Malignant melanoma: As an adjuvant treatment to surgery in adults with malignant melanoma who are free of disease but at high risk for systemic recurrence, within 56 days of surgery.

Follicular lymphoma: For initial treatment of clinically aggressive follicular non-Hodgkin lymphoma in conjunction with anthracycline-containing combination chemotherapy in patients 18 years of age and older. Efficacy of interferon alfa-2b in patients with low-grade, low-tumor burden follicular non-Hodgkin lymphoma has not been demonstrated.

Unlabeled Uses: Research in progress is assessing the role of interferon alfa-2b in treatment of the following: Superficial bladder cancer in situ (orphan designation August 10, 1988); basal cell carcinoma; chronic delta hepatitis (orphan designation May 4, 1990); acute hepatitis B (orphan designation November 17, 1988); delta hepatitis; chronic myelogenous leukemia (CML, orphan designation June 22, 1987); HIV infection in combination with zidovudine; respiratory (laryngeal) papillomatosis (orphan designation August 17, 1988); metastatic renal cell carcinoma (orphan designation June 22, 1987); ovarian carcinoma (orphan designation August 3, 1987); primary malignant brain tumors (orphan designation May 13, 1988); invasive carcinoma of the cervix (orphan designation April 18, 1988); mycosis fungoides (Sézary syndrome); and other conditions.

Various interferon alpha preparations are being investigated in the treatment of the following viral infections: Cutaneous warts, cytomegaloviruses, herpes keratoconjunctivitis, herpes simplex, rhinoviruses (1 set of causes of the "common cold"), vaccinia, and varicella-zoster. Investigational use of interferon alfa has shown significant activity in the treatment of the following conditions: Carcinoid tumor, cutaneous T-cell lymphoma, and essential thrombocythemia. Limited activity has been demonstrated in acute leukemia, chronic lymphocytic leukemia, Hodgkin disease, malignant gliomas, nasopharyngeal carcinoma, and osteosarcoma. Interferon alfa is also being investigated in the treatment of life-threatening hemangiomas of infancy and multiple sclerosis.

Limitations: No activity has been demonstrated by various interferon alpha preparations in breast cancer, colorectal carcinoma, gastric carcinoma, lung carcinoma, pancreatic carcinoma, prostatic carcinoma, or soft-tissue carcinoma.

Interferon Alfa-2b (Recombinant)

Contraindications:

Absolute: History of hypersensitivity to interferon alpha or any component of the injection.

Relative: Do not treat patients with a preexisting psychiatric condition or a history of severe psychiatric disorder with interferon alfa-2b. Discontinue interferon therapy for any patient developing severe depression during treatment. Patients with preexisting thyroid abnormalities may be treated if thyroid-stimulating hormone (TSH) levels can be maintained in the normal range by medication. Discontinue therapy in patients developing thyroid abnormalities during treatment whose thyroid function cannot be normalized by medication.

Immunodeficiency: Use may be indicated in certain immunodeficient conditions.

Elderly: No specific information is available about the use of interferon alfa-2b in elderly patients.

Fertility Impairment: Interferon alfa-2b can affect the menstrual cycle and decrease serum estradiol and progesterone levels. Do not give fertile women interferon alpha unless they use an effective form of contraception during therapy. Use interferon alpha with caution in fertile men.

Pregnancy: Category C. Use only if clearly needed. Recombinant interferons alfa-2a and alfa-2b induced a statistically significant increase in abortifacient activity in rhesus monkeys when given at tens or hundreds of times the standard human dose. Teratogenic activity in rhesus monkeys was not observed. Use interferon alpha in pregnant women only if the potential benefit justifies the potential risk to the fetus.

Lactation: It is not known if interferon alfa-2b is excreted in breast milk. In mice, murine interferons are excreted in milk. Because of the potential for serious adverse effects from interferon alfa-2b in nursing infants, decide whether to discontinue nursing or to discontinue the drug, taking into account the importance of the drug to the mother.

Children: For most of the indications for this drug, there is no experience in children and use is not typically recommended. The exception is in chronic hepatitis B virus infection, in which safety and efficacy for children 1 year of age and older have been established. Interferon alpha can affect the menstrual cycle and decrease serum estradiol and progesterone levels in females. Consider carefully whether to treat the adolescent patient.

Adverse Reactions: Most of the adverse reactions reported with interferon alfa-2b administration were mild to moderate and diminished in severity and number with continued therapy. Adverse reactions reported in patients with various dosage regimens included:

Malignant melanoma patients: In malignant melanoma, interferon alfa-2b dosing was modified because of adverse events in 65% of patients. Therapy was discontinued because of adverse events in 8% of patients during induction and 18% of patients during maintenance. The following is a list of most frequently reported adverse reactions: Fatigue (96%); neutropenia (92%); fever (81%); myalgia (75%); anorexia (69%); vomiting or nausea (66%); increased AST (63%); headache (62%); chills (54%); depression (40%); diarrhea (35%); alopecia (29%); altered taste sensation (24%); dizziness or vertigo (23%); anemia (22%); bleeding (8%). Adverse reactions classified as severe or life-threatening were recorded in 66% and 14% of interferon alfa-2b treated patients, respectively. Severe adverse reactions in treated patients included neutropenia or leukopenia (26%); fatigue (23%); fever (18%); myalgia, headache (17%); chills (16%); and increased AST (14%). Lethal hepatotoxicity occurred in 2 treated patients early in the clinical trial.

Cerebrovascular: Ischemic and hemorrhagic cerebrovascular events have occurred in patients treated with interferon alpha-based therapies. Events occurred in patients with few or no reported risk factors for stroke, including patients younger than 45 years of age. Because these are spontaneous reports, estimates of frequency cannot be made, and a causal relationship between therapies and these events is difficult to establish.

Cardiovascular: Cardiomyopathy, cardiac failure, atrial fibrillation, dysrhythmias, tachycardia, bradycardia, palpitations, extrasystoles, hypertension, postural hypotension, peripheral ischemia (less than 5%).

Cardiovascular adverse experiences may include significant hypotension, dysrhythmia, or tachycardia of 150 bpm and above. Hypotension may occur during administration or up to 2 days after therapy and may require supportive therapy including fluid replacement to maintain intravascular volume. Transient reversible cardiomyopathy has occurred. Supraventricular dysrhythmias occurred rarely and appeared to be correlated with preexisting conditions and prior therapy with cardiotoxic agents (eg, doxorubicin). These adverse experiences were controlled by modifying the dose or discontinuing treatment, but may require specific additional therapy. Closely monitor patients with a recent history of myocardial infarction or previous or current dysrhythmic disorder.

CNS: Fatigue (18% to 96%); depression (6% to 40%); dizziness (7% to 24%); paresthesia (3% to 21%); impaired concentration (3% to 14%); amnesia (14%); confusion (3% to 12%); hypoesthesia, irritability (10%); anxiety (1% to 9%); sleep disturbances (4% to 5%); tremor, poor coordination, extrapyramidal disorder, paresis, decreased libido, migraine, impaired consciousness, neuropathy, gait disturbance, aphasia, syncope, nervousness, agitation, emotional lability, vertigo, apathy, paroniria, neurosis (less than 5%).

CNS effects may be manifested by depression, confusion, and other alterations of mental status. More significant obtundation and coma have been observed in some patients, usually the elderly, treated at higher doses; these effects are usually rapidly reversible. Discontinuation of interferon alfa-2b therapy may be required. Narcotics, hypnotics, or sedatives may be used concurrently with caution.

Dermatologic: Alopecia (8% to 31%); rash (4% to 25%); increased sweating (4% to 21%); burning, itching, pain (3% to 20%); pruritus (4% to 11%); dry skin (9% to 10%); facial edema (less than 1% to 10%); dermatitis (8%); purpura, urticaria, acne, erythema, skin discoloration, vitiligo, peripheral edema, cyanosis, nail disorder, furunculosis, epidermal necrolysis, photosensitivity reaction, cold and clammy skin (less than 5%).

Interferon alfa-2b has been reported to exacerbate preexisting psoriasis. Use interferon alfa-2b in these patients only if the potential benefit justifies the potential risk.

GI: Anorexia (9% to 69%); nausea (1% to 66%); diarrhea (2% to 45%); vomiting (1% to 32%); dry mouth (4% to 28%); change in taste (10% to 24%); abdominal pain (4% to 21%); gingivitis (14%); constipation (1% to 14%); stomatitis, flatulence, dyspepsia, GI hemorrhage, eructation, cachexia, esophagitis, excessive thirst, excessive salivation, melena, rectal bleeding, oral leukoplakia, gum hyperplasia, dysphagia (less than 5%).

GU: Gynecomastia, virilism, uterine bleeding, menorrhagia, nocturia, polyuria, hematuria, micturition disorder, leukorrhea, impotence, herpes simplex (less than 5%).

Hepatic: Liver dysfunction, jaundice (less than 5%).

Hypersensitivity: Acute serious hypersensitivity reactions (eg, urticaria, angioedema, bronchoconstriction, anaphylaxis) have been reported rarely. If such an acute reaction occurs, discontinue the drug immediately and start appropriate medical therapy. Transient rashes have occurred in some patients following injection but have not necessitated treatment interruption.

Lab test abnormalities: Elevated AST and ALT; reductions in granulocyte and platelet counts; increased BUN (less than 5%). These abnormalities are usually mild to moderate and transient. Severe abnormalities are usually rapidly reversible upon cessation or reduction of interferon alfa-2b therapy.

A transient increase in ALT 2 or more times baseline values can occur during interferon alfa-2b for chronic hepatitis B. In clinical trials, this flare generally occurred 8 to 12 weeks after beginning therapy and was more frequent in responders than in nonresponders. Elevations in bilirubin of 3 mg/dL or more during therapy occurred infrequently. When

Interferon Alfa-2b (Recombinant)

ALT flare occurs, interferon alfa-2b can usually be continued unless signs and symptoms of liver failure are noted. During ALT flare, monitor clinical symptoms and liver function tests including ALT, prothrombin time, alkaline phosphatase, albumin, and bilirubin at approximately 2-week intervals.

Musculoskeletal: Myalgia (3% to 75%); arthralgia (8% to 19%); ataxia, hypertonia, leg cramps, arthrosis, right upper quadrant pain, hyperkinesia (less than 5%).

Ophthalmic: Visual disturbances (7%); eye pain, lacrimal gland disorder, conjunctivitis, photophobia (less than 5%).

Respiratory: Dyspnea (1% to 34%); coughing (6% to 31%); pharyngitis (1% to 31%); sinusitis (21%); nasal congestion (less than 1% to 10%); bronchospasm, wheezing, pneumonia, pleural pain, epistaxis (less than 5%).

Special Senses: Hearing disorder, tinnitus, earache, parosmia, speech disorder (less than 5%).

Miscellaneous: Fever (3% to 81%); unspecified symptoms (6% to 79%); asthenia (4% to 63%); headache (4% to 62%); chills (45% to 54%); rigors (14% to 30%); chest pain (1% to 28%); back pain (6% to 19%); unspecified pain (3% to 18%); moniliasis (17%); malaise (14%); weight decrease (less than 1% to 13%); lymphadenopathy, nonherpetic cold sores, abscess, hypercalcemia, weight loss, flushing, hot flashes, dehydration, sepsis, coma, viral and fungal infection (less than 5%).

Because of the fever and other flu-like symptoms associated with interferon alfa-2b administration, use cautiously in patients with debilitating medical conditions, such as those with a history of cardiovascular disease (eg, unstable angina, uncontrolled CHF), pulmonary disease (eg, COPD), or diabetes mellitus prone to ketoacidosis. Also observe caution in patients with coagulation disorders (eg, thrombophlebitis, pulmonary embolism) or severe myelosuppression.

Pharmacologic & Dosing Characteristics

Dosage: Variations in dosage, routes of administration, and adverse reactions exist among different brands of interferon. Therefore, do not use different brands of interferon in any single treatment regimen. Dosages also vary for each indication.

HCL: 2 million units/m^2 IM or subcutaneously 3 times/week for up to 6 months. Responding patients may benefit from continued treatment. Higher doses are not recommended. Normalization of 1 or more hematologic variable usually begins within 2 months of initiation of therapy. Improvement in all 3 hematologic variables (eg, red blood cells, white blood cells, platelets) may require more than 6 months of therapy. Maintain this dosage regimen unless the disease progresses rapidly or severe intolerance is manifested. If severe adverse reactions develop, reduce the dose by 50% or temporarily discontinue the drug until the adverse reactions abate. If persistent or recurrent intolerance develops after dosage adjustment, or if disease progresses, discontinue interferon alfa-2b treatment.

Condylomata acuminata: Reconstitute the 10 million unit vial with just 1 mL of diluent to provide the proper concentration of interferon alfa-2b for the treatment of condylomata; do not use more than 1 mL of the diluent provided in the package. Inject 1 million units/ 0.1 mL into each lesion 3 times/week on alternate days for 3 weeks.

Administer the injection intralesionally, using a tuberculin or similar syringe and a 25- to 30-gauge needle. Direct the needle at the center of the base of the wart and at an angle almost parallel to the plane of the skin (approximating the procedure for the commonly used PPD intradermal skin test). This will deliver the interferon to the dermal core of the lesion, infiltrating the lesion and causing a small induration. Take care not to go beneath the lesion too deeply; avoid subcutaneous injection, because this area is below the base of the lesion. Do not inject too superficially, because this will result in possible leakage, infiltrating only the keratinized layer and not the dermal core.

To reduce side effects, give interferon alfa-2b in the evening, when possible. Acetaminophen may be administered at the time of injection to alleviate some of the potential side effects.

The maximum response usually occurs 4 to 8 weeks after initiation of the first treatment course. When 12 to 16 weeks after the initial treatment course have passed and results are not satisfactory, give a second course of treatment using the above dosage schedule, providing that clinical symptoms and signs or changes in laboratory parameters do not preclude such a course of action. Patients with 6 or more condylomata may receive sequential courses of treatment at the above dosage schedule, treating up to 5 additional condylomata per course of treatment. Patients with more than 10 condylomata may receive additional sequences of treatment. Do not use containers other than the 10 million unit package for intralesional treatment because the dilution required for intralesional injection would result in a hypertonic solution or an inappropriate concentration.

AIDS-related Kaposi sarcoma: 30 million units/m^2 3 times/week subcutaneously or IM. Maintain the dosage regimen unless the disease progresses rapidly or severe intolerance develops. When patients initiate therapy at 30 million units/m^2 3 times/week, the average dose tolerated at the end of 12 weeks of therapy is 110 million units/week and 75 million units/week after 24 weeks. When disease stabilization or a response to treatment occurs, continue treatment until there is no further evidence of tumor or until discontinuation is required by evidence of a severe opportunistic infection or adverse effect. If severe adverse reactions develop, reduce the dose by 50% or temporarily discontinue treatment until adverse reactions abate.

Chronic hepatitis B: 30 to 35 million units/week subcutaneously or IM, either as 5 million units/day or 10 million units 3 times/week, for 16 weeks. If severe adverse reactions or laboratory abnormalities develop during interferon alfa-2b therapy, halve or discontinue the dose, if appropriate, until the adverse reactions abate. If intolerance persists after dose adjustment, discontinue therapy. Therapy has been resumed at up to 100% of the initial dose when granulocyte or platelet counts returned to normal or baseline values.

Chronic hepatitis C: 3 million units 3 times/week subcutaneously or IM. Normalization of ALT levels may occur in some patients as early as 2 weeks after initiation of therapy. Give patients responding to interferon alfa-2b therapy with a reduction in ALT level 6 months (24 weeks) of treatment. The optimal dose and duration of therapy are under investigation. Treatment for 18 to 24 months may be appropriate. Patients who relapse following interferon alfa-2b therapy may be retreated with the same dosage regimen to which they had responded previously. Patients who do not normalize their ALT values after 16 weeks of therapy rarely achieve a sustained response with extension of treatment. Consider discontinuing interferon therapy in these patients.

Moderate to severe adverse experiences may necessitate modification of the patient's dosage regimen (eg, a 50% reduction) or, in some cases, termination of therapy until adverse reactions abate. If persistent or recurrent intolerance develops following dosage adjustment or if disease progresses, discontinue treatment with interferon alfa-2b.

Malignant melanoma: Begin with induction treatment of 20 million units/m^2 5 consecutive days/week for 4 weeks as an IV infusion. Follow with maintenance therapy of 10 million units/m^2 3 times/week for 48 weeks as an subcutaneous injection. In the clinical trial, the median daily dose tolerated by patients was 19.1 million units/m^2 during the induction phase and 9.1 million units/m^2 during the maintenance phase.

Temporarily discontinue treatment if granulocyte counts fall below 500 cells/mm^3 or ALT/AST rises above 5 times the upper limit of normal. After adverse reactions abate, restart interferon alfa-2b treatment at 50% of the previous dose. If intolerance persists after dose adjustments or if granulocyte counts fall below 250 cells/mm^3 or ALT/AST rises above 10 times normal, discontinue interferon alfa-2b treatment. In the clinical trial, patients were able to achieve clinical benefit in conjunction with appropriate dose modifications. Maintain therapy for 1 year unless the disease progresses.

Follicular lymphoma: 5 million units subcutaneously 3 times/week for up to 18 months in conjunction with an anthracycline-containing chemotherapy regimen. In published reports, doses of myelosuppressive drugs were reduced by 25% from those used in a full-dose CHOP regimen and cycle length increased by 33% (eg, from 21 to 28 days) when an alpha interferon was added to the regimen. Modify the dose if serious toxicity occurs. For example, delay chemotherapy if either the neutrophil count is less than 1500 cells/mm^3 or the platelet count is less than 75,000 cells/mm^3. Temporarily interrupt interferon alfa-2b therapy for a neutrophil count less than 1,000 cells/mm^3 or a platelet count less than 50,000 cells/mm^3. Reduce the interferon dose by 50% to 2.5 million units 3 times/week for a neutrophil count between 1,000 and 1,500 cells/mm^3. Resuming the initial interferon alfa-2b dose has been tolerated after resolution of hematologic toxicity. Discontinue interferon alfa-2b therapy if AST exceeds 5 times the upper limit of normal or if serum creatinine is more than 2 mg/dL.

Route: The 3 million and 5 million units packages are for IM or subcutaneous injection only. The 10 million unit package is for IM, subcutaneous, IV, or intralesional injection. The 25 million and 50 million unit packages are for IM or subcutaneous injection or IV infusion. Do not give IM to patients with platelet counts more than 50,000 cells/mm^3. Administration by continuous or intermittent infusion and ophthalmic and intravaginal administration have also been described.

Missed Doses: Missing a dose of interferon alfa-2b will not have immediate consequences. Administer the missed dose as soon as possible. If more than 1 dose is missed, advise the clinician managing therapy.

Laboratory Tests: In addition to those tests normally required for monitoring patients, perform the following laboratory tests for all patients on interferon alfa-2b therapy prior to beginning treatment and then periodically thereafter:

(1) Standard hematologic tests (including CBC and differential as well as platelet counts) and

(2) blood chemistries (eg, electrolytes, liver function tests).

Give electrocardiograms prior to and during the course of treatment to patients with preexisting cardiac abnormalities or in advanced stages of cancer. Baseline and periodic chest radiographs may be indicated to assess the risk of cardiomyopathy.

Efficacy:

HCL: There was a depression of circulating red blood cells, white blood cells, and platelets during the first 1 to 2 months of treatment with interferon alfa-2b. Subsequently, most splenectomized and nonsplenectomized patients treated with interferon alfa-2b achieved substantial and sustained improvements in granulocytes, platelets, and hemoglobin levels in 75% of treated patients. At least some improvement occurred in 90%. Interferon alfa-2b also resulted in a decrease in bone-marrow hypercellularity and hairy cell infiltrates. The proportion of patients with a hairy-cell index (bone marrow cellularity multiplied by percentage of hairy cell infiltrate) was at least 50% in 87% of patients at the beginning of the study, but declined to 25% after 6 months of treatment and to 15% after 1 year. The percentage of patients with hairy cell leukemia who required red blood cell or platelet transfusions decreased significantly during treatment, as did the fraction of patients with confirmed or serious infections, as granulocyte counts improved. In nonsplenectomized patients, reversal of splenomegaly and of abnormalities in blood cell counts attributable to hypersplenism were also noted. When therapy among responding patients was continued for 6 months beyond the initial 12 months of therapy, 3% relapsed, compared with 18% of patients not treated for the additional 6 months.

Reduced risk of major complications of hairy cell leukemia (eg, serious infections, bleeding diatheses, transfusion requirements) were apparent within 3 months of initiation of treatment in comparisons of interferon alfa-2b-treated patients with a control group. No deaths occurred in patients treated with interferon alfa-2b during the subsequent 9 months of treatment and follow-up, while the mortality rate in the control group was 20% in the same time interval, based on probability-of-survival analysis. Subsequent follow-up (median observation, 40 months) demonstrated an overall survival of 87.8%. In a comparable historical control group (median observation, 24 months), overall median survival was approximately 40%.

Condylomata acuminata: Interferon alfa-2b is significantly more effective than placebo, as measured by disappearance of lesions, decreases in lesion size, and by an overall change in disease status. Among patients treated with interferon alfa-2b, 42% completely cleared all treated lesions, in contrast to 17% of placebo recipients. In another study, 81% of patients experiencing complete clearing of all treated lesions remained cleared 16 weeks after treatment began. Patients who did not achieve total clearing of all treated lesions had the same lesions treated with a second course of therapy. After the second course, 38% to 67% had clearing of all treated lesions. The overall proportion of patients who had cleared all treated lesions after 2 courses of treatment ranged from 57% to 85%. Patients having condylomata for a shorter duration had better responses to treatment with interferon alfa-2b than those with lesions of a longer duration. There was no difference in response to treatment of penile, vulvar, or perianal condylomata or of condylomata appearing in heavily or lightly keratinized areas.

Another study involved 97 patients in whom 3 lesions were treated with either intralesional injections of 1.5 million units of interferon alfa-2b per lesion followed by a topical application of 25% podophyllin, or a topical application of podophyllin alone. Treatment was given once a week for 3 weeks. Combination treatment was significantly more effective than podophyllin alone, as determined by the number of patients whose lesions cleared. This significant difference in response was evident after the second treatment and continued through 8 weeks after treatment. At the time of the patient's best response, 67% (33 of 49) of patients treated with both drugs had all 3 treated lesions clear, while 42% of podophyllin-treated patients had all 3 lesions clear.

AIDS-related Kaposi sarcoma: Interferon alfa-2b produced objective responses that were significantly greater in patients who were asymptomatic (ie, afebrile and without weight loss) than in those with systemic symptoms (44% to 57% vs 7% to 23%). The median time to response was 2 months, and the median duration of response was 3 to 5 months for asymptomatic patients, with 1 month to response and duration of 1 month in symptomatic patients. Similarly, the likelihood of response was greater in patients with relatively intact immune systems, as assessed by higher baseline T_4-lymphocyte (CD4) counts or T_4/T_8 ratios. The survival time was also longer in patients with T_4 counts more than 200 cells/mm^3 (median, 30.7 months) than in patients with lower T_4 counts (8.9 months) and greater in responders to therapy (median, 22.6 months) compared with nonresponders (9.7 months).

Chronic hepatitis B: Compared with untreated controls, a significantly greater proportion of interferon alfa-2b-treated patients lost HBeAg 1 to 6 months after therapy (7% vs 39% to 48%). Of responding patients who lost HBsAg, 58% did so 1 to 6 months after treatment. Similar normalization of serum ALT values was observed (12% vs 42% to 46%). The response to interferon alfa-2b was durable. Among 64 responding patients followed for 1.1 to 6.6 years after treatment, 95% remained serum HBeAg-negative, and 49% lost serum HBsAg.

Chronic hepatitis C: Interferon alfa-2b was shown to produce a statistically significant improvement in serum ALT levels. Of responders to therapy, 70% achieved a reduction in ALT levels to normal, 18% to near normal, and 12% achieved a partial response. Statistically significant histological improvement was also seen, evaluated by comparison of pre- and post-treatment liver biopsies. The improvement was primarily due to decreases in severity of necrosis and degeneration in the lobular and periportal regions. In patients with complete responses after 6 months of treatment, responses were less often sustained if interferon alfa-2b was discontinued (30%) than if it was continued for 18 to 24 months (56%). Of patients treated for 18 to 24 months, 24% achieved a durable sustained response, compared with 12.5% of patients treated for 6 months. Improvement in liver-cell inflammation and death rates was also seen with prolonged treatment.

Malignant melanoma: Safety and efficacy of interferon alfa-2b was evaluated as an adjuvant to surgical treatment in patients with melanoma who were free of disease after surgery, but at high risk for systemic recurrence. These included patients with lesions of Breslow thickness greater than 4 mm, or patients with lesions of any Breslow thickness with primary or recurrent nodal involvement. In a randomized, controlled trial involving 280 patients, 143 patients received interferon alfa-2b therapy at 20 million units/m^2 IV 5 times/week for 4 weeks (induction phase) followed by 10 million units/m^2 subcutaneously 3 times/week for 48 weeks (maintenance phase). Interferon alfa-2b therapy began up to 56 days after surgical resection. The remaining 137 patients were simply observed. Interferon alfa-2b therapy produced a significant increase in relapse-free and overall survival. Median time to relapse for the interferon group was 1.72 years vs 0.98 years for the observation group ($P < 0.01$). The estimated 5-year relapse-free survival rate, using the Kaplan-Meier method, was 37% for treated patients, compared with 26% for observation patients. Median overall survival time was 3.82 years vs 2.78 years, respectively ($P < 0.047$). The estimated 5-year overall survival rate was 46% vs 37%, respectively.

Follicular lymphoma: Safety and efficacy were evaluated in conjunction with CHVP chemotherapy (ie, cyclophosphamide, doxorubicin, teniposide, prednisone) as initial treatment in patients with clinically aggressive, large tumor burden, stage III/IV follicular non-Hodgkin lymphoma. Patients receiving CHVP plus interferon alfa-2b for 18 months had a significantly longer progression-free survival (2.9 vs 1.5 years), compared with CHVP alone. After a median follow-up of 6.1 years, the median survival of patients treated with CHVP alone was 5.5 years, whereas medial survival for combined therapy had not yet been reached.

Onset: Unknown

Duration: Unknown

Pharmacokinetics:

Absorption: The mean serum concentrations of interferon alfa-2b following IM and subcutaneous injections were comparable following 5 million units/m^2 doses. The peak concentrations achieved were 18 to 116 units/mL, occurring 3 to 12 hours after an IM or subcutaneous dose. After IV administration, serum concentrations peaked at 135 to 273 units/mL by the end of the infusion.

Elimination: The elimination half-lives were 2 to 3 hours after IM or subcutaneous administration and approximately 2 hours after IV infusion. Serum concentrations fell below detectable levels by 16 hours after the IM and subcutaneous injections. Concentrations declined at a slightly more rapid rate after IV administration, compared with the IM or subcutaneous routes, becoming undetectable 4 hours after infusion. Urine concentrations after a single 5 million units/m^2 dose were not detectable following administration by any of the parenteral routes. Alpha and beta interferons are metabolized or degraded primarily in the kidney. Catabolism of interferon is postulated to occur at the brush border or in the lysosomes of the tubular epithelium. Interferon alfa-2b is not dialyzed by either hemodialysis or peritoneal dialysis.

Serum neutralizing activity: Neutralizing IgG antibodies developed in less than 3% of 423 cancer patients, none of 90 HCL patients, and 15 of hepatitis C patients treated with parenteral interferon alfa-2b. Following intralesional therapy, 0.8% of recipients developed neutralizing antibodies. The clinical significance of these findings is unknown. In 1 analysis, 10 of 144 (6.9%) patients with hepatitis B or hepatitis C developed neutralizing antibodies against interferon alfa-2b.

Mechanism: Interferons exert their cellular effects by binding to specific membrane receptors on cell surfaces. The results of several studies suggest that once bound to the cell membrane, interferon initiates a complex sequence of intracellular events, including the induction of certain enzymes. This process is probably responsible, at least in part, for the various cellular responses to interferon, including inhibition of virus replication in virus-infected cells, suppression of cell proliferation and such immunomodulating activities as enhancement of the phagocytic activity of macrophages and augmentation of the specific cytotoxicity of lymphocytes for target cells.

Other postulated mechanisms include an effect on cell differentiation, including phenotype reversion, which may help to reestablish normal growth controls in cancer cells, and increased expression of Class I histocompatibility antigen, which may render a virus-infected cell susceptible to killing. Interferons may have a regulatory or suppressive effect on expression of oncogenes (genes that transform a host cell from a normal to a cancerous state). Some or all of these activities might contribute to interferon's therapeutic effects.

Drug Interactions: There may be synergistic adverse effects between interferon alfa-2b and zidovudine (AZT). Patients receiving both drugs have had a higher incidence of neutropenia than expected with zidovudine alone. Careful monitoring of WBC counts is indicated in all myelosuppressed patients and in all patients receiving other myelosuppressive medications. The effects of interferon alfa-2b when combined with other drugs used in the treatment of AIDS-related diseases is unknown.

Supraventricular dysrhythmias occurred rarely during interferon alfa-2b therapy and appeared to be correlated with preexisting conditions and prior therapy with cardiotoxic agents (eg, doxorubicin). These adverse experiences were controlled by modifying the dose or discontinuing treatment, but may require specific additional therapy.

Interferon alfa-2a can affect specific microsomal enzyme systems. Interferon alfa-2a has reduced hepatic clearance of theophylline or aminophylline by 33% to 81% in 8 of 9 subjects, apparently through inhibition of cytochrome P-450 microsomal enzymes. The clinical significance of this interaction has not been determined.

Interferons may inhibit the induction of an adequate antibody response following immunization with live virus vaccines (eg, measles, mumps, rubella, varicella, poliovirus). Avoid concurrent use.

As with other drugs administered by IM injection, give interferon alfa-2b with caution to patients receiving anticoagulant therapy.

Patient Information: The most common adverse experiences occurring with interferon alfa-2b therapy are flu-like symptoms, such as fever, headache, fatigue, anorexia, nausea, or vomiting, which appear to decrease in severity as treatment continues. Some of these symptoms may be minimized by bedtime administration. Acetaminophen may be used to prevent or partially alleviate fever and headache. Keep patients well hydrated, especially during the initial stages of treatment. Advise patients not to adjust the injected dose, except at the direction of the prescriber.

Pharmaceutical Characteristics

Concentration: 5 million, 6 million, 10 million, 15 million, 18 million, 25 million, or 50 million units/mL, after reconstitution according to instructions. Assuming interferon

Interferon Alfa-2b (Recombinant)

alfa-2b activity of 2.6 × 10⁸ units/mg protein, the 18 million or 50 million unit vials contain 125 mcg and 250 mcg protein, respectively.

Quality Assay: At least 90% of the molecules do not contain N-terminal methionine, an amino acid residue.

Packaging: 3, 5, 10, 18, 25, 50 million units packages of various volumes. Certain packages are inappropriate for some diagnoses or routes of administration. The multidose pen should not be used for intralesional injection. Solution forms should not be used for IV infusion. Consult product labeling for details.

Powder forms: Multidose vial of 10 million units powder with 2 mL vial of diluent (00085-0571-02); multidose vial of 18 million units powder with 1 mL vial of diluent (00085-1110-01); multidose vial of 50 million units powder with 1 mL vial of diluent (00085-0539-01).

Solution forms: 18 million units per 3 mL multidose vial (00085-1168-01); 25 million units/ 2.5 mL multidose vial (00085-1133-01).

Multidose pens: 3 million units/dose multidose pen containing 22.5 million units/1.5 mL, delivering 3 million units/0.2 mL dose (00085-1242-01); 5 million units/dose multidose pen containing 27.5 million units per 1.5 mL, delivering 5 million units per 0.2 mL dose (00085-1235-01); 10 million units/dose multidose pen containing 75 million units per 1.5 mL, delivering 10 million units per 0.2 mL dose (00085-1254-01). Each 6-dose pen is provided with 6 disposable 8 mm, 30-gauge needles and alcohol swabs.

Doseform: Solution or powder for solution

Appearance: Cream- to white-colored powder, yielding a colorless to light yellow clear solution

Solvent:

Solution forms: Phosphate-buffered solution

Diluent:

For reconstitution: Powder forms: Sterile water for injection. Either glass or plastic syringes may be used. Agitate gently, if desired, to hasten complete dissolution of the powder. If air bubbles form, wait until the solution has settled and all bubbles have risen to the top of the solution and disappeared before measuring the dose.

For infusion: Reconstitute and withdraw the appropriate dose of interferon alfa-2b powder. Inject it into a 100 mL bag of sodium chloride 0.9%. The final concentration of interferon alfa-2b should be at least 10 million units per 100 mL. Infuse the prepared solution over 20 minutes.

Adjuvant: None

Preservative:

Powder forms: None
Solution forms: 1.5 mg/mL m-cresol
Multidose pens: 1.5 mg/mL m-cresol

Allergens: Tetracycline, originally present during fermentation at 5 to 10 mg/L, is undetectable in the final product.

Excipients:

Powder forms: After reconstitution, human albumin 1 mg/mL, glycine 20 mg/mL, sodium phosphate dibasic 2.3 mg/mL, sodium phosphate monobasic 0.55 mg/mL
Solution forms: Human albumin 1 mg/mL, glycine 20 mg/mL, sodium phosphate dibasic 1.8 mg/mL, sodium phosphate monobasic 1.3 mg/mL, sodium chloride 7.5 mg/mL, edetate disodium 0.1 mg/mL, polysorbate 80 0.1 mg/mL
Multidose pens: Human albumin 1 mg/mL, glycine 20 mg/mL, sodium phosphate dibasic 1.8 mg/mL, sodium phosphate monobasic 1.3 mg/mL, sodium chloride 7.5 mg/mL, edetate disodium 0.1 mg/mL, polysorbate 80 0.1 mg/mL

pH: The pH of the powder forms is 7.2 after reconstitution. The pH of solution forms is 6.8. The isoelectric point of interferon alfa-2b is 6.

Shelf Life: Powder forms expire within 36 months. Multidose vials of solution expire within 24 months. Single-dose vials of solution expire within 18 months. Multidose pens expire within 12 months (additional experience pending).

Storage/Stability: Store at 2° to 8°C (35° to 46°F). Product is shipped from manufacturer to wholesaler in refrigerated trucks. For patient comfort, warm to room temperature before injection. Product can tolerate 18 months as powder at room temperature or up to 7 days at 45°C (113°F). Because the powder form has been lyophilized, it can withstand freezing temperatures if resultant solutions are clear and free of particulate matter. Diluent vials might crack if frozen, potentially compromising sterility. After reconstitution, product can tolerate 1 month in the refrigerator, 2 weeks at room temperature, or 7 days at 45°C (113°F). Do not freeze reconstituted product.

Solution forms provided in vials ranging from 3 to 25 million units/vial are stable at 35°C (95°F) for up to 7 days and at 30°C (86°F) for up to 14 days.

Multidose pens provided in strengths ranging from 18 to 60 million units/pen are stable at 30°C (86°F) for up to 2 days.

Handling: Interferon alfa-2b is compatible with glass and plastic syringes. Do not store the drug in syringes for long periods because the protein adheres to syringe surfaces. A study of biological activity suggests that interferon alfa-2b is stable for 42 days at 4°C (39°F) in polypropylene syringes at concentrations of 3 or 6 million units/mL, with or without albumin as a carrier protein. Interferon alfa-2b is also stable for 42 days at 4°C (39°F) in polypropylene syringes at 2 million units/mL in sterile water.

Production Process: Manufactured by recombinant DNA techniques, from the bacterial fermentation of a strain of *Escherichia coli* bearing a genetically engineered plasmid containing the gene coding for interferon alfa-2b, comparable with that produced by human leukocytes. Fermentation is conducted in a medium containing tetracycline 5 to 10 mg/L. Lysis of the bacteria is not required, but trace levels of *Escherichia coli* protein may be found after fermentation. Traditional physicochemical separation techniques are used to purify the final product, including ethanol extraction and a series of chromatographic procedures.

Media: *E. coli* in a defined nutrient medium

Disease Epidemiology

See Epidemiology of Diseases Treated with Interferon Alpha in the Interferon Alpha Summary.

Other Information

Perspective: See also Epidemiology of Diseases Treated with Interferon Alpha in the Interferon Alpha Summary.

1979: Human gene for interferon alfa cloned by recombinant DNA techniques.

1986: Interferon alfa-2b licensed June 4, 1986, for hairy cell leukemia; June 1988 for condylomata acuminata; November 1988 for AIDS-related Kaposi sarcoma; February 1991 for chronic non-A, non-B hepatitis; May 1992 for chronic hepatitis B (designated an orphan drug June 22, 1987).

Peginterferon Alfa-2b (Recombinant)

Interferons

Name: Manufacturer:
  PegIntron   Merck
  Sylatron   Merck

Synonyms: Peginterf A 2B, *Pegtron, Unitron PEG, Viraferonpeg*

Comparison: The various interferon alpha products are not generically interchangeable because of variations in dosage, routes of administration, and adverse events specific to different brands. Do not use different brands of interferon alpha in any single treatment regimen. For comparison of peginterferon alfa-2b and interferon alfa-2b, see the Efficacy section of this monograph.

Immunologic Characteristics

Antigen Source: Interferon alfa expressed from recombinant *Escherichia coli* bacteria

Viability: Not viable, but immunologically active

Antigenic Form: Interferon, human leukocyte

Antigenic Type: Protein, a covalent conjugate of recombinant interferon alfa-2b with monomethoxy polyethylene glycol (PEG). Interferon alfa-2b is a water-soluble protein with a molecular weight of 19,271 daltons produced by recombinant DNA techniques. The molecular weight of the PEG portion of the molecule is 12,000 daltons. The average molecular weight of the peginterferon alfa-2b molecule is approximately 31,000 daltons.

Strains: Interferon alfa-2b

Use Characteristics

Indications:

PegIntron: As part of a combination regimen, to treat chronic hepatitis C in patients with compensated liver disease.

In combination with ribavirin and an approved hepatitis C virus (HCV) NS3/4A protease inhibitor (eg, boceprevir, telaprevir) in adult patients (18 years of age and older) with HCV genotype 1 infection.

In combination with ribavirin in patients with genotypes other than 1, pediatric patients (3 to 17 years of age), or in patients with genotype 1 infection for whom use of an HCV NS3/4A protease inhibitor is not warranted based on tolerability, contraindications, or other clinical factors.

As monotherapy only in treating chronic hepatitis C in patients with compensated liver disease if there are contraindications to or significant intolerance of ribavirin, and for use only in previously untreated adult patients. Combination therapy provides substantially better response rates than monotherapy.

Sylatron: For adjuvant treatment of melanoma with microscopic or gross nodal involvement within 84 days of definitive surgical resection including complete lymphadenectomy.

Limitations: Peginterferon alfa-2b alone or in combination with ribavirin has not been studied in patients who have failed other alpha interferon treatments, as a treatment of HCV in patients who received liver or other organ transplants, or as a treatment of HCV in patients coinfected with HIV or HBV.

Patients with the following characteristics are less likely to benefit from re-treatment after failing a course of therapy: previous nonresponse, previous pegylated interferon treatment, significant bridging fibrosis or cirrhosis, and genotype 1 infection.

Contraindications:

Absolute: Patients with hypersensitivity to peginterferon alfa-2b or any component of the product. Patients with autoimmune hepatitis or decompensated liver disease (Child-Pugh score higher than 6 [class B and C]). Ribavirin therapy is contraindicated in pregnant women and in men whose female partners are pregnant or those with serious hemoglobinopathies (eg, thalassemia major, sickle-cell anemia).

Relative: Discontinue interferon therapy for any patient developing severe depression. Patients with preexisting thyroid abnormalities may be treated if thyroid-stimulating hormone (TSH) levels can be maintained in the normal range by medication. Discontinue therapy in patients who develop thyroid abnormalities and whose thyroid function cannot be normalized by medication. Do not use ribavirin in patients with creatinine clearance less than 50 mL/min.

Immunodeficiency: No impairment of effect is expected.

Elderly: Studies of peginterferon alfa-2b did not include enough subjects 65 years and older to determine whether they respond differently than younger subjects. Clinical experience has not identified differences in responses between elderly and younger patients. However, treatment with alpha interferons, including peginterferon alfa-2b, is associated with CNS, cardiac, and systemic (viral-like) adverse effects. Because these adverse reactions may be more severe in the elderly, exercise caution when using peginterferon alfa-2b in this population. This drug is substantially excreted by the kidney. The risk of toxic reactions may be greater in patients with impaired renal function.

Carcinogenicity: Has not been tested for carcinogenic potential. Consider ribavirin a potential carcinogen.

Mutagenicity: Neither peginterferon alfa-2b, nor its components interferon or methoxypolyethylene glycol, caused damage to DNA when tested in the standard battery of mutagenesis assays, nor in the presence and absence of metabolic activation. Ribavirin is genotoxic and mutogenic.

Fertility Impairment: Irregular menstrual cycles were observed in female cynomolgus monkeys given subcutaneous injections of 4,239 mcg/m^2 peginterferon alfa-2b every other day for 1 month, at approximately 345 times the recommended weekly human dose (based upon body surface area). These effects included transiently decreased serum levels of estradiol and progesterone, suggestive of anovulation. Normal menstrual cycles and serum hormone levels resumed in these animals 2 to 3 months after ceasing peginterferon alfa-2b treatment. Every-other-day dosing with 262 mcg/m^2 (approximately 21 times the weekly human dose) had no effects on cycle duration or reproductive hormone status. The effects of peginterferon alfa-2b on male fertility have not been studied.

Pregnancy: Category C. Nonpegylated interferon alfa-2b has been shown to have abortifacient effects in rhesus monkeys at 15 and 30 million units/kg (estimated human equivalent of 5 and 10 million units/kg, based on body surface area adjustment for a 60 kg adult). Peginterferon alfa-2b should be assumed to also have abortifacient potential. There are no adequate and well-controlled studies in pregnant women. Use peginterferon alfa-2b therapy during pregnancy only if the potential benefit to the mother outweighs the potential risk to the fetus. Therefore, peginterferon alfa-2b is recommended for use in fertile women only when they are using effective contraception during the treatment period.

Category X. Significant teratogenic or embryocidal effects have been demonstrated in all animal species exposed to ribavirin. Ribavirin may cause birth defects or the death of the unborn child. Ribavirin therapy is contraindicated in pregnant women and in men whose female partners are pregnant. Do not start ribavirin therapy until confirming a negative pregnancy test. Patients should use at least 2 forms of contraception and have monthly pregnancy tests during therapy.

Lactation: It is not known whether the components of peginterferon alfa-2b are excreted in human milk. Studies in mice have shown that mouse interferons are excreted in breast milk. Because of the potential for adverse reactions from the drug in nursing infants, decide whether to stop nursing or stop treatment, taking into account the importance of the product to the mother.

Children: Safety and efficacy in children younger than 18 years of age have not been established.

Adverse Reactions: Nearly all study patients experienced 1 or more adverse event. The incidence of serious adverse events was similar (approximately 12%) in all treatment groups. In many cases, events resolve after stopping peginterferon alfa-2b therapy. Some patients continue to experience adverse events for several months after stopping therapy. Overall, 10% of patients in the peginterferon alfa-2b groups stopped therapy due to adverse events, compared with 6% in the interferon alfa-2b group. Fourteen percent of patients in the peginterferon alfa-2b groups required dose reduction, compared with 6% in the interferon alfa-2b group.

Hepatitis C: The most common adverse events associated with peginterferon alfa-2b were flu-like symptoms in approximately 50% of patients, which may decrease in severity as treatment continues. Application site disorders occurred frequently (47%) and included injection-site inflammation and reaction (eg, bruise, itchiness, irritation). Injection-site pain was reported in 2% of patients receiving peginterferon alfa-2b. Alopecia is often associated with peginterferon alfa-2b. There was 1 death, a suicide, among patients receiving peginterferon alfa-2b and 2 deaths in the interferon alfa-2b group (1 murder/suicide and 1 sudden death).

Patients receiving peginterferon alfa-2b appeared to experience a greater number of adverse events (eg, injection-site reaction, fever, rigors, nausea) compared with patients receiving interferon alfa-2b. The number of adverse events was higher when receiving higher peginterferon alfa-2b dosages.

Fifty-seven percent of patients experienced psychiatric adverse events, most commonly depression (29%). Suicidal behavior (eg, ideation, attempts, suicides) occurred in 1% of patients during or shortly after treatment with peginterferon alfa-2b.

Adverse events that occurred at an incidence of 5% or more are provided in the following table. Because of ascertainment procedures, adverse event rate comparisons across studies should not be made.

Adverse Events Occurring in ≥ 5% of Patients[a]				
Adverse Events	Peginterferon alfa-2b 1 mcg/kg (n = 297)	Interferon alfa-2b 3 M units (n = 303)	Peginterferon alfa-2b 1.5 mcg/kg plus ribavirin (n = 511)	Interferon alfa-2b 3 M units plus ribavirin (n = 505)
Application Site				
Injection-site inflammation	47%	20%	75%	49%
Autonomic Nervous System				
Dry mouth	6%	7%	12%	8%
Flushing	6%	3%	4%	3%
Sweating, increased	6%	7%	11%	7%
Body as a Whole				
Headache	56%	52%	62%	58%
Fatigue	52%	54%	56%	63%
Viral-like symptoms	46%	38%	—	—
Rigors	23%	19%	48%	41%

Adverse Events Occurring in ≥ 5% of Patients[a]				
Adverse Events	Peginterferon alfa-2b 1 mcg/kg (n = 297)	Interferon alfa-2b 3 M units (n = 303)	Peginterferon alfa-2b 1.5 mcg/kg plus ribavirin (n = 511)	Interferon alfa-2b 3 M units plus ribavirin (n = 505)
Fever	22%	12%	46%	33%
Weight decrease	11%	13%	29%	20%
Right, upper quandrant pain	8%	8%	12%	6%
Malaise	7%	6%	4%	6%
Nervous System				
Dizziness	12%	10%	21%	17%
Endocrine				
Hypothyroidism	5%	3%	5%	4%
GI System				
Nausea	26%	20%	43%	33%
Anorexia	20%	17%	32%	27%
Diarrhea	18%	16%	22%	17%
Abdominal pain	15%	11%	13%	13%
Vomiting	7%	6%	14%	12%
Dyspepsia	6%	7%	9%	8%
Hematologic				
Neutropenia	6%	2%	26%	14%
Anemia	0%	0%	12%	17%
Leukopenia	< 1%	0%	6%	5%
Thrombocytopenia	7%	< 1%	5%	2%
Infectious				
Infection, viral	11%	10%	12%	12%
Liver and Biliary System				
Hepatomegaly	6%	5%	4%	4%
Musculoskeletal System				
Myalgia	56%	53%	56%	50%
Arthralgia	23%	27%	34%	28%
Musculoskeletal pain	28%	22%	21%	19%
Psychiatric				
Depression	29%	25%	31%	34%
Insomnia	23%	23%	40%	41%
Anxiety, emotional lability, irritability	28%	34%	47%	47%
Concentration impaired	10%	8%	17%	21%
Respiratory System				
Pharyngitis	10%	7%	12%	13%
Sinusitis	7%	7%	6%	5%
Coughing	6%	5%	23%	16%
Skin and Appendages				
Alopecia	22%	22%	36%	32%
Pruritus	12%	8%	29%	28%
Dry skin	11%	9%	24%	23%
Rash	6%	7%	24%	23%

a Patients reporting 1 or more adverse event. A patient may have reported 1 or more adverse event within a body system/ organ class category.

Numerous adverse events were observed at a frequency less than 5%. Without a nontreatment control group, the relationship to the study drug could not be determined. Individual serious adverse events occurred at a frequency 1% or less and included suicide attempt, suicidal ideation, severe depression, relapse of drug addiction/overdose, nerve palsy (eg, facial, oculomotor), cardiomyopathy, myocardial infarction, retinal ischemia, retinal vein thrombosis, transient ischemic attack, supraventricular arrhythmias, loss of consciousness, neutropenia, infection (eg, pneumonia, abscess), autoimmune thrombocytopenia, hyperthyroidism, rheumatoid arthritis, interstitial nephritis, lupus-like syndrome, aggravated psoriasis, and urticaria.

Metastatic Melanoma: The most common adverse reactions experienced by peginterferon alfa-2b–treated patients were fatigue (94%), increased ALT (77%), increased AST (77%), pyrexia (75%), headache (70%), anorexia (69%), myalgia (68%), nausea (64%), chills (63%), and injection-site reactions (62%). The most common serious adverse reactions were fatigue (7%), increased ALT (3%), increased AST (3%), and pyrexia (3%) in the peginterferon alfa-2b –treated group vs. < 1% in the observation group for these reactions. Thirty three percent of patients receiving peginterferon alfa-2b discontinued treatment due to adverse reactions. The most common adverse reactions present at the time of treatment discontinuation were fatigue (27%), depression (17%), anorexia (15%), increased ALT (14%), increased AST (14%), myalgia (13%), nausea (13%), headache (13%), and pyrexia (11%).

Cardiovascular: Cardiovascular events, which include hypotension, arrhythmia, bundlebranch block, tachycardia, cardiomyopathy, angina pectoris, and myocardial infarction developed in patients treated with peginterferon alfa-2b. Use peginterferon alfa-2b cautiously in patients with cardiovascular disease. Closely monitor patients with a history of myocardial infarction and arrhythmic disorder who require peginterferon alfa-2b therapy.

Autoimmune: Development or exacerbation of autoimmune disorders (eg, thyroiditis, thrombocytopenia, rheumatoid arthritis, interstitial nephritis, systemic lupus erythematosus, psoriasis) occurred in patients receiving peginterferon alfa-2b. Use peginterferon alfa-2b with caution in patients with autoimmune disorders.

CNS: Life-threatening or fatal neuropsychiatric events, including suicide, suicidal and homicidal ideation, depression, relapse of drug addiction/overdose, and aggressive behavior have occurred in patients with and without a previous psychiatric disorder during peginterferon alfa-2b treatment and follow-up. Psychoses and hallucinations developed in patients treated with alpha interferons. Use peginterferon alfa-2b with extreme caution in patients with a history of psychiatric disorders. Advise patients to report immediately any symptoms of depression or suicidal ideation. Monitor all patients for evidence of depression and other psychiatric symptoms. In severe cases, stop peginterferon alfa-2b immediately and institute psychiatric intervention.

Endocrine: Peginterferon alfa-2b causes or aggravates hypothyroidism and hyperthyroidism. Thyroid stimulating hormone (TSH) abnormalities developed in 16% of treated patients and were associated with clinically apparent hypothyroidism (5%) or hyperthyroidism (1%). Subjects developed new-onset TSH abnormalities while on treatment and during the follow-up period. At the end of the follow-up period, 7% of subjects still had abnormal TSH values.

Hyperglycemia has developed in patients treated with peginterferon alfa-2b. Diabetes mellitus has developed in patients treated with alpha interferons.

Patients with these conditions who cannot be effectively treated with medication should not begin peginterferon alfa-2b therapy. Patients who develop these conditions during treatment and cannot be controlled with medication should not continue peginterferon alfa-2b therapy.

GI: Fatal and nonfatal ulcerative and hemorrhagic colitis have developed within 12 weeks of beginning alpha interferon treatment. Abdominal pain, bloody diarrhea, and fever are typical manifestations. Stop peginterferon alfa-2b treatment immediately in patients who develop these signs and symptoms. Colitis usually resolves within 1 to 3 weeks after stopping alpha interferons.

Fatal and nonfatal pancreatitis have developed in patients treated with alpha interferon. Suspend peginterferon alfa-2b therapy in patients with signs and symptoms suggestive of pancreatitis; discontinue in patients diagnosed with pancreatitis.

Hematologic: Peginterferon alfa-2b suppresses bone marrow function, sometimes resulting in severe cytopenias. Rarely, alpha interferons may be associated with aplastic anemia. Peginterferon alfa-2b may cause severe decreases in neutrophil and platelet counts. Neutrophil counts decreased in 70% of patients. Severe and potentially life-threatening neutropenia (less than 0.5×10^9 cells/L) occurred in 1% of patients. Platelet counts decreased in 20% of patients. Severe decreases in platelet counts (less than 50,000 cells/mm^3) occurred in 1% of patients. The incidence and severity of thrombocytopenia and neutropenia were greater in the peginterferon alfa-2b groups compared with the interferon alfa group. Discontinue peginterferon alfa-2b in patients who develop severe decreases in neutrophil or platelet counts. Platelet and neutrophil counts generally returned to pretreatment levels within 4 weeks of the cessation of therapy.

Hepatic: In 10% of patients treated with peginterferon alfa-2b, ALT levels rose 2- to 5-fold above baseline. The elevations were transient and not associated with other liver functions.

Hypersensitivity: Serious, acute hypersensitivity reactions (eg, urticaria, angioedema, bronchoconstriction, anaphylaxis) developed rarely during alpha interferon therapy. If such a reaction develops, discontinue treatment with peginterferon alfa-2b and institute appropriate medical therapy immediately. Transient rashes do not require interrupting treatment.

Immunologic: Of patients receiving peginterferon alfa-2b, approximately 2% developed low-titer ($\leq$ 1:64) neutralizing antibodies to interferon alfa-2b. The clinical and pathological significance of the appearance of serum neutralizing antibodies is unknown. No apparent correlation of antibody development to clinical response or adverse events was observed. By using a Biacore assay to measure binding antibodies and an antiviral neutralization assay to measure serum neutralizing antibodies, the incidence of posttreatment binding antibody was approximately 10% for patients receiving peginterferon alfa-2b and approximately 15% for patients receiving interferon alfa-2b. Positive assays may be influenced by several factors, so that comparing the incidence of antibodies to various interferon products may be misleading.

Ophthalmic: Retinal hemorrhages, cotton wool spots, and retinal artery or vein obstruction developed after treatment with alpha interferons. Patients who have diabetes mellitus or hypertension should have eye examinations before beginning peginterferon alfa-2b treatment.

Renal: Closely monitor patients with impaired renal function for signs and symptoms of interferon toxicity. Adjust peginterferon alfa-2b dosing accordingly. Use peginterferon alfa-2b with caution in patients with creatinine clearance less than 50 mL/min.

Respiratory: Dyspnea, pulmonary infiltrates, pneumonitis, and pneumonia (sometimes resulting in patient deaths) have been associated with alpha interferon therapy. Closely monitor patients with pulmonary infiltrates or pulmonary function impairment.

Pharmacologic & Dosing Characteristics

Dosage:

Hepatitis C, Adults: The recommended dose of peginterferon alfa-2b is 1.5 mcg/kg/week subcutaneously in combination with ribavirin 800 to 1,400 mg orally based on patient body weight. The volume of peginterferon alfa-2b to be injected depends on drug concentration and the patient's body weight.

Duration of treatment:

Interferon alpha-naive patients: Treatment duration for patients with genotype 1 is 48 weeks. Consider stopping therapy in patients who do not achieve at least a 2 $\log_{10}$ drop or loss of HCV-RNA at 12 weeks, or if HCV-RNA remains detectable after 24 weeks of therapy. Treat patients with genotype 2 and 3 for 24 weeks.

Retreatment with peginterferon alfa-2b/ribavirin of prior treatment failures: Treatment duration for patients who previously failed therapy is 48 weeks, regardless of HCV genotype. Retreated patients who fail to achieve undetectable HCV-RNA at week 12 of therapy, or whose HCV-RNA remains detectable after 24 weeks of therapy, are highly unlikely to achieve sustained virologic response (SVR), so consider stopping therapy.

Recommended Peginterferon Alfa-2b Combination Therapy Dosing (Adults)					
Body weight kg (lbs)	Peginterferon alfa-2b ribavirin concentration	Amount of peginterferon alfa-2b to administer	Volume[a] (mL) of peginterferon alfa-2b	Ribavirin	
				Daily dose	Number of capsules
< 40 (< 88)	50 mcg per 0.5 mL	50	0.5	800 mg/day	Two 200 mg capsules AM Two 200 mg capsules PM
40 to 50 (88 to 111)	80 mcg per 0.5 mL	64	0.4	800 mg/day	Two 200 mg capsules AM Two 200 mg capsules PM
51 to 60 (112 to 133)		80	0.5	800 mg/day	Two 200 mg capsules AM Two 200 mg capsules PM
61 to 65 (134 to 144)	120 mcg per 0.5 mL	96	0.4	800 mg/day	Two 200 mg capsules AM Two 200 mg capsules PM
66 to 75 (145 to 166)		96	0.4	1,000 mg/day	Two 200 mg capsules AM Three 200 mg capsules PM
76 to 80 (167 to 177)		120	0.5	1,000 mg/day	Two 200 mg capsules AM Three 200 mg capsules PM
81 to 85 (178 to 187)		120	0.5	1,200 mg/day	Three 200 mg capsules AM Three 200 mg capsules PM

Peginterferon Alfa-2b (Recombinant)

Recommended Peginterferon Alfa-2b Combination Therapy Dosing (Adults)					
Body weight kg (lbs)	Peginterferon alfa-2b ribavirin concentration	Amount of peginterferon alfa-2b to administer	Volume[a] (mL) of peginterferon alfa-2b	Ribavirin	
				Daily dose	Number of capsules
86 to 105 (188 to 231)	150 mcg per 0.5 mL	150	0.5	1,200 mg/day	Three 200 mg capsules AM Three 200 mg capsules PM
> 105 (> 231)	b	b	b	1,400 mg/day	Three 200 mg capsules AM Four 200 mg capsules PM

a When reconstituted as directed.
b For patients weighing more than 105 kg (more than 231 pounds), calculate the peginterferon alfa-2b dose of 1.5 mcg/kg/week based on the individual patient weight. Two vials of peginterferon alfa-2b may be necessary to provide the dose.

Monotherapy: Treat adults as follows: Peginterferon alfa-2b 1 mcg/kg/week subcutaneously for 1 year, administered on the same day of the week. Consider stopping therapy in patients who do not achieve at least a 2 $\log_{10}$ drop or loss of HCV-RNA at 12 weeks of therapy, or whose HCV-RNA levels remain detectable after 24 weeks of therapy. Base the volume of peginterferon alfa-2b to be injected on patient weight, as follows.

Recommended Peginterferon Alfa-2b Monotherapy Dosing			
Body weight kg (lbs)	Peginterferon alfa-2b concentration to use	Amount (mcg) of peginterferon alfa-2b to administer	Volume (mL)[a] of peginterferon alfa-2b to administer
≤ 45 (≤ 100)	50 mcg per 0.5 mL	40	0.4
46 to 56 (101 to 124)	50 mcg per 0.5 mL	50	0.5
57 to 72 (125 to 159)	80 mcg per 0.5 mL	64	0.4
73 to 88 (160 to 195)	80 mcg per 0.5 mL	80	0.5
89 to 106 (196 to 234)	120 mcg per 0.5 mL	96	0.4
107 to 136 (235 to 300)	120 mcg per 0.5 mL	120	0.5
137 to 160 (301 to 353)	150 mcg per 0.5 mL	150	0.5

a When reconstituted as directed.

Children: Peginterferon alfa-2b 60 mcg/m^2/week subcutaneously in combination with ribavirin 15 mg/kg/day orally in 2 divided doses. Patients who reach their 18th birthday while receiving this combination therapy should remain on the pediatric dosing regimen. The treatment duration for patients with genotype 1 is 48 weeks. Patients with genotype 2 and 3 should be treated for 24 weeks.

The ribavirin dose for children based on body weight is as follows:

Ribavirin Dosing in Children		
Body weight kg (lbs)	Ribavirin daily dose	Ribavirin number of capsules
< 47 kg (< 103 lbs)	15 mg/kg/day	Use oral solution
47 to 59 kg (103 to 131 lbs)	800 mg/day	Two 200 mg capsules AM Two 200 mg capsules PM
60 to 73 kg (132 to 162 lbs)	1,000 mg/day	Two 200 mg capsules AM Three 200 mg capsules PM
> 73 kg (> 162 lbs)	1,200 mg/day	Three 200 mg capsules AM Three 200 mg capsules PM

Dose reduction: If a serious adverse event develops during the course of treatment, discontinue or modify the dosage of peginterferon alfa-2b and ribavirin until the adverse event abates or decreases in severity. If persistent or recurrent serious adverse events develop despite adequate dosage adjustment, discontinue treatment. For guidelines for dose modifications and discontinuation based on depression or laboratory parameters, see the following tables. Reduce dosage of peginterferon alfa-2b in adult patients on combination therapy in a 2-step process from the original starting dose of 1.5 mcg/kg/week to 1 mcg/kg/week, then to 0.5 mcg/kg/week, if needed. Reduce dosage in patients on monotherapy by reducing the original starting dose of 1 mcg/kg/week to 0.5 mcg/kg/week. Reduce dosage peginterferon alfa-2b in adults by using a lower-dose strength or administering a lesser volume.

In the adult combination therapy study 2, dose reductions occurred in 42% of subjects receiving peginterferon alfa-2b 1.5 mcg/kg plus ribavirin 800 mg daily including 57% of subjects weighing 60 kg or less. In study 4, 16% of subjects had a dose reduction of peginterferon alfa-2b to 1 mcg/kg in combination with ribavirin, with an additional 4% requiring the second dose reduction of peginterferon alfa-2b to 0.5 mcg/kg because of adverse events.

Reduce dosage in children by modifying the recommended dose in a 2-step process from the original starting dose of 60 mcg/m^2/wk to 40 mcg/m^2/wk, then to 20 mcg/m^2/wk, if needed. In the pediatric combination therapy trial, dose reductions occurred in 25% of subjects receiving peginterferon alfa-2b 60 mcg/m^2 weekly plus ribavirin 15 mg/kg daily.

Peginterferon Alfa-2b (Recombinant)

Guidelines for Modification or Discontinuation of Peginterferon Alfa-2b or Peginterferon Alfa-2b/Ribavirin and for Scheduling Visits for Patients With Depression					
	Initial management (4 to 8 weeks)			Depression status	
Depression severity[a]	Dose modification	Visit schedule	Remains stable	Improves	Worsens
Mild	No change	Evaluate once weekly by visit or phone.	Continue weekly visit schedule.	Resume normal visit schedule.	See moderate or severe depression.
Moderate	Adults: Adjust dose[b] Pediatrics: Decrease dose to 40 mcg/m²/ week, then to 20 mcg/m²/week, if needed.	Evaluate once weekly (office visit at least every other week).	Consider psychiatric consultation. Continue reduced dosing.	If symptoms improve and are stable for 4 weeks, may resume normal visit schedule. Continue reduced dosing or return to normal dose.	See severe depression.
Severe	Discontinue peginterferon alfa-2b/ribavirin permanently.	Obtain immediate psychiatric consultation.	Psychiatric therapy as necessary.		

a See *DSM-IV* for definitions.
b For patients on peginterferon alfa-2b/ribavirin combination therapy: 1st dose reduction of peginterferon alfa-2b is to 1 mcg/kg/week, 2nd dose reduction (if needed) of peginterferon alfa-2b is to 0.5 mcg/kg/week. For patients on peginterferon alfa-2b monotherapy: decrease peginterferon alfa-2b dose to 0.5 mcg/kg/week.

Guidelines for Dose Modification and Discontinuation of Peginterferon Alfa-2b or Peginterferon Alfa-2b/Ribavirin Based on Laboratory Parameters in Adults and Pediatrics				
	Peginterferon alfa-2b		Ribavirin	
Laboratory values	Adults	Pediatrics	Adults	Pediatrics
Hgb < 10 g/dL	For patients with cardiac disease, reduce by 50%[a]	See footnote[a]	Adjust dose[b]	1st reduction to 12 mg/kg/day 2nd reduction to 8 mg/kg/day
WBC < 1.5 × 10⁹/L Neutrophils < 0.75 × 10⁹/L Platelets < 50 × 10⁹/L (Adults) < 70 × 10⁹/L (Pediatrics)	Adjust dose[c]	1st reduction to 40 mcg/m²/week 2nd reduction to 20 mcg/m²/week	No dose change	No dose change
Hgb < 8.5 g/dL WBC < 1 × 10⁹/L Neutrophils < 0.5 × 10⁹/L Platelets < 25 × 10⁹/L (Adults) < 50 × 10⁹/L (Pediatrics) Creatinine > 2 mg/dL (Pediatrics)	Permanently discontinue	Permanently discontinue	Permanently discontinue	Permanently discontinue

a For adult patients with a history of stable cardiac disease receiving peginterferon alfa-2b in combination with ribavirin, reduce the peginterferon alfa-2b dose by half and the ribavirin dose by 200 mg/day if a > 2 g/dL decrease in hemoglobin is observed during any 4-week period. Permanently discontinue both peginterferon alfa-2b and ribavirin if patients have hemoglobin levels < 12 g/dL after this ribavirin dose reduction. Evaluate weekly children who have pre-existing cardiac conditions and experience a hemoglobin decrease ≥ 2 g/dL during any 4-week period during treatment.
b First dose reduction of ribavirin is by 200 mg/day, except by 400 mg/day in patients receiving the 1,400 mg dose; second dose reduction of ribavirin (if needed) is by an additional 200 mg/day.
c For patients on peginterferon alfa-2b/ribavirin combination therapy: first dose reduction of peginterferon alfa-2b is to 1 mcg/kg/week, second dose reduction (if needed) of peginterferon alfa-2b is to 0.5 mcg/kg/week. For patients on peginterferon alfa-2b monotherapy: decrease peginterferon alfa-2b dose to 0.5 mcg/kg/week.

Peginterferon Alfa-2b (Recombinant)

Reduced Peginterferon Alfa-2b Dose (0.5 mcg/kg) for (1 mcg/kg) Monotherapy in Adults			
Body weight kg (lbs)	Peginterferon alfa-2b concentration	Amount (mcg) of peginterferon alfa-2b to administer	Volume (mL)[a] of peginterferon alfa-2b to administer
≤ 45 (≤ 100)	50 mcg per 0.5 mL[b]	20	0.2
46 to 56 (101 to 124)	50 mcg per 0.5 mL[b]	25	0.25
57 to 72 (125 to 159)	50 mcg per 0.5 mL	30	0.3
73 to 88 (160 to 195)	50 mcg per 0.5 mL	40	0.4
89 to 106 (196 to 234)	50 mcg per 0.5 mL	50	0.5
107 to 136 (235 to 300)	80 mcg per 0.5 mL	64	0.4
≥ 137 (≥ 301)	80 mcg per 0.5 mL	80	0.5

a When reconstituted as directed.
b Must use vial. Minimum delivery for *Redipen* is 0.3 mL.

Two-Step Dose Reduction of Peginterferon Alfa-2b in Combination Therapy in Adults							
First dose reduction to peginterferon alfa-2b 1 mcg/kg				Second dose reduction to peginterferon alfa-2b 0.5 mcg/kg			
Body weight kg (lbs)	Peginterferon alfa-2b concentration	Amount (mcg) of peginterferon alfa-2b to administer	Volume (mL)[a] of peginterferon alfa-2b to administer	Body weight kg (lbs)	Peginterferon alfa-2b concentration	Amount (mcg) of peginterferon alfa-2b to administer	Volume (mL)[a] of peginterferon alfa-2b to administer
< 40 (< 88)	50 mcg per 0.5 mL	35	0.35	< 40 (< 88)	50 mcg per 0.5 mL[b]	20	0.2
40 to 50 (88 to 111)		45	0.45	40 to 50 (88 to 111)		25	0.25
51 to 60 (112 to 133)		50	0.5	51 to 60 (112 to 133)	50 mcg per 0.5 mL	30	0.3
61 to 75 (134 to 166)	80 mcg per 0.5 mL	64	0.4	61 to 75 (134 to 166)		35	0.35
76 to 85 (167 to 187)		80	0.5	76 to 85 (167 to 187)		45	0.45

a When reconstituted as directed.
b Must use vial. Minimum delivery for *Redipen* is 0.3 mL.

Discontinuation:

Adults: Discontinue therapy in HCV genotype 1 interferon-alfa-naive patients receiving peginterferon alfa-2b, alone or in combination with ribavirin, if there is not at least a 2 $\log_{10}$ drop or loss of HCV-RNA at 12 weeks of therapy, or whose HCV-RNA levels remain detectable after 24 weeks of therapy. Regardless of genotype, previously treated patients who have detectable HCV-RNA at week 12 or 24, are highly unlikely to achieve SVR, and discontinuation of therapy should be considered.

Children: Discontinue therapy in children receiving peginterferon alfa-2b/ribavirin combination (excluding those with HCV genotype 2 and 3) at 12 weeks if their treatment week-12 HCV RNA dropped below 2 $\log_{10}$ compared to pretreatment or at 24 weeks if they have detectable HCV RNA at treatment week 24.

Dosage based on renal function: In patients with moderate renal dysfunction (creatinine clearance 30 to 50 mL/min), reduce the peginterferon alfa-2b dose by 25%. Patients with severe renal dysfunction (creatinine clearance 10 to 29 mL/min), including those on hemodialysis, reduce the peginterferon alfa-2b dose by 50%. If renal function decreases during treatment, discontinue peginterferon alfa-2b therapy. When peginterferon alfa-2b is administered in combination with ribavirin, carefully monitor subjects with impaired renal function or those older than 50 years of age with respect to the development of anemia. Do not use peginterferon alfa-2b/ribavirin in patients with creatinine clearance less than 50 mL/min.

Metastatic melanoma: 6 mcg/kg/week SC for 8 doses followed by 3 mcg/kg/week SC for up to 5 years. Guidelines for dose modification are based on the National Cancer Institute Common Terminology Criteria for Adverse Events.

Permanently discontinue peginterferon alfa-2b for: Persistent or worsening severe neuropsychiatric disorders, grade 4 non-hematologic toxicity, inability to tolerate a dose of 1 mcg/kg/wk, new or worsening retinopathy

Withhold peginterferon alfa-2b dose for any of the following: Absolute neutrophil count (ANC) < 0.5×10^9 cells/L, platelet count < 50×10^9 cells/L, ECOG performance status ≥ 2, non-hematologic toxicity ≥ grade 3.

Resume dosing at a reduced dose when all of the following are present: Absolute neutrophil count ≥ 0.5×10^9 cells/L, platelet count ≥ 50×10^9 cells/L, ECOG performance status 0-1, non-hematologic toxicity completely resolved or improved to grade 1.

Dosage adjustment: Starting Dose of 6 mcg/kg/week: Modification of doses 1 to 8: First modification: 3 mcg/kg/week. Second modification: 2 mcg/kg/week. Third modification: 1 mcg/kg/week. Permanently discontinue if unable to tolerate 1 mcg/kg/week.

Starting Dose of 3 mcg/kg/week: Modification of doses 9 to 260: First modification: 2 mcg/kg/week. Second modification: 1 mcg/kg/week. Permanently discontinue if unable to tolerate 1 mcg/kg/week.

Route & Site: Subcutaneous. Rotate injection sites.

Overdosage: In clinical studies, a few patients accidentally received a dose greater than that prescribed. There were no instances in which a patient received more than 10.5 times the intended dose. The maximum dose received by any patient was 3.45 mcg/kg/week over a period of approximately 12 weeks. Patients who were overdosed experienced the following adverse reactions: severe fatigue, headache, myalgia, neutropenia, and thrombocytopenia. The highest single dose administered was 14 mcg/kg. The maximum known overdosage of ribavirin was an intentional ingestion of 10 g. There were no serious reactions attributed to these overdosages. In cases of overdosing, treat the patient symptomatically.

Missed Doses: Missing a dose of interferon alfa-2b will not have immediate consequences. Administer the missed dose as soon as possible and adjust weekly schedule. If more than 1 dose is missed, advise the clinician managing therapy.

Related Interventions: Perform ECGs in patients with preexisting cardiac abnormalities before treatment with peginterferon alfa-2b.

Premedicate with acetaminophen 500 to 1,000 mg orally 30 min before the first dose of peginterferon alfa-2b and as needed for subsequent doses.

Laboratory Tests: Conduct hematology and blood chemistry testing before starting treatment and periodically thereafter. In the clinical trial, CBC (including neutrophil and platelet counts) and chemistries (including AST, ALT, and bilirubin) were measured during the treatment period at weeks 2, 4, 8, and 12, and then at 6-week intervals, or more frequently if abnormalities developed. TSH levels were measured every 12 weeks during the treatment period. Consider dose reduction for neutrophil counts less than 0.75×10^9 cells/L or platelet counts less than 80×10^9 cells/L. Consider permanent discontinuation of therapy for neutrophil counts less than 0.50×10^9 cells/L or platelet counts less than 50×10^9 cells/L.

Assess serum HCV RNA levels after 24 weeks of treatment. Consider stopping treatment in any patient who has not achieved an HCV RNA level below the limit of detection of the assay after 24 weeks of therapy.

Peginterferon Alfa-2b (Recombinant)

Efficacy: A randomized study compared treatment with peginterferon alfa-2b (0.5, 1, or 1.5 mcg/kg once weekly subcutaneously) to treatment with interferon alfa-2b (3 million units 3 times weekly subcutaneously), in 1219 adults with chronic hepatitis from HCV infection. The patients were not previously treated with interferon alfa, had compensated liver disease, detectable HCV RNA, elevated ALT, and liver histopathology consistent with chronic hepatitis. Patients were treated for 48 weeks and followed for 24 weeks posttreatment. Seventy percent of all patients were infected with HCV genotype 1, and 74% of all patients had high baseline levels of HCV RNA (more than 2 million copies/mL of serum) — two factors known to predict poor response to treatment.

Response to treatment was defined as undetectable HCV RNA and normalization of ALT at 24 weeks posttreatment. The response rates to the 1 and 1.5 mcg/kg peginterferon alfa-2b doses were similar to each other and were both higher than response rates to interferon alfa-2b.

Response Rates to Peginterferon Alfa-2b				
	Peginterferon alfa-2b 0.5 mcg/kg (n = 315)	Peginterferon alfa-2b 1 mcg/kg (n = 298)	Interferon alfa-2b 3 M units TIW (n = 307)	Difference (95% CI) between Peginterferon alfa-2b 1 mcg/kg and interferon alfa-2b
Treatment response (Combined virologic response and ALT normalization)	17%	24%	12%	11 (5, 18)
Virologic responses[a]	18%	25%	12%	12 (6, 9)
ALT normalization	24%	29%	18%	11 (5, 18)

a Serum HCV RNA measured by a research-based polymerase chain reaction with a lower limit of detection of 100 copies/mL at National Genetics Institute, Los Angeles, CA.

Patients with both viral genotype 1 and high serum levels of HCV RNA at baseline were less likely to respond to treatment with peginterferon alfa-2b. Among patients with the 2 unfavorable prognostic variables, 8% (12/157) responded to peginterferon alfa-2b treatment and 2% (4/169) responded to interferon alfa-2b. Doses of peginterferon alfa-2b higher than the recommended dose did not result in higher response rates in these patients.

Patients receiving peginterferon alfa-2b with viral genotype 1 had a response rate of 14% (28/199) while patients with other viral genotypes had a 45% (43/96) response rate.

The treatment response rates were similar in men and women. Response rates were lower in black and Hispanic patients and higher in Asians, compared with whites. Although black patients had a higher proportion of poor prognostic factors compared with whites, the number of nonwhites studied (9% of the total) was insufficient to allow meaningful conclusions about differences in response rates after adjusting for prognostic factors.

Liver biopsies were obtained before and after treatment in 60% of patients. The modest reduction in inflammation compared with baseline was similar in all 4 treatment groups.

A second randomized study compared treatment with peginterferon alfa-2b (1.5 mcg/kg once weekly subcutaneously) plus ribavirin 800 mg daily to treatment with interferon alfa-2b (3 million units 3 times weekly subcutaneously) plus ribavirin 1,000 or 1,200 mg daily, in 1,530 adults with chronic HCV infection.

Response to treatment in the second study was defined as undetectable HCV RNA at 24 weeks post-treatment. The response rate to doses of peginterferon alfa-2b 1.5 mcg/kg plus ribavirin 800 mg was higher than the response rate to interferon alfa-2b/ribavirin. The response rate to peginterferon alfa-2b 1.5 mcg/kg for 4 weeks followed by 0.5 mcg/kg for 44 weeks (with ribavirin 800 mg throughout) was essentially the same as the response to interferon alfa-2b/ribavirin.

Response Rates of Peginterferon Alfa-2b in Combination with Ribavirin		
	Peginterferon alfa-2b 1.5 mcg/kg weekly plus ribavirin 800 mg daily	Interferon alfa-2b 3 M units 3 times a week plus ribavirin 1,000 or 1,200 mg daily
Overall response[a,b]	52% (264/511)	46% (231/505)
Genotype 1	41% (141/348)	33% (112/343)
Genotype 2-6	75% (123/163)	73% (119/162)

a Serum HCV RNA measured by a research-based polymerase chain reaction assay by a central laboratory.
b Difference in overall treatment response is 6% (95% CI: 0.2%, 11.6%) adjusted for viral genotype and presence of cirrhosis at baseline.

Patients with viral genotype 1, regardless of viral load, had a lower response rate compared with patients with other viral genotypes. Patients with both poor prognostic factors (genotype 1 and high viral load) had comparable response rates (30% and 29%) whether treated with peginterferon alfa-2b or interferon alfa-2b.

Patients with lower body weight tended to have higher adverse event rates and higher response rates than patients with higher body weights. Treatment response rates with peginterferon alfa-2b/ribavirin were 49% in men and 56% in women. Response rates were lower in black and Hispanic patients and higher in Asians, compared with whites. This analysis was unable to control for the effect of poor prognostic factors.

Liver biopsies were obtained before and after treatment in 68% of patients. The modest reduction in inflammation seen compared with baseline was similar in all treatment groups.

Metastatic melanoma: Safety and effectiveness of peginterferon alfa-2b were evaluated in an open-label, multicenter, randomized (1:1) study conducted in 1256 patients with surgically resected, AJCC Stage III melanoma within 84 days of regional lymph node dissection. Patients were randomized to observation (no therapy) (n = 629) or to peginterferon alfa-2b (n = 627) at a dose of 6 mcg/kg by SC injection once weekly for 8 doses followed by a 3 mcg/kg SC injection once weekly for a period of up to 5 years total treatment. The dose of peginterferon alfa-2b was adjusted to maintain an ECOG Performance Status of 0 to 1. The median age of the population was 50 years with 11% of patients 65 years or older, and 42% were female. Forty percent of the study population had microscopic, nonpalpable nodal involvement and 59% had clinically palpable nodes before lymphadenectomy. Eighty-four percent had an International Prognostic Index (IPI) score of 0 and 16% had an IPI score of 1. The main outcome measure was relapse-free survival (RFS), defined as time from randomization to earliest date of any relapse (local, regional, in-transit, or distant), or death from any cause. Secondary outcome measures included overall survival. Approximately one-third (36%) of patients required dose reductions and 29% of patients required a dose delay, with an average delay of 1.2 weeks, during the initial 8 weeks. Ninety-four patients (16%) did not continue on to the 3 mcg/kg/ week dosing regimen. Patients who continued after the initial 8 doses received 3 mcg/kg/ week for a median 14.3 months. Approximately half (52%) of the patients underwent dose reductions and 70% required dose delays (average delay 2.2 weeks). Based on 696 RFS events, determined by the Independent Review Committee, median RFS was 35 months (95% CI: 26, 47) and 26 months (95% CI: 20, 31) in the treatment and observation arms, respectively. The estimated hazard ratio for RFS was 0.82 (95% CI: 0.71, 0.96; unstratified log-rank P = 0.011) in favor of peginterferon alfa-2b.

Onset: Ninety-six percent of responders to peginterferon alfa-2b and 100% of responders to interferon alfa-2b first cleared their viral RNA by week 24 of treatment.

Duration: Unknown

Pharmacokinetics: Following a single subcutaneous dose of peginterferon alfa-2b, the mean absorption half-life ($t\frac{1}{2}k_a$) was 4.6 hours. Maximal serum concentrations (C_{max}) occur 15 to

44 hours post-dose and are sustained up to 48 to 72 hours. The C_{max} and AUC measurements of peginterferon alfa-2b increase in a dose-related manner. After multiple dosing, there is an increase in bioavailability of peginterferon alfa-2b. Week-48 mean trough concentrations (320 pg/mL; range, 0 to 2960) are approximately 3-fold higher than week-4 mean trough concentrations (94 pg/mL; range, 0 to 416). The mean peginterferon alfa-2b elimination half-life is approximately 40 hours (range, 22 to 60 hours) in patients with HCV infection. The apparent clearance of peginterferon alfa-2b is approximately 22 mL/hr•kg. Renal elimination accounts for 30% of clearance. Single-dose peginterferon alfa-2b pharmacokinetics following an subcutaneous 1 mcg/kg dose suggest the clearance of peginterferon alfa-2b is reduced approximately 50% in patients with impaired renal function (creatinine clearance less than 50 mL/min).

Pegylation of interferon alfa-2b produces a product (peginterferon alfa-2b) with clearance lower than that of nonpegylated interferon alfa-2b. When compared with interferon alfa-2b, peginterferon alfa-2b (1 mcg/kg) has approximately 7-fold lower mean apparent clearance and 5-fold greater mean half-life, permitting a reduced dosing frequency. At effective therapeutic doses, peginterferon alfa-2b has approximately 10-fold greater C_{max} and 50-fold greater AUC than interferon alfa-2b.

Pharmacokinetic data from geriatric patients (older than 65 years of age) treated with a single subcutaneous dose of 1 mcg/kg of peginterferon alfa-2b showed no remarkable differences in C_{max}, AUC, clearance, or elimination half-life from data obtained in younger patients.

During the 48-week treatment period with peginterferon alfa-2b, no differences in the pharmacokinetic profiles were observed between men and women with chronic HCV infection.

Metastatic melanoma: The pharmacokinetics were studied in 32 patients receiving adjuvant therapy for melanoma with peginterferon alfa-2b according to the recommended dose and schedule. At a dose of 6 mcg/kg/week once weekly, the geometric mean C_{max} was 4.4 ng/mL (CV 51%) and the geometric mean AUC was 430 ng•hr/mL (CV 35%) at week 8. The mean terminal half-life was $\approx$ 51 hours (CV 18%). The mean accumulation from week 1 to week 8 was 1.7. After administration of 3 mcg/kg/week once weekly, the mean geometric C_{max} was 2.5 ng/mL (CV 33%) and the geometric mean AUC was 228 ng•hr/mL (CV 24%) at week 4. The mean terminal half-life was approximately 43 hours (CV 19%).

Renal dysfunction: The disposition of peginterferon alfa-2b was studied in 26 subjects with varying degrees of renal function after administration of a single SC dose of peginterferon alfa-2b at 1 mcg/kg. The AUC increased by 1.3-, 1.7- and 1.9-fold in mild, moderate and severe renal impairment, respectively. The mean elimination half-life and maximal plasma concentration (C_{max}) increased in subjects with renal impairment. The mean AUC was similar in subjects with severe renal impairment on and not on hemodialysis, suggesting that no clinical meaningful amounts of peginterferon alfa-2b were removed during hemodialysis. After SC administration of 1 mcg/kg of peginterferon alfa-2b once weekly for four weeks in 21 subjects with varying degrees of renal function, AUC at week 4 increased 1.3-fold in moderate and 2.1-fold in severe renal impairment. The C_{max} at week 4 increased 1.8-fold in severe renal impairment, but no difference was observed in moderate renal impairment. Dose reductions of 25% and 50% are recommended in patients with moderate and severe renal impairment, respectively, receiving alpha interferons for chronic hepatitis C. The effect of varying degrees of renal impairment on the pharmacokinetics of peginterferon alfa-2b at the recommended doses of 3 mcg/kg or 6 mcg/kg for patients with melanoma has not been studied.

Mechanism: The biological activity of peginterferon alfa-2b derives from its interferon alfa-2b moiety. Interferons exert their cellular activities by binding to specific membrane receptors on the cell surface and initiating a complex sequence of intracellular events. These include the induction of certain enzymes, suppression of cell proliferation, immunomodulating activities such as enhancement of the phagocytic activity of macrophages and augmentation of the specific cytotoxicity of lymphocytes for target cells, and inhibition of virus replication in virus-infected cells. Interferon alfa regulates the Th1 T-helper cell subset in in vitro studies. The clinical relevance of these findings is not known.

Peginterferon alfa-2b raises concentrations of effector proteins such as serum neopterin and 2'5' oligoadenylate synthetase, raises body temperature, and causes reversible decreases in leukocyte and platelet counts. The correlation between the in vitro and in vivo pharmacologic and pharmacodynamic and clinical effects is unknown.

The mechanism by which peginterferon alfa-2b exerts its effects in patients with melanoma is unknown.

Drug Interactions: It is not known if peginterferon alfa-2b therapy causes clinically significant drug interactions with drugs metabolized by the liver in patients with HCV. In 12 healthy subjects known to be extensive CYP 2D6 metabolizers, a single subcutaneous dose of 1 mcg/kg peginterferon alfa-2b did not inhibit CYP 1A2, 2C8/9, 2D6, hepatic 3A4, or N-acetyltransferase; the effects of peginterferon alfa-2b on CYP 2C19 were not assessed. Nonetheless, exercise caution with drug by CYP2C8/9 (eg, warfarin, phenytoin) or CYP2D6 (eg, flecainide) as the therapeutic effect of these substrates may be decreased.

Monitor patients receiving methadone for signs and symptoms of increased narcotic effect. Peginterferon alfa-2b may increase methadone concentrations.

Closely monitor patients given nucleoside analogs for toxicities (especially hepatic decompensation and anemia). Discontinue nucleoside reverse-transcriptase inhibitors or reduce dose or discontinue interferon, ribavirin, or both with worsening toxicities. Concurrent use of didanosine with ribavirin is not recommended because fatal hepatic failure, peripheral neuropathy, pancreatitis, and symptomatic hyperlactactemia/lactic acidosis were reported in clinical trials.

Interferons may inhibit the induction of an adequate antibody response following immunization with live virus vaccines (eg, measles, mumps, rubella, varicella). Avoid concurrent use.

Lab Interference: None recognized.

Patient Information: Inform patients that there are no data evaluating whether peginterferon alfa-2b therapy will prevent transmission of HCV infection to others. Also, it is not known if treatment with peginterferon alfa-2b will cure HCV or prevent cirrhosis, liver failure, or liver cancer that may result from HCV virus. Patients should be well-hydrated, especially during the initial stages of treatment. Viral-like symptoms associated with administration of peginterferon alfa-2b may be minimized by bedtime administration of peginterferon alfa-2b or by use of antipyretics.

Pharmaceutical Characteristics

Concentration: The specific activity of peginterferon alfa-2b is approximately 0.7×10^8 units/mg protein.

Packaging:

PegIntron: Each 2 mL vial contains either 74, 118.4, 177.6, or 222 mcg of powdered peginterferon alfa-2b. Each box contains 2 syringes, one for reconstitution and one for injection. Pull the clear plastic safety sleeve over the needle after use. The syringe locks with an audible click when the green stripe on the safety sleeve covers the red stripe on the needle.

A box containing one 100 mcg/mL vial of peginterferon alfa-2b powder, one 5 mL vial of Sterile Water for Injection, 2 syringes with two 27-gauge, ½-inch needles and safety sleeves, and 2 alcohol swabs (NDC #: 00085-1368-01). Yields 50 mcg/0.5 mL.

A box containing one 160 mcg/mL vial of peginterferon alfa-2b powder, one 5 mL vial of Sterile Water for Injection, 2 syringes with two 27-gauge, ½-inch needles and safety sleeves, and 2 alcohol swabs (NDC #: 00085-1291-01). Yields 80 mcg/0.5 mL.

Peginterferon Alfa-2b (Recombinant)

A box containing one 240 mcg/mL vial of peginterferon alfa-2b powder, one 5 mL vial of Sterile Water for Injection, 2 syringes with two 27-gauge, ½-inch needles and safety sleeves, and 2 alcohol swabs (NDC #: 00085-1304-01). Yields 120 mcg/0.5 mL.

A box containing one 300 mcg/mL vial of peginterferon alfa-2b powder, one 5 mL vial of Sterile Water for Injection, 2 syringes with two 27-gauge, ½-inch needles and safety sleeves, and 2 alcohol swabs (NDC #: 00085-1279-01). Yields 150 mcg/0.5 mL.

Each *Redipen* is a dual-chamber glass cartridge containing peginterferon alfa-2b in the active chamber and sterile water in the diluent chamber. Each *Redipen* contains either 67.5 mcg, 108 mcg, 162 mcg, or 202.5 mcg of peginterferon alfa-2b. Because a small volume of solution is lost during preparation, each *Redipen* contains an excess amount of drug and diluent to ensure delivery of the labeled dose. Each box contains 1 *Redipen*, one 30-gauge, 8 mm needle and 2 alcohol swabs.

A box containing one 50 mcg/mL *Redipen* (NDC #: 00085-1323-01), box of four 50 mcg *Redipens* (00085-1323-02).

A box containing one 80 mcg/mL *Redipen* (NDC #: 00085-1316-01), box of four 80 mcg *Redipens* (00085-1316-02).

A box containing one 120 mcg/mL *Redipen* (NDC #: 00085-1297-01), box of four 120 mcg *Redipens* (00085-1297-02).

A box containing one 150 mcg/mL *Redipen* (NDC #: 00085-1370-01), box of four 150 mcg *Redipens* (00085-1370-02).

Sylatron: Each vial contains either 296, 444, or 888 mcg of powdered peginterferon alfa-2b. Each box contains one vial of powder, one vial of sterile water, 2 alcohol swabs, and 2 syringes (with safety sleeve), one for reconstitution and one for injection.

A box containing one 296-mcg vial of powder, yielding 40 mcg/0.1 mL (00085-1388-01, pack of four: 00085-1388-02)

A box containing one 444-mcg vial of powder, yielding 60 mcg/0.1 mL (00085-1287-02, pack of four: 00085-1287-03)

A box containing one 888-mcg vial of powder, yielding 120 mcg/0.1 mL (00085-1312-01, pack of four: 00085-1312-02)

Doseform: Powder for solution

Appearance: White to off-white lyophilized powder, yielding a clear and colorless solution

Diluent: Reconstitute each vial with only 0.7 mL sterile water for injection. Swirl gently to hasten complete dissolution of the powder. Discard the remaining diluent. Do not use other diluents.

To reconstitute the peginterferon alfa-2b in the *Redipen*, hold the *Redipen* upright (dose button down) and press the 2 halves of the pen together until there is an audible click. Gently invert the pen to mix the solution. Do not shake. Keeping the pen upright, attach the needle. Select the appropriate dose by pulling back on the dosing button until dark bands are visible and turning the button until the dark band is aligned with the correct dose. Each *Redipen* delivers up to 0.5 mL of reconstituted solution, with a concentration of either 50, 80, 120, or 150 mcg per 0.5 mL.

Adjuvant: None

Preservative: None

Allergens: None

Excipients: Each vial contains 1.11 mg dibasic sodium phosphate anhydrous, 1.11 mg monobasic sodium phosphate dihydrate, 59.2 mg sucrose, and 0.074 mg polysorbate 80.

Each *Redipen* contains 1.013 mg dibasic sodium phosphate anhydrous, 1.013 mg monobasic sodium phosphate dihydrate, 54 mg sucrose and 0.0675 mg polysorbate 80.

pH: Data not provided

Peginterferon Alfa-2b (Recombinant)

Shelf Life: Data not provided

Storage/Stability: Store *Redipen* at 2° to 8°C (36 to 46°F).

Store vials at 25°C (77°F). Discard frozen product. Product can tolerate short excursions at 15° to 30°C (59° to 86°F). Shipped at ambient temperature.

Use the reconstituted solution immediately. Solutions may be stored in a refrigerator up to 24 hours after reconstitution.

Do not add other medications to solutions containing peginterferon alfa-2b.

Discard used *Redipen*, as sterility of any remaining product cannot be guaranteed.

Production Process: Interferon alfa-2b is obtained from bacterial fermentation of a strain of *Escherichia coli* bearing a genetically engineered plasmid containing an interferon gene from human leukocytes. A 12-kilodalton monomethoxy polyethylene glycol moiety is attached covalently.

Media: *E. coli*

Other Information

First Licensed: January 19, 2001 (Schering Plough). To treat melanoma, April 11, 2011 (Merck).

References: Grace MJ, Cutler DL, Bordens RW. Pegylated IFNs for chronic hepatitis C: an update. *Expert Opin Drug Deliv.* 2005;2(2):219-226.

Interferon Alfa-n3 (Human Leukocyte Derived)

Interferons

Name:
Alferon N Injection

Manufacturer:
Hemispherx Biopharma, under license from
Hoffman-LaRoche

Synonyms: IFN-αn3

Comparison: The various interferon alpha products are not generically interchangeable, because variations in dosage, routes of administration, and adverse reactions exist among the different brands of interferon. Do not use different brands of interferon alpha in any single treatment regimen.

Immunologic Characteristics

Antigen Source: Interferon alpha expressed from human leukocytes challenged with avian Sendai virus.

Viability: Not viable, but immunologically active

Antigenic Form: Interferon, human leukocyte

Antigenic Type: Protein, natural source, containing at least 14 molecular subtypes. Consists of approximately 166 amino acids ranging in molecular weight from 16,000 to 27,000 daltons.

Strains: Interferon alfa-n3

Use Characteristics

Indications: For the intralesional treatment of refractory or recurring external condylomata acuminata (genital warts) in patients 18 years of age and older.

These warts are associated with infections of human papilloma virus (HPV), especially type 6 and possibly type 11. Select patients for treatment based on locations and sizes of the lesions, past treatment and response, and the patient's ability to comply with the treatment regimen. Interferon alfa-n3 is particularly useful for patients who have not responded satisfactorily to other treatment modalities (eg, podophyllin resin, surgery, laser, cryotherapy).

Unlabeled Uses: Interferon alpha is being investigated for efficacy in the treatment of mycosis fungoides (Sézary syndrome), non-Hodgkin lymphoma, multiple myeloma, cervical cancer, superficial bladder cancer, renal cancer, and malignant melanoma.

Various interferon alpha preparations are being investigated in the treatment of the following viral infections: cutaneous warts, cytomegaloviruses, herpes keratoconjunctivitis, herpes simplex, hepatitis C, human immunodeficiency virus, rhinoviruses, vaccinia, and varicella-zoster.

Investigational use of interferon alpha has shown significant activity in the treatment of the following conditions: carcinoid tumor, cutaneous T-cell lymphoma, and essential thrombocythemia. Limited activity has been demonstrated in acute leukemias, chronic lymphocytic leukemia, Hodgkin disease, malignant gliomas, nasopharyngeal carcinoma, osteosarcoma, and ovarian carcinoma. Interferon alpha is also being investigated in the treatment of life-threatening hemangiomas of infancy and multiple sclerosis.

Limitations: No activity has been demonstrated by various interferon alpha preparations in breast cancer, colorectal carcinoma, gastric carcinoma, lung carcinoma, pancreatic carcinoma, prostatic carcinoma, or soft tissue carcinoma.

Contraindications:

Absolute: Patients with known hypersensitivity to human interferon alpha or any component of the product, including mouse IgG, egg protein, or neomycin.

Relative: None

Immunodeficiency: Use may be indicated in certain immunodeficient conditions.

Elderly: No specific information is available about geriatric use of interferon alfa-n3.

Mutagenicity: Mutagenicity studies with interferon alfa-n3 have not been performed.

Fertility Impairment: In human clinical trials with interferon alfa-n3, menstrual cycle data were reported by 51 patients (36 recipients of active drug and 15 placebo recipients). There was no significant difference between the treatment groups with regard to menstrual cycle changes.

Interferon alfa-n3 can affect the menstrual cycle and decrease serum estradiol and progesterone levels in adult females. Caution fertile women to use effective contraception while being treated with interferon alfa-n3. Use interferon alfa-n3 with caution in fertile men.

Pregnancy: Category C. Use only if clearly needed. Recombinant interferons alfa-2a and alfa-2b induced a statistically significant increase in abortifacient activity in rhesus monkeys when given at tens or hundreds of times the standard human dose. Teratogenic activity in rhesus monkeys was not observed. Use interferon alfa-n3 in pregnant women only if the potential benefit justifies the potential risk to the fetus.

Lactation: It is not known if interferon alfa-n3 is excreted in breast milk. In mice, murine interferons are excreted in milk. Because of the potential for serious adverse effects from interferon alfa-n3 in nursing infants, decide whether to discontinue nursing or to discontinue the drug, considering the importance of the drug to the mother and the potential risks to the infant.

Children: Safety and efficacy have not been established in patients younger than 18 years of age. Interferon alfa-n3 can affect the menstrual cycle and decrease serum estradiol and progesterone levels in females. Interferon alfa-n3 is not recommended for use in patients younger than 18 years of age.

Adverse Reactions: After 4 weeks of treatment, the frequency of adverse reactions was similar in interferon alfa-n3 and placebo treatment groups (n = 104). The most frequent side effects were myalgias, fever, and headache, reported by 30% of patients after the first treatment session. In most cases, these effects were mild to moderate, transient, did not interfere with treatment, and diminished in severity and number with continued therapy. Application site disorders (eg, itching, pain) were reported more frequently by placebo recipients (26%) than by interferon alfa-n3 recipients (12%).

Other reactions reported by 5% or more of recipients included chills (14%), fatigue (14%), malaise (9%), and dizziness (9%). Other occasional or rare severe systemic adverse reactions include the following: back pain, insomnia, hypersensitivity to allergens, lymphadenopathy, tongue hyperesthesia, thirst, tingling of legs or feet, taste abnormalities, increased salivation, heat intolerance, visual disturbances, pharyngitis, muscle cramps, nose bleeds, throat tightness, papular rash, herpes labialis, hot flashes, nervousness, decrease in concentration, dysuria, and photosensitivity.

When administered by IM injection during clinical trials in cancer patients, interferon alfa-n3 exhibited a side effect profile similar to other alpha interferons.

Because of the viral-like symptoms associated with interferon alfa-n3 injection, use it cautiously in patients with debilitating medical conditions such as cardiovascular disease (eg, unstable angina and uncontrolled CHF), severe pulmonary disease (eg, COPD), or diabetes mellitus with ketoacidosis. Use interferon alfa-n3 cautiously in patients with coagulation disorders (eg, thrombophlebitis, pulmonary embolism, hemophilia), severe myelosuppression, or seizure disorders. Acute serious hypersensitivity reactions (eg, urticaria, angioedema, bronchoconstriction, anaphylaxis) have not been observed in recipients of interferon alfa-n3. If such reactions develop, however, discontinue interferon alfa-n3 immediately and start appropriate medical therapy.

Pharmacologic & Dosing Characteristics

Dosage: 0.05 mL (250,000 units) per wart, injected twice per week for up to 8 weeks. The maximum recommended dose per treatment session is 0.5 mL (2.5 million units).

Route & Site: Intralesional injection. Inject interferon alfa-n3 into the base of each wart, preferably using a 30-gauge needle attached to a syringe graduated in units of 0.01 mL. For large warts, interferon alfa-n3 may be injected at several points around the periphery of the wart, using a total dose of 0.05 mL per wart. The minimum effective dose of interferon alfa-n3 has not been established. Moderate to severe adverse experiences may require modification of the dosage regimen or, in some cases, termination of therapy.

Genital warts usually begin to disappear after several weeks of treatment with interferon alfa-n3. Continue treatment for a maximum of 8 weeks. Many patients who had partial resolution of warts during treatment experienced further resolution of their warts after cessation of treatment. Of the patients who had complete resolution of warts due to treatment, 48% had complete resolution of warts by the end of the treatment and 52% had complete resolution of warts during the 3 months after cessation of treatment. Thus, it is recommended that no further therapy (ie, interferon alfa-n3 or conventional therapy) be administered for 3 months after the initial 8-week course of treatment unless the warts enlarge or new warts appear. Studies to determine the safety and efficacy of a second course of treatment with interferon alfa-n3 have not been conducted.

Efficacy: Various controlled clinical trials have shown that therapy with interferon alfa-n3 resolves warts. Complete or partial resolution was noted in 80% of patients treated with interferon alfa-n3, compared with 44% for placebo-treated patients. Complete resolution was achieved in 54% of interferon alfa-n3 patients, compared with 20% in the placebo group. Of treated patients who achieved complete resolution, 48% achieved it by the end of treatment, and the remaining 52% experienced resolution during the 3 months following cessation of treatment. No recurrence developed in 76% of complete responders during a median of 48 weeks of follow-up observation. Interferon alfa-n3 was effective in treating lesions of all sizes, and there was no difference in resolution for perianal, penile, or vulvar lesions.

There was no difference in resolution for patients who had received prior treatment of their warts and for those who had not. Patients with primary occurrence of genital warts (ie, no prior treatment) had a similar resolution rate compared with the patients with recalcitrant warts.

Onset: Not known

Duration: Not known

Pharmacokinetics:

Absorption: In a study of the intralesional use of interferon alfa-n3, plasma concentrations of interferon were below detectable limits (3 units/mL or less). Minor side effects were noted, indicating that some of the injected interferon entered the systemic circulation.

Elimination: Systemically absorbed alpha and beta interferons are metabolized or degraded primarily in the kidney. Catabolism of interferon is postulated to occur at the brush border or in the lysosomes of the tubular epithelium. The mode of elimination after intralesional injection is unknown. Interferon alpha (human and recombinant) was not significantly cleared by hemodialysis.

Serum neutralizing activity: Few cases of human antibodies to interferon alfa-n3 or to the residual murine IgG antibodies in the formulation were detected during clinical trials.

Interferon Alfa-n3 (Human Leukocyte Derived)

Mechanism: Therapeutic effect may be due to inhibition of virus replication, suppression of cell proliferation, or immunomodulation. Interferon alfa-n3 binds to the same receptors as interferon alfa-2b. Binding of interferon to membrane receptors initiates a series of events that include induction of protein synthesis. These actions are followed by a variety of cellular responses, including inhibition of virus replication and suppression of cell proliferation, immunomodulation, enhancement of phagocytosis by macrophages, and augmentation of the cytotoxicity of lymphocytes. Enhancement of human-leukocyte-antigen expression occurs in response to exposure to interferons.

Drug Interactions: Systemic administration of interferon alfa-2a can affect specific microsomal enzyme systems. Interferon alfa-2a has reduced hepatic clearance of theophylline or aminophylline 33% to 81% in 8 of 9 subjects, apparently through inhibition of cytochrome P-450 microsomal enzymes. It is unknown if interferon alfa-n3 would exert a similar effect.

Synergistic toxicity has been observed when interferon alfa-2a is administered in combination with zidovudine (AZT), including a higher incidence of neutropenia. It is unknown if interferon alfa-n3 would exert a similar effect.

Interferons can inhibit the induction of an adequate antibody response following immunization with live virus vaccines (eg, measles, mumps, rubella, varicella). It is unknown if interferon alfa-n3 would exert a similar effect. Avoid concurrent use.

Pharmaceutical Characteristics

Concentration: 2×10^8 units per mg protein, 5 million units/mL

Quality Assay: Because interferon alfa-n3 is manufactured from human leukocytes, donor screening is performed to minimize the risk of transmitting infectious agents, in addition to viral-inactivation steps. There was no evidence of transmission of infection to drug recipients during clinical trials. Viral challenge showed that the manufacturing process inactivates model pathogenic viruses, yielding a 14-log volume reduction in a deliberate challenge of HIV-1, an 8-log reduction of hepatitis B virus, and a 9-log reduction of herpes simplex virus-1. No Sendai virus was present in the formulation during production tests, nor were cytomegalovirus, Epstein-Barr virus, or several other viruses.

Packaging: 5 million units/1 mL multidose vial

NDC Number: 54746-0001-01

Doseform: Solution

Appearance: Clear and colorless

Solvent: Phosphate-buffered saline: 8 mg/mL sodium chloride, 1.74 mg/mL sodium phosphate dibasic, 0.2 mg/mL potassium phosphate monobasic, and 0.2 mg/mL potassium chloride.

Adjuvant: None

Preservative: Phenol 3.3 mg/mL

Allergens: Residual neomycin less than 0.64 mcg/mL, residual murine IgG less than 8 ng/mL (usual range, 0.9 to 5.6 ng/mL), 1 mg/mL albumin human is added as a stabilizer.

Excipients: None

pH: 7.4

Shelf Life: Expires within 18 months.

Storage/Stability: Store at 2° to 8°C (35° to 46°F). Discard if frozen. To avoid foaming and protein degradation, do not shake. The product can tolerate incidental periods out of refrigeration during normal handling. Contact the manufacturer regarding individual stability scenarios. Shipped in insulated containers with coolant packs.

Production Process: Manufactured from pooled units of human leukocytes that have been induced by incomplete infection with avian Sendai virus to produce interferon alfa-n3. The process includes immunoaffinity chromatography with a murine monoclonal antibody, acidification at pH 2 for 5 days at 4°C (39°F), and gel-filtration chromatography. The acidification and purification steps also reduce the risk of viral transmission. The Sendai virus is grown in chicken eggs, but no egg protein has been detected in the initial stage of manufacture using an ELISA assay (limit of sensitivity, 16 ng/mL).

Media: Human leukocytes induced by incomplete infection with avian Sendai virus. The Sendai virus is grown in chicken eggs.

Disease Epidemiology

See Epidemiology of Diseases Treated with Interferon Alpha in the Interferon Alpha summary.

Other Information

Perspective: See also Epidemiology of Diseases Treated with Interferon Alpha in the Interferon Alpha summary.

1989: Interferon alfa-n3 licensed in October.

First Licensed: October 10, 1989

References: Friedman-Kien AE, et al. Natural interferon alfa for treatment of condylomata acuminata. *JAMA.* 1988;259:533-538.

Interferon Alfacon-1 (Recombinant)

Name:
Infergen

Manufacturer:
Boehringer Ingelheim Pharma,
distributed by Kadmon Pharmaceuticals

Synonyms: Alfacon refers to a "consensus" interferon that shares structural elements of both interferon-alfa and interferon-beta.

Comparison: The effects of interferon alfacon-1 display ranges of activity similar to other alfa interferons. Interferon alfacon-1 exhibits at least 5 times higher specific activity in vitro than interferon alfa-2a and interferon alfa-2b. Comparison of interferon alfacon-1 with an in vitro WHO potency standard for recombinant interferon alfa (83/514) reveals that the specific activity of interferon alfacon-1 in both an antiviral cytopathic effect assay and an antiproliferative assay is 1×10^9 units/mg. Correlation between in vitro activity and clinical activity of any interferon is unclear.

Immunologic Characteristics

Antigen Source: Interferon alfacon-1, a synthetic type-I interferon, expressed from recombinant *Escherichia coli* cells.

Viability: Not viable, but immunologically active

Antigenic Form: Interferon, type I

Antigenic Type: Protein. The 166-amino acid sequence of interferon alfacon-1 is derived by scanning several natural interferon-alpha subtypes and assigning the most common amino acid in each corresponding position. Four amino acid changes are made to facilitate synthesis, and the synthetic DNA sequence is constructed by chemical synthesis. Interferon alfacon-1 differs from interferon alfa-2 at 20/166 amino acids (88% homology). Comparison with interferon-beta shows identity at more than 30% of the amino acid positions, a greater similarity than any natural interferon-alpha subtype. This protein has a molecular weight of 19,434 daltons.

Strains: Interferon, consensus

Use Characteristics

Indications: For treating chronic hepatitis C virus (HCV) infection in patients 18 years and older with compensated liver disease. This indication is based on clinical trials conducted using interferon alfacon-1 alone at a time before combination treatment of chronic hepatitis C became standard of care, and on a single trial evaluating interferon alfacon-1 with ribavirin in patients who failed to respond to previous treatment with a pegylated interferon and ribavirin. Use of monotherapy with an interferon such as interferon alfacon-1 to treat hepatitis C is not recommended unless a patient is unable to take ribavirin. Patients with the following characteristics are less likely to benefit from retreatment with interferon alfacon-1/ribavirin combination therapy: response of $< 1 \log_{10}$ drop IN HCV RNA on previous treatment, Genotype 1, high viral load (> 850,000 IU/mL), African American race, and/or presence of cirrhosis.

Limitations: Rule out other causes of hepatitis, such as hepatitis B virus or autoimmune hepatitis, before starting therapy with interferon alfacon-1. No studies have been conducted in patients with decompensated hepatic disease. Do not treat them with interferon alfacon-1. Stop therapy in patients who develop symptoms of hepatic decompensation, such as jaundice, ascites, coagulopathy, or decreased serum albumin.

Interferon Alfacon-1 (Recombinant)

Contraindications:

Absolute: Patients with known hypersensitivity to interferon alphas, *E. coli*-derived products, or any component of the product.

Relative: Because type-I interferons are associated with depression, do not use interferon alfacon-1 in patients with severe psychiatric disorders. Discontinue therapy in patients who develop severe depression, suicidal ideation, or other severe psychiatric disorders.

Immunodeficiency: Use interferon alfacon-1 with caution in transplant patients or other chronically immunosuppressed patients.

Elderly: No specific information is available about geriatric use of interferon alfacon-1.

Pregnancy: Category C. Interferon alfacon-1 had embryocidal or abortifacient effects in golden Syrian hamsters when given at 135 times the human dose, and in cynomolgus and rhesus monkeys when given at 9 to 81 times the human dose. There are no adequate studies in pregnant women. Do not use interferon alfacon-1 during pregnancy. If a woman becomes pregnant or plans to become pregnant while taking interferon alfacon-1, inform her of the potential hazards to the fetus. Advise men and women treated with interferon alfacon-1 to use effective contraception.

Lactation: It is not known whether interferon alfacon-1 is excreted in breast milk. Use caution if interferon alfacon-1 is given to a nursing woman. The effect on the nursing child of oral interferon alfacon-1 in breast milk has not been evaluated.

Children: The safety and efficacy of interferon alfacon-1 have not been established in patients younger than 18 years of age. Interferon alfacon-1 therapy is not recommended in children.

Adverse Reactions: Most adverse events were mild to moderate in severity and abated when therapy ended. Unless otherwise specified, the adverse reactions listed below occurred in patients treated with 9 mcg interferon alfacon-1.

Body as a whole: Headache (82%); fatigue (69%); fever (61%); myalgia (58%); rigors (57%); body pain (54%); arthralgia (51%); influenza-like symptoms (presumed viral etiology, 15%); hot flushes, noncardiac chest pain (13%); increased sweating (12%); malaise (11%).

Most symptoms were short-lived and were treated symptomatically. While fever may be related to the flu-like symptoms reported in patients treated with interferon alfacon-1, rule out other possible causes of persistent fever.

Cardiovascular: Use interferon alfacon-1 with caution in patients with preexisting cardiac disease. Hypertension (5%), tachycardia (4%), and palpitation (3%) were the most common cardiovascular events reported for 9 mcg interferon alfacon-1 therapy, with 1% of patients reporting dose-limiting tachyarrhythmias. Supraventricular arrhythmias, chest pain, and MI are associated with interferon therapy.

CNS: Insomnia (39%); dizziness (22%); paresthesia (13%); amnesia, hypoesthesia (10%).

Dermatologic: Alopecia, pruritus (14%); rash (13%).

Endocrine: Give interferon alfacon-1 with caution to patients with a history of endocrine disorders. Abnormal thyroid stimulating hormone (TSH) and free thyroxine (T4) levels with hypothyroidism occurred in 4% of patients given 9 mcg interferon alfacon-1. Thyroid supplements were required by approximately 66% of those patients.

GI: Abdominal pain (41%); nausea (40%); diarrhea (29%); anorexia (24%); dyspepsia (21%); vomiting (12%).

Hematologic: Granulocytopenia (23%); thrombocytopenia (19%); leukopenia (15%).

Use interferon alfacon-1 cautiously in patients who have abnormally low peripheral blood cell counts or who are receiving agents that cause myelosuppression. Leukopenia, particularly granulocytopenia, may be severe in patients treated with interferon alphas. Leukopenia may require dose reduction or temporary cessation of therapy. In patients who received 15 mcg 3 times weekly, the higher dose was associated with a greater incidence of leukopenia and granulocytopenia. One or more dose reductions for any cause were required in 33% of patients. Do not treat patients who do not tolerate initial standard interferon therapy with 15 mcg 3 times weekly. Thrombocytopenia is a common, but less severe, event often associated with interferon-alfa. Withhold therapy if the absolute neutrophil count (ANC) is less than 500×10^6 cells/L or if the platelet count is less than 50×10^9 cells/L.

Hypersensitivity: Rarely, serious acute hypersensitivity reactions occur after treatment with interferon alphas. If hypersensitivity reactions (eg, urticaria, angioedema, bronchoconstriction, anaphylaxis) occur, discontinue the drug immediately and begin appropriate medical treatment.

Immunologic: Exacerbation of autoimmune disease has been reported in patients receiving type-I interferons. Do not use interferon alfacon-1 in patients with autoimmune hepatitis. Use with caution in patients with other autoimmune disorders.

Local: Injection-site erythema (23%).

Musculoskeletal: Back pain (42%); limb pain (26%); neck pain, skeletal pain (14%).

Ophthalmic: Ophthalmic disorders have been reported with interferon-alfa treatment. Investigators have reported retinal hemorrhages, cotton wool spots, and retinal artery or vein obstruction in rare cases. Conduct an eye examination on any patient complaining of loss of visual acuity or visual field. Because these events may occur in conjunction with other disease states, a visual exam before starting interferon therapy is recommended in patients with diabetes mellitus or hypertension.

Psychiatric: Nervousness (31%); depression (26%); anxiety (19%); emotional lability (12%).

Depression (usually mild to moderate), was the most common event resulting in drug discontinuation. Withdrawal from the study for adverse events occurred in 7% of patients treated with 9 mcg interferon alfacon-1 (including 4% because of psychiatric events).

Severe psychiatric events, including suicidal ideation and attempted suicide, may occur in patients treated with interferons. Suicidal ideation was rare (1%) for patients treated with 9 mcg interferon alfacon-1 compared with the overall incidence (55%) of psychiatric events. Use interferon alfacon-1 cautiously in patients who report a history of depression. Monitor all patients for depression. Other psychiatric events may also occur, including abnormal thinking, agitation, or apathy.

Respiratory: Pharyngitis (34%); upper respiratory infection (31%); cough (22%); sinusitis (17%); rhinitis (13%); respiratory tract congestion (12%); upper respiratory tract congestion (10%).

Pharmacologic & Dosing Characteristics

Dosage: The recommended dosage for treatment of chronic HCV infection is 9 mcg 3 times weekly for 24 weeks. Allow at least 48 hours to elapse between doses for interferon alfacon-1.

Patients who tolerated previous interferon therapy and did not respond or relapsed after its discontinuation may be treated with 15 mcg 3 times weekly for 6 months. Do not treat patients with 15 mcg 3 times weekly if they have not received, or have not tolerated, an initial course of interferon therapy.

For people who experience a severe adverse event while receiving interferon alfacon-1, temporarily withhold the drug. If the event does not become tolerable, discontinue therapy. Dose reduction to 7.5 mcg may be necessary. In the pivotal study, the doses for 11% of patients (26/231) who initially received 9 mcg interferon alfacon-1 were reduced to 7.5 mcg.

If reactions occur at the reduced dose, discontinue treatment or reduce the dose further. Decreased efficacy may result from treatment at doses less than 7.5 mcg. During subsequent treatment with 15 mcg, 33% of subjects required dose reductions in 3 mcg increments.

Interferon Alfacon-1 (Recombinant)

Route: Subcutaneous injection

Overdosage: The maximum overdose reported was 150 mcg given subcutaneously in a patient enrolled in a phase 1 advanced-malignancy trial. The patient received 10 times the prescribed dose for 3 days. The patient experienced a mild increase in anorexia, chills, fever, and myalgia. Increases in ALT (15 to 127 units/L), aspartate transaminase (AST, 15 to 164 units/L), and lactic dehydrogenase (LDH; 183 to 281 units/L) were reported. These values returned to normal or to baseline values within 30 days.

Laboratory Tests: Tests are recommended before beginning treatment (baseline), 2 weeks after starting therapy, and periodically thereafter during the 24 weeks of therapy, at the discretion of the prescriber. After the patient has completed therapy, periodically monitor any abnormal test values. Consider these entrance criteria used for clinical trials as guidelines to acceptable baseline values for initiating treatment: Platelet count 75×10^9 cells/L or more; hemoglobin 100 g/L or more; ANC more than $1,500 \times 10^6$ cells/L; serum creatinine concentration less than 180 mmol/L (less than 2 mg/dL) or creatinine clearance more than 0.83 mL/second (more than 50 mL/min); serum albumin more than 25 g/L; and bilirubin, TSH, and T_4 within normal limits.

Neutropenia, thrombocytopenia, hypertriglyceridemia, and thyroid disorders have been reported with interferon alfacon-1 therapy. Monitor these parameters closely. Withhold therapy if the ANC is less than 500×10^6 cells/L or if the platelet count is less than 50×10^9 cells/L.

The following variables were affected by therapy with interferon alfacon-1 in 231 patients treated with the 9 mcg dose:

Hemoglobin and hematocrit: Gradual decreases in mean values for hemoglobin and hematocrit occurred; hemoglobin and hematocrit were 4% and 5% below baseline, respectively, at the end of treatment. Decreases from baseline of 20% or more in hemoglobin or hematocrit were seen rarely (1% or less).

WBC: Decreases in mean values for both total white blood cell (WBC) count and ANC occurred within the first 2 weeks of treatment. By the end of treatment, mean decreases from baseline of 19% for WBCs and 23% for ANC were observed. These effects reversed during the posttreatment observation period. Decreases in ANC to levels less than 500×10^6 cells/L were seen in 2 subjects. In both cases, the ANC returned to clinically acceptable levels with a reduction of the interferon alfacon-1 dose. These transient decreases in neutrophils were not associated with infections.

Platelets: Decreases in mean platelet count by 16% compared with baseline were seen by the end of treatment but reversed during the posttreatment period. Values below normal were common during treatment; 3% of patients developed values less than 50×10^9 cells/L, which usually prompted dose reduction.

Triglycerides: Mean values for serum triglyceride increased shortly after the start of therapy, with increases of 41% compared with baseline observed at the end of treatment. Values at least 3 times pretreatment levels developed in 7% of subjects during treatment. This effect was promptly reversed after treatment stopped.

Thyroid function: Increases in TSH and decreases in T_4 mean values, consistent with hypothyroidism, occurred. Increases in TSH to more than 7 mU/L were seen in 10% of patients treated at the 9 mcg dose, either during treatment or during the post-treatment observation period. Thyroid supplements were instituted in approximately 33% of these people.

Laboratory values for subsequent treatment: Similar changes in the variables outlined above were observed among 165 patients treated with 15 mcg of interferon alfacon-1 after the failure of initial interferon therapy. However, mean decreases from baseline of 23% for WBC and 27% for ANC were observed, which was greater than those obscured during initial treatment. Reductions in WBCs and ANC resulted in alteration of doses in

11 patients (7%). Two patients experienced reversible reductions in ANC to less than 500×10^6 cells/L, which was not associated with infectious complications. No patient discontinued therapy because of hematologic toxicity.

Efficacy: The efficacy of interferon alfacon-1 in treating chronic HCV infection was examined among 704 patients previously untreated with interferon-alfa. Patients were at least 18 years old, had compensated liver disease, tested positive for HCV RNA, and had elevated ALT concentrations averaging more than 1.5 times the upper limit of normal. Other causes of chronic liver disease were ruled out. Efficacy was based on serum ALT concentrations at the end of therapy (24 weeks) and after 24 weeks of observation following the end of treatment to assess durability of response. HCV RNA was also assessed using a polymerase chain reaction assay. Liver histology was assessed by comparing a pretreatment biopsy specimen with a specimen obtained 24 weeks after stopping interferon therapy.

Subjects were randomized to receive 3 mcg interferon alfacon-1, 9 mcg interferon alfacon-1, or 3 million units interferon alfa-2b (IFN α-2b). All patients received the interferon subcutaneously 3 times weekly for 24 weeks. Complete response was defined as a decrease in ALT concentration to or below the upper limit of normal (48 unit/L) at the end of posttreatment observation. Reduction of HCV RNA to less than 100 copies/mL was measured as a secondary efficacy end point.

Sustained response rates are depicted in the following table. The 9 mcg interferon alfacon-1 dose arm showed efficacy similar to the IFN α-2b arm. The 3 mcg interferon alfacon-1 dose arm had lesser efficacy.

Rates (95% CI) of ALT Normalization and HCV RNA Reductions				
	End of 24-week Treatment		End of Observation (Sustained Response Rate)	
	Infergen (9 mcg)	IFN α-2b (3 million units)	*Infergen* (9 mcg)	IFN α-2b (3 million units)
Normalized ALT	39% (33%, 46%)	35% (29%, 41%)	17% (12%, 22%)	17% (13%, 22%)
HCV RNA Negative	33% (27%, 39%)	25% (19%, 31%)	9% (6%, 14%)	8% (5%, 13%)

Similar improvement in liver histology was observed in the 9 mcg interferon alfacon-1 (68%), 3 mcg interferon alfacon-1 (63%), and IFN α-2b (65%) dose arms.

Subsequent treatment with 15 mcg of interferon alfacon-1 was evaluated among 107 patients who had failed initial therapy with either 9 mcg interferon alfacon-1 or 3 million units (approximately 15 mcg) IFN α-2b. They were assessed for normalization of ALT and HCV RNA reduction after 24 weeks of observation. Overall, 15% had a sustained ALT response. Of patients who had relapsed after initial therapy, 30% (10/33) had a sustained ALT response. Eight percent (6/74) whose ALT concentration never normalized had a sustained ALT response. Of patients who had relapsed after initial therapy, 25% (8/32) had a sustained HCV response after subsequent treatment. Three percent (2/75) who never had a reduction in HCV RNA to less than 100 copies/mL had a sustained HCV response.

Onset: Not known

Duration: Not known

Pharmacokinetics: The pharmacokinetic properties of interferon alfacon-1 have not been evaluated in patients with chronic hepatitis C. Pharmacokinetics were evaluated in healthy volunteers after subcutaneous injection of 1, 3, or 9 mcg interferon alfacon-1. Plasma levels after subcutaneous administration of any dose were too low to be detected by either ELISA or by inhibition of viral cytopathic effect. However, analysis of levels of interferon alfacon-1-induced cellular products (eg, 2'5' oligoadenylate synthetase [OAS] and β-2 microglobulin) revealed a statistically significant, dose-related increase in the area under the curve (AUC)

($P < 0.001$ for all comparisons). Concentrations of 2'5' OAS peaked 24 hours after dosing, whereas levels of β-2 microglobulin peaked 24 to 36 hours after dosing.

All interferons are highly species-specific. Studies of interferon alfacon-1 in golden Syrian hamsters and rhesus monkeys demonstrated rapid absorption after subcutaneous injection. Peak serum concentrations of interferon alfacon-1 were observed at 1 hour and 4 hours after injection in golden Syrian hamsters and rhesus monkeys, respectively. Subcutaneous bioavailability was high in both species, averaging 99% in golden Syrian hamsters and 83% to 104% in rhesus monkeys. Clearance of interferon alfacon-1, averaging 1.99 mL/min/kg in golden Syrian hamsters and 0.71 to 0.92 mL/min/kg in rhesus monkeys, was due predominantly to catabolism and excretion by the kidneys. The terminal half-life of interferon alfacon-1 after subcutaneous dosing was 1.3 hours in golden Syrian hamsters and 3.4 hours in rhesus monkeys. Upon 7-day multiple subcutaneous dosing, no accumulation of serum levels was observed in golden Syrian hamsters.

Serum neutralizing activity: Serum antibody levels were measured in all patients using both an interferon alfacon-1-binding radioimmunoassay and an IFN α-2b-binding ELISA. A patient was considered to have developed binding antibodies if, using serum samples from 2 consecutive time points, a positive response was detected in either assay. The number of people developing positive binding-antibody responses was similar in the 9 mcg interferon alfacon-1 (11%) and 3 million units assay IFN α-2b (15%) groups. The titer of neutralizing antibodies to interferon was not measured. Sustained ALT response rates in patients treated with interferon alfacon-1 who developed binding antibodies (16%) were similar to rates in patients who did not develop detectable antibody titers (21%). The most frequently observed time to first antibody response was week 16 of interferon treatment. After interferon therapy was stopped, the number of patients with a positive antibody response declined during post-treatment observation.

Mechanism: Interferons exert cellular effects by binding to specific membrane receptors on cell surfaces. Once bound to the cell membrane, interferon may initiate a complex sequence of intracellular events that include the induction of certain enzymes. This process is probably responsible, at least in part, for cellular responses to interferon, including inhibition of virus replication in virus-infected cells, suppression of cell proliferation, enhancement of phagocytic activity of macrophages, and augmentation of specific cytotoxicity of lymphocytes for target cells.

Other postulated mechanisms for interferon's effect include an effect on cell differentiation (including phenotype reversion), which may help reestablish normal growth controls in cancer cells, and increased expression of class I histocompatibility antigen, which may render a virus-infected cell susceptible to killing. Interferons may have a regulatory or suppressive effect on expression of oncogenes. Some or all of these activities might contribute to interferon's therapeutic effects.

Drug Interactions: Use interferon alfacon-1 cautiously in patients receiving agents known to cause myelosuppression or agents known to be metabolized via the cytochrome P-450 pathway. Monitor patients taking drugs metabolized by this pathway closely for changes in the therapeutic or toxic levels of these drugs.

Interferons may inhibit the induction of an adequate antibody response following immunization with live virus vaccines (eg, measles, mumps, rubella, varicella). Avoid concurrent use.

Patient Information: If home use is prescribed, instruct the patient on proper dosage and administration. Explain the importance of proper disposal procedures. Caution against reuse of needles or syringes or reentry of the vial. Encourage use of a puncture-resistant container for disposal of used syringes and needles.

Inform the patient that the most common reactions occurring with interferon alfacon-1 therapy are flu-like symptoms, including fatigue, fever, rigors, headache, arthralgia, myalgia, and increased sweating. The use of nonnarcotic analgesics and bedtime administration of interferon alfacon-1 may prevent or lessen some of these symptoms. Inform patients of the possible development of depression with i nterferon alfacon-1 therapy. Ask patients to report any symptoms of depression immediately.

There are significant differences in specific activities among interferons. Changes in interferon brand may require adjustment of dosage or route of administration. Warn patients not to change brands of interferon without medical consultation. Also instruct them not to reduce the dose of interferon alfacon-1 without medical consultation.

Pharmaceutical Characteristics

Concentration: 0.03 mg/mL

Packaging: Single-dose vials containing 9 mcg (0.3 mL) in packs of 6 vials (NDC#: 66435-0202-09); single-dose vials containing 15 mcg (0.5 mL) in packs of 6 vials (66435-0201-15).

Doseform: Solution

Appearance: Clear, colorless liquid

Solvent: Phosphate-buffered saline

Adjuvant: None

Preservative: None

Allergens: None

Excipients: 100 mM sodium chloride (5.9 mg/mL), 25 mM sodium phosphate (3.8 mg/mL)

pH: 7 ± 0.2

Shelf Life: Data not provided.

Storage/Stability: Store at 2° to 8°C (36° to 46°F). Do not freeze. Contact manufacturer regarding exposure to extreme temperatures. Avoid vigorous shaking and exposure to direct sunlight. Just before injection, interferon alfacon-1 may be allowed to reach room temperature. Discard unused portions. Do not save unused drug for later administration. Shipping data not provided.

Production Process: Interferon alfacon-1 is produced in *E. coli* cells genetically altered by insertion of a synthetically constructed sequence that codes for interferon alfacon-1. Before final purification, the drug is allowed to oxidize to its native state. Its final purity is achieved by sequential passage over a series of chromatography columns.

Media: Genetically reengineered *E. coli* cells.

Disease Epidemiology

See Interferon Alpha Summary for details.

Other Information

Perspective:
1981: Amgen scientists synthesize interferon alfacon-1.

First Licensed: October 6, 1997

References: Blatt LM, et al. The biologic activity and molecular characterization of a novel synthetic interferon-alpha species, consensus interferon. *J Interferon Cytokine Res.* 1996;16(7):489-499.

Keeffe EB, et al. Therapy of hepatitis C: Consensus interferon trials. Consensus Interferon Study Group. *Hepatology.* 1997;26(3 Suppl 1):101S-107S.

Interferon Beta Summary

Interferons

Interferon Beta Comparisons			
	Avonex	*Rebif*	*Betaseron*, *Extavia*
	Interferon beta-1a	Interferon beta-1a	Interferon beta-1b
Manufacturer	Biogen Idec	Serono	Bayer
Distributor	Biogen Idec	Serono	Bayer, Novartis
Culture media	Chinese hamster ovary cells	Chinese hamster ovary cells	*Escherichia coli*
Form	Glycosylated	Glycosylated	Nonglycosylated
Concentration	Syringe: 15 mcg/0.5 mL Vial: 30 mcg/mL after reconstitution	22 mcg/0.5 mL or 44 mcg/0.5 mL	250 mcg or 8 million units/mL
Packaging	Four packs, each containing 1 vial or syringe, diluent, and supplies	Prefilled syringes	Vial of powder plus diluent
Doseform	Syringe: Solution Vial: Powder for solution	Solution	Powder for solution
Routine storage	Refrigerate	Refrigerate	Room temperature
Diluent	Sterile water without preservatives	N/A	Sodium chloride 0.54% without preservatives
Dose	30 mcg once a week	Begin with 8.8 mcg, escalating to 44 mcg, 3 times a week	250 mcg every other day
Route	IM	Subcutaneous	Subcutaneous
Selected side effects	Viral-like symptoms (61%), muscle ache (34%), fever (23%), injection-site reactions (3%), necrosis (3%)	Viral-like symptoms (59%), muscle ache (25%), fever (28%), injection-site reactions (92%), necrosis (3%)	Viral-like symptoms (76%), muscle ache (44%), fever (59%), injection-site reactions (85%), necrosis (5%)

Names:
  Avonex
  Rebif

Manufacturers:
  Biogen Idec
  EMD Serono

Synonyms: CAS 145258-61-3

Comparison: The amino acid sequence of both *Avonex* and *Rebif* are identical to that of natural fibroblast-derived human interferon beta. *Avonex* is less likely to be associated with injection-site reactions and necrosis than typically seen with *Betaseron* brand of interferon beta. The products also differ in dosage and route of administration. Differences in efficacy of *Avonex* and *Rebif* are discussed in the Efficacy section.

Immunologic Characteristics

Antigen Source: Interferon beta-1a, expressed from Chinese hamster ovary (CHO) cells containing the recombinant gene for human interferon beta.

Viability: Not viable, but immunologically active

Antigenic Form: Interferon, typically secreted by human fibroblasts

Antigenic Type: Glycosylated polypeptide (glycoprotein). Interferon beta-1a has 166 amino acids, weighing approximately 22,500 daltons. Glycosylation occurs at the asparagine residue at position 80. This glycoprotein is approximately 89% protein and 11% carbohydrate by weight. Interferon beta-1a contains a cysteine molecule at position 17, as does native interferon beta. Natural interferon beta and interferon beta-1a are glycosylated, with each containing a single N-linked complex carbohydrate moiety.

Strains: Interferon beta-1a

Use Characteristics

Indications: For the treatment of relapsing forms of multiple sclerosis (MS), to slow the accumulation of physical disability and decrease the frequency of clinical exacerbations. For *Avonex*, patients with MS in whom efficacy has been demonstrated include patients who experienced a first clinical episode and have magnetic resonance imaging (MRI) features consistent with MS.

Limitations: Safety and efficacy of treatment with interferon beta-1a after 2 years of therapy are not known. Safety and efficacy in patients with chronic progressive MS have not been evaluated.

The relationship between MRI findings and the clinical status of patients is not fully known. Changes in lesion area often do not correlate with changes in disability progression. The prognostic significance of the MRI findings in the pivotal interferon beta-1a study discussed in the Efficacy section has not been evaluated.

Contraindications:

Absolute: None

Relative: Patients with a history of hypersensitivity to natural or recombinant interferon beta, human albumin, or any other component of the formulation.

Use with caution in patients with depression. Depression and suicide have been reported in patients receiving other interferon compounds. Depression and suicidal ideation are known to occur at an increased frequency in the MS population. An equal incidence of depression was seen in the placebo-treated and interferon beta-1a–treated patients in the controlled MS study. Advise patients treated with interferon beta-1a to report immediately any symptoms of depression or suicidal ideation. If a patient develops depression, consider stopping interferon beta-1a therapy.

Immunodeficiency: Interferon beta-1a specifically has not been studied in immunocompromised patients.

Elderly: No specific information is available regarding use of interferon beta-1a in the elderly population. In general, dose selection for an elderly patient should be cautious, starting at the low end of the dosing range, reflecting the greater frequency of decreased hepatic, renal, or cardiac function, and of concomitant disease or other drug therapy.

Carcinogenicity: No carcinogenicity data for interferon beta-1a are available in animals or humans.

Mutagenicity: Interferon beta-1a was not mutagenic when tested in the Ames bacterial test and in an in vitro cytogenetic assay in human lymphocytes in the presence and absence of metabolic activation. These assays are designed to detect agents that interact directly with and cause damage to cellular DNA. Interferon beta-1a is a glycosylated protein that does not directly bind to DNA.

Fertility Impairment: It is not known whether interferon beta-1a can affect human reproductive capacity. Menstrual irregularities were observed in monkeys given interferon beta at a dose 100 times the recommended weekly human dose, based on body surface area. Anovulation and decreased serum progesterone levels were also noted transiently in some animals. These effects were reversible after stopping the drug. Treatment of monkeys with interferon beta at twice the recommended weekly human dose had no effects on cycle duration or ovulation.

The accuracy of extrapolating animal doses to human doses is not known. In the placebo-controlled study, 6% of patients receiving placebo and 5% of patients receiving *Avonex* experienced menstrual disorders. If menstrual irregularities occur in humans, it is not known how long they will persist following treatment.

Pregnancy: Category C. Use only if clearly needed. The reproductive toxicity of interferon beta-1a has not been studied in humans. In pregnant monkeys given interferon beta at 100 times the recommended weekly human dose, no teratogenic or other adverse effects on fetal development were observed. Abortifacient activity was evident following 3 to 5 doses at this level. No abortifacient effects were observed in monkeys treated at twice the recommended weekly human dose. *Rebif* was associated with significant embryolethal or abortifacient effects in cynomolgus monkeys administered doses approximately 2 times the cumulative weekly human dose, either during the period of organogenesis or later in pregnancy. There were no fetal malformations or other evidence of teratogenesis in these studies. There are no adequate and well-controlled studies with interferons in pregnant women. If a woman becomes pregnant or plans to become pregnant while taking interferon beta-1a, inform her of the potential hazards to the fetus and recommend that she discontinue therapy. The manufacturers recommend that women of childbearing age use birth control measures during interferon beta-1a therapy.

Lactation: It is not known if interferon beta-1a crosses into human breast milk. Because of the potential for serious adverse reactions in breast-feeding infants, decide whether to discontinue breast-feeding or to discontinue interferon beta-1a.

Children: Safety and efficacy of interferon beta-1a in children younger than 18 years of age have not been established.

Adverse Reactions: In a randomized, open-label, evaluator-blinded, active-comparator study, adverse events were generally similar between the *Rebif*-treated and *Avonex*-treated groups. Exceptions included injection-site disorders (*Rebif* [80%], *Avonex* [24%]), hepatic-function disorders (*Rebif* [14%], *Avonex* [7%]), and leukopenia (*Rebif* [3%], *Avonex* [less than 1%]).

The 5 most common adverse events associated (at $P \leq 0.075$) with *Avonex* treatment were viral-like symptoms, muscle ache, fever, chills, and asthenia. The incidence of all 5 adverse events diminished with continued treatment. Adverse events and laboratory abnormalities with *Avonex* treatment occurring at an incidence at least 4% more often among the 158 MS patients treated with interferon beta-1a 30 mcg once weekly by intramuscular (IM) injection, compared with patients treated with placebo, included the following: headache (67%), viral-like symptoms (61%), muscle ache (34%), nausea (33%), pain (24%), fever (23%), asthenia (21%), chills (21%), diarrhea (16%), dyspepsia (11%), infection (11%), arthralgia (9%), and anemia (8%).

The most frequently reported serious adverse reactions with *Rebif* were psychiatric disorders, including depression and suicidal ideation or attempt. The most common adverse reactions were injection-site disorders, influenza-like symptoms (eg, headache, fatigue, fever, rigors, chest pain, back pain, myalgia), abdominal pain, depression, elevation of liver enzymes, and hematologic abnormalities. The most frequent adverse reactions resulting in clinical intervention (eg, discontinuation of *Rebif*, dosage adjustment, concomitant medication to treat symptoms) were injection-site disorders, influenza-like symptoms, depression, and elevation of liver enzymes. Eight *Rebif*-treated patients developed injection-site necrosis during 2 years of therapy. All events resolved with conservative management; none required skin debridement or grafting. *Rebif* was continued in 7 of these patients and interrupted briefly in the eighth. Adverse events and laboratory abnormalities occurring with an incidence at least 4% more often among patients treated with *Rebif* 44 mcg, compared with placebo recipients, included injection-site reaction (92%), headache (70%), influenza-like symptoms (59%), fatigue (41%), leukopenia (36%), fever (28%), ALT increased (27%), myalgia (25%), back pain (25%), AST increased (17%), rigors (13%), vision abnormalities (13%), lymphadenopathy (12%), abnormal hepatic function (9%), thrombocytopenia (8%), dry mouth (5%), malaise (5%), and somnolence (5%).

Anaphylaxis is a rare complication of interferon use. Other allergic reactions included skin rash and urticaria, ranging from mild to severe without a clear relationship to dose or duration of exposure. Several allergic reactions, some severe, occurred after prolonged use.

Hepatic: Severe hepatic injury, including hepatic failure, has been reported rarely in patients taking interferon beta-1a. A case of fulminant hepatic failure requiring liver transplantation in a patient who initiated *Rebif* therapy while taking another hepatotoxic medication was reported. Symptomatic hepatic dysfunction, primarily presenting as jaundice, was reported as a rare complication of *Rebif*. Asymptomatic elevation of hepatic transaminases (particularly ALT) is common with interferon therapy. Start interferon beta-1a with caution in patients with active liver disease, alcohol abuse, increased serum ALT (more than 2.5 times the upper limit of normal [ULN]), or a history of significant liver disease. Consider dose reduction if ALT rises more than 5 times the ULN. The dose may be gradually re-escalated when enzyme levels normalize. Stop treatment with interferon beta-1a if jaundice or other clinical symptoms of liver dysfunction appear.

Avonex has also been evaluated in 290 patients with illnesses other than MS. The majority received 15 to 75 mcg subcutaneously 3 times per week for up to 6 months. The incidence of common adverse events was generally similar to those seen in the placebo-controlled MS study. In these non-MS studies, inflammation at the site of the subcutaneous injection was seen in 52% of treated patients. In contrast, IM injection-site inflammation was seen in 3% of MS patients. Subcutaneous injections were also associated with the following local reactions: injection-site necrosis, injection-site atrophy, injection-site edema, and injection-site hemorrhage. None of these was observed in the MS patients participating in the placebo-controlled study.

Throughout the placebo-controlled studies of *Avonex* and *Rebif*, serum samples from patients were monitored for the development of interferon beta-1 neutralizing activity. During the

Avonex study, 24% of interferon beta-1a–treated patients were found to have serum neutralizing activity at 1 or more time points tested. Fifteen percent of *Avonex*-treated patients tested positive for neutralizing activity at a level at which no placebo patient tested positive. In the *Rebif* study, 24% developed neutralizing antibodies at the 44 mcg dosage level. The significance of the appearance of serum neutralizing activity is unknown.

For both *Avonex* and *Rebif*, the incidence of depression was equal in the interferon and placebo arms (approximately 18% to 25%). However, because depression and suicide have been reported with these and other interferon products, use interferon beta-1a with caution in patients with depression.

In the *Avonex* placebo-controlled study, 4 patients receiving interferon beta-1a experienced seizures, while no seizures occurred in the placebo group. Three of these 4 patients had no history of seizure. Use caution when giving interferon beta-1a to patients with preexisting seizure disorder. For patients who develop seizures with no history, establish an etiologic basis and begin appropriate anticonvulsant therapy before considering resumption of interferon beta-1a treatment. The effect of interferon beta-1a on the medical management of patients with seizure disorder is unknown.

Closely monitor patients with cardiac disease, such as angina, congestive heart failure, or arrhythmia for worsening of their clinical condition during initial therapy with interferon beta-1a. Interferon beta-1a does not have any known direct-acting cardiac toxicity. However, viral-like symptoms seen with interferon beta-1a therapy may prove stressful to patients with severe cardiac conditions.

Many other events occurred during premarket evaluation of interferon beta-1a, administered either subcutaneously or IM, in all patient populations studied. Because most of the events were observed in open and uncontrolled studies, the role of interferon beta-1a in their causation cannot be reliably determined. The list is printed in the drug's product labeling.

There is no evidence that drug abuse or dependence occurs with interferon beta-1a therapy. However, the risk of dependence has not been systematically evaluated.

Pharmacologic & Dosing Characteristics

Dosage:

Avonex: For the treatment of relapsing forms of MS, 30 mcg injected IM once a week.

Rebif: For the treatment of relapsing forms of MS, 44 mcg 3 times weekly. Administer *Rebif*, if possible, at the same time (preferably the late afternoon or evening) on the same 3 days (eg, Monday, Wednesday, Friday) at least 48 hours apart. Generally, patients should start at 8.8 mg 3 times per week, increasing over a 4-week period to 44 mcg per dose, using the following table as a guide. Leukopenia or elevated liver function tests may warrant dose reductions of 20% to 50% until toxicity resolves.

Rebif Schedule for Patient Titration				
Interval	Recommended titration	*Rebif* dose	Volume	Syringe concentration
Weeks 1 to 2	20%	8.8 mcg	0.2 mL	22 mcg per 0.5 mL
Weeks 3 to 4	50%	22 mcg	0.5 mL	22 mcg per 0.5 mL
Weeks 5+	100%	44 mcg	0.5 mL	44 mcg per 0.5 mL

Route:

Avonex: IM

Rebif: Subcutaneous

Overdosage: Safety of doses higher than 60 mcg once a week (for *Avonex*) or 44 mcg 3 times a week (for *Rebif*) have not been evaluated adequately. The maximum safe dose has not been determined.

Missed Doses: Inject missed doses as soon as possible. Then resume the regular schedule, but do not give 2 injections within 2 days of each other.

Related Interventions: Acetaminophen 650 mg just before injection and for 24 hours after each injection has been used to reduce acute symptoms.

Laboratory Tests: Complete blood and differential white blood cell counts, platelet counts, and blood chemistries, including liver function tests, are recommended during interferon beta-1a therapy (eg, 1, 3, and 6 months, and periodically thereafter). There were no significant differences between the placebo and interferon beta-1a groups in the incidence of liver enzyme elevation, leukopenia, or thrombocytopenia. However, these are known to be dose-related laboratory abnormalities associated with the use of interferons. Patients with myelo-suppression may require more intensive monitoring of complete blood cell counts, with differential and platelet counts. Perform thyroid function tests every 6 months in patients with a history of thyroid dysfunction or as clinically indicated.

Efficacy:

Avonex: Avonex in MS was studied in a randomized, multicenter, double-blind placebo-controlled study in patients with relapsing (stable or progressive) MS. In this study, 301 patients received either 6 million units (30 mcg) of *Avonex* or placebo by IM injection once weekly. All patients had a definite diagnosis of at least 1-year duration. At entry, study participants had Kurtzke Expanded Disability Status Scale (EDSS) scores ranging from 1 to 3.5.

Time to onset of sustained progression in disability was significantly longer in patients treated with *Avonex* than in patients receiving placebo ($P = 0.02$). The Kaplan-Meier estimate of the percentage of patients progressing after 2 years was 34.9% for placebo-treated patients and 21.9% for *Avonex*-treated patients, indicating a slowing of the disease process. This is a 37% reduction in the risk of accumulating disability.

There was a statistically significant difference in confirmed change on the EDSS between groups, favoring those treated with *Avonex*. The mean change in EDSS from study entry to end of study was 0.5 among patients receiving placebo and 0.2 among those treated with *Avonex* ($P = 0.006$). For all patients included in the study, irrespective of time on study, the annual exacerbation rate was 0.67 per year in the *Avonex*-treated group and 0.82 per year in the placebo-treated group ($P = 0.04$).

Gadolinium (Gd)-enhancing lesions seen on brain MRI scans represent areas of break-down of the blood-brain barrier, thought to be secondary to inflammation. Patients treated with *Avonex* demonstrated significantly lower Gd-enhanced lesion numbers after 1 and 2 years of treatment ($P \leq 0.05$). The volume of Gd-enhanced lesions was also analyzed and showed similar treatment effects ($P \leq 0.03$). Percentage change in T2-weighted (proton density) lesion volume from study entry to year 1 was significantly lower in *Avonex*-treated patients than placebo-treated patients ($P = 0.02$).

Rebif: A head-to-head study involving 677 patients with relapsing-remitting MS compared the proportion of MS patients treated with either *Rebif* (44 mcg 3 times weekly subcutaneously) or *Avonex* (30 mcg once weekly IM) who were relapse free after 24 weeks (primary end point) and 48 weeks.

At 48 weeks, 62% of *Rebif* patients versus 52% of *Avonex* patients remained relapse free ($P = 0.009$). *Rebif* patients had a 19% relative increase in the risk to remain relapse free compared with *Avonex* patients. Other relapse measures, such as overall relapse rate, time to first relapse, and steroid use for relapses, were also significantly better in *Rebif* patients than in *Avonex* patients. Similarly, after 24 and 48 weeks of therapy, *Rebif* patients had a 12% and 10% increase in likelihood of remaining relapse free.

Regarding MRI activity, mean T2 active lesion count was 0.9 for *Rebif*-treated patients and 1.4 for *Avonex*-treated patients ($P < 0.001$); mean proportion of active scan per patient was 27% for *Rebif*-treated patients and 44% for *Avonex*-treated patients ($P < 0.001$); and the proportion of patients with no active scans was 58% for *Rebif*-treated patients and 38% for *Avonex*-treated patients ($P < 0.001$). The exact relationship between MRI findings and clinical outcomes for patients is unknown.

No new safety concerns were noted with comparable numbers of treatment discontinuations in both groups. Adverse events reported more frequently with *Rebif* were injection-site reactions, asymptomatic liver function test changes, and white blood cell abnormalities. Viral-like symptoms were reported in significantly more patients treated with *Avonex* than with *Rebif* ($P = 0.031$).

In a placebo-controlled study of 560 patients treated with *Rebif* 22 mcg or 44 mcg 3 times weekly for 2 years, 25% and 32% remained exacerbation free, respectively, compared with 15% in the placebo group. Median time to first exacerbation was 7.6 or 9.6 months, respectively, compared with 4.5 months for the placebo group. The median number of proton density T2-weighted MRI scans was 0.75 and 0.5, respectively, compared with 2.25 for the placebo group.

Onset: Not described.

Duration: How long therapy with interferon beta-1a can slow the accumulation of physical disability and decrease the frequency of clinical exacerbations is not yet known.

Pharmacokinetics: The relationships between serum interferon beta-1a levels and measurable pharmacodynamic activities to the mechanism(s) by which interferon beta-1a exerts its effects in MS are unknown.

Avonex: The pharmacokinetics of *Avonex* in MS patients have not been evaluated. Pharmacokinetics in healthy subjects after doses of 30 mcg to 75 mcg have been investigated. Serum levels of *Avonex*, as measured by antiviral activity, are slightly above detectable limits following a 30 mcg IM dose and increase with higher doses. When 60 mcg is given IM, the area under the curve (AUC) is 1,352 units•h/mL, the maximum concentration reached is 45 units/mL after 9.8 hours (range, 3 to 15 hours), with an elimination half-life of 10 hours. When 60 mcg is given subcutaneously, the AUC is 478 units•h/mL, the maximum concentration reached is 30 units/mL after 7.8 hours (range, 3 to 18 hours), with an elimination half-life of 8.6 hours. Serum levels of *Avonex* may be sustained after IM injection due to prolonged absorption from the IM site.

Biological response markers (eg, neopterin and β_2-microglobulin) are induced by *Avonex* after 15 mcg to 75 mcg parenteral doses in healthy subjects and treated patients. Marker levels increase within 12 hours of a dose and remain elevated for at least 4 days. Peak marker levels are usually seen 48 hours after dosing.

Rebif: Pharmacokinetics of *Rebif* in MS patients have not been evaluated. In healthy volunteers, a single subcutaneous injection of *Rebif* 60 mcg resulted in a peak serum concentration of 5.1 ± 1.7 units/mL, with a median time to peak serum concentration of 16 hours. The serum elimination half-life was 69 ± 37 hours, and the AUC from 0 to 96 hours was 294 ± 81 units• h/mL. Following every-other-day subcutaneous injections in healthy volunteers, the AUC increased approximately 240%, suggesting accumulation of interferon beta-1a after repeat administration. Total clearance is approximately 33 to 55 L/h. No gender-related effects on pharmacokinetics parameters were observed. Pharmacokinetics in pediatric or elderly patients or patients with renal or hepatic insufficiency have not been established. *Rebif* induces biological response markers after parenteral doses in both healthy volunteers and patients with MS. After one 60 mcg subcutaneous dose of *Rebif*, 2' to 5' oligoadenylate synthetase activity peaked between 12 to 24 hours. β_2-microglobulin and neopterin concentrations peaked at approximately 24 to 48 hours. All 3 markers remained elevated for up to 4 days. *Rebif* 222 mcg 3 times per week inhibited mitogen-induced release of proinflammatory cytokines (ie, interferon gamma, interleukin-1 and -6, and tumor necrosis factors alfa and beta) by peripheral blood mononuclear cells, on average, nearly double that observed with *Rebif* administered once per week at either 22 or 66 mcg.

Mechanism: Interferon beta exerts its biological effects by binding to specific receptors on the surface of human cells. This binding initiates a complex cascade of intracellular events that leads to the expression of numerous interferon-induced gene products and markers. These include 2', 5'oligoadenylate synthetase, β_2-microglobulin, and neopterin. These products have been measured in the serum and cellular fractions of blood collected from patients treated with interferon beta-1a. The specific interferon-induced proteins and mechanisms by which interferon beta-1a exerts its effects in MS have not been fully defined.

Drug Interactions: No unexpected adverse events were observed during clinical trials with concomitant therapies of MS exacerbations, including corticosteroids or ACTH. Some patients were treated with antidepressant therapy or oral contraceptive therapy without adverse effect.

Other interferons can reduce cytochrome P-450 oxidase-mediated drug metabolism. Formal hepatic drug metabolism studies with interferon beta-1a in humans have not been conducted. Hepatic microsomes isolated from interferon beta-1a–treated rhesus monkeys showed no influence of interferon beta-1a on P-450 enzyme metabolism activity.

As with all interferon products, proper monitoring of patients is required if interferon beta-1a is given in combination with myelosuppressive agents.

As with other drugs administered by IM injection, give *Avonex* with caution to patients receiving anticoagulant therapy.

Patient Information: Inform patients of the most common adverse events associated with interferon beta-1a. Symptoms of a viral-like syndrome are most prominent at the start of therapy and decrease in frequency with continued treatment. Acetaminophen 650 mg just before injection and for 24 hours after each injection has been used to reduce the acute symptoms associated with interferon beta-1a administration.

Caution patients to report depression or suicidal ideation.

Advise patients about the abortifacient potential of interferon beta.

Instruct people who will administer interferon beta-1a in reconstitution and injection. If a patient is to self-inject, assess the physical ability of that person to give an injection. Use a puncture-resistant container for disposal of needles and syringes. Caution patients against the reuse of these items.

Pharmaceutical Characteristics

Concentration:

Avonex, vial form: When reconstituted according to directions, each mL contains 30 mcg of interferon, equivalent to 6 million units of antiviral activity.

Avonex, syringe form: 30 mcg per 0.5 mL

Avonex, autoinjector: 30 mcg per .5 mL

Rebif: Either 22 mcg per 0.5 mL dose or 44 mcg per 0.5 mL dose, approximately 6 or 12 million units per 0.5 mL dose, respectively.

Quality Assay: Based on the World Health Organization's Second International Standard for Interferon, Human Fibroblast (Gb-23-902-531). The activity against other standards is not known.

Avonex: Specific activity of approximately 200 million international units of antiviral activity per mg, determined by an in vitro cytopathic effect bioassay using lung carcinoma cells (A549) and encephalomyocarditis virus. *Avonex* 30 mcg contains approximately 6 million units.

Rebif: Specific activity of approximately 270 M units of antiviral activity per mg. *Rebif* 44 mcg contains approximately 12 M units of antiviral activity, based on an in vitro cytopathic effect bioassay against vesicular stomatitis virus.

Packaging:

Avonex, vial form: Each "Administration Pack" contains 4 "Administration Dose Packs." Each Dose Pack contains 1 single-dose vial with 33 mcg (6.6 million units; the labeled quantity plus a 10% overfill) interferon beta-1a, one 10 mL diluent vial, 2 alcohol swabs, one 3 mL syringe, 1 *Micro Pin* (B. Braun Medical Inc) vial access pin, one 23-gauge, 1¼-inch needle, and 1 adhesive bandage (59627-0001-03).

Avonex, syringe form: Each "Administration Pack" contains 4 "Administration Dose Packs." Each Dose Pack contains 1 prefilled glass syringe with interferon beta-1a 30 mcg per 0.5 mL, with separate 23-gauge, 1¼-inch needle and a reclosable accessory pouch containing 4 alcohol pads, 4 gauze pads, and 4 adhesive bandages (59627-0002-05).

Avonex, autoinjector: Package of 4 "Administration Packs," each containing one 30 mcg per 0.5 mL autoinjector, one 25-gauge, ⅝-inch needle, and a pen cover; also includes reclosable accessory pouch containing 4 alcohol wipes, 4 gauze pads, and 4 adhesive bandages (59627-0003-04).

Rebif: Each "Titration Pack" contains six 8.8 mcg per 0.2 mL prefilled syringes with six 22 mcg per 0.5 mL prefilled syringes (44087-8822-01). Individual syringes: One 22 mcg per 0.5 mL prefilled syringe (44087-0022-01), twelve 22 mcg per 0.5 mL syringes (44087-0022-03). One 44 mcg per 0.5 mL prefilled syringe (44087-0044-01), twelve 44 mcg per 0.5 mL syringes (44087-0044-03). Each syringe has a 29-gauge, ½-inch needle.

Doseform:

Avonex: Syringe: solution. Vial: powder for solution

Rebif: Solution

Appearance:

Avonex, vial form: White to off-white lyophilized powder. Reconstituted solutions may appear slightly yellow.

Avonex, syringe form: Clear solution

Rebif: Clear solution

Diluent:

For reconstitution: Avonex: Sterile water for injection, preservative-free

Rebif: Sterile water for injection with sodium acetate and mannitol

Adjuvant: None

Preservative: None

Allergens: The prefilled syringe cap contains dry natural rubber.

Excipients:

Avonex, vial form: Albumin (human) 15 mg/mL, sodium chloride 5.8 mg, dibasic sodium phosphate 5.7 mg, and monobasic sodium phosphate 1.2 mg/mL.

Avonex, syringe form: Sodium acetate trihydrate 0.79 mg, acetic acid glacial 0.25 mg, arginine hydrochloride 15.8 mg, 0.025 mg of polysorbate 20 per 0.5 mL dose

Avonex, autoinjector: Sodium acetate trihydrate 0.79 mg, glacial acetic acid 0.25 mg, arginine hydrochloride 15.8 mg, and 0.025 mg of polysorbate-20 in water for injection

Rebif: Each 0.5 mL of solution contains albumin (human) 2 or 4 mg (for the 22 or 44 mcg product sizes, respectively), mannitol 27.3 mg, and sodium acetate 0.4 mg.

pH:
Avonex: Vial: 7.3. Syringe: 4.8
Rebif: Data not provided

Shelf Life:
Avonex: Expires within 15 months.
Rebif: Expires within 24 months.

Storage/Stability: Store routinely at 2° to 8°C (36° to 46°F). Discard frozen product. Remind patients not to store interferon beta-1a where high temperatures may be expected, such as in a glove compartment or on a windowsill. Contact the manufacturer regarding exposure to elevated temperatures. This product is shipped in insulated containers by second-day courier.

Avonex, vial form: Lyophilized product can tolerate 30 days at 25°C (77°F). After reconstitution, use the product as soon as possible within 6 hours, stored at 2° to 8°C (36° to 46°F). Protect from light.

Avonex, syringe form: Store at 2° to 8°C (36° to 46°F). After warming to room temperature, use within 7 days. Do not use external heat sources (eg, hot water) to warm *Avonex*. Protect from light.

Avonex, autoinjector: Store at 2° to 8°C (36° to 46°F). After warming to room temperature, use within 7 days. Do not use external heat sources (eg, hot water) to warm *Avonex*. Do not store above 25°C (77°F). Protect from light.

Rebif: If a refrigerator is unavailable (eg, while traveling), keep *Rebif* cool (ie, less than 25°C [77°F]) for up to 30 days and away from heat and light. Promptly discard syringe contents not used during administration.

Handling:
Avonex: Allow the vial of *Avonex* and the vial of diluent to reach room temperature before reconstitution. Use the blue *Micro Pin* vial access pin to transfer 1.1 mL of diluent to the medication vial. Rapid addition of the diluent may cause foaming, making it difficult to withdraw interferon beta-1a. Do not shake. After all of the interferon beta-1a cake is dissolved, slowly withdraw 1 mL of interferon beta-1a.

Production Process: Interferon beta-1a is produced in CHO cells, into which the human interferon beta gene has been introduced. The amino acid sequence of interferon beta-1a is identical to that of natural human interferon beta.

Media: CHO cells

Disease Epidemiology

See Disease Epidemiology section at the end of the Interferon Beta-1b monograph.

Other Information

Perspective:
1995: Avonex recommended for approval by the FDA's CNS Advisory Committee in December.

First Licensed:
Avonex: May 17, 1996
Rebif: March 7, 2002

Interferon Beta-1a (Recombinant)

References: Jacobs LD, Cookfair DL, Rudick RA, et al. Intramuscular interferon beta-1a for disease progression in relapsing multiple sclerosis [published correction appears in *Ann Neurol.* 1996;40(3):480]. *Ann Neurol.* 1996;39(3):285-294.

Goodin DS, Frohman EM, Garmany GP Jr, et al; Therapeutics and Technology Assessment Subcommittee of the American Academy of Neurology and the MS Council for Clinical Practice Guidelines. Disease modifying therapies in multiple sclerosis: report of the Therapeutics and Technology Assessment Subcommittee of the American Academy of Neurology and the MS Council for Clinical Practice Guidelines [published correction appears in *Neurology.* 2002;59(3):480]. *Neurology.* 2002;58(2):169-178.

Rutschmann OT, McCrory DC, Matchar DB; Immunization Panel of the Multiple Sclerosis Council for Clinical Practice Guidelines. Immunization and MS: a summary of published evidence and recommendations. *Neurology.* 2002;59(12):1837-1843.

Interferon Beta-1b (Recombinant)

Interferons

Name:
Betaseron
Extavia

Manufacturer:
Bayer HealthCare Pharmaceuticals
Novartis Pharmaceutical Corporation, manufactured by Bayer HealthCare Pharmaceuticals

Immunologic Characteristics

Antigen Source: Interferon beta-1b, expressed from recombinant *Escherichia coli* bacteria

Viability: Not viable, but immunologically active

Antigenic Form: Interferon, typically secreted by human fibroblasts

Antigenic Type: Glycoprotein. Interferon beta-1b has 165 amino acids, weighing 19.9 kilodaltons, whereas the natural form contains 166 amino acids, weighing 23 kilodaltons. Interferon beta-1b contains serine at position 17, rather than the cysteine molecule in native interferon beta. Interferon beta-1b does not contain the carbohydrate side chains found in the natural material.

Strains: The genetically engineered plasmid contains the gene for human interferon beta$_{ser17}$.

Use Characteristics

Indications: To treat relapsing forms of multiple sclerosis (MS) to reduce the frequency of clinical exacerbations. Patients with MS in whom efficacy has been demonstrated include patients who have experienced a first clinical episode and have MRI features consistent with MS.

MS patients with frequent attacks may be most likely to benefit from this drug. Postpartum patients who are not breastfeeding are another group likely to benefit.

Unlabeled Uses: Research in progress is assessing the role of interferon beta in the treatment of AIDS, AIDS-related Kaposi sarcoma, metastatic renal-cell carcinoma, malignant melanoma, cutaneous T-cell lymphoma and acute non-A/non-B hepatitis.

Limitations: While MS attack rates diminished in patients with relapsing forms of MS, almost all interferon beta-1b treated patients had attacks, and 1 in 4 patients deteriorated. The value of therapy for longer than 2 years has not yet been established. The safety and efficacy of interferon beta-1b in chronic progressive MS have not been established.

Contraindications:
Absolute: None
Relative: Patients with a history of hypersensitivity to natural or recombinant interferon beta, human albumin, or any other component of the formulation.

Immunodeficiency: Interferon beta-1b has not yet been studied in immunocompromised patients.

Elderly: No specific information is available about geriatric use of interferon beta-1b.

Carcinogenicity: The carcinogenic potential of interferon beta-1b was evaluated by studying its effect on the morphological transformation of the mammalian cell line BALBc-373. No significant increases in transformation frequency were noted. No carcinogenicity data are available in animals or humans. Interferon beta-1b was not mutagenic when assayed for genotoxicity in the Ames bacterial test in the presence or absence of metabolic activation.

1067

Interferon Beta-1b (Recombinant)

Fertility Impairment: Studies in rhesus monkeys at doses up to 0.33 mg (10.7 million units)/kg/day, to measure effects on menstrual cycle and hormone profiles, have not been completed. It is not known whether interferon beta-1b can affect human reproductive capacity.

Pregnancy: Category C. Use only if clearly needed. It is not known if interferon beta-1b crosses the human placenta.

Interferon beta-1b is not teratogenic at doses up to 0.42 mg (13.3 million units)/kg/day in rhesus monkeys, but demonstrated a dose-related abortifacient activity when administered at doses ranging from 0.25 to 0.42 mg (8 to 13.3 million units)/kg/day. Spontaneous abortions while on treatment were reported in 4 patients in clinical trials. Interferon beta-1b given to rhesus monkeys on gestation days 20 to 70 did not cause teratogenic effects; however, it is not known if teratogenic effects will occur in women. If the patient becomes pregnant or plans to become pregnant while taking interferon beta-1b, inform the patient of the potential hazard to the fetus and recommend that the patient discontinue therapy.

Lactation: It is not known if interferon beta-1b crosses into breast milk. Problems in humans have not been documented.

Children: Safety and efficacy of interferon beta-1b in children younger than 18 years of age have not been established.

Adverse Reactions: Experience with interferon beta-1b in patients with MS is limited to only a few hundred patients at the recommended dose of 0.25 mg (8 million units) every other day or more. Consequently, adverse reactions that occur with a low frequency may not yet have been observed.

Injection-site reactions (85%) and injection-site necrosis (5%) occurred after administration of interferon beta-1b. Most reactions were transient and did not require discontinuation of therapy. Incidence of injection site reactions declined over time, such that 79% of patients reported an event during the first 3 months, while 47% reported an event during the last 6 months of therapy. The median time to first occurrence of an injection-site reaction was 7 days. Patients with site reaction reported these events 183.7 days per year.

Flu-like symptoms complex was reported in 76% of patients treated with 0.25 mg (8 million units). Only myalgia (44%), fever (59%), and chills (46%) were reported as severe in more than 5% of patients. Incidence of flu-like symptoms declined over time, with 51% of patients reporting an event during the first 3 months, compared with 4% during the last 6 months of therapy. The median time to first occurrence was 3 days. The median duration per patient was 10.4 days per year.

Among 1,532 study patients who received interferon beta-1b, there were 3 suicides and 8 suicide attempts, compared with 1 suicide and 4 suicide attempts among 965 placebo recipients. All 5 patients received interferon beta-1b. Depression and suicide occurred in patients receiving interferon alpha, a related compound. Inform patients to be treated with interferon beta-1b that depression and suicidal ideation can be a side effect of treatment and to immediately report symptoms to the prescriber. Closely monitor patients exhibiting depression and consider stopping interferon therapy.

Neutralizing antibodies directed against interferon beta-1b were found at 1 or more time points in 45% of patients treated with 0.25 mg (8 million units) every other day. The relationship between antibody formation and clinical efficacy is not known.

Laboratory abnormalities included absolute neutrophil count (ANC) less than 1,500 cells/mm^3 (18%, none less than 500 cells/mm^3), WBC less than 3,000 cells/mm^3 (16%), ALT more than 5 times baseline (19%), and total bilirubin more than 2.5 times baseline (6%).

Hepatic: Severe hepatic injury, including hepatic failure, have been reported rarely in patients taking all beta-interferons. These cases include autoimmune hepatitis and severe liver damage leading to hepatic failure and transplant. Some cases occurred in patients taking other drugs or with comorbid medical illnesses associated with hepatic injury.

Injection-site: Injection-site necrosis occurred in 4% of patients in clinical trials, usually within the first 4 months of therapy. Generally, necrosis extended only to subcutaneous fat, typically 3 cm or less in diameter. Larger lesions have been reported, sometimes involving fascia overlying muscle. Do not inject into necrotic areas until fully healed; if multiple lesions occur, discontinue therapy until lesions heal.

Mild to moderate menstrual disorders (17%) were reported, including intermenstrual bleeding and spotting, early or delayed menses, decreased days of menstrual flow, and clotting and spotting during menstruation.

Other common adverse clinical and laboratory events associated with use of interferon beta-1b were: asthenia (49%); dizziness (35%); sweating (23%); malaise (15%); dyspnea, cystitis, palpitation (8%); breast pain, hypertension (7%); tachycardia, GI disorders, somnolence, laryngitis, pelvic pain, menorrhagia (6%); peripheral vascular disorders (5%).

Pharmacologic & Dosing Characteristics

Dosage: 0.25 mg (8 million units) every other day. Generally start patients at 0.0625 mg (0.25 mL) subcutaneously every other day and increase over a 6-week period to 0.25 mg (1 mL) every other day. Weeks 1 to 2: 0.0625 mg/0.25 mL; weeks 3 to 4: 1.25 mg/0.5 mL; weeks 5 to 6: 0.1875 mg/0.75 mL; weeks 7+: 0.25 mg/1 mL.

Route & Site: Subcutaneous, injected with a 27-gauge needle into an arm, abdomen, hip, or thigh.

Overdosage: Safety of doses greater than 0.25 mg every other day has not been adequately evaluated. The maximum amount that can be safely administered has not been determined.

Missed Doses: Resume therapy as soon as possible, with subsequent doses at 48-hour intervals after the delayed dose.

Laboratory Tests: Recommended laboratory tests prior to starting interferon beta-1b therapy and periodic intervals thereafter include: Hemoglobin; complete and differential blood cell counts; platelet counts; thyroid function (in patients with a history of thyroid dysfunction); blood chemistries, including liver function tests.

Consider discontinuing interferon beta-1b therapy if the ANC falls below 750 cells/mm^3. When the ANC returns to a value more than 750 cells/mm^3, restart therapy at a 50% reduced dose, if clinically appropriate.

Similarly, if hepatic transaminase levels (eg, AST, ALT) exceed 10 times the upper limit of normal, or if the serum bilirubin exceeds 5 times the upper limit of normal, consider discontinuing therapy. In each instance during clinical trials, hepatic enzyme abnormalities returned to normal following discontinuation of therapy. When measurements fall below this threshold, restart therapy at a 50% reduced dose, if clinically appropriate.

Efficacy: A double-blind, multi-clinic, randomized, placebo-controlled clinical investigation of 2 years duration was conducted with 372 ambulatory patients with RRMS, aged 18 to 50, with a Kurtzke expanded disability status scale (EDSS) of 5.5 or below. These patients exhibited a relapsing-remitting clinical course and had experienced 2 ore more exacerbations over 2 years preceding the trial without exacerbation in the preceding month. An exacerbation was defined as the appearance or clinical worsening of a clinical sign or symptom that persisted 24 or more hours. Volunteers received either 0.25 mg (8 million units), 0.05 mg (1.6 million units), or placebo.

After 2 years, there was a 31% reduction in annual exacerbation rate, from 1.31 in the placebo group to 0.9 in the 0.25 mg group. The proportion of patients free of exacerbations was 16% in the placebo group, compared with 25% in the 0.25 mg group.

Effects of Interferon beta-1b: 2-Year Study Results				
		Treatment groups		
Efficacy parameters		Placebo (n = 123)	0.25 mg (n = 124)	P value
Primary end points				
Annual exacerbation rate		1.31	0.9	0.0001
Percentage of exacerbation-free patients		16%	25%	0.094
Exacerbation frequency per patient	0	20	29	
	1	32	39	
	2	20	17	
	3	15	14	
	4	15	9	
	≥ 5	21	8	0.001
Secondary end points				
Median number of months to first on-study exacerbation		5	9	0.01
Rate of moderate or severe exacerbations per year		0.47	0.23	0.001
Mean number of moderate or severe exacerbation days per patient		44.1	19.5	0.001
Mean change in EDSS[a] score at end point		0.21	−0.07	0.144
Mean change in Scripps[b] score at end point		−0.53	0.66	0.126
Median duration in days per exacerbation		36	35.5	Not done
% change in mean MRI lesion area at end point		21.4%	−0.9%	0.0001

a EDSS scores range from 0 to 10, with higher scores reflecting greater disability.
b Scripps neurologic rating scores range from 0 to 100, with small scores reflecting greater disability.

Hospitalizations, lengths of hospital stays, and days of therapy with glucocorticoids were less frequent in treated patients compared with controls. Lesion area measured by magnetic-resonance imaging (MRI) increased by 16.5% in the placebo group, while it decreased by 1.1% in treated patients. Rate of appearance of active lesions and the number of new lesions also decreased. MRI scanning is viewed as a useful means to visualize changes in white matter that are believed to reflect pathologic changes that, appropriately located within the CNS, account for some of the signs and symptoms that typify RRMS. The relationship between MRI findings and the clinical status of patients is not fully known. Changes in lesion area often do not correlate with clinical exacerbations, probably because many of the lesions affect so-called "silent" regions of the CNS. Moreover, it is not clear what fraction of the lesions seen on MRI become foci of irreversible demyelinization (ie, classic white-matter plaques). The prognostic significance of MRI findings has not been evaluated.

Other analyses have shown that interferon beta-1b decreased the incidence of vision problems and improved motor coordination or tremors. Time to first exacerbation almost doubled.

Onset: Decline in attack frequency began 2 months after the start of treatment.

Duration: Decline in attack frequency has been sustained for at least 3 years in treated patients.

Pharmacokinetics: Because serum concentrations of interferon beta-1b are low or undetectable following subcutaneous administration of up to 0.25 mg (up to 8 million units), pharmacokinetic information in treated patients with MS is not available.

Following single and multiple daily subcutaneous doses of 0.5 mg (16 million units) to 12 healthy volunteers, serum concentrations were generally less than 100 units/mL. Peak serum concentrations occurred between 1 to 8 hours after administration, with a mean peak serum concentration of 40 units/mL. Bioavailability, based on a total dose of 0.5 mg (16 million units) given as 2 subcutaneous injections at different sites, was approximately 50%.

After IV administration of 0.006 to 2 mg (0.2 to 64 million units), similar pharmacokinetic profiles were seen in 12 healthy volunteers and in 142 patients with diseases other than MS. In patients receiving single IV doses, increases in serum concentrations were dose-proportional. Mean serum clearance values ranged from 9.4 to 28.9 mL/min/kg and were independent of dose. Mean terminal elimination half-life values ranged from 8 minutes to 4.3 hours, and mean steady-state volume of distribution values ranged from 0.25 to 2.88 L/kg. Three-times-weekly IV dosing for 2 weeks resulted in no accumulation of interferon beta-1b in serum. Pharmacokinetic parameters after single and multiple IV doses were comparable.

Mechanism: Interferon beta has both antiviral and immunoregulatory activity. The mechanisms by which interferon beta-1b exerts its actions in MS are not clearly understood, but do involve specific cell receptors on the surface of human cells. Binding to these receptors induces the expression of several interferon-induced gene products (eg, 2′, 5′-oligoadenylate synthetase, protein kinase, indolamine 2,3-dioxygenase), believed to mediate the biological actions of interferon beta-1b.

Interferon beta-1b decreases T-cell proliferation, blocks synthesis of interferon gamma, inhibits release of other cytokines that damage oligodendrocytes, and increases T-suppressor cell activity. Interferon gamma is thought to be involved in MS attacks.

Drug Interactions: No specific interactions between interferon beta-1b and other drugs have been fully evaluated.

In the placebo-controlled studies in MS, corticosteroids or ACTH were administered for treatment of relapses for periods of up to 28 days in 644 patients receiving interferon beta-1b.

Administration of 0.025 to 2.2 mg (0.8 to 71 million units) interferon beta-1b to 3 cancer patients led to a dose-dependent inhibition of antipyrine elimination. The effect of alternate-day administration of interferon beta-1b on drug metabolism in MS patients is unknown.

Therapeutic interferons may theoretically inhibit the induction of an adequate antibody response following immunization with live virus vaccines (eg, measles, mumps, rubella, varicella). Avoid concurrent use.

Patient Information: Instruct patients to store the drug in the refrigerator and to handle needles and syringes carefully. Advise patients to avoid pregnancy while taking this drug. Instruct patients not to inject into skin that is tender, red, or hard; the best areas for injection are loose and soft or flabby, away from joints and nerves. Instruct patients to rotate injection sites, not repeating the same site more often than weekly. Advise patients that taking interferon beta-1b at night may help lessen the severity of flu-like symptoms. Advise patients to contact their prescriber immediately if they experience depression.

Pharmaceutical Characteristics

Concentration: When properly reconstituted, 0.25 mg (8 million units) per mL. Each mg of interferon beta-1b contains approximately 32 million units.

Quality Assay: Activity is assayed on human fibroblast monolayers using a vesicular stomatitis virus challenge.

The current international standard of potency for recombinant interferon beta, adopted by WHO and others in 1993, supersedes an earlier standard developed by NIH for native interferon beta. Doses of 1.6 and 8 million units in the international system are equivalent to 9 and 45 million units in the supplanted system, respectively.

Packaging: 0.3 mg (9.6 million units) per single-dose clear glass vial, with separate 1.2 mL syringe of diluent, 2 alcohol pads, and 1 vial adapter with 27-gauge needle

NDC Number:
Bayer: 14 blister-wrapped packages, 50419-0523-35
Novartis: 15 blister-wrapped packages, 00078-0569-12

Interferon Beta-1b (Recombinant)

Doseform: Powder for solution

Appearance: White to off-white powder yielding a clear, colorless solution

Diluent:

> *For reconstitution:* Sodium chloride 0.54%. Add 1.2 mL of diluent to each vial of interferon. Gently swirl the vial to dissolve the drug completely; do not shake.

Adjuvant: None

Preservative: None

Allergens: None

Excipients: Human albumin 15 mg, mannitol 15 mg per vial

pH: Data not provided

Shelf Life: Expires within an unspecified period of time.

Storage/Stability: Store powder at room temperature (25°C, 77°F). Product may be exposed to 15° to 30°C (59° to 86°F) for short intervals. Do not freeze. Contact the manufacturer regarding exposure to extreme temperatures. Shipping data not provided.

> After reconstitution, the product can tolerate 3 hours in the refrigerator.

Handling: Drug is compatible with plastic syringes.

Production Process: Expressed from recombinant bacteria in a nonglycosylated form.

Media: *Escherichia coli* bacterial cell culture

Disease Epidemiology

Syndrome: MS is a degenerative disease in which the immune system is believed to attack myelin, a tissue that covers nerve fibers in the brain and spinal cord. The loss of myelin interferes with normal signals in the CNS. Symptoms of the disease range from very slight to crippling vision problems, muscle weakness, slurred speech, and poor coordination.

Incidence: MS usually strikes young adults 20 to 40 years of age. Women are affected twice as often as men. Some 200 new cases are diagnosed each week in the US.

Prevalence: An estimated 400,000 people in the US have physician-diagnosed MS. Another estimate suggests that 1 in 800 northern Europeans have clinically apparent MS, with many others subject to silent forms of the disease. Some 80% of cases are of the relapsing-remitting type, in which symptoms disappear totally or partially after a flare-up, followed by stability lasting months or years.

Other Information

Perspective:

1988: Orphan drug status granted for treating AIDS or MS.

1993: Interferon beta-1b licensed in the US on July 23, under accelerated approval procedures, the first product specifically approved for treatment of MS.

2009: Extavia brand of interferon beta-1b licensed to Novartis on August 20.

References: IFNB Multiple Sclerosis Study Group. Interferon beta-1b is effective in relapsing multiple sclerosis. I. Clinical results of a multicenter, randomized, double-blind, placebo-controlled trial. *Neurology.* 1993;43:655-661.

Goodin DS, Frohman EM, Garmany GP Jr, et al. Disease modifying therapies in multiple sclerosis: Report of the Therapeutics and Technology Assessment Subcommittee of the American Academy of Neurology and the MS Council for Clinical Practice Guidelines. *Neurology.* 2002;58(2):169-178.

Rutschmann OT, McCrory DC, Matchar DB, Immunization Panel of the Multiple Sclerosis Council for Clinical Practice Guidelines. Immunization and MS: a summary of published evidence and recommendations. *Neurology.* 2002;59(12):1837-1843.

Interferon Gamma-1b (Recombinant)

Interferons

Name:
Actimmune

Manufacturer:
InterMune Pharmaceuticals, under license
from Genentech

Synonyms: IFN-γ1b. Interferon gamma was previously called immune interferon or type II interferon. Known in Europe as *Imukine*. Note that previous dosage recommendations in units have been changed to international units.

Immunologic Characteristics

Antigen Source: Interferon gamma expressed from recombinant *Escherichia coli* bacteria

Viability: Not viable, but immunologically active

Antigenic Form: Interferon, typically secreted by T-lymphocytes and natural-killer lymphocytes

Antigenic Type: Glycoprotein, a single-chain polypeptide of 140 amino acids. Consists of non-covalent dimers of two identical 16,454 dalton monomers.

Strains: Interferon gamma-1b

Use Characteristics

Indications: For reducing the frequency and severity of serious infections associated with chronic granulomatous disease (CGD), an inherited disorder characterized by deficient phagocyte oxidative metabolism.

To delay the time to disease progression in patients with severe, malignant osteopetrosis, a life-threatening bone disorder.

Unlabeled Uses: Research in progress assesses the role of interferon gamma-1b in the treatment of ovarian cancer, small-cell lung cancer, atopic dermatitis, trauma-related infections, multi-drug resistant tuberculosis, cutaneous T-cell lymphoma, asthma, and allergies. Success has followed treatment of refractory leishmaniasis in conjunction with pentavalent antimony. Other research includes treatments for chronic myelogenous leukemia and AIDS.

Limitations: In clinical trials of patients with idiopathic pulmonary fibrosis, interferon gamma-1b offered no survival benefit compared with placebo.

Contraindications:
Absolute: Patients who develop or have known hypersensitivity to interferon gamma, *E. coli*-derived products, or any component of the formulation.
Relative: None

Immunodeficiency: Use may be indicated in certain immunodeficient conditions.

Elderly: No specific information is available about geriatric use of interferon gamma.

Carcinogenicity: Interferon gamma-1b has not been tested for carcinogenic potential.

Mutagenicity: No evidence of chromosomal damage was noted in the Ames test, nor in tests of murine bone marrow cells.

Fertility Impairment: Female cynomolgus monkeys treated with 150 mcg/kg/day subcutaneous doses of interferon gamma (approximately 100 times the human dose) exhibited irregular menstrual cycles during treatment. Similar findings were not observed in animals treated with 3 or 30 mcg/kg. No studies have been performed assessing any potential effects of interferon gamma on male fertility.

Interferon Gamma-1b (Recombinant)

Pregnancy: Category C. Use only if potential benefits justify potential risk to the fetus. The use of interferon gamma-1b increased the incidence of abortions in primates when given in doses approximately 100 times the human dose. Similar studies failed to demonstrate teratogenic activity for interferon gamma-1b.

Lactation: It is not known if interferon gamma-1b is excreted in breast milk. Because of the potential for serious adverse effects in nursing infants from interferon gamma-1b, decide whether to discontinue nursing or to discontinue the drug, taking into account the importance of the drug to the mother.

Children: Safety and efficacy in children younger than 1 year of age have not been established. The long-term effects of interferon gamma therapy on growth, development, and other parameters are not known.

Adverse Reactions: In patients with chronic granulomatous disease receiving interferon gamma-1b subcutaneous doses of 50 mcg/m^2 given 3 times weekly, adverse reactions from interferon gamma-1b that exceeded rates observed in placebo-treated patients included the following: fever (52%); headache (33%); rash (17%); chills, erythema or tenderness at the injection site, fatigue, diarrhea (14%); vomiting (13%); nausea (10%); myalgia (6%). No statistically significant differences between interferon gamma-1b and placebo groups were observed in hematologic, coagulation, hepatic, or renal laboratory studies.

Adverse reactions not observed in these patients, but seen rarely in patients with other diseases treated with doses greater than 100 mcg/m^2 by IM injection or IV infusion, included hypotension, syncope, tachydysrhythmia, heart block, heart failure, MI, confusion, disorientation, gait disturbance, parkinsonian symptoms, seizure, hallucinations, transient ischemic attacks, hepatic insufficiency, GI bleeding, pancreatitis, reversible renal insufficiency, deep venous thrombosis, pulmonary embolism, tachypnea, bronchospasm, interstitial pneumonitis, hyponatremia, hyperglycemia, and exacerbation of dermatomyositis.

Use interferon gamma-1b with caution in patients with preexisting cardiac disease, including symptoms of ischemia, CHF, or dysrhythmia. No direct cardiotoxic effect has been demonstrated, but it is possible that acute and transient flu-like or constitutional symptoms such as fever and chills, frequently associated with interferon gamma-1b administration at doses 250 mcg/m^2/day or more, may exacerbate preexisting cardiac conditions. Exercise caution when treating patients with known seizure disorders or compromised CNS function. Adverse CNS reactions, including decreased mental status, gait disturbance, and dizziness have been observed, particularly in recipients of doses 250 mcg/m^2/day or more. Most of these abnormalities were mild and reversible within a few days upon dose reduction or discontinuation of therapy.

Exercise caution when administering interferon gamma-1b to patients with myelosuppression. Reversible neutropenia and elevation of hepatic enzymes can be dose-limiting at doses more than 250 mcg/m^2/day. Thrombocytopenia and proteinuria occur rarely.

Acute serious hypersensitivity reactions have not been observed in patients receiving interferon gamma-1b. But if such an acute reaction develops, discontinue the drug immediately and start appropriate medical therapy. Transient cutaneous rashes have occurred in some patients following interferon gamma-1b injection, but have rarely necessitated treatment interruption.

Pharmacologic & Dosing Characteristics

Dosage: 50 mcg/m^2 (equivalent to 1 million International Units per m^2 or 1.5 million original units per m^2) for patients whose body surface area is more than 0.5 m^2 or 1.5 mcg/kg/dose for patients whose body surface area is 0.5 m^2 or less. (Error alert: If this medication is ordered in units, confirm with prescriber whether the order is based on units or original units.) Give injections 3 times per week (eg, Monday, Wednesday, Friday). Higher doses are not recommended. Safety and efficacy have not been established for interferon gamma-1b given in doses other than 50 mcg/m². The minimum effective dose of interferon gamma-1b has not been established. Give the drug at bedtime to minimize some of the most common flu-like symptoms. Acetaminophen may be used to prevent or partially alleviate fever and headache. If serious reactions occur, modify the dosage (eg, a 50% reduction) or discontinue therapy until the adverse reaction abates.

Route & Site: Subcutaneous injection, optimally in right and left deltoid and anterior thigh. Administration by IM injection or continuous (10-day to 8-week) or intermittent (at 1-, 6-, or 24-hour intervals) IV infusions have been reported.

Monitor: In addition to tests normally required to monitor chronic granulomatous disease, the following laboratory tests are recommended for all patients on interferon gamma-1b therapy, prior to therapy and at 3-month intervals during therapy: hematologic tests (eg, complete blood, differential, and platelet counts), blood chemistries (eg, renal and liver function tests), and urinalysis.

Efficacy: Interferon gamma-1b reduced the relative risk of serious infection 67% among chronic granulomatous disease patients 1 to 44 years of age (mean, 14.6 years), where serious infection was defined as a clinical event requiring hospitalization and parenteral antibiotics. There was a 2-fold reduction in the number of primary serious infections and in the total number and rate of serious infections, including recurrent events. In addition, the length of hospitalization for treatment of all clinical events was reduced 33% and the total number of hospital days for clinical events was reduced 67% compared with the placebo-treated group. The interferon gamma-1b treatment benefit with respect to time to serious infection was consistently demonstrated in all subgroup analyses, including stratification by pattern of inheritance, use of prophylactic antibiotics, and age.

In a randomized study, 16 patients with severe, malignant infantile osteopetrosis were randomized to receive interferon gamma-1b plus calcitriol or calcitriol alone. Disease progression was defined as death, reduction in hemoglobin or platelet counts, serious bacterial infection, a 50-decibel decrease in hearing, or progressive optic atrophy. The median time to progression for recipients of interferon gamma-1b was at least 165 days compared with 65 days in the control arm.

Onset: Unknown

Duration: Unknown

Pharmacokinetics: The IV, IM, and subcutaneous pharmacokinetics of interferon gamma-1b have been studied in healthy male subjects following single-dose administration of 100 mcg/m². Pharmacokinetic studies in patients with chronic granulomatous disease have not been performed.

Absorption: After IM or subcutaneous injection, the apparent fraction of dose absorbed was more than 89%. Peak plasma concentrations occurred approximately 4 hours after IM dosing (mean, 1.5 ng/mL) and 7 hours after subcutaneous dosing (mean, 0.6 ng/mL). There was no accumulation of interferon gamma-1b after 12 consecutive daily injections of 100 mcg/m².

Elimination: Interferon gamma-1b is rapidly cleared after IV administration (an apparent 1.4 L/min); the mean elimination half-life was 38 minutes. After IM and subcutaneous dosing, the mean elimination half-lives were 2.9 and 5.9 hours, respectively. Interferon gamma-1b was not detected in the urine of healthy human volunteers following 100 mcg/m² by IV, IM, or subcutaneous routes.

Serum neutralizing activity: No anti-interferon gamma-1b neutralizing antibodies in any patient with chronic granulomatous disease have been detected.

Mechanism: Gamma interferon has potent phagocyte-activating effects not seen with other interferons. These effects include generation of toxic oxygen metabolites within phagocytes. The metabolites are capable of mediating the killing of microorganisms such as *Staphylococcus aureus, Toxoplasma gondii, Leishmania donovani, Listeria monocytogenes*, and *Mycobacterium avium intracellulare*.

Clinical studies in patients with interferon gamma have revealed a broad range of biological activities, including enhancement of oxidative metabolism of tissue macrophages, enhancement of antibody-dependent cellular cytotoxicity (ADCC), and natural killer (NK) cell activity. Additionally, effects on Fc receptor expression on monocytes and major histocompatibility antigen expression have been noted. To the extent that interferon gamma is produced by antigen-stimulated T-lymphocytes and regulates the activity of immune cells, interferon gamma can be characterized as a lymphokine of the interleukin type. There is growing evidence that interferon gamma interacts functionally with other interleukin molecules, such as interleukin-2, and that all of the interleukins form part of a complex lymphokine regulatory network. For example, interferon gamma and interleukin-4 appear to reciprocally interact to regulate murine IgE levels. Interferon gamma can suppress IgE in humans. Interferon gamma also inhibits the production of collagen at the transcription level in human systems.

In chronic granulomatous disease, an inherited disorder characterized by deficient phagocyte oxidative mechanism, clinical trials provided evidence for a treatment-related enhancement of phagocyte function, including elevation of superoxide levels and improved killing of *Staphylococcus aureus*.

In severe, malignant osteopetrosis, an inherited disorder involving an osteoclast defect leading to bone overgrowth and deficient phagocyte oxidative mechanism, a treatment-related enhancement of superoxide production by phagocytes was observed in situ. Interferon gamma-1b enhances osteoclast function in vitro.

Drug Interactions: Use caution when administering interferon gamma-1b in combination with other potentially myelosuppressive agents. Studies in rodents using species-specific interferon gamma have demonstrated a decrease in hepatic microsomal cytochrome P-450 concentrations. If this phenomenon also occurs in humans, it could lead to a depression of the hepatic metabolism of certain drugs that use this degradation pathway (eg, theophylline). Interferons may inhibit the induction of an adequate antibody response following immunization with live virus vaccines (eg, measles, mumps, rubella). Avoid concurrent use.

Pharmaceutical Characteristics

Concentration: 100 mcg/0.5 mL. Equivalent to 2 million International Units per 0.5 mL. Formerly expressed as 3 million units per 0.5 mL. (Error alert: If this medication is ordered in units, confirm with prescriber whether the order is based on units or original units.)

Quality Assay: Purified by conventional column chromatography

Packaging: 0.5 mL single-dose vial

NDC Number: One single-dose vial (NDC #: 64116-0011-01), carton of 12 vials (64116-0011-12)

Doseform: Solution

Appearance: Clear, colorless solution

Solvent: Sterile water for injection

Adjuvant: None

Preservative: None

Allergens: None

Excipients: 20 mg mannitol, 0.36 mg sodium succinate, 0.05 mg polysorbate 20, each per 0.5 mL

pH: Not described

Shelf Life: Expires within an unspecified period of time

Storage/Stability: Store at 2° to 8°C (35° to 46°F) immediately upon receipt. Do not freeze. To avoid foaming and protein degradation, avoid excessive or vigorous agitation; do not shake. Either glass or plastic syringes are acceptable. The product cannot tolerate more than 12 hours at room temperature. Discard vials after this time. Contact the manufacturer regarding exposure to freezing temperatures. Shipping data not provided.

Handling: Interferon gamma-1b is compatible with glass and plastic syringes. The drug should not be stored in syringes for long periods because the protein adheres to syringe surfaces.

Production Process: Manufactured with recombinant DNA techniques, with fermentation of genetically engineered *E. coli* bacteria whose genes encode for this human protein. Purified by conventional column chromatography.

Media: *E. coli*

Disease Epidemiology

Prevalence: Chronic granulomatous disease affects approximately 400 Americans each year, primarily children. The estimated prevalence is 1 case per million people.

Other Information

Perspective: See also Epidemiology of Diseases Treated with Interferon Alpha in the Interferon Alpha Summary.

1965: Wheelock isolates interferon gamma.

1990: Interferon gamma-1b licensed on December 20 (designated an orphan drug September 30, 1988).

References: Bolinger AM, et al. Recombinant interferon gamma for treatment of chronic granulomatous disease and other disorders. *Clin Pharm.* 1992;11:834-850.

Gallin JI, et al. Interferon-gamma in the management of infectious diseases. *Ann Intern Med.* 1995;123:216-224.

Interleukins: General Statement

Interleukins

Nomenclature: The suffix "-kin" is used in naming interleukin-type substances except for interleukin 3 (IL-3), which was classified as a pleiotropic colony-stimulating factor and assigned the "plestim" stem (eg, daniplestim). The "kin" nomenclature series is divided into subgroups with an adjuvant stem representing the numerical class of the interleukin followed by the "kin" suffix.

The subgroups are:

-nakin for interleukin-1 derivatives
-onakin for interleukin-1a derivatives
-benakin for interleukin-1b derivatives
-leukin for interleukin-2 derivatives
-trakin for interleukin-4 derivatives
-penkin for interleukin-5 derivatives
-exakin for interleukin-6 derivatives
-eptakin for interleukin-7 derivatives
-octakin for interleukin-8 derivatives
-nonakin for interleukin-9 derivatives
-decakin for interleukin-10 derivatives
-elvekin for interleukin-11 derivatives
-dodekin for interleukin-12 derivatives

Aldesleukin (Recombinant)

Interleukins

Name:
Proleukin

Manufacturer:
Prometheus Laboratories,
for Novartis

Synonyms: Interleukin-2, IL-2, T-cell growth factor (TCGF), thymocyte-stimulating factor, lymphocyte mitogenic factor, epidermal thymocyte-activating factor, formerly called desalaleukin

Immunologic Characteristics

Antigen Source: Recombinant interleukin-2 expressed from *Escherichia coli* bacteria containing an analog of the human interleukin-2 gene.

Viability: Not viable, but immunologically active

Antigenic Form: Interleukin-2; des-alanyl-1, serine-125 human interleukin-2

Antigenic Type: Protein. A highly purified protein of 133 amino acids with an approximate molecular weight of 15,300 daltons. Unlike native interleukin-2, aldesleukin is not glycosylated, has no N-terminal alanine and has serine substituted for cysteine at amino acid position 125. Aldesleukin exists as biologically active, non-covalently bound microaggregates with an average size of 27 recombinant interleukin-2 molecules. This is in contrast to traditional aggregates in proteins that are irreversible, covalently bound structures and are often biologically inactive.

Use Characteristics

Indications: For the treatment of metastatic renal-cell carcinoma in adults. Also indicated for the treatment of metastatic melanoma in adults.

Unlabeled Uses: Research is underway on the use of aldesleukin for treatment of various cancers, including head and neck cancer, acute myelogenous leukemia, lymphoma, bladder and ovarian cancer; for treatment of primary immunodeficiency disease associated with T-cell defects (orphan designation, March 22, 1989); for cancer and Kaposi sarcoma in combination with zidovudine; for treatment of HIV-infected patients with more than 200 CD4 cells/mm^3.

Limitations: Carefully select candidates for aldesleukin treatment based on recommended cardiac and pulmonary function tests, laboratory tests of renal and hepatic function and performance and CNS status. The safety and efficacy of aldesleukin in combination with chemotherapy have not been established.

Contraindications:

Absolute: Patients with a history of hypersensitivity to interleukin-2 or any component of the formulation. Exclude patients with an abnormal thallium stress test or pulmonary function test from treatment with aldesleukin. Also exclude patients with organ allografts.

Relative: Patients who have had a nephrectomy are still eligible for treatment if they have serum creatinine levels up to 1.5 mg/dL.

Re-treatment with aldesleukin is permanently contraindicated in patients who experienced any of the following toxicities while receiving an earlier course of therapy: Sustained ventricular tachycardia (at least 5 beats); cardiac rhythm disturbances not controlled by or unresponsive to management; chest pain with ECG changes, consistent with angina or MI; cardiac tamponade; intubation required more than 72 hours; renal dysfunction requiring dialysis more than 72 hours; coma or toxic psychosis lasting longer than

Aldesleukin (Recombinant)

48 hours; repetitive or difficult-to-control seizures; bowel ischemia or perforation or GI bleeding requiring surgery.

Immunodeficiency: Use may be indicated in certain immunocompromised patients.

Elderly: No specific information is available about geriatric use of aldesleukin.

Carcinogenicity: No studies have been conducted assessing the carcinogenic or mutagenic potential of aldesleukin.

Fertility Impairment: No studies have been conducted assessing the effect of aldesleukin on fertility. The manufacturer recommends that aldesleukin not be administered to fertile people of either gender not practicing effective contraception.

Pregnancy: Category C. Given the adverse effect profile of this drug, use only with extreme caution, weighing the potential benefit with the risks associated with therapy. It is not known if aldesleukin crosses the placenta. Aldesleukin had embryolethal effects in rats when given in doses at 27 to 36 times the human dose. No evidence of teratogenicity was observed in the rats, other than that attributed to maternal toxicity.

Lactation: It is not known if aldesleukin is excreted in breast milk. Problems in humans have not been documented.

Children: Safety and efficacy have not been established in children younger than 18 years of age.

Adverse Reactions: The rate of drug-related deaths in 255 metastatic renal-cell carcinoma patients receiving single-agent aldesleukin was 4%. The rate of drug-related deaths in 270 metastatic melanoma patients receiving single-agent aldesleukin was 2%. Frequency and severity of adverse reactions is dose-related and schedule-dependent. Adverse events may require dose reduction or discontinuation. Most adverse reactions are self-limiting and are usually reversible within 2 to 3 days of discontinuation of therapy. Life-threatening toxicities have been ameliorated by IV dexamethasone administration, which may result in loss of the therapeutic effect of aldesleukin. Examples of adverse events with permanent sequelae include MI, bowel perforation or infarction and gangrene.

The following data on life-threatening adverse events reported in 1% or more of patients are based on 525 patients with renal-cell cancer or metastatic melanoma treated with the recommended infusion dosing regimen. Life-threatening events included: oliguria (6%); anuria (5%); hypotension, respiratory disorder (respiratory distress syndrome, respiratory failure, intubation) (3%); diarrhea, coma, bilirubinemia (2%); fever, infection, sepsis, supraventricular tachycardia, fluctuations in BP, MI, ventricular tachycardia, heart arrest, vomiting, thrombocytopenia, intravascular coagulopathy, increased creatinine, SGOT increase, acidosis, confusion, stupor, psychosis, dyspnea, apnea, acute kidney failure (1%).

Life-threatening events reported in less than 1% of the 525 patients included: hypothermia; shock; bradycardia; various dysrhythmias; myocardial ischemia; syncope; hemorrhage; phlebitis; endocarditis; pericardial effusion; peripheral gangrene; thrombosis; stomatitis; hematemesis; bloody diarrhea; intestinal perforation; pancreatitis; anemia; leukopenia; leukocytosis; hypocalcemia; hyperuricemia; respiratory acidosis; neuropathy; paranoid reaction; convulsion; delirium; lung edema; hyperventilation; hypoxia; hemoptysis; hypoventilation; pneumothorax; mydriasis; kidney failure; and acute tubular necrosis.

In a larger population of 1,800 patients treated with aldesleukin, other serious adverse events observed with a frequency of less than 1% under a variety of doses and schedules included: duodenal ulceration; bowel necrosis; myocarditis; supraventricular tachycardia; permanent or transient blindness secondary to optic neuritis; transient ischemic attack; meningitis; cerebral edema; pericarditis; allergic interstitial nephritis; and tracheo-esophageal fistula. Among these 1,800 patients, events that resulted in death included: liver or renal failure; intestinal perforation; cardiac arrest; malignant hyperthermia; pulmonary edema; respiratory arrest; stroke; pulmonary emboli; and severe depression leading to suicide.

In postmarketing experience, the following serious adverse events have been reported in a variety of treatment regimens that included interleukin-2: pneumonia; neutropenia; cholecystitis; colitis; gastritis; hepatitis; hepatosplenomegaly; intestinal obstruction; retroperitoneal hemorrhage; cerebral lesions and hemorrhage; encephalopathy; extrapyramidal syndrome; neuralgia; neuritis; neuropathy (demyelination); rhabdomyolysis; myopathy; myositis; hyperthyroidism; anaphylaxis; cellulitis; injection-site necrosis; persistent but nonprogressive vitiligo.

Aldesleukin has been associated with exacerbation of preexisting or initial presentation of autoimmune disease and inflammatory disorders. Exacerbation of Crohn disease, scleroderma, thyroiditis, inflammatory arthritis, diabetes mellitus, oculo-bulbar myasthenia gravis, crescentic IgA glomerulonephritis, cholecystitis, cerebral vasculitis, Stevens-Johnson syndrome and bullous pemphigoid have been reported following treatment with interleukin-2.

Aldesleukin therapy has been associated with capillary leak syndrome (CLS), resulting from extravasation of plasma proteins and fluid into the extravascular space and loss of vascular tone. CLS results in hypotension, specifically a drop in mean arterial blood pressure within 2 to 12 hours after the start of therapy. The resulting reduction in organ perfusion may be severe and may result in death. CLS may be associated with cardiac dysrhythmias (supraventricular and ventricular), angina, MI, respiratory insufficiency requiring intubation, GI bleeding or infarction, renal insufficiency and mental status changes. Extravasation of proteins and fluids into the extravascular space will lead to edema formation and creation of effusions. CLS management begins with careful monitoring of fluid and organ perfusion status. Frequently determine blood pressure and pulse, and monitor organ function, including assessment of mental status and urine output. Assess hypovolemia by catheterization and central pressure monitoring. Use extreme caution in patients with fixed requirements for large volumes of fluids (eg, patients with hypercalcemia).

Aldesleukin may exacerbate disease symptoms in patients with clinically unrecognized or untreated CNS metastases. Evaluate and treat CNS metastases in all patients prior to receiving aldesleukin therapy. They should be neurologically stable with a negative CT scan. In addition, use extreme caution in treating patients with a history of seizure disorder because aldesleukin may induce seizures.

Patients may experience mental status changes including irritability, confusion or depression while receiving aldesleukin. These changes may be indicators of bacteremia or early bacterial sepsis. Mental status changes solely due to aldesleukin are generally reversible after discontinuing the drug. However, alterations in mental status may progress for several days before recovery begins.

Intensive aldesleukin therapy is associated with impaired neutrophil function (reduced chemotaxis) and with an increased risk of disseminated infection, including sepsis and bacterial endocarditis, in treated patients.

Consequently, treat preexisting bacterial infections prior to initiation of aldesleukin therapy. Additionally, give all patients with in-dwelling central lines antibiotic prophylaxis effective against *Staphylococcus aureus*. Antibiotic prophylaxis associated with a reduced incidence of *Staphylococcus* infections in aldesleukin studies included use of oxacillin, nafcillin, ciprofloxacin or vancomycin. Disseminated infections acquired in the course of aldesleukin treatment contribute significantly to treatment morbidity. Use of antibiotic prophylaxis and aggressive treatment of suspected and documented infections may reduce the morbidity of aldesleukin treatment. Aldesleukin administration may cause anemia or thrombocytopenia. Packed red blood cell transfusions have been given both for relief of anemia and to ensure maximum oxygen-carrying capacity. Platelet transfusions have been given to resolve absolute thrombocytopenia and to reduce the risk of GI bleeding. In addition, leukopenia and neutropenia have been observed. Aldesleukin administration results in fever, chills, rigors, pruritus and GI adverse effects in most patients treated at recommended doses. Management of these effects is described below in "Concomitant Therapy."

Impairment of thyroid therapy has occurred following aldesleukin treatment. A small number of treated patients were subsequently prescribed thyroid-replacement therapy. This impairment of thyroid function may be a manifestation of autoimmunity; consequently, exercise extra caution when treating patients with known autoimmune disease.

Enhancement of cellular immune function by aldesleukin may increase the risk of allograft rejection in transplant patients.

The following data on common adverse events reported in more than 10% of patients (any grade of severity) are based on the same 525 patients with renal-cell cancer or metastatic melanoma described above.

Body as a whole: Chills (52%); fever (29%); malaise (27%); asthenia (23%); infection (13%); pain (12%); abdominal pain (11%); abdomen enlarged (10%).

Cardiovascular: Hypotension (71%); tachycardia (23%); vasodilation (13%); supraventricular tachycardia (12%); cardiovascular disorder (fluctuations in BP, asymptomatic EG changes, congestive heart failure; 11%); arrhythmia (10%).

CNS: Confusion (34%); somnolence (22%); anxiety (12%); dizziness (11%).

Dermatologic: Rash (42%); pruritus (24%); exfoliative dermatitis (18%).

GI: Diarrhea (67%); vomiting (50%); nausea (35%); stomatitis (22%); anorexia (20%); nausea and vomiting (19%).

GU: Oliguria (63%).

Hematologic/Lymphatic: Thrombocytopenia (37%); anemia (29%); leukopenia (16%).

Metabolic/Nutritional: Bilirubinemia (40%); increased creatinine (33%); peripheral edema (28%); SGOT increase (23%); weight gain (16%); edema (15%); acidosis, hypomagnesemia (12%); hypocalcemia (11%); alkaline phosphatase increase (10%).

Respiratory: Dyspnea (43%); lung disorder (physical findings associated with pulmonary congestion, rales, rhonchi; 24%); cough increase (11%); rhinitis (10%).

Pharmacologic & Dosing Characteristics

Dosage: To avoid foaming and protein degradation, do not shake this drug.

Renal-cell cancer: To treat patients with metastatic renal-cell carcinoma, give 600,000 units/kg (0.037 mg/kg) every 8 hours for a maximum of 14 doses. Following an aldesleukin-free interval ("rest period") of 9 days, repeat the same schedule for another 14 doses, for a maximum of 28 doses per course.

Some of the published doses and routes in metastatic renal-cell carcinoma include the following. Other dose regimens have been published as well, including intraperitoneal administration. These doses and routes are not included in the official product labeling:

Subcutaneous administration: 20 million units/m^2 on days 3 to 5 of weeks 1 and 4 of therapy, along with interferon alfa (and perhaps 5-fluorouracil) followed by 5 million units/m^2 subcutaneously on days 1, 3 and 5 of weeks 2, 3, 5, and 6. Treatment cycles are repeated every 8 weeks unless progressive disease occurs.

2-day pulse: 14.4 to 18 million units/m^2/day, along with interferon alfa, followed by 3.6 to 4.8 million units/m^2/day 5 days per week for 6 weeks.

Continuous IV administration: 3 to 6 million units/m^2/day for 5 days, along with interferon alfa.

6 million units/m^2/day on days 1 through 4, along with interferon alfa. Treat for 4 weeks, followed by 2 weeks rest, until progression, toxicity, or 6 courses are given.

12 million units/m^2/day for 4 days, along with interferon alfa.

Metastatic melanoma: Give 600,000 units/kg (0.037 mg/kg) every 8 hours for a maximum of 14 doses. Following an aldesleukin-free interval ("rest period") of 9 days, repeat the same schedule for another 14 doses, for a maximum of 28 doses per course.

Route: IV infusion over 15 minutes every 8 hours. Do not use in-line filters when administering aldesleukin.

Administration by continuous IV infusion and subcutaneous injection have also been reported, as noted above.

Additional Doses: Evaluate patients for response approximately 4 weeks after completion of a course of therapy and again immediately prior to the scheduled start of the next course. Give additional courses of therapy to patients only if there is some renal-cell tumor shrinkage following the last course and re-treatment is not contraindicated. Separate each treatment course by a rest period of at least 7 weeks from the date of hospital discharge. Renal-cell tumors have continued to regress up to 12 months following the initiation of aldesleukin therapy. Re-treatment with aldesleukin is permanently contraindicated in patients who experienced any of the following toxicities while receiving an earlier course of therapy: Sustained ventricular tachycardia (5 beats or more); cardiac rhythm disturbances not controlled or unresponsive to management; chest pain with ECG changes consistent with angina or MI; cardiac tamponade, intubation required more than 72 hours; renal dysfunction requiring dialysis more than 72 hours; coma or toxic psychosis lasting more than 48 hours; repetitive or difficult-to-control seizures; bowel ischemia or perforation; or GI bleeding requiring surgery.

Dose Modification: During clinical trials, doses were frequently withheld because of toxicity.

Renal-cell cancer: Patients treated with this schedule received a median of 20 of the 28 doses during the first course of therapy.

Metastatic melanoma: Patients received a median of 18 of 28 scheduled doses. Modify the dose by holding or interrupting a dose, rather than reducing the dose administered to avoid toxicity. Decide to stop, hold or restart aldesleukin therapy only after performing a comprehensive assessment of the patient.

Suggested Scheme for Holding and Restarting Aldesleukin Therapy		
Body system	Hold dose for:	Subsequent doses given if:
Cardiovascular	Atrial fibrillation, supraventricular tachycardia, or bradycardia that requires treatment or is recurrent or persistent.	Patient is asymptomatic with full recovery to normal sinus rhythm.
	Systolic blood pressure < 90 mm Hg with increasing requirements for pressors.	Systolic pressure ≥ 90 mm Hg and stable or improving requirements for pressors.
	Any ECG change consistent with MI or ischemia with or without chest pain; suspicion of cardiac ischemia.	Patient is asymptomatic, MI and myocarditis have been ruled out, clinical suspicion of angina is low and there is no evidence of ventricular hypokinesia.
Respiratory	Oxygen saturation < 94% on room air or ≤ 90% with 2 L oxygen by nasal prongs.	Oxygen saturation ≥ 94% on room air or > 90% with 2 L oxygen by nasal prongs.
CNS	Mental status changes, including moderate confusion or agitation.	Mental status changes completely resolved.
Body as a whole	Sepsis syndrome, patient is clinically unstable.	Sepsis syndrome has resolved, patient is clinically stable, infection is under treatment.

Aldesleukin (Recombinant)

Suggested Scheme for Holding and Restarting Aldesleukin Therapy		
Body system	Hold dose for:	Subsequent doses given if:
GU	Serum creatinine > 4.5 mg/dL or serum creatinine of ≥ 4 mg/dL in the presence of severe volume overload, acidosis or hyperkalemia.	Serum creatinine < 4 mg/dL and fluid and electrolyte status is stable.
	Persistent oliguria, urine output ≤ 10 mL/h for 16 to 24 hours with rising serum creatinine.	Urine output > 10 mL/h with a decrease of serum creatinine > 1.5 mg/dL or normalization of serum creatinine.
	Signs of hepatic failure, including encephalopathy, increasing ascites, liver pain or hypoglycemia.	All signs of hepatic failure have resolved. In such cases, discontinue all further treatment for that course of therapy. Consider starting a new course of therapy after waiting 7 weeks after cessation of adverse event and hospital discharge.
GI	Stool for blood repeatedly > 3 to 4+.	Stool for blood negative.
Dermatologic	Bullous dermatitis or marked worsening of preexisting skin condition (avoid topical steroid therapy because potential absorption through the skin may compromise the efficacy of aldesleukin therapy).	Resolution of all signs of bullous dermatitis.

Associated Tests: Conduct the following clinical evaluations on all patients prior to beginning treatment and then daily during drug administration: Standard hematologic tests (eg, CBC, differential and platelet counts), blood chemistries (eg, electrolytes, renal and hepatic function tests), and chest radiographs.

Give all patients baseline pulmonary function tests, including arterial blood gases. Document adequate pulmonary function (eg, FEV_1 more than 2 L or at least 75% of prediction for height and age) prior to initiating therapy. Screen all patients with a stress thallium study. Document normal ejection fraction and unimpaired wall motion. If a thallium stress test suggests minor wall motion abnormalities of questionable significance, a stress echocardiogram to document normal wall motion may be useful to exclude significant coronary artery disease.

Include vital signs (eg, temperature, pulse, blood pressure, respiration rate) and weight in daily monitoring during therapy. In a patient with a decreased blood pressure, especially less than 90 mm Hg, conduct constant cardiac monitoring for rhythm. If an abnormal complex or rhythm is seen, perform an ECG. Take vital signs in these hypotensive patients hourly and check central venous pressure.

Assess cardiac function daily by clinical examination and vital signs. Assess patients with signs or symptoms of chest pain, murmurs, gallops, irregular rhythm or palpitations with an ECG examination and CPK evaluation. If there is evidence of cardiac ischemia or CHF, repeat the thallium study.

During treatment, monitor pulmonary function on a regular basis by clinical examination, assessment of vital signs and pulse oximetry. Assess patients with dyspnea or clinical signs of respiratory impairment (eg, tachypnea, rales) with arterial blood gas determination. Repeat these tests as often as clinically indicated.

Concomitant Therapy: Several concomitant medications have been used during clinical trials to manage potential toxicities of aldesleukin. Acetaminophen and NSAIDs have been started immediately prior to aldesleukin therapy to reduce fever. Renal function was monitored because NSAIDs may cause synergistic nephrotoxicity. Meperidine was used to control the rigors associated with fever. An H_2 antagonist (eg, cimetidine, ranitidine) was given for prophylaxis of GI irritation and bleeding. Antiemetics and antidiarrheals were used to treat other GI adverse effects. These medications were discontinued 12 hours after the last dose of aldesleukin. An H_1 antagonist (eg, hydroxyzine, diphenhydramine) was used to control pruritic rashes and was continued until pruritus resolved. Manage patients with hypovolemia by administration of IV fluids, either colloids or crystalloids. Give oxygen if pulmonary function monitoring confirms reduced arterial oxygen saturation.

Early administration of dopamine (1 to 5 mcg/kg/min) to patients manifesting CLS, before the onset of hypotension, can help maintain organ perfusion, particularly to the kidney, and thus preserve urine output. Monitor weight and urine output carefully. If organ perfusion and blood pressure are not sustained by dopamine therapy, consider increasing the dopamine dose to 6 to 10 mcg/kg/min or adding phenylephrine 1 to 5 mcg/kg/min. Prolonged use of vasopressor drugs, either in combination or as individual agents, at relatively high doses may be associated with cardiac rhythm disturbances. Recovery from CLS begins soon after cessation of aldesleukin therapy. Usually, within a few hours, blood pressure rises, organ perfusion returns and resorption of extravasated fluid and proteins begin. If there has been excessive weight gain or edema formation (especially if associated with shortness of breath from pulmonary congestion), diuretic therapy after normalization of blood pressure hastens recovery.

Overdosage: Adverse effects from aldesleukin are dose-related. Administration of greater than the recommended dose has been associated with a more rapid onset of expected dose-limiting toxicities. Given the short half-life of aldesleukin, most adverse reactions will reverse shortly after discontinuing the drug. Treat any continuing symptoms supportively. Life-threatening toxicities have been ameliorated by IV administration of dexamethasone, which may result in loss of the therapeutic effect of aldesleukin.

Efficacy:

Renal-cell cancer: Objective response has been observed in 15% of 255 aldesleukin recipients (95% CI: 11% to 20%), with 4% complete response and 11% partial response. Durable responses were achieved with a median duration of objective (partial or complete) response of 23.2 months (range, 1 to 50 months or more). The median duration of objective partial response was 18.8 months. The proportion of responding patients who will have response durations of at least 12 months is projected by the Kaplan-Meier method to be 85% for all responders and 79% for patients with partial responses. Response was observed in both lung and non-lung sites (eg, liver, lymph node, renal bed recurrences, soft tissue). Patients with individual bulky lesions (more than 5 of at least 5 cm), as well as large cumulative tumor burden (more than 25 cm^2 tumor area), achieved durable responses.

Performance status as defined by the Eastern Cooperative Oncology Group (ECOG) is a significant predictor of response to aldesleukin. Stage 0 (Karnofsky scale 100, asymptomatic) patients had an 18% overall rate of objective response, including all 9 complete-response patients and 21 of 28 partial-response patients. Stage 1 (Karnofsky scale 80 to 90, symptomatic but fully ambulatory) patients had a 9% overall rate of objective response, all of whom were partial-response patients. Among stage 1 patients, 6 of 7 partial responders had resolution of tumor-related symptoms and improved performance status to stage 0.

Stage 0 patients also had lower rates of adverse events with fewer deaths (4% vs 6%), less frequent intubations (8% vs 25%), gangrene (0% vs 6%), coma (1% vs 6%), GI bleeding (4% vs 8%), and sepsis (6% vs 18%). These differences in toxicity are reflected in the shorter mean time to hospital discharge for stage 0 patients (2 vs 3 days), as well as the smaller percentage experiencing a delayed discharge (more than 7 days) from the hospital (8% vs 19%).

Aldesleukin (Recombinant)

ECOG and Karnofsky Performance Status Scale		
Performance Status Scale		Definition
ECOG	Karnofsky	
0	100	Asymptomatic
1	80-90	Symptomatic, fully ambulatory
2	60-70	Symptomatic, in bed < 50% of day
3	40-50	Symptomatic, in bed> 50% of day
4	20-30	Bedridden

Aldesleukin Response by Performance Status					
Pretreatment ECOG status	Patients treated	Extent of Response		Patients responding (%)	Death rate (%)
		Complete	Partial		
0	166	9	21	18	4
1	80	0	7	9	6
≥ 2	9	0	0	0	0

Metastatic melanoma: Eight clinical studies of 270 patients with metastatic melanoma were conducted. Objective response was seen in 16% (95% CI: 12% to 21%), with 6% complete and 10% partial responders. The median duration of objective (partial or complete) response was 9 months (1 to 122+ months); the median duration of objective complete responses has not been observed and the median duration for partial response was 6 months. The median progression-free survival for the 43 responding patients was 13 months. Responses in metastatic melanoma patients were observed in both visceral and non-visceral sites (eg, lung, liver, lymph node, soft tissue, adrenal, subcutaneous). Some patients with individual bulky lesions and large cumulative tumor burden achieved responses.

As with renal-cell carcinoma, among patients with metastatic melanoma, ECOG performance scale status is a significant predictor of higher response and lower toxicity to aldesleukin. Complete and partial response was achieved by 7% and 12%, respectively, of patients with ECOG performance status 0 but only by 4% and 5% among those with ECOG status 1 or more.

Onset: Onset of renal-cell tumor regression has been observed as early as 4 weeks after completion of the first course of treatment.

Duration: Renal-cell tumor regression may continue for up to 12 months after the start of treatment.

Pharmacokinetics: Aldesleukin exists as biologically active, noncovalently bound microaggregates with an average size of 27 molecules. The solubilizing agent, sodium dodecyl sulfate, may affect the kinetic properties of this drug.

Absorption: Aldesleukin achieves high plasma concentrations following a short IV infusion, with rapid distribution to extravascular, extracellular space. In sheep and humans, approximately 30% of the administered dose initially distributes to the plasma. In rats, approximately 70% of the drug is taken up into the liver, kidney and lung. The volume of distribution of the central compartment is 172 mL/kg.

Elimination: Aldesleukin is metabolized in the kidney with little or no bioactive protein excreted in the urine. Elimination involves both glomerular filtration and peritubular extraction in the kidney. Among 52 cancer patients receiving a 5-minute infusion of aldesleukin, the distribution and elimination half-lives were 13 and 85 minutes, respectively. Clearance is largely unaffected, even in patients with elevated serum creatinine values.

Greater than 80% of aldesleukin distributed to plasma, cleared from the circulation, and presented to the kidney is metabolized to amino acids in the cells lining the proximal convoluted tubules. In humans, the mean clearance rate in cancer patients is 268 mL/min.

Mechanism: In vitro studies of aldesleukin demonstrate enhancement of lymphocyte mitogenesis and stimulation of long-term growth of human interleukin-2 dependent cell lines; enhancement of lymphocyte cytotoxicity; induction of killer cell (lymphokine-activated [LAK] and natural [NK]) activity; and induction of gamma interferon production. In vivo murine tumor and human models indicate that aldesleukin activates cellular immunity with profound lymphocytosis, eosinophilia, and thrombocytopenia. Aldesleukin also activates the production of cytokines, including tumor necrosis factor, interleukin-1, and gamma interferon. In vivo experiments in murine tumor models have shown inhibition of tumor growth. The exact mechanism of the antitumor effect of aldesleukin is unknown.

Drug Interactions: Renal and hepatic function are impaired during aldesleukin therapy. Use of concomitant medications known to be nephrotoxic (eg, aminoglycosides, indomethacin), hepatotoxic (eg, asparginase, methotrexate), myelotoxic (eg, cytotoxic chemotherapy), or cardiotoxic (eg, doxorubicin) may further increase toxicity to these organs. Reduced kidney or liver function secondary to aldesleukin treatment may delay elimination of concomitant medications and increase the risk of adverse events from these drugs.

Aldesleukin may affect CNS function. Therefore, interactions could occur following concomitant administration of psychotropic drugs (eg, narcotics, analgesics, antiemetics, sedatives, tranquilizers).

Hypersensitivity reactions have been reported in patients receiving combination regimens containing sequential high-dose aldesleukin and antineoplastic agents, specifically dacarbazine, cisplatin, tamoxifen and interferon-alfa. These reactions consisted of erythema, pruritus and hypotension and occurred within hours of administration of chemotherapy. These events required medical intervention in some patients.

Myocardial injury, including MI, myocarditis, ventricular hypokinesia, and severe rhabdomyolysis, appear to be increased in patients receiving aldesleukin and interferon-alfa concurrently. Exacerbation or the initial presentation of several autoimmune and inflammatory disorders have been observed with concurrent use of interferon-alfa and aldesleukin, including crescentic IgA glomerulonephritis, oculo-bulbar myasthenia gravis, inflammatory arthritis, thyroiditis, bullous pemphigoid and Stevens-Johnson syndrome.

Corticosteroids reduce aldesleukin-induced adverse effects (eg, fever, renal insufficiency, hyperbilirubinemia, confusion, dyspnea). Avoid concomitant administration of these agents with aldesleukin, unless benefits of steroid use outweigh likely risks, because steroids may reduce the antitumor effectiveness of aldesleukin.

Beta-adrenergic antagonists (eg, propranolol) and other antihypertensive drugs may potentiate the hypotension seen with aldesleukin.

Natural interleukin-2 boosts systemic immune response to hepatitis B surface antigen in immunodeficient nonresponders to hepatitis B vaccination. But the recombinant interleukin-2 known as teceleukin did not augment response to hepatitis B vaccine in healthy adults in another study. The significance of these effects for aldesleukin is unknown. The effects of aldesleukin on cellular immunity and manifestations of delayed hypersensitivity (eg, anergy test, tuberculin test) responses are unknown at present.

Reactions to IV radiocontrast media may be increased in people who have received aldesleukin, especially in the previous 6 weeks. In one study, 12.6% of 501 patients treated with various interleukin-2 regimens experienced acute, atypical adverse reactions after receiving radiographic iodinated contrast media. These reactions most commonly occur 1 to 4 hours after giving the contrast media and may resemble earlier reactions to aldesleukin: hypersensi-

Aldesleukin (Recombinant)

tivity, fever, skin rash, joint pain, flushing, pruritus, emesis, hypotension, chills, edema, oliguria and dizziness.

Previous exposure to interleukin-2 can increase the likelihood of a type-I immediate hypersensitivity reaction to cisplatin. Hypersensitivity developed in 10 of 16 patients who received IL-2 before receiving cisplatin, but in none of the 15 patients who received cisplatin without IL-2. Other causes were ruled out in this analysis. The possibility that hypersensitivity to other drugs might also be enhanced cannot be discounted.

Pharmaceutical Characteristics

Concentration: After reconstitution with 1.2 mL diluent, 18 million units (1.1 mg) aldesleukin per mL

Quality Assay: Potency is measured by a lymphocyte proliferation bioassay; purity is assessed by electrophoresis and reversed-phase high-pressure liquid chromatography (RP-HPLC). In addition to units, 2 other potency systems have been used. One Roche Unit is approximately equivalent to 3 units; 1 Cetus Unit is approximately equivalent to 6 units. Use caution in interpreting medical orders.

Packaging: 22 million units (1.3 mg) aldesleukin per single-dose vial

NDC Number: 65483-0116-07

Doseform: Powder for solution

Appearance: White to off-white caked powder, yielding a clear, colorless to slightly yellow liquid

Diluent:

For reconstitution: 1.2 mL sterile water per vial. To avoid foaming and protein degradation, do not shake this drug.

For infusion: Pulse IV infusion: Dilute the dose of aldesleukin aseptically in 50 mL of 5% dextrose. If the dose is 1.5 mg or less (eg, a patient with a body weight less than 40 kg), dilute the aldesleukin dose in a smaller volume of 5% dextrose. Concentrations of aldesleukin less than 30 mcg/mL or more than 70 mcg/mL have shown increased variability in drug delivery. Avoid dilution and delivery of aldesleukin outside this concentration range.

Continuous IV infusion: For extended stability, add sufficient human serum albumin to the diluent container to yield a 0.1% concentration of albumin if the final concentration falls between 5 and 60 mcg/mL. Add the albumin to the fluid before adding the aldesleukin. Depending on the volume of diluent and concentration of source albumin, add the following volume:

Continuous IV Infusion		
Volume of IV diluent	For 5% albumin	For 25% albumin
50 mL	1 mL	0.2 mL
100 mL	2 mL	0.4 mL
150 mL	3 mL	0.6 mL

Under specific conditions of temperature, concentration, and pump environment, aldesleukin is physically and chemically stable for 6 days. These conditions are 32°C (90°F), 5 to 60 mcg/mL with albumin or 100 to 500 mcg/mL without albumin, using a Pharmacia Deltec CADD-1 pump system. Aldesleukin is not stable, with or without albumin, between 61 and 99 mcg/mL.

Although both glass bottles and plastic (ie, polyvinyl chloride) bags have been used in clinical trials with comparable results, use plastic bags for the dilution container because experimental studies suggest that use of plastic containers provides more consistent drug delivery. Do not use in-line filters when administering aldesleukin because the filter may produce a significant loss of bioactivity. Bring the solution to room temperature prior to infusion into the patient.

Subcutaneous: Avoid reconstitution or dilution with bacteriostatic water for injection or with 0.9% sodium chloride because of the likelihood of increased aggregation. Do not mix aldesleukin with other drugs.

Adjuvant: None

Preservative: None

Allergens: Tetracycline added during production is undetectable in the final product.

Excipients: When reconstituted to 18 million units/mL, each mL contains 50 mg mannitol, 0.18 mg sodium dodecyl sulfate, 0.17 mg monobasic sodium phosphate, and 0.89 mg dibasic sodium phosphate.

pH: 7.2 to 7.8

Shelf Life: Expires within 18 months.

Storage/Stability: Store unreconstituted powder at 2° to 8°C (36° to 46°F); do not freeze. Unopened vials were stored at 30°C (86°F) for 48 hours without loss of activity. Shipped in insulated containers with coolant packs. No data are available regarding the stability of frozen powder.

Reconstituted vials can be frozen for up to 7 days and thawed, for a single freeze-thaw cycle, without loss of activity. Multiple freeze-thaw cycles are not recommended because of an increased risk of turbidity.

Reconstituted or diluted aldesleukin can tolerate up to 48 hours at refrigerated and room temperatures. However, because this product contains no preservative, refrigerate any reconstituted and diluted solutions. Aldesleukin has been stored in a refrigerator for 5 days in 1 mL Bectin-Dickinson syringes with 20-gauge needles without loss of potency. Another test of 220 mcg/mL aldesleukin in 6 mL (1.2 mL reconstituted aldesleukin plus 4.8 mL dextrose 5%) was stable under refrigeration for up to 14 days. No data are available regarding freezing the product once diluted in an IV delivery container.

Handling: Drug is compatible with glass, polyvinyl chloride (PVC), and polypropylene syringes. The manufacturer indicates that PVC is preferred.

Production Process: Fermentation in a defined, reproducible medium containing tetracycline.

Media: *Escherichia coli*

Disease Epidemiology

Incidence: Approximately 26,000 Americans are diagnosed with renal-cell carcinoma each year. Nearly 50% have metastatic disease at presentation, and the median survival of patients with metastatic renal-cell carcinoma is approximately 12 months. The probability of survival for 2 years is less than 10%.

Other Information

Perspective:
1976: Morgan describes interleukin-2, then called T-cell growth factor.
1983: Taniguchi isolates complete complementary DNA for interleukin-2.
1992: Aldesleukin licensed on May 5, for treatment of renal-cell carcinoma.
1998: Aldesleukin licensed on January 9 for treatment of metastatic melanoma.

References: Kintzel PE, et al. Recombinant interleukin-2: A biological response modifier. *Clin Pharm.* 1991;10:110-128.

Schmidinger M, Hejna M, Zielinski CC. Aldesleukin in advanced renal cell carcinoma. *Expert Rev Anticancer Ther.* 2004;4(6):957-980.

Denileukin Diftitox (Recombinant)

Interleukins

Name:
  Ontak

Manufacturer:
  Eisai

Synonyms: $DAB_{486}IL\text{-}2$, IL-2 fusion protein

Immunologic Characteristics

Antigen Source: Expressed by recombinant *Escherichia coli*

Viability: Not viable, but immunologically active

Antigenic Form: DNA-derived cytotoxic protein composed of the amino acid sequences for diphtheria toxin fragments A and B ($Met_1\text{-}Thr_{387}$)-His followed by the sequences for interleukin-2 (IL-2; $Ala_1\text{-}Thr_{133}$), with a molecular weight of 58 kD.

Antigenic Type: Fusion protein. Diphtheria toxin in which the receptor-binding domain is replaced by IL-2 sequences.

Strains: Not applicable

Use Characteristics

Indications: For the treatment of persistent or recurrent cutaneous T-cell lymphoma whose malignant cells express the CD25 component of the IL-2 receptor.

Unlabeled Uses: Research in progress is assessing the role of denileukin diftitox in the treatment of severe rheumatoid arthritis, recent-onset type 1 diabetes, and IL-2 receptor-expressing leukemias and lymphomas.

Limitations: The safety and efficacy of denileukin diftitox in patients with CTCL whose malignant cells do not express the CD25 component of the IL-2 receptor have not been examined.

Contraindications:

Absolute: None

Relative: People with a known hypersensitivity to denileukin diftitox or any of its components: Diphtheria toxin, interleukin-2, or excipients.

Immunodeficiency: Because of risk of infection, use with caution in patients with compromised immune systems.

Elderly: Of patients enrolled in the randomized 2-dose study, 49% were at least 65 years of age. Those patients had response rates similar to those seen in younger patients. The following adverse events (regardless of causality) tended to be more frequent or more severe in lymphoma patients who were at least 65 years of age: anorexia, hypotension, anemia, confusion, rash, nausea, or vomiting.

Pregnancy: Category C. It is not known whether denileukin diftitox can cause fetal harm when administered to a pregnant woman or can affect reproductive capacity. Give denileukin diftitox to a pregnant woman only if clearly needed.

Lactation: It is not known whether denileukin diftitox crosses into breast milk. Because of the potential for serious adverse reactions in nursing infants, women receiving denileukin diftitox should discontinue nursing.

Children: Safety and efficacy in children younger than 18 years of age have not been established.

Adverse Reactions: Adverse reactions are based on 3 clinical studies in which 234 patients received denileukin diftitox 9 mcg/kg (n = 80) or 18 mcg/kg (n = 154) at the recommended schedule. Of these studies, one was placebo-controlled and dose-ranging (n = 100), one was a dose-comparison study of 9 and 18 mcg/kg (n = 71), and the third was a single-arm study assessing 18 mcg/kg (n = 63); all studies were limited to adult patients with CTCL (median age, 60 years; range, 23 to 91 years; 55% were men).

The most common reactions (at least 20%) were pyrexia, nausea, fatigue, rigors, vomiting, diarrhea, headache, peripheral edema, cough, dyspnea, and pruritus. The most common serious adverse reactions were capillary leak syndrome (11%), infusion reactions (8%), and visual changes, including loss of visual acuity (4%). Denileukin diftitox was discontinued in 28% (66/234) of patients because of adverse reactions.

The following table describes the experience of 100 patients administered denileukin diftitox as a single agent at the recommended dosing schedule in a randomized placebo-controlled trial. The median number of treatment cycles was 7 (range, 1 to 10) for the 9 mcg/kg cohort and 6 (range, 1 to 11) for the 18 mcg/kg cohort. The median age of patients was 59 years (range, 23 to 84 years of age).

Incidence of Adverse Reactions Occurring in ≥ 10% of Denileukin Diftitox-Treated Patients (18 mcg/kg group) and at a Higher Rate Than Placebo			
Event	Denileukin Diftitox 18 mcg/kg n = 55	Denileukin Diftitox 9 mcg/kg n = 45	Placebo
Pyrexia	35 (64%)	22 (49%)	7 (16%)
Nausea	33 (60%)	21 (47%)	10 (23%)
Rigors	26 (47%)	19 (42%)	9 (21%)
Fatigue	24 (44%)	21 (47%)	14 (32%)
Vomiting	19 (35%)	6 (13%)	3 (7%)
Headache	14 (26%)	13 (29%)	8 (18%)
Peripheral edema	14 (26%)	9 (20%)	10 (23%)
Diarrhea	12 (22%)	10 (22%)	4 (9%)
Anorexia	11 (20%)	4 (9%)	2 (5%)
Rash	11 (20%)	11 (24%)	2 (5%)
Myalgia	11 (20%)	8 (18%)	2 (5%)
Cough	10 (18%)	9 (20%)	3 (7%)
Pruritus	10 (18%)	7 (16%)	4 (9%)
Back pain	10 (18%)	7 (16%)	1 (2%)
Asthenia	10 (18%)	8 (18%)	2 (5%)
Hypotension	9 (16%)	3 (7%)	1 (2%)
Upper respiratory tract infection	7 (13%)	6 (13%)	5 (11%)
Dizziness	7 (13%)	5 (11%)	5 (11%)
Arthralgia	7 (13%)	7 (16%)	5 (11%)
Pain	7 (13%)	5 (11%)	3 (7%)
Chest pain	7 (13%)	2 (4%)	1 (2%)
Dysgeusia	6 (11%)	0 (0%)	1 (2%)
Dyspnea	6 (11%)	6 (13%)	2 (5%)

Infusion reactions: Infusion reactions that occurred within 24 hours of infusion and resolved within 48 hours of last infusion in that course were reported in 70.5% (165/234) of denileukin diftitox-treated patients. Serious infusion reactions were reported in 8.1% (19/234). There have been postmarketing reports of infusion reactions resulting in death. For patients completing at least 4 courses of denileukin diftitox, the incidence of infusion reactions was lower in the third and fourth cycles compared with the first and second cycles.

Capillary-leak syndrome: Capillary-leak syndrome was defined as occurrence of at least 2 of 3 symptoms (ie, hypotension, edema, serum albumin less than 3 g/dL) at any time during denileukin diftitox therapy. Capillary-leak syndrome was reported in 32.5% (76/234) of treated patients. Among these 76 patients, one-third required hospitalization or medical intervention to prevent hospitalization. There have been postmarketing reports of capillary-leak syndrome resulting in death. Onset of this syndrome may be delayed, occurring up to 2 weeks after infusion. Symptoms may persist or worsen after the cessation of therapy. Regularly assess patients for weight gain, new onset or worsening edema, and hypotension (including orthostatic changes), and monitor serum albumin levels before starting each course of therapy and more often as clinically indicated. Withhold denileukin diftitox when serum albumin levels are less than 3 g/dL.

Visual loss: Loss of visual acuity, usually with loss of color vision, with or without retinal pigment mottling, has been reported following administration of denileukin diftitox. Recovery was reported in some of the affected patients; however, most patients reported persistent visual impairment.

Immunogenicity: An immune response to denileukin diftitox was assessed using 2 enzyme-linked immunoassays. The first assay measured reactivity against intact denileukin diftitox calibrated against anti-diphtheria toxin. The second assay measured reactivity against the IL-2 portion of the protein. An additional in vitro cell-based assay measuring ability of serum antibodies to protect a human IL-2R–expressing cell line from toxicity by denileukin diftitox was used to detect the presence of neutralizing antibodies that inhibited functional activity. Immunogenicity data reflect the percentage of patients whose test results were considered positive for antibodies to the intact denileukin diftitox. Of 95 patients treated with denileukin diftitox in study 1, 66% tested positive for antibodies at baseline, probably because of prior exposure to diphtheria toxin or toxoid. After 1, 2, and 3 courses of treatment, 94%, 99%, and 100% of patients tested positive, respectively. Mean titers of anti-denileukin diftitox antibodies were similarly increased in the 9 and 18 mcg/kg/day dose groups after 2 courses of treatment. Meanwhile, pharmacokinetic parameters decreased substantially (peak plasma concentration, approximately 57%; area under the curve, approximately 80%), and clearance increased 2- to 8-fold. In study 2, 131 patients were assessed for binding antibodies. Of these, 51 (39%) patients had antibodies at baseline. Seventy-six percent of patients tested positive after 1 course of treatment and 97% after 3 courses of treatment. Neutralizing antibodies were assessed in 60 patients; 45%, 73%, and 97% had evidence of inhibited functional activity in the cellular assay at baseline and after 1 and 3 courses of treatment, respectively.

Hepatobiliary disorders: Increase in serum ALT or AST from baseline occurred in 84% (197/234) of subjects treated with *Ontak*. In the majority of subjects, these enzyme elevations occurred during the first or the second cycle; enzyme elevation resolved without medical intervention and did not require discontinuation of *Ontak*.

Pharmacologic & Dosing Characteristics

Dosage: The recommended treatment regimen (1 treatment cycle) is 9 or 18 mcg/kg/day administered for 5 consecutive days every 21 days for 8 cycles.

Route: IV infusion over 15 minutes. Do not administer as a bolus injection. If infusional adverse reactions occur, stop the infusion or reduce the rate, depending on the severity of the reaction. There is no clinical experience with prolonged infusion times (longer than 80 minutes).

Overdosage: There is no clinical experience with accidental denileukin diftitox overdosage and no known antidote. At a dose of 31 mcg/kg/day, the dose-limiting toxicities were moderate-to-severe nausea, vomiting, fever, chills, or persistent asthenia. Doses greater than

31 mcg/kg/day have not been evaluated. If overdose occurs, monitor hepatic and renal function and overall fluid balance closely.

Additional Doses: The optimal duration of therapy has not been determined; however, of patients who did not demonstrate a 25% or more decrease in tumor burden before the fourth course of treatment, only 2% (1 of 50) subsequently responded.

Laboratory Tests: Before administering this product, test the patient's malignant cells for CD25 expression. Perform a complete blood count and a blood chemistry panel, including liver and renal function and serum albumin levels, before initiating denileukin diftitox treatment, and weekly during therapy.

Of patients with lymphoma, 83% experienced hypoalbuminemia, which was considered moderate or severe in 17% of the affected patients. For most patients, the nadir for hypoalbuminemia occurs 1 to 2 weeks after denileukin diftitox administration. Monitor serum albumin levels before initiating each treatment course. Delay administration of denileukin diftitox until serum albumin levels are at least 3 g/dL.

Efficacy: Denileukin diftitox was evaluated among 71 patients with recurrent or persistent Stage Ib to IVa CTCL who had failed at least 1 other treatment, such as interferon, chemotherapy, or radiation. Entry to this study required demonstration of CD25 expression on at least 20% of the cells in any relevant skin biopsy or circulating cells. Denileukin diftitox was administered daily for 5 days every 3 weeks. Patients received a median of 6 courses of therapy (range 1 to 11). The study population had received a median of 5 prior therapies (range, 1 to 12), with 63% of patients entering the trial with Stage IIb or more advanced stage disease. Overall, 30% of patients treated with denileukin diftitox experienced an objective tumor response (50% reduction in tumor burden that was sustained for more than 6 weeks). Seven patients (10%) achieved a complete response, and 14 patients (20%) achieved a partial response. The overall median duration of response, measured from first day of response, was 4 months, with a median duration for complete response of 9 months and for partial response of 4 months.

In a phase I/II dose-escalation study, 35 patients with Stage Ia to IVb CTCL were treated. Denileukin diftitox was administered as an IV infusion at doses ranging from 3 to 31 mcg/kg/day for 5 days every 3 weeks. The overall response rate in patients with CTCL who expressed CD25 was 38%; the complete response rate was 16%; and the partial response rate was 22%. There were no responses in 21 patients with Hodgkin disease.

Denileukin diftitox was approved under an accelerated process that relied on surrogate endpoints. The manufacturer is currently conducting a blinded, placebo-controlled trial to assess the drug's effect on tumor-related symptoms, diminished use of rescue medications, and prolonged time to progression.

Pharmacokinetics: Pharmacokinetic parameters associated with denileukin diftitox were determined over a range of doses (3 to 31 mcg/kg/day) in patients with lymphoma. Denileukin diftitox was administered as an IV infusion on the schedule used in clinical trials. After the first dose, denileukin diftitox displayed 2-compartment behavior, with a distribution phase (half-life, approximately 2 to 5 minutes) and a terminal phase (half-life, approximately 70 to 80 minutes). Systemic exposure was variable but proportional to dose. Clearance was approximately 1.5 to 2 mL/min/kg. The volume of distribution was similar to that of circulating blood (0.06 to 0.08 L/kg). No accumulation was evident between the first and fifth doses. Development of antibodies to denileukin diftitox significantly impacts clearance rates.

Distribution: The biodistribution of radiolabeled denileukin diftitox was evaluated over 48 hours in rats. The liver and kidneys were the primary sites of distribution and accumulation of radiolabeled material outside of the vasculature.

Denileukin Diftitox (Recombinant)

Elimination: The excretion of denileukin diftitox was evaluated over 48 hours in rats. Denileukin diftitox was metabolized by proteolytic degradation. Excreted material was less than 25% of the total injected dose and consisted of low-molecular-weight metabolites.

Mechanism: Denileukin diftitox is a fusion protein designed to direct the cytocidal action of diphtheria toxin to cells that express the IL-2 receptor. The human IL-2 receptor exists in 3 forms, low (CD25), intermediate (CD122/CD132), and high (CD25/CD122/CD132) affinity. The high-affinity form of this receptor is usually found only on activated T-lymphocytes, activated B-lymphocytes, and activated macrophages. Malignant cells expressing at least 1 of the subunits of the IL-2 receptor are found in certain leukemias and lymphomas including cutaneous T-cell lymphoma (CTCL). Ex vivo studies suggest that denileukin diftitox interacts with the high-affinity IL-2 receptor on the cell surface and inhibits cellular protein synthesis, resulting in cell death within hours.

Pharmaceutical Characteristics

Concentration: 300 mcg/2 mL

Packaging: 300 mcg/2 mL single-use vial, 6 vials in a package

NDC Number: 62856-0603-01

Doseform: Frozen solution

Appearance: After thawing, a haze may be visible. This haze should clear when the solution is at room temperature. Denileukin diftitox solution must not be used unless the solution is clear, colorless, and without visible particulate matter.

Solvent: Water for injection

Diluent:

For infusion: Sodium chloride 0.9% without preservative. The concentration of denileukin diftitox must be at least 15 mcg/mL during all steps in preparing the solution for IV infusion. For each 1 mL of denileukin diftitox from the vial(s), no more than 9 mL of sodium chloride 0.9% without preservative should be added.

Adjuvant: None

Preservative: None

Allergens: Neomycin is used in fermentation, but is undetectable in the final product.

Excipients: 20 mM citric acid, 0.05 mM EDTA, less than 1% polysorbate 20.

pH: 6.9 to 7.2

Shelf Life: Expires within 12 months.

Storage/Stability: Store at −10°C (14°F) or colder. Bring denileukin diftitox to room temperature, up to 25°C (77°F) before preparing the dose. Vials may be thawed in a refrigerator at 2° to 8°C (36° to 46°F) for up to 24 hours or at room temperature for 1 to 2 hours. Do not heat or refreeze denileukin diftitox. Shipping data not provided.

Administer prepared solutions of denileukin diftitox within 6 hours, using a syringe pump or IV infusion bag. Do not administer denileukin diftitox through an in-line filter. Discard unused portions of denileukin diftitox immediately.

Handling: The concentration of denileukin diftitox must be at least 15 mcg/mL during all steps in preparing the solution for IV infusion. This is best accomplished by withdrawing the calculated dose from the vial(s) and injecting it into an empty IV infusion bag. For each 1 mL of denileukin diftitox from the vial(s), no more than 9 mL of sodium chloride 0.9% without preservative should then be added to the IV bag.

Denileukin Diftitox (Recombinant)

The solution in the vial may be mixed by gentle swirling. Do not vigorously shake denileukin diftitox solution. Prepare and hold diluted denileukin diftitox in plastic syringes or soft plastic IV bags. Do not use a glass container because adsorption to glass may occur in the dilute state.

Do not physically mix denileukin diftitox with other drugs.

Production Process: Expressed by recombinant *E. coli*. Neomycin is used in the fermentation process but is undetectable in the final product. The product is purified using reverse-phase chromatography followed by a multistep diafiltration process.

Media: Recombinant *E. coli*

Disease Epidemiology

Incidence: Approximately 1,000 people in the US are diagnosed with cutaneous T-cell lymphoma each year. It is often a slowly progressive disease, causing itchy, dry skin patches that can develop into tumors in the skin and other organs. Approximately 60% of patients with cutaneous T-cell lymphoma have IL-2 receptors on their tumors.

Other Information

Perspective:
1996: Denileukin diftitox granted orphan drug status.
1999: Denileukin diftitox licensed on February 5, 1999.

References: Eklund JW, Kuzel TM. Denileukin diftitox: A concise clinical review. *Expert Rev Anticancer Ther.* 2005;5(1):33-38.

LeMaistre CF, et al. Therapeutic effects of genetically engineered toxin (DAB$_{486}$IL-2) in patients with chronic lymphocytic leukemia. *Lancet.* 1991;337:1124-1125.

Winkelhake JK, Gauny SS. Human recombinant interleukin-2 as an experimental therapeutic. *Pharmacol Rev.* 1990;42:1-28.

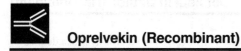

Oprelvekin (Recombinant)

Interleukins

Name:
Neumega

Manufacturer:
Genetics Institute, distributed by Pfizer

Immunologic Characteristics

Antigen Source: Recombinant interleukin-11 expressed by reengineered *Escherichia coli*.

Viability: Not viable, but immunologically active

Antigenic Form: Interleukin-11, recombinant

Antigenic Type: Protein. Oprelvekin has a molecular mass of approximately 19,000 daltons and is nonglycosylated. The polypeptide is 177 amino acids in length and differs from the 178 amino acid length of native IL-11 only in lacking the amino-terminal proline residue. This alteration has not resulted in measurable differences in bioactivity either in vitro or in vivo.

Use Characteristics

Indications: For the prevention of severe thrombocytopenia and reduction of need for platelet transfusions after myelosuppressive chemotherapy in patients with nonmyeloid malignancies who are at high risk of severe thrombocytopenia. Efficacy was demonstrated in people who had experienced severe thrombocytopenia following the previous chemotherapy cycle.

Limitations: Oprelvekin is not indicated following myeloablative chemotherapy. Oprelvekin has not been evaluated in people receiving chemotherapy regimens more than 5 days in duration or regimens associated with delayed myelosuppression (eg, nitrosoureas, mitomycin-C).

Contraindications:

Absolute: Patients with a history of hypersensitivity to oprelvekin or any component of the product.

Relative: None

Immunodeficiency: Use may be indicated in certain immunocompromised people.

Elderly: No specific information is available about geriatric use of oprelvekin.

Carcinogenicity: No studies have been performed to assess the carcinogenic potential of oprelvekin. In vitro, oprelvekin did not stimulate the growth of tumor colony-forming cells harvested from people with a variety of human malignancies.

Mutagenicity: Oprelvekin has been shown to be non-genotoxic in in vitro studies. These data suggest that oprelvekin is not mutagenic. Although prolonged estrus cycles have been noted at 2 to 20 times the human dose, no effects on fertility have been observed in rats treated with oprelvekin at doses up to 1,000 mcg/kg/day.

Pregnancy: Category C. Oprelvekin has embryocidal effects in pregnant rats and rabbits. There are no adequate studies of oprelvekin in pregnant women. Use oprelvekin during pregnancy only if the potential benefit justifies the potential risk to the fetus.

Lactation: It is not known if oprelvekin is excreted in human milk. Because many drugs are excreted in human milk and because of the potential for serious adverse reactions in nursing infants from oprelvekin, decide whether to discontinue nursing or to discontinue the drug, taking into account the importance of the drug to the mother.

Children: Efficacy trials have not been conducted among children. Preliminary data are available from an ongoing study in 28 children 8 months to 17 years of age treated with oprelvekin at doses of 25 to 100 mcg/kg following ICE (ifosfamide, carboplatin, etoposide) chemotherapy. Oprelvekin treatment was given daily for a maximum of 28 days in up to eight cycles. Based on this study, 75 to 100 mcg/kg in children will produce plasma levels consistent with those obtained in adults given 50 mcg/kg.

Adverse events in this study were generally similar to those observed using oprelvekin 50 mcg/kg in adults. Most adverse events associated with oprelvekin in adults occurred either with similar or lower frequency in the pediatric study. The rates of tachycardia (46%) and conjunctival injection (50%) in children were higher than in adults. There was no evidence of a dose-response relationship for any of the oprelvekin-associated adverse events among the pediatric patients.

No human studies have been performed to assess the long-term effects of oprelvekin on growth and development. In growing rodents treated with 100, 300 or 1,000 mcg/kg/day for a minimum of 28 days, thickening of femoral and tibial growth plates was noted, which did not completely resolve after a 28-day nontreatment period. In a nonhuman primate toxicology study of oprelvekin, animals treated for 2 to 13 weeks at doses of 10 to 1,000 mcg/kg showed partially reversible joint capsule and tendon fibrosis and periosteal hyperostosis. The clinical significance of these findings is not known. An asymptomatic, laminated periosteal reaction in the diaphyses of the femur, tibia, and fibula has been observed in one patient during pediatric trials involving multiple courses of oprelvekin treatment. The relationship of these findings to treatment with oprelvekin is unclear.

Adverse Reactions: In studies, 308 subjects 8 months to 75 years of age have been exposed to oprelvekin treatment. Subjects received up to six (eight in pediatric patients) courses of oprelvekin treatment, with each course lasting from 1 to 28 days. Other than sequelae of underlying malignancy or cytotoxic chemotherapy, most adverse events were mild or moderate in severity and reversed after stopping oprelvekin. Oprelvekin has caused serious allergic or hypersensitivity reactions, including anaphylaxis.

In general, the incidence and type of adverse events were similar between oprelvekin 50 mcg/kg and placebo groups. The following adverse events, occurring in 10% or more of people, were observed at equal or greater frequency in placebo-treated people: asthenia, pain, chills, abdominal pain, infection, anorexia, constipation, dyspepsia, ecchymosis, myalgia, bone pain, nervousness, and alopecia. Selected adverse events that occurred in oprelvekin-treated people are listed below. Events marked with * indicate that the event occurred in significantly more oprelvekin-treated than placebo-treated people.

Body as a whole: Edema* (59%), neutropenic fever (48%), headache (41%), fever (36%).

Cardiovascular: Tachycardia* (20%), vasodilation (19%), palpitations* (14%), syncope (13%), atrial fibrillation/flutter* (12%).

During oprelvekin therapy, monitor fluid balance. Patients receiving oprelvekin have commonly experienced mild to moderate fluid retention, as indicated by peripheral edema or dyspnea on exertion. Weight gain was uncommon. Fluid retention typically reverses within several days after stopping oprelvekin. In some people, preexisting pleural effusions increased during oprelvekin therapy. Monitor preexisting fluid collections, including pericardial effusions or ascites. Consider drainage if medically indicated. Capillary leak syndrome was not observed following treatment with oprelvekin. Use it with caution in people with clinically evident congestive heart failure (CHF) and those susceptible to developing CHF or patients with a history of heart failure. If a diuretic is used, monitor fluid and electrolyte balance carefully. Use cautiously in people who may retain fluids because of medical conditions or whose condition may be exacerbated by fluid retention. Sudden deaths have occurred in people receiving chronic diuretic therapy and ifosfamide who developed severe hypokalemia.

Use oprelvekin with caution in people with a history of atrial arrhythmia, and only after consideration of potential risks and anticipated benefit. Transient atrial arrhythmias (atrial fibrillation or atrial flutter) occurred in 10% of people after treatment with oprelvekin. In some people, this may be due to increased plasma volume associated with fluid retention; oprelvekin is not directly arrhythmogenic. Arrhythmias were usually transient and without clinical sequelae; some were asymptomatic. Conversion to sinus rhythm typically occurred spontaneously or after rate-control drug therapy. Most people continued to receive oprelvekin without recurrence of atrial arrhythmia. Clinical studies suggest that advancing age and other conditions associated with a risk of atrial arrhythmias, such as cardiac medications and a history of doxorubicin exposure, are risk factors for developing atrial fibrillation or atrial flutter in people receiving oprelvekin. Ventricular arrhythmias have not been attributed to oprelvekin.

CNS: Dizziness (38%), insomnia (33%).

Dermatologic: Rash (25%).

GI: Nausea/vomiting (77%); mucositis, diarrhea (43%); oral moniliasis* (14%).

Immunologic: Approximately 1% of people receiving oprelvekin developed antibodies to oprelvekin. Transient rashes were occasionally observed at the injection site. The presence of these antibodies or injection-site reactions have not been correlated with anaphylactoid reactions or loss of clinical response to oprelvekin. No anaphylactoid or other severe adverse allergic reactions were reported after single or repeated doses of oprelvekin.

Lab test abnormalities: Moderate decreases in hemoglobin concentration, hematocrit, and red blood cell count (approximately 10% to 15%) without a decrease in red blood cell mass have been observed. These changes are predominantly due to an increase in plasma volume (dilutional anemia), primarily related to renal sodium and water retention. The decrease in hemoglobin concentration typically begins within 3 to 5 days of starting oprelvekin, reversing within a week after stopping oprelvekin.

Ophthalmic: Transient, mild visual blurring has occasionally been reported by people treated with oprelvekin. Papilledema has been reported in 1.5% of subjects following repeated cycles of exposure. Nonhuman primates treated with oprelvekin 1,000 mcg/kg subcutaneously daily for 4 to 13 weeks developed papilledema not associated with inflammation or any other histologic abnormality; it reversed after stopping the drug. Use oprelvekin with caution in people with preexisting papilledema, or with tumors involving the CNS, because the papilledema could worsen or develop during treatment.

Respiratory: Dyspnea* (48%), rhinitis (42%), increased cough (29%), pharyngitis (25%), pleural effusions* (10%).

Special Senses: Conjunctival injection* (19%).

Cancer patients: The following adverse events also occurred more frequently in cancer patients receiving oprelvekin than in those receiving placebo: amblyopia, paresthesia, dehydration, skin discoloration, exfoliative dermatitis, and eye hemorrhage. A statistically significant association of oprelvekin to these events has not been established. Other than a higher incidence of severe asthenia in oprelvekin-treated people (14% vs 3% in placebo recipients), the rates of severe or life-threatening adverse events was comparable in the oprelvekin and placebo groups.

The incidence of fever, neutropenic fever, flu-like symptoms, thrombocytosis, thrombotic events, the average number of units of red blood cells transfused per patient, and the duration of neutropenia less than 500 cells/mcL were similar in the oprelvekin and placebo groups.

Two people with cancer treated with oprelvekin experienced sudden death, which the investigator considered possibly or probably related to oprelvekin. Both deaths occurred in people with severe hypokalemia (less than 3 mEq/L) who had received high doses of ifosfamide and were receiving daily doses of a diuretic. The relationship of these deaths to oprelvekin remains unclear.

Pharmacologic & Dosing Characteristics

Dosage:
> *Adult:* The recommended adult dose is 50 mcg/kg once daily. In clinical studies, doses were administered in courses of 10 to 21 days. Dosing beyond 21 days per treatment course is not recommended.
>
> *Children:* A dose of 75 to 100 mcg/kg in children produces plasma levels consistent with those obtained in adults given 50 mcg/kg.
>
> Begin dosing 6 to 24 hours after completing chemotherapy. The safety and efficacy of oprelvekin given immediately before or concurrently with cytotoxic chemotherapy have not been established. Stop oprelvekin at least 2 days before starting the next planned cycle of chemotherapy.

Route & Site: Subcutaneous injection in either the abdomen, thigh, or hip (or upper arm if not self-injecting).

Overdosage: Doses greater than 100 mcg/kg have not been given to humans. While clinical experience is limited, doses greater than 50 mcg/kg may be associated with an increased incidence of cardiovascular events in adults. If an overdose of oprelvekin is administered, discontinue oprelvekin and monitor the patient for signs of toxicity. Base resumption of oprelvekin upon individual factors (eg, evidence of toxicity, continued need for therapy).

Additional Doses: Oprelvekin has been given safely using the recommended dosing schedule for up to 6 cycles following chemotherapy. The safety and efficacy of chronic administration of oprelvekin have not been established. Continuous dosing (2 to 13 weeks) in nonhuman primates produced joint capsule and tendon fibrosis and periosteal hyperostosis. The relevance of these findings to humans is unclear.

Missed Doses: If a dose is missed, continue with the next scheduled dose.

Laboratory Tests: Obtain a complete blood count before and at regular intervals during oprelvekin therapy. Monitor platelet counts during the time of the expected nadir and until adequate recovery has occurred (post-nadir counts more than 50,000 cells/mcL).

The most common laboratory abnormality reported in clinical trials was a decrease in hemoglobin concentration, primarily resulting from plasma-volume expansion. The increase in plasma volume is also associated with a decrease in serum concentration of albumin and several other proteins (eg, transferrin, IgG). A corresponding decrease in calcium without clinical effects has been documented.

After daily subcutaneous injections, treatment with oprelvekin resulted in a 2-fold increase in plasma fibrinogen. Other acute-phase proteins also increased. These protein levels returned to normal after oprelvekin therapy ceased. Von Willebrand factor (vWF) concentrations increased with a normal multimer pattern in healthy subjects receiving oprelvekin.

Efficacy: In a study of oprelvekin in non-myelosuppressed cancer patients, daily subcutaneous dosing for 14 days increased the platelet count in a dose-dependent manner. No change in platelet reactivity has been observed in association with oprelvekin.

In a study in normal volunteers, subjects receiving oprelvekin had a mean increase in plasma volume greater than 20%. All subjects receiving oprelvekin increased plasma volume greater than 10%. Red blood cell volume decreased similarly, because of repeated phlebotomy, in the oprelvekin and placebo groups. As a result, whole-blood volume increased 10%, and hemoglobin concentration decreased 10% in subjects receiving oprelvekin, compared with placebo recipients. Mean 24-hour sodium excretion decreased, and potassium excretion did not increase, in subjects receiving oprelvekin.

Another study evaluated oprelvekin's effect on the need for platelet transfusions in people who had recovered from severe chemotherapy-induced thrombocytopenia and were to receive an additional cycle of the same chemotherapy without dose reduction. The results for the oprelvekin 50 mcg/kg and placebo groups are summarized below. More people avoided platelet transfusion in the oprelvekin 50 mcg/kg arm than in the placebo arm ($P = 0.04$). The difference in the proportion of people avoiding platelet transfusions in the oprelvekin 50 mcg/kg and placebo groups was 21% (95% CI: 2% to 40%).

Clinical Effect of Oprelvekin Therapy		
	Placebo (n = 30)	Oprelvekin 50 mcg/kg (n = 29)
Number (%) of patients avoiding platelet transfusion	2 (7%)	8 (28%)
Number (%) of patients requiring platelet transfusion	28 (93%)	21 (72%)
Median (mean) number of platelet transfusion events	2.5 (3.3)	1 (2.2)

A second study evaluated oprelvekin's effect on reducing platelet transfusions over two dose-intensive chemotherapy cycles in breast cancer patients who had not previously experienced severe chemotherapy-induced thrombocytopenia. Everyone received the same chemotherapy regimen (ie, cyclophosphamide 3200 mg/m^2, doxorubicin 75 mg/m^2). These patients received filgrastim (G-CSF) in all cycles. The primary endpoint was whether a patient required one or more platelet transfusions in the two study cycles. The results are summarized below:

Oprelvekin vs Placebo: Platelet Transfusions in Patients With and Without Prior Chemotherapy						
	Overall n = 77		No prior chemotherapy n = 54		Prior chemotherapy n = 23	
	Placebo n = 37	Oprelvekin n = 40	Placebo n = 27	Oprelvekin n = 27	Placebo n = 10	Oprelvekin n = 13
Number (%) of patients avoiding platelet transfusion	15 (41%)	26 (65%)	14 (52%)	19 (70%)	1 (10%)	7 (54%)
Number (%) of patients requiring platelet transfusion	16 (43%)	12 (30%)	9 (33%)	7 (26%)	7 (70%)	5 (38%)
Number (%) of patients not evaluable	6 (16%)	2 (5%)	4 (15%)	1 (4%)	2 (20%)	1 (8%)

This study showed a trend in favor of oprelvekin, particularly among people with prior chemotherapy. Treatment with oprelvekin was continued for up to four consecutive chemotherapy cycles without evidence of any adverse effect on the rate of neutrophil recovery or red blood cell transfusion requirements. Some people maintained platelet nadirs more than 20,000 cells/mcL for at least four sequential cycles of chemotherapy without the need for transfusions, chemotherapy dose reduction, or changes in treatment schedules.

Platelet activation studies done on a limited number of people showed no evidence of abnormal spontaneous platelet activation, or an abnormal response to adenosine diphosphate (ADP). Based on two studies, 19 of 69 people (28%) receiving oprelvekin 50 mcg/kg and 34 of 67 people (51%) receiving placebo reported at least one hemorrhagic adverse event that involved bleeding.

In a study among people who received autologus bone-marrow transplantation after myeloablative chemotherapy, the incidence of platelet transfusions and time to neutrophyil and platelet engraftment were similar in oprelvekin- and placebo-treated arms.

In long-term follow-up, the distribution of survival and progression-free survival times was similar between people randomized to oprelvekin therapy and those randomized to receive placebo.

Onset: In a clinical trial, platelet counts began to increase relative to baseline between 5 and 9 days after starting oprelvekin.

Duration: After cessation of treatment, platelet counts continued to increase for up to 7 days, then returned toward baseline within 14 days.

Pharmacokinetics: Oprelvekin was evaluated in healthy, adult subjects and oncology patients receiving chemotherapy. When a single 50 mcg/kg subcutaneous dose was given to 18 men, the peak serum concentration (C_{max}) of 17.4 ± 5.4 ng/mL (mean ± SD) was reached after 3.2 ± 2.4 hours (T_{max}). The terminal half-life was 6.9 ± 1.7 hours. When single 75 mcg/kg subcutaneous and IV doses were given to 24 healthy subjects, pharmacokinetic profiles were similar between men and women. The absolute bioavailability of oprelvekin was more than 80%. When multiple subcutaneous doses of 25 and 50 mcg/kg were given to cancer patients receiving chemotherapy, oprelvekin did not accumulate and clearance of oprelvekin was not impaired after multiple doses.

Oprelvekin was administered at doses ranging from 25 to 125 mcg/kg/day to 43 children (8 months to 18 years of age) and 1 adult patient receiving ICE (ifosfamide, carboplatin, etoposide) chemotherapy. Analysis of data from 40 children showed that C_{max}, T_{max}, and terminal half-life were comparable to that in adults. The mean area under the concentration-time curve (AUC) for children (8 months to 18 years of age) receiving 50 mcg/kg was approximately half that achieved in healthy adults receiving 50 mcg/kg. Available data suggest that clearance of oprelvekin decreases with increasing age in children.

Oprelvekin was administered as a single 50 mcg/kg subcutaneous dose to 48 healthy men and women 20 to 79 years of age; 18 subjects were 65 years of age and older. The pharmacokinetic profile of oprelvekin was similar between those 65 years of age and older and those younger than 65 years of age.

In preclinical studies in rats, radiolabeled oprelvekin was rapidly cleared from serum and distributed to highly perfused organs. The kidney was the primary route of elimination. The amount of intact oprelvekin in urine was low, indicating that the molecule was metabolized before excretion.

In a clinical study, a single dose of oprelvekin was administered to subjects with severely impaired renal function (creatinine clearance less than 30 mL/min). The mean ± SD values for C_{max} and AUC were 30.8 ± 8.6 ng/mL and 373 ± 106 ng•h/mL, respectively. When compared with control subjects in this study with normal renal function, the mean C_{max} was 2.2-fold higher and the mean AUC was 2.6-fold (95% CI, 1.7%-3.8%) higher in the subjects with severe renal impairment. In the subjects with severe renal impairment, clearance was approximately 40% of the value seen in subjects with normal renal function. The average terminal half-life was similar in subjects with severe renal impairment and those with normal renal function.

A second clinical study of 24 subjects with varying degrees of renal function was also performed and confirmed the results observed in the first study. Single 50 mcg/kg subcutaneous and IV doses were administered in a randomized fashion. As the degree of renal impairment increased, the oprelvekin AUC increased, although half-life remained unchanged. In the 6 patients with severe impairment, the mean ± SD C_{max} and AUC were 23.6 ± 6.7 ng/mL and 373 ± 55.2 ng•h/mL, respectively, compared with 13.1 ± 3.8 ng/mL and 195 ± 49.3 ng•h/mL, respectively, in the 6 subjects with normal renal function. A comparable increase in exposure was observed after intravenous administration of oprelvekin.

Oprelvekin (Recombinant)

The pharmacokinetic studies suggest that overall exposure to oprelvekin increases as renal function decreases, indicating that a 50% dose reduction of oprelvekin is warranted for patients with severe renal impairment. No dosage reduction is required for smaller changes in renal function.

In a study in which oprelvekin was administered to nonmyelosuppressed cancer patients, daily subcutaneous dosing for 14 days with oprelvekin increased the platelet count in a dose-dependent manner. Platelet counts began to increase relative to baseline between 5 and 9 days after the start of dosing with oprelvekin. After cessation of treatment, platelet counts continued to increase for up to 7 days, then returned toward baseline within 14 days. No change in platelet reactivity as measured by platelet activation in response to ADP, and platelet aggregation in response to ADP, epinephrine, collagen, ristocetin, and arachidonic acid has been observed in association with oprelvekin treatment.

In a randomized, double-blind, placebo-controlled study in normal volunteers, subjects receiving oprelvekin had a mean increase in plasma volume of more than 20%, and all subjects receiving oprelvekin had at least a 10% increase in plasma volume. Red blood cell volume decreased similarly (because of repeated phlebotomy) in the oprelvekin and placebo groups. As a result, whole blood volume increased approximately 10% and hemoglobin concentration decreased approximately 10% in subjects receiving oprelvekin compared with subjects receiving placebo. Mean 24-hour sodium excretion decreased, and potassium excretion did not increase in subjects receiving oprelvekin compared with subjects receiving placebo.

Mechanism: IL-11 is a thrombopoietic growth factor that directly stimulates proliferation of hematopoietic stem cells and megakaryocyte progenitor cells. It induces megakaryocyte maturation, increasing platelet production. The primary hematopoietic activity of oprelvekin is stimulation of megakaryocytopoiesis and thrombopoiesis. IL-11 is one of a family of human growth factors that includes human growth hormone, granulocyte colony-stimulating factor (G-CSF), and other growth factors.

Preclinical studies showed that mature megakaryocytes that develop during in vivo treatment with oprelvekin are ultrastructurally normal. Platelets produced in response to oprelvekin were morphologically and functionally normal and possessed a normal life-span.

IL-11 has nonhematopoietic activities in animals, including regulation of intestinal epithelium growth (eg, enhanced healing of GI lesions), inhibition of adipogenesis, induction of acute-phase protein synthesis, inhibition of pro-inflammatory cytokine production by macrophages, and stimulation of osteoclastogenesis and neurogenesis.

IL-11 is produced by bone-marrow stromal cells and is part of the cytokine family that shares the gp130 signal transducer. Primary osteoblasts and mature osteoclasts express mRNAs for both IL-11 receptor (IL-11R-alpha) and gp130. Both bone-forming and bone-resorbing cells are potential targets of IL-11.

Drug Interactions: Most people in trials evaluating oprelvekin were treated with filgrastim (G-CSF), with no adverse effect of oprelvekin on the activity of G-CSF. No information is currently available on the clinical use of sargramostim (GM-CSF) with oprelvekin. However, in a study in nonhuman primates in which oprelvekin and GM-CSF were coadministered, there were no adverse interactions between oprelvekin and GM-CSF and no apparent difference in the pharmacokinetic profile of oprelvekin.

Drug interactions between oprelvekin and other drugs have not been fully evaluated. Based on in vitro and nonclinical in vivo evaluations of oprelvekin, drug-drug interactions with known substrates of P-450 enzymes would not be predicted.

Patient Information: If oprelvekin is to be administered by a patient, instruct the patient regarding dosage and administration. Caution against the reuse of needles, syringes, vials and diluent. Recommend a puncture-resistant container for disposal of used needles and syringes.

Inform patients of the most common adverse reactions expected with oprelvekin, including symptoms related to fluid retention. These effects are generally mild or moderate and stop after treatment. The most common side effects seen in studies of oprelvekin were edema (swelling) of the arms or legs, shortness of breath when moving about, and anemia. These side effects are probably related to water retention. Edema and shortness of breath on exertion can occur within the first week of treatment and may continue throughout oprelvekin therapy. Patients may experience irregular heartbeats. If chest pain, shortness of breath, fatigue, blurred vision, or an irregular pulse that persists occur, contact the physician. For any other problems, whether or not related to oprelvekin, inform the physician. Advise female patients of childbearing potential of the possible risks of oprelvekin to the fetus.

Pharmaceutical Characteristics

Concentration: 5 mg/mL after reconstitution with 1 mL; specific activity of approximately 8×10^6 units/mg.

Packaging: Box of one 5 mg, single-dose vial and one prefilled syringe containing 1 mL sterile water (NDC #: 58394-0004-08)

Doseform: Lyophilized powder for reconstitution

Appearance: White lyophilized powder. The reconstituted oprelvekin solution is clear, colorless, and isotonic when reconstituted to 5 mg/1 mL.

Diluent:
For reconstitution: Sterile water for injection. During reconstitution, direct 1 mL of diluent toward the side of the vial. Swirl the contents gently. Avoid excessive or vigorous agitation.

Adjuvant: None

Preservative: None

Allergens: None

Excipients: 23 mg glycine, 1.6 mg dibasic sodium phosphate heptahydrate, 0.55 mg monobasic sodium phosphate monohydrate per vial

pH: 7

Shelf Life: Expires within 24 months.

Storage/Stability: Store at 2° to 8°C (36° to 46°F). If frozen, thaw before reconstitution. Discard unused portions. Storage for up to 3 days at room temperature should have no adverse effect on potency. Contact the manufacturer regarding exposure to extreme temperatures. Shipped in insulated, corrugated containers with coolant packs via overnight courier.

Oprelvekin may be used within 3 hours of reconstitution when stored either at 2° to 8°C (36° to 46°F) or at room temperature up to 25°C (77°F). Do not store the reconstituted solution in a syringe. Do not freeze or shake the reconstituted solution.

Production Process: Oprelvekin is synthesized in *Escherichia coli* as a thioredoxin/rhIL-11 fusion protein, which is then cleaved and purified to release the rhIL-11 protein. No blood products are employed during the manufacturing process.

Media: *E. coli*

Disease Epidemiology

Incidence: Approximately 25% of chemotherapy patients experienced the chemotherapy-induced thrombocytopenia for which oprelvekin is indicated. This amounts to 200,000 Americans and 500,000 chemotherapy-cycles.

Oprelvekin (Recombinant)

Other Information

Perspective:
1990: Human interleukin-11 first isolated and cloned.
1996: Designated an orphan drug.

First Licensed: November 25, 1997

References: Du X, Williams D. Interleukin-11: Review of molecular, cell biology and clinical use. *Blood.* 1997;89:3897-3908.

Sitaraman SV, Gewirtz AT. Oprelvekin. Genetics Institute. *Curr Opin Investig Drugs.* 2001;2(10):1395-1400.

Anakinra (Recombinant)

Interleukin Antagonists

Name:
  Kineret

Manufacturer:
  Amgen, under license to Biovitrum AB

Immunologic Characteristics

Antigen Source: Recombinant form of human interleukin-1 receptor antagonist (IL-1 Ra)

Viability: Not viable, but immunologically active

Antigenic Form: IL-1 Ra, recombinant, nonglycosylated

Antigenic Type: Protein. Anakinra differs from native human IL-1 Ra in the addition of a single methionine residue at its amino terminus. Anakinra consists of 153 amino acids, with a molecular weight of 17.3 kilodaltons.

Use Characteristics

Indications: To reduce signs and symptoms of moderate to severe active rheumatoid arthritis (RA) in patients 18 years of age and older who failed one or more disease-modifying antirheumatic drug (DMARDs). Anakinra can be used alone or in combination with DMARDs other than tumor necrosis factor (TNF)-blocking agents.

Contraindications:

Absolute: None

Relative: People with known hypersensitivity to *Escherichia coli*-derived proteins, anakinra, or any components of the product.

Immunodeficiency: The safety and efficacy of anakinra in immunosuppressed patients has not been evaluated.

Elderly: A total of 653 patients 65 years of age and older, including 135 patients 75 years of age and older, were studied in clinical trials. No differences in safety or effectiveness were observed between these patients and younger patients, but greater sensitivity of some older individuals cannot be ruled out. Because there is a higher incidence of infections in the elderly population in general, use caution in treating the elderly.

This drug is substantially excreted by the kidney. The risk of toxic reactions to this drug may be greater in patients with impaired renal function.

Carcinogenicity: Anakinra has not been evaluated for carcinogenic potential in animals.

Mutagenicity: Using a standard in vivo and in vitro battery of mutagenesis assays, anakinra did not induce gene mutations in either bacteria or mammalian cells.

Fertility Impairment: In rats and rabbits, anakinra at doses of up to 100-fold greater than the human dose had no adverse effects on male or female fertility.

Pregnancy: Category B. Reproductive studies have been conducted with anakinra on rats and rabbits at doses up to 100 times the human dose and have revealed no evidence of impaired fertility or harm to the fetus. However, there are no adequate and well-controlled studies in pregnant women. Because animal reproduction studies are not always predictive of human response, use anakinra during pregnancy only if clearly needed.

Lactation: It is not known if anakinra crosses into human breast milk. Because many drugs are secreted in human milk, use caution if anakinra is administered to nursing women.

Children: The safety and efficacy of anakinra in patients with juvenile rheumatoid arthritis (JRA) have not been established.

Adverse Reactions: The most serious adverse reactions were serious infections and neutropenia (particularly when used in combination with TNF-blocking agents). The most common adverse reaction with anakinra is injection-site reaction (ISR). These reactions were the most common reason for withdrawing from studies.

The data described herein reflect use of anakinra in 2,606 patients, including 1,812 exposed for at least 6 months and 570 exposed for at least 1 year. Studies 1 and 4 used the recommended dose of 100 mg/day. The patients studied were representative of the general population of patients with RA.

The following adverse events occurred in studies 1 and 4 at a frequency of at least 5% and a higher frequency in anakinra-treated patients.

Anakinra Adverse Reactions		
Adverse reaction	Placebo (n = 534)	Anakinra 100 mg/day (n = 1,366)
Injection site reaction	28%	71%
Infection	35%	40%
URI	13%	13%
Sinusitis	4%	6%
Influenza-like infection	4%	5%
Other	23%	26%
Headache	9%	12%
Nausea	6%	8%
Diarrhea	5%	7%
Sinusitis	6%	7%
Influenza-like symptoms	5%	6%
Abdominal pain	4%	5%

Injection-site reactions: The most common and consistently reported treatment-related adverse event associated with anakinra is ISR. Most ISRs were reported as mild, typically lasting 14 to 28 days, characterized by erythema, ecchymosis, inflammation, and pain. In studies 1 and 4, 71% of patients developed an ISR, typically reported within 4 weeks of therapy. ISRs in patients who had not previously experienced them were uncommon after the first month of therapy.

Infections: Combining studies 1 and 4, the incidence of infection was 40% in the anakinra-treated patients and 35% in placebo-treated patients. The incidence of serious infections in studies 1 and 4 was 1.8% in anakinra-treated patients and 0.6% in placebo-treated patients over 6 months. These infections consisted primarily of bacterial events such as cellulitis, pneumonia, and bone and joint infections, rather than unusual, opportunistic, fungal, or viral infections. Patients with asthma appeared to be at higher risk of developing serious infections (anakinra 5% vs placebo less than 1%). Most patients continued on study drug after the infection resolved. There were no on-study deaths due to serious infectious episodes in either study. In a study in which patients were receiving both etanercept and anakinra for up to 24 weeks, the incidence of serious infections was 7%. These infections consisted of bacterial pneumonia (2 cases) and cellulitis (2 cases), which were treated successfully with antibiotic therapy. Discontinue anakinra administration if a patient develops a serious infection. Do not begin anakinra treatment in patients with active infections. The safety and efficacy of anakinra in immunosuppressed patients or in patients with chronic infections have not been evaluated. Preliminary data suggest a higher rate of serious infections (7%, 4158) when anakinra and etanercept are used in combination compared with anakinra used alone. In this combination study, neutropenia (1,000 cells/mm^3

or less) was observed in 3% of patients (2/58). Use anakinra with TNF-blocking agents only with extreme caution and when no satisfactory alternative exists.

Malignancies: Twenty-one malignancies of various types were observed in 2,531 RA patients treated in clinical trials with anakinra for up to 50 months. The observed rates and incidences were similar to those expected for the population studied.

Hematologic: In placebo-controlled studies with anakinra, treatment was associated with small reductions in the mean values for total white blood count, platelets, and absolute neutrophil blood count (ANC), and a small increase in the mean eosinophil differential percentage. In all placebo-controlled studies, 8% of patients receiving anakinra had substantial decreases in ANC, compared with 2% of placebo patients. Six anakinra-treated patients (0.3%) developed neutropenia (ANC 1×10^9 cells/L). Additional patients treated with anakinra plus etanercept (2/58, 3%) developed ANC 1×10^9 cells/L. While neutropenic, 1 patient developed cellulitis and the other patient developed pneumonia. Both patients recovered with antibiotic therapy.

Hypersensitivity: Hypersensitivity reactions associated with anakinra administration are rare. If a severe hypersensitivity reaction occurs, discontinue anakinra and initiate appropriate therapy.

Pharmacologic & Dosing Characteristics

Dosage: 100 mg/day. Higher doses did not result in a higher response. Administer the dose at approximately the same time each day.

Route & Site: Subcutaneous

Overdosage: There have been no cases of overdose reported with anakinra in clinical trials of RA. In sepsis trials, no serious toxicities attributed to anakinra were seen when administered at mean calculated doses of up to 35 times those given to patients with RA over a 72-hour treatment period.

Efficacy: Safety and efficacy were evaluated in 3 randomized, double-blind, placebo-controlled trials of 1,392 patients (18 years of age and older with active RA). A fourth study assessed safety. In the efficacy trials, anakinra was studied in combination with other DMARDs (studies 1 and 2) or as a monotherapy (study 3).

Study 1 evaluated 501 patients with active RA on a stable dose of methotrexate (10 to 25 mg/week) for at least 8 weeks. They had at least 6 swollen/painful and 9 tender joints and either a C-reactive protein (CRP) of at least 1.5 mg/dL or an erythrocyte sedimentation rate (ESR) of at least 28 mm/h. Patients were randomized to anakinra or placebo in addition to their stable doses of methotrexate.

Study 2 evaluated 419 patients with active RA who had received methotrexate for at least 6 months including a stable dose (15 to 25 mg/week) for at least 3 months before enrollment. Patients were randomized to receive placebo or 1 of 5 doses of anakinra subcutaneously daily for 12 to 24 weeks in addition to their stable doses of methotrexate.

Study 3 evaluated 472 patients with active RA and similar inclusion criteria to study 1, except that these patients had received no DMARD for the previous 6 weeks or during the study. Patients were randomized to receive either anakinra or placebo. Patients were DMARD-naive or had failed no more than 3 DMARDs.

Study 4 was a placebo-controlled, randomized trial designed to assess the safety of anakinra in 1,414 patients receiving a variety of concurrent medications for their RA including some DMARD therapies, as well as patients who were DMARD-free. The TNF-blocking agents etanercept and infliximab were specifically excluded. Concurrent DMARDS included methotrexate, sulfasalazine, hydrochloroquine, gold, penicillamine, leflunomide, and azathioprine. Unlike studies 1, 2, and 3, patients predisposed to infection due to a history of underlying disease such as pneumonia, asthma, controlled diabetes, and chronic obstructive pulmonary disease (COPD) were also enrolled.

In studies 1, 2, and 3, signs and symptoms of RA were assessed using the American College of Rheumatology (ACR) response criteria (ACR20, ACR50, ACR70). In all 3 studies, patients treated with anakinra were more likely to achieve an ACR20 or higher magnitude of response (ACR50 and ACR70) than patients treated with placebo. The treatment response rates did not differ based on gender or ethnic group. Most clinical responses, both in patients receiving placebo and patients receiving anakinra, occurred within 12 weeks of enrollment.

	Proportion of Patients with ACR Responses in Studies 1 and 3				
	Study 1 (patients on methotrexate)		Study 3 (no DMARDs)		
Response	Placebo (n = 251)	Anakinra 100 mg/day (n = 250)	Placebo (n = 119)	Anakinra 75 mg/day (n = 115)	Anakinra 150 mg/day (n = 115)
ACR20					
Month 3	24%	34%[a]	23%	33%	33%
Month 6	22%	38%[b]	27%	34%	43%[a]
ACR50					
Month 3	6%	13%[c]	5%	10%	8%
Month 6	8%	17%[c]	8%	11%	19%[a]
ACR70					
Month 3	0%	3%[a]	0%	0%	0%
Month 6	2%	6%[a]	1%	1%	1%

a $P < 0.05$, anakinra vs placebo.
b $P < 0.001$, anakinra vs placebo.
c $P < 0.01$, anakinra vs placebo.

	Effect of Anakinra on Median ACR Component Scores in Study 1			
	Placebo/Methotrexate (n = 251)		Anakinra/Methotrexate (n = 250)	
Parameter (median)	Baseline	Month 6	Baseline	Month 6
Patient Reported Outcomes				
Disability index[a]	1.38	1.13	1.38	1
Patient global assessment[b]	51	41	51	29
Pain[b]	56	44	63	34
Objective Measures				
ESR (mm/h)	35	32	36	19
CRP (mg/dL)	2.2	1.6	2.2	0.5
Physician Assessments				
Tender/painful joints[c]	20	11	23	9
Physician global assessment[b]	59	31	59	26
Swollen joints[d]	18	10.5	17	9

a Health-assessment questionnaire; 0 = best, 3 = worst; includes dressing and grooming, arising, eating, walking, hygiene, reach, grip, and activities.
b Visual analog scale; 0 = best, 100 = worst.
c Scale 0 to 68.
d Scale 0 to 66.

Sensitization:

>*Immunogenicity:* In study 4, 28% of patients tested positive for anti-anakinra antibodies at month 6 in a highly sensitive, anakinra-binding biosensor assay. Of the 1,274 subjects with available data, less than 1% (n = 9) were seropositive in a cell-based bioassay for antibodies capable of neutralizing the biologic effects of anakinra. None of these 9 subjects were positive for neutralizing antibodies at more than 1 time point, and all of these subjects were negative for neutralizing antibodies by 9 months. No correlation between antibody development and clinical response or adverse events was observed. The long-term immunogenicity of anakinra is unknown.

Onset: Within 3 months

Pharmacokinetics: Bioavailability of anakinra after a 70 mg subcutaneous bolus injection in healthy subjects (n = 11) is 95%. In subjects with RA, maximum plasma concentrations of anakinra occurred 3 to 7 hours after subcutaneous administration of anakinra at clinically relevant doses (1 to 2 mg/kg; n = 18); the terminal half-life ranged from 4 to 6 hours. In RA patients, no unexpected accumulation of anakinra was observed after daily subcutaneous doses for up to 24 weeks.

>The influence of demographic factors on pharmacokinetics was studied among 341 patients receiving daily subcutaneous injection of anakinra at doses of 30, 75, and 150 mg for up to 24 weeks. The estimated anakinra clearance increased with increasing creatinine clearance and body weight. After adjusting for creatinine clearance and body weight, gender and age were not significant factors for mean plasma clearance.

>The mean plasma clearance of anakinra decreased 70% to 75% in normal subjects with severe or end-stage renal disease (creatinine clearance less than 30 mL/min). No formal studies have been conducted examining pharmacokinetics of anakinra administered subcutaneously in RA patients with renal impairment.

>No formal studies have been conducted examining pharmacokinetics of anakinra administered subcutaneously in RA patients with hepatic impairment.

Mechanism: Anakinra blocks the biologic activity of IL-1 by competitively inhibiting IL-1 from binding to the interleukin-1 type I receptor (IL-1 RI), which is expressed in a wide variety of tissues and organs.

>Inflammatory stimuli induce IL-1 production. IL-1 mediates various physiologic responses, including inflammatory and immunological responses. IL-1 has a broad range of activities, including cartilage degradation by induction of the rapid loss of proteoglycans, as well as stimulation of bone resorption. Naturally occurring IL-1 Ra levels in synovium and synovial fluid from RA patients are not sufficient to compete with the elevated amount of locally produced IL-1.

Drug Interactions: No data are available on the effects of vaccination in patients receiving anakinra. Do not give live vaccines concurrently with anakinra. No data are available on the secondary transmission of infection by live vaccines in patients receiving anakinra. Because anakinra interferes with normal immune response mechanisms to new antigens such as vaccines, vaccination may not be effective in patients receiving anakinra.

>No drug-drug interaction studies in human subjects have been conducted. Toxicologic and toxicokinetic studies in rats did not demonstrate any alterations in the clearance or toxicologic profile of either methotrexate or anakinra when the 2 agents were administered together.

>Preliminary data suggest a higher rate of serious infections (7%, 4158) when anakinra and etanercept are used, compared with anakinra alone. In this combination study, neutropenia (up to 1,000 cells/mm^3) was observed in 3% of patients (2/58). Use anakinra with TNF-blocking agents only with extreme caution and when no satisfactory alternative exists.

Anakinra (Recombinant)

Lab Interference: Patients receiving anakinra may experience a decrease in neutrophil counts. In clinical studies, 8% of patients receiving anakinra had substantial decreases in neutrophil counts, compared with 2% in the placebo group. Six anakinra-treated patients (0.3%) experienced neutropenia (ANC 1×10^9 cells/L). Assess neutrophil counts before starting anakinra treatment, and while the patient is receiving anakinra (monthly for 3 months, and thereafter quarterly for a period up to 1 year).

Patient Information: Inform patients of the signs and symptoms of allergic and other adverse drug reactions, as well as appropriate actions.

Pharmaceutical Characteristics

Concentration: 100 mg/0.67 mL anakinra

Packaging: Pack containing 28 single-use 1 mL prefilled glass syringes with 27-gauge, ½ inch needles (NDC #: 66658-0234-28).

Doseform: Solution

Appearance: Clear, colorless-to-white solution

Solvent: Water for injection

Adjuvant: None

Preservative: None. Discard unused portions.

Allergens: None

Excipients: 1.9 mg/mL sodium citrate, 8.22 mg/mL sodium chloride, 0.18 mg/mL disodium EDTA, and 1.05 mg/mL polysorbate 80.

pH: 6.5

Shelf Life: Expires within 24 months.

Storage/Stability: Store at 2° to 8°C (36° to 46°F). Do not freeze. Stable 72 hours if inadvertently frozen; thaw product in refrigerator if this occurs. Beyond 72 hours in the frozen state, discard product. Product can tolerate temperatures up to 30°C (86°F) for up to 2 days without adverse effect. Shipped in insulated containers to maintain appropriate temperature.

Handling: Do not shake. Protect from light.

Production Process: Produced by recombinant DNA technology using an *E. coli* bacterial expression system.

Media: *E. coli*

Disease Epidemiology

Prevalence: More than 2 million Americans have rheumatoid arthritis.

Other Information

First Licensed: November 14, 2001

References: Fleischmann R, Stern R, Iqbal I. Anakinra: an inhibitor of IL-1 for the treatment of rheumatoid arthritis. *Expert Opin Biol Ther.* 2004;4:1333-1344.

Furst DE. Anakinra: review of recombinant human interleukin-I receptor antagonist in the treatment of rheumatoid arthritis. *Clin Ther.* 2004;26:1960-1975.

Waugh J, Perry CM. Anakinra: a review of its use in the management of rheumatoid arthritis. *BioDrugs.* 2005;19:189-202.

Interleukin Antagonists

Name:
   Arcalyst

Manufacturer:
   Regeneron Pharmaceuticals

Immunologic Characteristics

Antigen Source: Dimeric fusion protein consisting of the ligand-binding domains of the extracellular portions of the human interleukin-1 receptor component (IL-1RI) and interleukin-1 receptor accessory protein (IL-1RAcP) linked in-line to the Fc portion of human IgG1

Viability: Not viable, but immunologically active

Antigenic Form: Soluble receptors linked to Fc portion of human IgG1 antibody

Antigenic Type: Protein. Dimeric fusion protein consisting of the ligand-binding domains of the extracellular portions of the human IL-1RI and IL-1RAcP linked in-line to the Fc portion of human IgG1. Rilonacept has a molecular weight of approximately 251 kDa.

Use Characteristics

Indications: To treat cryopyrin-associated periodic syndromes (CAPS), including familial cold autoinflammatory syndrome and Muckle-Wells syndrome in adults and children 12 years of age and older, by lessening signs and symptoms such as rash, joint pain, fever, and tiredness.

Contraindications:

Absolute: None

Relative: People hypersensitive to rilonacept or components of this preparation

Immunodeficiency: The effects of rilonacept in people with impaired immune systems are not known. Treatment with immunosuppressants, including rilonacept, may increase the risk of malignancies.

Elderly: Dosage modification based on advanced age is not required. In placebo-controlled studies in patients with CAPS and other indications, 70 patients randomized to treatment with rilonacept were 65 years of age and older and 6 were 75 years of age and older. In the CAPS trial, efficacy, safety, and tolerability were generally similar in elderly patients compared with younger adults; however, only 10 patients 65 years of age and older participated in the trial. In an open-label extension study of CAPS, a 71-year-old woman developed bacterial meningitis and died. Age did not appear to have a significant effect on steady-state trough rilonacept concentrations in the clinical study.

Carcinogenicity: Long-term animal studies have not been performed to evaluate the carcinogenic potential of rilonacept.

Mutagenicity: The mutagenic potential of rilonacept has not been evaluated.

Fertility Impairment: Male and female fertility was evaluated in a mouse surrogate model using a murine analog of rilonacept. Male mice were treated 8 weeks before mating and through female gestation day 15. Female mice were treated for 2 weeks before mating and on gestation days 0, 3, and 6. The murine analog of rilonacept did not alter male or female fertility parameters at doses up to 200 mg/kg (approximately 6-fold higher than the human 160 mg maintenance dose, based on body surface area).

Pregnancy: Category C. There are no adequate and well-controlled studies of rilonacept in pregnant women. Based on animal data, rilonacept may cause fetal harm. An embryo-fetal developmental toxicity study was performed in cynomolgus monkeys given 0, 5, 15, or 30 mg/kg twice a week (up to approximately 3.7-fold higher than the human 160 mg dose, based on body surface area). The fetus of the only monkey with exposure to rilonacept during the later period of gestation showed multiple fusions and absence of the ribs and thoracic vertebral bodies and arches. Exposure to rilonacept during this time period was below that expected clinically. Likewise, in the cynomolgus monkey, all doses of rilonacept reduced serum levels of estradiol up to 64% compared with controls and increased the incidence of lumbar ribs compared with both control animals and historical control incidences. In perinatal and postnatal developmental toxicology studies in the mouse model using a murine analog of rilonacept (0, 20, 100, or 200 mg/kg), there was a 3-fold increase in stillbirths in dams treated with 200 mg/kg 3 times per week (approximately 6-fold higher than the human 160 mg maintenance dose, based on body surface area). Use rilonacept during pregnancy only if the benefit justifies the potential risk to the fetus.

Lactation: It is not known if rilonacept crosses into human breast milk. Because many drugs are excreted in human milk, use caution when rilonacept is administered to a breast-feeding woman.

Children: Six children between 12 and 16 years of age with CAPS were treated with rilonacept at a weekly subcutaneous dose of 2.2 mg/kg (maximum, 160 mg) for 24 weeks during the open-label extension phase. These patients showed improvement from baseline in symptom scores and objective markers of inflammation (eg, serum amyloid A [SAA], C-reactive protein [CRP]). Adverse events included injection-site reactions and upper respiratory tract symptoms similar to those seen in adult participants. The trough drug levels for 4 pediatric patients measured at the end of the weekly dose interval (mean, 20 mcg/mL; range, 3.6 to 33 mcg/mL) were similar to adult patients with CAPS (mean, 24 mcg/mL; range, 7 to 56 mcg/mL). Safety and effectiveness in children younger than 12 years of age have not been established. When administered to pregnant primates, rilonacept treatment may have contributed to alterations in bone ossification in the fetus. It is not known if rilonacept will alter bone development in pediatric patients. Monitor pediatric patients treated with rilonacept for growth and development.

Adverse Reactions: These data reflect exposure to rilonacept in 600 patients, including 85 patients exposed for longer than 6 months and 65 patients exposed for 1 year or longer. These included patients with CAPS, patients with other diseases, and healthy volunteers. Approximately 60 patients with CAPS have been treated weekly with rilonacept 160 mg. The pivotal trial population included 47 patients with CAPS. These patients were 22 to 78 years of age (mean, 51 years). Thirty-one patients were women and 16 were men. All of the patients were white. Six children and adolescents (12 to 17 years of age) were enrolled directly into the open-label extension phase.

The most common adverse reactions reported by patients with CAPS treated with rilonacept were injection-site reactions and upper respiratory tract infections. The injection-site reactions included erythema, swelling, pruritus, bruising, inflammation, pain, edema, dermatitis, discomfort, urticaria, vesicles, warmth, and hemorrhage. Most injection-site reactions lasted for 1 to 2 days. None were assessed as severe, and no patient discontinued study participation because of an injection-site reaction. Six serious adverse reactions were reported by 4 patients during the clinical program. These serious adverse reactions were *Mycobacterium intracellulare* infection, GI bleeding and colitis, sinusitis and bronchitis, and *Streptococcus pneumoniae* meningitis.

Part A of the clinical trial was conducted in patients with CAPS naive to treatment with rilonacept as a randomized, double-blind, placebo-controlled, 6-week study comparing rilonacept with placebo. The following table shows the frequency of adverse events reported by at least 2 patients.

Most Frequent Adverse Reactions (Part A, Reported by ≥ 2 Patients)		
Adverse Event	Rilonacept 160 mg (n = 23)	Placebo (n = 24)
Any adverse event	17 (74%)	13 (54%)
Injection-site reactions	11 (48%)	3 (13%)
Upper respiratory tract infection	6 (26%)	1 (4%)
Sinusitis	2 (9%)	1 (4%)
Cough	2 (9%)	0
Hypesthesia	2 (9%)	0
Nausea	1 (4%)	3 (13%)
Diarrhea	1 (4%)	3 (13%)
Stomach discomfort	1 (4%)	1 (4%)
Urinary tract infection	1 (4%)	1 (4%)
Abdominal pain, upper	0	2 (8%)

Hematologic: One patient in a study for an unapproved indication developed transient neutropenia (absolute neutrophil count [ANC] less than 1×10^9 cells/L) after receiving a large dose (2,000 mg intravenously IV]) of rilonacept. The patient did not experience any infection associated with neutropenia.

Hepatic: No formal studies have been conducted to examine the pharmacokinetics of subcutaneous rilonacept in patients with hepatic function impairment.

Hypersensitivity: Hypersensitivity reactions associated with rilonacept are rare. If a hypersensitivity reaction occurs, discontinue rilonacept and initiate appropriate therapy.

Immunogenecity: Antibodies directed against the receptor domains of rilonacept were detected by enzyme-linked immunosorbent assay (ELISA) in patients with CAPS after rilonacept therapy. Nineteen of 55 subjects (35%) who received rilonacept for 6 weeks or longer tested positive for treatment-emergent binding antibodies on 1 or more occasions. Of the 19 subjects, 7 tested positive at the last assessment (week 18 or 24), and 5 subjects tested positive for neutralizing antibodies on more than 1 occasion. There was no correlation between antibody activity and either clinical effectiveness or safety. These data are highly dependent on the sensitivity and specificity of the specific assays used. Comparison with incidence of antibodies to other products may be misleading.

Infections: Interleukin-1 (IL-1) blockade may interfere with immune response to infections. Treatment with another medication that inhibits IL-1 is associated with an increased risk of serious infections, and serious infections have been reported in patients taking rilonacept. During part A of the rilonacept trial, the incidence of patients reporting infections was greater with rilonacept (48%) than placebo (17%). In part B (randomized withdrawal), the incidence of infections was similar in the 2 groups (18% and 22%, respectively). Part A started in winter months, while part B occurred mainly in summer months. In placebo-controlled studies across a variety of patient populations (360 patients treated with rilonacept and 179 treated with placebo), the incidence of infections was 34% and 27% (2.15 and 1.81 per patient-year) for rilonacept and placebo, respectively. One subject receiving rilonacept for an unapproved indication in another study developed an *M. intracellulare* infection in his olecranon bursa. The patient was on long-term glucocorticoid treatment. The infection occurred after an intra-articular glucocorticoid injection into the bursa with subsequent local exposure to a suspected source of mycobacteria. The patient recovered after appropriate antimicrobial therapy. One patient treated for another unapproved indication developed bronchitis/sinusitis, which resulted in hospitalization. One patient in an open-label CAPs study died from *S. pneumoniae* meningitis. Discontinue rilonacept if a patient develops a serious infection. Do not start treatment with rilonacept in patients with an active acute or chronic infection.

Lipid profiles: Cholesterol and lipid levels may be reduced in patients with chronic inflammation. Patients with CAPS treated with rilonacept experienced increases in mean total cholesterol, high-density lipoprotein (HDL) cholesterol, low-density lipoprotein (LDL) cholesterol, and triglycerides. The mean increases from baseline for total cholesterol, HDL cholesterol, LDL cholesterol, and triglycerides were 19, 2, 10, and 57 mg/dL, respectively, after 6 weeks of open-label therapy. Monitor lipid profiles of patients (eg, after 2 to 3 months) and consider lipid-lowering therapies as needed, based upon cardiovascular risk factors and current guidelines.

Renal: No formal studies have been conducted to examine the pharmacokinetics of subcutaneous rilonacept in patients with renal function impairment.

Pharmacologic & Dosing Characteristics

Dosage:

Adults 18 years of age and older: Start with a loading dose of 320 mg delivered as two 2 mL subcutaneous injections of 160 mg on the same day at different sites. Continue dosing with a once-weekly injection of 160 mg as a single subcutaneous injection. Do not administer rilonacept more often than once weekly. Dosage modification is not required based on advanced age or gender.

Children and adolescents 12 to 17 years of age: Start with a loading dose of 4.4 mg/kg (maximum, 320 mg) delivered as subcutaneous injection(s), with a maximum single-injection volume of 2 mL. Continue dosing with a weekly injection of 2.2 mg/kg (maximum, 160 mg) as a single subcutaneous injection, up to 2 mL. If the initial dose is given as 2 injections, give them on the same day at different sites. Do not administer rilonacept more often than once weekly.

Route & Site: Subcutaneous. Rotate sites (eg, abdomen, thigh, upper arm). Do not inject into sites that are bruised, red, tender, or hard.

Overdosage: There have been no reports of overdose with rilonacept. Maximum weekly subcutaneous doses up to 320 mg have been administered in clinical trials, without evidence of dose-limiting toxicities, for up to approximately 18 months in a small number of patients with CAPS and up to 6 months in patients with an unapproved indication. In addition, rilonacept doses up to 2,000 mg IV monthly for up to 6 months in another patient population were tolerated without dose-limiting toxicities. The maximum amount of rilonacept that can be safely administered has not been determined. In case of overdose, monitor the patient for signs or symptoms and start appropriate symptomatic treatment immediately.

Missed Doses: Interrupting the recommended schedule or delaying subsequent doses does not require restarting the series.

Laboratory Tests: Monitor patients for changes in lipid profiles. Provide medical treatment if warranted.

Efficacy: Safety and efficacy of rilonacept in treating CAPS was shown in a randomized, double-blind, placebo-controlled study with 2 parts (A and B) conducted sequentially in the same patients with familial cold autoinflammatory or Muckle-Wells syndromes. Part A was a 6-week, randomized, double-blind, parallel-group period comparing rilonacept at a dose of 160 mg weekly after an initial loading dose of 320 mg with placebo. Part B followed immediately after part A and consisted of a 9-week, patient-blind period, with all participants receiving rilonacept 160 mg weekly, followed by a 9-week, double-blind, randomized withdrawal period, during which patients were randomly assigned to remain on rilonacept 160 mg weekly or receive placebo. Patients were then given the option to enroll in a 24-week, open-label treatment extension phase, during which all patients were treated with rilonacept 160 mg weekly.

Using a daily diary questionnaire, patients rated the following 5 signs and symptoms of CAPS: joint pain, rash, feeling of fever or chills, eye redness or pain, and fatigue; each was rated on a scale of 0 (none, no severity) to 10 (very severe). The study evaluated the mean symptom scores using the change from baseline to the end of treatment.

The changes in mean symptom scores for the randomized, parallel-group period (part A) and the randomized withdrawal period (part B) of the study appear in the following table. Rilonacept-treated patients had a larger reduction in the mean symptom scores in part A than placebo-treated patients. In part B, mean symptom scores increased more in patients withdrawn to placebo than in patients who remained on rilonacept.

Mean Symptom Scores					
	Part A			Part B	
	Placebo (n = 24)	Rilonacept (n = 23)		Placebo (n = 23)	Rilonacept (n = 22)
Pretreatment baseline period (weeks −3 to 0)	2.4	3.1	Active rilonacept baseline period (weeks 13 to 15)	0.2	0.3
End point period (weeks 4 to 6)	2.1	0.5	End point period (weeks 22 to 24)	1.2	0.4
Mean change from baseline to end point	−30.5	−32.4	Mean change from baseline to end point	0.9	0.1
95% confidence interval for difference between treatment groups	(−32.4 to −31.3)		95% confidence interval for difference between treatment groups	(−31.3 to −30.4)	

In part A, patients treated with rilonacept experienced more improvement in each of the 5 components of the composite end point (joint pain, rash, feeling of fever/chills, eye redness/pain, and fatigue) than placebo-treated patients.

In part A, a higher proportion of patients in the rilonacept group experienced improvement from baseline in the composite score by at least 30% (96% vs 29% of patients), by at least 50% (87% vs 8%), and by at least 75% (70% vs 0%) compared with the placebo groups.

Onset: Improvement in symptom scores was noted within several days of initiation of rilonacept therapy in most patients.

Duration: During the open-label extension, reductions in mean symptom scores, serum CRP, and SAA levels were maintained for up to 1 year.

Pharmacokinetics: CRP and SAA are indicators of inflammatory disease activity elevated in patients with CAPS. Elevated SAA is associated with development of systemic amyloidosis in patients with CAPS. Compared with placebo, treatment with rilonacept resulted in sustained reductions from baseline in mean serum CRP and SAA to normal levels during the clinical trial. Rilonacept also normalized mean SAA from elevated levels.

The mean trough levels of rilonacept were approximately 24 mcg/mL at steady state after weekly 160 mg subcutaneous doses for up to 48 weeks in patients with CAPS. The steady state appeared to be reached by 6 weeks.

No study was conducted to evaluate the effect of age, gender, or body weight in response to rilonacept. Based on limited data, steady-state trough concentrations were similar between men and women. Age (26 to 78 years of age) and body weight (50 to 120 kg) did not appear to have a significant effect on trough rilonacept concentrations. The effect of race could not be assessed because only white patients participated in the clinical study, reflecting the epidemiology of the disease.

No pharmacokinetic data are available in patients with hepatic or renal function impairment.

Mechanism: In most cases, inflammation in CAPS is associated with mutations in the nucleotide-binding domain, leucine-rich family (NLR), pyrin-domain-containing 3 gene (NLRP-3 gene), which encodes the protein cryopyrin, an important component of the inflammasome. Cryopyrin regulates the protease caspase-1 and controls the activation of IL-1 beta. Mutations in NLRP-3 result in an overactive inflammasome, resulting in excessive release of activated IL-1 beta that drives inflammation. Rilonacept blocks IL-1 beta signaling by acting as a soluble decoy receptor that binds IL-1 beta and prevents its interaction with cell-surface receptors. Rilonacept also binds IL-1 alpha and IL-1 receptor antagonist (IL-1RA) with reduced affinity. The equilibrium dissociation constants for rilonacept binding to IL-1 beta, IL-1 alpha, and IL-1RA were 0.5, 1.4, and 6.1 pM, respectively.

SAA and CRP levels are acute-phase reactants typically elevated in patients with CAPS with active disease. During part A, mean levels of CRP decreased versus baseline for rilonacept-treated patients, while there was no change for placebo-treated patients. Rilonacept also led to a decrease in SAA versus baseline to levels within the normal range.

Mean SAA and CRP Levels Over Time in Part A		
Part A	Rilonacept	Placebo
SAA (normal range, 0.7 to 6.4 mg/L)	(n = 22)	(n = 24)
Pretreatment baseline	60	110
Week 6	4	110
CRP (normal range, 0 to 8.4 mg/L)	(n = 21)	(n = 24)
Pretreatment baseline	22	30
Week 6	2	28

Drug Interactions: No formal drug interaction studies have been conducted with rilonacept.

Concurrent administration of rilonacept with other drugs that block IL-1 has not been studied. Based upon the potential for pharmacologic interactions between rilonacept and a recombinant IL-1RA, concurrent administration of rilonacept and other agents that block IL-1 or its receptors is not recommended.

Concurrent administration of another drug that blocks IL-1 with a TNF-blocking agent in another patient population was associated with an increased risk of serious infections and neutropenia. Concurrent administration of rilonacept with TNF-blocking agents may also result in similar toxicities and is not recommended. Drugs that block TNF have been associated with an increased risk of reactivation of latent tuberculosis. Taking drugs, such as rilonacept, that block IL-1 may increase the risk of tuberculosis or other atypical or opportunistic infections. Follow current CDC guidelines to evaluate for and treat possible latent tuberculosis infections before initiating therapy with rilonacept.

The effects of rilonacept on active or chronic infections and the development of malignancies are not known. However, treatment with immunosuppressants, including rilonacept, may increase the risk of malignancies.

Formation of cytochrome P-450 enzymes is suppressed by increased levels of cytokines (eg, IL-1) during chronic inflammation. Thus, a molecule that binds to IL-1 (eg, rilonacept) could normalize the formation of cytochrome P-450 enzymes. This is clinically relevant for cytochrome P-450 substrates with a narrow therapeutic index, for which the dose is individually adjusted (eg, warfarin). Upon initiation of rilonacept in patients treated with these types of medications, monitor therapeutic effect or drug concentration and adjust medication doses as needed.

Because no data are available on the efficacy of live vaccines or the risks of secondary transmission of infection by live vaccines in patients receiving rilonacept, do not administer live vaccines concurrently with rilonacept. Because rilonacept may interfere with normal immune response to new antigens, vaccinations may not be effective in patients receiving rilonacept. No data are available on the effectiveness of vaccination with inactivated (killed) antigens in patients receiving rilonacept. Because IL-1 blockade may interfere with immune response to infections, adult and pediatric patients should receive recommended vaccinations before starting rilonacept therapy, including pneumococcal vaccine and inactivated influenza vaccine.

Pharmaceutical Characteristics

Concentration: 80 mg/mL after reconstitution

Packaging: Carton of 4 single-use 20 mL glass vials containing rilonacept 220 mg powder

NDC Number: 61755-0001-01

Doseform: Powder for reconstitution

Appearance: White to off-white powder. The reconstituted solution is viscous, clear, colorless to pale yellow, and essentially free from particulates.

Diluent:
For reconstitution: 2.3 mL of preservative-free sterile water per 220 mg vial

Adjuvant: None

Preservative: None

Allergens: None

Excipients: Histidine, arginine, polyethylene glycol 3350, sucrose, and glycine

pH: 6.2 to 6.8

Shelf Life: Expires within 12 months

Storage/Stability: Store at 2° to 8°C (36° to 46°F). Protect vials from light. After reconstitution, store rilonacept at room temperature, protect from light, and use within 3 hours. Contact the manufacturer regarding exposure to freezing or elevated temperatures. Shipping data are not provided. Patients should store cartons in a cool carrier with a cold pack and protect it from light when traveling.

Production Process: Rilonacept is expressed in recombinant Chinese hamster ovary (CHO) cells.

Media: Rilonacept is expressed in recombinant CHO cells.

Disease Epidemiology

Description: CAPS refers to rare genetic syndromes generally caused by mutations in the NLRP-3 gene (also known as cold-induced autoinflammatory syndrome-1). CAPS disorders are inherited in an autosomal dominant pattern, with male and female offspring equally affected. Features common to all disorders include fever, urticaria-like rash, arthralgia, myalgia, fatigue, and conjunctivitis.

Other Information

First Licensed: February 27, 2008

BCG Live (Intravesical)

General Immunostimulants

Names:
TheraCys
Tice BCG

Manufacturers:
Sanofi Pasteur
Merck

Synonyms: Bacille or Bacillus Calmette-Guérin, BCG. In other countries, *Tice BCG* is known as *OncoTice*.

Comparison: *TheraCys, Tice BCG, Pacis,* and other BCG products are not generically equivalent, because of differences in potency, route of administration, and indications. Refer to the BCG Vaccine monograph in the Vaccines/Toxoids section for a description of BCG for active vaccination against tuberculosis and for a table comparing BCG products (for all indications).

Immunologic Characteristics

Microorganism: Bacterium, *Mycobacterium bovis*, aerobic gram-positive rod, acid-fast bacillus (AFB), family Mycobacteriaceae. Also called *M. tuberculosis* variant *bovis* and the tubercle bacillus.

Viability: Live, attenuated

Antigenic Form: Whole bacterium

Antigenic Type: Protein

Strains:

Merck: Tice substrain of BCG strain of *Mycobacterium tuberculosis.*

Sanofi Pasteur: Connaught substrain of BCG strain of *Mycobacterium tuberculosis*

Use Characteristics

Indications: For treatment and prophylaxis of recurrent tumors in patients with carcinoma in situ of the urinary bladder and for the prophylaxis of primary or recurrent stage Ta and/or T1 papillary tumors following transurethral resection.

Limitations: Not recommended for stage TaG1 papillary tumors, unless judged to be at high risk of tumor recurrence. Not indicated for papillary tumors of stages higher than T1. Not approved for use as a vaccine for the prevention of tuberculosis. Not a vaccine for the prevention of cancer. Not indicated for treatment of papillary tumors occurring alone. No data are available regarding the effectiveness of intravesical instillation of BCG in the treatment of invasive bladder cancer. Small bladder capacity is associated with an increased risk of severe local reactions.

Contraindications:

Absolute: Do not use in immunodeficient patients, including those with congenital or acquired immune deficiencies, whether due to genetics, disease, or drug or radiation therapy. Contains live bacteria. Avoid use in patients infected with HIV. Do not administer to patients with active tuberculosis.

Relative: Do not administer BCG to patients with fever unless the cause of the fever is determined and evaluated. If the fever is due to an infection, withhold therapy until the patient is afebrile and off all corresponding therapy. Do not give BCG to patients with urinary tract infections. Postpone treatment until resolution of a concurrent febrile illness, urinary tract infection, or gross hematuria. Allow 7 to 14 days to elapse between biopsy, transurethral resection (TUR), or traumatic catheterization and BCG instillation. Instillation of BCG onto bleeding mucosa may promote systemic BCG infection. A positive tuberculin skin test is a contra-indication only if there is evidence of active tuberculosis infection.

Immunodeficiency: Do not use in nor allow handling of this product by immunodeficient patients. Do not use in those with congenital or acquired immune deficiencies, whether caused by genetics, disease, or drug or radiation therapy. Contains live bacteria. Avoid use in patients infected with HIV.

Elderly: Safety and efficacy of BCG have been established in geriatric patients.

Carcinogenicity: It is not known if BCG products are carcinogenic.

Mutagenicity: It is not known if BCG products are mutagenic.

Fertility Impairment: It is not known if BCG products can impair fertility.

Pregnancy: Category C. Use only if clearly needed. It is not known if BCG bacteria instilled into the urinary bladder can cross the placenta. Advise women not to become pregnant while on BCG therapy.

Lactation: It is not known if BCG mycobacteria are excreted in breast milk. Problems in humans have not been documented. It is advisable to discontinue nursing or discontinue the drug, taking into account the importance of the drug to the mother.

Children: Safety and efficacy of BCG for bladder carcinoma have not been established in children.

Adverse Reactions: Reactions are often localized to the bladder; 60% of recipients report bladder irritability beginning 3 to 4 hours after instillation and lasting 24 to 72 hours. The irritative side effects are usually seen after the third instillation, and tend to increase in severity after each administration. These irritative effects can usually be managed symptomatically with pyridium, propantheline bromide, or oxybutinin chloride, and acetaminophen or ibuprofen. The mechanism of action of the irritative side effects has not been studied, but is most consistent with an immunologic mechanism. There is no evidence that dose reduction or therapy with an antituberculous drug can prevent or lessen the irritative toxicity of BCG.

Local reactions during clinical trials included the following: dysuria (52% to 60%); urinary frequency (35% to 40%); hematuria (34% to 39%); cystitis (30%); urgency (18%); urinary tract infection (5% to 18%); nocturia (11%); urinary incontinence (6% to 7%); urinary retention (6%); cramps or pain (3% to 6%); decreased bladder capacity (5%); tissue in urine (1% to 2%); and local infections (1%). People with small bladder capacity are at increased risk of severe local irritation.

Systemic reactions such as malaise, fever, and chills may also occur. Systemic reactions during clinical trials included the following: malaise (40%); fever (13% to 38%); chills (1% to 34%); anemia (21%); nausea or vomiting (16%); viral-like syndrome (12%); anorexia (11%); myalgia, arthralgia, or arthritis (7%); diarrhea (3% to 6%); and, in less than 3% of cases, mild liver involvement, mild abdominal pain, systemic or pulmonary infection, cardiac effects, headache, hypersensitivity, skin rash, constipation, dizziness, fatigue, leukopenia, disseminated intravascular coagulation, thrombocytopenia, renal toxicity, genital pain, and flank pain.

Deaths have resulted from systemic BCG infection and sepsis. In addition, *M. bovis* infections have been reported in lung, liver, bone, bone marrow, kidney, regional lymph nodes, and prostate in patients who received intravesical BCG. Monitor patients for symptoms and signs of toxicity after each intravesical treatment. Febrile episodes with flu-like symptoms lasting more than 72 hours, fever 39°C (103°F) or higher, systemic manifestations increasing in intensity with repeated instillations, cough, or persistent abnormalities of liver function tests suggest systemic BCG infection and require antitubercular therapy. Use isoniazid (INH), rifampin, ethambutol, or streptomycin to antagonize disseminated BCG infection. BCG is not sensitive to pyrazinamide. Local symptoms (eg, prostatitis, epididymitis, orchitis) lasting longer than 2 to 3 days may also suggest active infection.

Lab Interference: BCG does not interfere with interferon gamma-release assays.

Occupational Exposure: Remind health care personnel to use appropriate precautions to avoid BCG exposure (eg, mask, gloves). PPD- or IGRA-negative health care personnel who routinely handle BCG vaccine should record annual PPD skin-test or IGRA results. In case of splashing BCG vaccine into an eye, flush affected eye(s) with copious amounts of water for 15 minutes while holding eyelid(s) open. In case of accidental self-inoculation, perform a PPD skin-test at the time of the accident and 6 weeks later to detect any skin-test conversion. Asymptomatic skin-test conversion is equivalent to BCG vaccination and does not require antituberculous medication.

Pharmacologic & Dosing Characteristics

Dosage: Begin intravesical treatment and prophylaxis for carcinoma in situ of the urinary bladder from 7 to 14 days after biopsy or transurethral resection, if performed. The patient refrains from drinking liquids for 4 hours before treatment and empties the bladder before BCG instillation.

Merck: Suspend the contents of one 50 mg vial in 50 mL of preservative-free 0.9% sodium chloride, delivered by gravity through a urethral catheter. Administer 1 instillation per week for 6 weeks.

Sanofi Pasteur: Instill the contents of one 81 mg vial in 50 mL preservative-free 0.9% sodium chloride, 1 instillation per week for 6 weeks.

The product is retained in the bladder for as long as possible up to 2 hours and then voided while the patient is seated, to avoid splashing of urine. Patients unable to retain the suspension for 2 hours should be allowed to void sooner, if necessary. During the first hour after instillation, the patient should lie for 15 minutes each in the prone and supine positions and on each side. During the second hour, the patient may select any posture.

Route: Intravesical

Overdosage: If the contents of more than 1 container are instilled, monitor patient carefully for signs of systemic BCG infection and treat if needed.

Additional Doses:

Merck: Continue treatment once monthly thereafter for up to 12 months. A longer maintenance was given in some cases.

Sanofi Pasteur: Follow induction therapy by 1 treatment given 3, 6, 12, 18, and 24 months after the initial treatment.

Missed Doses: If the clinician believes the bladder catheterization has been traumatic, do not administer BCG and delay treatment at least 1 week. Resume subsequent treatment as if no interruption in the schedule occurred.

Waste Disposal: Discard all materials contaminated during the use of BCG vaccine by autoclaving, incineration, or similar procedures. Instruct patients to void in a seated position into a toilet bowl containing approximately 2 cups of undiluted household bleach during the 6 hours after BCG instillation. Retain the voided urine in the bowl for 15 minutes before flushing. If the patient voids into a plastic urinal, add a mixture of household bleach diluted to one-tenth of its original strength to the urinal. Do not cap the urinal because gas can be generated by the solution.

Efficacy:

Merck: One-hundred and nineteen patients with mean age 69 years of age (range, 38 to 97 years) were available for efficacy evaluation. There were 2 categories of clinical response: complete histological response (CR), defined as complete resolution of carcinoma in situ documented by cystoscopy and cytology, with or without biopsy; and complete clinical response without cytology (CRNC), defined as an apparent complete disappearance of tumor upon cystoscopy. Fifty-four patients achieved CR and 36 patients achieved CRNC, for an overall response of 76%. When these patients were followed further, with a median duration of followup of 47 months, there was no significant difference in response rates between patients with or without prior intravesical chemotherapy. The median duration of response is estimated at at least 4 years. The incidence of cystectomy for 90 patients who achieved a complete response (CR or CRNC) was 11%. The median time to cystectomy in patients who achieved a complete response (CR or CRNC) exceeded 74 months. Efficacy of intravesical *Tice BCG* in preventing recurrence of TaT1 bladder cancer after complete transurethral resection of all papillary tumors was evaluated in 2 open-label, randomized clinical trials. Initial diagnosis of patients included in the studies was determined by cystoscopic biopsies. One was conducted by the Southwestern Oncology Group (SWOG) in patients at high risk of recurrence, defined as 2 occurrences of tumor within 56 weeks, any stage T1 tumor, or 3 or more tumors presenting simultaneously. The second study was conducted at Nijmegen University Hospital among patients not selected for high risk of recurrence. In each study, treatment started 1 to 2 weeks after TUR. In the SWOG trial (study 8795) patients were randomized to *Tice BCG* or mitomycin C (MMC). Both drugs were given intravesically weekly for 6 weeks, at 8 and 12 weeks, nd then monthly for a total duration of 1 year. Cystoscopy and urinary cytology were performed every 3 months for 2 years. Patients with progressive disease or residual or recurrent disease at or after the 6 month followup were removed from the study and were classified as treatment failures. The 2-year disease-free survival was 57% in the BCG-treated group and 45% in the MMC group. No statistically significant differences between the groups were noted in time to tumor progression, tumor invasion, or overall survival.

In the Nijmegen study, the efficacy of 3 treatments was compared: *Tice BCG*, RIVM substrain BCG (BCG-RIVM), and MMC. BCG was given intravesically weekly for 6 weeks, but maintenance BCG was not given. MMC was given intravesically weekly for 4 weeks and then monthly for a total duration of treatment of 6 months. Cystoscopy and urinary cytology were performed every 3 months until recurrence. A total of 387 patients were evaluable: 117 in the *Tice BCG* arm, 134 in the BCG-RIVM arm, and 136 in the MMC arm. Estimates of 2-year disease-free survival were 53%, 62%, and 64%, respectively. The differences in disease-free survival among the 3 groups were not statistically significant by the log-rank test ($P = 0.08$).

Sanofi Pasteur: In clinical trials, 74% of patients treated with BCG exhibited a complete response (negative by cystoscopic examination and by urine cytology), compared with 42% of patients treated with doxorubicin. For patients with some form of prior treatment other than these 2 drugs who where treated with either BCG or doxorubicin, the response rate was 81% or 53%, respectively. The response rates were 68% or 30%, respectively, if no prior treatment had been given. Responders demonstrate a median 48.4 months until treatment failure (eg, progression, tumor recurrence, death), compared with 5.9 months for patients treated with doxorubicin. However, there was no survival advantage, calculated as median time to death, for BCG over doxorubicin therapy.

Onset: Data not provided.

Duration: The estimated median duration of response is at least 48 months after BCG treatment. The median time to cystectomy in patients who achieved a complete response was longer than 74 months, whereas the median time to cystectomy for nonrespondents was 31 months.

Pharmacokinetics: Not systemically absorbed after bladder instillation. Excreted in urine.

Mechanism: Causes a local inflammatory reaction with histiocytic and leukocytic infiltration in the urothelium and lamina propria of the urinary bladder. The inflammatory effects are associated with an apparent elimination or reduction of superficial cancerous lesions. The antitumor activity of BCG may require a thymus-dependent immune response. T-lymphocyte mediated mechanisms may play an essential role.

Drug Interactions: Like all live bacterial vaccines, administration of BCG to patients receiving immunosuppressant drugs, including high-dose corticosteroids or radiation therapy, may predispose them to disseminated infection or insufficient response.

BCG therapy may induce hypersensitivity to tuberculin skin tests. This false-positive effect diminishes in probability as time since BCG exposure increases. It may be useful to determine tuberculin hypersensitivity prior to BCG therapy of bladder cancer.

Antitubercular therapy (eg, isoniazid) will antagonize disseminated BCG infections. Do not use antituberculosis drugs to prevent or treat local irritative toxicities of BCG. Other antimicrobial therapy may interfere with the effectiveness of BCG bladder cancer therapy. *TheraCys*-brand BCG is sensitive to most common antimycobacterial agents (eg, isoniazid, rifampin, ethambutol), but is not sensitive to pyrazinamide. Postpone intravesical instillations of BCG until after antibiotic treatment to avoid interference.

Patient Information: Instruct patients to increase fluid intake to "flush" the bladder in the hours after BCG treatment. Patients may experience burning with the first void after treatment. Instruct patients to report side effects, such as fever, chills, malaise, viral-like symptoms, or increased fatigue. If the patient experiences severe urinary side effects (eg, burning or painful urination, increased urgency or frequency of urination, blood in the urine), joint pain, cough, or skin rash, notify the physician immediately.

Pharmaceutical Characteristics

Concentration:
Merck: 1 to 8 $\times$ 10^8 CFU per 50 mg wet weight per vial, after reconstitution.
Sanofi Pasteur: 81 mg dry weight per vial, 1.7 to 19.2 $\times$ 10^8 CFU per vial. This is a higher dose than the Connaught product available in Canada for tuberculosis prophylaxis (8 to 32 $\times$ 10^5 CFU per 0.1 mL).

Quality Assay: Do not use any reconstituted product exhibiting flocculation or clumping that cannot be dispersed with gentle shaking. Tested for residual virulence, skin reactivity, and tuberculin sensitivity in guinea pigs.

Packaging:
Merck: 2 mL single-dose vial (without diluent) (NDC#: 00052-0602-02)
Sanofi Pasteur: One vial of 81 mg dry weight with one 3 mL vial of diluent; 50 mL vials of phosphate-buffered sodium chloride are available for use as final diluent (49281-0880-03)

Doseform: Powder for suspension

Appearance:
Merck: Beige, creamy white, buff, or light gray powder, yielding a cloudy suspension
Sanofi Pasteur: White powder in amber vial

Diluent: Store diluents at a temperature ranging from 2° to 25°C (35° to 77°F).
For reconstitution: Merck: 1 mL preservative-free 0.9% sodium chloride, to prepare for bladder instillation
    Sanofi Pasteur: 0.85% sodium chloride, 0.025% polysorbate 80, 0.06% sodium dihydrogen phosphate, 0.025% disodium hydrogen phosphate. Do not filter.
For instillation: Merck: For bladder instillation, dilute 1 mL of reconstituted product with 49 mL preservative-free 0.9% sodium chloride.
    Sanofi Pasteur: 50 mL of preservative-free 0.9% sodium chloride

Adjuvant: None
Preservative: None

Allergens: None

Excipients:

Merck: Lactose 125 mg/ampule

Sanofi Pasteur: Monosodium glutamate 5%

pH: Data not provided.

Shelf Life: Expires in 12 to 36 months.

Storage/Stability: Store at 2° to 8°C (35° to 46°F). Discard if frozen. After reconstitution, use within 2 hours. Do not expose solution to sunlight (direct or indirect); minimize exposure to artificial light.

Product can tolerate 1 occasion at up to 24°C (75°F) for up to 3 days if continuously stored in its package and protected from light. Shipped in insulated containers by second-day courier.

Handling: To avoid cross-contamination, do not prepare parenteral drugs in areas where BCG has been in use. Nosocomial infections have been reported in immunosuppressed patients receiving parenteral drugs prepared in areas where BCG was prepared. Handle all equipment, supplies, and receptacles in contact with BCG products as biohazardous.

Production Process: Cultured, lyophilized, and packaged.

Media:

Merck: Medium consists of glycerin, asparagine, citric acid, potassium phosphate, magnesium sulfate, and iron ammonium citrate.

Sanofi Pasteur: Glycerinized potato medium, followed by further passages on Sauton medium. Media components include potatoes, glycerin, asparagine, citric acid, potassium phosphate, magnesium sulfate, ferric ammonium citrate, calcium chloride, copper sulfate, and zinc sulfate.

Disease Epidemiology

Incidence: Bladder cancer is the sixth most common malignancy encountered in general medical practice, with its highest incidence in the sixth decade of life. It is 3 times more common in men than in women. Bladder cancer in situ is found in 20% to 30% of 53,000 new cases of bladder cancer in the US, with 12,000 related deaths annually.

Carcinoma in situ of the urinary bladder is a superficial neoplasm that is considered an aggressive precursor of invasive transitional cell carcinoma.

Prognosis: When detected early, the 5-year survival rate is 90%. For regional and distant disease, the survival rates are 45% and 9%, respectively.

Other Information

Perspective: Also see the BCG vaccine monograph in the Vaccines/Toxoids section.

1990: TheraCys licensed on May 21.

1998: Tice BCG licensed August 4.

2000: Pacis licensed on March 9.

Discontinued Products: *Pacis* (IAF Biovac, later Biochem Pharma, distributed by Shire).

References: Alexandroff AB, et al. BCG immunotherapy of bladder cancer: 20 years on. *Lancet.* 1999;353:1689-1694.

Fields LS, Waddell JA, Solimando DA Jr. Intravesical BCG live for superficial bladder cancer. *Hosp Pharm.* 2004;39:954-957.

Malmstrom PU. Advances in intravesical therapy of urinary bladder cancer. *Expert Rev Anticancer Ther.* 2004;4(6):1057-1067.

Immunosuppressants

Immunologic Modulators

Many drugs are intentionally used for their immunosuppressive effects. Such drugs may be beneficial in the treatment of certain cancers, autoimmune diseases, and hematologic disorders. Immune suppression is an essential tactic in organ transplantation.

Antineoplastic drugs are cytotoxic, not tumoricidal, and thus affect both normal and neoplastic cells. Although antineoplastic drugs are partially selective for malignant cells, they may still affect rapidly proliferating normal cells, such as in the bone marrow.

This section summarizes the interactions of immunosuppressive drugs with other immunologic drugs and reviews other pertinent characteristics of their use. For more detailed discussion of immunosuppressive drugs, refer to the current edition of *Drug Facts and Comparisons*.

Product Identification:
I. Alkylating Agents
   A. Nitrogen Mustards
      1. Bendamustine (*Treanda*, Cephalon)
      2. Chlorambucil (*Leukeran*, GlaxoSmithKline)
      3. Cyclophosphamide (*Cytoxan*, Mead Johnson; *Neosar*, Pfizer)
      4. Estramustine (*Emcyt*, Pfizer)
      5. Ifosfamide (generic; *Ifex*, Mead Johnson)
      6. Mechlorethamine (*Mustargen*, Ovation Pharmaceuticals)
      7. Melphalan (*Alkeran*, GlaxoSmithKline)
   B. Nitrosoureas
      1. Carmustine (BCNU; *BiCNU*, Bristol-Myers Squibb; *Gliadel*, Sanofi Aventis)
      2. Lomustine (CCNU; *CeeNu*, Bristol-Myers Squibb)
      3. Streptozocin (*Zanosar*, Pfizer)
   C. Busulfan (*Myleran*, GlaxoSmithKline; *Busulfex*, Orphan Medical)
   D. Cisplatin (CDDP; generic; *Platinol-AQ*, Bristol-Myers Squibb)
   E. Thiotepa (generic, Bedford; *Thioplex*, Immunex)
   F. Carboplatin (*Paraplatin*, Bristol-Myers Squibb)
II. Antimetabolites
   A. Azathioprine (generic; *Imuran*, Prometheus)
   B. Capecitabine (*Xeloda*, Roche)
   C. Cladribine (generic, Bedford; *Leustatin*, Ortho)
   D. Cytarabine (ARA-C; generic; *Cytosar-U*, Pfizer; *DepoCyt*, Novartis)
   E. Floxuridine (generic; *FUDR*, Roche)
   F. Fludarabine (*Fludara*, Berlex)
   G. Fluorouracil (generic; *Adrucil*, Pfizer)
   H. Gemcitabine (*Gemzar*, Lilly)
   I. Mercaptopurine (6-MP; *Purinethol*, GlaxoSmithKline)
   J. Methotrexate (amethoptherin; MTX; generic, various)
   K. Pentostatin (*Nipent*, Super Gen)
   L. Pralatrexate (*Folotyn*, Allos)
   M. Thioguanine (generic, GlaxoSmithKline)
III. Macrolide immunosuppressants
   A. Cyclosporine (generic; *Sandimmune*, Novartis; *Neoral*, Novartis)
   B. Sirolimus (*Rapamune*, Wyeth)
   C. Tacrolimus (FK-506; *Prograf*, Fujisawa)
   D. Temsirolimus (*Torisel*, Pfizer)
IV. Glucocorticosteroids (representative proprietary products)
   A. Corticotropin (ACTH; *Acthar*, Sanofi Aventis)
   B. Cortisone acetate (generic, various)
   C. Betamethasone, various salts (*Celestone*, Merck)
   D. Dexamethasone, various salts (generic, various; *Decadron*, Merck)

Immunosuppressants

E. Hydrocortisone, various salts (cortisol; generic; *Cortef* and *Solu-Cortef*, Pfizer)
F. Methylprednisolone, various salts (generic, various; *Medrol, Depo-Medrol*, and *Solu-Medrol*, Pfizer)
G. Prednisolone, various salts (generic)
H. Prednisone (generic; *Deltasone*, Pfizer)
I. Triamcinolone, various salts (generic; *Aristocort* and *Aristospan*, Fujisawa; *Kenacort, Kenaject*, and *Kenalog*, Apothecon)
V. Mitotic Inhibitors
  A. Cabazitaxel (*Jevtana*, Sanofi-Aventis)
  B. Docetaxel (*Taxotere*, Sanofi Aventis)
  C. Eribulin mesylate (*Halaven*, Eisai)
  D. Etoposide (VP-16; generic; *Toposar*, Pfizer; *VePesid*, Bristol-Myers Squibb)
  E. Ixabepilone (*Ixempra*, Bristol-Myers Squibb)
  F. Paclitaxel (*Onxol*, Zenith; *Taxol*, Bristol-Myers Squibb)
  G. Teniposide (*Vumon*, Bristol-Myers Squibb)
  H. Vinblastine (generic, various; *Velban*, Eli Lilly)
  I. Vincristine (generic; *Vincasar*, Pfizer)
  J. Vinorelbine (*Navelbine*, GlaxoSmithKline)
VI. Radiopharmaceuticals
  A. Chromic Phosphate 32-P (*Phosphocol P 32*, Mallinckrodt)
  B. Sodium Iodide 131-I (generic, Mallinckrodt; *Iodotope*, Bracco)
  C. Sodium Phosphate 32-P (generic, Mallinckrodt)
  D. Strontium-89 chloride Sr-89 (*Metastron*, Medi-Physics/Amersham)
  E. Samarium lexidronam Sm-153 (*Quadramet*, DuPont)
VII. Other Immunosuppressants
  A. Abiraterone acetate (*Zytiga*, Centocor Ortho Biotech)
  B. Altretamine (*Hexalen*, MGI Pharma)
  C. Dacarbazine (*DTIC-Dome*, Bayer)
  D. Dasatinib (*Sprycel*, Bristol-Myers Squibb)
  E. Glatiramer acetate (*Copaxone*, Teva)
  F. Gold Compounds
    1. Auranofin (*Ridaura*, GlaxoSmithKline)
    2. Gold sodium thiomalate (generic; *Aurolate*, Pasedena)
  G. Hydroxyurea (generic; *Hydrea*, Bristol-Myers Squibb)
  H. Irinotecan (*Camptosar*, Pfizer)
  I. Lapatinib (*Tykerb*, GlaxoSmithKline)
  J. Mycophenolate mofetil (*CellCept*, Roche)
  K. Nilotinib (*Tasigna*, Novartis Oncology)
  L. Pazopanib (*Votrient*, GlaxoSmithKline)
  M. Procarbazine (*Matulane*, Roche)
  N. Romidepsin (*Istodax*, Celgene)
  O. Temozolomide (*Temodar*, Merck)
  P. Topotecan (*Hycamtin*, GlaxoSmithKline)
  Q. Vandetanib (*Zactima*, AstraZeneca)
VIII. Immunologic Drugs with Monographs in this Volume
  A. Abatacept
  B. Adalimumab
  C. Aldesleukin
  D. Alefacept
  E. Alemtuzumab
  F. Anakinra
  G. Antithymocyte globulins
  H. Basiliximab
  I. Bevacizumab
  J. Daclizumab
  K. Denileukin diftitox
  L. Efalizumab
  M. Etanercept
  N. Ibritumomab

    O. Infliximab
    P. Interferon alfa
    Q. Interferon gamma
    R. Interleukin-2
    S. Ipilimumab (*Yervoy*, Bristol-Myers Squibb
    T. Muromonab-CD3
    U. Natalizumab
    V. Ofatumumab (*Arzerra*, GlaxoSmithKline)
    W. Omalizumab
    X. Rituximab
    Y. Sipuleucel-T (*Provenge*, Dendreon)
    Z. Tositumomab
    AA. Trastuzumab
IX. Other drugs that produce a predictable dose-related myelosuppression include
    A. Aminoquinolone Compounds
        1. Chloroquine (generic; *Aralen*, Winthrop-Breon)
        2. Hydroxychloroquine (generic; *Plaquenil*, Sanofi-Aventis)
    B. Amphotericin B (*Fungizone*, Bristol-Myers Squibb)
    C. Antibiotic Antineoplastic Agents
        1. Bleomycin (generic; *Blenoxane*, Bristol-Myers Squibb)
        2. Dactinomycin (*Cosmegen*, Ovation Pharmaceuticals)
        3. Daunorubicin (generic; *Cerubidine*, Bedford; *DaunoXome*, NeXstar)
        4. Doxorubicin (generic; *Adriamycin*, Pfizer; *Doxil*, Sequus)
        5. Epirubicin (*Ellence*, Pfizer)
        6. Idarubicin (*Idamycin*, Pfizer)
        7. Mitomycin (*Mutamycin*, Bristol-Myers Squibb)
        8. Plicamycin (*Mithracin*, Bayer)
        9. Valrubicin (*Valstar*, Medeva)
    D. Antithyroid Agents
        1. Carbamizole (*Neomercazole*, lagamed)
        2. Methimazole (generic; *Tapazole*, Eli Lilly)
        3. Propylthiouracil (generic, various)
    E. Antiviral Agents
        1. Abacavir/Lamivudine/Zidovudine (*Trizivir*, GlaxoSmithKline)
        2. Didanosine (*Videx*, Bristol-Myers Squibb)
        3. Ganciclovir (*Cytovene*, Roche)
        4. Lamivudine/Zidovudine (*Combivir*, GlaxoSmithKline)
        5. Valganciclovir (*Valcyte*, Roche)
        6. Zidovudine (*Retrovir*, GlaxoSmithKline)
    F. Bexarotene (*Targretin*, Ligand)
    G. Chloramphenicol (generic; *Chloromycetin*, Monarch Pharmaceuticals)
    H. Clozapine (*Clozaril*, Novartis)
    I. Colchicine (generic, various)
    J. Dapsone (generic, Jacobus)
    K. Eflornithine (*Ornidyl*, Sanofi Aventis)
    L. Enzymes
        1. Asparaginase (*Elspar*, Merck)
        2. Pegaspargase (*Oncaspar*, Enzon)
    M. Exemestane (*Aromasin*, Pfizer)
    N. Flucytosine (*Ancobon*, ICN)
    O. Imatinib (*Gleevec*, Novartis)
    P. Leflunomide (*Arava*, Sanofi Aventis)
    Q. Metamizole (*Dipyrone*, not available in USA)
    R. Mitoxantrone (*Novantrone*, Immunex)
    S. Penicillamine (*Cuprimine*, Merck; *Depen*, Wallace)
    T. Penicillin G (generic, various)
    U. Pentamidine (*NebuPent* and *Pentam 300*, LyphoMed)
    V. Procainamide (*Procanbid*, Monarch)

W. Sulfasalazine (*Azulfidine*, Pfizer)
X. Ticlopidine (*Ticlid*, Syntex)
Y. Zoledronic acid (*Zometa*, Novartis)

Immune Effects: Immunosuppression may be manifested as bone marrow depression, including leukopenia, lymphopenia, neutropenia, pancytopenia, granulocytopenia, or granulocytosis. These effects are often dose-related. Large cumulative doses may induce irreversible bone marrow damage. Therapy may be contraindicated in patients with preexisting drug-induced bone marrow suppression unless the benefit from such treatment warrants the risk. Other effects include suppression of humoral or cell-mediated immunity. Antibody response to antigenic challenge and T-cell function may be reduced. Immune tolerance may be induced. Expression of cell-mediated immunity (eg, response to delayed-hypersensitivity reagents) may be suppressed. Phagocyte number and function may also be reduced.

Immunosuppressive effects (eg, myelosuppression) may predispose the patient to bacterial, viral, fungal, or protozoal infections. Infections are more likely to occur when steroid and other immunosuppressive therapies are used concurrently. Infections may require dose modification or interruption.

The use of some immunosuppressive drugs (eg, cyclophosphamide) may predispose the patient to secondary neoplasms. Some immunosuppressants are carcinogenic (eg, azathioprine).

Other Immunosuppressants: Aminoquinolones (eg, chloroquine, hydroxychloroquine) fix DNA in its double strand form so that it cannot replicate or serve for the transcription of RNA. Protein synthesis is thus decreased through ribosomal destruction. In the treatment of rheumatoid arthritis, aminoquinolones may suppress formation of antigens responsible for hypersensitivity reactions that cause symptoms to develop. These drugs may induce hemolysis in individuals deficient in glucose-6-phosphate dehydrogenase (G-6-PD) in the presence of infection or stressful conditions.

Antibiotic antineoplastic drugs (eg, dactinomycin, daunorubicin, doxorubicin, mitomycin, plicamycin) can disrupt cellular functions of host mammalian tissues. Their primary mechanisms of action are to inhibit DNA-dependent RNA synthesis and to delay or inhibit mitosis. These antibiotics are cell cycle specific.

Colchicine is involved in leukocyte migration inhibition, reduction of lactic acid production by leukocytes, interference with kinin formation, and reduction of phagocytosis with inflammatory response abatement.

Gold compounds are taken up by macrophages with resultant inhibition of phagocytosis and inhibition of activity of lysosomal enzymes. Gold also decreases concentrations of rheumatoid factor and immunoglobulins. Hydroxyurea inhibits ribonucleotide reductase, thus interfering with RNA synthesis. It may also directly affect DNA.

Mitoxantrone appears to act by binding to DNA by intercalation between base pairs and by nonintercalative electrostatic interaction, resulting in inhibition of DNA and RNA synthesis.

Penicillamine lowers rheumatoid IgM factor, but produces no significant depression in absolute levels of serum immunoglobulins. In vitro it depresses T-cell activity but not B-cell activity and dissociates macroglobulins (rheumatoid factor).

Procarbazine produces toxic metabolites that induce chromosomal breakage. The mechanism of dacarbazine is unknown.

Zidovudine, in addition to antiviral and antibacterial effects, can bind to and inhibit some mammalian cellular DNA polymerases. The drug has a direct dose-dependent inhibitory effect on erythroid and myeloid function in vitro.

Pharmacologic & Dosing Characteristics

Mechanism: Alkylating agents form highly reactive carbonium ions that react with essential cellular components, altering normal biological function. Alkylating agents replace hydrogen atoms with an alkyl radical, causing cross-linking and abnormal base pairing in DNA molecules. These drugs also react with sulfhydryl, phosphate, and amine groups, resulting in multiple lesions in both dividing and nondividing cells. The defective DNA molecules are unable to carry out normal cellular reproductive functions.

Antimetabolites interfere with various metabolic functions, disrupting normal cellular functions. These drugs may act by two general mechanisms: (1) by incorporating the drug, rather than a normal cellular constituent, into an essential process or (2) by inhibiting a key enzyme from functioning normally. Their primary benefit is the ability to disrupt nucleic acid synthesis. These agents work only on dividing cells during the S phase of nucleic acid synthesis. The group includes methotrexate, which is a folic acid antagonist; fluorouracil, floxuridine, and cytarabine, which are pyrimidine analogs; and mercaptopurine and thioguanine, which are purine analogs. Antimetabolites are most effective on rapidly proliferating neoplasms.

Cyclosporine induces specific and reversible inhibition of immunocompetent lymphocytes in the G_0 (resting) or G_1 (postmitotic, presynthetic) phase of the cell cycle. T-lymphocytes are preferentially inhibited. The T-helper cell is the main target, although the T-suppressor cell may also be suppressed. Cyclosporine also inhibits lymphokine production and release (eg, interleukin-2, T-cell growth factor). This drug does not antagonize activation of antigen-specific suppressor T-cells. Cyclosporine does not cause bone marrow suppression. Immune tolerance toward vaccine antigens may potentially be induced by cyclosporine, raising the possibility of induction of tolerance to an infectious agent.

Glucocorticosteroids (also called corticosteroids) have both anti-inflammatory and immunomodulating properties, in addition to many other effects. These drugs decrease inflammation by stabilizing leukocyte lysosomal membranes, preventing release of destructive enzymes from leukocytes, antagonizing histamine activity, and other effects.

Corticosteroids suppress immune function by reducing the activity and volume of the lymphatic system, producing lymphocytopenia, decreasing immunoglobulin and complement concentrations, possibly by depressing reactivity of tissue to antigen-antibody interactions, and other effects. These drugs may mask signs of infection and new infections may appear during their use, perhaps due to decreased resistance and the inability of host defense mechanisms to prevent dissemination of the infection. Corticosteroids are not immunosuppressive when given as replacement therapy (eg, for Addison disease).

Mitotic inhibitors act as mitotic-spindle poisons, causing metaphase arrest. These agents are plant alkaloids derived from the periwinkle plant or the May-apple plant. They are M (mitosis) phase cell-cycle specific agents, but may also have some activity in the G_2 (postsynthetic, premitotic) and S (DNA synthesis) phases.

Radiopharmaceuticals exert a direct toxic effect on exposed tissue (eg, bone marrow) by radiation emission. Refer to Isotope-Conjugated Antibodies in the Immune Globulins section.

Drug Interactions:

Live Vaccines: Live, attenuated viral, or bacterial vaccines administered to patients receiving immunosuppressive therapy may not induce the expected antibody response. These vaccine recipients may remain susceptible despite immunization; protection against subsequent infection may not be obtained. In immunosuppressed persons, the risk of disseminated infection resulting from immunization may be increased. If both live and inactivated vaccines are available (eg, influenza, typhoid), select the inactivated vaccine.

Inactivated Vaccines: Inactivated viral and bacterial vaccines and toxoids administered to patients receiving immunosuppressive therapy may not induce the expected antibody response. These vaccine recipients may remain susceptible despite immunization; protection against subsequent infection may not be obtained. Response to immunization may be best if administered 10 to 14 days prior to immunosuppressive chemotherapy or radiation or 3 to 12 months after discontinuing immunosuppressive therapy. Similarly, antibody response to allergen extracts and *Hymenoptera* venoms may be impaired.

Delayed Hypersensitivity Reagents: Delayed hypersensitivity responses may be impaired in patients receiving immunosuppressive therapy. Tuberculin hypersensitivity may be suppressed, as well as reactions to histoplasmin, coccidioidin, *Candin*, and similar delayed-hypersensitivity reagents. When of diagnostic importance for a specific disease, accept a negative test as proof that hypersensitivity is absent only after normal reactivity has been demonstrated, as with an anergy-test panel. Reactivity to contact dermatitis allergen kits, poison ivy extracts, and similar drugs may also be impaired.

Colony-Stimulating Factors: Myeloid colony-stimulating factors (eg, filgrastim, sargramostim) used concurrently with immunosuppressive drugs may increase the potential for using higher doses of immunosuppressive chemotherapy (ie, full doses on the prescribed schedule). This may place the patient at greater risk of the hematopoietic consequences of chemotherapy. Because of the potential sensitivity of rapidly dividing hematopoietic progenitor cells to cytotoxic chemotherapeutic or radiologic therapies, do not administer sargramostim within 24 hours before or after chemotherapy or within 12 months before or after radiation therapy.

Multiple Immunosuppressive Agents: Concurrent use of multiple immunosuppressive drugs (eg, alkylating agents, azathioprine, corticosteroids, cyclosporine, interferons, muromonab-CD3) may increase the risk of infection or neoplasm. These effects are related to the intensity and duration of therapy.

Other Information

Perspective:
> *1935:* Kendall isolates cortisone from the human adrenal cortex. This and related work by Hench and Reichstein earn them the 1950 Nobel Prize for Physiology and Medicine.
> *1951:* Woodward synthesizes cortisone.
> *1960:* Küss and colleagues use 6-mercaptopurine, corticosteroids, and total body irradiation to prevent organ rejection in a kidney transplant, with the longest survival at that time (18 months) for unrelated donor and recipient.
> *1961:* Azathioprine developed, improving transplant success rates. Corticosteroids routinely added to immunosuppressive regimens in 1963.
> *1978:* Cyclosporine clinical trials begin in England; US trials start in 1979. The FDA approves cyclosporine in 1983.

Immunologic Adjuvants

Immunologic Adjuvants

An adjuvant is a substance that aids another substance in its action, derived from the Latin *adjuvare*, to help. In immunologic terms, adjuvants are added to a vaccine formulation to elicit an earlier, more potent, or more persistent immune response. Currently licensed adjuvants are primarily employed to improve antibody responses, but future adjuvants may evoke enhanced cell-mediated immunity (CMI) as well. Improved adjuvants will permit the use of antigens that are inherently less immunogenic.

Adjuvants work by a variety of mechanisms, such as (1) forming physical depots that slowly release antigen, (2) localizing and delivering antigen to immunocompetent cells, and (3) direct effects on macrophages and lymphocytes to release immune mediators (eg, interleukins, other messengers).

The ideal adjuvant acts without toxicity. In practical terms, an effective adjuvant must improve the efficacy of the vaccine formulation to which it is added, and the benefits of the adjuvant must outweigh its own risks.

Licensed Adjuvants

Aluminum Salts (including aluminum hydroxide, aluminum phosphate, and aluminum hydroxyphosphate sulfate): The term alum properly refers to aluminum potassium sulfate [$AlK(SO_4)_2 \cdot 12H_2O$ or alum potash], but is commonly misused to describe any of these aluminum salts.

The initial practice of protein precipitation in the presence of alum has been superseded, because of resultant variable potency. The more common method is mixture of antigen with preformed aluminum hydroxide or phosphate gels under controlled conditions. Such products are said to be adsorbed onto the salt.

To reduce batch-to-batch variation and increase potency uniformity, a specific preparation of aluminum hydroxide (*Alhydrogel*) was selected as the reference standard in 1988. Aluminum adjuvants are commonly used in vaccines containing antigens to protect against anthrax, diphtheria, *Haemophilus influenzae* type b, hepatitis B, pertussis, rabies, and tetanus. They are also used in some allergen extracts.

Aluminum adjuvants act by depot formation, slowing antigen excretion and prolonging the duration of interaction between antigen and antigen-presenting cells (eg, macrophages) and lymphocytes. Aluminum also attracts immunocompetent cells to the injection site, thus forming granulomas that contain antibody-secreting plasma cells. Development of B-cell memory may result from aluminum-induced complement activation. Rabbit studies suggest that aluminum may direct antigen to areas of regional lymph nodes that contain T-cells. Aluminum does not induce cell-mediated immunity.

Aluminum adjuvants are known to cause adverse events, especially local reactions such as erythema, persistent subcutaneous nodules, granulomatous inflammation, and contact hypersensitivity. Instability after lyophilizing and freezing are other disadvantages of aluminum adjuvants.

The only modern immunologic drug for which there is a choice between adsorbed and nonadsorbed (ie, fluid) forms is tetanus toxoid. While the rate of seroconversion and the promptness of antibody response are essentially equivalent for both the fluid and adsorbed forms of tetanus toxoid, adsorbed toxoids induce higher antitoxin titers, and, hence, more persistent antitoxin levels.

Therefore, adsorbed tetanus toxoid is strongly recommended for both primary and booster immunizations (preferably in combination with diphtheria toxoid). Use fluid tetanus toxoid to immunize the rare patient who is hypersensitive to the aluminum adjuvant. The only other rational use remaining for fluid tetanus toxoid is in compounding dilutions of a reagent for delayed-hypersensitivity skin-testing (refer to product monographs for details).

Reference:Vaccine. 2002 May 31; volume 20, supplement 3.

AS04: Adjuvant system #4, a combination of aluminum and 3-deacylated monophosphoryl lipid A. Included in *Cervarix* (GSK).

Protein Conjugates: The carrier proteins conjugated to *H. influenzae* type b polysaccharide antigens are considered adjuvants. These proteins (eg, diphtheria, meningococcal, tetanus proteins) overcome the inability of polysaccharide antigens to induce active immunity and T-cell immunologic memory in infants and young children.

Investigational Adjuvants

Much of the recent research into adjuvants shares the common feature of exploring the role of hydrophilic and lipophilic (ie, hydrophobic) character in immunologic processes. Among the following products that have been or are currently undergoing human clinical trials, the most promising candidates include immunostimulating complexes, liposomes, detoxified lipopolysaccharides, and derivatives of muramyl dipeptide.

Adjuvant 65: 86% peanut oil with 10% *Arlacel A* (an emulsifier), and 4% aluminum monostearate (a stabilizer), forming a metabolizable water-in-oil emulsion. Peanut oil can be broken down by lipases to glycerol and free fatty acids, but it can provoke granulomas or cysts at the injection site. Research was largely redirected to other candidate adjuvants when the carcinogenicity of *Arlacel A* (a poorly defined combination of fat and carbohydrate compounds with mannide monooleate) in several strains of mice was recognized.

AS02: Adjuvant system #2, a combination of monophosphoryl lipid A (MPL) and QS21, as an oil-in-water emulsion.

AS03: Adjuvant system #3, a combination of squalene, DL-α-tocopherol (a form of vitamin E), and polysorbate 80.

Cholera Toxin: Cholera toxin derivatives have been proposed as adjuvants for gastric mucosal immunity. The complete toxin molecule cannot be used itself because of its direct toxicity.

CpG: CpG is a sequence of DNA (an oligodeoxynucleotide, ODN) where cytosine (C) lies next to guanine (G), connected by a phosphodiester bond. Methylation of DNA occurs at any CpG site or motif. CpG-DNA elicits immunostimulatory signals with similarities to Toll-like receptor cascades. This can modulate innate as well as adaptive immune responses (Dalpke and Heeg, 2004).

Freund's Complete Adjuvant: An emulsion of mineral or paraffin oil with killed mycobacteria (also called complete Freund's adjuvant, FCA, or CFA), originally produced during tuberculosis research. One of the most potent adjuvants known, FCA promotes both cellular and humoral immunity. FCA is too toxic for routine human use because it contains nonmetabolizable mineral oil and because the mycobacterial components provoke pain, abscesses, granulomas, inflammation, and other severe reactions at the injection site. See also Muramyl Dipeptide.

Freund's Incomplete Adjuvant: A water-in-oil emulsion without mycobacteria, which primarily promotes humoral immunity. The preparation is also called incomplete Freund's adjuvant (FIA or IFA). FIA localizes antigen in the initial depot and disseminates to lymph nodes. Injection of FIA and antigen at separate sites does not affect the immune response. FIA is being evaluated by Immunization Products Limited with an investigational whole-virion HIV vaccine.

FIA was included with over 150,000 IM doses of influenza vaccine between 1951 and the late 1960s. It was administered widely to members of the US Armed Forces. In 1 study, anti-influenza antibody persisted for over 9 years, considerably longer than influenza vaccine without adjuvant. The most commonly used FIA-influenza product may have incorporated light mineral oil with *Arlacel A* as the emulsifier and only one-twentieth the usual influenza antigen dose.

The use of FIA with influenza vaccine was eventually abandoned because of infrequent abscesses, cysts (40 reported cases among 900,000 doses in 1963-64 in the United Kingdom), granulomas, or inflammation at the injection site. Long-term follow-up studies failed to show any increase in mortality, tumors, or autoimmune diseases attributable to this adjuvant, but the adjuvant may have sensitized some vaccine recipients to the trace quantities of penicillin added at that time to the eggs used for culturing the influenza virus.

Immunostimulating Complexes: ISCOMs are relatively stable, but not covalently bound, complexes of the saponin adjuvant *Quil-A*, cholesterol, phospholipid, and antigen in a specific molar ratio that can form cage-like structures approximately 40 nm in diameter. *Quil-A* is extracted from the bark of the *Quillaja saponaria molina* tree, harvested in the South American Andes. An ISCOM vaccine against equine influenza is licensed in Sweden, and a feline leukemia virus vaccine licensed in the US employs an ISCOM adjuvant system. ISCOMs appear to promote both cellular and humoral immunity, inducing cytotoxic T-lymphocytes. They may be effective as adjuvants both parenterally and orally. *Iscomatrix* is being developed by CSL.

Interleukins: Immunologic mediators, such as IL-1 and IL-2, may be direct adjuvants. IL-1 may have a role in augmenting proliferation of T-lymphocytes when antigen is present. IL-2, a T-cell growth factor, may also play a valuable role in modulating CMI.

Lipid A: Lipid A (also called Lipid IV_A) is a derivative of lipopolysaccharide, degraded to remove a phosphate group. Lipid A may promote both cellular and humoral immunity. Natural and synthetic forms and other derivatives are being tested.

Lipopolysaccharides: Lipopolysaccharide (LPS) adjuvants are usually derived from bacterial sources such as *Bordetella pertussis*, *Corynebacterium parvum* or other species, or various *Mycobacterium* or *Salmonella* species. Pertussis vaccine is known to exert an adjuvant effect on diphtheria and tetanus toxoids. LPS may stimulate production and release of immunologic mediators (eg, interleukin 1) and other mechanisms. LPS appears to promote both cellular and humoral immunity. To avoid toxicity, several LPS derivatives are being tested, including lipid A and P40. Isolated from *Corynebacterium granulosum*, P40 is an interesting cell-wall peptidoglycan associated with a glycoprotein.

Liposomes: Liposomes are microscopic vesicles, made of phospholipid bilayers alternating with aqueous compartments, that form an antigen depot. Liposomes have been constructed of lecithin, cholesterol, and stearylamine. Efficacy as an adjuvant is related to the number of layers, charge, composition, and method of preparation. Liposomes (eg, TLC A-60) with antigens entrapped within the aqueous phase are being evaluated by Elan Pharmaceuticals, including an investigational influenza A&B vaccine and an investigational HIV vaccine. Liposomes may promote both cellular and humoral immunity to both protein and carbohydrate antigens, perhaps related to antigen presentation in a hydrophobic microenvironment. Liposomes have been tested in combination with lipopolysaccharide, lipid A, or muramyl dipeptide. They may be effective as adjuvants both parenterally and orally.

MF59: Squalene/water emulsion, containing 43 mg/mL squalene, 2.5 mg/mL polyoxyethylene sorbitan monooleate (polysorbate 80), 2.4 mg/mL sorbitan trioleate (Span 85). A low-viscosity biodegradable aqueous emulsion, with an average particle size of 200 to 300 nm. A constituent of *Fluad*, an influenza vaccine widely used in Europe.

Microsphere Release Mechanisms: Microspheres of poly(lactic/glycolic) acid can incorporate a variety of proteins and release them slowly after injection or ingestion.

Mineral Salts: Mineral salts other than aluminum, such as calcium phosphate, cerium nitrate, zinc sulfate, colloidal iron hydroxide, and calcium chloride are also being investigated for use as adjuvants. None of these salts exhibit as strong an adjuvant effect as aluminum. Calcium phosphate was previously used with licensed vaccines in the US (eg, influenza vaccine from Parke-Davis in the late 1950s and early 1960s), and is still recommended for use around the world by the WHO.

Monophosphoryl Lipid A (*MPL*): *MPL* is derived from lipopolysaccharides of *Salmonella minnesota* R595 bacteria. Combined with *Mycobacterium phlei* cell-wall skeletons, it is being developed by Ribi ImmunoChem Research and GlaxoSmithKline as the *Detox* adjuvant for use with an investigational melanoma therapeutic vaccine. *Detox* appears to promote both cellular and humoral immunity. *MPL* is a component of *Cervarix* (HPV2) and is also included in the proprietary investigational adjuvant *Ovamid*.

Muramyl Dipeptide (MDP) Derivatives: MDP is the smallest component of FCA to possess humoral and cellular adjuvanticity. Structurally, MDP is N-acetylmuramyl-L-alanyl-D-isoglutamine. MDP induces an antibody response when given orally, even if the antigen is given by another route. Hydrophilic MDP induces several classes of antibodies, but not CMI. If MDP is administered with another product (eg, emulsion, liposome, glycerol mycolate) to increase lipophilicity, CMI develops. If MDP is given before antigen administration, antibody and CMI responses are diminished rather than enhanced, possibly because additional suppressor T-cells are present in the spleen, but not in lymph nodes. Derivatives, such as murabutide (NAcMur-L-Ala-D-Gln-a-n-butyl-ester) or murametide (NAcMur-L-Ala-D-Gln-OCH$_3$) are believed to have a more favorable therapeutic-toxic ratio.

Nonionic Block Copolymer (NBC) Surfactants: NBC surfactants are composed of chains or blocks of hydrophilic polyoxyethylene and hydrophobic polyoxypropylene, such as *Pluronic* polymer, in a 2% squalane-in-water emulsion. Insoluble polymers consisting of hydrophilic moieties adjoining hydrophobic moieties enhance chemotaxis, complement activation, and antibody formation. NBC adjuvants appear to promote humoral and cellular immunity. See Syntex Adjuvant Formulation-1.

Oil Emulsions: Oil emulsions (ie, water-in-oil emulsions) are believed to primarily promote humoral immunity. They may also provoke granulomas or cysts at the injection site. Antigen is typically trapped in the internal, aqueous phase of a water-in-oil (W/O) emulsion. Oil emulsions are currently used in some veterinary vaccines against brucellosis (strain 45/20) and foot-and-mouth disease. See Freund's Incomplete Adjuvant.

Polymannoacetate (acemannan): Derived from *Aloe vera* plants. Developed by Carrington Laboratories under proprietary name *ACM-1*. Available as a general immunostimulant for veterinary use.

Polymerization: Adjuvants can be formed by polymerizing antigen through treatment with glutaraldehyde (1,5-pentanedial). Glutaraldehyde appears to cross-link proteins, stabilize cell surfaces, and bind proteins to microspheres.

QS-21: *Stimulon*, Cambridge and GlaxoSmithKline

Saponins: Saponins (eg, QS-21) are mixtures of triterpine glycosides that classically form a soapy film when dissolved in water. Derived from the *Quillaja saponaria* tree, saponins act as surfactants and emulsifying agents. Saponin is currently being used in some veterinary vaccines (eg, anthrax, foot-and-mouth disease). Saponin may be hemolytic in humans. For veterinary anthrax vaccine, saponin is used to destroy tissue at the site of injection so anthrax spores may germinate.

Stearyl Tyrosine: This candidate adjuvant induces depot formation, like aluminum adjuvants, but does not induce IgE production.

Syntex Adjuvant Formulation-1: SAF-1 contains an emulsion of squalene and *Pluronic* L121 polymer, with polysorbate 80 as surfactant. Squalene is a threonyl oil derivative of muramyl dipeptide with low pyrogenicity. SAF-1 appears to promote both cellular and humoral immunity.

Thymosin Alpha-1: A synthetic form of thymosin, a group of peptide mediators secreted by the thymus gland, is licensed in Italy as an adjuvant for influenza vaccine. Thymosin is thought to work by exogenous replacement of thymic hormone.

Toll-like receptors (TLRs): Transmembrane proteins that recognize microbes after they breach physical barriers (eg, skin, intestinal mucosa) and activate immune cell responses. TLRs are a type of pattern-recognition receptors (PRRs) that play a key role in the innate immune system and recognize molecules that are broadly shared by pathogens but distinguishable from host molecules. These molecules are collectively referred to as pathogen-associated molecular patterns (PAMPs). TLRs are found in vertebrates (eg, fish, amphibians, reptiles, birds, mammals) as well as in invertebrates (eg, *Drosophila*). Toll refers to a receptor in the fruit fly *Drosophila melanogaster*, known for its role in the fly's immunity to fungal infection, by activating synthesis of antimicrobial peptides.

Trehalose Dimycolate: TDM is an immunostimulating component purified from Wax C of FCA.

Other Information

Perspective:

1916: LeMoignic & Pinoy use a mineral-oil emulsion as a vehicle for *Salmonella typhimurium* vaccination of humans.

1925: Ramon uses agar, tapioca, lecithin, saponin, starch oil, and bread crumbs to render diphtheria toxoid less soluble and augment immune response in humans. He is generally credited with introducing the concept of adjuvants. Tapioca had previously been used in France to enhance immune responses in immunized horses.

1925: Pope begins work on alum precipitation of diphtheria toxoid.

1926: Glenny et al report that alum precipitation enhances diphtheria toxoid activity.

1937: Freund et al report use of Freund's complete adjuvant.

1937: Aluminum-adsorbed form of tetanus toxoid licensed in the US.

1948: Aluminum-adsorbed form of diphtheria toxoid licensed in the US.

2010: HPV vaccine adjuvanted with AS04 licensed in the US.

References: Alving CR. Design and selection of vaccine adjuvants: animal models and human trials. *Vaccine*. 2002;20(suppl 3):S56-S64.

Baylor NW, Egan W, Richman P. Aluminum salts in vaccines: US perspective. *Vaccine* 2002; 20(Suppl 3):S18-23. Erratum 3428.

Cox JC, Coulter AR. Adjuvants—A classification and review of their modes of action. *Vaccine*. 1997;15:248-256.

Dalpke AH, Heeg K. CpG-DNA as immune response modifier. *Int J Med Microbiol*. 2004; 294:345-354.

Davenport FM. Seventeen years' experience with mineral oil adjuvant influenza vaccines. *Ann Allergy*. 1968;26:288-292.

Edelman R. Vaccine adjuvants. *Rev Infect Dis*. 1980;2:370-383.

Exley C, Siesjö P, Eriksson H. The immunobiology of aluminium adjuvants: How do they really work? *Trends Immunol*. 2010;31(Mar):103-109.

Gupta RK. Aluminum compounds as vaccine adjuvants. *Adv Drug Deliv Rev*. 1998; 32:155-172.

Gupta RK, et al. Adjuvants: A balance between toxicity and adjuvanticity. *Vaccine*. 1993;11:293-306.

Gupta RK, Rost BE, Relyveld E, Siber GR. Adjuvant properties of aluminum and calcium compounds. *Pharmaceut Biotechnol*. 1995;6:229-248.

Hem SL, White JL. Structure and properties of aluminum-containing adjuvants. *Pharmaceut Biotechnol.* 1995;6:249-276.

Lin R, Tarr PE, Jones TC. Present status of the use of cytokines as adjuvants with vaccines to protect against infectious diseases. *Clin Infect Dis.* 1995;21:1439-1449.

Marciani DJ. Vaccine adjuvants: role and mechanisms of action in vaccine immunogenicity. *Drug Discov Today.* 2003;8:934-943.

Myers KR, et al. Adjuvants for human vaccine usage: A rational design. In: Cryz SJ Jr. *Vaccines & Immunotherapy.* New York: Pergamon Press, 1991:404-411.

Page WF, Norman J, Benenson AS. Long-term follow-up of army recruits immunized with Freund's incomplete adjuvanted vaccine. *Vaccine Res.* 1993;2:141-149.

Pearse MJ, Drane D. ISCOMATRIX adjuvant: A potent inducer of humoral and cellular immune responses. *Vaccine.* 2004;22(19):2391-2395.

Tizard IR. *Veterinary Immunology: An Introduction,* 4th ed. Philadelphia: WB Saunders Co., 2000.

Warren HS, et al. Current status of immunological adjuvants. *Ann Rev Immunol.* 1986;4:369-388.

Naming Conventions

The United States Adopted Names (USAN) Council uses the following scheme to create non-proprietary names for cell therapy products. Under this nomenclature scheme for cell therapy products, the cell type/source and product manipulation or modification are parts of the cellular therapy product name, incorporated as infixes. The suffix *-cel* is used for all cell therapies, and *-imut* for noncellular immunotherapeutic products. The USAN Council sets a unique prefix (2 or 3 letters) for each name.

This naming scheme applies to cell therapy products, except minimally manipulated hematopoietic elements, combination products, and prophylactic vaccines. Because most cell therapy products are manipulated or modified in some way, the manipulation or modification is considered part of the product and thus part of the name. Such manipulation/modification includes transduction of cells with vectors or viruses, fusion of cells with tumor cell lines, or pulsing of cells with peptides, cell lysates, or other agents.

Name Elements: Product name composition: Prefix + Infix 1 + Infix 2 + Stem Qualifier. There may be more than one infix in the name.

Prefix: Established by USAN Council for uniqueness.

Infixes: May include:
- manipulation (*-gen* = transduced; *-pul* = pulsed with peptide or other agent; *-fus* = fused with peptide, cells, or other agent)
- cell type (*-myo* = myoblast, *-isle* = islet cell, *-den* = dendritic cell)

Suffixes:
- *-cel* (stem for all cell therapies)
- *-imut* (stem for all noncellular cell therapy products, including cell lysates, peptides, or proteins used for cancer vaccines).

Sub-stems for these vaccines include:

-*lisimut* (stem for cell lysates)

-*pepimut* (stem for peptides)

-*protimut* (stem for protein)

Qualifiers: Letter after hyphen at end of name
- T = Autologous
- L = Allogeneic
- X = Xenogeneic

Guidelines for Naming Cellular Therapies: The primary cell type in the product precedes the stem *-cel*. Residual or contaminating cells are not part of the name. Information on contaminating cells and reagents are included in prescribing information. Example: an autologous fibroblast cell product is *-fibrocel-T* or *-ficel-T*.

(1) Infixes for manipulation precede the infix for the cell type/category.

(2) If a product manipulation (eg, fusion to a tumor cell) has occurred, the infix *-fus* is part of the name. A description of the article(s) fused to the primary cell are provided in prescribing information. For example, a dendritic cell product fused with tumor cells would be *-fusdencel*.

(3) If a product manipulation (eg, pulsing) has occurred, the infix *-pul* alone is used. If more than one article or cell type has been used to pulse the product, only the pulsing manipulation infix *-pul* is part of the name. Details of the articles used to pulse the product

are provided in prescribing information. For example, a dendritic cell product pulsed with a tumor cell line or various tumor cell lines would be *-puldencel* or *-fuspuldencel.*

(4) If more than one article or cell type has been used to pulse the product, only the pulsing manipulation infix *-pul* is part of the name.

(5) In situations where one tumor cell line is used to pulse a product and another tumor cell line is fused to the primary cell, only infixes for the manipulations (ie, fused and pulsed) are included in the name. For example, *-pulfusdencel* (ie, pulsed and fused dendritic cell).

(6) If the primary cells have been transduced with a vector or virus, the infix *-gen-* is used. For example, plasmid DNA transduced retinal epithelial cells would be *-genretcel.*

(7) To distinguish various stem cell types, the infix for the cell type precedes the infix for progenitor *-tem.* For example, a neuronal stem cell is designated *-neurotemcel.*

(8) For tumor cancer cell lines used to prepare therapeutic immunomodulators (eg, cancer vaccines), the infix for the tumor cell type or source precedes the suffix *-tucel.* These products are cellular products. For example, a melanoma cell line used to prepare a therapeutic immunomodulating product (cancer vaccine) would be *-melatucel.* A melanoma cell product, pulsed or fused with other article(s), would be *-pulmeltucel* or *-fusmeltucel.* An autologous colon tumor therapeutic immunomodulator or vaccine would be *-coltucel.*

(9) Prophylactic vaccines are given descriptive names (eg, hepatitis B vaccine). This contrasts with therapeutic immunomodulators, frequently referred to as cancer vaccines, which is a misnomer. Therapeutic immunomodulators prepared using noncellular agents such as proteins, peptides, or cell lysates should have suffixes that set them apart from cellular immune modulators (cellular cancer or tumor vaccines). The suffix *-imut* (immunotherapeutics) is used. The infixes *-lis* (cell lysate), *-pep* (peptide), or *-pro* (protein) would precede the stem *-imut*, generating sub-stems for various noncellular vaccines: *-lisimut* (cell lysates), *-pepimut* (peptide), and *-protimut* (protein).

(10) The term immune cell or leukocyte (infix *-leu-*) will be used to describe hematopoietic cell preparations that do not fit a particular or specific cell type. Such cell preparations may contain a mixture of various blood cell elements. A subset of blood elements such as T-, B-, or NK-cells or antigen-presenting cells (APCs) that do not fit the definition of dendritic cells fall into this category.

(11) A product manipulation such as activation (eg, with cytokines) will be reflected in the name.

(12) Details of the manipulations and/or modifications will be described in prescribing information.

(13) The USAN Council will generate 2 or 3 letter prefixes for each name to provide uniqueness.

Proposed Infixes for Cellular Therapy Products:

Infixes for products:
- chondrocytes *-cho(n)-*
- dendritic cells *-den-*
- endothelial cell *-end(o)-*
- fibroblasts *-fi(b)-*
- hepatocytes *-hep(a)-*
- islets *-isle-*
- keratinocytes *-ker(a)-*
- myoblasts *-myo(b)-*

- renal tubular cells *-ren-*
- retinal epithelial cells *-ret-*
- tumor cells *-tucel*
    colon *-col-*
    glioma *-glio-*
    hepatic *-hep-*
    mammary *-mar-*
    melanoma *-mel-*
    nasopharyngeal *-naso-*
    prostate *-pros-*
    renal cell carcinoma *-ren-*
- gonad
    ovary *-ova-*
    testis *-tesi-*
- miscellaneous *-tum-*
- peripheral blood
    lymphocytes/monocytes/APC (white cells) *-leuco-*
    primary cord blood *-cor-*
- stem cells *-tem-*
    bone marrow *-myelotem-*
    mesenchymal *-mestem-*
    neuronal *-neurotem-*

Infixes for manipulation (used with the *-imut* stem):
- fused *-fus-*
- transduced with vector *-gen-*
- pulsed with tumor/peptide/virus *-pul-*

Infixes for therapeutic immunomodulators:
- cell lysate *-lis-*
- peptides *-pep-*
- protein *-pro(t)-*

Source: Cellular Therapies Working Group; United States Adopted Names Council. Cell therapy naming scheme. http://www.ama-assn.org/ama/pub/category/print/15395.html. Updated June 6, 2007. Accessed August 27, 2007.

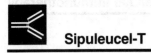

Sipuleucel-T

Cellular Immunotherapy

Name: *Manufacturer:*
  Provenge   Dendreon
Synonyms: APC8015

Immunologic Characteristics

Viability: Live human mononuclear cells harvested from the patient

Antigenic Type: Sipuleucel-T consists of autologous peripheral blood mononuclear cells, including antigen-presenting cells (APCs), that have been activated during a defined culture period with a recombinant human protein that consists of prostatic acid phosphatase (PAP), an antigen expressed in prostate cancer tissue, linked to granulocyte-macrophage colony-stimulating factor (GM-CSF), an immune cell activator. During culture, the recombinant antigen can bind to and be processed by APCs into smaller protein fragments. The recombinant antigen is designed to target APCs, and it may assist in directing the immune response to PAP. Minimal residual levels of intact PAP-GM-CSF are detectable in the final sipuleucel-T product. The cellular composition of sipuleucel-T is dependent on the cells obtained during leukapheresis. In addition to APCs, the final product contains T-cells, B-cells, natural killer cells, and other cells. The number of cells present and the cellular composition of each sipuleucel-T dose will vary.

Strains: Autologous to the patient from whom the cells were harvested

Use Characteristics

Indications: To treat asymptomatic or minimally symptomatic metastatic castrate-resistant (hormone-refractory) prostate cancer.

Contraindications: None

Immunodeficiency: Sipuleucel-T is designed to stimulate the immune system; concurrent use of immunosuppressive agents may alter the efficacy and/or safety of sipuleucel-T.

Elderly: In controlled trials, 72.6% (438/601) of patients in the sipuleucel-T group were 65 years of age and older. There were no apparent differences in safety of sipuleucel-T between patients 65 years of age and older and younger patients. In a survival analysis in metastatic castrate-resistant prostate cancer, 78% (382/488) of randomized patients were 65 years of age and older. The median survival of the sipuleucel-T group 65 years of age and older was 23.4 months (95% confidence interval [CI], 22-27.1), compared with 17.3 months in the control group (95% CI, 13.5-21.5).

Carcinogenicity: Sipuleucel-T has not been evaluated for carcinogenic potential.

Mutagenicity: Sipuleucel-T has not been evaluated for mutagenic potential.

Fertility Impairment: Sipuleucel-T has not been evaluated for impairment of fertility.

Children: Safety and efficacy of sipuleucel-T in children have not been established.

Adverse Reactions: The safety evaluation of sipuleucel-T is based on 601 patients with prostate cancer in the sipuleucel-T group who underwent at least 1 leukapheresis procedure in 4 randomized, controlled trials. The control was nonactivated autologous peripheral blood mononuclear cells. Almost all (98%) patients in the sipuleucel-T group and 96% in the control group reported an adverse event. The most common adverse events, reported in the sipuleucel-T group at a rate of at least 15%, were chills, fatigue, fever, back pain, nausea, joint ache, and headache. In 67% of the sipuleucel-T group, these adverse events were mild or moderate in severity. Severe (grade 3) and life-threatening (grade 4) adverse events were reported in 24% and 4% of the sipuleucel-T group, respectively, compared with 25% and 3% of the control group, respectively. Fatal (grade 5) adverse events were reported in 3.3% of the sipuleucel-T group, compared with 3.6% of the control group. The most common (at least 2%) grade 3 to 5 adverse events reported in the sipuleucel-T group were back pain and chills. Serious adverse events were reported in 24% of the sipuleucel-T group and 25% of the control group. Serious adverse events in the sipuleucel-T group included acute infusion reactions, cerebrovascular events, and single case reports of eosinophilia, rhabdomyolysis, myasthenia gravis, myositis, and tumor flare. Sipuleucel-T was discontinued in 1.5% of patients in study 1 because of adverse events. Some patients who required central venous catheters (CVCs) for treatment with sipuleucel-T developed infections, including sepsis. A small number of these patients discontinued treatment as a result. Monitor patients with CVCs for infectious sequelae.

Infusion reactions: Acute infusion reactions included fever, chills, respiratory events (eg, dyspnea, hypoxia, bronchospasm), nausea, vomiting, fatigue, hypertension, and tachycardia. In controlled trials, 71% of the sipuleucel-T group developed an acute infusion reaction. The most common events (20% or more) were chills, fever, and fatigue. In 95% of patients reporting acute infusion reactions, the events were mild or moderate. Fever and chills generally resolved within 2 days (72% and 89%, respectively). In controlled trials, severe (grade 3) acute infusion reactions were reported in 3.5% of patients in the sipuleucel-T group. The incidence of severe events was higher after the second infusion (2.1% vs 0.8% after first infusion), and decreased to 1.3% after the third infusion. Some (1.2%) patients in the sipuleucel-T group were hospitalized within 1 day of infusion to manage acute infusion reactions. No grade 4 or 5 acute infusion reactions were reported in the sipuleucel-T group. If an acute infusion reaction occurs, decrease or stop the infusion rate, depending on severity. Administer appropriate medical therapy as needed. Closely monitor patients with cardiac or pulmonary conditions.

Leukapheresis: Each dose of sipuleucel-T requires a standard leukapheresis procedure approximately 3 days before infusion. Adverse events reported 1 day or less after a leukapheresis procedure in 5% or more of patients included citrate toxicity (14%), oral paresthesia (13%), other paresthesia (11%), and fatigue (8%).

Cerebrovascular: In controlled trials, cerebrovascular events, including hemorrhagic and ischemic strokes, were observed in 3.5% of the sipuleucel-T group, compared with 2.6% of the control group.

Pharmacologic & Dosing Characteristics

Dosage: Before infusion, confirm that the patient's identity matches the identifiers on the infusion bag. Only use product prepared from cells of the same patient (autologous use only). Administer 3 doses at approximately 2-week intervals. Infuse the entire volume of the bag.

Route: Infuse intravenously (IV) over approximately 60 minutes. Do not use a cell filter. Interrupt or slow infusion for acute infusion reactions, depending on severity.

Overdosage: Each sipuleucel-T infusion comprises the maximum number of cells that can be processed from a single leukapheresis procedure. The number of cells in sipuleucel-T does not exceed the number of cells collected from the leukapheresis. There are no known instances of overdosage from either a single infusion or a full course of therapy with sipuleucel-T.

Missed Doses: In controlled trials, the median dosing interval between infusions was 2 weeks (range, 1 to 15 weeks). The maximum dosing interval has not been established. A patient who cannot receive a scheduled infusion of sipuleucel-T for any reason will need to undergo an additional leukapheresis procedure if treatment is to be continued. Advise patients of this possibility before starting treatment.

Sipuleucel-T

Related Interventions: To minimize acute infusion reactions, such as chills or fever, premedicate patients with oral acetaminophen and an antihistamine (eg, diphenhydramine) approximately 30 minutes before administering sipuleucel-T.

In controlled trials, symptoms of acute infusion reactions were treated with acetaminophen, IV histamine$_1$- and/or histamine$_2$-blockers, and low-dose IV meperidine.

Efficacy: The effect of sipuleucel-T on patients with metastatic castrate-resistant (hormone-refractory) prostate cancer was studied in 3 similar randomized, double-blind, placebo-controlled, multicenter trials. After randomization, patients from both treatment groups underwent a series of leukapheresis procedures (at approximately weeks 0, 2, and 4). Each leukapheresis procedure was followed approximately 3 days later by infusion of sipuleucel-T or control. The control was autologous peripheral blood mononuclear cells that had not been activated. Following disease progression, patients were treated at the health care provider's discretion with other anticancer interventions.

Study 1 assessed patients with asymptomatic or minimally symptomatic metastatic castrate-resistant (hormone-refractory) prostate cancer. Eligible patients had metastatic disease in soft tissue and/or bone, with evidence of progression at these sites or determined by serial prostate-specific antigen (PSA) measurements. Exclusion criteria included visceral (eg, liver, lung, brain) metastases, moderate to severe prostate cancer–related pain, and use of narcotics for cancer-related pain. A total of 512 patients were randomized in a 2:1 ratio to receive sipuleucel-T (n = 341) or control (n = 171). The median age was 71 years, and 90% of the patients were white. Thirty-five percent of patients had undergone radical prostatectomy, 54% had received local radiotherapy, and 82% had received combined androgen blockade. All patients had baseline testosterone levels less than 50 ng/mL. Forty-eight percent of patients were receiving bisphosphonates and 18% had received prior chemotherapy, including docetaxel. Eighty-two percent of patients had an Eastern Cooperative Oncology Group performance status of 0; 58% had primary Gleason scores of 4 or more; 44% had bone and soft tissue disease; 48% had bone-only disease; 7% had soft tissue-only disease; and 43% had more than 10 bony metastases.

In study 1, 237 of 512 randomized patients were evaluated for development of humoral and T-cell immune responses (proliferative and gamma-interferon *ELISpot* [enzyme-linked immunospot]) to the target antigens at baseline, and at weeks 6, 14, and 26. Antibody (immunoglobulin M and immunoglobulin G) responses against PAP-GM-CSF and PAP antigen alone were observed through the follow-up period in the sipuleucel-T group. Neutralizing antibody responses to GM-CSF were transient. T-cell proliferative and *ELISpot* responses to PAP-GM-CSF fusion protein were observed in cells collected from peripheral blood of patients through the follow-up period in the sipuleucel-T group, but not in controls. In some patients, a response to PAP antigen alone was observed. No conclusions could be made regarding the clinical significance of the observed immune responses.

Study 2 assessed patients with metastatic castrate-resistant prostate cancer and no cancer-related pain. The primary end point was time to disease progression; analysis of the primary end point did not reach statistical significance. All patients were to be followed for survival; however, the survival analysis was not prespecified. A third study similar in design to study 2 was terminated before completion of planned accrual.

Survival findings were consistent across multiple subgroups. Analyses of time to disease progression did not meet statistical significance in any phase 3 study of sipuleucel-T.

Summary of Overall Survival (All Patients as Randomized)				
	Study 1		Study 2	
	Sipuleucel-T (n = 341)	Control (n = 171)	Sipuleucel-T (n = 82)	Control (n = 45)
Overall survival median (95% CI)	25.8 months (22.8 to 27.7)	21.7 months (17.7 to 23.8)	25.9 months (20 to 32.4)	21.4 months (12.3 to 25.8)
HR (95% CI)	0.775[a] (0.614-0.979)		0.586[b] (0.388-0.884)	
P value	0.032[a]		0.01[c]	

a Hazard ratio (HR) and P value based on the Cox Model adjusted for PSA (ln) and lactate dehydrogenase (ln) and stratified by bisphosphonate use, number of bone metastases, and primary Gleason grade.
b HR based on the unadjusted Cox Model (not prespecified).
c P value based on a log-rank test (not prespecified).

Mechanism: Sipuleucel-T provides autologous cellular immunotherapy. While the mechanism of action is unknown, sipuleucel-T is designed to induce an immune response targeted against PAP, an antigen expressed in most prostate cancers. During ex-vivo culture with PAP-GM-CSF, APCs take up and process the recombinant target antigen into small peptides that are then displayed on the APC surface.

Drug Interactions: Use of either chemotherapy or immunosuppressive agents (eg, systemic corticosteroids) given concurrently with the leukapheresis procedure or sipuleucel-T has not been studied. Sipuleucel-T is designed to stimulate the immune system, and concurrent use of immunosuppressive agents may alter the efficacy and/or safety of sipuleucel-T. Therefore, evaluate patients to determine whether it is medically appropriate to reduce or discontinue immunosuppressive agents before treatment with sipuleucel-T.

Patient Information: Inform the patient or caregiver about the following:

- The recommended course of therapy for sipuleucel-T is 3 complete doses. Each infusion of sipuleucel-T is preceded by a leukapheresis procedure approximately 3 days beforehand. Patients will need to keep all scheduled appointments and arrive at each appointment on time because the leukapheresis and infusions must be appropriately spaced and the sipuleucel-T expiration time must not be exceeded.

- Patients who are unable to receive an infusion of sipuleucel-T will need to undergo an additional leukapheresis procedure if the treatment is to be continued.

- Counsel patients on the importance of adhering to preparation instructions for the leukapheresis procedure, the possible adverse effects of leukapheresis, and postprocedure care.

- If a patient does not have adequate peripheral venous access to accommodate the leukapheresis procedure and infusion of sipuleucel-T, a central venous catheter may be needed. Counsel patients on proper catheter care.

- Instruct patients to tell their health care provider if they are experiencing fever or any swelling or redness around the catheter site because these symptoms could be signs of an infection.

- Report signs and symptoms of acute infusion reactions such as fever, chills, fatigue, breathing problems, dizziness, high blood pressure, nausea, vomiting, headache, or muscle aches.

- Report any symptoms suggestive of a cardiac arrhythmia.

- Patients should inform their health care provider if they are taking immunosuppressive agents.

Pharmaceutical Characteristics

Concentration: Each dose of sipuleucel-T contains a minimum of 50 million autologous CD54+ cells activated with PAP-GM-CSF, suspended in 250 mL of Ringer's lactate injection in a sealed, patient-specific infusion bag.

Quality Assay: Potency is determined in part by measuring the increased expression of the CD54 molecule, also known as intercellular adhesion molecule 1, on the surface of APCs after culture with PAP-GM-CSF. CD54 is a cell-surface molecule that plays a role in the immunologic interactions between APCs and T-cells, and is considered a marker of immune cell activation.

Sipuleucel-T is released for infusion based on the microbial and sterility results from several tests: microbial contamination determination by gram stain, endotoxin content, and in-process sterility with a 2-day incubation to determine absence of microbial growth. The final (7-day incubation) sterility test results are not available at the time of infusion. If the sterility results become positive for microbial contamination after sipuleucel-T has been approved for infusion, Dendreon will notify the treating health care provider. Dendreon will attempt to identify the microorganism, perform antibiotic sensitivity testing on recovered microorganisms, and communicate the results to the treating health care provider. Additional information from the health care provider may be requested to determine the source of contamination.

Packaging: 250 mL patient-specific infusion bag (NDC #: none issued)

Doseform: Suspension

Appearance: Contents of the bag will be slightly cloudy, with a cream-to-pink color.

Solvent: Ringer's lactate injection (containing sodium chloride, sodium lactate, potassium chloride, and calcium chloride dihydrate)

Adjuvant: None

Preservative: None

Allergens: None

Excipients: None

pH: 6 to 7.5

Shelf Life: Data not provided.

Storage/Stability: Sipuleucel-T will arrive in a cardboard shipping box with a special insulated polyurethane container inside. The insulated container and gel packs within the container maintain the appropriate transportation and storage temperature of sipuleucel-T until infusion. Store the sipuleucel-T infusion bag within the insulated polyurethane container until administration. Do not remove the insulated polyurethane container from the outer cardboard shipping box. Contact the manufacturer regarding exposure to freezing or elevated temperatures.

Handling: Sipuleucel-T is not routinely tested for transmissible infectious diseases and may transmit diseases to people handling the product. Follow universal precautions. Sipuleucel-T is intended solely for autologous use.

(1) Sipuleucel-T is shipped directly to the infusing provider.

(2) Sipuleucel-T will arrive in a cardboard shipping box with a special insulated polyurethane container inside. The insulated container and gel packs maintain the appropriate temperature of sipuleucel-T until infusion.

(3) Upon receipt, open the outer cardboard shipping box to verify the product and patient-specific labels located on the top of the insulated container. Do not remove this insulated container from the shipping box or open the lid of the insulated container until the patient is ready for infusion.

(4) Do not infuse sipuleucel-T until confirmation of product release has been received from Dendreon. Dendreon will send a Cell Product Disposition Form containing the patient identifiers, expiration date and time, and the disposition status (approved for infusion or rejected) to the infusion site.

(5) Infusion must begin before the expiration date and time indicated on the Cell Product Disposition Form and Product Label. Do not initiate infusion of expired sipuleucel-T. Once the sipuleucel-T infusion bag is removed from the insulated container, it should remain at room temperature for no more than 3 hours. Do not return sipuleucel-T to the shipping container.

(6) After the patient is prepared for infusion and the Cell Product Disposition Form has been received, remove the sipuleucel-T infusion bag from the insulated container and inspect for signs of leakage. Contents of the bag will be slightly cloudy, with a cream-to-pink color. Gently mix and resuspend the contents of the bag, inspecting for clumps and clots. Small clumps of cellular material should disperse with gentle manual mixing. Do not administer if the bag leaks or if clumps remain in the bag.

(7) Before sipuleucel-T infusion, match the patient's identity with the patient identifiers on the Cell Product Disposition Form and the sipuleucel-T infusion bag. Observe the patient for at least 30 minutes after each infusion. If sipuleucel-T infusion must be interrupted, do not resume infusion if the infusion bag will be held at room temperature for more than 3 hours.

Production Process: Sipuleucel-T is made from the patient's own mononuclear cells. These cells are collected approximately 3 days before each scheduled infusion of sipuleucel-T at a leukapheresis center. The cells are sent to a special center where they are mixed with a protein to prepare them for infusion.

Media: Human mononuclear cells

Other Information

First Licensed: April 29, 2010

References: Harzstark AL, Small EJ. Sipuleucel-T for the treatment of prostate cancer. *Drugs Today (Barc).* 2008;44(4):271-278.

Higano CS, Schellhammer PF, Small EJ, et al. Integrated data from 2 randomized, double-blind, placebo-controlled, phase 3 trials of active cellular immunotherapy with sipuleucel-T in advanced prostate cancer. *Cancer.* 2009;115(16):3670-3679.

Sipuleucel-T Summary Table	
Generic name	Sipuleucel-T
Brand name	*Provenge*
Synonyms	APC8015
Manufacturer	Dendreon
Viability	Live human mononuclear cells
Indication	To treat asymptomatic or minimally symptomatic metastatic castrate-resistant (hormone-refractory) prostate cancer
Strains	Autologous to the patient
Concentration	Each dose contains at least 50 million autologous CD54+ cells activated with PAP-GM-CSF, suspended in 250 mL
Conjugating protein	None
Adjuvant	None
Preservative	None
Production medium	Autologous
Doseform	Suspension of cells
Solvent	Ringer's lactate injection
Packaging	Sealed, patient-specific infusion bag
Routine storage	2° to 8°C
Stability	Discard beyond the labeled infusion start time
Dosage	250 mL of patient-specific product
Standard schedule	Administer 3 doses at ≈ 2-week intervals
Route	Infuse over ≈ 60 minutes

Pertinent Nonimmunologic Drugs

Botulinum Toxins

Comparison of Botulinum Toxin Products[a]

	Type A			Type B
Generic name	OnabotulinumtoxinA	AbobotulinumtoxinA	IncobotulinumtoxinA	RimabotulinumtoxinB
Proprietary name	*Botox*	*Dysport*	*Xeomin*	*Myobloc*
Manufacturer	Allergan	Ipsen	Merz Pharmaceuticals	Elan
Labeled indications	Cervical dystonia, strabismus, blepharospasm associated with dystonia, or primary axillary hyperhidrosis; moderate to severe glabellar lines; muscle stiffness in adults with upper limb spasticity, urinary incontinence, chronic migraine	Cervical dystonia, and for temporary improvement in appearance of moderate to severe glabellar lines	Cervical dystonia, blepharospasm	Cervical dystonia
Strain	Hall strain	Hall strain	Hall strain	Bean strain
Dose[a]	*Strabismus/blepharospasm:* 1.25 to 5 type A units initially, later maximum 25 type A units per muscle *Cervical dystonia:* 200 to 300 type A units, customized to patient response *Glabellar lines:* 5 injections of 4 type A units each *Muscle spasticity:* 12.5 to 50 units per site *Detrusor overactivity:* Total 200 units, as 6.7 units per 1 mL injections across 30 sites *Chronic migraine:* Total 155 units, as 5 units per 0.1 mL injections across 7 muscles	*Cervical dystonia:* 500 units as a divided dose among affected muscles, repeated every 12 to 16 weeks or longer with doses between 250 and 1,000 units, based on patient response *Glabellar lines:* 50 units divided in 5 equal injections among affected muscles, repeated no more often than every 3 months	*Cervical dystonia:* 120 units per treatment *Blepharospasm:* Based on previous dose of onabotulinumtoxinA	2,500 to 5,000 type B units divided among affected muscles
Route	IM	IM	IM	IM
Standard schedule	Individualize therapy	Individualize therapy	Individualize therapy	Individualize therapy
Age range	≥ 12 years	*Cervical dystonia:* Adults *Glabellar lines:* Adults < 65 years	≥ 18 years	≥ 18 years
Doseform	Powder for solution	Powder for solution	Powder for solution	Solution
Concentration (units cannot be compared)[a]	100 type A units per vial	*Cervical dystonia:* 500 units/mL *Glabellar lines:* 120 to 200 units/mL	1.25 to 20 units per 0.1 mL	5,000 type B units/mL
Packaging[a]	100 type A units per vial	500 unit vial, 300 unit vial	50 unit vial, 100 unit vial	2,500 type B units per 0.5 mL, 5,000 type B units/mL, 10,000 type B units per 2 mL
Diluent	Sodium chloride 0.9%	Sodium chloride 0.9%	Sodium chloride 0.9%	Not applicable
Routine storage	Refrigerate at 2° to 8°C	Refrigerate at 2° to 8°C	Room temperature, refrigerator, or freezer	Refrigerate 2° to 8°C

a Dosage units follow different scales. Units of activity cannot be compared between botulinum toxin type A and type B products.

Botulinum Toxins Summary

Perspective:

1817-1822: Kerner describes disease now known as food-borne botulism and extracts botulinum toxin from sausage.

1870: Müller names sausage poisoning with the word botulism (from the Latin botulus, meaning "sausage").

1895: van Ermengem discovers *Bacillus botulinus*, later renamed *C. botulinum* bacteria

1977: Scott begins human trials of botulinum toxin.

Names: *Manufacturers:*
Dysport   Ipsen Biopharm, Ltd

Comparison: The potency units of various botulinum toxins are not interchangeable with other botulinum toxin products; therefore, units of biological activity cannot be compared with or converted into units of any other botulinum toxin product.

Immunologic Characteristics

Microorganism: Bacterium, *Clostridium botulinum*, anaerobic, endospore-forming gram-positive rod

Viability: Inactivated bacteriologically, but active toxin type A

Antigenic Form: Bacterial exotoxin type A neurotoxin complex

Antigenic Type: Protein

Strains: Hall strain

Use Characteristics

Indications: To treat adults with cervical dystonia to reduce the severity of abnormal head position and neck pain in both toxin-naive and previously treated patients.

For the temporary improvement in appearance of moderate to severe glabellar lines associated with procerus and corrugator muscle activity in adult patients younger than 65 years of age.

Limitations: Use caution when administering abobotulinumtoxinA to patients with surgical alterations to the facial anatomy, marked facial asymmetry, inflammation at the injection site(s), ptosis, excessive dermatochalasis, deep dermal scarring, or thick sebaceous skin. Concomitant neuromuscular disorder may exacerbate clinical effects of treatment. The safety of abobotulinumtoxinA for the treatment of hyperhidrosis has not been established.

Contraindications: Hypersensitivity to any botulinum-toxin product or excipients in this formulation. Allergy to cow's milk protein. Infection at the proposed injection site(s).

Immunodeficiency: No impairment of effect is likely.

Elderly:

Dystonia: There were insufficient patients 65 years or older in clinical studies to determine whether they respond differently than younger patients. Evaluate elderly patients for their greater frequency of concomitant disease and other drug therapy.

Glabellar lines: Of the subjects in placebo-controlled studies, 8 (1%) were 65 years and older. Efficacy was not observed in subjects 65 years and older. For the entire safety database of geriatric subjects, although there was no increase in the incidence of eyelid ptosis, geriatric subjects did have a higher rate of ocular events compared with younger subjects (11% vs 5%).

Carcinogenicity: AbobotulinumtoxinA has not been evaluated for carcinogenic potential.

Mutagenicity: AbobotulinumtoxinA has not been evaluated for mutagenic potential.

Fertility Impairment: In a fertility and early embryonic development study in rats in which either males (2.9, 7.2, 14.5, or 29 units/kg) or females (7.4, 20, 39, or 79 units/kg) received weekly IM injections before and after mating, dose-related increases in preimplantation loss and reduced numbers of corpora lutea were noted in treated females. Failure to mate was observed in males that received the high dose. The no-effect dose for effects on fertility was 7.4 units/kg in females and 14.5 units/kg in males (about half and equal to, respectively, the maximum recommended human dose [MRHD] of 1,000 units on a body-weight basis).

Pregnancy: Category C. AbobotulinumtoxinA produced embryo-fetal toxicity when given to pregnant rats at doses similar to or greater than the MRHD of 1,000 units on a body-weight (units/kg) basis. In an embryo-fetal development study in which pregnant rats received IM injections daily (2.2, 6.6, or 22 units/kg on gestation days 6 through 17) or intermittently (44 units/kg on gestation days 6 and 12 only) during organogenesis, increased early embryonic death was observed with both dosing schedules. The no-effect dose for embryo-fetal developmental toxicity was 2.2 units/kg (10% of MRHD). Maternal toxicity was seen at 22 and 44 units/kg. In a pre-and postnatal development study in which female rats received 6 weekly IM injections (4.4, 11, 22, or 44 units/kg) beginning on day 6 of gestation and continuing through parturition to weaning, an increase in stillbirths was observed at the highest dose, which was maternally toxic. The no-effect dose for pre- and postnatal developmental toxicity was 22 units/kg (comparable with MRHD). There are no adequate and well-controlled studies in pregnant women. Use abobotulinumtoxinA during pregnancy only if the potential benefit justifies the potential risk to the fetus.

Lactation: It is not known if botulinum toxin crosses into human breast milk.

Children: Safety and efficacy in children younger than 18 years have not been established.

Adverse Reactions: The effects of any botulinum-toxin product may spread from the injection area to produce symptoms consistent with botulinum toxin effects. These symptoms have been reported hours to weeks after injection, including asthenia, generalized muscle weakness, diplopia, blurred vision, ptosis, dysphagia, dysphonia, dysarthria, urinary incontinence, and breathing difficulties. Swallowing and breathing difficulties can be life-threatening, and there have been reports of death. The risk of symptoms is probably greatest in children treated for spasticity, but symptoms can also occur in adults treated for spasticity and other conditions, particularly in those who have underlying conditions that would predispose them to these symptoms. In unapproved uses, including spasticity in children and adults, and in approved indications, cases of spread of effect have been reported at doses comparable with those used to treat cervical dystonia and at lower doses.

Dystonia: Most commonly observed adverse reactions (more than 5% of patients) are muscular weakness, dysphagia, dry mouth, injection-site discomfort, fatigue, headache, neck pain, musculoskeletal pain, dysphonia, injection-site pain, and eye disorders.

Glabellar lines: The most frequently reported adverse events (2% or more) are nasopharyngitis, headache, injection-site pain, injection-site reaction, upper respiratory tract infection, eyelid edema, eyelid ptosis, sinusitis, and nausea.

Dysphagia and breathing: Treatment with botulinum-toxin products can result in swallowing or breathing difficulties. Patients with preexisting swallowing or breathing difficulties may be more susceptible. In most cases, this is a consequence of weakening of muscles in the area of injection that are involved in breathing or swallowing. When distant effects occur, additional respiratory muscles may be involved. Deaths as a complication of severe dysphagia have been reported. Dysphagia may persist for several weeks and require use of a feeding tube to maintain adequate nutrition and hydration. Aspiration may result from severe dysphagia and is a particular risk when treating patients in whom swallowing or respiratory function is already compromised. Treatment of cervical dystonia may weaken neck muscles that serve as accessory muscles of ventilation. This may result in a critical loss of breathing capacity in patients with respiratory disorders who may have become dependent upon these accessory muscles. Patients treated with botulinum toxin may require immediate medical attention if they develop problems with swallowing or speech or respiratory disorders. These reactions can occur within hours to weeks after injection with botulinum toxin.

Facial anatomy: Use caution in patients with surgical alterations to the facial anatomy, excessive weakness or atrophy in the target muscle(s), marked facial asymmetry, inflammation at the injection site(s), ptosis, excessive dermatochalasis, deep dermal scarring, thick seba-ceous skin, or the inability to substantially lessen glabellar lines by physically spreading them apart.

Neuromuscular: Monitor individuals with peripheral motor neuropathic diseases, amyotro-phic lateral sclerosis, or neuromuscular junction disorders (eg, myasthenia gravis or Lambert-Eaton syndrome) closely when given botulinum toxin. Patients with neuromuscu-lar disorders may be at increased risk of clinically significant effects, including severe dys-phagia and respiratory compromise from typical doses of abobotulinumtoxinA.

Dystonia: Data described below reflect 357 patients with cervical dystonia in 6 studies. Of these, 2 studies were randomized, double-blind, single-treatment, placebo-controlled studies with subsequent optional open-label treatment in which dose optimization (250 to 1,000 units per treatment) over the course of 5 treatment cycles was allowed. The popu-lation was almost entirely white (99%), with a median age of 51 years (range, 18 to 82 years). Most patients (87%) were younger than 65 years of age; 58% were women.

Common events: The most commonly reported adverse events (more than 5% of patients who received 500 units of abobotulinumtoxinA in the placebo-controlled clinical trials) in patients with cervical dystonia were muscular weakness, dysphagia, dry mouth, injection-site discomfort, fatigue, headache, neck pain, musculoskeletal pain, dysphonia, injection-site pain, and eye disorders (ie, blurred vision, diplopia, reduced visual acuity and accommodation). Most adverse events were mild or moderate in severity. Other than injection-site reactions, most adverse events became noticeable about 1 week after treat-ment and lasted several weeks. The rates of adverse events were higher in the combined controlled and open-label experience than in the placebo-controlled trials. During the clinical studies, 2 patients (less than 1%) experienced adverse events leading to with-drawal. One patient experienced disturbance in attention, eyelid disorder, feeling abnor-mal, and headache, and one patient experienced dysphagia. The following table compares the incidence of the most frequent treatment-emergent adverse events (TEAEs) from a single treatment cycle of 500 units of abobotulinumtoxinA compared with placebo.

Most Common TEAEs (> 5%) and Greater than Placebo: Double-Blind Phase of Clinical Trials		
System Organ Class Preferred Term	AbobotulinumtoxinA 500 units (N = 173)	Placebo (N = 182)
Any TEAE	61%	51%
General disorders and injection-site conditions	30%	23%
Injection-site discomfort	13%	8%
Fatigue	12%	10%
Injection-site pain	5%	4%
Musculoskeletal and connective-tissue disorders	30%	18%
Muscular weakness	16%	4%
Musculoskeletal pain	7%	3%
Gastrointestinal disorders	28%	15%
Dysphagia	15%	4%
Dry mouth	13%	7%
Nervous system disorders	16%	13%
Headache	11%	9%
Infections and infestations	13%	9%
Respiratory, thoracic and mediastinal disorders	12%	8%
Dysphonia	6%	2%
Eye disorders[a]	7%	2%

a The following preferred terms were reported: vision blurred, diplopia, visual acuity reduced, eye pain, eyelid disorder, accommodation disorder, dry eye, eye pruritus.

AbobotulinumtoxinA

Dose-response relationships for common adverse events in a randomized, multiple fixed-dose study in which the total dose was divided between 2 muscles (the sternocleidomastoid and splenius capitis) are shown in this table. Subjects who received a higher dose of abobotulinumtoxinA had an increased incidence of eyelid ptosis.

Common TEAEs by Dose in Fixed-Dose Study				
System organ class Preferred term	Placebo	AbobotulinumtoxinA dose		
		250 units	500 units	1,000 units
Any adverse event	30%	37%	65%	83%
Dysphagia	5%	21%	29%	39%
Dry mouth	10%	21%	18%	39%
Muscular weakness	0%	11%	12%	56%
Injection-site discomfort	10%	5%	18%	22%
Dysphonia	0%	0%	18%	28%
Facial paresis	0%	5%	0%	11%
Eye disorders	0%	0%	6%	17%

Injection site: Injection-site discomfort and injection-site pain were common adverse events following abobotulinumtoxinA administration. These events were mainly of mild or moderate intensity.

Less common events: The following selected adverse events were reported less frequently (less than 5%). Breathing difficulties were reported by approximately 3% of abobotulinumtoxinA–treated patients and in 1% of placebo patients during the double-blind phase. These consisted mainly of dyspnea and were generally mild in intensity. The median time to onset from last dose of abobotulinumtoxinA was approximately 1 week, and the median duration was approximately 3 weeks. Other selected adverse events with incidence less than 5% in the 500 unit group in the double-blind phase included dizziness (3.5% vs 1%) and muscle atrophy (1% vs 0%).

Laboratory findings: Subjects treated with abobotulinumtoxinA exhibited a small increase from baseline (0.23 mol/L) in mean blood glucose relative to placebo-treated subjects. This was not clinically significant among these subjects but could be a factor in patients whose diabetes is difficult to control.

Electrocardiography: Electrocardiographic (ECG) measurements were only recorded in a limited number of subjects in an open-label study without a placebo or active control. This study showed a statistically significant reduction in heart rate compared with baseline, averaging about 3 beats per minute, observed 30 minutes after injection.

Glabellar lines: In placebo-controlled trials, the most frequently reported adverse events (2% or more) after injection of abobotulinumtoxinA were nasopharyngitis, headache, injection-site pain, injection-site reaction, upper respiratory tract infection, eyelid edema, eyelid ptosis, sinusitis, and nausea. The following table reflects 398 subjects 19 to 75 years of age evaluated in randomized, placebo-controlled clinical studies that assessed use of abobotulinumtoxinA for temporary improvement of glabellar lines. Adverse events of any cause were reported for 48% of abobotulinumtoxinA-treated and 33% of placebo-treated subjects. TEAEs were generally mild to moderate in severity.

Treatment-Emergent Adverse Events With > 1% Incidence		
Adverse events by body system	AbobotulinumtoxinA n = 398 (%)[a]	Placebo n = 496 (%)[a]
Any treatment-emergent adverse event	191 (48%)	163 (33%)
Eye disorders		
Eyelid edema	8 (2%)	0
Eyelid ptosis	6 (2%)	1 (< 1%)
GI disorders		
Nausea	6 (2%)	5 (1%)
General disorders and injection-site conditions		
Injection-site pain	11 (3%)	8 (2%)
Injection-site reaction	12 (3%)	2 (< 1%)
Infections and infestations		
Nasopharyngitis	38 (10%)	21 (4%)
Upper respiratory tract infection	12 (3%)	9 (2%)
Sinusitis	8 (2%)	6 (1%)
Investigations		
Blood urine present	6 (2%)	1 (< 1%)
Nervous system disorders		
Headache	37 (9%)	23 (5%)

a Subjects who received treatment with placebo and abobotulinumtoxinA are counted in both treatment columns.

In the overall safety database, where some subjects received up to 12 treatments with abobotulinumtoxinA, adverse events were reported for 57% (1,425 per 2,491) of subjects. The most frequently reported events were headache, nasopharyngitis, injection-site pain, sinusitis, upper respiratory tract infection, injection-site bruising, and injection-site reaction (eg, numbness, discomfort, erythema, tenderness, tingling, itching, stinging, warmth, irritation, tightness, swelling).

Adverse events that emerged after repeated injections in 2% to 3% of the population included bronchitis, influenza, pharyngolaryngeal pain, cough, contact dermatitis, injection-site swelling, and injection-site discomfort.

The incidence of eyelid ptosis did not increase in the long-term safety studies with multiple re-treatments at intervals of 3 months or longer. Most eyelid ptosis events were mild to moderate in severity and resolved over several weeks.

There is extensive postlicensing experience outside the United States in treating glabellar lines. The following adverse events have been identified: vertigo, eyelid ptosis, diplopia, blurred vision, photophobia, dysphagia, nausea, injection-site reaction, malaise, influenza-like illness, hypersensitivity, sinusitis, amyotrophy, burning sensation, facial paresis, dizziness, headache, hypoesthesia, erythema, and excessive granulation tissue.

Immunogenicity: As with all therapeutic proteins, there is potential for immunogenicity. About 3% of dystonia subjects developed antibodies (binding or neutralizing) over time with abobotulinumtoxinA treatment. The significance of these antibodies is unknown because, in the presence of binding and neutralizing antibodies, some patients may continue to experience clinical benefit. Testing for antibodies to abobotulinumtoxinA was performed for 1,554 glabellar-line subjects who had up to 9 cycles of treatment. Two subjects (0.13%) tested positive for binding antibodies at baseline. Three additional subjects tested positive for binding antibodies after receiving abobotulinumtoxinA treatment. None of the subjects tested positive for neutralizing antibodies.

AbobotulinumtoxinA

Pharmacologic & Dosing Characteristics

Dosage: Do not exceed the recommended dosage and frequency of administration of abobotulinumtoxinA.

Dystonia: Initial dose of 500 units divided among the affected muscles. Limiting the dose injected into the sternocleidomastoid muscle may reduce the occurrence of dysphagia. Simultaneous electromyography (EMG)-guided application may be helpful in locating active muscles not identified by physical examination alone.

Glabellar lines: Give a total dose of 50 units, divided in 5 equal aliquots of 10 units each, to affected muscles to achieve clinical effect. Do not re-treat more frequently than every 3 months.

Route: IM

Overdosage: Excessive doses of abobotulinumtoxinA may produce neuromuscular weakness with a variety of symptoms. Respiratory support may be required where excessive doses cause paralysis of respiratory muscles. Symptoms of overdose are likely not to be present immediately following injection. If accidental injection or oral ingestion occurs, monitor the person for several weeks for signs and symptoms of excessive muscle weakness or paralysis. Symptomatic treatment may be necessary. Doses exceeding 1,000 units were rarely studied in clinical settings for any indication. In case of overdose, botulism antitoxin is available from the CDC. Antitoxin will not reverse any botulinum toxin-induced effects already apparent at time of antitoxin administration.

Additional Doses:

Dystonia: Re-treat every 12 to 16 weeks or longer, as necessary, based on return of clinical symptoms, with doses between 250 and 1,000 units to optimize clinical benefit. Do not re-treat at intervals less than 12 weeks. Titrate doses in 250 unit steps, according to patient response.

Glabellar lines: Administer no more frequently than every 3 months.

Efficacy:

Ethnicity: Exploratory analyses in trials for glabellar lines in African-American subjects with Fitzpatrick skin types IV, V, or VI and in Hispanic subjects, suggested that response rates at day 30 were comparable with, and no worse than, the overall population.

Dystonia: Efficacy was evaluated in 2 well-controlled, randomized, double-blind, placebo-controlled, single-dose, parallel-group studies in treatment-naive patients with cervical dystonia. The principal analyses involved 252 patients (121 on abobotulinumtoxinA, 131 on placebo) with 36% male, 64% female, and 99% white. In both placebo-controlled studies (study 1 and study 2), abobotulinumtoxinA 500 units IM was divided among 2 to 4 affected muscles. These studies were followed by long-term open-label extensions that allowed titration in 250 unit steps to subsequent doses ranging from 250 to 1,000 units. In extension studies, re-treatment was determined by clinical need after a minimum of 12 weeks. The median time to re-treatment was 14 weeks, with the 75th percentile at 18 weeks. The primary assessment of efficacy involved the Toronto Western Spasmodic Torticollis Rating Scale (TWSTRS) change from baseline at week 4 for both studies. The scale evaluates severity of dystonia, patient-perceived disability from dystonia, and pain. The adjusted mean change from baseline in the TWSTRS total score was significantly greater for the abobotulinumtoxinA group than for the placebo group at weeks 4 in both studies. Analyses by gender, weight, geographic region, underlying pain, cervical dystonia severity at baseline, and history of treatment with botulinum toxin showed no meaningful differences between groups. The following table indicates the average abobotulinumtoxinA dose, and percentage of total dose, injected into specific muscles in the pivotal clinical trials.

AbobotulinumtoxinA 500 Unit Starting Dose[a] by Unilateral Muscle Injected During Double-Blind Pivotal Phase 3, Studies 2 and 1 Combined					
		Dose injected		Percentage of the total abobotulinumtoxinA dose injected	
Number of patients injected per muscle[b]		Median units (min, max)	75th percentile	Median units (min, max)	75th percentile
Sternocleidomastoid	90	125 units (50, 350)	150 units	26.5% (10, 70)	30%
Splenius capitis	85	200 units (75, 450)	250 units	40% (15, 90)	50%
Trapezius	50	103 units (50, 300)	150 units	20.6% (10, 60)	30%
Levator scapulae	35	105 units (50, 200)	125 units	21.1% (10, 40)	25%
Scalenus (medius and anterior)	26	116 units (50, 300)	150 units	23.1% (10, 60)	30%
Semispinalis capitis	21	132 units (50, 250)	175 units	29.4% (10, 50)	35%
Longissimus	3	150 units (100, 200)	200 units	30% (20, 40)	40%

a Units and percent of total dose.
b Total number of patients in combined studies 2 and 1 who received initial treatment = 121.

Glabellar lines: Three double-blind, randomized, placebo-controlled, clinical studies evaluated efficacy in the temporary improvement of appearance of moderate to severe glabellar lines. These 3 studies enrolled healthy adults (19 to 75 years of age) with glabellar lines of at least moderate severity at maximum frown. Subjects were excluded if they had marked ptosis, deep dermal scarring, or a substantial inability to lessen glabellar lines, even by physically spreading them apart. The subjects in these studies received either abobotulinumtoxinA or placebo. The total dose was delivered in equally divided aliquots to specified injection sites. Investigators and subjects assessed efficacy at maximum frown by using a 4-point scale (none, mild, moderate, severe). Overall treatment success was defined as posttreatment glabellar line severity of none or mild with at least 2-grade improvement from baseline for the combined investigator and subject assessments (composite assessment) on day 30. Additional end points for each study were posttreatment glabellar-line severity of none or mild with at least a 1-grade improvement from baseline for the separate investigator and subject assessments on day 30. After the randomized studies, subjects were offered participation in a 2-year, open-label re-treatment study to assess the safety of multiple treatments.

Treatment Success at Day 30		
	2-grade improvement	
Study	AbobotulinumtoxinA n/N (%)	Placebo n/N (%)
GL-1	58/105 (55%)	0/53 (0%)
GL-2	37/71 (52%)	0/71 (0%)
GL-3	120/200 (60%)	0/100 (0%)

Study GL-1: Investigators' and Subjects' Assessment of Glabellar Line Severity at Maximum Frown Using a 4-Point Scale (% and Number of Subjects with Severity of None or Mild)

Day	Investigators' assessment		Subjects' assessment	
	AbobotulinumtoxinA (N = 105)	Placebo (N = 53)	AbobotulinumtoxinA (N = 105)	Placebo (N = 53)
14	90% (95)	17% (9)	77% (81)	9% (5)
30	88% (92)	4% (2)	74% (78)	9% (5)
60	64% (67)	2% (1)	60% (63)	6% (3)
90	43% (45)	6% (3)	36% (38)	6% (3)
120	23% (24)	4% (2)	19% (20)	6% (3)
150	9% (9)	2% (1)	8% (8)	4% (2)
180	6% (6)	0% (0)	7% (7)	8% (4)

Study GL-2 was a repeat-dose, double-blind, multicenter, placebo-controlled, randomized study. The study was initiated with 2 or 3 open-label treatment cycles of abobotulinumtoxinA administered in 5 aliquots of 10 units each. After the open-label treatments, subjects were randomized to receive either placebo or abobotulinumtoxinA 50 units. Subjects could receive up to 4 treatments through the course of the study. Efficacy was assessed in the final randomized treatment cycle. The study enrolled 311 subjects into the first treatment cycle and 142 subjects were randomized into the final treatment cycle.

Overall, the mean age was 47 years; most subjects were women (86%) and predominantly white (80%). At day 30, 52% of abobotulinumtoxinA-treated subjects achieved treatment success defined as composite 2-grade improvement of glabellar line severity at maximum frown. The proportion of responders in the final treatment cycle was comparable with the proportion of responders in all prior treatment cycles. After the final repeat treatment with abobotulinumtoxinA, the reduction of glabellar line severity at maximum frown was greater at day 30 in the abobotulinumtoxinA group compared with the placebo group as assessed by both investigators and subjects.

Study GL-3 was a single-dose, double-blind, multicenter, randomized, placebo-controlled study in which 300 previously untreated subjects received either placebo or abobotulinumtoxinA, administered in 5 aliquots of 10 units each. Subjects were followed for 150 days. The mean age was 44 years; most subjects were women (87%), and predominantly white (75%) or Hispanic (18%). At day 30, 60% of abobotulinumtoxinA–treated subjects achieved treatment success defined as composite 2-grade improvement of glabellar line severity at maximum frown. The reduction of glabellar line severity at maximum frown was greater at day 30 in the abobotulinumtoxinA group compared with the placebo group as assessed by both investigators and subjects.

Onset:

Dystonia: 2 to 4 weeks after injection.

Glabellar lines: Within 14 to 30 days.

Duration:

Dystonia: Typically 12 weeks or longer.

Glabellar lines: Clinical effect may last up to 4 months. Clinical studies demonstrated continued efficacy with up to 4 repeated administrations.

Pharmacokinetics: The primary pharmacodynamic effect of abobotulinumtoxinA is due to chemical denervation of the treated muscle, resulting in a measurable decrease of the compound muscle action potential, causing a localized reduction of muscle activity. Using currently available analytical technology, it is not possible to detect abobotulinumtoxinA in the peripheral blood after IM injection at the recommended doses.

Mechanism: Botulinum toxins inhibit release of the neurotransmitter acetylcholine from peripheral cholinergic nerve endings. Toxin activity occurs in the following sequence: toxin heavy chain-mediated binding to specific surface receptors on nerve endings, internalization of the toxin by receptor-mediated endocytosis, pH-induced translocation of the toxin light chain to the cell cytosol, and cleavage of SNAP25 leading to intracellular blockage of neurotransmitter exocytosis into the neuromuscular junction. This accounts for the therapeutic utility of the toxin in diseases characterized by excessive efferent activity in motor nerves. Recovery of transmission occurs gradually as the neuromuscular junction recovers from SNAP25 cleavage and as new nerve endings are formed.

Drug Interactions: No formal drug interaction studies have been conducted with abobotulinumtoxinA. Closely observe patients treated concomitantly with botulinum toxins and aminoglycosides or other agents interfering with neuromuscular transmission (eg, curare-like agents) because the effect of the botulinum toxin may be potentiated. Using anticholinergic drugs after administration of abobotulinumtoxinA may potentiate systemic anticholinergic effects such as blurred vision. The effect of administering different botulinum neurotoxin products at the same time or within several months of each other is unknown. Excessive weakness may be exacerbated by another administration of botulinum toxin before resolution of effects of previously administered botulinum toxin. Excessive weakness may also be exaggerated by administration of a muscle relaxant before or after administration of abobotulinumtoxinA.

Patient Information: Advise patients to inform their doctor or pharmacist if they develop any unusual symptoms (eg, difficulty with swallowing, speaking or breathing), or if any known symptom persists or worsens. Counsel patients that if loss of strength, muscle weakness, blurred vision, or drooping eyelids occur they should avoid driving a car or engaging in other potentially hazardous activities.

Pharmaceutical Characteristics

Concentration:

Dystonia: 300 unit and 500 unit vials, to be reconstituted with 0.6 mL and 1 mL of sodium chloride 0.9%, respectively, to yield a concentration of 500 units per mL.

Glabellar lines: 300 unit vial, to be reconstituted with 1.5 or 2.5 mL of sodium chloride 0.9%, to yield a concentration of 120 or 200 units per mL. Using 2.5 mL of diluent yields 10 units per 0.08 mL injection. Using 1.5 mL of diluent yields 10 units per 0.05 mL injection.

Quality Assay: One unit of abobotulinumtoxinA corresponds to the calculated median lethal intraperitoneal dose (LD_{50}) in mice. The method for performing the assay is specific to Ipsen's product abobotulinumtoxinA. Units of biological activity of botulinum toxin products are not interchangeable.

Packaging:

Cervical dystonia: Single-use glass vial: Box containing one 500 unit vial (NDC#: 15054-0500-01), box containing two 500 unit vials (15054-0500-02). Box containing one 300 unit vial (15054-0530-06)

Glabellar lines: 300 unit single-use glass vial (99207-0500-30)

Doseform: Powder for solution

Appearance: Powder yielding a clear, colorless solution

Diluent:

For reconstitution: Sodium chloride 0.9%

Adjuvant: None

Preservative: None

Allergens: None

AbobotulinumtoxinA

Excipients: Albumin human 125 mcg per vial, lactose 2.5 mg/vial

pH: Not described

Shelf Life: Expires within 12 months.

Storage/Stability: Store at 2° to 8°C (36° to 46°F). Protect vials from light. Do not freeze. Contact the manufacturer regarding exposure to freezing or elevated temperatures. Shipping data not provided. Swirl gently to dissolve. After reconstitution, store abobotulinumtoxinA at 2° to 8°C (36° to 46°F) and use within 4 hours. Do not freeze after reconstitution.

Dystonia: Use a 23- or 25-gauge needle for administration.

Glabellar lines: Use a 30-gauge needle for administration.

Handling:

Glabellar lines: Glabellar facial lines arise from the activity of the lateral corrugator and vertical procerus muscles. These can be readily identified by palpating the tensed muscle mass while having a patient frown. The corrugator depresses the skin, creating a "furrowed" vertical line surrounded by tensed muscle (ie, frown lines). The location, size, and use of the muscles vary markedly among individuals.

Physicians administering abobotulinumtoxinA must understand the relevant neuromuscular and/or orbital anatomy of the area involved and any alterations to the anatomy caused by prior surgical procedures.

Risk of ptosis can be mitigated by careful examination of the upper lid for separation or weakness of the levator palpebrae muscle (true ptosis), identification of last ptosis, and evaluation of the range of lid excursion while manually depressing the frontalis to assess compensation. To reduce the complication of ptosis, take the following steps:
- Avoid injection near the levator palpebrae superioris, particularly in patients with larger brow-depressor complexes.
- Place medial corrugator injections at least 1 cm above the bony supraorbital ridge.
- Ensure the injected volume/dose is accurate and minimized.
- Do not inject the toxin closer than 1 cm above the central eyebrow.

To inject abobotulinumtoxinA, advance the needle through the skin into the underlying muscle while applying finger pressure on the superior medial orbital rim. Inject patients with a total of 50 units in 5 equally divided aliquots. Using a 30-gauge needle, inject 10 units of abobotulinumtoxinA into each of 5 sites, 2 in each corrugator muscle, and one in the procerus muscle.

Production Process: Botulinum toxin type A, the active ingredient in abobotulinumtoxinA, is a purified neurotoxin type A complex produced by fermentation of *Clostridium botulinum* type A, Hall strain. It is purified from the culture supernatant by a series of precipitation, dialysis, and chromatography steps. The neurotoxin complex is composed of the neurotoxin, hemagglutinin proteins and nontoxin nonhemagglutinin protein.

Media: *Clostridium botulinum* cultures

Other Information

First Licensed: April 30, 2009

IncobotulinumtoxinA

Botulinum Toxins

Names: *Manufacturers:*
  Xeomin   Merz Pharmaceuticals

Comparison: The potency units of various botulinum toxins are not interchangeable with other botulinum toxin products; therefore, units of biological activity cannot be compared to or converted into units of any other botulinum toxin product.

Immunologic Characteristics

Antigen Source: Bacterium, *Clostridium botulinum* anaerobic, endospore-forming gram-positive rod

Viability: Inactivated bacteriologically, but active toxin type A

Antigenic Form: Bacterial exotoxin type A neurotoxin

Antigenic Type: Protein. The neurotoxic component has a molecular weight of 150,000 daltons.

Strains: *C. botulinum* type A, Hall strain

Use Characteristics

Indications: To treat adults with blepharospasm previously treated with onabotulinumtoxinA (*Botox*, Allergan)

To treat adults with cervical dystonia, to decrease the severity of abnormal head position and neck pain in both botulinum toxin–naive and previously treated patients

Contraindications: Hypersensitivity to any botulinum neurotoxin type A or to any excipient

Use in patients with an infection at an injection site could lead to severe local or disseminated infection.

Immunodeficiency: No impairment of effect is likely.

Elderly:

Blepharospasm: In a phase 3 study, 41 patients were older than 65 years, including 29 of 75 (39%) patients who received incobotulinumtoxinA and 12 of 34 (35%) patients who received placebo. Of these patients, 22 of the 29 (76%) incobotulinumtoxinA-treated patients, compared with 7 of the 12 (58%) placebo-treated patients, experienced an adverse event. One incobotulinumtoxinA-treated patient experienced severe dysphagia.

Cervical dystonia: In a phase 3 study, 29 patients were older than 65 years, including 19 patients who received incobotulinumtoxinA and 10 patients who received placebo. Of these, 10 (53%) incobotulinumtoxinA-treated patients and 4 (40%) placebo-treated patients experienced an adverse event. For patients older than 65 years treated with incobotulinumtoxinA, the most common adverse events were dysphagia (4 patients [21%]) and asthenia (2 patients [11%]). One (5%) incobotulinumtoxinA-treated patient experienced severe dizziness.

Carcinogenicity: IncobotulinumtoxinA has not been evaluated for carcinogenic potential.

Mutagenicity: IncobotulinumtoxinA has not been evaluated for mutagenic potential.

Fertility Impairment: In a fertility and early embryonic development study in rabbits, males and females were dosed with incobotulinumtoxinA (1.25, 2.5, or 3.5 units/kg) intramuscularly (IM) every 2 weeks for 5 and 3 doses, respectively, beginning 2 weeks before mating. No effects on mating or fertility were observed. The highest dose tested is approximately twice the maximum recommended human dose (MRHD) for cervical dystonia (120 units) on a body weight basis.

Pregnancy: Category C. There are no adequate and well-controlled studies in pregnant women. Use only if clearly needed. It is not known if incobotulinumtoxinA crosses the placenta. Incobotulinumtoxin A was embryotoxic in rats and increased abortions in rabbits when given at doses higher than the MRHD for cervical dystonia (120 units) on a body weight basis. When incobotulinumtoxinA was administered IM to pregnant rats during organogenesis (3, 10, or 30 units/kg on gestational days 6, 12, and 19; 7 units/kg on gestational days 6 to 19; or 2, 6, or 18 units/kg on gestational days 6, 9, 12, 16, and 19), decreases in fetal body weight and skeletal ossification were observed at doses that were also maternally toxic. The no-effect level for embryotoxicity in rats was 6 units/kg (3 times the MRHD for cervical dystonia on a body weight basis). IM administration to pregnant rabbits during organogenesis (1.25, 2.5, or 5 units/kg on gestational days 6, 18, and 28) resulted in an increased rate of abortion at the highest dose, which was also maternally toxic. In rabbits, the no-effect level for increased abortion was 2.5 units/kg (similar to the MRHD for cervical dystonia on a body weight basis).

Lactation: It is not known if botulinum toxin type A crosses into human breast milk. Problems in humans have not been documented.

Children: IncobotulinumtoxinA has not been studied in patients younger than 18 years and is therefore not recommended in pediatric patients.

Adverse Reactions:

Blepharospasm: The most common adverse events (occurred in at least 5% of patients and more frequently than with placebo) were eyelid ptosis, dry eye, dry mouth, diarrhea, headache, visual impairment, dyspnea, nasopharyngitis, and respiratory tract infection. Injection into the orbicularis oculi muscle may lead to reduced blinking and corneal exposure with possible ulceration or perforation. Do not repeat lower lid injections if diplopia occurred with previous botulinum toxin injections.

Cervical dystonia: The most common adverse events (occurred in at least 5% of patients and more frequently than with placebo) were dysphagia, neck pain, muscle weakness, injection-site pain, and musculoskeletal pain. Patients with smaller neck muscle mass and patients who require bilateral injections into the sternocleidomastoid muscles are at greater risk of dysphagia. Limiting the dose injected into the sternocleidomastoid muscle may decrease the occurrence of dysphagia.

Distant effect: Effects of incobotulinumtoxinA and other botulinum toxins may be observed beyond the site of local injection. Such symptoms are consistent with the mechanism of action of botulinum toxin and may include asthenia, generalized muscle weakness, diplopia, blurred vision, ptosis, dysphagia, dysphonia, dysarthria, urinary incontinence, and breathing difficulties. These symptoms have been reported hours to weeks after injection. Swallowing and breathing difficulties can be life-threatening, and there have been reports of death related to these effects. The risk of symptoms is probably greatest in children treated for spasticity, but symptoms can occur in adults treated for spasticity and other conditions, particularly in patients who have underlying conditions that would predispose them to these symptoms. In unapproved uses, symptoms consistent with spread of toxin effect have been reported at doses comparable to or lower than doses used to treat cervical dystonia. Advise patients or caregivers to seek immediate medical care if swallowing, speech, or respiratory disorders occur.

Airway: Botulinum toxin products can result in swallowing or breathing difficulties. Patients with preexisting swallowing or breathing difficulties may be more susceptible to these complications. In most cases, this is a consequence of weakening of muscles involved in breathing or swallowing. When distant effects occur, additional respiratory muscles may be involved. Death as a complication of severe dysphagia has been reported after treatment with botulinum toxin. Dysphagia may persist for several months and require use of a feeding tube to maintain adequate nutrition and hydration. Aspiration may result from severe dysphagia. Treatment of cervical dystonia with botulinum toxins may weaken neck muscles that serve as accessory muscles of ventilation. This may result in critical loss of breathing capacity in patients with respiratory disorders dependent on these accessory muscles. There have been reports of serious breathing difficulties, including respiratory failure, in patients with cervical dystonia treated with botulinum toxin products. Patients with smaller neck muscle mass and patients who require bilateral injections into the sternocleidomastoid muscles have been reported to be at greater risk of dysphagia. In general, limiting the dose injected into the sternocleidomastoid muscle may decrease the occurrence of dysphagia. Patients treated with botulinum toxin may require immediate medical attention to treat swallowing, speech, or respiratory disorders. These reactions can occur within hours to weeks after injection with botulinum toxin.

Hypersensitivity: Hypersensitivity reactions have been reported with botulinum toxin products (eg, anaphylaxis, serum sickness, urticaria, soft tissue edema, dyspnea).

Preexisting neuromuscular disorders: Closely monitor patients with peripheral motor neuropathic diseases, amyotrophic lateral sclerosis, or neuromuscular junctional disorders (eg, myasthenia gravis, Lambert-Eaton syndrome) when given botulinum toxin. Patients with neuromuscular disorders may be at increased risk of clinically significant effects, including severe dysphagia and respiratory compromise.

Ophthalmic: Reduced blinking from injection of botulinum toxin products in the orbicularis muscle can lead to corneal exposure, persistent epithelial defect, and corneal ulceration, especially in patients with VII nerve disorders. Carefully test corneal sensation in eyes previously operated upon, avoid injection into the lower lid area to prevent ectropion, and vigorously treat any epithelial defect. Protective drops, ointment, therapeutic soft contact lenses, or closure of the eye by patching or other means may be required. Because of its anticholinergic effects, use incobotulinumtoxinA with caution in patients at risk of developing narrow-angle glaucoma. To prevent ectropion, do not inject botulinum toxin products into the medial lower eyelid area. Ecchymosis easily occurs in the soft tissues of the eyelid. Immediate gentle pressure at the injection site can limit that risk.

Immunogenicity: As with all therapeutic proteins, there is a potential for immunogenicity. Neutralizing antibody titers were assessed in all clinical studies of incobotulinumtoxinA using the hemidiaphragm assay. In the incobotulinumtoxinA development program, 12 of 1,080 (1.1%) subjects who were antibody negative at baseline developed neutralizing antibodies to botulinum toxin during their study. Each of these 12 subjects had been treated with another botulinum toxin before exposure to incobotulinumtoxinA. Because the majority of patients had previously been exposed to other botulinum toxins, and because most trials were of short duration with controlled intervals between treatments, the potential for antibody formation has not been fully characterized. The significance of these antibodies is unknown because in the presence of neutralizing antibodies, some patients may continue to experience clinical benefit. A single subject with a 20-year history of cervical dystonia who was reported as botulinum toxin naive and treated with 240 units of incobotulinumtoxinA demonstrated transiently positive neutralizing antibodies that reverted to negative at study termination. This subject was determined to be a primary nonresponder.

Pharmacologic & Dosing Characteristics

Dosage: Individualize the dose and number of injection sites in treated muscle(s) for each patient based on the number and location of muscles involved, muscle mass, body weight, severity of disease, and response to any previous botulinum toxin injections. Inject carefully when close to sensitive structures, such as the carotid artery, lung apices, and esophagus. Before administering incobotulinumtoxinA, be familiar with the patient's anatomy and any anatomic alterations (eg, due to prior surgical procedures). Localization of the involved muscles with electromyographic guidance or nerve stimulation techniques may be useful. The number of injection sites varies with the size of the muscle to be treated and the volume of incobotulinumtoxinA injected.

The potency units of various botulinum toxins are not interchangeable. The units of biological activity of incobotulinumtoxinA cannot be compared to or converted into units of any other botulinum toxin.

Blepharospasm: When starting incobotulinumtoxinA therapy, base the dose on the previous dosing of onabotulinumtoxinA (*Botox*), although responses to the 2 products may differ in individual patients. In clinical trials for blepharospasm, incobotulinumtoxinA was not administered to patients who had not previously received onabotulinumtoxinA. In clinical trials, the mean dose per injection site was 5.6 units, the mean number of injections per eye was 6, and the mean dose per eye was 33.5 units (range, 10 to 50 units). In the controlled trial, few patients received a total dose of more than 75 units. The total initial dose of incobotulinumtoxinA in both eyes should not exceed 70 units (35 units per eye). If the previous dose of onabotulinumtoxinA is not known, the recommended starting dose is 1.25 to 2.5 units per injection site.

Cervical dystonia: The recommended initial total dose is 120 units per treatment session. Higher doses did not provide additional efficacy and were associated with an increased incidence of adverse reactions. IncobotulinumtoxinA is usually injected into sternocleidomastoid, splenius capitis, levator scapulae, scalenus, and/or trapezius muscle(s).

Route: IM. Use a suitable needle (eg, 26-gauge, 37 mm length for superficial muscles; 22-gauge, 75 mm length for deeper muscles).

Special Handling: Immediate medical attention may be required in cases of respiratory, speech, or swallowing difficulties.

Overdosage: Excessive doses of incobotulinumtoxinA may produce neuromuscular weakness with a variety of symptoms. Respiratory support may be required when excessive doses cause paralysis of the respiratory muscles. Monitor patients for symptoms of excessive muscle weakness or muscle paralysis. Symptomatic treatment may be necessary. Symptoms of overdose are not likely to be present immediately following injection. If accidental injection or oral ingestion occurs, monitor the patient for several weeks for signs and symptoms of excessive muscle weakness or paralysis. There is no significant information regarding overdose from clinical studies in cervical dystonia and blepharospasm. In the event of overdose, botulinum antitoxin is available from the Centers for Disease Control and Prevention (CDC). However, the antitoxin will not reverse any botulinum toxin–induced effects already apparent by the time of antitoxin administration.

Additional Doses: Determine the frequency of repeat treatments by clinical response, but generally treatment is no more frequent than every 12 weeks.

Blepharospasm: Tailor subsequent dosing to patient response, to a maximum dose of 35 units per eye.

Missed Doses: Interrupting the recommended schedule or delaying subsequent doses does not require restarting the series.

Efficacy:

Blepharospasm: IncobotulinumtoxinA was investigated in 109 patients with blepharospasm. At least 10 weeks had elapsed since the most recent onabotulinumtoxinA dose. Patients were randomized to receive a single administration of incobotulinumtoxinA (n = 75) or placebo (n = 34). The primary efficacy end point was the change in the Jankovic Rating Scale (JRS) severity subscore from baseline to week 6 postinjection. The difference between the incobotulinumtoxinA group and the placebo group was −1 point (95% CI, −1.4 to −0.5; $P < 0.001$). Neither age nor gender subgroups differed in response to incobotulinumtoxinA.

Cervical dystonia: IncobotulinumtoxinA was studied in 233 patients with cervical dystonia. For patients previously treated with a botulinum toxin, the trial required that at least 10 weeks had passed since the most recent botulinum toxin administration. Patients were randomized to receive a single administration of incobotulinumtoxinA 240 units (n = 81), incobotulinumtoxinA 120 units (n = 78), or placebo (n = 74). Most patients received 2 to 10 injections into selected muscles. At study baseline, 61% of patients had previously received a botulinum toxin as treatment for cervical dystonia. The primary efficacy end point was the change in the Toronto Western Spasmodic Torticollis Rating Scale (TWSTRS) total score from baseline to week 4 postinjection. The difference between the group receiving incobotulinumtoxinA 240 units and the placebo group in change of TWSTRS total score from baseline to week 4 was −9 points (95% CI, −12 to −5.9 points). The difference between the group receiving incobotulinumtoxinA 120 units and the placebo group from baseline to week 4 was −7.5 points (95% CI, −10.4 to −4.6 points). Patients assigned to either placebo or incobotulinumtoxinA had a wide range of responses, but the active treatment groups were more likely to show greater improvements. Initial incobotulinumtoxinA doses of 120 units and 240 units demonstrated no significant difference in effectiveness between the doses. The efficacy of incobotulinumtoxinA was similar in patients who were botulinum toxin naive and those who had received botulinum toxin before the study. Neither age nor gender subgroups differed in response to incobotulinumtoxinA.

Onset: The median first onset of effect occurs within 7 days after injection.

Duration: The typical duration of effect of each treatment is up to 3 months; however, the effect may last significantly longer, or shorter, in individual patients.

Pharmacokinetics: In rodents, the degree and duration of hindlimb muscle paralysis is dose dependent. In humans, recovery from paralysis after IM injection occurs within 3 to 4 months as nerve terminals sprout and reconnect with the muscle endplate.

Using currently available analytical technology, it is not possible to detect incobotulinumtoxinA in peripheral blood after IM injection at recommended doses.

Mechanism: IncobotulinumtoxinA blocks cholinergic transmission at the neuromuscular junction by inhibiting the release of acetylcholine from peripheral cholinergic nerve endings. This inhibition occurs in the following sequence: neurotoxin binding to cholinergic nerve terminals, internalization of neurotoxin into the nerve terminal, translocation of the light-chain part of the molecule into the cytosol of the nerve terminal, and enzymatic cleavage of SNAP25, a presynaptic target protein essential for the release of acetylcholine. Impulse transmission is reestablished by formation of new nerve endings.

Drug Interactions: No formal drug interaction studies have been conducted with incobotulinumtoxinA. Observe patients treated concomitantly with incobotulinumtoxinA and aminoglycoside antibiotics, spectinomycin, or other agents that interfere with neuromuscular transmission (eg, tubocurarine-like agents); or muscle relaxants because the effect of incobotulinumtoxinA may be potentiated.

Use of anticholinergic drugs after administration of incobotulinumtoxinA may potentiate systemic anticholinergic effects.

Patient Information: Seek immediate medical care if swallowing, speech, or respiratory disorders arise. Injections of incobotulinumtoxinA may cause dyspnea or mild to severe dysphagia, with the risk of aspiration. If loss of strength, muscle weakness, blurred vision, or drooping eyelids occurs, avoid driving or engaging in other hazardous activities. Injections of incobotulinumtoxinA may cause reduced blinking or effectiveness of blinking.

Pharmaceutical Characteristics

Concentration: Concentration varies with diluent added to either vial

IncobotulinumtoxinA

Diluent Volumes for Reconstituting IncobotulinumtoxinA		
Volume of preservative-free sodium chloride 0.9%	50 unit vial (units per 0.1 mL)	100 unit vial (units per 0.1 mL)
0.25 mL	20 units	
0.5 mL	10 units	20 units
1 mL	5 units	10 units
2 mL	2.5 units	5 units
4 mL	1.25 units	2.5 units
8 mL		1.25 units

Quality Assay: Each unit corresponds to the mouse median lethal dose (LD_{50}) when the reconstituted product is injected intraperitoneally into mice under defined conditions.

Packaging: Borosilicate glass single-use vials with latex-free bromobutyl rubber closures and tamper-proof aluminum seals in the following pack sizes: 50 unit vial (NDC#: 00259-1605-01), 100 unit vial (00259-1610-01)

Doseform: Powder yielding solution

Appearance: White to off-white powder, yielding clear, colorless solution. Do not use if cloudy or if floccular or particulate matter is present.

Diluent:

For reconstitution: Sodium chloride 0.9%. Gently mix by rotating the vial.

Adjuvant: None

Preservative: None

Allergens: None

Excipients: Human albumin 1 mg/vial and sucrose 4.7 mg/vial

pH: 7.4

Shelf Life: Expires within 36 months

Storage/Stability: Store unopened vials at room temperature (20° to 25°C [68° to 77° F]), in a refrigerator (2° to 8°C [36° to 46°F]), or in a freezer (−20° to −10°C [−4° to 14°F]). Protect vials from light. Do not freeze.

Store reconstituted incobotulinumtoxinA at 2° to 8°C (36° to 46°F) and administer within 24 hours.

Handling: Discard vial if vacuum is not present before reconstitution. After reconstitution, use incobotulinumtoxinA for only one injection session and for only one patient. If proposed injection sites are marked with a pen, do not inject through the marks, as a permanent tattooing effect may occur.

Production Process: IncobotulinumtoxinA is produced from fermentation of Hall strain *C. botulinum* serotype A. The botulinum toxin complex is purified from the culture supernatant and then the active ingredient is separated from the proteins (hemagglutinin and non-hemagglutinin) through a series of steps yielding the active neurotoxin with molecular weight of 150 kDa, without accessory proteins.

Media: Data not provided

Other Information

First Licensed: August 2, 2010

Botulinum Toxins

Names:
> Botox
> Botox Cosmetic

Manufacturer:
> Allergan Pharmaceuticals

Synonyms: Also known as botulinum toxin type A

Comparison: The potency units of various botulinum toxins are not interchangeable with other botulinum toxin products; therefore units of biological activity cannot be compared to or converted into units of any other botulinum toxin product.

Immunologic Characteristics

Microorganism: Bacterium, *Clostridium botulinum*, anaerobic, endospore-forming gram-positive rod

Viability: Inactivated bacteriologically, but active toxin type A

Antigenic Form: Bacterial exotoxin type A neurotoxin complex

Antigenic Type: Protein. The neurotoxic component has a molecular weight of 150,000 daltons.

Strains: *C. botulinum* type A, Hall strain

Use Characteristics

Indications: Primary hyperhidrosis, a severe form of underarm sweating, in patients whose condition cannot be adequately managed with topical agents, including prescription antiperspirants.

Treatment of strabismus and blepharospasm associated with dystonia, including benign essential blepharospasm or VII nerve disorders in patients 12 years of age and older. For treatment of cervical dystonia in adults to decrease the severity of abnormal head position and neck pain associated with cervical dystonia.

To prevent headaches in adult patients with chronic migraine (at least 15 days per month, with headache lasting 4 or more hours per day). Safety and effectiveness have not been established in preventing episodic migraine (up to 14 headache days per month) in 7 placebo-controlled studies.

To treat urinary incontinence due to detrusor overactivity associated with a neurologic condition (eg, spinal cord injury, multiple sclerosis [MS]) in adults who have an inadequate response to or who are intolerant of an anticholinergic medication.

The cosmetic formulation is indicated for the temporary improvement in the appearance of moderate to severe glabellar lines associated with corrugator or procerus muscle activity in adults up to 65 years of age.

To treat upper limb spasticity in adult patients to decrease severity of increased muscle tone in elbow flexors (biceps), wrist flexors (flexor carpi radialis and flexor carpi ulnaris), and finger flexors (flexor digitorum profundus and flexor digitorum sublimis).

Unlabeled Uses: Treatment of hemifacial spasms, spasmodic torticollis (ie, clonic twisting of the head), oromandibular dystonia, spasmodic dysphonia (laryngeal dystonia), and other dystonia (eg, writer's cramp, focal task-specific dystonias). Botulinum toxin is being assessed in the treatment of head and neck tremor unresponsive to pharmacologic therapy. Designated an orphan drug for the treatment of dynamic muscle contracture in pediatric cerebral palsy patients (December 6, 1991).

Limitations: Efficacy in deviations larger than 50 prism diopters, in restrictive strabismus, in Duane syndrome with lateral rectus weakness, and in secondary strabismus caused by prior surgical over-recession of the antagonist is doubtful, or multiple injections over a period of time may be required. Botulinum toxin is ineffective in chronic paralytic strabismus except to reduce antagonist contracture in conjunction with surgical repair.

Safety and effectiveness of onabotulinumtoxinA have not been established in treating other upper limb muscle groups, or in treating lower limb spasticity. Safety and effectiveness have not been established in treating spasticity in patients younger than 18 years. Onabotulinum-toxinA has not been shown to improve upper extremity functional abilities, or range of motion at a joint affected by a fixed contracture. Treatment with OnabotulinumtoxinA is not intended to substitute for usual standard of care rehabilitation regimens.

The presence of type A botulinum antitoxin antibodies may reduce the effectiveness of botulinum toxin therapy. In clinical studies, reduction in effectiveness due to antibody production occurred in 1 patient with blepharospasm who received 3 doses of toxin over a 6-week period totaling 92 units, and in several patients with torticollis who received multiple doses experimentally, totaling more than 300 units in a 1-month period. For this reason, keep the dose of botulinum toxin for strabismus and blepharospasm as low as possible, in any case less than 200 units per 1-month period.

Clinicians administering botulinum toxin must understand the relevant neuromuscular and orbital anatomy and any alterations to the anatomy due to prior surgical procedures, and must have an understanding of standard electromyographic techniques.

Use caution when botulinum toxin is used in the presence of inflammation at the proposed injection site(s) or when excessive weakness or atrophy is present in the target muscle(s).

Contraindications:

Absolute: Individuals with a known hypersensitivity to any ingredient in the formulation.

Relative: The presence of infection at the proposed injection site(s). Intradetrusor injection is contraindicated in patients who have an acute urinary tract infection, and in patients with acute urinary retention who are not routinely performing clean intermittent self-catheterization.

Immunodeficiency: No impairment of effect is likely.

Elderly: Little specific information is available about use of botulinum toxin in the elderly population.

Glabellar lines: Clinical studies did not include sufficient subjects older than 65 years of age to determine whether they respond differently from younger people. Available data show that people 50 years of age and younger respond at higher rates than people 65 years of age and older. Compared with the placebo group (22%), people 65 years of age and older were more likely to respond according to investigator assessment at day 30 (39%), but the difference was not statistically significant. By subject global assessment among people 65 years of age and older, response was greater for *Botox*-treated people than placebo recipients at all time points except day 120 ($P = 0.036$).

Carcinogenicity: Long-term studies in animals have not been performed to assess the carcinogenic potential of onabotulinumtoxinA.

Fertility Impairment: When onabotulinumtoxinA (4, 8, or 16 units/kg intramuscularly [IM]) was administered to pregnant mice or rats 2 times during organogenesis, reductions in fetal body weight and decreased fetal skeletal ossification occurred with the 2 highest doses. The no-effect dose for developmental toxicity in these studies (4 units/kg) is approximately 1.5 times the average high human dose for upper limb spasticity of 360 units on a body weight basis (units/kg). When onabotulinumtoxinA was administered to pregnant rats (0.125, 0.25,

0.5, 1, 4, or 8 units/kg IM) or rabbits (0.063, 0.125, 0.25, or 0.5 units/kg IM) daily during organogenesis, reduced fetal body weights and decreased fetal skeletal ossification were observed at the 2 highest doses in rats and at the highest dose in rabbits. These doses were also associated with significant maternal toxicity, including abortions, early deliveries, and maternal death. The developmental no-effect doses in these studies are less than the average high human dose based on units/kg. When pregnant rats received single injections (1, 4, or 16 units/kg IM) at 3 different periods of development (before implantation, implantation, or organogenesis), no adverse effects on fetal development were observed. The developmental no-effect level for a single maternal dose in rats (16 units/kg) is approximately 3 times the average high human dose based on units/kg.

Pregnancy: Category C. Use for ophthalmic indications only if clearly needed. Not recommended for cosmetic use during pregnancy. When pregnant mice and rats were injected IM during organogenesis, the drug had no observed developmental effect at 4 units/kg. Higher doses were associated with reductions in fetal body weight or delayed ossification. In rabbits, daily injection of 0.125 units/kg (days 6 to 18 of gestation) and 2 units/kg (days 6 and 13 of gestation) produced severe maternal toxicity, abortions, and fetal malformations. Higher doses resulted in death of the dams. It is not known if botulinum toxin crosses the placenta.

Lactation: It is not known if botulinum toxin is excreted in breast milk. Problems in humans have not been documented.

Children:

Glabellar lines: OnabotulinumtoxinA has not been studied in children younger than 18 years of age.

Ophthalmic uses: Not indicated for use in children 12 years of age and younger.

Adverse Reactions: The most serious adverse events include rare reports of death, sometimes associated with dysphagia, pneumonia, or other significant debility. Rare reports involved the cardiovascular system, including arrhythmia and myocardial infarction, sometimes fatal. Some of these patients had preexisting risk factors such as cardiovascular disease. Postmarketing surveillance identified reports of skin rash (eg, erythema multiforme, urticaria, psoriasiform eruption), pruritus, allergic reaction, and local swelling of the eyelid. Spontaneous reports of serious adverse events since 1990 included anaphylactic reaction, myasthenia gravis, decreased hearing, ear noise and local numbness, blurred vision and retinal vein occlusion, glaucoma, and vertigo with nystagmus.

Distant effect: Botulinum-toxin effects may, in some cases, be observed beyond the injection area. Symptoms are consistent with the mechanism of action of botulinum toxin and may include asthenia, generalized muscle weakness, diplopia, blurred vision, ptosis, dysphagia, dysphonia, dysarthria, urinary incontinence, and breathing difficulties. These symptoms have been reported hours to weeks after the injection. Swallowing and breathing difficulties can be life-threatening, and there have been reports of death related to spread of toxin effects. The risk of the symptoms is probably greatest in children treated for spasticity, but symptoms can also occur in adults treated for spasticity and other conditions, and particularly in those patients who have underlying conditions that would predispose them to these symptoms. In unapproved uses, including spasticity in children and adults, and in approved indications, symptoms consistent with spread of toxin effect have been reported at doses comparable with or lower than doses used to treat cervical dystonia.

Strabismus: Inducing paralysis in 1 or more extraocular muscles may produce spatial disorientation, double vision, or past pointing. Covering the affected eye may alleviate these symptoms. Extraocular muscles adjacent to the injection site may also be affected, causing ptosis or vertical deviation, especially with higher doses of botulinum toxin. In 2,058 adults who received 3,650 injections for horizontal strabismus, 15.7% of recipients developed ptosis and 16.9% developed vertical deviation. The incidence of ptosis was much less after inferior rectus injection (0.9%) and much greater after superior rectus injection (37.7%). Among 3,104 patients who received 5,587 injections, 0.3% of the patients developed ptosis that lasted more than 180 days and 2.1% developed vertical deviation greater than 2 prism diopters that lasted more than 180 days. In these patients, the injection procedure itself caused 9 scleral perforations. A vitreous hemorrhage occurred and later resolved in 1 patient. No retinal detachment or visual loss occurred in any case. Sixteen retrobulbar hemorrhages occurred. Decompression of the orbit after 5 minutes was performed in 1 case to restore retinal circulation. No eye lost vision from retrobulbar hemorrhage. Five eyes had pupillary change consistent with ciliary ganglion damage (Adie pupil).

During the administration of botulinum toxin for the treatment of strabismus, retrobulbar hemorrhages sufficient to compromise retinal circulation have occurred from needle penetrations into the orbit. Access to appropriate instruments to decompress the orbit is recommended. Ocular (globe) penetrations by needles have also occurred. Keep an ophthalmoscope available to diagnose this condition.

Blepharospasm: In a study of blepharospasm patients who received an average dose per eye of 33 units of the currently manufactured *Botox*, injected at 3 to 5 sites, the most frequent adverse reactions were ptosis (21%), superficial punctate keratitis (6%), and eye dryness (6%). This rate of ptosis is higher than that seen with the original *Botox*-treated group (4%). Other events reported in prior clinical studies in decreasing order of incidence include irritation, tearing, lagophthalmos, photophobia, ectropion, keratitis, diplopia and entropian, diffuse skin rash, and local swelling of the eyelid skin lasting for several days following eyelid injection. One case involved acute angle-closure glaucoma 1 day after receiving botulinum toxin for blepharospasm, with recovery 4 months later after laser iridotomy and trabeculectomy. Focal facial paralysis, syncope, and exacerbation of myasthenia gravis were reported after treatment of blepharospasm. Ecchymosis occurs easily in the soft eyelid tissues. It can be prevented by applying pressure at the injection site immediately after injection. In 2 cases of VII nerve disorder (1 case with an aphakic eye), reduced blinking from botulinum toxin injection of the orbicularis muscle led to serious corneal exposure, persistent epithelial defect, and corneal ulceration. Perforation requiring corneal grafting occurred in 1 case, an aphakic eye. Use careful testing of corneal sensation in eyes previously operated upon. Avoiding injection into the lower lid area to avoid ectropion may reduce this hazard. Vigorously treat any corneal epithelial defect. This may require protective drops, ointment, therapeutic soft contact lenses, or closure of the eye by patching or other means. Two patients previously incapacitated by blepharospasm experienced cardiac collapse attributed to overexertion within 3 weeks following botulinum toxin therapy. Caution sedentary patients to resume activity slowly and carefully.

Cervical dystonia: The most frequent adverse reactions were dysphagia (19%), upper respiratory infection (12%), neck pain (11%), and headache (11%). Other events reported in 2% to 10% of patients in decreasing order of incidence include increased cough, influenza-like syndrome, back pain, rhinitis, dizziness, hypertonia, injection-site soreness, asthenia, oral dryness, speech disorder, fever, nausea, and drowsiness. Stiffness, numbness, diplopia, ptosis, and dyspnea have been reported rarely. The literature includes a report of a woman who developed brachial plexopathy 2 days after injection of *Botox* 120 units to treat cervical dystonia. Dysphonia has been reported.

Glabellar lines: The most frequent adverse events were headache, respiratory infection, influenza-like syndrome, blepharoptosis (droopy eyelids), and nausea. Less frequent (less than 3%) adverse events included facial pain, injection-site erythema, and muscle weakness. While local weakness of the injected muscle(s) is representative of the expected action of botulinum toxin, weakness of adjacent muscles may occur as a result of the spread of toxin. These events are considered to be associated with injection, occurring within the first week. The events were generally transient but some lasted several months. In the placebo-controlled clinical study, adverse events occurring greater than 1% more often in the *Botox*-treated group included blepharoptosis (3.2%), facial pain (2.2%), muscle weakness (2%), skin tightness (1%), dyspepsia (1%), tooth disorder (1%), and hypertension (1%). In an open-label study evaluating safety of repeated injections, blepharoptosis occurred in 2.1% of subjects in the first treatment cycle and 1.2% in the second cycle. One case has been published of diplopia, which resolved completely in 3 weeks. Transient ptosis, the most frequently reported complication, has been reported in the literature in approximately 5% of patients.

Axillary hyperhidrosis: Evaluate patients for potential causes of secondary hyperhidrosis (eg, hyperthyroidism) to avoid symptomatic treatment with the diagnosis of the underlying disease. The safety and efficacy of botulinum toxin for hyperhidrosis in other body areas have not been established. Weakness of hand muscles or blepharoptosis may occur in patients who receive botulinum toxin for palmar hyperhidrosis or facial hyperhidrosis, respectively. The most frequent adverse events (3% to 10%) after botulinum toxin in double-blind studies included injection-site pain and hemorrhage, nonaxillary sweating, infection, pharyngitis, viral-like syndrome, headache, fever, neck or back pain, itching, and anxiety.

Immunogenicity: Treatment with botulinum toxin may elicit neutralizing antibodies that reduce the effectiveness of subsequent treatments by inactivating the biological activity of the toxin. The rate of formation of neutralizing antibodies has not been well studied. Botulinum toxin injections at more frequent intervals or at higher doses may lead to greater incidence of antibody formation. In the cervical dystonia study that enrolled only patients with a history of receiving *Botox* at multiple treatment sessions, 17% of patients at study entry had a positive murine-based assay for neutralizing activity. Of those without neutralizing activity at the start of the study, 2% converted to positive by the end of the study. Conflicting data exist on whether neutralizing activity predicts clinical response.

Neuromuscular disorders: Exercise caution when administering onabotulinumtoxinA to people with peripheral motor naturopathic diseases (eg, amyotrophic lateral sclerosis) or neuromuscular junctional disorders (eg, myasthenia gravis, Lambert-Eaton syndrome). Patients with neuromuscular disorders may be at increased risk of clinically significant systemic effects, including severe dysphagia and respiratory compromise. In some cases, dysphagia lasted several months and required placement of a gastric feeding tube. Dysphagia is a commonly reported adverse event after treatment with botulinum toxins in cervical dystonia patients, especially patients with smaller neck muscle mass and patients who require bilateral injections into the sternocleidomastoid muscle. Injections into the levator scapulae may be associated with an increased risk of upper respiratory infection and dysphagia.

Upper limb spasticity: Closely monitor patients with compromised respiratory status treated with onabotulinumtoxinA for upper limb spasticity. In a placebo-controlled study in patients with stable reduced pulmonary function (defined as forced expiratory volume in the first second of expiration [FEV_1] 40% to 80% of predicted value and FEV_1/forced vital capacity (FVC) less than or equal to 0.75), the event rate in change of FVC greater than or equal to 15% or greater than or equal to 20% was generally greater in patients treated with onabotulinumtoxinA than in patients treated with placebo. Differences from placebo were not statistically significant. In patients with reduce lung function, upper respiratory infections were also reported more frequently as adverse reactions in patients treated with onabotulinumtoxinA.

Detrusor overactivity: Autonomic dysreflexia associated with intradetrusor injections could occur in patients treated for detrusor overactivity associated with a neurologic condition and may require prompt medical therapy. In clinical trials, the incidence of autonomic dysreflexia was greater in patients treated with onabotulinumtoxinA 200 units compared with placebo (1.5% and 0.4%, respectively). In placebo-controlled trials, the proportion of subjects who were not using clean intermittent catheterization before injection and who

OnabotulinumtoxinA

subsequently required catheterization for urinary retention after treatment was 31% for onabotulinumtoxinA and 7% for placebo. The duration of postinjection catheterization was 289 and 358 days, respectively. Given the risk of urinary retention, consider only patients willing and able to initiate catheterization posttreatment if required. In patients who are not catheterizing, assess postvoid residual (PVR) urine volume within 2 weeks after treatment and periodically for up to 12 weeks. Start catheterization if PVR urine volume exceeds 200 mL and continue until PVR falls below 200 mL. Instruct patients to contact their physician if they experience difficulty in voiding, as catheterization may be required.

Chronic migraine: In efficacy trials (study 1 and study 2), the most frequent adverse events leading to discontinuation in the onabotulinumtoxinA group were neck pain, headache, worsening migraine, muscular weakness, and eyelid ptosis.

Vulnerable anatomy: Take care when injecting in or near vulnerable anatomic structures. Serious adverse events, including fatal outcomes, have been reported in patients who received botulinum toxin directly into salivary glands, the orolingual pharyngeal region, esophagus, and stomach. Some patients had preexisting dysphagia or significant debility. Pneumothorax associated with the injection procedure has been reported following the administration of botulinum toxin near the thorax. Use caution when injecting near the lung, particularly the apices.

Consultation: For overdose or accident management information, call Allergan Pharmaceuticals at (800) 433-8871 from 8 AM to 4 PM Pacific time or (714) 246-5954 for a recorded message at other times.

Pharmacologic & Dosing Characteristics

Dosage:

Axillary hyperhidrosis: 50 type A units per axilla. Define the hyperhidrotic area to be injected using standard staining techniques (eg, Minor's iodine-starch test). Using a 30-gauge needle, inject 50 units intradermally in 0.1 to 0.2 mL aliquots to each axilla, evenly distributed among 10 to 15 sites approximately 1 to 2 cm apart (eg, in a honeycomb-like pattern). Each injection site has a ring of effect of up to 2 cm in diameter. Inject each dose to a depth of approximately 2 mm, at a 45° angle to the skin surface, with the needle's bevel side up to minimize leakage. Administer repeat injections for hyperhidrosis when the clinical effect of a previous injection diminishes. If injection sites are marked in ink, do not inject botulinum toxin directly through the ink mark to avoid a permanent tattoo effect.

Minor's Iodine-Starch Test: Shave underarms and abstain from use of deodorants or antiperspirants for 24 hours before the test. Patient should rest comfortably without exercise or hot drinks for approximately 30 minutes before the test. Dry the underarm area and then immediately paint it with iodine solution. Allow the area to dry, then lightly sprinkle the area with starch powder. Gently blow off any excess starch powder. The hyperhidrotic area will develop a deep blue-black color over approximately 10 minutes.

Blepharospasm: Inject 1.25 to 2.5 type A units (0.05 to 0.1 mL at each site) using a 27- to 30-gauge needle. Each treatment lasts approximately 3 months, following which the procedure can be repeated indefinitely. At repeat treatment sessions, the dose may be increased up to 2-fold if the response from the initial treatment is insufficient, usually defined as an effect that does not last more than 2 months. However, there appears to be little benefit from injecting more than 5 units per site. Some tolerance may be found when botulinum toxin is used in treating blepharospasm if treatments are given more frequently than every 3 months, and it is rare for the effect to be permanent. To avoid development of type A botulinum antitoxin antibodies, keep the dose of botulinum toxin for both strabismus and blepharospasm as low as possible. Do not allow the cumulative dose of botulinum toxin in a 30-day period to exceed 200 units.

Cervical dystonia: In the placebo-controlled trial, the median total dose was 236 type A units (25th to 75th percentile range: 198 to 300 units). In that trial, the mean percentages of the total dose per muscle were as follows: splenius capitus/cervicis (38%), trapezius (29%), longissimus (29%), sternocleidomastoid (25%), semispinalis (21%), levator scapulae (20%), scalene (15%). Dosing in initial and subsequent treatment sessions should be customized to the patient, based on head and neck position, localization of pain, muscle hypertrophy, patient response, and adverse event history. The initial dose should be at a lower dose, with subsequent dosing adjusted based on individual response. Limiting the total dose injected into the sternocleidomastoid muscles to less than or equal to 100 units may decrease the risk of dysphagia.

Chronic migraine: Inject 155 units IM using a 30-gauge, ½-inch needle, with 5 units per 0.1 mL per site. Divide the injections across 7 specific head/neck muscle areas. A 1-inch needle may be needed in the neck region for patients with thick neck muscles. Except for the procerus muscle, which should be injected at one midline site, inject all muscles bilaterally, with half of the injection sites on each side of midline. The recommended retreatment schedule is every 12 weeks.

Dosing by Muscle for Chronic Migraine	
Head/Neck area	Recommended dose (number of sites[a])
Frontalis[b]	20 units divided among 4 sites
Corrugator[b]	10 units divided among 2 sites
Procerus	5 units in 1 site
Occipitalis[b]	30 units divided among 6 sites
Temporalis[b]	40 units divided among 8 sites
Trapezius[b]	30 units divided among 6 sites
Cervical paraspinal muscle group[b]	20 units divided among 4 sites
Total dose	155 units divided among 31 sites

a Each IM injection site = 5 units per 0.1 mL.
b Distribute doses bilaterally.

Detrusor overactivity: Not more than 200 units per treatment.

Glabellar lines: An effective dose for facial lines is determined by gross observation of the patient's ability to activate the superficial muscles injected. Using a 30-gauge needle, inject 4 type A units per 0.1 mL into each of 5 sites, 2 in each corrugator muscle and 1 in the procerus muscle, for a total dose of 20 units. Do not inject more often than every 3 months.

Strabismus: Initial doses: Use the smaller doses listed below for treatment of small deviations. Use the larger doses only for large deviations. For vertical muscles and for horizontal strabismus of more than 20 prism diopters, inject 1.25 to 2.5 type A units into any one muscle. For horizontal strabismus of 20 to 50 prism diopters, inject 2.5 to 5 type A units into any one muscle. For persistent VI nerve palsy of 1 month or longer duration, inject 1.25 to 2.5 type A units into the medial rectus muscle.

Subsequent doses: Reexamine patients 7 to 14 days after each injection to assess the effect of that dose and any residual or recurrent strabismus. Give patients experiencing adequate paralysis of the target muscle who require subsequent injections a dose comparable with the initial dose. Subsequent doses may be increased up to twice the quantity of the previously administered dose for patients experiencing incomplete paralysis of the target muscle. Do not administer subsequent injections until the effects of the previous dose have dissipated, as evidenced by substantial function in the injected and adjacent muscles. The maximum recommended dose in a single injection for any one muscle is 25 units.

Upper limb spasticity: Customize dose for initial and sequential treatment sessions based on the size, number, and location of muscles involved; severity of spasticity; presence of local muscle weakness; the patient's response to previous treatment; or adverse event history with onabotulinumtoxinA. In trials, doses from 75 to 360 units were divided among selected muscles at a given treatment session. Recommended dose ranges per muscle are as follows:

- Biceps brachii: 100 to 200 units divided among 4 sites
- Flexor carpi radialis: 12.5 to 50 units at 1 site
- Flexor carpi ulnaris: 12.5 to 50 units at 1 site
- Flexor digitorum profundus: 30 to 50 units at 1 site
- Flexor digitorum sublimis: 30 to 50 units at 1 site

Repeat the dose when the effect of a previous dose has diminished, but generally no sooner than 12 weeks later. The degree and pattern of muscle spasticity at time of re-injection may require altering the dose and muscles to be injected.

Route & Site:

Blepharospasm: Inject diluted botulinum toxin using a 27- to 30-gauge needle without electromyographic guidance into the medial and lateral pretarsal orbicularis oculi of the upper lid and into the lateral pretarsal orbicularis oculi of the lower lid.

Cervical dystonia: A 25-, 27-, or 30-gauge needle may be used for superficial muscles, and a longer 22-gauge needle for deeper musculature. Localization of involved muscles with electromyographic guidance may be useful. To reduce the complication of ptosis, avoid injection near the levator palpebrae superioris. To reduce the complication of diplopia, avoid medial lower lid injections, thereby reducing diffusion into the inferior oblique. To avoid ecchymosis, apply pressure at the injection site immediately after injection.

Detrusor overactivity: Instill the bladder with enough saline to achieve adequate visualization for the injections, but avoid overdistension. Inject onabotulinumtoxinA 200 units per 30 mL into the detrusor muscle via a flexible or rigid cystoscope, avoiding the trigone. Fill (prime) the injection needle with approximately 1 mL of toxin solution before starting the injections (depending on needle length) to remove any air. Insert the needle approximately 2 mm into the detrusor. Space 30 injections of 6.7 units per 1 mL each approximately 1 cm apart. For the final injection, inject approximately 1 mL of sterile saline so the full dose is delivered. After giving the injections, drain the saline used for bladder wall visualization. Observe the patient for at least 30 minutes postinjection. Consider reinjection when the clinical effect of the previous injections diminishes (median time to qualification for retreatment in the double-blind, placebo-controlled clinical studies was 295 to 337 days [42 to 48 weeks]), but no sooner than 12 weeks from the prior bladder injection.

Glabellar lines: Inject into each of 5 sites, 2 in each corrugator muscle and 1 in the procerus muscle. Glabellar facial lines arise from the activity of the corrugator and orbicularis oculi muscles. These muscles move the brow medially, and the procerus and depressor supercilii pull the brow inferiorly. This creates a frown or "furrowed brow." The location, size, and use of the muscles vary markedly among individuals. Lines induced by facial expression occur perpendicular to the direction of action of contracting facial muscles. To reduce the complication of ptosis, avoid injection near the levator palpebrae superioris, place the medial corrugator injection at least 1 cm above the bony supraorbital ridge, ensure the injected dose is accurate and minimized, and do not inject toxin less than 1 cm above the central eyebrow.

Strabismus: Botulinum toxin is intended for injection into extraocular muscles using the electrical activity recorded from the tip of the injection needle as a guide to placement within the target muscle. Do not attempt to inject without surgical exposure or electromyographic guidance. Prepare injection of botulinum toxin by drawing into a syringe an amount of the properly diluted toxin slightly greater than the intended dose. Expel air bubbles in the syringe barrel and attach the syringe to the electromyographic injection needle, preferably a 1½-inch, 27-gauge needle. Expel fluid volume in excess of the intended dose through the needle into a waste container to ensure patency of the needle and confirm that there is no leakage.

Use new needles and syringes each time the vial is entered for dilution or removal of botulinum toxin. To prepare the eye for botulinum toxin, place several drops of a local anesthetic and an ocular decongestant solution several minutes prior to injection. The volume of botulinum toxin injected for treatment of strabismus ranges from 0.05 to 0.15 mL per muscle.

Upper limb spasticity: Use an appropriate needle size (eg, 25- to 30-gauge) for superficial muscles, and use a longer 22-gauge needle for deeper musculature. Localize involved muscles with electromyographic guidance or nerve stimulation techniques.

Dilution: Use a 2½-inch, 21-gauge needle with syringe to add an appropriate amount of sodium chloride 0.9% without preservative to a vial of botulinum toxin. Because the toxin is denatured by bubbling and similar violent agitation, inject the diluent into the vial gently. Discard the vial if a vacuum does not pull the diluent into the vial.

Chronic migraine: The recommended dilution is 200 units per 4 mL or 100 units per 2 mL, with a final concentration of 5 units per 0.1 mL.

Detrusor overactivity: Add 6 mL of nonpreserved sodium chloride 0.9% solution to a 200 unit vial and mix gently. Draw 2 mL into each of three 10 mL syringes. Complete reconstitution by adding 8 mL of sodium chloride 0.9% into each 10 mL syringe and mix gently. This will result in three 10 mL syringes, each containing 6.7 units/mL and totaling 200 units. Use immediately after reconstitution.

Alternatively, reconstitute two 100 unit vials, each with 6 mL of nonpreserved sodium chloride 0.9% solution and mix gently. Draw 4 mL into each of two 10 mL syringes. Draw the remaining 2 mL from each vial into a third 10 mL syringe. Complete reconstitution by adding 6 mL of sodium chloride 0.9% into each 10 mL syringe, and mix gently. This will result in three 10 mL syringes, each containing 6.7 units/mL and totaling 200 units. Use immediately after reconstitution.

Glabellar lines: Add 2.5 mL of sodium chloride 0.9% to the 100 unit vial, to yield 4 units per 0.1 mL.

Ophthalmic: Adding 1 mL of diluent to the vial yields a concentration of 10 units per 0.1 mL. Similarly, addition of 2, 4, or 8 mL to the vial yields concentrations of 5 units per 0.1 mL, 2.5 units per 0.1 mL, or 1.25 units per 0.1 mL, respectively. Adjustment of the toxin dose is also possible by administering a smaller or larger injection volume, from 0.05 mL (a 50% decrease in dose, compared with 0.1 mL) to 0.15 mL (a 50% increase in dose).

Upper limb spasticity: The recommended dilution is 200 units per 4 mL or 100 units per 2 mL with nonpreserved sodium chloride 0.9%. Use the lowest dose to start, generally administering no more than 50 units per site.

Toxicity: There have been no reported instances of systemic toxicity or clinical botulism resulting from accidental injection or oral ingestion of botulinum toxin. If accidental injection or oral ingestion occurs, supervise the patient for several days on an ambulatory basis for signs or symptoms of systemic weakness or muscle paralysis. The entire content of a vial is less than the estimated dose for systemic toxicity in humans weighing 6 kg or more.

Overdosage: Signs and symptoms of overdose are not apparent immediately postinjection. Should accidental injection or oral ingestion occur, medically supervise the patient for up to several weeks for signs or symptoms of systemic weakness or muscle paralysis. An antitoxin is available from the Centers for Disease Control and Prevention (CDC) in the event of immediate knowledge of an overdose or misinjection. The antitoxin will not reverse any botulinum toxin–induced muscle weakness already apparent by the time of antitoxin administration.

Related Interventions: Administer prophylactic antibiotics (except aminoglycosides) 1 to 3 days pretreatment, on treatment day, and 1 to 3 days posttreatment. Discontinue any antiplatelet therapy at least 3 days before injection. Counsel patients on anticoagulant therapy to decrease the risk of bleeding. Use caution when performing a cystoscopy. An intravesical instillation of diluted local anesthetic, with or without sedation, or general anesthesia may be used before injection. If a local anesthetic instillation is performed, drain the bladder and irrigate with sterile saline before injection.

Efficacy:

Axillary hyperhidrosis: Efficacy and safety were evaluated in 2 placebo-controlled trials. Study 1 included adult patients who scored 3 or 4 on the 4-point Hyperhidrosis Disease Severity Scale (HDSS) and who produced at least 50 mg of sweat in each axilla at rest over 5 minutes. The percentage of responders based on at least a 2-grade decrease from baseline HDSS score, or based on a more than 50% decrease from baseline in axillary sweat production, was greater in both the 50-unit and 75-unit *Botox* groups, compared with the placebo group ($P < 0.001$). However, the percentage of responders was not significantly different between the 2 *Botox* dosage groups. The median duration of response following the first treatment with either dose was 201 days. Among those who received a second *Botox* injection, the median duration of response was similar to that observed after the first treatment.

Blepharospasm: A study of 26 of 27 patients (96.3%) with essential blepharospasm refractory to other forms of treatment reported improvement within 48 hours after injection of botulinum toxin. In another study, 12 patients with blepharospasm were evaluated in a double-blind, placebo-controlled study. Patients receiving botulinum toxin improved, compared with the placebo group. The mean dystonia score improved by 72%, the self-assessment score rating improved by 61%, and a videotape evaluation rating improved by 39%. The effects of treatment lasted a mean of 12.5 weeks.

Cervical dystonia: A randomized, double-blind, placebo-controlled study of patients with a history of receiving *Botox* in an open-label manner evaluated efficacy in cervical dystonia. Patients treated with *Botox* (median total dose, 236 units) were more likely to improve on a Physician Global Assessment scale than placebo recipients. Similarly, *Botox*-treated patients had significant reductions in pain intensity and pain frequency compared to baseline measurements. Female patients may receive somewhat greater benefit than males. There is a consistent treatment-associated effect between subsets older than and younger than 65 years of age.

Chronic migraine: OnabotulinumtoxinA was evaluated in two 24-week, 2-injection–cycle studies. Study 1 and study 2 included chronic migraine adults who were not using any concurrent headache prophylaxis, and during a 28-day baseline period had more than 15 headache days lasting 4 hours or more, with more than 50% being migraine/probable migraine. In both studies, patients were randomized to receive placebo or onabotulinumtoxinA 155 to 195 units every 12 weeks for the 2-cycle, double-blind phase. Patients were allowed to use acute headache treatments during the study. Treatment demonstrated statistically significant and clinically meaningful improvements from baseline for key efficacy variables compared with placebo.

Detrusor overactivity: Two clinical studies were conducted in patients with urinary incontinence due to detrusor overactivity associated with a neurologic condition who were either spontaneously voiding or using catheterization. A total of 691 spinal cord injury (T1 or below) or MS patients who had an inadequate response to or were intolerant of at least 1 anticholinergic medication were enrolled. These patients were randomized to receive either onabotulinumtoxinA 200 units (n = 227), 300 units (n = 223), or placebo (n = 241). In both studies, when compared with placebo, significant improvements in the primary efficacy variable of change from baseline in weekly frequency of incontinence episodes were observed for the 200 unit group at the primary efficacy time point at week 6. Increases in maximum cystometric capacity and reductions in maximum detrusor pressure during the first involuntary detrusor contraction were also observed. No additional benefit of 300 units over 200 units was demonstrated.

Glabellar lines: Two randomized, double-blind, placebo-controlled studies evaluated the cosmetic formulation on glabellar facial lines. Volunteers were excluded if they had an infection or skin problem at the injection site, history of facial nerve palsy, marked facial asymmetry, ptosis, excessive dermatochalasis, deep dermal scarring, thick sebaceous skin, inability to substantially lessen glabellar lines even by physically spreading them apart, or had a known history of disorder involving the neuromuscular system. Subjects received a single IM injection of 0.1 mL per injection site, with 4 units per site in the active treatment group. There were 5 injection sites: 1 in the procerus muscle and 2 in each corrugator supercilii muscle. In these studies, the severity of glabellar lines was reduced for up to 120 days in the onabotulinumtoxinA group compared with the placebo group, based on both investigator rating of severity at maximum frown and at rest and by subject global assessment of change in appearance. By day 7, 74% of subjects had achieved a significant reduction in frown severity score based on investigator assessment. This increased to 80% by day 30, compared with 3% for the placebo group. The corresponding values for the subjects' assessments were 83% and 89%, compared with 7% for the placebo group. The responder rates were higher for subjects 50 years of age or younger, compared with those 51 to 64 years of age. Efficacy for both of these groups was higher than for subjects 65 years of age or older. Exploratory analyses by gender suggest that both genders receive benefit, although women may be somewhat more likely to respond than men (85% to 93% response for women, compared with 59% to 72% for men, at day 30).

Strabismus: Of 677 patients with strabismus treated with 1 or more injections of botulinum toxin, 55% improved to an alignment of 10 or fewer prism diopters when evaluated 6 months or more following injection.

Upper limb spasticity: Efficacy and safety to treat upper limb spasticity were evaluated in 3 double-blind, placebo-controlled studies. Patients treated with onabotulinumtoxinA improved on Ashworth scale (a clinical measure of force required to move an extremity around a joint) and on a physician global assessment of response to treatment.

Onset:

Blepharospasm: Initial effect is seen within 3 days and peaks 1 to 2 weeks after treatment.

Cervical dystonia: Clinical improvement generally begins within the first 2 weeks after injection, with maximum clinical benefit at approximately 6 weeks postinjection.

Glabellar lines: Typically, botulinum toxin induces chemical denervation 1 to 2 days after injection, increasing in intensity during the first week. By day 7, 74% to 83% of subjects respond. By day 30, 80% to 89% of subjects respond.

Strabismus: Initial dose typically induces paralysis beginning 1 to 2 days after injection and increasing in intensity during the first week.

Duration:

Blepharospasm: Each treatment lasts approximately 3 months, after which the procedure can be repeated indefinitely.

Cervical dystonia: Most patients who showed a beneficial response by week 6 returned to baseline status by 3 months after treatment.

Glabellar lines: 90 to 120 days.

Strabismus: The paralysis lasts for 2 to 6 weeks and gradually resolves over a similar period. Overcorrections lasting more than 6 months are rare. Half of patients will require subsequent doses because of inadequate paralytic response to the initial dose, or because of mechanical factors, such as large deviations or restrictions, or because of the lack of binocular motor fusion to stabilize the alignment.

Pharmacokinetics: Botulinum toxin is not expected to be present in peripheral blood at measurable levels after IM injection at recommended doses. The recommended quantities of neurotoxin administered at each treatment session are not expected to result in systemic, overt distant clinical effects in patients without other neuromuscular dysfunction. However, subclinical systemic effects have been shown by single-fiber electromyography after IM doses of botulinum toxins appropriate to produce clinically observable local muscle weakness. These adverse effects may be due to local spread of toxin from the injection site or misplaced injections. Spread could occur via circulation, retrograde or orthograde axonal transport, or some action of the toxin at a third, central, or unidentified site.

Mechanism: Botulinum toxin blocks neuromuscular conduction by binding to receptor sites on motor nerve terminals, entering the nerve terminals and inhibiting the release of acetylcholine. This inhibition occurs as the neurotoxin cleaves SNAP-25, a protein integral to successful docking and release of acetylcholine from vesicles situated within nerve endings. When injected IM, botulinum toxin produces a localized chemical-denervation muscle paralysis. When the muscle is chemically denervated, it atrophies and may develop extrajunctional acetylcholine receptors. There is evidence that the axonal nerve can sprout and extrajunctional acetylcholine receptors may develop. There is evidence that reinnervation of the muscle may occur, thus slowly reversing muscle denervation produced by the botulinum toxin.

The paralytic effect on muscles injected with botulinum toxin is useful in reducing excessive abnormal contractions associated with blepharospasm.

When used for the treatment of strabismus, it is postulated that the administration of botulinum toxin affects muscle pairs by inducing an atrophic lengthening of the injected muscle and a corresponding shortening of the opposing muscle. Following periocular injection of botulinum toxin, distant muscles show electrophysiologic changes but no clinical weakness or other clinical change for a period of several weeks or months, parallel to the duration of local clinical paralysis.

When injected intradermally, onabotulinumtoxinA produces temporary chemical denervation of the sweat gland by stopping release of acetylcholine, resulting in local reduction in sweating.

Drug Interactions: The presence of type A botulinum antitoxin antibodies may reduce the effectiveness of botulinum toxin therapy.

The effect of botulinum toxin may be potentiated by aminoglycoside antibiotics (eg, amikacin, gentamicin, tobramycin) or any other drugs that interfere with neuromuscular transmission (eg, curare-like nondepolarizing blockers, lincosamines, polymyxins, quinidine, magnesium sulfate, anticholinesterases, succinylcholine chloride).

The effect of administering different botulinum neurotoxin serotypes at the same time or within several months of each other is unknown. Excessive neuromuscular weakness may be exacerbated by administration of another botulinum toxin before resolution of the effects of a previously administered botulinum toxin. Exercise caution when botulinum toxin is used in patients taking any of these drugs.

Patient Information: Patients with blepharospasm may have been extremely sedentary for a long time. Caution sedentary patients to resume activity slowly and carefully following the administration of botulinum toxin. Advise patients and caregivers to seek immediate medical attention if swallowing, speech, or respiratory disorders arise.

Pharmaceutical Characteristics

Concentration: 100 type A units per vial

Quality Assay: One type A unit corresponds to the calculated median lethal intraperitoneal dose (LD_{50}) in mice. The specific activity is approximately 20 units per nanogram of neurotoxin protein complex. The method for measuring the potency of *Botox* is unique to that product. Units of biological activity of various botulinum toxins cannot be compared with or converted into units of other botulinum toxins. Differences in species sensitivities to various botulinum neurotoxin serotypes preclude extrapolation of animal dose-activity relationships to human dose relationships.

Packaging:
Botox: Vial of 100 units (NDC#: 00023-1145-01); vial of 200 units (00023-3921-02)
Botox Cosmetic: Vial of 50 units (00023-3919-50); vial of 100 units (00023-9232-01)

Doseform: Powder for solution

Appearance: White powder, yielding a clear, colorless liquid, free of particulate matter.

Diluent:
For reconstitution: Sodium chloride 0.9% without preservative

Adjuvant: None

Preservative: None

Allergens: None

Excipients: Albumin (human) 0.5 mg per 100 units and sodium chloride 0.9 mg per 100 units

pH: 6.5 to 7 in sodium chloride 0.9% without preservative

Shelf Life: Expires within 24 months (200 unit vials) or 36 months (100 unit vials).

Storage/Stability: Refrigerate at 2°C to 8°C (36°F to 46°F). The product can tolerate up to 5 days at 30°C (86°F). Shipped via overnight courier in insulated containers.

After reconstitution, refrigerate and discard within 24 hours. Do not freeze reconstituted solution.

Production Process: Purified from the culture solution by dialysis and a series of acid precipitations to a crystalline complex, consisting of the neurotoxin and several accessory proteins (eg, hemagglutinin protein). The crystalline complex is redissolved in a solution containing sodium chloride and albumin and then sterile-filtered through a 0.2 micron filter prior to lyophilization.

Media: A medium containing casein hydrolysate, glucose, and yeast extract.

Disease Epidemiology

Incidence: An estimated 25,000 cases of blepharospasm and 5,000 to 10,000 cases of strabismus occur in the United States per year. Cervical dystonia affects approximately 75,000 people in North America.

Other Information

Perspective:
1984: Botulinum toxin type A designated an orphan drug for blepharospasm and strabismus.
1989: Oculinum licensed on December 29. Renamed *Botox* in 1992.
2000: Botox licensed to treat cervical dystonia on December 21.
2002: Botox Cosmetic licensed on April 15, 2002, for temporary improvement in the appearance of glabellar lines.

Discontinued Products: *Oculinum* (Oculinum Inc and Allergan)

References: Cheng CM, Chen JS, Patel RP. Unlabeled uses of botulinum toxins: a review, part 1. *Am J Health Syst Pharm.* 2006;63(2):145-152.

Cheng CM, Chen JS, Patel RP. Unlabeled uses of botulinum toxins: a review, part 2. *Am J Health Syst Pharm.* 2006;63(3):225-232.

Erbguth FJ, Naumann M. Historical aspects of botulinum toxin: Justinus Kerner (1786-1862) and the "sausage poison." *Neurology.* 1999;53(8):1850-1853.

Jankovic J, Brin MF. Therapeutic uses of botulinum toxin. *N Engl J Med.* 1991;324(17):1186-1194.

Pearce LB, First ER, Borodic GE. Botulinum toxin potency: a mystery resolved by the median paralysis. *J R Soc Med.* 1994;87(9):571-572.

Wang YC, Burr DH, Korthals GJ, Sugiyama H. Acute toxicity of aminoglycoside antibiotics as an aid in detecting botulism. *Appl Environ Microbiol.* 1984;48(5):951-955.

RimabotulinumtoxinB

Botulinum Toxins

Name:
Myobloc

Manufacturer:
Solstice Neurosciences

Synonyms: Also known as botulinum toxin type B, *NeuroBloc*, or *AN-072*.

Comparison: The potency units of various botulinum toxins are not interchangeable with other botulinum toxin products, therefore units of biological activity cannot be compared to or converted into units of any other botulinum toxin product.

Immunologic Characteristics

Microorganism: Bacterium, *Clostridium botulinum*, anaerobic, endospore-forming gram-positive rod

Viability: Inactivated bacteriologically, but active toxin type B

Antigenic Form: Bacterial exotoxin type B neurotoxin

Antigenic Type: Protein. The seven serologically distinct botulinum neurotoxins, designated A through G, share a common structural organization consisting of one heavy chain and one light chain polypeptide linked by a single disulfide bond.

Strains: *Clostridium botulinum* type B, Bean strain

Use Characteristics

Indications: To treat patients with cervical dystonia and to reduce the severity of abnormal head position and neck pain associated with cervical dystonia.

Contraindications:

Absolute: People with a known hypersensitivity to any ingredient in the formulation.

Relative: None

Immunodeficiency: No impairment of effect is likely.

Elderly: In controlled studies for rimabotulinumtoxinB treated patients, 152 (74.5%) were older than 65, and 52 (25.5%) were 65 years of age or older. The most frequent reported adverse events occurred at similar rates in both age groups. Efficacy results did not suggest any large differences between these age groups. Very few patients 75 years of age or older were enrolled, therefore no conclusions regarding the safety and efficacy of rimabotulinumtoxinB within this age group can be determined.

Carcinogenicity: No long-term carcinogenicity studies in animals have been performed.

Pregnancy: Category C. Animal reproduction studies have not been conducted with rimabotulinumtoxinB. It is also not known whether rimabotulinumtoxinB can cause fetal harm when administered to a pregnant woman or can affect reproduction capacity. RimabotulinumtoxinB should be given to a pregnant woman only if clearly needed.

Lactation: It is not known if botulinum toxin crosses into human breast milk. Because many drugs are excreted in human milk, caution should be exercised when rimabotulinumtoxinB is administered to a nursing woman.

Children: Safety and effectiveness in pediatric patients have not been established.

Adverse Reactions: The most commonly reported adverse reactions associated with rimabotulinumtoxinB treatment in all studies were dry mouth, dysphagia, dyspepsia, and injection-site pain. Dry mouth and dysphagia were the adverse reactions most frequently resulting in discontinuation of treatment. There was an increased incidence of dysphagia with increased dose in the sternocleidomastoid muscle. The incidence of dry mouth showed some dose-related increase with doses injected into the splenius capitis, trapezius and sternocleidomastoid muscles.

Distant effect: Botulinum-toxin effects may, in some cases, be observed beyond the injection area. Symptoms are consistent with the mechanism of action of botulinum toxin and may include asthenia, generalized muscle weakness, diplopia, blurred vision, ptosis, dysphagia, dysphonia, dysarthria, urinary incontinence, and breathing difficulties. These symptoms have been reported hours to weeks after injection. Swallowing and breathing difficulties can be life-threatening, and there have been reports of death related to spread of toxin effects. The risk of the symptoms is probably greatest in children treated for spasticity, but symptoms can also occur in adults treated for spasticity and other conditions, and particularly in those patients who have underlying conditions that would predispose them to these symptoms. In unapproved uses, including spasticity in children and adults, and in approved indications, symptoms consistent with spread of toxin effect have been reported at doses comparable with or lower than doses used to treat cervical dystonia.

Only 9 subjects without history of tolerating injections of type A botulinum toxin have been studied. Adverse reaction rates have not been adequately evaluated in these patients and may be higher than those here.

RimabotulinumtoxinB was studied in both placebo-controlled single treatment studies and uncontrolled repeated treatment studies; most treatment sessions and patients were in the uncontrolled studies. These data reflect exposure to rimabotulinumtoxinB at varying doses in 570 subjects, including more than 300 patients with 4 or more treatment sessions. Most treatment sessions were at doses of 12,500 units or less. There were 57 patients administered a dose of 20,000 or 25,000 units.

The rates of adverse events and association with rimabotulinumtoxinB are best assessed in the results from the placebo-controlled studies of a single treatment session with active monitoring. The data below reflect those adverse events occurring in 5% or more of patients exposed to rimabotulinumtoxinB treatment. Annual rates of adverse events are higher in the overall data, which includes longer duration follow-up of patients with repeated treatment experience. The mean age of the population in these studies was 55 years with approximately 66% being female. Most of the patients studied were white and all had cervical dystonia that was rated as moderate to severe in severity.

Treatment-Emergent Adverse Events by Dose Group, Following Single Treatment Session				
	Dose Groups			
Adverse events	Placebo (n = 104)	2,500 units (n = 31)	5,000 units (n = 67)	10,000 units (n = 106)
Dry mouth	3 (3%)	1 (3%)	8 (12%)	36 (34%)
Dysphagia	3 (3%)	5 (16%)	7 (10%)	27 (25%)
Neck pain related to cervical dystonia	17 (16%)	0 (0%)	11 (16%)	18 (17%)
Injection site pain	9 (9%)	5 (16%)	8 (12%)	16 (15%)
Infection	16 (15%)	4 (13%)	13 (19%)	16 (15%)
Pain	10 (10%)	2 (6%)	4 (6%)	14 (13%)
Headache	8 (8%)	3 (10%)	11 (16%)	12 (11%)
Dyspepsia	5 (5%)	1 (3%)	0 (0%)	11 (10%)
Nausea	5 (5%)	3 (10%)	2 (3%)	9 (8%)
Viral-like syndrome	4 (4%)	2 (6%)	6 (9%)	9 (8%)
Torticollis	7 (7%)	0 (0%)	3 (4%)	9 (8%)
Pain-related to cervical dystonia/torticollis	4 (4%)	3 (10%)	3 (4%)	7 (7%)

RimabotulinumtoxinB

Treatment-Emergent Adverse Events by Dose Group, Following Single Treatment Session				
	Dose Groups			
Adverse events	Placebo (n = 104)	2,500 units (n = 31)	5,000 units (n = 67)	10,000 units (n = 106)
Arthralgia	5 (5%)	0 (0%)	1 (1%)	7 (7%)
Back pain	3 (3%)	1 (3%)	3 (4%)	7(7%)
Cough increased	3 (3%)	1 (3%)	4 (6%)	7 (7%)
Myasthenia	3 (3%)	1 (3%)	3 (4%)	6 (6%)
Asthenia	4 (4%)	1 (3%)	0 (0%)	6 (6%)
Dizziness	2 (2%)	1 (3%)	2 (3%)	6 (6%)
Accidental injury	4 (4%)	0 (0%)	3 (4%)	5 (5%)
Rhinitis	6 (6%)	1 (3%)	1 (1%)	5 (5%)

In the overall clinical-trial experience with rimabotulinumtoxinB, most cases of dry mouth or dysphagia were reported as mild or moderate in severity. Severe dysphagia was reported by 3% of patients, with none requiring medical intervention. Severe dry mouth was reported by 6%. Dysphagia and dry mouth were the most frequent adverse reactions leading to discontinuation from repeated treatment studies.

The following additional adverse reactions were reported in 2% or more of patients participating in any of the clinical studies:

Cardiovascular: Migraine.

CNS: Anxiety, tremor, hyperesthesia, somnolence, confusion; pain related to cervical dystonia/torticollis, vertigo, vasodilation.

Dermatologic: Pruritus.

GI: Gastrointestinal disorder, vomiting, glossitis, stomatitis, tooth disorder.

GU: Urinary tract infection, cystitis, vaginal moniliasis.

Hematologic/Lymphatic: Ecchymosis.

Metabolic: Peripheral edema, edema, hypercholesterolemia.

Musculoskeletal: Arthritis, joint disorder.

Respiratory: Dyspnea, lung disorder; pneumonia.

Special Senses: Amblyopia, otitis media, abnormal vision, taste perversion, tinnitus.

Miscellaneous: Allergic reaction, fever, headache related to injection, chest pain, chills, hernia, malaise, abscess, cyst, neoplasm, viral infection.

Immunogenicity: During the repeated treatment studies, subjects were followed for development of antibody responses against rimabotulinumtoxinB. Only patients who showed a positive ELISA assay were subsequently tested for the presence of neutralizing activity against rimabotulinumtoxinB in the mouse neutralization assay (MNA). Among 446 subjects, 12% had positive ELISA assays at baseline. Patients began to develop new ELISA responses after a single treatment session with rimabotulinumtoxinB. By six months after initiating treatment, estimates for the ELISA-positive rate were 20%, rising to 36% at one year and 50% status at 18 months. Serum neutralizing activity was primarily not seen in patients until after 6 months. Estimated rates of development were 10% at 1 year and 18% at 18 months in the overall group of patients, based on analysis of samples from ELISA-positive individuals. The effect of conversion to ELISA- or MNA-positive status on efficacy was not evaluated in these studies, and the clinical significance of development of antibodies has not been determined. The data reflect the percentage of patients whose test results were considered positive for antibodies to rimabotulinumtoxinB in both an in vitro and in viva assay. The results of these antibody tests are highly dependent on the sensitivity and specificity of the assays. Comparison of the incidence of antibodies to rimabotulinumtoxinB with the incidence of antibodies to other products may be misleading.

Use caution when administering rimabotulinumtoxinB to people with peripheral motor neuropathic diseases (eg, amyotrophic lateral sclerosis, motor neuropathy) or neuromuscular junctional disorders (eg, myasthenia gravis, Lambert-Eaton syndrome). Patients with neuromuscular disorders may be at increased risk of clinically significant systemic effects including severe dysphagia and respiratory compromise from typical doses of rimabotulinumtoxinB. Rarely, administering a botulinum toxin to patients with known or unrecognized neuromuscular disorders resulted in extreme sensitivity to the systemic effects of typical clinical doses. In some cases, dysphagia lasted months and required placement of a gastric feeding tube. Dysphagia is a commonly reported adverse event after treatment with all botulinum toxins in cervical dystonia patients. In other rare cases, patients developed aspiration pneumonia and died after the finding of dysphagia.

There were no documented cases of botulism resulting from the IM injection of rimabotulinumtoxinB in patients with cervical dystonia treated in clinical trials. If, however, botulism is clinically suspected, hospitalization for the monitoring of systemic weakness or paralysis and respiratory function (incipient respiratory failure) may be required.

This product contains albumin, a derivative of human blood. Based on effective donor screening and product manufacturing processes, it carries an extremely remote risk for transmission of viral diseases. A theoretical risk for transmission of Creutzfeldt-Jakob disease (CJD) also is considered extremely remote. No cases of transmission of viral diseases or CJD have ever been identified for albumin.

Pharmacologic & Dosing Characteristics

Dosage: The recommended initial dose of rimabotulinumtoxinB for patients with a prior history of tolerating botulinum toxin injections is 2,500 to 5,000 units divided among affected muscles. Give patients without a prior history of tolerating botulinum toxin injections a lower initial dose.

Route & Site: Into muscle to be chemically denervated, typically the splenius capitus, sternocleidomastoid, levator scapulae, trapezius, semispinalis capitus, or scalene muscles. Chemodenervation of specific muscles reduces neck pain and the severity of abnormal head position characteristic of cervical dystonia.

Overdosage: Symptoms of overdose are likely not to present immediately following injections. Should a patient ingest the product or be accidentally overdosed, monitor that person for up to several weeks for signs and symptoms of systemic weakness or paralysis. After an overdose, an antitoxin may be administered.

Contact Elan Pharmaceuticals at (888) 638-7605 for additional information and the state health department to process a request for antitoxin through the CDC. The antitoxin will not reverse any botulinum toxin induced muscle weakness effects already apparent by the time of antitoxin administration.

Additional Doses: Optimize subsequent dosing according to the patient's individual response.

Missed Doses: Interrupting the recommended schedule or delaying subsequent doses does not require restarting the series.

Waste Disposal: Discard according to standard medical waste practices.

Efficacy: Two randomized, multi-center, double-blind, placebo-controlled studies of the treatment of cervical dystonia enrolled only adult patients with a history of receiving onabotulinumtoxinA in an open-label manner, with a perceived good response and tolerable adverse effects.

Study #301 enrolled patients who had an acceptable response to type A toxin, while Study #302 enrolled only patients who had lost responsiveness to type A toxin. All subjects had moderate or greater severity of cervical dystonia with 2 or more muscles involved, no neck contractures or other causes of decreased neck range of motion, and no history of any other neuromuscular disorder. Subjects in Study #301 were randomized to receive placebo, 5,000 units, or 10,000 units of rimabotulinumtoxinB. Subjects in Study #302 received placebo or 10,000 units of rimabotulinumtoxinB. Subjects received toxin type B in a single treatment session into 2 to 4 muscles per subject from the following: splenius capitus, sternocleidomastoid, levator scapulae, trapezius, semispinalis capitus, and scalene muscles. The total dose was divided between the selected muscles, and from 1 to 5 injections were made per muscle.

The primary outcome for both studies was the Toronto Western Spasmodic Torticollis Rating Scale (TWSTRS)-Total Score (scale range of possible scores is 0 to 87) at week 4. TWSTRS is comprised of three sub-scales which examine 1) Severity—severity of abnormal head position; 2) Pain—severity and duration of pain caused by dystonia; and 3) Disability—effects of abnormal head position and pain on patient's activities. The secondary end points were the Patient Global and Physician Global Assessments of change at Week 4. Both Global Assessments used a 100 point visual analog scale (VAS). The Patient Global Assessment allows a patient to indicate how they feel at the time of evaluation, compared to the pre-injection baseline. Likewise, the Physician Global Assessment indicates the patient's change from baseline to Week 4. Scores of 50 indicate no change, 0 much worse, and 100 much better. Results of comparisons of the primary and secondary efficacy variables are summarized on the following page.

Efficacy Results From Two Phase 3 RimabotulinumtoxinB Studies[a]					
	Study 301			Study 302	
Assessments	Placebo n = 36	5,000 units n = 36	10,000 units n = 37	Placebo n = 38	10,000 units n = 39
TWSTRS Total					
Mean at baseline	43.6	46.4	46.9	51.2	52.8
Change from baseline	-4.3	-9.3	-11.7	-2	-11.1
95% confidence interval		(-8.9, -1.2)	(-11.1, -3.3)		(-12.1, -5.2)
P value		0.012	0.0004		0.0001
Patient Global					
Mean at week 4	43.6	60.6	64.6	39.5	60.2
95% confidence interval		(7, 26.9)	(11.3, 31.1)		(11.2, 29.1)
P value		0.001	0.0001		0.0001
Physician Global					
Mean at week 4	52	65.3	64.2	47.9	60.6
95% confidence interval		(5.5, 21.3)	(3.9, 19.7)		(7.4, 18.1)
P value		0.001	0.004		0.0001
TWSTRS-Subscales					
Severity					
Mean at baseline	18.4	20.2	20.2	22.1	22.6
Change from baseline	-2.3	-3.2	-4.8	-1.2	22.6
95% confidence interval		(-2.5, 0.6)	(-4.0, -1)		(-3.9, -1)
P value		0.22	0.002		0.001

Efficacy Results From Two Phase 3 RimabotulinumtoxinB Studies[a]					
	Study 301			Study 302	
Assessments	Placebo n = 36	5,000 units n = 36	10,000 units n = 37	Placebo n = 38	10,000 units n = 39
Pain					
Mean at baseline	10.9	11.8	12.4	12.2	11.9
Change from baseline	-0.5	-3.6	-4.2	-0.2	-3.6
95% confidence interval		(-4.7, -1.1)	(-5.1, -1.4)		(-5, -2.1)
P value		0.002	0.0008		0.0001
Disability					
Mean at baseline	14.3	14.4	14.4	16.9	18.3
Change from baseline	-1.6	-2.5	-2.7	0.8	-3.8
95% confidence interval		(-2.7, 0.7)	(-2.8, 0.6)		(-4.1, -1)
P value		0.26	0.19		0.002

a 95% CI are for differences between active and placebo groups. The *P* values compare active dose and placebo. For TWSTRS-Total and TWSTRS-subscale scores, *P* values are for each variable with center and treatment in the model and the baseline value of the variable included as a covariate. For the Patient Global and Physician Global Assessments, *P* values are from ANOVA for each variable with center and treatment in the model.

There were no statistically significant differences in results between 5,000 units and 10,000 unit doses in Study #301. Although there was a rimabotulinumtoxinB-associated decrease in pain, there remained many patients who experienced an increase in dystonia-related neck pain irrespective of treatment group.

In rimabotulinumtoxinB-injected patients, 19% had 2 muscles injected, 48% had 3 muscles injected, and 33% had 4 muscles injected. The next table indicates the frequency of use for each of the permitted muscles, and the fraction of the total dose of the treatment injected into each muscle, for those patients in whom the muscle was injected.

Studies 301 and 302 Combined Data: Fraction of Total Dose Injected Into Involved Muscles				
		Fraction of Total Dose Injected by Percentiles		
Muscle injected	Percent frequency injected[a]	25th	50th	75th
Splenius capitus	88	0.3	0.4	0.5
Sternocleidomastoid	80	0.2	0.25	0.3
Semispinalis capitus	52	0.3	0.36	0.5
Levator scapulae	46	0.13	0.2	0.2
Trapezius	38	0.2	0.25	0.35
Scalene complex	13	0.2	0.25	0.3

a Percent frequency of patients in whom each muscle was injected

Onset: Within 1 to 7 days

Duration: The duration of effect in patients responding to rimabotulinumtoxinB treatment ranges from 12 to 16 weeks at doses of 5,000 units or 10,000 units.

Pharmacokinetics: Although pharmacokinetic and pharmacodynamic studies were not performed, rimabotulinumtoxinB is not expected to be present in peripheral blood at measurable levels following IM injection at recommended doses. Recommended quantities of neurotoxin administered at each dosing session are not expected to result in systemic, distant overt clinical effects in patients without other neuromuscular dysfunction. While rimabotulinumtoxinB has not been assessed for systemic effects, systemic effects have been shown by electromyography after IM doses of other botulinum toxins appropriate to produce clinically observable local muscle weakness.

Mechanism: RimabotulinumtoxinB acts at the neuromuscular junction to produce flaccid paralysis. Botulinum toxin interrupts cholinergic transmission between a nerve and affected muscle, causing relaxation. Cervical dystonia is a neurologic movement disorder in which neck and shoulder muscles contract, forcing the head and neck into abnormal, and sometimes painful, positions that can interfere with normal daily activities.

These toxins inhibit acetylcholine release at the neuromuscular junction via a three-stage process: 1) Heavy-chain mediated neurospecific binding of the toxin, 2) internalization of the toxin by receptor-mediated endocytosis, and 3) ATP and pH dependent translocation of the light chain to the neuronal cytosol where it acts as a zinc-dependent endoprotease cleaving polypeptides essential for neurotransmitter release. RimabotulinumtoxinB cleaves synaptic Vesicle Associated Membrane Protein (VAMP, also known as synaptobrevin), a component of the protein complex responsible for docking and fusion of the synaptic vesicle to the presynaptic membrane, a necessary step to neurotransmitter release.

Drug Interactions: Coadminister rimabotulinumtoxinB with aminoglycosides or other agents interfering with neuromuscular transmission (eg, curare-like compounds) only with caution, as the effect of the toxin may be potentiated.

The effect of administering different botulinum neurotoxin serotypes at the same time or within less than 4 months of each other is unknown. However, neuromuscular paralysis may be potentiated by coadministration or overlapping administration of different botulinum toxin serotypes.

Pharmaceutical Characteristics

Concentration: 5,000 type B units of botulinum toxin per mL

Quality Assay: One unit of rimabotulinumtoxinB corresponds to the calculated median lethal intraperitoneal dose (LD_{50}) in mice. The method for performing the assay is specific to Elan Pharmaceutical's manufacture of rimabotulinumtoxinB. Due to differences in specific details such as the vehicle, dilution scheme and laboratory protocols for various mouse LD_{50} assays, units of biological activity of rimabotulinumtoxinB cannot be compared to or converted into units of any other botulinum toxin or any toxin assessed with any other specific assay method. Therefore, differences in species sensitivity to different botulinum neurotoxin serotypes precludes extrapolation of animal dose-activity relationships to human dose estimates. The specific activity of rimabotulinumtoxinB ranges between 70 to 130 units/ng.

Packaging: 2,500 type B units per 0.5 mL (NDC #: 10454-0710-10), 5,000 units per 1 mL (10454-0711-10), 10,000 units per 2 mL (10454 -0712-10), each in 3.5 mL glass vials

Doseform: Solution

Appearance: Clear and colorless to light-yellow solution

Solvent: 0.1 molar sodium chloride

Adjuvant: None

Preservative: None

Allergens: None

Excipients: 0.05% human serum albumin, 0.01 molar sodium succinate

pH: Approximately pH 5.6

Shelf Life: Expires within 21 months

Storage/Stability: Store at 2° to 8°C (36° to 46°F). Discard if frozen. Contact the manufacturer regarding exposure to elevated temperatures. Shipping data not provided.

RimabotulinumtoxinB solution may be diluted with sodium chloride 0.9%. After dilution, use the product within 4 hours, as the formulation does not contain a preservative.

Handling: Do not shake.

Production Process: RimabotulinumtoxinB is produced by fermentation of the bacterium *Clostridium botulinum* type B (Bean strain). This toxin exists in noncovalent association with hemagglutinin and nonhemagglutinin proteins as a neurotoxin complex. The neurotoxin complex is recovered from the fermentation process and purified through a series of precipitation and chromatography steps.

Disease Epidemiology

Prevalence: Cervical dystonia affects some 75,000 people in North America.

Other Information

Perspective:
1992: Designated orphan drug January 16.
2000: Botulinum toxin type B (*Myobloc*) licensed on December 8, 2000.

References: Brashear A, et al. Safety and efficacy of *NeuroBloc* (botulinum toxin type B) in type A-responsive cervical dystonia. *Neurology.* 1999;53:1439-1446.

Brin MF, Lew MF, Alder CH DD, et al. Safety and efficacy of *NeuroBloc* (botulinum toxin type B) in type A-responsive cervical dystonia. *Neurology.* 1999;53:1431-1438.

Cheng CM, Chen JS, Patel RP. Unlabeled uses of botulinum toxins: A review, part 1. *Am J Health Syst Pharm.* 2006;63:145-152.

Cheng CM, Chen JS, Patel RP. Unlabeled uses of botulinum toxins: A review, part 2. *Am J Health Syst Pharm.* 2006;63:225-232.

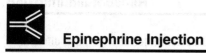 **Epinephrine Injection**

Pertinent Nonimmunologic Drugs

Names:
For self administration:

Adrenaclick
(1:1,000 w/v)

EpiPen, EpiPen Jr. auto-injectors
(1:1,000 w/v or 1:2,000 w/v),
EpiPen training device

Twinject auto-injectors
(1:1,000 w/v),
Twinject demonstrator

For professional administration:
Adrenalin Chloride Solution
Epinephrine Injection

Manufacturers:

Shionogi Pharma (formerly Sciele Pharma)
(also distributed by Greenstone, LLC)

Meridian Medical Technologies,
distributed by Dey Pharma

Shionogi Pharma

Monarch Pharmaceuticals
Adamis Laboratories

Synonyms: *Epi, Adrenalin,* adrenaline
Comparison: Generically equivalent, adjusting for concentration

---

Immunologic Characteristics

Viability: Not viable

Antigenic Form: Chemical

Strains: Levorotary 4-1-hydroxy-2-(methylamino) ethyl-,(R)-1,2-benzenediol. Also described as (-)-3,4-dihydroxy-alpha-[methylamino) methyl] benzyl alcohol, and beta-(3,4-dihydroxyphenyl)- alpha-methylaminoethanol. The empiric formula of epinephrine is $C_9O_3H_{13}N$.

Use Characteristics

Indications: Emergency treatment of severe allergic reactions, including anaphylaxis, induced by insect stings or bites, foods, drugs, and other allergens. Epinephrine is widely considered the drug of choice for treatment of such emergencies. It can also be used in the treatment of idiopathic or exercise-induced anaphylaxis. Severe immediate hypersensitivity reactions, including anaphylaxis, may be induced by the administration of allergen extracts or any biological agent.

Adrenaclick, EpiPen, and *Twinject* products are intended for self-administration by a person with a history of an anaphylactic reaction. Such reactions may occur within minutes after exposure and consist of flushing, apprehension, syncope, tachycardia, thready or unobtainable pulse associated with a fall in blood pressure, convulsions, vomiting, diarrhea and abdominal cramps, involuntary urination, wheezing, dyspnea due to laryngeal spasm, pruritus, rashes, urticaria, or angioedema. Products for self-administration are designed as emergency supportive therapy only and do not substitute for immediate medical or hospital care.

Limitations: Epinephrine is the preferred treatment for serious allergic situations. It is preferred, even though some doseforms may contain bisulfites as an antioxidant, an agent that in other products has caused allergic-type reactions in certain susceptible patients. Alternatives to epinephrine in a life-threatening situation (eg, terbutaline, ephedrine) may not be satisfactory. The presence of a sulfite should not deter administration of the drug for treatment of serious allergic or other emergency situations.

Do not use epinephrine to counteract circulatory collapse or hypotension due to phenothiazines (eg, chlorpromazine), because such agents may reverse the vasopressor effect of epinephrine, leading to a further lowering of blood pressure.

Contraindications:

Absolute: None, in a life-threatening situation.

Relative: Use epinephrine with extreme caution in patients who have heart disease. Use of epinephrine with drugs that may sensitize the heart to dysrhythmias (eg, digitalis, mercurial diuretics, quinidine) ordinarily is not recommended. Anginal pain may be induced by epinephrine in patients with coronary insufficiency, including angina pectoris. The effects of epinephrine may be potentiated by tricyclic antidepressants and monoamine oxidase (MAO) inhibitors. Hyperthyroid patients, patients with cardiovascular disease, hypertension, diabetes, organic brain damage, psychoneurotic disorders, elderly individuals, pregnant women, and children weighing less than 30 kg (for *EpiPen Jr.* and *Twinject* 0.15 mg products, children weighing less than 15 kg) may be theoretically at greater risk of developing adverse reactions after epinephrine administration.

Epinephrine may aggravate narrow-angle (congestive) glaucoma. Despite these concerns, epinephrine is essential for the treatment of anaphylaxis.

Immunodeficiency: No impairment of effect is likely.

Elderly: Elderly patients may theoretically be at greater risk of developing adverse reactions after epinephrine administration.

Pregnancy: Category C. Use only if clearly needed. Pregnant women may be theoretically at greater risk of developing adverse reactions after epinephrine administration. Epinephrine crosses the placenta and may cause anoxia in the fetus. Use only if the potential benefit justifies the potential risk to the fetus.

Lactation: Epinephrine is excreted in breast milk. Use by nursing mothers may cause serious adverse reactions in the infant. Because of this potential, decide whether to discontinue nursing or to withhold epinephrine, taking into account the importance of the drug to the mother.

Children: Children weighing less than 30 kg (for *Adrenaclick*, *EpiPen Jr.*, and *Twinject* 0.15 mg products, children weighing less than 15 kg) may be at greater risk of developing adverse reactions after epinephrine administration. Syncope has occurred following administration of epinephrine in asthmatic children. Epinephrine may be given safely to children at a dosage appropriate to body weight.

Adverse Reactions: Palpitations, tachycardia, sweating, nausea and vomiting, respiratory difficulty, pallor, dizziness, weakness, tremor, headache, apprehension, nervousness, and anxiety. These effects are more likely to occur, and in an exaggerated form, in those with hypertension or hyperthyroidism. Cardiac dysrhythmias may follow epinephrine administration. Excessive doses may cause acute hypertension and cardiac dysrhythmia.

Pharmacologic & Dosing Characteristics

Dosage: Usual dosage of epinephrine 1:1,000 w/v solution in allergic emergencies:

Adults and children older than 12 years: 0.3 to 0.5 mg, 0.3 to 0.5 mL of a 1:1,000 w/v solution

Children 6 to 12 years: 0.2 mg, 0.2 mL of a 1:1,000 w/v solution

Children 2 to 6 years: 0.15 mg, 0.15 mL of a 1:1,000 w/v solution

Infants younger than 2 years: 0.05 mg per 0.05 mL to 0.1 mg per 0.1 mL of a 1:1,000 w/v solution

Give more or less, based on individual assessment of the patient. With severe persistent ana-phylaxis, repeat injections if necessary every 5 to 15 minutes according to patient response. The general dose in children is 0.01 mg/kg.

Epinephrine Dosing[a,b] (dosing by body mass preferred)			
Age group	Mass (kg)[c]	Mass (lbs)[c]	Epinephrine dose (1 mg/mL = 1:1,000 w/v)
1-6 mo	4-7 kg	9-15 lbs	0.05 mg per 0.05 mL
7-18 mo	7-11 kg	15-24 lbs	0.1 mg per 0.1 mL
19-36 mo	11-14 kg	24-31 lbs	0.13 mg per 0.13 mL
37-48 mo	14-17 kg	31-37 lbs	0.16 mg per 0.16 mL
49-59 mo	17-19 kg	37-42 lbs	0.18 mg per 0.18 mL
5-7 y	19-23 kg	42-51 lbs	0.2 mg per 0.2 mL
8-10 y	23-35 kg	51-77 lbs	0.3 mg per 0.3 mL
11-12 y	35-45 kg	77-99 lbs	0.4 mg per 0.4 mL
> 12 y	> 45 kg	> 99 lbs	0.5 mg per 0.5 mL

a Standard dose is 0.01 mg/kg body mass, up to 0.5 mg.
b Preferably by IM injection.
c Mass reflects 50th percentile for corresponding ages.

Route & Site: Preferably IM or alternatively subcutaneously, when given for allergic emer-gency treatment. Epinephrine may be administered intracardially or IV diluted to 0.1 mg/mL or less.

Instruct patients prescribed epinephrine for self-administration to inject into the anterolateral aspect of the thigh, not the buttock. *Adrenaclick, EpiPen,* and*Twinject* products may be administered through a thin layer of clothing, if necessary.

Accidental injection of epinephrine into hands or feet may result in loss of blood flow to the affected area and should be avoided. In case of accidental injection into these areas, instruct the patient to go immediately to the nearest emergency room for treatment.

Diluted epinephrine 1:10,000 w/v may be administered through an endotracheal tube, if no other parenteral access is available, directly into the bronchial tree. It is rapidly absorbed there from the capillary bed of the lung.

Waste Disposal: After using an auto-injector, take care not to allow the used needle to be involved in an accidental stick. Give the used device to a healthcare worker for proper dis-posal.

Overdosage: Large doses or inadvertent IV injection of epinephrine may result in cerebral hemorrhage due to a sharp rise in blood pressure, bradycardia, tachycardia, or other dysrhyth-mias. Overdosage sometimes results in extreme pallor and coldness of the skin, metabolic aci-dosis, and kidney failure. Fatalities may result from pulmonary edema caused by peripheral vasoconstriction together with cardiac stimulation. Rapidly acting vasodilators (eg, nitrates, alpha-adrenergic antagonists) can counteract the vasopressor effects of epinephrine. If pro-longed hypotension follows such measures, it may be necessary to administer another pres-sor drug (eg, dopamine, norepinephrine). Epinephrine is rapidly inactivated in the body, and its use in treatment is primarily supportive.

Additional Doses: In severe persistent anaphylaxis, if symptoms are not noticeably improved, repeat injections if necessary at 10- to 15-minute intervals.

Efficacy: Very high

Onset:

Solutions: Rapid. Subcutaneous administration produces bronchodilation within 5 to 10 min-utes, with maximal effects occurring within 20 minutes.

Duration:
Solutions: Short. Additional doses may be warranted at 10- to 15-minute intervals.

Pharmacokinetics: Epinephrine is poorly absorbed from the GI tract and is ineffective if given orally. It is rapidly metabolized by the liver and other tissues to metanephrine or normetanephrine, which are subsequently conjugated and excreted in the urine in the form of sulfates and glucuronides.

Epinephrine crosses the placenta, but not in the blood-brain barrier.

Mechanism: Epinephrine, the active principle secreted from the adrenal medulla, is a sympathomimetic catecholamine drug, acting on both alpha- and beta-adrenergic receptors. The strong vasoconstrictor action of epinephrine through its effect on alpha-adrenergic receptors acts quickly to counter vasodilation and increased vascular permeability induced by histamine and other mediators that can lead to loss of intravascular fluid volume and hypotension during anaphylactic reactions.

Through its action on beta-adrenergic receptors on bronchial smooth muscle, epinephrine causes bronchial smooth muscle relaxation, which alleviates bronchospasm, wheezing and dyspnea. Epinephrine also relaxes smooth muscle of the stomach, intestine, pregnant uterus and urinary bladder wall, and is a cardiac stimulant, thus increasing cardiac output. This drug mobilizes liver glycogen, resulting in hyperglycemia and possibly glycosuria. Epinephrine alleviates pruritus, urticaria and angioedema and may be effective in relieving GI and GU symptoms associated with anaphylaxis.

Drug Interactions: Rapidly acting vasodilators (eg, nitrates, alpha-adrenergic antagonists) can counteract the vasopressor effects of epinephrine.

The $beta_1$- and $beta_2$-adrenergic-agonist effects of epinephrine are antagonized by beta-adrenergic antagonists (ie, "beta blockers"), while the alpha-adrenergic effects of epinephrine predominate. This may result in increased systolic and diastolic blood pressure and decreased heart rate. Most patients on beta blockers receiving epinephrine to treat anaphylaxis survived the experience, but difficulty in maintaining blood pressure and pulse often lasted hours longer than in uncomplicated anaphylactic treatment.

Do not use epinephrine to counteract circulatory collapse or hypotension due to phenothiazines (eg, chlorpromazine). Because phenothiazines may reverse the vasopressor effect of epinephrine, such an act could lead to a further lowering of blood pressure.

Use of epinephrine with drugs that may sensitize the heart to dysrhythmias (eg, digitalis, mercurial diuretics, quinidine) ordinarily is not recommended. The effects of epinephrine may be potentiated by tricyclic antidepressants, monoamine oxidase (MAO) inhibitors, levothyroxine and certain antihistamines (eg, chlorpheniramine, tripelennamine, diphenhydramine).

Because epinephrine may cause hyperglycemia, diabetic patients receiving epinephrine may require an increased dosage of insulin or oral hypoglycemic agents.

If epinephrine and sodium bicarbonate are to be coadministered, inject individually at separate sites. Epinephrine is unstable in alkaline solutions.

Patient Information: Advise patients prescribed epinephrine for self-administration (eg, *Adrenaclick*, *EpiPen*, *Twinject*) to read and understand thoroughly the patient instructions before any emergency arises.

Counsel patients chronically treated with beta-adrenergic antagonists or other drugs that may potentially interact with epinephrine (eg, MAO inhibitors), for whom repeated injections of allergen extracts are indicated, regarding the increased risk of such immunotherapy because of the added difficulty in treating possible anaphylactoid reactions.

Twinject: To prepare to deliver the second dose, unscrew and remove the gray cap, avoiding the exposed needle. Holding the blue hub at the needle base, pull the syringe from the barrel. Slide the yellow collar off the plunger. If symptoms have not improved within about

10 minutes, insert the needle into the upper leg (anterolateral thigh) and push the plunger down all the way. Then remove the device from the skin, bend the needle back against a hard surface, put the syringe (needle first) into the blue case, and put on the other half of the case.

Pharmaceutical Characteristics

Concentration: 1:1,000 w/v solution (1 mg epinephrine base per mL, 0.1%) or 1:2,000 w/v solution (0.5 mg/mL, 0.05%), as the hydrochloride salt

Other epinephrine formulations are described at the end of this monograph.

Quality Assay: USP monograph.

Packaging:

Adrenaclick: 0.3 mg: Spring-loaded auto-injector, containing 1.1 mL of 1:1,000 w/v epinephrine, delivering a single dose of epinephrine 0.3 mg per 0.3 mL through a 25-gauge, ½-inch needle, when activated with pressure at the tip, with patient instructions, in a plastic tube; 1 auto-injector (59630-0804-01, Greenstone 59762-0171-01), 2 auto-injectors (59630-0804-02, Greenstone 59762-0171-02).

    0.15 mg: Spring-loaded auto-injector, containing 1.1 mL of 1:1,000 w/v epinephrine, delivering a single dose of 0.15 mg per 0.15 mL epinephrine through a 25-gague, ½-inch needle, when activated with pressure at the tip, with patient instructions, in a plastic tube; 1 auto-injector (59630-0803-01, Greenstone 59762-0172-01), 2 auto-injectors (59630-0803-02, Greenstone 59762-0172-02).

Adrenalin: 1:1,000 w/v epinephrine: Ten 1 mg per 1 mL ampules (NDC #: 00071-4188-03); 30 mL multidose vial (00071-4011-13).

EpiPen: Spring-loaded auto-injector, containing 2 mL of 1:1,000 w/v epinephrine, delivering a single dose of 0.3 mg per 0.3 mL epinephrine through a 23-gauge, ½-inch needle, when activated with 2 to 8 pounds of pressure at the tip, with patient instructions, in a clear plastic tube; 2 auto-injectors and trainer (49502-0500-02).

EpiPen Jr.: Spring-loaded auto-injector, containing 2 mL of 1:2,000 w/v epinephrine, delivering a single dose of 0.15 mg per 0.3 mL epinephrine through a 23-gauge, ½-inch needle, when activated with 2 to 8 pounds of pressure at the tip, with patient instructions, in a plastic tube; 2 auto-injectors and trainer (49502-0501-02).

EpiPen Trainer: Spring-loaded simulator that simulates the action of an auto-injector but contains no needle or drug. Includes a resetting device for repeated use (NDC #: none assigned).

Twinject 0.3 mg: Spring-loaded auto-injector, containing 1.1 mL of 1:1,000 w/v epinephrine, delivering a single dose of 0.3 mg per 0.3 mL epinephrine through a 25-gauge, ½-inch needle, when activated with 2 to 8 pounds of pressure at the tip, and a second 0.3 mg per 0.3 mL dose by manual action, with patient instructions, in a blue plastic tube; single-unit carton (13436-0700-01); 2-pack carton containing 2 injectors and 1 demonstrator (13436-0700-02).

Twinject 0.15 mg: Spring-loaded auto-injector, containing 1.1 mL of 1:1,000 w/v epinephrine, delivering a single dose of 0.15 mg per 0.15 mL epinephrine through a 25-gauge, ½-inch needle, when activated with 2 to 8 pounds of pressure at the tip, and a second 0.15 mg per 0.15 mL dose by manual action, with patient instructions, in a blue plastic tube; single-unit carton (13436-0701-01); 2-pack carton containing two injectors and one demonstrator (13436-0701-02).

Twinject Demonstrator: Spring-loaded simulator that mimics the action of an auto-injector but contains no needle or drug.

Adamis: 1:1,000 w/v epinephrine: 0.3 mg per 0.3 mL prefilled, single-use syringe with 25-gauge, ⅝-inch needle in a carrying case (38739-0030- 01).

Doseform: Various solutions

Appearance: Solutions are clear and colorless. Discard any epinephrine product that is discolored or contains a precipitate. Discoloration indicates the oxidation of epinephrine and possible loss of potency. A pink color indicates oxidation to adrenochrome and brown from the formation of melanin.

Solvent: Sterile water with various excipients added to adjust tonicity and pH.

Diluent:

For infusion: For direct IV infusion, epinephrine must be diluted to 1 mg per 250 mL. In extreme emergencies, epinephrine 0.1 mg/mL (1:10,000) can be administered intracardially or through an endotracheal tube.

Adjuvant: None

Preservative: None, except multidose containers include chlorobutanol 5 mg/mL (a derivative of chloroform and chloral).

Allergens: None. Although not allergenic, sulfites in some formulations may cause bronchoconstriction in sensitive recipients; nonetheless, use in emergency situations.

Excipients:

Adrenaclick products: Sodium chloride, chlorobutanol, and sodium bisulfate, all sealed under nitrogen.

Adrenalin: Sodium chloride for tonicity, 0.1% or less sodium bisulfite in ampules or 0.15% in multidose vials.

EpiPen products: 6 mg/mL sodium chloride, 1.67 mg/mL sodium metabisulfite, hydrochloric acid to adjust pH.

Twinject: Sodium chloride 8.67 mg/mL, chlorobutanol 5 mg/mL or less, sodium bisulfite 1.5 mg/mL, sealed under nitrogen.

Adamis: Sodium chloride 1.8 mg, sodium metabisulfite 0.5 mg, hydrochloric acid to adjust pH, each per 0.3 mL.

pH: 2.2 to 5

Shelf Life:

EpiPen products: expire within 24 months.

Twinject products: expire within 18 months.

Adrenaclick products: expire within 18 months.

Other injections generally expire within 15 months.

Storage/Stability: Epinephrine deteriorates rapidly on exposure to air or light, turning pink from oxidation to adrenochrome and brown from the formation of melanin. Protect from light. Protect from excessive heat.

Solutions: Store at room temperature, approximately 25°C (77°F), 30°C (86°F) or less. Do not expose to temperatures greater than 40°C (104°F). Do not refrigerate, because this may lead to precipitation. Discard if frozen. Frozen auto-injectors may malfunction. Shipped at ambient temperature.

Production Process: The naturally occurring levorotary isomer, which is 20 times as potent as the dextrorotary form, is obtained in pure form by separation from the synthetically produced racemate. Air in epinephrine ampules is displaced with nitrogen.

Threat Epidemiology

Incidence: In a study of a mixed group of patients with allergies to insects, foods, and other allergens, a mean of 0.38 epinephrine uses per patient year (PPY) was recorded, with the frequencies of individual patients ranging from 0 to 2.82 doses PPY. Antihistamine uses averaged 0.69 PPY, ranging from 0 to 4.47 doses PPY. Food-allergic patients administered antihistamines or epinephrine more frequently to themselves than did insect-allergic patients.

Epinephrine Injection

Other Information

Perspective:

1856: Vulpian discovers epinephrine in the human adrenal gland.

1897: Abel isolates and calls the "blood-pressure raising constituent of the suprarenal capsule" by the name "epinephrine."

1901: Takamine names the pressor substance of the adrenal gland "adrenaline." Aldrich isolates the product in crystalline form and determines its chemical formula.

1965: Ana-Kit introduced on July 31.

1980: Epi-Pen introduced in the United States.

2003: Twinject products approved in the United States on June 6 for Hollister-Stier Laboratories.

2005: Twinject responsibility shifts to Verus Pharmaceuticals.

2009: Adrenaclick approved on November 25 .

Other Doseforms of Epinephrine:

Dilute Solutions for Injection: Epinephrine 1:10,000 w/v (0.1 mg/mL, adult), 10 mL prefilled syringe with 18-gauge, 3.5-inch needle; 10 mL prefilled syringe with 21-gauge, 1.5-inch needle; various manufacturers.

Epinephrine 1:100,000 w/v (0.01 mg/mL, pediatric), 5 mL prefilled syringe with 21-gauge, 1.5-inch needle, various manufacturers.

Ophthalmic Solutions: Various salts equivalent to 0.25% to 2% epinephrine base: *Epifrin* (Allergan), *Glaucon* (Alcon).

Solutions for Nebulization: 1% to 2.25% epinephrine base: *Adrenalin* (Monarch), *microNefrin* (Bird; Palm Springs, CA), *Nephron* (Nephron; Tacoma, WA), *S2* (Nephron; Tacoma, WA).

Metered-Dose Inhalers: 0.22 mg epinephrine base per inhalation: *Primatene Mist* (Whitehall Robins).

Discontinued Products:
AnaKit (Miles, later Bayer) containing 2-dose epinephrine manual syringe and 4 chewable chlorpheniramine 2 mg tablets in a case; *EpiE-ZPen* and *EpiE-ZPen Jr.* (Survival Technology, Center Laboratories) auto-injectors activated by pressing gray button at top of device; *Sus-Phrine* ampules (Steris Laboratories, distributed by Forest Laboratories) 1:200 w/v suspension.

References:
Grabenstein JD. Anaphylaxis: Epinephrine and emergency responses. *Hosp Pharm.* 1997;32:1377–1378, 1382–1389.

Joint Task Force on Practice Parameters; American Academy of Allergy, Asthma, and Immunology; American College of Allergy, Asthma, and Immunology; Joint Council of Allergy, Asthma, and Immunology. The diagnosis and management of anaphylaxis: An updated practice parameter. *J Allergy Clin Immunol.* 2005; 115(3 Suppl):S483-523.

Kemp SF, Lockey RF. Anaphylaxis: A review of causes and mechanisms. *J Allergy Clin Immunol.* 2002;110:341–348.

Sampson HA, Muñoz-Furlong A, Bock SA, et al. Symposium on the definition and management of anaphylaxis: Summary report. *J Allergy Clin Immunol.* 2005;115:584-591.

Epinephrine Comparisons, for Self-Administration			
Proprietary Name	*EpiPen,* *EpiPen Jr.*	*Twinject* 0.3 or 0.15 mg	*Adrenaclick* 0.3 or 0.15 mg
Manufacturer	Meridian, Dey	Shionogi Pharma	Shionogi Pharma
Concentration	1:1,000 w/v, 1 mg/mL or 1:2,000, 0.5 mg/mL	1:1,000 w/v, 1 mg/mL	1:1,000 w/v, 1 mg/mL
Packaging	Auto-injector	Auto-injector	Auto-injector
Number of epinephrine doses per device	1	2	1
Doses delivered	1 spring-loaded dose of either 0.3 mg per 0.3 mL or 0.15mg per 0.3 mL	1 spring-loaded and 1 manual dose of either 0.3 mg per 0.3 mL or 0.15 mg per 0.15 mL	1 spring-loaded dose of either 0.3 mg per 0.3mL or 0.15 mg per 0.15 mL
Needle	23-gauge, ½-inch	25-gauge, ½-inch for first dose, ⅝-inch for second dose	25-gauge ½-inch
Shelf life	24 months	18 months	18 months

Histamine Injection

Pertinent Nonimmunologic Drugs

Names:
Positive skin test control
Histamine dihydrochloride
Histamine phosphate
Histatrol (histamine phosphate)

Manufacturers:

Hollister-Stier Laboratories
Allermed Laboratories
ALK Abelló

Comparison: Generically equivalent, adjusting for concentration

---

Immunologic Characteristics

Viability: Not viable

Antigenic Form: Chemical

Antigenic Type:

Description: The empiric formula of histamine dihydrochloride is $C_5H_9N_3 \cdot 2HCl$; its molecular weight is approximately 185 daltons. The empiric formula of histamine phosphate is $C_5H_9N_3 \cdot 2H_3PO_4$. The molecular weight of histamine base is 111.15 daltons.

Use Characteristics

Indications: For use as a positive-control reagent in evaluation of allergenic skin testing.

Unlabeled Uses: An earlier product manufactured by Eli Lilly was labeled only for diagnosis of pheochromocytoma or to test the ability of gastric mucosa to secrete hydrochloric acid. Nonetheless, it was frequently used as a skin test reagent, diluted as necessary. *Histatrol* is labeled for use as a skin test reagent, but not for the GI uses.

Contraindications:

Absolute: None

Relative: Do not inject histamine into individuals with hypotension, severe hypertension, or severe cardiac, pulmonary, or renal disease.

Immunodeficiency: Skin test reactivity to histamine will not likely be diminished in immuno-compromised patients, because histamine destabilizes mast cells directly.

Elderly: Skin test reactivity declines with advancing age, more rapidly after 60 years of age.

Pregnancy: Category C. Use only if clearly needed. Histamine can induce contractions of uterine muscle. Limit exposure to histamine during pregnancy; use it during pregnancy only if the potential benefit outweighs the potential risk to the fetus or mother.

Lactation: It is not known if histamine is excreted in breast milk. Problems in humans have not been documented.

Children: Histamine solutions for percutaneous skin testing have been used safely and effectively in infants and young children. Neonates and infants have lower skin test reactivity to histamine, and to common allergens, than older children. Approximately 20% of infants younger than 6 months of age have a negative reaction to percutaneous histamine base 1 mg/mL. Expect relatively small skin test reactions in children younger than 6 years of age. Safety and effectiveness of ID testing in children younger than 6 years of age have not been established.

Adverse Reactions: Following injection of large doses of histamine, systemic reactions may occur: flushing, dizziness, headache, bronchial constriction, urticaria, asthma, marked hypertension or hypotension, abdominal cramps, vomiting, metallic taste, and local or generalized allergic manifestations. Small histamine doses by any route may precipitate asthma in patients with bronchial disease.

Pharmacologic & Dosing Characteristics

Route & Site:
Scratch/Prick/Puncture tests: Use histamine base 1 to 6 g/mL for scratch, prick, or puncture testing.

ID tests: For tests, inject 0.02 to 0.05 mL of histamine base 0.1 mg/mL or 0.01 mg/mL.

Do not inject into a venule or capillary. Histamine is not intended for inhalation or subcutaneous use.

Overdosage: A large subcutaneous dose of histamine may cause severe occipital headache, blurred vision, anginal pain, a rapid drop in blood pressure, and cyanosis of the face. Epinephrine or antihistamines may be used to treat these reactions.

Efficacy: Extremely reliable

Interpretation: Response is based on the size of erythema or induration that appears after 15 to 20 minutes. Interpret all positive reactions in comparison with the reaction to an appropriate negative control (eg, 0.9% sodium chloride).

Negative reactions to both the positive- and negative-control reagents suggest that some agent is suppressing the patient's ability to respond to the histamine (eg, recent administration of an antihistamine). If the patient responds to the histamine, but not the negative control, the patient's responsiveness to other allergens can be considered unimpaired. If the patient responds to both the positive- and negative-control tests, assess the patient for dermatographism.

Onset: 10 to 20 minutes

Duration: 1 to 2 hours

Pharmacokinetics: Histamine is degraded either by oxidative deamination or by methylation and oxidative deamination, so that the principle excretion products are imidazoleacetic acid-riboside and 1-methyl imidazoleacetic acid, respectively.

Mechanism: Histamine is a direct mast-cell degranulator. It acts as a potent vasodilator when released from mast cells during an allergic reaction. It is largely responsible for the immediate skin test reaction of a hypersensitive patient when challenged with an offending allergen.

Drug Interactions: H_1 antihistamines (eg, diphenhydramine, hydroxyzine, promethazine) suppress skin test reactivity to histamine, although the potency and duration of skin test suppression vary.

Long-acting H_1 antihistamines (eg, astemizole, terfenadine) may interfere for as long as 6 weeks. Other drugs with H_1 antihistamine effects, such as tricyclic antidepressants (TCAs), may also suppress reactions; discontinue them at least 7 days before skin testing. H_2 antihistamines (eg, cimetidine, ranitidine) do not decrease skin test responsiveness alone, but may increase skin test suppression synergistically in combination with H_1 antihistamines.

Topical corticosteroids also suppress local dermal reactivity to histamine; discontinue use of topical corticosteroids at the skin test site for at least 2 to 3 weeks before skin testing. Oral corticosteroids appear to have no immediate effect on skin test reactivity. Administer negative-control reagents (eg, 0.9% sodium chloride) to all subjects, to assess the patient's level of dermatographism.

Histamine Injection

Concentration:

ALK and Allermed: 1 mg/mL is equivalent to 5.43 millimoles/L.

Hollister-Stier: 10 mg/mL of histamine dihydrochloride equivalent to 6 mg/mL histamine base.

Quality Assay: USP monograph.

Packaging:

Scratch/Prick/Puncture/Percutaneous test reagents: ALK: 2.75 mg/mL histamine phosphate, equivalent to 1 mg/mL histamine base, in 50% glycerin w/v; 5 mL vial (NDC #: 00268-0247-05); available in a *Multitest* dosage form or dropper bottle.

Allermed: 5 mg/mL histamine phosphate, equivalent to 1.8 mg histamine base, in 50% glycerin; 1, 2, 4, and 5 mL vials (NDC #: none assigned).

Hollister-Stier: 5 mL vial with dropper assembly for percutaneous (scratch, prick, or puncture) administration (65044-9998-01).

ID test reagents: ALK: 0.275 mg/mL histamine phosphate, equivalent to 0.1 mg/mL histamine base; 5 mL vial (00268-0248-05).

Allermed: 0.01 mg/mL histamine phosphate, equivalent to 0.0036 mg histamine base, in an aqueous solution; 2 and 5 mL vials (NDC #: none assigned).

Doseform: Solution

Appearance: Clear and colorless

Solvent:

ALK: Prick: 50% glycerin, 0.45% sodium chloride, 0.4% phenol

ID: 0.9% sodium chloride

Allermed: Prick: 50% glycerin, 0.25% sodium chloride, 0.125% sodium bicarbonate

ID: 0.5% sodium chloride, 0.25% sodium bicarbonate

Hollister-Stier: Prick: 50% glycerin, 0.5% sodium chloride, and 0.275% sodium bicarbonate

Diluent: Compound dilutions with the same diluent used for the allergenic drug being assessed. For allergen extracts, this is optimally a solution containing 0.03% human serum albumin with 0.9% sodium chloride and 0.4% phenol (HSA, also called albumin saline).

Adjuvant: None

Preservative:

ALK: Prick: 50% glycerin

ID: 0.4% phenol

Allermed: Prick: 50% glycerin

ID: 0.4% phenol

Hollister-Stier: Prick: 50% glycerin

Allergens: None. Histamine destabilizes mast cells directly.

Excipients: None

pH: 3 to 6

Shelf Life: Expires within 36 months.

Storage/Stability: Store at 2° to 8°C (35° to 46°F). Protect from prolonged exposure to light. In 1 study, exposure to ultraviolet irradiation for 4 hours caused significantly more decomposition (-27%) than boiling at 100°C (212°F) for 4.5 hours (-11.5%). Histamine is not adversely affected by freezing.

ALK: Product can tolerate 1 month at elevated temperatures (30° to 32°C [86° to 90°F]). Shipping data not provided.

Allermed: Product can tolerate 10 days at room temperature and 7 days at 40°C (104°F). Shipped via second-day courier at ambient temperature.

Production Process: Obtained by decarboxylation of the amino acid histidine.

Other Information

Perspective:
1907: Windhaus synthesizes histamine.
1910: Barger and Dale isolate histamine from ergot and later from animal intestinal mucosa.
1932: Dragstedt and Gebauer-Fuelnegg describe release of histamine into circulation as a result of an anaphylactic reaction.

First Licensed:
ALK: October 1989
Allermed: January 1983, revised February 14, 1992

Discontinued Products: Generic (Eli Lilly)

References: Joint Council of Allergy, Asthma, & Immunology. Practice parameters for allergy diagnostic testing. *Ann Allergy Asthma Immunol.* 1995;75:543–625. http://www.jcaai.org/Param/Aller.htm.

Histamine Comparisons		
Route	Scratch, prick, puncture, or percutaneous	ID
Proprietary name	generic, *Histatrol*	generic, *Histatrol*
Manufacturers	ALK, Allermed, Hollister-Stier	ALK, Allermed, Hollister-Stier
Concentration	1 or 1.8 mg/mL histamine base equivalent to 2.75 or 5 mg/mL histamine phosphate	0.0036 or 0.1 mg/mL histamine base equivalent to 0.01 or 0.275 mg/mL histamine phosphate
Packaging	1, 2, 4, 5 mL vials	2, 5 mL vials

Miscellaneous Nonimmunologic Drugs

Pertinent Nonimmunologic Drugs

Codeine & Morphine: Codeine and similar opiate drugs (eg, morphine), like histamine, directly degranulate mast cells and may be used as positive-control reagents in the assessment of allergenic skin tests. Codeine phosphate 3 to 50 mg/mL in aqueous media or a 5% to 9% solution in 50% glycerin has been used for prick or puncture tests. Concentrations of 0.001 to 2 mg/mL have been used for ID tests. Morphine base 1 mg/mL has been used for prick or puncture tests and 0.1 to 1 mg/mL for ID tests.

Compound 48/80: Compound 48/80, like histamine, directly degranulates mast cells and has been used experimentally as a positive-control reagent in the assessment of allergenic skin tests. Compound 48/80 has been described as an N-methylhomoanisyl-formaldehyde condensation product. It is not a licensed drug in the US. Concentrations of 0.2 to 450 mg/mL have been used for prick or puncture tests and 0.1 mg/mL for ID tests.

2,4-Dinitrochlorobenzene, Chemical Grade:

Synonym: DNCB

License Status: Not licensed by the FDA for use as a human drug.

Viability: Not viable

Antigenic Form: Synthetic chemical not found in nature

Antigenic Type: Chemical sensitizer. Skin tests assess delayed (type IV) hypersensitivity.

Diluent for Reconstitution: Acetone or alcohol

Unlicensed Use: DNCB has been used as a contact sensitizer to assess a patient's capacity to mount a delayed hypersensitivity response to allergens. DNCB is not a licensed drug in the US, implying that safety and efficacy have not been established. Use of this drug in this way is not approved by the FDA.

Dosage: 0.1 mL of 20 mg/mL DNCB has been applied to a measured area of skin, then occluded with paper tape for 24 hours. At least 90% of nonatopic people will become allergic to DNCB so that application of 0.1 mL of 1 mg/mL DNCB 14 to 21 days later will produce a positive reaction to an open-patch test. The second concentration must be lower than the induction concentration to avoid irritant reactions.

Interpretation: A positive response to the second application implies a valid capacity to mount a delayed hypersensitivity response. A nonspecific irritant response may occur 1 to 5 days after test application.

If the second application does not elicit a response, some clinicians have used a 24-hour, closed-patch test with 10% aqueous solution of the irritant chemical sodium laurel sulfate to assess the afferent limb (eg, antigen processing, recognition, memory) or efferent limb (eg, inflammation) of the immune response. If inflammation results from the sodium laurel sulfate, the inflammatory system may be considered at least grossly intact.

References: Bates SE, et al. Immunological skin testing and interpretation: A plea for uniformity. *Cancer.* 1979;43:2306-2314.

Demoly P, Piette V, Bousquet J. In vivo methods for study of allergy: Skin tests, techniques, and interpretation. In: Adkinson NF Jr., Yunginger JW, Busse WW, Bochner B, Holgate S, Simons FER. *Middleton's Allergy: Principles and Practice.* 6th ed. St. Louis: Elsevier, 2003:631-643.

Pertinent Nonimmunologic Drugs

Diluents are important to the clinician for reconstituting lyophilized drugs and for compounding reagent dilutions for hypersensitivity testing and immunotherapy. Various sterile diluents are available in 1.8, 4, 4.5, 9, 30, and 100 mL vials. Manufacturers and resellers include ALK-Abelló, Allergy Laboratories, Allermed, Antigen Laboratories, Greer Laboratories, Hollister-Stier, Nelco Laboratories, and others.

Preferred Diluents:

Human Albumin: Aqueous allergen extracts are commonly diluted with a solution containing 0.03% human serum albumin (HSA) as a protein preservative, 0.9% sodium chloride for isotonicity, and 0.4% phenol as an antimicrobial agent. Dilute *Hymenoptera* venoms with HSA diluent.

Glycerin: Dilution in 50% glycerin in sterile water for injection provides a higher degree of protein preservation than HSA, but glycerin injections may cause local irritation or sterile abscesses. Glycerin is often used as the diluent for prick skin test dilutions, because the viscosity of the glycerin retards the flow of 1 prick-test reagent into neighboring reagents. Glycerin may increase the incidence of false-positive skin test reactions, especially in the higher dose associated with ID injection. Injections more than 0.2 mL of a 50% glycerin product may be painful.

Various concentrations of sterile parenteral glycerin, ranging from 10% to 50%, diluted with either sterile water or various combinations of sodium chloride or phosphate or bicarbonate buffers, are available from ALK-Abello, Allergy Laboratories, Greer Laboratories, Hollister-Stier, Meridian Division, and other manufacturers. Undiluted sterile parenteral glycerin, with a glycerin content 95% or more, is available from Hollister-Stier and perhaps other manufacturers.

Sodium Chloride: Isotonic 0.9% sodium chloride can serve as an effective diluent, although dilutions are not stable for more than several hours to days.

The presence of preservatives (eg, thimerosal, phenol) in sodium chloride diluents generally poses no problems, except in the extraordinary patient who may be hypersensitive to the preservative. "Phenol-saline" (0.9% sodium chloride with 0.4% phenol) is the preferred diluent for alum-precipitated allergen extracts (eg, *Center-Al*).

Inadequate Diluents:
Several diluents are sold by allergen-extract manufacturers that provide less than optimal protein stability. Use of suboptimal diluents may cause allergen extracts to lose potency faster and may cause a greater differential in potency when beginning a new treatment formula.

Suboptimal fluids for diluting aqueous allergen extracts and other immunologic drugs include: Phenol-saline (0.9% sodium chloride with 0.4% phenol).

Phosphate-buffered saline (0.5% sodium chloride with 0.08% to 0.11% Na_2HPO_4, 0.036% to 0.04% K_2HPO_4, and 0.4% phenol).

Coca's solution, also called buffered saline (bicarbonate-saline: 0.5% sodium chloride, 0.275% sodium bicarbonate, 0.4% phenol).

Various glycero-saline solutions (eg, 10% glycerin, 0.5% sodium chloride, 0.4% phenol; 25% glycerin, 0.5% sodium chloride, sodium phosphate, potassium phosphate, 0.4% phenol).

Diluents

References: Anderson MC, et al. Antigenic and allergenic changes during storage of a pollen extract. *J Allergy Clin Immunol.* 1982;69:3-10.

Grabenstein JD. Immunologic necessities: diluents, adjuvents, and excipients. *Hosp Pharm.* 1996; 31:1387-1388, 1390-1398, 1401.

Nelson HS. Effect of preservatives and conditions of storage on the potency of allergy extracts. *J Allergy Clin Immunol.* 1981;67:64-69.

Investigational Drugs

Drug Development and Approval Process

The United States Food and Drug Administration does not itself test new drugs, but it does monitor and review clinical trials conducted by private and corporate researchers or other government agencies. During clinical investigation, as scientists work to determine the value of a new chemical or biological drug, drugs are legally available under Investigational New Drug (IND) exemptions to the 1938 Food, Drug, and Cosmetic Act, with the 1963 Harris-Kefauver amendments. An IND permit exempts the sponsor from the usual prohibition against shipping unlicensed drugs in interstate commerce. Although no absolute lines delineate the stages of clinical investigation, the progress of drug research is usually conceived in the following manner:

Preclinical Testing: Laboratory and animal studies are conducted to assess safety and biological activity. This stage requires 1 to 6.5 years.

Phase 1 (Clinical Pharmacology): Safety testing and pharmacologic profiling of the safe dosage range in 20 to 80 healthy human volunteers, especially men to avoid any potential teratogenic effects in unexpected pregnancies. These studies determine how the drug is absorbed into the body, distributed, metabolized, and eliminated, as well as its duration of action and organs of toxicity. This phase requires about 1 year; 50% to 70% of candidate drugs tested at this stage progress to the next step.

Phase 2 (First Controlled Studies): Effectiveness testing for 1 or more specific diseases or conditions in several dozen to several hundred volunteers with the disease or condition of interest. The objective of phase 2 studies is to define proper doses and regimens, assess efficacy and safety in patients, and provide information on comparative efficacy. This phase requires about 2 years; about 33% of candidate drugs progress to the next step.

Phase 3 (Expanded Clinical Trials): Extensive clinical trials in 1,000 to 5,000 patient volunteers. Vaccine trials often include tens of thousands of healthy volunteers. The objective of these trials is to provide sufficient evidence of safety and efficacy in "adequate and well-controlled clinical trials." This phase requires about 3 years; roughly 27% of candidate drugs tested at this stage progress to the next step. For serious and life-threatening diseases, phases 2 and 3 can be combined to shorten the approval process in an expedited review.

FDA Review Process: When a sponsor believes it has scientifically established the safety and efficacy of an investigational biological drug, the sponsor submits a Biologics License Application (BLA) to the FDA's Center for Biologics Evaluation and Review (CBER). BLAs are analogous to New Drug Applications (NDAs) submitted to the Center for Drug Evaluation and Review (CDER) for approval of new chemical entities. But BLAs also describe a validated manufacturing process and facility, in greater detail than with chemical entities because uniform biological manufacturing processes are critical to the product quality of biological drugs. CBER reviews vaccines, blood derivatives, allergens, and similar products. CDER reviews monoclonal antibodies and therapeutic biologicals. The BLA or NDA requests a license to market the drug in the United States. Review by the FDA takes 2 months to 7 years (mean, 2.5 years). About 20% of candidate drugs submitted to FDA review are eventually licensed. From the start of the investigational drug pipeline to its finish, only 1 in 4,000 drug candidates is accepted as safe and effective. In the proper bureaucratic parlance, chemical drugs are approved, while biological drugs are licensed.

Phase 4 ("Postmarketing Surveillance"): After approval or licensing, additional studies may be undertaken to obtain information about other uses of the drug, to compare a drug to similar drugs, procedures, or therapies, or to assess adverse effects in greater detail. Such postmarketing surveillance may take the form of deliberate clinical studies or retrospective pharmacoepidemiologic research into automated clinical databases.

Prior to approval or licensing, an investigational drug may be granted orphan drug status under provisions of the Orphan Drug Act (PL 97-414), enacted in January 1983 as an amendment to the Food, Drug, and Cosmetic Act.

The Orphan Drug Act provides the technical assistance and economic incentives to pharmaceutical manufacturers to develop and market drugs for prevention, diagnosis, or treatment of rare diseases and conditions. The Orphan Drug Act was amended in 1984 (PL 98-551) to define a rare disease or condition as one occurring in less than 200,000 individuals in the United States; the amendment provides similar incentives for more prevalent conditions if it is reasonable to expect the cost of developing and marketing the drug in the United States would not be recovered from sales in the United States. In the case of vaccines, other prophylactic drugs, or diagnostic agents, the number of expected recipients must generally be less than 200,000 people.

Orphan drug status, by itself, does not imply safety or efficacy. To obtain orphan status, a scientific rationale for use of the drug must be provided. If the orphan drug is ultimately licensed by the FDA, the drug's sponsor receives 7 years of exclusive license to market that product. In addition, the sponsor may claim a substantial portion of clinical-trial costs for a federal tax credit. The list of designated orphan drugs (both biological and chemical), is updated quarterly and publicized by the FDA's Office of Orphan Products Development.

Drug Development & Approval Process: It takes 15 years on average for an experimental drug to travel from lab to medicine chest. Only 5 in 5,000 compounds screened in preclinical testing make it to human testing. Only 1 of these 5 drugs tested in people is approved.

Drug Development and Approval Process							
	Preclinical Testing		Phase 1	Phase 2	Phase 3		FDA	Approval
Years	6.5		1.5	2	3.5		1.5	Total = 15
Test populations	Laboratory and animal studies	F i l e	20 to 80 Healthy volunteers	100 to 500 Patient volunteers	1,000 to 5,000 volunteers (vaccines: 10,000+)	F i l e	Review process	Postmarketing safety monitoring
Purpose	Assess safety and biological activity	I N D	Determine safety and dosage	Evaluate effectiveness. Look for side effects.	Verify effectiveness. Monitor adverse reactions from long-term use.	B L A o r N D A		Large-scale manufacturing
				Expedited Review: Phases 2 and 3 combined to shorten approval process on new medicines for serious and life-threatening diseases.				Distribution
								Education
% of all new drugs that pass			70% of INDs	33% of INDs	27% of INDs		20% of INDs	
Success rate	5,000 compounds evaluated		5 enter trials				1 approved	

Adapted with permission from publications of the Pharmaceutical Research and Manufacturers Association, Washington, DC.

The average new biological drug requires a median 35 to 40 months after BLA submission, compared to 20 to 25 months for the average new chemical drug, to be reviewed for safety and efficacy. Some 3,000 biotechnology products were designated investigational new drugs in 1991, but an average of only 6 to 16 are approved annually (these are products that entered the investigational pipeline about 5 or more years earlier).

Emergency Use Authorization (EUA): EUA is a special authority under section 564 of the Federal Food, Drug, and Cosmetic Act, as amended by the Project BioShield Act of 2004 (Public Law 108-276, 21 USC 360bbb-3; http://www.fda.gov/opacom/laws/fdcact/ fdcact5e.htm). Congress gave the FDA authority to issue an EUA to allow use of medications during a declared emergency involving a heightened risk of attack on the public or US military forces. An EUA can be issued for either an unapproved medical product or an unapproved use of an approved medical product. For more information, see http://www.fda.gov/ EmergencyPreparedness/Counterterrorism/ucm182568.htm.

References: Asbury CH. The orphan drug act: The first 7 years. *JAMA*. 1991;265:893-897.

Beatrice MG. Regulation, licensing, and inspection of biological products. *Pharm Eng*. 1991;10:29-35.

Haffner ME. Adopting orphan drugs—two dozen years of treating rare diseases. *N Engl J Med*. 2006;354:445-447.

Kessler DA. The regulation of investigational drugs. *N Engl J Med*. 1989;320:281-288.

Miller HI, Young FE. The drug approval process at the Food and Drug Administration: New biotechnology as a paradigm of a science-based activist approach. *Arch Intern Med*. 1989;149:655-657. 21 CFR 312.

The following section of *ImmunoFacts* describes immunologic drugs in various stages of clinical investigation in human subjects. In general, investigational drugs are not reported here until they have demonstrated some preliminary evidence of efficacy and are in phases 2 or 3. Investigational immunologic drugs are grouped by immunopharmacologic type (eg, vaccines, immune globulins, immunodiagnostics). Products about to be licensed are intermixed with products just beginning clinical assessment.

Investigational Vaccines & Toxoids

Investigational Drugs

Products in this section are listed in alphabetic sequence by proper name. For cases where the proper name would not imply the investigated use of a product, refer to the following table:

Purpose Being Investigated	Product(s)
Cancers, various	Gonadotropin-Releasing Hormone Vaccine, Therapeutic Vaccines for Cancer
Smoking cessation	Nicotine-Binding Vaccine

Anthrax Vaccine (Recombinant)

Sponsors: Avecia, Dynport Vaccine Company with Avant

Trade Name: *Thraxine (Avecia)*

Antigenic Type: Recombinant protective antigen (rPA), aluminum adjuvanted.

Media: Avant—grown in *Escherichia coli*; Avecia—grown in *Escherichia coli*

Botulinum Toxoids

Microbiology: *Clostridium botulinum*, anaerobic, endospore-forming, gram-positive rod

Indications: Investigated for use in prevention of botulinum intoxication, especially among high-risk laboratory workers.

Dosage: 0.5 mL deep subcutaneous. The vaccination series consists of 4 injections (at 0, 2, 12, and 24 weeks), then a booster dose 12 months after the first injection of a basic series. Annual boosters are given for sustained immunity. Examine recipients' arms 48 hours after each inoculation for delayed-hypersensitivity reactions.

Efficacy: After the initial series and at least 1 booster dose, more than 90% of recipients develop protective antitoxin levels.

Adverse Reactions: Safety estimates are based on more than 12,000 injections administered since 1970. During the first 48 hours, 5% to 7% of recipients experience minor side effects such as mild or moderate local reactions at the site of injection. Usually this is limited to erythema, but swelling, edema, induration, or limitation of arm movement may occur. In less than 1% of cases, more generalized reactions may occur (eg, general malaise, fever or chills, headache, sore joints, stiff neck, dizziness, nausea, vomiting, double vision, or prickling sensation on face and body). Adverse effects are more frequent following booster doses than after the initial series.

Protective Level: A titer of 1:16 (0.15 to 0.3 units antitoxin/mL) for B or E antitoxin is satisfactory for deferring a booster dose for 2 more years. Some 44% of people considered for a subsequent booster dose in 1 series had adequate immunity and booster doses were deferred.

Disease Epidemiology: Botulism is a serious intoxication characterized by weakness, extreme dryness of the mouth, and nerve paralysis. With treatment the case-fatality rate is about 8%.

Perspective: See also the botulinum antitoxin and botulinum toxin monographs.

1947: Nigg, Reames, and colleagues develop botulinum A and B toxoid.

1991: Administered to about 6,000 American troops deployed for the Persian Gulf War; some immunization records called the product "Vaccine B."

References: Arnon SS, Schechter R, Inglesby TV, et al. Botulinum toxin as a biological weapon: medical and public health management. *JAMA*. 2001;285(8):1059-70.

CDC. New telephone number to report botulism cases and request antitoxin. *MMWR*. 2003;52:774.

CDC. Notice of CDC's discontinuation of investigational pentavalent (ABCDE) botulinum toxoid vaccine for workers at risk for occupational exposure to botulinum toxins. *MMWR*. 2011;60(42):1454-1455.

Siegel LS. Human immune response to botulinum pentavalent (ABCDE) toxoid determined by a neutralization test and by an enzyme-linked immunosorbent assay. *J Clin Microbiol*. 1988;26:2351-2356.

Botulinum Toxoid Pentavalent Types A, B, C, D, E Adsorbed

Sponsors: Manufactured by Michigan Department of Public Health, distributed by the Centers for Disease Control and Prevention

Antigenic Type: Inactivated toxoid, types A, B, C, D, and E. Toxin is inactivated with formalin, then partially purified. Aluminum-phosphate adsorbed suspension, preserved with 0.034% or 0.022% formaldehyde and thimerosal 1:10,000.

Botulinum Toxoid Heptavalent Types A, B, C, D, E, F, G Adsorbed

Sponsors: US Army Medical Research and Materiel Command
Antigenic Type: Inactivated toxoids, types A, B, C, D, E, F, and G

Campylobacter Vaccine

Sponsors: BioPort, Antex, Emergent BioSolutions
Trade Name: *Campyvax*
Antigenic Type: Oral vaccine with mucosal adjuvant (a recombinant molecule similar to the heat-labile enterotoxin of *E. coli*-LTRI 92G).
Microbiology: *Campylobacter jejuni* or *Campylobacter coli*. Aerobic, gram-negative, spirally curved rods.
Indications: Investigated for use in inducing active immunity against *Campylobacter enteritis*, an important cause of traveler's diarrhea.
Disease Epidemiology: Disease is characterized by diarrhea, abdominal pain, malaise, fever, nausea, and vomiting.

Chikungunya Virus Vaccine

Sponsors: US Army Medical Research and Materiel Command
Antigenic Type: Live, attenuated virus
Microbiology: Single-stranded RNA virus, genus *Alphavirus*, family Togaviridae
Indications: Investigated for use in induction of active immunity against chikungunya virus.
Transmission: Aedes mosquito vector. Virus is endemic to sub-Saharan Africa and to the Asian tropics.
References: Edelman R, Tacket CO, Wasserman SS, Bodison SA, Perry JG, Mangiafico JA. Phase II safety and immunogenicity study of live chikungunya virus vaccine TSI-GSD-218. *Am J Trop Med Hyg*. 2000;62:681-685.

Lahariya C, Pradhan SK. Emergence of chikungunya virus in Indian subcontinent after 32 years: A review. *J Vector Borne Dis*. 2006;43(4):151-160.

Levitt NH, Ramsburg HH, Hasty SE, et al. Development of an attenuated strain of chikungunya virus for use in vaccine production. *Vaccine*. 1986;4:157-162.

Cholera Vaccines
Inactivated Vaccine

Antigenic Type: Various types of killed cholera vaccine are being tested. These include killed whole *Vibrio cholerae* O1 (called whole-cell or WC vaccines) alone or with the B subunit of cholera toxin (the immunogenic nontoxin portion of cholera toxin; BS). A killed WC/BS vaccine is licensed in Sweden and other European countries. The vaccine is mixed with a bicarbonate antacid before oral administration. Another candidate vaccine contains a cholera lipopolysaccharide-toxin conjugate. Candidate vaccines against both the classical O1 and O139 types are being tested.

Indications: Investigated for use in oral induction of active immunity against the causative organism. The B subunit may confer some short-lived cross-protection against enterotoxigenic *Escherichia coli* (ETEC), another common cause of diarrheal disease.

References: Levine MM. Enteric infections. *Lancet*. 1990;335:958-961.

WHO. Cholera vaccines: WHO position paper—Recommendations. *Vaccine*. 2010;28 (Jul 5):4687-4688.

Live, Attenuated Vaccine

Sponsors: Berna Biotech with University of Maryland

Synonym: CVD103-HgR

Antigenic Type: Live, attenuated. Three approaches have been used: (1) Expression of *Vibrio cholerae* O1 antigens by attenuated strains of *Salmonella typhi* (eg, Ty21a strain), (2) attenuation of *Vibrio cholerae* O1 by deletion mutations that reduce virulence, or (3) attenuation of *Vibrio cholerae* O1 by mutations that affect nutritional requirements.

Indications: Investigated for use in oral induction of active immunity against the causative organism. The Ty21a vector also induces antibodies against *Salmonella typhi*.

License Status: The CVD103-HgR live, oral cholera vaccine was licensed in Switzerland in 1994.

References: Tacket CO, Losonsky G, Nataro JP, et al. Onset and duration of protective immunity in challenged volunteers after vaccination with live, oral cholera vaccine CVD 103-HgR. *J Infect Dis*. 1992;166:837-841.

Clostridium difficile Vaccine

Sponsors: Acambis

Trade Name: *CdVax*

Indications: Investigated for prevention of antibiotic-associated colitis caused by *Clostridium difficile*.

Cytomegalovirus Vaccine

Antigenic Type: Live, attenuated virus

Indications: Investigated for use in induction of active immunity against cytomegalovirus.

Perspective:

1974: Elek and Stern develop AD-169 cytomegalovirus-lysate vaccine strain.

1975: Plotkin and colleagues develop attenuated Towne vaccine strain on the 125 passage in WI-38 human diploid cells, using virus harvested from a congenitally-infected infant named Towne.

References: Arvin AM, Fast P, Myers M, Plotkin S, Rabinovich R; National Vaccine Advisory Committee. Vaccine development to prevent cytomegalovirus disease: report from the National Vaccine Advisory Committee. *Clin Infect Dis.* 2004;39:233-239.

Marshall GS, Plotkin SA. Progress toward developing a cytomegalovirus vaccine. *Infect Dis Clin N Amer.* 1990;4:283-298.

Paston SJ, Dodi IA, Madrigal JA. Progress made towards the development of a CMV peptide vaccine. *Hum Immunol.* 2004;65:544-549.

Plotkin SA, Starr SE, Friedman HM, Gönczöl E, Brayman K. Vaccines for the prevention of human cytomegalovirus infection. *Rev Infect Dis.* 1990;12:S827-S838.

Dengue-Fever Vaccine

Synonym: Disease also known as breakbone fever.

Antigenic Type: Live, attenuated virus, serotype 2. Disease occurs in 4 serotypes: 1, 2, 3, and 4.

Microbiology: Single-stranded RNA virus, family Flaviviridae

Indications: Investigated for use in induction of active immunity against the causative virus.

Incidence: An estimated 35 million cases occur annually around the world, with 15,000 deaths. Case-fatality rate: Up to 20% during the shock crisis. Endemic to New and Old World tropical and subtropical regions, with major outbreaks in Southeast Asia and on Pacific islands. The incidence of dengue fever is increasing in tropical regions, including Puerto Rico and the Virgin Islands.

Transmission: Mosquito vector (*Aedes aegypti* and *Aedes albopictus*)

Perspective:

1906: US Army Tropical Disease Board confirms mosquito vector.

1922: Dengue hemorrhagic fever epidemics in Texas and Louisiana.

1944: Sabin isolates dengue-1 and dengue-2 viruses.

1956: Hammon and colleagues isolate dengue-3 and dengue-4 viruses.

1981: Dengue outbreak in Havana causes more than 344,000 illnesses and 158 deaths.

References: CDC. Imported Dengue — United States, 1999 and 2000. *MMWR.* 2002;51:281-283. http://www.cdc.gov/mmwr/PDF/wk/mm5113.pdf

Innis BL, Eckels KH. Progress in development of a live-attenuated, tetravalent dengue virus vaccine by the United States Army Medical Research and Materiel Command. *Am J Trop Med Hyg.* 2003;69(6 suppl):1-4. Erratum in: *Am J Trop Med Hyg.* 2004;70:336.

Sponsors: US Army Medical Research and Materiel Command

Sponsors: Acambis, Sanofi-Aventis

Trade Name: *ChimeriVax-Dengue*

Eastern Equine Encephalitis Vaccine

Sponsors: US Army Medical Research and Materiel Command

Synonym: EEE vaccine

Antigenic Type: Formalin-inactivated, whole virus, grown in tissue culture

Microbiology: Single-stranded RNA virus, genus *Alphavirus*, family Togaviridae, WRAIR PE-6 strain

Indications: Investigated for use in induction of active immunity against the causative virus.

Dosage: Two 0.5 mL doses 28 days apart, which protects for about 1 year.

Incidence: Case-fatality rate: Nearly 50%.

Transmission: *Aedes*, *Culiseta* mosquito vectors. The virus is endemic to parts of the United States, Canada, the Caribbean, and South America.

Incubation: 5 to 10 days

References: Borio L, Inglesby T, Peters CJ, et al. Hemorrhagic fever viruses as biological weapons: medical and public health management. *JAMA*. 2002;287(18):2391-2405.

Davis LE, Beckham JD, Tyler KL. North American encephalitic arboviruses. *Neurol Clin*. 2008;26:727-757, ix.

Escherichia coli Vaccines

Synonym: *E. coli*, enteropathogenic *E. coli* (EPEG), enterotoxigenic *E. coli* (ETEC)

Microbiology: *Escherichia coli*, facultative, anaerobic gram-negative rods

Indications: Investigated for use in oral induction of active immunity against the causative organism.

Incidence: Some 630 million cases occur annually around the world, with 775,000 deaths.

Perspective:

1886: Escherich describes organism, initially named *Bacterium coli*.

References: Katz DE, DeLorimier AJ, Wolf MK, et al. Oral immunization of adult volunteers with microencapsulated enterotoxigenic *Escherichia coli* (ETEC) CS6 antigen. *Vaccine*. 2003;21:341-346.

Toxoid

Antigenic Type: Inactivated heat-labile toxin (LT) and heat-stable toxin (ST) toxin. There is strong antigenic similarity between LT and cholera toxin.

Inactivated Vaccine

Antigenic Type: Inactivated bacteria. Candidate vaccines have used as antigens: (1) purified fimbrae, or (2) inactivated fimbriated whole bacteria with or without accompanying toxoid. Novavax Inc. is testing an oral, lipid vesicle-based liquid formulation against *E. coli* O157:H7.

Live, Attenuated Vaccine

Antigenic Type: Live, attenuated bacteria. Candidate vaccines have used as antigens: (1) nonenterotoxigenic fimbriated strains of bacteria, (2) attenuated strains engineered to express colonization factor antigens and LT and ST toxoid antigens, or (3) expression of *Escherichia coli* antigens by attenuated Ty21a strain *Salmonella typhi*.

Gonadotropin-Releasing Hormone Vaccine

Sponsors: Aphton with GlaxoSmithKline

Trade Name: *Gonadimmune*

Indications: Investigated for use in treating various cancers.

Hantaan Vaccine

Sponsors: US Army Medical Research and Development Command and The Salk Institute

Antigenic Type: Live, attenuated vaccinia virus, expressing immunogenic Korean hemorrhagic fever (KHF) antigens.

Microbiology: Hantavirus, a 3-segmented RNA virus

Incidence: About 200,000 cases of kidney disease related to hanta virus occur each year, mainly in China, North and South Korea, and Russia. Infections occur with a case-fatality rate of 5% to 10%.

Transmission: Several antigenic subtypes exist, each associated with a single species of rodent: *Apodemus* field mice with Hantaan virus, rats with Seoul virus, and Puumala virus with *Clethrionmys* species of bank voles.

Perspective:

1951-54: 2,500 American soldiers in Korea develop hemorrhagic fever; 121 die.

1993: Hanta virus outbreak in the four-corners area of New Mexico, Utah, Colorado, and Arizona.

References: McClain DJ, Summers PL, Harrison SA, Schmaljohn AL, Schmaljohn CS. Clinical evaluation of a vaccinia-vectored Hantaan virus vaccine. *J Med Virol*. 2000;60:77-85.

Schmaljohn CS, Hasty SE, Dalrymple JM. Preparation of candidate vaccinia-vectored vaccines for hemorrhagic fever with renal syndrome. *Vaccine*. 1992;10:10-13.

Helicobacter pylori Vaccine

Sponsors: Novartis, Acambis, others

Indications: Investigated for use in inducing active immunity against *Helicobacter pylori*, the cause of some ulcers. Some vaccine candidates of this type target urease, an enzyme that facilitates colonization of the gastric mucosa.

Hepatitis B Vaccines

Sponsors: Amgen
Antigenic Type: Purified hepatitis B surface antigen
Indications: Investigated for use in induction of active immunity against hepatitis B.

Sponsors: Cytel
Trade Name: *Theradigm-HBV*
Indications: Investigated for use in treating chronically-infected hepatitis B patients. The putative mechanism involves induction of cytotoxic T-lymphocytes to reduce hepatitis B viral DNA and HBeAg.
References: Bennett RG, Powers DC, Remsburg RE, Scheve A, Clements ML. Hepatitis B vaccination for older adults. *J Am Geriatr Soc*. 1996;44:699-703.

Sponsors: Dynavax
Trade Name: *Heplisav*
Antigenic Type: HBsAg 20 mcg with 1018 ISS adjuvant 3 mg (a TLR9 agonist). ISS refers to DNA immunostimulatory sequences, which are CpG motifs containing bacterial DNA components that have potent NK cell-activating and interferon-inducing properties.
Indications: To induce active immunity against hepatitis B.
References: Cooper C, Mackie D. Hepatitis B surface antigen-1018 ISS adjuvant-containing vaccine: a review of HEPLISAV safety and efficacy. *Expert Rev Vaccines*. 2011;10(4):417-427.

Hepatitis C Vaccine

Sponsors: Various, including Novartis, Genelabs
Microbiology: Double-stranded DNA, family Hepadnaviridae
Indications: Investigated for use in induction of active immunity against hepatitis C.

Hepatitis E Vaccine

Sponsors: Genelabs, GlaxoSmithKline

Antigenic Type: Hepatitis E antigen

Indications: Investigated for use in induction of active immunity against hepatitis E.

Incidence: The disease is fatal in 15% to 20% of infected pregnant women. The highest incidence of hepatitis E is in Asia, Africa, Latin America, and Russia. Studies of the US blood supply suggest that more than 2% of the population (about 4.8 million people) has been exposed to the virus, although endemic transmission in the United States has not been documented.

Transmission: A water-borne disease, by the fecal-oral route, with debilitating and potentially fatal sequelae.

Incubation: 2 to 9 weeks (mean: 45 days)

Perspective:
   1955: First documented outbreak of hepatitis E, diagnosed retrospectively, occurs in New Delhi with 29,000 cases.

References: CDC. Hepatitis E among US travelers, 1989-1992. *MMWR*. 1993;42:1-4.

   Emerson SU, Purcell RH. Hepatitis E virus. *Rev Med Virol*. 2003;13:145-154.

   Shrestha MP, Scott RM, Joshi DM, et al. Safety and efficacy of a recombinant hepatitis E vaccine. *N Engl J Med*. 2007;356(9):895-903.

Herpes Simplex Types 1 & 2 Vaccine

Sponsors: GlaxoSmithKline, Apollon with Wyeth

Synonym: HSV-1, HSV-2

Trade Name: *Simplirix*

Antigenic Type: Viral vaccine, using glycoproteins gD2 and gB2 combined with MPL or other adjuvants.

Incidence: Herpes simplex type 2 causes 600,000 new cases in the United States each year. Some 10 to 25 million Americans experience chronic recurrent genital HSV infections. About 20% of the general population has evidence of HSV-2 infection.

References: Koelle DM, Corey L. Herpes simplex: insights on pathogenesis and possible vaccines. *Annu Rev M ed*. 2008;59:381-395.

   Langenberg AGM, Burke RL, Adair SF, Sekulovich R, Tigges M, Dekker CL, Corey L. A recombinant glycoprotein vaccine for herpes simplex type 2: Safety and efficacy. *Ann Intern Med*. 1995;122:889-898.

   Roizman B. Introduction: Objectives of herpes simplex virus vaccines seen from a historical perspective. *Rev Infect Dis*. 1991;13(Suppl 11):S892-S894.

Herpes Simplex 2 Vaccine

Sponsors: Novartis

Synonym: HSV-2, gD2

Antigenic Type: Viral vaccine

Microbiology: Double-stranded DNA virus, herpes simplex viruses types 1 and 2 (*Herpesvirus hominis*), genus *Simplexvirus*, subfamily Alphaherpesvirinae, family Herpesvirdae

Indications: Investigated for use in induction of active immunity against herpes simplex virus 2, a cause of genital herpes.

References: Roizman B. Introduction: Objectives of herpes simplex virus vaccines seen from a historical perspective. *Rev Infect Dis.* 1991;13(Suppl 11):S892-S894.

Human Immunodeficiency Virus (HIV) Vaccines

Various products are under investigation for the treatment or prevention of disease

Microbiology: Single-stranded RNA virus, subfamily Lentivirinae, family Retroviridae. While many investigational vaccine formulations were initially prepared with the IIIb strain, the MN strain is more common in the United States and many sponsors are considering shifting their products to that strain.

Indications: Investigated for use in secondary prevention of progression to AIDS in HIV-infected people. Research is also underway to assess effectiveness for primary prevention of HIV infection.

Perspective:

1981: Acquired immune deficiency syndrome (AIDS) first reported, although there were US cases in 1978 or earlier.

1983-84: Human T-cell lymphotropic (leukemia) virus type III/lymphadenopathy-associated virus (HTLV-III/LAV) identified as the causative organism by Montagnier at the Institut Pasteur in Paris and Robert Gallo at the US National Institutes of Health.

1985: Screening tests of human serum for the presence of antibodies against this virus become available.

1986: HTLV-III/LAV renamed the human immunodeficiency virus type 1 (HIV-1).

1988: Zidovudine (azidothymidine, AZT, *Retrovir*) licensed in the United States. The drug was first synthesized in 1964; antiviral activity against HIV noted in 1985; advanced clinical trials began in 1986.

Sponsors: MicroGeneSys

Synonym: HIV-1 (rgp 160)

Trade Name: *VaxSyn*

Antigenic Type: Recombinant HIV-1 envelope glycoprotein, gp160, strain IIIb, with an aluminum-phosphate adjuvant, containing epitopes against which anti-HIV neutralizing antibodies have been detected. The antigen is expressed from a recombinant baculovirus produced in cells of the lepidopteran insect, *Spodoptera frugiperda*.

References: Redfield RR, Birx DL, Ketter N, et al. A phase I evaluation of the safety and immunogenicity of vaccination with recombinant gp160 in patients with early human immunodeficiency virus infection. *N Engl J Med.* 1991;324:1677-1684.

Sponsors: Novartis
Antigenic Type: Env 2-3. gp120 antigen (strain undescribed), produced in either Chinese hamster ovary (CHO) cells or yeast cells

Sponsors: Genentech
Antigenic Type: gp120, strains IIIB or MN, with aluminum adjuvant
References: Belshe RB, et al. Neutralizing antibodies to HIV-1 in seronegative volunteers immunized with recombinant gp120 from the MN strain of HIV-1. *JAMA.* 1994;272:475-480.

Sponsors: Baxter, National Institutes of Health
Antigenic Type: r-gp160 antigen, produced by mammalian cells, retaining glycosylation and 3-dimensional configuration (IIIb strain), using a live, recombinant vaccinia virus vector.

Sponsors: Immune Response Corporation
Synonym: Salk HIV Immunogen, HIV Immunotherapeutic vaccine (RG-83894)
Trade Name: *Remune*
Antigenic Type: Gamma-irradiated and chemically-inactivated envelope-depleted, whole HIV virus in incomplete Freund's adjuvant (IFA), strain HZ321.

Sponsors: MicroGeneSys
Synonym: HIV-1 (rp24 antigen)
Trade Name: *VaxSyn*
Antigenic Type: rp24 core antigen (strain undescribed)

Sponsors: Viral Technologies, a joint venture of Cel-Sci Corporation and Alpha 1 Biomedicals
Synonym: HGP-3
Antigenic Type: p17 core protein, HGP-30, a highly conceived sequence based on the SF2 strain

Sponsors: Biogen Idec
Trade Name: *Theravir*
Antigenic Type: Murine monoclonal anti-idiotype antibody vaccine

Sponsors: Repligen
Synonym: RP400c
Antigenic Type: HIV V3 loop-segment antigen, a primary target for neutralizing antibodies.

Sponsors: Sanofi-Aventis
Synonym: ALVAC-HIV-1 (E120TMG-vCP1521, MN120TMG-vCP205, MN120TMGNP-vCP1452)
Antigenic Type: Live recombinant canarypox virus (ALVAC) expressing gp160, MN strain

Influenza Vaccines

Perspective:
1937: Francis develops experimental attenuated vaccine for human use.
References: Ruben FL. Now and future influenza vaccines. *Infect Dis Clin N Amer.* 1990;4:1-10.

Adjuvanted

Sponsors: Novartis, GlaxoSmithKline, VaxInnate, others

Antigenic Type: Traditional whole- or split-virion influenza vaccines with various adjuvants, such as aluminum salts, MF59, AS03, or flagellin. See "Immunologic Adjuvants" section for more detail.

Liposomal

Sponsors: Elan Pharmaceuticals

Antigenic Type: Inactivated, protein with a liposome adjuvant (TLC A-60)

Indications: Investigated for use in induction of active immunity against the causative organism.

Recombinant, Inactivated

Sponsors: MicroGeneSys with National Institute of Allergy and Infectious Diseases

Antigenic Type: Recombinant hemagglutinin antigens harvested from moth cells. Higher than usual doses are more immunogenic but induce side effects no more frequently than traditional vaccines.

Indications: Investigated for use in induction of active immunity; production is faster than in traditional, fertilized chicken-egg methods.

References: Powers DC, et al. Influenza A virus vaccines containing purified recombinant H3 hemagglutinin are well tolerated and induce protective immune responses in healthy adults. *J Infect Dis.* 1995;171:1595-1599.

Japanese Encephalitis Vaccine

Sponsors: Acambis
Trade Name: *ChimerVax-JE*

Junín Virus Vaccine

Sponsors: Government of Argentina, Pan American Health Organization, US Army Medical Research and Materiel Command

Synonym: Argentine hemorrhagic fever (AHF) vaccine

Antigenic Type: Live, attenuated virus

Microbiology: Single-stranded RNA virus, Junín virus, Tacaribe group, family Arenaviridae. Similar to Machupo virus causing Bolivian hemorrhagic fever.

Indications: Investigated for use in induction of active immunity against the causative virus.

Media: Fetal rhesus monkey lung cells

Incidence: In typical years, 300 to 600 cases are reported from endemic areas of the Argentine pampas. AHF has a case-fatality rate of 5% to 30%.

Transmission: Rodent vector

Perspective:
1955: Syndrome of hemorrhagic fever described in Junín, Argentina, by Aribalzaga.
1988-90: Randomized, controlled vaccine trial demonstrates 95% efficacy.
1991: Widespread immunization of susceptibles begins. Through 1997, more than 160,000 Argentinean people have been vaccinated.

References: Maiztegui JI, McKee KT Jr., Barrera Oro JG, et al. Protective efficacy of a live attenuated vaccine against Argentine hemorrhagic fever. *J Infect Dis.* 1998;177:277-283.

Klebsiella Vaccine

Sponsors: Berna Biotech

Antigenic Type: Inactivated. Capsular polysaccharides of 24 different serotypes of *Klebsiella*, 50 mcg of each type.

Microbiology: *Klebsiella*, facultative, anaerobic gram-negative rods, family Enterobacteriacae

Indications: Investigated for use in induction of active immunity against the causative organism.

Perspective:
1883: Friedlander isolates *Klebsiella pneumoniae*, initially named Friedlander's bacillus.

References: Cross AS, Sadoff JC, Furer E, et al. *Escherichia coli* and *Klebsiella* vaccines and immunotherapy. *Infect Dis Clin N Amer.* 1990;4:271-282.

Leishmaniasis Vaccine

Synonym: Disease is also known as Aleppo boil, Baghdad boil, Delhi boil, Oriental sore, Espundia, Uta, Chiclero ulcer. Kala-azar ("black fever" in Hindu) is caused by *Leishmania donovani*.

Antigenic Type: Convit and colleagues tested a vaccine combining live BCG mycobacteria with killed leishmanial promastigotes.

Microbiology: Hemoflagellate protozoa, including mucocutaneous forms (eg, *Leishmania braziliensis*), dermal forms (eg, *Leishmania tropica*, *Leishmania mexicana*), and visceral forms (eg, *Leishmania donovani*, *Leishmania infantum*, *Leishmania chagasi*).

Indications: Investigated for use in induction of active immunity against leishmaniasis.

Transmission: Sandfly bites

References: Playfair JHL, Blackwell JM, Miller HRP. Modern vaccines: Parasitic diseases. *Lancet.* 1990;335:1263-1266.

Leprosy Vaccine

Synonym: Leprosy is also known as Hansen disease.

Antigenic Type: Most candidate vaccines have combined live BCG mycobacteria with killed leprosy bacilli.

Microbiology: Mycobacteria, *Mycobacterium leprae*, aerobic gram-positive rod, acid-fast bacilli, family Mycobacteriaceae

Indications: Investigated for use in induction of active immunity against lepromatous infections.

Perspective: See also lepromin monograph.

1970: Mycobacterium leprae grown in armadillo cell culture.

References: Fine P, Dockrell H. Leprosy vaccines. *Vaccine.* 1991;7:291-293.

Malaria Vaccine

Sponsors: GlaxoSmithKline, US Army Medical Research and Materiel Command, Novartis; others

Synonym: LSA-1

Antigenic Type: Recombinant protein vaccine, using an outer-surface protein, Osp-A. Candidate vaccines are targeted against the various stages of the protozoan life-cycle, primarily the first (1) sporozoite (exoerythrocytic), (2) merozoite (eg, schizogonic, asexual, erythrocytic), and (3) gametocyte.

Liver stage antigen-1 (LSA-1), made by fusing part of the *Plasmodium falciparum* circumsporozite (CS) protein to HBsAg protein, formulated with RTS,S/AS02A adjuvant

Microbiology: Sporozoate protozoa, *Plasmodium vivax*, *Plasmodium malariae*, *Plasmodium falciparum*, and *Plasmodium ovale*. Mixed infections are not infrequent.

Indications: Investigated for use in induction of active immunity against malaria.

Efficacy: In a study of LSA-1 vaccine in 2,022 children in Mozambique, vaccine efficacy against clinical malaria attack was 30%. Efficacy against primary infection with *Plasmodium falciparum* was 45% and against severe disease was 58%.

Incidence: Malaria arguably causes more deaths than any other infectious disease in the world. Over 2.1 billion people live in malarious areas. An estimated 489 million cases of malaria occurred in 1986, of which 234 million were caused by *Plasmodium falciparum*, with more than 2.3 million fatalities. From 1950 to 1992, only 23 outbreaks of malaria had been reported in the United States, more than half in California.

Transmission: 50 to 60 species of *Anopheles* mosquito

Incubation: 10 to 17 days (range, 1 to more than 35 days)

Perspective:

1781: Cornwallis loses 2,000 of his 8,000 troops to malarial fever near Yorktown, Virginia; surrenders to the Continental Army.

1820s: Quinine identified in bark of the Peruvian guina-guina tree. Quinine is also found in cinchona bark.

1860s: During the Civil War, more than 1.2 million recorded malaria cases occurred among Confederate and Union troops, with more than 8,000 deaths.

Early 1900s: 500,000 cases of malaria reported annually in the United States.

1950s: Chloroquine used for malaria prophylaxis.

References: Alonso PL, Sacarlal J, Aponte JJ, et al. Efficacy of the RTS,S/AS02A vaccine against *Plasmodium falciparum* infection and disease in young African children: randomised controlled trial. *Lancet.* 2004;364:1411-1420.

Alonso PL, Sacarlal J, Aponte JJ, et al. Duration of protection with RTS,S/AS02A malaria vaccine in prevention of Plasmodium falciparum disease in Mozambican children: single-blind extended follow-up of a randomised controlled trial. *Lancet.* 2005;366:2012-2018.

Heppner DG Jr, Kester KE, Ockenhouse CF, et al. Towards an RTS,S-based, multi-stage, multi-antigen vaccine against falciparum malaria: progress at the Walter Reed Army Institute of Research. *Vaccine.* 2005;23:2243-2250.

Measles Vaccine (Edmonston-Zagreb Strain)

Sponsors: Institute of Immunology, Zagreb, Croatia

Antigenic Type: Live, attenuated virus cultured in human diploid cells

Indications: Investigated for use in induction of active immunity against the causative organism. The Edmonston-Zagreb strain may exhibit superior immunogenicity, compared to the Schwarz strain, in young infants in developing countries.

Dosage: High-titer measles vaccines (at least $10^{4.7-5.0}$ $TCID_{50}$ per dose) have been withdrawn from clinical study in developing countries because of increased mortality compared with standard-titer vaccines. The effect may be caused by temporary suppression of cell-mediated immunity after vaccination. Standard vaccines, such as those used in North America, contain 10^{3-4} $TCID_{50}$ per dose.

Melanoma Vaccines

Incidence: In 1991, the lifetime risk of malignant melanoma in the United States was 1 in 105 people. The rate of melanoma death is about 2.2 per 100,000 people. Melanoma causes about 75% of all deaths from skin cancer. More than 200,000 Americans are affected by malignant melanoma. In 1997, an estimated 43,000 cases were diagnosed, and about 7,300 melanoma-associated deaths occurred. The 5-year survival rate is 87% for those with localized disease, but only 16% for those with metastatic melanoma.

References: Hersey P. Melanoma vaccines: Current status and future prospects. *Drugs.* 1994;47:373-382.

Sponsors: Ribi ImmunoChem Research, Corixa, and GlaxoSmithKline

Synonym: Melanoma theraccine. Ribi uses the term theraccine to describe its therapeutic vaccines and distinguish its therapeutic application against existing disease from the classic preventive use of a vaccine.

Trade Name: *Melacine*

Antigenic Type: Melanoma tumor lysate (from 2 broadly antigenic cell lines) combined with bacterially-derived *DETOX* adjuvant (MPL immunostimulant from *Salmonella minnesota* R595 and mycobacterial cell-wall skeleton).

Indications: Investigated for use in treatment of stage III to IV melanoma; potential adjunct to surgical removal of primary lesions in stage II patients to prevent recurrence of disease.

Orphan Status: December 20, 1989

References: Sondak VK, Sosman JA. Results of clinical trials with an allogenic melanoma tumor cell lysate vaccine: Melacine. *Sem Cancer Biol.* 2003;13:409-415.

Sponsors: Bristol-Myers Squibb with Progenics (licensed from Memorial Sloan-Kettering Cancer Center)

Synonym: GMK vaccine

Antigenic Type: Ganglioside GM2 conjugate therapeutic vaccine

Indications: Investigated for use in treatment of malignant melanoma.

Sponsors: Biogen Idec
Trade Name: *Melimmune-1, Melimmune-2*
Indications: Investigated for use in treatment of malignant melanoma.

Sponsors: Sanofi Pasteur
Antigenic Type: Vaccinia virus-infected allogenic malignant cell lines, lysate subfraction
Indications: Investigated for use in treatment of malignant melanoma.

Sponsors: Biomira
Trade Name: *Theratope GM2-KLH*
Antigenic Type: Sialyl-Tn-KLH synthetic carbohydrate with QS-21 adjuvant
Indications: Investigated for use in treatment of malignant melanoma.

Sponsors: Bristol-Myers Squibb/Oncogen
Synonym: BMY-35047
Indications: Investigated for use in treatment of malignant melonoma.

Sponsors: Sanofi Pasteur
Synonym: VMO
Antigenic Type: Vaccinia melanoma oncolysates (VMO)
Indications: Investigated for use as an adjuvant or postsurgical therapy for prevention of recurrence of stage III melanoma.

Sponsors: Avax Technologies and Thomas Jefferson University
Trade Name: *M-Vax*
Antigenic Type: Autologous cellular vaccine. A patient's tumor cells, removed during surgery, are modified with hapten DNP and combined with cyclophosphamide and BCG adjuvants. The modified cells are then readministered to that patient on an outpatient basis in a series of IV injections.
References: Melanoma vaccine — AVAX Technologies: DNP-VACC, M-Vax. *BioDrugs.* 2003;17(1):69-72.

Meningococcal Group B Vaccine

Sponsors: Sanofi Pasteur, Novartis, and others

Antigenic Type: Meningococcal group B polysaccharide vaccines are not inherently immunogenic. Various attempts have been made to conjugate group B polysaccharide to protein carriers (eg, outer membrane proteins, tetanus toxoid). Sanofi Pasteur's formulation conjugates an outer membrane protein of group B meningococcus to a group C polysaccharide.

Indications: Investigated for use in induction of active immunity against the causative organism.

Incidence: Group B meningococcal infection accounts for more than half of the meningococcal meningitis in many developed countries.

References: Frasch CE. Vaccines for prevention of meningococcal disease. *Clin Microbiol Rev.* 1989;2(Suppl):S134-S138.

Granoff DM. Review of meningococcal group B vaccines. *Clin Infect Dis.* 2010;50(suppl 2): S54-S65.

Ruijne N, Lea RA, O'Hallahan J, Oster P, Martin D. Understanding the immune responses to the meningococcal strain-specific vaccine MeNZB measured in studies of infants. *Clin Vaccine Immunol.* 2006;13(7):797-801.

Silva Junior FC, Gioia CA, Oliveira JM, Cruz SC, Frasch CE, Milagres LG. Differential capacities of outer membrane proteins from Neisseria meningitidis B to prime the murine immune system after vaccination. *Scand J Immunol.* 2007;65(1):1-7.

Zimmer SM, Stephens DS. Serogroup B meningococcal vaccines. *Curr Opin Investig Drugs.* 2006;7(8):733-739.

Nicotine-Binding Vaccine

Sponsors: Scripps Research Institute; Nabi Biopharmaceuticals

Synonym: NicVax

Indications: Investigated for use as an aid to smoking cessation, by binding nicotine in the bloodstream, before it reaches the brain.

References: Hatsukami DK, Rennard S, Jorenby D, et al. Safety and immunogenicity of a nicotine conjugate vaccine in current smokers. *Clin Pharmacol Ther.* 2005;78(5):456-467. Erratum in: *Clin Pharmacol Ther.* 2006;79(4):396.

Parainfluenza-3 Virus Vaccine

Sponsors: MicroGeneSys; Sanofi Pasteur; MedImmune

Virology: Single-stranded RNA virus, genus *Paramyxovirus*, family Paramyxoviridae

Q Fever Vaccine

Sponsors: US Army Medical Research and Materiel Command

Synonym: Q stands for "query" or Queensland

Antigenic Type: Formalin-inactivated, whole bacteria vaccine, or a vaccine produced by chloroform-methanol extraction followed by gamma irradiation.

Microbiology: Pleomorphic intracellular bacteria, *Coxiella burnetii* (formerly *Rickettsia burneti*), intracellular parasites, gram-negative rods, family Rickettsiaceae, phase 1, Henzerling strain. Treat active infections with a tetracycline.

Indications: Investigated for use in induction of active immunity against *Coxiella burnetii*.

Media: Phase 1 (natural state) organisms grown in egg-yolk sac culture.

Transmission: Humans are usually infected by inhalation of aerosolized particles from contaminated environment; cattle, sheep, goats, and ticks are primary reservoirs.

Incubation: 20 days (range, 14 to 39 days)

Perspective:
1937: Derrick recognizes Q fever as a clinical entity in Australia. Disease named "Q" for query or Queensland fever caused by lack of information surrounding the etiology and nature of the disease. Burnet subsequently identified the causative organism.

1956: Tigertt and Benenson develop vaccine.

References: Ackland JR, Worswick DA, Marmion BP. Vaccine prophylaxis of Q fever: A follow-up study of the efficacy of Q-Vax (CSL) 1985-1990. *Med J Austral.* 1994;160:704-708.

Gidding HF, Wallace C, Lawrence GL, McIntyre PB. Australia's national Q fever vaccination program. *Vaccine.* 2009;27(14):2037-2041.

Sawyer LA, Fishbein DB, McDade JE. Q fever: Current concepts. *Rev Infect Dis.* 1987;9:935-946.

Respiratory Syncytial Virus Vaccine

Sponsors: Molecular Vaccines, Wyeth, Sanofi Pasteur

Synonym: RSV

Antigenic Type: Two forms: split virus, inactivated, IM and live attenuated vaccine, intranasal

Microbiology: Respiratory syncytial virus, genus *Pneumovirus*, family Paramyxoviridae

Indications: Investigated for use in induction of active immunity against RSV.

Incidence: 90,000 infants are hospitalized each year in the United States with RSV infection; 2,000 to 4,500 of these infants die from the infection. An estimated 65 million cases occur annually around the world with 160,000 deaths. RSV is the most common cause of bronchiolitis and pneumonia in infants and young children worldwide. In the United States, most cases occur between November and April.

Perspective:
1956: Morris and colleagues isolate RSV from a chimpanzee.
1969: Investigational inactivated RSV vaccine causes worse bronchiolitis and pneumonia, with more severe morbidity and death, in vaccine recipients than in placebo recipient.

References: Piedra PA. Clinical experience with respiratory syncytial virus vaccines. *Pediatr Infect Dis J.* 2003;22(2 suppl):S94-S99.

Power UF. Respiratory syncytial virus (RSV) vaccines—two steps back for one leap forward. *J Clin Virol.* 2008;41(1):38-44.

Rheumatoid Arthritis Therapeutic Vaccine

Prevalence: 2 million people in the United States

Sponsors: Immune Response Corporation

Antigenic Type: Vaccine targeted against aberrant T cells, using Vβ14T and Vβ17T cell-receptor peptides. Comparable products against other types of T cells may be effective in other autoimmune diseases, such as multiple sclerosis and Type 1 (insulin-dependent) diabetes mellitus.

Sponsors: Anergen

Trade Name: *AnervaX*

Antigenic Type: DR4/1-peptide vaccine. Derived from a human rheumatoid arthritis-associated leukocyte antigen (HLA), believed to aid in presentation of rheumatoid antigens to T cells.

Rift Valley Fever Vaccine

Sponsors: US Army Medical Research and Materiel Command

Antigenic Type: Both formalin-inactivated and live, attenuated whole virus vaccines

Virology: Rift Valley fever (RVF) virus, genus *Phlebovirus*, family Bunyaviridae

Indications: Investigated for use in induction of active immunity against the causative virus.

Transmission: RVF is a viral disease characterized by fever and occasionally ocular disease, encephalitis, and hemorrhagic fever. RVF is both a zoonotic and a human threat. The Great Rift Valley is a major geological feature of Africa, extending from the lakes of east Africa north to the Jordan River valley. Transmitted by mosquitoes and direct contact. RVF is typically endemic to northeastern, southern, and eastern Africa.

Perspective:
1977: An RVF epidemic unexpectedly strikes the Nile Valley of Egypt, with higher than usual rates of serious complications. People most at risk are those visiting rural areas or working with domestic livestock. While efforts are underway to perfect a live, attenuated RVF vaccine, an inactivated RVF vaccine has been available on a limited scale to laboratory workers since 1967. This latter vaccine was given to 2,000 Swedish peacekeeping soldiers stationed in the Sinai peninsula at the time. The vaccine was subsequently refined in the late 1970s; both are inactivated with formalin.

References: Meadors GF III, Gibbs PH, Peters CJ. Evaluation of a new Rift Valley fever vaccine: Safety and immunogenicity trials. *Vaccine.* 1986;4:179-184.

Pittman PR, Liu CT, Cannon TL, et al. Immunogenicity of an inactivated Rift Valley fever vaccine in humans: a 12-year experience. *Vaccine.* 1999;18:181-189.

Schistosomiasis Vaccine

Synonym: The disease is also called bilharziasis or snail fever.

Microbiology: Trematode form of helminth: *Schistosoma mansoni, S. haemotobium, S. japonicum, S. mekongi,* and *S. intercalatum.*

References: Dunne DW, Hagan P, Abath FGC. Prospects for immunological control of schistosomiasis. *Lancet.* 1995;345:1488-1492.

Playfair JHL, Blackwell JM, Miller HRP. Modern vaccines: Parasitic diseases. *Lancet.* 1990;335:1263-1266.

Shigella Vaccine

Sponsors: US Army Medical Research and Materiel Command, Acambis, and others

Synonym: Disease is known as bacillary dysentery or shigellosis.

Antigenic Type: Live, attenuated. Antigen has been produced by: (1) Insertion of the plasmid that contains genes for synthesis of *Shigella sonnei* O antigen into attenuated Ty21a strain *Salmonella typhi,* and (2) insertion of the plasmid that contains genes for synthesis of *Shigella flexneri* 2a O antigen into *Escherichia coli* K-12 strain. *Shigella sonnei* O-specific polysaccharide conjugated to *Pseudomonas aeruginosa* recombinant exoprotein A. Other candidate vaccines use *Shigella flexneri* 2a strain bacteria genetically altered to reduce reproductive or metabolic capacity.

Microbiology: *Shigella flexneri* 2a and *Shigella sonnei,* facultative, anaerobic gram-negative rods, family Enterobacteriaceae

Indications: Investigated for use in induction of active immunity against the causative organisms. The Ty21a vector also induces antibodies against *Salmonella typhi.*

Incidence: An estimated 250 million cases occur annually around the world, with 654,000 deaths.

Perspective:
1914: Sonne describes *Shigella sonnei.*

References: Cohen D, Askenazi S, Green MS, et al. Double-blind, vaccine-controlled, randomized efficacy trial of an investigational *Shigella sonnei* conjugate vaccine in young adults. *Lancet.* 1997;349:155-159.

Katz DE, Coster TS, Wolf MK, et al. Two studies evaluating the safety and immunogenicity of a live, attenuated Shigella flexneri 2a vaccine (SC602) and excretion of vaccine organisms in North American volunteers. *Infect Immun.* 2004;72:923-930.

Levine MM. Enteric infections. *Lancet.* 1990;335:958-961.

Staphylococcus aureus Vaccine

Sponsors: NABI

Trade Name: *StaphVAX*

Antigenic Type: Bivalent polysaccharide-protein conjugate vaccine, types 5 and 8

Indications: Investigated for prevention of *Staphylococcus aureus* infections in patients with end-stage renal disease.

Streptococcus Group A Vaccine

Sponsors: ID Biomedical

Synonym: "Strep throat" vaccine

Trade Name: *StrepAvax*

Antigenic Type: Streptococcal antigens expressed from vaccinia virus or *Salmonella typhimurium* vector

Microbiology: Homofermentative gram-positive cocci, family Micrococcaceae

Indications: Investigated for use in intranasal induction of active immunity against the causative organisms. Indirectly, an effective vaccine would also reduce the incidence of acute rheumatic fever and, thus, CHF.

Incidence: An estimated 3 million cases occur annually around the world, with 52,000 deaths.

Streptococcus Group B Polysaccharide Vaccine

Synonym: GBS vaccine

Antigenic Type: Inactivated, purified polysaccharides

Microbiology: *Streptococcus*, homofermentative gram-positive cocci, family Micrococcaceae

Indications: Investigated for use in induction of active immunity against the causative organisms.

Incidence: Invasive group B streptococcal infection develops in approximately 3 neonates per 1,000 live births; approximately 11,000 cases annually in the United States, with 2,500 deaths and 1,350 cases of permanent neurologic sequelae.

References: Baker CJ. Immunization to prevent group B streptococcal disease: Victories and vexations. *J Infect Dis.* 1990;161:917-921.

CDC. Prevention of perinatal group B streptococcal disease: A public health perspective. *MMWR.* 1996;45(RR-7):1-24.

Schuchat A, Wenger JD. Epidemiology of group B streptococcal disease: Risk factors, prevention strategies, and vaccine development. *Epidemiol Rev.* 1994;15:374-402.

Therapeutic Vaccines for Cancer

Sponsors: Somatix

Synonym: Granulocyte-macrophage colony-stimulating factor-transduced autologous tumor cells

Trade Name: *GVAX*

Indications: Investigated for use in treating metastatic renal cell carcinoma, colorectal cancer, lung and breast cancers, prostate cancer, melanoma, and other cancers.

Sponsors: Biomira

Trade Name: *Theratope MUC-1*

Indications: Investigated for use in treating breast cancer.

Sponsors: Biomira

Trade Name: *Theratope STn-KLH*

Indications: Investigated for use in treating breast, colorectal, ovarian, or pancreatic cancers.

Tick-Borne Central European Encephalitis Vaccine

Sponsors: Baxter (of Austria), Novartis (of Germany)

Synonym: TBE vaccine

Trade Name: *FSME-Immun Inject* (Baxter), *Encepur* (Novartis)

Antigenic Type: Inactivated, purified whole virus with aluminum adjuvant

Microbiology: Flavivirus, single-stranded RNA

Indications: Investigated for use in the induction of active immunity against the causative virus. The following data refer to the *FSME-Immun Inject* formulation:

Dosage: Three 0.5 mL doses, with the second 1 to 3 months after the first and the third dose 9 to 12 months after the second. Accelerated schedules are being investigated. To achieve immunity before the beginning of tick activity, give the first 2 doses during the winter months. The second dose can be given as soon as 2 weeks after the first dose to hasten immunity during summer months.

Adverse Reactions: Erythema and swelling around the injection site may occur, as may swelling of the regional lymph glands or general reactions such as fatigue, pain in a limb, nausea, or headache. Rarely, fever higher than 38°C (higher than 100.4°F), vomiting, or temporary rash occurs. Very rarely, neuritis in varying degrees occurs.

Route: Intramuscular

Booster Dose: A booster dose is recommended 3 years after the primary series.

Efficacy: Over 90% of vaccine recipients are protected against the TBE for 1 year after the second injection. Efficacy increases to 97% for the year following the third dose.

Drug Interactions: TBE immune globulin (*FSME-Bulin*) given within 4 weeks before active immunization may impair vaccine effect. If antibody titers after vaccination are inadequate after the third dose, repeat that dose.

Concentration: At least 1 mcg/0.5 mL

Packaging: 0.5 mL prefilled, single-dose syringe with needle of unspecified gauge and length

Doseform: Suspension

Adjuvant: Aluminum hydroxide 1 mg/0.5 mL

Allergens: Human albumin 0.5 mg/0.5 mL

Excipients: Formaldehyde less than 0.01 mg/0.5 mL

Shelf Life: Expires within 12 months

Storage/Stability: Store at 2° to 8°C (35° to 45°F). Discard frozen vaccine.

Medium: Chick-embryo cells

Incidence: Tick-borne encephalitis (TBE) is a complex of diseases caused by the TBE virus complex. The primary forms of TBE are Central European encephalitis (CEE) and Russian spring-summer encephalitis (RSSE). Others include Omsk hemorrhagic fever, Kyasanur Forest disease, Negishi, Powassan, and louping ill.

CEE occurs in Russia, other former Soviet republics, and elsewhere in Europe, from Scandinavia to Greece. It is also known as Frühssommer-Meningoencephalitis (FSME) or the Sofyn strain. CEE occurs chiefly from April through August or September, when *Ixodes ricinus*, the principal tick vector, is active. The incidence of TBE is highest in Austria, Russia, other former Soviet republics, the republics of Czech and Slovak, Germany, Hungary, Poland, Switzerland, and northern areas of the former Yugoslavia (ie, Slovenia, Croatia, and Serbia). The disease occurs less frequently in Bulgaria, Romania, Denmark, France, the Aland Islands and neighboring Finnish coastline, and along the coastline of southern Sweden, from Uppsala to Karlshamn. Incidence in endemic areas of Austria, Russia, and other former Soviet republics vary from 10 to 50 cases per 100,000 population. Disease usually begins with an influenza-like illness, after a 7- to 14-day incubation, developing into generally benign meningoencephalitis. Some 20% of disease survivors have minor sequelae. Case-fatality rates are estimated to be 1% to 5%.

RSSE, transmitted by *Ixodes persulcatus* ticks, occurs in China, Korea, and eastern areas of former Soviet republics and Russia, including Siberia. It may also be called the Neudoerfl strain. Severity of disease, incidence of sequelae and case-fatality rates are higher in the Far East and eastern regions of former Soviet republics and Russia and lower in western and central Europe. The prodromal syndrome of RSSE is more severe than CEE. Neurologic sequelae occur in 30% to 60% of survivors. Death may occur in 20% to 40% of recognized, untreated cases.

Susceptible Pools: Human infections most often occur in persons who visit or work in forested areas. Infection also may be acquired by consuming unpasteurized dairy products from infected cows, goats, or sheep. Travelers should avoid tick-infested endemic areas and protect themselves from tick bites by dressing appropriately and using insect repellents (eg, DEET).

Transmission: *Ixodes* and *Dermacentor* tick vectors. Transmission via contaminated milk is possible.

Perspective:
1989: FSME vaccine offered to intermediate nuclear forces (INF) treaty inspectors visiting rural and forested areas of the Soviet Union.

1993: FSME vaccine recommended to American troops deployed to provinces of the former Yugoslavia.

References: Canadian Committee to Advise on Tropical Medicine and Travel. Statement on tick-borne encephalitis. *Can Commun Dis Rep.* 2006;32(ACS-3):1-18.

Gunther G, Haglund M. Tick-borne encephalopathies: epidemiology, diagnosis, treatment and prevention. *CNS Drugs.* 2005;19:1009-1032.

Harbacz I, Bock H, Jungst C, et al. A randomized phase II study of new tick-borne encephalitis vaccine using three different doses and two immunization regimens. *Vaccine.* 1992;10:145-150.

Kunz C, Heinz FX, Hofmann H. Immunogenicity and reactogenicity of a highly purified vaccine against tick-borne encephalitis. *J Med Virol.* 1980;6:103-109.

McNeil JG, Lednar WM, Stansfield SK, et al. Central European tick-borne encephalitis: Assessment of risk for persons in the Armed Services and vacationers. *J Infect Dis.* 1985;152:650-651.

WHO. Vaccines against tick-borne encephalitis: WHO position paper-recommendations. *Vaccine.* 2011;29(48):8769-8770.

Tuberculosis Vaccine

References: Kamath AT, Fruth U, Brennan MJ, et al; AERAS Global TB Vaccine Foundation; World Health Organization. New live mycobacterial vaccines: the Geneva consensus on essential steps towards clinical development. *Vaccine*. 2005;23(29):3753.

Orme IM. Tuberculosis vaccines: current progress. *Drugs*. 2005;65:2437-2444.

Skeiky YA, Sadoff JC. Advances in tuberculosis vaccine strategies. *Nat Rev Microbiol*. 2006;4(6):469-476.

Dobbelaer R, et al. The second Geneva Consensus: Recommendations for novel live TB vaccines. *Vaccine*. 2010;28:2259-2270.

Sponsors: Aeras Global TB Vaccine Foundation
Antigenic Type: RBCG30 that overexpresses ag85B

Sponsors: GlaxoSmithKline and Corixa
Antigenic Type: Mtb72f, consisting of fusion protein of antigenic domains from *M. tuberculosis* with adjuvants

Sponsors: University of Oxford
Antigenic Type: MVA85A—MVA expressing Ag85A

Tularemia Vaccine

Sponsors: US Army Medical Research and Materiel Command
Synonym: Disease is known as rabbit fever, deerfly fever, and O'Hara disease.
Antigenic Type: Live, attenuated bacteria
Microbiology: *Francisella tularensis*, aerobic gram-negative coccobacillus, strain LVS
Indications: Investigated for use in induction of active immunity against *Francisella tularensis*, primarily for protection of laboratory workers and animal caretakers. Vaccine prevents disease or reduces severity.
Dosage: 1 to 20 drops, through which 15 to 30 impressions are made to just prick the skin. Allow site to air dry for 5 minutes, then wipe off excess fluid with sterile, dry gauze; apply no dressing.
Route: Scarification, deltoid area
Incidence: At least 157 cases of tularemia were reported in the United States in 1992.
Perspective:
  1912: Chapin and McCoy isolate *Bacterium tularense*, cause of plague-like disease of squirrels, named for Tulare County, California.
  1950: Kadull and colleagues reduce tularemia morbidity with phenol-inactivated vaccine.
  1961: Eigelsback describes attenuated vaccine.
References: CDC. Tularemia—United States, 1990-2000. *MMWR*. 2002;51:182-184. http://www.cdc.gov/mmwr/preview/mmwrhtml/mm5109a1.htm.

Dennis DT, Inglesby TV, Henderson DA, et al. Tularemia as a biological weapon: Medical and public health management. *JAMA*. 2001;285:2763-2773. http://www.jama.ama-assn.org/issues/v285n21/rpdf/jst10001.pdf.

Koskela P. Humoral immunity induced by a live *Francisella tularensis* vaccine: Complement-fixing antibodies determined by an enzyme-linked immunosorbent assay (CF-ELISA). *Vaccine*. 1985;3:389-391.

Vaccinia Vaccine (Cell Culture-Produced)

Sponsors: Bavarian Nordic

Trade Name: *Imvamune*

Indications: Investigated for prevention of smallpox infection in immune-compromised people.

Strain: Modified Vaccinia Ankara (MVA), replication-deficient strain

Route: IM

Sponsors: Vaxgen, in partnership with the Chemo-Sero Research Institute (Kaketsuken) of Kumamoto, Japan

Indications: Investigated for prevention of smallpox infection in immune-compromised people.

Strain: LC16m8 attenuated strain (licensed in Japan)

References: Kenner J, Cameron F, Empig C, Jobes DV, Gurwith M. LC16m8: an attenuated smallpox vaccine. *Vaccine*. 2006;24(47-48):7009-7022.

Venezuelan Equine Encephalitis Vaccines

Sponsors: US Army Research And Materiel Command

Microbiology: Single-stranded RNA virus, genus *Alphavirus*, family Togaviridae

Indications: Investigated for use in induction of active immunity against the causative virus.

Incidence: Case-fatality rate: Normally less than 1%, except that 15% of cases with encephalitis die.

Transmission: Transmitted by *Aedes, Culex, Mansonia, Psorophora* mosquito vectors. Virus is endemic to northern South America and Central America.

Perspective:
1965: US Army develops TC-83 vaccine.
1967: Outbreak in Columbia kills more than 100,000 horses.
1971: 2.25 million doses given to horses in Central America and Texas. At least 84 human cases of VEE occurred in Texas.

References: Borio L, Inglesby T, Peters CJ, et al. Hemorrhagic fever viruses as biological weapons: medical and public health management. *JAMA*. 2002;287(18):2391-2405.

McClain DJ, Pittman PR, Ramsburg HH, et al. Immunologic interference from sequential administration of live attenuated alphavirus vaccines. *J Infect Dis*. 1998;177:634-641.

Tsai TF. Arboviral infections in the United States. *Infect Dis Clin N Amer*. 1991;5:73-102.

Attenuated

Synonym: VEE vaccine, attenuated

Antigenic Type: Live, attenuated virus, TC-83 strain

Dosage: 0.5 mL, subcutaneously. Immunity persists for about 5 years. The optimal regimen seems to be initial immunization with the attenuated vaccine (strain TC-83), followed by boosters with the inactivated vaccine (strain C-84).

Inactivated

Synonym: VEE vaccine, inactivated

Antigenic Type: Formalin inactivated, whole virus, C-84 strain

Pharmaceutics: Attenuated virus strain TC-83 inactivated with formalin to form C-84 strain.

Western Equine Encephalitis Vaccine

Sponsors: US Army Medical Research and Materiel Command

Synonym: WEE vaccine

Antigenic Type: Formalin-inactivated, whole virus, grown in tissue culture

Microbiology: Single-stranded RNA virus, genus *Alphavirus*, family Togaviride

Indications: Investigated for use in induction of active immunity against the causative virus.

Dosage: Two 0.5 mL doses 28 days apart, with booster doses after 6 months and then annually

Incidence: 41 cases (1 fatal) in 1987. Case-fatality rate: 3%.

Transmission: Transmitted by *Culex tarsalis*, *Culiseta* mosquito vectors, avian reservoir. Virus is endemic throughout North and South America; outbreaks occur most commonly in the western United States, Uruguay, and Argentina.

References: Borio L, Inglesby T, Peters CJ, et al. Hemorrhagic fever viruses as biological weapons: medical and public health management. *JAMA*. 2002;287(18):2391-2405.

Davis LE, Beckham JD, Tyler KL. North American encephalitic arboviruses. *Neurol Clin*. 2008;26:727-7 57, ix.

Investigational Drugs

Products in this section are listed in alphabetic sequence by proper name. For cases where the proper name would not imply the investigated use of a product, refer to the following table:

Purpose Being Investigated	Product(s)
Anthrax	Raxibacumab
Candidiasis	Efungumab
Cytomegalovirus	Sevirumab
Hepatitis B	Tuvirumab
Human immunodeficiency virus	Ibalizumab
Respiratory syncytial virus	Motavizumab Reslivizumab
Staphylococcus aureus	Tefibazumab
Staphylococcus epidermidis	Pagibaximab
Shiga toxin–producing *Escherichia coli* (STEC)	Urtoxazumab

Anthrax Immune Globulin (Monoclonal)

Sponsors: Elusys Therapeutics

Synonym: *Anthim*, ETI-204

References: Mohamed N, Clagett M, Li J, et al. A high-affinity monoclonal antibody to anthrax protective antigen passively protects rabbits before and after aerosolized *Bacillus anthracis* spore challenge. *Infect Immun.* 2005;73(2):795-802.

Sponsors: Medarex and PharmAthene

Synonym: MDX-1303, *Valtorim*

References: Vitale L, Blanset D, Lowy I, et al. Prophylaxis and therapy of inhalational anthrax by a novel monoclonal antibody to protective antigen that mimics vaccine-induced immunity. *Infect Immun.* 2006;74(10):5840-5847.

Anthrax Immune Globulin (Polyclonal)

Sponsors: Cangene; Emergent BioSolutions

Antigenic Type: Hyperimmune globulin, IgG, polyclonal, polymeric

Bavituximab

Sponsors: Peregrine Pharmaceuticals

Synonym: ch3G4, *Tarvacin*

Antigenic Type: IgG1 anti-(phosphatidylserine) (human-mouse monoclonal ch3G4 heavy chain) with disulfide bond to human-mouse ch3G4 K-chain, dimer. Molecular weight 145,300 daltons. Binds to a phospholipid called phosphatidylserine (PS), normally located on the inside of cells, but which becomes exposed on the outside of cells that line the blood vessels of tumors.

Indications: Investigated for treatment of solid cancers (eg, brain, prostate, breast, lung) or chronic hepatitis C.

Clostridium difficile Antitoxin (Unspecified Source)

Sponsors: Eli Lilly
Synonym: LY 355636
Antigenic Type: Antitoxin for oral administration
Indications: Investigated for *Clostridium difficile*-associated disease.

Clostridium difficile Hyperimmune Globulin (Bovine)

Sponsors: ImmuCell
Trade Name: *DiffGAM*
Antigenic Type: Hyperimmune globulin from bovine milk; enteric-coated for oral administration
Indications: Investigated for treatment and prevention of diarrhea and colitis caused by *Clostridium difficile*.

Efungumab

Sponsors: NeuTec Pharma
Synonym: *Mycograb*, anti-HSP90
Antigenic Type: Immunoglobulin scFv fragment, anti-(heat shock protein 90 homolog from *Candida albicans*), methionylalanyl-[hman HSP90mab VH domain]-tris[(tetraglycyl)seryl]-[HSP90mab V-Kappa domain]-[arginyl-trialanyl-leucyl-glutamyl]-hexahistidine
Indications: Investigated for treatment of invasive candidiasis.
References: Pachl J, Svoboda P, Jacobs F, et al; Mycograb Invasive Candidiasis Study Group. A randomized, blinded, multicenter trial of lipid-associated amphotericin B alone versus in combination with an antibody-based inhibitor of heat shock protein 90 in patients with invasive candidiasis. *Clin Infect Dis.* 2006;42(10):1404-1413.

Ibalizumab

Sponsors: Biogen Idec, Tanox
Synonym: 5A8, Hu-5A8, TNX-355
Antigenic Type: Humanized version of murine anti-CD4 IgG4
Indications: Investigated for treatment of HIV infection.
References: Dimitrov A. Ibalizumab, a CD4-specific mAb to inhibit HIV-1 infection. *Curr Opin Investig Drugs.* 2007;8(8):653-661.

Klebsiella/*Pseudomonas* Intravenous Immunoglobulin (Human)

Sponsors: Berna Biotech

Synonym: K/PIG

Antigenic Type: IgG, polyclonal, primarily monomeric. This drug is harvested from human volunteers immunized with the capsular polysaccharides of 24 different serotypes of *Klebsiella* and an 8-valent *Pseudomonas aeruginosa* vaccine in which the type-specific O-polysaccharides have been conjugated to *Pseudomonas* toxin A.

Bacteriology: *Klebsiella*, facultative, anaerobic gram-negative rod; *Pseudomonas aeruginosa*, aerobic gram-negative rod, family Pseudomonadaceae

Indications: Investigated for use in treating bacterial infections involving *Klebsiella* species or *Pseudomonas aeruginosa*.

References: Cross AS, et al. *Escherichia coli* and *Klebsiella* vaccines and immunotherapy. *Infect Dis Clin N Amer*. 1990;4:271-282.

McClain JB, Edelman R, Shmuklarsky M, Que J, Cryz SJ, Cross AS. Unusual persistence in healthy volunteers and ill patients of hyperimmune immunoglobulin directed against multiple *Pseudomonas* O-chain and *Klebsiella* serotypes after intravenous infusion. *Vaccine*. 2001;19:3499-3508.

Motavizumab (Humanized)

Sponsors: MedImmune

Synonym: MEDI-524

Trade Name: *Numax*

Antigenic Type: IgG1 anti-(respiratory syncytial virus glycoprotein F) (human-mouse monoclonal MEDI-524 γ1-chain) with disulfide bond to human-mouse MIDE-524 K-chain, dimer. Molecular weight 148,000 daltons.

Indications: Investigated for prevention of serious lower respiratory tract disease caused by RSV virus in children.

References: Mejias A, Chavez-Bueno S, Rios AM, et al. Comparative effects of two neutralizing anti-respiratory syncytial virus (RSV) monoclonal antibodies in the RSV murine model: time versus potency. *Antimicrob Agents Chemother*. 2005;49:4700-4707.

Pagibaximab (Chimeric)

Sponsors: GlaxoSmithKline

Synonym: A110, HU96-110

Antigenic Type: IgG1, anti-*Staphylococcus epidermidis* lipoteichoic acid (human-mouse monoclonal HU96-110 heavy chain) with disulfide bond to human-mouse HU96-110 K-chain, dimer. Molecular weight 146,100 daltons.

Indications: Investigated for prevention of staphylococcal sepsis in premature infants.

Raxibacumab

Sponsors: Human Genome Sciences

Trade Name: *ABthrax*

Antigenic Type: IgG1, anti-anthrax protective antigen, PA heavy chain with disulfide bond to PA λ-chain, dimer. Molecular weight 142,900 daltons.

Indications: Investigated for the treatment of anthrax infection.

Production Medium: Mouse myeloma cell line

References: Subramanian GM, Cronin PW, Poley G, et al. A phase 1 study of PAmAb, a fully human monoclonal antibody against *Bacillus anthracis* protective antigen, in healthy volunteers. *Clin Infect Dis*. 2005;41(1):12-20.

Migone TS, et al. Raxibacumab for the treatment of inhalational anthrax. *N Engl J Med*. 2009;361(Jul 9):135-144.

Reslivizumab (Humanized)

Sponsors: Merck

Synonym: SCH 55700

Antigenic Type: IgG4, anti-human interleukin-5 (human-rat monoclonal SCH 55700 γ4-chain) with disulfide bond to human-rat SCH 55700 light chain, dimer. Molecular weight 150,000 daltons.

Indications: Investigated for treatment of bronchial asthma and prevention of serious lower respiratory tract disease caused by respiratory syncytial virus (RSV) in pediatric patients at high risk of RSV disease.

Sevirumab (Human)

Sponsors: Novartis with Protein Design Labs

Synonym: Cytomegalovirus monoclonal IgG antibodies, EV2-7, SDZ MSL 109, CAS 138660-96-5

Trade Name: *Protovir*

Antigenic Type: IgG1 human monoclonal antibody, kappa type, 150,000 daltons

Indications: Investigated for treating cytomegalovirus retinitis in patients with AIDS. Clinical trials are focusing on extending time to remission or progression to retinitis.

References: Borucki MJ, Spritzler J, Asmuth DM, et al; AACTG 266 Team. A phase II, double-masked, randomized, placebo-controlled evaluation of a human monoclonal anti-Cytomegalovirus antibody (MSL-109) in combination with standard therapy versus standard therapy alone in the treatment of AIDS patients with Cytomegalovirus retinitis. *Antiviral Res*. 2004;64:103-111.

Tefibazumab

Sponsors: Avid Bioservices, Inhibitex

Synonym: INH-H2002, *Aurexis*

Antigenic Type: IgG1, anti-*Staphylococcus aureus* protein ClfA (clumping factor A) (human-mouse monoclonal Aurexis heavy chain) with disulfide bond to human-mouse Aurexis κ-chain, dimer. Molecular weight 147,590 daltons.

Indications: Investigated for treatment of *Staphylococcus aureus* infections.

References: Domanski PJ, Patel PR, Bayer AS, et al. Characterization of a humanized monoclonal antibody recognizing clumping factor A expressed by Staphylococcus aureus. *Infect Immun*. 2005;73:5229-5232.

Reilley S, Wenzel E, Reynolds L, Bennet B, Patti JM, Hetherington S. Open-label, dose escalation study of the safety and pharmacokinetic profile of tefibazumab in healthy volunteers. *Antimicrob Agents Chemother*. 2005;49:959-962.

Tuvirumab (Human)

Sponsors: Novartis, Protein Design Labs

Synonym: PE1-1, SDZ OST 577, CAS 138660-97-6

Antigenic Type: Antiviral monoclonal antibody, IgG1, lambda type, 150,000 daltons, targeted against the hepatitis B surface antigen

Indications: Investigated for use in treating reinfections in patients undergoing liver transplantation because of chronic hepatitis B infection.

Urtoxazumab

Sponsors: Teijin Pharma

Antigenic Type: Humanized monoclonal antibody directed against Shiga-like toxin 2 (Stx2)

Indications: Investigated for treatment of hemolytic uremic syndrome due to Shiga-like toxin-producing Escherichia coli (STEC) infection.

References: López EL, et al. Safety and pharmacokinetics of urtoxazumab, a humanized monoclonal antibody, against Shiga-like toxin 2 in healthy adults and in pediatric patients infected with Shiga-like toxin-producing *Escherichia coli. Antimicrob Agents Chemother*. 2010;54:239-243.

Varicella-Zoster Immune Globulin (Human)

Sponsors: Cangene Corporation

Synonym: VZIG-IM

Trade Name: *VariZIG*

Antigenic Type: IgG, human, polyclonal

Indications: For postexposure prophylaxis of varicella, principally immunocompromised patients; neonates whose mothers have signs and symptoms of varicella around the time of delivery (ie, 5 days before to 2 days after); premature infants born at 28 weeks' gestation or more who are exposed during the neonatal period and whose mothers do not have evidence of immunity; premature infants born at less than 28 weeks' gestation or who weigh 1,000 g or less at birth and were exposed during the neonatal period, regardless of maternal history of varicella disease or vaccination; and pregnant women.

VZIG-IM is expected to provide maximum benefit when administered as soon as possible after exposure. Although it can be effective if administered as late as 10 days after exposure; treatment after 10 days is of uncertain value.

Dosage: 125 units per 10 kg body weight, up to a maximum of 625 units (5 vials). The minimum dose is 125 units.

Route: IM

Packaging: 125 unit vials

Doseform: Powder yielding 5% solution

Drug Interactions: Delay varicella vaccination until 5 months after VZIG-IM administration.

Perspective:
1962: Ross shows that varicella antibodies in gamma globulin could modify disease.
1969: Zoster immune globulin (ZIG), prepared from patients convalescing from herpes zoster, shown to be effective in preventing clinical varicella in susceptible healthy children.
1978: VZIG available as an IND.
1980: VZIG licensed in the United States to Massachusetts PHBL on December 23, 1980, but initial distribution limited to ensure availability for the most urgent cases. Distribution discontinued in 2006.

References: Canadian National Advisory Committee on Immunization. VariZIG as the varicella-zoster immune globulin for the prevention of varicella in at-risk patients. *Can Comm Dis Resp.* 2006;32(ACS-8):1-8. http://www.phac-aspc.gc.ca/publicat/ccdr-rmtc/06pdf/acs-32-08.pdf.

CDC. A new product (VariZIG) for postexposure prophylaxis of varicella available under an investigational new drug application expanded access protocol. *MMWR.* 2006;55:209-210.

West Nile Virus Immune Globulin

Sponsors: Omrix Biopharmaceuticals

Trade Name: *Omr-IgG-am*

Antigenic Type: Polyvalent IgG, 5% solution for IV infusion, manufactured with solvent-detergent treatment and nanofiltration at pH 4.

Indications: Investigated for treatment of West Nile virus infection.

Investigational Immune Globulins, Immunoantidotes

Investigational Drugs

Botulinum F(ab')$_2$ Antitoxin Types A, B, C, D, E, F, G (Equine)

Sponsors: Cangene Corporation

Synonym: NP-018 H-BAT, HBAT, heptavalent botulinum antitoxin

Antigenic Type: IgG F(ab')$_2$ and Fab fragments, equine, polyclonal

Indications: To treat botulinum intoxication, by neutralizing circulating botulinum toxin.

Dosage: Adult and pediatric dosing guidance appears in the protocol provided with the product.

Route: IV infusion, after dilution

Consultation: For infant cases, contact the Infant Botulism Treatment and Prevention Program (IBTPP) at (510) 231-7600 or http://www.infantbotulism.org. For other cases, consult state health department, which can access CDC botulism experts.

Concentration: Total protein 30 to 70 mg/mL, consisting of $\geq$ 90% F(ab')$_2$ and F(ab')$_2$-related fragments and Fab; $\leq$ 2% high molecular weight fragments, $\leq$ 2% monomeric IgG; $\leq$ 7% low molecular weight fragments. Potency is expressed in units based on the amount of toxin-specific neutralizing antibodies to a specific toxin serotype in the mouse neutralization assay. By definition, 1 U of antitoxin neutralizes 10,000 LD$_{50}$ of types A, B, C, D, F, and G toxins and 1,000 LD$_{50}$ of type E toxin. The nominal potency of NP-018 H-BAT mimics the previously licensed Sanofi Pasteur antitoxin for serotypes A, B, and E, while similar amounts of serotypes C, D, F, and G were filled based on the supply of equine plasma. Potency per container: 7,500 units anti-A, 5,500 units anti-B, 5,000 units anti-C, 1,000 units anti-D, 8,500 units anti-E, 5,000 units anti-F, and 1,000 units anti-G.

Packaging: 20 mL or 50 mL glass vial containing various fill quantities

Doseform: Liquid

Appearance: Clear to opalescent liquid, essentially free of foreign particles.

Preservative: None

Excipients: Maltose 10%, polysorbate-80 0.03%, residual tri-n-butyl phosphate $\leq$ 0.001%, octylphenol ethoxylate (*Triton X-100*) $\leq$ 0.001%, and pepsin $\leq$ 0.005 units/mL.

Storage/Handling: Stored for long-term storage in a freezer set at $-15°C$ (5°F) at CDC's Strategic National Stockpile (SNS). When released for patient use, product is shipped at 2° to 8°C (35° to 46°F) and must be refrigerated at 2° to 8°C (35° to 46°F) upon receipt, until ready to be prepared for IV infusion. Do not refreeze.

If received frozen, product can be thawed expeditiously at 37°C (99°F) in a water bath. Do not shake vial, avoid foaming. Dilute each ml of antitoxin in 10 ml of sodium chloride 0.9% for injection. The unused IV bag can be refrigerated for use within approximately 8 to 10 h. In-line filtration is optional. Begin infusion slowly, at 0.5 mL/min for first 30 min. Infusion rate may be increased to 2 ml/min, if tolerated.

Production Process: Equine plasma harvested from horses immunized with botulism toxoids and toxins, then modified by enzymatic digestion with pepsin. Bulk product is mixed with tri-n-butyl phosphate (TNBP) 1% and octylphenol ethoxylate (*Triton X-100*) 1% in the solvent/detergent (SD) viral-inactivation step.

References: CDC. Investigational heptavalent botulinum antitoxin (HBAT) to replace licensed botulinum antitoxin AB and investigational botulinum antitoxin E. *MMWR* 2010;59:299.

Arnon SS, Schechter R, Inglesby TV, et al. Botulinum toxin as a biological weapon: Medical and public health management. *JAMA*. 2001;285:1059-1070.

Hibbs RG, et al. Experience with the use of investigational F(ab')$_2$ heptavalent botulism immune globulin of equine origin during an outbreak of type E botulism in Egypt. *Clin Infect Dis*. 1996;23:337-340.

Other Antichemical Antidotes in Research

The basic immunologic principles that permit digoxin Fab to be effective in reducing the morbidity and mortality of toxicity may also provide other antibodies or antibody fragments to antagonize the adverse or undesired effects of a wide variety of chemical compounds.

Experimental work in animals has been conducted that successfully antagonized renin, thus correcting renin-dependent hypertension. Similar antibodies have successfully antagonized the effects of colchicine, desipramine, gastrin, histamine, mescaline, morphine, oxytocin, steroid hormones, vasopressin, and other drugs.

It will likely be quite a few years before any of these specific antichemical antibodies are licensed for general use in the United States, but progress is being made.

Investigational Immune Globulins, Isoantibodies

Investigational Drugs

Products in this section are listed in alphabetic sequence by proper name. For cases where the proper name would not imply the investigated use of a product, refer to the following table:

Purpose Being Investigated	Product(s)
Alzheimer disease	Bapineuzumab, Gantenerumab, Ponezumab, Solanezumab
Allergies	Talizumab
Asthma	Anrukinzumab, Benralizumab, Gomiliximab, Lebrikizumab, Mepolizumab, Pascolizumab, Tralokinumab
Autoimmune diseases, various	Briakinumab, Briobacept, Cedelizumab, Fontolizumab, Priliximab
Cancers and lymphomas, various	Abagovomab, Apolizumab, Atacicept, Bivatuzumab, Blinatumomab, Cantuzumab, Cantuzumab mertansine, Catumaxomab, Cixutumomab, Conatumumab, Dacetuzumab, Dalotuzumab, Drozitumab, Ecromeximab, Edrecolomab, Elotuzumab, Ensituximab, Epratuzumab, Farletuzumab, Fresolimumab, Ganitumab, Girentuximab, Glembatumumab, Intetumumab, Ipilimumab, Iratumumab, Labetuzumab, Lexatumumab, Lintuzumab, Lorvotuzumab mertansine, Lucatumumab, Lumiliximab, Mapatumumab, Matuzumab, Milatuzumab, Mitumomab, Necitumumab, Nimotuzumab, Olaratumab, Oregovomab, Pemtumomab, Ramucirumab, Rilotumumab, Robatumumab, Samalizumab, Sibrotuzumab, Siltuximab, Siplizumab, Sontuzumab, Teprotumumab, Toralizumab, Trastuzumab emtansine, Tremelimumab, Tucotuzumab celmoleukin, Veltuzumab, Volociximab, Zalutumumab, Zanolimumab
Coronary interventions	Tadocizumab
Diabetes, insulin-dependent	Otelixizumab, Teplimab
Glomerulosclerosis	Fresolimumab
Inflammatory diseases	Fezakinumab, Sfalimumab, Tralokinumab, Vedolizumab
Lupus erythematosus	Rontalizumab, Sifalimumab
Macular degeneration	Volociximab
Multiple sclerosis	Priliximab
Muscular dystrophy	Stamulumab
Myelodysplastic syndrome	Aflibercept
Myocardial infarction	Pexelizumab
Osteoporosis	Sotatercept
Psoriasis	Otelixizumab, Zanolimumab
Pulmonary fibrosis	Fresolimumab
Rheumatoid arthritis	Atacicept, Keliximab, Ocrelizumab, Zanolimumab
Sepsis, septic shock	Afelimomab, Nerelimomab
Thrombocytopenic purpura	Toralizumab
Transplantation	Cedelizumab, Clenoliximab, Enlimomab, Inolimumab, Odulimomab, Teneliximab, Visilizumab

Abagovomab

Antigenic Type: IgG1, anti-idiotype anti-[anti-CA125] human-mouse clone 3D5 γ-1 heavy chain with disulfide bond to human-mouse clone 3D5 κ light chain, tridisulfide dimer.

Indications: Investigated for treatment of ovarian and other cancers.

References: Sabbatini P, Dupont J, Aghajanian C, et al. Phase I study of abagovomab in patients with epithelial ovarian, fallopian tube, or primary peritoneal cancer. *Clin Cancer Res.* 2006;12(18):5503-5510.

Afelimomab

Sponsors: Abbott Laboratories

Antigenic Type: Anti-tumor necrosis factor F(ab′)2 fragment

Indications: Investigated for treatment of severe sepsis or septic shock.

References: Panacek EA, Marshall JC, Albertson TE, et al; Monoclonal Anti-TNF: a Random-ized Controlled Sepsis Study Investigators. Efficacy and safety of the monoclonal anti-tumor necrosis factor antibody F(ab′)2 fragment afelimomab in patients with severe sepsis and elevated interleukin-6 levels. *Crit Care Med.* 2004;32(11):2173-2182.

Aflibercept

Sponsors: Regeneron

Antigenic Type: des-432-lysine-[VEGF receptor 1-(103-204)-peptide (containing Ig-like C2-type domain) fusion protein with VEGF receptor 2(206-308)-peptide (containing Ig-like C2-type 3 domain fragment) fusion protein with IgG1-peptide (Fc fragment)], bisdisulfide dimer

Indications: Investigated for treatment of myelodysplastic syndrome.

References: Chu QS. Aflibercept (AVE0005): An alternative strategy for inhibiting tumour angiogenesis by vascular endothelial growth factors. *Expert Opin Biol Ther.* 2009;9:263-271.

Moroney JW, et al. Aflibercept in epithelial ovarian carcinoma. *Future Oncol.* 2009;5:591-600.

Anrukinzumab

Sponsors: Wyeth

Synonym: IMA-638

Antigenic Type: IgG1, anti-(human IL-13) (human-mouse heavy chain) with disulfide bridge to human-mouse κ-chain, dimer. Molecular weight 145.4 kDa.

Indications: Investigated for treatment of asthma.

Apolizumab

Sponsors: Protein Design Labs

Synonym: Hu1D10

Trade Name: *Remitogen*

Antigenic Type: IgG1 anti-human histocompatibility antigen HLA-DR (human-mouse monoclonal Hu1D10 γ1-chain) with disulfide bond to human-mouse Hu1D10 light chain, dimer. Molecular weight approximately 150,000 daltons.

Indications: Investigated for treatment of B-cell malignancies.

References: Mone AP, Huang P, Pelicano H, et al. Hu1D10 induces apoptosis concurrent with activation of the AKT survival pathway in human chronic lymphocytic leukemia cells. *Blood.* 2004;103:1846-1854.

Atacicept

Antigenic Type: [86-serine, 101-glutamic acid, 196-serine, 197-serine, 222-aspartic acid, 224-leucine] [TNF receptor superfamily 13B-(30-110)-peptide (transmembrane activator and CAML interactor [TACI] fragment containing TNFR-Cys 1 and TNFR-Cys 2) fusion protein with IgG1-peptide (gamma-1-chain Fc fragment)], bidisulfide dimer

Indications: Investigated for treatment of rheumatoid arthritis, B-cell non-Hodgkin lymphoma, and autoimmune diseases.

References: Munafo A, Priestley A, Nestorov I, Visich J, Rogge M. Safety, pharmacokinetics and pharmacodynamics of atacicept in healthy volunteers. *Eur J Clin Pharmacol.* 2007;63(7):647-656.

Nestorov I, Munafo A, Papasouliotis O, Visich J. Pharmacokinetics and biological activity of atacicept in patients with rheumatoid arthritis. *J Clin Pharmacol.* 2008;48(4):406-417.

Bapineuzumab

Sponsors: Wyeth

Synonym: AAB-001, humanized 3D-6 monoclonal antibody

Antigenic Type: IgG1, anti-human beta-amyloid (human-mouse monoclonal heavy chain) with disulfide bond to human-mouse light chain, dimer. Molecular weight 148,800 daltons.

Indications: Investigated for prevention of Alzheimer disease.

Benralizumab

Sponsors: MedImmune

Synonym: MEDI-563

Antigenic Type: IgG1, anti-IL-5 receptor α-chain (human-mouse monoclonal MEDI-563 heavy chain) with disulfide bond to human-mouse monoclonal MEDI-563 κ-chain, dimer.

Indications: Investigated for treatment of asthma.

Bivatuzumab

Sponsors: Boehringer Ingelheim

Synonym: CD44v6, BIWA4

References: Sauter A, Kloft C, Gronau S, et al. Pharmacokinetics, immunogenicity and safety of bivatuzumab mertansine, a novel CD44v6-targeting immunoconjugate, in patients with squamous cell carcinoma of the head and neck. *Int J Oncol.* 2007;30(4):927-935.

Blinatumomab

Sponsors: MedImmune

Synonym: MEDI-538, MT-103

Antigenic Type: IgG anti-(human B-lymphocyte antigen CD19) (single-chain) fusion protein with IgG anti-(human T-cell surface glycoprotein CD3 ε-chain) (clone 1 single-chain) with hexa-L-histamine. Molecular weight 54.1 kDa.

Indications: Investigated for treatment of cancer.

References: Nagorsen D, et al. Immunotherapy of lymphoma and leukemia with T-cell engaging BiTE antibody blinatumomab. *Leuk Lymphoma.* 2009;50:886-891.

Briakinumab

Sponsors: Abbott Laboratories

Synonym: ABT-874, BSF 415977

Antigenic Type: IgG1, anti-human IL-12 subunit beta (p40, CLMF p40 or NKSF2). Molecular weight 146.5 kDa.

Indications: Investigated for treatment of autoimmune disorders.

References: Lima XT, et al. Briakinumab. *Expert Opin Biol Ther.* 2009;9:1107-1113.

Briobacept

Antigenic Type: Cytokine receptor BAFF-R (human extracellular domain-containing fragment BR3) fusion protein with IgG1 (human Fc domain-containing fragment), dimer.

Indications: Investigated for treatment of autoimmune diseases.

Cantuzumab (Chimeric Human-Murine)

Sponsors: ImmunoGen, GlaxoSmithKline

Synonym: huC242-DMI/SB408075

Indications: Investigated for treatment of colorectal cancer, non-small cell lung cancer, and pancreatic cancers.

Cantuzumab Mertansine (Chimeric Human-Murine)

Sponsors: GlaxoSmithKline, Chemsyn Laboratories, Unisyn Technologies, ImmunoGen

Synonym: SB-408075, C242-DM1

Antigenic Type: IgG1, anti-mucin CanAg (human-mouse monoclonal C242 heavy chain) with disulfide bond to human-mouse C242 light chain, dimer, linked to $N^{2'}$-deacetyl-$N^{2'}$-(3-mercapto-1-oxopropyl) maytansine.

Indications: Investigated for treatment of colorectal, pancreatic, and other solid tumor types that express C242 antigen.

References: Smith SV. Technology evaluation: cantuzumab mertansine, ImmunoGen. *Curr Opin Mol Ther.* 2004;6(6):666-674.

Catumaxomab

Sponsors: Fresenius Biotech North America

Synonym: Removab

Antigenic Type: Bispecific monoclonal antibody targeting epithelial cell adhesion molecule (EpCAM) and CD3.

Indications: Investigated for treatment of various cancers.

References: Sebastian M, Passlick B, Friccius-Quecke H, et al. Treatment of non-small cell lung cancer patients with the trifunctional monoclonal antibody catumaxomab (anti-EpCAM x anti-CD3): a phase I study. *Cancer Immunol Immunother.* 2007;56(10):1637-1644.

Cedelizumab (Chimeric Human-Murine)

Sponsors: Ortho-McNeil Pharmaceutical

Synonym: OKT4, OKT4a, RWJ 49004, CAS 156586-90-2

Antigenic Type: Monoclonal IgG4 against OKTcdr4a (complementary-determining region-grafted anti-human CD4 antigen)

Indications: Investigated for use in prophylaxis of rejection of solid organ allograft and as a disease-modifying agent in autoimmune disease.

Cixutumomab

Sponsors: ImClone Systems

Synonym: IMC-A12

Antigenic Type: IgG1, anti-human insulin-like growth factor I receptor (EC 2.7.10.1 or CD221 antigen; human monoclonal IMC-A12 γ-chain). Molecular weight 146.3 kDa.

Indications: Investigated for treatment of solid tumors.

References: McKian KP, Haluska P. Cixutumumab. *Expert Opin Investig Drugs.* 2009;18:1025-1033.

Clenoliximab (Chimeric Human-Murine)

Sponsors: Biogen Idec with GlaxoSmithKline
Synonym: IDEC-151
Antigenic Type: Anti-CD4 IgG, monoclonal, "primatized"
Indications: Investigated for use in prevention of organ transplant rejection.

Conatumumab

Sponsors: Amgen
Synonym: AMG 655, XG1-048, TRAIL-R2, anti-CD262
Antigenic Type: IgG1, anti-(human cytokine receptor DR5 (death receptor 5)) (human monoclonal XG1-048 v w heavy chain) with disulfide bridge to human monoclonal XG1-048 v w light chain, dimer. Molecular weight 145.65 kDa.
Indications: Investigated for treatment of certain cancers.

Dacetuzumab

Sponsors: Seattle Genetics
Synonym: SGN-40, huS2C6
Antigenic Type: IgG1, anti-(human CD40) (human-mouse monoclonal SGN-40 γ1-chain) with disulfide bridge to human-mouse monoclonal SGN-40 κ-chain, dimer. Molecular weight 145.1 kDa (for the peptide)
Indications: Investigated for treatment of CD40-positive cancers.
References: Khubchandani S, et al. Dacetuzumab, a humanized mAb against CD40 for the treatment of hematological malignancies. *Curr Opin Investig Drugs.* 2009;10:579-587.

Dalotuzumab

Sponsors: Merck
Synonym: MK-0646
Antigenic Type: IgG1, anti-insulin-like growth factor I receptor (human-mouse monoclonal heavy chain) with disulfide bond to human-mouse monoclonal κ-chain, dimer.
Indications: Investigated for treatment of certain cancers.

Drozitumab

Sponsors: Genentech
Synonym: PRO95780, anti-DR5, rhuMAb DR5
Antigenic Type: IgG1, anti-citokine receptor DR5 (death receptor 5) (human monoclonal heavy chain) with disulfide bond to human λ3-chain, dimer.
Indications: Investigated for treatment of certain cancers.

Ecromeximab

Sponsors: Kyowa Hakko Kogyo Company

Synonym: KW-2871, KM871

Antigenic Type: IgG1, anti-GD3 ganglioside (human-mouse monoclonal KM871 γ1-chain) with disulfide bond to human-mouse KM871 κ-chain, dimer. Molecular weight 145,255 daltons.

Indications: Investigated for treatment of malignant melanoma.

Edrecolomab (Murine)

Sponsors: Centocor

Synonym: 17-1A, CAS 156586-89-9

Trade Name: *Panorex*

Antigenic Type: IgG2a, monoclonal, 148-kilodalton protein, targeting a 37 to 40 kilodalton cell-surface glycoprotein associated with human colon cancers.

Indications: Investigated for use as adjuvant therapy in the treatment of postoperative colorectal cancer.

Incidence: In 1991 in the United States, 28,300 new cases of pancreatic cancer were diagnosed and 25,000 deaths occurred; this is the fifth leading cause of cancer death. Only 3% of patients survive more than 5 years after diagnosis.

Orphan Status: April 4, 1988

References: Adkins JC, et al. Edrecolomab (monoclonal antibody 17-1A). *Drugs.* 1998;56:619-626.

Hartung G, Hofheinz RD, Dencausse Y, et al. Adjuvant therapy with edrecolomab versus observation in stage II colon cancer: a multicenter randomized phase III study. *Onkologie.* 2005;28:347-350.

Elotuzumab

Sponsors: PDL BioPharma

Synonym: PDL-063

Antigenic Type: IgG1, anti-human protein CS1 (human SLAM family member 7 (CD2-like receptor activating cytotoxic cells, CD319 antigen); human-mouse HuLuc63 heavy chain). Molecular weight 145.5 kDa.

Indications: Investigated for treatment of certain cancers.

References: van Rhee F, et al. Combinatorial efficacy of anti-CS1 monoclonal antibody elotuzumab (HuLuc63) and bortezomib against multiple myeloma. *Mol Cancer Ther.* 2009;8:2616-2624.

Enlimomab (Murine)

Sponsors: Boehringer-Ingelheim

Synonym: BI-RR-1, anti-ICAM-1 Mab, CAS 142864-19-5

Antigenic Type: IgG2a, monoclonal, anti-human antigen CD-54, 150,000 daltons

Indications: Investigated for use in prevention of acute allograft rejection and delayed graft rejection.

References: Mileski WJ, Burkhart D, Hunt JL, et al. Clinical effects of inhibiting leukocyte adhesion with monoclonal antibody to intercellular adhesion molecule-1 (enlimomab) in the treatment of partial-thickness burn injury. *J Trauma*. 2003;54:950-958.

Ensituximab

Sponsors: Neogenix Oncology

Synonym: NPC-1C

Antigenic Type: IgG1, anti-(colorectal and pancreatic carcinoma-associated antigen) (human-mouse monoclonal NPC-1C heavy chain) with disulfide bond to human-mouse monoclonal NPC-1C κ-chain, dimer

Indications: Investigated for treatment of certain cancers.

Epratuzumab

Sponsors: Amgen, Immunomedics

Synonym: AMG-412, IMMU-103, IMMU-hLL2

Trade Name: *LymphoCide*

Indications: Investigated for treatment of non-Hodgkin B-cell lymphoma.

References: Davies SL. Epratuzumab. *Drugs Future*. 2005;30:683-687.

Ertumaxomab

Sponsors: Fresenius Biotech GmbH

Synonym: *Rexomun*

Antigenic Type: Bispecific monoclonal antibody targeting HER2/neu and CD3 with selective binding to activatory Fc gamma type I/III receptors, based on mouse IgG_{2a} and rat IgG_{2b}. These antibodies may redirect T cells and accessory immune effector cells (eg, macrophages, dendritic cells [DCs] and natural killer [NK] cells) to the tumor site. According to preclinical data, trifunctional antibodies activate these immune cells, which can trigger a complex antitumor immune response.

Indications: Investigated for use in treating metastatic breast cancer.

References: Friedländer E, Barok M, Szöllosi J, Vereb G. ErbB-directed immunotherapy: antibodies in current practice and promising new agents. *Immunol Lett*. 2008;116(2):126-140.

Farletuzumab

Sponsors: Morphotek

Synonym: MORAb-003

Antigenic Type: IgG1, anti-human folate receptor α (ovarian tumor-associated antigen Mov18; human-mouse monoclonal MORAb-003 heavy chain). Molecular weight 145.4 kDa.

Indications: Investigated for treatment of certain cancers.

References: Spannuth WA, et al. Farletuzumab in epithelial ovarian carcinoma. *Expert Opin Biol Ther*. 2010;10:431-437.

Fezakinumab

Sponsors: Wyeth

Synonym: ILV-094

Antigenic Type: IgG1, anti-human IL-22 (human monoclonal heavy chain). Molecular weight 144.5 kDa.

Indications: Investigated for treatment of inflammatory diseases.

Fontolizumab

Sponsors: Protein Design Labs

Synonym: HuZAF

Antigenic Type: IgG1, anti-human interferon gamma (human-mouse monoclonal HuZAF γ1-chain) with disulfide bond to human-mouse HuZAF light chain, dimer. Molecular weight approximately 150,000 daltons.

Indications: Investigated for treatment of autoimmune diseases.

References: Reinisch W, Hommes DW, Van Assche G, et al. A dose-escalating, placebo-controlled, double-blind, single-dose and multi-dose, safety and tolerability study of fontolizumab, a humanised anti-interferon-gamma antibody, in patients with moderate-to-severe Crohn's disease. *Gut*. 2006;55(8):1138-1144.

Fresolimumab

Sponsors: Genzyme

Synonym: GC1008

Antigenic Type: IgG4, anti-(transforming growth factor β or cetermin) (human monoclonal GC-1008 heavy chain) with disulfide bond to human monoclonal GC-1008 light chain, dimer.

Indications: Investigated for treatment of idiopathic pulmonary fibrosis, focal segmental glomerulosclerosis, and cancer.

Galiximab

Sponsors: Biogen Idec

Synonym: IDEC-114

Antigenic Type: IgG1, anti-human CD80 antigen (human-macaque monoclonal IDEC-114 heavy chain) with disulfide bond to human-macaque IDEC-114 λ-chain, dimer.

Indications: Investigated for treatment of psoriasis.

References: Czuczman MS, Thall A, Witzig TE, et al. Phase I/II study of galiximab, an anti-CD80 antibody, for relapsed or refractory follicular lymphoma. *J Clin Oncol.* 2005;23:4390-4398.

Ganitumab

Sponsors: Amgen

Synonym: AMG 479

Antigenic Type: IgG, anti-human insulin-like growth factor I receptor) (human monoclonal heavy chain) with disulfide bond to human monoclonal light chain, dimer.

Indications: Investigated for treatment of certain cancers.

Gantenerumab

Sponsors: Hoffmann-LaRoche

Synonym: R1450, R04909832

Antigenic Type: IgG1 anti-(human beta-amyloid proteins 42 and 40 monoclonal heavy chain) with disulfide bond to κ light chain, dimer. Molecular weight 146.3 kDa.

Indications: Investigated for treatment of Alzheimer disease.

Girentuximab

Sponsors: WILEX AG

Synonym: Rencarex, WX-G250, cG250

Antigenic Type: IgG1, anti-(human antigen MN) (human-mouse monoclonal cG250 heavy chain) with disulfide bond to human-mouse monoclonal cG250 κ-chain, dimer

Indications: Investigated for treatment of renal cell cancer.

Glembatumumab

Sponsors: CuraGen

Synonym: CR011, CR011-vcMMAE

Antigenic Type: IgG, anti-(glycoprotein NMB extracellular domain) (human monoclonal CR011 heavy chain) with disulfide bond to human monoclonal CR011 γ2 κ-chain, dimer.

Indications: Investigated for treatment of certain cancers.

References: Naumovski L, Junutula JR. Glembatumumab vedotin, a conjugate of an anti-glycoprotein non-metastatic melanoma protein B mAb and monomethyl auristatin E for the treatment of melanoma and breast cancer. *Curr Opin Mol Ther.* 2010;12:248-257.

Gomiliximab

Sponsors: Biogen Idec

Synonym: IDEC-152

Antigenic Type: IgG1, anti-human IgE receptor type II (human-macaque monoclonal IDEC-152 γ1-chain) with disulfide bond to human-macaque IDEC-152 κ-chain, dimer.

Indications: Investigated for treatment of allergic asthma.

Inolimomab (Murine)

Sponsors: Biotest Pharma

Synonym: Anti-CD25 Mab, anti-IL2 Mab, BT 563

Trade Name: *Leukotac*

Antigenic Type: Murine IgG1-kappa directed against alpha-chain of human IL-2 receptor (CD25)

Indications: Investigated for suppression or reversal of graft vs host disorders and treatment or prophylaxis of acute transplant rejection.

References: Bay JO, Dhedin N, Goerner M, et al. Inolimomab in steroid-refractory acute graft-versus-host disease following allogeneic hematopoietic stem cell transplantation: retrospective analysis and comparison with other interleukin-2 receptor antibodies. *Transplantation.* 2005;80:782-788.

Intetumumab

Sponsors: Centocor

Synonym: CNTO-95

Antigenic Type: IgG1, anti-human integrin alpha-V (vitronectin receptor subunit alpha or CD51). Molecular weight 145.6 kDa.

Indications: Investigated for treatment of solid tumors.

Iratumumab

Sponsors: Medarex

Synonym: MDX-060

Antigenic Type: IgG1 anti-human CD30 antigen, dimer. Molecular weight 170,000 daltons.

Indications: Investigated for treatment of relapsed or refractory CD30-positive lymphoma including Hodgkin disease.

Keliximab (Chimeric)

Sponsors: GlaxoSmithKline

Synonym: IDEC CE9.1, SB 210396 Anti-CD4 Monoclonal Antibody Antigenic

Antigenic Type: IgG1, monoclonal, "primatized"

Indications: Investigated for treating rheumatoid arthritis.

Labetuzumab

Sponsors: Immunomedics
Trade Name: *CEA-Cide*
Indications: Investigated for treatment of colorectal cancer.

Lebrikizumab

Sponsors: Genentech
Synonym: MILR1444A, PRO301444
Antigenic Type: IgG4, anti-IL-13 (human-mouse monoclonal MILR1444A γ4-chain) with disulfide bond to human-mouse monoclonal MILR1444A κ-chain, dimer
Indications: Investigated for treatment of asthma.

Lexatumumab

Sponsors: Human Genome Sciences
Synonym: HGS-ETR2, HGs1018
Antigenic Type: IgG1 anti-human tumor necrosis factor receptor superfamily member 10B (death receptor 5 or RAIL-R2) (human monoclonal HGS-ETR2 heavy chain), with disulfide bond to human monoclonal HGS-ETR2 λ-chain, dimer. Molecular weight 143,600 daltons.
Indications: Investigated for treatment of cancer.
References: Marini P. Drug evaluation: lexatumumab, an intravenous human agonistic mAb targeting TRAIL receptor 2. *Curr Opin Mol Ther.* 2006;8(6):539-546.

Lintuzumab

Sponsors: Protein Design Labs
Synonym: SGN-33
Antigenic Type: Humanized anti-CD33 IgG
Indications: Investigated for treatment of acute myelogenous leukemia.
References: Feldman EJ, Brandwein J, Stone R, et al. Phase III randomized multicenter study of a humanized anti-CD33 monoclonal antibody, lintuzumab, in combination with chemotherapy, versus chemotherapy alone in patients with refractory or first-relapsed acute myeloid leukemia. *J Clin Oncol.* 2005;23(18):4110-4116.

Lorvotuzumab Mertansine

Sponsors: ImmunoGen

Synonym: huN901-DM1, BB-10901, IMGN901

Antigenic Type: IgG1, anti-(human cell adhesion molecule NCAM [neural cell adhesion molecule]) (human-mouse monoclonal huN901 heavy chain) with disulfide bond to human-mouse monoclonal huN901 light chain, dimer, tetraamide with N2′-<3-<(3- carboxy-1-methylpropyl)dithio]-1-oxopropyl]-N2′-deacetylmaytansine

Indications: Investigated for treatment of certain cancers.

Lucatumumab

Sponsors: Novartis Pharmaceuticals

Synonym: CHIR-12.12, HCD-122

Antigenic Type: IgG1, anti-(human CD40) (human monoclonal CHIR-12.12 heavy chain) with disulfide bridge to human monoclonal CHIR-12.12 light chain, dimer. Molecular weight 146 kDa.

Indications: Investigated for treatment of certain cancers.

Lumiliximab

Sponsors: Biogen Idec

Antigenic Type: Anti-CD23 antibody

Indications: Investigated for treatment of chronic lymphocytic leukemia.

References: Rosenwasser LJ, Meng J. Anti-CD23. *Clin Rev Allergy Immunol.* 2005;29(1):61-72.

Mapatumumab

Sponsors: Human Genome Sciences

Synonym: TRAIL-R1 mAb, TRM-1, HGS-ETR1

Antigenic Type: IgG1, anti-human cytokine receptor DR4 (death receptor 4) (human monoclonal TRM-1 heavy chain), with disulfide bond to human monoclonal TRM-1 λ-chain, dimer.

Indications: Investigated for treatment of cancer.

References: Vulfovich M, Saba N. Technology evaluation: mapatumumab, Human Genome Sciences/GlaxoSmithKline/Takeda. *Curr Opin Mol Ther.* 2005;7(5):502-510.

Matuzumab

Sponsors: Merck KGaA

Synonym: EMD72000

Antigenic Type: Anti-EGFR monoclonal antibody formulated in a liposomal vehicle

Indications: Investigated for treatment of colorectal cancer.

References: Mamot C, Ritschard R, Kung W, Park JW, Herrmann R, Rochlitz CF. EGFR-targeted immunoliposomes derived from the monoclonal antibody EMD72000 mediate specific and efficient drug delivery to a variety of colorectal cancer cells. *J Drug Target.* 2006;14(4):215-223.

Mepolizumab (Humanized)

Sponsors: GlaxoSmithKline

Synonym: SB240563

Antigenic Type: Anti-interleukin-5 monoclonal antibody

Indications: Investigated for treatment of asthma and atopic dermatitis.

References: Oldhoff JM, Darsow U, Werfel T, et al. Anti-IL-5 recombinant humanized monoclonal antibody (mepolizumab) for the treatment of atopic dermatitis. *Allergy.* 2005;60:693-696.

Milatuzumab

Sponsors: Immunomedics

Synonym: IMMU-115

Antigenic Type: IgG1, anti-(human HLA class II antigen invariant chain) (human-mouse monoclonal hLL1 heavy chain) with disulfide bridge to human-mouse monoclonal hLL1 κ-chain, dimer. Molecular weight 146.7 kDa.

Indications: Investigated for treatment of multiple myeloma and other hematological malignancies.

References: Stein R, Mattes MJ, Cardillo TM, et al. CD74: A new candidate target for the immunotherapy of B-cell neoplasms. *Clin Cancer Res.* 2007;13(18 pt 2):5556s-5563s.

Mitumomab

Sponsors: ImClone Systems

Synonym: BEC2, anti-CD3

Indications: Investigated for treatment of small-cell lung cancer.

Necitumumab

Sponsors: ImClone Systems

Synonym: IMC-11F8

Antigenic Type: IgG1, anti-(human epidermal growth factor receptor) (human monoclonal IMC-11F8 γ1-chain) with disulfide bond to human monoclonal IMC-11F8 κ-chain, dimer

Indications: Investigated for treatment of certain cancers.

Nerelimomab (Murine)

Sponsors: Novartis with Bayer and Celltech

Synonym: BAY-x-1351, anti-cachectin, CAS 162774-06-3

Antigenic Type: IgG1

Indications: Investigated for use in treating septic shock by neutralizing tumor necrosis factor.

References: Abraham E, et al. Efficacy and safety of monoclonal antibody to human tumor necrosis factor alfa in patients with sepsis syndrome. *JAMA*. 1995;273:934-941.

Nimotuzumab

Sponsors: YM Biosciences

Bacteriology: IgG1 anti-(hR3 B1 chain anti-EGFR) with disulfide bond to humanized-mouse hR3 K-chain, dimer

Indications: Investigated in the treatment of glioma, metastatic pancreatic cancer, and non-small cell lung cancer.

References: Spicer J. Technology evaluation: nimotuzumab, the Center of Molecular Immunology/YM BioSciences/Oncoscience. *Curr Opin Mol Ther*. 2005;7(2):182-191.

Ocrelizumab

Sponsors: Genentech

Synonym: PR070769

Antigenic Type: IgG1, anti-human CD20 antigen (human-mouse monoclonal 2H7 γ1-chain), with disulfide bond to human-mouse monoclonal 2H7 κ-chain, dimer. Molecular weight 148,000 daltons.

Indications: Investigated for treatment of rheumatoid arthritis.

References: Kausar F, et al. Ocrelizumab: A step forward in the evolution of B-cell therapy. *Expert Opin Biol Ther*. 2009;9:889-895.

Odulimomab (Murine)

Sponsors: Sanofi-Aventis

Antigenic Type: IgG murine monoclonal antibody against leukocyte function antigen-1 or CD11a

Indications: Investigated for preventing rejection of kidney transplants and for rejection of certain bone marrow transplants.

Olaratumab

Sponsors: Imclone Systems

Synonym: IMC-3G3, IMC3G3

Antigenic Type: IgG1, anti-(human platelet-derived growth factor receptor α) (human monoclonal 3G3 γ) with disulfide bond to human monoclonal 3G3 κ-chain, dimer

Indications: Investigated for treatment of solid tumors.

Oregovomab (Murine)

Sponsors: AltaRex Corporation

Synonym: B43.13

Trade Name: *OvaRex*

Antigenic Type: IgG1, anti-human CA125 carbohydrate antigen (mouse monoclonal B43.13 γ1-chain) with disulfide bond to mouse B43.13 κ-chain, dimer. Molecular weight approximately 150,000 daltons.

Indications: Investigated for treatment of ovarian cancer.

Orphan Status: 1996

References: Ehlen TG, Hoskins PJ, Miller D, et al. A pilot phase 2 study of oregovomab murine monoclonal antibody to CA125 as an immunotherapeutic agent for recurrent ovarian cancer. *Int J Gynecol Cancer*. 2005;15:1023-1034.

Otelixizumab

Sponsors: TolerRx

Synonym: TRX4, ChAglyCD3

Antigenic Type: IgG1, anti-(human CD3) (human-rat monoclonal heavy chain) with disulfide bridge to human-rat monoclonal λ-chain, dimer. Molecular weight 145.1 kDa.

Indications: Investigated for treatment of type 1 diabetes and psoriasis.

Pascolizumab

Sponsors: GlaxoSmithKline

Synonym: SB-240683

Antigenic Type: IgG1, anti-human interleukin 4 (human-mouse monoclonal SB-240683 γ1-chain) with disulfide bond to human-mouse SB-240683 κ-chain, dimer. Molecular weight approximately 149,000 daltons.

Indications: Investigated for treatment of asthma.

References: Hart TK, Blackburn MN, Brigham-Burke M, et al. Preclinical efficacy and safety of pascolizumab (SB 240683): a humanized anti-interleukin-4 antibody with therapeutic potential in asthma. *Clin Exp Immunol.* 2002;130:93-100.

Pemtumomab

Sponsors: Abbott Laboratories, Antisoma

Indications: Investigated for treatment of ovarian cancer.

References: Verheijen RH, Massuger LF, Benigno BB, et al. Phase III trial of intraperitoneal therapy with yttrium-90-labeled HMFG1 murine monoclonal antibody in patients with epithelial ovarian cancer after a surgically defined complete remission. *J Clin Oncol.* 2006;24:571-578.

Pexelizumab

Sponsors: Alexion Pharmaceuticals, Procter & Gamble Pharmaceuticals

Synonym: 5G1.1 scFv, h5G1.1 scFv

Antigenic Type: IgG, anti-human complement C5 α-chain, human-mouse monoclonal 5G1.1-SC single chain. Molecular weight 26,500 daltons.

Indications: Investigated for treatment of cardiopulmonary bypass and acute myocardial infarction.

References: Carrier M, Menasche P, Levy JH, et al. Inhibition of complement activation by pexelizumab reduces death in patients undergoing combined aortic valve replacement and coronary artery bypass surgery. *J Thorac Cardiovasc Surg.* 2006;131:352-356.

Ponezumab

Sponsors: Pfizer

Synonym: PF-04360365, RN-1219

Antigenic Type: IgG2, anti-(human β-amyloid) (human-mouse monoclonal PF-04360365 clone 9TL heavy chain) with disulfide bond to human-mouse monoclonal PF-04360365 clone 9TL light chain, dimer

Indications: Investigated for treatment of Alzheimer disease.

Priliximab (Chimeric Human-Murine)

Sponsors: Centocor

Synonym: Anti-CD4 cM-T412 antibody, CAS 147191-91-1

Trade Name: *Centara*

Antigenic Type: IgG1, monoclonal, 150 kilodalton antibody

Indications: Investigated for use in treating multiple sclerosis.

Other Research: Investigated for use in treating rheumatoid arthritis (epidemiology: about 2 million affected persons in the United States), Crohn disease (epidemiology: 235,000 affected persons in the United States), lupus erythematosus (epidemiology: 175,000 affected persons in the United States), psoriasis, and transplant rejection.

Incidence: In the United States, approximately 250,000 people suffer from multiple sclerosis.

Orphan Status: June 5, 1991

References: [No authors listed]. Priliximab. Anti-CD4 MAb, CEN 000029, MT 412, cMT 412, *Centara. Drugs R D*. 1999;1(1):95-96.

Ramucirumab

Sponsors: ImClone Systems

Synonym: IMC-1121B

Antigenic Type: IgG1, anti-human vascular endothelial growth factor receptor type VEGFR-2 extracellular domain (EC 2.7.10.1 or protein-tyrosine kinase receptor Flk-1 or CD309 antigen; human monoclonal IMC-1121B γ-chain receptor 2 extracellular domain). Molecular weight 143.6 kDa.

Indications: Investigated for treatment of solid tumors.

References: Krupitskaya Y, Wakelee HA. Ramucirumab, a fully human mAb to the transmembrane signaling tyrosine kinase VEGFR-2 for the potential treatment of cancer. *Curr Opin Investig Drugs*. 2009;10:597-605.

Rilotumumab

Sponsors: Amgen

Synonym: AMG 102

Antigenic Type: IgG2, anti-human hepatocyte growth factor (Scatter factor or hepatopoeitin-A; human monoclonal 2.12.1 heavy chain). Molecular weight 145.2 kDa.

Indications: Investigated for treatment of solid tumors.

References: Giordano S. Rilotumumab, a mAb against human hepatocyte growth factor for the treatment of cancer. *Curr Opin Mol Ther*. 2009;11:448-455.

Robatumumab

Sponsors: Schering-Plough

Synonym: SCH 717454

Antigenic Type: IgG1, anti-human insulin-like growth factor I receptor (EC 2.7.10.1 or CD221 antigen; human monoclonal SCH 717454 heavy chain). Molecular weight 144.6 kDa.

Indications: Investigated for treatment of certain cancers.

References: Wang Y, et al. A fully human insulin-like growth factor-I receptor antibody SCH 717454 (Robatumumab) has antitumor activity as a single agent and in combination with cytotoxics in pediatric tumor xenografts. *Mol Cancer Ther.* 2010;9:410-418.

Rontalizumab

Sponsors: Genentech

Synonym: RhuMAb IFNalpha

Antigenic Type: IgG1, anti-interferon α (human-mouse monoclonal rhuMAb IFN-alpha heavy chain) with disulfide bond to human-mouse monoclonal rhuMAb IFNalpha κ-chain, dimer

Indications: Investigated for treatment of systemic lupus erythematosus.

Samalizumab

Sponsors: Alexion Pharmaceuticals

Synonym: ALXN6000

Antigenic Type: IgG2/4, anti-CD200 (antigen) (human-mouse monoclonal ALXN6000 heavy chain) with disulfide bond to human-mouse monoclonal ALXN6000 κ-chain, dimer

Indications: Investigated for treatment of certain cancers.

Sibrotuzumab

Sponsors: Life Science Pharmaceuticals

Indications: Investigated for treatment of colorectal, head and neck, and lung cancers.

References: Kloft C, Graefe EU, Tanswell P, et al. Population pharmacokinetics of sibrotuzumab, a novel therapeutic monoclonal antibody, in cancer patients. *Invest New Drugs.* 2004;22(1):39-52.

Sifalimumab

Sponsors: MedImmune

Synonym: MEDI-545, MDX-1103

Antigenic Type: IgG1, anti-interferon α (human monoclonal MEDI-545 heavy chain) with disulfide bond to human monoclonal MEDI-545 κ-chain, dimer

Indications: Investigated for treatment of systemic lupus erythematosus, dermatomyositis, and polymyositis.

Siltuximab

Sponsors: Johnson & Johnson

Synonym: CNTO-328

Antigenic Type: IgG1, anti-IL-6) (human-mouse monoclonal CNTO 328 heavy chain) with disulfide bond to human-mouse monoclonal CNTO 328 κ-chain, dimer

Indications: Investigated for treatment of certain cancers.

References: Puchalski T, Prabhakar U, Jiao Q, Berns B, Davis HM. Pharmacokinetic and pharmacodynamic modeling of an anti-interleukin-6 chimeric monoclonal antibody (siltuximab) in patients with metastatic renal cell carcinoma. *Clin Cancer Res.* 2010;16:1652-1661.

Siplizumab

Sponsors: MedImmune

Synonym: MEDI-507

Antigenic Type: IgG1, anti-human CD2 antigen (human-rat monoclonal MEDI-507 γ1-chain) with disulfide bond to mouse MEDI-507 light chain, dimer. Molecular weight approximately 150,000 daltons.

Indications: Investigated for treatment of T-cell lymphoma, binding to CD2 antigen.

Solanezumab

Sponsors: Eli Lilly and Company

Synonym: LY2062430

Antigenic Type: IgG1, anti-(human β-amyloid) (human-mouse monoclonal LY2062430 heavy chain) with disulfide bond to human-mouse monoclonal LY2062430 light chain, dimer

Indications: Investigated for treatment of Alzheimer disease.

References: Siemers ER, et al. Safety and changes in plasma and cerebrospinal fluid amyloid beta after a single administration of an amyloid beta monoclonal antibody in subjects with Alzheimer disease. *Clin Neuropharmacol.* 2010;33:67-73.

Sontuzumab

Sponsors: Hangzhou Onicon

Antigenic Type: IgG1 anti-(human episialin) (human-mouse monoclonal HMFG-1 gamma-1-chain) with disulfide bond to human-mouse HMFG-1 dimer

Indications: Investigated for treatment of certain cancers.

Sotatercept

Sponsors: Acceleron Pharma

Synonym: ACE-011

Antigenic Type: Activin receptor type IIA (synthetic human extracellular domain-containing fragment) fusion protein with immunoglobulin G1 (synthetic human heavy chain Fc fragment), dimer

Indications: Investigated as red-cell maturation agent for the treatment of anemia, and bone anabolic agent for the treatment of cancer-related bone loss.

Stamulumab

Sponsors: Wyeth

Synonym: MYO-029

Antigenic Type: IgG1, anti-human growth differentiation factor 8 (human MYO-029 heavy chain), with disulfide bond to human MYO-029 λ-chain, dimer

Indications: Investigated for treatment of muscular dystrophy and age-related sarcopenia or frailty.

Tadocizumab

Sponsors: Yamanouchi Pharma America

Synonym: YM337, C4G1

Antigenic Type: IgG1 anti-(human integrin-α IIbβ3) Fab fragment (human-mouse monoclonal C4G1 γ1-chain) with disulfide bond to human-mouse C4G1 K-chain, dimer

Indications: Investigated for treatment of patients undergoing percutaneous coronary interventions.

Talizumab

Sponsors: Tanox

Synonym: TNX-901

Antigenic Type: IgG, anti-human IgE Fc region (human-mouse monoclonal Hu901 λ-chain) with disulfide bond to human-mouse Hu901 κ-chain, dimer. Molecular weight 146,348 daltons.

Indications: Investigated for treatment of peanut-induced hypersensitivity.

Teneliximab

Sponsors: Bristol-Myers Squibb

Synonym: BMS-224819, chi220

Antigenic Type: IgG1, anti-human CD40 antigen (human-mouse monoclonal chi220 γ1-chain) with disulfide bond to human-mouse chi220 light chain. Molecular weight 73,046 daltons.

Indications: Investigated for treatment of autoimmune diseases or to prevent transplant rejection.

Teplimab

Sponsors: MacroGenics

Synonym: MGA031

Antigenic Type: IgG1 anti-(human CD3 E-chain) (human-mouse monoclonal MGA031 heavy chain) with disulfide bond to human-mouse MGA031 light chain, dimer. Molecular weight 145,800 daltons.

Indications: Investigated for treatment of insulin-dependent diabetes.

Teprotumumab

Sponsors: Roche

Synonym: RO4858696-000

Antigenic Type: IgG1k, anti-(insulin-like growth factor I receptor)(human monoclonal heavy chain) with disulfide bond to human monoclonal light chain, dimer

Indications: Investigated for treatment of solid and hematologic tumors.

Toralizumab

Sponsors: Biogen Idec

Synonym: IDEC-131, anti-g39, anti-CD40L, anti-CD154

Antigenic Type: IgG1 anti-human CD40 ligand (human-mouse monoclonal IDEC-131 γ1-chain) with disulfide bond to human-mouse IDEC-131 κ-chain. Molecular weight 148,426 daltons.

Indications: Investigated for treatment of immune thrombocytopenic purpura, T-cell mediated diseases, and B-cell malignancies.

Tralokinumab

Sponsors: MedImmune

Synonym: CAT-354

Antigenic Type: IgG4, anti-IL-13) (human monoclonal CAT-354 heavy chain) with disulfide bond to human monoclonal CAT-354 light chain, dimer

Indications: Investigated for treatment of asthma and inflammatory diseases.

Trastuzumab Emtansine

Sponsors: Genentech

Synonym: PRO132365, trastuzumab-MCC-DM1, T-DM1

Antigenic Type: IgG1, anti-(p185neu receptor) (human-mouse monoclonal rhuMab HER2 γ1-chain) with disulfide bond to human-mouse monoclonal rhuMab HER2 light chain, dimer, tetraamide with N2'-[3-[[1-[(4-carboxycyclohexyl)methyl]-2,5-dioxo-3-pyrrolidinyl]thio]-1-oxopropyl]-N2'-deacetylmaytansine

Indications: Investigated for treatment of certain cancers.

Tremelimumab

Sponsors: Boehringer Ingelheim, Pfizer

Synonym: CP-675,206, anti-CD152; previously referred to as ticilimumab

Antigenic Type: IgG2 anti-(human CTLA-4) (human monoclonal CP675206 clone 11.2.1 heavy chain) with disulfide bond to human CP675206 clone 11.2.1 light chain, dimer. Molecular weight 150,000 daltons.

Indications: Investigated for treatment of metastatic melanoma and pancreatic cancer.

Tucotuzumab Celmoleukin

Sponsors: EMD Lexigen

Synonym: EMD273066, KS-IL2

Antigenic Type: IgG1 anti-(human antigen 17-1A) (human mouse monoclonal huKS-IL2 heavy chain) fusion protein with interleukin 2 (human), with disulfide bond to human-mouse huKS-IL2 light, dimer

Indications: Investigated for treatment of colorectal, non-small cell lung, ovarian, and prostate cancers.

Vedolizumab

Sponsors: Millennium Pharmaceuticals

Synonym: MLN02, LDP02

Antigenic Type: IgG1, anti-human integrin LPAM-1 (lymphocyte Peyer patch adhesion molecule 1) (human-mouse heavy chain). Molecular weight 146.8 kDa.

Indications: Investigated for treatment of ulcerative colitis and Crohn disease.

Veltuzumab

Sponsors: Immunomedics
Synonym: IMMU-106
Antigenic Type: IgG1, anti-(human CD20) (human-mouse monoclonal hA20 heavy chain) with disulfide bridge to human-mouse monoclonal hA20 κ-chain, dimer. Molecular weight 145.3 kDa.
Indications: Investigated for treatment of non-Hodgkin lymphoma.
References: Qu Z, Goldenberg DM, Cardillo TM, Shi V, Hansen HJ, Chang CH. Bispecific anti-CD20/22 antibodies inhibit B-cell lymphoma proliferation by a unique mechanism of action. *Blood.* 2008;111(4):2211-2219.

Goldenberg DM, et al. Veltuzumab (humanized anti-CD20 monoclonal antibody): Characterization, current clinical results, and future prospects. *Leuk Lymphoma.* 2010;51:747-755.

Visilizumab

Sponsors: Protein Design Labs
Trade Name: *Nuvion*
Indications: Investigated for treatment of ulcerative colitis, transplantation, and steroid-refractory graft versus host disease.
References: Carpenter PA, Lowder J, Johnston L, et al. A phase II multicenter study of visilizumab, humanized anti-CD3 antibody, to treat steroid-refractory acute graft-versus-host disease. *Biol Blood Marrow Transplant.* 2005;11:465-471.

Volociximab

Sponsors: Icos Corporation, Protein Design Labs, Biogen Idec
Synonym: M200
Antigenic Type: IgG4, anti-human α5β1 integrin (human-mouse clone p200-M heavy chain), with disulfide bond to human-mouse clone p200-M κ-chain, dimer. Molecular weight 145,500 daltons.
Indications: Investigated as an antiangiogenic agent to treat solid tumors and age-related macular degeneration.
References: Kuwada SK. Drug evaluation: Volociximab, an angiogenesis-inhibiting chimeric monoclonal antibody. *Curr Opin Mol Ther.* 2007;9(1):92-98.

Zalutumumab

Sponsors: Medarex, Genmab
Synonym: HuMax-EGFr, 2F8
Antigenic Type: IgG1, anti-(human epidermal growth factor receptor) (human monoclonal 2F8 heavy chain) with disulfide bond to human monoclonal 2F8 K-chain, dimer
Indications: Investigated for treatment of head and neck cancer.
References: Rivera F, Salcedo M, Vega N, Blanco Y, Ló pez C. Current situation of zalutumumab. *Expert Opin Biol Ther.* 2009;9:667-674.

Zanolimumab

Sponsors: DSM Biologics, Statens Serum Institute of Denmark, Genmab A/S

Synonym: MDX-016, HuMax-CD4

Antigenic Type: IgG, anti-human CD4 antigen (human monoclonal 6G5 heavy chain), with disulfide bond to human monoclonal 6G5 light chain, dimer. Molecular weight 147,000 daltons.

Indications: Investigated for treatment of rheumatoid arthritis, psoriasis, and cutaneous T-cell lymphoma.

References: Kim YH, Duvic M, Obitz E, et al. Clinical efficacy of zanolimumab (HuMax-CD4): two phase 2 studies in refractory cutaneous T-cell lymphoma. *Blood.* 2007;109(11):4655-4662.

Investigational Drugs

Products in this section are listed in alphabetical sequence by isotope and then proper name. For cases where the proper name would not imply the investigated use of a product, refer to the following table:

Purpose Being Investigated	Product(s)
Cancers and lymphomas, various	Altumomab, Bectumomab, Clivatuzumab tetraxetan, CR49, Epratuzumab, Labetuzumab, Pemtumomab, Rituxumab, Tacatuzumab, Votumumab
Infection, imaging of	Sulesomab

For a discussion of isotope-conjugated antibodies and the principles of imaging using isotopes, see the text toward the end of the Immune Globulins section.

References: Harwood SJ, et al. The use of monoclonal antibodies for immunoscintigraphic detection of cancer. *J Pharm Pract.* 1994;7:93-116.

Indium In 111 Altumomab Pentetate (Murine)

Sponsors: Hybritech

Synonym: Anti-CEA monoclonal antibody type ZCE 025 (murine), MAB 35, ZCE025, CAS 139039-70-6 (antibody alone), or CAS 139039-69-3 (antibody conjugate)

Trade Name: *Hybri-CEAker*

Antigenic Type: IgG1, monoclonal, dimer, 150,000 daltons

Indications: Investigated for detection of suspected and previously unidentified tumor foci of recurrent colorectal carcinoma.

Orphan Status: February 6, 1990

References: Lofberg M, Liewendahl K, Lamminen A, Korhola O, Somer H. Antimyosin scintigraphy compared with magnetic resonance imaging in inflammatory myopathies. *Arch Neurol.* 1998;55:987-993.

Indium In 111 Immunoglobulin G (Human)

Sponsors: Novartis

Antigenic Type: IgG, all 4 subtypes, polyclonal

Indications: Investigated for imaging infectious and inflammatory foci.

References: Oyen WJG, et al. Indium-111-labeled human nonspecific immunoglobulin G: a new radiopharmaceutical for imaging infectious and inflammatory foci. *Clin Infect Dis.* 1992;14:1110-1118.

Sponsors: Ortho-McNeil

Synonym: CAS 145464-27-3

Trade Name: *Macroscint*

Antigenic Type: IgG, polyclonal, pentetate form (N,N-bis[2-(bis[carboxymethyl]amino)-ethyl] glycine conjugate)

Indications: Investigated for use as an imaging agent for occult infection and inflammation.

Indium In 111 Rituximab (Chimeric Human-Murine)

Sponsors: Biogen Idec
Synonym: Engineered pan-B cell anti-CD20, In2B8
Antigenic Type: Monoclonal IgG1 antibodies formed with murine variable regions and human constant regions
Indications: Investigated for imaging non-Hodgkin B-cell lymphoma.

Iodine I 124 Girentuximab

Sponsors: IBA Molecular
Synonym: 124IcG250, Redectane
Antigenic Type: IgG1, anti-(human antigen MN) (human-mouse monoclonal cG250 heavy chain) with disulfide bond to human-mouse monoclonal cG250 κ-chain, dimer, labeled with iodine-124
Indications: Investigated for diagnosis of clear-cell renal cancer.

Iodine I 125 CR49 Monoclonal Antibody (Unspecified Source)

Sponsors: Neoprobe
Trade Name: *RIGScan CR49*
Antigenic Type: Radio-labeled monoclonal antibody that binds to specific antigen on colorectal cancer cells.
Indications: Investigated for use in guiding surgical resection of colorectal cancer. The radio-tagged monoclonal antibody would be coupled with a proprietary hand-held radiation detector to quantitate gamma emissions, enabling more complete removal of cancerous cells. RIGS stands for radio-immuno-guided surgery.
References: Anonymous. RIGScan CR: RIGScan CR49. *Drugs R D*. 2004;5:240-241.

Iodine I 131 Labetuzumab (Chimeric Human-Murine)

Sponsors: Immunomedics
Synonym: hMN-14
Trade Name: *CEA-Cide*
Antigenic Type: IgG1, anti-human CEA (human-mouse hMN-14 γ-chain) with disulfide bond to human-mouse hMN-14 κ-chain, dimer, chelated to 131-I. Molecular weight approximately 150,000 daltons.
References: Liersch T, Meller J, Kulle B, et al. Phase II trial of carcinoembryonic antigen radio-immunotherapy with 131I-labetuzumab after salvage resection of colorectal metastases in the liver: five-year safety and efficacy results. *J Clin Oncol*. 2005;23:6763-6370.

Technetium Tc 99m Bectumomab (Murine)

Sponsors: Immunomedics

Synonym: IMMU-LL2, CAS 158318-63-9

Trade Name: *ImmuRAID-LL2, LymphoScan*

Antigenic Type: IgG2a monoclonal Fab' binding fragments, 48 to 50 kilodaltons, targeting human antigen CD22

Indications: Investigated for diagnostic imaging in the evaluation of the extent of disease in patients with histologically confirmed diagnosis of non-Hodgkin B-cell lymphoma, acute B-cell lymphoblastic leukemia (in children and adults), AIDS-related lymphoma, and chronic B-cell lymphocytic leukemia.

Orphan Status: April 7, 1992

References: Lamonica D, Czuczman M, Nabi H, Klippenstein D, Grossman Z. Radioimmunoscintigraphy (RIS) with bectumomab (Tc99m labeled IMMU-LL2, Lymphoscan) in the assessment of recurrent non-Hodgkin's lymphoma (NHL). *Cancer Biother Radiopharm.* 2002;17:689-697.

Technetium Tc 99m Sulesomab (Murine)

Sponsors: Immunomedics

Synonym: CAS 167747-19-5

Trade Name: *ImmuRAID-MN3, LeukoScan*

Antigenic Type: IgG1 monoclonal Fab' binding fragments of 50 kilodaltons against human NCA-90 granulocyte cell antigens

Indications: Investigated for detection of location and extent of suspected infections affecting prosthetic joints, bones, and foot ulcers in patients with diabetes; appendicitis; osteomyelitis.

References: Delcourt A, Huglo D, Prangere T, et al. Comparison between Leukoscan (Sulesomab) and Gallium-67 for the diagnosis of osteomyelitis in the diabetic foot. *Diabetes Metab.* 2005;31:125-133.

Vicente AG, Almoguera M, Alonso JC, et al. Diagnosis of orthopedic infection in clinical practice using Tc-99m sulesomab (antigranulocyte monoclonal antibody fragment Fab'2). *Clin Nucl Med.* 2004;29:781-785.

Technetium Tc 99m Votumumab (Human)

Sponsors: Organon Teknika

Synonym: 88BV59, CAS 148189-70-2

Trade Name: *OncoSpect, HumaSPECT*

Antigenic Type: IgG3, monoclonal, kappa type, 170,000 daltons, targeting human carcinoma-associated antigen.

Indications: Investigated for diagnostic imaging and therapy of cancer.

References: Elgqvist J, Bernhardt P, Hultborn R, et al. Myelotoxicity and RBE of 211At-conjugated monoclonal antibodies compared with 99mTc-conjugated monoclonal antibodies and 60Co irradiation in nude mice. *J Nucl Med.* 2005;46(3):464-471.

Yttrium Y 90 Clivatuzumab Tetraxetan

Sponsors: Immunomedics
Synonym: hPAM4-DOTA, IMMU-107, 90hY-PAM4, hPAM4-Cide
Antigenic Type: IgG1, anti-(human mucin MUC1) (human-mouse monoclonal hPAM4 heavy chain) with disulfide bond to human-mouse monoclonal hPAM4 κ-chain, dimer, 1,4,7,10-tetraazacyclododecane-1,4,7,10-tetraacetic acid conjugate, yttrium-90Y chelate
Indications: Investigated for treatment of pancreatic cancer.

Yttrium Y 90 Epratuzumab Tetraxetan

Sponsors: Amgen, Immunomedics
Synonym: hLL2
Trade Name: *LymphoCide*
Indications: Investigated for radioimmunotherapy of non-Hodgkin B-cell lymphoma.
References: Davies SL. Epratuzumab. *Drugs Future.* 2005;30:683-687.

Yttrium Y 90 Labetuzumab Tetraxetan (Chimeric Human-Murine)

Sponsors: Immunomedics
Synonym: hMN-14
Trade Name: *CEA-Cide*
Antigenic Type: IgG1, anti-human CEA (human-mouse hMN-14 γ-chain) with disulfide bond to human-mouse hMN-14 κ-chain, dimer, chelated to 90-Y. Molecular weight approximately 150,000 daltons.
Indications: Investigated for treatment of gastrointestinal cancer and pancreatic cancer.
References: Govindan SV, Cardillo TM, Moon SJ, Hansen HJ, Goldenberg DM. CEACAM5-targeted therapy of human colonic and pancreatic cancer xenografts with potent labetuzumab-SN-38 immunoconjugates. *Clin Cancer Res.* 2009;15:6052-6061.

Yttrium Y 90 Pemtumomab

Sponsors: Abbott Laboratories, Antisoma
Synonym: R-1549, 90Y-muHMFG1
Trade Name: *Theragyn*
Antigenic Type: IgG, murine monoclonal. The antibody component, HMFG1 (human milk-fat globulin-1), targets and binds to a tumor antigen called MUC1. This is a protein found on the surface of cancer cells in many types of epithelial tumor, including ovarian, stomach, pancreatic, breast, lung, and colorectal cancers.
Indications: Investigated for targeted radiotherapy of ovarian cancer and gastric cancer.
References: Verheijen RH, Massuger LF, Benigno BB, et al. Phase III trial of intraperitoneal therapy with yttrium-90-labeled HMFG1 murine monoclonal antibody in patients with epithelial ovarian cancer after a surgically defined complete remission. *J Clin Oncol.* 2006;24:571-578.

Yttrium Y 90 Tacatuzumab (Chimeric Human-Murine)

Sponsors: Immunomedics

Synonym: hAFP-31

Trade Name: *AFP-Cide*

Antigenic Type: IgG1, anti-human α-fetoprotein (human-mouse hAFP-31 γ1-chain) with disulfide bond to human-mouse hAFP-31 κ-chain, dimer, chelated to 90-Y

Indications: Investigated as antineoplastic treatment.

Investigational Immune Globulins, Isoantibodies (Toxin-Conjugated)

Investigational Drugs

A wide variety of immunotoxins are in advanced clinical trials, have achieved orphan drug status, and are undergoing review of safety and efficacy by FDA.

Most of these investigational antibodies will serve as therapeutic agents, using the specificity of antibodies and the cytotoxicity of organic toxins to aid treatment of a wide variety of diseases. A brief description of various products under investigation follows. One of the most commonly studied toxins, ricin, was the subject of crystallography experiments on the space shuttle *Columbia* during a July 1992 mission.

References: Ghetie V, et al. Immunotoxins in the therapy of cancer: From bench to clinic. *Pharmacol Ther*. 1994;63:209-234.

Pai LH. Immunotoxin therapy for cancer. *JAMA*. 1993;269:78-81.

Inotuzumab Ozogamicin (Chimeric Human-Murine)

Sponsors: Wyeth

Synonym: CMC-544, WAY-207294, G544

Antigenic Type: IgG4 anti-human CD22 (human-mouse monoclonal G544 heavy chain) with disulfide bond to human-mouse G544 κ-chain, dimer, linked with ozogamicin. Molecular weight approximately 150,000 daltons.

Indications: Indicated for treatment of various cancers.

References: DiJoseph JF, Dougher MM, Kalyandrug LB, et al. Antitumor efficacy of a combination of CMC-544 (inotuzumab ozogamicin), a CD22-targeted cytotoxic immunoconjugate of calicheamicin, and rituximab against non-Hodgkin's B-cell lymphoma. *Clin Cancer Res*. 2006;12:242-249.

Nofetumomab with *Pseudomonas* Exotoxin (Chimeric Human-Murine)

Sponsors: NeoRx Corporation

Trade Name: *OncoPurge*

Antigenic Type: NR-LU-10 monoclonal antibodies conjugated to *Pseudomonas* exotoxin

Indications: Investigated for use in eliminating tumor cells harvested for autologous bone marrow transplantation for breast cancer patients undergoing high-dose chemotherapy.

Investigational Drugs

Research into a variety of novel forms of allergen extracts has been underway for well over a decade. These studies aim to increase efficacy and decrease adverse effects associated with immunotherapy. None of these products has as yet been licensed in the United States, although some are available in other countries.

Promising investigational forms of allergen extracts include formalin-treated allergens ("allergoids"), glutaraldehyde-treated allergens (ie, polymerized allergens), and a polypeptide that mimics IgE. Polymerized allergens are in phase 3 studies sponsored by Schering Laboratories.

ImmuLogic Pharmaceutical Corporation is investigating specific epitopes that would provide immunotherapy without allergenic effects. ImmuLogic's *CatVax* consists of 2 peptide epitopes and is in phase II trials. Other epitopes in the *Allervax* series are being developed for various ragweed (*RagVax*), cedar, grass, and dust mite allergens.

References: Grammer LC, Shaughnessy MA. Immunotherapy with modified allergens. *Immunol Allergy Clin N Amer.* 1992;12:95-105.

Allergen Extracts with MPL

Sponsors: Allergy Therapeutics

Trade Name: *Pollinex Quattro*

Antigenic Type: Natural allergens (eg, grasses, trees, ragweed) are chemically modified, then combined with a depot technology using tyrosine and adjuvanted with monophosphoryl lipid A (MPL), a TLR4 agonist.

Indications: Investigated for treatment of specific allergies as an ultra-short course of 4 injections over 3 weeks.

References: Patel P, Salapatek AM. Pollinex Quattro: a novel and well-tolerated, ultra short-course allergy vaccine. *Expert Rev Vaccines.* 2006;5(5):617-629.

Investigational Immunodiagnostics

Investigational Drugs

Candida albicans Antigen

Sponsors: Greer Laboratories

Trade Name: *CASTA*

Antigenic Type: Fungal antigen. Skin tests assess delayed (type IV) hypersensitivity.

Indications: Investigated for use in assessment of delayed-type hypersensitivity and cellular immune responsiveness.

Mycology: *Candida albicans*, ATCC #10231. Subdivision Deuteromycotina (formerly called Fungi imperfecti), class Blastomyces

References: Esch RE, Buckley CE III. A novel *Candida albicans* skin test antigen: Efficacy and safety in man. *J Biol Standard.* 1988;16:33-43.

Mycobacterium avium Skin Test Antigen

Sponsors: Statens Seruminstitut (Copenhagen, Denmark)

Synonym: *Mycobacterium avium* sensitin (MAS) RS-10

Antigenic Type: Bacterial antigen. Skin tests assess type IV hypersensitivity.

Microbiology: Bacterium, *Mycobacterium avium*

Indications: Investigated for use in assessing *Mycobacterium avium* infection.

References: von Reyn CF, Williams DE, Horsburgh CR Jr., et al. Dual skin testing with *Mycobacterium avium* sensitin and purified protein derivative to discriminate pulmonary disease due to *M. avium* complex from pulmonary due to *Mycobacterium tuberculosis*. *J Infect Dis.* 1998;177:730-736.

Patch Testing Reagents & Devices

Compared with the licensed contact dermatitis reagents, these investigational products and devices are purported to reduce the likelihood of errors in application and the amount of time required to prepare and apply the patches to the skin.

Epiquick, manufactured by Hermal Kurt Herrmann, consists of measured amounts of allergen suspended in petrolatum or other vehicle and placed in *Finn Chambers*, attached to a foil backing, and sealed with a polyethylene plastic covering.

Accupatch, manufactured by Dermx, incorporates allergen into the adhesive matrix of a patch. In preliminary studies with paraphenylenediamine (PPD), the allergen in permanent hair dye, *Accupatch* demonstrated comparable hypersensitivity compared with *Finn Chambers*.

References: Adams RM. Recent advances in contact dermatitis. *Ann Allergy.* 1991;67:552-567.

Marks JG Jr., DeLeo VA. *Contact and Occupational Dermatology.* St. Louis: Mosby Year Book; 1992.

Marks JG Jr. The *Accupatch*: A new patch testing device. *Am J Contact Dermatitis.* 1991;2:98-101.

Investigational Drugs

Products in this section are listed in alphabetic sequence by proper name. For cases where the proper name would not imply the function or investigated use of a product, refer to the following table:

Category	Product(s)
Bactericidal/permeability factors	Opebacan
Colony-stimulating factors	Lanimostim, Lenograstim
Interferon-alfa analog	Albinterferon Alfa-2b
Interleukin-2 analogs	Teceleukin
Interleukin-3 analogs	Daniplestim, Milodistim
Interleukin-18 analogs	Iboctadekin
Stem-cell factors	Ancestim, Garnocestim
Tumor-necrosis factor analogs	Onercept, Pegsunercept

Albinterferon Alfa-2b

Sponsors: Human Genome Sciences

Synonym: Albuferon

Antigenic Type: Inteferon alfa-2b fused to albumin

Indications: Investigated for treatment of chronic hepatitis C.

References: Chemmanur AT, Wu GY. Drug evlauation: Albuferon-alpha—an antiviral interferon-alpha/albumin fusion protein. *Curr Opin Investig Drugs.* 2006;7(8):750-758.

Ancestim

Sponsors: Amgen

Trade Name: *Stemgen*

Indications: Investigated for treatment of bone metastases.

References: da Silva MG, Pimentel P, Carvalhais A, et al. Ancestim (recombinant human stem cell factor, SCF) in association with filgrastim does not enhance chemotherapy and/or growth factor-induced peripheral blood progenitor cell (PBPC) mobilization inpatients with a prior insufficient PBPC collection. *Bone Marrow Transplant.* 2004;34:683-691. Letters in: *Bone Marrow Transplant.* 2005;35:1019-1020.

Daniplestim (Recombinant)

Sponsors: Searle, Schering

Synonym: SC-55494, CAS 161753-30-6

Trade Name: *Synthakine*

Antigenic Type: Synthetic human variant interleukin-3

Indications: Investigated for use in stimulating bone marrow to produce and release early-stage or precursor blood cells; for hematopoietic restoration following high-dose chemotherapy.

References: Patel SD, Guo R, Miller WM, et al. Clinical-scale production of granulocyte progenitor and post-progenitor cells using daniplestim, leridistim, progenipoietin, promegapoietin and autologous plasma. *Cytotherapy.* 2000;2:85-94. Erratum in: *Cytotherapy.* 2000;2:405.

Garnocestim

Sponsors: GlaxoSmithKline
Synonym: SB-251353
Antigenic Type: 5-73-macrophage inflammatory protein 2α (human gene gro2)
Indications: Investigated for peripheral blood stem-cell mobilization to reduce incidence, duration, and severity of chemotherapy-induced cytopenias.

Granulocyte-Macrophage Colony-Stimulating Factor (Recombinant)

Indications: Investigated for treatment of low blood cell counts; for treatment of AIDS patients with neutropenia caused by the disease, zidovudine (AZT), or ganciclovir; for treatment of severe thermal injuries in patients with more than 40% full or partial thickness burns; for treatment of patients with myelodysplastic syndrome; for treatment of patients with aplastic anemia; for treatment of neutropenia associated with bone marrow transplants; for treatment of neutropenia caused by hairy cell leukemia; for treatment of chronic lymphocytic leukemia to increase granulocyte count. Also seeking an indication for CMV retinitis.

Sponsors: Schering and Novartis
Synonym: Molgramostim, GM-CSF
Trade Name: *Leucomax*
Description: GM-CSF produced from recombinant bacterial cultures (*Escherichia coli*)
References: Kopf B, De Giorgi U, Vertogen B, et al. A randomized study comparing filgrastim versus lenograstim versus molgramostim plus chemotherapy for peripheral blood progenitor cell mobilization. *Bone Marrow Transplant.* 2006;38(6):407-412.

Sponsors: Novartis and Chugai
Synonym: Ecogramostim, Regramostim, GM-CSF
Description: GM-CSF produced from Chinese hamster ovary (CHO) cell culture
References: Hussein AM, Ross M, Vredenburgh J, et al. Effects of granulocyte-macrophage colony stimulating factor produced in Chinese hamster ovary cells (regramostim), *Escherichia coli* (molgramostim) and yeast (sargramostim) on priming peripheral blood progenitor cells for use with autologous bone marrow after high-dose chemotherapy. *Eur J Haematol.* 1995;55(5):348-356.

Sponsors: Cangene
Trade Name: *Leucotropin*

Iboctadekin

Sponsors: GlaxoSmithKline
Synonym: SB-485232, Interferon-gamma-inducing factor
Antigenic Type: Human interleukin-18, recombinant. Molecular weight 18,217 daltons, 157 amino acids, single polypeptide chain that is not glycosylated.
Indications: Investigated for treatment of disseminated solid tumors.
Production Method: Expressed in *Escherichia coli*. Formed in vivo following activation of proIL-18 by caspase-4.

Interleukin-2 (Recombinant)

Sponsors: Cel-Sci Corporation and Chesapeake Biological Labs
Trade Name: *Multikine*
Indications: Investigated for use in treating cancers or immune deficiencies.
References: Timar J, Forster-Horvath C, Lukits J, et al. The effect of leukocyte interleukin injection (*Multikine*) treatment on the peritumoral and intratumoral subpopulation of mononuclear cells and on tumor epithelia: a possible new approach to augmenting sensitivity to radiation therapy and chemotherapy in oral cancer--a multicenter phase I/II clinical trial. *Laryngoscope.* 2003;113(12):2206-2217.

Interleukin-3 (Recombinant)

Sponsors: Sanofi-Aventis with Immunex Corporation
Synonym: IL-3, multilineage CSF
Indications: Designated an orphan drug for promotion of erythropoiesis in Diamond-Blackfan anemia (congenital pure red-cell aplasia).
Other Research: Seeking indications for bone marrow failure, platelet deficiencies, autologous bone marrow transplantation, adjuvant to chemotherapy, and peripheral stem-cell transplant.
Orphan Status: May 20, 1991

Sponsors: Genetics Institute with Novartis
Synonym: SDZ ILE-964, CAS 148641-02-5
Trade Name: *Muplestim, Hemokine*
Antigenic Type: Interleukin-3 expressed by recombinant *Escherichia coli*
Indications: Investigated for use in treatment of breast, ovarian, and lung cancers and lymphoma.

Interleukin-4 (Recombinant)

Sponsors: Schering-Plough
Indications: Seeking indications for treatment of immunodeficient diseases, for cancer therapy, and as a vaccine adjuvant.

Sponsors: Sterling Drug with Immunex Corporation
Indications: Seeking indications for cancer immunomodulation.

Interleukin-6 (Recombinant)

Sponsors: Novartis with Genetics Institute; Serono Laboratories

Synonym: SDZ ILE-969

Trade Name: *Sigosix*

Antigenic Type: Interleukin-6 expressed by recombinant *Escherichia coli* or Chinese hamster ovary cells (glycosylated).

Indications: Investigated for use in treatment of breast, lung, renal, and ovarian cancers and lymphoma. Also investigated for treatment of thrombocytopenia in bone marrow transplantation and chemotherapy.

Interleukin-10

Sponsors: Schering

Trade Name: *Pleioten, Tenovil*

Antigenic Type: Interleukin-10

Interleukin-12 (Recombinant)

Sponsors: Genetics Institute with Roche

Indications: Investigated for use in treatment of kidney cancer.

Interleukin-18

Sponsors: Serono

Indications: Investigated for treatment of rheumatoid arthritis or Crohn disease.

Lanimostim

Sponsors: Eximias Pharmaceutical Corporation

Synonym: 4-221-CSF-1, p3ACSF-69

Antigenic Type: Colony-stimulating factor, an anti-infective growth factor that acts on both progenitor and mature cells of the macrophage line. Molecuar weight 49,033 daltons.

Indications: Investigated as antineoplastic treatment and for the treatment of serious fungal infections.

Lenograstim

Sponsors: Sanofi-Aventis, Chugai

Synonym: G-CSF, Lenograstim

Trade Name: *Granocyte, Neutrogin*

Antigenic Type: Granulocyte colony-stimulating factor

Description: Glycosylated polypeptide consisting of 174 amino acids produced from cultured Chinese hamster ovary (CHO) cells containing the recombinant gene for human G-CSF. Glycosylation occurs at a threonine molecule at position 133. Lenograstim's amino acid sequence is identical to the natural product, with a molecular weight of 20 kilodaltons. Its biological half-life after subcutaneous dosing is 3 to 6 hours.

References: Dunn CJ, Goa KL. Lenograstim: an update of its pharmacological properties and use in chemotherapy-induced neutropenia and related clinical settings. *Drugs.* 2000;59:681-717.

Frampton JE, Yarker YE, Goa KL. Lenograstim: A review of its pharmacologic properties and therapeutic efficacy in neutropenia and related clinical settings. *Drugs.* 1995;49:767-793.

Kopf B, De Giorgi U, Vertogen B, et al. A randomized study comparing filgrastim versus lenograstim versus molgramostim plus chemotherapy for peripheral blood progenitor cell mobilization. *Bone Marrow Transplant.* 2006;38(6):407-412.

Macrophage Colony-Stimulating Factor

Sponsors: Biogen Idec, Novartis

Synonym: M-CSF

Trade Name: *Macrolin*

Indications: Investigated for treatment of certain cancers and fungal diseases.

Sponsors: Genetics Institute with Scigenics and Schering-Plough

Trade Name: *Macstim*

Indications: Investigated for treatment of cancer, infectious disease, and elevated serum cholesterol.

Milodistim (Recombinant)

Sponsors: Immunex

Synonym: PIXY-321, GM-CSF/IL3, CAS 137463-76-4

Trade Name: *Pixykine*

Antigenic Type: A fusion molecule with an interleukin-3 domain attached to a granulocyte-macrophage colony-stimulating factor domain, expressed from *Saccharomyces cerevisiae*.

Comment: PIXY-321 is reported to have enhanced biological effects in vitro compared with GM-CSF or IL-3 alone.

References: Williams DE, Park LS. Hematopoietic effects of a granulocyte-macrophage colony-stimulating factor/interleukin-3 fusion protein. *Cancer.* 1991;67:2705-2707.

Onercept

Sponsors: Serono
Antigenic Type: Tumor-necrosis factor binding protein-1.
Indications: Investigated for the treatment of psoriasis and psoriatic arthritis.
References: Nikas SN, Drosos AA. Onercept. Serono. *Curr Opin Investig Drugs*. 2003;4:1369-1376.

Opebacan (Recombinant)

Sponsors: Xoma Corporation
Synonym: rBPI21
Trade Name: *Neuprex*
Antigenic Type: N-terminal fragment of bactericidal/permeability-increasing protein (BPI), 21,000 daltons
Indications: Investigated for concurrent use with antibiotics to enhance bactericidal activity and to enhance survival in severe sepsis. BPI is a human host-defense protein made by polymorphonuclear leukocytes. BPI kills gram-negative bacteria, enhances the activity of antibiotics, neutralizes gram-negative endotoxin, and inhibits angiogenesis.

Pegsunercept

Sponsors: Amgen
Synonym: sTNF-RI
Antigenic Type: 1-105-Tumor necrosis factor p55 (L-methionyl) (human), 30 kilodalton pegylated. Tumor necrosis factor-alfa receptor type 1.
Indications: Investigated for treatment of ovarian cancer.
References: Furst DE, Fleischmann R, Kopp E, et al; 990136 Study Group. A phase 2 dose-finding study of PEGylated recombinant methionyl human soluble tumor necrosis factor type I in patients with rheumatoid arthritis. *J Rheumatol*. 2005;32:2303-2310.

Pitrakinra

Sponsors: Aerovance
Synonym: Binetrakin
Trade Name: *Aerovant*
Antigenic Type: IL-4 and IL-13 inhibitor
Indications: Investigated for treatment of atopic asthma
References: Wenzel S, Wilbraham D, Fuller R, Getz EB, Longphre M. Effect of an interleukin-4 variant on late phase asthmatic response to allergen challenge in asthmatic patients: Results of two phase 2a studies. *Lancet*. 2007;370(9596):1422-1431.

Polyribonucleotide

Sponsors: Hemispherx Biopharma

Synonym: Poly(I)$_n$:poly(C$_{12}$Un)(poly I:C$_{12}$U), polyriboinosinic: polyribocytidylic-polyribouridylic acid, a synthetic double-stranded RNA

Trade Name: *Ampligen*

Indications: Designated an orphan drug for treatment of AIDS; for treatment of renal cell carcinoma.

Orphan Status: July 19, 1988; May 20, 1991

References: Armstrong JA, McMahon D, Huang XL, et al. A phase I study of *Ampligen* in human immunodeficiency virus-infected subjects. *J Infect Dis.* 1992;166:717-722.

Teceleukin (Recombinant)

Sponsors: Hoffmann-La Roche with Immunex Corporation

Trade Name: *Tecin*

Antigenic Type: Interleukin-2. Unlike native interleukin-2, teceleukin is not glycosylated, and includes a methionine residue at the amino terminus.

Indications: Designated an orphan drug for treatment of metastatic renal cell carcinoma (February 5, 1990); for treatment of metastatic malignant melanoma (February 6, 1990); for use in combination with interferon alfa-2a for treatment of metastatic renal cell carcinoma (May 3, 1990); for use in combination with interferon alfa-2a for treatment of metastatic malignant melanoma (May 11, 1990).

Orphan Status: February 5, 1990

References: Kintzel PE, Calis KA. Recombinant interleukin-2: A biological response modifier. *Clin Pharm.* 1991;10:110-128.

Thymalfasin

Sponsors: SciClone Pharmaceuticals

Synonym: Thymosin alfa-1, CAS 69521-94-4

Trade Name: *Zadaxin*

Antigenic Type: Synthetic form of polypeptide extract of the thymus gland, 28-amino acid peptide, molecular weight 3,100 daltons

Indications: Investigated for use in treating chronic hepatitis B, chronic active hepatitis C, non-small cell lung cancer, and DiGeorge syndrome (absent or underdeveloped thymus gland).

Comment: In Italy, thymosin-alpha-1 (*Zadaxin*, SciClone) was licensed in 1998 as an adjuvant to influenza vaccine. Several doses of thymosin alpha-1 improved the immune response to hepatitis B vaccine in previous nonresponders and to influenza vaccine in elderly veterans in small studies.

Orphan Status: May 3, 1991

References: Billich A. Thymosin alpha 1. SciClone Pharmaceuticals. *Curr Opin Investig Drugs*. 2002;3:698-707.

Gravenstein S, Duthie EH, Miller BA, et al. Augmentation of influenza antibody response in elderly men by thymosin alpha 1: A double-blind, placebo-controlled clinical study. *J Am Geriatr Soc*. 1989;37:1-8.

Mutchnick MG, et al. Thymosin treatment of chronic hepatitis B: A placebo-controlled pilot trial. *Hepatology*. 1991;14:409-415.

Shen SY, Josselson J, McRoy C, Sadler J, Chretien P. Effects of thymosin alpha 1 (TA1) on peripheral T-cell and *Hepatavax-B* vaccination (V) in previously nonresponsive hemodialysis (HD) patients. *Hepatology*. 1987;7:1120.

Thymopentin

Sponsors: Immunobiology Research Institute

Synonym: CAS 96558-55-0

Trade Name: *Timunox*

Antigenic Type: Synthetic pentapeptide, corresponding to amino acids 32 to 36 of the thymic hormone thymopoietin, not immunogenic

Indications: Investigated for use in treating HIV infection.

References: Donati D, Gastaldi L. Controlled trial of thymopentin in hemodialysis patients who fail to respond to hepatitis B vaccination. *Nephron*. 1988;50:133-136.

Fabrizi F, Dixit V, Martin P. Meta-analysis: the adjuvant role of thymopentin on immunological response to hepatitis B virus vaccine in end-stage renal disease. *Aliment Pharmacol Ther*. 2006;23(11):1559-1566.

Thymosin Fraction 5

Sponsors: SciClone Pharmaceuticals

Indications: Investigated for treatment of chronic active hepatitis and as an adjuvant to influenza vaccine.

References: Goldstein AL, Badamchian M. Thymosins: chemistry and biological properties in health and disease. *Expert Opin Biol Ther.* 2004;4:559-573.

Investigational Drugs

Alvircept Sudotox

Sponsors: Pfizer, NIH

Synonym: U-85, 855, sCD4-PE40, CAS 137487-62-8

Antigenic Type: Chimeric protein linking the first 178 amino acids of the extracellular domain of CD4 via 2 linker residues to amino acids 1 to 3 and 253-613 of *Pseudomonas aeruginosa* exotoxin A.

Indications: Investigated for use in treatment of HIV infection.

Cintredekin Besudotox

Sponsors: NeoPharm

Synonym: IL13-PE38, hIL13-PE8QQR (plasmid phuIL13-Tx)

Antigenic Type: Human interleukin-13 linked with *Pseudomonas aeruginosa* exotoxin A. Molecular weight 50,700 daltons.

Indications: Investigated for treatment of malignant glioma, including glioblastoma multiforme and anaplastic astrocytoma.

References: Rainov NG, Soling A. Technology evaluation: cintredekin besudotox, NeoPharm/Nippon. *Curr Opin Mol Ther*. 2005;7:170-181.

Pseudomonas aeruginosa Extract

Sponsors: DynaGen (Cambridge, MA)

Trade Name: *ImmuDyn*

Antigenic Type: Purified bacterial extract

Indications: Investigated for use in treating immune thrombocytopenia purpura as required to increase platelet counts.

Trisaccharides A & B

Sponsors: Chembiomed

Trade Name: *Biosynject*

Antigenic Type: Oligosaccharide

Indications: Investigated for use in treating moderate to severe clinical forms of hemolytic disease of the newborn arising from placental transfer of antibodies against blood group substances A and B (April 12, 1987); for use in ABO-incompatible solid organ transplantation, including kidney, heart, liver, and pancreas (April 20, 1987); for treatment of moderate to severe clinical forms of transfusion reactions arising from ABO-incompatible transfusion of blood, blood products, and blood derivatives (August 3, 1987); for prevention of ABO-medial hemolytic reactions arising from ABO-incompatible bone marrow transplantation (April 15, 1988).

Mechanism: Synthetic oligosaccharides representing blood groups' specificities (eg, blood group A and B) appear to cause dissociation of anti-A antibody bound to RBCs. At concentration of 1 mg/mL, the rate of dissociation of ^{125}-I-anti-A-antibody from red blood cells at 37° was accelerated. This effect may be caused by prevention of spontaneously dissociated antibodies from reassociating with RBCs. In another study, trisaccharide A competed with group A red blood cells for binding antibodies of IgG and IgM. Trisaccharide A can effectively immunoadsorb anti-A agglutinins found in group O donor sera.

Orphan Status: April 12, 1987

Investigational Drugs

Botulinum Toxin Type F

Sponsors: Porton International

Antigenic Type: Bacterial exotoxin type F excreted by *Clostridium botulinum*, an anaerobic, endospore-forming gram-positive rod. The toxin has a molecular weight of about 300 kilodaltons, has no hemagglutinin activity, and is antigenically distinct from toxin type A.

Indications: For treatment of spasmodic torticollis (cervical dystonia); for treatment of essential blepharospasm.

Orphan Status: First designated an orphan drug on October 24, 1991.

Belangenpumatucel-L

Sponsors: NovaRx Corporation

Synonym: *Lucanix*

Antigenic Type: Allogeneic vaccine cocktail of TGF-β blocked, whole non-small cell lung cancer tumor cells

Indications: Investigated for treatment of non-small cell lung cancer.

Galgenprostucel-L

Sponsors: Cell Genesys

Synonym: CG1940, part of *GVAX Prostate*

Antigenic Type: Galgenprostucel-L is 1 of 2 components of a prostate cancer cellular immunotherapy. CG1940 consists of a prostate adenocarcinoma cell line, PC-3, modified to secrete human granulocyte-macrophage colony-stimulating factor (GM-CSF) and irradiated to prevent cellular replication.

Indications: Investigated for treatment of prostate cancer.

Lapuleucel-T

Sponsors: Dendreon Corporation

Synonym: *Neuvenge*, APC8024

Antigenic Type: Specific active immunotherapeutic composed of antigen-loaded autologous antigen-presenting cells to stimulate T-cell immune response specific for tumor-associated antigen Her2/neu.

Indications: Investigated for treatment of cancers overexpressing Her2/neu.

Litgenprostucel-L

Sponsors: Cell Genesys

Synonym: CG8711, part of *GVAX Prostate*

Antigenic Type: Litgenprostucel-L is 1 of 2 components of a prostate cancer cellular immunotherapy. CG1940 consists of a prostate adenocarcinoma cell line, LNCaP, modified to secrete human granulocyte-macrophage colony-stimulating factor (GM-CSF) and irradiated to prevent cellular replication.

Indications: Investigated for treatment of prostate cancer.

Onamelatucel-L

Sponsors: CancerVax Corporation

Antigenic Type: Specific active immunotherapeutic composed of similar numbers of viable, gamma-irradiated, replication-incompetent whole cells derived from 3 human melanoma cell lines designated M10-VACC, M24-VACC, and M101-VACC.

Indications: Investigated for treatment of cancer, principally melanoma

Viral Vectors of Gene Therapy

Investigational Drugs

One of the most specific means of introducing therapeutic genes into human cells involves recombinant viruses (eg, adenoviruses, retroviruses, vaccinia). These vectors are capable of carrying new genetic material into cells of the virus recipient. Once inside human cells, the recombination of viral and host genetic material permits expression of new proteins the recipient is not otherwise able to synthesize.

Proteins expressed from recombinant genes may be helpful in restoring metabolic balance (eg, replacement of adenosine deaminase), treating cancer (eg, causing a tumor to make itself more immunogenic, causing expression of cytokines like IL-2 within the tumor, creating antisense oligonucleotides), or other diseases such as AIDS (eg, synthesizing genetic decoys directed at reverse transcriptase). It may even be possible to treat HIV-infected people by rearranging and administering recombinant HIV-1 viruses that contain anti-HIV genes.

Immunizing patients with their own tumor cells whose genes have been modified has been called tumor vaccination, although it is actually a form of immunotherapy. If gene coding for common tumor antigens is identified, true primary or secondary prevention of cancer may be possible in the future.

On September 14, 1990, a 4-year-old girl with severe combined immunodeficiency syndrome (SCID), secondary to adenosine deaminase (ADA) deficiency, was the first human treated with gene therapy. Her peripheral-blood T-lymphocytes were removed and treated ex vivo by retrovirally mediated gene transfer of the gene encoding normal human ADA. The experiment succeeded; she experienced fewer infections and a much more normal life.

Other patients are treated by systemic in vivo delivery of the recombinant viruses. An adenovirus vector is being studied with a human cystic fibrosis transmembrane-conductance-regulator gene administered by intratracheal instillation to airway epithelial cells.

Viral vectors work by entering target cells, integrating into the cell, and delivering genetic information to the nucleus. Retroviral vectors have been the most extensively studied. For optimal safety, viral vectors must be rendered incapable of replicating, a state called replication-defective, often by means of several discrete steps. Viral vectors must also be free of contamination with pathogens or toxins. The process of introduction of a virus into a host cell is traditionally referred to as infection, but the introduction of a vector virus that does not spread beyond the target cell is called transduction.

All gene-therapy work to date has involved somatic cells. Recombination of germinal cells will not be explored until further experience is gained, since the implications of recombination errors on the progeny of such gene-therapy recipients has not been fully explored.

References: Goldspiel BR, Green L, Calis KA. Human gene therapy. *Clin Pharm.* 1993;12:488-505.

Kessler DA, Siegel JP, Noguchi PD, Zoon KC, Feiden KL, Woodcock J. Regulation of somatic-cell therapy and gene therapy by the Food and Drug Administration. *N Engl J Med.* 1993;329:1169-1175.

Morsy MA, Mitani K, Clemens P, Caskey CT. Progress toward human gene therapy. *JAMA.* 1993;270:2338-2345.

Rodgers JR, Rich RR. Molecular biology and immunology: an introduction. *J Allergy Clin Immunol.* 1991;88:534-550.

Adenoviruses

Description: Double-stranded DNA viruses, genome of 36 to 38 kilobases

Transport Capacity: Can introduce genes of 7 to 8 kilobases. High titers, 10^{11} to 10^{12} plaque-forming units per mL, are possible.

Targets: Delivery into both dividing and nondividing cells. Specific targets include airway epithelial cells (which reproduce slowly), hepatocytes, neurons, and hematopoietic (eg, lymphoid, myeloid) cells.

Mechanism: DNA functions outside the chromosomes (episomal) rather than by insertion into the genome itself, further reducing any potential for malignant transformation.

Persistence: Transient, short-term expression, since the modified gene is not passed on to progeny of the transduced cell.

Safety: Live oral adenovirus vaccines have been used to vaccinate millions of human adults (eg, military trainees) for more than 15 years without apparent problems.

Herpes Viruses

Description: Double-stranded DNA viruses, genome of 150 kilobases

Transport Capacity: Can introduce genes larger than 10 kilobases.

Targets: Delivery into both dividing and nondividing cells. Innate affinity or tropism for neural cells. Specific targets include lymphoid cells and nondividing cells (eg, differentiated neurons, hepatocytes).

Mechanism: DNA functions outside the chromosomes (episomal) rather than by insertion into the genome itself, further reducing any potential for malignant transformation.

Persistence: Transient, short-term expression, since the modified gene is not passed onto progeny of the transduced cell.

Sponsors: Genetic Therapy, Inc.

Indications: Investigated for treatment of primary and metastatic brain tumors.

Orphan Status: Designated an orphan drug on October 16, 1992.

Parvoviruses

Example: Adeno-associated virus (AAV)

Description: Double-stranded DNA virus, genome of unspecified kilobases

Transport Capacity: Can introduce genes of 4.7 kilobases.

Targets: Specific targets include hematopoietic cells, fibroblasts, epithelial cells, and cells of the CNS.

Mechanism: DNA functions outside the chromosomes rather than by insertion into the genome itself, further reducing any potential for malignant transformation. AAV specifically integrates into the genome at a certain site on chromosome 19. The ability of AAV to enter latency is considered an advantage for this viral type.

Persistence: Transient, short-term expression, since the modified gene is not passed onto progeny of the transduced cell.

Retroviruses

Example: Moloney murine leukemia virus

Description: Single-stranded RNA virus, genome of 10 kilobases

Transport Capacity: Can introduce small genes, from 8 to 9 kilobases. Up to 90% efficient.

Targets: Delivery only into replicating cells. Retroviruses do not integrate into nondividing cells. Specific targets include hematopoietic cells, fibroblasts, endothelial cells, myoblasts, smooth muscle cells, and hepatocytes.

Mechanism: Retroviruses stably integrate a foreign gene into the host genome.

Persistence: Permanent expression of the implanted gene is possible, since the genome is itself changed.

Sponsors: Genetic Therapy, Inc.

Indications: Vector to produce glucocerebrosidase. Investigated for use as enzyme replacement therapy for patients with types I, II, or III Gaucher disease.

Orphan Status: Designated an orphan drug in 1993.

Falimarev

Sponsors: Therion Biologics Corporation

Synonym: Panvac-F

Indications: Investigated in treatment of CEA-bearing or MUC-1-expressing tumors of pancreatic cancer.

Type: Fowlpox virus, CEA, MUC-1. Genome size = 290 ± 50 kilobase pairs

---

Inalimarev

Sponsors: Therion Biologics Corporation

Synonym: Panvac-V

Indications: Investigated in treatment of CEA-bearing tumors or MUC-1-expressing tumors of pancreatic cancer.

Type: Vaccinia virus, CEA, MUC-1. Genome size = 290 ± 50 kilobase pairs

---

Investigational Drugs

To facilitate the treatment of diseases unusual in the United States, the Drug Service of the Centers for Disease Control and Prevention (CDC) makes available to clinicians a variety of special drug products. Some of these drugs have been licensed by the FDA, but use has fallen to the point where they are not commercially profitable (eg, diphtheria antitoxin, botulism antitoxin). Others are considered experimental in the United States, even though they may be available in other countries. Unlicensed drugs may be used in the United States under an Investigational New Drug (IND) exemption to the Food Drug and Cosmetic Act, as amended.

The CDC Drug Service formulary is posted at http://www.cdc.gov/ncidod/srp/drugs/drug-service.html. For current information about availability of special immunologic and other drugs from the CDC Drug Service, call (404) 329-3670; after normal duty hours, call (404) 329-2888. Physicians requesting an investigational drug stocked at CDC must register as coinvestigators and provide the CDC Drug Service with data on product efficacy and adverse reactions.

References: Becher JA, Parvin RM, Van Assendelft OW. Immunobiologics and drugs available from the Centers for Disease Control. *J Pharm Technol.* 1989;5:181-186.

CDC. Management of patients with suspected viral hemorrhagic fever. *MMWR.* 1988;37 (S-3):1-16.

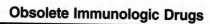
Obsolete Immunologic Drugs

Just as new drug products are continually developed, outmoded and less effective drugs fall into disfavor and obsolescence. Few reference books devote much space to obsolete drug products. But the effects of vaccines and immunologic drugs and questions about vaccine use can persist for years and even decades in some cases.

Questions periodically arise: What is this name entered 20 years ago into my vaccination record? When did I last get a dose of tetanus antigen? What immunizations did I receive as a child? How do measles vaccine policies of the 1960s influence present day disease epidemiology? How far have we come? What have we learned along the way?

This section reviews products previously available in the United States. It will be expanded as additional research reveals additional entries. Availability dates are based on specific citations of licensure or revocation dates, if available, or from citations in historic drug references (such references may not reflect actual availability). Readers are invited to share written or pictorial information about other obsolete immunologic drugs with the editor. Proprietary names of contemporary products that are no longer manufactured have also been included within individual monographs.

References:

Multiple editions of *American Drug Index*, *Modern Drug Encyclopedia*, the American Medical Association's *New and Nonofficial Drugs*, *Pharmacopeia of the United States*, *Physician's Desk Reference*, *Remington's Pharmaceutical Sciences*, and *United States Dispensatory*.

Obsolete Vaccines & Toxoids			
Generic name	Proprietary or product names	Manufacturer	Estimated availability
Acne Vaccine	*Acne mixed UBA* (Undenatured Bacterial Antigen)	Eli Lilly	1910s-1960s
	Acne Serobacterin	Sharp & Dohme	
	Acolac	US Standard	
	Furunculosis Bacterin	Abbott	
	Furunculosis Vaccine	Parke-Davis-Sherman	
	Staphylo-Acne Bacterin	Abbott	
	Staphylo-Acne Vaccine	Squibb	
Adenovirus Vaccine Inactivated	Generic	Parke-Davis	1957-1965
Adenovirus & Influenza Vaccine Inactivated	*Resprogen*	Parke-Davis	1959-1966
Arthritis Vaccine	Crowe Vaccine	Sherman	1938-1952
	Rheumatoid Arthritis Vaccine	Lederle	
	Rheumatism Phylacogen	Parke-Davis	
	Sherwood's Formula Arthritis Vaccine	Cutter	
Autogenous Vaccines	Individually prepared for each patient		1900-1968

Obsolete Immunologic Drugs

	Obsolete Vaccines & Toxoids		
Generic name	Proprietary or product names	Manufacturer	Estimated availability
Bacillus influenzae Vaccine (Pfeiffer's bacillus)	generic	various	1918, 1920s
Brucella Vaccine	*Brucellin*	Merck Sharp & Dohme	1938-1952
Cholera Vaccine (whole-cell)	generic	various	1900s-2001
	generic	Wyeth Laboratories	1941-2001
Diphtheria Toxin-Antitoxin Mixture	generic	various	1925-1945
Diphtheria-Pertussis Toxoid-Vaccine, USP XIV	*Diptussis*	Cutter	1949-1955
	Perdipigen	Eli Lilly	
Diphtheria-Tetanus-Pertussis-Polio	*Tetravax*	Merck Sharp & Dohme	1959-1965
Diphtheria-Tetanus-Pertussis-Poliovirus Toxoid-Vaccine, USP XVI	*Tetra-Solgen*	Eli Lilly	1959-1968
	Quadrigen	Parke-Davis	
Diphtheria-Tetanus-Poliovirus Toxoid-Vaccine	*Trinfagen No. 1*	Pitman-Moore	early 1960s
Escherichia coli Vaccines	generic	various	1900s-1950s
Gonococcal Vaccines	*Gonorrhea Phylacogen*	Parke-Davis	1934-1952
	Gono-Yatren	Winthrop	
	Neisser Serobacterin	Mulford	
	Neiso-Lysate	Eli Lilly	
Haemophilus influenzae (Influenza bacillus) Vaccine	generic	various	1910s to 1960s
Haemophilus influenzae type b Polysaccharide Vaccine	*b-CAPSA-I*	Praxis/Mead-Johnson	1985-1989
	HIB-Vax	Connaught	
	HIB-Immune	Lederle	
Haemophilus influenzae type b Polysaccharide Protein Conjugate Vaccine	*ProHIBit*	Connaught, Aventis Pasteur	1987-2000
Hepatitis B Vaccine (Plasma-Derived), USP XXII	*Heptavax-B*	Merck Sharp & Dohme	1981-1990
Japanese Encephalitis Vaccine (Mouse Brain Derived)	*JE-Vax*	Sanofi Pasteur	1992-2011
Klebsiella pneumoniae Vaccine	Friedlander vaccine	various	1910s-1950s
Lyme Disease Vaccine	*Lymerix*	GlaxoSmithKline	1998-2002
Measles Vaccine Inactivated, Adsorbed	*Pfizer-Vax Measles-K*	Pfizer	1963-1968
Measles-Mumps Attenuated Vaccine, USP XXII	*M-M-Vax*	Merck Sharp & Dohme	1973
Measles-Smallpox Vaccine	*Attenuvax-Smallpox*	Merck Sharp & Dohme	1967
Meningococcal Vaccine (whole cell)	generic	various	1910s-1950s
Mumps Vaccine Inactivated, USP XX	generic	various	1951-1975

Obsolete Vaccines & Toxoids			
Generic name	Proprietary or product names	Manufacturer	Estimated availability
Pertussis Vaccine	generic	various	1910s-1950s
Pertussis Vaccine- Antitoxin Mixture	generic	various	late 1940s
Pertussis-Tetanus Toxoid Vaccine	generic	various	early 1950s
Plague Vaccine	generic	Cutter Laboratories and Miles Pharmaceutical Division	1942-1999
		Greer Laboratories	1994-1999
		various	1900s-1930s
Pneumococcus Vaccine (whole cell)	generic	various	1900s-1940s
Pneumococcal 14-valent Polysaccharide Vaccine	*Pneumovax*	Merck	1977-1983
	Pnu-Imune	Lederle	
Pneumococcal 23-valent Polysaccharide Vaccine	*Pnu-Imune 23*	Wyeth Lederle	
Poliovirus Vaccine Inactivated, original potency	*Purivax* and generic	various	1983-2002
			1954-1989
Poliovirus Vaccine Inactivated, enhanced-potency, MRC-5 human diploid-cell	*Poliovax*	Connaught	1988-1991
Poliovirus Vaccine Live Oral Trivalent	*Orimune*	Wyeth-Lederle Vaccines	1961-2000
Pseudomonas Vaccine	*Pseudogen*	Parke-Davis	1970s (never licensed)
Rabies Vaccine (Nerve Tissue), USP XIX	*Rabies Iradogen*	Parke-Davis	1908-1957
Rabies Vaccine (Duck Embryo), USP XX Minimum dose: 0.5 mL NTV or 1 mL DEV daily for 14 days. After severe exposure, 21 doses, either as 21 daily doses or as 14 doses on the first 7 days (either 2 separate injections or a double dose), followed by 7 daily doses.	generic	Eli Lilly	1957-1981
Rabies Vaccine (Split Virion, WI-38 Human-Diploid Cell), USP XXI	*Wyvac*	Wyeth	1982-1985
Rocky Mountain Spotted Fever Vaccine, USP XXI	generic	various	1942-1975
Rotavirus Vaccine Live Oral Tetravalent	*RotaShield*	Wyeth-Lederle Vaccines	1998-1999
Rubella Vaccine Attenuated	*Rubelogen*	Parke-Davis	1969-1979
	Lirubel	Dow	
	Meruvax	Merck Sharp & Dohme	
	Cendevax	RIT-SKF	

Obsolete Immunologic Drugs

Obsolete Vaccines & Toxoids			
Generic name	Proprietary or product names	Manufacturer	Estimated availability
Shiga (Dysentery) Vaccine	generic	Parke-Davis	1941-1949
		various	1920s-1950s
Staphylococcus Toxoid	generic	various	1933-1980
Staphylococcus Toxoid-Vaccine Mixture	*Vatox Staphylococcus Toxoid Vaccine*	National Drug Company	1941-1952
	Ambotoxoid	Squibb	
Staphylococcus Vaccine	*Staphylo-Serobacterin*	Mulford	1925-1952
	generic	various	1900s-1930s
Streptococcus (Scarlet Fever) Toxin, USP XIII	generic	various	1924-1950s
Streptococcal Vaccine	*Strepto-Serobacterin*	Mulford	1925-1952
	Ulcerative colitis streptococcus vaccine	Parke-Davis	
Streptococcal (Erysipelas) Vaccine	*Erysipelas Bacterin*	Abbott	1934-1952
	Erysipelas Phylacogen	Parke-Davis	
	Erysipelas Streptococcus Immunogen	Parke-Davis	
Streptococcal Toxin with Staphylococcal Vaccine	*Strepto-Staphylo Vatox*	National Drug Company	1941-1952
Tularemia Vaccine	generic	various	1940s to 1950s
Typhoid H Antigen	generic	Eli Lilly	1949-1952
Typhoid-Paratyphoid A&B Vaccine, USP XVII	*Typho-Bacterin Mixed*	Mulford	1925-1969
Typhoid-Paratyphoid A&B Tetanus Vaccine	generic	Parke-Davis	1940s
Typhoid Vaccine (Whole Cell)	generic	various	1900s-1940s
Typhus Vaccine, USP XXI	generic	various	1941-1981

Influenza Vaccine Strains Distributed in the US Since 1943, with Antigen Quantity per Dose

*Formulas composed of 15 mcg hemagglutinin antigen per influenza type per 0.5 mL dose.

Note that historical references to H0N0, H1N1, H1swN1, and A' influenza viruses would be considered H1N1 viruses by current terminology.

2012-2013 Trivalent: A/California/7/2009-like (H1N1), A/Victoria/361/2011 (H3N2), and B/Wisconsin/1/2010.

2011-2012 Trivalent: A/California/7/2009-like (H1N1), A/Perth/16/2009-like (H3N2), and B/Brisbane/60/2008-like.

2010-2011 Trivalent: A/California/7/2009 (H1N1), A/Perth/16/2009-like (H3N2), and B/Brisbane/60/2008.*

2009-2010 Monovalent: A/California/7/2009 (H1N1) ("swine origin").

2009-2010 Trivalent: A/Brisbane/59/2007 (H1N1), A/Brisbane/10/2007–like (eg, A/Uruguay/716/2007) (H3N2), and B/Brisbane/60/2008.*

2008-2009 Trivalent: A/Brisbane/59/2007 (H1N1), A/Brisbane/10/2007-like strain (eg, A/Uruguay/716/2007) (H3N2), and B/Florida/04/2006.*

2007-2008 Trivalent: A/Solomon Islands/3/2006-like (H1N1), A Wisconsin/67/2005-like (H3N2), and B/Malaysia/2506/2004-like (eg, B/Ohio/1/2005).*

2006-2007 Trivalent: A/New Caledonia/20/99-like (H1N1, eg, A/Hiroshima/52/2005), A/Wisconsin/67/2005-like (H3N2), and B/Malaysia/2506/2004-like (eg, B/Ohio/1/2005).*

2005-2006 Trivalent: A/New Caledonia/20/99-like (H1N1), A/California/7/2004-like (H3N2, eg, A/New York/55/2004), and B/Shanghai/361/2002-like (eg, B/Jilin/20/2003).*

2004-2005 Trivalent: A/New Caledonia/20/99 (H1N1), A/Fujian/411/2002-like (H3N2, eg, A/Wyoming/3/2003, A/Kumamoto/102/2002), B/Shanghai/361/2002-like (eg, B/Jilin/20/2003).*

2002-2004 Trivalent: A/New Caledonia/20/99 (H1N1), A/Panama/2007/99 (H3N2) (A/Moscow/10/99-like), B/Hong Kong/1434/2002 (B/Hong Kong/330/2001-like).*

2001-2002 Trivalent: A/New Caledonia/20/99-like (H1N1), A/Panama/2007/99 (H3N2) (A/Moscow/10/99-like), B/Victoria/504/2000 or B/Guangdong/120/2000 (B/Sichuan/379/99-like).*

2000-2001 Trivalent: A/New Caledonia/20/99 (H1N1), A/Panama/2007/99 (H3N2) (A/Moscow/10/99-like), B/Yamanashi/16/98.*

1999-2000 Trivalent: A/Beijing/262/95 (H1N1), A/Sydney/5/97 (H3N2), B/Yamanashi/16/98.*

1998-1999 Trivalent: A/Beijing/262/95 (H1N1), A/Sydney/5/97 (H3N2), B/Harbin/07/94.*

1997-1998 Trivalent: A/Johannesburg/82/96 (H1N1) (A/Bayern/7/95-like), A/Nanchang/933/95 (H3N2) (A/Wuhan/359/95-like), B/Harbin/07/94.*

1996-1997 Trivalent: A/Texas/36/91 (H1N1), A/Nanchang/933/95 (H3N2), (A/Wuhan/359/95-like), B/Harbin/07/94.*

1995-1996 Trivalent: A/Texas/36/91 (H1N1), A/Johannesburg/33/94, B/Harbin/07/94.*

1994-1995 Trivalent: A/Texas/36/91 (H1N1), A/Shangdong/9/93 (H3N2), B/Panama/45/90.*

1993-1994 Trivalent: A/Texas/36/91 (H1N1), A/Beijing/32/92 (H3N2), B/Panama/45/90.*

1991-1993 Trivalent: A/Texas/36/91 (H1N1), A/Beijing/353/89 (H3N2), B/Panama/45/90.*

1989-1991 Trivalent: A/Taiwan/1/86 (H1N1) (A/Singapore/6/86-like), A/Shanghai/16/89 (H3N2) (A/Shanghai/11/87-like and A/Guizhou/54/89-like), B/Yamagata/16/88.*

1988-1989 Trivalent: A/Taiwan/1/86 (H1N1) (A/Singapore/6/86-like), A/Sichuan/2/87 (H3N2), B/Victoria/2/87.*

1987-1988 Trivalent: A/Taiwan/1/86 (H1N1) (A/Singapore/6/86-like), A/Leningrad/360/86 (H3N2), B/Ann Arbor/1/86.*

1986-1987 Trivalent: A/Chile/1/83 (H1N1), A/Mississippi/1/85 (H3N2) (A/Christchurch/4/85-like), B/Ann Arbor/1/86.*

1986-1987 Supplemental monovalent formulation: A/Taiwan/1/86 (H1N1) 15 mcg/0.5 mL.*

1984-1986 Trivalent: A/Chile/1/83 (H1N1), A/Philippines/2/82 (H3N2), B/USSR/100/83.*

1983-1984 Trivalent: A/Brazil/11/78 (H1N1), A/Philippines/2/82 (H3N2), B/Singapore/222/79.*

1981-1983 Trivalent: A/Brazil/11/78 (H1N1), A/Bangkok/1/79 (H3N2), B/Singapore/222/79.*

1980-1981 Trivalent: A/Brazil/11/78 (H1N1), A/Bangkok/1/79 (H3N2), B/Singapore/222/79. Contained 7 mcg of each hemagglutinin antigen.

1979-1980 Trivalent: A/Brazil/11/78 (H1N1), A/Texas/1/77 (H3N2), B/Hong Kong/5/72. Contained 7 mcg of each hemagglutinin antigen.

1978-1979 Trivalent: A/USSR/90/77 (H1N1), A/Texas/1/77 (H3N2), B/Hong Kong/5/72. Youth (younger than 26 years of age): 20 mcg, 7 mcg, 7 mcg. Adult (26 years of age and older): 7 mcg of each type. First formula standardized by hemagglutinin antigen content.

1977-1978 Bivalent: A/Victoria/3/75 (H3N2), B/Hong Kong/5/72. Last annual formula to be standardized in chick-cell agglutination u, 200 of each type per 0.5 mL.

1976-1977 Bivalent: A/Victoria/3/75 (H3N2), 200 CCA u, A/Swine/New Jersey/8/76 (H1N1) 200 CCA u. The original recommendation, before H1N1 virus detected, was for 700 CCA of A/Victoria/3/75 (H3N2) and 500 CCA of B/Hong Kong/5/72.

1976-1977 Monovalent: A/Swine/New Jersey/8/76 (H1N1) 200 CCA u.

1976-1977 Monovalent: B/Hong Kong/5/72 500 CCA u.

1975-1976 Trivalent: A/Port Chalmers/1/73 (H3N2) 350 CCA u, A/Scotland/840/74 (H3N2) 350 CCA u, B/Hong Kong/5/72 500 CCA u.

1974-1975 Bivalent: A/Port Chalmers/1/73 (H3N2) 700 CCA u, B/Hong Kong/5/72 500 CCA u.

1973-1974 Monovalent: B/Hong Kong/5/72 500 CCA u.

1973-1974 Bivalent: A/England/42/72 (H3N2) 700 CCA u, B/Massachusetts/1/71 300 CCA u.

1972-1973 Bivalent: A2/Aichi/2/68/X-31 (A/Hong Kong/1/68-like) (H3N2) 700 CCA u, B/Massachusetts/1/71 300 CCA u.

1970-1972 Bivalent: A2/Aichi/2/68/X-31 (A/Hong Kong/1/68-like) (H3N2) 600 CCA u, B/Massachusetts/3/66 400 CCA u.

1969-1972 Bivalent: A2/Aichi/2/68/X-31 (A/Hong Kong/1/68-like) (H3N2) 400 CCA u, B/Massachusetts/3/66 300 CCA u.

1969-1970 Trivalent: A2/Ann Arbor/7/67 (H2N2) 200 CCA u, A2/Aichi/2/68/X-31 (A/Hong Kong/1/68-like) (H3N2) 400 CCA u, B/Massachusetts/3/66 400 CCA u.

1968-1969 Supplemental monovalent formulation: A2/Aichi/2/68/X-31 ("Hong Kong variant," A/Hong Kong/1/68-like) (H3N2) 400 CCA u.

1968-1969 Hexavalent: A/Puerto Rico/8/34 (H1N1) 100 CCA u, A1/Ann Arbor/1/57 (H1N1) 100 CCA u, A/Ann Arbor/7/67 (H2N2) 400 CCA u, A'/Swine/Iowa/1976/31 (H1N1) 100 CCA u, B/Massachusetts/3/66 200 CCA u, B/Lee/40 100 CCA u.

1967-1969 Pentavalent: A/Puerto Rico/8/34 (H1N1) 100 CCA u, A1/Ann Arbor/1/57 (H1N1) 100 CCA u, A2/Taiwan/1/64 (H2N2) 100 CCA u, A2/Japan/170/62 (H2N2) 100 CCA u, B/Massachusetts/3/66 200 CCA u.

1967-1969 Trivalent: A2/Taiwan/1/64 (H2N2) 150 CCA u, A2/Japan/170/62 (H2N2) 150 CCA u, B/Massachusetts/3/66 300 CCA u.

1966-1968 Hexavalent: A/Puerto Rico/8/34 (H1N1) 100 CCA u, A1/Ann Arbor/1/57 (H1N1) 100 CCA u, A2/Taiwan/1/64 (H2N2) 400 CCA u, A'/Swine/Iowa/1976/31 (H1N1) 100 CCA u, B/Maryland/1/59 200 CCA u, B/Lee/40 100 CCA u.

1965-1967 Pentavalent: A/Puerto Rico/8/34 (H1N1) 100 CCA u, A1/Ann Arbor/1/57 (H1N1) 100 CCA u, A2/Taiwan/1/64 (H2N2) 100 CCA u, A2/Japan/170/62 (H2N2) 100 CCA u, B/Maryland/1/59 200 CCA u.

1964-1965 Quadrivalent: A/Puerto Rico/8/34 (H1N1) 100 CCA u, A1/Ann Arbor/1/57 (H1N1) 100 CCA u, A2/Japan/170/62 (H2N2) 200 CCA u, B/Maryland/1/59 200 CCA u.

1963-1966 Hexavalent: A/Puerto Rico/8/34 (H1N1) 100 CCA u, A1/Ann Arbor/1/57 (H1N1) 100 CCA u, A2/Japan/170/62 (H2N2) 400 CCA u, A'/Swine/Iowa/1976/31 (H1N1) 100 CCA u, B/Maryland/1/59 200 CCA u, B/Great Lakes/1739/54 100 CCA u.

1963-1964 Hexavalent: A/Puerto Rico/8/34 (H1N1) 100 CCA u, A1/Ann Arbor/1/57 (H1N1) 100 CCA u, A2/Japan/170/62 (H2N2) 100 CCA u, A2/Japan/305/57 (H2N2) 100 CCA u, B/Maryland/1/59 100 CCA u, B/Great Lakes/1739/54 100 CCA u.

1960-1963 Quadrivalent: A/Puerto Rico/8/34 (H1N1) 100 CCA u, A1/Ann Arbor/1/57 (H1N1) 100 CCA u, A2/Japan/305/57 (H2N2, "Asian" or "Far East") 100 CCA u, A'/Swine/Iowa/1976/31 (H1N1) 100 CCA u. Dose: 1 mL for adults, 0.5 mL for children 6 to 12 years of age, and 0.1 to 0.2 mL for children 3 months to 5 years.

1959-1963 Hexavalent: A/Puerto Rico/8/34 (H1N1) 100 CCA u, A1/Ann Arbor/1/57 (H1N1) 100 CCA u, A2/Japan/305/57 (H2N2, "Asian" or "Far East") 400 CCA u, A'/Swine/Iowa/1976/31 (H1N1) 100 CCA u, B/Great Lakes/1739/54 200 CCA u, B/Lee/40 100 CCA u.

1959-1963 Quadrivalent: A/Puerto Rico/8/34 (H1N1) 100 CCA u, A1/Ann Arbor/1/57 (H1N1) 100 CCA u, A2/Japan/305/57 (H2N2, "Asian" or "Far East") 200 CCA u, B/Great Lakes/1739/54 100 CCA u.

1957-1959 Pentavalent: A/Puerto Rico/8/34 (H1N1) 200 CCA u, A2/Japan/305/57 (H2N2, "Asian" or "Far East") 200 CCA u, A'/Swine/Iowa/1976/31 (H1N1) 200 CCA u, B/Great Lakes/1739/54 200 CCA u.

1957-1959 Pentavalent: A/Puerto Rico/8/34 (H1N1) 75 CCA u, A/Puerto Rico/301/54 (H1N1) 75 CCA u, A2/Japan/305/57 (H2N2, "Asian" or "Far East") 200 CCA u, A'/Swine/Iowa/1976/31 (H1N1) 75 CCA u, B/Great Lakes/1739/54 75 CCA u.

1957-1959 Quadrivalent: A/Puerto Rico/8/34 (H1N1) 100 CCA u, A/Puerto Rico/301/54 (H1N1) 100 CCA u, A2/Japan/305/57 (H2N2, "Asian" or "Far East") 200 CCA u, B/Great Lakes/1739/54 100 CCA u.

1957-1958 Quadrivalent: A/Puerto Rico/8/34 (H1N1) 200 CCA u, A/Puerto Rico/301/54 (H1N1) 200 CCA u, A'/Swine/Iowa/1976/31 (H1N1) 200 CCA u, B/Great Lakes/1739/54 200 CCA u.

1957-1958 Monovalent: A2/Japan/305/57 (H2N2, "Asian" or "Far East") either 200 or 400 CCA u.

1956-1957 Pentavalent: A/Puerto Rico/8/34 (H1N1) 75 CCA u, A/Puerto Rico/301/54 (H1N1) 75 CCA u, A2/Japan/305/57 (H2N2, "Asian" or "Far East") 200 CCA u, A'/Swine/Iowa/1976/31 (H1N1) 75 CCA u, B/Great Lakes/1739/54 75 CCA u.

1956-1957 Pentavalent: A/Puerto Rico/8/34 (H1N1) 22%, A/Puerto Rico/301/54 (H1N1) 22%, A'/Swine/Iowa/1976/31 (H1N1) 22%, B/Great Lakes/1739/54 17%, B/Lee/40 17%.

1956-1957 Pentavalent: A/Puerto Rico/8/34 (H1N1) 500 CCA u, A/Puerto Rico/301/54 (H1N1) 500 CCA u, A'/Swine/Iowa/1976/31 (H1N1) 500 CCA u, B/Great Lakes/1739/54 500 CCA u, B/Lee/40 500 CCA u.

1955-1957 Trivalent: A1/FM/1/47 (H1N1) 750 CCA u, A'/Swine/Iowa/1976/31 (H1N1) 750 CCA u, B/Great Lakes/1739/54 750 CCA u.

1954-1955 Quadrivalent: A/Puerto Rico/8/34 (H1N1) 22%, A1/FM/1/47 (H1N1) 22%, A1/Conley/50 (H1N1) 22%, B/Lee/40 33%.

1954-1955 Quadrivalent: A/Puerto Rico/8/34 (H1N1) 500 CCA u, A1/FM/1/47 (H1N1) 500 CCA u, A1/Conley/50 (H1N1) 500 CCA u, B/Lee/40 500 CCA u.

1953-1955 Trivalent: A1/FM/1/47 (H1N1) 750 CCA u, A1/Conley/50 (H1N1) 750 CCA u, B/Lee/40 750 CCA u.

1951-1954 Quadrivalent: A/Puerto Rico/8/34 (H1N1) 22%, A1/FM/1/47 (H1N1) 22%, A1/Cuppett/50 (H1N1) 22%, B/Lee/40 33%.

1950-1951 Quadrivalent: A/Puerto Rico/8/34 (H1N1) 500 CCA u, A1/FM/1/47 (H1N1) 500 CCA u, A1/Cuppett/50 (H1N1) 500 CCA u, B/Lee/40 500 CCA u.

1948-1951 Trivalent: A/Puerto Rico/8/34 (H1N1) 25%, A1/FM/1/47 (H1N1) 25%, B/Lee/40 50%.

1947-1948 Quadrivalent: A/Puerto Rico/8/34 (H1N1) 12.5%, A/Weiss/43 (H1N1) 25%, A1/FM/1/47 (H1N1) 25%, B/Lee/40 50%.

1946-1950 Trivalent: A/Puerto Rico/8/34 (H1N1) 450 CCA u, A1/FM/1/47 (H1N1) 300 CCA u, B/Lee/40 300 CCA u.

1944-1946 Trivalent: A/Puerto Rico/8/34 (H1N1) 450 CCA u, A/Weiss/43 (H1N1) 300 CCA u, B/Lee/40 300 CCA u.

1943-1946 Trivalent: A/Puerto Rico/8/34 (H1N1) 25%, A/Weiss/43 (H1N1) 25%, B/Lee/40 50%.

Sources: FDA archives.

Physician's Desk Reference, serial editions.

Top F. Influenza—General discussion. I. *J Infect Dis.* 1977;136(Supplement):S555-S562.

World Health Organization. *WHO Report on Global Surveillance of Epidemic prone Infectious Diseases* (WHO/CDS/CSR/ISR/2000.1). Geneva:WHO, 2000.

Obsolete Polyvalent Bacterial Vaccines, Various

Various combinations of killed whole or extracted bacteria, used for prophylaxis or treatment of bacterial infections caused by organisms represented in the formulation. Common uses included infections of the respiratory tract or sinuses. First licensed in the US in 1914. Eventually withdrawn because of questionable efficacy and limited spectrum. Most licenses were revoked in the late 1970s.

Representative Parenteral & Oral Products

Bacterial Antigen Complexes (BAC, Polyvalent Acellular): Respiratory BAC; Gram-Negative BAC, Pooled Stock BAC #1; Pooled Stock BAC #2; Staphylococcal BAC, Pooled Skin BAC, Hoffman Laboratories, containing antigens from various species of *Streptococcus, Diplococcus, Staphylococcus, Neisseria, Haemophilus, Klebsiella, Proteus, Pseudomonas, Escherichia,* and *Aerobacter.*

Bacterial Intravenous Protein (BIP), Cutter Laboratories, containing streptococci, staphylococci, pneumococci, *Neisseria catarrhalis, Bacillus friedlanderiae,* and *Bacillus influenzae.*

Catarrhalis Serobacterin Vaccine Mixed, Sharpe & Dohme, containing *Neisseria catarrhalis, Diplococcus pneumoniae, Klebsiella pneumoniae, Staphylococcus aureus, Staphylococcus albus,* and various streptococci.

Catarrhalis Vaccine Combined, No. 4, Eli Lilly, containing *Neisseria catarrhalis, Klebsiella pneumoniae, Staphylococcus aureus, Staphylococcus albus,* and various pneumococci and streptococci.

Entoral oral capsules, Eli Lilly, containing *Diplococcus pneumoniae, Haemophilus influenzae* type b, *Neisseria catarrhalis,* and various streptococci.

Haemophilus influenzae Mixed Vaccine, No. 4, Eli Lilly, containing *Haemophilus influenzae, Neisseria catarrhalis, Klebsiella pneumoniae, Staphylococcus aureus, Staphylococcus albus,* and various pneumococci and streptococci.

Haemophilus influenzae Serobacterin Vaccine Mixed, Sharp & Dohme, containing *Haemophilus influenzae, Klebsiella pneumoniae, Staphylococcus albus, Staphylococcus aureus, Diplococcus pneumoniae, Neisseria catarrhalis,* and various streptococci.

Immunovac (parenteral injection and enteric coated oral tablets), Parke-Davis, containing *Bacillus friedlanderiae, Diplococcus pneumoniae, Neisseria catarrhalis,* hemolytic and nonhemolytic streptococci (including viridans), *Staphylococcus aureus, Staphylococcus albus, Pseudodiphtheria bacillus* and *Haemophilus influenzae.*

Inflolac, US Standard, containing *Haemophilus influenzae, Streptococcus hemolyticus, Streptococcus viridans, Neisseria catarrhalis*, and type I, II, and III pneumococci.

Influenza-Pneumonia Vaccine, Parke-Davis, containing *Haemophilus influenzae, Staphylococcus aureus*, hemolytic and nonhemolytic streptococci, and pneumococci types I, II, III, V, VII, VIII, and XIV.

Influenza-Pneumonia Vaccine, Pitman-Moore, containing *Haemophilus influenzae, Klebsiella pneumoniae, Neisseria catarrhalis, Staphylococcus aureus, Streptococcus viridans*, hemolytic and nonhemolytic streptococci, and pneumococci types I, II, III, IV, VII, VIII, and XIV.

Mixed Infection Phylacogen, Parke-Davis, containing *Escherichia coli, Diplococcus pneumoniae, Staphylococcus albus, Staphylococcus aureus*, and various streptococci.

Mixed Respiratory Vaccine (MRV), Hollister-Stier Laboratories (later Miles Pharmaceutical Division), containing antigens from various species of *Staphylococcus, Streptococcus, Moraxella catarrhalis, Klebsiella pneumoniae*, and *Haemophilus influenzae*.

MVRI No. 4. (Mixed Vaccine Respiratory Infections), Cutter Laboratories, containing staphylococci, pathogenic streptococci, pneumococci, *Streptococcus pyogenes, Klebsiella pneumoniae, Haemophilus influenzae*, and *Neisseria catarrhalis*.

Neovacagen, Sharp & Dohme, a combination of the antihistamine methapyrilene and bacterial antigens.

Omnadin, Winthrop-Stearns, containing protein obtained from nonpathogenic bacteria, various animal fats, and lipoids derived from bile.

Piromen, Travenol Laboratories, containing *Pseudomonas* polysaccharides and nucleic acids.

Pneumo-Strep-Bacterin, Mulford, containing pneumococci types, I, II, and III, *Streptococcus hemolyticus*, nonhemolyticus, and *Streptococcus viridans*.

Pyorrhea Serobacterin, Mulford, containing various species of pneumococci, staphylococci and streptococci, plus *Bacillus diphtheroid, Haemophilus influenzae*, and *Neisseria catarrhalis*.

Respiratory UBA (Undenatured Bacterial Antigen), Eli Lilly, containing various species of pneumococci, staphylococci, streptococci, plus *Haemophilus influenzae*, and *Neisseria catarrhalis*.

Urethritis Vaccine, Abbott, Lederle, Parke-Davis, containing various species of gonococci, pneumococci, staphylococci, streptococci, plus *Bacillus pseudodiphtheriae, Escherichia coli*, and *Neisseria catarrhalis*.

Vacagen, Sharp & Dohme, containing *Haemophilus influenzae, Klebsiella pneumoniae, Neisseria catarrhalis, Staphylococcus aureus, Streptococcus pneumoniae*, and various other streptococci.

Other products included bronchitis vaccine (Sherman), *Colac* (US Standard), *Catolac* (US Standard), *Friedländer Vaccine* (Sherman), influenza vaccine (sic, various), pertussis mixed vaccine (various), *Shervac* (Sherman), *Stapholac* (US Standard), *Streptolac* (US Standard), ulcerative colitis streptococcus vaccine (Parke-Davis), and Van Cott vaccines (various).

Representative Topical Products

Some mixed bacterial preparations were compounded to treat bacterial skin eruptions, including:

Antipeol bacterial antigen ointment and liquid (Bio-Therapeutic, 1947), topical doseforms containing various staphylococci, streptococci, and *Bacillus pyocyaneus*, in a vehicle containing zinc oxide, lanolin, and other ingredients.

Bio-Cream (Sherman, 1949), a topical product containing various pneumococci, staphylococci, streptococci, and *Escherichia coli* in a greaseless base.

Colo-Jel, Eli Lilly, containing bacteriophage-lysed *Escherichia coli*, pneumococci, staphylococci, and streptococci in a water-soluble jelly base.

Ento-Jel, Eli Lilly, containing bacteriophage-lysed *Neisseria catarrhalis*, pneumococci, staphylococci and streptococci in a water-soluble jelly base.

Staphylo-Jel, Eli Lilly, containing bacteriophage-lysed staphylococci and streptococci in a water-soluble jelly base.

Strepto-Jel, Eli Lilly, containing bacteriophage-lysed staphylococci and streptococci in a water-soluble jelly base.

Representative Bacteriophage Products

Bacteriophages are viruses that cause transmissible lysis of bacteria. They were commonly used alone or in combination with killed bacteria for a variety of uses.

A-Vee 11 Preparation, Sherman, containing various strains of staphylococci and corresponding bacteriophages in liquid form.

A-Vee 12 Preparation, Sherman, containing various strains of pyogenic organisms and corresponding bacteriophages in liquid form.

A-Vee 51 Preparation, Sherman, containing various strains of staphylococci and corresponding bacteriophages in a face cream.

A-Vee 52 Preparation, Sherman, containing various strains of pyogenic organisms and corresponding bacteriophages in cream form.

Bacteriophage-Staphylococcus, Abbott, containing various strains of staphylococci and corresponding bacteriophages.

Bacteriophage-Staphylococcus-Coli, Abbott, containing various strains of staphylococci and coliform bacilli and corresponding bacteriophages.

Bacte-Coli-Phage, Anglo-French, containing *Bacillus coli* and *paracoli* and corresponding bacteriophages.

Bacte-Dysenteri-Phage, Anglo-French, containing *Bacilli dysentery* and *Bacilli paradysentery* and corresponding bacteriophages.

Bacte-Intesti-Phage, Anglo-French, containing various strains of enterococci, staphylococci, streptococci, *Bacilli dysentery*, *Bacilli paradysentery*, *Bacillus proteus*, *Bacillus pyocyaneous*, *Bacillus coli*, and corresponding bacteriophages.

Bacte-Pyo-Phage Polyvalent, Anglo-French, containing various strains of enterococci, pneumococci, staphylococci, streptococci, *Bacillus proteus*, *Bacillus pyocyaneous*, *Bacillus coli*, and corresponding bacteriophages.

Bacte-Rhino-Phage, Anglo-French, containing various strains of pneumococci, staphylococci, streptococci, *Bacillus proteus*, *Bacillus pyocyaneous*, *Bacillus paracoli*, and corresponding bacteriophages.

Bacte-Staphy-Phage, Anglo-French, containing various strains of staphylococci and corresponding bacteriophages.

Colo-Lysate, Eli Lilly, containing various strains of pneumococci, staphylococci, streptococci, and corresponding bacteriophages.

Ento-Lysate Bacteriophage-Lysed Respiratory Antigen, Eli Lilly, containing bacteriophage-lysed *Neisseria catarrhalis*, pneumococci, staphylococci, and streptococci.

Staphylo-Lysate, Eli Lilly, containing various strains of staphylococci, streptococci, and corresponding bacteriophages.

Strepto-Lysate, Eli Lilly, containing various strains of staphylococci, streptococci, and corresponding bacteriophages.

Obsolete Immune Plasmas

Until the early 1980s, CDC periodically harvested immune plasma from patients convalescing from unusual diseases, mostly of viral origin. This practice has largely ceased, given the concern over transmission of blood-borne pathogens such as HIV and hepatitis C. Recent advances in antiviral therapy have also provided therapeutic options other than infusion of exogenous immune plasma. The following list reviews products previously harvested by CDC. In an isolated case of one of these diseases, contact the CDC Drug Service regarding availability of residual supplies of the immunologic product or alternative therapies.

> African Hemorrhagic Fever Immune Plasma against Ebola or Marburg viruses
> California Encephalitis Immune Plasma
> Herpes Simian B Immune Plasma
> Junin (Argentinean Hemorrhagic Fever) Immune Plasma
> Lassa Fever Immune Plasma
> Machupo (Bolivian Hemorrhagic Fever, Green Monkey Disease) Immune Plasma
> Russian Spring-Summer Encephalitis (RSSE) Immune Plasma
> Saint Louis Encephalitis Immune Plasma
> Venezuelan Equine Encephalitis Immune Plasma
> Western Equine Encephalitis Immune Plasma

Other obsolete immune globulins that were more broadly distributed appear in the following table.

Obsolete Immune Globulins

Generic name	Proprietary or product names	Manufacturer	Estimated availability
Anthrax Antiserum	generic	various	1910s-1951
Antivenin Crotalidae Polyvalent (Equine)	generic	Wyeth	1950s-2002
Arcitumomab	CEA-Scan	Immunomedics	1996-2000s
Brucella Antiserum	generic	Mulford	1910s-1950s
Dysentery Antiserum	Anti-dysenteric antiserum (Shiga bacillus)	Mulford	1900s-1940s
Fanolesomab	NeutroSpec	Palatin, Mallinckrodt	2004-2005
Gas Gangrene Antitoxin (Equine), USP XIII	generic	various	1917-1976
Gas Gangrene & Tetanus Antitoxin (Equine), USP XIV	generic	various	1940-1965
Gemtuzumab Ozogamicin	Mylotarg	Wyeth (later Pfizer)	2000-2010
Gonococcal Antiserum	generic	Parke-Davis	1924-1941
Haemophilus influenzae type b Antiserum (Rabbit)	generic	various	1941-1970s
Imciromab Pentetate	Myoscint	Centocor	1996-2000
Immune Globulin IV (Human)	Gammagee-V	Merck Sharp & Dohme	1969
Measles Immune Globulin (Human), USP XIX	generic	Parke-Davis	1963-1977
Measles Immune Serum (Human), USP XII	generic	Cutter	1945-1965
Meningococcal Antiserum (Equine), USP XII	generic	various	1925-1952

Obsolete Immunologic Drugs

Obsolete Immune Globulins			
Generic name	Proprietary or product names	Manufacturer	Estimated availability
Mumps Immune Globulin	*Hyparotin*	Cutter	1945-1980
Mumps Immune Serum	*Hyparotin*	Cutter	1940s-1965
Nofetumomab	*Verluma*	DuPont, Dr. Karl Thomae GmbH, Boehringer Ingelheim Pharma KG	1996-2000s
Pertussis Antiserum	generic	Wyeth	1949-1952
Pertussis Immune Globulin (Human), USP XXII	*HyperTussis*	Cutter	1958-1988
Pertussis Immune Serum (Human), USP XVI	*HyperTussis*	Cutter	1947-1965
Plague Antiserum	generic	no data	1926-1937
Pneumococcal Antiserum, USP XII	generic	various	1910s-1965
Poliomyelitis Immune Globulin (Human)	*Gamulin*	Pitman-Moore	1950s-1960s
Rabies Antiserum, (Equine), USP XXI	generic	various	1951-1989
Respiratory Syncytial Virus Immune Globulin	*Respigam*	MedImmune	1996-2005
Rocky Mountain Spotted Fever Antiserum	generic	Lederle	1949-1951
Satutumomab Pendetide	*OncoScint CR/OV*	Cytogen	1992-2000
Shigella or Dysenteric Antiserum (Equine)	generic	various	1925-1951
Staphylococcal Antitoxin (Equine)	generic	Squibb	1941-1951
Streptococcal Antiserum	generic	various	1925-1941
Streptococcus (Erysipelas) Antiserum	generic	various	1925-1952
Streptococcus (Scarlet Fever) Antitoxin (Equine), USP XIII	generic	various	1924-1951
Streptococcus (Scarlet Fever) Immune Serum (Human), USP XII	generic	no data	1945-1965
Tetanus Antitoxin (Equine), USP XXII	generic	various	1907-1957
Tuberculosis Antiserum	Anti-tubercle Serum	Mulford	1890s-1940s
Tularemia Antiserum	generic	Sharp & Dohme	1933-1941
Typhus Antiserum	generic	various	1940s
Varicella-zoster immune globulin	generic	Massachusetts Biological Laboratory	1980-2005

Obsolete Immunodiagnostics			
Generic name	Proprietary or product names	Manufacturer	Estimated availability
Blastomycin, USP XVIII	generic	Parke-Davis	1950-1970
Brucella Skin Test	*Brucellergen*	Merck Sharp & Dohme	1941-1970
Colostrum (Human, Primiparae)	*Primicol*	Sherman	1949-1952
Ducrey Vaccine (Test)	generic	Lederle	1941-1952
Diphtheria Toxin for Schick Test, USP XXII	generic	various	1913-1974
Echinococcin (Casoni's Test)	generic	no data	1950
Kveim Antigen	generic	no data	1935
Leishmanin	generic	no data	no data
Leutin	generic	no data	1937
Lymphogranuloma Venereum Antigen, USP XXII	*Lygranum-ST*	Lederle	1925-1967
Mallein	generic	no data	1937-1951
Multiple Skin Test Antigen Device	*Multitest CMI*	Connaught	1982-1990s
Mumps Skin Test Antigen	*MSTA*	Aventis-Pasteur	before 1960s-2000
Oidiomycin	*Dermatophytin "O"*	Hollister-Stier	until 1990s
Streptococcus (Scarlet Fever) Antitoxin for Schultz-Charlton Test	generic	various	1941-1952
Streptococcus (Scarlet Fever) Toxin for Dick Test	generic	various	1924-1950
Streptokinase-Streptodornase	*Varidase*	Lederle	1957-1981
Trichinella Extract, USP	generic	various	1938-1952
Trichophytin	*Dermatophytin*	Hollister-Stier	until 1990s
Tuberculin, Old (OT)	*MonoVacc, Tine Test*	Connaught, Lederle, others	before 1960s-2000

Miscellaneous Obsolete Immunologic Drugs			
Generic Name	Proprietary or product names	Manufacturer	Estimated availability
Allergen Extract, Alum-precipitated	*Allpyral*	Hollister-Stier	1970s to 1990s
Erysipelas & Prodigiosus Toxins	generic	Parke-Davis	1925-1951
Histamine Azoprotein	*Hapamine*	Parke-Davis	1950s-1960s
Interferon alfa-n1	*Wellferon*	GlaxoSmithKline	1999-2002
Penicillinase Injection	*Neutrapen*	SchenLabs, Riker	1960s
Poison Ivy Extract, Oral	generic	Miles	until 1990s
Poison Ivy and Oak Extracts, Parenteral	generic	Miles, Parke-Davis	until 1990s
	Ivyol	Mulford	1925–1960
Poison Ivy and Oak Extracts, Patch Test	generic	Hollister-Stier	until 1990s

International Immunologic Drugs

International Immunologic Drugs

This section reviews immunologic drugs available in countries other than the United States. The first list features proprietary names of products also available in the United States. The second identifies novel drugs not currently available within the United States. Separate indices of Canadian and Mexican immunologic drugs also appear in this section. Another feature of this section is a set of tables that translate common disease and product terms into several other languages.

While most of these products are available today, some may no longer be manufactured. These lists will be expanded as additional research reveals additional entries. Immunologic drug names that are translations of the generic name in the local, vernacular language are not generally included in this list. Means of legally importing drugs from other names are described elsewhere. Readers are invited to share written or pictorial information from additional international immunologic drugs with the editor.

Vaccines, Toxoids, & Immunogens			
Proprietary name	Manufacturer	Region	Composition
Abhayrab	Human Biologicals Institute	India	Rabies vaccine (Vero cell)
Acelluvax	Novartis	Europe	Recombinant acellular pertussis vaccine
Actacel	Sanofi Pasteur	Canada, Mexico	Diphtheria-tetanus-acellular-pertussis-Hib vaccine
ACVax	GlaxoSmithKline	United Kingdom	Meningococcal A & C vaccine
ACWYVax	GlaxoSmithKline	United Kingdom	Meningococcal ACYW-135 vaccine
Adifteper	Ism	Italy	Diphtheria & tetanus toxoids with pertussis vaccine
Adinvira A + B	Imuna	Czechoslovakia	Influenza A & B vaccine
Adiugrip	Sanofi Pasteur	Europe	Influenza A & B Vaccine
Admun	Duncan	United Kingdom	Influenza A & B vaccine
Admune GB	Duncan	United Kingdom	Influenza A & B vaccine
ADT vaccine	CSL Limited	Australia	Diphtheria & tetanus toxoids (for adult use)
AgB	Laboratorio Pablo Cassará	South America	Hepatitis B vaccine (*Hansenula polymorpha*-derived)
Agrippal	Novartis	Italy	Influenza A & B vaccine
Agrippal S1	Novartis	Europe	Influenza A & B vaccine
Aimmugen	Japanese Chemo-Sero Therapeutic Research Institute (Kaketsuken)	Japan	Hepatitis A vaccine
AKDS	unspecified	Russia	Diphtheria & tetanus toxoids with whole-cell pertussis vaccine
Aldiana	Sevac	Czech Republic	Diphtheria toxoid
Alditeana	Sevac	Czech Republic	Diphtheria & tetanus toxoids
Alditepera	Sevac	Czech Republic	Diphtheria & tetanus toxoids with pertussis vaccine
Almevax	Novartis	United Kingdom	Rubella vaccine (RA 27/3 strain)
Alpharix	GlaxoSmithKline	Europe	Influenza A & B vaccine (split)
Alorbat	Asta Pharma	Europe	Influenza A & B vaccine
Alteana	Imuna Pharm	Europe	Tetanus toxoid
Amaril	Sanofi Pasteur	Europe	Yellow fever vaccine

Vaccines, Toxoids, & Immunogens			
Proprietary name	Manufacturer	Region	Composition
AmBirix	GlaxoSmithKline	Europe	Hepatitis A and hepatitis B vaccine
AMC	not specified	Cuba	*Haemophilus influenzae* type b vaccine
Anadifterall	Novartis	Italy	Diphtheria toxoid
Anatetall	Novartis	Italy	Tetanus toxoid adsorbed
Anatoxal Di Te	Crucell	Europe	Diphtheria & tetanus toxoids (for adult use)
Anatoxal Di Te Per	Crucell	Europe	Diphtheria & tetanus toxoids with pertussis vaccine
Anflu	Sinovac Biotech	China	Influenza vaccine (split virion)
Anthrax vaccine live spore	Kirov Institute of Microbiology, Tblisi Scientific Research Institute of Vaccines & Serums	Russia, Georgia	Live spore vaccine, strain STI-1 (Sterne) nonencapsulated, without adjuvant. Scarification: 10^{8-9} spores/mL Subcutaneous: 10^8 spores/mL
	Lanzhou Institute of Biological Products	China	Live spore vaccine, Sterne-like A16R strain
Anthrax vaccine precipitated	Centre for Applied Microbiology & Research	United Kingdom	Inactivated, acellular filtrate of Sterne strain $34F_2$, capsulating
Antisarampion	Leti	Spain	Measles vaccine (Schwarz strain)
Arepanrix	GlaxoSmithKline	Europe, Japan	Influenza vaccine, pandemic strain
Arilvax	Novartis	United Kingdom	Yellow fever vaccine
Avaxim	Sanofi Pasteur	Europe	Hepatitis A vaccine
B-Hepavac II	Merck	Singapore	Hepatitis B vaccine (recombinant)
Begrivac	Novartis	Germany	Influenza A & B vaccine
Betagen	Sanofi Pasteur	Canada	Hepatitis B vaccine (mammalian cell, investigational)
BETT	Biological E	India	Tetanus toxoid
Bevac	Biological E	India	Hepatitis B vaccine
Biaflu Zonale	Farmabiagini	Italy	Influenza A & B vaccine
Biken-HB	Biken	Japan	Hepatitis B vaccine
Bilive	Sinovac Biotech	China	Hepatitis A and hepatitis B vaccine (inactivated)
Bimmugen	Japanese Chemo-Sero Therapeutic Research Institute (Kaketsuken)	Japan	Hepatitis B vaccine
BioPolio	Bharat Biotech	Asia	Poliovirus vaccine, live, oral (Sabin strains, primary monkey kidney cells)
Biviraten	Crucell	Switzerland	Measles & mumps vaccine (EZ19 & Rubini strains)
Boostrix	GlaxoSmithKline	Canada, Mexico	Tdap (adult)
Bubo-KOK	Combiotech Science-Industry Company	Russia	Diphtheria-tetanus-pertussis-hepatitis B
Bubo-M	Combiotech Science-Industry Company	Russia	Diphtheria-tetanus-hepatitis B (unspecified source)
Buccapol Berna	Crucell	Europe	Poliovirus vaccine, oral (Sabin strains)
Cacar	not specified	Indonesia	Smallpox vaccine
Campak Kerig	Pasteur Institute	Indonesia	Measles vaccine

Vaccines, Toxoids, & Immunogens			
Proprietary name	Manufacturer	Region	Composition
CDT Vaccine	CSL Limited	Australia	Diphtheria & tetanus toxoids (for pediatric use)
CEF	Novartis	Italy	Measles vaccine (Schwarz strain)
Celvapan	Baxter	Europe	Influenza A vaccine, pandemic strain (whole virion, without adjuvant)
Certiva	Baxter	Europe	Diphtheria-tetanus-acellular pertussis vaccine
Cinquerix	GlaxoSmithKline	Europe	Diphtheria-tetanus-pertussis-Hib-poliovirus vaccine
Covaxis	Sanofi Pasteur	Europe	Diphtheria and tetanus toxoids with acellular pertussis vaccine
D-Immun	Österreichisches Institut	Austria	Diphtheria toxoid
Di Anatoxal	Crucell	Europe	Diphtheria toxoid
Di Te Anatoxal	Crucell	Switzerland	Diphtheria & tetanus toxoids (for pediatric use)
Di Te Per Anatoxal	Crucell	Switzerland	Diphtheria & tetanus toxoids with pertussis vaccine
Di Te Per Pol Anatoxal	Crucell	Europe	Diphtheria & tetanus toxoids with pertussis and poliovirus vaccine
Di Te Pol SSI	Statens Seruminstitut	Denmark	Diphtheria & tetanus toxoids with poliovirus vaccine
Dif-Per-Tet-All	Novartis	Italy	Diphtheria & tetanus toxoids with pertussis vaccine
Dif-Tet-All	Novartis	Italy	Diphtheria & tetanus toxoids (for adult use)
Diftavax	Sanofi Pasteur	Mexico	Tetanus-diphtheria toxoids (Td)
Diftet	Bul Bio - National Center of Infectious and Parasitic Diseases (BB-NCIPD)	Bulgaria	Diphtheria and tetanus toxoids
Diftetkok	Bul Bio - National Center of Infectious and Parasitic Diseases (BB-NCIPD)	Bulgaria	Diphtheria and tetanus toxoids with whole-cell pertussis vaccine
Ditanrix	GlaxoSmithKline	Europe	Diphtheria & tetanus toxoids adsorbed
Ditoxim	Dong Shin	Korea	Diphtheria & tetanus toxoids (for adult use)
Double Antigen BI	Bengal Immunity Co.	India	Diphtheria & tetanus toxoids (unspecified potency)
DSDPT	Dong Shin	Korea	Diphtheria & tetanus toxoids with whole-cell pertussis vaccine
D.T. Adulte	Sanofi Pasteur	France	Diphtheria & tetanus toxoids (for adult use)
D.T. Bis	Sanofi Pasteur	France	Diphtheria & tetanus toxoids (for booster injections)
D.T. Coq	Sanofi Pasteur	France	Diphtheria & tetanus toxoids with pertussis vaccine
D.T. Vax	Sanofi Pasteur	France	Diphtheria & tetanus toxoids (for pediatric use)

Vaccines, Toxoids, & Immunogens			
Proprietary name	Manufacturer	Region	Composition
DT Wellcovax	Novartis	United Kingdom	Diphtheria & tetanus toxoids (for pediatric use)
Dual Antigen	Serum Institute of India	India	Diphtheria & tetanus toxoids (for pediatric use)
Dupla	Instituto Butantan	Brazil	Diphtheria & tetanus toxoids
Duplex	unspecified	Sweden	Diphtheria & tetanus toxoids (unspecified potency)
Easyfive	Panacea Biotec	India	Diphtheria and tetanus toxoids with whole-cell pertussis, hepatitis B, and Hib vaccines
Easyfour	Panacea Biotec	India	Diphtheria and tetanus toxoids with whole-cell pertussis and Hib vaccines
Ecolarix	GlaxoSmithKline	Europe	Measles & rubella vaccine (Schwarz & RA 27/3 strains)
Ecovac-4	Panacea Biotec	India	Diphtheria and tetanus toxoids with whole-cell pertussis and hepatitis B vaccines
Elvarix	VEB Sachsisches Serumwerk Dresden	Germany	Influenza vaccine, split
Enivac HB	Panacea Biotec	India	Hepatitis B vaccine
Enterovaccino	Isi	Italy	Typhoid vaccine
Enzira	CSL/Pfizer	Europe	Influenza A & B vaccine trivalent
Eolarix	GlaxoSmithKline	Europe	Measles & rubella vaccine (Schwarz & RA 27/3 strains)
Epaxal	Crucell	Switzerland	Hepatitis A vaccine, virosome technology
Ervax	GlaxoSmithKline	Mexico	Rubella vaccine (RA 27/3 strain)
Ervevax	GlaxoSmithKline	Europe, Australia	Rubella vaccine (RA 27/3 strain)
Euvax B	LG Life Sciences, Sanofi Pasteur	Korea, Europe	Hepatitis B vaccine
Fendrix	GlaxoSmithKline	Europe	Hepatitis B vaccine with AS04 adjuvant (dialysis formulation)
Fluad	Novartis	Europe	Influenza A & B vaccine, with MF-59 adjuvant
Fluarix	VEB Sachsisches Serumwerk Dresden	Europe, Australia	Influenza vaccine, split
FluBlok	Protein Sciences	India	Influenza trivalent hemagglutinin antigens
Flubron	Pfizer	United Kingdom	Influenza A & B vaccine
Flugen	unspecified	United Kingdom	Influenza A & B vaccine
Fluval AB	Omnivest	Hungary	Influenza A & B vaccine
Fluvax	CSL	Australia	Influenza A & B vaccine
Fluviral S/F	Shire	Canada	Influenza A & B vaccine
Fluvirin	Servier	United Kingdom	Influenza A & B vaccine
Focetria	Novartis	Europe	Influenza A/H5N1 vaccine with MF-59 adjuvant
FunED-Ceme	FunED	Brazil	Diphtheria & tetanus toxoids with pertussis vaccine
Gen H-B-Vax	Merck	Europe	Hepatitis B vaccine (recombinant)

Vaccines, Toxoids, & Immunogens			
Proprietary name	Manufacturer	Region	Composition
Gene Vac-B	Serum Institute of India	India	Hepatitis B vaccine
GenHevac B	Sanofi Pasteur	Singapore	Hepatitis B vaccine (mammal cell)
Gripax	Hebrew University	Israel	Influenza A & B vaccine
Gripovax	GlaxoSmithKline	Belgium	Influenza A & B vaccine
Grippol	Mikrogen	Russia	Influenza vaccine, inactivated
Gunevax	Novartis	Italy	Rubella vaccine (RA 27/3 strain)
H-Adiftal	Ism	Italy	Diphtheria toxoid adsorbed
H-Adiftetal	Ism	Italy	Diphtheria & tetanus toxoids (for adult use)
H-Atetal	Ism	Italy	Tetanus toxoid adsorbed
H-B-Vax	MSD-Novartis	Europe, Australia	Hepatitis B vaccine (serum)
H-B-Vax-DNA	Merck	Netherlands	Hepatitis B vaccine (recombinant)
H-B-Vax II	Merck	Worldwide	Hepatitis B vaccine (recombinant)
H-B-Vax II DNA	Merck	Worldwide	Hepatitis B vaccine (recombinant)
H-B-Vax Pro	Sanofi Pasteur MSD	Europe	Hepatitis B vaccine (recombinant)
Havax	Vabiotech	Asia	Hepatitis A vaccine
HAVpur	Novartis	Europe	Hepatitis A vaccine (virosome)
HBY	Green Cross	Japan	Hepatitis B vaccine
Healive	Sinovac Biotech	China	Hepatitis A vaccine (recombinant)
Heberbiovac HB	Centro de Ingeniería y Genética Biotecnología	Cuba	Hepatitis B vaccine (recombinant)
Hepabest	Sanofi Pasteur	Mexico	Hepatitis A vaccine
Hepacare	Novartis	Europe	Hepatitis B (pre-S1, pre-S2 proteins) vaccine
Hepaccine-B	Cheil Jedang	Asia	Hepatitis B vaccine (plasma derived)
Hepagene	Novartis	Europe	Hepatitis B vaccine (multiple antigens)
Hepamun	SK Chemicals Life Science	Asia	Hepatitis B vaccine (unspecified source)
Hepativax	Sanofi Pasteur	Mexico	Hepatitis B vaccine
Hepavax-Gene	Crucell	Europe	Hepatitis B vaccine, Hansenula polymorpha medium
Hepcare	Novartis	Europe	Hepatitis B vaccine
Heprecomb	Crucell	Europe	Hepatitis B vaccine
Heptavax-II	Merck	Worldwide	Hepatitis B vaccine (recombinant)
Heptis-B	Boryung Biopharma	Asia	Hepatitis B vaccine (recombinant, unspecified source)
Hevac B	Sanofi Pasteur	Europe	Hepatitis B vaccine (serum)
Hexavax	Sanofi Pasteur	Europe	DTaP-IPV-Hep B-Hib vaccine
Hexaxim	Sanofi Pasteur	Europe	Diphtheria and tetanus toxoids with acellular pertussis, inactivated poliovirus, Haemophilus, and hepatitis B vaccines
Hiberix	GlaxoSmithKline	Europe, Australia	Hib vaccine (PRP-TT)
HIBest	Sanofi Pasteur	Mexico	Hib vaccine (PRP-T)
HibPRO	Serum Institute of India	Asia	Hib vaccine (unspecified conjugating protein)

Vaccines, Toxoids, & Immunogens			
Proprietary name	Manufacturer	Region	Composition
Hinkuys karokote	National Public Health Institute	Finland	Pertussis vaccine
HIS	Serbian Institute	Yugoslavia (sic)	Influenza A & B vaccine
Humenza	Sanofi Pasteur	Europe	Influenza vaccine, pandemic strain
Immravax	Sanofi Pasteur	Europe	Measles-mumps-rubella vaccine (Schwarz, Urabe Am-3, & RA 27/3 strains)
Immunil	Sidus	Brazil	Pneumococcal vaccine
Imovax D.T. Adult	Sanofi Pasteur	Europe	Tetanus & diphtheria toxoids (for adult use)
Imovax Gripe	Sanofi Pasteur	Europe	Influenza A & B vaccine
Imovax Neumo	Sanofi Pasteur	Mexico	Pneumococcal polysaccharide vaccine 23-valent
Imovax Oreillons	Sanofi Pasteur	Europe	Mumps vaccine (Urabe strain)
Imovax Parotiditis	Sanofi Pasteur	Europe	Mumps vaccine
Imovax Pneumo	Sanofi Pasteur	Mexico	Pneumococcal polysaccharide vaccine 23-valent
Imovax Polio	Sanofi Pasteur	Europe	Poliovirus vaccine, inactivated
Imovax Rage	Sanofi Pasteur	Europe	Rabies vaccine
Imovax ROR	Sanofi Pasteur	Europe	Measles-mumps-rubella vaccine (Schwarz, Urabe Am-3, & RA 27/3 strains)
Imovax Sarampion	Sanofi Pasteur	Europe	Measles vaccine
Imovax Tetano	Sanofi Pasteur	Europe	Tetanus toxoid adsorbed
IndiRab	Bharat Biotech	Asia	Rabies vaccine (Pitman Moore strain, Vero cells)
Infanrix Hexa	GlaxoSmithKline	Europe	DTaP-IPV-Hep B-Hib vaccine
Infanrix Penta	GlaxoSmithKline	Europe	Diphtheria-tetanus-acellular pertussis-hepatitis B-poliovirus vaccine
Infanrix Quinta	GlaxoSmithKline	Europe	Diphtheria-tetanus-acellular pertussis-inactivated poliovirus-Hib vaccine-toxoid
Inflexal	Crucell	Switzerland	Influenza A & B vaccine
Inflexal V	Crucell	Europe	Virosomal influenza A & B vaccine
Influmix	Schiapparelli	Europe	Influenza A & B vaccine
Influpozzi Zonale	Ivp	Italy	Influenza A & B vaccine
Influsplit SSW	VEB Sachsisches Serumwerk Dresden	Germany	Influenza vaccine, split
Influvac	Duphar	Europe, Australia	Influenza A & B vaccine
Influvirus	Ism	Italy	Influenza A & B vaccine
Instivac	Sanofi Pasteur	Southern hemisphere	Influenza A & B vaccine, intradermal
Intanza	Sanofi Pasteur	Europe	Influenza A & B vaccine trivalent, intra-dermal
Invirin	GlaxoSmithKline	United Kingdom	Influenza A & B vaccine
Invivac	Solvay	Europe	Influenza vaccine virosomal
Ipad TP	Sanofi Pasteur	Europe	Tetanus-polio vaccine (unspecified type)
IPV-Virelon	Novartis	Europe	Inactivated poliovirus vaccine

Vaccines, Toxoids, & Immunogens			
Proprietary name	Manufacturer	Region	Composition
Isiflu Zonale	Isi	Italy	Influenza A & B vaccine
Istivac	Sanofi Pasteur	Europe	Influenza A & B vaccine
Kaksoisrokote	National Public Health Institute	Finland	Diphtheria & tetanus toxoids (for pediatric use)
Kikhoste	Statens Institut for Folkehelse	Norway	Pertussis vaccine
Komenotex	Combiotech Science-Industry Company	Russia	Hepatitis B vaccine (unspecified source *Pichia pastoris*)
Koplivac	Philips-Duphar	Australia	Measles vaccine (Edmonston strain)
Kotipa	Perum Bio Farma	Indonesia	Cholera-typhoid-paratyphoid A-B-C vaccine
Lancy Vaxina	Crucell	Switzerland	Smallpox vaccine
Lavantuutirokote	Central Public Health Laboratory	Finland	Typhoid vaccine
Liomorbillo	Ism	Italy	Measles vaccine (unspecified strain)
Liovaxs	Novartis	Italy	Smallpox vaccine
LM-2 Vaccine	Dong Shin	Korea	Measles & mumps vaccine (unspecified strains)
LM-3 Vaccine	Dong Shin	Korea	Measles-mumps-rubella vaccine (unspecified strains)
Lteanas Imuna	Imuna	Slovakia	Tetanus toxoid adsorbed
Lyssavac N	Crucell	Europe	Rabies vaccine (purified duck embryo)
M-M-Rvax	Sanofi Pasteur MSD	Europe	Measles-mumps-rubella vaccine (Moraten, Jeryl Lynn B, RA 27/3 strains)
M-M-Vax	Merck	Europe	Measles & mumps vaccine (Moraten & Jeryl Lynn strains)
M-Mvax	Novartis	Europe	Measles-mumps vaccine
M-Vac	Serum Institute of India	India	Measles vaccine live (Edmonston-Zagreb strain)
Masern-Virus-Impstoff	Novartis	Europe	Measles vaccine
Measavac	Pfizer	United Kingdom	Measles vaccine (Edmonston strain)
Mencevax	GlaxoSmithKline	Europe, Australia	Meningococcal polysaccharide vaccine
Mengivax A/C	Sanofi Pasteur	Europe	Meningococcal groups A/C conjugate vaccine
Meningtec	Wyeth	Canada	Meningococcal group C, CRM197-conjugate
Menjugate	Novartis	Europe	Meningococcal group C conjugate vaccine
Menpovax 4	Novartis	Europe	Meningococcal A,C,Y,W-135 vaccine
Menpovax A+C	Novartis	Europe	Meningococcal A and C vaccine
Mesavac	Pfizer	United Kingdom	Measles vaccine (Edmonston strain)
Mevilin-L	Novartis	United Kingdom	Measles vaccine (Schwarz strain)
MFR	Statens Serum Institute	Denmark	Measles-mumps-rubella vaccine
MFV	Servier	United Kingdom	Influenza A & B vaccine
MFV-Ject	Sanofi Pasteur	United Kingdom	Influenza A & B vaccine
Miniflu	Schiapparelli	Italy	Influenza A & B vaccine

International Names for Immunologic Drugs Licensed in the US

Vaccines, Toxoids, & Immunogens			
Proprietary name	Manufacturer	Region	Composition
MMRvaxpro	Sanofi Pasteur MSD	Europe	Measles-mumps-rubella vaccine (Moraten, Jeryl Lynn B, Wistar RA 27/3 strains)
Moniarix	SmithKline Beecham	Europe	Pneumococcal polysaccharide vaccine, 17-valent (1980s)
Monovax	Sanofi Pasteur	France	BCG vaccine
Mopavac	Sevac	Czech Republic	Measles & mumps vaccine (Schwarz & Jeryl Lynn strains)
Moraten	Crucell	Europe	Measles vaccine (Edmonston-Zagreb strain)
Morbilvax	Novartis	Italy	Measles vaccine (Schwarz strain)
MoRu-Viraten	Crucell	Canada	Measles-rubella vaccine (unspecified measles & RA 27/3 strains)
Morubel	Novartis	Italy	Measles-rubella vaccine (Schwarz, RA27/3 strains)
Morupar	Novartis	Italy	Measles-mumps-rubella vaccine (Schwarz, Urabe Am 9, RA27/3 strains)
Movivac	Sevac	Czech Republic	Measles vaccine (Schwarz strain)
Mumaten	Crucell	Switzerland	Mumps vaccine (Rubini strain)
Munevan	Novartis	United Kingdom	Influenza A & B vaccine
Mutagrip	Sanofi Pasteur	Germany	Influenza A & B vaccine
Nasoflu	GlaxoSmithKline	Europe	Influenza vaccine live intranasal
NeisVac-C	Baxter	Europe, Canada	Meningococcal conjugate vaccine serogroup C
Neotyf	Novartis	Italy	Typhoid vaccine, capsules
Nilgrip	CSL, Instituto Biológico Argentino	South America	Influenza A & B vaccine (subunit)
Nimenrix	GlaxoSmithKline	Europe	Meningococcal groups A/C/Y/W-135 conjugate (tetanus toxoid) vaccine
Nivgrip	Nicolau Institute of Virology	Romania	Influenza vaccine, whole
Nothav	Novartis	Europe	Hepatitis A vaccine
Okavax	Sanofi Pasteur	Japan, Europe	Varicella vaccine (Oka strain)
Optaflu	Novartis	Europe	Influenza A & B vaccine (cell culture)
Oral-Virelon	Novartis	Germany	Poliovirus vaccine, oral
PanBlok	Protein Sciences	India	Influenza A/H5N1
Pandemrix	GlaxoSmithKline	Europe	Influenza vaccine, pandemic strain
Panvax	CSL	Australia	Influenza A/H1N1/2009/California
Pariorix	GlaxoSmithKline	Mexico, Europe	Mumps vaccine (Urabe Am-3 strain)
Pavivac	Sevac	Czech Republic	Mumps vaccine (Jeryl Lynn strain)
Penta	Sanofi Pasteur	Europe	Diphtheria-tetanus-pertussis-Hib-poliovirus vaccine
Pentacoq	Sanofi Pasteur	Europe	Diphtheria-tetanus-pertussis-Hib-poliovirus vaccine
PentActHib	Sanofi Pasteur	Europe	Diphtheria-tetanus-pertussis-Hib-poliovirus vaccine
Pentavac	Sanofi Pasteur	Europe	Diphtheria and tetanus toxoids with acellular pertussis, inactivated poliovirus, and *Haemophilus* vaccines

Vaccines, Toxoids, & Immunogens			
Proprietary name	Manufacturer	Region	Composition
Pentaxim	Sanofi Pasteur	Europe	Diphtheria and tetanus toxoids with acellular pertussis, inactivated polio-virus, and *Haemophilus* vaccines
Pertuvac	Novartis	Europe	Acellular pertussis vaccine
Pluserix	GlaxoSmithKline	Mexico, Europe	Measles-rubella vaccine (unspecified measles & RA 27/3 strains)
Pneumo 23	Sanofi Pasteur	France	Pneumococcal vaccine, 23-valent
PneumoNovum	Sanofi Pasteur	Europe	Pneumococcal polysaccharide vaccine, 23-valent
Pneumopur	Novartis	Europe	Pneumococcal polysaccharide vaccine polyvalent
Pneumovax II	Merck	Europe	Pneumococcal polysaccharide vaccine, 23-valent
Pneumovax N	Merck	Europe	Pneumococcal polysaccharide vaccine, 23-valent
Polio Sabin	GlaxoSmithKline	Europe	Poliovirus vaccine, oral
Polio-Vaccinol A	Roehm Pharma	Germany	Poliovirus vaccine, oral
Polioral	Novartis	Italy	Poliovirus vaccine, oral
Poliovax-IN	Novartis	Europe	Inactivated poliovirus vaccine
Poloral	Crucell	Europe	Poliovirus vaccine, oral
Preflucel	Baxter	India	Influenza trivalent IM vaccine (cell culture)
Prepandrix	GlaxoSmithKline	Europe	Influenza A/H5N1 vaccine
Primavax	Sanofi Pasteur	Europe	Diphtheria & tetanus toxoids adsorbed with hepatitis B vaccine
Priorix	GlaxoSmithKline	Europe, Australia	Measles-mumps-rubella vaccine
Priorix-Tetra	GlaxoSmithKline	Europe	Measles (Schwarz strain)-mumps (RIT 4385 strain)-rubella (RA 27/3 strain)-varicella (Oka strain) vaccine
Procomvax	Merck, Sanofi Pasteur	Europe	*Haemophilus* influenzae type b-hepatitis B vaccine
Prodiax 23	Merck	Korea	Pneumococcal polysaccharide vaccine, 23-valent
Pulmovax	Merck	Europe	Pneumococcal polysaccharide vaccine, 23-valent
Pumarix	GlaxoSmithKline	Europe	Influenza A/H5N1 vaccine
Quadracel	Sanofi Pasteur	Mexico	Diphtheria-tetanus-acellular pertussis-inactivated poliovirus vaccine
Quadrimeningo	Bio-Med	India	Meningococcal polysaccharide vaccine (groups A, C, Y, and W-135)
Quatro-Virelon	Novartis	Europe	Diphtheria-tetanus-pertussis-poliovirus vaccine
Quattvaxem	Novartis	Europe	Diphtheria and tetanus toxoids with acellular pertussis and Hib vaccines
Quinivax-IN	Valda Laboratori	Europe	Diphtheria-tetanus-acellular pertussis-Hib-poliovirus vaccine
Quintanrix	GlaxoSmithKline	Europe	Diphtheria and tetanus toxoids with acellular pertussis, hepatitis B, and Hib vaccines

Vaccines, Toxoids, & Immunogens			
Proprietary name	Manufacturer	Region	Composition
Quinvaxem	Crucell	Europe	Diphtheria and tetanus toxoids with acellular pertussis, *Haemophilus*, and hepatitis B vaccines
R-HB vaccine	Merck (Banyu)	Japan	Hepatitis B vaccine (recombinant)
R-Vac	Serum Institute of India	India	Rubella vaccine (RA27/3 strain)
Rabdomune	Impfstofwerke	Germany	Rabies vaccine
Rabipur	Novartis	Germany	Rabies vaccine (Flury LEP strain)
Rabirix	Bharat Biotech	Asia	Vero cell culture
Rabivac	Novartis	Germany	Rabies vaccine (Pitman-Moore strain)
Rabivax	Serum Institute of India	Asia	Rabies vaccine (Pitman-Moore strain, human diploid cell culture)
Rasilvax	Novartis	Italy	Rabies vaccine
Repevax	Sanofi Pasteur	Europe	Tetanus and diphtheria toxoids with acellular pertussis and inactivated poliovirus vaccines (for adults)
Revac-B	Bharat-Biotech	Asia	Hepatitis B vaccine (*Pichia pastoris*)
Revac-B mcf	Bharat-Biotech	Asia	Hepatitis B vaccine (*Pichia pastoris*), thimerosal free
Revaxis	Sanofi Pasteur	Europe	Diphtheria-tetanus-pertussis-poliovirus vaccine
Rimevax	GlaxoSmithKline	Mexico, Europe	Measles vaccine (Schwarz strain)
Rimparix	GlaxoSmithKline	Europe	Measles & mumps vaccine (Schwarz & Urabe Am-3 strains)
Rorvax	Sanofi Pasteur	Europe, Brazil	Measles-mumps-rubella vaccine (Moraten, Jeryl Lynn, RA27/3 strains)
Rosovax	Ism	Italy	Rubella vaccine (unspecified strain)
Rouvax	Sanofi Pasteur	Europe	Measles vaccine (Schwarz strain)
Rubavax	Sanofi Pasteur	United Kingdom	Rubella vaccine (RA 27/3 strain)
Rubeaten	Crucell	Europe	Rubella vaccine (RA 27/3 strain)
Rubella vaccine	Kitasato Institute	Japan	Rubella vaccine (Takahashi strain)
Rubellovac	Novartis	Germany	Rubella vaccine
Rubilin	Novartis	United Kingdom	Rubella vaccine (RA 27/3 strain)
Rudi-Rouvax	Sanofi Pasteur	France	Measles & rubella vaccines (Schwarz & RA 27/3 strains)
Rudivax	Sanofi Pasteur	Europe	Rubella vaccine (RA 27/3 strain)
Sampar	Sanofi Pasteur	Indonesia	Plague vaccine
Sandovac	Sandoz	Austria	Influenza A & B vaccine
Sci-B-Vac	SciGen	Singapore	Hepatitis B vaccine
Serap	Perum Bio Farma	Indonesia	Diphtheria-tetanus-pertussis vaccine
Shantetra	Shantha Biotech	India	Diphtheria and tetanus toxoids with whole-cell pertussis and hepatitis B vaccines
Shanvac-B	Shantha Biotech	India	Hepatitis B vaccine (via *Pichia pastoris*)
SII Q-Vac	Serum Institute of India	India	Diphtheria and tetanus toxoids with whole-cell pertussis and hepatitis B vaccines
SII Rabivax	Serum Institute of India	India	Rabies vaccine (Pitman-Moore strain)

Vaccines, Toxoids, & Immunogens			
Proprietary name	Manufacturer	Region	Composition
SMBV	Sanofi Pasteur	Europe	Rabies vaccine (suckling mouse-brain culture; PV-11 strain)
Stafal Sevac	Sevac	Czech Republic	Staphylococcus phage lysate
Stamaril	Sanofi Pasteur	Europe	Yellow fever vaccine
Streptopur	Novartis	Europe	Pneumococcal polysaccharide vaccine polyvalent
Subinvira	Imuna	Czech Republic	Influenza A & B vaccine, split
Suduvax	Green Cross	South America, Asia	Varicella vaccine (Korean strain, like Oka)
T-Immun	Baxter	Germany	Tetanus toxoid adsorbed
T-Vaccinol	Roehm Pharma	Germany	Tetanus toxoid adsorbed
T-Wellcovax	Wellcopharm	Germany	Tetanus toxoid adsorbed
Tanrix	GlaxoSmithKline	Europe	Tetanus toxoid adsorbed
Td-Pur	Novartis	Europe	Tetanus & diphtheria toxoids adsorbed
Td-Rix	GlaxoSmithKline	Europe	Tetanus and diphtheria toxoids (adult)
Td-Virelon	Novartis	Europe	Tetanus & diphtheria toxoids adsorbed with inactivated poliovirus vaccine
Te Anatoxal	Crucell	Switzerland	Tetanus toxoid adsorbed
Tedivax	GlaxoSmithKline	Europe	Tetanus-diphtheria toxoids (adult)
Tet-Aktiv	Tropon-Cutter	Germany	Tetanus toxoid adsorbed
Tet-Tox	CSL Limited	Australia	Tetanus toxoid adsorbed
Tetadif	Bul Bio - National Center of Infectious and Parasitic Diseases (BB-NCIPD)	Bulgaria	Tetanus and diphtheria toxoids
Tetamun SSW	VEB Sachsisches Serumwerk Dresden	Germany	Tetanus toxoid, fluid
Tetamyn	Bioclon	Mexico	Tetanus toxoid
Tetanol	Novartis, Sanofi Pasteur	Europe, Mexico	Tetanus toxoid adsorbed
Tetanol pur	Novartis	Europe	Tetanus toxoid
Tetanovac	Sanofi Pasteur	Mexico	Tetanus toxoid
Tetasorbat SSW	VEB Sachsisches Serumwerk Dresden	Germany	Tetanus toxoid adsorbed
Tetatox	Crucell	Italy	Tetanus toxoid adsorbed
Tetavax	Sanofi Pasteur	Europe	Tetanus toxoid adsorbed
TETRAct-HIB	Sanofi Pasteur	Europe	Tetanus-diphtheria-pertussis-Hib vaccine
Tetravac	Sanofi Pasteur	Europe	Diphtheria-tetanus-pertussis-poliovirus vaccine
Tetraxim	Sanofi Pasteur	Europe	Tetanus-diphtheria-pertussis-IPV vaccine
Te/Vac/Ptap	Unknown	Yugoslavia (sic)	Tetanus toxoid adsorbed
Tevax	GlaxoSmithKline	Europe	Tetanus toxoid
Thybar	Bharat Biotech	Asia	Typhoid Vi polysaccharide vaccine
Tifovax	Sanofi Pasteur	Mexico	Vi polysaccharide
Tresivac	Serum Institute of India	India	Measles-mumps-rubella vaccine live (Edmonston-Zagreb, L-Zagreb, RA 27/3 strains)

Vaccines, Toxoids, & Immunogens			
Proprietary name	Manufacturer	Region	Composition
Triacel	Sanofi Pasteur	Europe, Mexico	Diphtheria-tetanus-acellular pertussis vaccine
Triacelluvax	Novartis	Europe	Diphtheria-tetanus-acellular pertussis vaccine
Trimovax ("ROR")	Sanofi Pasteur	Europe	Measles-mumps-rubella vaccine (Schwarz, Urabe Am-3, & RA 27/3 strains)
Tripacel	Sanofi Pasteur	Europe, Australia	Diphtheria-tetanus-acellular pertussis vaccine
Triple Antigen	CSL Limited, Serum Institute	Australia, India	Diphtheria & tetanus toxoids with pertussis vaccine
Triplice (VT)	Instituto Butantan	Brazil	Diphtheria-tetanus- pertussis vaccine
Triplice Viral (VTV)	Instituto Butantan	Brazil	Measles-mumps-rubella vaccine
Triplovax	Sanofi Pasteur	Europe, Brazil	Measles-mumps-rubella vaccine (Moraten, Jeryl Lynn, RA27/3 strains)
Tripvac DTP	Biological E	India	Diphtheria and tetanus toxoids with whole-cell pertussis vaccine
Tritanrix HepB	GlaxoSmithKline	Mexico	Diphtheria-tetanus-pertussis-hepatitis B vaccine
Tritanrix HepB-Hib	GlaxoSmithKline	Europe	Diphtheria-tetanus-pertussis-hepatitis B-*Haemophilus b* vaccine
Trivacuna Leti	Lab. Leti	Spain	Diphtheria & tetanus toxoids with pertussis vaccine
Trivax	Novartis	United Kingdom	Fluid diphtheria & tetanus toxoids with pertussis vaccine
Trivax-AD	Novartis	United Kingdom	Adsorbed diphtheria & tetanus toxoids with pertussis vaccine
Trivax Hib	GlaxoSmithKline	Europe	Diphtheria-tetanus-acellular pertussis-Hib vaccine
Trivb	Unknown	Brazil	Diphtheria & tetanus toxoids with pertussis vaccine
Triviraten	Crucell	Switzerland	Measles-mumps-rubella vaccine (EZ19, Rubini, & RA 27/3 strains)
Trivivac	Sevac	Czech Republic	Measles-mumps-rubella vaccine (Schwarz, Jeryl Lynn, RA 27/3 strains)
Trivivax	Sanofi Pasteur	Mexico	Measles-mumps-rubella vaccine
Tussitrupin Forte	Unknown	Germany	Pertussis vaccine
Typbar	Bharat Biotech	Asia	Typhoid Vi polysaccharide vaccine
Tyne	not specified	Sweden	BCG vaccine
Typh-Vax	CSL Limited	Australia	Typhoid vaccine, oral
Typherix	GlaxoSmithKline	Europe, Australia	Typhoid Vi polysaccharide vaccine
Typhoral-L	Crucell	Germany	Typhoid Ty21a vaccine, oral
Unifive	Sanofi Pasteur	Europe	Diphtheria and tetanus toxoids with acellular pertussis, *Haemophilus*, and hepatitis B vaccines
Va-Diftet	Finlay Vacunas & Sueros	Cuba	Diphtheria & tetanus toxoids
Vac-DPT	Bioclon	Mexico	Diphtheria & tetanus toxoids with pertussis vaccine

Vaccines, Toxoids, & Immunogens			
Proprietary name	Manufacturer	Region	Composition
Vaccin tuberculeux atténué lyophilisé	Sanofi Pasteur	France	BCG vaccine, ID
Vacina Dupla	Butantan	Brazil	Tetanus & diphtheria toxoids (adult or pediatric strengths)
Vacina Triplice	Butantan	Brazil	Diphtheria & tetanus toxoids with pertussis vaccine
Vacunol	Temis-Lostalo	Brazil	Tetanus toxoid adsorbed
Vakcin Sampar	Perum Bio Farma	Indonesia	Plague vaccine
Vaksin Campak Kerig	Perum	Indonesia	Measles vaccine (Schwarz strain)
Vari-L	SK Chemicals Life Science	Asia	Varicella zoster virus (chickenpox) vaccine
Varicella-RIT	GlaxoSmithKline	Europe	Varicella vaccine
Varie	Institute of Sera and Vaccine	Czechoslovakia	Smallpox vaccine
Varilrix	GlaxoSmithKline	Europe, Mexico	Varicella vaccine
Vax-TyVi	Finlay Vacunas & Sueros	Cuba	Typhoid Vi polysaccharide vaccine oral Ty21a
Vax-Tet	Finlay Vacunas & Sueros	Cuba	Tetanus toxoid
Vaxem-Hib	Novartis	Europe	*Haemophilus influenzae* type b vaccine
Vaxicoq	Sanofi Pasteur	France	Pertussis vaccine
Vaxigrip	Sanofi Pasteur	Europe, Australia	Influenza A & B vaccine
Vaxihaler-Flu	Riker	United Kingdom	Influenza A & B vaccine, inhaler
Vaxipar	Novartis	Italy	Mumps vaccine (Urabe AM-9 strain)
VaxiRab	Zydus Cadila	India	Rabies vaccine (duck-embryo)
VCDT	Cantacuzino Institute	Romania	Diphtheria & tetanus toxoids (for pediatric use)
Vepacel	Baxter	Europe	Influenza A/H5N1 vaccine
Verorab	Sanofi Pasteur	France	Rabies vaccine (Vero cell)
Vibriomune	Duncan, Flockhart	United Kingdom	Cholera vaccine
Virelon C	Novartis	Germany	Poliovirus vaccine, subcutaneously
Virelon T 20	Novartis	Germany	Poliovirus vaccine, oral
Virivac	Sanofi Pasteur MSD	Europe	Measles-mumps-rubella vaccine (Moraten, Jeryl Lynn B, RA 27/3 strains)
Virohep	Europe	Virohep	Hepatitis A vaccine (virosome)
VVR	Cantacuzino Institute	Romania	Measles vaccine (Schwarz strain)
Welltrivax	not specified	Spain	Diphtheria-tetanus-pertussis vaccine
X-flu	CSL	Asia	Influenza A & B vaccine trivalent
Zaditeadvax	Imunoloski Zavod	Croatia	Diphtheria & tetanus toxoids (for adult use, 5/7.5 Lfu)
Zaditevax	Imunoloski Zavod	Croatia	Diphtheria & tetanus toxoids (for pediatric use, 30/7.5 Lfu)
Zamevax A+C	Imunoloski Zavod	Croatia	Meningococcal A+C vaccine
Zamovax	Imunoloski Zavod	Croatia	Measles vaccine (Edmonston-Zagreb strain)
Zampavax	Imunoloski Zavod	Croatia	Measles-mumps vaccine (Edmonston-Zagreb & HDC or L-Zagreb CEF strains)

Vaccines, Toxoids, & Immunogens			
Proprietary name	Manufacturer	Region	Composition
Zamruvax	Imunoloski Zavod	Croatia	Measles-rubella vaccine (Edmonston-Zagreb & RA 27/3 strains)
Zapavax	Imunoloski Zavod	Croatia	Mumps vaccine (L-Zagreb CEF strain)
Zaruvax	Imunoloski Zavod	Croatia	Rubella vaccine (RA 27/3 strain)
Zatevax	Imunoloski Zavod	Croatia	Tetanus toxoid adsorbed
Zatribavax	Imunoloski Zavod	Croatia	Diphtheria & tetanus toxoids with pertussis vaccine
Zatrivax	Imunoloski Zavod	Croatia	Measles-mumps-rubella vaccine (Edmonston-Zagreb, RA 27/3, & L-Zagreb CEF strains)
Zerotyph	Boryung Biopharma	Asia	Typhoid vaccine oral capsules (Ty21a strain)

Immune Globulins			
Proprietary name	Manufacturer	Region	Composition
Abhayrig	Human Biologicals Institute	India	Rabies antiserum (equine)
Alphaglobulin	Alpha	United Kingdom	Immune globulin IM and IV
AntiHep	Combiotech Science-Industry Company	Russia	Hepatitis B immune globulin (human)
ATG-Fresenius	Fresenius	Europe	Antithymocyte globulin (canine)
Aunativ	Kabi	Germany	Hepatitis B immune globulin
BEATS	Biological E	India	Tetanus antitoxin
Beriglobin	Novartis	Germany	Immune globulin IM or oral
Berirab	Novartis	Germany	Rabies immune globulin
Bharglob	Bharat Serums & Vaccines	Asia	Immune globulin IM
Biaven IV	Farmabiagini	Italy	Immune globulin IV
Carig	Zydus Cadila	Asia	Rabies antiserum (equine)
Clotinab	Isu Abxis	Korea	Abciximab (biosimilar) Fab
Cutterglobin	Tropon-Cutter	Germany	Immune globulin IM
Cytoglobin	Tropon-Cutter	Germany	Cytomegalovirus immune globulin IV
Cytotect	Biotest	Europe	Cytomegalovirus immune globulin IV
Endobulin	Baxter	Europe	Immune globulin IV
Endogamma	Ism	Italy	Immune globulin IV
EquiRab	Bharat Serums & Vaccines	Asia	Rabies antiserum (equine)
Gamaffine	Haffkine Bio-Pharmaceutical Corporation	India	Immune globulin IM
Gamma 16	Sanofi Pasteur	France	Immune globulin IM
Gamma Anti-D	Grifols	Europe	$Rh_o(D)$ immune globulin
Gamma Anti-Hepatitis B	Grifols	Europe	Hepatitis B immune globulin
Gamma Anti-Tétanos	Grifols	Europe	Tetanus immune globulin
Gamma IV	Bharat Serums & Vaccines	Asia	Immune globulin IV
Gammabulin	Baxter	Europe	Immune globulin IM
Gammabyk	Altana	Europe	Immune globulin IM
Gammamen	Ism	Italy	$Rh_o(D)$ immune globulin
Gammanorm	Biovitrum	Europe	Immune globulin subcutaneous
Gammaprotect	Biotest	Germany	Hepatitis B immune globulin
Gammatet	Novartis	Europe	Tetanus immune globulin
GammaVenin	Novartis	Europe	Immune globulin IV
GammoNativ	Kabi	Europe	Immune globulin IV
Globuman P IM	Crucell	Europe	Immune globulin IM
Glogama	unspecified	Spain	Immune globulin IM
Haima-D	Aima	Italy	$Rh_o(D)$ immune globulin
Haimabig	Aima	Italy	Hepatitis B immune globulin
Haimarab	Aima	Italy	Rabies immune globulin
Haimatetanus	Aima	Italy	Tetanus immune globulin
Haimaven IV	Aima	Italy	Immune globulin IV

Immune Globulins			
Proprietary name	Manufacturer	Region	Composition
Haimazig	Aima	Italy	Varicella-zoster immune globulin
Hemogamma	Baxter	Germany	Immune globulin IM
Hepaga	Sevac	Czech Republic	Hepatitis B immune globulin
Hepaglobin	Tropon-Cutter	Germany	Hepatitis B immune globulin
Hepatect IV	Biotest	Europe	Hepatitis B immune globulin IV
Hepatothera	Japanese Chemo-Sero Therapeutic Research Institute (Kaketsuken)	Japan	Hapatitis B immune globulin
Hepuman P IM	Crucell	Europe	Hepatitis B immune globulin
Humotet	Wellcome	United Kingdom	Tetanus immune globulin
IgGa	Bio-Transfusion	France	Immune globulin IM
Igamad	Instituto Grifols	Europe	$Rh_o(D)$ immune globulin IM
Igantet	Instituto Grifols	Europe	Tetanus immune globulin IM
Igantibe	Instituto Grifols	Europe	Hepatitis B immune globulin IM
Igantid	Instituto Grifols	Europe	$Rh_o(D)$ immune globulin IM
Iggamma	Novartis	Italy	Immune globulin IM
Igrho	Novartis	Italy	$Rh_o(D)$ immune globulin
Igtetano	Novartis	Italy	Tetanus immune globulin
Igvena N	Novartis	Italy	Immune globulin IV
Immossar	Choay Laboratories	France	Lymphocyte immune globulin
Immunar	Armour	Europe	Immune globulin IM
Immunoglobulin 7S	Armour	Europe	Immune globulin IV
Immunohbs	Isi	Italy	Hepatitis B immune globulin
Immunomorb	Isi	Italy	Immune globulin IM
ImmunoRho	Isi	Italy	$Rh_o(D)$ immune globulin
Immunotetan	Isi	Italy	Tetanus immune globulin
Immunozig	Isi	Italy	Varicella-zoster immune globulin
Imogam 16	Sanofi Pasteur	Italy	Immune globulin IM
Imogam Rab	Sanofi Pasteur	Worldwide	Rabies immune globulin
Indobulin	Baxter	Austria	Immune globulin IV
Intragam	Serotherpaeutisches	Austria	Immune globulin IV
Intraglobin	Biotest	Europe	Immune globulin IV
Isiven IV	Isi	Italy	Immune globulin IV
Kabiglobin	Pharmacia	Europe	Immune globulin IV
KamRAB	Kamada	Israel	Rabies immune globulin
KamRho-D	Kamada	Israel	$Rh_o(D)$ immune globulin IM or IV
Kenketsu Jochu-globulin	Japanese Chemo-Sero Therapeutic Research Institute (Kaketsuken)	Japan	Immune globulin IV pepsin-treated
Kenketsu Venilon-I	Japanese Chemo-Sero Therapeutic Research Institute (Kaketsuken)	Japan	Immune globulin S-sulfonated
Liosiero Antibotulinicum	Ism	Italy	Botulinum immune serum
Lymphoglobuline	Sanofi Pasteur	Europe	Lymphocyte immune globulin
Lymphoser	Crucell	Switzerland	Lymphocyte immune globulin

Immune Globulins			
Proprietary name	Manufacturer	Region	Composition
MabThera	Genentech/IDEC	Europe	Rituximab
Normagamma	Ism	Italy	Immune globulin IM
Partobulin	Baxter	Europe	$Rh_o(D)$ immune globulin
Partogamma	Farmabiagini	Italy	$Rh_o(D)$ immune globulin
Partogloman	unspecified	Europe	$Rh_o(D)$ immune globulin IM
Polyglobin N	Tropon-Cutter	International	Immune globulin IV
Polyglobin R	Tropon-Cutter	International	Cytomegalovirus immune globulin
Probi-Rho D	unspecified	Mexico	$Rh_o(D)$ immune globulin IM
Pressimmun	Novartis	Europe	Lymphocyte immune globulin
Purimmune	Armour Pharma	Germany	Immune globulin IV
Rabglob	Bharat Serums & Vaccines	Asia	Rabies immune globulin
Rabiabulin	Baxter	Brazil	Rabies immune globulin
Rabies Gamma	Farmabiagini	Italy	Rabies immune globulin
Rabuman	Crucell	Europe	Rabies immune globulin
Rhega	Sevac	Czech Republic	$Rh_o(D)$ immune globulin
Rhega	Spofa	Poland	$Rh_o(D)$ immune globulin
Rhesogam	Novartis	Germany	$Rh_o(D)$ immune globulin
Rhesogamma	unspecified	Europe	$Rh_o(D)$ immune globulin IM
Rhesonativ	Biovitrun	Europe	$Rh_o(D)$ immune globulin IM
Rhesuman P IM	Crucell	Europe	$Rh_o(D)$ immune globulin
Rhesuman-iv	Crucell	Switzerland	$Rh_o(D)$ immune globulin
Rhobulin	Green Cross	Japan	$Rh_o(D)$ immune globulin
Rhodiglobin	Sanofi Pasteur	Europe	Immune globulin IM or IV
Riclanin	Inprofarm	Spain	Immune globulin IM
Sanglopor	Aventis Behring	Japan	Immune globulin IV
Seroglubin	Cutter	Mexico	Immune globulin IM
Suduvax	Korean Green Cross	Korea	Varicella vaccine
Tega	Imuna	Slovakia	Tetanus immune globulin
Tetabulin	Baxter	Europe	Tetanus immune globulin
Tetagam	Novartis	Germany	Tetanus immune globulin
Tetagamma	Ism	Italy	Tetanus immune globulin
Tetaglobulina	Sanofi Pasteur	Brazil	Tetanus immune globulin
Tetaglobuline	Sanofi Pasteur	Europe	Tetanus immune globulin
Tetamyn	Bioclon	Mexico	Tetanus immune globulin
Tetanobulin	Baxter	Germany	Tetanus immune globulin
Tetanothera	Japanese Chemo-Sero Therapeutic Research Institute (Kaketsuken)	Japan	Tetanus immune globulin
Tetanus Gamma	Farmabiagini	Italy	Tetanus immune globulin
Tetaven-IV	Baxter	Italy	Tetanus immune globulin IV
Tetavenin	Baxter	Italy	Tetanus immune globulin
Tetglob	Bharat Serums & Vaccines	Asia	Rabies immune globulin
Tetuman	Crucell	Europe	Tetanus immune globulin

Immune Globulins			
Proprietary name	Manufacturer	Region	Composition
Thymogam	Bharat Serums & Vaccines	Asia	Antithymocyte globulin (equine)
Thymoglobuline	Sanofi Pasteur	Europe	Antithymocyte globulin (rabbit)
Uman-Big	Farmabiagini	Italy	Hepatitis B immune globulin
Uman-Cig	Farmabiagini	Italy	Cytomegalovirus immune globulin
Uman-Gal E	Farmabiagini	Italy	Lymphocyte immune globulin
Uman-Gamma	Farmabiagini	Italy	Immune globulin IM
Uman-Vzig	Farmabiagini	Italy	Varicella-zoster immune globulin
Vacciniabulin	Green Cross	Japan	Vaccinia immune globulin
Vacuman	Crucell	Europe	Vaccinia immune globulin
Var Zeta IM	Schiapparelli	Italy	Varicella-zoster immune globulin
Var Zeta IV	Schiapparelli	Italy	Varicella-zoster immune globulin
Varicellon	Novartis	Germany	Varicella-zoster immune globulin
Varitect	Biotest	Germany	Varicella-zoster immune globulin
VariZIG	Cangene	Canada	Varicella-zoster immune globulin (human)
Veinoglobuline	Sanofi Pasteur	France	Immune globulin IV
Venbig	Farmabiagini	Italy	Hepatitis B immune globulin
Venilon	Teijin	Japan	Immune globulin IV
Venimmun	Novartis	Europe	Immune globulin IV
Venogamma	Schiapparelli	Italy	Immune globulin IV
Venogamma Antirho D	Schiapparelli	Italy	$Rh_o(D)$ immune globulin IV
Venoglobulina	Sanofi Pasteur	Italy	Immune globulin IV
Vigam-S	Bioproducts Laboratory	United Kingdom	Varicella-zoster immune globulin
Vinobulin	Bharat Serums & Vaccines	Asia	Anti-$Rh_o(D)$ immune globulin
WellcoTIG	Wellcopharm	Germany	Tetanus immune globulin
Zaantide	Imunoloski Zavod	Croatia	Diphtheria antitoxin (equine)
Zaantite	Imunoloski Zavod	Croatia	Tetanus antitoxin (equine)
Zahuhebig	Imunoloski Zavod	Croatia	Hepatitis B immune globulin
Zahuigim	Imunoloski Zavod	Croatia	Immune globulin IM
Zahuigiv	Imunoloski Zavod	Croatia	Immune globulin IV
Zahurig	Imunoloski Zavod	Croatia	Rabies immune globulin
Zahutig	Imunoloski Zavod	Croatia	Tetanus immune globulin
Zoster immune globulin	CSL Limited	Australia	Varicella-zoster immune globulin
Zyrig	Zydus Cadila	Asia	Rabies antiserum (equine)

Immediate Hypersensitivity Antigens			
Proprietary name	Manufacturer	Region	Composition
Alavac	Bencard	Europe	Allergen extracts (various)
Alipagène	Unknown	France	$Al(OH)_3$-precipitated allergen extract
Alpha-Test	Hollister-Stier	United Kingdom	Allergen extracts (various)
Alutard SQ	ALK-Abelló	Europe	Alum-precipitated allergen extract
Anjuvac	Dome	Denmark	Allergen extracts (various)
Aquagen	ALK-Abelló	Europe	Allergen extract aqueous
Desalerga	Sevac	Czech Republic	Allergen extracts (various)
Dialerga	Sevac	Czech Republic	Allergen extracts (various)
Haygen	Beecham	United Kingdom	Allergen extracts (various)
Migen	Bencard	Europe	Allergen extracts (various)
Norisen	E. Merck	United Kingdom	Allergen extracts (various)
Paspat	Luitpold	Australia	Allergen extracts (various)
Pen-Kit	Actipharm	Switzerland	Benzylpenicilloic acid, penicillin sodium, & penicilloyl polylysine
Phazet	Pharmacia	Denmark	Allergen extracts (various)
Pollinex	Beecham-Bencard	Canada, Europe	Allergen extracts (various)
Polvac+	Bencard	Europe	Allergen extracts (various)
Promiten	Pharmacia	Europe	Dextran-1
Reless	Pharmacia	Europe	*Hymenoptera* venoms (various)
Soluprick	ALK	Denmark	Allergen extracts (various)
Spectralgen	Pharmacia	United Kingdom	Allergen extracts (various)
Testarpen	Polfa	Poland	Penicilloyl polylysine
Tyrivac	unspecified	Europe	Allergen extracts (various)

Delayed Hypersensitivity Antigens			
Proprietary name	Manufacturer	Region	Composition
Esferulina	ALK	Mexico	Spherule-derived Coccidioidin
Imotest tuberculosis	Sanofi Pasteur	France	PPD multipuncture device
Leukotest	Beiersdorf	Germany	Patch test allergens in petrolatum
Montest	Sanofi Pasteur	France	PPD multipuncture device
Trolab	Hermal	Germany	Patch test allergens in petrolatum
Tubergen	Novartis	Europe	Tuberculin (unspecified)

Immunologic Mediators			
Proprietary name	Manufacturer	Region	Composition
Beneferson	Unknown	Germany	Interferon beta
Berofor	Basotherm	Germany	Interferon alfa-2c
Canferon A	Takeda	Japan	Interferon alfa
Celleron 5 Mio	Unknown	Europe	Interferon alfa, unspecified
Cibian	Yamanochi	Japan	Interferon beta
Feron	Toray	Japan	Interferon beta
Fiblaferon 3,4,5 IV	Rentschler	Germany	Interferon beta
Frone	Serono	Italy	Interferon beta
Heberón Alfa R	Centro de Ingeniería Genética y Biotecnología	Cuba	Interferon alfa-2b (recombinant)
Heberón Gamma R	Centro de Ingeniería Genética y Biotecnología	Cuba	Interferon gamma (recombinant)
Humoferon	Unknown	Italy	Interferon alfa-n1
Immulin	Unknown	Australia	Interferon (unspecified)
Immuneron	Biogen Idec	United Kingdom	Interferon gamma
Imufor Gamma	Unknown	Germany	Interferon gamma-1b
Imukin	Unknown	France	Interferon gamma
Imunovax-gamma	Shionogi	Japan	Interferon gamma-1a
Kombiferon	Acad Med Sci	Russia	Alpha & beta interferons
Laroferon	Roche	Europe	Interferon alfa-2a
Naferon	Chiron	Italy	Interferon beta
Neutrofil	Laborotorio Pablo Cassará	South America	Filgrastim
Reaferon	Acad Med Sci	Russia	Beta interferon
Shanferon	Shantha Biotech	India	Interferon alfa 2b (recombinant)
Sumiferon	Sumitomo	Japan	Beta interferon
Viraferon	Schering	Europe	Interferon alfa-2b
Wellferon	Novartis	Canada	Interferon alfa-n1

Immunomodulating Drugs			
Proprietary name	Manufacturer	Region	Composition
Alexan	Mack, Illert	Germany	Cytarabine
Azalan	Quimica y Farmacia	Mexico	Azathioprine
Carmubris	Bristol	Germany	BCNU
Cyclostin	Farmitalia	Germany	Cyclophosphamide
Endoxin	Asta Pharma	Germany	Cyclophosphamide
Farmitrexat	Farmitalia	Germany	Methotrexate
Fluroblastin	Farmitalia	Germany	Fluorouracil
Immunol	Sarm	Italy	Levamisole
Imurek	Wellcome	Germany	Azathioprine
Platiblastin	Farmitalia	Germany	Cisplatin
Puri-Nethol	Wellcome	Germany	Mercaptopurine
Udicil	Upjohn	Germany	Cytarabine
Velbe	Lilly	Germany	Vinblastine
Wormex	Pfizer	Europe	Levamisole

Other Drugs			
Proprietary name	Manufacturer	Region	Composition
Ana-Help	Stallergenes	France	Epinephrine autoinjector
Dysport	Porton	United Kingdom	Botulinum A toxin
Fastjekt	Allergopharma	Germany	Epinephrine autoinjector
ImmuCyst	Sanofi Pasteur	Canada	BCG for bladder cancer

Unique Vaccines & Immunologic Drugs Not Available Within the US

International Immunologic Drugs

In other countries, patients may receive foreign licensed vaccines against brucellosis, leptospirosis, *Pseudomonas*, and perhaps other diseases for which protection is unavailable in the United States. Inclusion in this list, however, is no guarantee of safety or efficacy. Readers aware of additional novel products not listed here are encouraged to notify the editor.

Vaccines			
Generic contents	Manufacturer	Region	Proprietary or common name
Autologous tumor vaccine (based on heat-shock protein technology)	Antigenics	Russia	*Oncophage*
BCG vaccine, INH-resistant strain	Novartis	United Kingdom	
BCG vaccine, oral	Butantan	Brazil	*Onco BCG Oral*
Brucella vaccine	Sanofi Pasteur	France	*Vaccin brucellique*
Candida albicans & *Klebsiella pneumoniae* ribosomes, oral	Pierre Fabre	France	*Globene*
Cholera, typhoid, & paratyphoid A, B, & C vaccines	Perum Bio Farma	Indonesia	*Vakcin Kotipa*
Cholera-typhoid-paratyphoid A & B vaccine	Institute of Immunology & Virology Torlak	Yugoslavia (sic)	*Ty AB Cholera*
Cholera-typhoid vaccine	National Institute of Health	Pakistan	*TC Vaccine*
Cholera vaccine, oral, inactivated (whole-cell components with toxin-coregulated pilus)	Vabiotech	Asia	*ORC-Vax*
Cholera vaccine, oral, inactivated (with ETEC labile toxin)	Crucell	Europe, Mexico	*Dukoral*
Cholera vaccine, oral, live (CVD 103-HgR)	Crucell	Europe	*Mutachol Berna, Orochol Berna*
Cholera vaccine, whole-cell, inactivated, oral (bivalent 01 [Inaba and Ogawa] and 0139)	Shantha Biotech	Asia	*Shanchol*
Clostridium welchii type C toxoid	Novartis	United Kingdom	*Pigbel*
Colibacilosis porcina vaccine	Centre for Genetic Engineering & Biotechnology	Cuba	
Crimean hemorrhagic fever vaccine, inactivated	Bul Bio - National Center of Infectious and Parasitic Diseases (BB-NCIPD)	Bulgaria	Anti-CHF vaccine
Diphtheria and tetanus toxoids with acellular pertussis, *Haemophilus*, hepatitis B, and meningcoccal A&C vaccines	GlaxoSmithKline	Europe	*Globorix*
Diphtheria-tetanus-acellular pertussis-hepatitis B	GlaxoSmithKline	Europe	*Zilbrix*

Vaccines			
Generic contents	Manufacturer	Region	Proprietary or common name
Diphtheria-tetanus-acellular pertussis-hepatitis B-Hib	GlaxoSmithKline	Europe	*Zilbrix Hib*
Diphtheria-tetanus-acellular pertussis-hepatitis B-inactivated poliovirus-Hib vaccine-toxoid	GlaxoSmithKline	Europe	*Infanrix Hexa*
Diphtheria-tetanus-pertussis-parapertussis	Imunoloski Zavod	Croatia	*Zatetravax*
Diphtheria-tetanus-pertussis-parapertussis vaccine-toxoid	Zagreb Institute for Immunology	Croatia	
Diphtheria-tetanus-poliovirus vaccine-toxoid (for pediatric use)	Sanofi Pasteur	France	*D.T. Polio, Dultavax, Revaxis*
Diphtheria-tetanus-poliovirus vaccine	Sanofi Pasteur	Europe	*Diftavax*
Diphtheria-tetanus-rubella vaccine-toxoid (for adult use)	Sanofi Pasteur	France	*D.T. Bis Rudivax*
Diphtheria-tetanus-typhoid-paratyphoid A & B	Sanofi Pasteur	Europe	*DT-TAB*
Diphtheria-tetanus-whole-cell pertussis-IPV-Hib	Sanofi Pasteur	Canada, Europe	*Penta, Pentacoq, PentActHib*
Diphtheria-tetanus-whole-cell pertussis-poliovirus vaccine-toxoid	Sanofi Pasteur	Europe	*Tetracoq, TETRAct-HIB*
	Berna Biotech	Switzerland	*Di Te Per Pol Impf-stoff*
Diphtheria toxoid (25 Lf units/dose)	Sanofi Pasteur	Canada	
Dysentery lysate	Bioclon	Mexico	*Disenterolisin*
Eastern & western encephalomyelitis vaccine	Ivanovskij Institute	Russia	
Encephalomyelitis aviar vaccine	Labiofam	Cuba	
Encephalomyocarditis vaccine	Labiofam	Cuba	
Gonococcus vaccine	Biomed	Russia	
Haemophilus influenzae type b-Meningococcal serogroup C conjugate vaccine	GlaxoSmithKline	Europe	*Menitorix*
Haemophilus influenzae type b-Meningococcal serogroups C and Y, with tetanus toxoid-conjugate	GlaxoSmithKline	Europe	*MenHibrix*
Hemorrhagic fever with renal syndrome vaccine	Green Cross	Korea	
Hepatitis A-typhoid vaccine	GlaxoSmithKline	Europe	*Hepatyrix*
Hepatitis A-typhoid Vi vaccine	Sanofi Pasteur	Europe, Mexico	*Viatim, Vivaxim*
Hepatitis A vaccine, live	Chongqing Zhifei	China	*Donggan Jiaxing Ganyan Jiandu Huoyimiao*
Hepatitis B, diphtheria, tetanus vaccine (for infant use)	Sanofi Pasteur	Europe	*Primavax*

Vaccines			
Generic contents	Manufacturer	Region	Proprietary or common name
Herpes simplex virus type 1 vaccine, inactivated	Hermal	Europe	*Lupidon G*
Herpes simplex virus type 2 vaccine, inactivated	Hermal	Europe	*Lupidon H*
Herpes virus vaccine, types 1 & 2	MA-Research Institute of Infectious & Parasitic Diseases	Bulgaria	
Lactobacillus acidophilus vaccine	Solco	Europe	*Ginatren, Gynatren, SolcoTrichovac*
Leptospira vaccine	Sanofi Pasteur	France	*Leptospires ictero-haemorrhagiae*
Leptospira vaccine	Finlay Vacunas & Sueros	Cuba	*Vax-spiral*
Leptospira vaccine	Ism	Italy	*Leptospires interrogans*
Leptospira vaccine (Weil disease & Akiaymi)	Denka Seiken	Japan	
Lungworm vaccine	Allen & Hanbury's	United Kingdom	*Dictol*
Measles-mumps vaccine (E-Zagreb/L-Zagreb, CEF strains)	Institute of Immunology	Croatia	*Vamoavax*
Meningococcal B & C vaccine	Finlay Vacunas & Sueros	Cuba	*Va-Mengoc-BC*
Meningococcal serogroup A vaccine, with tetanus toxoid-conjugate	Serum Institute of India	Africa	*MenAfriVax*
Meningococcal serogroup B, New Zealand strain outer membrane vesicle vaccine	Novartis	New Zealand	*MeNZB*
Plague vaccine, live	Central Asiatic Research Institute for Plague Control	Kazakhstan	
Plague vaccine, live	Stravropol Research Antiplague Institute	Russia	
Pneumococcal and nontypable *Haemophilus influenzae* vaccines	GlaxoSmithKline	Europe	*Synflorix*
Pseudomonas aeruginosa vaccine	Argentina Quimica	Argentina	*Etiopax*
Pseudomonas aeruginosa vaccine	Biomed	Poland	*Pseudovac*
Pseudomonas vaccine	Sevac	Czech Republic	*Psaeva*
Q fever vaccine	CSL Limited	Australia	*Q-Vax*
Rickettsia rickettsii vaccine (Rocky Mountain spotted fever)	Butantan	Brazil	*Vacina Contra a Febre Maculosa*
Rotavirus vaccine (attenuated human virus strain G1)	GlaxoSmithKline	Mexico, Latin America	*Rotarix*
Smallpox (modified Vaccinia Ankara)	Bavarian Nordic	Europe	*Ivamune*
Staphylococcus toxoid	Butantan	Brazil	*Anatoxina Estafilocócica*
	Sevac	Czech Republic	*Polystafana*
Staphylococcus vaccine	Instituto Biológico Argentino (BIOL)	South America	*Stavacin*

Vaccines			
Generic contents	Manufacturer	Region	Proprietary or common name
Staphylococcus vaccine & toxoid	Sanofi Pasteur	France	*Divasta*
	Crucell	Switzerland	*Staphypan Berna*
Tetanus-diphtheria-acellular pertussis-IPV (adult use)	GlaxoSmithKline	Europe	*Boostrix Polio*
Tetanus-diphtheria-IPV (adult use)	Sanofi Pasteur	Canada	*Td-Polio*
	Sanofi Pasteur	Europe	*Dultavax, Revaxis*
Tetanus-influenza vaccine	Sanofi Pasteur	France	*Tetagrip* (composition changes annually)
Tetanus-poliovirus vaccine-toxoid	Sanofi Pasteur	Canada	T. Polio
Tick-borne encephalitis vaccine	Novartis	Europe	*Encepur, FSME-Vaccine*
	Baxter	Europe	*FSME-Immun, Ticovac*
Tularemia vaccine	Omsk Bacteriological Preparations Company	Russia	
Typhoid-paratyphoid A & B vaccine	Ism	Italy	*Vimona*
	Novartis	Italy	*Typhidrall*
Typhoid-paratyphoid A, B, & C vaccine	Perum Bio Farma	Indonesia	*Vakcin Tipa*
Typhoid-tetanus vaccine	Isi	Italy	*Vaccini Tab Te*
	Zagreb Institute for Immunology	Europe	
Typhoid-tetanus-paratyphoid A & B vaccine	Institute of Immunology & Virology Torlak	Yugoslavia (sic)	
Typhus E vaccine	Biomed	Russia	
Venezuelan encephalomyelitis vaccine	Ivanovskij Institut	Russia	

Individual Stock Bacterial Vaccines			
Generic contents	Manufacturer	Region	Proprietary or common name
Bacillus M.U. 345	Sanum-Kehlbeck	Germany	*Utilin*
Bacillus Sa. C 501	Sanum-Kehlbeck	Germany	*Recarcin*
Bacillus subtilis lysate	Germania Apotheke	Austria	*Immunergon*
	Sanum-Kehlbeck	Germany	*Latensin*
	Biotest	Germany	*Subtivaccin*
Escherichia coli	Symbiopharm	Germany	*Symbioflor-Antigen*
Mycobacterium phlei F.U. 36	Sanum-Kehlbeck	Germany	*Utilin S*
Streptococcus faecalis	Symbiopharm	Germany	*Symbioflor 1*

Mixed Stock Bacterial Vaccines			
Generic contents	Manufacturer	Region	Proprietary or common name
	Millot-Solac	France	*Ampho-Vaccin*
	Crucell	Italy	*Annexine Berna*
	Bruschetti	Italy	*Apiocolina*
	Reuffer	Mexico	*Biocord*
	Cassenne	France	*Biostim*
	Crucell	Europe	*Broncasma Berna*
	Byk Gulden	Europe	*Broncho-Vaxom*
	Crucell	Europe	*Buccalin*
	Bouty	Italy	*Carbotiol*
	Abc-To	Italy	*Colifagina*
	Scharper	Italy	*Colopten*
	Bouty	Italy	*Dentovac*
	Lipha	Switzerland	*Diribiotin CK*
	Bioclón	Mexico	*Disenterolisin*
	Crucell	Italy	*Duplovac*
	Bioclón	Mexico	*Enterocolisin*
	Southon-Horton	United Kingdom	*Esobactulin*
	Labs Fournier	France	*Imocur* (polyvalent bacteria)
	Sarbach	France	*Imudon*
	Hefa-Frenon	Europe	*I.R.S. 19*
Various complex mixtures	Crucell	Italy	*Katar Berna*
	Ashe	Europe	*Lantigen B*
	Disprovent	Argentina	*Larcoral*
	Lifepharma	Italy	*Liobifar*
	Lisapharma	Italy	*Lisenteral*
	Omega	Canada	*Megavac*
	Hermanl	Germany	*Omnadin*
	Byk Gulden-Luitpold	Australia, Europe, Mexico	*Paspat*
	Crucell	Italy	*Pethic Berna*
	Rudefsa	Mexico	*Pulmonar OM*
	Debat	France	*Rhinopten*
	Sauba	France	*Rhinovac*
	Inava	Europe	*Ribomunyl*
	Solco	Europe	*SolcoUrovac*
	Stallergènes	France	*Stallergènes MRV*
	Crucell	Europe	*Staphypan Berna*
	Cassenne	France	*Stimugene*
	Midy	Europe	*Uro-Vaxom*
	Pharmuka	France	*Vaccin Antipyogene Bruschettini*
	Sanofi Pasteur	France	*Vaccine CCB*
	Bouty	Italy	*Vaxitiol*

Immune Globulins			
Generic contents	Manufacturer	Region	Proprietary or common name
Anthrax antiserum	MA-Research Institute of Infectious & Parasitic Diseases	Bulgaria	
Antiallergic IgG	Association Nationale	France	*Allergama*
	Landerlan	Spain	*Lergiabul*
	Sanofi Pasteur	Argentina	*Alergamma*
	Sanofi Pasteur	France	*Allerglobuline*
	Sidus	Brazil	*Afilaxina*
Antiendotoxin IgM antibodies	Centocor	Europe	HA-1A, *Centoxin*
Candida albicans equine IgG suppository	Gibipharma	Italy	*Anti-Candida*
Diphtheria immune globulin, human	Crucell	Switzerland	*Diphuman*
Frühsommer-Meningoenzephalitis immune globulin	Baxter, Behring	Europe	*FSME-Bulin*
	Novartis	Europe	*Encegam*
Gas-gangrene antitoxin	Bharat Serums & Vaccines	Asia	AGGS
	Butantan	Brazil	*Soro Antigangrenoso*
	Czech Institute of Sera & Vaccines	Czech Republic	*Gasea*
	Novartis	Germany	*Gasbrand-Antitoxin*
IgA, oral	Baxter	Europe	*IgAbulin*
IgA-IgG, oral	Baxter	Austria	*IgAbulin*
IgA-IgG-IgM, IM	CHI	France	*IgGAM*
IgA-IgG-IgM, IV	Biotest	Germany	*Pentaglobulin*
IgG-IgM, IM	Novartis	Germany	*Gamma-M-Konzentrat*
IgG from horses primed with cartilage & parathyroid	Labs Morrith	Spain	*Artroglobina*
IgG from horses primed with embryonic extract	Labs Morrith	Spain	*Embrioglobina*
IgG from horses primed with histamine	Labs Morrith	Spain	*Femiglobina*
IgG with histamine	Bharat Serums & Vaccines	Asia	*Histoglob*
	Chinoin	Italy	*Istaglobina*
	Kaken	Japan	*Linovin*
	Promedica	France	*Histoglobine*
Measles immune globulin	Crucell	Europe	*Moruman*
	Farmabiagini	Italy	*Morbilgamma*
	Baxter	Europe	*Morbulin*
	Novartis	Italy	*Imgorbillo*

Immune Globulins			
Generic contents	Manufacturer	Region	Proprietary or common name
Mumps immune globulin	Aima	Italy	*Haimaparot*
	Crucell	Europe	*Mumaten*
	Crucell	Europe	*Paruman*
	Farmabiagini	Italy	*Pargamma*
	Baxter	Germany	*Mumps immunoglobulin*
	Isi	Italy	*Immunoparot*
	Landerlan	Spain	*Paperbulina*
	Novartis	Italy	*Igparotite*
Pertussis immune globulin	Aima	Italy	*Haimapertus*
	Association Nationale	France	*GammaCOQ*
	Novartis	Germany	*Tussoglobin*
	Crucell	Europe	*Tosuman*
	Farmabiagini	Italy	*Pertus-Gamma*
	Isi	Italy	*Immunopertox*
	Ism	Italy	*Pertoglobulin*
	PMC	France	*Serocoq*
	Novartis	Italy	*Igpertosse*
Pseudomonas immune globulin	Tropon-Cutter	Germany	*Psomaglobin*
Rabies immune globulin equine F(ab')2	Sanofi Pasteur	Asia	*Favirab*
Rh$_o$(D)-neutralizing monoclonal antibody (IgG1 human-mouse)	Bharat Serums & Vaccines	Asia	*Rhoclone*
Rubella immune globulin	Novartis	Germany	*Röteln-Immunoglobulins*
	Crucell	Europe	*Rubeuman*
	Farmabiagini	Italy	*Rosol-Gamma*
	Baxter	Brazil	*Rubeolabulin*
	Baxter	Europe	*Rubellabulin*
	Isi	Italy	*Immunoros*
	Novartis	Italy	*Igrosolia*
Staphylococcus aureus & *Streptococcus pyogenes* equine IgG suppository	Gibipharma	Italy	*Anti-Piogeni*
Zoster immune globulin	CSL Limited	Australia	

Immunodiagnostics			
Generic contents	Manufacturer	Region	Proprietary or common name
Battery Antigen (PPD-B) (*Mycobacterium intracellulare*)	Connaught	Canada	
Brucellosis skin test reagent	Sanofi Pasteur	France	*Test Brucellique PS*
Mallein	Institut d'Etat	Iran	
PPD tuberculin patch test, normal strength (10 units)	Sanofi Pasteur	France	*Neotest Normal*
PPD tuberculin patch test, higher strength (50 units)	Sanofi Pasteur	France	*Neotest Fort*
Tuberculin ointment	Fresenius	Germany	*Perkutan-Tuberculin-Salbe "S"*

Immunologic Mediators			
Generic contents	Manufacturer	Region	Proprietary or common name
Celmoleukin (Interleukin-2 recombinant)	Takeda	Asia	*Celeuk*
Interferon alfa (ointment, ophthalmic, & vaginal doseforms)	Zagreb Institute for Immunology	Croatia	
Interferon beta	Rentschler	Germany	*Fiblaferon 3,4,5, I.V.*
	Novartis	Italy	*Naferon*
	Serono	Italy	*Frone*
	Toray	Japan	*Feron*
	Yamanochi	Japan	*Cibian*
Lenograstim	Unknown	Europe	*Granocyte, Neutrogin*
Molgramostim	Unknown	Germany	*Leucomax*
Transfer factor	Sevac	Czech Republic	

Other Immunologic Drugs			
Generic contents	Manufacturer	Region	Proprietary or common name
Allergen extract, preseasonal	ALK-Abelló	Europe	*ALK7*
Allergen extracts, sublingual	ALK-Abelló	Europe	*Pangramin SLIT*
	Stallergenes	Europe	*Oralair*
Corynebacterium parvum immunostimulant	Sanofi Pasteur	Europe	*Coparvax*
Inosiplex	Several	Canada, Europe	*Aviral, Isoprinosin, Delimmun, Imunovir, Modimmunal, Virustop*
Neisseria perflavia lysate	LTM	Europe	*Ducton*
Thymopentin	Cilag	Germany	*Timunox*
	Italfarmco	Italy	*Sintomodulina*
Thymostimulin	Serono	Europe	*TP-1*

Unique Vaccines & Immunologic Drugs Not Available Within the US

Combination Products			
Generic contents	Manufacturer	Region	Proprietary or common name
Ampicillin with IgG	Algonga	Spain	*Pleoampicilin*
Bacterial antigens & IgG	Instituto Massone	Brazil	*Mucogamm-A-11 Compuesto*
Chloramphenicol, streptomycin, betamethasone, IgG	Prem	Spain	*Tumisan Globulina*
Chloramphenicol with IgG in a collyrium	Labs H. Faure	France	*Gammaphenicol*
IgG, ampicillin, & streptomycin	Castillon	Spain	*Gammaproin*
IgG & interferon	Bernabo	Brazil	*Immunogamma 5*
IgG, histamine, serotonin	Crinos	Italy	*Trilergan*
Secretory IgA & interferon	Cassara	Brazil	*A-Virostat*

References: Citations on preceding pages were derived from multiple sources, including the following:

Australia's *Immunisation Procedures Handbook*; Britain's *Immunisation Against Infectious Diseases*; Canada's *Compendium of Pharmaeuticals and Specialties* and *Canadian Immunization Guide*; France's *Dictionnaire Vidal*; Germany's *Rote Liste*; Italy's *L'Informatore Farmaceutica*; Mexico's *Diccionario de Especialidades Farmaceuticas-PLM*; Switzerland's *Arzneimittel Kompendium der Sweiz*; Muller's *European Drug Index, Martindale: The Extra Pharmacopoeia*; Schlesser's *Drugs Available Abroad, Unlisted Drugs Index - Guide 9*; the World Health Organization's *International List of Availability of Vaccines*; Geneva, February 1996, the *World Pharmaceutical Directory*; and various product catalogs and product information provided by manufacturers.

Pertinent journal articles include: Shirk MB, et al. Obtaining drugs from foreign markets. *Am J Hosp Pharm.* 1992;49:2731-2739.

Generic Names: Generic names do not always translate predictably into other languages. A partial glossary of immunologic synonyms in a few languages is provided in the international glossary in this section. This glossary is admittedly biased toward languages of European origin (in contrast with complex Asian characters), but still provides useful information. Readers aware of additional synonyms in these or other languages are invited to share them. For languages that do not use the Roman alphabet, phonetic spellings will be needed.

Take care with abbreviations, too. In France and in French-speaking Canada, DTP refers to the "vaccin diphtérique-tétanique-poliomyélitique." Our own combination of diphtheria and tetanus toxoids with pertussis vaccine is abbreviated DCT there. Similarly, MMR would translate into Spanish or Portuguese as SPR (Sarampión-parotiditis-Rubéola in Español) and ROR in French (Rougeole-Oreillons-Rubéole).

In the United Kingdom and to a lesser extent in other parts of the British Commonwealth, a series of common abbreviations has been adopted to describe vaccines and immune globulins. For example, DTPer/Vac/Ads refers to the adsorbed vaccine that immunizes against diphtheria, tetanus, and pertussis. Vaccinia (smallpox) vaccine is abbreviated Var/Vac, referring to variola vaccine, not to varicella. Tet/Vac/FT is the term for the fluid toxoid of tetanus, while Pol/Vac/Oral refers to the oral poliovirus vaccine.

References: Perry WLM, et al. Abbreviated titles for serologic products. *BMJ.* 1956;2:38-40, reprinted in *Bull Am Soc Hosp Pharm.* 1956;13:576-578.

Canadian Immunologic Drugs [Index du Médicament Canadian]: Additional products beyond those described here may also be available. Information about current product availability in other nations is inevitably delayed and may not be reflected here. Contact local health departments, pharmacies, manufacturers, and other suppliers for details.

Bacterial Vaccines & Toxoids			
Product [French translation]	Manufacturer	Proprietary name	Comment
Bacillus Calmette-Guérin (BCG) vaccine [Vaccin BCG]	Sanofi Pasteur		Intradermal, Connaught strain, 8 to 30 × 10⁵ CFU/0.1 mL dose
Cholera & typhoid vaccine [Vaccin vivant typhi Ty21a; cholérique CVD 103-HgR]	Berna	*Colertif*	Oral; CVD 103-HgR, Ty21a strains
Cholera vaccine [Vaccin anticholérique]	Sanofi Pasteur (Curcell)	*Dukoral*	Oral, inactivated (with ETEC labile toxin)
	Berna	*Mutachol*	Oral vaccine (CVD 103-HgR)
Diphtheria & tetanus toxoids, pediatric (DT) [Anatoxines diphtérique et tétanique adsorbées (DT)]	Sanofi Pasteur		D25/T5 Lf/0.5 mL adsorbed, pediatric
Diphtheria & tetanus toxoids with acellular (component) pertussis vaccine (DTaP) [Vaccin anticoquelucheux, anatoxines diphtérique et tétanique adsorbées (CPDT)]	Sanofi Pasteur	*Tripacel*	D15/T5/P20/0.5 mL adsorbed, pediatric
	GlaxoSmithKline	*Infanrix*	
Diphtheria & tetanus toxoids with pertussis & conjugated *Haemophilus influenzae* type b vaccines (DTP-Hib) [Anatoxines diphtérique et tétanique et vaccins anticoquelucheux et conjugué contre *Haemophilus* b (DTP-Hib ou DCT-Hib)]	Sanofi Pasteur	*ACTacel*	Hybrid, ActHIB/DTP
Haemophilus influenzae type b (Hib) vaccine [Vaccin conjugué contre *Haemophilus* b]	Sanofi Pasteur	*ActHIB*	Tetanus toxoid conjugate
	GlaxoSmithKline	*Hiberix*	Tetanus toxoid conjugate
	Merck Frosst	*PedvaxHIB*	Meningococcal OMP conjugate

Bacterial Vaccines & Toxoids			
Product [French translation]	Manufacturer	Proprietary name	Comment
Haemophilus influenzae type b (Hib) vaccine reconstituted with DTcP vaccine [Vaccin conjugué contre l'*haemophilus* b (Hib), reconstitué avec un composant du vaccin anticoquelucheux combiné, anatoxines diphtérique et tétanique adsorbées (CPDT)]	Sanofi Pasteur	*Actacel* (classic or hybrid)	Hib-20 mcg, D15/T5/P20/ 0.5 mL adsorbed, pediatric
	GlaxoSmithKline	*Infanrix HIB*	
Meningococcal group C conjugate vaccine [Vaccin conjugué meningo-coccique]	Merck Frosst, Novartis	*Menjugate*	Diphtheria CRM$_{197}$ conjugate
	Shire Biologics	*NeisVac-C*	Tetanus toxoid conjugate
	Wyeth Canada	*Meningitec*	Diphtheria CRM$_{197}$ conjugate
Meningococcal groups A, C vaccine [Vaccin polysaccharidique meningococcique]	Sanofi Pasteur	*Menomune A/C*	Polysaccharide
	GlaxoSmithKline	*Mencevax AC*	Polysaccharide
Meningococcal groups A, C, Y, W-135 vaccine [Vaccin polysaccharidique meningoccocique]	Sanofi Pasteur	*Menomune A/C/Y/W-135*	A/C/Y/W-135
Meningococcal groups A, C, Y, W-135 conjugate vaccine [Vaccin conjugué meningo-coccique groups A, C, Y, W-135]	Sanofi Pasteur	*Menactra*	Diphtheria toxoid conjugate vaccine
	Novartis	*Menveo*	A/C/Y/W-135
Pertussis vaccine, acellular (component) [Vaccin anticoquelucheux]	Sanofi Pasteur		
Pneumococcal conjugate vaccine, 7-valent [Saccharides capsulaires de *S. pneumoniae*]	Pfizer	*Prevnar*	
Pneumococcal conjugate vaccine, 13-valent [Saccharides capsulaires de *S. pneumoniae*]	Pfizer	*Prevnar 13*	
Pneumococcal conjugate vaccine, 10-valent [Saccharides capsulaires de *S. pneumoniae*, sérotypes 1, 4, 5, 6B, 7F, 9V, 14, 18C, 19F, et 23F]	GlaxoSmithKline	*Synflorix*	Conjugated to protein D carrier
Pneumococcal vaccine, 23-valent [Vaccin polyvalent pneumo-coccique polysaccharidique]	Merck Frosst	*Pneumovax 23*	
	Sanofi Pasteur	*Pneumo 23*	

Bacterial Vaccines & Toxoids			
Product [French translation]	Manufacturer	Proprietary name	Comment
Tetanus & diphtheria toxoids, adult (Td) [Anatoxines tétanique diphtérique adsorbées (Td)]	Wyeth Canada		
Tetanus & diphtheria toxoids and acellular pertussis (Tdap) [Anatoxines tétanique diphtérique adsorbées et vaccin anticoquelucheux component]	GlaxoSmithKline	*Boostrix*	d2/T20/P8–8–2.5/0.5 mL adsorbed, age > 7 years
	Sanofi Pasteur	*Adacel*	D2/T5/P15.5/0.5 mL adsorbed, pediatric
Tetanus toxoid adsorbed (TT) [Anatoxine tétanique adsorbée]	Sanofi Pasteur		T5 Lf/0.5 mL adsorbed
Typhoid vaccine, oral [Vaccin antityphoïdique oral atténué Ty21a]	Berna	*Vivotif Berna L*	Attenuated, Ty-21a strain; capsules or oral sachets
Typhoid Vi capsular polysaccharide vaccine (parenteral, inactivated) [Vaccin polysaccharidique capsulaire Vi *Salmonella typhi*]	Sanofi Pasteur	*Typhim Vi*	Polysaccharide vaccine
	GlaxoSmithKline	*Typherix*	25 mcg/0.5 mL

Combined Bacterial & Viral Vaccines & Toxoids			
Product [French translation]	Manufacturer	Proprietary name	Comment
Diphtheria & tetanus toxoids with component pertussis vaccine, combined with hepatitis B surface antigen and inactivated poliovirus [Anatoxines diphtérique et tétanique et vaccin anticoquelucheux adsorbés (cellulaire), hépatite B, et antipoliomyélitique inactivé]	GlaxoSmithKline	*Pediarix*	
Diphtheria & tetanus toxoids with component pertussis vaccine, combined with inactivated poliomyelitis [Vaccin anti poliomyélite adsorbée, inactivé, anatoxines diphtérique et tétanique adsorbée, vaccin anticoquelucheux adsorbée]	Sanofi Pasteur	*Quadracel*	D15/T5/Pert20/Pol40-8-32/0.5 mL
	GlaxoSmithKline	*Infanrix IPV*	

Combined Bacterial & Viral Vaccines & Toxoids			
Product [French translation]	Manufacturer	Proprietary name	Comment
Diphtheria & tetanus toxoids with component pertussis vaccine, combined with inactivated poliomyelitis & Hib conjugate vaccines [Vaccin anticoquelucheux combiné et anatoxines diphtérique et tétanique adsorbées et combinées au vaccin anti-poliomyélitique inactivé et vaccin conjugué contre *Haemophilus* b]	GlaxoSmithKline	*Infanrix IPV/Hib*	
	Sanofi Pasteur	*Pediacel*	
Diphtheria & tetanus toxoids with component pertussis vaccine, combined with inactivated poliovirus, Hib, and hepatitis B vaccines [Anatoxine diphthérique, anatoxine tétanique, anatoxine coquelucheuse, hémagglutinine filamenteuse, pertactine, antigéne de contact de l'hépatite B, poliovirus de type I, II, et III inactivé, PRP d'haemophilus influenzae type B]	GlaxoSmithKline	*Infanrix Hexa*	
Diphtheria & tetanus toxoids with inactivated poliovirus vaccine adsorbed (DT-Polio) [Anatoxines diphtérique et tétanique et vaccin antipoliomyélitique inactivé adsorbées (DT-Polio)]	Sanofi Pasteur		D25/T5 Lf/0.5 mL adsorbed, pediatric
Diphtheria & tetanus toxoids with pertussis, poliovirus, & conjugated *Haemophilus influenzae* type b vaccines (DTaP-Polio-Hib) [Anatoxines diphtérique et tétanique et vaccins anticoquelucheux, antipoliomyélitique inactivé, et conjugué contre *Haemophilus* b (DTaP-Polio-Hib ou DCT-Polio-Hib)]	Sanofi Pasteur	*Pentacel*	
Hepatitis A and typhoid Vi polysaccharide vaccine [Vaccin de l'hépatite A et polysaccharidique capsulaire Vi Salmonella typhi]	Sanofi Pasteur	*Vivaxim*	

Combined Bacterial & Viral Vaccines & Toxoids			
Product [French translation]	Manufacturer	Proprietary name	Comment
Tetanus and diphtheria toxoids with component pertussis vaccine, combined with inactivated poliovirus vaccine [Anatoxine tétanique, anatoxine diphtérique, anatoxine coquelucheuse, hémagglutinine filamenteuse, pertactine, poliovirus de type I, II, et III inactivé adsorbées (Tdap-Polio)]	GlaxoSmithKline	*Boostrix-Polio*	
	Sanofi Pasteur	*Adacel-Polio*	
Tetanus and diphtheria toxoids with inactivated poliovirus vaccine adsorbed (Td-Polio) [Anatoxine tétanique et diphtériqe et vaccin antipoliomyélitique inactivé adsorbées (Td-Polio)]	Sanofi Pasteur	Td Polio Adsorbed	

Viral Vaccines			
Product [French translation]	Manufacturer	Proprietary name	Comment
Hepatitis A vaccine (HAV) [Vaccin de l'hépatite A]	Sanofi Pasteur	*Avaxim*	160 units/0.5 mL
			80 units/0.5 mL
	Crucell	*Epaxal*	500 units/0.5 mL
	GlaxoSmithKline	*Havrix 1440*	1,440 units/mL
		Havrix 720 Jr.	720 units/mL
	Merck Frosst	*Vaqta*	50 units/mL
Hepatitis A & hepatitis B vaccine [Vaccin bivalent contre l'hépatite A et l'hépatite B]	GlaxoSmithKline	*Twinrix*	720 units/20 mcg/mL
		Twinrix Junior	360 units/10 mcg/mL
Hepatitis B vaccine (HBV) [Vaccin de l'hépatite B]	Merck Frosst	*Recombivax HB*	10 mcg/mL, 40 mcg/mL (dialysis)
	GlaxoSmithKline	*Engerix-B*	20 mcg/mL
Human papillomavirus bivalent (types 16, 18) recombinant vaccine [Vaccin recombinant bivalent contre le virus du papillome humain (types 16 et 18)]	GlaxoSmithKline	*Ceravix*	Recombinant viral L1 proteins
Human papillomavirus quadrivalent (types 6, 11, 16, 18) recombinant vaccine [Vaaccin recombinant quadrivalent contre le virus du papillome humain (types 6, 11, 16 et 18)]	Merck Frosst	*Gardasil*	Recombinant viral L1 proteins

Viral Vaccines			
Product [French translation]	Manufacturer	Proprietary name	Comment
Influenza A & B vaccine [Vaccin viral contre la grippe ou vaccin grippal]	Sanofi Pasteur	*Fluzone, Vaxigrip*	Split or whole virus
	GlaxoSmithKline	*Fluviral S/F*	Split or whole virus
	Solvay Pharma	*Influvac*	
	Sanofi Pasteur	*Intanza*	Intradermal
Influenza A & B vaccine, intranasal [Vaccin anti-grippal (vivant, atténué) vaporisateur nasal]	AstraZeneca Canada	*FluMist*	
Japanese encephalitis vaccine [Vaccin contre encephalitis Japonique]	Intercell	*Ixiaro*	
Measles-mumps-rubella vaccine [Virus vivant de la rubé-ole, des oreillons, et de la rougeole atténuée]	Merck Frosst	*M-M-R II*	Moraten, Jeryl Lynn, RA 27/3 strains
	GlaxoSmithKline	*Priorix*	Schwarz, RIT 4385, and RA 27/3 strains
Measles-mumps-rubella-varicella vaccine [Virus vivant de la rubé-ole, des oreillons, de la rougeole, et de la varicella atténuée]	GlaxoSmithKline	*Priorix-Tetra*	Schwarz, Jeryl Lynn, RA 27/3, Oka strains
Measles-rubella vaccine [Vaccin antirougeoleux et antirubéoleux]	Sanofi Pasteur	*Rudi-Rouvax*	
	GlaxoSmithKline	*Eolarix*	
Poliovirus vaccine, inactivated [Vaccin antipoliomyéli-tique inactivé]	Sanofi Pasteur	*Imovax Polio*	Vero cell culture
	Sanofi Pasteur	generic	Human diploid cell culture
Rabies vaccine [Vaccin antirabique inactivé]	Novartis, Merck Frosst	*RabAvert*	Chick embryonic fibro-blasts
	Sanofi Pasteur	*Imovax Rabies*	Human diploid cell culture
Rotavirus vaccine, live, oral, monovalent [Vaccin monovalent oral à virus vivant contre le rota-virus]	GlaxoSmithKline	*Rotarix*	Type G1P[8], RIX4414 strain
Rotavirus vaccine, live, oral, pentavalent [Vaccin pentavalent oral à virus vivant contre le rota-virus]	Merck Frosst Canada	*RotaTeq*	Types G1, G2, G3, G4, P1[8]

Viral Vaccines			
Product [French translation]	Manufacturer	Proprietary name	Comment
Tick-borne encephalitis vaccine inactivated [Vaccin contre le virus de l'encéphalite à tiques (inactivé)]	Baxter Corporation	*FSME-Immun*	2.4 mcg/0.5 mL
Vaccinia (smallpox) vaccine [Vaccin antivariolique]	Sanofi Pasteur		Available only from Canadian LCDC
Varicella vaccine [Vaccin á virus vivant, atténué, contre la varicella]	GlaxoSmithKline	*Varilrix*	2,000 units/0.5 mL
	Merck Frosst Canada	*Varivax III*	1,350 units/0.5 mL, stored in refrigerator
Yellow fever vaccine [Vaccin contre la fiévre jaune]	Sanofi Pasteur	*YF-Vax*	
Zoster vaccine live [Vaccin vivant atténué contre le virus varicelle-zona]	Merck Frosst Canada	*Zostavax*	

Broad-Spectrum Immune Globulins			
Product [French translation]	Manufacturer	Proprietary name	Comment
Immune globulin IM (IGIM) [Immunoglobulines poly-valentes humaines pour injection intramusculaire]	Sanofi Pasteur	*Imogam*	
	Talecris	*Gamastan S/D*	
Immune globulin IV (IGIV) [Immunoglobulines poly-valentes humaines pour injection intraveineuse]	Baxter	*Gammagard S/D*	
	CSL Behring Canada	*Privigen, Sando-globulin NF*	
	Octapharma Pharmazeutika	*Octagam*	
	Talecris	*Gamunex*	
	Talecris	*IGIVnex*	
Immune globulin subcutane-ous (IGSC) [Immunoglobulines poly-valentes humaines pour injection sous-cutaré]	CSL Behring Canada	*Vivaglobin*	

Anti-Infective Immune Globulins			
Product [French translation]	Manufacturer	Proprietary name	Comment
Cytomegalovirus immune globulin, IV [Cytomegalovirus immu-noglobuline IV (humaine)]	CSL Behring Canada	*CytoGam*	50 mg/mL
Hepatitis B immune globulin (HBIG) [Immunoglobulines humaines spécifiques anti-hépatite B]	Cangene	*HepaGam B*	Intravenous
	Talecris	*HyperHep B S/D*	
Palivizumab	Abbott Laboratories	*Synagis*	50 or 100 mg/vial
Pertussis immune globulin [Immunoglobulines humaines spécifiques anti-coqueluche]	Österreichisches Institut für Hämoderivate		
Rabies immune globulin (RIG) [Immunoglobulines humaines spécifiques anti-rabiques]	Sanofi Pasteur	*Imogam Rabies*	
	Talecris	*HyperRab S/D*	
Vaccinia immune globulin, IV [Immunoglobulines humaines spécifiques anti-vaccin-variole]	Cangene	CNJ-016	
Varicella-zoster immune globulin (VZIG) [Immunoglobuline intra-veineuse varicella (humaine)]	Cangene	*VariZIG*	125 units/vial

Immunoantidotes: Antitoxins			
Product [French translation]	Manufacturer	Proprietary name	Comment
Botulinum antitoxin (equine) [Antitoxine botulinique (équine)]	ZLB Behring		Trivalent Types ABE or Monovalent Type E
Diphtheria antitoxin (equine) [Antitoxine diphtérique (équine)]	ZLB Behring		
Tetanus immune globulin (TIG) [Immunoglobulines humaines spécifiques anti-tétanos]	Talecris	*HyperTet S/D*	
	Österréichisches Institut für Hämoderivate		
	Cangene		Tetanus plasma (human)

Immunoantidotes: Antivenins			
Product [French translation]	Manufacturer	Proprietary name	Comment
Antivenin *Latrodectus mactans* (black widow spider) (equine) [Antivenin *Latrodectus mactans* trousse]	Merck Frosst		

Isoantibodies: Erythrocytic			
Product [French translation]	Manufacturer	Proprietary name	Comment
$Rh_o(D)$ immune globulin (RhIG) [Immunoglobulines humaines spécifiques anti-D]	Cangene	*WinRho SDF*	IV infusion or IM
	Talecris	*HyperRho S/D Full Dose*	

Isoantibodies: Lymphocytic			
Product [French translation]	Manufacturer	Proprietary name	Comment
Antithymocyte globulin (ATG) [Immunoglobulines humaines spécifiques anti-lymphocytaire]	Pfizer Canada	*Atgam*	
Antithymocyte globulin (rabbit) [Globuline antithymocytes (lapin)]	Genzyme	*Thymoglobulin*	
Basiliximab	Novartis	*Simulect*	20 mg/vial
Daclizumab	Hoffmann-LaRoche	*Zenapax*	5 mg/mL
Muromonab-CD3 (OKT-3) [Muromonab CD3]	Janssen-Ortho	*Orthoclone OKT3*	

Isoantibodies: Other			
Product [French translation]	Manufacturer	Proprietary name	Comment
Abatacept	Bristol-Myers Squibb Canada	*Orencia*	250 mg/vial
Abciximab	Centocor	*ReoPro*	2 mg/mL
Adalimumab	Abbott Laboratories	*Humira*	40 mg per 0.8 mL
Alefacept	Astellas Pharma Canada	*Amevive*	
Alemtuzumab	Genzyme	*MabCampath*	30 mg/mL
Anakinra	Amgen Canada	*Kineret*	150 mg/mL
Bevacizumab	Hoffman-LaRoche	*Avastin*	25 mg/mL
Canakinumab	Novartis	*Ilaris*	150 mg/mL
Certolizumab pegol	Nektar Therapeutics and UCB	*Cimzia*	200 mg/vial
Cetuximab	ImClone Systems	*Erbitux*	2 mg/mL
Denosumab	Angen Canada	*Prolia*	60 mg/mL syringe
Eculizumab	Alexion Pharmaceuticals	*Soliris*	10 mg/mL
Efalizumab	Serono Canada	*Raptiva*	150 mg/vial
Etanercept	Immunex	*Enbrel*	25 mg/vial
Golimumab	Centocor	*Simponi*	50 mg per 0.5 mL
Infliximab	Centocor, Schering Canada	*Remicade*	100 mg/vial
Natalizumab	Biogen Idec Canada	*Tysabri*	300 mg per 15 mL
Omalizumab	Novartis Pharmaceuticals (Canada)	*Xolair*	150 mg/vial
Panitumumab	Amgen Canada	*Vectibix*	100 mg per 5 mL, 200 mg per 10 mL, 400 mg per 20 mL IV
Ranibizumab	Novartis Pharmaceuticals (Canada)	*Lucentis*	10 mg/mL
Rituximab	Hoffmann-LaRoche	*Rituxan*	10 mg/mL
Tocilizumab	Hoffmann-LaRoche	*Actemra*	20 mg/mL
Trastuzumab	Hoffmann-LaRoche	*Herceptin*	440 mg/vial
Ustekinumab	Janssen-Ortho	*Stelara*	90 mg/mL

Digoxin-Binding Antibodies			
Product [French translation]	Manufacturer	Proprietary name	Comment
Digoxin immune Fab (ovine) [Fragments d'anticorps spécifiques de la digoxine Fab (ovins)]	GlaxoSmithKline	*Digibind*	

Isoantibodies: Radiodiagnostic			
Product [French translation]	Manufacturer	Proprietary name	Comment
Capromab pendetide	Cytogen	*ProstaScint*	with In-111
Imciromab pentetate	Centocor	*Myoscint*	with 99m-Tc

Isoantibodies: Radiotherapeutic			
Product [French translation]	Manufacturer	Proprietary name	Comment
Ibritumomab tiuxetan	Bayer	*Zevalin*	
Satumomab pendetide	Hospira Healthcare Corporation	*Oncoscint CR/OV*	1 mg/vial
Tositumomab	GlaxoSmithKline	*Bexxar*	

Antibody-Mediated Allergens & Antigens: Allergen Extracts			
Product [French translation]	Manufacturer	Proprietary name	Comment
Aqueous & glycerinated doseforms [Extraits d'allergénes]	Allergy Laboratories		
	Western Allergy Services	*Pollinex*	
	Nelco Laboratories		
	Omega Laboratories		
	Pfizer	*Pharmalgen*	
Alum-precipitated doseforms	Western Allergy Services	*Pollinex, Center-AI*	
	Bayer	*Allpyral*	
Tyrosine-absorbed dose-forms	Western Allergy Services	*Pollinex R*	Ragweed extract (PNU)

Antibody-Mediated Allergens & Antigens: *Hymenoptera* Allergens			
Product [French translation]	Manufacturer	Proprietary name	Comment
Purified bee & vespid venoms [Extrait de protéine de venim]	Bayer	*Albay, Venomil*	
	ALK-Abelló	*Pharmalgen*	

Antibody-Mediated Allergens & Antigens: Other Antibody-Mediated Drugs			
Product [French translation]	Manufacturer	Proprietary name	Comment
Benzylpenicilloyl polylysine (BPL)	AllerQuest	*Pre-Pen*	

Index of Canadian Immunologic Drugs

T-Lymphocyte-Mediated Allergens: Mycobacterial Antigens			
Product [French translation]	Manufacturer	Proprietary name	Comment
Purified protein derivative (PPD) solution [Tuberculine dérivée de protéines Purifiées (PPD, mantoux, antigéne diag-nostique)]	Sanofi Pasteur	*Tubersol*	

T-Lymphocyte-Mediated Allergens: Ubiquitous Antigens			
Product [French translation]	Manufacturer	Proprietary name	Comment
Diphtheria toxoid [Anatoxine diphtérique]	Sanofi Pasteur		D 0.2 Lf/mL for reaction test
Tetanus toxoid, fluid (TT) [Anatoxine tétanique liq-uide]	Sanofi Pasteur		T10 Lf/mL

Immunologic Mediators: Colony-Stimulating Factors			
Product [French translation]	Manufacturer	Proprietary name	Comment
Ancestim stem-cell growth factor [Agent hématopoïétique]	Biovitrum	*Stemgen*	1,875 or 2,500 mcg/mL
Filgrastim	Amgen	*Neupogen*	300 mcg/mL
Molgramostim [Molgramostime]	Schering/Novartis	*Leucomax*	
Pegfilgrastim	Amgen Canada	*Neulasta*	10 mg/mL
Romiplostim	Amgen Canada	*Nplate*	500 mcg/mL
Sargramostim [Sargramostime]	Wyeth Canada	*Leukine*	

Immunologic Mediators: Interferons & Interleukins			
Product [French translation]	Manufacturer	Proprietary name	Comment
Aldesleukin [Aldesleukine]	Novartis Pharmaceuti-cals Canada	*Proleukin*	25 million units/vial
Interferon alfa-2a [Interféron alfa-2a]	Hoffmann-LaRoche Limited	*Roferon-A*	
Interferon alfa-2b [Interféron alfa-2b]	Schering Canada	*Intron A*	
Interferon alfa-n1 [Interféron alfa-n1]	Wellcome	*Wellferon*	
Interferon alfacon-1 [Interféron alfacon-1]	Three Rivers Pharma-ceuticals	*Infergen*	0.03 mg/mL
Interferon beta-1a [Interféron bêta-1a]	Biogen Canada	*Avonex*	
	Serono Canada	*Rebif*	

Immunologic Mediators: Interferons & Interleukins

Product [French translation]	Manufacturer	Proprietary name	Comment
Interferon beta-1b [Interféron bêta-1b]	Bayer	*Ferona*	
	Berlex Canada	*Betaseron*	
	Novartis	*Extavia*	
Peginterferon alfa-2a [Peginterféron alfa 2-a]	Hoffmann-LaRoche Limited	*Pegasys*	
Peginterferon alfa-2b [Peginterféron alfa 2-b]	Schering Canada	*PEG-Intron, Unitron Peg, Pegetron*	

Immunomodulators: Broad Immunostimulants

Product [French translation]	Manufacturer	Proprietary name	Comment
BCG therapeutic [BCG thérapeutique]	Sanofi Pasteur	*ImmuCyst*	Intravesical, Connaught strain 0.4 to 6.4×10^8 CFU per vial
	Organon Canada	*OncoTice*	800 million units/vial
	Shire Biologics	*Pacis*	120 mg/vial
Melanoma lysate [Fraction des allules de melanone]	Corixa Corporation	*Melacine*	Immunostimulating agent

Pertinent Nonimmunologic Drugs

Product [French translation]	Manufacturer	Proprietary name	Comment
Botulinum toxin type A [Toxine botulinique de type A]	Allergan	*Botox*	100 units/vial
	Merz Pharmaceuticals	*Xeomin*	100 units/vial
Botulinum toxin type B [Toxine botulinique de type B]	Solstice	*Myobloc*	
Epinephrine	Allerex	*EpiPen, EpiPen Jr.*	For Meridian Medical Technologies
	Monarch	*Adrenalin*	

References: Canadian Health Protection Branch. Notices of Compliance. http://www.hc-sc.gc.ca/hpfb-dgpsa/tpd-dpt/index_drugs_noc_e.html.

Canadian Pharmacists Association. *Compendium of Pharmaceuticals and Specialties (CPS)*, 39th ed. Ottawa: Canadian Pharmacists Association, 2004.

Public Health Agency of Canada. *Canadian Immunization Guide, 7th ed.* Ottawa: Public Health Agency of Canada, 2006. Erratum *Can Comm Dis Rep.* 2008;34(May):16-25. http://www.phac-aspc.gc.ca/publicat/cig-gci/index.html.

International Immunologic Drugs

Additional products beyond those described here may also be available. Information about current product availability in other nations is inevitably delayed and may not be reflected here. Contact local health departments, pharmacies, distributors, and other suppliers for details.

Bacterial Vaccines & Toxoids			
Product [Spanish translation]	Distributor	Proprietary name	Comment
BCG Vaccine [Vacuna BCG]	Birmex for Serum Institute of India		Danish substrain
	Organizacion de Reactivos, Biologicos e Immunologia		Danish substrain
	Laboratorios Imperiales for Japan BCG Laboratory	*Tuvax*	
	Sanofi Pasteur		
Cholera vaccine, oral, inactivated (with ETEC labile toxin) [Vacuna Atenuada Oral Contra El Cólera]	Sanofi Pasteur (Crucell)	*Dukoral*	
Diphtheria & tetanus toxoids with acellular pertussis vaccine (DTaP) [Vacuna contra difteria, tosferina (acelular), y tétanos, DPaT]	Sanofi Pasteur	*Triacel*	Pediatric strength
	GlaxoSmithKline	*Infanrix*	Pediatric strength
Diphtheria & tetanus toxoids with whole-cell pertussis vaccine (DTwP) [Vacuna antipertussis con toxoides difterico y tétanico, DPwT]	Laboratorios de Biologicos y Reactivos de Mexico (Birmex)		
	Laboratorios Imperiales	*ShanTrip*	Shantha Biotechnics
	Ivax Pharmaceuticals Mexico for Novartis	*Trenin DPT*	
	Sanofi Pasteur	*DPTvac*	
Diphtheria & tetanus toxoids with pertussis and *Haemophilus* vaccines (DTaP-Hib) [Vacuna contra difteria, tosferina, tétanos y *Haemophilus*, DTP-Hib]	Sanofi Pasteur	*Actacel*	Hib powder + DTaP diluent
Diphtheria & tetanus toxoids [Toxoides contra difteria y tétanos (DT)]	Various	Generic	

Bacterial Vaccines & Toxoids			
Product [Spanish translation]	Distributor	Proprietary name	Comment
Haemophilus influenzae type b (Hib) conjugated vaccine [Vacuna conjugada de *Haemophilus influenzae* tipo b (conjugada a la proteína)]	Sanofi Pasteur	*HIBest, ActHIB*	
	GlaxoSmithKline	*Hiberix*	
	MSD (Merck)	*PedvaxHIB*	
Meningococcal vaccine [Vacuna meningococcica]	Sanofi Pasteur	*Imovax Meningo A+C*	
	GlaxoSmithKline	*Mencevax AC*	
Meningococcal A/C/Y/W-135 conjugate vaccine [Vacuna antimeningocóccica de los serotipos A, C, Y, y W-135 conjugada a toxoide diftérico]	Sanofi Pasteur	*Menactra*	
Meningococcal C conjugate vaccine [Vacuna anti-meningocóccica del serotipo C conjugada a proteina diftérico	Baxter	*Neis-Vac C*	Tetanus conjugate
	Novartis	*Menjugate*	Diphtheria conjugate
Pneumococcal conjugate vaccine 7-valent [Vacuna antineumococcica conjugada con proteina 7-valente]	Pfizer	*Prevenar*	Diphtheria protein
Pneumococcal conjugate vaccine 10-valent [Vacuna antineumococcica conjugada con proteina 10-valente]	GlaxoSmithKline	*Synflorix*	Haemophilus D protein
Pneumococcal conjugate vaccine 13-valent [Vacuna antineumococcica conjugada con proteina 13-valente]	Pfizer	*Prevenar 13*	
Pneumococcal polysaccharide vaccine 23-valent [Vacuna antineumococcica polivalente]	MSD (Merck)	*Pulmovax*	
	Sanofi Pasteur	*Imovax Neumo 23*	
Tetanus & diphtheria toxoids (Td) [Vacuna contra tétanus y difteria, Td]	Birmex	Generic	
	Sanofi Pasteur	*Diftavax T*	
	Sanofi Pasteur	*Imovax DT Adulto*	

Bacterial Vaccines & Toxoids			
Product [Spanish translation]	Distributor	Proprietary name	Comment
Tetanus & diphtheria toxoids with acellular pertussis vaccine for adolescents and adults [Vacuna combinada contra tétanus, difteria, y tosferia acelular]	GlaxoSmithKline	*Boostrix*	
Tetanus toxoid adsorbed (TT) [Toxoide tetánico]	Sanofi Pasteur	*Tetanovac*	
		Tetanol	
	Bioclón	*Tetinox*	
		Toxoide Tetánico Myn	
	Gerencia General		
Typhoid Vi polysaccharide vaccine [Vacuna de polisacárido capsular Vi contra la fiebre tifoidea]	Sanofi Pasteur	*Tifovax, Typhim Vi*	
Typhoid oral, attenuated vaccine [Vacuna oral, atuenado contra la fiebre tifoidea]	Progela	*Zerotyph*	Boryung Biopharma, Korea
Typhoid whole-cell vaccine (subcutaneous) [Vacuna antitifoidica]	Gerencia General		

Viral Vaccines			
Product [Spanish translation]	Distributor	Proprietary name	Comment
Hepatitis A vaccine [Vacuna contra la hepatitis A]	Sanofi Pasteur	*Avaxim*	
	GlaxoSmithKline	*Havrix*	720 or 1,440 ELU
	Ivax Pharmaceuticals Mexico for Biken, Japan	*Nothav*	
	MSD (Merck)	*Vaqta*	
Hepatitis A & hepatitis B vaccine [Vacuna contra la hepatitis A y hepatitis B]	GlaxoSmithKline	*Twinrix*	

Viral Vaccines			
Product [Spanish translation]	Distributor	Proprietary name	Comment
Hepatitis B vaccine (HBV) [Vacuna contra hepatitis B]	Sanofi Pasteur	*Hepativax*	
	Berna Biotech	*Heprecomb*	
	GlaxoSmithKline	*Engerix-B*	
	Ivax Pharmaceuticals Mexico	*Viralinte*	
	Laboratorio Farma-cológico Nutrimedi for Heberbiotec, Cuba	*Heberbiovac HB*	
	Laboratorios Imperiales	*Shanvac-B*	Shantha Biotechnics
	Laboratorios Pisa for LG Life Sciences, Korea	*Euvax-B*	
	Laboratorios Pisa for Laboratorios Pablo Cas-sara, Argentina	*B-Vaxin*	
	MSD (Merck)	*H-B-Vax II*	
	Probiomed	*Probivac-B*	
	Grupo Carbel	*Hepavax-Gene*	
Human papillomavirus biva-lent (types 16, 18) recombi-nant vaccine [Vacuna contra el virus del pap-iloma humano (VPH) tipos 16 y 18]	GlaxoSmithKline	*Cervarix*	
Human papillomavirus quadrivalent (types 6, 11, 16, 18) recombinant vaccine [Vacuna contra el virus del papiloma humano (VPH) tipos 6, 11, 16, 18]	MSD Mexico	*Gardasil*	
Influenza vaccine [Vacuna contra gripe]	Birmex	*Inflexel Berna V*	
	GlaxoSmithKline	*Fluarix*	
	Ivax Pharmaceuticals for Novartis	*Agrippal S1*	
	Landsteiner	*Influvac*	
	Novartis	*Fluvirene*	
	Sanofi Pasteur	*Fluzone, Imovax Gripe, Vaxigrip*	
Influenza vaccine with adju-vant [Vacuna contra gripe con adyuvante]	Novartis	*FluAd*	MF59
Measles-mumps-rubella vaccine [Vacuna contra el sarampión, parotidis, y la rubéola (SRP)]	Berna Biotech	*Triviraten*	
	GlaxoSmithKline	*Priorix*	Schwarz, Urabe Am-3, & RA 27/3 strains
	Ivax Pharmaceuticals Mexico for Novartis	*Morupar*	
	MSD Mexico	*M-M-R II*	
	Sanofi Pasteur	*Trimovax, Trivivax*	

Viral Vaccines			
Product [Spanish translation]	Distributor	Proprietary name	Comment
Measles-rubella vaccine [Vacuna contra sarampión y rubéola]	Birmex for Berna Biotech	*MoRu-Viraten*	
	GlaxoSmithKline	*Pluserix*	
	Sanofi Pasteur	*Rudi-Rouvax*	
Measles-mumps-rubella-varicella vaccine (MMRV) [Vacuna contra sarampión, las paperas, rubéola, y varicea (SPRV)]	MSD (Merck)	*ProQuad*	
Measles vaccine [Vacuna contra sarampión]	Sanofi Pasteur	*Rouvax*	
	GlaxoSmithKline	*Rimevax*	Schwarz strain
Mumps vaccine [Vacuna contra parotidis]	GlaxoSmithKline	*Pariorix*	Urabe Am-3 strain
Poliovirus vaccine inactivated [Vacuna antipoliomielitica inactivada, IPV]	GlaxoSmithKline	*Ipoliorix*	
	Sanofi Pasteur	*Enpovax HDC*	
	Sanofi Pasteur	*Imovax Polio*	
Poliovirus vaccine, oral, attenuated (OPV) [Vacuna contra poliomyelitis]	GlaxoSmithKline	*Polio Sabin*	
	Laboratorios Imperiales for PT Biofarma, Indonesia	*Vopix*	
	Novartis	*Polioral*	
Rabies vaccine [Vacuna antirabica]	Teva for Novartis	*Rabipur, Rabivac*	
	Sanofi Pasteur	*Imovax Rabia Vero, Verorab*	
Rotavirus vaccine live oral pentavalent [Vacuna contra el rotavirus]	GlaxoSmithKline	*Rotarix*	G1P[8]
	MSD Mexico	*RotaTeq*	Types G1, G2, G3, G4, P1[8]
Rubella vaccine [Vacuna contra rubéola]	Sanofi Pasteur	*Imovax Rubéola*	
	Sanofi Pasteur	*Rudivax*	
	GlaxoSmithKline	*Ervevax*	RA 27/3 strain
Varicella vaccine [Vacuna contra varicela]	Sanofi Pasteur	*Okavax*	
	GlaxoSmithKline	*Varilrix*	
	MSD (Merck)	*Varivax III*	
Yellow fever vaccine [Vacuna contra la fiebre amarilla]	Sanofi Pasteur	*Stamaril*	

Combined Bacterial & Viral Vaccines			
Product [Spanish translation]	Distributor	Proprietary name	Comment
Diphtheria & tetanus toxoids with acellular pertussis vaccine, combined with inactivated poliomyelitis vaccine [Vacuna contra difteria, tosferina (acelular), tétanos y poliomielitis, DTaP-IPV]	GlaxoSmithKline	*Infanrix IPV*	
	Sanofi Pasteur	*Imovax DTP Polio*	
Diphtheria & tetanus toxoids with acellular pertussis vaccine, combined with poliovirus and Hib vaccines [Vacuna combinada contra difteria, tétanus, tosferia acelular, poliomielitis inactivada y Hib]	GlaxoSmithKline Mexico	*Pediacel*	
	Sanofi Pasteur	*Pentaxim*	
Diphtheria & tetanus toxoids with component pertussis vaccine, combined with inactivated poliomyelitis vaccine [Vacuna contra difteria, tosferina, tétanos y poliomielitis, DTP-IPV]	Sanofi Pasteur	*Quadracel*	D15/T5/Pert20/Pol40-8-32/0.5 mL
Diphtheria & tetanus toxoids with inactivated poliomyelitis vaccine [Vacuna contra difteria, tosferina, y poliomielitis, DT-IPV]	Sanofi Pasteur	*Dultavax*	
Diphtheria & tetanus toxoids with pertussis vaccine, combined with hepatitis B vaccine [Vacuna contra difteria, tosferina, tétanos y hepatitis B, DTP-Hep B]	GlaxoSmithKline	*Tritanrix HB (DTP-HB 10)*	
Diphtheria & tetanus toxoids with whole cell pertussis vaccine, combined with hepatitis B and Hib vaccines [Vacuna combinada contra difteria, tétanus, tosferia de célula complete, hepatitis B, y Hib]	GlaxoSmithKline	*Tritanrix HB + Hiberix*	

Combined Bacterial & Viral Vaccines			
Product [Spanish translation]	Distributor	Proprietary name	Comment
Diphtheria & tetanus toxoids with acellular pertussis vaccine, combined with hepatitis B poliovirus, and Hib vaccines [Vacuna combinada contra difteria, tétanus, tosferia acelular, hepatitis B, polio-mielitis inactivada y Hib]	GlaxoSmithKline	*Infanrix Hexa*	
	Sanofi Pasteur	*Hexavac*	
Haemophilus influenzae type b conjugate and hepatitis B vaccine [Vacuna conjugada con proteina meningocócica contra *Haemophilus* b y vacuna por recombinación contra la hepatitis B]	MSD (Merck)	*Comvax*	
Bacterial antigens polyvalent [Antigenos bacterianos lisados o Fracciones ribo-somales y membranarias]	Altana	*Luivac*	
	Altana	*Paspat*	
	Grunenthal	*Broncho-Vaxom*	
	Grunenthal	*Uro-Vaxom*	
	Pierre Fabre	*Ribovac*	
	Sanofi Pasteur	*Biostim*	

Broad-Spectrum Immune Globulins			
Product [Spanish translation]	Distributor	Proprietary name	Comment
Hepatitis B immune globulin (HBIG) [Immunoglobulina anti-hepatitis B]	CSL Behring	*Gammaglobulina*	
Immune globulin intramuscular (IGIM) [Immunoglobulina, gamma globulina]	Berna Biotech	*Gamma globulina*	
	CSL Behring	*Beriglobina P*	distributed for Behring-werke
	Octapharma	*Seroglubin*	distributed for Bayer
Immune globulin intravenous (IGIV) [Immunoglobulina, gamma globulina, intravenosa]	Baxter	*Gammagard S/D*	
	Berna Biotech	*Immunoglobulina-G B 5%*	
	CSL Behring	*Gamma Venin P*	
	Grifols	*Flebogamma*	
	Landsteiner	*Vigam*	
	Novartis	*Sandoglobulina*	
	Octapharma	*Octagam*	
Immune globulin IgG-IgM-IgA IV [Immunoglobulina humana enriquecida con IgM]	Laboratorios Pisa	*Pentaglobin*	

Anti-Infective Immune Globulins

Product [Spanish translation]	Distributor	Proprietary name	Comment
Rabies immune globulin (RIG) [Immunoglobulina antirrábica]	Sanofi Pasteur	*Imogam Rabia*	
	Probifasa	*Hyperab*	distributed for Bayer
	Octapharma	*BayRab*	
	CSL Behring	*Berirab P*	
	Landsteiner	*KamRAB*	

Immunoantidotes: Antitoxins

Product [Spanish translation]	Distributor	Proprietary name	Comment
Tetanus immune globulin (TIG) [Immunoglobulina contra el tétanos]	CSL Behring	*Tetanogamma P*	distributed for Behring-werke
	Probifasa	*HyperTet*	distributed for Bayer
	Octapharma	*Baytet*	
	Probiomed	*Probitet*	

Immunoantidotes: Antivenins

Product [Spanish translation]	Distributor	Proprietary name	Comment
Suero antiviperino polyvalent snake antivenin against *Bothrops atrox asper* and *Crotalus basilicus basilicus*	Gerencia General		
Antivip-DL polyvalent snake antivenin against *Bothrops atrox asper* and *Crotalus durissus terrificus*	Bioclón		
Suero antiofídico polivalente "Myn" snake antivenin against *Bothrops atrox asper* and *Crotalus durissus terrificus*	Bioclón	*Alacramyn*	Fab
Alacramyn polyvalent scorpion antivenin against *Centruroides limpidus limpidus*, *Centruroides noxius*, and *Centruroides suffusus suffusus*	Bioclón	*Antivipmyn*	Fab
Antialacrán-DL polyvalent Scorpion antivenin against *Centruroides* species	Bioclón		
Suero antialacrá polyvalent Scorpion antivenin against *Centruroides* species	Gerencia General		
Anticoral snake Fab antivenin [Faboterápico polivalente anticoral]	Bioclón	*Coralmyn*	Fab (*Micrurus* sp)
Antispider Fab antivenin [Faboterápico polivalente anttoarácnido]	Bioclón	*Aracmyn*	Fab (*Latrodectus mactans* and *Loxosceles* species)

Isoantibodies: Erythrocytic			
Product [Spanish translation]	Distributor	Proprietary name	Comment
Rh$_o$(D) immune globulin (RhIG) [Immunoglobulina Rh$_o$(D)]	Berna Biotech	Rh$_o$(D) Humana Berna	
	ISI Medifarm	ImmunoRho	
	Probifasa	Anti Rh$_o$(D)	distributed for Bayer
	Aventis Behring	Rhesogamma P	
	Ivax	Rhophylac	
	Landsteiner	D-Gam	
	Octopharma	Octaglob-D	
	Probiomed	Probi-Rho D	

Isoantibodies: Lymphocytic			
Product [Spanish translation]	Distributor	Proprietary name	Comment
Antithymocyte globulin	Sanofi Pasteur	Linfoglobulina	
	Pfizer	Atgam	
Basiliximab	Novartis	Simulect	
Daclizumab	Roche	Zenapax	
Globulina antilinfocito	Laboratorios Pisa	Tecelac	
Muromonab-CD3 (OKT–3)	Cilag	Orthoclone OKT3	distributed for Ortho

Isoantibodies: Other			
Product [Spanish translation]	Distributor	Proprietary name	Comment
Abciximab	Lilly	ReoPro	
Adalimumab	Abbott	Humira	
Cetuximab	MSD (Merck)	Ertibux	
Etanercept	Wyeth	Enbrel	
Infliximab	Schering Plough	Remicade	
Rituximab	Roche	MabThera	
Trastuzumab	Genentech	Herceptin	

Immunologic Mediators			
Product [Spanish translation]	Distributor	Proprietary name	Comment
Aldesleukin [Aldesleukina]	Chiron, Asofarma	*Proleukin*	
Filgrastim	Roche	*Neupogen*	G-CSF
	Landsteiner	*Biofilgran*	
Interferon alfa-2a	Probiomed	*Proquiferón*	
	Cryopharma	*Alferon*	
Peginterferon alfa-2a	Roche	*Pegasys*	
Interferon alfa-2b	Armstrong	*FNI 2B*	
	Roche	*Roferon-A*	
	Schering	*Viraferon*	
	Schering-Plough	*Intron A*	
	Probiomed	*Urifron*	
	Lemery	*Lemeron*	
Interferon alfa-2b with riba-virin	Schering	*Hepatron C*	
	Probiomed	*Urifron*	
Interferon alfa mixture	Pisa Laboratorios	*Multiferon*	
Peginterferon alfa-2b	Schering	*Pegtrón*	
Interferon beta [Interferon de fibroblastos humanos]	Serono	*Frone*	
Interferon beta-1a	Abbott	*Avonex*	Manufactured by Biogen Idec
	Landsteiner	*Xerfelan*	
	Probiomed	*Emaxem*	
	Probiomed	*Jumtab*	
	Serono	*Rebif*	
Interferon beta-1b	Probiomed	*Uribeta*	
	Schering	*Betaferon*	
Molgramostim	Schering	*Leucomax*	GM-CSF
	Schering	*Mielogen*	GM-CSF
	Probiomed	*Gramal*	
Oprelvekin [Oprelvekina, interleucina-11]	Wyeth	*Neumega*	
Tuberculin purified protein derivative (PPD) [Tuberculina PPD]	Sanofi Pasteur	*Tubersol*	

Index of Mexican Immunologic Drugs

Immunostimulants			
Product [Spanish translation]	Distributor	Proprietary name	Comment
BCG for bladder instillation [BCG intravesical para Ca. vesical in situ]	Teva	*Cultivo BCG SSI*	
	Organon	*OncoTice*	
	Sanofi Pasteur	*Theracys*	

Other			
Product [Spanish translation]	Distributor	Proprietary name	Comment
Botulinum toxin type A	Allergan	*Botox*	
	Antipar	*Novag Infancia*	

References: PLM Staff. *Diccionario de Especialidades Farmaceuticas-PLM*. Montvale, NJ: Thomson PDR, 2004.

México Secretariá de Salud. *Manual de Vacunación 2008-2009*. Districo Federal de México, 2008. http://www.censia.salud.gob.mx/interior/vacunacion/vacunacion_index.html.

International Immunologic Drugs

International Immunologic Terms

United States	German	French	Spanish	Dutch	Italian	Portuguese
Immune Globulin	Sera, Immunoglobulin	Immunoglobulins	Immunoglobulina, Suero	Serum, bloedwei	Siero	Sérum, Soro
Vaccine	Impfstoffe	Vaccin	Vacuna	Vaccine	Vaccino	Vacina
Toxoid	Toxoid	Anatoxine	Toxoide	Toxoid	Anatossina, Tossoide	Anatoxina, Toxóide
Polysaccharide	Polysaccharid	Polyosidique	Polisacárido	Meervoudig suiker	Polisaccaride	Polissacáride
Cholera	Choler	Choléra	Cólera	Cholera	Colera	Cólera
Hepatitis A	Übertragbare Gelbsucht	Hépatite épidémique	Hepatitis epidémico	Lever ontsteking A	Epatite pidemica	Hepatite epidémica
Influenza	Grippe	Grippe	Gripe	Griep	Influenzae	Gripe
Malaria	Malaria	Malaria, paludisme	Paludismo	Malaria	Malaria	Malária, paludismo
Measles	Masern	Rougeole	Sarampión	Mazelen	Morbillo	Rúbéola, Sarampo
Mumps	Mumps	Oreillons	Paperas	Bof	Parotite, Sclerosi multipla	Paratidite epidémica, Papeira
Pertussis	Keuchhusten	Coqueluche	Tosferina	Kinkhoest	Pertosse	Pertussis
Pneumonia	Lungenentzündung	Pneumonie	Neumonía, pulmonia	Longontsteking	Polmonite	Pneumonia
Poliomyelitis	Kinderlähmung	Poliomyélite	Poliomielitis	Kinderverlamming	Paralisi infantile	Poliomielite
Rabies	Tollwut	Rage, Rabique	Rabia	Hondsdolheid	Rabbia	Raiva, Rábico
Rubella	Röteln	Rubéole	Rubéola	Rode hond, Roodvonk	Rosolia	Rubela

International Glossary of Immunologic Terms

	International Immunologic Terms					
United States	German	French	Spanish	Dutch	Italian	Portuguese
Tetanus	Wundstarrkrampf	Tétanos	Tétano	Tetanus, wondklem	Tetano	Tétano
Tuberculin PPD	Gereinigtes tuberculin (GT)	Tuberculine purifée	Tuberculina PPD	Huidtest voor Tuberculoses	Tubercolina PPD	Tuberculina PPD
Tuberculosis	Schwindsucht	Tuberculose	Tuberculosis	Tuberculoses	Tuberculosi	Tuberculose
Typhoid fever	Typhus	Fiévre typhoïde	Fiebre Tifoidea	Buiktyphus, typheuse koorts	Febbre tifoide, tifo	Febre tifóide
Typhus	Fleckfieber	Typhus	Tifo, tifus	Vlektyphus	Tifo petecchiale	Tifo enxatemático
Varicella	Windpocken	Varicelle-zona	Varicela, viruela buena	Waterpokken	Varicella	Varicela
Yellow fever	Gelbfieber	Fièvre jaune	Fiebre amarilla	Gele Koorts	Febbre gialla	Febre amarela
Zoster (Shingles)	Herpes zoster	Zona	Culebrilla	Herpes zoster	Fuoco di S. Antonio	Herpes zóster
Allergic	Überempfindlich, Allergisch	Allergique	Alérgico	Overgevoeligheids reactie	Allergia	Alérgico

International Immunologic Drugs

General Comments: The distribution of infectious disease risk is quite volatile around the world. To inform travelers of current disease risks, the Centers for Disease Control and Prevention (CDC) revises *Health Information for International Travel* every 2 years. Updates appear at http://www.cdc.gov/travel.

Definitive travel health recommendations are available from state and some local health departments, travel clinics (specialists in "emporiatrics"), and the CDC 24 hour international travel information hotline (877- FYI-TRIP). Obtain malaria information from CDC's fax information service (888–232–3299) or its Web site. Both lines are designed for either travelers or health professionals. Advise callers to use a touch-tone telephone, although rotary calls can be directed to an operator during normal business hours. Have pen and paper available to write down drug and vaccine names and other advice.

Risk Factors of Preventable Diseases: The following section reviews major risk factors affecting the health of international travelers. These remarks only address health risks that can be modified by vaccination or malaria chemoprophylaxis. They do not address other potential bacterial, viral, fungal, or protozoal infections that are not vaccine-preventable, nor are environmental and other hazards discussed (eg, heat injury).

Since health risks are not uniform within any country, the medial threat is a function of not only the destination country, but also the specific destination(s), as well as business activities and recreation conducted while in that country. Risk also varies by season of year, altitude, mode of travel, and other factors.

Food & Drink: Food and drink can be tainted by contamination before preparation, during improper preparation, or by improper storage. Cholera, typhoid, and hepatitis A are well known food- and water-borne diseases. Since cholera and typhoid vaccines are only marginally effective, good food and beverage discipline is the best way to avoid these and other diseases, even in vaccine recipients.

Eat meats and vegetables well-cooked and piping hot. Raw meat, seafood, and salads are especially hazardous. Lettuce grown in developing countries may be fertilized with human excrement or irrigated with water polluted with parasites and other pathogens. Dairy products may be unpasteurized or improperly handled after pasteurization. Food from street vendors is particularly risky. Thick-skinned peelable fruits (eg, oranges) are usually safe if peeled by the traveler. A simple rule of thumb is "Boil it, cook it, peel it, or forget it." The safest food for infants is breast milk.

"Don't drink the water" is another well known aphorism; extend this caution also to consuming ice cubes, brushing teeth, cleaning contact lenses, and other personal hygiene activities. Alcohol content has little effect on sterility. Avoid fresh milk.

Water can be purified in several ways. Boiling for 5 minutes (adding 1 minute for each 1,000 feet above 5,000 feet elevation) is the most effective method, but may be impractical. The most readily accessible method is to carry a dropper bottle of either household chlorine bleach or 2% tincture of iodine. Four drops of bleach or 5 drops of iodine in a quart of clear, room temperature water will kill most organisms within 30 minutes. Iodine can be hazardous during pregnancy. For cloudy or cold water, double both the dose of the chemical and the contact time. Canned or bottled carbonated beverages, hot coffee and tea from boiled water, beer, and wine are generally safe. Bottled water does not necessarily come from a safe source.

Insect Control: Disease-carrying mosquitoes and other insects are usually most active from dusk to dawn, although the dengue-carrying *Aedes* mosquito is active at midday. Reduce risk by avoiding outdoor exposure during hours of peak activity, minimizing exposed skin surface by wearing long-sleeved shirts and long pants, sleeping in screened areas, and properly using insecticides (eg, spraying pyrethrin before occupying a sleeping area). Urban travel is generally associated with less mosquito exposure than rural travel.

Insect repellents containing DEET (N,N-diethylmetatoluamide) are quite effective, although products containing more than 32% DEET may cause skin rashes. Use high concentration repellents sparingly, if at all, on infants and children, because of risk of systemic absorption leading to seizures and neurologic damage. Do not apply repellent to broken skin; keep it away from eyes and mouths. Apply tick repellents (eg, permethrin, *Permanone*) only to clothing, not to skin.

Malaria is arguably the most widespread and destructive infectious disease in the world. More than 2.1 billion people live in malarial areas, 270 million people are infected each year, and 1 million people die of malaria annually around the world. Use appropriate chemoprophylaxis.

Medical Access: Rabies is enzootic in animal populations in Latin America, the Far East, and Africa. Cleanse any animal bites promptly and thoroughly; obtain postexposure prophylaxis promptly if the animal is likely to harbor the virus. Advise travelers planning to hike the mountains of India or engage in other activities far removed from modern medical facilities to consider pre-exposure rabies prophylaxis. Equine antirabies serum (ARS), with its attendant side effects, is more likely to be used in developing countries than human rabies immune globulin (RIG) for passive postexposure immunity.

Pretravel and post-travel tuberculin skin tests may be appropriate for visitors to areas with high tuberculosis infection rates (eg, Africa, Asia). BCG vaccination is not generally recommended for travelers.

Advise travelers to observe several general medication precautions. Take along a list of the generic and proprietary names of medications, as well as an adequate supply. Plan ahead for storage options for heat-sensitive items and any special needs for insect sting kits, medical alert bracelets, extra eyeglasses, and ophthalmic prescriptions. Carry critical items; do not stow them with luggage.

In general, early treatment is preferable to prophylaxis in the management of traveler's diarrhea. The most common cause of such diarrhea is enterotoxigenic *Escherichia coli*, with *Campylobacter*, *Shigella*, *Salmonella* viruses, and parasites also contributing.

Prophylactic antibiotics can alter the gastrointestinal flora and actually increase the risk of certain invasive diarrheal infections. Loperamide (*Imodium*) or bismuth subsalicylate (*Pepto-Bismol*) are often used in mild cases of 2 to 3 loose stools per day. For more severe cases, products such as doxycycline 100 mg, sulfamethoxazole/trimethoprim 800 mg/160 mg, and ciprofloxacin 500 mg have been used. When prescribed, antibiotics are usually taken twice daily for just 3 days. Blood or mucus in the stool or fever suggests the need for more aggressive evaluation. Oral rehydration solutions are helpful in the management of severe diarrhea. The more readily available alternative of fruit juices, caffeine-free soft drinks, and salted crackers is often sufficient to meet fluid, glucose, and electrolyte needs.

Lodging & Social Contact: Disease risk obviously varies between a traveler who stays in a 5-star resort hotel and another traveler who backpacks through jungle and wilderness, even if they are in the same exotic country. Choice of lodging often influences the types of meals the traveler eats. The experiences of many international travelers at popular tourist attractions in exotic locations should allow accurate assessment of disease risk. Those who travel off the beaten track accept a greater risk, since quantitatively and qualitatively less is known about the health threats they face.

The risk of sexually transmitted diseases (STDs) may affect international travelers. Heterosexual transmission of HIV-1 and HIV-2 predominates in Africa and some other parts of the world. Also consider the risk of hepatitis B, gonorrhea, syphilis, and other STDs. Hepatitis B can be prevented by vaccination.

Occupational & Recreational Risks: Health care workers can acquire blood-borne infections at least as readily in foreign locales as they can in this country. Complete a hepatitis B vaccine series before departing.

Swimming or wading in contaminated fresh water increases the risk of schistosomiasis or leptospirosis in some tropical settings. Close or frequent contact with animals increases the risk of zoonotic diseases.

Immunization Needs: Because some vaccines may require more than 1 dose to induce complete immunity, travelers should seek medical advice about 6 weeks before departure. International immunization practices may differ from US standards, including the possibility of reuse of needles without effective sterilization. To avoid the risk of HIV, hepatitis B, and other blood-borne infections, travelers should never be immunized under circumstances where there is doubt about the quality of the vaccines and the use of sterile needles.

While travelers usually focus on the need for protection against exotic diseases, it is no less important to ensure they are immune to tetanus, measles, rubella, influenza, hepatitis B, poliovirus, and other vaccine-preventable infections more commonly associated with domestic life. Measles, rubella, hepatitis B, tetanus, and mumps occur far more frequently in the developing countries than in the United States or Canada.

Adequate tetanus immunity precludes the need for administration of equine tetanus antitoxin, with its attendant side effects, in event of trauma. Human hyperimmune tetanus immune globulin (TIG) is not generally available in developing countries. The prime seasons for influenza in the Southern Hemisphere is opposite our own (April through September, rather than November through March). Influenza transmission occurs in tropical areas through the year.

Prevent hepatitis A in travelers to areas where hygiene is poor, particularly those traveling away from standard tourist routes, by giving hepatitis A vaccine. Hepatitis A antibody tests for susceptibility are now widely available. Hepatitis A vaccines may be licensed in the near future.

Consider typhoid vaccine for travelers to rural areas of countries with endemic disease involving stays longer than 1 week. Oral cholera vaccines may be licensed in the future. Vaccination is also indicated for travelers with a compromised gastric acid barrier (eg, chronic users of antacids, cimetidine, ranitidine, omeprazole).

Give yellow fever vaccine in accordance with specific instructions provided for individual countries.

Meningococcal meningitis is a risk in savanna regions of sub-Saharan Africa during the dry season from December to June. Meningitis outbreaks may extend up the Nile Valley into northern Egypt. In recent years, epidemics have been reported in Kenya, Tanzania, Nepal, and India. Vaccination is warranted for travelers at such times and places. Muslim pilgrims to the Hajj or Umrah to Saudi Arabia may be required to demonstrate meningococcal vaccination for entry into that country.

For travel to most developing countries, consider a pretravel and post-travel tuberculin skin test. BCG vaccination is not generally recommended for travelers.

For travel to rural areas of Vietnam and some other Southeast Asian countries, consider plague vaccine.

Consider Japanese encephalitis vaccine if a month or longer stay is anticipated in rice-growing areas of rural Asia with extensive mosquito exposure.

The data that follow on certificate requirements were accurate when printed, but may be invalidated by more recent policy changes. Always consult the most current detailed references when assessing the immunization and chemoprophylaxis needs of individual travelers.

Vaccination Certificate Requirements: Under provisions of International Health Regulations adopted by the World Health Organization (WHO), a country may require an International Certificate of Vaccination for certain diseases before allowing a traveler to enter. Americans use Public Health Service (PHS) Form 731, International Certificates of Vaccination, commonly called the "yellow shot record," to record these immunizations. This form can also serve as a personal immunization record (see Section V). The 1969 edition of the International Health Regulations has been revised, with the new version taking effect in 2007.

Yellow Fever: Under International Health Regulations, a country under certain conditions may require an "International Certificate of Vaccination Against Yellow Fever" from international travelers. The certificate is valid for 10 years beginning 10 days after a single-dose primary vaccination or on the date of revaccination if within 10 years of previous injection.

Cholera: A certificate of cholera immunization is no longer required by any country or territory. Some earlier governmental requirements were in excess of International Health Regulations. The certificate is valid for 6 months beginning 6 days after 1 injection of cholera vaccine or on the date of revaccination if within 6 months of a previous injection. Epidemiologically, a cholera vaccination certificate will not prevent the introduction of the disease into any country.

Smallpox: Smallpox was deleted from diseases subject to International Health Regulations, effective January 1, 1982. With new concerns regarding release of smallpox virus as a bioterrorist weapon, recent smallpox vaccinations should be documented on PHS 731, to facilitate international travel.

Quarantine: For the purposes of the International Health Regulations, the incubation periods of the quarantinable diseases are: Cholera, 5 days; plague, 6 days; yellow fever, 6 days.

Direct Travel from the United States: For direct travel from the United States, only the following countries require an International Certificate of Vaccination:

Countries Requiring an International Certificate of Vaccination	
Cholera	
None	
Yellow Fever	
Benin	Ghana
Burkino Faso	Liberia
Cameroon	Mali
Central African Republic	Mauritania (stay > 2 weeks)
Congo	Niger
Côte d'Ivoire	Rwanda
Democratic Republic of Congo	São Tomé & Príncipe
French Guiana	Togo
Gabon	

For travel to and between other countries, check individual country requirements.

Return to the United States: No vaccinations are required to enter or return to the United States.

References: Canadian Committee to Advise on Tropical Medicine and Travel. Statement on motion sickness. *Can Comm Dis Rep.* 2003;29(ACS-11):1-12.

Canadian Committee to Advise on Tropical Medicine and Travel. Travel statement on jet lag. *Can Comm Dis Rep*. 2003;29(ACS-3):4-8.

Canadian National Advisory Committee. The immunocompromised traveller. *Can Comm Dis Rep*. 2007;33(ACS-4):1-24.

Canadian National Advisory Committee on Immunization. Statement on personal protective measures to prevent arthropod bites. *Can Comm Dis Rep*. 2005:31(ACS-4):1-20.

CDC. *Health Information for International Travel*. Washington, DC: GPO, revised annually. http://www.cdc.gov/travel.

CDC. Revised international health regulations effective for the United States. *MMWR*. 2007;56(28):712-713.

Hill DR, Pearson RD. Health advice for international travel. *Ann Intern Med*. 1988;108:839-852.

Kelly PW. Practicing travel medicine. *J US Army Med Dept*. 1991;(Nov-Dec):14-21.

Mackell SM. Vaccinations for the pediatric traveler. *Clin Infect Dis*. 2003;37:1508-1516.

Nahlen BL, Parsonnet J, Preblud SR, et al. International travel and the child younger than two years: II. Recommendations for prevention of travelers' diarrhea and malaria chemoprophylaxis. *Pediatr Infect Dis J*. 1989;8:735-739.

Preblud SR, Tsai TF, Brink EW, et al. International travel and the child younger than two years: I. Recommendations for immunization. *Pediatr Infect Dis J*. 1989;8:416-425.

Ryan ET, Wilson ME, Kain KC. Illness after international travel. *N Engl J Med*. 2002;347:505-516.

Stauffer W, Christenson JC, Fischer PR. Preparing children for international travel. *Travel Med Infect Dis*. 2008;6(3):101-113.

US State Department Citizens' Emergency Center [when traveling abroad], 202-647-5225, http://www.state.gov/www/servies.html.

World Health Organization. International Health Regulations. http:/www./who.int/topics/international_health_regulations/en/.

World Health Organization. *International Travel and Health: Vaccination Requirements and Health Advice*. Albany, NY: WHO, revised annually. http://www.who.int/ith/en.

Zwerling A, Behr MA, Verma A, Brewer TF, Menzies D, Pai M. The BCG World Atlas: a database of global BCG vaccination policies and practices. *PLoS Med*. 2011;8(3):e1001012.

Checklist for International Travel Needs

International Immunologic Drugs

General information:
Date of birth:_____
Activity during travel:_____
Occupation:_____
Recreational Habits:_____
Drug hypersensitivities:_____
  Describe reactions:_____
  When did they occur?_____
Current medications:_____
Previous malaria prophylaxis?_____
  Reactions?_____

Requirement for an International Certificate of Vaccination?
List traveler's itinerary in sequence, check current incidence of cholera and yellow fever in the "Blue Sheet," then check WHO or CDC table.
(1) cholera prophylaxis:_____
(2) yellow fever vaccine:_____

Sanitation at destination(s)? Good____ Poor____
(1) If poor, consider vaccination for hepatitis A:_____
(2) For those living more than 1 week in smaller cities or villages or in rural areas off the usual tourist routes, or those with a compromised gastric acid barrier (eg, chronic users of antacids, cimetidine, ranitidine, omeprazole), consider typhoid vaccine:_____

Adequacy of "domestic" vaccines?
tetanus-diphtheria-pertussis:_____
measles-mumps-rubella:_____
poliovirus:_____
influenza:_____
hepatitis B:_____
meningococcal:_____
rotavirus:_____
Haemophilus, pneumococcal:_____

Specific immunization needs by destination:
(1) Sub-Saharan Africa, Nepal, India, Saudi Arabia: Consider meningococcal vaccine for travel from December to June:_____
(2) Sub-Saharan Africa, southeast Asia, the interior Amazon basin: Consider hepatitis B vaccine if staying more than 6 months, expecting close contact or sexual contact with the local population, or a health care worker:_____
(3) South and southeast Asia (including India, Thailand, and China): consider Japanese encephalitis vaccine if staying more than 1 month in rural areas:_____
(4) Most developing countries: Consider a pretravel and post-travel tuberculin skin test:____

1374

Ready access to medical care?

meningococcal vaccine:_____

rabies vaccine:_____

Patient education checklist:

(1) Food and beverage precautions:_____

(2) Insect control:_____

(3) Environmental risks (eg, heat, snakes):_____

(4) Other health risks (eg, schistosomiasis, drugs procured in other countries, rabies prevention, avoidance of sexually transmitted diseases [STDs], surveillance after return):_____

Generic considerations for travelers:

- *Record-Keeping:* Make a list of all prescription and nonprescription medications you use. Include brand and generic names, strength, purpose, and directions. Keep a list of medication and food allergies, describing what type of reactions you've had. Take a list of your doctors' and pharmacist's names, addresses, and telephone numbers.
- *Handling:* Keep all medications with you in carry-on baggage. Carry all medications in originally labeled containers. Do not store medications in vehicles or in other places that get extremely hot. Carry an extra copy of each prescription. Take an extra pair of eyeglasses and your prescription.
- *Dehydration:* Drink plenty of fluids from reliable sources during your travel, especially in hot climates and on long airline flights.
- *Sun Sensitivity:* Use plenty of sunscreen and lip balm to protect your skin.
- *Crossing Time Zones:* Long flights eastbound or westbound can make medication dosing confusing. For once or twice a day medications, you may want to continue taking your drugs on your "home" time while in flight. When you arrive, set your watch to the new time and count the number of hours that have elapsed since your last dose and add enough hours to the present time to add up to 12 or 24 hours. Use this as your new dosage time, give or take an hour for convenience. Ask your physician or pharmacist for specific information for you. If you have diabetes, crossing at least 2 time zones may call for adjusting your insulin dose. Flying west makes your day longer; you may need more insulin. If you fly east, your day is shorter; you may need less insulin. If you draw up your insulin dose while in the air, you will only need to inject half as much air into the insulin vial. Consider also the changes in eating habits and activity that travel causes. Test your blood sugar often.

Malaria Checklist:

(1) *Risk of Malaria:* Inform travelers about the risk of malaria infection and the presence of drug-resistant *Plasmodium falciparum* malaria at their destinations.

(2) *Anti-Mosquito Measures:* Advise travelers how to protect themselves against mosquito bites.

(3) *Chemoprophylaxis:*
- Advise travelers to use prophylaxis continuously while in malaria-endemic areas and for 4 weeks after leaving such areas.
- Question travelers about drug allergies and other contraindications for use of drugs to prevent malaria.
- Advise travelers which drug to use for prophylaxis and, if chloroquine is used, whether *Fansidar* should be carried for presumptive self-treatment.
- Inform travelers that antimalarial drugs can cause side effects; if these side effects are serious, seek medical help promptly and discontinue use of the drug.
- Warn travelers they may acquire malaria even if they use malaria chemoprophylaxis.

(4) *In case of illness:*
- Inform travelers that symptoms of malaria may be mild and that they should suspect malaria if they experience unexplained fever or other symptoms such as persistent headaches, muscular aching and weakness, vomiting, or diarrhea.
- Inform travelers that malaria may be fatal if treatment is delayed.
- Seek medical help promptly if malaria is suspected and a blood sample should be taken on 1 or more occasions and examined for malaria parasites.
- Remind travelers that self-treatment should be taken only if prompt medical care is not available and that medical advice should still be sought as soon as possible after self-treatment.

(5) *Special considerations:*
- Pregnant women and young children require special attention because they cannot use some drugs (eg, mefloquine, doxycycline).
- Concurrent use of other drugs (eg, beta adrenergic blockers) may be a contraindication to use of mefloquine.

Adapted from *International Travel and Health*, World Health Organization, Geneva.

Travel Health Checklist:

(1) Learn about the destination (eg, accommodations, food and water quality, geography, medical services). Gather maps and informative documents.

(2) Seek expert travel-health advice at least 4 weeks before departure.

(3) Begin appropriate immunizations. Obtain International Certificate of Vaccination (PHS Form 731, the "yellow shot record") and keep it with passport.

(4) Obtain dental check-up and medical examination (especially before prolonged travel.

(5) Obtain adequate supply of current prescription medication(s).

(6) Obtain a medical-alert bracelet for conditions such as diabetes or drug allergies.

(7) Purchase extra pair of eyeglasses or contact lenses, plus sunglasses.

(8) Collect items for travel first-aid kit (especially if traveling off usual tourist routes).

(9) Check health insurance plan for international coverage.

(10) Buy additional insurance, as needed.

This form may be reproduced for individual patients if credit is given to *ImmunoFacts*.

Synonyms: *Mal'aria* ("bad" or "evil" air in Italian), ague, intermittent fever, swamp fever, paludism, Roman fever

Epidemiology: Malaria is arguably the most widespread and destructive infectious disease in the world. More than 2.5 billion people live in malarial areas, more than half the planet's human population. An estimated 100 to 300 million people are newly infected annually, and 1 to 3 million people die of malaria each year around the world.

An estimated 15 million Americans travel abroad each year, half to developing countries. About 25 to 30 million people travel annually to malaria-endemic areas. Two million Americans travel to areas endemic with *Plasmodium falciparum* each year. Well over 1,000 imported malaria infections are reported each year; from 1980 to 1987, 35 US citizens died of malaria. Up to 30,000 North American and European travelers contract malaria each year. Between 0.4% and 7% of these infections are fatal.

Parasitology: Plasmodia are protozoa. Female anophiline mosquitoes inject sporozoites stored in salivary glands during the act of feeding. The sporozoites are carried in the human bloodstream to the liver, where the sporozoite transforms itself into a merozoite. It replicates repeatedly for about 2 weeks, by a process called schizogony. The patient develops intense fever when the cell bursts to release thousands of merozoites into the bloodstream. Each merozoite enters a red blood cell, where it appears as a minute circlet with a small nucleus, the ring stage. The parasite grows, consuming the red cell's hemoglobin until it fills more than half the red cell, the trophozoite stage. The parasitic nucleus then reorganizes into several merozoites. The demolished red cell bursts and the merozoites seek new red cells.

These cycles occur in concert, so that fevers peak every 48 hours for *Plasmodium falciparum* (malignant tertian malaria), *Plasmodium ovale*, and *Plasmodium vivax* (tertian malaria) or every 72 hours for *Plasmodium malariae* (quartan malaria). After several asexual cycles, some of the merozoites become male or female gametocytes. The sexual merozoite invades a red blood cell for the ring stage, but becomes greatly enlarged. The gametocytes circulate in the bloodstream unchanged until taken into the stomach of a feeding female anophiline mosquito. There, the male gametocytes develop flagella, swim to the female gametes, penetrate, and fertilize them. From the female develops an oocyst that yields thousands of sporozoites after 14 to 21 days.

Patient Counseling: Malaria occurs as headaches, malaise, fever, chills, and sweats. Sometimes the symptoms are described as a flu-like illness. It may cause anemia and jaundice; in some cases, infections may cause heart or kidney failure, coma, or even death. Deaths and illnesses caused by malaria are largely preventable.

Symptoms of malaria may develop as soon as 8 days after infection, or there may be a delay of several months or years. If fever develops within 6 months (possibly up to 4 years) after traveling in an endemic area, the possibility of malaria should be considered. Generally, there is a greater risk in rural areas than in cities, but risk may still exist in cities. All travelers to areas infested with malaria, regardless of their age, should take prophylactic medications, even for visits as brief as 1 night.

Specific advice includes the following:

(1) Avoid mosquito bites, especially after sunset. That is when the mosquitos responsible for transmitting malaria are most active. Long trousers, sleeves, netting or screens on windows, and mosquito nets over beds help prevent bites. Tuck the edges of mosquito nets under the mattress; increased protection may result from impregnating the net with per-

methrin (*Permanone*) or deltamethrin. Avoid dark-colored clothing, which attracts mosquitoes.

(2) Use insect repellent on exposed skin. Repellents containing DEET (N,N diethyl-meta-toluamide) or dimethyl phthalate are the most effective.

(3) Even the measures above are unlikely to be fully protective, so be sure to take medications for prophylaxis regularly. Prophylaxis should start 1 to 2 weeks before arriving in the malaria-endemic region and continue during and for 4 weeks after exposure.

Pregnancy & Lactation: Malaria is more dangerous to the pregnant woman than chloroquine. It is recommended that pregnant women take chloroquine if needed for prophylaxis.

Mefloquine, if indicated, may be used in nonpregnant women of childbearing potential, but pregnancy should be avoided for 3 months after stopping the drug. Similarly, doxycycline may be used if indicated, but avoid pregnancy for 1 week after stopping the drug.

Chloroquine is excreted into breast milk, but is generally safe in infants and children. Breast-fed babies, as well as bottle-fed babies, should receive chemoprophylaxis, if indicated.

Children: Chloroquine is quite toxic to children in overdoses, so take caution to keep it out of the reach of children. Doxycycline should not be given to children younger than 8 years of age. Consult detailed references for complete dosing details.

Consultation: Professional advice on the diagnosis and management of malaria is available from CDC. Clinicians should telephone (404) 332-4555 or (404) 639-1610.

History:

1630s: Quinine introduced into Europe, harvested from bark of South American cinchona trees by Jesuit missionaries.

1878: Viennese pharmacist Ziedler synthesizes dichlorodiphenyl trichloroethylene (DDT).

1880: Laveran isolates the malaria parasite *Plasmodium falciparum*, initially called *Oscillaria malariae*. He received the 1907 Nobel Prize for this work and related work on protozoology.

1898: Ross in India demonstrates that avian malaria is transmitted by mosquitoes to chickens. Grassi in Italy demonstrates transmission to humans. Ross receives the 1902 Nobel Prize.

1945: Early large-scale field trial of DDT insecticide conducted along the Tennessee River. Muller receives 1948 Nobel Prize for developing DDT.

National Policy: Centers for Disease Control & Prevention. *Health Information for International Travel, 2005-2006.* Washington, DC: Government Printing Office [revised regularly].

References: Keystone JS. Prevention of malaria. *Drugs.* 1990;39:337-354.

Lobel HO, Koxarsky PE. Update on prevention of malaria for travelers. *JAMA.* 1997;278:1767–1771.

Wolfe MS. Protection of travelers. *Clin Infect Dis.* 1997;25:177–186.

Wyler DJ. Malaria: Overview and update. *Clin Infect Dis.* 1993;16:449-458.

Typical Drug Dosages in the Prophylaxis of Malaria		
Drug	Adult dose	Pediatric dose
Chloroquine phosphate (*Aralen*)	300 mg base (500 mg salt) orally, weekly beginning 2 weeks before arrival, continuing until 4 weeks after departure	In general, 5 mg/kg base (8.3 mg/kg salt) orally, weekly, up to 300 mg base
Mefloquine hydrochloride (*Lariam*)	228 mg base (250 mg salt) orally, weekly beginning 1 week before arrival, continuing until 4 weeks after departure	In general, 5 mg/kg. *15-19 kg:* 62.5 mg *20-30 kg:* 125 mg *31-45 kg:* 187.5 mg *> 45 kg:* 250 mg weekly
Doxycycline (*Vibramycin*)	100 mg orally, daily during exposure, continuing until 4 weeks after departure	In general, 1.5 mg/kg. *> 8 years of age:* 2 mg/kg orally per day, up to 100 mg/day
Hydroxychloroquine sulfate (*Plaquenil*)	310 mg base (400 mg salt) orally, weekly	In general, 5 mg/kg base (6.5 mg/kg salt) orally, weekly, up to 310 mg base
Proguanil (*Paludrine*)	200 mg orally, daily in combination with weekly chloroquine	In general, 3 mg/kg. *< 2 years:* 50 mg/day *2-6 years:* 100 mg/day *7-10 years:* 150 mg/day *> 10 years:* 200 mg/day
Primaquine[a]	15 mg base (26.3 mg salt) orally, daily for 14 days as terminal prophylaxis after departure	In general, 0.3 mg/kg base (0.5 mg/kg salt) orally, daily for 14 days

a Check glucose-6-phosphate dehydrogenase (G6PD) levels in appropriate patients prior to primaquine therapy.

Timing: Begin chloroquine 1 to 2 weeks or doxycycline 1 to 2 days before travel. Continue all prophylactic regimens during and for 4 weeks after exposure.

Drugs Potentially Used for Presumptive Treatment of Malaria		
Drug	Adult dose	Pediatric dose
Pyrimethamine-sulfadoxine (*Fansidar*)	3 tablets (each tablet contains 25 mg pyrimethamine and 500 mg sulfadoxine) orally as a single dose	*5-10 kg:* 0.5 tablet *11-20 kg:* 1 tablet *21-30 kg:* 1.5 tablets *31-45 kg:* 2 tablets *> 45 kg:* 3 tablets
Mefloquine hydrochloride (*Lariam*)	1,000 mg single dose. May not result in radical cure in all cases. Seek medical care.	In general, 15 mg/kg
Halofantrine (*Halfan*)	500 mg every 6 hours for 3 doses (1,500 mg total). A second full course should be taken 1 week after the first course.	3 doses of 8 mg/kg at 6-hour intervals

Generic & Proprietary Names of Antimalarial Drugs Around The World	
Generic & colloquial names	Proprietary names
amodiachin	see amodiaquine
amodiaquine	*Basoquin, Camoquine, Flavoquine*
amodiquine with primaquine	*Camoprim*
arteannuin	see artemisinin
artemether and lumefantrine	*Coartem*
artemisinin	generic
bigumal	see proguanil
chlorguanide	see proguanil
chloroquine diphosphate	*Cidanchin, Dichinalex*
chloroquine hydrochloride	*Aralen HCl*
chloroquine phosphate	*Aralen Phosphate, Avlochlor*, generic, *Klorokinfosfat, Malarex, Malarivon*[a]*, Resochin, Weimerquin*, and many others
chloroquine sulfate	*Bemasulph, Nivaquine*[a]
chloroquine, unnamed salts	*Delagil, Lagaquin, Malatets*
chloroquine with bismuth glycollylarsanilate	*Aralis, Milibis with Aralen*
chloroquine with chlorproguanil	*Lapaquin*
chloroquine with prednisone and aspirin	*Elestol*
chloroquine phosphate with primaquine phosphate (C-P tablets)	*Aralen with Primaquine*
chloroquine with pyrimethamine	*Darachlor*
chlorproquanil	*Lapudrine*
cycloguanil embonate	*Camolar*
doxycycline	*Abadox, Doryx, Doxy, Doxy Caps, Doxychel, Ecodox, Liomycin, Monocline, Nordox, Roximycin, Vibramycin, Vibra-Tabs, Vivox*, Generic, and many others
halofantrine	*Halfan*
hydroxychloroquine sulfate	*Ercoquin, Plaquenil, Quensyl*
mefloquine hydrochloride	*Lariam, Mephaquine*
mepacrine	see quinacrine
primaquine phosphate	Generic
proguanide	see proguanil
proguanil	*Chloriquane, Paludrine, Paludrinol*
pyrimethamine	*Daraprim, Erbaprelina, Malocide, Pirimecidan, Tindurin*
pyrimethamine with dapsone	*Maloprim*
pyrimethamine with sulfadoxine	*Falcidar, Fansidar*
pyrimethamine with sulfadoxine and mefloquine	*Fansimef*
pyrimethamine with sulfalene	*Metakelfin*
qinghaosu	see artemisinin
quinacrine	*Acranil, Atabrine*
quinidine gluconate injection	Generic

Generic & Proprietary Names of Antimalarial Drugs Around The World	
Generic & colloquial names	Proprietary names
quinine, various salts	*Adaquine, Adquin, Bichinine, Biquin, Biquinate, Chinine, Dentojel, Formula-Q, Grisotets, Kinin, Kinine, Legatrin, M-KYA, Myoquine, QM-260, Quin-amm, Quinate, Quinbisan, Quinbisul, Quindan, Quine, Quinoctal, Quinoforme, Quiphile, Quinsan, Quinsul, Q-vel, Strema,* Generic, and many others

a Available in an oral liquid dosage form.

Hepatitis A and Hepatitis B Endemicity by Region		
Geographic region	Hepatitis A	Hepatitis B
Africa	High	High (most)
Caribbean	High	Intermediate
Central America	High	Intermediate
Eastern Europe	Intermediate	Intermediate
Middle East[a]	High	High
Russian Federation	Intermediate	Intermediate
South America (temperate)	High	Intermediate
South America (tropical)	High	High
South and Southeast Asia[b]	High	High
Southern Europe	Intermediate	Intermediate

a Israel: Intermediate HBV endemicity.
b Japan: Low HAV and intermediate HBV endemicity.

Summary of Travel-Related Vaccine Recommendations

International Immunologic Drugs

(See detailed references for complete guidance.)

Summary of Travel-Related Vaccine Recommendations[a]							
Vaccine	North America, N&W Europe, Australia, New Zealand, Japan	Eastern (Asian) Mediterranean, North Africa	Tropical Africa	Middle East	Asia	Mexico, Central & South America	Caribbean & Pacific Islands
Hepatitis A		needed	needed	needed	needed	needed	needed
Hepatitis B		prolonged visits	prolonged visits	prolonged visits	prolonged visits	optional	prolonged visits
Japanese encephalitis					prolonged visits, rural areas		
Meningococcal meningitis		needed for North Africa	Meningitis belt, outbreaks, prolonged visits	Pilgrimage to Mecca, outbreaks	Parts of India, Nepal, trekking	outbreaks	
Polio		needed	needed	needed	needed		needed (Pacific)
Rabies			prolonged visits	prolonged visits	prolonged visits		prolonged visits
Td or Tdap	needed	needed	needed	needed	needed	needed	needed
Typhoid	needed	needed	needed	needed	needed	needed	needed
Yellow Fever			needed for Central, East, and West Africa			depends on destination (eg, equatorial countries)	

a Source: US Public Health Service. Also ensure immunity to "domestic" diseases before departure (eg, measles, mumps, rubella, varicella).

Resources

Vaccine Indications Based on Age and Other Factors

The following tables summarize authoritative guidelines on recommended childhood vaccinations; vaccine needs based on the patient's age; and vaccines indicated (and immunity needed) by the patient's occupation, health status, lifestyle, or other factors.

These summaries condense a large volume of information. Readers must consider all notes carefully and apply their clinical skills in assessing each patient individually. Consult authoritative references for complete information about dosage schedules, booster doses and intervals, contraindications, and other use factors. Many of the notes in the tables are mnemonic devices to aid in their repeated use. For example, T corresponds to travelers, CC refers to contacts of pathogen carriers or infectious cases, and CS refers to close contacts of susceptible patients.

Vaccine recommendations change from time to time, and clinicians should stay up-to-date by reading professional literature (eg, *MMWR*, summaries in other journals). Subsequent revisions of authoritative guidelines on which these tables were based obviously take precedence.

How to Use the Immunization Summary Tables

(1) Consider the individual patient.

(2) For the age range pertaining to this patient, read down the column looking for indicated vaccines. Read all pertinent footnotes. Compare these recommendations with the patient's actual vaccination and medical history. Consider possible contraindications.

(3) Repeat with each appropriate column in the Immunization Recommendations Based on Personal Factors table.

(4) Remember that vaccine recommendations change periodically. Read professional literature to stay up-to-date.

References: ACIP. General recommendations on immunization. *MMWR*. 2011;60(RR-2):1-61.

American College of Physicians. *Guide to Adult Immunization: A Team-Based Manual*. 4th ed. Philadelphia, PA: American College of Physicians; 2011.

Canadian National Advisory Committee on Immunization. *Canadian Immunization Guide*. 7th ed. Ottawa, ON: Public Health Agency of Canada; 2006. http://www.phac-aspc.gc.ca/publicat/cig-gci/index.html.

CDC. *Health Information for International Travel*. Washington, DC: Government Printing Office (revised biennially). http://wwwn.cdc.gov/travel/ (supplements).

CDC. Recommended adult immunization schedule. Current version available at: http://www.cdc.gov/vaccines/schedules/hcp/adult.html.

CDC. Recommended childhood and adolescent immunization schedule. Current version available at: http://www.cdc.gov/vaccines/schedules/hcp/child-adolescent.html.

Pickering LK, Baker CJ, Kimberlin DW, Long SS, eds. *Red Book: 2009 Report of the Committee on Infectious Diseases*. 28th ed. Elk Grove Village, IL: American Academy of Pediatrics; 2009.

WHO. *International Travel and Health: Vaccination Requirements and Health Advice*. Geneva, Switzerland: World Health Organization (revised annually). http://www.who.int/ith/en/.

Immunization Schedules for Children and Adolescents

For those who fall behind or start late, see the catch-up schedule.

Recommended Immunization Schedule for Children 0 to 6 Years of Age — United States, 2012[a]

Vaccine	Birth	1 mo	2 mo	4 mo	6 mo	9 mo	12 mo	15 mo	18 mo	19 to 23 mo	2 to 3 y	4 to 6 y
									Age			
Hepatitis B[b]	HepB	HepB					HepB					
Rotavirus[c]			RV	RV	RV[c]							
Diphtheria, tetanus, pertussis[d]			DTaP	DTaP	DTaP		[d]	DTaP				DTaP
Haemophilus influenzae type b[e]			Hib	Hib	Hib[e]		Hib					
Pneumococcal[f]			PCV	PCV	PCV		PCV					PPSV
Inactivated poliovirus[g]			IPV	IPV			IPV					IPV
Influenza[h]							Influenza (yearly)					
Measles, mumps, rubella[i]							MMR		[i]			MMR
Varicella[j]							Varicella		[j]			Varicella
Hepatitis A[k]							Dose 1[k]				HepA series	
Meningococcal[l]							MCV4[l]					

☐ Range of recommended ages for all children

▨ Range of recommended ages for certain high-risk groups

■ Range of recommended ages for all children and certain high-risk groups

a This schedule includes recommendations in effect as of December 23, 2011. Any dose not administered at the recommended age should be administered at a subsequent visit, when indicated and feasible. The use of a combination vaccine generally is preferred over separate injections of its equivalent component vaccines. Providers should consult the relevant Advisory Committee on Immunization Practices (ACIP) statement for detailed recommendations available at: http://www.cdc.gov/vaccines/pubs/acip-list.htm. Clinically significant adverse events that follow immunization should be reported to the Vaccine Adverse Event Reporting System (VAERS) at http://www.vaers.hhs.gov or by telephone, 1-800-822-7967.

b **Hepatitis B vaccine (HepB)** *(minimum age: birth)*
   At birth –
   • Administer monovalent HepB vaccine to all newborns prior to hospital discharge.
   • If mother is hepatitis B surface antigen (HBsAg)–positive, administer HepB vaccine and 0.5 mL of hepatitis B immune globulin (HBIG) within 12 hours of birth. These infants should be tested for HBsAg and antibody to HBsAg (anti-HBs) 1 to 2 months after receiving the last dose of the series.
   • If mother's HBsAg status is unknown, administer HepB vaccine within 12 hours of birth to infants weighing 2,000 g or more and HepB vaccine plus HBIG to infants weighing less than 2,000 g. Determine mother's HBsAg status as soon as possible, and, if HBsAg-positive, administer HBIG for infants weighing 2,000 g or more (no later than 1 week of age).
   Doses after the birth dose –
   • The second dose should be administered at age 1 or 2 months. Monovalent HepB vaccine should be used for doses administered before age 6 weeks.
   • Administration of a total of 4 doses of HepB vaccine is permissible when a combination vaccine containing HepB is administered after the birth dose.
   • Infants who did not receive a birth dose should receive 3 doses of a HepB-containing vaccine starting as soon as feasible.
   • The minimal interval between dose 1 and 2 is 4 weeks, and between dose 2 and 3 is 8 weeks. The final (third or fourth) dose in the HepB vaccine series should be administered no earlier than age 24 weeks and at least 16 weeks after the first dose.

c **Rotavirus vaccine (RV)** *(minimum age: 6 weeks for both RV-1 [Rotarix] and RV-5 [RotaTeq])*
  - Maximum age for the first dose in the series is 14 weeks 6 days, and 8 months 0 days for the final dose in the series. Vaccination should not be initiated for infants 15 weeks 0 days or older.
  - If RV-1 (*Rotarix*) is administered at 2 and 4 months of age, a dose at 6 months is not indicated.

d **Diphtheria and tetanus toxoids and acellular pertussis vaccine (DTaP)** *(minimum age: 6 weeks)*
  - The fourth dose may be administered as early as 12 months of age, provided at least 6 months have elapsed since the third dose.

e *Haemophilus influenzae* **type b conjugate vaccine (Hib)** *(minimum age: 6 weeks)*
  - If PRP-OMP (*PedvaxHIB* or *ComVax* [HepB-Hib]) is administered at 2 and 4 months of age, a dose at 6 months of age is not indicated.
  - *Hiberix* should only be used for the booster (final) dose in children 12 months through 4 years of age.

f **Pneumococcal vaccine** *(minimum age: 6 weeks for pneumococcal conjugate vaccine [PCV]; 2 years for pneumococcal polysaccharide vaccine [PPSV])*
  - Administer 1 dose of PCV to all healthy children 24 through 59 months of age who are not completely vaccinated for their age.
  - For children who have received an age-appropriate series of 7-valent PCV (PCV7), a single supplemental dose of 13-valent PCV (PCV13) is recommended for: all children 14 through 59 months of age and children 60 through 71 months of age with underlying medical conditions.
  - Administer PPSV at least 8 weeks after last dose of PCV to children 2 years or older with certain underlying medical conditions, including a cochlear implant. See *MMWR* 2010;59(RR-11) available at http://www.cdc.gov/mmwr/pdf/rr/rr5911.pdf.

g **Inactivated poliovirus vaccine (IPV)** *(minimum age: 6 weeks)*
  - If 4 or more doses are administered before 4 years of age, an additional dose should be administered at 4 to 6 years of age.
  - The final dose in the series should be administered on or after the fourth birthday and at least 6 months after the previous dose.

h **Influenza vaccine** *(minimum age: 6 months for trivalent inactivated influenza vaccine [TIV]; 2 years for live, attenuated influenza vaccine [LAIV])*
  - For most healthy children 2 years and older, either LAIV or TIV may be used. However, LAIV should not be administered to some children, including 1) children with asthma, 2) children 2 through 4 years of age who have had wheezing in the past 12 months, or 3) children who have any other underlying medical conditions that predispose them to influenza complications. For all other contraindications to use of LAIV, see *MMWR* 2010;59(RR-8) available at http://www.cdc.gov/mmwr/pdf/rr/rr5908.pdf.
  - For children 6 months through 8 years of age: For the 2011-12 season, administer 2 doses (separated by at least 4 weeks) to those who did not receive at least 1 dose of the 2010-11 vaccine. Those who received at least 1 dose of the 2010-11 vaccine require 1 dose for the 2011-12 season. For the 2012-13 season, follow dosing guidelines in the 2012 ACIP influenza vaccine recommendations.

i **Measles, mumps, and rubella vaccine (MMR)** *(minimum age: 12 months)*
  - The second dose may be administered before 4 years of age, provided at least 4 weeks have elapsed since the first dose.
  - Administer MMR vaccine to infants 6 through 11 months of age who are traveling internationally. These children should be revaccinated with 2 doses of MMR vaccine, the first at ages 12 through 15 months and at least 4 weeks after the previous dose, and the second at ages 4 through 6 years.

j **Varicella vaccine** *(minimum age: 12 months)*
  - The second dose may be administered before 4 years of age, provided at least 3 months have elapsed since the first dose.
  - For children 12 months to 12 years of age, the recommended minimum interval between doses is 3 months. However, if the second dose was administered at least 4 weeks after the first dose, it can be accepted as valid.

k **Hepatitis A vaccine (HepA)** *(minimum age: 12 months)*
  - Administer the second (final) dose 6 to 18 months after the first.
  - Unvaccinated children 24 months and older at high risk should be vaccinated. See *MMWR* 2006;55(RR-7) available at http://www.cdc.gov/mmwr/pdf/rr/rr5507.pdf.
  - A 2-dose HepA vaccine series is recommended for anyone 24 months and older, previously unvaccinated, for whom immunity against hepatitis A virus infection is desired.

l **Meningococcal conjugate vaccine, quadrivalent (MCV4)** *(minimum age: 9 months for Menactra [MCV4-D]; 2 years for Menveo [MCV4-CRM])*
  - For children 9 through 23 months of age 1) with persistent complement component deficiency; 2) who are residents of or travelers to countries with hyperendemic or epidemic disease; or 3) who are present during outbreaks caused by a vaccine serogroup, administer 2 primary doses of MCV4-D, ideally at ages 9 months and 12 months or at least 8 weeks apart.
  - For children 24 months and older with 1) persistent complement component deficiency who have not been previously vaccinated; or 2) anatomic/functional asplenia, administer 2 primary doses of either MCV4 at least 8 weeks apart.
  - For children with anatomic/functional asplenia, if MCV4-D (*Menactra*) is used, administer at a minimum age of 2 years and at least 4 weeks after completion of all PCV doses.
  - See *MMWR* 2011;60(3):72-76 available at http://www.cdc.gov/mmwr/pdf/wk/mm6003.pdf and Vaccines for Children Program resolution No. 6/11-1 available at http://www.cdc.gov/vaccines/programs/vfc/downloads/resolutions/06-11-mening-mcv.pdf and *MMWR* 2011;60(40):1391-1392 available at http://www.cdc.gov/mmwr/pdf/wk/mm6040.pdf for further guidance, including revaccination guidelines.

For those who fall behind or start late, see the catch-up schedule.

Recommended Immunization Schedule for Children 7 to 18 Years of Age — United States, 2012[a]			
Vaccine	Age		
	7 to 10 y	11 to 12 y	13 to 18 y
Tetanus, diphtheria, pertussis[b]	1 dose (if indicated)	1 dose	1 dose (if indicated)
Human papillomavirus[c]	c	3 doses	HPV series
Meningococcal[d]	d	Dose 1	Booster at 16 y
Influenza[e]	Influenza (yearly)		
Pneumococcal[f]	f		
Hepatitis A[g]	HepA series		
Hepatitis B[h]	HepB series		
Inactivated poliovirus[i]	IPV series		
Measles, mumps, rubella[j]	MMR series		
Varicella[k]	Varicella series		

Range of recommended ages for all children

Range of recommended ages for catch-up immunization

Range of recommended ages for certain high-risk groups

a This schedule includes recommendations in effect as of December 23, 2011. Any dose not administered at the recommended age should be administered at a subsequent visit, when indicated and feasible. The use of a combination vaccine generally is preferred over separate injections of its equivalent component vaccines. Providers should consult the relevant ACIP statement for detailed recommendations available at http://www.cdc.gov/vaccines/pubs/acip-list.htm. Clinically significant adverse events that follow immunization should be reported to VAERS at http://www.vaers.hhs.gov or by telephone, 1-800-822-7967.

b **Tetanus and diphtheria toxoids and acellular pertussis vaccine (Tdap)** *(minimum age: 10 years for Boostrix and 11 years for Adacel)*
   • Persons 11 to 18 years of age who have not received Tdap vaccine should receive a dose followed by Td booster doses every 10 years thereafter.
   • Tdap vaccine should be substituted for a single dose of Td in the catch-up series for children 7 through 10 years of age. Refer to the catch-up schedule if additional doses of tetanus and diphtheria toxoid–containing vaccine are needed.
   • Tdap can be administered regardless of the interval since the last tetanus and diphtheria toxoid–containing vaccine.

c **Human papillomavirus vaccine (HPV) (HPV4 [*Gardasil*] and HPV2 [*Cervarix*])** *(minimum age: 9 years)*
   • Either HPV4 or HPV2 is recommended in a 3-dose series for females 11 or 12 years of age. HPV4 is recommended in a 3-dose series for males 11 or 12 years of age.
   • The vaccine series can be started beginning at 9 years of age.
   • Administer the second dose 1 to 2 months after the first dose and the third dose 6 months after the first dose (at least 24 weeks after the first dose).
   • See *MMWR* 2010;59(20):626-632 available at http://www.cdc.gov/mmwr/pdf/wk/mm5920.pdf.

d **Meningococcal conjugate vaccine, quadrivalent (MCV4)**
   • Administer MCV4 at 11 through 12 years of age with a booster dose at 16 years of age.
   • Administer MCV4 at 13 through 18 years of age if patient is not previously vaccinated.
   • If the first dose is administered at 13 through 15 years of age, a booster dose should be administered at 16 through 18 years of age with a minimum interval of at least 8 weeks after the preceding dose.
   • If the first dose is administered at 16 years or older, a booster dose is not needed.
   • Administer 2 primary doses at least 8 weeks apart to previously unvaccinated persons with persistent complement component deficiency or anatomic/functional asplenia, and 1 dose every 5 years thereafter.
   • Adolescents 11 through 18 years of age with human immunodeficiency virus (HIV) infections should receive a 2-dose primary series of MCV4 at least 8 weeks apart.
   • See *MMWR* 2011;60(3):72-76 available at http://www.cdc.gov/mmwr/pdf/wk/mm6003.pdf and Vaccines for Children Program resolution No. 6/11-1 available at http://www.cdc.gov/vaccines/programs/vfc/downloads/resolutions/06-11-mening-mcv.pdf for further guidelines.

e **Influenza vaccine (trivalent inactivated influenza vaccine [TIV] and live, attenuated influenza vaccine [LAIV])**
   • For most healthy, nonpregnant persons, either LAIV or TIV may be used, except LAIV should not be used for some persons, including those with asthma or any other underlying medical conditions that predispose them to influenza complications. For all other contraindications to use of LAIV, see *MMWR* 2010;59(RR-8) available at http://www.cdc.gov/mmwr/pdf/rr/rr5908.pdf.
   • Administer 1 dose to persons 9 years and older.

- For children 6 months through 8 years of age: For the 2011-12 season, administer 2 doses (separated by at least 4 weeks) to those who did not receive at least 1 dose of the 2010-11 vaccine. Those who received at least 1 dose of the 2010-11 vaccine require 1 dose for the 2011-12 season. For the 2012-13 season, follow dosing guidelines in the 2012 ACIP influenza recommendations.

f **Pneumococcal vaccine (pneumococcal conjugate vaccine [PCV] and pneumococcal polysaccharide vaccine [PPSV])**
- A single dose of PCV may be administered to children 6 through 18 years of age who have anatomic/functional asplenia, HIV infection or other immunocompromising condition, cochlear implant, or cerebral spinal fluid leak. See *MMWR* 2010;59(RR-11) available at http://www.cdc.gov/mmwr/pdf/rr/rr5911.pdf.
- Administer PPSV at least 8 weeks after the previous dose of PCV to children 2 years or older with certain underlying medical conditions, including a cochlear implant. A single revaccination should be administered after 5 years to children with anatomic/functional asplenia or an immunocompromising condition.

g **Hepatitis A vaccine (HepA)**
- HepA vaccine is recommended for children older than 23 months of age who live in areas where vaccination programs target older children, who are at increased risk of infection, or for whom immunity against hepatitis A virus is desired. See *MMWR* 2006:55(RR-7) available at http://www.cdc.gov/mmwr/pdf/rr/rr5507.pdf.
- Administer 2 doses at least 6 months apart to unvaccinated persons.

h **Hepatitis B vaccine (HepB)**
- Administer the 3-dose series to those not previously vaccinated.
- For those with incomplete vaccination, follow the catch-up recommendations.
- A 2-dose series (separated by at least 4 months) of adult formulation *Recombivax HB* is licensed for use in children 11 to 15 years of age.

i **Inactivated poliovirus vaccine (IPV)**
- The final dose in the series should be administered at least 6 months after the previous dose.
- If both OPV and IPV were administered as part of a series, a total of 4 doses should be administered, regardless of the child's current age.
- IPV is not routinely recommended for US residents 18 years or older.

j **Measles, mumps, and rubella vaccine (MMR)**
- The minimum interval between the 2 doses of MMR vaccine is 4 weeks.

k **Varicella vaccine**
- For persons without evidence of immunity (see *MMWR*. 2007;56[RR-4] available at http://www.cdc.gov/mmwr/pdf/rr/rr5504.pdf), administer 2 doses if not previously vaccinated or the second dose if only 1 dose has been administered.
- For persons 7 to 12 years of age, the recommended minimum interval between doses is 3 months. However, if the second dose was administered at least 4 weeks after the first dose, it can be accepted as valid.
- For persons 13 years of age or older, the minimum interval between doses is 4 weeks.

References:

ACIP. Recommended immunization schedules for persons aged 0 through 18 years– United States, 2012. *MMWR*. 2012;61(5):QG1-QG4.

Catch-up Immunization Schedule for Persons 4 Months to 18 Years of Age Who Start Late or Who Are More Than 1 Month Behind

The following table provides catch-up schedules and minimum intervals between doses for children whose vaccinations have been delayed. A vaccine series does not need to be restarted, regardless of the time that has elapsed between doses. Use the section appropriate for the child's age.

Catch-Up Schedule for Persons 4 Months to 6 Years of Age — United States, 2012					
Vaccine	Minimum age for dose 1	Minimum interval between doses			
		Dose 1 to 2	Dose 2 to 3	Dose 3 to 4	Dose 4 to 5
HepB	**Birth**	**4 weeks**	**8 weeks** and ≥ 16 weeks after first dose; minimum age for final dose is 24 weeks		
Rotavirus[a]	**6 weeks**	**4 weeks**	**4 weeks**[a]		
DTaP[b]	**6 weeks**	**4 weeks**	**4 weeks**	**6 months**	**6 months**[b]
Hib[c]	**6 weeks**	**4 weeks** if first dose administered at younger than 12 months of age **8 weeks** (as final dose) if first dose administered at 12 to 14 months of age **No further doses needed** if first dose administered at 15 months of age or older	**4 weeks**[c] if current age is younger than 12 months **8 weeks** (as final dose)[c] if current age is 12 months or older and first dose administered at younger than 12 months of age and second dose administered at younger than 15 months of age **No further doses needed** if previous dose administered at 15 months of age or older	**8 weeks** (as final dose) This dose only necessary for children 12 to 59 months of age who received 3 doses before 12 months of age	

Catch-Up Schedule for Persons 4 Months to 6 Years of Age — United States, 2012				
	Minimum age for dose 1	Minimum interval between doses		
Vaccine		Dose 1 to 2	Dose 2 to 3	Dose 3 to 4	Dose 4 to 5
Pneumo-coccal[d]	6 weeks	**4 weeks** if first dose administered at younger than 12 months of age **8 weeks** (as final dose for healthy children) if first dose administered at 12 months of age or older or current age is 24 to 59 months **No further doses needed** for healthy children if first dose administered at 24 months of age or older	**4 weeks** if current age is younger than 12 months **8 weeks** (as final dose for healthy children) if current age is 12 months or older **No further doses needed** for healthy children if previous dose administered at 24 months of age or older	**8 weeks** (as final dose) This dose only necessary for children 12 to 59 months of age who received 3 doses before 12 months of age or for high-risk children who received 3 doses at any age	
IPV[e]	6 weeks	**4 weeks**	**4 weeks**	**6 months**[e] minimum age 4 years for final dose	
Meningo-coccal[f]	9 months	**8 weeks**[f]			
MMR[g]	12 months	**4 weeks**			
Varicella[h]	12 months	**3 months**			
HepA	12 months	**6 months**			

Catch-Up Schedule for Children 7 to 18 Years of Age — United States, 2012					
Vaccine	Minimum age for dose 1	Minimum interval between doses			
		Dose 1 to 2	Dose 2 to 3	Dose 3 to 4	Dose 4 to 5
Td/Tdap[j]	7 years[j]	4 weeks	4 weeks if first dose administered at younger than 12 months of age 6 months if first dose administered at 12 months of age or older	6 months if first dose administered at younger than 12 months of age	
HPV[k]	9 years	Routine dosing intervals are recommended[k]			
HepA	12 months	6 months			
HepB	Birth	4 weeks	8 weeks (and at least 16 weeks after first dose)		
IPV[e]	6 weeks	4 weeks	4 weeks[e]	6 months[e]	
Meningococcal[f]	9 months	8 weeks[f]			
MMR[g]	12 months	4 weeks			
Varicella[h]	12 months	3 months if person is younger than 13 years of age 4 weeks if person is 13 years of age or older			

a **Rotavirus vaccine (RV) (RV-1 [*Rotarix*] and RV-5 [*RotaTeq*])**
- The maximum age for the first dose is 14 weeks 6 days; and 8 months 0 days for the final dose in the series. Vaccination should not be initiated for infants 15 weeks 0 days of age or older.
- If RV-1 was administered for the first and second doses, a third dose is not indicated.

b **Diphtheria and tetanus toxoids and acellular pertussis vaccine (DTaP)**
- The fifth dose is not necessary if the fourth dose was administered at 4 years or older.

c **Haemophilus influenzae type b conjugate vaccine (Hib)**
- Hib vaccine should be considered for unvaccinated persons 5 years or older who have sickle cell disease, leukemia, human immunodeficiency virus (HIV) infection, or anatomic/functional asplenia.
- If the first 2 doses were PRP-OMP (*PedvaxHIB* or *Comvax*), and administered at 11 months or younger, the third (and final) dose should be administered at 12 to 15 months of age and at least 8 weeks after the second dose.
- If the first dose was administered at 7 to 11 months of age, administer the second dose at least 4 weeks later and a final dose at 12 to 15 months of age.

d **Pneumococcal vaccine** *(minimum age: 6 weeks for pneumococcal conjugate vaccine [PCV]; 2 years for pneumococcal polysaccharide vaccine [PPSV])*
- For children 24 through 71 months of age with underlying medical conditions, administer 1 dose of PCV if 3 doses of PCV were received previously, or administer 2 doses of PCV at least 8 weeks apart if fewer than 3 doses of PCV were received previously.
- A single dose of PCV may be administered to certain children 6 through 18 years of age with underlying medical conditions. See age-specific schedules for details.
- Administer PPSV to children 2 years or older with certain underlying medical conditions. See *MMWR* 2010;59(RR-11) available at http://www.cdc.gov/mmwr/pdf/rr/rr5911.pdf.

e **Inactivated poliovirus vaccine (IPV)**
- A fourth dose is not necessary if the third dose was administered at 4 years or older and at least 6 months after the previous dose.
- In the first 6 months of life, minimum age and minimum intervals are only recommended if the person is at risk for imminent exposure to circulating poliovirus (ie, travel to a polio-endemic region or during an outbreak).
- IPV is not routinely recommended for US residents 18 years or older.

f **Meningococcal conjugate vaccine, quadrivalent (MCV4)** *(minimum age: 9 months for Menactra [MCV4-D]; 2 years for Menveo [MCV4-CRM])*
- See Recommended Immunization Schedule for Children 0 to 6 Years of Age — United States, 2012 table and Recommended Immunization Schedule for Children 7 to 18 Years of Age — United States, 2012 table for further guidance.

g **Measles, mumps, and rubella vaccine (MMR)**
- Administer the second dose routinely at 4 to 6 years of age.

h **Varicella vaccine**
- Administer the second dose routinely at 4 to 6 years of age. If the second dose was administered at least 4 weeks after the first dose, it can be accepted as valid.

j **Tetanus and diphtheria toxoids vaccine (Td) and tetanus and diphtheria toxoids and acellular pertussis vaccine (Tdap)**
- For children 7 through 10 years of age who are not fully immunized with the childhood DTaP vaccine series, Tdap vaccine should be substituted for a single dose of Td vaccine in the catch-up series; if additional doses are needed, use Td vaccine. For these children, an adolescent Tdap vaccine dose should not be given.
- An inadvertent dose of DTaP vaccine administered to children 7 through 10 years of age can count as part of the catch-up series. This dose can count as the adolescent Tdap dose, or the child can later receive a Tdap booster dose at 11 through 12 years of age.

k **Human papillomavirus vaccine (HPV) (HPV4 [*Gardasil*] and HPV2 [*Cervarix*])**
- Administer the vaccine series to females (either HPV2 or HPV4) and males (HPV4) at 13 to 18 years of age if not previously vaccinated.
- Use recommended routine dosing intervals for vaccine series catch-up; see Recommended Immunization Schedule for Children 7 to 18 Years of Age — United States, 2012 table.

References:

ACIP. Recommended immunization schedules for persons aged 0 through 18 years–United States, 2012. *MMWR*. 2011;60(5):QG1-QG4. http://www.cdc.gov/mmwr/pdf/wk/mm6005.pdf.

Immunization Schedules for Adults

These schedules indicated the recommended age groups and medical indications for which administration of currently licensed vaccines is commonly indicated for adults 19 years and older, as of January 1, 2012. For all vaccines being recommended on the Adult Immunization Schedule: a vaccine series does not need to be restarted, regardless of the time that has elapsed between doses. Licensed combination vaccines may be used whenever any components of the combination are indicated and when the vaccine's other components are not contraindicated. For detailed recommendations on all vaccines, including those used primarily for travelers or that are issued during the year, consult the manufacturer's package inserts and the complete statements from the ACIP (http://www.cdc.gov/vaccines/pubs/acip-list.htm). Use of trade names and commercial sources is for identification only and does not imply endorsement.

ACIP vaccine recommendations and additional resources are available at http://www.cdc.gov/vaccines/pubs/acip-list.htm.

Information on travel vaccine requirements and recommendations (eg; for hepatitis A and B, meningococcal, and other vaccines) is available at http://wwwnc.cdc.gov/travel/page/vaccinations.htm.

NOTE: These recommendations must be read along with the footnotes that follow containing number of doses, intervals between doses, and other important information.

Recommended Adult Immunization Schedule by Vaccine and Age Group – United States, 2012

Vaccine	Age group (y)					
	19 to 21	22 to 26	27 to 49	50 to 59	60 to 64	≥ 65
Influenza[a]	1 dose annually					
Td/Tdap[b,*]	Substitute 1-time dose of Tdap for Td booster; then boost with Td every 10 y				Td/Tdap[c]	
Varicella[d,*]	2 doses					
HPV female[e,*]	3 doses					
HPV male[e,*]	3 doses					
Zoster[f]					1 dose	
MMR[g,*]	1 or 2 doses					1 dose
Pneumococcal (polysaccharide)[h,i]			1 or 2 doses			1 dose
Meningococcal[j,*]			1 or more doses			
Hepatitis A[k,*]			2 doses			
Hepatitis B[l,*]			3 doses			

For all persons in this category who meet the age requirements and who lack documentation of vaccination or have no evidence of previous infection.

Recommended if some other risk factor is present (eg, based on medical, occupational, lifestyle, or other indications).

No recommendation.

Vaccines That Might Be Indicated for Adults Based on Medical and Other Indications – United States, 2012

Indication

Vaccine	Pregnancy	Immuno-compromis-ing conditions (excluding HIV)^d,f,g,n	HIV infection CD4+ T lymphocyte count <200 cells/mcL	HIV infection CD4+ T lymphocyte count ≥200 cells/mcL	Men who have sex with men	Heart disease, chronic lung disease, chronic alcoholism	Asplenia^m (including elective splenectomy and persistent complement component deficiencies)	Chronic liver disease	Diabetes, kidney failure, end-stage renal disease, receipt of hemodialysis	Health care personnel
Influenza^a	1 dose TIV annually	1 dose TIV annually	1 dose TIV annually		1 dose TIV or LAIV annually		1 dose TIV annually	1 dose TIV annually		1 dose TIV or LAIV annually
Td/Tdap^b,*	Substitute 1-time dose of Tdap for Td booster; then boost with Td every 10 y									
Varicella^d,*	Contraindicated	Contraindicated	Contraindicated	2 doses	2 doses	2 doses	2 doses	2 doses	2 doses	2 doses
HPV female^e,*	3 doses through 26 y of age	3 doses through 26 y of age	3 doses through 26 y of age	3 doses through 26 y of age	3 doses through 26 y of age	3 doses through 26 y of age	3 doses through 26 y of age	3 doses through 26 y of age	3 doses through 26 y of age	
HPV male^e,*		3 doses through 26 y of age	3 doses through 26 y of age	3 doses through 26 y of age	3 doses through 21 y of age	3 doses through 21 y of age	3 doses through 21 y of age	3 doses through 21 y of age	3 doses through 21 y of age	
Zoster^f	Contraindicated	Contraindicated	Contraindicated		1 dose	1 dose	1 dose	1 dose	1 dose	1 dose
MMR^g,*	Contraindicated	Contraindicated	Contraindicated		1 or 2 doses	1 or 2 doses	1 or 2 doses	1 or 2 doses	1 or 2 doses	1 or 2 doses
Pneumococcal (polysac-charide)^h,i		1 or 2 doses	1 or 2 doses	1 or 2 doses	1 or 2 doses	1 or 2 doses	1 or 2 doses	1 or 2 doses	1 or 2 doses	
Meningococcal^j,*	1 or more doses	1 or more doses	1 or more doses	1 or more doses	1 or more doses	1 or more doses	1 or more doses	1 or more doses	1 or more doses	
Hepatitis A^k,*	2 doses	2 doses	2 doses	2 doses	2 doses	2 doses	2 doses	2 doses	2 doses	
Hepatitis B^l,*	3 doses	3 doses	3 doses	3 doses	3 doses	3 doses	3 doses	3 doses	3 doses	

For all persons in this category who meet the age requirements and who lack documentation of vaccination or have no evidence of previous infection.

Recommended if some other risk factor is present (eg, based on medical, occupational, lifestyle, or other indications).

Contraindicated.

No recommendation.

* Covered by the Vaccine Injury Compensation Program.

a **Influenza vaccination**
- Annual vaccination against influenza is recommended for all persons 6 months and older.
- Persons 6 months and older, including pregnant women, can receive the trivalent inactivated vaccine (TIV).
- Healthy, nonpregnant adults younger than 50 years without high-risk medical conditions can receive either intranasally administered live, attenuated influenza vaccine (LAIV) (*Flu-Mist*) or TIV. Health care personnel who care for severely immunocompromised persons (ie, those who require care in a protected environment) should receive TIV rather than LAIV. Other persons should receive TIV.
- The intramuscular or intradermal administered TIV are options for adults 18 through 64 years of age.
- Adults 65 years and older can receive the standard dose TIV or the high-dose TIV (*Fluzone High-Dose*).

b **Tetanus, diphtheria, and acellular pertussis (Td/Tdap) vaccination**
- Administer a 1-time dose of Tdap to adults younger than 65 years who have not received Tdap previously or for whom vaccine status is unknown to replace 1 of the 10-year Td boosters.
- Tdap is specifically recommended for the following persons: 1) pregnant women more than 20 weeks' gestation, 2) adults, regardless of age, who are close contacts of infants younger than 12 months (eg, parents, grandparents, or child care providers), and 3) health care personnel.
- Tdap can be administered regardless of interval since the most recent tetanus or diphtheria–containing vaccine.
- Pregnant women not vaccinated during pregnancy should receive Tdap immediately postpartum.
- Adults 65 years and older may receive Tdap.
- Adults with unknown or incomplete history of completing a 3-dose primary vaccination series with Td-containing vaccines should begin or complete a primary vaccination series. Tdap should be substituted for a single dose of Td in the vaccination series with Tdap preferred as the first dose.
- For unvaccinated adults, administer the first 2 doses at least 4 weeks apart and the third dose 6 to 12 months after the second.
- If incompletely vaccinated (ie, less than 3 doses), administer remaining doses.

c Refer to the ACIP statement for recommendations for administering Td/Tdap as prophylaxis in wound management.

d **Varicella vaccination**
- Tdap is recommended for adults 65 and older who have contact with children younger than 12 months of age. Either Td or Tdap can be used if there is no infant contact.
- All adults without evidence of immunity to varicella (as defined below) should receive 2 doses of single-antigen varicella vaccine or a second dose if they have received only 1 dose.
- Special consideration should be given to those who: 1) have close contact with persons at high risk for severe disease (eg, health care personnel and family contacts of persons with immunocompromising conditions) or 2) are at high risk for exposure or transmission (eg, teachers; child care employees; residents and staff members of institutional settings, including correctional institutions; college students; military personnel; adolescents and adults living in households with children; nonpregnant women of childbearing age; and international travelers).
- Pregnant women should be assessed for evidence of varicella immunity. Women who do not have evidence of immunity should receive the first dose of varicella vaccine upon completion or termination of pregnancy and before discharge from the health care facility. The second dose should be administered 4 to 8 weeks after the first dose.
- Evidence of immunity to varicella in adults includes any of the following: 1) documentation of 2 doses of varicella vaccine at least 4 weeks apart; 2) US-born before 1980 (although for health care personnel and pregnant women, birth before 1980 should not be considered evidence of immunity); 3) history of varicella based on diagnosis or verification of varicella by a health care provider (for a patient reporting a history of or having an atypical case, a mild case, or both, health care providers should seek either an epidemiologic link with a typical varicella case or to a laboratory-confirmed case or evidence of laboratory confirmation, if it was performed at the time of acute disease); 4) history of herpes zoster based on diagnosis or verification of herpes zoster by a health care provider; or 5) laboratory evidence of immunity or laboratory confirmation of disease.

e **Human papillomavirus (HPV) vaccination**
- Two vaccines are licensed for use in females, bivalent HPV vaccine (HPV2) and quadrivalent HPV vaccine (HPV4), and one HPV vaccine for use in males (HPV4).
- For females, either HPV4 or HPV2 is recommended in a 3-dose series for routine vaccination at 11 or 12 years of age, and for those 13 through 26 years of age, if not previously vaccinated.
- For males, HPV4 is recommended in a 3-dose series for routine vaccination at 11 or 12 years of age, and for those 13 through 21 years of age, and for those 13 through 21 years of age, if not previously vaccinated. Males 22 through 26 years of age may be vaccinated.
- HPV vaccines are not live vaccines and can be administered to persons who are immunocompromised as a result of infection (including HIV infection), disease, or medications. Vaccine is recommended for immunocompromised persons through 26 years of age who did not get any or all doses when they were younger. The immune response and vaccine efficacy might be less than that in immunocompetent persons.

- Men who have sex with men might especially benefit from vaccination to prevent condyloma and anal cancer. HPV4 is recommended for men who have sex with men through age 26 years who did not get any or all doses when they were younger.
- Ideally, vaccine should be administered before potential exposure to HPV through sexual activity; however, persons who are sexually active should still be vaccinated consistent with age-based recommendations. HPV vaccine can be administered to persons with a history of genital warts, abnormal Papanicolaou test, or positive HPV DNA test.
- A complete series for either HPV4 or HPV2 consists of 3 doses. The second dose should be administered 1 to 2 months after the first dose; the third dose should be administered 6 months after the first dose (at least 24 weeks after the first dose).
- Although HPV vaccination is not specifically recommended for health care personnel based on their occupation, health care personnel should receive the HPV vaccine if they are in the recommended age group.

f **Zoster vaccination**

- A single dose of zoster vaccine is recommended for adults 60 years and older regardless of whether they report a prior episode of herpes zoster. Although the vaccine is licensed by the FDA for use among and can be administered to persons 50 years and older, the ACIP recommends that vaccination begin at 60 years of age.
- Persons with chronic medical conditions may be vaccinated unless their condition constitutes a contraindication, such as pregnancy or severe immunodeficiency.
- Although zoster vaccination is not specifically recommended for health care personnel, health care personnel should receive the vaccine if they are in the recommended age group.

g **Measles, mumps, rubella (MMR) vaccination**

- Adults born before 1957 generally are considered immune to measles and mumps. All adults born in 1957 or later should have documentation of 1 or more doses of MMR vaccine unless they have a medical contraindication to the vaccine, laboratory evidence of immunity to each of the 3 diseases, or documentation of provider-diagnosed measles or mumps disease. For rubella, documentation of provider-diagnosed disease is not considered acceptable evidence of immunity.

Measles component –

- A routine second dose of MMR vaccine, administered a minimum of 28 days after the first dose, is recommended for adults who: 1) are students in postsecondary educational institutions; 2) work in a health care facility; or 3) plan to travel internationally.
- Persons who received inactivated (killed) measles vaccine or measles vaccine of unknown type from 1963 to 1967 should be revaccinated with 2 doses of MMR vaccine.

Mumps component –

- A routine second dose of MMR vaccine, administered a minimum of 28 days after the first dose, is recommended for adults who: 1) are students in postsecondary educational institutions; 2) work in a health care facility; or 3) plan to travel internationally.
- Persons vaccinated before 1979 with either killed mumps vaccine or mumps vaccine of unknown type who are at high risk for mumps infection (eg, persons who are working in a health care facility) should be revaccinated with 2 doses of MMR vaccine.

Rubella component –

- For women of childbearing age, regardless of birth year, rubella immunity should be determined. If there is no evidence of immunity, women who are not pregnant should be vaccinated. Pregnant women who do not have evidence of immunity should receive MMR vaccine upon completion or termination of pregnancy and before discharge from the health care facility.

Health care personnel born before 1957 –

- For unvaccinated health care personnel born before 1957 who lack laboratory evidence of measles, mumps, and/or rubella immunity or laboratory confirmation of disease, health care facilities should consider routinely vaccinating personnel with 2 doses of MMR vaccine at the appropriate interval for measles and mumps or 1 dose of MMR vaccine for rubella.

h **Pneumococcal polysaccharide vaccination (PPSV)**

- Vaccinate all persons with the following indications: 1) 65 years and older without a history of PPSV vaccination; 2) adults younger than 65 years of age with chronic lung disease (including chronic obstructive pulmonary disease, emphysema, and asthma); chronic cardiovascular diseases; diabetes mellitus; chronic liver disease (including cirrhosis); alcoholism; cochlear implants, chronic cerebrospinal fluid leaks; immunocompromising conditions; and functional or anatomic asplenia (eg, sickle cell disease and other hemoglobinopathies, congenital or acquired asplenia, splenic dysfunction, or splenectomy [if elective splenectomy is planned, vaccinate at least 2 weeks before surgery]); 3) residents of nursing homes or long-term care facilities; and 4) adults who smoke cigarettes.
- Persons with asymptomatic or symptomatic HIV infection should be vaccinated as soon as possible after their diagnosis.
- When cancer chemotherapy or other immunosuppressive therapy is being considered, the interval between vaccination and initiation of immunosuppressive therapy should be at least 2 weeks. vaccination during chemotherapy or radiation therapy should be avoided.

- Routine use of PPSV is not recommended for American Indians/Alaska Natives or other persons younger than 65 years unless they have underlying medical conditions that are PPSV indications. However, public health authorities may consider recommending PPSV for American Indians/Alaska Natives who are living in areas where the risk for invasive pneumococcal disease is increased.

i **Revaccination with PPSV**

- One-time revaccination 5 years after the first dose is recommended for persons 19 through 64 years of age with chronic renal failure or nephrotic syndrome; functional or anatomic asplenia (eg, sickle cell disease or splenectomy); and for persons with immunocompromising conditions.
- Persons who received PPSV before age 65 years for any indication should receive another dose of the vaccine at age 65 years or later if at least 5 years have passed since their previous dose.
- No further doses are needed for persons vaccinated with PPSV at or after age 65 years.

j **Meningococcal vaccination**

- Administer 2 doses of meningococcal conjugate vaccine quadrivalent (MCV4) at least 2 months apart to adults with functional asplenia or persistent complement component deficiencies.
- HIV-infected persons who are vaccinated should also receive 2 doses.
- Administer a single dose of meningococcal vaccine to microbiologists routinely exposed to isolates of *Neisseria meningitidis*; military recruits; and persons who travel to or live in countries in which meningococcal disease is hyperendemic or epidemic.
- First-year college students up through age 21 years who are living in residence halls should be vaccinated if they have not received a dose on or after their sixteenth birthday.
- MCV4 is preferred for adults with any of the preceding indications who are 55 years and younger; meningococcal polysaccharide vaccine (MPSV4) is preferred for adults 56 years and older.
- Revaccination with MCV4 every 5 years for adults previously vaccinated with MCV4 or MPSV4 who remain at increased risk for infection (eg, adults with anatomic or functional asplenia or persistent complement component deficiencies).

k **Hepatitis A vaccination**

- Vaccinate any person seeking protection from hepatitis A virus (HAV) infection and persons with any of the following indications: 1) men who have sex with men or persons who use injection drugs; 2) persons working with HAV-infected primates or with HAV in a research laboratory setting; 3) persons with chronic liver disease and persons who receive clotting-factor concentrates; 4) persons traveling to or working in countries that have high or intermediate endemicity of hepatitis A; and 5) unvaccinated persons who anticipate close personal contact (eg, household or regular babysitting) with an international adoptee during the first 60 days after arrival in the United States from a country with high or intermediate endemicity. The first dose of the 2-dose hepatitis A vaccine series should be administered as soon as adoption is planned, ideally 2 or more weeks before the arrival of the adoptee.
- Single-antigen vaccine formulations should be administered in a 2-dose schedule at either 0 and 6 to 12 months (*Havrix*), or 0 and 6 to 18 months (*Vaqta*). If the combined hepatitis A and hepatitis B vaccine (*Twinrix*) is used, administer 3 doses at 0, 1, and 6 months; alternatively, a 4-dose schedule may be used, administered on days 0, 7, and 21 to 30, followed by a booster dose at month 12.

l **Hepatitis B vaccination**

- Vaccinate persons with any of the following indications and any person seeking protection from hepatitis B virus (HBV) infection: 1) sexually active persons who are not in a long-term, mutually monogamous relationship (eg, persons with more than 1 sex partner during the previous 6 months); persons seeking evaluation or treatment for a sexually transmitted disease (STD); current or recent injection-drug users; and men who have sex with men; 2) health care personnel and public safety workers who are exposed to blood or other potentially infectious body fluids; 3) persons with diabetes younger than 60 years as soon as feasible after diagnosis; persons with diabetes who are 60 years or older at the discretion of the treating clinician based on increased need for assisted blood glucose monitoring in long-term care facilities, likelihood of acquiring hepatitis B infection, its complications or chronic sequelae, and likelihood of immune response to vaccination; 4) persons with end-stage renal disease, including patients receiving hemodialysis; persons with HIV infection; and persons with chronic liver disease; 5) household contacts and sex partners of persons with chronic HBV infection; clients and staff members of institutions for persons with developmental disabilities; and international travelers to countries with high or intermediate prevalence of chronic HBV infection; and 6) all adults in the following settings: STD treatment facilities; HIV testing and treatment facilities; facilities providing drug-abuse treatment and prevention services; health care settings targeting services to injection-drug users or men who have sex with men; correctional facilities; end-stage renal disease programs and facilities for chronic hemodialysis patients; and institutions and nonresidential daycare facilities for persons with developmental disabilities.

- Administer missing doses to complete a 3-dose series of hepatitis B vaccine to those persons not vaccinated or not completely vaccinated. The second dose should be administered 1 month after the first dose; the third dose should be given at least 2 months after the second dose (and at least 4 months after the first dose). If the combined hepatitis A and hepatitis B vaccine (*Twinrix*) is used, administer 3 doses at 0, 1, and 6 months; alternatively, a 4-dose *Twinrix* schedule, administered on days 0, 7, and 21 to 30, followed by a booster dose at month 12 may be used.
- Adult patients receiving hemodialysis or with other immunocompromising conditions should receive 1 dose of 40 mcg/mL (*Recombivax HB*) administered on a 3-dose schedule or 2 doses of 20 mcg/mL (*Engerix-B*) administered simultaneously on a 4-dose schedule at 0, 1, 2, and 6 months.

m **Selected conditions for which *Haemophilus influenzae* type b (Hib) vaccine may be used**

- One dose of Hib vaccine should be considered for persons who have sickle cell disease, leukemia, or HIV infection, or who have anatomic or functional asplenia if they have not previously received Hib vaccine.

n **Immunocompromising conditions**

- Inactivated vaccines are generally acceptable (eg, pneumococcal, meningococcal, influenza [inactivated influenza vaccine]), and live vaccines generally are avoided in persons with immune deficiencies or immunocompromising conditions. Information on specific conditions is available at http://www.cdc.gov/vaccines/pubs/acip-list.htm.

References:

ACIP. Recommended adult immunization schedule-United States, 2012. *MMWR.* 2012;61(4):QG1-QG4. http://www.cdc.gov/mmwr/pdf/wk/mm6004.pdf.

Vaccine Indications by Risk Group

Immunization Recommendations Based on Personal Factors

Immunologic drug	Occupation: Health care workers	Day care workers	Essential workers (police, fire, etc.)	Animal/Lab workers	Military personnel	Health Status: HIV-infected people	Other immunodeficiencies	Pregnant women	People with chronic illness	Lifestyle and Other Factors: Travelers and Immigrants	Nursing home and institutional residents or staff	Ethnic and social groups	Other groups
Routine													
Diphtheria and tetanus	Tdap	Tdap	Tdap	Tdap	Tdap	Tdap	Tdap	Tdap	Tdap	Tdap	Tdap	Tdap	Tdap
Measles	+	+			+	HC	0	0		T,I		H	
Mumps	+	+			+	HC	0	0		T,I		H	
Rubella	+	+			+	HC	0	0, RT		T,I		H	
Haemophilus influenzae type b						+	AS	NC	S	I		H	
Hepatitis A	SR	SR		L	T	S	S	NC		T,I	SR	H,SR	PE,SR
Hepatitis B	BX		BX	L (BX)	BX,T	+	HD	HP	HD	T,I	BX,MR,PI	APH, LS	BX,CC, PE
Human papillomavirus										S		S	S
Influenza A & B	+	+	+		+	+	+	NC+	+	T,I	+	H	CS
Pneumococcal						+	+	NC	+	SR	SR	H	
Poliovirus	IPV	IPV		L	IPV	IPV	IPV	NC		T,I		H	CS
Rotavirus						0	0	0				H	S
Varicella	SV	SV		SV	SV	0	SV	0		T,I		H	
Zoster						0	0				+		S

A-18

| Immunization Recommendations Based on Personal Factors | | | | | | | | | | | | |
| Occupation | | | | | Health Status | | | | Lifestyle and Other Factors | | | |
Health care workers	Day care workers	Essential workers (police, fire, etc.)	Animal /Lab workers	Military personnel	HIV-infected people	Other immunodeficiencies	Pregnant women	People with chronic illness	Travelers and Immigrants	Nursing home and institutional residents or staff	Ethnic and social groups	Other groups
Immunologic drug												
Specific scenarios												
Anthrax			A,L	T			RB					
Japanese encephalitis									T			
Meningococcal			L	BT,T	NC	AS	NC		T			
Rabies			A,L	T	0	0	NC		T			PE
Smallpox			L	T			RB	0				
Typhoid			L	T	Vi	Vi	Vi,RB		T			CC
Yellow fever			L	T	0	0	RB					
BCG					0	0	0				B,H	
Tuberculin skin test	TST				TST	TST	SR	NC	SR	T,I	TST	H,SR	ADU CC

A-19

Vaccine Indications by Risk Group

Key for Table

+ – Immunity needed. Vaccine indicated if patient is susceptible. Prescriber must still consider possible contraindications, as well as vaccination history.

O – Vaccine generally contraindicated. Certain isolated individuals may benefit from this vaccine. Consult detailed references.

A – Animal workers, including veterinarians and their assistants.

ADU – Alcoholics, IV drug abusers, and medically under-served, low-income populations.

AP – Alaskan natives, Pacific Islanders, immigrants, and refugees from hepatitis B endemic areas (particularly Haiti, Africa, and Eastern Asia).

AS – Asplenic patients.

B – BCG is indicated in the United States for infants and children at high risk of intimate exposure to persistently untreated or ineffectively treated patients with infectious pulmonary tuberculosis (TB) who cannot be placed on long-term preventative therapy, or those continuously exposed to people with TB who have bacilli resistant to isoniazid and rifampin, or infants and children in groups in which the rate of new infections is 1% per year.

BT – Military recruits at basic training.

BX – If exposed to blood or other contaminated body fluids.

C – Chronic illnesses include: hemodynamically significant cardiovascular disease, pulmonary disease (eg, asthma, active tuberculosis, myasthenia gravis, cystic fibrosis, chronic obstructive pulmonary disease), diabetes mellitus, renal or hepatic dysfunction, sickle-cell and chronic hemolytic anemia, chronic alcoholism, or cirrhosis and others.

CC – Close contacts of pathogen carriers or close contacts of infectious cases.

CS – Close contacts of susceptible patients.

H – When assessing the homeless, review status for all routine vaccines.

HC – HIV-infected children.

HD – Hemophilia, thalassemia, dialysis, and renal failure patients.

HIV – Human immunodeficiency virus.

HP – Screen all pregnant women for HBsAg; vaccinate the newborn infants of mothers who are HBsAg positive.

I – Selected immigrants based on origin, age, and health; includes refugees, guest workers, foreign students, and internationally adopted children.

IPV – Enhanced-potency inactivated poliovirus vaccine (e-IPV), if not vaccinated as a child.

L – Laboratory workers potentially exposed to the corresponding pathogen.

LS – Homosexual and bisexual men, intravenous drug abusers, prostitutes, heterosexually-active people, or recently acquired sexually transmitted disease.

MR – Clients and staff or institutions for the mentally or developmentally retarded.

NC – Not contraindicated.

P – Includes women planning to become pregnant within 3 months.

PE – Used for postexposure prophylaxis.

PI – Prison inmates.

RB – Consider the risk-benefit ratio; vaccinate only if clearly needed.

RT – Screen all pregnant women for rubella antibody titer. If vaccine needed, administer after delivery, but before patient's discharge. $Rh_o(D)$ immune globulin does not interfere with rubella vaccine.

S – Vaccine indicated for selected individuals in this category. See diagnosis and drug tables on following pages.

SR – Many in this category warrant vaccinations, based on other risk factors. See diagnosis and drug tables on following pages.

SV – Women of childbearing potential if seronegative for varicella.

T – Selected travelers, depending on destinations and itinerary. For further information, telephone CDC's international health requirements and recommendations 24-hour hotline: (800) 356-4674.

Td – Adult strength tetanus-diphtheria toxoids (Td) indicated at 10-year intervals. Wound-management guidelines are cited elsewhere.

Tdap – Adult strength tetanus-diphtheria toxoids with acellular pertussis vaccine indicated at 10-year intervals. Wound management guidelines are cited elsewhere.

TST – Many in this category warrant testing.

Vi – Use typhoid Vi injectable vaccine rather than typhoid live attenuated vaccine in capsules.

Diseases and Diagnoses Warranting Immunization	
Disease/Diagnosis	Vaccine(s) indicated
Age ≥ 50 years or ≥ 65 years (even if healthy)	Influenza, pneumococcal
Alcoholism, chronic	Pneumonia
Anemia, chronic, severe (including sickle cell and chronic hemolytic)	Influenza, pneumococcal
Antibiotic allergies, multiple (especially penicillin and erythromycin)	Influenza, pneumococcal
Aspirin therapy, long-term, in children	Influenza
Asplenia	Influenza, pneumococcal
Asthma	Influenza, pneumococcal
Atherosclerosis	Influenza, pneumococcal
Azotemia	Influenza
Bedridden, chronically	Influenza, pneumococcal
Cancer	Influenza, pneumococcal
Cardiovascular disease (altered circulatory dynamics)	Influenza, pneumococcal
Cerebrospinal fluid leaks	Pneumococcal
Cirrhosis	Pneumococcal
Claudication, intermittent	Influenza, pneumococcal
Conditions that compromise respiratory function or handling respiratory secretions	Influenza
Congestive heart failure	Influenza, pneumococcal
Cystic fibrosis	Influenza, pneumococcal
Diabetes mellitus	Influenza, pneumococcal
Dialysis, kidney	Hepatitis B, influenza, pneumococcal
Heart valve, artificial	Influenza, pneumococcal
Hemophilia	Hepatitis A, hepatitis B
Hepatitis B, chronic carriers of	Hepatitis A
Hepatitis C infection	Hepatitis A, hepatitis B
HIV infection	Influenza, pneumococcal
Immunodeficiency, natural or induced	Influenza, pneumococcal
Kidney disease, chronic	Influenza, pneumococcal
Liver failure	Hepatitis A, influenza
Mitral stenosis	Influenza, pneumococcal
Myasthenia gravis	Influenza, pneumococcal
Nephrotic syndrome	Influenza, pneumococcal
Panacinar emphysema (with use of alpha$_1$-proteinase inhibitor)	Hepatitis B
Protein C deficiency, severe congenital (with use of protein C concentrate [human])	Hepatitis A, hepatitis B
Pulmonary disease	Influenza, pneumococcal
Renal failure	Influenza, pneumococcal
Septal defect	Influenza, pneumococcal
Sexually transmitted diseases, repeated	Hepatitis A, hepatitis B
Smoke tobacco, adults who	Pneumococcal
Splenic dysfunction, asplenia	Influenza, pneumococcal
Thalassemia	Hepatitis B
Transplantation, organ	Influenza, pneumococcal
Tuberculosis, active	Influenza, pneumococcal

Drugs Indicative of Disease Warranting Immunization		
Category title	Representative drugs	Immunization-indicating disease states
Anti-Infective Drugs		
Antifungal antibiotics	Ketoconazole	Hyperadrenocorticism
Anti-influenza agents	Amantadine	Influenza A prophylaxis
Antimalarial agents	Chloroquine, hydroxychloroquine	Rheumatoid arthritis, travel to hepatitis-B endemic area
Antitubercular agents	Rifampin, pyrazinamide	Tuberculosis treatment
Antivirals	Zidovudine, didanosine	HIV infection
Sulfonamides	Sulfasalazine	Crohn disease
Antineoplastic Drugs		
Alkylating agents	Cyclophosphamide	Cancer, various
Antimetabolites	Azathioprine	Glomerulonephritis, immunosuppression, nephrotic syndrome, cirrhosis
Interferons	Interferon-alfa	Cancer, hepatitis, various
Mitotic inhibitors	Etoposide	Cancer, various
Blood Modifiers		
Anticoagulants	Heparin, warfarin	Cardiovascular disease
Folic acid products	Leucovorin	Antagonist rescue, anemia
Hemorrheologic agents	Pentoxifylline	Cardiovascular disease
Hemostatics	Coagulation factors VII, IX	Hemophilia
Thrombolytic agents	Alteplase, streptokinase	Cardiovascular disease
Cardiovascular Drugs		
Cardiac drugs	Digoxin, disopyramide	Cardiovascular disease
Diuretics	Furosemide	Congestive heart failure
Vasodilating agents	Dipyridamole, isosorbide nitroglycerin	Cardiovascular disease
CNS Drugs		
Gold compounds	Auranofin	Rheumatoid arthritis
Heavy metal antagonists	Penicillamine	Rheumatoid arthritis
GI Drugs		
Digestants	Pancreatin, pancrelipase	Cystic fibrosis
Miscellaneous GI drugs	Mesalamine	Crohn disease
	Colchicine	Cirrhosis

Drugs Indicative of Disease Warranting Immunization		
Category title	Representative drugs	Immunization-indicating disease states
Hormones		
Adrenal hormones	Corticosteroids	Asthma, certain anemias, immunosuppression
Adrenal steroid inhibitors	Aminoglutethimide, trilostane	Hyperadrenocorticism
Insulins	Insulins	Diabetes mellitus
Sulfonylureas	Glyburide	Diabetes mellitus
Immunologic Drugs		
Immune globulins	IV immune globulin	Immunodeficiency
	Antithymocyte globulin	Organ transplant
	Muromonab-CD3	Organ transplant
Immunosuppressants	Cyclosporine	Organ transplant
Radioisotopes		
Therapeutic isotopes	NaI-131, NaP-32	Certain cancers
Renal Drugs		
Agents for gout	Allopurinol	Renal calculi
Ammonia detoxicants	Potassium acid phosphate	Renal calculi
Respiratory Drugs		
Anticholinergic agents	Ipratropium	Pulmonary disease
Leukotriene receptor antagonists	Zafirlukast	Asthma
Parasympathomimetics	Pyridostigmine bromide	Myasthenia gravis
Respiratory smooth muscle relaxants	Aminophylline, theophylline	Pulmonary disease
Sympathomimetic agents	Albuterol	Pulmonary disease
Enzyme replacements	Alpha$_1$-proteinase inhibitor	Congenital panacinar emphysema

Interviewing & Counseling About Immunizations

Through effective interviewing and counseling, clinicians can increase vaccine acceptance. Interviewing comes first. The only way to determine a patient's needs is to question and evaluate that patient's health risks. In a good interview, which might last just 1 to 5 minutes, the clinician solicits pertinent information regarding medical and immunization history. This information is used in subsequent decisions about vaccines or immunologic tests needed by the patient.

Counseling is the second step, educating patients to change their immunization behavior. Effective counseling of any type requires that the health care professional provide information individualized to the patient's needs. Conduct educational counseling in an understandable manner that enables the patient to accept and carry out immunization recommendations. In this regard, counseling about vaccines is very similar to counseling patients about other medications.

Behavior experts report that there are four primary factors involved in patients' decisions whether or not to be vaccinated:

(1) Perceived barriers to vaccination (eg, expense, ease of access, knowledge),

(2) Belief in the effectiveness of the vaccine,

(3) Perceptions of susceptibility to disease, and

(4) Perceptions of severity of disease if they contract it.

Counseling patients about vaccination should center around these four issues. The simple act of advising patients of their susceptibility and informing them where vaccine is available can dramatically increase vaccine-acceptance rates.

The patient's perceptions of disease susceptibility and vaccine efficacy may not correspond with scientifically accepted fact. In such cases, education can serve a real need. Barriers to vaccination include factors such as fear, anxiety, inconvenience, pain, and expense. If the person considers barriers to be relatively weak and their readiness to be vaccinated is great, then he or she is likely to be immunized. Conversely, if the person's readiness is low and the perceived barriers are strong, then the desired behavior is less likely to occur.

In many cases, the clinician will counsel not the patient, but the patient's agent. For example, parents make immunization decisions for their children and many adults assist with immunization decisions for their aging parents. Viewing the immunization decision through the eyes of the decision maker is important. The key elements in a patient's immunization decision are perceptions of disease susceptibility, disease severity, barriers, and vaccine efficacy. Knowing this, clinicians can target their counsel to improve the probability of influencing the decision-making process regarding immunization.

Minimize suggestive or leading inquiries when interviewing and counseling. Such questions tend to include the desired response within the question itself and often reflect the opinions of the person asking the questions. For example, asking "You've had all your shots, haven't you?" is likely to prejudice the response. One exception to this rule might be in taking a patient's history of prior tetanus immunization. "Have you been treated in an emergency room in the last few years, where you may have received a tetanus booster?" can be helpful in interviewing. Leading questions can be useful to test how closely the counselor and patient agree but, overall, this type of question tends to bias answers.

An important role of the immunization counselor is to dispel misconceptions and misinformation about particular vaccines. For example, be prepared to counter common misconceptions about influenza vaccine with facts regarding its safety and low incidence of side effects. Similarly, the risks of encephalopathy following pertussis vaccine are now recognized to be much lower than earlier thought, if there is any casual link at all, and fears of human immunodeficiency virus (HIV) transmission from hepatitis B vaccine have been conclusively put to rest. The key issue whenever confronted with side-effect disputes is to ask if the risk of side effects does or does not outweigh the risk of the disease to be prevented.

Before the counseling phase, gather enough data to identify diseases to which the patient is susceptible. Clinicians can then suggest a set of immunizations to protect the patient against potential infections. The goal is to inform the patient of his or her immunization needs and convince the individual to accept these vaccines, in light of the risks and benefits involved.

In developing an immunization plan, consider the individual's age, occupation, place of residence, travel plans, lifestyle, underlying disease states, and other individual factors. Then, in consultation with detailed immunization references, construct a specific list and schedule of needed vaccines. The immunization advice may be communicated verbally if it is simple, but written recommendations may make it easier for the patient to follow complex schedules. Providing written handouts or appointment cards can remind patients of important data or dates after they leave the counseling session. Handouts are available from the CDC (404-639-1836), many vaccine manufacturers, and other sources. Be prepared to explain specifically when and where immunizations are available and what costs to expect.

The final part of the counseling process is the evaluation phase. By asking the patient to summarize the material communicated, the counselor can determine if the patient understands the ideas discussed. The ultimate success of immunization counseling is determined by whether or not the patient actually is immunized. Immunization is favored if convenience can be enhanced: suggest the patient get influenza vaccine along with a friend who also needs it. Ask for the promise of a parent to obtain a child's immunizations by a certain date. Remind the patient that the small inconvenience involved in getting immunized is an investment in health that pays dividends for years to come. Congratulate vaccinees on their wise decision and suggest that they encourage family or friends with similar vaccine needs to be vaccinated as well.

References

Kirk JK, Grabenstein JD. Interviewing and counseling patients about immunizations. *Hosp Pharm.* 1991;26(11):1006-1010.

Activities for Immunization Advocacy

The Need for Advocacy

Advocacy of immunizations is needed because as many as 50,000 Americans die of vaccine-preventable infections every year, primarily from influenza, pneumococcal disease, hepatitis B, and measles. The vast majority of these persons visited health care providers in the year preceding their death, either as inpatients or outpatients, but were not vaccinated.

Tens of millions of Americans are susceptible to these infections, despite the availability of effective vaccines. About 30% to 40% of American children from 2 to 6 years of age are inadequately immunized with routine vaccines, although over 95% of children are vaccinated in compliance with regulations before entry into kindergarten or elementary school (the so-called-school-entry gate). The majority of American adults are inadequately vaccinated, especially against influenza, pneumococcal disease, hepatitis B, tetanus, and diphtheria.

Influenza and pneumonia combined are the sixth leading cause of premature mortality in the United States: 36,000 people die of influenza in an average year, and 172,000 excess hospitalizations because of pneumonia or influenza occur with each moderate influenza epidemic, costing millions of dollars. Patients older than 64 years of age account for 80% of pneumonia or influenza deaths.

Remarkably, 40% to 55% of patients who die following influenza receive medical care at a hospital during the year preceding their death; 75% of those who will die visit an outpatient clinic in the year before their death. Despite this access to health care, less than 30% of high-risk groups are immunized. Although influenza vaccine has been recommended for all members of high-risk groups since 1960, a half of a century, many clinicians fail to offer vaccine to those most at risk. Over 40 million Americans should receive influenza vaccine each year because of their increased susceptibility. Increased use of influenza vaccine, assuming 70% efficacy and 70% coverage, could prevent 20,000 deaths and 80,000 hospitalizations each year in the United States. Canadians appear to be more successful at delivering influenza vaccine to high-risk groups than their southern neighbors.

Similarly, for pneumococcal disease, only 10% to 20% of a likely 48 million vaccine candidates have been immunized. The mortality rate from this infection (5% for pneumonia, 15% to 40% for bacteremia, 30% to 50% for pneumococcal meningitis) has not changed substantially since the 1950s, despite advances in antibiotic therapy. At least two-thirds of patients with serious pneumococcal infections have been hospitalized at least once within 3 to 5 years before the illness, but had not been vaccinated.

Specific Advocacy Activities

Methods for Determining Immunization Needs: Methods of screening for immunization needs may be organized in several ways and model screening forms have been included in the Immunization Documents Appendix. Clinicians can be involved in some or all of the following forms of immunization surveillance:

(1) Occurrence screening identifies vaccine needs at the time of particular events, such as hospital or nursing home admission or discharge, an ambulatory or emergency-room visit, mid-decade birthdays (years 25, 35, 45, and so forth), and any contact with the health care delivery system for any patient younger than 8 years or older than 64 years of age.

(2) Diagnosis screening reviews vaccine needs among patients with conditions that place them at increased risk of preventable infections. Diagnoses such as hemophilia, thalassemia, most types of cancer, sickle cell anemia, chronic alcoholism, cirrhosis, cerebrospinal fluid leaks, human immunodeficiency virus (HIV) infection, multiple antibiotic allergies, and other disorders should prompt specific attention to the patients' vaccine needs.

(3) Procedure screening identifies vaccine needs on the basis of medical or surgical procedures. These include splenectomy, heart or lung surgery, organ transplant, chemotherapy, radiation therapy, immunosuppression of other types, dialysis, and prescription of certain medications.

(4) Periodic mass screening can be conducted during autumn influenza programs and during programs to control outbreaks (eg, local measles epidemics). Schools and other institutions can perform such screening when registering new cohorts of students, residents, or other groups. Mass screening also may be appropriate where no comprehensive immunization program has been conducted in the past few years. Mass screenings help improve vaccine-coverage rates acutely, but long-term benefits are much greater when such intermittent programs are combined with ongoing, comprehensive screening efforts.

Once patients in need of immunization have been identified, they must be advised of their infection risk and encouraged to accept the immunizations they need. If appropriate, also remind the patients' physician(s) of the patients' need for vaccination. Do not reschedule patients needing immunizations to a future appointment that may be missed. Rather, vaccinate them during the current health care contact unless valid contraindications exist. In general, mild fevers or mild diarrheal illness do not contraindicate immunization, nor do current antimicrobial therapy, convalescence, prematurity, pregnancy, recent exposure to an infectious disease, breastfeeding, history of nonspecific allergies, or family history of allergies, convulsions, sudden infant death syndrome, or adverse events following vaccination.

Advising patients of their need for immunization can take several forms. In the ambulatory setting, individualized or form letters or postcards can be mailed to patients, patients can be telephoned, or an insert can be included with prescriptions informing patients of their infection risk and the availability and efficacy of vaccines.

Adhesive warning labels also can be affixed to prescription containers for drugs that indicate need for vaccination against influenza and pneumococcal disease (eg, digoxin, warfarin, theophylline, insulin). These labels would be analogous to labels currently in widespread use (eg, "shake well," "take with food or milk"). Such labels might read "You May Need Flu or Pneumococcal Vaccine: Ask Your Doctor or Pharmacist." For inpatients and institutional residents, chart notes, consultations, messages to patients, and similar means can be used.

While most of the screening criteria described above are specific for indications of influenza or pneumococcal vaccines, conduct comprehensive screening on the patients thus identified. In other words, interest in a patient might be initiated because of his or her need for pneumococcal vaccine, but while assessing that patient, take the opportunity to check for needs for any vaccine: influenza, pneumococcal, or hepatitis B vaccine, tetanus-diphtheria (Td) bivalent or with acellular pertussis (Tdap) vaccine boosters, etc.

Administrative Matters

Infection-control committees can prevent infections among staff and patients by encouraging sound institutional policies on:

(1) Hepatitis B preexposure prophylaxis, to provide immunity to health care workers exposed to blood products and other contaminated items.

(2) Hepatitis B postexposure (eg, needle-stick) prophylaxis, to protect previously unvaccinated patients from infection.

(3) Rabies pre- and postexposure prophylaxis, to protect individuals at occupational risk of rabies or following exposures to potentially rabid animals. Rabies vaccine is the only overused immunization in the United States; sound policies can minimize unneeded vaccinations.

(4) Wound-management guidelines, to prevent tetanus and diphtheria in patients with trauma.

(5) Pertussis contraindications, to minimize inappropriate exclusions from vaccination and to maximize the number of people protected.

(6) Employee immunization requirements (against measles, rubella, influenza, hepatitis A, hepatitis B, and other diseases), to reduce disease transmission from patient to employee and from employee to patient.

(7) Tuberculosis screening of patients and staff, to conduct rational surveillance of high-risk populations served by the institution and to preclude nosocomial infection.

Adopt quality indicators and monitoring systems to assure that all patients are assessed for immunization adequacy prior to leaving the facility. In some settings, standing orders to this effect may be helpful. Drug-use evaluation (DUE) criteria for drugs that indicate need for influenza and pneumococcal vaccine should include immunization of these patients. For example, immunize all patients on digoxin, warfarin, insulin, or chronic theophylline therapy against influenza and pneumococcal disease.

Institutional policies on the administration of immunizations should include immediate availability of epinephrine and other products used to treat adverse events. Similarly, have Advanced Cardiac Life Support (ACLS) trained providers readily available when immunizations are offered.

Planning Influenza Vaccination Programs

(1) Assure that adequate vaccine supplies have been ordered.

(2) Name one or two primary vaccine advocates on the staff to coordinate department activities. Charge these people with developing an outreach program to identify patients at risk of influenza and pneumococcal disease.

(3) Work with the employee health department to encourage vaccination of the staff of the whole institution, since nosocomial transmission of influenza from staff to immunosuppressed patients can be fatal.

(4) Prepare for ill-founded excuses. Explain to the unwilling that modern influenza vaccines cause far fewer side effects than vaccines produced in the 1960s and 1970s, and are far more effective at preventing disease and death. A recent double-blind, placebo-controlled study demonstrated no difference between modern influenza vaccine and saline placebo in terms of disability or systemic symptoms.

(5) Fight the myth that influenza vaccine can cause influenza. The malaise some persons experience following vaccination is common to many vaccines and is not an infectious process. People who develop true influenza within a few days after being vaccinated were certainly incubating the virus at the time of injection and would have gotten sick whether they were vaccinated or not. In the American vernacular, "flu" is casually used as a generic term for a wide class of viral illnesses, including "stomach flu," that have nothing to do with influenzae. Avoid using the term "flu," favoring the specific term influenza instead.

(6) Expand your vaccine offerings beyond just influenza vaccine. Consider all the vaccine needs of your clientele.

Model Activities for National Adult Immunization Awareness Week

(1) Lead your infection-control committee in declaring a local observation of National Adult Immunization Awareness Week. Invite the print, radio, and television media to a ceremony marking the week to see what a good job you do protecting the public health. Vaccinate a local celebrity in front of their cameras.

(2) Lead your Pharmacy and Therapeutics (P&T) committee in recommending influenza and pneumococcal vaccine for patients receiving appropriate medications.

(3) Devote an issue of the pharmacy or hospital newsletter to explaining the need to protect adults against preventable infections. Or review a vaccine-preventable disease every issue or two.

(4) For every admission with a vaccine-indicating diagnosis, recommend influenza and pneumococcal vaccination just prior to discharge. Use any medium that communicates: *Post-It* notes, index cards, letters, chart notes, preprinted forms.

(5) Start screening for vaccine needs by medication use; send an individualized, preprinted message to the physician recommending vaccination.

(6) As you take medication histories, start taking immunization histories as well. Add this information to computerized patient profiles so that dates for booster doses can be generated.

(7) Encourage good documentation of immunizations (eg, state form, PHS Form 731), computerized immunization profiles, inpatient and outpatient chart entries.

(8) Codify your vaccine-use policies, following national guidelines: hepatitis B (preexposure and needle-stick), rabies prophylaxis (to preclude unneeded vaccination), DTP to DT conversion in pediatrics (strict criteria, to maximize pertussis prophylaxis), and wound management.

(9) Order immunization references for your drug-information center and libraries.

(10) Conduct educational programs for pharmacy staff, nurses, physicians, patients, and other groups. Incorporate immunization routines into diabetic, asthmatic, and heart disease clinics. Give talks at local civic and retirement centers and to other groups.

(11) Encourage your own parents and older relatives to be vaccinated.

(12) Obtain pamphlets, videotapes, and additional information from the Immunization Action Coalition (http://www.immunize.org), the National Foundation for Infectious Diseases (301-656-0003), or from Technical Information Services, Centers for Disease Control and Prevention (404-639-1836).

(13) Encourage recognition that buying vaccines saves total costs to the health care system by reducing the number of hospital admissions and the number of deaths.

Drug-Product Selection

(1) Delete tetanus toxoid from formularies in favor of combined tetanus-diphtheria toxoids (Td) bivalent or with acellular pertussis vaccine (Tdap) for wound prophylaxis in order to sustain diphtheria immunity in the population. If this decision is not accepted, purchase adsorbed tetanus toxoid in place of fluid tetanus toxoid.

(2) Favor trivalent measles-mumps-rubella (MMR) vaccine over single- or double-antigen formulations in order to boost immunity against each of the three diseases. Change requests for single- or double-antigen vaccines to trivalent MMR, in consultation with the prescriber, as frequently as possible.

(3) Reassess agents and doses used in anergy skin-test batteries (refer to Rational Anergy Test Batteries in the Hypersensitivity Agents section).

(4) Ensure sufficient vials of crotalid antivenin are stocked to treat the entire course of severe envenomation in a pit viper snakebite victim (8 to 15 vials).

Ten Things to Do First in Immunization Advocacy

(1) Increase use of influenza and pneumococcal vaccines by staff and patients.

(2) Start screening for vaccine needs on admission, on discharge, by drug use, etc. Use any medium that communicates: *Post-It* notes, index cards, letters, chart notes, preprinted forms.

(3) Codify vaccine use policies: hepatitis B (preexposure and needle-stick) rabies (to preclude unneeded immunization), DTP to DT switch (to maximize pertussis vaccination), wound management (Td or Tdap, rather than TT).

(4) Delete tetanus toxoid, in favor of Td or Tdap.

(5) Assure use of current guidelines regarding rational tuberculin skin testing.

(6) Conduct educational programs for pharmacy, nursing, physicians, patients, and other groups (eg, classes, newsletters). Conduct an education program (eg, ground rounds, in-service) on patient immunization or occupational immunization; publish a newsletter on immunizations.

(7) Start keeping vaccine profiles and taking vaccine histories.

(8) Build immunization advocacy into continuous quality-improvement (CQI) activities or drug-use evaluation (DUE) programs.

(9) Encourage your own parents and older relatives to be vaccinated against influenza and pneumococcal disease.

(10) Do something special for the National Adult Immunization Awareness Week, the last full week of each October.

Inappropriate Contraindications

Conditions often inappropriately regarded as contraindications are printed below. Do NOT routinely withhold immunization in the following instances:

(1) Reaction to a previous dose of diphtheria and tetanus toxoids with pertussis (DTP) vaccine that involved only soreness, redness, or swelling in the immediate vicinity of the vaccination site or temperature below 40.5°C (105°F).

(2) Mild acute illness with low-grade fever or mild diarrheal illness in an otherwise well child.

(3) Current antimicrobial therapy or the convalescent phase of an illness.

(4) Prematurity. The appropriate age to initiate immunization of the prematurely born infant is the usual chronologic age from birth. Do not reduce vaccine doses for preterm infants.

(5) Pregnancy in the patient or a household contact.

(6) Recent exposure to an infectious disease.

(7) Breastfeeding. The only vaccine virus that has been isolated from breast milk is rubella vaccine virus. There is no good evidence that breast milk from women immunized against rubella is harmful to infants.

(8) A history of nonspecific allergies or relatives with allergies.

(9) Allergies to penicillin or any other antibiotic, except anaphylactic reactions to neomycin (pertinent for MMR-containing vaccine) or streptomycin (pertinent for oral poliovirus vaccine). No vaccine licensed in the United States or Canada contains penicillin.

(10) Allergies to duck meat or duck feathers. No vaccine available in the United States or Canada is produced in substrates containing duck antigens.

(11) A family history of convulsions in persons considered for pertussis or measles vaccination.

(12) A family history of sudden infant death syndrome (SIDS) in children considered for DTP vaccination.

(13) A family history of an adverse event, unrelated to immunosuppression, following vaccination.

(14) History of an adverse reaction to one of the older influenza vaccines prior to the zonal centrifuge (1960s) and improved purification (1970s).

References

ACIP. General recommendations on immunization: recommendations of the Advisory Committee on Immunization Practices (ACIP). *MMWR.* 2006;55(RR-15):1-48. Erratum in: *MMWR.* 2006;55(48):1303. *MMWR.* 2007;56(11):256. http://www.cdc.gov/mmwr/pdf/rr/rr5515.pdf.

Standards for Pediatric Immunization Practices

(1) Immunization services are readily available.

(2) There are no barriers or unnecessary prerequisites to the receipt of vaccines.

(3) Immunization services are available free or for a minimal fee.

(4) Providers utilize all clinical encounters to screen and, when indicated, immunize children.

(5) Providers educate parents and guardians about immunization in general terms.

(6) Providers question parents or guardians about contraindications and, before immunizing a child, inform them in specific terms about the risks and benefits of the immunizations their child is to receive.

(7) Providers follow only true contraindications.

(8) Providers administer simultaneously all vaccine doses for which a child is eligible at the time of each visit.

(9) Providers use accurate and complete recording procedures.

(10) Providers coschedule immunization appointments in conjunction with appointments for other child health services.

(11) Providers report adverse events following immunization promptly, accurately, and completely.

(12) Providers operate a tracking system.

(13) Providers adhere to appropriate procedures for vaccine management.

(14) Providers conduct semiannual audits to assess immunization coverage levels and to review immunization records in the patient populations they serve.

(15) Providers maintain up-to-date, easily retrievable medical protocols at all locations where vaccines are administered.

(16) Providers operate with patient-oriented and community-based approaches.

(17) Vaccines are administered by properly trained individuals.

(18) Providers receive ongoing education and training on current immunization recommendations.

Reference

American Academy of Pediatrics: Standards for child and adolescent immunization practices. *Pediatrics*. 2003;112:958-963.

Vaccine Recommendations for Persons Infected with HIV

Special immunization recommendations are appropriate for persons infected with the human immunodeficiency virus (HIV):

Live Bacterial or Viral Vaccines:

Persons infected with HIV and persons who have developed the acquired immunodeficiency syndrome (AIDS) are theoretically at risk of disseminated infection following immunization with a live, albeit attenuated, bacterial or viral vaccine. Specific recommendations follow:

BCG (injection or instillation): Disseminated mycobacterial infection may result from exposure to this drug. Do not expose HIV-infected persons in the United States to BCG.

BCG vaccination of children who are born to HIV-infected mothers in developing nations and who are vaccinated shortly after birth appears to be relatively safe but questionably effective. WHO recommends that only HIV-infected infants who are asymptomatic and live in areas with high tuberculosis risk receive BCG. Waiting to immunize children at 1 year of age has also been suggested for developing countries.

Measles, mumps, and rubella (MMR): Vaccinate both symptomatic and asymptomatic children and adults according to routine schedules; consider the possibility of less than optimal immunogenicity.

Poliovirus (oral form, OPV): Do not administer live, oral poliovirus vaccine to any HIV-infected child or adult in the United States, nor to their household contacts. Give inactivated poliovirus vaccine (e-IPV) injection instead. WHO continues to recommend routine use of OPV, a rational approach in developing nations with a substantial risk of endemic poliomyelitis.

Rotavirus: There are insufficient data from clinical trials to support rotavirus vaccination of infants with indeterminate HIV status who are born to mothers with HIV/AIDS.

Typhoid (capsule form): Do not administer live, oral typhoid vaccine to any HIV-infected child or adult. Inactivated typhoid vaccine injection may be used if needed.

Vaccinia (smallpox): Do not administer live vaccinia (smallpox) vaccine to any HIV-infected child or adult, except in an outbreak, based on personal risk of exposure.

Varicella (chickenpox) and zoster (shingles): Do not administer live varicella vaccine to any HIV-infected child or adult, until results of ongoing studies are published. Consider the value of VZIG for immunocompromised people.

Yellow fever: Base decisions to administer live yellow fever vaccine to a HIV-infected child or adult on an assessment of the patient's state of immunosuppression and the risk of exposure to the yellow fever virus. Offer the option of immunization to asymptomatic persons infected with HIV who cannot avoid potential exposure to yellow fever virus.

Inactivated Vaccines or Toxoids:

In general, immunization with an inactivated vaccine or toxoid poses no additional risk to persons infected with HIV and persons who have developed AIDS. But these persons may be less likely to develop an adequate immune response to vaccination and may remain susceptible to the disease at issue. While HIV-infected persons and AIDS patients may develop less than optimal immunity, compared with uninfected persons, immunization is often still recommended to confer at least partial protection. Optimally, complete the immunization of HIV-infected persons before they meet the criteria for AIDS. Specific recommendations follow:

Diphtheria and tetanus toxoids with pertussis vaccine (DTP): Observe routine pediatric DTP vaccination schedules among HIV-infected children; consider the possibility of less than optimal immunogenicity.

Diphtheria and tetanus toxoids (pediatric): Observe routine pediatric DT vaccination schedules among HIV-infected children; consider the possibility of less than optimal immunogenicity. DTP is the preferred drug for most children.

Haemophilus influenzae type b (Hib): Observe routine pediatric Hib vaccination schedules among HIV-infected children; consider the possibility of less than optimal immunogenicity. Routine Hib vaccination of all HIV-infected adults is generally recommended to decrease susceptibility to Hib infections. Optimally, complete immunization of HIV-infected persons before they meet the criteria for AIDS.

Hepatitis A: Observe standard recommendations; consider the possibility of less than optimal immunogenicity.

Hepatitis B: Observe routine pediatric hepatitis B vaccination schedules among HIV-infected children; consider the possibility of less than optimal immunogenicity. Routine hepatitis B vaccination of all HIV-infected adults (unless known to already be infected with hepatitis B) is generally recommended to decrease susceptibility to hepatitis B infections. Optimally, complete immunization of HIV-infected persons before they meet the criteria for AIDS.

Human papillomavirus: Observe standard recommendations; consider the possibility of less than optimal immunogenicity.

Influenza: Routine influenza vaccination of all HIV-infected persons is generally recommended (using inactivated vaccine) to decrease susceptibility to influenza infections; consider the possibility of less than optimal immunogenicity. Chemical antiviral prophylaxis (eg, amantadine) may be appropriate during periods of increased influenza A activity in a community.

Meningococcal A/C/Y/W-135: Observe standard recommendations; consider the possibility of less than optimal immunogenicity.

Pneumococcal: Routine pneumococcal vaccination of all HIV-infected persons is generally recommended to decrease susceptibility to pneumococcal infections; consider the possibility of less than optimal immunogenicity. Optimally, complete immunization of HIV-infected persons before they meet the criteria for AIDS.

Poliovirus (injection, e-IPV): Observe standard recommendations; consider the possibility of less than optimal immunogenicity. Use of e-IPV is preferred over the oral, attenuated poliovirus vaccine.

Rabies: Observe standard recommendations; consider the possibility of less than optimal immunogenicity.

Tetanus and diphtheria (Td adult bivalent or with acellular pertussis vaccine, Tdap): Routine Td vaccination of all HIV-infected adults is recommended to decrease susceptibility to tetanus and diphtheria infections; consider the possibility of less than optimal immunogenicity. Furste has suggested a lower threshold for deciding to use TIG in wounded HIV-infected persons, under the assumption that their circulating antitetanus antitoxin level may be lower than among uninfected persons.

Typhoid (injection): Observe standard recommendations; consider the possibility of less than optimal immunogenicity. Encourage standard food and water precautions.

Safety of Immunizing HIV-Infected Persons:

In vitro studies show that proliferating CD4 cells are more susceptible to infection with HIV than nonproliferating cells, raising the possibility that immunization may be a cofactor in exacerbating the progression of HIV infection to AIDS. Published reports show temporary increases in plasma HIV viremia after injection of tetanus toxoid or influenza or hepatitis B vaccines. These increases lasted up to 6 weeks. Is this clinically important? No clinical data have substantiated the concern about antigenic stimulation causing deterioration of clinical status. We encounter natural antigenic stimulation innumerable times during our lives. Actual infections may be riskier than an immunization, because of more prolonged antigenic value of induction of specific antibodies. CDC and WHO continue to recommend immunization of HIV-infected persons as described above, when the benefits of immunization outweigh the risks of infection.

Drug/Vaccine	Summary of Recommendations for Immunization of HIV-Infected Persons in the United States	
	Known asymptomatic	Symptomatic
BCG	No	No
DTP/Td/Tdap	Yes	Yes
e-IPV[a]	Yes	Yes
Hepatitis A	Yes	Yes
Hepatitis B	Yes	Yes
Hib[b]	Yes	Yes
Human papillomavirus	Yes	Yes
Influenza, inactivated	Yes	Yes
Japanese encephalitis	Yes	Yes
Meningococcal	Yes	Yes
MMR	Yes	Yes[c]
Pneumococcal	Yes	Yes
Poliovirus	Yes (IPV only)	Yes (IPV only)
Rabies	Yes	Yes
Rotavirus	No	No
Typhoid	Yes (injection only)	Yes (injection only)
Vaccinia[d]	No	No
Varicella[e]	Yes	No
Yellow fever	Yes, if high risk	No
Zoster	No	No

a For adults 18 years of age or older, use only if indicated.
b Also consider for HIV-infected adults.
c Consider risk and benefit.
d Except in an outbreak setting.
e Consult detailed references.

References

CDC. Update on adult immunization: recommendations of the Immunization Practices Advisory Committee (ACIP). *MMWR*. 1991;40(RR-12):1-94.

Hibberd PL, et al. Approach to immunization in the immunosuppressed host. *Infect Dis Clin N Amer*. 1990;4:123-142.

Jewett JF, et al. Preventive health care for adults with HIV infection. *JAMA*. 1993;269:1144-1153.

Onorato IM, et al. Childhood immunization, vaccine-preventable diseases and infection with human immunodeficiency virus. *Pediatr Infect Dis J*. 1988;7:588-595.

Pau AK, et al. Active immunization with HIV-infected patients. *Pharmacotherapy*. 1996;16:163-170.

Spach DH. Immunizations for HIV-infected adults: indications, timing, and response. *Top HIV Med*. 2006;14(5):154-158.

Records of medical care and pharmaceutical care are kept because human memory is not perfect. Additionally, data about care and progress need to be readily available to the many health professionals from many disciplines and specialties who contribute to any one patient's care. Like records for other prescription drugs, accurate immunization records are essential to document immunization delivery, to establish the proper timing for "refills" (ie, booster doses), and to preclude unneeded immunization.

Immunization data are needed by all health professionals who aid health maintenance and disease prevention, including pharmacists, physicians, nurses and public-health workers. In order to assist patient-care decisions, information about the presence or absence of a history of previous immunizations must be readily available to vaccine prescribers. Usually, data is recorded in medical records, although pharmacy records are increasingly reflecting use of the preventive medicines. Standardization of records improves the efficiency and accuracy of data retrieval.

Two hazards threaten the accuracy of immunization records: Forgetting actual immunizations and imagining nonexistent ones. The two hazards have different causes but a common solution: Centralized and complete documentation.

Forgetfulness is a characteristic both of individual people and of the health care system as a whole. Individual forgetfulness is well known to all of us. The system forgets when one clinician is unaware that another clinician has immunized a patient.

Adults may be especially vulnerable to both individual and collective forgetfulness. Adults are more likely to have complicated medical histories. Pieces of their medical records are often located with multiple office-based physicians, plus at hospitals where care has been provided. Clearly, centralization of immunization documentation is helpful to ensure complete access to such data.

Fictional immunizations may be recorded if patients are asked biased questions, such as "You've had all your vaccinations, haven't you?" Undocumented claims of previous infection or vaccination may come from susceptible persons and claims of susceptibility may come from immune persons. In one study, college freshmen were more likely to provide "I don't know" answers than were their mothers; offspring and parents also tend to report histories differently. These findings reinforce the importance of documenting immunization records so they are available to subsequent vaccine prescribers.

Decision-Making with Inadequate Immunization Records

Despite the best efforts in taking immunization histories, doubt about previous doses will often persist. In many cases, patients should be vaccinated in the face of doubt, since risk of infection often outweighs the minor risk of an adverse event in an immune person receiving vaccine.

The National Advisory Committee on Immunization of Canada issued recommendations in 1990 that all children lacking written documentation of immunizations be started on a routine immunization schedule for children not immunized in early infancy. The American Academy of Pediatrics offers similar recommendations (1991). The Canadian recommendations suggest that children who develop a serious adverse reaction during a primary immunization series with diphtheria, tetanus and pertussis antigens be assessed individually before receiving additional doses of these agents.

Document Types

Only through accurate immunization records, readily available to clinicians and patients alike, can the shortcoming of memory and recall be solved. Four basic types of immunization records are needed in clinical practice:

a. Forms to determine which immunizations a patient needs (eg, screening forms, needs assessment),

b. Forms to educate patients or guardians about the need for immunization and obtain their agreement (eg, consent forms),

c. Forms to document the patient's vaccination history (eg, immunization records, patient profiles), and

d. Forms to advise the FDA and other authorities of problems associated with vaccine use.The following sections discuss each type of immunization record in detail.

Forms to Determine Immunization Needs

Screening Form for Immunization Needs

The first step in any immunization-delivery program is to determine what immunizations each patient needs. This step may be more important in assessing adults than children, since immunization recommendations for adults are more individualized to specific risk factors. To determine needs, the clinician must collect relevant medication information about the patient's personal indications and contraindications to vaccination. To help organize the process of taking patients' immunization histories, a screening form may be helpful.

An immunization-screening form is reprinted here with instructions for use. The form is appropriate for:

a. Assessing the immunization needs of persons admitted to hospital or an emergency room or entering nursing home, schools or other institutions,

b. Assessing the immunization needs of clients of private physicians and public health clinics,

c. Assessing employees' immunization needs, helping immunization programs run by occupational-health personnel, and

d. Screening patients for vaccination during influenza seasons or other infectious outbreaks (eg, measles, mumps, rubella).

Although the form is intended to consider pediatric patients as well as adults, it is not specifically designed for well-baby screening. Another more specific form may be appropriate in such cases.

Most significantly, this form allows individual assessment of a patient's indications and contraindications for vaccination. In fact, use of this instrument can turn what would have been a mass vaccination program into an individualized immunization encounter. This tool serves both as a summary of immunization history to date, as well as a record of immunizations ordered and administered as a result of that day's immunization assessment. In addition to immunizations, data about tuberculin skin tests can also be recorded. This screening form was refined in the course of several thousand patient encounters.

As automation of patient medical records becomes more prevalent, the immunization data gathered on forms such as the one proposed here should be entered into automated medical records. For example, "smart cards" that record the patient's diagnoses, current medications, laboratory values, and other pertinent information should also record the patient's immunization history.

When querying patients about their immunization history, memory cues are often helpful for patients trying to remember vaccinations and their timing. For tetanus-diphtheria boosters, patients can be asked about their last visit to an emergency room (ER) for wound management.

To establish timing, ask whether vaccinations occurred before or after major life events (eg, births, marriages, deaths). If time is available for more thorough inquiry, ask the patient's family to check records that may be kept at home.

Line-by-line instructions for using the immunization-screening form follow. The form, which follows the list of instructions, may be freely reproduced for individual patients, if credit is given to *ImmunoFacts*.

Instructions

This immunization-screening form is divided into four major segments. The first solicits patient-specific medical information from the patient or the patient's family. The second part summarizes the immunization history of the patient. The third section identifies the immunizations ordered for each patient and subsequent information about the administration of those doses. The final part records any reactions to vaccination or a tuberculin skin test.

Part 1: To Be Completed by Patient or Family

Items 1-2. Annual influenza is recommended for everyone 50 years of age and older. Initial pneumococcal vaccination is recommended for everyone 65 years of age and older. Influenza vaccination is contraindicated for children younger than 6 months of age.

Item 3. If the patient is definitely or possibly pregnant, defer live vaccines (eg, BCG, measles, mumps, rubella, oral typhoid, yellow fever) until after delivery, counsel to avoid pregnancy, or consider risk/benefit ratio.

Item 4. In moderate to severe febrile illness, defer vaccination until after fever abates. Low-grade fever is not a contraindication to vaccination.

Item 5. Telephone numbers are useful for reminding patients to return for all vaccines needed or to have a tuberculin skin test (TST) read.

Item 6.
   a. If eating eggs causes laryngeal swelling or other severe systemic reactions, do not give influenza or yellow-fever vaccines.
   b. If thimerosal or mercury allergy is noted, consider waiving vaccines containing thimerosal as a preservative (eg, some forms of hepatitis B, Td or Tdap, influenza). But confirm that the allergy involves the airway, in contrast to contact dermatitis.
   c. Avoid certain vaccines if severe antibiotic allergy to streptomycin (ie, poliovirus) or neomycin (eg, poliovirus, measles, mumps, rubella) is claimed. No vaccine currently available in US or Canada contains penicillin.
   d. Hypersensitivity to tetanus antitoxin (containing equine serum) may be erroneously reported as allergy to tetanus toxoid; clarify the circumstances, type, and onset of reaction.

Item 7. If patient has a history of positive tuberculin skin test, do not rechallenge with PPD. Do not give BCG vaccine.

Item 8.
   a. If the patient has cancer, annual influenza vaccine and initial pneumococcal vaccine are generally recommended. Patients on chemotherapy may have diminished response, but still warrant immunization. Do not give these patients live vaccines, due to the patients' immunosuppression. See also other comments in this section.
   b. If children have a personal history of convulsions, see detailed references for full discussion.
   c. If the patient is diabetic, give annual influenza and initial pneumococcal vaccination.
   d. If the patient has heart or vascular disease (eg, congestive heart failure, septal defect, ischemic heart disease, atherosclerosis, intermittent claudication), give annual influenza and initial pneumococcal vaccination.
   e. If the patient has Hodgkin disease, give annual influenza and initial pneumococcal vaccination 2 weeks before or 1 to 3 months after radiation or chemotherapy.

f. If the patient is immunosuppressed by drugs (eg, azathioprine, cyclosporine, steroids greater than 20 mg prednisone-equivalent per day for more than 2 weeks [for children, more than 2 mg/kg]), radiation, or any other means, follow guidelines in sections (e) and (i).

g. If an adult patient has chronic pulmonary disease (eg, asthma, tuberculosis, cystic fibrosis, myasthenia gravis, bronchitis), give annual influenza and initial pneumococcal vaccination. Give children with chronic pulmonary disease influenza vaccine; if older than 2 years of age, give pneumococcal vaccine.

h. If the patient is asplenic or has bone-marrow problems, treat as if immunosuppressed [see sections (e), (f), and (i)].

i. If the patient has a defective immune system, avoid most live vaccines. Give annual influenza and initial pneumococcal vaccination. Give influenza and pneumococcal vaccines to persons infected with HIV. They should receive MMR and hepatitis B if needed, but do not give them BCG or yellow-fever vaccines.

j. Deal with other conditions on an individual basis; refer to authoritative guidelines. If patient has chronic kidney disease (eg, dialysis, transplant, erythropoietin therapy), cerebrospinal fluid leaks, chronic alcoholism, cirrhosis, sickle-cell anemia, hepatic failure or some other chronic conditions, give annual influenza and initial pneumococcal vaccination. Hemophilia and thalassemia are indications for hepatitis B vaccine.

Item 9. Give influenza vaccine to children on chronic aspirin therapy. Other drugs are often indicators of an underlying chronic illness that warrants vaccination against influenza, pneumococci, or hepatitis B (eg, insulin, theophylline, digoxin, coagulation factors).

Item 10. Give hepatitis B vaccine to persons exposed to blood products (eg, health care workers, dialysis patients, hemophiliacs), as well as the institutionalized mentally retarded, actively homosexual or bisexual men, intravenous drug abusers, and other groups.

Item 11. Serious reactions may suggest avoiding certain specific repeat vaccinations. But be wary of inappropriate contraindications that tempt exclusion of patients who should properly be vaccinated.

Part 2: To Be Completed by Clinical Personnel

Item 12. For patients 8 years of age and younger who have not received influenza vaccine before, give a second dose of split-virus at least 1 month after the first.

Item 13. Booster doses of pneumococcal vaccine are now recommended after 5 years have elapsed for adult patients at highest risk of fatal pneumococcal infection (eg, those with asplenia, nephrotic syndrome, renal failure, transplant recipients). Revaccinate children with nephrotic syndrome, asplenia, or sickle-cell anemia after 3 to 5 years, if they would be 10 years of age and younger at revaccination. For children older than 10 years of age with nephrotic syndrome, asplenia, or sickle-cell anemia, give a single revaccination if more than 5 years have elapsed. If child is younger than 10 years of age, consider revaccination 3 years later.

Item 14. If the patient's tetanus-diphtheria series is not complete, schedule appropriate return visits. If the patient's most recent tetanus-diphtheria dose was more than 10 years ago, give a booster dose. After the seventh birthday, use adult-strength tetanus-diphtheria toxoids (Td) bivalent or with acellular pertussis vaccine (Tdap), not plain tetanus toxoid. Asking patients to remember their last ER visit is an effective means of recalling the date of a Td or Tdap booster.

Item 15. Assuming the patient is tuberculin-negative, recommend a new test for newly arrived immigrants, new residents of nursing homes, new prison inmates, and employees of nursing homes and hospitals.

Item 16. Consider the patient's individual risk of other preventable diseases, as well as categorical assessment by age, travel plans, occupation, and life-style risk factors.

Part 3: Immunization Orders
Items 17-22. Use the "Dose" column to order vaccinations and tests. For influenza, Td or Tdap, and tuberculin, choose the desired formulation. Record doses administered in the following columns: Site, lot number, name of person administering the dose, and date.

Item 23. Signature of prescriber authorizing these immunologic agents.

Part 4: Clinical Observations
Item 24. Record immediate and delayed hypersensitivity reactions here. Note date and time of onset of reaction.

Item 25. Record response to tuberculin skin tests here.

Item 26. Record other pertinent remarks and observations here. The preceding information reflects a summary of common vaccine indications and contraindications. Assess each patient individually. Consult detailed references for full information on use and dosage.

Screening Form for Vaccines & Immunologic Tests[*]

PART 1: To be completed by PATIENT or Family:

1. Age
2. Date of Birth:
3. Are you pregnant? (circle one)   Yes   No   Maybe
4. Do you have a fever today? (circle one)   Yes   No
5. What is your daytime telephone number?
6. Do you have drug or food allergies?   No   Yes   egg   mercury   antibiotic: _____
   other: _____
   Describe reaction: _____
7. Have you ever had a positive tuberculosis (TB) test?   No   Yes   When? _____
8. Are you being treated by a doctor for: (circle all that apply to you)
   a. cancer (type): _____
   b. convulsions or other neurologic problems
   c. diabetes
   d. heart or vascular disease (CHF, etc.)
   e. Hodgkin disease
   f. immunosuppression (from drugs, radiation, etc.)
   g. lung disease (asthma, COPD, active TB, etc.)
   h. spleen or bone marrow problems (asplenia, etc.)
   i. weakened immune system
   j. other:
9. What drugs and medications do you take? _____
10. Are you ever exposed to blood, blood products, or infectious materials? (circle one) Yes   No
11. Describe any serious immunization reaction you have had: _____

PART 2: To be completed by CLINICAL PERSONNEL

12. Influenza A & B Vaccine History:
   a. from oral history/from records
   b. date of last dose: _____
   c. vaccine last used; injection/nasal
   d. is today patient's first dose?   Yes   No   unknown
   e. is a second dose needed?   No   Yes   (< 9 yo)
13. Pneumococcal Vaccine History:
   a. from oral history/from records
   b. previous dose?   no data   No   Yes   7/14/23/?-valent
   c. date of previous dose: _____
14. Tetanus Diphtheria Toxoids History:
   a. from oral history/from records
   b. basic series complete? Yes No no data
   c. date of last dose: _____
   d. product last used: Plain tetanus toxoid (TT); adult-strength Td; Tdap; pediatric-strength DT; pediatric DTP; unknown
15. Tuberculin Skin Test History:
   a. date of last test: _____
   b. reaction: ___ mm x ___ mm/NEGATIVE
   c. old tuberculin (OT, Tine, MonoVacc)/ ___ tu PPD
16. Other Needs: consider hepatitis A and B, HPV, measles, mumps, rubella, varicella, polio, *Haemophilus*, rabies, zoster, others. Ask about travel, occupation, life-style, and other risk factors

PART 3: IMMUNIZATION ORDER:

	Dose:	Route:	Site:	Lot #:	Admin by:	Date:
17. Influenza A&B Vaccine: Inj/Nasal	___ mL					
18. Pneumococcal Vaccine:	___ mL ___ IM/SC					
19. Tetanus/Diphtheria: adult Td/Tdap/ped DT	___ mL ___ IM					
20. Tuberculin Test: PPD	___ mL ___ ID					
21. Other:	___ mL					
22. Other	___ mL					
23. Ordered by:	Date:					

PART 4: CLINICAL OBSERVATIONS:

24. Reactions to these vaccines:
   Date/time noted: _____
   Immediate: _____
   Delayed: _____
25. Reaction to this tuberculin test:
   ___ mm x ___ mm   Read by: _____
   Date read: _____
26. REMARKS:

Patient Identification Stamp:

[*] This form may be enlarged and reproduced for individual patients, if credit is given to *ImmunoFacts*.

Immunization Self-Assessment Form

Another approach to determine immunization needs is to have the patient assess his or her own needs. The following form might be distributed at health fairs, in waiting rooms, as enclosures with paycheck or prescriptions, or in other ways that put the form in front of persons likely to be deficient in immune protection.

Adult Immunization Self-Assessment Form
(for people 15 years of age or older)

Name: _____ Date: _____

Everybody needs to keep his or her immunizations up-to-date. Preventable diseases can be stopped if we get vaccinated. Take this quiz to see if it's time for you to get any booster shots.

Don't just use your memory. Check your "yellow shot record" (PHS Form 731) or other immunization records you keep. These records might be in your medical record or with your doctor, pharmacist, parents, or school(s). If you think you may need extra immunizations after reading this and noting the cautions, check with your regular doctor or health care provider.

Give copies of this quiz to your friends or relatives who might need extra vaccinations too.

1. When was your last tetanus and diphtheria "shot"?

  a. These shots might be listed at TT, Tet Txd, Td, Tdap, Tet/Diph or similar names in your immunization records. If you find no entry, try to remember your last visit to an emergency room, when you may have received a dose.

  b. If more than 10 years have passed, consider getting a booster today. Most cases of tetanus occur in people 50 years of age or older.

2. Have you ever received the pneumococcal vaccine? When?

  a. It might be listed in your records as "Pneumovax." The people who need this vaccine usually need just 1 dose, but check with your doctor if you have trouble with infections.

  b. If you have any of the following, you might need pneumococcal vaccine:

  ____ diabetes   ____ anemia
  ____ alcoholism   ____ problems of the spleen
  ____ asthma   ____ chronic heart, lung, liver or kidney disease
  ____ cirrhosis   ____ 65 years of age and older, even if healthy
  ____ other chronic illnesses:

  c. If you circled any of the items above, you probably also need an influenza vaccine every fall, beginning next October or November.

  d. If you have any of the following conditions, you'll need to talk with a doctor before getting pneumococcal vaccine (check all those that apply):

  ____ Hodgkin disease
  ____ immunodeficiency

3. To the best of your knowledge, did you receive all your childhood immunizations?

  ____ YES ____ NO ____ NOT SURE   SOME: _____

  Preventing measles, mumps, rubella and polio are still important matters, even for adults. Almost everybody born in 1957 or more recently should get two MMR shots after their first birthday.

4. Do you have contact with blood, blood products, or contaminated materials at work or elsewhere?

  ____ YES ____ NO

  If so, you may need protection against hepatitis B virus. This vaccine is needed by many hospital workers, IV drug users, homosexual and bisexual men, immigrants from Asia or Pacific islands, and others.

5. For women: Have you received the complete series of HPV (human papillomavirus) vaccine (3 doses)?

  ____ YES ____ NO

  If not, you may need to complete this series to get the fullest protection.

6. Have you recently arrived in the US from another country, recently moved into a nursing home, or are you employed by a nursing home or hospital?

_____ YES _____ NO

If so, you should be screened for tuberculosis (TB). You should not be retested if you have ever tested positive to a previous TB test (also called *MonoVacc*, *PPD*, *Tine*, *Aplitest*, and similar names).

7. Are you planning a trip to other countries, such as Asia, Africa, the Caribbean, South or Central America, or the Pacific? _____ YES _____ NO

If so, plan a review of needed immunizations 3 months before departure.

8. Check below if any of the following pertain to you:

_____ I have a fever today.

_____ I take these drugs regularly:

_____ I am now, or I might be, pregnant.

_____ I have had a positive tuberculin skin test in the past.

_____ I am allergic to: _____ eggs _____ mercury _____ neomycin _____ other:

Describe the reaction: _____ When? _____

_____ I am taking steroids or other drugs that suppress the immune system.

_____ I had serious reactions to immunizations before. Describe:

_____ My spleen does not work properly or I have some other problem with my immune system

_____ I am receiving radiation therapy.

_____ I have had problems with my nervous system before, such as seizures or Guillain-Barré syndrome.

_____ List any other serious medical problem:

* This form may be enlarged and reproduced for individual patients, if credit is given to *ImmunoFacts*.

The Prescription for Protection

Bring this form, your outpatient medical records, and your immunization records when you go to see your doctor. If you have any questions, talk to your health care provider. If you have any difficulty in reading or understanding your records, please don't hesitate to call your doctor or health clinic.

Key Questions to Ask Before Immunizing

Following is a list of general questions to ask before immunization. Additional questions may be appropriate in some settings.

1. How do you feel today? Do you have diarrhea or a substantial fever, or are you vomiting today?
2. Do you have any drug or food allergies?
3. Have you ever had a reaction to any vaccine? If yes, describe it.
4. Are you being treated by a doctor for any condition? Which medications do you take?

For live vaccines

1. Do you have any form of immune suppression? Do you have cancer or any disease that affects the immune system?
2. Have you received blood or antibodies (immune globulins) in the past 3 to 11 months?
3. Are you pregnant or planning a pregnancy in the next month or so?

For pertussis vaccine for children

1. Does the infant or child have any neurologic problems (eg, seizures) that is not resolved or stabilized?

Immunization Documents

Immunization Records

Personal

The ideal personal immunization record for a patient spans both his or her inpatient and outpatient immunization experiences, involves the patient in the health-promotion/disease-prevention process, and provides insurance against loss of clinicians' immunization records. Several personal immunization records are available, including those of the various state health departments and Public Health Service (PHS) Form 731, International Certificates of Vaccination, commonly called the "yellow shot record."

Each state and the District of Columbia prints its own immunization record, often designed for both pediatric and adult immunizations, providing lifelong patient records. Canadian authorities specifically recommend that adults carry their personal immunization record in their wallets.

As its title implies, PHS Form 731 documents vaccines indicated for international travel, but can also serve as a convenient common document for a life's worth of vaccinations. PHS Form 731 is used by the US Department of Defense and the Coast Guard for military personnel and their family members, and by the US State Department for diplomats and their families. PHS Form 731 is available from the Government Printing Office (GPO, telephone 866-512-1800, stock number 017-001-00-440-5). It may also be available from local health departments.

Advances in electronics may soon make "smart cards," portable electronic medical records the size of credit cards, common forms of health documentation. As these miniature patient databases are developed and refined, include special immunization sections in their design.

Clinic, Office & Pharmacy

Clinicians need proper evidence of their patients' immunization experiences. These records may take either paper or electronic form. Immunizations may be recorded in the progress notes, treatment or encounter sections of a medical record. But data retrieval is more efficient if a dedicated form is used to consolidate all immunization records, rather than have them intermingled among other records of care. For example, federal hospitals and clinics may use Standard Form (SF) 601, Immunization Record, as the common document to record immunizations. The American College of Physicians advocates a similar form they call the Patient Immunization Record Form.

Even the position of immunization documents within a medical record is important. Simply moving a health-maintenance inventory that included recommendations for routine adult immunizations from the back toward the front of an encounter record increased health-promotion activities.

While paper records are adequate, electronic medical records offer advantages of faster, more complete retrieval and automated screening. Several studies have shown the efficacy of automatic reminder messages, introspective medical records, and screening by diagnosis or drug therapy for indicators for influenza or pneumococcal immunization in increasing immunization-delivery rates.

Pharmacies may be prime locations to centralize immunizations records, given the multiple physicians caring for many patients. Recording immunizations in pharmacy databases can aid screening for immunologic drugs interactions. Given the need to maintain immunization records for the decades of a patient's life and the need to archive automated prescription files periodically, it may be advisable for pharmacies to maintain a separate data file of immunization records that can be compared to the master drug file.

Electronic records also make it easier to screen immunization files for needed booster doses or to screen prescription files for drugs that suggest immunization indications. For example, prescriptions for insulin, oral hypoglycemic agents, digoxin, nitroglycerin, warfarin, theophylline, beta-adrenergic agonists, and other drugs indicate diabetes, heart disease, and lung disease. These and other diagnoses are themselves indications for annual influenza and periodic pneumococcal immunization.

Immunization records can be automated in simple databases (eg, Access) or in more sophisticated databases integrated with other clinical functions (eg, prescription profiles, drug-interaction screening).

Optimal immunization profiles include the following data elements.

Demographic Data

Patient name, gender, date of birth, occupation, telephone number, identification number, primary physician(s) and other health care provider(s).

Clinical Data

Previous hypersensitivity reactions, allergies or serum sickness; pregnancy (current or planned); current fever; any immunodeficiency in the household; previous positive tuberculin skin tests; regular medications; any chronic illnesses.

Travel History

International travel concluded, international travel planned.

Immunization History Table

Vaccine names along one axis. Along other axis: Dose, site, route of administration, date given, manufacturer and lot number, date next dose due and any reactions noted (local or systemic).

A prototype immunization profile is provided on the following page. This form may be freely reproduced for individual patients, if credit is given to *ImmunoFacts*.

Patient Immunization Record*							
Patient name:			Gender:		Occupation:		
Identification #:				Birth date:			
Daytime telephone #:							
Previous hypersensitivity reaction to:							
Agent:			Describe reaction:			When?	
Agent:			Describe reaction:			When?	
Heath care provider(s):							
Address:							
Phone:							
Questions to ask during each encounter: Pregnancy? Fever? Regular medications? Chronic illness? Previous reactions? Travel plans? Immunodeficiency in household?							
Immunologic drug	Dose, site, route of administration	Date given	Manufacturer	Lot #	Name, title of person giving drug	Date next dose due	Note
DTP,							5 doses
DT, or							5 doses
Td or Tdap							q 10 y
Haemophilus influenzae b							
Pneumococcal							all ≥ 65 y
Rotavirus							3 doses
Influenza							
Measles, Mumps, Rubella							2 doses if > 1957
Human papillomavirus							3 doses
Varicella/Zoster							
Hepatitis B							3 doses
Tuberculin Skin Test							Reaction:
Other Vaccines							

* This form may be enlarged and reproduced for individual patients if credit is given to *ImmunoFacts*.

Record Requirements for The National Childhood Vaccine Injury Act

Since March 21, 1988, the National Childhood Vaccine Injury Act has required health care providers to maintain certain records of immunizations. These records are intended to consolidate information about vaccine use and to provide information relevant to any claims pursuant to the act. Any vaccine product containing any of the following antigens is subject to the record-keeping requirement: Diphtheria, tetanus, pertussis, measles, mumps, rubella, poliovirus, *Haemophilus influenzae* type b, hepatitis A, hepatitis B, varicella, rotavirus, meningococcal (both conjugate and polysaccharide), human papillomavirus (HPV), annual trivalent influenza, and pneumococcal conjugate vaccines. Despite the title of this law, the record-keeping requirements pertain to both adult and pediatric recipients of the vaccines covered.

Clinicians are required to record certain data in the vaccine recipient's permanent medical record or in a permanent office log:
1. The manufacturer and lot number of the vaccine,
2. The date of administration of the vaccine and
3. The name, address and title of the person administering the vaccine.

The Act further requires the health care provider to report to a health department or to the FDA any occurrence following immunization of any event set forth in the Vaccine Injury Table (http://www.hrsa.gov/osp/vicp/table.htm).

The US Department of Health and Human Services has established the Vaccine Adverse Event Reporting System (VAERS) to collect all reports of suspected adverse events after the administration of any vaccine, including but not limited to the reporting of events required by the National Childhood Vaccine Injury Act of 1986. The VAERS toll-free telephone number for forms and information is (800) 822-7967, http://www.vaers.hhs.gov.

Additional information is available from the National Vaccine Injury Compensation Program (http://www.hrsa.gov/osp/vicp/index.htm), Health Resources & Services Administration, Parklawn Building, 5600 Fishers Lane, Room 16C-17, Rockville, MD 20857; (800) 338-2382.

To file a claim for vaccine injury, call or write to the US Court of Federal Claims, 717 Madison Place NW, Washington, DC 20005; (202) 219-9657.

Problem Reporting Mechanisms

Vaccine Adverse Events Reporting System (VAERS) & Adverse Drug Experience Reporting Program (MedWatch)

Despite all precautions to the contrary, adverse events temporally associated with immunization do rarely occur. To monitor the safety of vaccines, the FDA and CDC rely on clinicians to report adverse events. Clinicians have been required by law since 1988 to report events listed under "Record Requirements for the National Childhood Vaccine Injury Act." The Vaccine Adverse Events Reporting System (VAERS) took effect in November 1990, replacing separate systems at the CDC and FDA. FDA Form 3500 continues to be used to report adverse events for other drugs (eg, immune globulins, interferons, tuberculins). The form can be accessed online at http://www.vaers.hhs.gov, or call (800) FDA-1088 for forms or other information.

The FDA's MedWatch program is used to report adverse events and product problems with human drug products, biological products, medical devices (including in vitro diagnostics), special nutritional products (eg, dietary supplements, medical foods, infant formulas) and other products regulated by the FDA. MedWatch is intended to simplify and standardize previous reporting systems, producing a faster and more effective surveillance system.

One version of the single-page MedWatch reporting form is for voluntary reporting by health professionals and consumers (FDA Form 3500), while the other version (FDA Form 3500A) is used by distributors and manufacturers for reporting required by statute or FDA regulations. Completed forms can be mailed to the FDA, faxed to (800) FDA-0178, or filled out online at http://www.fda.gov/medwatch. The FDA is most interested in hearing from clinicians about cases in which a medical product was associated with a serious outcome: Death, life-threatening condition, initial or prolonged hospitalization, disability or congenital anomaly. The FDA is particularly interested in reports on products on the market for less than 3 years, because historically that is when most critical problems are discovered.

Actions taken by the FDA after analysis of safety data can include "Dear Health Professional" letters, product labeling changes (eg, boxed warnings), manufacturer-sponsored postmarketing studies and, if needed, product withdrawals. FDA experience with silicone breast implants, temafloxacin and use of angiotensin-converting enzyme (ACE) inhibitors during pregnancy highlight the vital role that reports from health professionals play in the identification of suspected adverse events.

FDA Drug Quality Reporting System

If problems are noted with the quality of drug products, report the problems to surveillance systems operated by the FDA (www.fda.gov/AboutFDA/CentersOffices/CDER/ucm082071.htm). The program relies on voluntary reports to monitor the quality of prescription products available to the US public. Reports are categorized according to problem type: Adverse drug experiences, contamination, drug claims, deterioration, labeling, packaging, physical or chemical variation, reconstitution problems, tampering, and therapeutic effect problems.

Reported problems are correlated with reports from other health professionals, to allow trend analysis of medical products on the market. The larger the number of reports, the more accurate such analysis becomes.

Medication Error Reporting Program

Just as drug products can have defects, drug use can be associated with mishaps. The Institute for Safe Medication Practices compiles information about medication errors in an effort to educate clinicians and prevent subsequent errors. The Institute for Safe Medication Practices (ISMP) has been certified as a Patient Safety Organization by the U.S. Department of Health and Human Services under the Patient Safety Act of 2005. Information reported to a PSO in the form of a "patient safety work product" is considered privileged and confidential under the Patient Safety Act and Patient Safety Rule (http://www.pso.ahrq.gov/psos/fastfacts.htm#ff21). The causes of errors are many: Lack of product knowledge; poor communication; ambiguities in product names, directions for use, or abbreviations; or patient misuse.

It is important to know that some good can come from medication errors. By informing others of the error, the chance of recurrence may be reduced. Reports to ISMP are forwarded to the FDA's MedWatch program. For product-related errors, ISMP notifies manufacturers. Reporters can choose whether or not they would like to be identified. Names and locations are handled in confidence by all the parties. Submissions to the ISMP Medication Errors Reporting Program (800-FAIL-SAFE or https://www.ismp.org/orderforms/reporterrortoismp.asp) can be completely anonymous. An iPhone application (Practice Rx) is also available on iTunes.

Types of errors or near-errors reported to the program include administering the wrong drug, strength, or dose; confusion over look-alike or sound-alike drugs; incorrect routes of administration; miscalculations; and errors in prescribing and transcribing. Your experiences and observations can help others. By sharing your encounters, you can have a positive impact on the quality of future patient care and the improvement of drug standards.

Report Forms & Additional Information

Toll-free telephone numbers for additional forms and information for the various problem-reporting systems are provided below:

Vaccine Adverse Events Reporting System (VAERS)	(800) 822-7967
FDA Medical Products Reporting Program (MedWatch)	(800) FDA-1088
Institute for Safe Medication Practices (ISMP)	(800) FAIL-SAFE, 215-947-7797

References

Bolger GR, et al. FDA's drug quality reporting system. *Consult Pharm.* 1992;7:28-31.

CDC. Immunization information systems progress - - United States, 2006. *MMWR.* 2008;57:289-291. http://www.cdc.gov/mmwr/PDF/wk/mm5711.pdf.

CDC. Surveillance for safety after immunization: Vaccine Adverse Event Reporting System (VAERS)- - United States, 1991-2001. *MMWR.* 2003;52(SS-01):1-24. Errata 52:113.

CDC. Vaccine adverse event reporting system - United States. *MMWR.* 1990;39:730-733.

Cohen MR, ed. *Medication Errors.* 2nd ed. Washington, DC: American Pharmaceutical Association; 2006.

CDC. National Childhood Vaccine Injury Act: Requirements for permanent vaccination records and for reporting of selected events after vaccination. *MMWR.*1988;37:197-200.

Clayton EW, et al. Compensation under the National Childhood Vaccine Injury Act. *J Pediatr.* 1990;116:508-513.

FDA. New vaccine adverse event reporting system. *FDA Drug Bulletin.* 1990;20:7-8, 11-12.

Grabenstein JD, Proulx SM, Cohen MR. Recognizing and preventing errors with immunologic drugs. *Hosp Pharm.* 1996;31:791-794, 799, 803-804.

Grabenstein JD. Compensation for vaccine injury: Balancing society's need and personal risk. *Hosp Pharm.* 1995;30:831-32, 834-836.

Grabenstein JD. Get it in writing: Documenting immunizations. *Hosp Pharm.* 1991;26:901-904.

Grabenstein JD. Screening patients for need of vaccines and immunologic tests: Using a standardized form. *Consult Pharm.* 1991;5:735-739.

Kapit RM, Grabenstein JD. Adverse events after immunization: Reports & results. *Hosp Pharm.* 1995;30:1031-1032, 1035-36, 1038, 1041.

Kessler DA. Introducing MedWatch: A new approach to reporting medication and device adverse effects and product problems. *JAMA.* 1993;269:2765-2768.

Kessler DA. MedWatch: The new FDA medical products reporting program. *Am J Hosp Pharm.* 1993;50:1151-1152.

Kirk JK, et al. Interviewing and counseling patients about immunizations. *Hosp Pharm.* 1991;26:1006-1010.

Landwirth J. Medical-legal aspects of immunization: Policy and practices. *Pediatr Clin N Amer.* 1990; 37:771-784.

Marwick C. Congress to simplify those complex, anxiety-provoking immunization booklets. *JAMA.* 1992;268:3413.

Perkins LD. Complying with the National Childhood Vaccine Injury Act. *Am J Hosp Pharm.* 1990;47:1260, 1262, 1266.

PHS. Vaccine information materials. *Fed Reg.* 1991(Oct 15);56:51798-51818.

Title 42. *United States Code*, Section 300.

Summary of the National Childhood Vaccine Injury Act Table (Effective November 10, 2008)		
Vaccine or Toxoid	Illness, Disability, Injury or Condition Covered	Time of First Symptom or Manifestation of Onset or of Significant Aggravation after Administration
Tetanus toxoid-containing vaccines (eg, DTaP, DTP-Hib, DT, Td, Tdap, TT)	A. Anaphylaxis or anaphylactic shock	0 to 4 hours
	B. Brachial neuritis	2 to 28 days
	C. Any acute sequelae (including death) of above events	Not applicable
Pertussis antigen-containing vaccines (eg, DTaP, DTP, P, DTP-Hib, Tdap)	A. Anaphylaxis or anaphylactic shock	0 to 4 hours
	B. Encephalopathy (or encephalitis)	0 to 72 hours
	C. Any acute complication or sequelae (including death) of above events	Not applicable
Measles, mumps, and rubella virus-containing vaccines in any combination (eg, MMR, MR, M, R)	A. Anaphylaxis or anaphylactic shock	0 to 4 hours
	B. Encephalopathy (or encephalitis)	5 to 15 days
	C. Any acute complication or sequelae (including death) of above events	Not applicable
Rubella virus-containing vaccines (eg, MMR, MR, R)	A. Chronic arthritis	7 to 42 days
	B. Any acute complication or sequelae (including death) of above events	Not applicable
Measles virus-containing vaccines (eg, MMR, MR, M)	A. Thrombocytopenic purpura	7 to 30 days
	B. Vaccine-strain measles viral infection in an immunodeficient recipient	0 to 6 months
	C. Any acute complication or sequelae (including death) of events above	Not applicable
Polio live virus-containing vaccines (OPV)	A. Paralytic poliomyelitis:	
	— in a nonimmunodeficient recipient	0 to 30 days
	— in an immunodeficient recipient	0 to 6 months
	— in a vaccine-associated community case	Not applicable
	B. Vaccine-strain polio viral infection:	
	— in a nonimmunodeficient recipient	0 to 30 days
	— in an immunodeficient recipient	0 to 6 months
	— in a vaccine-associated community case	Not applicable
	C. Any acute complication or sequelae (including death) of events above	Not applicable
Polio inactivated-virus containing vaccines (eg, IPV)	A. Anaphylaxis or anaphylactic shock	0 to 4 hours
	B. Any acute complication or sequelae (including death) of above event	Not applicable
Hepatitis A antigen-containing vaccines	No condition specified	Not applicable
Hepatitis B antigen-containing vaccines	A. Anaphylaxis or anaphylactic shock	0 to 4 hours
	B. Any acute complication or sequelae (including death) of above events above	Not applicable
Haemophilus influenzae type b polysaccharide conjugate vaccines	No condition specified	Not applicable
Influenza vaccines, trivalent	No condition specified	Not applicable
Varicella vaccine	No condition specified	Not applicable
Rotavirus vaccine	No condition specified	Not applicable

Summary of the National Childhood Vaccine Injury Act Table (Effective November 10, 2008)		
Vaccine or Toxoid	Illness, Disability, Injury or Condition Covered	Time of First Symptom or Manifestation of Onset or of Significant Aggravation after Administration
Vaccines containing live, oral, rhesus-based rotavirus	A. Intussusception	0 to 30 days
	B. Any acute complication or sequelae (including death) of above events	Not applicable
Pneumococcal conjugate vaccines	No condition specified	Not applicable
Any new vaccine recommended by the CDC for routine administration to children after publication of a notice of coverage by the Secretary of HHS	No condition specified	Not applicable

National Vaccine Injury Compensation Program

Qualifications & Aids to Interpretation

The following qualifications and aids to interpretation apply to the Vaccine Injury Table:

I. Anaphylaxis or anaphylactic shock: For purposes of this section, anaphylaxis and anaphylactic shock mean an acute, severe, and potentially lethal systemic allergic reaction. Most cases resolve without sequelae. Signs and symptoms begin minutes to a few hours after exposure. Death, if it occurs, usually results from airway obstruction caused by laryngeal edema or bronchospasm and may be associated with cardiovascular collapse. Other significant clinical signs and symptoms may include the following: Cyanosis; hypotension; bradycardia; tachycardia; arrhythmia; edema of the pharynx, trachea, or larynx with stridor and dyspnea. Autopsy findings may include acute emphysema, which results from lower respiratory tract obstruction; edema of the hypopharynx, epiglottis, larynx, or trachea; and minimal findings of eosinophilia in the liver, spleen, and lungs. When death occurs within minutes of exposure and without signs of respiratory distress, there may not be significant pathologic findings.

II. Encephalopathy: For purposes of this section, a vaccine recipient shall be considered to have suffered an encephalopathy only if such recipient manifests, within the applicable period, an injury meeting the description below, and then a chronic encephalopathy persists in such person for more than 6 months beyond the date of vaccination.

    A. An acute encephalopathy is one that is sufficiently severe so as to require hospitalization (whether or not hospitalization occurred).

        1. For children younger than 18 months of age who present without an associated seizure event, an acute encephalopathy is indicated by a significantly decreased level of consciousness lasting for 24 or more hours. Those children younger than 18 months of age who present following a seizure shall be viewed as having an acute encephalopathy if their significantly decreased level of consciousness persists longer than 24 hours and cannot be attributed to a postictal state (seizure) or medication.

        2. For adults and children 18 months of age and older, an acute encephalopathy is one that persists for 24 hours or more and is characterized by 2 or more of the following:

            a. A significant change in mental status that is not medication related; specifically a confusional state, delirium, or psychosis;

            b. A significantly decreased level of consciousness, which is independent of a seizure and cannot be attributed to the effects of medication; and

            c. A seizure associated with loss of consciousness.

        3. Increased intracranial pressure may be a clinical feature of acute encephalopathy in any age group.

        4. A "significantly decreased level of consciousness" is indicated by the presence of 1 or more of the following clinical signs for at least 24 hours (see paragraphs II.A.1 and II.A.2 of this section for applicable time frames):

            a. Decreased or absent response to environment (responds, if at all, only to loud voice or painful stimuli);

b. Decreased or absent eye contact (does not fix gaze upon family members or other individuals); or

c. Inconsistent or absent responses to external stimuli (does not recognize familiar people or things).

5. The following clinical features alone, or in combination, do not demonstrate an acute encephalopathy or a significant change in either mental status or level of consciousness as described above: Sleepiness, irritability (fussiness), high-pitched and unusual screaming, persistent inconsolable crying, and bulging fontanelle. Seizures alone are not sufficient to constitute a diagnosis of encephalopathy. In the absence of other evidence of an acute encephalopathy, seizures shall not be viewed as the first symptom or manifestation of the onset of an acute encephalopathy

B. Chronic encephalopathy occurs when a change in mental or neurologic status, first manifested during the applicable time period, persists for a period of at least 6 months from the date of vaccination. Individuals who return to a normal neurologic state after the acute encephalopathy shall not be presumed to have suffered residual neurologic damage from that event; any subsequent chronic encephalopathy shall not be presumed to be a sequelae of the acute encephalopathy. If a preponderance of the evidence indicates that a child's chronic encephalopathy is secondary to genetic, prenatal, or perinatal factors, that chronic encephalopathy shall not be considered to be a condition set forth in the table.

C. An encephalopathy shall not be considered to be a condition set forth in the table if in a proceeding on a petition it is shown by a preponderance of the evidence that the encephalopathy was caused by an infection, a toxin, a metabolic disturbance, a structural lesion, a genetic disorder, or trauma (without regard to whether the cause of the infection, toxin, trauma, metabolic disturbance, structural lesion, or genetic disorder is known). The encephalopathy shall be considered to be a condition set forth in the table if it is not possible to determine the cause by a preponderance of the evidence of an encephalopathy at the time a decision is made on a petition filed under section 2111(b) of the Act for a vaccine-related injury or death.

D. In determining whether or not an encephalopathy is a condition set forth in the table, the court shall consider the entire medical record.

III. Seizure and convulsion: For purposes of paragraph II of this section, the terms "seizure" and "convulsion" include myoclonic, generalized tonic-clonic (grand mal), and simple and complex partial seizures. Absence (petit mal) seizures shall not be considered to be a condition set forth in the table. Jerking movements or staring episodes alone are not necessarily an indication of seizure activity.

IV. Sequela: The term "sequela" means a condition or event that was actually caused by a condition listed in the Vaccine Injury Table.

V. Chronic arthritis:

A. For purposes of this section, chronic arthritis may be found in a person with no history of arthropathy (joint disease) in the 3 years prior to vaccination on the basis of:

1. Medical documentation, recorded within 30 days after the onset, of objective signs of acute arthritis (joint swelling) that occurred between 7 and 42 days after a rubella vaccination;

2. Medical documentation (recorded within 3 years after the onset of acute arthritis) of the persistence of objective signs of intermittent or continuous arthritis for more than 6 months following vaccination; and

3. Medical documentation of an antibody response to the rubella virus.

B. For purposes of this section, the following shall not be considered as chronic arthritis: Musculoskeletal disorders, such as diffuse connective tissue diseases (including, but not limited to, rheumatoid arthritis, juvenile rheumatoid arthritis, systemic lupus erythematosus, systemic sclerosis, mixed connective tissue disease, polymyositis/dermatomyositis, fibromyalgia, necrotizing vasculitis and vasculopathies, Sjögren syndrome), degenerative joint disease, infectious agents other than rubella (whether by direct invasion or as an immune reaction), metabolic and endocrine diseases, trauma, neoplasms, neuropathic disorders, bone and cartilage disorders, arthritis associated with ankylosing spondylitis, psoriasis, inflammatory bowel disease, Reiter syndrome, or blood disorders.

C. Arthralgia (joint pain) or stiffness without joint swelling shall not be viewed as chronic arthritis for purposes of this section.

VI. Brachial neuritis:

A. This term is defined as dysfunction limited to the upper extremity nerve plexus (ie, its trunks, divisions, or cords) without involvement of other peripheral (eg, nerve roots or a single peripheral nerve) or central (eg, spinal cord) nervous system structures. A deep, steady, often severe aching pain in the shoulder and upper arm usually heralds onset of the condition. The pain is followed in days or weeks by weakness and atrophy in upper extremity muscle groups. Sensory loss may accompany the motor deficits, but is generally a less notable clinical feature. The neuritis, or plexopathy, may be present on the same side as or on the opposite side of the injection; it is sometimes bilateral, affecting both upper extremities.

B. Weakness is required before the diagnosis can be made. Motor, sensory, and reflex findings on physical examination and the results of nerve conduction and electromyographic studies must be consistent in confirming that dysfunction is attributable to the brachial plexus. The condition should thereby be distinguishable from conditions that may give rise to dysfunction of nerve roots (ie, radiculopathies) and peripheral nerves (ie, including multiple mononeuropathies), as well as other peripheral and CNS structures (eg, cranial neuropathies and myelopathies).

VII. Thrombocytopenic purpura: This term is defined by a serum platelet count less than 50,000 cells/mm^3. Thrombocytopenic purpura does not include cases of thrombocytopenia associated with other causes such as hypersplenism, autoimmune disorders (including alloantibodies from previous transfusions), myelodysplasias, lymphoproliferative disorders, congenital thrombocytopenia, or hemolytic uremic syndrome. This does not include cases of immune (formerly called idiopathic) thrombocytopenic purpura (ITP) that are mediated, for example, by viral or fungal infections, toxins, or drugs. Thrombocytopenic purpura does not include cases of thrombocytopenia associated with disseminated intravascular coagulation, as observed with bacterial and viral infections. Viral infections include, for example, those infections secondary to Epstein-Barr virus, cytomegalovirus, hepatitis A and B, rhinovirus, HIV, adenovirus, and dengue virus. An antecedent viral infection may be demonstrated by clinical signs and symptoms and need not be confirmed by culture or serologic testing. Bone marrow examination, if performed, must reveal a normal or an increased number of megakaryocytes in an otherwise normal marrow.

VIII. Vaccine-strain measles infection: This term is defined as a disease caused by the vaccine-strain that should be determined by vaccine-specific monoclonal antibody or polymerase chain reaction tests.

IX. Vaccine-strain poliovirus infection: This term is defined as a disease caused by poliovirus that is isolated from the affected tissue and should be determined to be the vaccine-strain by oligonucleotide or polymerase chain reaction. Isolation of poliovirus from the stool is not sufficient to establish a tissue-specific infection or disease caused by vaccine-strain poliovirus.

Principles for Handling, Shipping, & Storing Immunologic Drugs

Most of the vaccines and immunologic drugs described in *ImmunoFacts* are sensitive to extreme temperatures. Exposure to heat or freezing can dramatically reduce the potency of these drugs, even though the change may not be readily noticeable. Immunologic drugs are usually mixtures of complex molecules for which no simple potency tests are available. Mishandling vaccines and other biologicals not only wastes the intrinsic value of these drugs, it wastes the money used to buy them. But, even worse may be the human effects of invalidated immunologic drugs.

If these damaged drugs are administered, the recipients may get little if any benefit from them. This is true whether the immunologic drug will be used for diagnosis, prevention, or therapy. This means that you might not know whether to believe a skin test result. Or that the person you vaccinate may not gain immunity and thus remain susceptible to infection. Or the person given the impotent antibodies might get the disease you hope to avoid. Or the person given an inadequate therapy may not be cured or successfully treated.

Follow these principles to enhance the quality of the immunologic drugs you administer. For simplicity, the term vaccines may be used below, even when the same concepts apply to other immunologic drugs as well.

General Principles

If you are responsible for shipping, handling, or storing immunologic drugs, be sure to keep the following principles in mind. The guiding principle is maintaining the "cold chain." The cold chain extends from the refrigerators or freezers at the manufacturing plant, all the way to the pharmacy, clinic, ward, or office, until the product is actually administered to the patient. If you maintain the cold chain, keeping cold things cold and frozen things frozen, you can be confident in the quality of the vaccines, antibodies, and other immunologic drugs you use.

- Have good routine and emergency procedures. Designating primary and alternate people to be responsible for receiving, handling, and shipping immunologic drugs lets you focus training efficiently. It also helps you achieve standards of quality.
- Use good equipment.
- Size matters. If possible, use separate commercial refrigerators and freezers. For storage of smaller volumes, use a full-size refrigerator-freezer. Refrigerator units lacking a separate freezer, often intended for dormitories or mini-bars, do not keep consistent frozen temperatures.
- Frost-free freezers are preferred, because ice buildup interferes with the freezer's ability to maintain very low temperatures. The ice actually acts as in insulator. As little as ¼-inch of ice can disrupt the cold chain. If you have to defrost the freezer, place the drugs inside temporary cold storage until the unit returns to the proper cold temperature.
- Stabilization. For new refrigerators and freezers, 2 to 7 days may be required for temperatures to stabilize.
- Allow enough space. Refrigerators and freezers cool by convection. That means that cool air must be allowed to circulate around the boxes of vaccines and other drugs to cool them. Packing a refrigerator too full can lead to subtle increases in temperature.
- Keep refrigerator doors closed as much as possible. Close doors promptly after retrieving an item. Storing immunologic drugs in the body of the refrigerator, not on the shelves in the doors themselves, reduces temperature variation. In the doors, store only diluents or bottles of water to provide insulation and a thermal reserve. Do not store food, drinks, or patient specimens in the same refrigerator you use for medications.

- Do not leave refrigerated items out at room temperature for too long. If your practice requires vials to stay out for more than a few minutes, keep them in an insulated container with coolant packs fresh from the refrigerator. Cover them with a form-fitting lid. Coolant packs might also be called thermal packs, gel packs, blue-ice packs, or chemical packs. Coolant packs filled with water have roughly the same thermal capacity as those filled with ethylene glycol or other fluids. Alternately, plastic bottles filled with water, then chilled, can be used. Do not let medication vials touch frozen coolant packs directly. Use a towel or sheet of cardboard to separate them. During lunch and breaks, return the vials to the refrigerator and the coolant packs to the refrigerator. Reassemble the insulated tray when you return.

- Test the refrigerators. Refrigerators should maintain a temperature between 2° and 8°C (36° to 46°F). Set the thermostat in the middle of that range. Keep a log on the front or side of each refrigerator and check the thermometer inside at the same time each day (preferably early in the day). If you forget to check the temperature, leave that space blank. Do not just assume the temperature was the same as the day before or after. If the thermometer does not fluctuate at least a little, test the thermometer to make sure it is working properly. Maximum/minimum thermometers are available that can record a unit's temperature range.

- Test the freezers. Standard freezers should maintain a temperature well below 0°C (32°F), such as -15°C (5°F). Use the same method as you did to test the refrigerators, but you will need a thermometer that reliably reads temperatures at freezing temperatures.

- Test the shipping methods. Send out test shipments with temperature monitors to assess handling procedures along the route of travel.

- Plan ahead for electrical and mechanical problems. An inventory of vaccines and antibodies often represents a significant economic investment. For example, Health Care Logistics (Circleville, OH: 800-848-1633) offers electric and battery-powered temperature and temperature/humidity recording kits. Placing temperature probes in glycerin or similar material can reduce detection sensitivity slightly, such as during brief intervals when doors are open. Consider an alarm system that warns if the power goes off or the machines malfunction. Simple systems record temperatures and sound audible alarms. Sophisticated systems can alert a guard or attendant or even telephone a designated number. For large inventories, a backup generator may be justified, to provide emergency power in case of electrical interruptions. Test these generators periodically. Install locks or guards on electrical plugs so that they are not accidentally unplugged by maintenance or other workers. Do not use electrical outlets controlled by a wall switch. Place signs in circuit breaker panels, warning not to disrupt power to refrigerators and freezers. Clean coils and replace door seals as needed.

- Storing coolant packs in the refrigerator not only keeps them ready for use in shipping, they can provide additional insulation and cooling power in case of a power outage.

- Plan ahead for shortages or unusual demand. Who will you contact for out-of-the-ordinary vaccines, antibodies, or antivenins? Do those parties know that you are depending on them? Coordinate your plans with those other parties.

- Train everyone who handles vaccines and immunologic drugs in good storage and handling procedures. You can use this section of *ImmunoFacts* as a rough lesson plan for in-service training. Conduct training once a year or so and include it in the orientation of new personnel. Collect samples of expired or empty packages, monitoring devices, and related items for use as training aids. Post signs and pictures on refrigerator doors that show how medications inside should be arranged. Training reduces waste and improves the quality of the immunologic drugs you use.

- If you lock the refrigerator, designate primary and alternate people to keep the key to the lock.

- Inform all workers about the importance of reporting any breach of proper handling guidelines. Tell them you would prefer them admitting mistakes and throwing away impotent vaccines, rather than injecting useless vaccines into people. Make sure that workers are not penalized for reporting problems.

Handling Procedures

- When receiving deliveries, check the contents of the boxes you receive against the invoice or other shipping documents that accompany them. Move these products into the appropriate refrigerator or freezer promptly. You may also want to check the contents against the original ordering documents too. Report any discrepancies according to institutional policies.
- If the packages you receive contain temperature monitors, check to see if the package you receive has been exposed to temperatures that are either too hot or too cold. Several kinds of monitoring devices are used. Instructions for reading them are usually attached. Usually these monitors are disposable, but some should be returned to the sender. The most common kinds include:
    - Recording thermometers that produce linear or circular charts of temperature variation. These monitors have the advantage of showing both how extreme a temperature was reached and how long that extreme persisted.
    - In color-change monitors, a dye is released if the temperature crosses a predetermined threshold, most of these monitors do not return to their original color when temperatures moderate. For example, some turn color if the temperature drops below 0°C (32°F), such as the "32°F Freeze Watch." They are relatively inexpensive, but do not report the highest or lowest temperature reached. Some do not disclose whether the extreme lasted for minutes or hours. Others turn color if the temperature rises above certain thresholds. Most of these monitors do not return to their original color. For example, the monitor might not report whether the temperature reached merely 100°F or 120°F, nor whether the extreme lasted for 10 minutes or 10 hours.
    - Similar to simple color-change monitors are window monitors that show a bit more information. For example, some show which of 5 temperature levels was reached, such as the "10-I-Time-Temperature-Monitor."
- Whenever the monitor shows that the package reached an unacceptable temperature, place the vaccine in quarantine, such as putting it into a paper bag marked "Do Not Use." Move the vaccine to a refrigerator or freezer, as appropriate, until the question about the usability of the vaccine is resolved. Then contact the manufacturer immediately for instructions about further handling or replacement. You can reuse some undisturbed monitors, by using them when you ship out perishable packages or by keeping them in the refrigerators and freezers to reveal any temperature abnormalities.
- Store containers of the same vaccine together. To avoid choosing the wrong vial, it may be helpful to separate products that have similar packaging or similar names. For example, placing the adult and pediatric strengths of tetanus-diphtheria (Td, Tdap, and DT) toxoids in separate locations may be wise. Similarly, as more combination vaccines become available, it will become increasingly important to clearly label which section of the refrigerator is intended for which product.
- Be sure to read labels when removing products from the shelf; do not rely solely on its proper location. Too often, practitioners easily confuse look-alike packaging. Even experienced professionals commit this error. The phenomenon is called confirmation bias. People too often rely on familiar evidence (the color and shape of the vials) while missing contrary evidence (the drug names on the containers). One way to reduce error potential of this type is to tell yourself the name of the drug you need ("I need 0.5 mL of hepatitis B vaccine") and then read the container label to yourself ("I see 0.5 mL of hepatitis B vaccine in my hand").
- Arrange the shelves so that the products with the closest expiration dates are in front. Place vaccines and other products with longer potency in the back. Check 100% of the shelving of the refrigerator and freezer for expired medications at least monthly. Remove those containers and dispose of them properly. Return unused products for credit, if possible. Dispose of live vaccines (eg, typhoid, BCG, live viruses) as hazardous waste.
- Order sensibly and routinely. Do not overstock. Keep records of wastage by expiration and adjust order quantities appropriately.

- Consensus on how long to retain a multidose vial after it is first entered is beginning to form. Many institutions use a 30-day policy, after which they discard the remaining portion. But this policy is not based on any firm evidence of hazard to patients after 30 days; it may have arisen in concert with frequency of pharmacy inspections of medication stations in hospitals. Many institutions allow multidose vials to be used until the original expiration date marked on the container, unless contamination is apparent or suspected. Such guidelines are consistent with recommendations of the Centers for Disease Control & Prevention. This policy will reduce waste without harm to patients. All multidose vials describe on their labels the preservative included, such as thimerosal, phenol, benzyl alcohol, parabens (eg, methylparabens, propylparabens), or benzethonium chloride.
- Filling syringes: When drawing vaccines into syringes, two issues are important: sterility and stability. Good aseptic technique is needed at all times to prevent the contamination of the vaccine as it is transferred from the vial to the syringe, and then again when injected into the patient. Reusing needles or syringes has led directly to the transmission of hepatitis B virus and perhaps other blood-borne pathogens. Some drugs can attach themselves to the polymers in plastic syringes, although the physical and chemical stability of individual vaccines when stored in syringes for prolonged periods has not generally been studied. Avoid situations where you draw up vaccines and store them for more than a day, if possible. Even then, the filled syringes should be stored under the same conditions as the vials would have been. For more specific information, consult detailed references or call manufacturers.
- Using diluents at temperatures above room temperature can inactivate live virus (eg, varicella, MMR). Reconstitute these vaccines only with diluents at room temperature or refrigerated diluents.
- Examples of vendors of products for quality shipping and handling
  - Endurotherm shipping containers insulated with polyurethane foam (various sizes), SCA, ThermoSafe, Phoenix, AZ.
  - VaxiCool refrigerator/freezer with storage area approximately 1 cubic foot (power supply options: AC, attached battery, car battery, solar panels), AcuTemp, Dayton, OH.
  - VaxiPak shipping container with storage area for 1 to 24 vials, AcuTemp, Dayton, OH.
  - TempTale-3 and TempTale-4 multiple-use temperature monitors, Sensitech, Beverly, MA.

Shipping Procedures

- In shipping, use boxes of appropriate size, neither too large nor too small. Boxes that are too large contain too much air space that must be cooled before the contents can be kept cool. The warmest part of any package is on the top or side farthest away from the coolant packs.
- Several types of insulated shipping containers are manufactured. The most common kinds include:
  - Individual panels of rigid expanded polyurethane, usually white, lining the top, bottom, and all four sides of the type of box that is blown into place. This type of container has the least insulating capacity.
  - Molded expanded polystyrene (eg, Styrofoam), often used in insulated coolers, fits snugly against the walls of a cardboard box. This material is crisp or brittle when flexed.
  - Foil- and plastic-lined panels of isocyanurate with angled joints at the corners.
  - Polyurethane with foam molded between layers of cardboard.
- For vaccines that do not need to be frozen: Place the medications and coolant packs in the container in a consistent and systematic way. For maximum protection against heat, use cold packs on the bottom, on all sides, and on the top. Coolant packs taken directly from a freezer should be allowed to warm to about to 5°C (41°F) before packing. This recommendation is especially important during cold weather, as they may freeze vaccines. For this reason, refrigerated coolant packs are preferred over frozen ones. Fill all remaining empty space with some kind of filling material, such as Styrofoam pellets, brown 2-ply, or wrapping paper. Fillers

have little or no insulating value. Seal the box with strong tape so that it remains tightly closed during the entire journey.

- Ship via a courier that will get the box to the destination before the contents are exposed to extreme temperatures. Usually, this means within 48 hours. Consider the distance to be covered and the day the shipment leaves the facility. Do not routinely ship on Thursdays or Fridays, to reduce the likelihood that medications will sit idle at ambient temperatures over a weekend. In most cases, overnight or second-day courier services are justified.
- Display shipping labels prominently with clear, detailed addresses. Add additional labels to advise shippers of the perishable nature of the contents.
- After packing, sealing, and labeling the box, return it to a refrigerator until picked up by the shipping company if a delay of several hours is expected.
- Ask recipients to reuse or return undamaged boxes and coolant packs for reuse. For this purpose, the lowest cost class of transport may be used. Reuse saves money and is ecologically sound.

Storage Procedures

Drugs Normally Frozen

Normal storage: Only live viral vaccines can be stored in a freezer without damaging the product. Continuous freezing (below $-20°C$ or $-4°F$) is the preferred condition for varicella vaccine, except for a short period in the refrigerator just before use. Freezing is optional for vaccines containing measles, mumps, and rubella antigens.

Diluents: Do not freeze diluents for these vaccines. There is a theoretical risk that vial seals might contract, breaching the sterility of the container. Either store these diluents at room temperature or in a refrigerator.

Shipping during warm weather: Ship frozen drugs separately from refrigerated drugs. Use dry ice (ie, frozen carbon dioxide) to make sure that vaccines arrive in a frozen state. To avoid skin damage, handle dry ice with gloves, not with bare hands. In addition, wear eye shields. Blocks of dry ice stay cold longer than an equivalent weight of dry ice pellets. Use at least 2.3 kg (5 pounds) of dry ice per package. When dry ice evaporates, it releases gaseous carbon dioxide. Technically, dry ice undergoes sublimation, changing from a solid directly to a gas, without existing as a liquid. Keep it only in well-ventilated areas.

Shipping during cold weather: Follow the same principles as in paragraph above. No special considerations are required, although somewhat less dry ice may be needed.

Traveling with these drugs: Individual or small supplies of medications that need to be frozen can be transported in similar insulated containers, such as personal food or beverage containers. Coolants can include frozen water (ie, "wet" ice, frozen water) or chemical coolants, as appropriate. Seal medications in water-tight bags or containers to keep them dry, if they might be immersed in water. Do not leave these vaccines in a vehicle parked in the sun or in other locations subject to extreme temperatures.

Drugs Normally Refrigerated

Normal handling: Pack the most temperature-sensitive vaccines closest to the coolant packs. The warmest part of any package is on the top or side farthest away from the coolant packs. To avoid freezing, store coolant packs in the refrigerator, rather than a freezer. This recommendation is especially important during cold weather.

Specific products:

- Measles, mumps, and rubella vaccines (eg, MMR): Attenuated measles, mumps, and rubella viruses in modern reconstituted vaccines can be inactivated by as little as 5 minutes in sunlight. Incandescent and fluorescent lighting will also produce this effect, but after an indeterminate longer period of time. This phenomenon was noted when people vaccinated with later doses from a 50-dose vial were found to be more likely to contract measles than people who received the first few doses from that vial. At one time, 50-dose vials were tinted red to reduce light exposure. Protect reconstituted MMR vaccines from light with an opaque covering before administration. Use within 8 hours after reconstitution.

- DTP (and its component) vaccines and hepatitis B vaccine are the vaccines most susceptible to damage after freezing.

Shipping during warm weather: Use refrigerated coolant packs to make sure the medications arrive in a cold, but not frozen, state. In especially warm weather, additional coolants may be needed.

Shipping during cold weather: Follow the same principles as in the paragraph above, except that less coolant may be needed.

Traveling with these drugs: Individual or small supplies of medications can be transported in smaller insulated containers, such as personal food or beverage containers. Coolants can include refrigerated water or chemical coolants, as appropriate. Wrap medications to keep them dry. Seal medications in water-tight bags or containers to keep them dry, if they might be immersed in water. Do not leave these vaccines in locations subject to extreme temperatures.

Drugs Normally Stored at Room Temperature

Normal storage: No special requirements.

Traveling with these drugs: Individual or small supplies of medications can be transported without special packaging. But do not leave these products in automobiles during warm weather, where the temperature inside the vehicle can be far higher than the ambient temperature.

Other Physical Properties

Solutions freeze at a point lower than the freezing point of pure water, one of the so-called colligative properties. Thus, liquid vaccines may actually freeze at $-1°$ to $-5°C$ (23° to 28°F), rather than 0°C (32°F). But this characteristic is not consistent, and should not generally be relied on. Therefore, do not subject drugs properly stored in a refrigerator to storage conditions below 0°C (32°F). The so-called "shake-test" to assess resuspension of frozen vaccines is not reliable.

Room temperature coolant packs have been evaluated as "heat sinks" to absorb heat and protect vaccines from freezing. Unfortunately, the packs often exhibit a supercooling phenomenon, where the temperature falls to about $-4°C$ (25°F) before rising to nearly 0°C (32°F). This situation was too erratic to be used reliably to protect vaccines from freezing.

When Severe Weather Threatens

The following procedures are prudent steps to take before a hurricane, blizzard, or other severe weather system threatens a geographic area. To protect vaccine in storage and to minimize the potential monetary loss, implement emergency procedures at both the depot and provider level. Part of these procedures should include messages to all providers who receive public-purchased vaccines, or at least to those in the geographic areas of highest risk.

In advance of the emergency, ensure the following:

(1) Identify an alternative storage facility (eg, hospital, packing plant, state depot), with backup power (ie, generator), where the vaccine can be properly stored and monitored for the duration of the storm

(2) Assign staff to pack and move the vaccine

(3) Use appropriate packing containers, coolant packs (for most vaccines), and dry ice (for varicella and yellow fever vaccines)

(4) Transport the vaccine to the secure storage facility. Providers should suspend vaccinations before weather conditions deteriorate. Allow sufficient time for packing and transporting vaccine before the storm can adversely affect local conditions.

The following are other precautions and appropriate measures to protect vaccine inventories:

I. Emergency Procedures
  A. List emergency phone numbers, companies, and points of contact for:
    1. Electrical power company
    2. Refrigeration repair company
    3. Temperature alarm monitoring company
    4. Perimeter alarm repair company
    5. Perimeter alarm monitoring company
    6. Backup storage facility
    7. Transportation to backup storage
    8. Dry ice vendor
    9. Emergency generator repair company
    10. National Weather Service (local office)
    11. National Hurricane Center Web site: http://www.nhc.noaa.gov/
    12. Vaccine and Immune Globulin Manufacturers: See Appendix G.
      a. Sanofi Pasteur: 800-VACCINE (800-822-2463)
      b. GlaxoSmithKline: 800-366-8900
      c. Wyeth Laboratories: 800-820-2815
  B. Support to providers storing vaccine:
    1. Identify hospitals, health departments or other facilities that could serve as emergency vaccine storage facilities and communicate this information. This might also be done at the regional or county level or with the assistance of Bioterrorism or Emergency Preparedness Units.
    2. Prioritize assistance and communication to providers in areas at highest risk, eg, low lying coastal or floodplain areas.
  C. Entering vaccine storage spaces:
    Describe how to enter vaccine storage spaces in an emergency if the building is closed. Include a floor diagram and the locations of: doors, flash lights, spare batteries, light switches, keys, locks, alarms, circuit breakers, packing materials, etc.
  D. Identify who on staff to call for the following issues:
    1. Equipment problems
    2. Backup storage
    3. Backup transportation
    4. Security
  E. Identify what vaccines to pack first in an emergency, perhaps while the power is still working:
    1. Pack refrigerated vaccines first, with an adequate supply of coolant packs.
    2. Remove and pack frozen vaccines (eg, varicella, yellow fever), using dry ice, immediately before they are to be transported.
  F. Pack and transport all vaccine inventory. If that is not possible, determine the types and amounts to save. For example, save only the most expensive vaccines, to minimize dollar loss or save some portion of all vaccines to ensure a short-term, complete supply for resuming vaccination of the served population. Assuming prompt resupply from outside the emergency area, first priority may favor the vaccines most expensive to replace.
  G. Follow vaccine packing procedures for transport to backup storage facilities:
    1. Open refrigerated units only when absolutely necessary and only after you have made all preparations for packing and moving the vaccine to alternative storage sites.
    2. Use properly insulated containers or the best available expedient materials.
  H. Move vaccine to backup storage according to prearranged plans: how to load transportation vehicle (away from heating ducts); routes to take; time en route.

References

CDC. *Vaccine Management: Recommendations for Storage and Handling of Selected Biologicals*. http://www.cdc.gov/vaccines/pubs/downloads/bk_vac_mgt.pdf. Published January 2007. Accessed August 29, 2007.

Canadian National Advisory Committee on Immunization. National guidelines for vaccine storage and transportation. *Can Comm Dis Rep*. 1995;21:93-97.

Kartoglu U, Ozgüler NK, Wolfson LJ, Kurzatkowski W. Validation of the shake test for detecting freeze damage to adsorbed vaccines. *Bull WHO*. 2010;88:624-631.

World Health Organization. *Guidelines on the International Packaging and Shipping of Vaccines*. http://www.who.int/vaccines-documents/DocsPDF06/818.pdf. Published December 2005. Accessed August 29, 2007.

Immunizations & Civil Emergencies

Despite public demand to the contrary, few additional vaccinations are needed following a natural disaster in the United States. Outbreaks of communicable diseases are rare after floods and earthquakes here. Nonetheless, individuals whose immunities have lapsed may be more likely to be identified during and following a catastrophe than under normal conditions.

Public health planners must ensure that mass immunization programs do not divert limited labor from more valuable relief activities. Immunization programs may also give the public a false sense of security, potentially leading to neglect of basic rules of hygiene and sanitation that are far more important than immunizations in preventing infection. If resources are available, public concern about immunity may provide a useful opportunity to reach adults who might not otherwise be vaccinated.

In general, rates of diseases present in a community before a disaster may increase because of decreased sanitation or overcrowding of displaced persons. Infectious diseases that were not present in the community before the disaster are not usually a problem.

Share the information in this section with the news media, if appropriate, to educate the public.

Routine Immunizations

Continue routine pediatric and adult immunization plans unabated during the course of the civic emergency and cleanup. Remember that millions of American adults are inadequately vaccinated, especially against influenza, pneumococcal disease, hepatitis B, tetanus, diphtheria, and pertussis. The interval following a natural disaster may be an opportune time to bring their immune protection up to where it should be.

Vaccinate every person assessed for immunization adequacy against all diseases that pose a threat. In other words, interest in a patient might be initiated because of his or her need for a tetanus-diphtheria toxoid booster. But while assessing the patient, take the opportunity to check for needs for other vaccines: Influenza, pneumococcal, or hepatitis B vaccine, or any immunization need.

Revaccinate adults against tetanus, diphtheria, and pertussis at 10-year or appropriate intervals. Revaccinate persons with open wounds who are exposed to flood waters or debris if more than 5 years have passed since their most recent booster dose. Include assessing the adequacy of each patient's personal immunity against diseases to which he or she is exposed as routine procedures within acute-care clinics and hospital emergency departments. Begin influenza and pneumococcal vaccination programs on schedule in the fall.

Extraordinary Immunizations

In disaster situations, extraordinary risk of preventable infections varies with exposure to water, debris, and other vectors, increased periods of time outdoors, and other occupational or vocational risks.

- Emergency Workers: Vaccinate those who are likely to be exposed to blood against hepatitis B.
- Sanitation and Water-Treatment Workers: Generally no greater risk of hepatitis B or tetanus than the general population. Vaccinate against hepatitis A, if possible.
- Relief workers (eg, those working on levees): Generally require no greater protection than standard immunity against influenza (seasonally), tetanus, diphtheria, and pertussis.
- National Guard and Military Reserve Personnel: Military personnel require an assortment of immunizations to comply with standards of military readiness, beyond the needs of a present disaster (eg, hepatitis A). These requirements may exceed needs of other citizens in the area of the disaster.

Seek local expert opinion to determine specific requirements in your setting. Your city, county, and state health departments are good places to seek advice.

Principles Involved in Hasty Immunity

Inducing active immunity by vaccination generally takes 1 to 2 weeks or more. It takes this much time for the body to produce protective quantities of antibodies. If a patient needs more acute protection, use preformed antibodies in the form of an immune globulin product (eg, tetanus immune globulin).

Active immunity develops in a person in response to infection or after administration of a vaccine or toxoid. Sufficient active immunity to protect the host may take several weeks or months to induce, especially if several doses of a basic series are needed. But active immunity is long-lasting. A vaccine is a formulation of whole or fractional microorganisms (eg, bacteria, viruses) or portions of them. Toxoids are a subset of vaccines. Toxoids are modified bacterial toxins, rendered nontoxic themselves while retaining the ability to stimulate antitoxin formation (ie, specific antibodies against the natural toxin).

Passive immunity, on the other hand, is temporary immunity provided in the form of preformed, donated antitoxins or antibodies (ie, immune globulins) from another living host (either human or animal). Passive immunity protects almost immediately but only persists with the biological half-life of IgG, usually measured in weeks. For delayed but more prolonged immunity, active vaccination may be appropriate in addition to passive immunization.

Both active and passive immunization strategies are discussed below, organized by specific disease threats.

Tetanus: Tetanus toxoid provides active immunity against the disease. Combined tetanus and diphtheria toxoids (Td) bivalent or with acellular pertussis vaccine (Tdap) is the preferred product for persons 7 years of age or older. Prompt-acting tetanus immune globulin (TIG) is reserved for treating serious wounds in persons with unknown or inadequate immunity. Follow the CDC's wound-management guidelines to prevent tetanus, provided in the Bacterial Vaccines & Toxoids section of *ImmunoFacts*.

Hepatitis A: To prevent hepatitis A, passive immunity with immune globulin intramuscular (IGIM) or active hepatitis A vaccination may be recommended, although this is unusual in disaster settings in the US. Human waste from sewage plants is a potential source of viral infection. But such sewage is typically diluted by flood waters to a point where it is no longer hazardous and frequent handwashing is sufficient protection.

Hepatitis B: The vaccine actively induces the recipient's own circulating antibodies against the hepatitis B virus (HBV), as well as stimulating the production of memory B-cells that permit an accelerated response upon rechallenge. Giving hepatitis B immune globulin (HBIG), on the other hand, is essentially the loan of someone else's antibodies. If an HBIG recipient does not develop any of his or her own specific anti-HBV antibody-producing plasma cells through active vaccination, the loaned antibodies are eventually catabolized and not replaced. In this respect, the immunity provided by HBIG is only temporary. In some cases of postexposure prophylaxis, both vaccine and HBIG are given, to provide immediate but transient protection while the delayed but long-lasting immunity develops.

Personal Hygiene & Water Sanitation

To prevent water-borne diseases, the most important consideration for public health workers is to restore the public water supply. Until this happens, only consume water that is bottled or trucked in from a safe source or disinfected before use. This caution pertains to water used in any form of beverage, making ice, brushing teeth, and cooking. Water brought to a vigorous boil for at least 5 minutes will be reliably disinfected. Water boiled for shorter times or heated to lower temperatures will be less completely disinfected.

Chemical treatment of water is less reliable than boiling as a means of disinfection. Two to 4 drops of full strength (4% to 6%) household bleach or 8 drops of 2% iodine tincture will disinfect a liter of water after 20 to 30 minutes. More time or more chemical is needed if the water is cold or turbid.

Washing hands for at least 10 seconds with soap and safe water is extremely valuable in stopping transmission of microbes. Washing is especially important before preparing or eating food, after toilet use, and after handling potentially contaminated items.

No Action Generally Needed

No additional immunization or prophylaxis is generally needed or possible for diseases described below. Health professionals should calm the populace and news media, as appropriate, citing these facts:

Cholera: Cholera is not typically found in the US, although the risk in Latin America is growing. While it is true that the causative bacterium is transmitted through food, water, and inadequate sanitation, disease risk in the US is negligible. Cholera occasionally infects fisherman off the Texas and Louisiana coasts. The parenteral cholera vaccine confers only limited immunity of short duration and is no longer manufactured in the United States.

Malaria: The parasites that cause malaria are not native to the US. Even if increased time spent outdoors increases the number of mosquito bites a person receives, the bites do not transmit malaria.

St. Louis Encephalitis (SLE): This disease is caused by a mosquito-borne flavivirus. In 1992, only 14 isolated cases of SLE were reported in the US. Twelve of these cases occurred in Texas, with the balance in California. In the last few decades, most cases occurred in Texas, Illinois, Ohio, Indiana, Mississippi, and bordering states. The virus is transmitted by the *Culex tarsalis* mosquito. No vaccine against this virus is available. The SLE immune plasma, previously available from the CDC, was withdrawn in the early 1980s. Incidence of SLE did not increase in Florida or Louisiana following Hurricane Andrew in 1992.

Other Arthropod-Borne Viruses (Arboviruses): Arthropods include insects that transmit disease, such as mosquitoes and ticks. Several other arboviruses cause human illness, most notably the Western Equine Encephalitis (WEE) alphavirus, but these are rare. WEE causes fewer than 20 reported cases in the US in the average year, most frequently in Colorado, Texas, North Dakota, and bordering states. The WEE immune plasma previously available from the CDC was withdrawn in the early 1980s. LaCrosse bunyavirus is endemic in the eastern US, causing 100 to 300 reported cases per year. Despite its name, California encephalitis has been reported most often in Ohio, Wisconsin, Minnesota, and bordering states. Time spent outdoors increases exposure to disease-transmitting mosquitoes, but disease incidence is still remarkably rare in most years.

Typhoid Fever: The bacterium causing typhoid is no longer routinely found in the US. When present, the bacterium is transmitted through food, water, and inadequate sanitation, but disease risk is negligible in its absence. Several effective vaccines are available, if recommended by health authorities, administered either by injection or by swallowing capsules. Vaccination is of limited value since protective levels of antibodies do not develop until several weeks after the final dose. By this time, adequate sanitation in the US is usually restored.

Other Communicable Diseases: Enterotoxigenic *Escherichia coli*, *Shigella*, *Salmonella*, and *Campylobacter* bacteria, the Norwalk virus, *Giardia* and *Cryptosporidium* parasites, the agents that cause leptospirosis and tularemia, and other infectious microbes may be transmitted by contaminated water, but no means of immunoprophylaxis are currently available. Appropriate food and water discipline and personal hygiene will minimize the threat of these diseases.

Major Causes of Morbidity During Flooding

During the summer 1993 flooding of the Mississippi and Missouri Rivers, the most common conditions prompting visits to emergency rooms in Missouri included injuries (47.7%) and illnesses (44.5%). The most common injuries were sprains, lacerations, and abrasions or contusions. The most common illnesses were gastrointestinal, rashes or dermatitis, and heat-related problems. No acute infectious disease outbreaks were noted.

Infectious disease outbreaks after flooding in the US are rare. Health professionals should help control unsubstantiated rumors of disease outbreaks.

Note

Recommendations for prophylaxis printed in this volume are intended to assist in the prevention of disease. They do not take the place of appropriate acute clinical care provided by patients' physicians and other health care providers to treat disease. Consult public health authorities for specific recommendations.

References

American College of Physicians. *Guide for Adult Immunization*. 3rd ed. Philadelphia: American College of Physicians; 1994.

CDC. Flood disasters and immunization—California. *MMWR*. 1983;32:171-172,178.

CDC. Emergency mosquito control associated with Hurricane Andrew—Florida and Louisiana, 1992. *MMWR*. 1993;42:240-242.

CDC. Arboviral diseases—United States, 1992. *MMWR*. 1993;42:467-468.

CDC. Public health consequences of a flood disaster—Iowa, 1993. *MMWR*. 1993;42:653-656.

CDC. Morbidity surveillance following the Midwest flood—Missouri, 1993. *MMWR*. 1993;42:797-798.

CDC. Infectious disease and dermatologic conditions in evacuees and rescue workers after hurricane Katrina—Multiple States, August—September, 2005. *MMWR*. 2005;54:961-964.

CDC. Public health response to hurricanes Katrina and Rita—United States, 2005. *MMWR*. 2006;55:229-231.

CDC. Natural disaster and severe weather. http://www.bt.cdc.gov/disasters/index.asp.

CDC. Recommendations for post-exposure interventions to prevent infection with hepatitis B virus, hepatitis C virus, or human immunodeficiency virus, and tetanus in persons wounded during bombings and other mass-casualty events. *MMWR*. 2008;57(RR-6):1-21. www.cdc.gov/mmwr/PDF/rr/rr5706.pdf.

French JG, Holt KW. Floods. In: Gregg MB, ed. *The Public Health Consequences of Disasters, 1989*. Atlanta, GA: US Dept. of Health and Human Services, Public Health Service, Centers for Disease Control;1989:69-78.

Heymann DL, ed. *Control of Communicable Diseases Manual*. 19th ed. Washington, DC: American Public Health Association, 2008.

Tsai TF. Arboviral infections in the United States. *Infect Dis Clin North Am*. 1991;5:73-102.

Watson JT, Gayer M, Connolly MA. Epidemics after natural disasters. *Emerg Infect Dis*. 2007;13(1):1-5. http://www.cdc.gov/ncidod/EID/13/1/pdfs/1.pdf

Terrorism Preparedness: Key Resources

Anthrax: Advisory Committee on Immunization Practices. Use of anthrax vaccine in the United States. *MMWR.* 2010;59(RR-6):1-30. http://www.cdc.gov/mmwr/PDF/rr/rr5906.pdf

Inglesby TV, O'Toole T, Henderson DA, et al. Anthrax as a biological weapon, 2002: updated recommendations for management. *JAMA.* 2002;287:2236-2252.

Botulism: Arnon SS, Schechter R, Inglesby TV, et al. Botulinum toxin as a biological weapon: medical and public health management. *JAMA.* 2001;285:1059-1070.

Shapiro RL, Hatheway C, Becher J, Swerdlow DL. Botulism surveillance and emergency response. A public health strategy for a global challenge. *JAMA.* 1997;278:433-435.

Hemorrhagic Fevers: Borio L, Inglesby T, Peters CJ, et al. Hemorrhagic fever viruses as biological weapons: medical and public health management. *JAMA.* 2002;287:2391-2405.

Plague: Inglesby TV, Dennis DT, Henderson DA, et al. Plague as a biological weapon: medical and public health management. *JAMA.* 2000;283:2281-2290.

Smallpox (Variola): ACIP, HICPAC. Recommendations for using smallpox vaccine in preevent vaccination program: Supplemental recommendations. MMWR. 2003;52(RR-7):1-16. http://www.cdc.gov/mmwr/PDF/rr/rr5207.pdf

Advisory Committee on Immunization Practices. Vaccinia (smallpox) vaccine. *MMWR.* 2001;50(RR-10):1-25. http://www.cdc.gov/mmwr/PDF/RR/RR5010.pdf

CDC. Surveillance guidelines for smallpox vaccine (vaccinia) adverse reactions. *MMWR.* 2006;55(RR-1):1-16. http://www.cdc.gov/mmwr/PDF/rr/rr5501.pdf

CDC. Smallpox Vaccination Clinic Guide. http://www.bt.cdc.gov/agent/smallpox/vaccination/pdf/smallpox-vax-clinic-guide.pdf

CDC. Smallpox vaccination and adverse events: Guidance for clinicians. *MMWR.* 2003;52(RR-4):1-30. http://www.cdc.gov/mmwr/PDF/rr/rr5204.pdf

Fenner F, Henderson DA, Arita I, Jezek Z, Ladnyi ID. *Smallpox and Its Eradication.* Geneva: World Health Organization; 1988. http://www.who.int/emc/diseases/smallpox/Smallpoxeradication.html

Henderson DA, Inglesby TV, Bartlett JG, et al. Smallpox as a biological weapon: medical and public health management. *JAMA.* 1999;281:2127-2137.

Tularemia: Dennis DT, Inglesby TV, Henderson DA, et al. Tularemia as a biological weapon: medical and public health management. *JAMA.* 2001;285:2763-2773.

Centers for Disease Control and Prevention. Tularemia—United States, 1990-2000. *MMWR.* 2002;51:182-184. http://www.cdc.gov/mmwr/preview/mmwrhtml/mm5109a1.htm.

Broad-Based Bioterrorism Resources

Centers for Disease Control and Prevention: *Public Health Emergency Preparedness and Response*. http://www.bt.cdc.gov

Christopher GW, Cieslak TJ, Pavlin JA, Eitzen EM Jr. Biological warfare. A historical perspective. *JAMA*. 1997;278:412-417.

Franz DR, Jahrling PB, Friedlander AM, et al. Clinical recognition and management of patients exposed to biological warfare agents. *JAMA*. 1997;278:339-411.

US Army Center for Health Promotion and Preventive Medicine. *The Medical NBC Battlebook. USACHPPM Tech Guide 244*. August 2002. chppm-www.apgea.army.mil/documents/TG/TECHGUID/tg244.pdf

US Army Medical Research Institute of Infectious Diseases. *Medical Management of Biological Casualties*, 6th ed. Fort Detrick, MD: US Army Medical Research Institute of Infectious Diseases, Apr 2005. usamriid.detrick.army.mil/education/instruct.htm

Barbera J, Macintyre A, Gostin L, et al. Large-scale quarantine following biological terrorism in the United States: scientific examination, logistic and legal limits, and possible consequences. *JAMA*. 2001;286:2711-2717.

Chemical Weapon Casualties

Field Management of Chemical Casualties Handbook. 2nd ed. Aberdeen Proving Ground, MD: 2000. US Army Medical Research Institute of Chemical Defense. https://ccc.apgea.army.mil/products/info/products.htm

Medical Management of Chemical Casualties Handbook, 3rd ed. Aberdeen Proving Ground, MD: 1999. US Army Medical Research Institute of Chemical Defense. https://ccc.apgea.army.mil/products/info/products.htm

Radiologic Casualties

Medical Management of Radiologic Casualties Handbook. 2nd ed. Betheseda, MD: Military Medical Operations Office, Armed Forces Radiobiology Research Institute; April 2003. http://www.afrri.usuhs.mil/www/outreach/pdf/2edmmrchandbook.pdf

This section begins with a summary of the excipients included in licensed vaccines in the United States, as of the revision date at the bottom of the page.

Excipients are inactive ingredients of a drug product necessary for production of a finished pharmaceutical formulation.

After the list of excipients is a list of culture media used in the manufacturing process of vaccines licensed in the United States.

Growth media are culture materials used to produce mass quantities of a microorganism antibody, or other immunologic agent, suitable for further processing into a finished pharmaceutical product.

All reasonable efforts have been made to ensure the accuracy of this information, but manufacturers may change product contents before that information is reflected here.

Excipients Included in US Licensed Vaccines[a]		
Excipient	Use	Vaccine
Acetone	Solvent	Adenovirus 4 & 7 vaccine
Albumin, egg (Ovalbumin)	Growth medium	Influenza (*Fluarix, FluLaval*), Rabies (*RabAvert*)
Albumin, human serum	Component of growth medium, protein stabilizer	Adenovirus 4 & 7, Measles (*Attenuvax*), MMR (*MMR-II*), MMRV (*ProQuad*), Mumps (*Mumpsvax*), Rabies (*Imovax*), Rubella (*Meruvax II*)
Albumin or serum, bovine	Component of growth medium, protein stabilizer	Adenovirus 4 & 7, Hepatitis A (*Havrix, Vaqta*), JE (*Ixiaro*), MMR (*MMR-II*), MMRV (*ProQuad*), Rabies (*Imovax, RabAvert*), Rotavirus (*RotaTeq*), Varicella (*Varivax*), Zoster (*Zostavax*)
Aluminum hydroxide	Adjuvant	Anthrax (*BioThrax*), DTaP (*Infanrix*), DTaP-Hep B-IPV (*Pediarix*), Hepatitis A (*Havrix*), Hepatitis A-Hepatitis B (*Twinrix*), Hepatitis B (*Engerix-B*), Human papillomavirus (*Cervarix*), JE (*Ixiaro*), Td (Massachusetts), Tdap (*Boostrix*)
Aluminum hydroxyphosphate sulfate	Adjuvant	Hepatitis A (*Vaqta*), Hepatitis B (*Recombivax HB*), Hib (*PedvaxHIB*), Hib-Hepatitis B (*Comvax*), Human papillomavirus (*Gardasil*)
Aluminum phosphate	Adjuvant	DTaP (*Daptacel*), Hepatitis A-Hepatitis B (*Twinrix*), Pneumococcal (*Prevnar*), Rabies (*BioRab*), Td (*Decavac*), Td (Massachusetts), Tdap (*Adacel*)
Aluminum potassium sulfate	Adjuvant	DTaP (*Daptacel, Tripedia*), DTaP-Hib (*TriHIBit*), DT (Sanofi Pasteur)
Amino acids	Component of growth medium	Anthrax (*BioThrax*), Hepatitis A (*Havrix*), Hepatitis A-Hepatitis B (*Twinrix*), Rotavirus (*Rotarix*), Td (Aventis Pasteur), Typhoid oral (*Vivotif*)
Ammonium sulfate	Protein fractionation	DTaP-Hib (*TriHIBit*), Hib (Act-HIB)
Amphotericin B	Antibacterial	Rabies (*RabAvert*)
Ascorbic acid	Antioxidant	Typhoid oral (*Vivotif*)

Vaccine Excipient & Media Summary

Excipients Included in US Licensed Vaccines[a]		
Excipient	**Use**	**Vaccine**
Bactopeptone	Component of growth medium	Influenza (varies seasonally)
Beta-propiolactone	Viral inactivator	Influenza (*Fluvirin*), Rabies (*Imovax, RabAvert*)
Benzethonium chloride	Preservative	Anthrax (*BioThrax*)
Brilliant green	Dye	Vaccinia (*Dryvax-historic*)
Calcium carbonate	Antacid	Rotavirus (*Rotarix*)
Calcium chloride	Medium nutrient	Rotavirus (*Rotarix*)
Castor oil	Nonionic surfactant	Adenovirus 4 & 7 vaccine
Cellulose acetate phthalate	Binding agent	Adenovirus 4 & 7 vaccine
Cellulose microcrystalline	Binding agent	Adenovirus 4 & 7 vaccine
Chlortetracycline	Antibacterial	Rabies (*RabAvert*), Vaccinia (*Dryvax*)
Cystine	Medium nutrient	Rotavirus (*Rotarix*)
Dextran	Medium nutrient	Rotavirus (*Rotarix*)
Dextrose	Sugar	Adenovirus 4 & 7 vaccine
DNA	Manufacturing residue	Hepatitis A (*Vaqta*), JE (*Ixiaro*)
Dulbecco's Modified Eagle Medium (DMEM)	Growth medium	Rotavirus (*Rotarix*)
Ethylenediamine-tetraacetic acid sodium (EDTA)	Preservative	Rabies (*RabAvert*), Varicella (*Varivax*)
Egg protein	Manufacturing residue	Influenza (all brands), Yellow fever (*YF-Vax*)
FD&C yellow #6 aluminum lake dye	Dye	Adenovirus 4 & 7 vaccine
Ferric (III) nitrate	Medium nutrient	Rotavirus (*Rotarix*)
Formaldehyde, formalin	Antimicrobial, toxin inactivator, stabilizier	Anthrax (*BioThrax*), DTaP (all brands), DTaP-Hep B-IPV (*Pediarix*), DTaP-Hib (*TriHIBit*), DT (all brands), Hepatitis A (*Havrix, Vaqta*), Hepatitis A-Hepatitis B (*Twinrix*), Hib (*ActHIB*), Hib-Hepatitis B (*Comvax*), Influenza (*Fluzone, Fluarix, FluLaval*), JE (*Ixiaro*), Meningococcal (*Menveo*), Poliovirus inactivated (*Ipol*), Td (all brands), Tdap (*Adacel, Boostrix*)
Fructose	Sugar	Adenovirus 4 & 7 vaccine
Gelatin	Stabilizer in freeze-drying, solvent	Influenza (*Fluarix, FluMist, Fluzone*), MMR (*MMR-II*), MMRV (*ProQuad*), Rabies (*RabAvert*), Rubella (*Meruvax II*), Typhoid oral (*Vivotif*), Varicella (*Varivax*), Yellow fever (*YF-Vax*), Zoster (*Zostavax*)
Gentamicin	Antibacterial	Influenza (*Fluarix, FluMist*)
Glucose	Medium nutrient	Rotavirus (*Rotarix*)
Glutamine	Medium nutrient	Rotavirus (*Rotarix*)
Glutaraldehyde	Toxin detoxifier	DTaP (*Infanrix*), DTaP-Hep B-IPV (*Pediarix*), Tdap (*Boostrix*)
Glycerin	Solvent	Vaccinia (*DryVax*)
Glycine	Protein stabilizer	DT (most brands), Td (most brands)

Excipients Included in US Licensed Vaccines[a]		
Excipient	Use	Vaccine
Histidine	Stabilizer	Human papillomavirus (*Gardasil*)
Hydrochloric acid	Adjust pH	DT (most brands), DTaP (most brands)
Hydrocortisone	Component of growth medium	Influenza (*Fluarix*)
Lactose	Stabilizer in freeze-drying, filling	Adenovirus 4 & 7 vaccine, BCG (*Tice*), Hib (some packages), Meningococcal (*Menomune*), Typhoid oral (*Vivotif*)
Magnesium stearate	Lubricant for capsule or tablet filling	Adenovirus 4 & 7 vaccine, Typhoid oral (*Vivotif*)
Magnesium sulfate	Medium nutrient	Rotavirus (*Rotarix*)
Mannose	Sugar	Adenovirus 4 & 7 vaccine
Monophosphoryl lipid A (MPL)	Adjuvant	Human papillomavirus (*Cervarix*)
Monosodium glutamate	Stabilizer	Influenza (*FluMist*), MMRV (*ProQuad*), Varicella (*Varivax*), Zoster (*Zostavax*)
MRC-5 cellular protein	Manufacturing residue	Hepatitis A (*Havrix*, *Vaqta*), Hepatitis A-Hepatitis B (*Twinrix*), MMRV (*ProQuad*), Poliovirus inactivated (*Poliovax*), Rabies (*Imovax*), Varicella (*Varivax*)
Neomycin	Antibacterial	DTaP-Hep B-IPV (*Pediarix*), Hepatitis A-Hepatitis B (*Twinrix*), Influenza (*Fluvirin*), Measles (*Attenuvax*), MMR (*MMR-II*), MMRV (*ProQuad*), Mumps (*Mumpsvax*), Poliovirus inactivated (*Ipol*), Rabies (*Imovax*, *RabAvert*), Rubella (*Meruvax II*), Vaccinia (*DryVax*), Varicella (*Varivax*), Zoster (*Zostavax*)
Phenol	Preservative, antibacterial	Pneumococcal (*Pneumovax-23*), Typhoid inactivated (*Typhim Vi*), Vaccinia (*Dryvax*)
Phenol red (phenolsulfon-phthalein)	pH indicator, dye	Rabies (*Imovax*), Rotavirus (*Rotarix*)
2-Phenoxyethanol	Preservative, stabilizer	DTaP (*Infanrix*, *Daptacel*), DTaP-Hep B-IPV (*Pediarix*), Hepatitis A (*Havrix*), Hepatitis A-Hepatitis B (*Twinrix*), Poliovirus inactivated (*Ipol*), Td (Sanofi Pasteur)
Phosphate buffers (eg, disodium, monosodium, potassium, sodium dihydrogenphosphate)	Adjust pH	DT (most brands), DTaP (most brands), Hepatitis A (*Havrix*), Hepatitis A-Hepatitis B (*Twinrix*), Hepatitis B (*Engerix-B*), Hib (*Act-Hib*), Human papillomavirus (*Cervarix*), Influenza (*Fluarix*, *FluMist*, *FluLaval*), Measles (*Attenuvax*), Meningococcal (*Menactra*, *Menveo*), MMR (*MMR-II*), MMRV (*ProQuad*), Mumps (*Mumpsvax*), Poliovirus inactivated (*Ipol*), Rabies (*BioRab*), Rotavirus (*RotaTeq*), Rubella (*Meruvax II*), Typhoid inactivated (*Typhim Vi*), Varicella (*Varivax*), Zoster (*Zostavax*)
Plasdone C	Film forming	Adenovirus 4 & 7 vaccine
Polacrilin potassium	Resin to mask taste	Adenovirus 4 & 7 vaccine

Vaccine Excipient & Media Summary

Excipients Included in US Licensed Vaccines[a]		
Excipient	**Use**	**Vaccine**
Polydimethylsilozone	Antifoaming agent	Typhoid inactivated (*Typhim Vi*)
Polymyxin B	Antibacterial	DTaP-Hep B-IPV (*Pediarix*), Influenza (*Fluvirin*), Poliovirus inactivated (*Ipol*), Vaccinia (*Dryvax*)
Polyoxyethylene9-10 nonyl phenol (Triton N-101, octoxynol 9)	Nonionic surfactant (viral inactivation)	Influenza (*Fluvirin*)
Polyoxyethylated octyl phenol (also called ethylene glycol octyl phenyl ether, octoxynol-10, octyl-phenoxypolyethoxyethanol, p-isooctyphenyl ether, Triton X-100)	Nonionic surfactant (viral inactivation)	Influenza (*Fluarix, Fluzone*)
Polysorbate 20	Surfactant	Hepatitis A (*Havrix*), Hepatitis A-Hepatitis B (*Twinrix*)
Polysorbate 80	Surfactant	DTaP (*Infanrix, Tripedia*), DTaP-Hep B-IPV (*Pediarix*), DTaP-Hib (*TriHIBit*), Human papillomavirus (*Gardasil*), Influenza (*Fluarix*), Meningococcal (*Menveo*), Rotavirus (*RotaTeq*), Tdap (*Adacel, Boostrix*)
Potassium chloride	Adjust pH, tonicity, medium nutrient	MMRV (*ProQuad*), Rotavirus (*Rotarix*), Zoster (*Zostavax*)
Potassium glutamate	Stabilizer	Rabies (*RabAvert*)
Potassium phosphate	Adjust pH	Adenovirus 4 & 7 vaccine
Protamine sulfate		JE (*Ixiaro*)
Sodium acetate	Adjust pH	DT (some brands), Td (some brands)
Sodium bicarbonate	Adjust pH	Adenovirus 4 & 7 vaccine, MMRV (*ProQuad*)
Sodium borate	Adjust pH	Hepatitis A (*Vaqta*), Hib-Hepatitis B (*Comvax*), Human papillomavirus (*Gardasil*)
Sodium chloride	Adjust tonicity	Most vaccines, including Anthrax, BCG, Human papillomavirus (*Gardasil, Cervarix*), Influenza (*Fluarix*), Measles, Meningococcal (*Menactra*), MMR, MMRV, Mumps, Pneumococcal, Polio inactivated, Rabies, Rotavirus (*Rotarix*), Rubella, Typhoid inactivated, Varicella, Yellow fever, Tdap (*Boostrix*), Zoster (*Zostavax*)
Sodium citrate	Adjust pH	Rotavirus (*RotaTeq*)
Sodium deoxycholate	Anionic surfactant (viral inactivation)	Influenza (*Fluarix, FluLaval*)
Sodium hydrogenocarbonate	Medium nutrient	Rotavirus (*Rotarix*)
Sodium hydroxide	Adjust pH	DT (most brands), Rotavirus (*RotaTeq*), Td (most brands)
Sodium metabisulphite		JE (*Ixiaro*)
Sodium phosphate	Medium nutrient	Rotavirus (*Rotarix*)
Sodium pyruvate	Medium nutrient	Rotavirus (*Rotarix*)

Excipients Included in US Licensed Vaccines[a]		
Excipient	Use	Vaccine
Sorbitol	Stabilizer, solvent	Measles (*Attenuvax*), MMR (*MMR-II*), MMRV (*ProQuad*), Mumps (*Mumpsvax*), Rotavirus (*Rotarix*), Rubella (*Meruvax II*), Yellow fever (*YF-Vax*)
Streptomycin	Antibacterial	Poliovirus inactivated (*Ipol*), Vaccinia (*Dryvax*)
Succinate buffer	Adjust pH	Meningococcal (*Menveo*)
Sucrose	Stabilizer	Adenovirus 4 & 7 vaccine, DTaP-Hib (*TriHIBit*), Hib (*Act-HIB*), Influenza (*FluMist*), Measles (*Attenuvax*), MMR (*MMR-II*), MMRV (*ProQuad*), Mumps (*Mumpsvax*), Rotavirus (*RotaTeq*), Typhoid oral (*Vivotif*), Varicella (*Varivax*), Zoster (*Zostavax*)
Sucrose	Medium nutrient	Rotavirus (*Rotarix*)
Thimerosal	Preservative in some multi-dose containers (see package labeling for precise content)	Influenza (some multidose containers), Meningococcal (*Menomune*). Some single-dose containers contain trace amounts of thimerosal from the production process, but substantially lower concentrations than if used as a preservative. Consult product monographs and labeling for details.
Tocopheryl hydrogen succinate	Component of growth medium	Influenza (*Fluarix*)
Trypsin	Separates cells from culture containers	Rotavirus (*Rotarix*, *RotaTeq*)
Tyrosine	Medium nutrient	Rotavirus (*Rotarix*)
Urea	Stabilizer	Varicella vaccine (*Varivax*, refrigerator stable)
Vitamins unspecified	Component of growth medium	Anthrax (*BioThrax*), Rabies (*Imovax*), Rotavirus (*Rotarix*), Td (Sanofi Pasteur)
Xanthan	Thickening agent	Rotavirus (*Rotarix*)
Yeast protein	Component of growth medium	DTaP-Hep B-IPV (*Pediarix*), Hepatitis A-Hepatitis B (*Twinrix*), Hepatitis B (*Engerix-B*, *Recombivax-HB*), Hib (*HibTiter*), Hib-Hepatitis B (*Comvax*)

a Proprietary names appear in italics.

Vaccine Excipient & Media Summary

Vaccine-Production Media[a]	
Vaccine Culture Media	**Vaccine(s)**
Bovine protein	DTaP-Hep B-IPV (poliovirus component, *Pediarix*), Pneumococcal (*Pneumovax-23*), Typhoid oral (*Vivotif*)
Baculovirus expression-vector system (rod-shaped double-stranded DNA viruses)	Human papillomavirus (*Cervarix*)
Calf skin	Vaccinia (*Dryvax*)
Chick embryo fibroblast tissue culture	Measles (*Attenuvax*), Mumps (*Mumpsvax*), combination vaccines containing them, MMRV (*ProQuad*), Rabies (*RabAvert*)
Chick kidney cells	Influenza (master viruses for *FluMist*)
Chicken embryo (fertilized egg)	Influenza (all brands), Yellow fever (*YF-Vax*)
Cohen-Wheeler, modified (pertussis components)	DTaP (alternate is Stainer-Scholte media)
Dulbecco's modified Eagle's medium (including amino acids, mineral salts, glucose, vitamins, iron, phenol red)	Adenovirus 4 & 7 vaccine
Fenton media containing bovine casein	Tdap (*Boostrix*)
Franz complete medium	Meningococcal (*Menveo*)
Human diploid tissue culture, MRC-5	Hepatitis A (*Havrix, Vaqta*), Hepatitis A-Hepatitis B (*Twinrix*), MMRV (*ProQuad*), Poliovirus inactivated (*Poliovax*), Rabies (*Imovax*), Varicella (*Varivax*), Zoster (*Zostavax*)
Human diploid tissue culture, WI-38	Adenovirus 4&7 vaccine, MMRV (*ProQuad*), Rubella (*Meruvax II*), combination vaccines containing it, Varicella (*Varivax*), Zoster (*Zostavax*)
Lathan medium derived from bovine casein	DTaP (*Infanrix*, tetanus component), DTaP-Hep B-IPV (*Pediarix*), Tdap (*Boostrix*)
Linggoud-Fenton medium containing bovine extract	DTaP (*Infanrix* diphtheria component), DTaP-Hep B-IPV (*Pediarix*), Tdap (*Boostrix*)
Medium 199 (including amino acids, vitamins, sucrose, phosphate, glutamate, human albumin, fetal bovine serum)	Measles (*Attenuvax*), Mumps (*Mumpsvax*), combination vaccines containing them
Minimum essential medium (including amino acids, vitamins, fetal bovine serum, human albumin)	Rubella (*Meruvax II*), combination vaccines containing it
Monkey kidney tissue culture, Vero (Vervet or African green monkeys)	DTaP-Hep B-IPV (poliovirus component, *Pediarix*), JE (*Ixiaro*), Poliovirus inactivated (*Ipol*), Rotavirus (*RotaTeq*)
Mueller-Hinton agar medium (including beef infusion, caesin hydrolysate, starch, agar)	Meningococcal conjugate (*Menactra*)
Mueller-Miller medium	Diphtheria and tetanus vaccines (most brands), meningococcal conjugate (*Menactra*)
Puziss-Wright medium 1095	Anthrax (*BioThrax*)
Rhesus fetal lung tissue culture	Rabies (*BioRab*)
Stainer-Scholte medium	DTaP (*Daptacel, Infanrix*, pertussis component), DTaP-Hep B-IPV (*Pediarix*), Tdap (*Boostrix*)
Soy peptone broth	Pneumococcal (*Prevnar*)
Synthetic/semi-synthetic	Anthrax (*BioThrax*), BCG (*Tice*), DT (all brands), Hib (all brands), Meningococcal (*Menomune*), Pneumococcal (*Pneumovax-23*), Td (all brands), Typhoid inactivated (*Typhim Vi*)

Vaccine-Production Media[a]	
Vaccine Culture Media	Vaccine(s)
Trichoplusia ni insect cells (member of moth family *Noctuidae*) in serum-free culture media composed of chemically-defined lipids, vitamins, amino acids, and mineral salts	Human papillomavirus (*Cervarix*)
Watson-Scherp medium	Meningococcal conjugate (*Menactra*)
Yeast or yeast extract (typically *Saccharomyces cerevisiae*)	Hepatitis A-Hepatitis B (*Twinrix*), Hepatitis B (*Engerix-B, Recombivax-HB*), Hib (*HibTiter, PedvaxHIB*), Hib-Hepatitis B (*Comvax*), Human papillomavirus (*Gardasil*), Medium for growing *Corynebacterium diphtheriae* strain C7 (b197) to obtain CRM_{197} protein for conjugation to polysaccharides (*HibTiter, Prevnar*).

a Proprietary names appear in italics.

References

Burke CJ, Hsu TA, Volkin DB. Formulation, stability, and delivery of live attenuated vaccines for human use. *Crit Rev Ther Drug Carrier Syst*. 1999;16(1):1-83.

Canadian National Advisory Committee on Immunization. Statement on thimerosal. *Can Comm Dis Rep*. 2003;29(ACS-1):1-10.

CDC. Thimerosal in vaccines: a joint statement of the American Academy of Pediatrics and the Public Health Service. *MMWR*. 1999;48:563-565.

Fletcher MA, Hessel L, Plotkin SA. Human diploid cell strains (HDCS) viral vaccines. *Dev Biol Stand*. 1998;93:97-107.

Grabenstein JD. Immunologic necessities: Diluents, adjuvants, and excipients. *Hosp Pharm*. 1996;31:1387-92,1397-1401.

Grabenstein JD. Clinical management of hypersensitivities to vaccine components. *Hosp Pharm*. 1997;32:77-84,87.

Hayflick L. The limited in vitro lifetime of human diploid cell strains. *Exp Cell Res*. 1965;37:614-636.

Jacobs JP, Jones CM, Baille JP. Characteristics of a human diploid cell designated MRC-5. *Nature*. 1970;227(5254):168-170.

Jacobs JP. The status of human diploid cell strain MRC-5 as an approved substrate for the production of viral vaccines. *J Biol Stand*. 1976;4(2):97-99.

Offit PA, Jew RK. Addressing parents's concerns: Do vaccines contain harmful preservatives, adjuvants, additives, or residuals. *Pediatrics*. 2003;112:1394-1401.

Immunologic Drug Interactions

Significance is based on the consequences of infection or toxicity and their epidemiologic probability (within the US, except for drugs frequently associated with international travel).

Validity is based on the strength of evidence of published reports, with consideration of biological plausibility.

Frequency is based on published reports, with consideration of present understanding of biological mechanisms.

Each interaction is discussed in detail within the text of each monograph and in the following references:

Gizurarson S. Clinically relevant vaccine-vaccine interactions: A guide for practitioners. *BioDrugs*. 1998;9:443-453.

Grabenstein JD. Drug interactions involving immunologic agents. I. Vaccine-vaccine, vaccine-immunoglobulin, and vaccine-drug interactions. *DICP*. 1990;24:62-81.

Grabenstein JD. Drug interactions involving immunologic agents. II. Immunodiagnostic & other immunologic drug interactions. *DICP*. 1990;24:186-193. Review.

Hilleman MR. Experiences with combined viral vaccines. *Symp Series Immunobiol Standard*. 1967;7:7-20.

Vaccine-Vaccine Interactions

Individual interactions

Precipitant drug	Object drug	Effect (possible mechanism)	Management	Significance	Validity	Frequency
Cholera vaccine, parenteral	Oral poliovirus type-1 vaccine	Reduced seroconversion rate	Separate vaccine doses by 1 month, if possible.	Moderate	Possible	Some recipients
Cholera vaccine, parenteral*	Yellow fever vaccine*	Reduced seroconversion rate to both vaccines	Separate vaccines by ≥ 3 weeks, if possible, or give on the same day.	Major	Probable	Most recipients
Hepatitis B vaccine	Yellow fever vaccine	Resultant antibody levels reduced; may reduce duration of immunity	Separate vaccine doses by 1 month, if possible.	Major	Possible	Some recipients
Measles vaccine	Meningococcal A & C vaccine	Reduced seroconversion rate	Separate vaccine doses by 1 month, if possible.	Major	Possible	Some recipients
Oral poliovirus vaccine	Oral rotavirus vaccine (RIT 4237 strain)	Reduced seroconversion rate (antigenic or viral competition)	Separate vaccine doses by 1 month, if possible.	Minimal	Probable	Most recipients

Categorical interactions

Precipitant drug	Object drug	Effect (possible mechanism)	Management	Significance	Validity	Frequency
Live vaccines* (exceptions are known)	Live vaccines* (exceptions are known)	Impaired antibody response (antigenic competition)	Give simultaneously or separate doses by 1 month unless specific data are available.	Moderate	Possible	Some recipients

* Reciprocal effects on each interacting agent.

Refer to text for complete description of each interaction.

Immunologic Drug Interactions

Vaccine-Immunoglobulin Interactions

Precipitant drug	Object drug	Effect (possible mechanism)	Management	Significance	Validity	Frequency
Individual interactions						
Diphtheria antitoxin	Diphtheria toxoid	Impaired active immunity (partial antigen [Ag]-antibody [Ab] antagonism)	Wait 3 weeks after antitoxin before giving toxoid.	Moderate	Probable	Most recipients
Immune globulin IM	Hepatitis A vaccine	Anti-hepatitis A antibody titers reduced (partial Ag-Ab antagonism)	Use only vaccine unless prompt protection is needed.	Moderate	Established	Most recipients
Rabies immune globulin & antirabies serum	Rabies vaccines	Active immunity delayed several days (partial Ag-Ab antagonism)	Follow CDC rabies-management guidelines.	Insignificant	Probable	Most recipients
Tetanus immune globulin & antitoxin	Tetanus toxoid	Active immunity delayed several days (partial Ag-Ab antagonism)	Follow CDC wound-management guidelines.	Insignificant	Possible	Most recipients
Vaccinia immune globulin	Vaccinia (smallpox) vaccine	Effective as antidote (antagonism to viral replication)	Use VIG as antidote for adverse vaccine reactions.	Major	Established	Most recipients
Varicella-zoster immune globulin	Varicella vaccine	Effects incompletely described (possible Ag-Ab antagonism or reduced viral replication)	Avoid concurrent use.	Major	Possible	Undetermined
Categorical interactions						
Anti–TNF-alfa inhibiting antibodies	Vaccines, live	Antibody response may be impaired; microbial replication may be potentiated and adverse effects increased.	Avoid concurrent use. Vaccinate 1 or more months before TNF-alfa inhibitor use begins.	Moderate	Possible	Some recipients
Lymphocyte immune globulins	Vaccines & toxoids	Antibody response may be fully or partially impaired (ie, suppressed antibody production, impaired T-cell function, induction of immune tolerance)	Vaccinate prior to inducing immuno-suppression or wait 3 to 12 months after discontinuing immunosuppressant therapy.	Major	Probable	Most recipients

Vaccine-Immunoglobulin Interactions

Categorical interactions (continued)

Precipitant drug	Object drug	Effect (possible mechanism)	Management	Significance	Validity	Frequency
Lymphocyte immune globulins	Live vaccines	Antibody response may be impaired; microbial reproduction may be potentiated, and adverse effects increased. Other possible effects include impaired T-cell function or induction of immune tolerance.	Vaccinate prior to inducing immunosuppression or wait 3 to 12 months after discontinuing immunosuppressant therapy.	Major	Probable	Most recipients
Immune globulin (IG) (IM and IV), hyperimmune globulins, or blood products	Live vaccines	Diminished active immunity (Ag-Ab antagonism from donated antibodies)	Administer vaccine 14 days before or 3 to 11 months after IG depending on IG dose; or repeat vaccine after recommended interval. Recommended intervals: 3 months after HBIG, TIG, RhIG, or IGIM for hepatitis A; 4 months after RIG; 5 months after IGIM 0.25 mL/kg; 6 months after IGIM 0.5 mL/kg; 8 months after IGIV 400 mg/kg; 8 to 11 months after high-dose IGIV; 10 months after RSV-IG.*	Major	Established	Most recipients

* After transfusing blood products, the interval depends on the product (assuming 10 mL/kg throughout): Washed red blood cells (RBCs)—no wait required; RBCs with adenine-saline added—3 months; packed RBCs—5 months; whole blood—6 months; plasma or platelet products—7 months. (AAP. *Pediatrics*. 1994;93:682–685.)

Refer to text for complete description of each interaction.

Vaccine-Drug Interactions

Individual interactions

Precipitant drug	Object drug	Effect (possible mechanism)	Management	Significance	Validity	Frequency
Acyclovir	Varicella vaccine	Impaired active immunity (antagonizes viral replication)	Avoid concurrent use.	Major	Probable	Many recipients
Anti-herpesvirus drugs (eg, acyclovir, valacyclovir)	Zoster vaccine, live	Impaired active immunity (antagonizes viral replication.	Avoid concurrent use.	Major	Probable	Most recipients
Anti-infective drugs (eg, amoxicillin, chloramphenicol, sulfonamides, proguanil)	Typhoid oral vaccine (Ty21a)	Impaired active immunity (antagonizes bacterial reproduction)	Avoid concurrent use.	Major	Probable	Most recipients
Antitubercular drugs (eg, isoniazid)	BCG vaccine	Impaired active immunity (antagonizes bacterial reproduction)	Follow CDC guidelines for BCG indications.	Major	Established	Most recipients
BCG vaccine	Theophylline	Decreased elimination, increased half-life	Observe patient for drug toxicity.	Moderate	Possible	Some recipients
Chloramphenicol	Tetanus toxoid	Impaired anamnestic response (humoral or cellular immune suppression)	Avoid concurrent use.	Moderate	Possible	Many recipients
Chloroquine	Rabies vaccine–HDCV (ID)	Depressed antibody response if vaccine is given ID to patients on long-term chloroquine therapy	Complete vaccination 1 to 2 months before exposure, or draw titer to confirm antibody production.	Major	Probable	Many recipients
Indomethacin	Vaccinia (smallpox) vaccine	Exaggerated cutaneous reaction	Avoid concurrent use.	Minimal	Possible	Isolated case
Influenza vaccine	Aminopyrine	Decreased elimination, increased half-life (P450-pathway inhibition)	Aminopyrine is not used therapeutically.	Insignificant	Established	Most recipients
Influenza vaccine	Carbamazepine	Decreased elimination, increased half-life	Observe patient for drug toxicity.	Major	Possible	Some recipients
Influenza vaccine	Clorazepate	Decreased elimination (P450-pathway inhibition)	Observe patient for drug toxicity.	Moderate	Possible	Isolated case
Influenza vaccine	Phenobarbital	Decreased elimination, increased half-life (P450-pathway inhibition)	Observe patient for drug toxicity.	Moderate	Possible	Some recipients

Vaccine-Drug Interactions

Precipitant drug	Object drug	Effect (possible mechanism)	Management	Significance	Validity	Frequency
Individual interactions (continued)						
Influenza vaccine	Phenytoin	Contradictory data: Increased, decreased serum levels (P450-pathway inhibition)	Observe patient for toxicity or increased seizures.	Moderate	Possible	Some recipients
Influenza vaccine	Theophylline	Decreased elimination, increased half-life (P450-pathway inhibition)	Observe patient for drug toxicity.	Minimal to moderate	Possible	Isolated cases
Influenza vaccine	Warfarin	Prolonged prothrombin time (PT) (decreased procoagulant synthesis)	Observe patient for bleeding or increased PT.	Minimal to moderate	Unlikely	Isolated cases
Interleukin-2	Hepatitis B vaccine	Seroconversion of previous nonresponders	Beneficial effect	Major	Probable	Most recipients
Phenytoin	Typhoid vaccine (parenteral)	Decreased antibody response	Anticipate suboptimal antibody response.	Moderate	Possible	Some recipients
Categorical interactions						
Antimicrobial preservatives (eg, benzyl alcohol, parabens, phenol, thimerosal)	Live vaccines	Inhibition or death of viruses and bacteria	Avoid use. Use appropriate preservative-free diluent.	Major	Established	Most recipients
Corticosteroids, systemic	Varicella vaccine	Increased incidence of rash among children with acute lymphocytic leukemia	Withhold steroids for 1 week before and 2 weeks after vaccination.	Moderate	Probable	Some recipients
Immunosuppressants (eg, alkylating agents, antimetabolites, corticosteroids, cyclosporine, radioisotopes)	All vaccines & toxoids	Antibody response may be fully or partially impaired (ie, suppressed antibody production, impaired T-cell function, induction of immune tolerance)	Vaccinate prior to inducing immunosuppression, or wait 3 to 12 months after discontinuing immunosuppressant therapy.	Major	Established	Most recipients

Vaccine-Drug Interactions

Precipitant drug	Object drug	Effect (possible mechanism)	Management	Significance	Validity	Frequency
		Categorical interactions (continued)				
Immunosuppressants (eg, alkylating agents, antimetabolites, corticosteroids, cyclosporine, radioisotopes)	Live vaccines	Antibody response may be impaired; microbial reproduction may be potentiated, and adverse effects increased. Other possible effects include impaired T-cell function and induction of immune tolerance	Vaccinate prior to inducing immunosuppression, or wait 3 to 12 months after discontinuing immunosuppressant therapy.	Major	Established	Most recipients
Levamisole	Vaccines & toxoids	Increased protective effect	Beneficial effect	Moderate	Possible	Some recipients
Thymosin alfa-1	Vaccines (eg, influenza, hepatitis B)	Increased antibody titers among immunodeficient vaccine recipients	Beneficial effect	Moderate	Probable	Many recipients
Interferons	Live vaccines (eg, vaccinia)	Inhibition of antibody response	Avoid concurrent use (including interferon-inducing drugs).	Major	Possible	Some recipients

Refer to text for complete description of each interaction.

Immunoglobulin-Drug Interactions

Precipitant drug	Object drug	Effect (possible mechanism)	Management	Significance	Validity	Frequency
Individual interactions						
Digoxin immune Fab	Digoxin, digitoxin	Drug inactivation and elimination (immune-complex formation)	Intended effect. Use according to manufacturer's instructions.	Major	Established	Most recipients
IG, Factor VIII & cyclophosphamide	Anti-Factor VIII antibodies	Immune tolerance to Factor VIII	Beneficial effect	Major	Probable	Most recipients
Categorical interactions						
Lymphocyte immune globulins*	Immunosuppressants, other*	Increased risk of infections and neoplasms (decreased cellular and humoral immunity)	Use smallest effective dose of each agent.	Major	Probable	Some recipients

* Reciprocal effects on each interacting agent.

Refer to text for complete description of each interaction.

Diagnostic Drug Interactions

Precipitant drug	Object drug	Effect (possible mechanism)	Management	Significance	Validity	Frequency
Individual interactions						
BCG vaccine	Tuberculin skin tests	Possible false-positive test (corresponding cellular immunity)	Evaluate test carefully. Effect may persist for months to years, although it dissipates over time.	Major	Established	Most recipients
Histamine H₂ antagonists (eg, cimetidine, ranitidine)	Delayed-hypersensitivity reagents (eg, coccidioidin, histoplasmin)	Increased skin-test responsiveness (antagonizes suppression of cellular immunity)	Beneficial effect. Effect dissipates shortly after discontinuing drug.	Moderate	Possible	Some recipients
Levamisole	Delayed-hypersensitivity reagents (eg, coccidioidin, histoplasmin)	Increased skin-test responsiveness (antagonizes suppression of cellular immunity)	Beneficial effect. Effect dissipates shortly after discontinuing drug.	Moderate	Possible	Some recipients
Live-virus vaccines	Tuberculin skin tests	Possible false-negative test (decreased cellular immunity)	Evaluate test carefully. Test before, with, or 6 weeks after vaccination.	Major	Established	Many recipients
Live-virus vaccines	Delayed-hypersensitivity reagents (eg, coccidioidin, histoplasmin)	Possible false-negative test (decreased cellular immunity)	Evaluate test carefully. Effect may persist for weeks after vaccination.	Moderate	Probable	Many recipients
Lymphocyte immune globulins	Delayed-hypersensitivity reagents (eg, coccidioidin, histoplasmin)	Possible false-negative test (decreased cellular immunity)	Evaluate test carefully. Effect may persist for weeks after vaccination.	Moderate	Probable	Many recipients
Viral vaccines (eg, influenza)	Methacholine inhalation	False-positive test possible (increased bronchial sensitivity to methacholine)	Evaluate test knowingly. Effect may persist for days after vaccination.	Moderate	Established	Many recipients

Diagnostic Drug Interactions

Precipitant drug	Object drug	Effect (possible mechanism)	Management	Significance	Validity	Frequency
Categorical interactions						
Antihistamines (H₁ alone or H₁ and H₂ jointly)	Immediate-hypersensitivity reagents (eg, venoms, allergen extracts)	False-negative test possible (histamine-receptor antagonism)	Evaluate test knowingly. Effect may persist for days or weeks after vaccination.	Major	Established	Most recipients
Corticosteroids, systemic	Delayed-hypersensitivity reagents (eg, PPD, coccidioidin)	False-negative test possible after prolonged therapy (decreased cellular immunity).	Evaluate test knowingly. Effect may persist for weeks after cessation.	Major	Established	Many recipients
Corticosteroids, topical	Immediate-hypersensitivity reagents (eg, venoms, allergen extracts)	False-negative test possible after prolonged therapy	Evaluate test knowingly. Effect may persist for weeks after cessation.	Major	Probable	Many recipients
Immunosuppressants (eg, alkylating agents, antimetabolites)	Delayed-hypersensitivity reagents (eg, PPD, coccidioidin)	False-negative test possible (decreased cellular immunity)	Evaluate test knowingly. Effect may persist for weeks after cessation.	Major	Probable	Many recipients
Tricyclic antidepressants (eg, amitriptyline)	Immediate-hypersensitivity reagents (eg, venoms, allergen extracts)	False-negative test possible	Evaluate test knowingly. Effect may persist for days after cessation.	Major	Established	Most recipients.

Other Immunologic Drug Interactions

Effecter drug	Affected drug	Effect (possible mechanism)	Management	Significance	Validity	Frequency
Individual interactions						
Corticosteroids	Sargramostin (GM-CSF)	Potentiated myeloproliferative effects	Use with caution.	Major	Probable	Some recipients
Ethanol	Levamisole	Disulfiram-like adverse reactions	Avoid concurrent use.	Moderate	Probable	Some recipients
Interferon-alfa[*]	Zidovudine[*]	Synergistic toxicity	Consider risk/benefit ration for concurrent use; monitor for toxicity.	Major	Probable	Some recipients
Levamisole with 5-Fluorouracil	Phenytoin	Elevated plasma phenytoin concentrations	Observe for toxicity; counsel to seek assistance if needed.	Moderate	Probable	Some recipients
Levamisole	Warfarin	Prolonged prothrombin time (PT) (decreased procoagulant synthesis)	Observe for bleeding or increased PT; counsel to seek assistance if needed.	Moderate	Possible	Some recipients
Lithium	Sargramostim (GM-CSF)	Potentiated myeloproliferative effects	Use with caution.	Major	Probable	Some recipients
Categorical interactions						
Anticoagulant drugs (eg, warfarin)	Drugs administered intramuscularly	Increased risk of bleeding (diminished capacity to coagulate)	Observe for bleeding or increased PT; counsel to seek assistance if needed.	Moderate	Unlikely	Isolated cases
Immunosuppressants (eg, alkylating agents, antimetabolites)	Interferons	Potentiated myelosuppression	Use with caution	Major	Probable	Some recipients
Interferons	Theophylline, aminophylline	Decreased elimination, increased half-life (P450-pathway inhibition)	Observe for drug toxicity; counsel to seek assistance if needed.	Moderate	Probable	Most recipients

Other Immunologic Drug Interactions

Effecter drug	Affected drug	Effect (possible mechanism)	Management	Significance	Validity	Frequency
Categorical interactions (continued)						
Myelosuppressive agents (eg, cytotoxic chemo-therapy, radiation therapy)	Sargramostim (GM-CSF)	Potentiated myeloproliferative effects	Avoid sargramostim use within 24 hours before or after chemotherapy or 12 hours before or after radia-tion.	Major	Probable	Some recipients

* Reciprocal effects on each interacting agent

Refer to text for complete description of each interaction.

Other Drug Interactions Affecting Immunologic Drugs

Effecter drug	Affected drug	Effect (possible mechanism)	Management	Significance	Validity	Frequency
Beta-adrenergic antagonists (eg, atenolol, propranolol)	Epinephrine	Hypotension, or hypertension with tachycardia; prolonged difficulty in managing blood pressure (blockade of beta-adrenergic receptors or decreased c-AMP)	Supportive therapy. Counsel patients about additional difficulty in treating anaphylaxis.	Major	Established	Most recipients
Monamine oxidase inhibitors (eg, phenelzine, pargyline)	Epinephrine	Enhanced pressor effect, hypertensive crisis (metabolic antagonism)	Supportive therapy. Effect may persist for weeks after MAOI cessation. Counsel patients about additional difficulty in treating anaphylaxis.	Moderate	Established	Many recipients
Tricyclic antidepressants (eg, amitriptyline)	Epinephrine infusions	Enhanced pressor effect, dysrhythmias	Supportive therapy. Counsel patients about additional difficulty in treating anaphylaxis.	Moderate	Probable	Many recipients

Refer to text for complete description of each interaction.

Laboratory Tests Affected by Immunologic Drugs

Effecter drug	Affected drug	Effect (possible mechanism)	Management	Significance	Validity	Frequency
Coccidioidin, mycelial (ie, *BioCox*)	Complement-fixing antibodies to *Emmonsiella capsulata* and *Coccidioides immitis*	Increased titer	Use spherule-derived coccidioidin or draw blood sample before test administration.	Moderate	Established	Many recipients
Dextran-1	Bilirubin assays using alcohol	Turbidity that may invalidate assays	Draw blood samples before dextran administration.	Moderate	Established	Many recipients
Dextran-1	Blood glucose assays using sulfuric acid or acetic acid hydrolysis	Falsely elevated glucose values	Draw blood samples before dextran administration.	Moderate	Established	Many recipients
Dextran-1	Blood typing by proteolytic enzyme techniques	Rouleaux formation	Draw blood samples before dextran administration.	Moderate	Established	Many recipients
Dextran-1	Total protein assays using biuret reagent	Turbidity that may invalidate assays	Draw blood samples before dextran administration.	Moderate	Established	Many recipients
Digoxin Fab fragments	Test of serum digoxin concentration	Misleading readings possible	Evaluate test knowingly	Moderate	Established	Some recipients
Digoxin immune fab	Digitalis immunoassays	Falsely high values possible (bound digoxin assessed as bioavailable)	Evaluate test knowingly. Effect may persist for days.	Major	Established	Most recipients
Haemophilus influenzae type vaccines	Hib antigenuria (by latex agglutination)	False-positive test possible	Evaluate test knowingly. Effect may persist for 1 to 2 weeks.	Moderate	Established	Many recipients
Histoplasmin, mycelial (Various, eg, Parke-Davis)	Complement-fixing antibodies to *Emmonsiella capsulata*	Increased titer	Use yeast-lysate histoplasmin to draw blood sample not more than 48 to 96 hours after test administration.	Moderate	Established	Many recipients

Laboratory Tests Affected by Immunologic Drugs

Effecter drug	Affected drug	Effect (possible mechanism)	Management	Significance	Validity	Frequency
Human IG products	Tests to assess immunity based on serum antibody concentrations (eg, anti-HBs, anti-varicella-zoster)	False-positive readings possible	Evaluate test knowingly	Moderate	Established	Some recipients
IG products containing maltose	Glucose concentrations based on glucose dehydrogenase pyrroloquinolinequinone (GDH-PQQ) method	Falsely elevated readings possible	Evaluate test knowingly	Moderate	Established	Some recipients
Murine antibody products	Tests using murine monoclonal antibodies (eg, some serum pregnancy tests)	Falsely elevated or depressed readings possible	Evaluate test knowingly	Moderate	Established	Some recipients
Omalizumab	Tests of total serum IgE concentration	Elevated readings possible	Evaluate test knowingly	Moderate	Established	Some recipients
Rh$_o$(D)IG	Rh$_o$(D)IG immunoassays	False-positive test in recipients (exogenous supplementation)	Evaluate test knowingly.	Moderate	Established	Most recipients
Rh$_o$(D)IG and other IG products	Antiglobulin (Coombs) test in newborns	Weakly positive test possible	Evaluate test knowingly.	Moderate	Established	Some recipients

Refer to text for complete description of each interaction.

Abbott Laboratories
100 Abbott Park Road
Abbott Park, IL 60064-3500
847-937-6100
http://www.abbott.com

Acambis
See Sanofi Pasteur

Alexion Pharmaceuticals
352 Knotter Drive
Cheshire, CT 06410
203-272-2596
http://www.alxn.com

ALK Abelló
1700 Royston Lane
Round Rock, TX 78664
512-251-0037
http://www.alk-abello.com

Allerderm Laboratories
3400 E. McDowell Road
Phoenix, AZ 85008-7899
800-365-6868
http://www.allerderm.com

Allergan
PO Box 19534
Irvine, CA 92623-9534
714-246-4500
800-433-8871
http://www.allergan.com

Allergy Laboratories
PO Box 348
Oklahoma City, OK 73109
405-235-1451
800-654-3971
http://www.allergylabs.com

AllerMed
7203 Convoy Court
San Diego, CA 92111-1020
858-292-1060
800-221-2748
http://www.allermed.com

AllerQuest
http://www.allerquest.com

American Red Cross (International Headquarters)
2025 E Street, NW
Washington, DC 20006
202-303-5000
800-733-2767
http://www.redcross.org

Amgen
One Amgen Center Drive
Thousand Oaks, CA 91320-1799
805-447-1000
800-772-6436
http://www.amgen.com

Antigen Laboratories
PO Box 123
Liberty, MO 64069
800-821-7013
http://www.antigenlab.com

Antivenin Production Laboratory, Department of Microbiology
Arizona State University
Tempe, AZ 85287
480-965-1457

Armour Pharmaceutical Company
See CSL Behring

Astellas
3 Parkway North
Deerfield, IL 60015
800-695-4321
http://www.us.astellas.com

AstraZeneca
1800 Concord Pike
Wilmington, DE 19803
800-236-9933
http://www.astrazeneca-us.com

Athena Neurosciences
See Elan Pharmaceuticals

Aventis Behring
See CSL Behring

Baxter
One Baxter Parkway
Deerfield, IL 60015
800-422-9837
847-948-2000
http://www.baxter.com

Directory of Manufacturers & Sponsors

Bayer Biological
See Bayer HealthCare

Bayer HealthCare
100 Bayer Road
Pittsburgh, PA 15205-9741
800-468-0894
203-812-2000
http://www.bayerhealthcare.com

Berlex Laboratories
See Bayer HealthCare

Berna Biotech
See Crucell

Berna Products
See Crucell

Biocine
See Novartis Pharmaceuticals

Biogen Idec
14 Cambridge Center
Cambridge, MA 02142
617-679-2000
http://www.biogenidec.com

Biotest Pharmaceuticals Corporation
5800 Park of Commerce Boulevard NW
Boca Raton, FL 33487
561-989-5800
800-327-7106
http://www.biotestpharma.com

Bristol-Myers Squibb
345 Park Avenue
New York, NY 10154
800-332-2056
http://www.bms.com

BTG International
5 Tower Bridge, Suite 800
300 Barr Harbor Drive
West Conshohocken, PA 19428
610-278-1660
http://www.btgplc.com

Burroughs Wellcome
See GlaxoSmithKline

California Department of Health Care Services
PO Box 997413
Sacramento, CA 95899-7413
916-445-4171
http://www.dhcs.ca.gov

Cangene
155 Innovation Drive
Winnipeg, Manitoba Canada R3T 5Y3
204-275-4300
800-768-2304
http://www.cangene.com

Celltech Pharmaceutical
See UCB Pharmaceuticals

Center Laboratories
See ALK Abelló

Centers for Disease Control and Prevention
1600 Clifton Road NE
Atlanta, GA 30333
800-232-4636
http://www.cdc.gov

Centocor Ortho Biotech
800 Ridgeview Road
Horsham, PA 19044
610-651-6000
800-457-6399
http://www.centocor.com

Cetus Oncology Corporation
See Novartis Pharmaceuticals

Chiron Therapeutics
See Novartis Pharmaceuticals

Ciba-Geigy Corporation
See Novartis Pharmaceuticals

Connaught Laboratories
See Sanofi Pasteur

Crucell
PO Box 2048
Leiden, The Netherlands 2301 CA
http://www.crucell.com

CSL Behring
1020 First Avenue
PO Box 61501
King of Prussia, PA 19406-0901
610-878-4000
http://www.cslbehring-us.com/homepage

CSL Limited
45 Poplar Road
Parkville, Victoria, Australia 3052
http://www.csl.com.au

Cutter Biologicals
See Bayer HealthCare

Cytogen Corporation
See EUSA Pharma

Delmont Laboratories
715 Harvard Avenue
PO Box 269
Swarthmore, PA 19081
610-543-3365
800-562-5541
http://www.delmont.com

Dendreon
3005 First Avenue
Seattle, WA 98121
877-256-4545
http://www.dendreon.com

Eisai
100 Tice Boulevard
Woodcliff Lake, NJ 07677
201-692-1100
http://www.eisai.com

Elan Pharmaceuticals
1300 Gould Drive
Gainesville, GA 30504
770-534-8239
http://www.elan.com

Eli Lilly and Company
Lilly Corporate Center
Indianapolis, IN 46285
317-276-2000
800-545-5979
http://www.lilly.com

Elkins-Sinn
See Wyeth

EUSA Pharma
One Summit Square
1717 Langhorne-Newton Road
Suite 201
Langhorne, PA 19047
215-867-4900
800-833-3533
http://www.eusapharma.com

Forest Laboratories
909 Third Avenue
New York, NY 10022
212-421-7850
800-947-5227
http://www.frx.com

Forest Pharmaceuticals
13600 Shoreline Drive
St. Louis, MO 63045
314-493-7000
800-678-1605
http://www.forestpharm.com

Fujisawa Healthcare
See Astellas

Genentech
1 DNA Way
South San Francisco, CA 94080-4990
650-225-1000
800-551-2231
800-821-8590
http://www.gene.com

Genetics Institute
87 Cambridge Park Drive
Cambridge, MA 02140
617-876-1170

Genzyme Corporation
500 Kendall Street
Cambridge, MA 02142
617-252-7500
http://www.genzyme.com

GlaxoSmithKline
5 Moore Drive
PO Box 13398
Research Triangle Park, NC 27709
888-825-5249
http://www.gsk.com

Greer Laboratories
639 Nuway Circle NE
PO Box 800
Lenoir, NC 28645-0800
828-754-5327
800-378-3906
http://www.greerlabs.com

Grifols USA
2410 Lillyvale Avenue
Los Angeles, CA 90032-3514
888-474-3657
http://www.grifolsusa.com

Hemispherx Biopharma
1 Penn Center
1617 John F. Kennedy Boulevard
Suite 660
Philadelphia, PA 19103
215-988-0080
http://www.hemispherx.net

Hoechst-Marion Roussel
See Sanofi-Aventis

Hollister-Stier
3525 N. Regal
Spokane, WA 99207
800-992-1120
509-489-5656
http://www.hollister-stier.com

Hyland Immuno
See Baxter HealthCare

ICI Pharmaceuticals Group
See AstraZeneca

ID Biomedical Corporation
See GlaxoSmithKline

Idec Pharmaceuticals
See Biogen Idec

ImClone Systems Incorporated
180 Varick Street, 6th Floor
New York, NY 10014
212-645-1405
http://www.imclone.com

Immunex Corporation
See Amgen

Immuno US
See Baxter HealthCare

ImmunoGen
830 Winter Street
Waltham, MA 02451-1477
781-895-0600
http://www.immunogen.com

Immunomedics
300 American Road
Morris Plains, NJ 07950
973-605-8200
http://www.immunomedics.com

Interferon Sciences
See Hemispherx Biopharma

InterMune
3280 Bayshore Boulevard
Brisbane, CA 94005
415-466-2200
http://www.intermune.com

Knoll Pharmaceuticals
See Abbott Laboratories

Lederle Laboratories
See Pfizer

Lederle-Praxis Biologicals
See Pfizer

Legere Pharmaceuticals
7326 E. Evans Road
Scottsdale, AZ 85260
480-991-4033
800-528-3144

Liposome Company
See Elan Pharmaceuticals

Mallinckrodt
675 McDonnell Boulevard
Hazelwood, MO 63042
314-654-2000
http://www.mallinckrodt.com

Massachusetts Biological Laboratories
55 Lake Avenue North
Worcester, MA 01655
508-856-2000
http://www.umassmed.edu/massbiolabs

Mead Johnson Nutritionals
2701 Patriot Boulevard, 4th Floor
Glenview, IL 60026
847-832-2420
http://www.mjn.com

Medarex
See Bristol-Myers Squibb

MedImmune
One MedImmune Way
Gaithersburg, MD 20878
301-398-0000
http://www.medimmune.com

Merck & Co
1 Merck Drive
PO Box 100
Whitehouse Station, NJ 08889-0100
908-423-1000
http://www.merck.com

Merck Vaccines
PO Box 4
770 Sumneytown Pike
West Point, PA 19486-0004
800-672-6372
http://www.merckvaccines.com

Meridian Medical Technologies
10240 Old Columbia Road
Columbia, MD 21046
800-638-8093
http://www.meridianmeds.com

Millennium
40 Landsdowne Street
Cambridge, MA 02139
800-390-5663
617-679-7000
http://www.millennium.com

Nabi Biopharmaceuticals
12276 Wilkins Avenue
Rockville, MD 20852
800-685-5579
http://www.nabi.com

Nektar Therapeutics
201 Industrial Road
San Carlos, CA 94070
650-631-3100
http://www.nektar.com

Nelco Laboratories
154 Brook Avenue, PO Box 58
Deer Park, NY 11729
631-242-3662
800-541-0790
http://www.nelcolabs.com

Novartis Pharmaceuticals
One Health Plaza
East Hanover, NJ 07936-1080
800-277-2254
888-669-6682
http://www.pharma.us.novartis.com

Octapharma USA
121 River Street, 12th Floor
Hoboken, NJ 07032
201-604-1130
http://www.octapharma.com

Organon
See Merck

Organon Teknika
See Merck

Ortho Biotech Products
See Centocor Ortho Biotech

Ortho-Clinical Diagnostics
100 Indigo Creek Drive
Rochester, NY 14626
800-828-6316
http://www.orthoclinical.com

**Österreichisches Institut für
    Häemoderivate**
See Baxter HealthCare

Parke-Davis
See Pfizer US Pharmaceutical Group

Pasteur-Mérieux-Connaught
See Sanofi Pasteur

Pfizer US Pharmaceutical Group
235 E. 42nd Street
New York, NY 10017
212-733-2323
http://www.pfizer.com

Pharmacia
See Pfizer US Pharmaceutical Group

Praxis Biologics
See Pfizer

Protein Sciences
1000 Research Parkway
Meriden, CT 06450
203-686-0800
800-488-7099
http://www.proteinsciences.com

Protherics
See BTG International

Purdue Frederick
One Stamford Forum
201 Tresser Boulevard.
Stamford, CT 06901
203-588-8000
800-877-5666
http://www.purduepharma.com

Regeneron
777 Old Saw Mill River Road
Tarrytown, NY 10591
914-345-7400
http://www.regeneron.com

**Research Institute for Microbial Diseases,
    Osaka University**
    (Biken is a transliterated acronym
    for the preceding phrase)
3-1 Yamadaoka, Suita-shi
Osaka, Japan 565-0871
06-6879-8264
http://www.biken.osaka-u.ac.jp

Rhône-Poulenc Rorer Pharmaceuticals
See Sanofi Pasteur

Ribi ImmunoChem Research
See GlaxoSmithKline

Roche Laboratories
340 Kingsland Street
Nutley, NJ 07110
973-235-5000
http://www.rocheusa.com

Sandoz Pharmaceuticals
See Novartis Pharmaceuticals

Sanofi-Aventis Pharmaceuticals
55 Corporate Drive
Bridgewater, NJ 08807
800-981-2491
http://www.sanofi-aventis.us

Sanofi Pasteur
Box 187 Discovery Drive
Swiftwater, PA 18370
570-839-7187
http://www.sanofipasteur.us

Schering-Plough
See Merck

Sclavo
See Novartis Pharmaceuticals

Seragen
See Ligand Pharmaceuticals

Serono Laboratories
One Technology Place
Rockland, MA 02370
800-283-8088
http://www.emdserono.com

Shionogi Pharma
Five Concourse Parkway, Suite 1800
Atlanta, GA 30328
800-461-3696
http://www.Shionogi-inc.com

SmithKline Beecham Pharmaceuticals
See GlaxoSmithKline

Solstice Neurosciences
40 General Warren Boulevard, Suite 160
Malvern, PA 19355
866-220–5042
http://www.solsticeneuro.com

Spectrum Pharmaceuticals
157 Technology Drive
Irvine, CA 92618
949-788-6700
http://www.spectrumpharm.com

Survival Technology
See Meridian Medical Technologies

Swiss Serum & Vaccine Institute Berne
See Crucell

Takeda Chemical Industries, Limited
1-1 Doshomachi 4-Chome
Chuo-Ku, Osaka, Japan 540-8645
81-6-6204-2111
http://www.takeda.com

Takeda Pharmaceuticals North America
One Takeda Parkway
Deerfield, IL 60015
224-554-6500
http://www.tpna.com

Talecris Biotherapeutics
4101 Research Commons
79 T.W. Alexander Drive
Research Triangle Park, NC 27709
919-316-6300
http://www.talecris.com

Three Rivers Pharmaceuticals
119 Commonwealth Drive
Warrendale, PA 15086
800-405-8506
http://www.3riverspharma.com

Triton Biosciences
See Bayer HealthCare

UCB Pharmaceuticals
1950 Lake Park Drive
Smyrna, GA 30080
770-970-7500
www.ucbpharma.com

**United States Army Medical Materiel
    Development Activity**
1430 Veterans Drive
Fort Detrick, MD 21702-5009
301-619-7056
http://www.usammda.army.mil

**United States Army Medical Research
    Institute of Infectious Diseases**
1425 Porter Street
Frederick, MD 21702-5011
http://www.usamriid.army.mil

Univax Biologics
See Nabi

Upjohn Company
See Pfizer US Pharmaceutical Group

Wellcome Foundation Limited
See GlaxoSmithKline

Winthrop Pharmaceuticals
See Sanofi-Aventis Pharmaceuticals

Wyeth
See Pfizer

Xoma
2910 Seventh Street
Berkeley, CA 94710
510-201-7200
http://www.xoma.com

ZLB Behring
See CSL Behring

Advisory Committee on Immunization Practices (ACIP)
Centers for Disease Control and Prevention
1600 Clifton Road, NE
Mailstop E-05
Atlanta, GA 30333
404-639-8836
http://www.cdc.gov/vaccines/recs/acip

American Academy of Allergy, Asthma & Immunology (AAAAI)
555 East Wells Street, Suite 1100
Milwaukee, WI 53202
414-272-6071
http://www.aaaai.org

American Academy of Dermatology (AAD)
PO Box 4014
Schaumburg, IL 60168-4014
866-503-7546
http://www.aad.org

American Academy of Pediatrics (AAP)
141 Northwest Point Boulevard
Elk Grove Village, IL 60007-1098
847-434-4000
http://www.aap.org

American Association of Immunologists
9650 Rockville Pike
Bethesda, MD 20814-3994
301-634-7178
http://www.aai.org

American Cancer Society (ACS)
1599 Clifton Road NE
Atlanta, GA 30329
800-ACS-2345
http://www.cancer.org

American College of Allergy, Asthma & Immunology (ACAAI)
85 West Algonquin Road, Suite 550
Arlington Heights, IL 60005
http://www.acaai.org

American College Health Association (ACHA)
891 Elkridge Landing Road, Suite 100
Linthicum, MD 21090
410-859-1500
http://www.acha.org

American College of Obstetricians and Gynecologists (ACOG)
409 12th Street SW
PO Box 96920
Washington, DC 20090-6920
202-638-5577
http://www.acog.org

American College of Physicians (ACP)
190 N Independence Mall West
Philadelphia, PA 19106-1572
800-523-1546
215-351-2400
http://www.acponline.org

American College of Preventive Medicine (ACPM)
1307 New York Avenue, NW
Suite 200
Washington, DC 20005
202-466-2044
http://www.acpm.org

American Diabetes Association (ADA)
ATTN: National Call Center
1701 North Beauregard Street
Alexandria, VA 22311
800-342-2383
http://www.diabetes.org

American Heart Association (AHA)
National Center
7272 Greenville Avenue
Dallas, TX 75231
800-242-8721
http://www.americanheart.org

American Lung Association (ALA)
1301 Pennsylvania Avenue NW
Suite 800
Washington, DC 20004
800-586-4872
212-315-8700
http://www.lungusa.org

American Medical Association (AMA)
515 North State Street
Chicago, IL 60610
800-621-8335
http://www.ama-assn.org

American Nurses Association (ANA)
8515 Georgia Avenue, Suite 400
Silver Spring, MD 20910-3492
301-628-5000
http://www.nursingworld.org

American Pharmacists Association (APhA)
2215 Constitution Avenue NW
Washington, DC 20037-2985
202-628-4410
800-237-2742
http://www.pharmacist.com

American Public Health Association (APHA)
800 I Street NW
Washington, DC 20001-3710
202-777-2742
http://www.apha.org

American Society of Consultant Pharmacists (ASCP)
1321 Duke Street
Alexandria, VA 22314
703-739-1300
800-355-2727
http://www.ascp.com

American Society of Health-System Pharmacists (ASHP)
7272 Wisconsin Avenue
Bethesda, MD 20814
301-657-3000
866-279-0681
http://www.ashp.org

American Society of Tropical Medicine and Hygiene (ASTMH)
111 Deer Lake Road, Suite 100
Deerfield, IL 60015
847-480-9592
http://www.astmh.org

American Thoracic Society (ATS)
61 Broadway
New York, NY 10006-2755
212-315-8600
http://www.thoracic.org

American Veterinary Medical Association (AVMA)
1931 North Meacham Road, Suite 100
Schaumburg, IL 60173
800-248-2862
http://www.avma.org

Animal and Plant Health Inspection Service (APHIS)
Center for Veterinary Biologics
1920 Dayton Avenue
Ames, IA 50010
515-337-6100
515-232-5785
http://www.aphis.usda.gov

Association of State and Territorial Health Officials
2231 Crystal Drive, Suite 450
Arlington, VA 22202
202-371-9090
http://www.astho.org

(Australian) National Health and Medical Research Council
GPO Box 1421
Canberra, ACT 1421
Australia
+61-2 6217-9100
http://www.nhmrc.gov.au

Biotechnology Industry Organization (BIO)
1201 Maryland Avenue SW, Suite 900
Washington, DC 20024
202-962-9200
http://www.bio.org

Canada's Research-Based Pharmaceutical Companies (Rx&D)
55 Metcalfe Street, Suite 1220
Ottawa, Ontario K1P 6L5
Canada
613-236-0455
http://www.canadapharma.org

Canadian Medical Association
1867 Alta Vista Drive
Ottawa, Ontario K1G 5W8
Canada
888-855-2555
http://www.cma.ca

Canadian Pharmacists Association (CPhA)
1785 Alta Vista Drive
Ottawa, Ontario K1G 3Y6
Canada
800-917-9489
613-523-7877
http://www.pharmacists.ca

Centers for Disease Control and Prevention (CDC)
1600 Clifton Road
Atlanta, GA 30333
888-232-6348
800-232-4636
http://www.cdc.gov

Division of Global Migration and Quarantine
http://www.cdc.gov/ncidod/dq

Division of Tuberculosis Elimination
http://www.cdc.gov/tb

Drug Service
404-639-3670
http://www.cdc.gov/ncidod/srp/drugs/
formulary.html

Emergency Operations Center (EOC)
770-488-7100

Influenza Information
http://www.cdc.gov/flu

Malaria Case Management Hotline
770-488-7788
http://www.cdc.gov/malaria

Morbidity and Mortality Weekly Report
(MMWR)
404-498-1150
http://www.cdc.gov/mmwr

National Center for Injury Prevention and
Control
770-488-1506
http://www.cdc.gov/ncipc

National Immunization Hotline
800-232-2522 (English)
800-232-0233 (Spanish)

Traveler's Health Hotline
877-394-8747
http://www.cdc.gov/travel/

Vaccine Adverse Event Reporting System
(VAERS)
800-822-7967
http://www.vaers.hhs.gov

Every Child by Two
666 11th Street, N.W. Suite 202
Washington, DC 20005-3806
202-783-7034
http://www.ecbt.org

(US) Food and Drug Administration (FDA)
10903 New Hampshire Avenue
Silver Spring, MD 20993
888-INFO-FDA
http://www.fda.gov

Center for Biologics Evaluation and
Research (CBER)
1401 Rockville Pike
Rockville, MD 20852-1448
301-827-1800
800-835-4709
http://www.fda.gov/cber

Center for Drug Evaluation and Research
(CDER)
301-796-3400
888-463-6332
http://www.fda.gov/cder

Center for Veterinary Medicine
240-276-9300
http://www.fda.gov/cvm

MedWatch Program
800-FDA-1088
http://www.fda.gov/medwatch/

Office of Orphan Products Development
800-300-7469
http://www.fda.gov/orphan

Office of Public Affairs
301-796-4540

Office of Regulatory Affairs
800-300-7469
http://www.fda.gov/ora

Vaccine Adverse Event Reporting System
(VAERS)
800-822-7967
http://www.vaers.hhs.gov

Health Canada
A. L. 0900C2
Ottawa, Ontario K1A 0K9
Canada
613-946-8081
http://www.hc-sc.gc.ca

Canada Communicable Disease Report
(CCDR)
http://www.phac-aspc.gc.ca/publicat/
ccdr-rmtc

Health Products and Food Branch
http://www.hc-sc.gc.ca/ahc-asc/
branch-dirgen/hpfb-dgpsa

Sources of Additional Information

Travel Health
http://www.phac-aspc.gc.ca/tmp-pmv

National Advisory Committee on
Immunization (NACI)
http://www.phac-aspc.gc.ca/naci-ccni

Health Departments, State and Local
Consult your telephone book.

Immune Deficiency Foundation (IDF)
40 W Chesapeake Avenue, Suite 308
Towson, MD 21204
800-296-4433
http://www.primaryimmune.org

Immunization Action Coalition
1573 Selby Avenue, Suite 234
St. Paul, MN 55104
651-647-9009
http://www.immunize.org

Vaccine Information
http://www.vaccineinformation.org

**Infectious Diseases Society of America
(IDSA)**
1300 Wilson Boulevard, Suite 300
Arlington, VA 22209
703-299-0200
http://www.idsociety.org

**Institute for Safe Medication Practices
(ISMP)**
200 Lakeside Drive, Suite 200
Horsham, PA 19044
215-947-7797
http://www.ismp.org

Manufacturers of immunologic drugs
See Directory of Manufacturers and
Sponsors

MedicAlert Foundation International
2323 Colorado Avenue
Turlock, CA 95382
888-633-4298
http://www.medicalert.org

Mexican Secretariat of Health
(Secretaría de Salud de Mexico)
Lieja 7
Col. Juárez
06696-México D.F.
http://www.salud.gob.mx

Military Vaccine Agency (MILVAX)
5111 Leesburg Pike
Falls Church, VA 22041
877-GET-VACC
http://www.vaccines.mil

**National Coordinating Council for Medica-
tion Error Reporting and Prevention
(MERP)**
800-223-7767
800-23-ERROR
http://www.nccmerp.org

**National Council on Patient Information
and Education (NCPIE)**
4915 Saint Elmo Avenue, Suite 505
Bethesda, MD 20814-6082
301-656-8565
http://www.talkaboutrx.org

**National Foundation for Infectious
Diseases (NFID)**
4733 Bethesda Avenue, Suite 750
Bethesda, MD 20814
301-656-0003
http://www.nfid.org

National Immunization Hotline
800-232-2522 (English)
800-232-0233 (Spanish)

**National Institute of Allergy and
Infectious Diseases (NIAID)**
6610 Rockledge Drive
MSC 6612
Bethesda, MD 20892-6612
866-284-4107
301-496-5717
http://www.niaid.nih.gov

National Institutes of Health (NIH)
9000 Rockville Pike
Bethesda, MD 20892
301-496-4000
http://www.nih.gov

**National Organization for Rare Disorders
(NORD)**
55 Kenosia Avenue
PO Box 1968
Danbury, CT 06813-1968
800-999-6673
203-744-0100
http://rarediseases.org

National Vaccine Injury Compensation Program (VICP)
Parklawn Building
Room 16C-26
5600 Fishers Lane
Rockville, MD 20857
800-338-2382
http://www.hrsa.gov/vaccinecompensation

Office of Disease Prevention and Health Promotion (ODPHP)
U.S. Department of Health and Human Services
Office of Disease Prevention and Health Promotion
Office of Public Health and Science, Office of the Secretary
1101 Wootton Parkway, Suite LL100
Rockville, MD 20852
240-453-8280
http://www.odphp.osophs.dhhs.gov

Pan American Health Organization
(PAHO, a regional office of the World Health Organization)
525 23rd Street NW
Washington, DC 20037
202-974-3000
http://www.paho.org

Pharmaceutical Research and Manufacturers of America (PhRMA)
950 F Street, NW
Washington, DC 20004
202-835-3400
http://www.phrma.org

State and Selected Local Health Departments
Consult your telephone book.

United States Pharmacopeia (USP)
12601 Twinbrook Parkway
Rockville, MD 20852
800-227-8772
http://www.usp.org

US Department of Health & Human Services (HHS)
200 Independence Avenue SW
Washington, DC 20201
202-619-0257
877-696-6775
http://www.hhs.gov

National Vaccine Advisory Committee (NVAC)
http://www.hhs.gov/nvpo/nvac

National Vaccine Program Office
http://www.hhs.gov/nvpo

US Government Printing Office (GPO)
732 North Capital Street NW
Washington, DC 20401
202-512-0000
866-512-1800
http://www.gpo.gov

Vaccine Adverse Event Reporting System (VAERS)
PO Box 1100
Rockville, MD 20849-1100
800-822-7967
http://www.vaers.hhs.gov

World Health Organization (WHO)
Headquarters
Avenue Appia 20
1211 Geneva 27
Switzerland
+41 22-791-21-11
http://www.who.int/immunization/en

This glossary includes succinct versions of standardized, consensus definitions developed by the Brighton Collaboration of clinicians and scientists to facilitate the development, evaluation, and dissemination of high-quality information about the safety of human vaccines. Such entries include the phrase "See Brighton Collaboration definition." The full versions of these definitions are available at http://www.brightoncollaboration.org.

abscess: Localized soft-tissue collection of fluid. (See Brighton Collaboration definition.)

acellular vaccine: Vaccine containing purified components of bacteria, but not whole cells nor the full cellular components.

acquired immunity: Immunity resulting from development of active or passive immunity. Opposite of natural or innate immunity.

active immunity: Immunity produced in response to the administration of a vaccine or toxoid, or, generally, in response to natural infection. Active immunity may take several weeks or months to induce, but is generally long-lasting.

active immunization: Administration of a vaccine or toxoid. Such immunity may not be fully developed for several weeks to months after vaccination, but remains protective usually for a number of years.

acute disseminated encephalomyelitis (ADEM): Focal or multifocal findings referable to the CNS. (See Brighton Collaboration definition.)

adaptive immunity: The ability to mount a specific immune response against a microbe or antigen. Contrast with innate immunity.

adjunct: An auxiliary treatment, secondary to the main treatment.

adjuvant: A substance that aids another substance in its action (eg, aluminum phosphate in vaccine formulations).

Adrenalin: Parke-Davis's proprietary name for epinephrine.

adverse event: An undesirable health event that may be causally or coincidentally related to use of a medication. For example, an adverse event may occur after vaccination but not be caused by the vaccination.

adverse reaction: An undesirable health event that is presumed to be caused by use of a medication. Also called a side effect or complication.

affinity: The intrinsic binding power of an antibody-combining site with an antigenic substrate binding site.

agglutination: Clumping together of bacteria when exposed to antibodies, as when bacterial cells are added to serum.

agglutinin: An antibody that causes agglutination.

agglutinogen: A substance that stimulates development of a specific agglutinin, thereby acting as an antigen.

agonist: A drug capable of combining with receptors to evoke a pharmacologic effect, possessing affinity and intrinsic activity.

alastrim: Variola minor.

alexin: Complement.

aliquot: A portion of a liquid or solid substance.

allergen: Any substance that indicates a state of, or brings on manifestations of, allergy. It may or may not be a protein or an antigen.

allergy: An altered reaction of body tissues to a specific substance (an allergen), which in nonsensitive persons produces no reaction. It is generally an antibody-antigen reaction, but antibody cannot be demonstrated in all cases. The reaction may be due to the release of histamine or similar mediators from affected cells.

allodynia: Pain resulting from a nonpainful stimulus to normal skin.

allogeneic: Obtained from another individual, thus having immunologically distinct cell types.

allograft: A graft of tissue or an organ from a member of the same species.

alloimmunization: The result of a blood transfusion that immunizes the recipient against donor antigens the recipient lacks.

Glossary

allotype: The protein portion of an allele that may be discerned as an antigen by another member of the same species.

Ames test: A mutant strain of *Salmonella typhimurium* that lacks the ability to synthesize histidine is inoculated into a growth medium deficient in histidine but containing a test compound. If the compound causes DNA damage resulting in mutation, some of the bacteria may regain the ability to synthesize histidine and will proliferate to form colonies. The ability to cause mutations indicate that the substance may be carcinogenic. The test is limited by the potential for false-negative results: Mutations that do not affect histidine synthesis.

anamnestic response: Literally, a memory response. A vigorous antibody response to an antigen to which the body has previously been exposed.

anaphylaxis: A clinical syndrome that may include urticaria with swelling of the mouth, difficulty breathing, hypotension, shock or other symptoms. Largely synonymous with anaphylactic reaction. Hypersensitivity reaction characterized by sudden onset, rapid progression of signs and symptoms, involvement of two or more organ systems (eg, dermatologic, cardiovascular, respiratory). (See Brighton Collaboration definition.)

anatoxine: Ramon's term for toxoid (French).

anergy: Lack of responsiveness to delayed-hypersensitivity antigens.

angioedema: Local allergic wheals accompanied by swelling of subcutaneous or submucosal tissue. Synonymous with angioneurotic edema, giant urticaria, hives, Quincke disease, urticaria.

angioneurotic edema: Angioedema.

antibodies: Proteins synthesized by plasma cells, often in response to an immunogen that has gained access to the body. These proteins react specifically with an antigen in a demonstrable way. Most antibodies consist of 2 light chains and 2 heavy chains, although some are found as dimers, trimers, or pentamers. Major antibody isotypes include IgA, IgD, IgE, IgG and IgM. Functional examples of IgG antibodies include antitoxins, bacteriolysins (antibodies that lyse bacteria), opsonins (antibodies that make invasive bacteria subject to phagocytosis or engulfment and destruction by white blood cells), agglutinins (antibodies that combine with specific antigens and cause them to agglutinate or clump).

antigen: A substance that can elicit and/or combine with an antibody.

antiglobulin: A precipitin that precipitates globulin (ie, an antibody that agglutinates other antibodies). Also called the Coombs test. A direct antiglobulin test detects antibodies bound to circulating red blood cells in vivo (eg, in hemolytic disease of the newborn). The indirect antiglobulin test detects serum antibodies that bind to red cells in vitro.

anti-idiotypic antibodies: Antibodies that may function as antigens since their variable regions resemble the antigenic determinants of a given antigen and are also the configurational complement to an idiotypic antibody that would bind both the antigen and the anti-idiotypic antibody.

antioxidant: An agent that prevents oxidation, usually intended to serve as a preservative. Example: Metabisulfite.

antitoxin: Any antibody that binds and inactivates a toxin.

arthralgia: Pain in one or more joints.

Arthus response: A severe local inflammatory reaction that occurs at the site of repeated injection of an antigenic substance. Arthus reactions occur hours after antigen challenge, persist for several days, involve primary neutrophils, and require complement-fixing antibodies. Arthus is pronounced ahr-TOOS.

aseptic meningitis: Inflammation of the meninges in which common microbes cannot be identified in cerebrospinal fluid. (See Brighton Collaboration definition.)

asthenia: Weakness or tiring of eyes due to muscle fatigue.

asthma: An inflammatory disorder of respiration, characterized by airway narrowing, bronchospasm, wheezing and difficulty in expiration.

ataxis: Failure of muscle coordination; irregularity of muscle action.

atopic: Pertaining to a person with atopy.

atopic dermatitis: Itchy, red, scaly rash that lasts more than 2 weeks. It may occur in the folds of the arms or legs. It often comes and goes.

atopy: The tendency to manifest allergic diseases such as asthma, eczema, hay fever, urticaria or food allergy, associated with specific IgE directed toward an allergen.

attack rate: The proportion of people within a defined population who develop a particular disease within a specified period of time.

attenuated vaccine: A vaccine containing live, weakened bacteria or viruses that induce active immunity. These vaccines can be dangerous in an immunocompromised patient who cannot mount an effective defense against even weakened microorganisms.

autoantibody: An antibody directed against one of the host's own antigens.

autoimmune disease: A response against self-antigen(s) involving T cells, B cells, or autoantibodies that causes injury systemically or at a specific organ. Autoimmune disease is an unusual consequence of autoimmunity.

autoimmunity: Autoantibodies or self-reactive T cells or B cells that bind to self-antigens. A certain level of autoimmunity is a natural process, but autoimmunity also can be triggered by infection or other processes.

autologous vaccine: Bacterial vaccine produced from microorganisms isolated from the individual to be vaccinated.

avidity: The combining power of an antibody with the corresponding antigen; related to the affinity and valenne of the antibody and its antigen.

B-cell: See B-lymphocyte.

bacterin: The veterinary term for a killed bacterial vaccine. Live bacterial and live and killed viral veterinary immunogens are referred to as vaccines.

bacteriolysin: A type of antibody that lyses bacteria.

bacteriophage: A virus that causes transmissible lysis of bacteria.

basic series: A set of several vaccine or toxoid doses needed to initially establish protective immunity.

Bell palsy: Unilateral facial weakness.

bevel: The inclined opening at the tip of needle.

bifurcated: Two-pronged, as in the needle used to administer smallpox vaccine by scarification.

biologicals: Category of complex drug products derived from biological sources (eg, from plant, animal, microbial sources); members of the category. In US law and regulation, refers to viruses, therapeutic sera, toxins, antitoxins, vaccines, blood, blood components or derivatives, allergenic products or analogous products. Sometimes misapplied as a category name for immunologic drugs. Synonymous with biologics.

biological weapon: Biological agents (eg, viruses, bacteria, toxins, molds) intended to kill or injure military personnel or civilians.

biologics: See biologicals.

biotechnology: A technique that uses living organisms or a part of a living organism to produce or modify a product, to improve a plant or animal, or to develop a microorganism to be used for a specific purpose.

birth cohort: The number of children born in one particular year.

bleb: Elevation of the epidermis.

blepharospasm: Intermittent or sustained closure of the eyes due to involuntary contractions of the orbicularis oculi muscle.

B-lymphocyte: A type of immune cell that serves as the precursor of plasma cells that produce specific antibody; primarily responsible for cellular immunity.

booster response: The substantially increased response to vaccination, greater than the response to an earlier immunization. Synonymous with anamnestic response. Typically limited to protein-based vaccines, rather than polysaccharide vaccines.

Brill disease: Rat flea-borne typhus.

bubonic: Characterized by inflamed swollen or enlarged lymph nodes, often with suppuration. Such nodes are called buboes. Example: Bubonic plague.

bulbar: Pertaining to the medulla oblongata.

bullous: Characterized by blisters.

caprine: Pertaining to goats.

caprylate: A saturated medium-chain fatty acid of plant origin, subjected to rapid beta-oxidation. Used pharmaceutically to refer to caprylic acid solutions. Caprylic acid is also known as octanoic acid.

capsid: Protein outer coat around the nucleic-acid core of a virus.

carrier: A person who harbors a specific pathogenic organism without discernible symptoms or signs of disease and who is capable of spreading the organism to others. Also, an immunogenic molecule that is recognized by T-cells in an antibody response.

case-fatality rate: The proportion of people with a particular condition (the cases) that die from that condition within a specific period of time. The denominator is the number of incident cases; the numerator is the number of cause-specific deaths among those cases.

catabolize: The destructive phase of metabolism, in which complex substances are broken down into simpler components. The opposite of anabolism.

catarrhal: Associated with catarrh, inflammation of mucous membranes.

CD: Abbreviation for "cluster of differentiation," referring to molecules on cell surfaces that distinguish different kinds of immune cells.

cell-mediated immunity: See cellular immunity.

cellular immunity: Immunity mediated primarily by T-lymphocytes and secondarily by B-lymphocytes, as opposed to immunity mediated by antibodies. Cellular immunity is generally considered to be responsible for immune memory responses. Also called cell-mediated immunity.

cellulitis: Acute, infectious, expanding inflammatory condition of the skin that may include localized pain, tenderness, erythema, induration, swelling, or warmth. Cellulitis may be accompanied by fever and/or regional lymphadenopathy. (See Brighton Collaboration definition.)

cetylpyridinium: A quaternary cationic surfactant.

challenge: In vaccine testing, the deliberate exposure of animals or people to an infectious agent.

chemical vaccine: Literally, a purely synthesized or synthetic vaccine. Broadly, any purified, nonviable, non-whole cell, subunit vaccine.

chimeric: Involving components of two different species.

chromosomes: Discrete units of the genome that carry many genes, found in the nucleus of all cells.

clone: A genetically identical series of molecules, cells or organisms asexually descended from a common ancestor.

coalescence: Gathering together; fusion.

cohort: Any group of like items.

collyrium: A solution used as a cleanser for the eyes.

colonization: Habitation of microorganisms within a part of the body without necessarily causing pathology. Largely synonymous with infection.

colony-stimulating factors: Growth factors that support survival, clonal expansion, and differentiation of hematopoietic progenitor cells.

colostrum: Secretion from the breast before the onset of true lactation 2 to 3 days after delivery. Contains mainly serum and white blood cells, rich in IgA, although it may also contain IgM and IgG.

combination vaccine: A medication that immunizes against more than one disease (or more than one serotype of the disease) at a time.

communicability: Capacity to be transmitted to other persons.

communicable: Capable of spreading infection, spreading disease.

complement: Complex group of serum proteins involved in inflammation, activation of phagocytes, and bacteriolysis and hemolysis.

condylomata acuminata: Venereal or genital warts. Associated with infections of human papillomavirus (HPV), especially HPV type 6 and possibly type 11.

confidence interval: A range in which a measurement or value (ie, point estimate) falls with some probability.

congenital rubella syndrome: A syndrome in a developing fetus of a woman who contracted rubella infection during pregnancy, often characterized by impairments of ears, eyes, heart, brain, and nervous system. The fetus may be miscarried, stillborn, or born with profound birth defects or mental retardation.

conidia: Asexual spores of fungi.

conjugate: A reagent formed by covalently coupling two molecules together.

conjugate vaccine: A vaccine containing a saccharide linked by a covalent bond to a protein "carrier."

contact: A person who has been in such association with an infected person or animal or a contaminated environment as to have had opportunity to acquire the infection.

contagious: Capable of being transmitted from one person to another by contact or close proximity.

contraindication: A circumstance that renders the use of a medication inadvisable, usually because of elevated risk of harm.

convalescent serum: Human serum with a high titer of antibodies against a particular microorganism, harvested from patients recuperating from a disease; an early form of therapy for specific infections. Related term: Convalescent plasma.

Coombs & Gell system: A categorization system used to describe various immunopathologic reactions. The system is helpful but somewhat simplistic in that many immunologic diseases involve a combination of these reaction types. See definition of types I through IV.

Coombs' test: See antiglobulin.

correlate of protection: An immune marker statistically correlated with vaccine efficacy (equivalently predictive of vaccine efficacy) that may or may not be a mechanistic causal agent of protection. Synonymous with predictor of protection. This marker can be used to accurately predict the level of vaccine efficacy conferred to vaccine recipients (individuals or subgroups defined by the immune marker level). A correlate of protection is either a mechanistic or a nonmechanistic correlate of protection.

cresol: An alkyl-phenolic surface-active antimicrobial disinfectant.

crying, persistent: Crying that is continuous and unaltered for 3 or more hours. (See Brighton Collaboration definition.)

cytokines: Soluble intercellular mediators of immunity that mediate interactions between cells (eg, interferons, interleukins, hematopoietic growth factors). Some cytokines activate macrophages to destroy intracellular pathogens; others activate inflammatory or repair processes or regulate normal cell growth and differentiation.

cytoplasm: The living matter within a cell, excluding the nucleus, that is responsible for cell function (eg, protein synthesis).

cytotoxic reaction: A type II immunopathologic reaction involving IgG, IgM and complement. It is characterized by lysis or phagocytosis of circulating antigens and acute inflammation of tissues. Examples include autoimmune hemolytic anemia and Goodpasture syndrome.

cytotoxic T-lymphocytes (CTL): Immune cell that can destroy cancerous cells and cells infected with viruses, fungi, or certain bacteria. Also known as killer T-cells, because they kill infected cells, CTLs carry the CD8 marker on their surfaces.

Dalton: A unit of measure for molecular weight, formerly called the atomic mass unit (AMU). Named for John Dalton, the English chemist who proposed the atomic theory and established the existence of atoms.

dehiscence: Bursting open.

delayed hypersensitivity: A type IV immunopathologic reaction involving T lymphocytes, lymphokines and monokines. It is characterized by a delayed (after 24 to 72 hours) mononuclear cell infiltrate. Examples include tuberculosis, sarcoidosis and polymyositis.

demyelinating disorder: A condition that results in damage to the protective myelin sheath that covers nerves in the brain and spinal cord. In this disorder, nerve impulses slow or stop, causing neurologic problems. Specific examples include multiple sclerosis, transverse myelitis, optic neuritis, and acute disseminated encephalomyelitis.

denature: To change the physical properties of a substance, such as by heat or chemicals that alter tertiary structure.

dermatographism: A form of urticaria in which induration develops in response to pressure.

dermatome: The area of skin supplied by the sensory nerve of a single dorsal root ganglion.

diafiltration: A method of dialysis by filtration, removing salts and low molecular weight components using water.

Dick method: Injection of a combined toxin-antitoxin to prevent scarlet fever.

Dick test: A skin test to ascertain sensitivity to scarlet fever, using a toxin of *Streptococcus hemolyticus*.

dimorphic: Characteristic of certain fungi, capable of growth as a yeast or as a mold under different environmental conditions.

disease: Any abnormal condition that interferes with normal physiological processes.

distal: Farther from center, from a medial line, or from the trunk. Opposite of proximal.

DNA (deoxyribonucleic acid): Double-stranded helical molecule found in nucleus of each cell. Carries genetic information that encodes proteins and enables cells to reproduce and perform their functions.

DNA vaccine: A vaccine containing fragments of DNA encoding genes for key microbial antigens (proteins). The host, in turn, expresses the genes, producing the protein, yielding a significant immunologic response.

Dohle bodies: Light blue cytoplasmic inclusions in leukocytes.

dorsal: Pertaining to the back, or a position toward a rear part. Opposite of ventral.

doseforms: The form in which a drug product is provided (eg, tablets, capsules, lyophilized powders for reconstitution, adsorbed suspensions, fluid solutions).

eczema vaccinatum: Presence of lesions 4 to 28 days after exposure to vaccinia virus that are papules, vesicles or pustules and are concentrated in localized areas (severe cases may involve the entire body). (See Brighton Collaboration definition.)

effective: Capable of preventing, treating, diagnosing, or curing a disease or health problem. See efficacy.

effectiveness: A reasonable expectation that, in a significant proportion of the target population, the pharmacological or other effect of a medication, when used under adequate direction, for use and warnings against unsafe use, will serve a clinically significant function in the diagnosis, cure, mitigation, treatment, or prevention of disease in man (see also 21 CFR 601.25 (d) (2)).

efficacy: The construct used by FDA to indicate that a given drug can produce a desired beneficial effect in preventing, treating, diagnosing, or otherwise managing a disease or other medical condition.

Emergency Use Authorization: Category of medications issued by FDA for use during a declared emergency involving a heightened risk of attack on the public or US military forces.

emulsion: A 2-phase system prepared by combining 2 immiscible liquids, 1 of which is uniformly dispersed throughout the other.

encephalitis: A syndrome characterized by confusion, irritability, severe or continuing headache, stiff neck, and vomiting. Acute inflammation of central nervous system parenchyma, with or without involvement of the meninges. Can also involve encephalopathy lasting more than 24 hours and other neurologic manifestations. (See Brighton Collaboration definition.)

encephalomyelitis: Inflammation of the brain and spinal cord.

endemic: Characteristic of a disease that recurs among people in a locality or a population.

endemic disease: The continuous prevalence of a disease or infectious agent within a given geographic area or population group; may also refer to the usual prevalence of a given disease within such area or group.

endotoxin: A lipopolysaccharide contained in the cell wall of Gram-negative bacteria that is released when these bacteria rupture, associated with septic shock and tissue damage.

enzootic: Characteristic of a disease that recurs among animals in a locality or a population. Corresponds to endemic in humans.

epidemic: An infectious disease or condition that attacks many people at the same time in the same geographical location.

epidemiology: The study of the distribution of disease or a condition in a population of people.

epitope: An antigenic determinant, the site on an antigen to which an antibody binds.

epizootic: An infectious disease or condition that attacks many animals at the same time in the same geographical location. Corresponds to epidemic in humans.

equine: Pertaining to horses.

erythema: An area of diffused redness of the skin, caused by capillary congestion. Frequently referred to as the flare of an allergic skin response.

erythema nodosum: Red and painful nodules on legs.

erythrocytes: Mature red blood cells.

erythroid: Pertaining to red blood cells, erythrocytes.

etiology: Origin or cause.

excipients: Inactive ingredients of a drug product necessary for production.

Expanded Programme of Immunization: A WHO program to immunize children against prevalent diseases.

exposure: Contact with infectious or other agents in a way that can lead to a disease or health problem.

expression: In genetic engineering, the result of inserting a gene into a cell, so that the cell manufactures a desired protein.

ex vivo: Outside the body (Latin).

Fab: The portion of an antibody that contains the antigen-combining site.

facultative: Capable of living under more than one set of environmental conditions.

false-negative result: A negative result to a diagnostic test when the patient truly has the disease or outcome in question.

false-positive result: A positive result to a diagnostic test when the patient is truly devoid of the disease or outcome in question.

fatigue: A new symptom of fatigue that is the primary complaint and is not relieved by rest and interferes with the patient's function. (See Brighton Collaboration definition.)

Fc: The portion of an antibody that is responsible for binding to antibody receptors on cells and the C1q component of the complement system.

fever: An elevation of body temperature 38°C or more. (See Brighton Collaboration definition.)

Fisher syndrome: Clinical syndrome of ataxia, ophthalmoplegia, and areflexia (without limb weakness), described by Fisher in 1956, considered a form of Guillain-Barré syndrome. Considered a benign, self-limited illness, with favorable prognosis for resolution of symptoms and signs within 6 months. Like, frequently associated with a preceding antigenic stimulus such as infectious illness (most commonly *Campylobacter jejuni*). (See Brighton Collaboration definition.)

flare: Erythema; an area of redness.

flexor: A muscle that bends a part in a generally proximal direction. Opposite of extensor.

formaldehyde: An alkylating antimicrobial agent.

formalin: Solution of 37% formaldehyde in water.

formulation: The mixture of ingredients that constitutes a medication. For a vaccine, this may include an antigen, a diluent, excipients, and perhaps an adjuvant or preservative.

freeze: For the storage of drugs, generally defined as −5°C (23°F) or colder.

Freund complete adjuvant: Freund incomplete adjuvant plus heat-killed whole mycobacteria. Causes high fevers and severe abscesses at injection sites. Used to enhance antibody formation to an antigen.

Freund incomplete adjuvant: Mixture of mineral oil and an aqueous emulsifying agent. Used to enhance antibody formation to an antigen.

Frei test: Test used to confirm diagnosis of lymphogranuloma inguinale; an intradermal injection of an extract of lymph nodes of lymphogranulomatous patients.

gamma globulin: An obsolete term for immunoglobulins, especially IgG. The term refers to the presence of immunoglobulins in the gamma region of serum separated by electrophoresis. Gamma globulin is a misnomer since some antibodies are found in the beta region and hence are beta globulins. IgG and IgA primarily exist as gamma globulins, although some are beta globulins. To further confound the issue, although most IgM and IgD molecules are beta globulins, some are gamma globulins. Nonetheless, common usage usually equates gamma globulin with IgG and often with IGIM.

GAVI Alliance (GAVI): Formerly the Global Alliance for Vaccines and Immunization. An alliance of stakeholders in both the private and public sectors, to save children's lives and protecting people's health through the worldwide expansion of mass vaccination programs.

Gell & Coombs system: See Coombs & Gell system.

gene: A unit of genetic material (DNA), a segment of DNA encoding a protein, a segment of DNA that contains information for a specific function.

gene therapy: Therapy at the intracellular level to replace or inactivate the effects of disease-causing genes or to augment normal gene functions to overcome illness.

generalized vaccinia: Vesicles and/or pustules at 4 or more distinct areas of the body at sites removed from the initial smallpox vaccination site, between 4 and 21 days after exposure. (See Brighton Collaboration definition.)

genetic engineering: Manipulation of genetic material to produce proteins.

genome: The complete set of genes present in a cell or virus.

geometric mean titer: A measure of central tendency for antibody response. To calculate a geometric mean titer, the common logarithm (base 10) of each antibody titer is determined, the mean of these log values is calculated, and then the antilogarithm of the mean is determined.

glucose: Dextrose.

glycerin: $C_3H_8O_3$, a trihydric alcohol, trihydroxypropane. A syrupy colorless liquid, soluble in all proportions in water and alcohol. Used as a solvent, preservative and an emollient.

glycerine: Glycerin.

glycerol: Glycerin.

glycine: The simplest of amino acids, alpha-aminoacetic acid. A stabilizer that protects proteins from aggregation and decomposition.

glycoprotein: A protein with sugar side chains.

glycosylation: Addition of sugar molecules to another molecule (usually an antigen). Glycosylation may change the 3-dimentional configuration of epitopes and affect antigen-antibody binding.

graft vs host disease: A pathological reaction between a host and a tissue graft; a natural reaction that may be intentionally suppressed in organ transplantation.

granulocyte: A type of white blood cell, subcategorized into neutrophils, basophils and eosinophils.

growth factors: Responsible for regulating cell proliferation (rapid and repeated reproduction), function and differentiation.

Guillain-Barré syndrome (GBS): Acute idiopathic polyneuritis. An uncommon illness characterized by ascending paralysis (ie, bilateral and flaccid weakness of the limbs without deep tendon reflexes in weak limbs) that is usually self-limited and reversible. Frequently associated with a preceding antigenic stimulus such as infectious illness (most commonly *Campylobacter jejuni*). Though most persons with GBS recover without residual weakness, approximately 5% of cases are fatal. Also known as Landry-Guillain-Barré syndrome, Landry-Guillain-Barré-Strohl syndrome, and polyradiculoneuropathy. (See Brighton Collaboration definition.)

hapten: A low molecular weight chemical that, when conjugated to a carrier (eg, poly-l-lysine), has the properties under appropriate conditions of an antigen with the hapten's specificity. Synonymous with haptene. Haptens do not generate antibody formation themselves.

helper T-lymphocytes: Lymphocytes carrying CD4 marker on their surfaces that act as chief regulatory cells of immune response. Responsible for many immune-system functions, including turning antibody production on and off.

hematopoiesis: The process of blood cell development.

herd immunity: The relative degree of resistance of a group or community to a disease. The resistance of a community to infection and spread of an infectious agent, derived from the resistance to infection of a high proportion of individual members of the community.

homofermentative: Producing a fermentation that results in one end product.

host: An organism that harbors another organism or tissue.

humanized antibodies: Monoclonal antibodies that contain 100% human protein sequences, although not of purely human origin.

humoral: Pertaining to molecules in solution in the extracellular fluids (eg, antibody, complement). The term corresponds to the ancient practice of describing the body's fluids as humors.

humoral immunity: Immunity mediated by antibodies (ie, immunoglobulins).

hybridoma: A cell culture derived from a clone of fused cells of different kinds, one of which is a tumor cell.

hyperemic area: A congested area, such as red areas on the skin that disappear with application of pressure.

hypersensitivity: An adaptive response in an exaggerated or inappropriate form that causes tissue damage. hypha: Bunches of branching cylindrical tubules of mold growth. Plural: Hyphae.

hypotonic-hyporesponsive episode (HHE): A clinical condition involving sudden onset of reduced muscle tone, reduced responsiveness and change of skin color (ie, paleness or cyanosis). (See Brighton Collaboration definition.)

idiotope: A single antigenic determinant, several of which compose the antigenic structure of an idiotype on an antibody.

idiotype: Antigenic structure associated with the surface of the variable region of an antibody.

immediate hypersensitivity: A type I immunopathologic reaction often involving IgE, IgG, basophils, and/or mast cells. It is characterized by an immediate (within 15 minutes or less) induration and erythema reaction, smooth muscle constriction, and/or anaphylaxis. Examples include atopy, anaphylaxis and asthma.

immune complex: Antigen-antibody complex.

immune-complex reaction: A type III immunopathologic reaction involving IgG, IgM, IgA and complement. It is characterized by accumulation of polymorphonuclear leukocytes and macrophages. Examples include serum sickness, rheumatoid arthritis and systemic lupus erythematosus.

immune globulin: A sterile solution containing antibodies, generally used for maintenance of certain immunodeficiencies or for passive immunization against specific diseases.

immune plasma: Human blood plasma with a high titer of antibodies against a particular microorganism; an early form of therapy for specific infections.

immune response: The reaction of the immune system to foreign substances.

immune system: Complex network of specialized organs, cells, molecules, and signals responsible for fighting disease. Primary function is to identify foreign substances and develop a defense against them.

immunity: Resistance to infectious agents, usually associated with antibodies or cells active against the agent or its toxin.

immunization: Process by which a person or animal becomes protected against a disease. Process of inducing immunity by administering an antigen (part of a vaccine) to allow the immune system to prevent infection or illness when it later encounters an infectious agent. Usually interchangeable with vaccination.

immunocompetent: Possessing the ability to mount a normal immune response.

immunocompromised: To have an immune response reduced by one or more of several causes, such as disease, radiation, medication, malnutrition, or an infection.

immunogen: A substance that stimulates the formation of antibodies.

immunogenicity: Capacity to stimulate formation of antibodies.

immunoglobulin: One of a family of proteins capable of acting as antibodies. An obsolete term is gamma globulin, referring to the presence of immunoglobulins in the gamma region of serum separated by electrophoresis. Some antibodies are beta globulins.

immunomodulators: A substance that causes a change in immune response, either stimulant or suppressant.

immunopharmaceutics: The study of the characteristics of immunologic dose-forms and immunologic drug delivery.

immunopharmacology: The study of effects of immunologic drugs on living organisms.

immunostimulant: A substance that promotes, accelerates or increases an immune response.

immunosuppressant: A substance that suppresses, slows or reduces an immune response.

inactivated vaccine: A vaccine composed of killed microorganisms or isolated microbial components that will induce active immunity. Note, it is the microbe that is inactivated, not the vaccine. In contemporary use, inactivated vaccines are more properly termed subunit vaccines.

inadvertent inoculation of vaccinia: Cutaneous or mucosal lesion or corneal ulceration at an anatomical site other than a vaccination site. (See Brighton Collaboration definition).

incidence: The frequency of occurrence of any event or condition for a certain population over a defined period of time. Contrast with prevalence.

incubation: Maintenance of a culture at the optimal conditions for growth.

incubation period: The time between inoculation (exposure) and clinical manifestations of disease.

induration: Palpable thickening, firmness, or hardening of soft tissue. (See Brighton Collaboration definition).

infection: Habitation of microorganisms within a part of the body without necessarily causing pathology. Largely synonymous with colonization.

infectious: Capable of being transferred to another cell or organism.

influenza-like illness (ILI): A term not uniformly defined by clinicians or the public, but that includes symptoms such as sudden-onset febrile illness, body aches (eg, myalgia, arthralgia) headache, sore throat, chills, extreme fatigue, cough, dizziness, neck pain, malaise, and lack of appetite. Nausea and vomiting are usually secondary to infections other than influenza. The CDC ILI surveillance case definition involves fever (greater than or equal to 37.8 degrees C, [100 degrees F]) plus cough, sore throat, or both in the absence of another known cause of illness.

injection-site reaction: Any description of morphological or physiological change at or near an injection site. This includes the injection site, areas adjacent to the injection site, or a reaction that may shift slightly away from the injection site because of gravity (eg, swelling, hematoma). (See Brighton Collaboration definition.)

innate immunity: The initial, nonspecific immune response in defense of the body against an infection. Includes barriers to infection, such as skin, stomach acid, mucus, the cough reflex, and enzymes in tears, saliva, and skin oils.

inoculation: Injection of a microorganism, serum or toxoid into the body, not necessarily for the purpose of immunization.

inoculum: The quantity of substance introduced by inoculation.

interferon: One of a group of glycoproteins formed by cells exposed to viruses.

interleukin: One of a group of proteins that serve as immunologic messenger between immune cells.

International Finance Facility (IFF): A mechanism to provide funds for development assistance.

International Finance Facility for Immunization: An IFF-style mechanism to secure funding for vaccines and immunization services in the poorest countries.

intracutaneous: Intradermal.

intussusception: The invagination of 1 segment of intestine into a segment of distal intestine. (See Brighton Collaboration definition.)

investigational new drug: Regulatory status of a drug before licensing, before safety and effectiveness have been confirmed.

in vitro: Literally, in glass (Latin). Broadly, in the laboratory.

in vivo: In the body (Latin).

isoagglutinin: Antibody in serum that agglutinates blood cells of members of the species from which it is derived.

isoantibody: An antibody produced against an isoantigen.

isoantigen: A substance present in certain individuals that stimulates production of antibodies in other members of the same species, but not in the donor.

isohemagglutinin: Substance normally present in most human serum, responsible for clumping of red blood cells when incompatible blood are mixed.

isoimmunization: Immunization of an individual against antigens of an individual of the same species.

isologous: Genetically identical.

isotonic: Having the same osmotic pressure. Products isotonic with blood do not induce hemolysis.

isotopes: Elements containing the same number of protons (ie, same atomic number), but a different number of neutrons (and hence a different mass number).

isotype: Major group of immune globulins (eg, IgA, IgD, IgE, IgG, IgM).

jet injection: The technique of injecting a drug through the skin without puncturing it, by use of a nozzle that ejects a fine spray of liquid with sufficient speed and pressure to penetrate the skin. This method is capable of immunizing large numbers of people quickly and economically, but is capable of disease transmission if performed improperly.

keloid: Scar formation in the skin following trauma or incision.

killer cells: See T-cytotoxic cell.

Kjeldahl method: A method to determine the amount of nitrogen in an organic compound, by heating the strong sulfuric acid.

Klebs-Löffler bacillus: *Corynebacterium diphtheriae.*

labeled: Included in the product insert for a given drug. In order to be labeled, an entry must meet FDA criteria for safety and efficacy.

latency period: A period of subclinical or inapparent pathologic changes following exposure, ending with the onset of symptoms of disease.

latent: Dormant.

leukocyte: A white blood cell, subcategorized into granulocytes and agranulocytes. Granulocytes include neutrophils, basophils and eosinophils. Agranulocytes include lymphocytes and monocytes.

Lf: Limit of flocculation, a unit of measure; 1 Lf is the amount of toxoid giving the most rapid flocculation with 1 standard unit of antitoxin when mixed and incubate in vitro.

liberty measles: Patriotic name in the United States for rubella during World War I (otherwise called "German measles").

ligand: A molecule or ion that can bind to a protein.

liposomes: Tiny spheres composed of phospholipids.

live vaccine: A vaccine containing live, weakened bacteria or viruses that induces active immunity. These vaccines can be dangerous in an immunocompromised patient who cannot mount an effective defense against even weakened microorganisms.

local reaction: See injection-site reaction.

logarithm: The exponent expressing the power to which a fixed number (the base) must be raised in order to produce a given number (the antilogarithm).

lupus erythematosus: An autoimmune disorder in which people produce antibodies to their own tissues.

lymph node: A rounded body consisting of accumulations of lymphatic tissue, found at intervals in the course of lymphatic vessels. Lymph nodes store special cells that can trap cancerous cells or microbes traveling through the body in lymph. Also called lymph glands.

lymphadenopathy: Selling of lymph glands in neck.

lymphoblast: An enlarged lymphocyte activated by contact with an antigen; capable of proliferating and differentiating into memory or effecter cell types.

lymphocyte: An immune cell; any of the mononuclear, nonphagocytic leukocytes found in blood, lymph and lymphoid tissues. The two major classes, B- and T-lymphocytes are responsible for humoral and cellular immunity, respectively.

lymphokines: Mediators secreted by lymphocytes that, alone or in combination, may participate in antitumor responses of the cellular immune system (eg, interferon gamma, interleukin-2, tumor necrosis factor).

lyophilization: Process of rapidly freezing a substance at an extremely low temperature, followed by dehydration in a high vacuum. Also called freeze-drying.

lyophilize: Freeze dry.

macrophage: Phagocytic mononuclear cells found in tissue; those found in blood are called monocytes.

macule: A colored spot on the skin, not elevated above the surface of the skin.

maculopapular: A rash consisting of both macules and papules.

magic bullets: Paul Ehrlich's term for chemicals formulated to seek out and destroy germs without harming tissue or organs.

major histocompatibility complex (MHC): The gene cluster that controls parts of the immune response. Among the products of these genes are the histocompatability antigens, such as HLA class I antigens, which are present on every cell with a nucleus and which serve as markers to distinguish self from non-self.

maltose: A disaccharide sugar formed from two units of glucose. Added to some antibody preparations as a protein stabilizer and osmotic agent.

Mantoux method: Intradermal tuberculin skin test.

mast cells: A tissue cell that has high-affinity receptors for IgE, generating inflammatory mediators (eg, histamine) in allergy. Distinct mast cells are found in mucosa and in connective tissue.

mechanistic correlate of protection: A correlate of protection that is mechanistically and causally responsible for protection.

memory cells: Sensitized T and B cells generated during an immune response to a specific antigen. Memory cells are long lived and enable an accelerated immune response when the host is challenged again by the same antigen.

meningitis: Inflammation of the membranes (meninges) that cover the brain and spinal cord.

meningitis, aseptic: Clinical evidence of acute meningitis (eg, fever, headache, vomiting, bulging fontanelle, nuchal rigidity), with pleocytosis in CSF and negative test for bacteria in CSF. (See Brighton Collaboration definition.)

Merthiolate: Lilly's proprietary name for thimerosal.

metabisulfite: A type of antioxidant associated with bronchospasm in some sensitive persons.

microarray: A technique that simultaneously evaluates expression levels of thousands of genes.

minor determinants: Nonbenzylpenicilloyl haptens. Designated as minor determinants, in that they are present in lesser amounts than the major determinant, benzylpenicilloyl. The minor determinants may nevertheless be associated with examples of significant clinical hypersensitivity.

moiety: An entity; a part.

molar: A measure of concentration. A 1 molar (1 M) solution contains one mole of a substance per liter.

mold: Fungus in the form of multicellular filamentous colonies.

mole: The unit of measure for molecular weight of a compound expressed in grams. Also called gram molecular weight (GMW).

Moloney test: Intradermal test of diphtheria toxoid to determine disease susceptibility.

monoclonal antibodies: Antibodies with the same specificity, produced by a single clone of identical plasma cells, a hybridoma, that can be produced in essentially unlimited quantities.

monocytes: Phagocytic mononuclear cells found in blood; those found in tissue are called macrophages.

monokine: Substance released from a macrophage or monocyte that affects the function of another cell.

monomeric: Consisting of a single unit.

morbidity: Any departure from a state of physiological or psychological well-being.

mucosal immunity: Resistance to infection across mucous membranes. Mucosal immunity depends on immune cells and antibodies in the linings of the respiratory tract, reproductive tract, gastrointestinal tract, and other moist surfaces of the body exposed to the outside environment.

murine: Pertaining to a mouse or mice.

mycelium: A mass of intertwined hyphae that accumulates during active growth in the mold form.

myelitis: Acute spinal cord inflammation, with or without involvement of the meninges. Can also involve myelopathy and other neurologic manifestations. (See Brighton Collaboration definition.)

nadir: The lowest point; the least value.

National Drug Code: An 11-digit number that uniquely identifies a drug product. The first 5 digits describe the manufacturer, labeler or other distributor. The next 4 digits identify the generic drug entity and the final 2 digits identify the package size.

National Immunization Days: Organized programs within nations to deliver immunizations on a large scale.

natural-killer cells: Lymphocytes that have the ability to recognize and destroy tumor cells and some virally infected cells without prior sensitization.

negative control: A skin test reagent used to assess the nonallergic skin response to irritation or dermatographism (eg, sodium chloride 0.9%).

negative-predictive value: A mathematical estimate of the probability that a patient will not have a disease or outcome in question, given that a diagnostic test has yielded a negative result.

neutralizing antibodies: Antibodies that bind to microbes and prevent them from binding to cellular receptors.

Ninhydrin: Proprietary name for a preparation of triketohydrindene hydrate, used to determine protein nitrogen.

nodule: The presence of a discrete or well-demarcated soft tissue mass or lump that is firm and at the injection site. (See Brighton Collaboration definition.)

nonmechanistic correlate of protection: A correlate of protection that is not a mechanistic causal agent of protection.

normal saline: Sodium chloride 0.9%; a solution isotonic with human plasma.

notifiable disease: A disease that law or regulation requires be reported to the public health or other authority in the pertinent jurisdiction when the diagnosis is made.

nuclides: A collective term for isotopes of all the elements.

occlusion: Closure of a passage.

oleoresin: The oily residue remaining after evaporation of the solvent used in the extraction process.

oncogenic: Leading to the formation and development of tumors.

opsonin: A class of circulating antibodies that help phagocytes destroy invading bacteria.

opsonization: Increase in susceptibility to phagocytosis by deposition of antibody and C3b on an antigen.

osmolality: Osmotic concentration of a solution, determined by the ionic concentration of the dissolved substance per unit mass of solvent.

osmolarity: Osmotic concentration of a solution, determined by the ionic dissolved substance per unit volume of solvent.

outbreak: Epidemic. Alternatively, an epidemic limited to a localized increase in the incidence of a disease, as opposed to a generalized epidemic.

ovine: Pertaining to sheep.

pandemic: A disease or condition affecting the majority of the population of a large region, or which is epidemic at the same time in many different parts of the world. In the context of influenza, pandemics typically involve both wide geographic dispersion and greater than usual morbidity and mortality.

papule: A small, solid elevation of the skin ("bump").

papulovesicular: A rash consisting of both papules and vesicles.

parasite: An organism that lives on or in an organism of another species, from which it obtains nourishment.

paratope: The internal antigen binding site on an antibody.

parenteral: Administered in a way to avoid the enteral tract, typically by injection into a vein or into the skin.

paresthesia: An abnormal sensation, such as burning, pricking, tickling, or tingling.

paroxysmal: Characterized by sudden, periodic attacks or symptoms.

passage: Sequential culture of bacteria or viruses in a laboratory growth medium, usually in an effort to reduce virulence. The passage number is the number of serial times the microbe is grown in separate cultures.

passive immunity: Temporary immunity provided by preformed, donated antitoxin or antibodies (ie, immune globulins). Most passive immunity is protective almost immediately, but only persists for a few weeks.

passive immunization: An immediate, although short-lived, immunity provided by injection of antibodies synthesized in another host (either human or animal).

passive transfer: The conferring of immunity to a nonimmune host by injection of antibody from an immune donor.

PATH: Program for Appropriate Technology in Health, an international, nonprofit organization. PATH uses funding from the Bill and Melinda Gates Foundation, GAVI, and other sources to work on emerging and persistent global health issues such as vaccines and immunization.

pathogenicity: The capacity of an infectious agent to cause disease in a susceptible host.

pegylation: Addition of polyethylene glycol (PEG) to a protein drug, to prolong that drug's half life.

pellicle: A thin piece of cuticle or skin; a film or surface on a liquid; a thin nonliving sheath forming the surface layer of certain one-celled organisms. Synonymous with scum.

peptide: A compound containing two or more amino acids.

peste: Plague (French), caused by *Yersinia pestis*. Also a book by Albert Camus.

Pfeiffer bacillus: *Haemophilus influenzae.*

phagocyte: A cell that has the ability to ingest and destroy particulate substances such as bacteria and protozoa.

phagocytosis: Engulfment and digestion of bacteria and other particles by leukocytes circulating in serum. Usually mediated by opsonic antibodies that combine with the surface antigens of microbes to make them more susceptible to phagocytosis. Protective actions of phagocytosis are further enhanced by complement.

pharmaceutics: The study of the characteristics of drug dosage forms and drug delivery.

pharmacokinetics: The processes of absorption, distribution, metabolism, and excretion of a medication.

pharmacology: The study of the effects of drugs on living organisms.

pharmacoepidemiology: The study of the distribution of use and the effects of medications in one or more populations of people.

phenolsulfonphthalein: The chemical name of phenol red.

phenol red: A phenolic compound used as an indicator of hydrogen ion concentration, from pH 6.8 to 8.4.

phylactic: Pertaining to the active defense of the body against infection.

placebo: An inactive substance administered to some study participants, while others receive an active substance, to provide an objective basis for measuring effects of the active substance.

plasma: The liquid part of the lymph and blood.

plasma cells: Derived from B-lymphocytes, plasma cells are the major producers of immunoglobulins.

plasmid: A small, self-reproducing piece of DNA that exists outside the chromosome. It can alter a hereditary characteristic when inserted into a foreign bacterium. Plasmids can be used in recombinant DNA technology as acceptors of foreign DNA.

pneumonic: Concerning or involving the lungs or pneumonia (eg, pneumonic plague).

polyclonal antibodies: Antibodies with differing specificities, derived from multiple cell types.

polymerase chain reaction (PCR): A technique for specifically amplifying trace amounts of DNA to make them readily detectable.

polymeric: Consisting of multiple units.

polysaccharide vaccine: A vaccine composed of purified bacterial capsule carbohydrate fragments. T-cell memory response to polysaccharide vaccines, as compared with proteinaceous antigens, may be reduced or absent in immunodeficient hosts.

polysorbate-80: Nonionic surfactant, sorbitan monoleate polyoxyalkylene derivative. Proprietary name: *Tween-80.*

positive control: A skin test reagent (eg, histamine) used to ensure skin reactivity and the absence of suppressive pharmacotherapy (eg, antihistamines).

positive-predictive value: A mathematical estimate of the probability that a patient will have a disease or outcome in question, given that a diagnostic test has yielded a positive result.

precipitin: A class of antibodies that reacts with its specific antigen to form an insoluble precipitate.

prevalence: The number of cases of a disease or condition present in a specified population at a given time. Contrast with incidence.

prick test: An epicutaneous or transcutaneous test of immediate hypersensitivity (allergy). A sharp needle is used to puncture the skin, but not to draw blood. Also called a puncture or percutaneous test.

primary series: A set of several vaccine or toxoid doses needed to initially establish protective immunity.

prime: To give an initial sensitization to an antigen.

prodromal: Pertaining to the initial stage of a disease, the interval between the earliest symptoms and the appearance of a rash or fever.

progressive vaccinia: A vaccinia virus lesion that fails to heal and/or progresses to necrosis. *Vaccine.* 2007;25:5735-5744. (See Brighton Collaboration definition.)

properdin: A serum globulin that in the presence of both complement and magnesium ions, combines with and kills invading bacteria. One of the components of the human inborn host defense system against microorganisms.

prophylaxis: Prevention.

protein vaccine: A vaccine composed of proteins, usually in the form of whole or fragmented bacteria or viruses. Protein vaccines tend to induce more persistent immunity than polysaccharide vaccines.

proteomics: The scientific study of the role of proteins in the structure, growth, health, and disease of organisms.

protozoa: The phylum of the animal kingdom that includes the simplest animals. Most are unicellular, although some are colonial. Most reproduce asexually by fission, although conjugation and sexual reproduction may occur.

proximal: Nearest the point of attachment, center of the body, or point of reference. Opposite of distal.

pruritus: Itching.

pseudopods: Irregular projections, as of erythema.

puncture test: An epicutaneous or transcutaneous test of immediate hypersensitivity (allergy). A sharp needle is used to puncture the skin, but not to draw blood. Also called a prick or percutaneous test.

pustule: Collection of pus within or beneath the epidermis.

pyrogen: Any substance that produces fever.

racemate: A salt or ester of an optically inactive mixture of equal proportions of dextrorotary and levorotary isomers.

radioactive: Capable of giving off radiant energy, such as alpha or beta particles or gamma rays.

radioimmunoscintigraphy: Gamma-camera imaging with radioactively labeled antibodies.

radioisotope: An isotope possessing the characteristic of radioactivity.

radionuclide: A nuclide possessing the characteristic of radioactivity.

rash: A skin or mucosal change consisting of a clearly indetified primary lesion (morphology) and/or secondary skin change. (See Brighton Collaboration definition.)

reactogenicity: The capacity or degree to which a medication causes adverse reactions.

reagent: Any chemical or other substance used in a test.

reagin: IgE.

reassortant: A bacterium or virus containing 2 or more pieces of nucleic acid from different parents.

recall antigen: An antigen, to which the patient is assumed to have been exposed previously, administered as part of an anergy skin test battery, to which the patient is expected to respond.

receptors: Proteinaceous structures often found at cell surfaces that bind specific molecules.

recombinant DNA: DNA produced by combining pieces of DNA from different sources.

recombinant vaccine: A vaccine containing proteins derived from recombinant DNA technology.

refrigerate: For the storage of drugs, defined in the *USP* as storage at 2° to 8°C (36° to 46°F).

relative risk: The ratio of the risk of an outcome among an exposed group to the risk among an unexposed group.

replicon: A self-replicating DNA or RNA molecule or fragment that cannot form infectious particles but does express proteins of interest. Replicons can act as vectors to deliver genes that express proteins useful as vaccine antigens. Replicons are a type of artificial virus-like particle.

reservoir: The human or animal population, or the environment in which the infectious agent exists, and from which it can be transmitted.

replication: The mode of viral reproduction, in which copies of DNA or RNA are made.

Rh agglutinogen: A specific substance, also called the Rh factor, present in some red blood cells. The term Rh derives from the rhesus monkey in which the substance was first identified. When Rh agglutinogen enters the circulation of a person who naturally lacks the factor, that person develops anti-Rh agglutinin antibodies. Subsequent transfusions of Rh-positive blood may result in serious transfusion reactions, characterized by massive agglutination and hemolysis of red blood cells.

rheumatoid factor: An anti-immunoglobulin antibody directed against denatured IgG in the serum of patients with rheumatoid arthritis and other rheumatoid diseases.

ribozymes: Enzymes that cut RNA at a specific site.

ricin: A poisonous substance derived from the seed of the castor oil plant that agglutinates erythrocytes.

RNA vaccine: A vaccine containing fragments of RNA encoding genes for key microbial antigens (proteins). The host, in turn, expresses the genes, producing the protein, yielding a significant immunologic response.

robust take–vaccinia: Erythema or induration 7.5 cm or more in diameter, with tenderness or warmth, occurring 8 to 12 days after smallpox vaccination, that begins to resolve within 72 hours of onset. (See Brighton Collaboration definition.)

room temperature: For the storage of drugs, defined in the *USP* as less than 40°C (104°F), preferably between 15° and 30°C (59° and 86°F).

rosette: A cluster (eg, a central cell surrounded by bound cells).

rosetting: Technique for identifying cells by mixing them with particles or other cells to which they bind.

rusts: An order of fungi parasitic on plants. Many are allergenic.

safe: For medications, the condition of having reasonable risk of harm, given the patient's condition, the magnitude of the benefit expected, and the alternatives available. In 21 CFR 600.3, the relative freedom from harmful effect when prudently administered, taking into consideration the character of the product in relation to the condition of the recipient.

saline: Containing sodium chloride.

scarification: The process of making numerous superficial incisions in the skin. A technique used for smallpox and tularemia immunization.

scarifier: A tool used for scarification.

scratch test: A transcutaneous test of immediate hypersensitivity (allergy). A sterile scarifier is used to carefully break or scratch the skin, about 2 to 4 mm in length.

secondary attack rate: The number of new cases among contacts of a primary case within the accepted incubation period of the disease. The denominator is the total number of exposed contacts during the same period of time.

secondary response: The immune response that follows a second or subsequent encounter with a particular antigen.

secretory IgA: A dimer of IgA molecules with secretory component, linked by a J chain.

seizure: Episode of neuronal hyperactivity most commonly resulting in sudden, involuntary muscular contractions. (See Brighton Collaboration definition.)

sensitivity: A mathematical estimate of the probability that a diagnostic test will yield a positive result when the patient truly has the disease or outcome in question.

sepsis: The presence of bacteria and/or their toxins in the blood or tissues.

septic shock: Blood poisoning with a sudden drop in blood pressure and increased heart rate and temperature.

sequela: A condition following as a consequence of a previous event.

seroconversion: Development of laboratory evidence of antibody response to a disease or a vaccine. Usually defined empirically as a certain change in reciprocal antibody titer or a certain concentration of serum antibody.

serogroup: The kind of microbe, characterized by testing for antigens recognizable by serum. A serogroup is more specific than a species, but less specific than a serotype or strain.

seroprotection: Development of laboratory evidence of antibody response to a disease or a vaccine. Usually defined empirically as a certain change in reciprocal antibody titer or a concentration of serum antibody that is correlated in clinical studies with protection from disease.

serotype: The kind of microbe, characterized by testing for antigens recognizable by serum. A serotype is more specific than a serogroup or a species, but less specific than a strain.

serovar: Serological variant, comparable to serogroup or serotype.

serum: The watery portion of blood after coagulation; plasma minus fibrinogen.

serum sickness: Adverse immunologic response to an antigen, usually a heterologous protein, characterized by a type III immune-complex reaction. Typically involves a syndrome of rash, edema, joint pains, and fever following a few days after repeated doses of heterologous proteins (eg, animal antibody products).

Schick test: A skin test to ascertain sensitivity to diphtheria, using a toxin of *Corynebacterium diphtheriae.*

sic: From the Latin, thus. Used to indicate that an apparent error or questionable entry has been printed properly.

side effect: An undesirable health event that is presumed to be caused by use of a medication.

smuts: An order of fungi parasitic on plants. Many are allergenic.

specificity: A mathematical estimate of the probability that a diagnostic test will yield a negative result when the patient truly is devoid of the disease or outcome in question.

spherule: A form of yeast consisting of spherical thick-walled structures filled with a few to several hundred endospores.

Glossary

split-virion vaccine: A vaccine composed of chemically disrupted viruses. The smaller viral particle size generally reduces the incidence of adverse reactions, but may also reduce the induction of protective antibodies. Synonymous with subvirion.

statistical significance: The probability that an event or a difference occurred as the result of an intervention (eg, medication administration) rather than by chance.

stem cell: A cell found in the bone marrow, believed to be able to differentiate into any of the blood cell types.

sterilizing immunity: An immune response that completely prevents establishment of an infection.

strabismus: A squinting disorder of the eye in which optic axes cannot be directed at the same object, due to lack of muscular coordination.

strain: The kind of microbe, characterized by testing for antigens recognizable by serum. A strain is more specific than a type, subtype, or serotype.

stratification: Separation of a study group into subgroups according to specific characteristics.

stroma: Foundation-supporting tissues of an organ. Opposite of parenchyma.

subunit vaccine: A vaccine containing portions of a bacterium or virus.

subvirion vaccine: Synonymous with split-virion.

surfactant: A surface-active agent that reduces surface tension. Surfactants act as detergents.

surrogate of protection: See correlate of protection.

surrogate marker: An indirect measure of disease status.

susceptible: Not possessing sufficient resistance against a pathogenic agent to prevent contracting infection or disease if exposed to the agent.

swelling: Enlargement of an anatomic site, may be accompanied by erythema and tenderness. (See Brighton Collaboration definition.)

synergistic: Characterized by an increased effect associated with 2 agents in combination not produced alone, or an effect greater than the total effects of each agent operating by itself.

systemic: Beyond the injection site. Affecting the whole body.

T-cell: See T-lymphocyte.

T-cytotoxic cells: A subset of T-cells that recognizes and induces lysis of target cells bearing specific antigens. Also called killer cells or killer T-cells.

T-helper cells: A subset of T-cells that produces lymphokines, stimulates antibody production by B cells and facilitates the production of antigen-specific cytotoxic killer T-cells.

T-lymphocyte: A thymus-derived immune cell that participates in a variety of cell-mediated immune reactions. T-lymphocytes include T-helper, T-suppressor and T-cytotoxic cells.

T-suppressor cells: A subset of T-cells that reduces the activity of T and B cells.

thimerosal: An antimicrobial preservative, sodium ethylercurithiosalicylate, containing about 50% mercury. Acts by modifying functional groups of proteins and nucleic acids through enzyme inhibition. Lilly's proprietary name is *Merthiolate*.

thrombocytopenia: Platelet count less than 150×10^9 cells/L. (See Brighton Collaboration definition.)

thymocyte: An immune cell originating in the thymus; a T-lymphocyte.

thymus: A glandular structure composed mainly of lymphoid tissue that contributes to cell-mediated immunity by being the site where T-cells develop.

tines: Prongs.

Tine Test: Lederle's proprietary name for a multipuncture device, often used to refer to a multipuncture tuberculin test.

titer: A measurement of the amount or concentration of a substance in a solution. It usually refers to the amount of medication or antibodies found in a patient's blood and serum.

toll-like receptors: A class of single membrane-spanning noncatalytic receptors that recognize structurally conserved molecules derived from microbes once they breach physical barriers (eg, skin, intestinal mucosa) and activate immune cells (from German, "toll," unusual). Believed to play a key role in innate immunity.

toxoid: An inactivated bacterial toxin, rendered nontoxic while retaining the ability to stimulate the formation of antitoxin (ie, specific antibodies against the unaltered toxin).

transfer factor: A factor present in lymphocytes that have been sensitized to antigens and which can be transferred to a nonsensitized recipient. The recipient will then react to the same antigen(s) originally used to sensitize the donor's lymphocytes. In humans, the factor can be transferred by injecting the recipient with either intact lymphocytes or extracts of disrupted cells.

transmission: The act of spreading of an infectious agent to a receptive portal of entry through which infection may take place.

transverse myelitis: A neurologic disorder caused by inflammation across both sides of one level, or segment, of the spinal cord.

Triton W-30: An anionic surfactant.

tumor necrosis factor: One of a group of peptides that permits cells to transmit signals to each other.

turbid: Cloudy, not clear.

Tween 80: See polysorbate-80.

type I: Immediate, allergic hypersensitivity reactions, primarily mediated by immunoglobulins (eg, atopy, asthma, anaphylaxis).

type II: Cytotoxic reactions (eg, autoimmune diseases).

type III: Immune-complex reaction (eg, serum sickness).

type IV: Delayed hypersensitivity cell-mediated immunity, primarily mediated by T-lymphocytes (eg, tuberculosis, granulomatous diseases).

ubiquitous: Commonly encountered.

ultrafiltered: Filtration of a colloidal substance in which the dispersed particles, but not the liquid, are retained.

unexplained sudden infant death: Sudden death of a child younger than 2 years old that remains unexplained after excluding other causes of death by review of clinical history, history of final events, and complete autopsy report with various tissue sampling and radiologic studies. (See Brighton Collaboration definition.)

unlabeled use: A use not included in the product insert for a given drug. Lack of inclusion neither confirms nor rules out safety and efficacy.

urticaria: A vascular reaction of the skin characterized by eruption of pale evanescent wheals, which may be associated with severe itching. Synonymous with angioedema or hives.

urushiol: The principal toxic irritant substance of plants such as poison ivy that produces severe dermatitis upon contact.

vaccination: Literally, inoculation with cowpox virus (originally called vaccine virus) to prevent smallpox. Broadly, to deliver any vaccine to develop active immunity.

vaccine: The category of drugs used to induce active immunity.

Vaccine Fund, The: A nonprofit financing resource created to support the GAVI immunization goals, providing financial support directly to low-income countries to strengthen their health delivery and immunization services and to purchase new and under-used vaccines.

vaccine vial monitors: A label on a vaccine vial that changes color when exposed to heat over time. If the VVM indicates a color change, health workers should not use the vaccine inside.

vaccinia: Cowpox virus, the active ingredient in modern smallpox vaccine.

valence: The combining power of a molecule or product.

variola: Smallpox virus.

variolation: Intentional inoculation with smallpox virus (usually in the form of scabs) to prevent more severe infections.

vector: An animate intermediary in the indirect transmission of an infectious agent that carries the agent from a reservoir to a susceptible host.

Vero cells: African green monkey kidney cells, a cell line initiated from a normal adult monkey in 1962.

vesicle: A small, circumscribed epidermal elevation of the skin containing clear fluid. Blister.

virion: A complete viral particle, consisting of RNA or DNA surrounded by a protein shell or capsid. An infectious virus.

virosomes: Tiny spherical vesicles that contain viral proteins embedded in their membranes. When the membranes consist of phospholipids, the spheres also can be called liposomes.

virulence: The degree of pathogenicity of an infectious agent, indicated by case-fatality rates or ability to invade and damage host tissues.

virus: A tiny organism that multiplies within cells and causes disease.

volume of distribution: A measure of the extent of distribution of a drug in bodily fluids, the dilution space. Apparent volumes of distribution greater than 3 liters suggest distribution of a drug outside the plasma compartment.

wheal: A smooth, hardened, slightly elevated area. Frequently referred to as the wheal of an allergic skin response. Synonymous with induration.

whole-virion vaccine: A vaccine composed of intact viruses. Contrast with split-virion vaccines.

yeast: Unicellular growth of fungi; most reproduce by budding.

zoonosis: An infection transmissible under natural conditions from vertebrate animals to humans. Plural: Zoonoses.

References

Kohl KS, Bonhoeffer J, Chen R, et al. The Brighton Collaboration: enhancing comparability of vaccine safety data. *Pharmacoepidemiol Drug Saf.* 2003;12(4):335-340.

Jefferson T. A basic glossary of vaccinology. *J Epidemiol Community Health.* 2001;55(5):294-295.

Ofosu-amaah S, Shah KP. Immunization glossary. *Assignment Child.* 1985;(69-72):455-462.

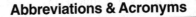
The following is a list of abbreviations that are used throughout this book.

7S: Synonym for IgG, referring to 7 Svedberg units

19S: Synonym for IgM, referring to 19 Svedberg units

69-kd: 69-kilodalton protein

AAFP: American Academy of Family Physicians

AAP: American Academy of Pediatrics

Ab: antibody

ACIP: Advisory Committee on Immunization Practices

ACLS: Advanced Cardiac Life Support

ACOG: American College of Obstetricians and Gynecologists

ACP: American College of Physicians

ACR: American College of Rheumatology

ACR##: ACR response level

ACTH: adrenocorticotropic hormone (use corticotropin)

ADCC: antibody-dependent cellular cytotoxicity

ADEM: acute disseminated encephalomyelitis

AFB: acid-fast bacilli

AFI: acute febrile illness

AFIP: Armed Forces Institute of Pathology

AFP: alpha-fetoprotein

Ag: antigen

AIDS: acquired immunodeficiency syndrome

ALA: American Lung Association

ALG: antilymphoblast globulin

ALL: acute lymphocytic leukemia

ALT: alanine aminotransferase

AML: acute myelogenous leukemia

AMP: adenosine monophosphate

ANC: absolute neutrophil count

ANT: anthrax vaccine

anti-HBc: antibody to HB_cAg, indicative of prior infection with hepatitis B virus at some undefined time

anti-HBe: antibody to HB_cAg, indicative of lower titer of hepatitis B virus

anti-HBs: antibody to HB_sAg, indicative of past infection with and immunity to hepatitis B virus, passive antibody from HBIG, or immune response from hepatitis B vaccine

APC: antigen-presenting cells

APDT: acellular pertussis vaccine with diphtheria and tetanus toxoids, DTaP

APhA: American Pharmacists Association

APHIS: Animal and Plant Health Inspection Service (USDA)

APTT: activated partial thromboplastin time

ARC: AIDS-related complex (use symptomatic HIV infection); American Red Cross

ARDS: acute respiratory distress syndrome

ARS: antirabies serum

ATCC: American Type Culture Collection

ATG: antithymocyte globulin

ATS: American Thoracic Society

AU: allergy unit

AUC: area under the curve

AvP: Aventis Pasteur

AZT: azidothymidine, the proper generic name for which is zidovudine

BAU: bioequivalent allergy units

BB-IND: investigational new drug number issued by CBER (formerly BoB)

BCG: Bacille Calmette-Guérin tuberculosis vaccine (see TUB)

BUN: blood urea nitrogen (use serum urea nitrogen)

BoB: Bureau of Biologics, CBER (FDA) since 1982

BPIG: bacterial polysaccharide immune globulin

BPL: benzylpenicilloyl polylysine

BRM: biological response modifier

c.: *circa*, approximately

C: Centigrade, Celsius

CAS: Chemical Abstracts Service (a numeric system of nomenclature for chemical compounds)

CATMAT: Committee to Advise on Tropical Medicine and Travel (Public Health Agency of Canada)

CBC: complete blood cell count

CBER: Center for Biologics Evaluation and Research (FDA)

CD: clusters of differentiation

CDAI: Crohn disease activity index

CD3: Antigenic marker on T cell associated with T-cell receptor

CD4: Antigenic marker on helper/inducer T cells (also called OKT 4, T4, and Leu 3)

CD8: Antigenic marker on suppressor/cytotoxic T cells (also called OKT8, T8, and Leu 8)

CDC: Centers for Disease Control and Prevention

CDER: Center for Drug Evaluation and Research (FDA)

CEA: carcinoembryonic antigen

CF: complement fixation

CFA: complete Freund adjuvant

CFR: *Code of Federal Regulations*

CFU: colony-forming unit

CFU-GEMM: colony-forming unit of granulocytes, erythrocytes, monocytes, and megakaryocytes

CFU-GM: colony-forming unit of granulocytes and macrophages

CGD: chronic granulomatous disease

CHF: congestive heart failure

CHO: carbohydrate; Chinese hamster ovary cell culture

CI: confidence interval

CIS: carcinoma in situ

CK: creatine kinase

CLL: chronic lymphocytic leukemia

CLS: capillary leak syndrome

CMI: cell-mediated immunity

CML: chronic myelocytic leukemia

CMS: Centers for Medicare & Medicaid Services

CMV: cytomegalovirus

CNS: central nervous system

COPD: chronic obstructive pulmonary disease

CPM: counts per minute

CPT: Current Procedural Terminology (American Medical Association)

CR: complete response

CRIE: crossed radioimmunoelectrophoresis

CRM: cross-reacting mutant

CRP: C-reactive protein

CRS: congenital rubella syndrome; cytokine-release syndrome

CSF: colony-stimulating factor; cerebrospinal fluid

CT: computed tomography

CTLA-4: cytotoxic T-lymphocyte-associated antigen-4

CVS: Challenge Virus Standard

DAT: diphtheria antitoxin

DEAE: diethyaminoethyl

DEV: duck embryo (rabies) vaccine

DH: delayed hypersensitivity

DHHS: US Department of Health and Human Services

DIC: disseminated intravascular coagulation

DIN: Deutsche Industrie Normen (German standards)

DK: dog kidney

dL: deciliter

DMARD: disease-modifying antirheumatic drug

DNA: deoxyribonucleic acid

DNCB: 2, 4-dinitrochlorobenzene

DoD: US Department of Defense

DrTPar: diphtheria toxoid (reduced antigen quantity for adults), tetanus toxoid, and acellular pertussis (reduced antigen quantity for adults) vaccine, for adult use

DT: diphtheria toxoid and tetanus toxoid, adsorbed, for pediatric use

DTaP: diphtheria and tetanus toxoids with acellular pertussis vaccine

DTH: delayed-type hypersensitivity

DTP: diphtheria toxoid, tetanus toxoid, and pertussis (antigens unspecified) vaccine

DTPa: diphtheria toxoid, tetanus toxoid, and acellular pertussis vaccine, for pediatric use

DTPa-HIB-IPV: diphtheria toxoid, tetanus toxoid, acellular pertussis, *Haemophilus influenzae* type b conjugate, poliovirus inactivated vaccine

DTwP: diphtheria and tetanus toxoids with whole-cell pertussis vaccine

D5W: dextrose 5% solution in water

EBV: Epstein-Barr virus

ECG: electrocardiogram

EEE: eastern equine encephalitis

EGFR: epidermal growth factor receptor

EIA: enzyme immunoassay

e-IPV: enhanced-potency inactivated poliovirus vaccine

ELISA: enzyme-linked immunosorbent assay

ElU: ELISA unit

EPEG: enteropathogenic *Escherichia coli*

EPI: Expanded Programme on Immunization (WHO)

ESR: erythrocyte sedimentation rate

EST: equine skin-test reagent

ETAF: epidermal thymocyte-activating factor

EUA: Emergency Use Authorization

F: Fahrenheit

FA: direct fluorescent or immunofluorescent antibody test

Fab: antigen-binding fragment of an immunoglobulin molecule

Fc: constant fragment of an immunoglobulin molecule

FcεRI: high-affinity IgE receptor

FDA: US Food and Drug Administration

FeLV: feline leukemia virus

FEV$_1$: forced expiratory volume in the first second of expiration

FHA: filamentous hemagglutinin

FRhL: fetal rhesus lung

FSME: Frühsommer-Meningoenzephalitis

g: gram

G6PD: glucose-6-phosphate dehydrogenase

GAVI: Global Alliance for Vaccines and Immunisation

GBS: Guillain-Barré syndrome; group B streptococci

G-CSF: granulocyte colony-stimulating factor

GDH-PQQ: glucose dehydrogenase pyrroloquinolinequinone

GG: gamma globulin, an obsolete term for IG

GM-CSF: granulocyte-macrophage colony-stimulating factor

gp: glycoprotein

gpELISA: glycoprotein enzyme-linked immunosorbent assay

GPIIb/IIIa: glycoprotein IIb/IIIa (receptor on human platelets)

GSAP: greatest single allergen present

GVHD: graft-vs-host disease

GSK: GlaxoSmithKline

H: hemagglutinin

HA: hemagglutination

HACA: human antichimeric antibody

HAHA: human antihuman antibody

HAHTGG: horse antihuman thymocyte gamma globulin

HAI: hemagglutination inhibition

HAMA: human antimouse antibody

HAV: hepatitis A virus vaccine

HAV-HBV: hepatitis A virus and hepatitis B virus vaccine

HB$_c$Ab: hepatitis B core antibody, see also anti-HBc

HB$_c$Ag: hepatitis B core antigen

HbCV: *Haemophilus influenzae* type b conjugate vaccine

HB$_e$Ag: hepatitis B e antigen, correlates with HBV replication, high serum viral titers, and serum infectivity

HBIG: hepatitis B immune globulin. *H-BIG* is the registered trademark of Abbott Laboratories.

HbOC: *Haemophilus influenzae* type b oligosaccharide conjugate

HbPs: *Haemophilus influenzae* type b polysaccharide

HB$_s$Ab: hepatitis B surface antibody, see also anti-HBs

HB$_s$Ag: hepatitis B surface antigen

HBV: hepatitis B virus vaccine

HBVig: hepatitis B virus immune globulin

hCG: human chorionic gonadotropin

HCIG: hepatitis C immune globulin

HCL: hairy cell leukemia

HCPCS: Healthcare Common Procedure Coding System

HCV: hepatitis C virus

HDCV: human diploid cell (rabies) vaccine

HDN: hemolytic disease of the newborn

HEL: *Helicobacter pylori* vaccine

HER2: human epidermal growth factor receptor 2

Hg: elemental symbol for mercury

HHS: US Department of Health & Human Services

HI: hemagglutination inhibition

Hib: *Haemophilus influenzae* type b

HIB: *Haemophilus influenzae* type b vaccine, not otherwise specified

HIB-HbOC: *Haemophilus influenzae* type b conjugate vaccine (diphtheria CRM197 protein conjugate) (oligosaccharides conjugated to diphtheria CRM197 toxin protein)

HIBcn: *Haemophilus influenzae* type b conjugate vaccine

HICPAC: Healthcare Infection Control Practices Advisory Committee

HIPAA: Health Insurance Portability and Accountability Act of 1996

HIV: human immunodeficiency virus

HLA: human leukocyte antigen

H-P: heat- and phenol-inactivated (typhoid) vaccine

HPV: human papilloma virus, high passage (rubella) virus

h: hour

HSA: human serum albumin

HSV: herpes simplex virus

HTLV-III: human T-cell lymphotropic or leukemia virus type III, an early name for HIV type 1

IAC: Immunization Action Coalition

ICAM: intracellular adhesion molecule

ICD: International Classification of Diseases

ID: intradermal; idiotype

IDCF: immunodiffusion complement fixation

IDTP: immunodiffusion tube precipitin

IEF: isoelectric focusing

IF: immunofluorescent test

IFA: incomplete Freund's adjuvant

IFF: International Finance Facility

IFFIm: International Finance Facility for Immunisation

IFN: interferon

Ig: immune globulin, synonymous with immunoglobulin

IgA: immunoglobulin A, a monomer, dimer, or trimer associated with secretory immunity, agglutination, and immune-complex formation

IgD: immunoglobulin D, a monomer, function unknown

IgE: immunoglobulin E, a monomer associated with allergy, hypersensitivity, and fixation to mast cells

IgG: immunoglobulin G, a monomer associated with humoral immunity, agglutination, complement fixation, and cytotoxicity

IGIM: immune globulin, intramuscular

IGIV: immune globulin, intravenous

IgM: immunoglobulin M, a pentamer associated with secretory immunity, agglutination, complement fixation, cytotoxicity, and immune-complex formation

IGSC: immune globulin subcutaneous

IH: infectious hepatitis

IL: interleukin

IL-1Ra: interleukin-1 receptor antagonist

IL-2Ra: interleukin-2 receptor α-chain

ILI: influenza-like illness

IM: intramuscular

IMIG: intramuscular preparation of immunoglobulin G

IND: investigational new drug

INF: influenza virus vaccine, not otherwise specified

INFa: influenza virus attenuated live vaccine

INFan: influenza virus attenuated live vaccine, intranasal

INFi: influenza virus inactivated vaccine

INFs: influenza virus vaccine, split virion

INFs-AB3: influenza virus vaccine, split virion, types A and B, trivalent

INFw: influenza virus vaccine, whole virion

INH: isoniazid

IOM: Institute of Medicine

IPV: poliovirus inactivated (injectable) vaccine

ISCOM: immunostimulating complex

ISG: immune serum globulin, an obsolete term for IGIM

ITLC: instant thin-layer chromatography

ITP: immune thrombocytopenic purpura

IU: international unit

IV: intravenous

IVIg: immune globulin intravenous preparation

JE: Japanese encephalitis

JRA: juvenile rheumatoid arthritis

keV: kilo-electron volt

kg: kilogram

KMV: killed measles vaccine

KS: Kaposi sarcoma

L: liter

LAIV: live attenuated influenza vaccine

LAK cell: lymphocyte-activated killer cell

LAV: lymphadenopathy-associated virus, an early name for HIV-1

LCDC: Laboratory Centre for Disease Control, now the Public Health Agency of Canada's Infectious Disease Prevention and Control Branch (IDPCB)

LD$_{50}$: median lethal dose

LDH: lactate dehydrogenase

Lf unit: limit of flocculation unit

LFA: leukocyte function antigen

LIG: lymphocyte immune globulin

LPF: lymphocytosis-promoting factor

LPS: lipopolysaccharide

LT: heat-labile toxin of *Escherichia coli*

m: meter

M: molar

Mab: monoclonal antibody

MAE: medically attended event

MAI: *Mycobacterium avium intracellulare*

MAO: monoamine oxidase

MAOI: monoamine oxidase inhibitor

MBq: megabecquerel (unit of radiation)

MCA: monoclonal antibody

mcg: microgram

mcGy: microGray

mCi: millicurie (unit of radiation)

M-CSF: monocyte-macrophage colony-stimulating factor

MDCK: Madin-Darby canine kidney cell culture

MEN: meningococcal (*Neisseria meningitidis*) vaccine, not otherwise specified

MENcn: meningococcal (*Neisseria meningitidis*) conjugate vaccine, serogroup(s) not otherwise specified

MENcn-AC: meningococcal (*Neisseria meningitidis*) conjugate vaccine, serogroups A, C

MENps-ACYW: meningococcal (*Neisseria meningitidis*) polysaccharide vaccine, serogroups A, C, Y, W-135

mEq: milliequivalent

MER: methanol-extracted residue (of phenol-treated BCG)

MeV: million electron volts

mg: milligram

MHC: major histocompatibility complex

MI: myocardial infarction

MIG: measles immune globulin, an obsolete product

min: minute

MIRD: medical internal radiation dosimetry

mIU: milli-international unit

mL: milliliter

mm: millimeter

MMP: matrix metalloproteinases; also a proprietary process for extracting mold allergens

MMR: measles virus, mumps virus, rubella virus vaccine

MMRV: measles-mumps-rubella-varicella vaccine

M-M-R II: measles-mumps-rubella vaccine

MMR-VAR: measles virus, mumps virus, rubella virus, and varicella virus vaccine

mo: month

MoAb: monoclonal antibody

MonAb: monoclonal antibody

mOsm: milliosmole

M-R: measles-rubella vaccine

MRV: mixed respiratory vaccine, a trademark of Hollister-Stier

MS: multiple sclerosis

MSD: Merck Sharp & Dohme Corp., a subsidiary of Merck & Co., Inc.

MSTA: mumps skin-test antigen, a trademark of Aventis Pasteur

MTX: methotrexate

MVD: Merck Vaccine Division

MVRI: mixed vaccine respiratory infections

NABI: North American Biologicals, now Nabi Biopharmaceuticals

NaCl: sodium chloride

NANB: non-A, non-B hepatitis

NAT: nucleic acid testing

NF: *National Formulary*, also a designation for compliance with NF standards

ng: nanogram

NHL: non-Hodgkin lymphoma

NID: National Immunization Day (WHO)

NIH: National Institutes of Health

NIP: National Immunization Program, now National Center for Immunization and Respiratory Diseases (NCIRD)

NK cell: natural killer cell

NPV: negative predictive value

NSAID: nonsteroidal anti-inflammatory drug

NSCLC: non–small-cell lung cancer

NTM: nontuberculous mycobacteria

OBRR: Office of Blood Research and Review, now CBER (FDA)

OKT: Ortho-Kung T cell, designation for a series of antigens

OoB: Office of Biologics, now CBER (FDA)

OPV: poliovirus attenuated live oral trivalent vaccine

OR: odds ratio; overall response

ORR: overall or objective response rate (complete response + partial response)

OSHA: Occupational Safety and Health Administration

OspA: outer surface protein A (in Lyme disease vaccine)

OT: old tuberculin

PATH: (Program for Appropriate Technology in Health), now PATH

PCP: *Pneumocystis carinii* pneumonia

PCR: polymerase chain reaction

PCV7: pneumococcal conjugate vaccine, 7-valent

PEG: polyethylene glycol

PFU: plaque-forming units

pg: picogram

pH: hydrogen-ion concentration

PHS: US Public Health Service

PID: primary immune deficiency

PIG: pertussis immune globulin or poliovirus immune globulin, both obsolete products

PKA: prekallikrein activity

pKi: isoelectric point

PL: public law

PLA: product license application

PMC: Pasteur Mérieux Connaught, now Aventis Pasteur

PNU: pneumococcal (*Streptococcus pneu-*

moniae) vaccine, not otherwise specified

PNUcn-7: pneumococcal (*Streptococcus pneumoniae*) conjugate vaccine, 7-valent

PNUps-23: pneumococcal (*Streptococcus pneumoniae*) polysaccharide, 23-valent vaccine

POL: poliovirus vaccine, not otherwise specified

PPD: purified protein derivative of tuberculin; also p-phenylenediamine mix

PPD-B: PPD-Battery, an atypical nontuberculous mycobacterial (NTM) antigen

PPD-S: the US reference standard for purified protein derivative of tuberculin

PPL: penicilloyl polylysine, more commonly called benzylpenicilloyl polylysine

PPV: positive predictive value

PRP: polyribosyl-ribitol-phosphate, a polysaccharide antigen of *Haemophilus influenzae* type b

PRR: partial response rate

PSA: prostate-specific antigen

PSMA: prostate-specific membrane antigen

PT: pertussis toxin

PTCA: percutaneous transluminal coronary angioplasty

PVC: polyvinyl chloride

R: Roentgen (unit of radiation)

RA: rheumatoid arthritis

RAB: rabies vaccine, not otherwise specified

RAB-HDCV: rabies vaccine, human diploid cell culture

RABig: rabies immune globulin

RAB-PCEC: rabies vaccine, purified chick embryo cell culture

RAST: radioallergosorbent test

RAST-I: radioallergosorbent test inhibition

RBC: red blood cell

RCP: radiochemical purity

RES: reticuloendothelial system

RF: rheumatoid factor

RFFIT: rapid fluorescent focus inhibition test

RhIG: Rh$_o$(D) immune globulin

RhoIG: Rh$_o$(D) immune globulin

RIA: radioimmune assay

RIG: rabies immune globulin

RIT: Recherche et Industrie Therapeutiques, a Belgian institution

RMSF: Rocky Mountain spotted fever

RNA: ribonucleic acid

ROR: the French acronym for MMR

RRMS: relapsing-remitting multiple sclerosis

RSSE: Russian spring-summer encephalitis

RSV: respiratory syncytial virus vaccine

RSVigiv: respiratory syncytial virus immune globulin, intravenous

RSVmab: respiratory syncytial virus monoclonal antibody (palivizumab)

RTA: ricin toxin A chain

RVA: rabies vaccine adsorbed (BioPort Corporation)

S: sedimentation coefficient

SC: a dangerous abbreviation for subcutaneous (use subcutaneous); secretory component

SCLC: small-cell lung cancer

SCN: severe chronic neutropenia

SD: standard deviation; solvent-detergent treatment

SES: socioeconomic status

SGOT: serum glutamic oxaloacetic transaminase, now commonly known as aspartate transaminase (AST)

SGPT: serum glutamic pyruvic transaminase, now commonly known as serum alanine transaminase (ALT)

SIDS: sudden infant death syndrome

sIgA: secretory IgA

SKB: SmithKline Biologicals, SmithKline Beecham Pharmaceuticals

SK-SD: streptokinase-streptodornase

SLE: St. Louis encephalitis; systemic lupus erythematosus

SMA: smallpox vaccine, not otherwise specified

SMAvac: smallpox (vaccinia virus) vaccine

SMX/TMP: sulfamethoxazole with trimethoprim

sp.: species

SPECT: single-photon emission computed tomography

SPF: specific pathogen-free

SPL: Staphage Lysate, a trademark of Delmont Laboratories

SQ: a dangerous abbreviation for subcutaneous (subcutaneous is preferred)

SRU: sample ratio units

SSPE: subacute sclerosing panencephalitis

STD: sexually transmitted disease

SV$_{40}$: simian vacuolating agent #40, a member of the family Papovaviridae

SWFI: sterile water for injection, USP

TAB: typhoid-paratyphoid A and B vaccine

TAC: total allergen content

TAG: tumor-associated glycoprotein

TAT: tetanus antitoxin

TBE: tick-borne encephalitis

TCGF: T-cell growth factor (interleukin-2)

TCID$_{50}$: tissue culture infective doses

Td: tetanus toxoid and diphtheria toxoid (reduced antigen quantity for adults) vaccine, for adolescent and adult use

Tdap: tetanus toxoid and diphtheria toxoid with acellular pertussis vaccine (reduced diphtheria and pertussis antigen quantity for adults), for adolescent and adult use

TETig: tetanus immune globulin

TIG: tetanus immune globulin

TIV: trivalent (injectable) inactivated influenza vaccine

TLS: tumor lysis syndrome

TMP/SMX: trimethoprim with sulfamethoxazole

TNBP: tri-n-butylphosphate

TNF: tumor necrosis factor

TNFR: tumor necrosis factor receptor

TOPV: trivalent oral poliovirus vaccine, synonymous with OPV

TOX: toxoplasmosis (*Toxoplasma gondii*) vaccine

TP: tube precipitin

TPD: typhoid (*Salmonella typhi*) vaccine, not otherwise specified

TPDa: typhoid (*Salmonella typhi*) vaccine, attenuated live (oral Ty21a strain)

TPD-HP: typhoid (*Salmonella typhi*) vaccine, heat and phenol inactivated, dried

TPD-Vi: typhoid (*Salmonella typhi*) vaccine, Vi capsular polysaccharide

TRUE Test: thin-layer rapid-use epicutaneous test

TSH: thyroid-stimulating hormone

TSI-GSD: The Salk Institute-Government Service Division

TST: tuberculin skin test

TT: tetanus (*Clostridium tetani*) toxoid vaccine

TU: tuberculin unit

TUB: tuberculosis (*Mycobacterium tuberculosis*) vaccine, not BCG

TUR: transurethral resection

U: unit

UNICEF: United Nations Children's Fund

URI: upper respiratory infection

USAMMDA: US Army Medical Materiel Development Activity

USAMRIID: US Army Medical Research Institute of Infectious Diseases

USAN: US Adopted Names (Council)

USDA: US Department of Agriculture

USP: *United States Pharmacopeia*, also a designation for compliance with USP standards

VA: Department of Veterans Affairs

VACig: vaccinia virus (smallpox vaccine) immune globulin (for smallpox vaccine, see SMA)

VAERS: Vaccine Adverse Event Reporting System

VAPP: vaccine-associated paralytic poliomyelitis

VAR: varicella (chickenpox) (varicella zoster virus) vaccine

VARig: varicella-zoster immune globulin

Vd: apparent volume of distribution

VEE: Venezuelan equine encephalitis

VEGF: vascular endothelial growth factor

VICP: (National) Vaccine Injury Compensation Program

VIG: vaccinia immune globulin

v/v, vol/vol: volume-to-volume dilution

VVM: vaccine vial monitors

VZIG: varicella-zoster immune globulin

VZV: varicella-zoster virus

WBC: white blood cell

WBE: whole-body (insect) extract

WEE: western equine encephalitis

WHO: World Health Organization

WRAIR: Walter Reed Army Institute of Research

WRAMC: Walter Reed Army Medical Center

w/v, wt/vol: weight-to-volume dilution

y: year

ZIG: zoster immune globulin

ZLB: Swiss initials for central blood laboratory (now CSL Behring, formerly ZLB Behring)

Abrutyn E, Berlin JA. Intrathecal therapy in tetanus. A meta-analysis. *JAMA*. 1991;266:2262-2267.

Adams WG, Deaver KA, Cochi SL, et al. Decline of childhood *Haemophilus influenzae* type b (Hib) disease in the Hib vaccine era. *JAMA*. 1993;269:221-226.

American College of Obstetricians and Gynecologists. ACOG Committee Opinion. Immunization during pregnancy. *Obstet Gynecol*. 2003;101:207-212.

Andrew M, Blanchette VS, Adams M, et al. A multicenter study of the treatment of childhood chronic idiopathic thrombocytopenic purpura with anti-D. *J Pediatr*. 1992;120(4 pt 1):522-527.

Antonelli G, Currenti M, Turriziani O, Dianzani F. Neutralizing antibodies to interferon-alpha: relative frequency in patients treated with different interferon preparations. *J Infect Dis*. 1991;163:882-885.

Arbeter AM, Baker L, Starr SE, Levine BL, Books E, Plotkin SA. Combination measles, mumps, rubella and varicella vaccine. *Pediatrics*. 1986;78(4 pt 2):742-747.

Archer JD. The FDA does not approve uses of drugs. *JAMA*. 1984;252:1054-1055.

Arthurs B, Flanders M, Codere F, Gauthier S, Dresner S, Stone L. Treatment of blepharospasm with medication, surgery and type A botulinum toxin. *Can J Ophthalmol*. 1987;22:24-28.

Athale UH, Luo-Mutti C, Chintu C. How safe is BCG vaccination in children born to HIV-positive mothers? *Lancet*. 1992;340:434-435.

Badaro R, Falcoff E, Badaro FS, et al. Treatment of visceral leishmaniasis with pentavalent antimony and interferon gamma. *N Engl J Med*. 1990;322:16-21.

Baker CJ, Melish ME, Hall RT, Casto DT, Vasan U, Givner LB. Intravenous immune globulin for the prevention of nosocomial infection in low-birth-weight neonates. The Multicenter Group for the Study of Immune Globulin in Neonates. *N Engl J Med*. 1992;327:213-219.

Benenson AS. Immunization and military medicine. *Rev Infect Dis*. 1984;6:1-12.

Bernard KW, Fishbein DB, Miller KD, et al. Pre-exposure rabies immunization with human diploid cell vaccine: decreased antibody responses in persons immunized in developing countries. *Am J Trop Med Hyg*. 1985;34:633-647.

Bielory L, Wright R, Nienhuis AW, Young NS, Kaliner MA. Antithymocyte globulin hypersensitivity in bone marrow failure patients. *JAMA*. 1988;260:3164-3167.

Blumhardt R, Pappano JE Jr, Moyer DG. Depression of poison ivy skin tests by measles vaccine. *JAMA*. 1968;206:2739-2741.

Bolaños R, Cerdas L, Abalos JW. Venoms of coral snakes (*Micrurus* spp.): report on a multivalent antivenin for the Americas. *Bull Pan Am Health Organ*. 1978;12:23-27.

Braun MM, Cauthen G. Relationship of the human immunodeficiency virus epidemic to pediatric tuberculosis and Bacillus Calmette-Guérin immunization. *Pediatr Infect Dis J*. 1992;11:220-227.

Bryan JP, Sjogren MH, Macarthy P, Cox B, Kao TC, Perine PL. Dosing schedule for recombinant hepatitis B vaccine. *J Infect Dis*. 1991;163:1384-1385.

Centers for Disease Control and Prevention. Hepatitis B associated with jet gun injection—California. *MMWR*. 1986;35:373-376.

Centers for Disease Control and Prevention. Inadequate immune response among public safety workers receiving intradermal vaccination against hepatitis B—United States, 1990-1991. *MMWR*. 1991;40:569-572.

Crawford J, Ozer H, Stoller R, et al. Reduction by granulocyte colony-stimulating factor of fever and neutropenia induced by chemotherapy in patients with small-cell lung cancer. *N Engl J Med.* 1991;325:164-170.

Cupit GC, Self TH, Bekemeyer WB. The effect of pneumococcal vaccine on the disposition of theophylline. *Eur J Clin Pharmacol.* 1988;34:505-507.

Decker MD, Edwards KM, Bradley R, Palmer P. Comparative trial in infants of four conjugate *Haemophilus influenzae* type b vaccines. *J Pediatr.* 1992;120(2 pt 1):184-189.

Diaz W, Salamone FR, Muller RJ. Aplastic anemia: focus on treatment with anti-thymocyte globulin. *Hosp Pharm.* 1989;24:737-741, 754.

Edsall G. Specific prophylaxis of tetanus. *JAMA.* 1959;171:417-427.

Edwards KM. Diphtheria, tetanus, and pertussis immunizations in adults. *Infect Dis Clin North Am.* 1990;4:85-103.

Edwards KM, Decker MD, Graham BS, Mezzatesta J, Scott J, Hackell J. Adult immunization with acellular pertussis vaccine. *JAMA.* 1993;269:53-56.

Edwards KM, Decker MD, Halsey NA, et al. Differences in antibody response to whole-cell pertussis vaccines. *Pediatrics.* 1991;88:1019-1023.

Eibl MM, Wolf HM, Furnkranz H, Rosenkranz A. Prophylaxis of necrotizing enterocolitis by oral IgA-IgG: review of a clinical study in low birth weight infants and discussion of the pathogenic role of infection. *J Clin Immunol.* 1990;10(6 suppl):72S-77S, discussion 77S-79S.

English PC. Therapeutic strategies to combat pneumococcal disease: repeated failure of physicians to adopt pneumococcal vaccine, 1900-1945. *Perspect Biol Med.* 1987;30:170-185.

Fine PE, Rodrigues LC. Modern vaccines. Mycobacterial diseases. *Lancet.* 1990;335:1016-1020.

Furcolow ML, Mantz HL, Lewis I. The roentgenographic appearance of persistent pulmonary infiltrates associated with sensitivity to histoplasmin. *Pub Health Rep.* 1947;62:1711-1718.

Furste W. The potential development of tetanus in wounded patients with AIDS: tetanus toxoid and tetanus immune globulin. *Arch Surg.* 1986;121:367.

Gaillat J, Zmirou D, Mallaret MR, et al. Clinical trial of an antipneumococcal vaccine in elderly subjects living in institutions [in French]. *Rev Epidémiol Santé Publique.* 1985;33:437-444.

Gheorghiu M. The present and future role of BCG vaccine in tuberculosis control. *Biologicals.* 1990;18:135-141.

Giammanco G, De Grandi V, Lupo L, et al. Interference of oral poliovirus vaccine on RIT 4237 oral rotavirus vaccine. *Eur J Epidemiol.* 1988;4:121-123.

Grabenstein JD. Comment on anaphylactic shock. *Drug Intell Clin Pharm.* 1984;18:646-647.

Grabenstein JD. Drug interactions involving immunologic agents. Part I. Vaccine-vaccine, vaccine-immunoglobulin, and vaccine-drug interactions. *DICP.* 1990;24:67-81.

Grabenstein JD. Drug interactions involving immunologic agents. Part II. Immunodiagnostic and other immunologic drug interactions. *DICP.* 1990;24:186-193.

Grabenstein JD, Baker JR Jr. Comment: Cyclosporine and vaccination. *Drug Intell Clin Pharm.* 1985;19:679-680.

Grabenstein JD, Smith LJ. Incidence of anaphylactic self-treatment in an outpatient population. *Ann Allergy.* 1989;63:184-188.

Greenberg MA, Birx DL. Safe administration of mumps-measles-rubella vaccine in egg-allergic children. *J Pediatr.* 1988;113:504-506.

Greenberg PD, Lax KG, Schechter CB. Tuberculosis in house staff. A decision analysis comparing the tuberculin screening strategy with the BCG vaccination. *Am Rev Respir Dis.* 1991;143:490-495.

Gross PA, Ennis FA. Influenza vaccine: split-product versus whole-virus types—how do they differ. *N Engl J Med.* 1977;296:567-568.

Halsey NA, Klein D. Maternal immunization. *Pediatr Infect Dis J.* 1990;9:574-581.

Hanson CV, Nishiyama Y, Paul S. Catalytic antibodies and their applications. *Curr Opin Biotechnol.* 2005;16:631-636.

Hardy IR, Gershon AA. Prospects for use of a varicella vaccine in adults. *Infect Dis Clin North Am.* 1990;4:159-173.

Herman JJ, Radin R, Schneiderman R. Allergic reactions to measles (rubeola) vaccine in patients hypersensitive to egg protein. *J Pediatr.* 1983;102:196-199.

Herwaldt LA. Pertussis and pertussis vaccines in adults. *JAMA.* 1993;269:93-94.

Hibberd PL, Rubin RH. Approach to immunization in the immunosuppressed host. *Infect Dis Clin North Am.* 1990;4:123-142.

Howard PA, Haley C. Duration of immunity from hepatitis B vaccine. *Drug Intell Clin Pharm.* 1988;22:985-987.

Howard TP, Solomon DA. Reading the tuberculin skin test. Who, when, and how? *Arch Intern Med.* 1988;148:2457-2459.

Insel RA. Maternal immunization to prevent neonatal infections. *N Engl J Med.* 1988;319:1219-1220.

Ippoliti C, Williams LA, Huber S. Toxicity of rapidly infused concentrated intravenous immune globulin. *Clin Pharm.* 1992;11:1022-1026.

Janeway CA, Merler E, Rosen FS, Salmon S, Crain JD. Metabolism of gamma globulin fragments in normal and agammaglobulinemic persons. *N Engl J Med.* 1968;278:919-923.

Jilg W, Schmidt M, Deinhardt F. Vaccination against hepatitis B: comparison of three different vaccination schedules. *J Infect Dis.* 1989;160:766-769.

Juntunen-Backman K, Peltola H, Backman A, Salo OP. Safe immunization of allergic children against measles, mumps, and rubella. *Am J Dis Child.* 1987;141:1103-1105.

Kaplan JE, Nelson DB, Schonberger LB, et al. The effect of immune globulin on the response to trivalent oral poliovirus and yellow fever vaccinations. *Bull World Health Organ.* 1984;62:585-590.

Karzon DT, Edwards KM. Diphtheria outbreaks in immunized populations. *N Engl J Med.* 1988;318:41-43.

Kletz MR, Holland CL, Mendelson JS, Bielory L. Administration of egg-derived vaccines in patients with history of egg sensitivity. *Ann Allergy.* 1990;64:527-529.

Krotoski WA, Mroczkowski TF, Rea TH, et al. Lepromin skin testing in the classification of Hansen's disease in the United States. *Am J Med Sci.* 1993;305:18-24.

Kumar A. Cimetidine: an immunomodulator. *DICP.* 1990;24:289-295.

Lavi S, Zimmerman B, Koren G, Gold R. Administration of measles, mumps, and rubella virus vaccine (live) to egg-allergic children. *JAMA.* 1990;263:269-271.

Leavengood DC, Renard RL, Martin BG, Nelson HS. Cross allergenicity among grasses determined by tissue threshold changes. *J Allergy Clin Immunol.* 1985;76:789-794.

Levin MJ, Murray M, Rotbart HA, Zerbe GO, White CJ, Hayward AR. Immune response of elderly individuals to a live attenuated varicella vaccine. *J Infect Dis.* 1992;166:253-259.

Levine HB, Scalarone GM, Campbell GD, Graybill JR, Kelly PC, Chaparas SD. Histoplasmin-CYL, a yeast phase reagent in skin test studies with humans. *Am Rev Respir Dis.* 1979;119:629-636.

Livengood JR, Mullen JR, White JW, Brink EW, Orenstein WA. Family history of convulsions and use of pertussis vaccine. *J Pediatr.* 1989;115:527-531.

Bibliography

Losonsky GA, Fishaut JM, Strussenberg J, Ogra PL. Effect of immunization against rubella on lactation products. I. Development and characterization of specific immunologic reactivity in breast milk. *J Infect Dis.* 1982;145:654-660.

Losonsky GA, Fishaut JM, Strussenberg J, Ogra PL. Effect of immunization against rubella on lactation products. II. Maternal-neonatal interactions. *J Infect Dis.* 1982;145:661-666.

Losonsky GA, Johnson JP, Winkelstein JA, Yolken RH. Oral administration of human serum immunoglobulin in immunodeficient patients with viral gastroenteritis. A pharmacokinetic and functional analysis. *J Clin Invest.* 1985;76:2362-2367.

Lucas GS, Jobbins K, Bloom AL. Intravenous immunoglobulin and blood group antibodies. *Lancet.* 1987;2:742.

MacKenzie WR, Davis JP, Peterson DE, Hibbard AJ, Baker G, Zarvan BS. Multiple false-positive serologic tests for HIV, HTLV-1, and hepatitis C following influenza vaccination, 1991. *JAMA.* 1992;268:1015-1017.

Margolis KL, Nichol KL, Poland GA, Pluhar RE. Frequency of adverse reactions to influenza vaccine in the elderly. A randomized, placebo-controlled trial. *JAMA.* 1990;264:1139-1141.

Marsh DG, Goodfriend L, King TP, Lowenstein H, Platts-Mills TA. Allergen nomenclature [in English, French]. *Bull World Heath Organ.* 1986;64:764-774.

McCluskey DR, Boyd NA. Anaphylaxis with intravenous gammaglobulin. *Lancet.* 1990;336:874.

McCollough NC, Gennaro JF Jr. Diagnosis, symptoms, treatment and sequelae of envenomation by *Crotalus adamanteus* and genus *Ancistrodon*. *J Fla Med Assoc.* 1968;55:327-329.

Mertin J, Rudge P, Kremer M, et al. Double-blind controlled trial of immunosuppression in the treatment of multiple sclerosis: final report. *Lancet.* 1982;2:351-354.

Meuer SC, Dumann H, Meyer zum Buschenfelde KH, Kohler H. Low-dose interleukin-2 induces systemic immune responses against HBsAg in immunodeficient non-responders to hepatitis B vaccination. *Lancet.* 1989;1:15-18.

Miller JR, Orgel HA, Meltzer EO. The safety of egg-containing vaccines for egg-allergic patients. *J Allergy Clin Immunol.* 1983;71:568-573.

Moore DA, Hopkins RS. Assessment of a school exclusion policy during a chickenpox outbreak. *Am J Epidemiol.* 1991;133:1161-1167.

Mueller JH, Miller PA. Variable factors influencing the production of tetanus toxin. *J Bacteriol.* 1954;67:271-277.

Murphy KR, Strunk RC. Safe administration of influenza vaccine in asthmatic children hypersensitive to egg proteins. *J Pediatr.* 1985;106:931-933.

Nelson BK. Snake envenomation. Incidence, clinical presentation and management. *Med Toxicol Adverse Drug Exp.* 1989;4:17-31.

Nesbitt GH. Canine allergic inhalant dermatitis: a review of 230 cases. *J Am Vet Med Assoc.* 1978;172:55-60.

Nightingale SL. The FDA and drug uses: reprise. *JAMA.* 1985;253:632.

Noble GR, Bernier RH, Esber EC, et al. Acellular and whole-cell pertussis vaccines in Japan. Report of a visit by US scientists. *JAMA.* 1987;257:1351-1356.

Oren I, Hershow RC, Ben-Porath E, et al. A common-source outbreak of fulminant hepatitis B in a hospital. *Ann Intern Med.* 1989;110:691-698.

Ozawa N, Shimizu M, Imai M, Miyakawa Y, Mayumi M. Selective absence of immunoglobulin A1 or A2 among blood donors and hospital patients. *Transfusion.* 1986;26:73-76.

Pabst HF, Godel J, Grace M, Cho H, Spady DW. Effect of breast-feeding on immune response to BCG vaccination. *Lancet.* 1989;1:295-297.

Palevsky PM, Rendulic D, Diven WF. Maltose-induced hyponatremia. *Ann Intern Med.* 1993;118:526-528.

Parrish HM, Hayes RH. Hospital management of pit viper venenations. *Clin Toxicol.* 1970;3:501-511.

Parrish HM, Khan MS. Bites by coral snakes: report of 11 representative cases. *Am J Med Sci.* 1967;253:561-568.

Pillemer L, Grossberg DB, Wittler RG. The immunochemistry of toxins and toxoids. II. The preparation and immunological evaluation of purified tetanal toxoid. *J Immunol.* 1946;54:213-224.

Pirofsky B, Reid RH, Bardana EJ Jr, Baker RL. Myasthenia gravis treated with purified antithymocyte antiserum. *Neurology.* 1979;29:112-116.

Podolsky SH. The changing fate of pneumonia as a public health concern in 20th-century America and beyond. *Am J Public Health.* 2005;95:2144-2154.

Pollack W. Rh hemolytic disease of the newborn: its cause and prevention. *Prog Clin Biol Res.* 1981;70:185-302.

Polmar SH, Smith TF, Pirofsky B, et al. Rapid infusion of intravenous immunoglobulin in patients with primary immunodeficiency disease. *J Allergy Clin Immunol.* 1992;89:86A.

Prince HE. Molds and bacteria in the etiology of respiratory allergic diseases. XXI. Studies with mold extracts produced from cultures grown in modified synthetic media. A preliminary report. *Ann Allergy.* 1961;19:259-267.

Radosevich CA, Gordon LI, Weil SC, Marder RJ, Rosen ST. Complete resolution of pure red cell aplasia in a patient with chronic lymphocytic leukemia following antithymocyte globulin therapy. *JAMA.* 1988;259:723-725.

Redfield RR, Wright DC, James WD, Jones TS, Brown C, Burke DS. Disseminated vaccinia in a military recruit with human immunodeficiency virus (HIV) disease. *N Engl J Med.* 1987;316:673-676.

Reisman RE. Venom immunotherapy: when is it reasonable to stop. *J Allergy Clin Immunol.* 1991;87:618-620.

Rietschel RL, Fowler JF, eds. *Fisher's Contact Dermatitis.* 5th ed. Philadelphia, PA: Lippincott Williams & Wilkins; 2001.

Robbins JB, Schneerson R. Polysaccharide-protein conjugates: a new generation of vaccines. *J Infect Dis.* 1990;161:821-832.

Rodney WM, Chopivsky P, Quan M. Adult immunization: the medical record design as a facilitator for physician compliance. *J Med Educ.* 1983;58:576-580.

Rodwell JD, Alvarez VL, Lee C, et al. Site-specific covalent modification of monoclonal antibodies: in vitro and in vivo evaluations. *Proc Natl Acad Sci USA.* 1986;83:2632-2636.

Rose RM, Rey-Martinez J, Croteau C, et al. Failure of recombinant interleukin-2 to augment the primary humoral response to a recombinant hepatitis B vaccine in healthy adults. *J Infect Dis.* 1992;165:775-777.

Russell FE, Carlson RW, Wainschel J, Osborne AH. Snake venom poisoning in the United States. Experiences with 550 cases. *JAMA.* 1975;233:341-344.

Schiff RI, Sedlak D, Buckley RH. Rapid infusion of Sandoglobulin in patients with primary humoral immunodeficiency. *J Allergy Clin Immunol.* 1991;88:61-67.

Schmidt JO. Allergy to *Hymenoptera* venoms. In: Piek T, ed. *Venoms of the Hymenoptera.* London, England: Academic Press; 1986:509-549.

Schmidt JO. Chemistry, pharmacology, and chemical ecology of ant venoms. In: Piek T, ed. *Venoms of the Hymenoptera.* London, England: Academic Press; 1986:425-508.

Schwarz JA, Koch W, Buhler V, Kaumeier S. Pharmacokinetics of low molecular (monovalent) dextran (Dx 1) in volunteers. *Int J Clin Pharmacol Ther Toxicol.* 1981;19:358-367.

Bibliography

Seeff LB, Wright EC, Finkelstein JD, et al. Efficacy of hepatitis B immune serum globulin after accidental exposure. Preliminary report of the Veterans Administration Cooperative Study. *Lancet.* 1975;2:939-941.

Seibert FB. The isolation and properties of the purified protein derivative of tuberculin. *Am Rev Tuberc.* 1934;30:713-720.

Shapiro GG, Anderson JA. Controversial techniques in allergy. *Pediatrics.* 1988;82:935-937.

Shaw FE Jr, Guess HA, Roets JM, et al. Effect of anatomic injection site, age and smoking on the immune response to hepatitis B vaccination. *Vaccine.* 1989;7:425-430.

Shirk MB, Hale KN. Obtaining drugs from foreign markets. *Am J Hosp Pharm.* 1992;49:2731-2739.

Siber GR. Immune globulin to prevent nosocomial infections. *N Engl J Med.* 1992;327:269-271.

Slade HB, Schwartz SA. Mucosal immunity: the immunology of breast milk. *J Allergy Clin Immunol.* 1987;80(3 pt 1):348-358.

Smith TA II, Figge HL. Treatment of snakebite poisoning. *Am J Hosp Pharm.* 1991;48:2190-2196.

Spaite DW, Dart RC, Hurlbut K, et al. Skin testing: implications in the management of pit-viper envenomation. *Ann Emerg Med.* 1988;17:389.

Steinhart R, Reingold AL, Taylor F, Anderson G, Wenger JD. Invasive *Haemophilus influenzae* infections in men with HIV infection. *JAMA.* 1992;268:3350-3352.

Steinhoff MC, Auerbach BS, Nelson KE, et al. Antibody responses to *Haemophilus influenzae* type B vaccines in men with human immunodeficiency virus infection. *N Engl J Med.* 1991;325:1837-1842.

Stevens DA, Levine HB, Deresinski SC, et al. Spherulin in clinical coccidioidomycosis: comparison with coccidioidin. *Chest.* 1975;68:697-702.

Stiehm ER. Skin testing prior to measles vaccination for egg-sensitive patients. *Am J Dis Child.* 1990;144:32.

Tacket CO, Shandera WX, Mann JM, Hargrett NT, Blake PA. Equine antitoxin use and other factors that predict outcome in type A foodborne botulism. *Am J Med.* 1984;76:794-798.

Temianka D. Pneumococcal vaccination: when in doubt, go ahead. *JAMA.* 1991;265:211-212.

Todd PA, Brogden RN. Muromonab CD3. A review of its pharmacology and therapeutic potential. *Drugs.* 1989;37:871-899.

Trissel LA, Martinez JF. Sargramostim incompatibility. *Hosp Pharm.* 1992;27:929.

Ujhelyi MR, Colucci RD, Cummings DM, et al. Monitoring serum digoxin concentrations during digoxin immune Fab therapy. *DICP.* 1991;25:1047-1049.

Ujhelyi MR, Green PJ, Cummings DM, Robert S, Vlasses PH, Zarowitz BJ. Determination of free serum digoxin concentrations in digoxin toxic patients after administration of digoxin fab antibodies. *Ther Drug Monit.* 1992;14:147-154.

Ujhelyi MR, Robert S, Cummings DM, et al. Disposition of digoxin immune Fab in patients with kidney failure. *Clin Pharmacol Ther.* 1993;54:388-394.

Wainwright RB, McMahon BJ, Bulkow LR, et al. Duration of immunogenicity and efficacy of hepatitis B vaccine in a Yupik Eskimo population. *JAMA.* 1989;261:2362-2366.

Watt C, Gennaro J. Pit viper bites in south Georgia and north Florida. *Trans South Surg Assoc.* 1966;77:378.

Weber RW, Nelson HS. Pollen allergens and their interrelationships. *Clin Rev Allergy.* 1985;3:291-318.

Weiss ME, Adkinson NF. Immediate hypersensitivity reactions to penicillin and related antibiotics. *Clin Allergy.* 1988;18:515-540.

Wingert WA, Wainschel J. Diagnosis and management of envenomation by poisonous snakes. *South Med J.* 1975;68:1015-1026.

Additional Sources

General References

American Society of Microbiology. *Vaccine Development: Current Status & Future Needs*. Washington, DC: American Society of Microbiology, 2005. http://www.asm.org/Academy/index.asp?bid=38323.

Atkinson W, Wolfe S, Hamborsky J, McIntyre L, eds. *Epidemiology and Prevention of Vaccine-Preventable Disease*, 11th ed. Atlanta: Centers for Disease Control and Prevention, April 2009.

Australian Immunisation Handbook. 9th ed. National Health & Medical Research Council. Australian Government Department of Health and Ageing. Canberra: National Capital Printers; 2008. http://www1.health.gov.au/immhandbook

British Joint Committee on Vaccination & Immunisation. *Immunisation Against Infectious Disease*, 3rd ed. London: Her Majesty's Stationary Office, 2006. http://www.dh.gov.uk/assetRoot/04/14/17/61/04141761.pdf

Canadian National Advisory Committee on Immunization. *Canadian Immunization Guide*. 7th ed. Ottawa, Canada: Public Health Agency of Canada, 2006. http://www.phac-aspc.gc.ca/publicat/cig-gci/index.html

Cancer Facts & Figures/American Cancer Society. Atlanta, GA: The Society; 2009. http://www.cancer.org/downloads/STT/500809web.pdf

Centers for Disease Control and Prevention. *Health Information for International Travel 2010*. Atlanta, GA: US Department of Health and Human Services, Public Health Service; 2010. Revised biennially. http://www.cdc.gov/travel/index.htm#Reference

Centers for Disease Control and Prevention. Immunization of health-care workers: recommendations of the Advisory Committee on Immunization Practices and the Hospital Infection Control Practices Advisory Committee (HICPAC). *MMWR*. 1997;46(RR-18):1-42. http://www.cdc.gov/mmwr/PDF/rr/rr4618.pdf

Centers for Disease Control and Prevention. Recommendations of the Advisory Committee on Immunization Practices: use of vaccines and immune globulins in persons with altered immunocompetence. *MMWR*. 1993;42(RR-4):1-18. http://www.cdc.gov/mmwr/PDF/rr/rr4204.pdf

Gizurarson S. Optimal delivery of vaccines: clinical pharmacokinetic considerations. *Clin Pharmacokinet*. 1996;30:1-15.

Grabenstein JD, Pittman Pr, Greenwood JT, Engler RJM. Immunization to protect the U.S. Armed Forces: Heritage, current practice, prospects. *Epidemiol Rev*. 2006;28:3-26. http://www.vaccines.mil/documents/library/MilitaryImztn2005fulc.pdf

Guide for Adult Immunization/ACP Task Force on Adult Immunization and Infectious Diseases Society of America. 3rd ed. Philadelphia, PA: American College of Physicians; 1994.

Heymann DL, ed. *Control of Communicable Diseases Manual*. 19th ed. Washington, DC: American Public Health Association; 2008.

National Institute of Allergy & Infectious Diseases. *The Jordan report: Accelerated development of vaccines 2007*. Bethesda, MD: NIH, May 2007. http://www3.niaid.nih.gov/about/organization/dmid/pdf/jordan2007.pdf.

Kelso JM, Li JT, Niklas RA, et al; Adverse reactions to vaccines: A practice parameter. *Ann Allergy Asthma Immunol*. 2009;103 (suppl 2):S1-S14.

Kroger AT, Atkinson WL, Marcuse EK, Pickering LK; Advisory Committee on Immunization Practices (ACIP) Centers for Disease Control and Prevention (CDC). General recommendations on immunization: Recommendations of the Advisory Committee on Immunization Practices (ACIP). *MMWR Recomm Rep*. 2006;55 (RR-15):1-48.

National Vaccine Advisory Committee. *Adult Immunization*. Washington, DC: Department of Health and Human Services; 1994.

New Zealand Ministry of Health. *New Zealand Immunisation Handbook—2006*. Wellington, New Zealand: New Zealand Ministry of Health; April 2006. http://www.moh.govt.nz

Pickering LK, ed. *2009 Red Book: Report of the Committee on Infectious Diseases*. 28th ed. Elk Grove Village, IL: American Academy of Pediatrics; 2009.

Plotkin SA, Orenstein WA, Offit PA. *Vaccines*. 5th ed. Philadelphia, PA: Saunders; 2008.

Rosenthal KS. Vaccines make good immune theater: Immunization described as a three-act play. *Infect Dis Clin Pract*. 2006;14:35-45.

Russell FE. *Snake Venom Poisoning*. Great Neck, NY: Scholium International; 1983.

U.S. Army Regulation 40-562, Navy Bureau of Medicine and Surgery Instruction 6230.15, Air Force Joint Instruction 48-110, Coast Guard Commandant Instruction M6230.4F. *Immunizations and Chemoprophylaxis*. Washington, DC; September 29, 2006. http://www.apd.army.mil/pdffiles/r40_562.pdf.

van den Oever R, de Graeve D, Hepp B, et al. Pharmacoeconomics of immunisation: a review. *Pharmacoeconomics*. 1993;3:286-308.

WHO. *International Travel & Health: Vaccination Requirements & Health Advice*. Albany, NY: WHO; revised annually. http://www.who.int/ith/en

Vaccine Advocacy & Delivery Methods

Centers for Disease Control and Prevention. Immunization of health-care workers: recommendations of the Advisory Committee on Immunization Practices and the Hospital Infection Control Practices Advisory Committee (HICPAC). *MMWR*. 1997;46(RR-18):1-42. http://www.cdc.gov/mmwr/PDF/rr/rr4618.pdf

Centers for Disease Control and Prevention. Use of standing orders programs to increase adult vaccination rates: recommendations of the Advisory Committee on Immunization Practices. *MMWR*. 2000;49(RR-1):15-26. http://www.cdc.gov/mmwr/PDF/rr/rr4901.pdf

Fedson DS. Adult immunization. Summary of the National Vaccine Advisory Committee Report. *JAMA*. 1994;272:1133-1137.

Grabenstein JD, Wilson JP. Are vaccines safe? Risk communication applied to vaccines. *Hosp Pharm*. 1999;34:713-718, 731-723, 727-729.

Standards for Vaccine Delivery

American Academy of Pediatrics. Standards for child and adolescent immunization practices. National Vaccine Advisory Committee. *Pediatrics*. 2003; 112(4):958-963.

American Pharmaceutical Association. Guidelines for pharmacy-based immunization delivery, Aug 1997. http://www.aphanet.org/pharmcare/immguide/html

American Society of Consultant Pharmacists. Guidelines for immunization advocacy by consultant pharmacists, Aug 1998. http://www.ascp.com/public/r/immunization

American Society of Health-System Pharmacists. ASHP guidelines on the pharmacist's role in immunization. *Am J Health-Syst Pharm*. 2003;60:1371-1377. http://www.ashp.org/public/pubs/ajhpopen/ASHPAdv-ASHP-guidelines.pdf

Centers for Disease Control and Prevention. Adult immunization programs in nontraditional settings: quality standards and guidance for program evaluation: a report of the National Vaccine Advisory Committee. *MMWR*. 2000;49(RR-1):1-13. http://www.cdc.gov/mmwr/PDF/rr/rr4901.pdf

Gershon AA, Gardner P, Peter G, Nichols K, Orenstein W. Quality standards for immunization. Guidelines from the Infectious Diseases Society of America. *Clin Infect Dis*. 1997;25:782-786. http://www.journals.uchicago.edu/IDSA/guide/OC31_782.pdf

National Coalition for Adult Immunization. Standards for adult immunization practice. *Am J Infect Control*. 1993;21:331-332. http://www.nfid.org/ncai/publications/standards

Pickering LK, Baker CJ, Freed GL, et al. Immunization programs for infants, children, adolescents, and adults: Clinical practice guidelines by the Infectious Diseases Society of America. *Clin Infect Dis.* 2009;49(6):817-840

Poland GA, Shefer AM, McCauley M, Webster PS, Whitley-Williams PN, Peter G; National Vaccine Advisory Committee, Ad Hoc Working Group for the Development of Standards for Adult Immunization Practices. Standards for adult immunization practices. *Am J Prev Med.* 2003;25:144-150. http://www.aphanet.org/pharmcare/AdultStandards.pdf

Pregnancy, Breast-feeding & Immunizations

Advisory Committee on Immunization Practices. Guiding principles for development of ACIP recommendations for vaccination during pregnancy and breastfeeding. *MMWR.* 2008;57(21):580.

American College of Obstetricians and Gynecologists. ACOG Committee Opinion. Immunization during pregnancy. *Obstet Gynecol.* 2003;101:207-212.

American College of Obstetricians and Gynecologists. ACOG educational bulletin. Management of isoimmunization in pregnancy. *Int J Gynaecol Obstet.* 1996;55:183-190.

American College of Obstetricians and Gynecologists. ACOG practice bulletin #4. Prevention of Rh D alloimmunization. Clinical management guidelines for obstetrician-gynecologists. *Int J Gynaecol Obstet.* 1999;66:63-70.

Centers for Disease Control and Prevention. *Health Information for International Travel 2009-2010.* Atlanta, GA: US Department of Health and Human Services, Public Health Service; 2009-2010. Revised biennially. http://www.cdc.gov/travel

Grabenstein JD. Vaccines and antibodies in relation to pregnancy and lactation. *Hosp Pharm.* 1999;34:949-952, 955-956, 959-960.

Halsey NA, Klein D. Maternal immunization. *Pediatr Infect Dis J.* 1990;9:574-581.

Insel RA. Maternal immunization to prevent neonatal infections. *N Engl J Med.* 1988;319:1219-1220.

Saari TN. Immunization of preterm and low birth weight infants. *Pediatrics.* 2003;112(1 Pt 1):193-198.

Slade HB, Schwartz SA. Mucosal immunity: the immunology of breast milk. *J Allergy Clin Immunol.* 1987;80(3 pt 1): 348-358.

Immunocompromised Hosts & Immunizations

Centers for Disease Control and Prevention. Anergy skin testing and preventive therapy for HIV-infected persons: revised recommendations. *MMWR.* 1997;46(RR-15):1-10. http://www.cdc.gov/mmwr/PDF/rr/rr4615.pdf

Centers for Disease Control and Prevention. Guidelines for preventing opportunistic infections among hematopoietic stem cell transplant recipients: recommendations of Centers for Disease Control and Prevention, the Infectious Diseases Society of America, and the American Society of Blood and Marrow Transplantation. *MMWR.* 2000;49(RR-10):1-135. http://www.cdc.gov/mmwr/PDF/rr/rr4910.pdf

Centers for Disease Control and Prevention. Recommendations of the Advisory Committee on Immunization Practices: use of vaccines and immune globulins in persons with altered immunocompetence. *MMWR.* 1993;42(RR-4):1-18. http://www.cdc.gov/mmwr/PDF/rr/rr4204.pdf

Ozer H, Armitage JO, Bennett CL, et al; American Society of Clinical Oncology. 2000 update of recommendations for the use of hematopoietic colony-stimulating factors: evidence-based, clinical practice guidelines. American Society of Clinical Oncology Growth Factors Expert Panel. *J Clin Oncol.* 2000;18:3558-3585.

Bibliography

Historical Summaries

Allen A. Vaccine: *The Controversial Story of Medicine's Greatest Lifesaver*. New York: WW Norton & Co., 2007.

Artenstein AW, Opal JM, Opal SM, Tramont EC, Peter G, Russell PK. History of U.S. military contributions to the study of vaccines against infectious diseases. *Mil Med*. 2005;170 (4 Suppl):3-11.

Bibel DJ, ed. *Milestones in Immunology*. Madison, WI: Science Tech; 1988.

Chase A. *Magic Shots: A Human and Scientific Account of the Long and Continuing Struggle to Eradicate Infectious Diseases by Vaccination*. New York, NY: Morrow; 1982.

Clark WR. *At War Within: The Double-Edged Sword of Immunity*. New York, NY: Oxford University Press; 1995.

Collier R. *The Plague of the Spanish Lady: The Influenza Pandemic of 1918-1919*. London, England: Allison & Busby; 1996.

Coombs RR, Gell PG. The classification of allergic reactions underlying disease. In: Gell PG, Coombs RR, eds. *Clinical Aspects of Immunology*. Philadelphia, PA: FA Davis; 1963:317-337.

Crosby AW. *America's Forgotten Pandemic: The Influenza of 1918*. 2nd ed. New York, NY: Cambridge University Press; 2003.

Crosby MC. *The American Plague: The Untold Story of Yellow Fever, The Epidemic That Shaped Our History*. Berkley Press, 2006.

Desowitz RS. *The Malaria Capers: More Tales of Parasites and People, Research and Reality*. New York, NY: W.W. Norton; 1991.

Desowitz RS. *The Thorn in the Starfish: How the Immune System Works*. New York, NY: W.W. Norton; 1987.

Etheridge EW. *Sentinel for Health: A History of the Centers for Disease Control*. Berkeley: University of California Press; 1992.

Galambos L, Sewell JE. *Networks of Innovation: Vaccine Development at Merck, Sharp & Dohme, and Mulford, 1895-1995*. New York, NY: Cambridge University Press; 1995.

Garrett L. *The Coming Plague, Newly Emerging Diseases in a World Out of Balance*. New York, NY: Farrar, Straus and Giroux; 1994.

Geison GL. *The Private Science of Louis Pasteur*. Princeton, NJ: Princeton University Press; 1995.

Gould T. *A Summer Plague: Polio and Its Survivors*. New Haven, CT: Yale University Press; 1995.

Grabenstein JD, Pittman PR, Greenwood JT, Engler RJM. Immunization to protect the US Armed Forces: heritage, current practice, prospects. *Epidemiol Rev*. 2006;28:3-26.

Gregg CT. *Plague: An Ancient Disease in the Twentieth Century*. Rev. ed. Albuquerque: University of New Mexico Press; 1985.

Neustadt RE, Fineberg HV. *The Epidemic That Never Was: Policy-Making and the Swine Flu Scare*. New York, NY: Vintage Books; 1983.

Nigrovic LE, Thompson KM. The Lyme vaccine: A cautionary tale. *Epidemiol Infect*. 2007;135(1):1-8.

Offit PA. *Vaccinated: One Man's Quest to Defeat the World's Deadliest Diseases*. Washington, DC: Smithsonian Books, 2007.

Parish HJ. *A History of Immunization*. Baltimore, MD: Williams & Wilkins; 1965.

Parish HJ. *Victory with Vaccines: The Story of Immunization*. Edinburgh, London: E & S Livingstone Ltd.; 1968.

Parrino J, Graham BS. Smallpox vaccines: Past, present, and future. *J Allergy Clin Immunol*. 2006;118(6):1320-1326.

Rosenberg CE. *The Cholera Years: The United States in 1832, 1849, and 1866.* Chicago, IL: University of Chicago Press; 1987.

Ryan F. *The Forgotten Plague: How the Battle Against Tuberculosis was Won—and Lost.* Boston, MA: Little, Brown; 1993.

Silverstein AM. *Pure Politics and Impure Science: The Swine Flu Affair.* Baltimore, MD: Johns Hopkins University Press; 1981.

Smith JS. *Patenting the Sun: Polio and the Salk Vaccine.* New York, NY: Morrow; 1990.

Starzl TE. The *Puzzle People: Memoirs of a Transplant Surgeon.* Pittsburgh, PA: University of Pittsburgh Press; 2003.

FDA Advisory Review Panel Reports

Food and Drug Administration, HHS. Biological products; blood and blood derivatives; implementation of efficacy review. *Fed Regist.* 1985 Dec 24;50:52602-52723.

Food and Drug Administration, HHS. Biological products; bacterial vaccines and toxoids; implementation of efficacy review. Final rule and final order. *Fed Regist.* 2004 Jan 5;69:255-267.

Food and Drug Administration, HHS. Biological products; bacterial vaccines and toxoids; implementation of efficacy review; proposed rule. *Fed Regist.* 1985 Dec 13;50:51002-51117.

Food and Drug Administration, HHS. Biological products; allergenic extracts; opportunity for hearing. *Fed Regist.* 1985 Aug 9;50:32314-32318.

Food and Drug Administration, HHS. Biological products; allergenic extracts; implementation of efficacy review; proposed rule. *Fed Regist.* 1985 Jan 23;50:3082-3287.

Food and Drug Administration, HHS. Viral and rickettsial vaccines; proposed implementation of efficacy review. *Fed Regist.* 1980 Apr 15;45:25652-25758.

Food and Drug Administration, HHS. Skin test antigens; implementation of efficacy review. *Fed Regist.* 1979 Jul 10;44:40284-40290, 45617.

Food and Drug Administration, HHS. Skin test antigens; proposed implementation of efficacy review. *Fed Regist.* 1997 Sep 30;42:52674-52723, 61613.

Institute of Medicine Reports

Institute of Medicine. *Immunization Safety Review: Influenza Vaccines and Neurological Complications.* Washington, DC: National Academy of Sciences; October 2003. http://www.nap.edu/catalog/10822.html

Institute of Medicine. *Immunization Safety Review: Measles-Mumps-Rubella Vaccine and Autism.* Washington, DC: National Academy of Sciences; April 2001. http://www.nap.edu/catalog/10101.html

Institute of Medicine. *Immunization Safety Review: Simian Virus-40 Contaminiation of Polio Vaccine and Cancer.* Washington, DC: National Academy of Sciences; October 2002. http://www.nap.edu/catalog/10534.html

Institute of Medicine. *Immunization Safety Review: Thimerosal-Containing Vaccines and Neurodevelopmental Outcomes.* Washington, DC: National Academy of Sciences; October 2001. http://www.nap.edu/catalog/10208.html

Institute of Medicine. *Immunization Safety Review: Vaccinations and Sudden Unexpected Death in Infancy.* Washington, DC: National Academy of Sciences; March 2003. http://www.nap.edu/catalog/10649.html

Institute of Medicine. *Immunization Safety Review: Vaccines and Autism.* Washington, DC: National Academy of Sciences; May 2004. http://www.nap.edu/catalog/10997.html

This index lists all generic, proprietary, and group names included in *ImmunoFacts*®. Additionally, many synonyms, abbreviations, and other terms are included.

Index

Index

Index

Index

Meningococcal serogroup B, New Zealand strain outer membrane vesicle vaccine, 1336
Meningococcal serogroups C and Y, *Haemophilus influenzae,* tetanus toxoid-conjugate, 1335
Meningococcal vaccine, 152, 1357
  travel-related recommendations for, 1371, 1382
  whole cell, 1298
Meningtec, 1319
Menitorix, 1335
Menjugate, 1319, 1344, 1357
Menomune A/C, 1344
Menomune-A/C/Y/W-135, 38, 152, 153, 1344
Menpovax 4, 1319
Menpovax A+C, 1319
MENps, 152, 153
Menveo, 38, 152, 158, 1344
MeNZB, 1336
Mepacrine, 1380
Mephaquine, 1380
Mepolizumab, 1244
Mepolizumab (humanized), 1257
Mercapto mix, 938, 939
Mercaptobenzothiazole, 938, 939
Mercaptopurine, 1124, 1128, 1332
Meruvax, 1299
Mesavac, 1319
Mescaline, 1243
Metakelfin, 1380
Metamizole, 1126
Metastron, 1125
Metavert, 773
Methimazole, 1126
Methotrexate, 1124, 1128, 1332
Methyl-parahydroxybenzoate, 938
Methylprednisolone, 1125

Mevilin-L, 1319
Mexican immunologic drugs, 1356
MF59, 1132
MFR, 1319
MFV, 1319
MFV-Ject, 1319
MGA031, 1265
MGC, 153
MICRhoGAM, 401, 522, 523
Microsphere release mechanisms, 1133
Micruroides euryxanthus antivenin, 489
Micruroides fulvius tenere antivenin, 489
Micrurus antivenin, 1363
Micrurus fulvius antivenin (equine), 405, 496
Micrurus fulvius fulvius antivenin, 489
Mielogen, 1365
Migen, 1331
Milatuzumab, 1244, 1257
Milibis with Aralen, 1380
Milodistim, 1277
Milodistim (recombinant), 1281
MILR 1444A, 1255
Mineral salts, 1133
Miniflu, 1319
Missed doses, 26
Mithracin, 1126
Mitomycin, 1126, 1127
Mitotic inhibitors, 1125, 1128
Mitoxantrone, 1126, 1127
Mitumomab, 1244, 1257
Mixed Infection Phylacogen, 1305
Mixed respiratory vaccine, 1305
Mixed stock bacterial vaccines, 1338
Mixed vaccine respiratory infections, 1305
Mixed-vespid venoms, 901

MK-0646, 1249
MLN02, 1266
MMR, 299
MMRV, 299, 310, 1360
MMRvaxpro, 1320
MN120TMGNP-vCP205, 1219
MN120TMGNP-vCP1452, 1219
Modimmunal, 1341
Modulators, 965
  Canadian, 1354
  colony-stimulating factors, 966
  general immunostimulants, 1118
  immunologic adjuvants, 1130
  immunosuppressants, 1124
  interferons, 997
  interleukin antagonists, 1105
  interleukins, 1078
  international names for, 1332
Molgramostim, 1278, 1341, 1354, 1365
Molgramostime, 1354
Moloney murine leukemia virus, 1292
Moniarix, 1320
Monilia, 933
Monocline, 1380
Monoclonal antibodies, 14
  naming conventions for, 397
Monokines, 965
Monomeric antibodies, 14
Monophosphoryl lipid A, 1131, 1133
Monophosphoryl lipid A, allergen extracts with, 1275
MonoVacc, 1309
Monovax, 1320
Montest, 1331
Mopavac, 1320

Index

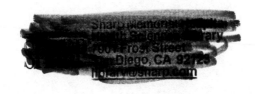